WEIGHT LOSS SECRET REVEALED

DR. YUCAN DEWITT

To Matty and Bunny
"Look beyond what you see"

Foreword

Time passing can suggest many things. It may indicate that we are late, behind or that we just missed the mark. Time passing to some may mean that we are stagnant, or unproductive. It may also indicate that we have arrived! "I did it and it is my time to shine"! No matter what the perspective, there is still one constant. We have 24 hours in a day. Wow! A day to rest and maintain. A day to leap and explore. A day to help someone and effect a change. Today. "Can I have it all right now"? "Is there a short cut or a direct path"? "I've got a scheduling conflict, will you do it for me?" Hmmm......And just like that, we are at the top of another 24 hour set --- wandering, searching, hoping. Everybody's searching for something. And if we look close enough, we will find the answer within.

WEIGHT LOSS SECRET REVEALED

Eat less. Exercise more. Eat less. Exercise more.
Eat less. Exercise more. Eat less. Exercise more.
Eat less. Exercise more. Eat less. Exercise more.
Eat less. Exercise more. Eat less. Exercise more.
Eat less. Exercise more. Eat less. Exercise more.
Eat less. Exercise more. Eat less. Exercise more.
Eat less. Exercise more. Eat less. Exercise more.
Eat less. Exercise more. Eat less. Exercise more.
Eat less. Exercise more. Eat less. Exercise more.
Eat less. Exercise more. Eat less. Exercise more.
Eat less. Exercise more. Eat less. Exercise more.
Eat less. Exercise more. Eat less. Exercise more.
Eat less. Exercise more. Eat less. Exercise more.
Eat less. Exercise more. Eat less. Exercise more.
Eat less. Exercise more. Eat less. Exercise more.
Eat less. Exercise more. Eat less. Exercise more.
Eat less. Exercise more. Eat less. Exercise more.
Eat less. Exercise more. Eat less. Exercise more.
Eat less. Exercise more. Eat less. Exercise more.
Eat less. Exercise more. Eat less. Exercise more.
Eat less. Exercise more. Eat less. Exercise more.
Eat less. Exercise more. Eat less. Exercise more.
Eat less. Exercise more. Eat less. Exercise more.
Eat less. Exercise more. Eat less. Exercise more.
Eat less. Exercise more. Eat less. Exercise more.
Eat less. Exercise more. Eat less. Exercise more.
Eat less. Exercise more. Eat less. Exercise more.
Eat less. Exercise more. Eat less. Exercise more.
Eat less. Exercise more. Eat less. Exercise more.
Eat less. Exercise more. Eat less. Exercise more.
Eat less. Exercise more. Eat less. Exercise more.
Eat less. Exercise more. Eat less. Exercise more.
Eat less. Exercise more. Eat less. Exercise more.
Eat less. Exercise more. Eat less. Exercise more.
Eat less. Exercise more. Eat less. Exercise more.

Eat less. Exercise more. Eat less. Exercise more.
Eat less. Exercise more. Eat less. Exercise more.
Eat less. Exercise more. Eat less. Exercise more.
Eat less. Exercise more. Eat less. Exercise more.
Eat less. Exercise more. Eat less. Exercise more.
Eat less. Exercise more. Eat less. Exercise more.
Eat less. Exercise more. Eat less. Exercise more.
Eat less. Exercise more. Eat less. Exercise more.
Eat less. Exercise more. Eat less. Exercise more.
Eat less. Exercise more. Eat less. Exercise more.
Eat less. Exercise more. Eat less. Exercise more.
Eat less. Exercise more. Eat less. Exercise more.
Eat less. Exercise more. Eat less. Exercise more.
Eat less. Exercise more. Eat less. Exercise more.
Eat less. Exercise more. Eat less. Exercise more.
Eat less. Exercise more. Eat less. Exercise more.
Eat less. Exercise more. Eat less. Exercise more.
Eat less. Exercise more. Eat less. Exercise more.
Eat less. Exercise more. Eat less. Exercise more.
Eat less. Exercise more. Eat less. Exercise more.
Eat less. Exercise more. Eat less. Exercise more.
Eat less. Exercise more. Eat less. Exercise more.
Eat less. Exercise more. Eat less. Exercise more.
Eat less. Exercise more. Eat less. Exercise more.
Eat less. Exercise more. Eat less. Exercise more.
Eat less. Exercise more. Eat less. Exercise more.
Eat less. Exercise more. Eat less. Exercise more.
Eat less. Exercise more. Eat less. Exercise more.
Eat less. Exercise more. Eat less. Exercise more.
Eat less. Exercise more. Eat less. Exercise more.
Eat less. Exercise more. Eat less. Exercise more.
Eat less. Exercise more. Eat less. Exercise more.
Eat less. Exercise more. Eat less. Exercise more.
Eat less. Exercise more. Eat less. Exercise more.

Eat less. Exercise more. Eat less. Exercise more.
Eat less. Exercise more. Eat less. Exercise more.
Eat less. Exercise more. Eat less. Exercise more.
Eat less. Exercise more. Eat less. Exercise more.
Eat less. Exercise more. Eat less. Exercise more.
Eat less. Exercise more. Eat less. Exercise more.
Eat less. Exercise more. Eat less. Exercise more.
Eat less. Exercise more. Eat less. Exercise more.
Eat less. Exercise more. Eat less. Exercise more.
Eat less. Exercise more. Eat less. Exercise more.
Eat less. Exercise more. Eat less. Exercise more.
Eat less. Exercise more. Eat less. Exercise more.
Eat less. Exercise more. Eat less. Exercise more.
Eat less. Exercise more. Eat less. Exercise more.
Eat less. Exercise more. Eat less. Exercise more.
Eat less. Exercise more. Eat less. Exercise more.
Eat less. Exercise more. Eat less. Exercise more.
Eat less. Exercise more. Eat less. Exercise more.
Eat less. Exercise more. Eat less. Exercise more.
Eat less. Exercise more. Eat less. Exercise more.
Eat less. Exercise more. Eat less. Exercise more.
Eat less. Exercise more. Eat less. Exercise more.
Eat less. Exercise more. Eat less. Exercise more.
Eat less. Exercise more. Eat less. Exercise more.
Eat less. Exercise more. Eat less. Exercise more.
Eat less. Exercise more. Eat less. Exercise more.
Eat less. Exercise more. Eat less. Exercise more.
Eat less. Exercise more. Eat less. Exercise more.
Eat less. Exercise more. Eat less. Exercise more.
Eat less. Exercise more. Eat less. Exercise more.
Eat less. Exercise more. Eat less. Exercise more.
Eat less. Exercise more. Eat less. Exercise more.
Eat less. Exercise more. Eat less. Exercise more.

Eat less. Exercise more. Eat less. Exercise more.
Eat less. Exercise more. Eat less. Exercise more.
Eat less. Exercise more. Eat less. Exercise more.
Eat less. Exercise more. Eat less. Exercise more.
Eat less. Exercise more. Eat less. Exercise more.
Eat less. Exercise more. Eat less. Exercise more.
Eat less. Exercise more. Eat less. Exercise more.
Eat less. Exercise more. Eat less. Exercise more.
Eat less. Exercise more. Eat less. Exercise more.
Eat less. Exercise more. Eat less. Exercise more.
Eat less. Exercise more. Eat less. Exercise more.
Eat less. Exercise more. Eat less. Exercise more.
Eat less. Exercise more. Eat less. Exercise more.
Eat less. Exercise more. Eat less. Exercise more.
Eat less. Exercise more. Eat less. Exercise more.
Eat less. Exercise more. Eat less. Exercise more.
Eat less. Exercise more. Eat less. Exercise more.
Eat less. Exercise more. Eat less. Exercise more.
Eat less. Exercise more. Eat less. Exercise more.
Eat less. Exercise more. Eat less. Exercise more.
Eat less. Exercise more. Eat less. Exercise more.
Eat less. Exercise more. Eat less. Exercise more.
Eat less. Exercise more. Eat less. Exercise more.
Eat less. Exercise more. Eat less. Exercise more.
Eat less. Exercise more. Eat less. Exercise more.
Eat less. Exercise more. Eat less. Exercise more.
Eat less. Exercise more. Eat less. Exercise more.
Eat less. Exercise more. Eat less. Exercise more.
Eat less. Exercise more. Eat less. Exercise more.
Eat less. Exercise more. Eat less. Exercise more.
Eat less. Exercise more. Eat less. Exercise more.
Eat less. Exercise more. Eat less. Exercise more.
Eat less. Exercise more. Eat less. Exercise more.

Eat less. Exercise more. Eat less. Exercise more.
Eat less. Exercise more. Eat less. Exercise more.
Eat less. Exercise more. Eat less. Exercise more.
Eat less. Exercise more. Eat less. Exercise more.
Eat less. Exercise more. Eat less. Exercise more.
Eat less. Exercise more. Eat less. Exercise more.
Eat less. Exercise more. Eat less. Exercise more.
Eat less. Exercise more. Eat less. Exercise more.
Eat less. Exercise more. Eat less. Exercise more.
Eat less. Exercise more. Eat less. Exercise more.
Eat less. Exercise more. Eat less. Exercise more.
Eat less. Exercise more. Eat less. Exercise more.
Eat less. Exercise more. Eat less. Exercise more.
Eat less. Exercise more. Eat less. Exercise more.
Eat less. Exercise more. Eat less. Exercise more.
Eat less. Exercise more. Eat less. Exercise more.
Eat less. Exercise more. Eat less. Exercise more.
Eat less. Exercise more. Eat less. Exercise more.
Eat less. Exercise more. Eat less. Exercise more.
Eat less. Exercise more. Eat less. Exercise more.
Eat less. Exercise more. Eat less. Exercise more.
Eat less. Exercise more. Eat less. Exercise more.
Eat less. Exercise more. Eat less. Exercise more.
Eat less. Exercise more. Eat less. Exercise more.
Eat less. Exercise more. Eat less. Exercise more.
Eat less. Exercise more. Eat less. Exercise more.
Eat less. Exercise more. Eat less. Exercise more.
Eat less. Exercise more. Eat less. Exercise more.
Eat less. Exercise more. Eat less. Exercise more.
Eat less. Exercise more. Eat less. Exercise more.
Eat less. Exercise more. Eat less. Exercise more.
Eat less. Exercise more. Eat less. Exercise more.
Eat less. Exercise more. Eat less. Exercise more.
Eat less. Exercise more. Eat less. Exercise more.
Eat less. Exercise more. Eat less. Exercise more.

Eat less. Exercise more. Eat less. Exercise more.
Eat less. Exercise more. Eat less. Exercise more.
Eat less. Exercise more. Eat less. Exercise more.
Eat less. Exercise more. Eat less. Exercise more.
Eat less. Exercise more. Eat less. Exercise more.
Eat less. Exercise more. Eat less. Exercise more.
Eat less. Exercise more. Eat less. Exercise more.
Eat less. Exercise more. Eat less. Exercise more.
Eat less. Exercise more. Eat less. Exercise more.
Eat less. Exercise more. Eat less. Exercise more.
Eat less. Exercise more. Eat less. Exercise more.
Eat less. Exercise more. Eat less. Exercise more.
Eat less. Exercise more. Eat less. Exercise more.
Eat less. Exercise more. Eat less. Exercise more.
Eat less. Exercise more. Eat less. Exercise more.
Eat less. Exercise more. Eat less. Exercise more.
Eat less. Exercise more. Eat less. Exercise more.
Eat less. Exercise more. Eat less. Exercise more.
Eat less. Exercise more. Eat less. Exercise more.
Eat less. Exercise more. Eat less. Exercise more.
Eat less. Exercise more. Eat less. Exercise more.
Eat less. Exercise more. Eat less. Exercise more.
Eat less. Exercise more. Eat less. Exercise more.
Eat less. Exercise more. Eat less. Exercise more.
Eat less. Exercise more. Eat less. Exercise more.
Eat less. Exercise more. Eat less. Exercise more.
Eat less. Exercise more. Eat less. Exercise more.
Eat less. Exercise more. Eat less. Exercise more.
Eat less. Exercise more. Eat less. Exercise more.
Eat less. Exercise more. Eat less. Exercise more.
Eat less. Exercise more. Eat less. Exercise more.
Eat less. Exercise more. Eat less. Exercise more.
Eat less. Exercise more. Eat less. Exercise more.

Eat less. Exercise more. Eat less. Exercise more.
Eat less. Exercise more. Eat less. Exercise more.
Eat less. Exercise more. Eat less. Exercise more.
Eat less. Exercise more. Eat less. Exercise more.
Eat less. Exercise more. Eat less. Exercise more.
Eat less. Exercise more. Eat less. Exercise more.
Eat less. Exercise more. Eat less. Exercise more.
Eat less. Exercise more. Eat less. Exercise more.
Eat less. Exercise more. Eat less. Exercise more.
Eat less. Exercise more. Eat less. Exercise more.
Eat less. Exercise more. Eat less. Exercise more.
Eat less. Exercise more. Eat less. Exercise more.
Eat less. Exercise more. Eat less. Exercise more.
Eat less. Exercise more. Eat less. Exercise more.
Eat less. Exercise more. Eat less. Exercise more.
Eat less. Exercise more. Eat less. Exercise more.
Eat less. Exercise more. Eat less. Exercise more.
Eat less. Exercise more. Eat less. Exercise more.
Eat less. Exercise more. Eat less. Exercise more.
Eat less. Exercise more. Eat less. Exercise more.
Eat less. Exercise more. Eat less. Exercise more.
Eat less. Exercise more. Eat less. Exercise more.
Eat less. Exercise more. Eat less. Exercise more.
Eat less. Exercise more. Eat less. Exercise more.
Eat less. Exercise more. Eat less. Exercise more.
Eat less. Exercise more. Eat less. Exercise more.
Eat less. Exercise more. Eat less. Exercise more.
Eat less. Exercise more. Eat less. Exercise more.
Eat less. Exercise more. Eat less. Exercise more.
Eat less. Exercise more. Eat less. Exercise more.
Eat less. Exercise more. Eat less. Exercise more.
Eat less. Exercise more. Eat less. Exercise more.
Eat less. Exercise more. Eat less. Exercise more.

Eat less. Exercise more. Eat less. Exercise more.
Eat less. Exercise more. Eat less. Exercise more.
Eat less. Exercise more. Eat less. Exercise more.
Eat less. Exercise more. Eat less. Exercise more.
Eat less. Exercise more. Eat less. Exercise more.
Eat less. Exercise more. Eat less. Exercise more.
Eat less. Exercise more. Eat less. Exercise more.
Eat less. Exercise more. Eat less. Exercise more.
Eat less. Exercise more. Eat less. Exercise more.
Eat less. Exercise more. Eat less. Exercise more.
Eat less. Exercise more. Eat less. Exercise more.
Eat less. Exercise more. Eat less. Exercise more.
Eat less. Exercise more. Eat less. Exercise more.
Eat less. Exercise more. Eat less. Exercise more.
Eat less. Exercise more. Eat less. Exercise more.
Eat less. Exercise more. Eat less. Exercise more.
Eat less. Exercise more. Eat less. Exercise more.
Eat less. Exercise more. Eat less. Exercise more.
Eat less. Exercise more. Eat less. Exercise more.
Eat less. Exercise more. Eat less. Exercise more.
Eat less. Exercise more. Eat less. Exercise more.
Eat less. Exercise more. Eat less. Exercise more.
Eat less. Exercise more. Eat less. Exercise more.
Eat less. Exercise more. Eat less. Exercise more.
Eat less. Exercise more. Eat less. Exercise more.
Eat less. Exercise more. Eat less. Exercise more.
Eat less. Exercise more. Eat less. Exercise more.
Eat less. Exercise more. Eat less. Exercise more.
Eat less. Exercise more. Eat less. Exercise more.
Eat less. Exercise more. Eat less. Exercise more.
Eat less. Exercise more. Eat less. Exercise more.
Eat less. Exercise more. Eat less. Exercise more.
Eat less. Exercise more. Eat less. Exercise more.
Eat less. Exercise more. Eat less. Exercise more.

Eat less. Exercise more. Eat less. Exercise more.
Eat less. Exercise more. Eat less. Exercise more.
Eat less. Exercise more. Eat less. Exercise more.
Eat less. Exercise more. Eat less. Exercise more.
Eat less. Exercise more. Eat less. Exercise more.
Eat less. Exercise more. Eat less. Exercise more.
Eat less. Exercise more. Eat less. Exercise more.
Eat less. Exercise more. Eat less. Exercise more.
Eat less. Exercise more. Eat less. Exercise more.
Eat less. Exercise more. Eat less. Exercise more.
Eat less. Exercise more. Eat less. Exercise more.
Eat less. Exercise more. Eat less. Exercise more.
Eat less. Exercise more. Eat less. Exercise more.
Eat less. Exercise more. Eat less. Exercise more.
Eat less. Exercise more. Eat less. Exercise more.
Eat less. Exercise more. Eat less. Exercise more.
Eat less. Exercise more. Eat less. Exercise more.
Eat less. Exercise more. Eat less. Exercise more.
Eat less. Exercise more. Eat less. Exercise more.
Eat less. Exercise more. Eat less. Exercise more.
Eat less. Exercise more. Eat less. Exercise more.
Eat less. Exercise more. Eat less. Exercise more.
Eat less. Exercise more. Eat less. Exercise more.
Eat less. Exercise more. Eat less. Exercise more.
Eat less. Exercise more. Eat less. Exercise more.
Eat less. Exercise more. Eat less. Exercise more.
Eat less. Exercise more. Eat less. Exercise more.
Eat less. Exercise more. Eat less. Exercise more.
Eat less. Exercise more. Eat less. Exercise more.
Eat less. Exercise more. Eat less. Exercise more.
Eat less. Exercise more. Eat less. Exercise more.
Eat less. Exercise more. Eat less. Exercise more.
Eat less. Exercise more. Eat less. Exercise more.

Eat less. Exercise more. Eat less. Exercise more.
Eat less. Exercise more. Eat less. Exercise more.
Eat less. Exercise more. Eat less. Exercise more.
Eat less. Exercise more. Eat less. Exercise more.
Eat less. Exercise more. Eat less. Exercise more.
Eat less. Exercise more. Eat less. Exercise more.
Eat less. Exercise more. Eat less. Exercise more.
Eat less. Exercise more. Eat less. Exercise more.
Eat less. Exercise more. Eat less. Exercise more.
Eat less. Exercise more. Eat less. Exercise more.
Eat less. Exercise more. Eat less. Exercise more.
Eat less. Exercise more. Eat less. Exercise more.
Eat less. Exercise more. Eat less. Exercise more.
Eat less. Exercise more. Eat less. Exercise more.
Eat less. Exercise more. Eat less. Exercise more.
Eat less. Exercise more. Eat less. Exercise more.
Eat less. Exercise more. Eat less. Exercise more.
Eat less. Exercise more. Eat less. Exercise more.
Eat less. Exercise more. Eat less. Exercise more.
Eat less. Exercise more. Eat less. Exercise more.
Eat less. Exercise more. Eat less. Exercise more.
Eat less. Exercise more. Eat less. Exercise more.
Eat less. Exercise more. Eat less. Exercise more.
Eat less. Exercise more. Eat less. Exercise more.
Eat less. Exercise more. Eat less. Exercise more.
Eat less. Exercise more. Eat less. Exercise more.
Eat less. Exercise more. Eat less. Exercise more.
Eat less. Exercise more. Eat less. Exercise more.
Eat less. Exercise more. Eat less. Exercise more.
Eat less. Exercise more. Eat less. Exercise more.
Eat less. Exercise more. Eat less. Exercise more.
Eat less. Exercise more. Eat less. Exercise more.
Eat less. Exercise more. Eat less. Exercise more.
Eat less. Exercise more. Eat less. Exercise more.

Eat less. Exercise more. Eat less. Exercise more.
Eat less. Exercise more. Eat less. Exercise more.
Eat less. Exercise more. Eat less. Exercise more.
Eat less. Exercise more. Eat less. Exercise more.
Eat less. Exercise more. Eat less. Exercise more.
Eat less. Exercise more. Eat less. Exercise more.
Eat less. Exercise more. Eat less. Exercise more.
Eat less. Exercise more. Eat less. Exercise more.
Eat less. Exercise more. Eat less. Exercise more.
Eat less. Exercise more. Eat less. Exercise more.
Eat less. Exercise more. Eat less. Exercise more.
Eat less. Exercise more. Eat less. Exercise more.
Eat less. Exercise more. Eat less. Exercise more.
Eat less. Exercise more. Eat less. Exercise more.
Eat less. Exercise more. Eat less. Exercise more.
Eat less. Exercise more. Eat less. Exercise more.
Eat less. Exercise more. Eat less. Exercise more.
Eat less. Exercise more. Eat less. Exercise more.
Eat less. Exercise more. Eat less. Exercise more.
Eat less. Exercise more. Eat less. Exercise more.
Eat less. Exercise more. Eat less. Exercise more.
Eat less. Exercise more. Eat less. Exercise more.
Eat less. Exercise more. Eat less. Exercise more.
Eat less. Exercise more. Eat less. Exercise more.
Eat less. Exercise more. Eat less. Exercise more.
Eat less. Exercise more. Eat less. Exercise more.
Eat less. Exercise more. Eat less. Exercise more.
Eat less. Exercise more. Eat less. Exercise more.
Eat less. Exercise more. Eat less. Exercise more.
Eat less. Exercise more. Eat less. Exercise more.
Eat less. Exercise more. Eat less. Exercise more.
Eat less. Exercise more. Eat less. Exercise more.
Eat less. Exercise more. Eat less. Exercise more.
Eat less. Exercise more. Eat less. Exercise more.
Eat less. Exercise more. Eat less. Exercise more.

Eat less. Exercise more. Eat less. Exercise more.
Eat less. Exercise more. Eat less. Exercise more.
Eat less. Exercise more. Eat less. Exercise more.
Eat less. Exercise more. Eat less. Exercise more.
Eat less. Exercise more. Eat less. Exercise more.
Eat less. Exercise more. Eat less. Exercise more.
Eat less. Exercise more. Eat less. Exercise more.
Eat less. Exercise more. Eat less. Exercise more.
Eat less. Exercise more. Eat less. Exercise more.
Eat less. Exercise more. Eat less. Exercise more.
Eat less. Exercise more. Eat less. Exercise more.
Eat less. Exercise more. Eat less. Exercise more.
Eat less. Exercise more. Eat less. Exercise more.
Eat less. Exercise more. Eat less. Exercise more.
Eat less. Exercise more. Eat less. Exercise more.
Eat less. Exercise more. Eat less. Exercise more.
Eat less. Exercise more. Eat less. Exercise more.
Eat less. Exercise more. Eat less. Exercise more.
Eat less. Exercise more. Eat less. Exercise more.
Eat less. Exercise more. Eat less. Exercise more.
Eat less. Exercise more. Eat less. Exercise more.
Eat less. Exercise more. Eat less. Exercise more.
Eat less. Exercise more. Eat less. Exercise more.
Eat less. Exercise more. Eat less. Exercise more.
Eat less. Exercise more. Eat less. Exercise more.
Eat less. Exercise more. Eat less. Exercise more.
Eat less. Exercise more. Eat less. Exercise more.
Eat less. Exercise more. Eat less. Exercise more.
Eat less. Exercise more. Eat less. Exercise more.
Eat less. Exercise more. Eat less. Exercise more.
Eat less. Exercise more. Eat less. Exercise more.
Eat less. Exercise more. Eat less. Exercise more.
Eat less. Exercise more. Eat less. Exercise more.

Eat less. Exercise more. Eat less. Exercise more.
Eat less. Exercise more. Eat less. Exercise more.
Eat less. Exercise more. Eat less. Exercise more.
Eat less. Exercise more. Eat less. Exercise more.
Eat less. Exercise more. Eat less. Exercise more.
Eat less. Exercise more. Eat less. Exercise more.
Eat less. Exercise more. Eat less. Exercise more.
Eat less. Exercise more. Eat less. Exercise more.
Eat less. Exercise more. Eat less. Exercise more.
Eat less. Exercise more. Eat less. Exercise more.
Eat less. Exercise more. Eat less. Exercise more.
Eat less. Exercise more. Eat less. Exercise more.
Eat less. Exercise more. Eat less. Exercise more.
Eat less. Exercise more. Eat less. Exercise more.
Eat less. Exercise more. Eat less. Exercise more.
Eat less. Exercise more. Eat less. Exercise more.
Eat less. Exercise more. Eat less. Exercise more.
Eat less. Exercise more. Eat less. Exercise more.
Eat less. Exercise more. Eat less. Exercise more.
Eat less. Exercise more. Eat less. Exercise more.
Eat less. Exercise more. Eat less. Exercise more.
Eat less. Exercise more. Eat less. Exercise more.
Eat less. Exercise more. Eat less. Exercise more.
Eat less. Exercise more. Eat less. Exercise more.
Eat less. Exercise more. Eat less. Exercise more.
Eat less. Exercise more. Eat less. Exercise more.
Eat less. Exercise more. Eat less. Exercise more.
Eat less. Exercise more. Eat less. Exercise more.
Eat less. Exercise more. Eat less. Exercise more.
Eat less. Exercise more. Eat less. Exercise more.
Eat less. Exercise more. Eat less. Exercise more.
Eat less. Exercise more. Eat less. Exercise more.
Eat less. Exercise more. Eat less. Exercise more.

Eat less. Exercise more. Eat less. Exercise more.
Eat less. Exercise more. Eat less. Exercise more.
Eat less. Exercise more. Eat less. Exercise more.
Eat less. Exercise more. Eat less. Exercise more.
Eat less. Exercise more. Eat less. Exercise more.
Eat less. Exercise more. Eat less. Exercise more.
Eat less. Exercise more. Eat less. Exercise more.
Eat less. Exercise more. Eat less. Exercise more.
Eat less. Exercise more. Eat less. Exercise more.
Eat less. Exercise more. Eat less. Exercise more.
Eat less. Exercise more. Eat less. Exercise more.
Eat less. Exercise more. Eat less. Exercise more.
Eat less. Exercise more. Eat less. Exercise more.
Eat less. Exercise more. Eat less. Exercise more.
Eat less. Exercise more. Eat less. Exercise more.
Eat less. Exercise more. Eat less. Exercise more.
Eat less. Exercise more. Eat less. Exercise more.
Eat less. Exercise more. Eat less. Exercise more.
Eat less. Exercise more. Eat less. Exercise more.
Eat less. Exercise more. Eat less. Exercise more.
Eat less. Exercise more. Eat less. Exercise more.
Eat less. Exercise more. Eat less. Exercise more.
Eat less. Exercise more. Eat less. Exercise more.
Eat less. Exercise more. Eat less. Exercise more.
Eat less. Exercise more. Eat less. Exercise more.
Eat less. Exercise more. Eat less. Exercise more.
Eat less. Exercise more. Eat less. Exercise more.
Eat less. Exercise more. Eat less. Exercise more.
Eat less. Exercise more. Eat less. Exercise more.
Eat less. Exercise more. Eat less. Exercise more.
Eat less. Exercise more. Eat less. Exercise more.
Eat less. Exercise more. Eat less. Exercise more.
Eat less. Exercise more. Eat less. Exercise more.
Eat less. Exercise more. Eat less. Exercise more.

Eat less. Exercise more. Eat less. Exercise more.
Eat less. Exercise more. Eat less. Exercise more.
Eat less. Exercise more. Eat less. Exercise more.
Eat less. Exercise more. Eat less. Exercise more.
Eat less. Exercise more. Eat less. Exercise more.
Eat less. Exercise more. Eat less. Exercise more.
Eat less. Exercise more. Eat less. Exercise more.
Eat less. Exercise more. Eat less. Exercise more.
Eat less. Exercise more. Eat less. Exercise more.
Eat less. Exercise more. Eat less. Exercise more.
Eat less. Exercise more. Eat less. Exercise more.
Eat less. Exercise more. Eat less. Exercise more.
Eat less. Exercise more. Eat less. Exercise more.
Eat less. Exercise more. Eat less. Exercise more.
Eat less. Exercise more. Eat less. Exercise more.
Eat less. Exercise more. Eat less. Exercise more.
Eat less. Exercise more. Eat less. Exercise more.
Eat less. Exercise more. Eat less. Exercise more.
Eat less. Exercise more. Eat less. Exercise more.
Eat less. Exercise more. Eat less. Exercise more.
Eat less. Exercise more. Eat less. Exercise more.
Eat less. Exercise more. Eat less. Exercise more.
Eat less. Exercise more. Eat less. Exercise more.
Eat less. Exercise more. Eat less. Exercise more.
Eat less. Exercise more. Eat less. Exercise more.
Eat less. Exercise more. Eat less. Exercise more.
Eat less. Exercise more. Eat less. Exercise more.
Eat less. Exercise more. Eat less. Exercise more.
Eat less. Exercise more. Eat less. Exercise more.
Eat less. Exercise more. Eat less. Exercise more.
Eat less. Exercise more. Eat less. Exercise more.
Eat less. Exercise more. Eat less. Exercise more.
Eat less. Exercise more. Eat less. Exercise more.

Eat less. Exercise more. Eat less. Exercise more.
Eat less. Exercise more. Eat less. Exercise more.
Eat less. Exercise more. Eat less. Exercise more.
Eat less. Exercise more. Eat less. Exercise more.
Eat less. Exercise more. Eat less. Exercise more.
Eat less. Exercise more. Eat less. Exercise more.
Eat less. Exercise more. Eat less. Exercise more.
Eat less. Exercise more. Eat less. Exercise more.
Eat less. Exercise more. Eat less. Exercise more.
Eat less. Exercise more. Eat less. Exercise more.
Eat less. Exercise more. Eat less. Exercise more.
Eat less. Exercise more. Eat less. Exercise more.
Eat less. Exercise more. Eat less. Exercise more.
Eat less. Exercise more. Eat less. Exercise more.
Eat less. Exercise more. Eat less. Exercise more.
Eat less. Exercise more. Eat less. Exercise more.
Eat less. Exercise more. Eat less. Exercise more.
Eat less. Exercise more. Eat less. Exercise more.
Eat less. Exercise more. Eat less. Exercise more.
Eat less. Exercise more. Eat less. Exercise more.
Eat less. Exercise more. Eat less. Exercise more.
Eat less. Exercise more. Eat less. Exercise more.
Eat less. Exercise more. Eat less. Exercise more.
Eat less. Exercise more. Eat less. Exercise more.
Eat less. Exercise more. Eat less. Exercise more.
Eat less. Exercise more. Eat less. Exercise more.
Eat less. Exercise more. Eat less. Exercise more.
Eat less. Exercise more. Eat less. Exercise more.
Eat less. Exercise more. Eat less. Exercise more.
Eat less. Exercise more. Eat less. Exercise more.
Eat less. Exercise more. Eat less. Exercise more.
Eat less. Exercise more. Eat less. Exercise more.
Eat less. Exercise more. Eat less. Exercise more.
Eat less. Exercise more. Eat less. Exercise more.
Eat less. Exercise more. Eat less. Exercise more.

Eat less. Exercise more. Eat less. Exercise more.
Eat less. Exercise more. Eat less. Exercise more.
Eat less. Exercise more. Eat less. Exercise more.
Eat less. Exercise more. Eat less. Exercise more.
Eat less. Exercise more. Eat less. Exercise more.
Eat less. Exercise more. Eat less. Exercise more.
Eat less. Exercise more. Eat less. Exercise more.
Eat less. Exercise more. Eat less. Exercise more.
Eat less. Exercise more. Eat less. Exercise more.
Eat less. Exercise more. Eat less. Exercise more.
Eat less. Exercise more. Eat less. Exercise more.
Eat less. Exercise more. Eat less. Exercise more.
Eat less. Exercise more. Eat less. Exercise more.
Eat less. Exercise more. Eat less. Exercise more.
Eat less. Exercise more. Eat less. Exercise more.
Eat less. Exercise more. Eat less. Exercise more.
Eat less. Exercise more. Eat less. Exercise more.
Eat less. Exercise more. Eat less. Exercise more.
Eat less. Exercise more. Eat less. Exercise more.
Eat less. Exercise more. Eat less. Exercise more.
Eat less. Exercise more. Eat less. Exercise more.
Eat less. Exercise more. Eat less. Exercise more.
Eat less. Exercise more. Eat less. Exercise more.
Eat less. Exercise more. Eat less. Exercise more.
Eat less. Exercise more. Eat less. Exercise more.
Eat less. Exercise more. Eat less. Exercise more.
Eat less. Exercise more. Eat less. Exercise more.
Eat less. Exercise more. Eat less. Exercise more.
Eat less. Exercise more. Eat less. Exercise more.
Eat less. Exercise more. Eat less. Exercise more.
Eat less. Exercise more. Eat less. Exercise more.
Eat less. Exercise more. Eat less. Exercise more.
Eat less. Exercise more. Eat less. Exercise more.

Eat less. Exercise more. Eat less. Exercise more.
Eat less. Exercise more. Eat less. Exercise more.
Eat less. Exercise more. Eat less. Exercise more.
Eat less. Exercise more. Eat less. Exercise more.
Eat less. Exercise more. Eat less. Exercise more.
Eat less. Exercise more. Eat less. Exercise more.
Eat less. Exercise more. Eat less. Exercise more.
Eat less. Exercise more. Eat less. Exercise more.
Eat less. Exercise more. Eat less. Exercise more.
Eat less. Exercise more. Eat less. Exercise more.
Eat less. Exercise more. Eat less. Exercise more.
Eat less. Exercise more. Eat less. Exercise more.
Eat less. Exercise more. Eat less. Exercise more.
Eat less. Exercise more. Eat less. Exercise more.
Eat less. Exercise more. Eat less. Exercise more.
Eat less. Exercise more. Eat less. Exercise more.
Eat less. Exercise more. Eat less. Exercise more.
Eat less. Exercise more. Eat less. Exercise more.
Eat less. Exercise more. Eat less. Exercise more.
Eat less. Exercise more. Eat less. Exercise more.
Eat less. Exercise more. Eat less. Exercise more.
Eat less. Exercise more. Eat less. Exercise more.
Eat less. Exercise more. Eat less. Exercise more.
Eat less. Exercise more. Eat less. Exercise more.
Eat less. Exercise more. Eat less. Exercise more.
Eat less. Exercise more. Eat less. Exercise more.
Eat less. Exercise more. Eat less. Exercise more.
Eat less. Exercise more. Eat less. Exercise more.
Eat less. Exercise more. Eat less. Exercise more.
Eat less. Exercise more. Eat less. Exercise more.
Eat less. Exercise more. Eat less. Exercise more.
Eat less. Exercise more. Eat less. Exercise more.
Eat less. Exercise more. Eat less. Exercise more.

Eat less. Exercise more. Eat less. Exercise more.
Eat less. Exercise more. Eat less. Exercise more.
Eat less. Exercise more. Eat less. Exercise more.
Eat less. Exercise more. Eat less. Exercise more.
Eat less. Exercise more. Eat less. Exercise more.
Eat less. Exercise more. Eat less. Exercise more.
Eat less. Exercise more. Eat less. Exercise more.
Eat less. Exercise more. Eat less. Exercise more.
Eat less. Exercise more. Eat less. Exercise more.
Eat less. Exercise more. Eat less. Exercise more.
Eat less. Exercise more. Eat less. Exercise more.
Eat less. Exercise more. Eat less. Exercise more.
Eat less. Exercise more. Eat less. Exercise more.
Eat less. Exercise more. Eat less. Exercise more.
Eat less. Exercise more. Eat less. Exercise more.
Eat less. Exercise more. Eat less. Exercise more.
Eat less. Exercise more. Eat less. Exercise more.
Eat less. Exercise more. Eat less. Exercise more.
Eat less. Exercise more. Eat less. Exercise more.
Eat less. Exercise more. Eat less. Exercise more.
Eat less. Exercise more. Eat less. Exercise more.
Eat less. Exercise more. Eat less. Exercise more.
Eat less. Exercise more. Eat less. Exercise more.
Eat less. Exercise more. Eat less. Exercise more.
Eat less. Exercise more. Eat less. Exercise more.
Eat less. Exercise more. Eat less. Exercise more.
Eat less. Exercise more. Eat less. Exercise more.
Eat less. Exercise more. Eat less. Exercise more.
Eat less. Exercise more. Eat less. Exercise more.
Eat less. Exercise more. Eat less. Exercise more.
Eat less. Exercise more. Eat less. Exercise more.
Eat less. Exercise more. Eat less. Exercise more.
Eat less. Exercise more. Eat less. Exercise more.

Eat less. Exercise more. Eat less. Exercise more.
Eat less. Exercise more. Eat less. Exercise more.
Eat less. Exercise more. Eat less. Exercise more.
Eat less. Exercise more. Eat less. Exercise more.
Eat less. Exercise more. Eat less. Exercise more.
Eat less. Exercise more. Eat less. Exercise more.
Eat less. Exercise more. Eat less. Exercise more.
Eat less. Exercise more. Eat less. Exercise more.
Eat less. Exercise more. Eat less. Exercise more.
Eat less. Exercise more. Eat less. Exercise more.
Eat less. Exercise more. Eat less. Exercise more.
Eat less. Exercise more. Eat less. Exercise more.
Eat less. Exercise more. Eat less. Exercise more.
Eat less. Exercise more. Eat less. Exercise more.
Eat less. Exercise more. Eat less. Exercise more.
Eat less. Exercise more. Eat less. Exercise more.
Eat less. Exercise more. Eat less. Exercise more.
Eat less. Exercise more. Eat less. Exercise more.
Eat less. Exercise more. Eat less. Exercise more.
Eat less. Exercise more. Eat less. Exercise more.
Eat less. Exercise more. Eat less. Exercise more.
Eat less. Exercise more. Eat less. Exercise more.
Eat less. Exercise more. Eat less. Exercise more.
Eat less. Exercise more. Eat less. Exercise more.
Eat less. Exercise more. Eat less. Exercise more.
Eat less. Exercise more. Eat less. Exercise more.
Eat less. Exercise more. Eat less. Exercise more.
Eat less. Exercise more. Eat less. Exercise more.
Eat less. Exercise more. Eat less. Exercise more.
Eat less. Exercise more. Eat less. Exercise more.
Eat less. Exercise more. Eat less. Exercise more.
Eat less. Exercise more. Eat less. Exercise more.
Eat less. Exercise more. Eat less. Exercise more.
Eat less. Exercise more. Eat less. Exercise more.

Eat less. Exercise more. Eat less. Exercise more.
Eat less. Exercise more. Eat less. Exercise more.
Eat less. Exercise more. Eat less. Exercise more.
Eat less. Exercise more. Eat less. Exercise more.
Eat less. Exercise more. Eat less. Exercise more.
Eat less. Exercise more. Eat less. Exercise more.
Eat less. Exercise more. Eat less. Exercise more.
Eat less. Exercise more. Eat less. Exercise more.
Eat less. Exercise more. Eat less. Exercise more.
Eat less. Exercise more. Eat less. Exercise more.
Eat less. Exercise more. Eat less. Exercise more.
Eat less. Exercise more. Eat less. Exercise more.
Eat less. Exercise more. Eat less. Exercise more.
Eat less. Exercise more. Eat less. Exercise more.
Eat less. Exercise more. Eat less. Exercise more.
Eat less. Exercise more. Eat less. Exercise more.
Eat less. Exercise more. Eat less. Exercise more.
Eat less. Exercise more. Eat less. Exercise more.
Eat less. Exercise more. Eat less. Exercise more.
Eat less. Exercise more. Eat less. Exercise more.
Eat less. Exercise more. Eat less. Exercise more.
Eat less. Exercise more. Eat less. Exercise more.
Eat less. Exercise more. Eat less. Exercise more.
Eat less. Exercise more. Eat less. Exercise more.
Eat less. Exercise more. Eat less. Exercise more.
Eat less. Exercise more. Eat less. Exercise more.
Eat less. Exercise more. Eat less. Exercise more.
Eat less. Exercise more. Eat less. Exercise more.
Eat less. Exercise more. Eat less. Exercise more.
Eat less. Exercise more. Eat less. Exercise more.
Eat less. Exercise more. Eat less. Exercise more.
Eat less. Exercise more. Eat less. Exercise more.
Eat less. Exercise more. Eat less. Exercise more.

Eat less. Exercise more. Eat less. Exercise more.
Eat less. Exercise more. Eat less. Exercise more.
Eat less. Exercise more. Eat less. Exercise more.
Eat less. Exercise more. Eat less. Exercise more.
Eat less. Exercise more. Eat less. Exercise more.
Eat less. Exercise more. Eat less. Exercise more.
Eat less. Exercise more. Eat less. Exercise more.
Eat less. Exercise more. Eat less. Exercise more.
Eat less. Exercise more. Eat less. Exercise more.
Eat less. Exercise more. Eat less. Exercise more.
Eat less. Exercise more. Eat less. Exercise more.
Eat less. Exercise more. Eat less. Exercise more.
Eat less. Exercise more. Eat less. Exercise more.
Eat less. Exercise more. Eat less. Exercise more.
Eat less. Exercise more. Eat less. Exercise more.
Eat less. Exercise more. Eat less. Exercise more.
Eat less. Exercise more. Eat less. Exercise more.
Eat less. Exercise more. Eat less. Exercise more.
Eat less. Exercise more. Eat less. Exercise more.
Eat less. Exercise more. Eat less. Exercise more.
Eat less. Exercise more. Eat less. Exercise more.
Eat less. Exercise more. Eat less. Exercise more.
Eat less. Exercise more. Eat less. Exercise more.
Eat less. Exercise more. Eat less. Exercise more.
Eat less. Exercise more. Eat less. Exercise more.
Eat less. Exercise more. Eat less. Exercise more.
Eat less. Exercise more. Eat less. Exercise more.
Eat less. Exercise more. Eat less. Exercise more.
Eat less. Exercise more. Eat less. Exercise more.
Eat less. Exercise more. Eat less. Exercise more.
Eat less. Exercise more. Eat less. Exercise more.
Eat less. Exercise more. Eat less. Exercise more.
Eat less. Exercise more. Eat less. Exercise more.
Eat less. Exercise more. Eat less. Exercise more.
Eat less. Exercise more. Eat less. Exercise more.

Eat less. Exercise more. Eat less. Exercise more.
Eat less. Exercise more. Eat less. Exercise more.
Eat less. Exercise more. Eat less. Exercise more.
Eat less. Exercise more. Eat less. Exercise more.
Eat less. Exercise more. Eat less. Exercise more.
Eat less. Exercise more. Eat less. Exercise more.
Eat less. Exercise more. Eat less. Exercise more.
Eat less. Exercise more. Eat less. Exercise more.
Eat less. Exercise more. Eat less. Exercise more.
Eat less. Exercise more. Eat less. Exercise more.
Eat less. Exercise more. Eat less. Exercise more.
Eat less. Exercise more. Eat less. Exercise more.
Eat less. Exercise more. Eat less. Exercise more.
Eat less. Exercise more. Eat less. Exercise more.
Eat less. Exercise more. Eat less. Exercise more.
Eat less. Exercise more. Eat less. Exercise more.
Eat less. Exercise more. Eat less. Exercise more.
Eat less. Exercise more. Eat less. Exercise more.
Eat less. Exercise more. Eat less. Exercise more.
Eat less. Exercise more. Eat less. Exercise more.
Eat less. Exercise more. Eat less. Exercise more.
Eat less. Exercise more. Eat less. Exercise more.
Eat less. Exercise more. Eat less. Exercise more.
Eat less. Exercise more. Eat less. Exercise more.
Eat less. Exercise more. Eat less. Exercise more.
Eat less. Exercise more. Eat less. Exercise more.
Eat less. Exercise more. Eat less. Exercise more.
Eat less. Exercise more. Eat less. Exercise more.
Eat less. Exercise more. Eat less. Exercise more.
Eat less. Exercise more. Eat less. Exercise more.
Eat less. Exercise more. Eat less. Exercise more.
Eat less. Exercise more. Eat less. Exercise more.
Eat less. Exercise more. Eat less. Exercise more.
Eat less. Exercise more. Eat less. Exercise more.
Eat less. Exercise more. Eat less. Exercise more.

Eat less. Exercise more. Eat less. Exercise more.
Eat less. Exercise more. Eat less. Exercise more.
Eat less. Exercise more. Eat less. Exercise more.
Eat less. Exercise more. Eat less. Exercise more.
Eat less. Exercise more. Eat less. Exercise more.
Eat less. Exercise more. Eat less. Exercise more.
Eat less. Exercise more. Eat less. Exercise more.
Eat less. Exercise more. Eat less. Exercise more.
Eat less. Exercise more. Eat less. Exercise more.
Eat less. Exercise more. Eat less. Exercise more.
Eat less. Exercise more. Eat less. Exercise more.
Eat less. Exercise more. Eat less. Exercise more.
Eat less. Exercise more. Eat less. Exercise more.
Eat less. Exercise more. Eat less. Exercise more.
Eat less. Exercise more. Eat less. Exercise more.
Eat less. Exercise more. Eat less. Exercise more.
Eat less. Exercise more. Eat less. Exercise more.
Eat less. Exercise more. Eat less. Exercise more.
Eat less. Exercise more. Eat less. Exercise more.
Eat less. Exercise more. Eat less. Exercise more.
Eat less. Exercise more. Eat less. Exercise more.
Eat less. Exercise more. Eat less. Exercise more.
Eat less. Exercise more. Eat less. Exercise more.
Eat less. Exercise more. Eat less. Exercise more.
Eat less. Exercise more. Eat less. Exercise more.
Eat less. Exercise more. Eat less. Exercise more.
Eat less. Exercise more. Eat less. Exercise more.
Eat less. Exercise more. Eat less. Exercise more.
Eat less. Exercise more. Eat less. Exercise more.
Eat less. Exercise more. Eat less. Exercise more.
Eat less. Exercise more. Eat less. Exercise more.
Eat less. Exercise more. Eat less. Exercise more.
Eat less. Exercise more. Eat less. Exercise more.

Eat less. Exercise more. Eat less. Exercise more.
Eat less. Exercise more. Eat less. Exercise more.
Eat less. Exercise more. Eat less. Exercise more.
Eat less. Exercise more. Eat less. Exercise more.
Eat less. Exercise more. Eat less. Exercise more.
Eat less. Exercise more. Eat less. Exercise more.
Eat less. Exercise more. Eat less. Exercise more.
Eat less. Exercise more. Eat less. Exercise more.
Eat less. Exercise more. Eat less. Exercise more.
Eat less. Exercise more. Eat less. Exercise more.
Eat less. Exercise more. Eat less. Exercise more.
Eat less. Exercise more. Eat less. Exercise more.
Eat less. Exercise more. Eat less. Exercise more.
Eat less. Exercise more. Eat less. Exercise more.
Eat less. Exercise more. Eat less. Exercise more.
Eat less. Exercise more. Eat less. Exercise more.
Eat less. Exercise more. Eat less. Exercise more.
Eat less. Exercise more. Eat less. Exercise more.
Eat less. Exercise more. Eat less. Exercise more.
Eat less. Exercise more. Eat less. Exercise more.
Eat less. Exercise more. Eat less. Exercise more.
Eat less. Exercise more. Eat less. Exercise more.
Eat less. Exercise more. Eat less. Exercise more.
Eat less. Exercise more. Eat less. Exercise more.
Eat less. Exercise more. Eat less. Exercise more.
Eat less. Exercise more. Eat less. Exercise more.
Eat less. Exercise more. Eat less. Exercise more.
Eat less. Exercise more. Eat less. Exercise more.
Eat less. Exercise more. Eat less. Exercise more.
Eat less. Exercise more. Eat less. Exercise more.
Eat less. Exercise more. Eat less. Exercise more.
Eat less. Exercise more. Eat less. Exercise more.
Eat less. Exercise more. Eat less. Exercise more.
Eat less. Exercise more. Eat less. Exercise more.

Eat less. Exercise more. Eat less. Exercise more.
Eat less. Exercise more. Eat less. Exercise more.
Eat less. Exercise more. Eat less. Exercise more.
Eat less. Exercise more. Eat less. Exercise more.
Eat less. Exercise more. Eat less. Exercise more.
Eat less. Exercise more. Eat less. Exercise more.
Eat less. Exercise more. Eat less. Exercise more.
Eat less. Exercise more. Eat less. Exercise more.
Eat less. Exercise more. Eat less. Exercise more.
Eat less. Exercise more. Eat less. Exercise more.
Eat less. Exercise more. Eat less. Exercise more.
Eat less. Exercise more. Eat less. Exercise more.
Eat less. Exercise more. Eat less. Exercise more.
Eat less. Exercise more. Eat less. Exercise more.
Eat less. Exercise more. Eat less. Exercise more.
Eat less. Exercise more. Eat less. Exercise more.
Eat less. Exercise more. Eat less. Exercise more.
Eat less. Exercise more. Eat less. Exercise more.
Eat less. Exercise more. Eat less. Exercise more.
Eat less. Exercise more. Eat less. Exercise more.
Eat less. Exercise more. Eat less. Exercise more.
Eat less. Exercise more. Eat less. Exercise more.
Eat less. Exercise more. Eat less. Exercise more.
Eat less. Exercise more. Eat less. Exercise more.
Eat less. Exercise more. Eat less. Exercise more.
Eat less. Exercise more. Eat less. Exercise more.
Eat less. Exercise more. Eat less. Exercise more.
Eat less. Exercise more. Eat less. Exercise more.
Eat less. Exercise more. Eat less. Exercise more.
Eat less. Exercise more. Eat less. Exercise more.
Eat less. Exercise more. Eat less. Exercise more.
Eat less. Exercise more. Eat less. Exercise more.
Eat less. Exercise more. Eat less. Exercise more.

Eat less. Exercise more. Eat less. Exercise more.
Eat less. Exercise more. Eat less. Exercise more.
Eat less. Exercise more. Eat less. Exercise more.
Eat less. Exercise more. Eat less. Exercise more.
Eat less. Exercise more. Eat less. Exercise more.
Eat less. Exercise more. Eat less. Exercise more.
Eat less. Exercise more. Eat less. Exercise more.
Eat less. Exercise more. Eat less. Exercise more.
Eat less. Exercise more. Eat less. Exercise more.
Eat less. Exercise more. Eat less. Exercise more.
Eat less. Exercise more. Eat less. Exercise more.
Eat less. Exercise more. Eat less. Exercise more.
Eat less. Exercise more. Eat less. Exercise more.
Eat less. Exercise more. Eat less. Exercise more.
Eat less. Exercise more. Eat less. Exercise more.
Eat less. Exercise more. Eat less. Exercise more.
Eat less. Exercise more. Eat less. Exercise more.
Eat less. Exercise more. Eat less. Exercise more.
Eat less. Exercise more. Eat less. Exercise more.
Eat less. Exercise more. Eat less. Exercise more.
Eat less. Exercise more. Eat less. Exercise more.
Eat less. Exercise more. Eat less. Exercise more.
Eat less. Exercise more. Eat less. Exercise more.
Eat less. Exercise more. Eat less. Exercise more.
Eat less. Exercise more. Eat less. Exercise more.
Eat less. Exercise more. Eat less. Exercise more.
Eat less. Exercise more. Eat less. Exercise more.
Eat less. Exercise more. Eat less. Exercise more.
Eat less. Exercise more. Eat less. Exercise more.
Eat less. Exercise more. Eat less. Exercise more.
Eat less. Exercise more. Eat less. Exercise more.
Eat less. Exercise more. Eat less. Exercise more.
Eat less. Exercise more. Eat less. Exercise more.
Eat less. Exercise more. Eat less. Exercise more.
Eat less. Exercise more. Eat less. Exercise more.

Eat less. Exercise more. Eat less. Exercise more.
Eat less. Exercise more. Eat less. Exercise more.
Eat less. Exercise more. Eat less. Exercise more.
Eat less. Exercise more. Eat less. Exercise more.
Eat less. Exercise more. Eat less. Exercise more.
Eat less. Exercise more. Eat less. Exercise more.
Eat less. Exercise more. Eat less. Exercise more.
Eat less. Exercise more. Eat less. Exercise more.
Eat less. Exercise more. Eat less. Exercise more.
Eat less. Exercise more. Eat less. Exercise more.
Eat less. Exercise more. Eat less. Exercise more.
Eat less. Exercise more. Eat less. Exercise more.
Eat less. Exercise more. Eat less. Exercise more.
Eat less. Exercise more. Eat less. Exercise more.
Eat less. Exercise more. Eat less. Exercise more.
Eat less. Exercise more. Eat less. Exercise more.
Eat less. Exercise more. Eat less. Exercise more.
Eat less. Exercise more. Eat less. Exercise more.
Eat less. Exercise more. Eat less. Exercise more.
Eat less. Exercise more. Eat less. Exercise more.
Eat less. Exercise more. Eat less. Exercise more.
Eat less. Exercise more. Eat less. Exercise more.
Eat less. Exercise more. Eat less. Exercise more.
Eat less. Exercise more. Eat less. Exercise more.
Eat less. Exercise more. Eat less. Exercise more.
Eat less. Exercise more. Eat less. Exercise more.
Eat less. Exercise more. Eat less. Exercise more.
Eat less. Exercise more. Eat less. Exercise more.
Eat less. Exercise more. Eat less. Exercise more.
Eat less. Exercise more. Eat less. Exercise more.
Eat less. Exercise more. Eat less. Exercise more.
Eat less. Exercise more. Eat less. Exercise more.
Eat less. Exercise more. Eat less. Exercise more.
Eat less. Exercise more. Eat less. Exercise more.

Eat less. Exercise more. Eat less. Exercise more.
Eat less. Exercise more. Eat less. Exercise more.
Eat less. Exercise more. Eat less. Exercise more.
Eat less. Exercise more. Eat less. Exercise more.
Eat less. Exercise more. Eat less. Exercise more.
Eat less. Exercise more. Eat less. Exercise more.
Eat less. Exercise more. Eat less. Exercise more.
Eat less. Exercise more. Eat less. Exercise more.
Eat less. Exercise more. Eat less. Exercise more.
Eat less. Exercise more. Eat less. Exercise more.
Eat less. Exercise more. Eat less. Exercise more.
Eat less. Exercise more. Eat less. Exercise more.
Eat less. Exercise more. Eat less. Exercise more.
Eat less. Exercise more. Eat less. Exercise more.
Eat less. Exercise more. Eat less. Exercise more.
Eat less. Exercise more. Eat less. Exercise more.
Eat less. Exercise more. Eat less. Exercise more.
Eat less. Exercise more. Eat less. Exercise more.
Eat less. Exercise more. Eat less. Exercise more.
Eat less. Exercise more. Eat less. Exercise more.
Eat less. Exercise more. Eat less. Exercise more.
Eat less. Exercise more. Eat less. Exercise more.
Eat less. Exercise more. Eat less. Exercise more.
Eat less. Exercise more. Eat less. Exercise more.
Eat less. Exercise more. Eat less. Exercise more.
Eat less. Exercise more. Eat less. Exercise more.
Eat less. Exercise more. Eat less. Exercise more.
Eat less. Exercise more. Eat less. Exercise more.
Eat less. Exercise more. Eat less. Exercise more.
Eat less. Exercise more. Eat less. Exercise more.
Eat less. Exercise more. Eat less. Exercise more.
Eat less. Exercise more. Eat less. Exercise more.
Eat less. Exercise more. Eat less. Exercise more.
Eat less. Exercise more. Eat less. Exercise more.
Eat less. Exercise more. Eat less. Exercise more.

Eat less. Exercise more. Eat less. Exercise more.
Eat less. Exercise more. Eat less. Exercise more.
Eat less. Exercise more. Eat less. Exercise more.
Eat less. Exercise more. Eat less. Exercise more.
Eat less. Exercise more. Eat less. Exercise more.
Eat less. Exercise more. Eat less. Exercise more.
Eat less. Exercise more. Eat less. Exercise more.
Eat less. Exercise more. Eat less. Exercise more.
Eat less. Exercise more. Eat less. Exercise more.
Eat less. Exercise more. Eat less. Exercise more.
Eat less. Exercise more. Eat less. Exercise more.
Eat less. Exercise more. Eat less. Exercise more.
Eat less. Exercise more. Eat less. Exercise more.
Eat less. Exercise more. Eat less. Exercise more.
Eat less. Exercise more. Eat less. Exercise more.
Eat less. Exercise more. Eat less. Exercise more.
Eat less. Exercise more. Eat less. Exercise more.
Eat less. Exercise more. Eat less. Exercise more.
Eat less. Exercise more. Eat less. Exercise more.
Eat less. Exercise more. Eat less. Exercise more.
Eat less. Exercise more. Eat less. Exercise more.
Eat less. Exercise more. Eat less. Exercise more.
Eat less. Exercise more. Eat less. Exercise more.
Eat less. Exercise more. Eat less. Exercise more.
Eat less. Exercise more. Eat less. Exercise more.
Eat less. Exercise more. Eat less. Exercise more.
Eat less. Exercise more. Eat less. Exercise more.
Eat less. Exercise more. Eat less. Exercise more.
Eat less. Exercise more. Eat less. Exercise more.
Eat less. Exercise more. Eat less. Exercise more.
Eat less. Exercise more. Eat less. Exercise more.
Eat less. Exercise more. Eat less. Exercise more.

Eat less. Exercise more. Eat less. Exercise more.
Eat less. Exercise more. Eat less. Exercise more.
Eat less. Exercise more. Eat less. Exercise more.
Eat less. Exercise more. Eat less. Exercise more.
Eat less. Exercise more. Eat less. Exercise more.
Eat less. Exercise more. Eat less. Exercise more.
Eat less. Exercise more. Eat less. Exercise more.
Eat less. Exercise more. Eat less. Exercise more.
Eat less. Exercise more. Eat less. Exercise more.
Eat less. Exercise more. Eat less. Exercise more.
Eat less. Exercise more. Eat less. Exercise more.
Eat less. Exercise more. Eat less. Exercise more.
Eat less. Exercise more. Eat less. Exercise more.
Eat less. Exercise more. Eat less. Exercise more.
Eat less. Exercise more. Eat less. Exercise more.
Eat less. Exercise more. Eat less. Exercise more.
Eat less. Exercise more. Eat less. Exercise more.
Eat less. Exercise more. Eat less. Exercise more.
Eat less. Exercise more. Eat less. Exercise more.
Eat less. Exercise more. Eat less. Exercise more.
Eat less. Exercise more. Eat less. Exercise more.
Eat less. Exercise more. Eat less. Exercise more.
Eat less. Exercise more. Eat less. Exercise more.
Eat less. Exercise more. Eat less. Exercise more.
Eat less. Exercise more. Eat less. Exercise more.
Eat less. Exercise more. Eat less. Exercise more.
Eat less. Exercise more. Eat less. Exercise more.
Eat less. Exercise more. Eat less. Exercise more.
Eat less. Exercise more. Eat less. Exercise more.
Eat less. Exercise more. Eat less. Exercise more.
Eat less. Exercise more. Eat less. Exercise more.
Eat less. Exercise more. Eat less. Exercise more.
Eat less. Exercise more. Eat less. Exercise more.

Eat less. Exercise more. Eat less. Exercise more.
Eat less. Exercise more. Eat less. Exercise more.
Eat less. Exercise more. Eat less. Exercise more.
Eat less. Exercise more. Eat less. Exercise more.
Eat less. Exercise more. Eat less. Exercise more.
Eat less. Exercise more. Eat less. Exercise more.
Eat less. Exercise more. Eat less. Exercise more.
Eat less. Exercise more. Eat less. Exercise more.
Eat less. Exercise more. Eat less. Exercise more.
Eat less. Exercise more. Eat less. Exercise more.
Eat less. Exercise more. Eat less. Exercise more.
Eat less. Exercise more. Eat less. Exercise more.
Eat less. Exercise more. Eat less. Exercise more.
Eat less. Exercise more. Eat less. Exercise more.
Eat less. Exercise more. Eat less. Exercise more.
Eat less. Exercise more. Eat less. Exercise more.
Eat less. Exercise more. Eat less. Exercise more.
Eat less. Exercise more. Eat less. Exercise more.
Eat less. Exercise more. Eat less. Exercise more.
Eat less. Exercise more. Eat less. Exercise more.
Eat less. Exercise more. Eat less. Exercise more.
Eat less. Exercise more. Eat less. Exercise more.
Eat less. Exercise more. Eat less. Exercise more.
Eat less. Exercise more. Eat less. Exercise more.
Eat less. Exercise more. Eat less. Exercise more.
Eat less. Exercise more. Eat less. Exercise more.
Eat less. Exercise more. Eat less. Exercise more.
Eat less. Exercise more. Eat less. Exercise more.
Eat less. Exercise more. Eat less. Exercise more.
Eat less. Exercise more. Eat less. Exercise more.
Eat less. Exercise more. Eat less. Exercise more.
Eat less. Exercise more. Eat less. Exercise more.
Eat less. Exercise more. Eat less. Exercise more.
Eat less. Exercise more. Eat less. Exercise more.

Eat less. Exercise more. Eat less. Exercise more.
Eat less. Exercise more. Eat less. Exercise more.
Eat less. Exercise more. Eat less. Exercise more.
Eat less. Exercise more. Eat less. Exercise more.
Eat less. Exercise more. Eat less. Exercise more.
Eat less. Exercise more. Eat less. Exercise more.
Eat less. Exercise more. Eat less. Exercise more.
Eat less. Exercise more. Eat less. Exercise more.
Eat less. Exercise more. Eat less. Exercise more.
Eat less. Exercise more. Eat less. Exercise more.
Eat less. Exercise more. Eat less. Exercise more.
Eat less. Exercise more. Eat less. Exercise more.
Eat less. Exercise more. Eat less. Exercise more.
Eat less. Exercise more. Eat less. Exercise more.
Eat less. Exercise more. Eat less. Exercise more.
Eat less. Exercise more. Eat less. Exercise more.
Eat less. Exercise more. Eat less. Exercise more.
Eat less. Exercise more. Eat less. Exercise more.
Eat less. Exercise more. Eat less. Exercise more.
Eat less. Exercise more. Eat less. Exercise more.
Eat less. Exercise more. Eat less. Exercise more.
Eat less. Exercise more. Eat less. Exercise more.
Eat less. Exercise more. Eat less. Exercise more.
Eat less. Exercise more. Eat less. Exercise more.
Eat less. Exercise more. Eat less. Exercise more.
Eat less. Exercise more. Eat less. Exercise more.
Eat less. Exercise more. Eat less. Exercise more.
Eat less. Exercise more. Eat less. Exercise more.
Eat less. Exercise more. Eat less. Exercise more.
Eat less. Exercise more. Eat less. Exercise more.
Eat less. Exercise more. Eat less. Exercise more.
Eat less. Exercise more. Eat less. Exercise more.
Eat less. Exercise more. Eat less. Exercise more.
Eat less. Exercise more. Eat less. Exercise more.

Eat less. Exercise more. Eat less. Exercise more.
Eat less. Exercise more. Eat less. Exercise more.
Eat less. Exercise more. Eat less. Exercise more.
Eat less. Exercise more. Eat less. Exercise more.
Eat less. Exercise more. Eat less. Exercise more.
Eat less. Exercise more. Eat less. Exercise more.
Eat less. Exercise more. Eat less. Exercise more.
Eat less. Exercise more. Eat less. Exercise more.
Eat less. Exercise more. Eat less. Exercise more.
Eat less. Exercise more. Eat less. Exercise more.
Eat less. Exercise more. Eat less. Exercise more.
Eat less. Exercise more. Eat less. Exercise more.
Eat less. Exercise more. Eat less. Exercise more.
Eat less. Exercise more. Eat less. Exercise more.
Eat less. Exercise more. Eat less. Exercise more.
Eat less. Exercise more. Eat less. Exercise more.
Eat less. Exercise more. Eat less. Exercise more.
Eat less. Exercise more. Eat less. Exercise more.
Eat less. Exercise more. Eat less. Exercise more.
Eat less. Exercise more. Eat less. Exercise more.
Eat less. Exercise more. Eat less. Exercise more.
Eat less. Exercise more. Eat less. Exercise more.
Eat less. Exercise more. Eat less. Exercise more.
Eat less. Exercise more. Eat less. Exercise more.
Eat less. Exercise more. Eat less. Exercise more.
Eat less. Exercise more. Eat less. Exercise more.
Eat less. Exercise more. Eat less. Exercise more.
Eat less. Exercise more. Eat less. Exercise more.
Eat less. Exercise more. Eat less. Exercise more.
Eat less. Exercise more. Eat less. Exercise more.
Eat less. Exercise more. Eat less. Exercise more.
Eat less. Exercise more. Eat less. Exercise more.
Eat less. Exercise more. Eat less. Exercise more.

Eat less. Exercise more. Eat less. Exercise more.
Eat less. Exercise more. Eat less. Exercise more.
Eat less. Exercise more. Eat less. Exercise more.
Eat less. Exercise more. Eat less. Exercise more.
Eat less. Exercise more. Eat less. Exercise more.
Eat less. Exercise more. Eat less. Exercise more.
Eat less. Exercise more. Eat less. Exercise more.
Eat less. Exercise more. Eat less. Exercise more.
Eat less. Exercise more. Eat less. Exercise more.
Eat less. Exercise more. Eat less. Exercise more.
Eat less. Exercise more. Eat less. Exercise more.
Eat less. Exercise more. Eat less. Exercise more.
Eat less. Exercise more. Eat less. Exercise more.
Eat less. Exercise more. Eat less. Exercise more.
Eat less. Exercise more. Eat less. Exercise more.
Eat less. Exercise more. Eat less. Exercise more.
Eat less. Exercise more. Eat less. Exercise more.
Eat less. Exercise more. Eat less. Exercise more.
Eat less. Exercise more. Eat less. Exercise more.
Eat less. Exercise more. Eat less. Exercise more.
Eat less. Exercise more. Eat less. Exercise more.
Eat less. Exercise more. Eat less. Exercise more.
Eat less. Exercise more. Eat less. Exercise more.
Eat less. Exercise more. Eat less. Exercise more.
Eat less. Exercise more. Eat less. Exercise more.
Eat less. Exercise more. Eat less. Exercise more.
Eat less. Exercise more. Eat less. Exercise more.
Eat less. Exercise more. Eat less. Exercise more.
Eat less. Exercise more. Eat less. Exercise more.
Eat less. Exercise more. Eat less. Exercise more.
Eat less. Exercise more. Eat less. Exercise more.
Eat less. Exercise more. Eat less. Exercise more.
Eat less. Exercise more. Eat less. Exercise more.
Eat less. Exercise more. Eat less. Exercise more.

Eat less. Exercise more. Eat less. Exercise more.
Eat less. Exercise more. Eat less. Exercise more.
Eat less. Exercise more. Eat less. Exercise more.
Eat less. Exercise more. Eat less. Exercise more.
Eat less. Exercise more. Eat less. Exercise more.
Eat less. Exercise more. Eat less. Exercise more.
Eat less. Exercise more. Eat less. Exercise more.
Eat less. Exercise more. Eat less. Exercise more.
Eat less. Exercise more. Eat less. Exercise more.
Eat less. Exercise more. Eat less. Exercise more.
Eat less. Exercise more. Eat less. Exercise more.
Eat less. Exercise more. Eat less. Exercise more.
Eat less. Exercise more. Eat less. Exercise more.
Eat less. Exercise more. Eat less. Exercise more.
Eat less. Exercise more. Eat less. Exercise more.
Eat less. Exercise more. Eat less. Exercise more.
Eat less. Exercise more. Eat less. Exercise more.
Eat less. Exercise more. Eat less. Exercise more.
Eat less. Exercise more. Eat less. Exercise more.
Eat less. Exercise more. Eat less. Exercise more.
Eat less. Exercise more. Eat less. Exercise more.
Eat less. Exercise more. Eat less. Exercise more.
Eat less. Exercise more. Eat less. Exercise more.
Eat less. Exercise more. Eat less. Exercise more.
Eat less. Exercise more. Eat less. Exercise more.
Eat less. Exercise more. Eat less. Exercise more.
Eat less. Exercise more. Eat less. Exercise more.
Eat less. Exercise more. Eat less. Exercise more.
Eat less. Exercise more. Eat less. Exercise more.
Eat less. Exercise more. Eat less. Exercise more.
Eat less. Exercise more. Eat less. Exercise more.
Eat less. Exercise more. Eat less. Exercise more.
Eat less. Exercise more. Eat less. Exercise more.

Eat less. Exercise more. Eat less. Exercise more.
Eat less. Exercise more. Eat less. Exercise more.
Eat less. Exercise more. Eat less. Exercise more.
Eat less. Exercise more. Eat less. Exercise more.
Eat less. Exercise more. Eat less. Exercise more.
Eat less. Exercise more. Eat less. Exercise more.
Eat less. Exercise more. Eat less. Exercise more.
Eat less. Exercise more. Eat less. Exercise more.
Eat less. Exercise more. Eat less. Exercise more.
Eat less. Exercise more. Eat less. Exercise more.
Eat less. Exercise more. Eat less. Exercise more.
Eat less. Exercise more. Eat less. Exercise more.
Eat less. Exercise more. Eat less. Exercise more.
Eat less. Exercise more. Eat less. Exercise more.
Eat less. Exercise more. Eat less. Exercise more.
Eat less. Exercise more. Eat less. Exercise more.
Eat less. Exercise more. Eat less. Exercise more.
Eat less. Exercise more. Eat less. Exercise more.
Eat less. Exercise more. Eat less. Exercise more.
Eat less. Exercise more. Eat less. Exercise more.
Eat less. Exercise more. Eat less. Exercise more.
Eat less. Exercise more. Eat less. Exercise more.
Eat less. Exercise more. Eat less. Exercise more.
Eat less. Exercise more. Eat less. Exercise more.
Eat less. Exercise more. Eat less. Exercise more.
Eat less. Exercise more. Eat less. Exercise more.
Eat less. Exercise more. Eat less. Exercise more.
Eat less. Exercise more. Eat less. Exercise more.
Eat less. Exercise more. Eat less. Exercise more.
Eat less. Exercise more. Eat less. Exercise more.
Eat less. Exercise more. Eat less. Exercise more.
Eat less. Exercise more. Eat less. Exercise more.
Eat less. Exercise more. Eat less. Exercise more.
Eat less. Exercise more. Eat less. Exercise more.

Eat less. Exercise more. Eat less. Exercise more.
Eat less. Exercise more. Eat less. Exercise more.
Eat less. Exercise more. Eat less. Exercise more.
Eat less. Exercise more. Eat less. Exercise more.
Eat less. Exercise more. Eat less. Exercise more.
Eat less. Exercise more. Eat less. Exercise more.
Eat less. Exercise more. Eat less. Exercise more.
Eat less. Exercise more. Eat less. Exercise more.
Eat less. Exercise more. Eat less. Exercise more.
Eat less. Exercise more. Eat less. Exercise more.
Eat less. Exercise more. Eat less. Exercise more.
Eat less. Exercise more. Eat less. Exercise more.
Eat less. Exercise more. Eat less. Exercise more.
Eat less. Exercise more. Eat less. Exercise more.
Eat less. Exercise more. Eat less. Exercise more.
Eat less. Exercise more. Eat less. Exercise more.
Eat less. Exercise more. Eat less. Exercise more.
Eat less. Exercise more. Eat less. Exercise more.
Eat less. Exercise more. Eat less. Exercise more.
Eat less. Exercise more. Eat less. Exercise more.
Eat less. Exercise more. Eat less. Exercise more.
Eat less. Exercise more. Eat less. Exercise more.
Eat less. Exercise more. Eat less. Exercise more.
Eat less. Exercise more. Eat less. Exercise more.
Eat less. Exercise more. Eat less. Exercise more.
Eat less. Exercise more. Eat less. Exercise more.
Eat less. Exercise more. Eat less. Exercise more.
Eat less. Exercise more. Eat less. Exercise more.
Eat less. Exercise more. Eat less. Exercise more.
Eat less. Exercise more. Eat less. Exercise more.
Eat less. Exercise more. Eat less. Exercise more.
Eat less. Exercise more. Eat less. Exercise more.
Eat less. Exercise more. Eat less. Exercise more.
Eat less. Exercise more. Eat less. Exercise more.
Eat less. Exercise more. Eat less. Exercise more.

Eat less. Exercise more. Eat less. Exercise more.
Eat less. Exercise more. Eat less. Exercise more.
Eat less. Exercise more. Eat less. Exercise more.
Eat less. Exercise more. Eat less. Exercise more.
Eat less. Exercise more. Eat less. Exercise more.
Eat less. Exercise more. Eat less. Exercise more.
Eat less. Exercise more. Eat less. Exercise more.
Eat less. Exercise more. Eat less. Exercise more.
Eat less. Exercise more. Eat less. Exercise more.
Eat less. Exercise more. Eat less. Exercise more.
Eat less. Exercise more. Eat less. Exercise more.
Eat less. Exercise more. Eat less. Exercise more.
Eat less. Exercise more. Eat less. Exercise more.
Eat less. Exercise more. Eat less. Exercise more.
Eat less. Exercise more. Eat less. Exercise more.
Eat less. Exercise more. Eat less. Exercise more.
Eat less. Exercise more. Eat less. Exercise more.
Eat less. Exercise more. Eat less. Exercise more.
Eat less. Exercise more. Eat less. Exercise more.
Eat less. Exercise more. Eat less. Exercise more.
Eat less. Exercise more. Eat less. Exercise more.
Eat less. Exercise more. Eat less. Exercise more.
Eat less. Exercise more. Eat less. Exercise more.
Eat less. Exercise more. Eat less. Exercise more.
Eat less. Exercise more. Eat less. Exercise more.
Eat less. Exercise more. Eat less. Exercise more.
Eat less. Exercise more. Eat less. Exercise more.
Eat less. Exercise more. Eat less. Exercise more.
Eat less. Exercise more. Eat less. Exercise more.
Eat less. Exercise more. Eat less. Exercise more.
Eat less. Exercise more. Eat less. Exercise more.
Eat less. Exercise more. Eat less. Exercise more.
Eat less. Exercise more. Eat less. Exercise more.
Eat less. Exercise more. Eat less. Exercise more.

Eat less. Exercise more. Eat less. Exercise more.
Eat less. Exercise more. Eat less. Exercise more.
Eat less. Exercise more. Eat less. Exercise more.
Eat less. Exercise more. Eat less. Exercise more.
Eat less. Exercise more. Eat less. Exercise more.
Eat less. Exercise more. Eat less. Exercise more.
Eat less. Exercise more. Eat less. Exercise more.
Eat less. Exercise more. Eat less. Exercise more.
Eat less. Exercise more. Eat less. Exercise more.
Eat less. Exercise more. Eat less. Exercise more.
Eat less. Exercise more. Eat less. Exercise more.
Eat less. Exercise more. Eat less. Exercise more.
Eat less. Exercise more. Eat less. Exercise more.
Eat less. Exercise more. Eat less. Exercise more.
Eat less. Exercise more. Eat less. Exercise more.
Eat less. Exercise more. Eat less. Exercise more.
Eat less. Exercise more. Eat less. Exercise more.
Eat less. Exercise more. Eat less. Exercise more.
Eat less. Exercise more. Eat less. Exercise more.
Eat less. Exercise more. Eat less. Exercise more.
Eat less. Exercise more. Eat less. Exercise more.
Eat less. Exercise more. Eat less. Exercise more.
Eat less. Exercise more. Eat less. Exercise more.
Eat less. Exercise more. Eat less. Exercise more.
Eat less. Exercise more. Eat less. Exercise more.
Eat less. Exercise more. Eat less. Exercise more.
Eat less. Exercise more. Eat less. Exercise more.
Eat less. Exercise more. Eat less. Exercise more.
Eat less. Exercise more. Eat less. Exercise more.
Eat less. Exercise more. Eat less. Exercise more.
Eat less. Exercise more. Eat less. Exercise more.
Eat less. Exercise more. Eat less. Exercise more.
Eat less. Exercise more. Eat less. Exercise more.

Eat less. Exercise more. Eat less. Exercise more.
Eat less. Exercise more. Eat less. Exercise more.
Eat less. Exercise more. Eat less. Exercise more.
Eat less. Exercise more. Eat less. Exercise more.
Eat less. Exercise more. Eat less. Exercise more.
Eat less. Exercise more. Eat less. Exercise more.
Eat less. Exercise more. Eat less. Exercise more.
Eat less. Exercise more. Eat less. Exercise more.
Eat less. Exercise more. Eat less. Exercise more.
Eat less. Exercise more. Eat less. Exercise more.
Eat less. Exercise more. Eat less. Exercise more.
Eat less. Exercise more. Eat less. Exercise more.
Eat less. Exercise more. Eat less. Exercise more.
Eat less. Exercise more. Eat less. Exercise more.
Eat less. Exercise more. Eat less. Exercise more.
Eat less. Exercise more. Eat less. Exercise more.
Eat less. Exercise more. Eat less. Exercise more.
Eat less. Exercise more. Eat less. Exercise more.
Eat less. Exercise more. Eat less. Exercise more.
Eat less. Exercise more. Eat less. Exercise more.
Eat less. Exercise more. Eat less. Exercise more.
Eat less. Exercise more. Eat less. Exercise more.
Eat less. Exercise more. Eat less. Exercise more.
Eat less. Exercise more. Eat less. Exercise more.
Eat less. Exercise more. Eat less. Exercise more.
Eat less. Exercise more. Eat less. Exercise more.
Eat less. Exercise more. Eat less. Exercise more.
Eat less. Exercise more. Eat less. Exercise more.
Eat less. Exercise more. Eat less. Exercise more.
Eat less. Exercise more. Eat less. Exercise more.
Eat less. Exercise more. Eat less. Exercise more.
Eat less. Exercise more. Eat less. Exercise more.
Eat less. Exercise more. Eat less. Exercise more.
Eat less. Exercise more. Eat less. Exercise more.

Eat less. Exercise more. Eat less. Exercise more.
Eat less. Exercise more. Eat less. Exercise more.
Eat less. Exercise more. Eat less. Exercise more.
Eat less. Exercise more. Eat less. Exercise more.
Eat less. Exercise more. Eat less. Exercise more.
Eat less. Exercise more. Eat less. Exercise more.
Eat less. Exercise more. Eat less. Exercise more.
Eat less. Exercise more. Eat less. Exercise more.
Eat less. Exercise more. Eat less. Exercise more.
Eat less. Exercise more. Eat less. Exercise more.
Eat less. Exercise more. Eat less. Exercise more.
Eat less. Exercise more. Eat less. Exercise more.
Eat less. Exercise more. Eat less. Exercise more.
Eat less. Exercise more. Eat less. Exercise more.
Eat less. Exercise more. Eat less. Exercise more.
Eat less. Exercise more. Eat less. Exercise more.
Eat less. Exercise more. Eat less. Exercise more.
Eat less. Exercise more. Eat less. Exercise more.
Eat less. Exercise more. Eat less. Exercise more.
Eat less. Exercise more. Eat less. Exercise more.
Eat less. Exercise more. Eat less. Exercise more.
Eat less. Exercise more. Eat less. Exercise more.
Eat less. Exercise more. Eat less. Exercise more.
Eat less. Exercise more. Eat less. Exercise more.
Eat less. Exercise more. Eat less. Exercise more.
Eat less. Exercise more. Eat less. Exercise more.
Eat less. Exercise more. Eat less. Exercise more.
Eat less. Exercise more. Eat less. Exercise more.
Eat less. Exercise more. Eat less. Exercise more.
Eat less. Exercise more. Eat less. Exercise more.
Eat less. Exercise more. Eat less. Exercise more.
Eat less. Exercise more. Eat less. Exercise more.
Eat less. Exercise more. Eat less. Exercise more.

Eat less. Exercise more. Eat less. Exercise more.
Eat less. Exercise more. Eat less. Exercise more.
Eat less. Exercise more. Eat less. Exercise more.
Eat less. Exercise more. Eat less. Exercise more.
Eat less. Exercise more. Eat less. Exercise more.
Eat less. Exercise more. Eat less. Exercise more.
Eat less. Exercise more. Eat less. Exercise more.
Eat less. Exercise more. Eat less. Exercise more.
Eat less. Exercise more. Eat less. Exercise more.
Eat less. Exercise more. Eat less. Exercise more.
Eat less. Exercise more. Eat less. Exercise more.
Eat less. Exercise more. Eat less. Exercise more.
Eat less. Exercise more. Eat less. Exercise more.
Eat less. Exercise more. Eat less. Exercise more.
Eat less. Exercise more. Eat less. Exercise more.
Eat less. Exercise more. Eat less. Exercise more.
Eat less. Exercise more. Eat less. Exercise more.
Eat less. Exercise more. Eat less. Exercise more.
Eat less. Exercise more. Eat less. Exercise more.
Eat less. Exercise more. Eat less. Exercise more.
Eat less. Exercise more. Eat less. Exercise more.
Eat less. Exercise more. Eat less. Exercise more.
Eat less. Exercise more. Eat less. Exercise more.
Eat less. Exercise more. Eat less. Exercise more.
Eat less. Exercise more. Eat less. Exercise more.
Eat less. Exercise more. Eat less. Exercise more.
Eat less. Exercise more. Eat less. Exercise more.
Eat less. Exercise more. Eat less. Exercise more.
Eat less. Exercise more. Eat less. Exercise more.
Eat less. Exercise more. Eat less. Exercise more.
Eat less. Exercise more. Eat less. Exercise more.
Eat less. Exercise more. Eat less. Exercise more.
Eat less. Exercise more. Eat less. Exercise more.

Eat less. Exercise more. Eat less. Exercise more.
Eat less. Exercise more. Eat less. Exercise more.
Eat less. Exercise more. Eat less. Exercise more.
Eat less. Exercise more. Eat less. Exercise more.
Eat less. Exercise more. Eat less. Exercise more.
Eat less. Exercise more. Eat less. Exercise more.
Eat less. Exercise more. Eat less. Exercise more.
Eat less. Exercise more. Eat less. Exercise more.
Eat less. Exercise more. Eat less. Exercise more.
Eat less. Exercise more. Eat less. Exercise more.
Eat less. Exercise more. Eat less. Exercise more.
Eat less. Exercise more. Eat less. Exercise more.
Eat less. Exercise more. Eat less. Exercise more.
Eat less. Exercise more. Eat less. Exercise more.
Eat less. Exercise more. Eat less. Exercise more.
Eat less. Exercise more. Eat less. Exercise more.
Eat less. Exercise more. Eat less. Exercise more.
Eat less. Exercise more. Eat less. Exercise more.
Eat less. Exercise more. Eat less. Exercise more.
Eat less. Exercise more. Eat less. Exercise more.
Eat less. Exercise more. Eat less. Exercise more.
Eat less. Exercise more. Eat less. Exercise more.
Eat less. Exercise more. Eat less. Exercise more.
Eat less. Exercise more. Eat less. Exercise more.
Eat less. Exercise more. Eat less. Exercise more.
Eat less. Exercise more. Eat less. Exercise more.
Eat less. Exercise more. Eat less. Exercise more.
Eat less. Exercise more. Eat less. Exercise more.
Eat less. Exercise more. Eat less. Exercise more.
Eat less. Exercise more. Eat less. Exercise more.
Eat less. Exercise more. Eat less. Exercise more.
Eat less. Exercise more. Eat less. Exercise more.
Eat less. Exercise more. Eat less. Exercise more.
Eat less. Exercise more. Eat less. Exercise more.

Eat less. Exercise more. Eat less. Exercise more.
Eat less. Exercise more. Eat less. Exercise more.
Eat less. Exercise more. Eat less. Exercise more.
Eat less. Exercise more. Eat less. Exercise more.
Eat less. Exercise more. Eat less. Exercise more.
Eat less. Exercise more. Eat less. Exercise more.
Eat less. Exercise more. Eat less. Exercise more.
Eat less. Exercise more. Eat less. Exercise more.
Eat less. Exercise more. Eat less. Exercise more.
Eat less. Exercise more. Eat less. Exercise more.
Eat less. Exercise more. Eat less. Exercise more.
Eat less. Exercise more. Eat less. Exercise more.
Eat less. Exercise more. Eat less. Exercise more.
Eat less. Exercise more. Eat less. Exercise more.
Eat less. Exercise more. Eat less. Exercise more.
Eat less. Exercise more. Eat less. Exercise more.
Eat less. Exercise more. Eat less. Exercise more.
Eat less. Exercise more. Eat less. Exercise more.
Eat less. Exercise more. Eat less. Exercise more.
Eat less. Exercise more. Eat less. Exercise more.
Eat less. Exercise more. Eat less. Exercise more.
Eat less. Exercise more. Eat less. Exercise more.
Eat less. Exercise more. Eat less. Exercise more.
Eat less. Exercise more. Eat less. Exercise more.
Eat less. Exercise more. Eat less. Exercise more.
Eat less. Exercise more. Eat less. Exercise more.
Eat less. Exercise more. Eat less. Exercise more.
Eat less. Exercise more. Eat less. Exercise more.
Eat less. Exercise more. Eat less. Exercise more.
Eat less. Exercise more. Eat less. Exercise more.
Eat less. Exercise more. Eat less. Exercise more.
Eat less. Exercise more. Eat less. Exercise more.
Eat less. Exercise more. Eat less. Exercise more.

Eat less. Exercise more. Eat less. Exercise more.
Eat less. Exercise more. Eat less. Exercise more.
Eat less. Exercise more. Eat less. Exercise more.
Eat less. Exercise more. Eat less. Exercise more.
Eat less. Exercise more. Eat less. Exercise more.
Eat less. Exercise more. Eat less. Exercise more.
Eat less. Exercise more. Eat less. Exercise more.
Eat less. Exercise more. Eat less. Exercise more.
Eat less. Exercise more. Eat less. Exercise more.
Eat less. Exercise more. Eat less. Exercise more.
Eat less. Exercise more. Eat less. Exercise more.
Eat less. Exercise more. Eat less. Exercise more.
Eat less. Exercise more. Eat less. Exercise more.
Eat less. Exercise more. Eat less. Exercise more.
Eat less. Exercise more. Eat less. Exercise more.
Eat less. Exercise more. Eat less. Exercise more.
Eat less. Exercise more. Eat less. Exercise more.
Eat less. Exercise more. Eat less. Exercise more.
Eat less. Exercise more. Eat less. Exercise more.
Eat less. Exercise more. Eat less. Exercise more.
Eat less. Exercise more. Eat less. Exercise more.
Eat less. Exercise more. Eat less. Exercise more.
Eat less. Exercise more. Eat less. Exercise more.
Eat less. Exercise more. Eat less. Exercise more.
Eat less. Exercise more. Eat less. Exercise more.
Eat less. Exercise more. Eat less. Exercise more.
Eat less. Exercise more. Eat less. Exercise more.
Eat less. Exercise more. Eat less. Exercise more.
Eat less. Exercise more. Eat less. Exercise more.
Eat less. Exercise more. Eat less. Exercise more.
Eat less. Exercise more. Eat less. Exercise more.
Eat less. Exercise more. Eat less. Exercise more.
Eat less. Exercise more. Eat less. Exercise more.
Eat less. Exercise more. Eat less. Exercise more.

Eat less. Exercise more. Eat less. Exercise more.
Eat less. Exercise more. Eat less. Exercise more.
Eat less. Exercise more. Eat less. Exercise more.
Eat less. Exercise more. Eat less. Exercise more.
Eat less. Exercise more. Eat less. Exercise more.
Eat less. Exercise more. Eat less. Exercise more.
Eat less. Exercise more. Eat less. Exercise more.
Eat less. Exercise more. Eat less. Exercise more.
Eat less. Exercise more. Eat less. Exercise more.
Eat less. Exercise more. Eat less. Exercise more.
Eat less. Exercise more. Eat less. Exercise more.
Eat less. Exercise more. Eat less. Exercise more.
Eat less. Exercise more. Eat less. Exercise more.
Eat less. Exercise more. Eat less. Exercise more.
Eat less. Exercise more. Eat less. Exercise more.
Eat less. Exercise more. Eat less. Exercise more.
Eat less. Exercise more. Eat less. Exercise more.
Eat less. Exercise more. Eat less. Exercise more.
Eat less. Exercise more. Eat less. Exercise more.
Eat less. Exercise more. Eat less. Exercise more.
Eat less. Exercise more. Eat less. Exercise more.
Eat less. Exercise more. Eat less. Exercise more.
Eat less. Exercise more. Eat less. Exercise more.
Eat less. Exercise more. Eat less. Exercise more.
Eat less. Exercise more. Eat less. Exercise more.
Eat less. Exercise more. Eat less. Exercise more.
Eat less. Exercise more. Eat less. Exercise more.
Eat less. Exercise more. Eat less. Exercise more.
Eat less. Exercise more. Eat less. Exercise more.
Eat less. Exercise more. Eat less. Exercise more.
Eat less. Exercise more. Eat less. Exercise more.
Eat less. Exercise more. Eat less. Exercise more.
Eat less. Exercise more. Eat less. Exercise more.
Eat less. Exercise more. Eat less. Exercise more.
Eat less. Exercise more. Eat less. Exercise more.

Eat less. Exercise more. Eat less. Exercise more.
Eat less. Exercise more. Eat less. Exercise more.
Eat less. Exercise more. Eat less. Exercise more.
Eat less. Exercise more. Eat less. Exercise more.
Eat less. Exercise more. Eat less. Exercise more.
Eat less. Exercise more. Eat less. Exercise more.
Eat less. Exercise more. Eat less. Exercise more.
Eat less. Exercise more. Eat less. Exercise more.
Eat less. Exercise more. Eat less. Exercise more.
Eat less. Exercise more. Eat less. Exercise more.
Eat less. Exercise more. Eat less. Exercise more.
Eat less. Exercise more. Eat less. Exercise more.
Eat less. Exercise more. Eat less. Exercise more.
Eat less. Exercise more. Eat less. Exercise more.
Eat less. Exercise more. Eat less. Exercise more.
Eat less. Exercise more. Eat less. Exercise more.
Eat less. Exercise more. Eat less. Exercise more.
Eat less. Exercise more. Eat less. Exercise more.
Eat less. Exercise more. Eat less. Exercise more.
Eat less. Exercise more. Eat less. Exercise more.
Eat less. Exercise more. Eat less. Exercise more.
Eat less. Exercise more. Eat less. Exercise more.
Eat less. Exercise more. Eat less. Exercise more.
Eat less. Exercise more. Eat less. Exercise more.
Eat less. Exercise more. Eat less. Exercise more.
Eat less. Exercise more. Eat less. Exercise more.
Eat less. Exercise more. Eat less. Exercise more.
Eat less. Exercise more. Eat less. Exercise more.
Eat less. Exercise more. Eat less. Exercise more.
Eat less. Exercise more. Eat less. Exercise more.
Eat less. Exercise more. Eat less. Exercise more.
Eat less. Exercise more. Eat less. Exercise more.
Eat less. Exercise more. Eat less. Exercise more.

Eat less. Exercise more. Eat less. Exercise more.
Eat less. Exercise more. Eat less. Exercise more.
Eat less. Exercise more. Eat less. Exercise more.
Eat less. Exercise more. Eat less. Exercise more.
Eat less. Exercise more. Eat less. Exercise more.
Eat less. Exercise more. Eat less. Exercise more.
Eat less. Exercise more. Eat less. Exercise more.
Eat less. Exercise more. Eat less. Exercise more.
Eat less. Exercise more. Eat less. Exercise more.
Eat less. Exercise more. Eat less. Exercise more.
Eat less. Exercise more. Eat less. Exercise more.
Eat less. Exercise more. Eat less. Exercise more.
Eat less. Exercise more. Eat less. Exercise more.
Eat less. Exercise more. Eat less. Exercise more.
Eat less. Exercise more. Eat less. Exercise more.
Eat less. Exercise more. Eat less. Exercise more.
Eat less. Exercise more. Eat less. Exercise more.
Eat less. Exercise more. Eat less. Exercise more.
Eat less. Exercise more. Eat less. Exercise more.
Eat less. Exercise more. Eat less. Exercise more.
Eat less. Exercise more. Eat less. Exercise more.
Eat less. Exercise more. Eat less. Exercise more.
Eat less. Exercise more. Eat less. Exercise more.
Eat less. Exercise more. Eat less. Exercise more.
Eat less. Exercise more. Eat less. Exercise more.
Eat less. Exercise more. Eat less. Exercise more.
Eat less. Exercise more. Eat less. Exercise more.
Eat less. Exercise more. Eat less. Exercise more.
Eat less. Exercise more. Eat less. Exercise more.
Eat less. Exercise more. Eat less. Exercise more.
Eat less. Exercise more. Eat less. Exercise more.
Eat less. Exercise more. Eat less. Exercise more.
Eat less. Exercise more. Eat less. Exercise more.

Eat less. Exercise more. Eat less. Exercise more.
Eat less. Exercise more. Eat less. Exercise more.
Eat less. Exercise more. Eat less. Exercise more.
Eat less. Exercise more. Eat less. Exercise more.
Eat less. Exercise more. Eat less. Exercise more.
Eat less. Exercise more. Eat less. Exercise more.
Eat less. Exercise more. Eat less. Exercise more.
Eat less. Exercise more. Eat less. Exercise more.
Eat less. Exercise more. Eat less. Exercise more.
Eat less. Exercise more. Eat less. Exercise more.
Eat less. Exercise more. Eat less. Exercise more.
Eat less. Exercise more. Eat less. Exercise more.
Eat less. Exercise more. Eat less. Exercise more.
Eat less. Exercise more. Eat less. Exercise more.
Eat less. Exercise more. Eat less. Exercise more.
Eat less. Exercise more. Eat less. Exercise more.
Eat less. Exercise more. Eat less. Exercise more.
Eat less. Exercise more. Eat less. Exercise more.
Eat less. Exercise more. Eat less. Exercise more.
Eat less. Exercise more. Eat less. Exercise more.
Eat less. Exercise more. Eat less. Exercise more.
Eat less. Exercise more. Eat less. Exercise more.
Eat less. Exercise more. Eat less. Exercise more.
Eat less. Exercise more. Eat less. Exercise more.
Eat less. Exercise more. Eat less. Exercise more.
Eat less. Exercise more. Eat less. Exercise more.
Eat less. Exercise more. Eat less. Exercise more.
Eat less. Exercise more. Eat less. Exercise more.
Eat less. Exercise more. Eat less. Exercise more.
Eat less. Exercise more. Eat less. Exercise more.
Eat less. Exercise more. Eat less. Exercise more.
Eat less. Exercise more. Eat less. Exercise more.
Eat less. Exercise more. Eat less. Exercise more.
Eat less. Exercise more. Eat less. Exercise more.

Eat less. Exercise more. Eat less. Exercise more.
Eat less. Exercise more. Eat less. Exercise more.
Eat less. Exercise more. Eat less. Exercise more.
Eat less. Exercise more. Eat less. Exercise more.
Eat less. Exercise more. Eat less. Exercise more.
Eat less. Exercise more. Eat less. Exercise more.
Eat less. Exercise more. Eat less. Exercise more.
Eat less. Exercise more. Eat less. Exercise more.
Eat less. Exercise more. Eat less. Exercise more.
Eat less. Exercise more. Eat less. Exercise more.
Eat less. Exercise more. Eat less. Exercise more.
Eat less. Exercise more. Eat less. Exercise more.
Eat less. Exercise more. Eat less. Exercise more.
Eat less. Exercise more. Eat less. Exercise more.
Eat less. Exercise more. Eat less. Exercise more.
Eat less. Exercise more. Eat less. Exercise more.
Eat less. Exercise more. Eat less. Exercise more.
Eat less. Exercise more. Eat less. Exercise more.
Eat less. Exercise more. Eat less. Exercise more.
Eat less. Exercise more. Eat less. Exercise more.
Eat less. Exercise more. Eat less. Exercise more.
Eat less. Exercise more. Eat less. Exercise more.
Eat less. Exercise more. Eat less. Exercise more.
Eat less. Exercise more. Eat less. Exercise more.
Eat less. Exercise more. Eat less. Exercise more.
Eat less. Exercise more. Eat less. Exercise more.
Eat less. Exercise more. Eat less. Exercise more.
Eat less. Exercise more. Eat less. Exercise more.
Eat less. Exercise more. Eat less. Exercise more.
Eat less. Exercise more. Eat less. Exercise more.
Eat less. Exercise more. Eat less. Exercise more.
Eat less. Exercise more. Eat less. Exercise more.
Eat less. Exercise more. Eat less. Exercise more.

Eat less. Exercise more. Eat less. Exercise more.
Eat less. Exercise more. Eat less. Exercise more.
Eat less. Exercise more. Eat less. Exercise more.
Eat less. Exercise more. Eat less. Exercise more.
Eat less. Exercise more. Eat less. Exercise more.
Eat less. Exercise more. Eat less. Exercise more.
Eat less. Exercise more. Eat less. Exercise more.
Eat less. Exercise more. Eat less. Exercise more.
Eat less. Exercise more. Eat less. Exercise more.
Eat less. Exercise more. Eat less. Exercise more.
Eat less. Exercise more. Eat less. Exercise more.
Eat less. Exercise more. Eat less. Exercise more.
Eat less. Exercise more. Eat less. Exercise more.
Eat less. Exercise more. Eat less. Exercise more.
Eat less. Exercise more. Eat less. Exercise more.
Eat less. Exercise more. Eat less. Exercise more.
Eat less. Exercise more. Eat less. Exercise more.
Eat less. Exercise more. Eat less. Exercise more.
Eat less. Exercise more. Eat less. Exercise more.
Eat less. Exercise more. Eat less. Exercise more.
Eat less. Exercise more. Eat less. Exercise more.
Eat less. Exercise more. Eat less. Exercise more.
Eat less. Exercise more. Eat less. Exercise more.
Eat less. Exercise more. Eat less. Exercise more.
Eat less. Exercise more. Eat less. Exercise more.
Eat less. Exercise more. Eat less. Exercise more.
Eat less. Exercise more. Eat less. Exercise more.
Eat less. Exercise more. Eat less. Exercise more.
Eat less. Exercise more. Eat less. Exercise more.
Eat less. Exercise more. Eat less. Exercise more.
Eat less. Exercise more. Eat less. Exercise more.
Eat less. Exercise more. Eat less. Exercise more.
Eat less. Exercise more. Eat less. Exercise more.

Eat less. Exercise more. Eat less. Exercise more.
Eat less. Exercise more. Eat less. Exercise more.
Eat less. Exercise more. Eat less. Exercise more.
Eat less. Exercise more. Eat less. Exercise more.
Eat less. Exercise more. Eat less. Exercise more.
Eat less. Exercise more. Eat less. Exercise more.
Eat less. Exercise more. Eat less. Exercise more.
Eat less. Exercise more. Eat less. Exercise more.
Eat less. Exercise more. Eat less. Exercise more.
Eat less. Exercise more. Eat less. Exercise more.
Eat less. Exercise more. Eat less. Exercise more.
Eat less. Exercise more. Eat less. Exercise more.
Eat less. Exercise more. Eat less. Exercise more.
Eat less. Exercise more. Eat less. Exercise more.
Eat less. Exercise more. Eat less. Exercise more.
Eat less. Exercise more. Eat less. Exercise more.
Eat less. Exercise more. Eat less. Exercise more.
Eat less. Exercise more. Eat less. Exercise more.
Eat less. Exercise more. Eat less. Exercise more.
Eat less. Exercise more. Eat less. Exercise more.
Eat less. Exercise more. Eat less. Exercise more.
Eat less. Exercise more. Eat less. Exercise more.
Eat less. Exercise more. Eat less. Exercise more.
Eat less. Exercise more. Eat less. Exercise more.
Eat less. Exercise more. Eat less. Exercise more.
Eat less. Exercise more. Eat less. Exercise more.
Eat less. Exercise more. Eat less. Exercise more.
Eat less. Exercise more. Eat less. Exercise more.
Eat less. Exercise more. Eat less. Exercise more.
Eat less. Exercise more. Eat less. Exercise more.
Eat less. Exercise more. Eat less. Exercise more.
Eat less. Exercise more. Eat less. Exercise more.
Eat less. Exercise more. Eat less. Exercise more.
Eat less. Exercise more. Eat less. Exercise more.

Eat less. Exercise more. Eat less. Exercise more.
Eat less. Exercise more. Eat less. Exercise more.
Eat less. Exercise more. Eat less. Exercise more.
Eat less. Exercise more. Eat less. Exercise more.
Eat less. Exercise more. Eat less. Exercise more.
Eat less. Exercise more. Eat less. Exercise more.
Eat less. Exercise more. Eat less. Exercise more.
Eat less. Exercise more. Eat less. Exercise more.
Eat less. Exercise more. Eat less. Exercise more.
Eat less. Exercise more. Eat less. Exercise more.
Eat less. Exercise more. Eat less. Exercise more.
Eat less. Exercise more. Eat less. Exercise more.
Eat less. Exercise more. Eat less. Exercise more.
Eat less. Exercise more. Eat less. Exercise more.
Eat less. Exercise more. Eat less. Exercise more.
Eat less. Exercise more. Eat less. Exercise more.
Eat less. Exercise more. Eat less. Exercise more.
Eat less. Exercise more. Eat less. Exercise more.
Eat less. Exercise more. Eat less. Exercise more.
Eat less. Exercise more. Eat less. Exercise more.
Eat less. Exercise more. Eat less. Exercise more.
Eat less. Exercise more. Eat less. Exercise more.
Eat less. Exercise more. Eat less. Exercise more.
Eat less. Exercise more. Eat less. Exercise more.
Eat less. Exercise more. Eat less. Exercise more.
Eat less. Exercise more. Eat less. Exercise more.
Eat less. Exercise more. Eat less. Exercise more.
Eat less. Exercise more. Eat less. Exercise more.
Eat less. Exercise more. Eat less. Exercise more.
Eat less. Exercise more. Eat less. Exercise more.
Eat less. Exercise more. Eat less. Exercise more.
Eat less. Exercise more. Eat less. Exercise more.
Eat less. Exercise more. Eat less. Exercise more.

Eat less. Exercise more. Eat less. Exercise more.
Eat less. Exercise more. Eat less. Exercise more.
Eat less. Exercise more. Eat less. Exercise more.
Eat less. Exercise more. Eat less. Exercise more.
Eat less. Exercise more. Eat less. Exercise more.
Eat less. Exercise more. Eat less. Exercise more.
Eat less. Exercise more. Eat less. Exercise more.
Eat less. Exercise more. Eat less. Exercise more.
Eat less. Exercise more. Eat less. Exercise more.
Eat less. Exercise more. Eat less. Exercise more.
Eat less. Exercise more. Eat less. Exercise more.
Eat less. Exercise more. Eat less. Exercise more.
Eat less. Exercise more. Eat less. Exercise more.
Eat less. Exercise more. Eat less. Exercise more.
Eat less. Exercise more. Eat less. Exercise more.
Eat less. Exercise more. Eat less. Exercise more.
Eat less. Exercise more. Eat less. Exercise more.
Eat less. Exercise more. Eat less. Exercise more.
Eat less. Exercise more. Eat less. Exercise more.
Eat less. Exercise more. Eat less. Exercise more.
Eat less. Exercise more. Eat less. Exercise more.
Eat less. Exercise more. Eat less. Exercise more.
Eat less. Exercise more. Eat less. Exercise more.
Eat less. Exercise more. Eat less. Exercise more.
Eat less. Exercise more. Eat less. Exercise more.
Eat less. Exercise more. Eat less. Exercise more.
Eat less. Exercise more. Eat less. Exercise more.
Eat less. Exercise more. Eat less. Exercise more.
Eat less. Exercise more. Eat less. Exercise more.
Eat less. Exercise more. Eat less. Exercise more.
Eat less. Exercise more. Eat less. Exercise more.
Eat less. Exercise more. Eat less. Exercise more.
Eat less. Exercise more. Eat less. Exercise more.

Eat less. Exercise more. Eat less. Exercise more.
Eat less. Exercise more. Eat less. Exercise more.
Eat less. Exercise more. Eat less. Exercise more.
Eat less. Exercise more. Eat less. Exercise more.
Eat less. Exercise more. Eat less. Exercise more.
Eat less. Exercise more. Eat less. Exercise more.
Eat less. Exercise more. Eat less. Exercise more.
Eat less. Exercise more. Eat less. Exercise more.
Eat less. Exercise more. Eat less. Exercise more.
Eat less. Exercise more. Eat less. Exercise more.
Eat less. Exercise more. Eat less. Exercise more.
Eat less. Exercise more. Eat less. Exercise more.
Eat less. Exercise more. Eat less. Exercise more.
Eat less. Exercise more. Eat less. Exercise more.
Eat less. Exercise more. Eat less. Exercise more.
Eat less. Exercise more. Eat less. Exercise more.
Eat less. Exercise more. Eat less. Exercise more.
Eat less. Exercise more. Eat less. Exercise more.
Eat less. Exercise more. Eat less. Exercise more.
Eat less. Exercise more. Eat less. Exercise more.
Eat less. Exercise more. Eat less. Exercise more.
Eat less. Exercise more. Eat less. Exercise more.
Eat less. Exercise more. Eat less. Exercise more.
Eat less. Exercise more. Eat less. Exercise more.
Eat less. Exercise more. Eat less. Exercise more.
Eat less. Exercise more. Eat less. Exercise more.
Eat less. Exercise more. Eat less. Exercise more.
Eat less. Exercise more. Eat less. Exercise more.
Eat less. Exercise more. Eat less. Exercise more.
Eat less. Exercise more. Eat less. Exercise more.
Eat less. Exercise more. Eat less. Exercise more.
Eat less. Exercise more. Eat less. Exercise more.
Eat less. Exercise more. Eat less. Exercise more.
Eat less. Exercise more. Eat less. Exercise more.
Eat less. Exercise more. Eat less. Exercise more.

Eat less. Exercise more. Eat less. Exercise more.
Eat less. Exercise more. Eat less. Exercise more.
Eat less. Exercise more. Eat less. Exercise more.
Eat less. Exercise more. Eat less. Exercise more.
Eat less. Exercise more. Eat less. Exercise more.
Eat less. Exercise more. Eat less. Exercise more.
Eat less. Exercise more. Eat less. Exercise more.
Eat less. Exercise more. Eat less. Exercise more.
Eat less. Exercise more. Eat less. Exercise more.
Eat less. Exercise more. Eat less. Exercise more.
Eat less. Exercise more. Eat less. Exercise more.
Eat less. Exercise more. Eat less. Exercise more.
Eat less. Exercise more. Eat less. Exercise more.
Eat less. Exercise more. Eat less. Exercise more.
Eat less. Exercise more. Eat less. Exercise more.
Eat less. Exercise more. Eat less. Exercise more.
Eat less. Exercise more. Eat less. Exercise more.
Eat less. Exercise more. Eat less. Exercise more.
Eat less. Exercise more. Eat less. Exercise more.
Eat less. Exercise more. Eat less. Exercise more.
Eat less. Exercise more. Eat less. Exercise more.
Eat less. Exercise more. Eat less. Exercise more.
Eat less. Exercise more. Eat less. Exercise more.
Eat less. Exercise more. Eat less. Exercise more.
Eat less. Exercise more. Eat less. Exercise more.
Eat less. Exercise more. Eat less. Exercise more.
Eat less. Exercise more. Eat less. Exercise more.
Eat less. Exercise more. Eat less. Exercise more.
Eat less. Exercise more. Eat less. Exercise more.
Eat less. Exercise more. Eat less. Exercise more.
Eat less. Exercise more. Eat less. Exercise more.
Eat less. Exercise more. Eat less. Exercise more.
Eat less. Exercise more. Eat less. Exercise more.
Eat less. Exercise more. Eat less. Exercise more.
Eat less. Exercise more. Eat less. Exercise more.
Eat less. Exercise more. Eat less. Exercise more.

Eat less. Exercise more. Eat less. Exercise more.
Eat less. Exercise more. Eat less. Exercise more.
Eat less. Exercise more. Eat less. Exercise more.
Eat less. Exercise more. Eat less. Exercise more.
Eat less. Exercise more. Eat less. Exercise more.
Eat less. Exercise more. Eat less. Exercise more.
Eat less. Exercise more. Eat less. Exercise more.
Eat less. Exercise more. Eat less. Exercise more.
Eat less. Exercise more. Eat less. Exercise more.
Eat less. Exercise more. Eat less. Exercise more.
Eat less. Exercise more. Eat less. Exercise more.
Eat less. Exercise more. Eat less. Exercise more.
Eat less. Exercise more. Eat less. Exercise more.
Eat less. Exercise more. Eat less. Exercise more.
Eat less. Exercise more. Eat less. Exercise more.
Eat less. Exercise more. Eat less. Exercise more.
Eat less. Exercise more. Eat less. Exercise more.
Eat less. Exercise more. Eat less. Exercise more.
Eat less. Exercise more. Eat less. Exercise more.
Eat less. Exercise more. Eat less. Exercise more.
Eat less. Exercise more. Eat less. Exercise more.
Eat less. Exercise more. Eat less. Exercise more.
Eat less. Exercise more. Eat less. Exercise more.
Eat less. Exercise more. Eat less. Exercise more.
Eat less. Exercise more. Eat less. Exercise more.
Eat less. Exercise more. Eat less. Exercise more.
Eat less. Exercise more. Eat less. Exercise more.
Eat less. Exercise more. Eat less. Exercise more.
Eat less. Exercise more. Eat less. Exercise more.
Eat less. Exercise more. Eat less. Exercise more.
Eat less. Exercise more. Eat less. Exercise more.
Eat less. Exercise more. Eat less. Exercise more.
Eat less. Exercise more. Eat less. Exercise more.
Eat less. Exercise more. Eat less. Exercise more.

Eat less. Exercise more. Eat less. Exercise more.
Eat less. Exercise more. Eat less. Exercise more.
Eat less. Exercise more. Eat less. Exercise more.
Eat less. Exercise more. Eat less. Exercise more.
Eat less. Exercise more. Eat less. Exercise more.
Eat less. Exercise more. Eat less. Exercise more.
Eat less. Exercise more. Eat less. Exercise more.
Eat less. Exercise more. Eat less. Exercise more.
Eat less. Exercise more. Eat less. Exercise more.
Eat less. Exercise more. Eat less. Exercise more.
Eat less. Exercise more. Eat less. Exercise more.
Eat less. Exercise more. Eat less. Exercise more.
Eat less. Exercise more. Eat less. Exercise more.
Eat less. Exercise more. Eat less. Exercise more.
Eat less. Exercise more. Eat less. Exercise more.
Eat less. Exercise more. Eat less. Exercise more.
Eat less. Exercise more. Eat less. Exercise more.
Eat less. Exercise more. Eat less. Exercise more.
Eat less. Exercise more. Eat less. Exercise more.
Eat less. Exercise more. Eat less. Exercise more.
Eat less. Exercise more. Eat less. Exercise more.
Eat less. Exercise more. Eat less. Exercise more.
Eat less. Exercise more. Eat less. Exercise more.
Eat less. Exercise more. Eat less. Exercise more.
Eat less. Exercise more. Eat less. Exercise more.
Eat less. Exercise more. Eat less. Exercise more.
Eat less. Exercise more. Eat less. Exercise more.
Eat less. Exercise more. Eat less. Exercise more.
Eat less. Exercise more. Eat less. Exercise more.
Eat less. Exercise more. Eat less. Exercise more.
Eat less. Exercise more. Eat less. Exercise more.
Eat less. Exercise more. Eat less. Exercise more.
Eat less. Exercise more. Eat less. Exercise more.
Eat less. Exercise more. Eat less. Exercise more.

Eat less. Exercise more. Eat less. Exercise more.
Eat less. Exercise more. Eat less. Exercise more.
Eat less. Exercise more. Eat less. Exercise more.
Eat less. Exercise more. Eat less. Exercise more.
Eat less. Exercise more. Eat less. Exercise more.
Eat less. Exercise more. Eat less. Exercise more.
Eat less. Exercise more. Eat less. Exercise more.
Eat less. Exercise more. Eat less. Exercise more.
Eat less. Exercise more. Eat less. Exercise more.
Eat less. Exercise more. Eat less. Exercise more.
Eat less. Exercise more. Eat less. Exercise more.
Eat less. Exercise more. Eat less. Exercise more.
Eat less. Exercise more. Eat less. Exercise more.
Eat less. Exercise more. Eat less. Exercise more.
Eat less. Exercise more. Eat less. Exercise more.
Eat less. Exercise more. Eat less. Exercise more.
Eat less. Exercise more. Eat less. Exercise more.
Eat less. Exercise more. Eat less. Exercise more.
Eat less. Exercise more. Eat less. Exercise more.
Eat less. Exercise more. Eat less. Exercise more.
Eat less. Exercise more. Eat less. Exercise more.
Eat less. Exercise more. Eat less. Exercise more.
Eat less. Exercise more. Eat less. Exercise more.
Eat less. Exercise more. Eat less. Exercise more.
Eat less. Exercise more. Eat less. Exercise more.
Eat less. Exercise more. Eat less. Exercise more.
Eat less. Exercise more. Eat less. Exercise more.
Eat less. Exercise more. Eat less. Exercise more.
Eat less. Exercise more. Eat less. Exercise more.
Eat less. Exercise more. Eat less. Exercise more.
Eat less. Exercise more. Eat less. Exercise more.
Eat less. Exercise more. Eat less. Exercise more.
Eat less. Exercise more. Eat less. Exercise more.

Eat less. Exercise more. Eat less. Exercise more.
Eat less. Exercise more. Eat less. Exercise more.
Eat less. Exercise more. Eat less. Exercise more.
Eat less. Exercise more. Eat less. Exercise more.
Eat less. Exercise more. Eat less. Exercise more.
Eat less. Exercise more. Eat less. Exercise more.
Eat less. Exercise more. Eat less. Exercise more.
Eat less. Exercise more. Eat less. Exercise more.
Eat less. Exercise more. Eat less. Exercise more.
Eat less. Exercise more. Eat less. Exercise more.
Eat less. Exercise more. Eat less. Exercise more.
Eat less. Exercise more. Eat less. Exercise more.
Eat less. Exercise more. Eat less. Exercise more.
Eat less. Exercise more. Eat less. Exercise more.
Eat less. Exercise more. Eat less. Exercise more.
Eat less. Exercise more. Eat less. Exercise more.
Eat less. Exercise more. Eat less. Exercise more.
Eat less. Exercise more. Eat less. Exercise more.
Eat less. Exercise more. Eat less. Exercise more.
Eat less. Exercise more. Eat less. Exercise more.
Eat less. Exercise more. Eat less. Exercise more.
Eat less. Exercise more. Eat less. Exercise more.
Eat less. Exercise more. Eat less. Exercise more.
Eat less. Exercise more. Eat less. Exercise more.
Eat less. Exercise more. Eat less. Exercise more.
Eat less. Exercise more. Eat less. Exercise more.
Eat less. Exercise more. Eat less. Exercise more.
Eat less. Exercise more. Eat less. Exercise more.
Eat less. Exercise more. Eat less. Exercise more.
Eat less. Exercise more. Eat less. Exercise more.
Eat less. Exercise more. Eat less. Exercise more.
Eat less. Exercise more. Eat less. Exercise more.
Eat less. Exercise more. Eat less. Exercise more.

Eat less. Exercise more. Eat less. Exercise more.
Eat less. Exercise more. Eat less. Exercise more.
Eat less. Exercise more. Eat less. Exercise more.
Eat less. Exercise more. Eat less. Exercise more.
Eat less. Exercise more. Eat less. Exercise more.
Eat less. Exercise more. Eat less. Exercise more.
Eat less. Exercise more. Eat less. Exercise more.
Eat less. Exercise more. Eat less. Exercise more.
Eat less. Exercise more. Eat less. Exercise more.
Eat less. Exercise more. Eat less. Exercise more.
Eat less. Exercise more. Eat less. Exercise more.
Eat less. Exercise more. Eat less. Exercise more.
Eat less. Exercise more. Eat less. Exercise more.
Eat less. Exercise more. Eat less. Exercise more.
Eat less. Exercise more. Eat less. Exercise more.
Eat less. Exercise more. Eat less. Exercise more.
Eat less. Exercise more. Eat less. Exercise more.
Eat less. Exercise more. Eat less. Exercise more.
Eat less. Exercise more. Eat less. Exercise more.
Eat less. Exercise more. Eat less. Exercise more.
Eat less. Exercise more. Eat less. Exercise more.
Eat less. Exercise more. Eat less. Exercise more.
Eat less. Exercise more. Eat less. Exercise more.
Eat less. Exercise more. Eat less. Exercise more.
Eat less. Exercise more. Eat less. Exercise more.
Eat less. Exercise more. Eat less. Exercise more.
Eat less. Exercise more. Eat less. Exercise more.
Eat less. Exercise more. Eat less. Exercise more.
Eat less. Exercise more. Eat less. Exercise more.
Eat less. Exercise more. Eat less. Exercise more.
Eat less. Exercise more. Eat less. Exercise more.
Eat less. Exercise more. Eat less. Exercise more.
Eat less. Exercise more. Eat less. Exercise more.
Eat less. Exercise more. Eat less. Exercise more.

Eat less. Exercise more. Eat less. Exercise more.
Eat less. Exercise more. Eat less. Exercise more.
Eat less. Exercise more. Eat less. Exercise more.
Eat less. Exercise more. Eat less. Exercise more.
Eat less. Exercise more. Eat less. Exercise more.
Eat less. Exercise more. Eat less. Exercise more.
Eat less. Exercise more. Eat less. Exercise more.
Eat less. Exercise more. Eat less. Exercise more.
Eat less. Exercise more. Eat less. Exercise more.
Eat less. Exercise more. Eat less. Exercise more.
Eat less. Exercise more. Eat less. Exercise more.
Eat less. Exercise more. Eat less. Exercise more.
Eat less. Exercise more. Eat less. Exercise more.
Eat less. Exercise more. Eat less. Exercise more.
Eat less. Exercise more. Eat less. Exercise more.
Eat less. Exercise more. Eat less. Exercise more.
Eat less. Exercise more. Eat less. Exercise more.
Eat less. Exercise more. Eat less. Exercise more.
Eat less. Exercise more. Eat less. Exercise more.
Eat less. Exercise more. Eat less. Exercise more.
Eat less. Exercise more. Eat less. Exercise more.
Eat less. Exercise more. Eat less. Exercise more.
Eat less. Exercise more. Eat less. Exercise more.
Eat less. Exercise more. Eat less. Exercise more.
Eat less. Exercise more. Eat less. Exercise more.
Eat less. Exercise more. Eat less. Exercise more.
Eat less. Exercise more. Eat less. Exercise more.
Eat less. Exercise more. Eat less. Exercise more.
Eat less. Exercise more. Eat less. Exercise more.
Eat less. Exercise more. Eat less. Exercise more.
Eat less. Exercise more. Eat less. Exercise more.
Eat less. Exercise more. Eat less. Exercise more.
Eat less. Exercise more. Eat less. Exercise more.

Eat less. Exercise more. Eat less. Exercise more.
Eat less. Exercise more. Eat less. Exercise more.
Eat less. Exercise more. Eat less. Exercise more.
Eat less. Exercise more. Eat less. Exercise more.
Eat less. Exercise more. Eat less. Exercise more.
Eat less. Exercise more. Eat less. Exercise more.
Eat less. Exercise more. Eat less. Exercise more.
Eat less. Exercise more. Eat less. Exercise more.
Eat less. Exercise more. Eat less. Exercise more.
Eat less. Exercise more. Eat less. Exercise more.
Eat less. Exercise more. Eat less. Exercise more.
Eat less. Exercise more. Eat less. Exercise more.
Eat less. Exercise more. Eat less. Exercise more.
Eat less. Exercise more. Eat less. Exercise more.
Eat less. Exercise more. Eat less. Exercise more.
Eat less. Exercise more. Eat less. Exercise more.
Eat less. Exercise more. Eat less. Exercise more.
Eat less. Exercise more. Eat less. Exercise more.
Eat less. Exercise more. Eat less. Exercise more.
Eat less. Exercise more. Eat less. Exercise more.
Eat less. Exercise more. Eat less. Exercise more.
Eat less. Exercise more. Eat less. Exercise more.
Eat less. Exercise more. Eat less. Exercise more.
Eat less. Exercise more. Eat less. Exercise more.
Eat less. Exercise more. Eat less. Exercise more.
Eat less. Exercise more. Eat less. Exercise more.
Eat less. Exercise more. Eat less. Exercise more.
Eat less. Exercise more. Eat less. Exercise more.
Eat less. Exercise more. Eat less. Exercise more.
Eat less. Exercise more. Eat less. Exercise more.
Eat less. Exercise more. Eat less. Exercise more.
Eat less. Exercise more. Eat less. Exercise more.

Eat less. Exercise more. Eat less. Exercise more.
Eat less. Exercise more. Eat less. Exercise more.
Eat less. Exercise more. Eat less. Exercise more.
Eat less. Exercise more. Eat less. Exercise more.
Eat less. Exercise more. Eat less. Exercise more.
Eat less. Exercise more. Eat less. Exercise more.
Eat less. Exercise more. Eat less. Exercise more.
Eat less. Exercise more. Eat less. Exercise more.
Eat less. Exercise more. Eat less. Exercise more.
Eat less. Exercise more. Eat less. Exercise more.
Eat less. Exercise more. Eat less. Exercise more.
Eat less. Exercise more. Eat less. Exercise more.
Eat less. Exercise more. Eat less. Exercise more.
Eat less. Exercise more. Eat less. Exercise more.
Eat less. Exercise more. Eat less. Exercise more.
Eat less. Exercise more. Eat less. Exercise more.
Eat less. Exercise more. Eat less. Exercise more.
Eat less. Exercise more. Eat less. Exercise more.
Eat less. Exercise more. Eat less. Exercise more.
Eat less. Exercise more. Eat less. Exercise more.
Eat less. Exercise more. Eat less. Exercise more.
Eat less. Exercise more. Eat less. Exercise more.
Eat less. Exercise more. Eat less. Exercise more.
Eat less. Exercise more. Eat less. Exercise more.
Eat less. Exercise more. Eat less. Exercise more.
Eat less. Exercise more. Eat less. Exercise more.
Eat less. Exercise more. Eat less. Exercise more.
Eat less. Exercise more. Eat less. Exercise more.
Eat less. Exercise more. Eat less. Exercise more.
Eat less. Exercise more. Eat less. Exercise more.
Eat less. Exercise more. Eat less. Exercise more.
Eat less. Exercise more. Eat less. Exercise more.
Eat less. Exercise more. Eat less. Exercise more.
Eat less. Exercise more. Eat less. Exercise more.

Eat less. Exercise more. Eat less. Exercise more.
Eat less. Exercise more. Eat less. Exercise more.
Eat less. Exercise more. Eat less. Exercise more.
Eat less. Exercise more. Eat less. Exercise more.
Eat less. Exercise more. Eat less. Exercise more.
Eat less. Exercise more. Eat less. Exercise more.
Eat less. Exercise more. Eat less. Exercise more.
Eat less. Exercise more. Eat less. Exercise more.
Eat less. Exercise more. Eat less. Exercise more.
Eat less. Exercise more. Eat less. Exercise more.
Eat less. Exercise more. Eat less. Exercise more.
Eat less. Exercise more. Eat less. Exercise more.
Eat less. Exercise more. Eat less. Exercise more.
Eat less. Exercise more. Eat less. Exercise more.
Eat less. Exercise more. Eat less. Exercise more.
Eat less. Exercise more. Eat less. Exercise more.
Eat less. Exercise more. Eat less. Exercise more.
Eat less. Exercise more. Eat less. Exercise more.
Eat less. Exercise more. Eat less. Exercise more.
Eat less. Exercise more. Eat less. Exercise more.
Eat less. Exercise more. Eat less. Exercise more.
Eat less. Exercise more. Eat less. Exercise more.
Eat less. Exercise more. Eat less. Exercise more.
Eat less. Exercise more. Eat less. Exercise more.
Eat less. Exercise more. Eat less. Exercise more.
Eat less. Exercise more. Eat less. Exercise more.
Eat less. Exercise more. Eat less. Exercise more.
Eat less. Exercise more. Eat less. Exercise more.
Eat less. Exercise more. Eat less. Exercise more.
Eat less. Exercise more. Eat less. Exercise more.
Eat less. Exercise more. Eat less. Exercise more.
Eat less. Exercise more. Eat less. Exercise more.
Eat less. Exercise more. Eat less. Exercise more.

Eat less. Exercise more. Eat less. Exercise more.
Eat less. Exercise more. Eat less. Exercise more.
Eat less. Exercise more. Eat less. Exercise more.
Eat less. Exercise more. Eat less. Exercise more.
Eat less. Exercise more. Eat less. Exercise more.
Eat less. Exercise more. Eat less. Exercise more.
Eat less. Exercise more. Eat less. Exercise more.
Eat less. Exercise more. Eat less. Exercise more.
Eat less. Exercise more. Eat less. Exercise more.
Eat less. Exercise more. Eat less. Exercise more.
Eat less. Exercise more. Eat less. Exercise more.
Eat less. Exercise more. Eat less. Exercise more.
Eat less. Exercise more. Eat less. Exercise more.
Eat less. Exercise more. Eat less. Exercise more.
Eat less. Exercise more. Eat less. Exercise more.
Eat less. Exercise more. Eat less. Exercise more.
Eat less. Exercise more. Eat less. Exercise more.
Eat less. Exercise more. Eat less. Exercise more.
Eat less. Exercise more. Eat less. Exercise more.
Eat less. Exercise more. Eat less. Exercise more.
Eat less. Exercise more. Eat less. Exercise more.
Eat less. Exercise more. Eat less. Exercise more.
Eat less. Exercise more. Eat less. Exercise more.
Eat less. Exercise more. Eat less. Exercise more.
Eat less. Exercise more. Eat less. Exercise more.
Eat less. Exercise more. Eat less. Exercise more.
Eat less. Exercise more. Eat less. Exercise more.
Eat less. Exercise more. Eat less. Exercise more.
Eat less. Exercise more. Eat less. Exercise more.
Eat less. Exercise more. Eat less. Exercise more.
Eat less. Exercise more. Eat less. Exercise more.
Eat less. Exercise more. Eat less. Exercise more.
Eat less. Exercise more. Eat less. Exercise more.

Eat less. Exercise more. Eat less. Exercise more.
Eat less. Exercise more. Eat less. Exercise more.
Eat less. Exercise more. Eat less. Exercise more.
Eat less. Exercise more. Eat less. Exercise more.
Eat less. Exercise more. Eat less. Exercise more.
Eat less. Exercise more. Eat less. Exercise more.
Eat less. Exercise more. Eat less. Exercise more.
Eat less. Exercise more. Eat less. Exercise more.
Eat less. Exercise more. Eat less. Exercise more.
Eat less. Exercise more. Eat less. Exercise more.
Eat less. Exercise more. Eat less. Exercise more.
Eat less. Exercise more. Eat less. Exercise more.
Eat less. Exercise more. Eat less. Exercise more.
Eat less. Exercise more. Eat less. Exercise more.
Eat less. Exercise more. Eat less. Exercise more.
Eat less. Exercise more. Eat less. Exercise more.
Eat less. Exercise more. Eat less. Exercise more.
Eat less. Exercise more. Eat less. Exercise more.
Eat less. Exercise more. Eat less. Exercise more.
Eat less. Exercise more. Eat less. Exercise more.
Eat less. Exercise more. Eat less. Exercise more.
Eat less. Exercise more. Eat less. Exercise more.
Eat less. Exercise more. Eat less. Exercise more.
Eat less. Exercise more. Eat less. Exercise more.
Eat less. Exercise more. Eat less. Exercise more.
Eat less. Exercise more. Eat less. Exercise more.
Eat less. Exercise more. Eat less. Exercise more.
Eat less. Exercise more. Eat less. Exercise more.
Eat less. Exercise more. Eat less. Exercise more.
Eat less. Exercise more. Eat less. Exercise more.
Eat less. Exercise more. Eat less. Exercise more.
Eat less. Exercise more. Eat less. Exercise more.
Eat less. Exercise more. Eat less. Exercise more.
Eat less. Exercise more. Eat less. Exercise more.

Eat less. Exercise more. Eat less. Exercise more.
Eat less. Exercise more. Eat less. Exercise more.
Eat less. Exercise more. Eat less. Exercise more.
Eat less. Exercise more. Eat less. Exercise more.
Eat less. Exercise more. Eat less. Exercise more.
Eat less. Exercise more. Eat less. Exercise more.
Eat less. Exercise more. Eat less. Exercise more.
Eat less. Exercise more. Eat less. Exercise more.
Eat less. Exercise more. Eat less. Exercise more.
Eat less. Exercise more. Eat less. Exercise more.
Eat less. Exercise more. Eat less. Exercise more.
Eat less. Exercise more. Eat less. Exercise more.
Eat less. Exercise more. Eat less. Exercise more.
Eat less. Exercise more. Eat less. Exercise more.
Eat less. Exercise more. Eat less. Exercise more.
Eat less. Exercise more. Eat less. Exercise more.
Eat less. Exercise more. Eat less. Exercise more.
Eat less. Exercise more. Eat less. Exercise more.
Eat less. Exercise more. Eat less. Exercise more.
Eat less. Exercise more. Eat less. Exercise more.
Eat less. Exercise more. Eat less. Exercise more.
Eat less. Exercise more. Eat less. Exercise more.
Eat less. Exercise more. Eat less. Exercise more.
Eat less. Exercise more. Eat less. Exercise more.
Eat less. Exercise more. Eat less. Exercise more.
Eat less. Exercise more. Eat less. Exercise more.
Eat less. Exercise more. Eat less. Exercise more.
Eat less. Exercise more. Eat less. Exercise more.
Eat less. Exercise more. Eat less. Exercise more.
Eat less. Exercise more. Eat less. Exercise more.
Eat less. Exercise more. Eat less. Exercise more.
Eat less. Exercise more. Eat less. Exercise more.
Eat less. Exercise more. Eat less. Exercise more.
Eat less. Exercise more. Eat less. Exercise more.

Eat less. Exercise more. Eat less. Exercise more.
Eat less. Exercise more. Eat less. Exercise more.
Eat less. Exercise more. Eat less. Exercise more.
Eat less. Exercise more. Eat less. Exercise more.
Eat less. Exercise more. Eat less. Exercise more.
Eat less. Exercise more. Eat less. Exercise more.
Eat less. Exercise more. Eat less. Exercise more.
Eat less. Exercise more. Eat less. Exercise more.
Eat less. Exercise more. Eat less. Exercise more.
Eat less. Exercise more. Eat less. Exercise more.
Eat less. Exercise more. Eat less. Exercise more.
Eat less. Exercise more. Eat less. Exercise more.
Eat less. Exercise more. Eat less. Exercise more.
Eat less. Exercise more. Eat less. Exercise more.
Eat less. Exercise more. Eat less. Exercise more.
Eat less. Exercise more. Eat less. Exercise more.
Eat less. Exercise more. Eat less. Exercise more.
Eat less. Exercise more. Eat less. Exercise more.
Eat less. Exercise more. Eat less. Exercise more.
Eat less. Exercise more. Eat less. Exercise more.
Eat less. Exercise more. Eat less. Exercise more.
Eat less. Exercise more. Eat less. Exercise more.
Eat less. Exercise more. Eat less. Exercise more.
Eat less. Exercise more. Eat less. Exercise more.
Eat less. Exercise more. Eat less. Exercise more.
Eat less. Exercise more. Eat less. Exercise more.
Eat less. Exercise more. Eat less. Exercise more.
Eat less. Exercise more. Eat less. Exercise more.
Eat less. Exercise more. Eat less. Exercise more.
Eat less. Exercise more. Eat less. Exercise more.
Eat less. Exercise more. Eat less. Exercise more.
Eat less. Exercise more. Eat less. Exercise more.
Eat less. Exercise more. Eat less. Exercise more.
Eat less. Exercise more. Eat less. Exercise more.

Eat less. Exercise more. Eat less. Exercise more.
Eat less. Exercise more. Eat less. Exercise more.
Eat less. Exercise more. Eat less. Exercise more.
Eat less. Exercise more. Eat less. Exercise more.
Eat less. Exercise more. Eat less. Exercise more.
Eat less. Exercise more. Eat less. Exercise more.
Eat less. Exercise more. Eat less. Exercise more.
Eat less. Exercise more. Eat less. Exercise more.
Eat less. Exercise more. Eat less. Exercise more.
Eat less. Exercise more. Eat less. Exercise more.
Eat less. Exercise more. Eat less. Exercise more.
Eat less. Exercise more. Eat less. Exercise more.
Eat less. Exercise more. Eat less. Exercise more.
Eat less. Exercise more. Eat less. Exercise more.
Eat less. Exercise more. Eat less. Exercise more.
Eat less. Exercise more. Eat less. Exercise more.
Eat less. Exercise more. Eat less. Exercise more.
Eat less. Exercise more. Eat less. Exercise more.
Eat less. Exercise more. Eat less. Exercise more.
Eat less. Exercise more. Eat less. Exercise more.
Eat less. Exercise more. Eat less. Exercise more.
Eat less. Exercise more. Eat less. Exercise more.
Eat less. Exercise more. Eat less. Exercise more.
Eat less. Exercise more. Eat less. Exercise more.
Eat less. Exercise more. Eat less. Exercise more.
Eat less. Exercise more. Eat less. Exercise more.
Eat less. Exercise more. Eat less. Exercise more.
Eat less. Exercise more. Eat less. Exercise more.
Eat less. Exercise more. Eat less. Exercise more.
Eat less. Exercise more. Eat less. Exercise more.
Eat less. Exercise more. Eat less. Exercise more.
Eat less. Exercise more. Eat less. Exercise more.
Eat less. Exercise more. Eat less. Exercise more.
Eat less. Exercise more. Eat less. Exercise more.

Eat less. Exercise more. Eat less. Exercise more.
Eat less. Exercise more. Eat less. Exercise more.
Eat less. Exercise more. Eat less. Exercise more.
Eat less. Exercise more. Eat less. Exercise more.
Eat less. Exercise more. Eat less. Exercise more.
Eat less. Exercise more. Eat less. Exercise more.
Eat less. Exercise more. Eat less. Exercise more.
Eat less. Exercise more. Eat less. Exercise more.
Eat less. Exercise more. Eat less. Exercise more.
Eat less. Exercise more. Eat less. Exercise more.
Eat less. Exercise more. Eat less. Exercise more.
Eat less. Exercise more. Eat less. Exercise more.
Eat less. Exercise more. Eat less. Exercise more.
Eat less. Exercise more. Eat less. Exercise more.
Eat less. Exercise more. Eat less. Exercise more.
Eat less. Exercise more. Eat less. Exercise more.
Eat less. Exercise more. Eat less. Exercise more.
Eat less. Exercise more. Eat less. Exercise more.
Eat less. Exercise more. Eat less. Exercise more.
Eat less. Exercise more. Eat less. Exercise more.
Eat less. Exercise more. Eat less. Exercise more.
Eat less. Exercise more. Eat less. Exercise more.
Eat less. Exercise more. Eat less. Exercise more.
Eat less. Exercise more. Eat less. Exercise more.
Eat less. Exercise more. Eat less. Exercise more.
Eat less. Exercise more. Eat less. Exercise more.
Eat less. Exercise more. Eat less. Exercise more.
Eat less. Exercise more. Eat less. Exercise more.
Eat less. Exercise more. Eat less. Exercise more.
Eat less. Exercise more. Eat less. Exercise more.
Eat less. Exercise more. Eat less. Exercise more.
Eat less. Exercise more. Eat less. Exercise more.
Eat less. Exercise more. Eat less. Exercise more.
Eat less. Exercise more. Eat less. Exercise more.

Eat less. Exercise more. Eat less. Exercise more.
Eat less. Exercise more. Eat less. Exercise more.
Eat less. Exercise more. Eat less. Exercise more.
Eat less. Exercise more. Eat less. Exercise more.
Eat less. Exercise more. Eat less. Exercise more.
Eat less. Exercise more. Eat less. Exercise more.
Eat less. Exercise more. Eat less. Exercise more.
Eat less. Exercise more. Eat less. Exercise more.
Eat less. Exercise more. Eat less. Exercise more.
Eat less. Exercise more. Eat less. Exercise more.
Eat less. Exercise more. Eat less. Exercise more.
Eat less. Exercise more. Eat less. Exercise more.
Eat less. Exercise more. Eat less. Exercise more.
Eat less. Exercise more. Eat less. Exercise more.
Eat less. Exercise more. Eat less. Exercise more.
Eat less. Exercise more. Eat less. Exercise more.
Eat less. Exercise more. Eat less. Exercise more.
Eat less. Exercise more. Eat less. Exercise more.
Eat less. Exercise more. Eat less. Exercise more.
Eat less. Exercise more. Eat less. Exercise more.
Eat less. Exercise more. Eat less. Exercise more.
Eat less. Exercise more. Eat less. Exercise more.
Eat less. Exercise more. Eat less. Exercise more.
Eat less. Exercise more. Eat less. Exercise more.
Eat less. Exercise more. Eat less. Exercise more.
Eat less. Exercise more. Eat less. Exercise more.
Eat less. Exercise more. Eat less. Exercise more.
Eat less. Exercise more. Eat less. Exercise more.
Eat less. Exercise more. Eat less. Exercise more.
Eat less. Exercise more. Eat less. Exercise more.
Eat less. Exercise more. Eat less. Exercise more.
Eat less. Exercise more. Eat less. Exercise more.
Eat less. Exercise more. Eat less. Exercise more.

Eat less. Exercise more. Eat less. Exercise more.
Eat less. Exercise more. Eat less. Exercise more.
Eat less. Exercise more. Eat less. Exercise more.
Eat less. Exercise more. Eat less. Exercise more.
Eat less. Exercise more. Eat less. Exercise more.
Eat less. Exercise more. Eat less. Exercise more.
Eat less. Exercise more. Eat less. Exercise more.
Eat less. Exercise more. Eat less. Exercise more.
Eat less. Exercise more. Eat less. Exercise more.
Eat less. Exercise more. Eat less. Exercise more.
Eat less. Exercise more. Eat less. Exercise more.
Eat less. Exercise more. Eat less. Exercise more.
Eat less. Exercise more. Eat less. Exercise more.
Eat less. Exercise more. Eat less. Exercise more.
Eat less. Exercise more. Eat less. Exercise more.
Eat less. Exercise more. Eat less. Exercise more.
Eat less. Exercise more. Eat less. Exercise more.
Eat less. Exercise more. Eat less. Exercise more.
Eat less. Exercise more. Eat less. Exercise more.
Eat less. Exercise more. Eat less. Exercise more.
Eat less. Exercise more. Eat less. Exercise more.
Eat less. Exercise more. Eat less. Exercise more.
Eat less. Exercise more. Eat less. Exercise more.
Eat less. Exercise more. Eat less. Exercise more.
Eat less. Exercise more. Eat less. Exercise more.
Eat less. Exercise more. Eat less. Exercise more.
Eat less. Exercise more. Eat less. Exercise more.
Eat less. Exercise more. Eat less. Exercise more.
Eat less. Exercise more. Eat less. Exercise more.
Eat less. Exercise more. Eat less. Exercise more.
Eat less. Exercise more. Eat less. Exercise more.
Eat less. Exercise more. Eat less. Exercise more.
Eat less. Exercise more. Eat less. Exercise more.
Eat less. Exercise more. Eat less. Exercise more.

Eat less. Exercise more. Eat less. Exercise more.
Eat less. Exercise more. Eat less. Exercise more.
Eat less. Exercise more. Eat less. Exercise more.
Eat less. Exercise more. Eat less. Exercise more.
Eat less. Exercise more. Eat less. Exercise more.
Eat less. Exercise more. Eat less. Exercise more.
Eat less. Exercise more. Eat less. Exercise more.
Eat less. Exercise more. Eat less. Exercise more.
Eat less. Exercise more. Eat less. Exercise more.
Eat less. Exercise more. Eat less. Exercise more.
Eat less. Exercise more. Eat less. Exercise more.
Eat less. Exercise more. Eat less. Exercise more.
Eat less. Exercise more. Eat less. Exercise more.
Eat less. Exercise more. Eat less. Exercise more.
Eat less. Exercise more. Eat less. Exercise more.
Eat less. Exercise more. Eat less. Exercise more.
Eat less. Exercise more. Eat less. Exercise more.
Eat less. Exercise more. Eat less. Exercise more.
Eat less. Exercise more. Eat less. Exercise more.
Eat less. Exercise more. Eat less. Exercise more.
Eat less. Exercise more. Eat less. Exercise more.
Eat less. Exercise more. Eat less. Exercise more.
Eat less. Exercise more. Eat less. Exercise more.
Eat less. Exercise more. Eat less. Exercise more.
Eat less. Exercise more. Eat less. Exercise more.
Eat less. Exercise more. Eat less. Exercise more.
Eat less. Exercise more. Eat less. Exercise more.
Eat less. Exercise more. Eat less. Exercise more.
Eat less. Exercise more. Eat less. Exercise more.
Eat less. Exercise more. Eat less. Exercise more.
Eat less. Exercise more. Eat less. Exercise more.
Eat less. Exercise more. Eat less. Exercise more.
Eat less. Exercise more. Eat less. Exercise more.
Eat less. Exercise more. Eat less. Exercise more.

Eat less. Exercise more. Eat less. Exercise more.
Eat less. Exercise more. Eat less. Exercise more.
Eat less. Exercise more. Eat less. Exercise more.
Eat less. Exercise more. Eat less. Exercise more.
Eat less. Exercise more. Eat less. Exercise more.
Eat less. Exercise more. Eat less. Exercise more.
Eat less. Exercise more. Eat less. Exercise more.
Eat less. Exercise more. Eat less. Exercise more.
Eat less. Exercise more. Eat less. Exercise more.
Eat less. Exercise more. Eat less. Exercise more.
Eat less. Exercise more. Eat less. Exercise more.
Eat less. Exercise more. Eat less. Exercise more.
Eat less. Exercise more. Eat less. Exercise more.
Eat less. Exercise more. Eat less. Exercise more.
Eat less. Exercise more. Eat less. Exercise more.
Eat less. Exercise more. Eat less. Exercise more.
Eat less. Exercise more. Eat less. Exercise more.
Eat less. Exercise more. Eat less. Exercise more.
Eat less. Exercise more. Eat less. Exercise more.
Eat less. Exercise more. Eat less. Exercise more.
Eat less. Exercise more. Eat less. Exercise more.
Eat less. Exercise more. Eat less. Exercise more.
Eat less. Exercise more. Eat less. Exercise more.
Eat less. Exercise more. Eat less. Exercise more.
Eat less. Exercise more. Eat less. Exercise more.
Eat less. Exercise more. Eat less. Exercise more.
Eat less. Exercise more. Eat less. Exercise more.
Eat less. Exercise more. Eat less. Exercise more.
Eat less. Exercise more. Eat less. Exercise more.
Eat less. Exercise more. Eat less. Exercise more.
Eat less. Exercise more. Eat less. Exercise more.
Eat less. Exercise more. Eat less. Exercise more.
Eat less. Exercise more. Eat less. Exercise more.

Eat less. Exercise more. Eat less. Exercise more.
Eat less. Exercise more. Eat less. Exercise more.
Eat less. Exercise more. Eat less. Exercise more.
Eat less. Exercise more. Eat less. Exercise more.
Eat less. Exercise more. Eat less. Exercise more.
Eat less. Exercise more. Eat less. Exercise more.
Eat less. Exercise more. Eat less. Exercise more.
Eat less. Exercise more. Eat less. Exercise more.
Eat less. Exercise more. Eat less. Exercise more.
Eat less. Exercise more. Eat less. Exercise more.
Eat less. Exercise more. Eat less. Exercise more.
Eat less. Exercise more. Eat less. Exercise more.
Eat less. Exercise more. Eat less. Exercise more.
Eat less. Exercise more. Eat less. Exercise more.
Eat less. Exercise more. Eat less. Exercise more.
Eat less. Exercise more. Eat less. Exercise more.
Eat less. Exercise more. Eat less. Exercise more.
Eat less. Exercise more. Eat less. Exercise more.
Eat less. Exercise more. Eat less. Exercise more.
Eat less. Exercise more. Eat less. Exercise more.
Eat less. Exercise more. Eat less. Exercise more.
Eat less. Exercise more. Eat less. Exercise more.
Eat less. Exercise more. Eat less. Exercise more.
Eat less. Exercise more. Eat less. Exercise more.
Eat less. Exercise more. Eat less. Exercise more.
Eat less. Exercise more. Eat less. Exercise more.
Eat less. Exercise more. Eat less. Exercise more.
Eat less. Exercise more. Eat less. Exercise more.
Eat less. Exercise more. Eat less. Exercise more.
Eat less. Exercise more. Eat less. Exercise more.
Eat less. Exercise more. Eat less. Exercise more.
Eat less. Exercise more. Eat less. Exercise more.
Eat less. Exercise more. Eat less. Exercise more.

Eat less. Exercise more. Eat less. Exercise more.
Eat less. Exercise more. Eat less. Exercise more.
Eat less. Exercise more. Eat less. Exercise more.
Eat less. Exercise more. Eat less. Exercise more.
Eat less. Exercise more. Eat less. Exercise more.
Eat less. Exercise more. Eat less. Exercise more.
Eat less. Exercise more. Eat less. Exercise more.
Eat less. Exercise more. Eat less. Exercise more.
Eat less. Exercise more. Eat less. Exercise more.
Eat less. Exercise more. Eat less. Exercise more.
Eat less. Exercise more. Eat less. Exercise more.
Eat less. Exercise more. Eat less. Exercise more.
Eat less. Exercise more. Eat less. Exercise more.
Eat less. Exercise more. Eat less. Exercise more.
Eat less. Exercise more. Eat less. Exercise more.
Eat less. Exercise more. Eat less. Exercise more.
Eat less. Exercise more. Eat less. Exercise more.
Eat less. Exercise more. Eat less. Exercise more.
Eat less. Exercise more. Eat less. Exercise more.
Eat less. Exercise more. Eat less. Exercise more.
Eat less. Exercise more. Eat less. Exercise more.
Eat less. Exercise more. Eat less. Exercise more.
Eat less. Exercise more. Eat less. Exercise more.
Eat less. Exercise more. Eat less. Exercise more.
Eat less. Exercise more. Eat less. Exercise more.
Eat less. Exercise more. Eat less. Exercise more.
Eat less. Exercise more. Eat less. Exercise more.
Eat less. Exercise more. Eat less. Exercise more.
Eat less. Exercise more. Eat less. Exercise more.
Eat less. Exercise more. Eat less. Exercise more.
Eat less. Exercise more. Eat less. Exercise more.
Eat less. Exercise more. Eat less. Exercise more.
Eat less. Exercise more. Eat less. Exercise more.

Eat less. Exercise more. Eat less. Exercise more.
Eat less. Exercise more. Eat less. Exercise more.
Eat less. Exercise more. Eat less. Exercise more.
Eat less. Exercise more. Eat less. Exercise more.
Eat less. Exercise more. Eat less. Exercise more.
Eat less. Exercise more. Eat less. Exercise more.
Eat less. Exercise more. Eat less. Exercise more.
Eat less. Exercise more. Eat less. Exercise more.
Eat less. Exercise more. Eat less. Exercise more.
Eat less. Exercise more. Eat less. Exercise more.
Eat less. Exercise more. Eat less. Exercise more.
Eat less. Exercise more. Eat less. Exercise more.
Eat less. Exercise more. Eat less. Exercise more.
Eat less. Exercise more. Eat less. Exercise more.
Eat less. Exercise more. Eat less. Exercise more.
Eat less. Exercise more. Eat less. Exercise more.
Eat less. Exercise more. Eat less. Exercise more.
Eat less. Exercise more. Eat less. Exercise more.
Eat less. Exercise more. Eat less. Exercise more.
Eat less. Exercise more. Eat less. Exercise more.
Eat less. Exercise more. Eat less. Exercise more.
Eat less. Exercise more. Eat less. Exercise more.
Eat less. Exercise more. Eat less. Exercise more.
Eat less. Exercise more. Eat less. Exercise more.
Eat less. Exercise more. Eat less. Exercise more.
Eat less. Exercise more. Eat less. Exercise more.
Eat less. Exercise more. Eat less. Exercise more.
Eat less. Exercise more. Eat less. Exercise more.
Eat less. Exercise more. Eat less. Exercise more.
Eat less. Exercise more. Eat less. Exercise more.
Eat less. Exercise more. Eat less. Exercise more.
Eat less. Exercise more. Eat less. Exercise more.
Eat less. Exercise more. Eat less. Exercise more.

Eat less. Exercise more. Eat less. Exercise more.
Eat less. Exercise more. Eat less. Exercise more.
Eat less. Exercise more. Eat less. Exercise more.
Eat less. Exercise more. Eat less. Exercise more.
Eat less. Exercise more. Eat less. Exercise more.
Eat less. Exercise more. Eat less. Exercise more.
Eat less. Exercise more. Eat less. Exercise more.
Eat less. Exercise more. Eat less. Exercise more.
Eat less. Exercise more. Eat less. Exercise more.
Eat less. Exercise more. Eat less. Exercise more.
Eat less. Exercise more. Eat less. Exercise more.
Eat less. Exercise more. Eat less. Exercise more.
Eat less. Exercise more. Eat less. Exercise more.
Eat less. Exercise more. Eat less. Exercise more.
Eat less. Exercise more. Eat less. Exercise more.
Eat less. Exercise more. Eat less. Exercise more.
Eat less. Exercise more. Eat less. Exercise more.
Eat less. Exercise more. Eat less. Exercise more.
Eat less. Exercise more. Eat less. Exercise more.
Eat less. Exercise more. Eat less. Exercise more.
Eat less. Exercise more. Eat less. Exercise more.
Eat less. Exercise more. Eat less. Exercise more.
Eat less. Exercise more. Eat less. Exercise more.
Eat less. Exercise more. Eat less. Exercise more.
Eat less. Exercise more. Eat less. Exercise more.
Eat less. Exercise more. Eat less. Exercise more.
Eat less. Exercise more. Eat less. Exercise more.
Eat less. Exercise more. Eat less. Exercise more.
Eat less. Exercise more. Eat less. Exercise more.
Eat less. Exercise more. Eat less. Exercise more.
Eat less. Exercise more. Eat less. Exercise more.
Eat less. Exercise more. Eat less. Exercise more.
Eat less. Exercise more. Eat less. Exercise more.

Eat less. Exercise more. Eat less. Exercise more.
Eat less. Exercise more. Eat less. Exercise more.
Eat less. Exercise more. Eat less. Exercise more.
Eat less. Exercise more. Eat less. Exercise more.
Eat less. Exercise more. Eat less. Exercise more.
Eat less. Exercise more. Eat less. Exercise more.
Eat less. Exercise more. Eat less. Exercise more.
Eat less. Exercise more. Eat less. Exercise more.
Eat less. Exercise more. Eat less. Exercise more.
Eat less. Exercise more. Eat less. Exercise more.
Eat less. Exercise more. Eat less. Exercise more.
Eat less. Exercise more. Eat less. Exercise more.
Eat less. Exercise more. Eat less. Exercise more.
Eat less. Exercise more. Eat less. Exercise more.
Eat less. Exercise more. Eat less. Exercise more.
Eat less. Exercise more. Eat less. Exercise more.
Eat less. Exercise more. Eat less. Exercise more.
Eat less. Exercise more. Eat less. Exercise more.
Eat less. Exercise more. Eat less. Exercise more.
Eat less. Exercise more. Eat less. Exercise more.
Eat less. Exercise more. Eat less. Exercise more.
Eat less. Exercise more. Eat less. Exercise more.
Eat less. Exercise more. Eat less. Exercise more.
Eat less. Exercise more. Eat less. Exercise more.
Eat less. Exercise more. Eat less. Exercise more.
Eat less. Exercise more. Eat less. Exercise more.
Eat less. Exercise more. Eat less. Exercise more.
Eat less. Exercise more. Eat less. Exercise more.
Eat less. Exercise more. Eat less. Exercise more.
Eat less. Exercise more. Eat less. Exercise more.
Eat less. Exercise more. Eat less. Exercise more.
Eat less. Exercise more. Eat less. Exercise more.
Eat less. Exercise more. Eat less. Exercise more.
Eat less. Exercise more. Eat less. Exercise more.
Eat less. Exercise more. Eat less. Exercise more.

Eat less. Exercise more. Eat less. Exercise more.
Eat less. Exercise more. Eat less. Exercise more.
Eat less. Exercise more. Eat less. Exercise more.
Eat less. Exercise more. Eat less. Exercise more.
Eat less. Exercise more. Eat less. Exercise more.
Eat less. Exercise more. Eat less. Exercise more.
Eat less. Exercise more. Eat less. Exercise more.
Eat less. Exercise more. Eat less. Exercise more.
Eat less. Exercise more. Eat less. Exercise more.
Eat less. Exercise more. Eat less. Exercise more.
Eat less. Exercise more. Eat less. Exercise more.
Eat less. Exercise more. Eat less. Exercise more.
Eat less. Exercise more. Eat less. Exercise more.
Eat less. Exercise more. Eat less. Exercise more.
Eat less. Exercise more. Eat less. Exercise more.
Eat less. Exercise more. Eat less. Exercise more.
Eat less. Exercise more. Eat less. Exercise more.
Eat less. Exercise more. Eat less. Exercise more.
Eat less. Exercise more. Eat less. Exercise more.
Eat less. Exercise more. Eat less. Exercise more.
Eat less. Exercise more. Eat less. Exercise more.
Eat less. Exercise more. Eat less. Exercise more.
Eat less. Exercise more. Eat less. Exercise more.
Eat less. Exercise more. Eat less. Exercise more.
Eat less. Exercise more. Eat less. Exercise more.
Eat less. Exercise more. Eat less. Exercise more.
Eat less. Exercise more. Eat less. Exercise more.
Eat less. Exercise more. Eat less. Exercise more.
Eat less. Exercise more. Eat less. Exercise more.
Eat less. Exercise more. Eat less. Exercise more.
Eat less. Exercise more. Eat less. Exercise more.
Eat less. Exercise more. Eat less. Exercise more.

Eat less. Exercise more. Eat less. Exercise more.
Eat less. Exercise more. Eat less. Exercise more.
Eat less. Exercise more. Eat less. Exercise more.
Eat less. Exercise more. Eat less. Exercise more.
Eat less. Exercise more. Eat less. Exercise more.
Eat less. Exercise more. Eat less. Exercise more.
Eat less. Exercise more. Eat less. Exercise more.
Eat less. Exercise more. Eat less. Exercise more.
Eat less. Exercise more. Eat less. Exercise more.
Eat less. Exercise more. Eat less. Exercise more.
Eat less. Exercise more. Eat less. Exercise more.
Eat less. Exercise more. Eat less. Exercise more.
Eat less. Exercise more. Eat less. Exercise more.
Eat less. Exercise more. Eat less. Exercise more.
Eat less. Exercise more. Eat less. Exercise more.
Eat less. Exercise more. Eat less. Exercise more.
Eat less. Exercise more. Eat less. Exercise more.
Eat less. Exercise more. Eat less. Exercise more.
Eat less. Exercise more. Eat less. Exercise more.
Eat less. Exercise more. Eat less. Exercise more.
Eat less. Exercise more. Eat less. Exercise more.
Eat less. Exercise more. Eat less. Exercise more.
Eat less. Exercise more. Eat less. Exercise more.
Eat less. Exercise more. Eat less. Exercise more.
Eat less. Exercise more. Eat less. Exercise more.
Eat less. Exercise more. Eat less. Exercise more.
Eat less. Exercise more. Eat less. Exercise more.
Eat less. Exercise more. Eat less. Exercise more.
Eat less. Exercise more. Eat less. Exercise more.
Eat less. Exercise more. Eat less. Exercise more.
Eat less. Exercise more. Eat less. Exercise more.
Eat less. Exercise more. Eat less. Exercise more.
Eat less. Exercise more. Eat less. Exercise more.
Eat less. Exercise more. Eat less. Exercise more.

Eat less. Exercise more. Eat less. Exercise more.
Eat less. Exercise more. Eat less. Exercise more.
Eat less. Exercise more. Eat less. Exercise more.
Eat less. Exercise more. Eat less. Exercise more.
Eat less. Exercise more. Eat less. Exercise more.
Eat less. Exercise more. Eat less. Exercise more.
Eat less. Exercise more. Eat less. Exercise more.
Eat less. Exercise more. Eat less. Exercise more.
Eat less. Exercise more. Eat less. Exercise more.
Eat less. Exercise more. Eat less. Exercise more.
Eat less. Exercise more. Eat less. Exercise more.
Eat less. Exercise more. Eat less. Exercise more.
Eat less. Exercise more. Eat less. Exercise more.
Eat less. Exercise more. Eat less. Exercise more.
Eat less. Exercise more. Eat less. Exercise more.
Eat less. Exercise more. Eat less. Exercise more.
Eat less. Exercise more. Eat less. Exercise more.
Eat less. Exercise more. Eat less. Exercise more.
Eat less. Exercise more. Eat less. Exercise more.
Eat less. Exercise more. Eat less. Exercise more.
Eat less. Exercise more. Eat less. Exercise more.
Eat less. Exercise more. Eat less. Exercise more.
Eat less. Exercise more. Eat less. Exercise more.
Eat less. Exercise more. Eat less. Exercise more.
Eat less. Exercise more. Eat less. Exercise more.
Eat less. Exercise more. Eat less. Exercise more.
Eat less. Exercise more. Eat less. Exercise more.
Eat less. Exercise more. Eat less. Exercise more.
Eat less. Exercise more. Eat less. Exercise more.
Eat less. Exercise more. Eat less. Exercise more.
Eat less. Exercise more. Eat less. Exercise more.
Eat less. Exercise more. Eat less. Exercise more.
Eat less. Exercise more. Eat less. Exercise more.

Eat less. Exercise more. Eat less. Exercise more.
Eat less. Exercise more. Eat less. Exercise more.
Eat less. Exercise more. Eat less. Exercise more.
Eat less. Exercise more. Eat less. Exercise more.
Eat less. Exercise more. Eat less. Exercise more.
Eat less. Exercise more. Eat less. Exercise more.
Eat less. Exercise more. Eat less. Exercise more.
Eat less. Exercise more. Eat less. Exercise more.
Eat less. Exercise more. Eat less. Exercise more.
Eat less. Exercise more. Eat less. Exercise more.
Eat less. Exercise more. Eat less. Exercise more.
Eat less. Exercise more. Eat less. Exercise more.
Eat less. Exercise more. Eat less. Exercise more.
Eat less. Exercise more. Eat less. Exercise more.
Eat less. Exercise more. Eat less. Exercise more.
Eat less. Exercise more. Eat less. Exercise more.
Eat less. Exercise more. Eat less. Exercise more.
Eat less. Exercise more. Eat less. Exercise more.
Eat less. Exercise more. Eat less. Exercise more.
Eat less. Exercise more. Eat less. Exercise more.
Eat less. Exercise more. Eat less. Exercise more.
Eat less. Exercise more. Eat less. Exercise more.
Eat less. Exercise more. Eat less. Exercise more.
Eat less. Exercise more. Eat less. Exercise more.
Eat less. Exercise more. Eat less. Exercise more.
Eat less. Exercise more. Eat less. Exercise more.
Eat less. Exercise more. Eat less. Exercise more.
Eat less. Exercise more. Eat less. Exercise more.
Eat less. Exercise more. Eat less. Exercise more.
Eat less. Exercise more. Eat less. Exercise more.
Eat less. Exercise more. Eat less. Exercise more.
Eat less. Exercise more. Eat less. Exercise more.
Eat less. Exercise more. Eat less. Exercise more.

Eat less. Exercise more. Eat less. Exercise more.
Eat less. Exercise more. Eat less. Exercise more.
Eat less. Exercise more. Eat less. Exercise more.
Eat less. Exercise more. Eat less. Exercise more.
Eat less. Exercise more. Eat less. Exercise more.
Eat less. Exercise more. Eat less. Exercise more.
Eat less. Exercise more. Eat less. Exercise more.
Eat less. Exercise more. Eat less. Exercise more.
Eat less. Exercise more. Eat less. Exercise more.
Eat less. Exercise more. Eat less. Exercise more.
Eat less. Exercise more. Eat less. Exercise more.
Eat less. Exercise more. Eat less. Exercise more.
Eat less. Exercise more. Eat less. Exercise more.
Eat less. Exercise more. Eat less. Exercise more.
Eat less. Exercise more. Eat less. Exercise more.
Eat less. Exercise more. Eat less. Exercise more.
Eat less. Exercise more. Eat less. Exercise more.
Eat less. Exercise more. Eat less. Exercise more.
Eat less. Exercise more. Eat less. Exercise more.
Eat less. Exercise more. Eat less. Exercise more.
Eat less. Exercise more. Eat less. Exercise more.
Eat less. Exercise more. Eat less. Exercise more.
Eat less. Exercise more. Eat less. Exercise more.
Eat less. Exercise more. Eat less. Exercise more.
Eat less. Exercise more. Eat less. Exercise more.
Eat less. Exercise more. Eat less. Exercise more.
Eat less. Exercise more. Eat less. Exercise more.
Eat less. Exercise more. Eat less. Exercise more.
Eat less. Exercise more. Eat less. Exercise more.
Eat less. Exercise more. Eat less. Exercise more.
Eat less. Exercise more. Eat less. Exercise more.
Eat less. Exercise more. Eat less. Exercise more.
Eat less. Exercise more. Eat less. Exercise more.
Eat less. Exercise more. Eat less. Exercise more.

Eat less. Exercise more. Eat less. Exercise more.
Eat less. Exercise more. Eat less. Exercise more.
Eat less. Exercise more. Eat less. Exercise more.
Eat less. Exercise more. Eat less. Exercise more.
Eat less. Exercise more. Eat less. Exercise more.
Eat less. Exercise more. Eat less. Exercise more.
Eat less. Exercise more. Eat less. Exercise more.
Eat less. Exercise more. Eat less. Exercise more.
Eat less. Exercise more. Eat less. Exercise more.
Eat less. Exercise more. Eat less. Exercise more.
Eat less. Exercise more. Eat less. Exercise more.
Eat less. Exercise more. Eat less. Exercise more.
Eat less. Exercise more. Eat less. Exercise more.
Eat less. Exercise more. Eat less. Exercise more.
Eat less. Exercise more. Eat less. Exercise more.
Eat less. Exercise more. Eat less. Exercise more.
Eat less. Exercise more. Eat less. Exercise more.
Eat less. Exercise more. Eat less. Exercise more.
Eat less. Exercise more. Eat less. Exercise more.
Eat less. Exercise more. Eat less. Exercise more.
Eat less. Exercise more. Eat less. Exercise more.
Eat less. Exercise more. Eat less. Exercise more.
Eat less. Exercise more. Eat less. Exercise more.
Eat less. Exercise more. Eat less. Exercise more.
Eat less. Exercise more. Eat less. Exercise more.
Eat less. Exercise more. Eat less. Exercise more.
Eat less. Exercise more. Eat less. Exercise more.
Eat less. Exercise more. Eat less. Exercise more.
Eat less. Exercise more. Eat less. Exercise more.
Eat less. Exercise more. Eat less. Exercise more.
Eat less. Exercise more. Eat less. Exercise more.
Eat less. Exercise more. Eat less. Exercise more.
Eat less. Exercise more. Eat less. Exercise more.

Eat less. Exercise more. Eat less. Exercise more.
Eat less. Exercise more. Eat less. Exercise more.
Eat less. Exercise more. Eat less. Exercise more.
Eat less. Exercise more. Eat less. Exercise more.
Eat less. Exercise more. Eat less. Exercise more.
Eat less. Exercise more. Eat less. Exercise more.
Eat less. Exercise more. Eat less. Exercise more.
Eat less. Exercise more. Eat less. Exercise more.
Eat less. Exercise more. Eat less. Exercise more.
Eat less. Exercise more. Eat less. Exercise more.
Eat less. Exercise more. Eat less. Exercise more.
Eat less. Exercise more. Eat less. Exercise more.
Eat less. Exercise more. Eat less. Exercise more.
Eat less. Exercise more. Eat less. Exercise more.
Eat less. Exercise more. Eat less. Exercise more.
Eat less. Exercise more. Eat less. Exercise more.
Eat less. Exercise more. Eat less. Exercise more.
Eat less. Exercise more. Eat less. Exercise more.
Eat less. Exercise more. Eat less. Exercise more.
Eat less. Exercise more. Eat less. Exercise more.
Eat less. Exercise more. Eat less. Exercise more.
Eat less. Exercise more. Eat less. Exercise more.
Eat less. Exercise more. Eat less. Exercise more.
Eat less. Exercise more. Eat less. Exercise more.
Eat less. Exercise more. Eat less. Exercise more.
Eat less. Exercise more. Eat less. Exercise more.
Eat less. Exercise more. Eat less. Exercise more.
Eat less. Exercise more. Eat less. Exercise more.
Eat less. Exercise more. Eat less. Exercise more.
Eat less. Exercise more. Eat less. Exercise more.
Eat less. Exercise more. Eat less. Exercise more.
Eat less. Exercise more. Eat less. Exercise more.
Eat less. Exercise more. Eat less. Exercise more.
Eat less. Exercise more. Eat less. Exercise more.

Eat less. Exercise more. Eat less. Exercise more.
Eat less. Exercise more. Eat less. Exercise more.
Eat less. Exercise more. Eat less. Exercise more.
Eat less. Exercise more. Eat less. Exercise more.
Eat less. Exercise more. Eat less. Exercise more.
Eat less. Exercise more. Eat less. Exercise more.
Eat less. Exercise more. Eat less. Exercise more.
Eat less. Exercise more. Eat less. Exercise more.
Eat less. Exercise more. Eat less. Exercise more.
Eat less. Exercise more. Eat less. Exercise more.
Eat less. Exercise more. Eat less. Exercise more.
Eat less. Exercise more. Eat less. Exercise more.
Eat less. Exercise more. Eat less. Exercise more.
Eat less. Exercise more. Eat less. Exercise more.
Eat less. Exercise more. Eat less. Exercise more.
Eat less. Exercise more. Eat less. Exercise more.
Eat less. Exercise more. Eat less. Exercise more.
Eat less. Exercise more. Eat less. Exercise more.
Eat less. Exercise more. Eat less. Exercise more.
Eat less. Exercise more. Eat less. Exercise more.
Eat less. Exercise more. Eat less. Exercise more.
Eat less. Exercise more. Eat less. Exercise more.
Eat less. Exercise more. Eat less. Exercise more.
Eat less. Exercise more. Eat less. Exercise more.
Eat less. Exercise more. Eat less. Exercise more.
Eat less. Exercise more. Eat less. Exercise more.
Eat less. Exercise more. Eat less. Exercise more.
Eat less. Exercise more. Eat less. Exercise more.
Eat less. Exercise more. Eat less. Exercise more.
Eat less. Exercise more. Eat less. Exercise more.
Eat less. Exercise more. Eat less. Exercise more.
Eat less. Exercise more. Eat less. Exercise more.
Eat less. Exercise more. Eat less. Exercise more.
Eat less. Exercise more. Eat less. Exercise more.

Eat less. Exercise more. Eat less. Exercise more.
Eat less. Exercise more. Eat less. Exercise more.
Eat less. Exercise more. Eat less. Exercise more.
Eat less. Exercise more. Eat less. Exercise more.
Eat less. Exercise more. Eat less. Exercise more.
Eat less. Exercise more. Eat less. Exercise more.
Eat less. Exercise more. Eat less. Exercise more.
Eat less. Exercise more. Eat less. Exercise more.
Eat less. Exercise more. Eat less. Exercise more.
Eat less. Exercise more. Eat less. Exercise more.
Eat less. Exercise more. Eat less. Exercise more.
Eat less. Exercise more. Eat less. Exercise more.
Eat less. Exercise more. Eat less. Exercise more.
Eat less. Exercise more. Eat less. Exercise more.
Eat less. Exercise more. Eat less. Exercise more.
Eat less. Exercise more. Eat less. Exercise more.
Eat less. Exercise more. Eat less. Exercise more.
Eat less. Exercise more. Eat less. Exercise more.
Eat less. Exercise more. Eat less. Exercise more.
Eat less. Exercise more. Eat less. Exercise more.
Eat less. Exercise more. Eat less. Exercise more.
Eat less. Exercise more. Eat less. Exercise more.
Eat less. Exercise more. Eat less. Exercise more.
Eat less. Exercise more. Eat less. Exercise more.
Eat less. Exercise more. Eat less. Exercise more.
Eat less. Exercise more. Eat less. Exercise more.
Eat less. Exercise more. Eat less. Exercise more.
Eat less. Exercise more. Eat less. Exercise more.
Eat less. Exercise more. Eat less. Exercise more.
Eat less. Exercise more. Eat less. Exercise more.
Eat less. Exercise more. Eat less. Exercise more.
Eat less. Exercise more. Eat less. Exercise more.
Eat less. Exercise more. Eat less. Exercise more.
Eat less. Exercise more. Eat less. Exercise more.

Eat less. Exercise more. Eat less. Exercise more.
Eat less. Exercise more. Eat less. Exercise more.
Eat less. Exercise more. Eat less. Exercise more.
Eat less. Exercise more. Eat less. Exercise more.
Eat less. Exercise more. Eat less. Exercise more.
Eat less. Exercise more. Eat less. Exercise more.
Eat less. Exercise more. Eat less. Exercise more.
Eat less. Exercise more. Eat less. Exercise more.
Eat less. Exercise more. Eat less. Exercise more.
Eat less. Exercise more. Eat less. Exercise more.
Eat less. Exercise more. Eat less. Exercise more.
Eat less. Exercise more. Eat less. Exercise more.
Eat less. Exercise more. Eat less. Exercise more.
Eat less. Exercise more. Eat less. Exercise more.
Eat less. Exercise more. Eat less. Exercise more.
Eat less. Exercise more. Eat less. Exercise more.
Eat less. Exercise more. Eat less. Exercise more.
Eat less. Exercise more. Eat less. Exercise more.
Eat less. Exercise more. Eat less. Exercise more.
Eat less. Exercise more. Eat less. Exercise more.
Eat less. Exercise more. Eat less. Exercise more.
Eat less. Exercise more. Eat less. Exercise more.
Eat less. Exercise more. Eat less. Exercise more.
Eat less. Exercise more. Eat less. Exercise more.
Eat less. Exercise more. Eat less. Exercise more.
Eat less. Exercise more. Eat less. Exercise more.
Eat less. Exercise more. Eat less. Exercise more.
Eat less. Exercise more. Eat less. Exercise more.
Eat less. Exercise more. Eat less. Exercise more.
Eat less. Exercise more. Eat less. Exercise more.
Eat less. Exercise more. Eat less. Exercise more.
Eat less. Exercise more. Eat less. Exercise more.
Eat less. Exercise more. Eat less. Exercise more.

Eat less. Exercise more. Eat less. Exercise more.
Eat less. Exercise more. Eat less. Exercise more.
Eat less. Exercise more. Eat less. Exercise more.
Eat less. Exercise more. Eat less. Exercise more.
Eat less. Exercise more. Eat less. Exercise more.
Eat less. Exercise more. Eat less. Exercise more.
Eat less. Exercise more. Eat less. Exercise more.
Eat less. Exercise more. Eat less. Exercise more.
Eat less. Exercise more. Eat less. Exercise more.
Eat less. Exercise more. Eat less. Exercise more.
Eat less. Exercise more. Eat less. Exercise more.
Eat less. Exercise more. Eat less. Exercise more.
Eat less. Exercise more. Eat less. Exercise more.
Eat less. Exercise more. Eat less. Exercise more.
Eat less. Exercise more. Eat less. Exercise more.
Eat less. Exercise more. Eat less. Exercise more.
Eat less. Exercise more. Eat less. Exercise more.
Eat less. Exercise more. Eat less. Exercise more.
Eat less. Exercise more. Eat less. Exercise more.
Eat less. Exercise more. Eat less. Exercise more.
Eat less. Exercise more. Eat less. Exercise more.
Eat less. Exercise more. Eat less. Exercise more.
Eat less. Exercise more. Eat less. Exercise more.
Eat less. Exercise more. Eat less. Exercise more.
Eat less. Exercise more. Eat less. Exercise more.
Eat less. Exercise more. Eat less. Exercise more.
Eat less. Exercise more. Eat less. Exercise more.
Eat less. Exercise more. Eat less. Exercise more.
Eat less. Exercise more. Eat less. Exercise more.
Eat less. Exercise more. Eat less. Exercise more.
Eat less. Exercise more. Eat less. Exercise more.
Eat less. Exercise more. Eat less. Exercise more.
Eat less. Exercise more. Eat less. Exercise more.
Eat less. Exercise more. Eat less. Exercise more.

Eat less. Exercise more. Eat less. Exercise more.
Eat less. Exercise more. Eat less. Exercise more.
Eat less. Exercise more. Eat less. Exercise more.
Eat less. Exercise more. Eat less. Exercise more.
Eat less. Exercise more. Eat less. Exercise more.
Eat less. Exercise more. Eat less. Exercise more.
Eat less. Exercise more. Eat less. Exercise more.
Eat less. Exercise more. Eat less. Exercise more.
Eat less. Exercise more. Eat less. Exercise more.
Eat less. Exercise more. Eat less. Exercise more.
Eat less. Exercise more. Eat less. Exercise more.
Eat less. Exercise more. Eat less. Exercise more.
Eat less. Exercise more. Eat less. Exercise more.
Eat less. Exercise more. Eat less. Exercise more.
Eat less. Exercise more. Eat less. Exercise more.
Eat less. Exercise more. Eat less. Exercise more.
Eat less. Exercise more. Eat less. Exercise more.
Eat less. Exercise more. Eat less. Exercise more.
Eat less. Exercise more. Eat less. Exercise more.
Eat less. Exercise more. Eat less. Exercise more.
Eat less. Exercise more. Eat less. Exercise more.
Eat less. Exercise more. Eat less. Exercise more.
Eat less. Exercise more. Eat less. Exercise more.
Eat less. Exercise more. Eat less. Exercise more.
Eat less. Exercise more. Eat less. Exercise more.
Eat less. Exercise more. Eat less. Exercise more.
Eat less. Exercise more. Eat less. Exercise more.
Eat less. Exercise more. Eat less. Exercise more.
Eat less. Exercise more. Eat less. Exercise more.
Eat less. Exercise more. Eat less. Exercise more.
Eat less. Exercise more. Eat less. Exercise more.
Eat less. Exercise more. Eat less. Exercise more.
Eat less. Exercise more. Eat less. Exercise more.
Eat less. Exercise more. Eat less. Exercise more.

Eat less. Exercise more. Eat less. Exercise more.
Eat less. Exercise more. Eat less. Exercise more.
Eat less. Exercise more. Eat less. Exercise more.
Eat less. Exercise more. Eat less. Exercise more.
Eat less. Exercise more. Eat less. Exercise more.
Eat less. Exercise more. Eat less. Exercise more.
Eat less. Exercise more. Eat less. Exercise more.
Eat less. Exercise more. Eat less. Exercise more.
Eat less. Exercise more. Eat less. Exercise more.
Eat less. Exercise more. Eat less. Exercise more.
Eat less. Exercise more. Eat less. Exercise more.
Eat less. Exercise more. Eat less. Exercise more.
Eat less. Exercise more. Eat less. Exercise more.
Eat less. Exercise more. Eat less. Exercise more.
Eat less. Exercise more. Eat less. Exercise more.
Eat less. Exercise more. Eat less. Exercise more.
Eat less. Exercise more. Eat less. Exercise more.
Eat less. Exercise more. Eat less. Exercise more.
Eat less. Exercise more. Eat less. Exercise more.
Eat less. Exercise more. Eat less. Exercise more.
Eat less. Exercise more. Eat less. Exercise more.
Eat less. Exercise more. Eat less. Exercise more.
Eat less. Exercise more. Eat less. Exercise more.
Eat less. Exercise more. Eat less. Exercise more.
Eat less. Exercise more. Eat less. Exercise more.
Eat less. Exercise more. Eat less. Exercise more.
Eat less. Exercise more. Eat less. Exercise more.
Eat less. Exercise more. Eat less. Exercise more.
Eat less. Exercise more. Eat less. Exercise more.
Eat less. Exercise more. Eat less. Exercise more.
Eat less. Exercise more. Eat less. Exercise more.
Eat less. Exercise more. Eat less. Exercise more.
Eat less. Exercise more. Eat less. Exercise more.
Eat less. Exercise more. Eat less. Exercise more.

Eat less. Exercise more. Eat less. Exercise more.
Eat less. Exercise more. Eat less. Exercise more.
Eat less. Exercise more. Eat less. Exercise more.
Eat less. Exercise more. Eat less. Exercise more.
Eat less. Exercise more. Eat less. Exercise more.
Eat less. Exercise more. Eat less. Exercise more.
Eat less. Exercise more. Eat less. Exercise more.
Eat less. Exercise more. Eat less. Exercise more.
Eat less. Exercise more. Eat less. Exercise more.
Eat less. Exercise more. Eat less. Exercise more.
Eat less. Exercise more. Eat less. Exercise more.
Eat less. Exercise more. Eat less. Exercise more.
Eat less. Exercise more. Eat less. Exercise more.
Eat less. Exercise more. Eat less. Exercise more.
Eat less. Exercise more. Eat less. Exercise more.
Eat less. Exercise more. Eat less. Exercise more.
Eat less. Exercise more. Eat less. Exercise more.
Eat less. Exercise more. Eat less. Exercise more.
Eat less. Exercise more. Eat less. Exercise more.
Eat less. Exercise more. Eat less. Exercise more.
Eat less. Exercise more. Eat less. Exercise more.
Eat less. Exercise more. Eat less. Exercise more.
Eat less. Exercise more. Eat less. Exercise more.
Eat less. Exercise more. Eat less. Exercise more.
Eat less. Exercise more. Eat less. Exercise more.
Eat less. Exercise more. Eat less. Exercise more.
Eat less. Exercise more. Eat less. Exercise more.
Eat less. Exercise more. Eat less. Exercise more.
Eat less. Exercise more. Eat less. Exercise more.
Eat less. Exercise more. Eat less. Exercise more.
Eat less. Exercise more. Eat less. Exercise more.
Eat less. Exercise more. Eat less. Exercise more.
Eat less. Exercise more. Eat less. Exercise more.
Eat less. Exercise more. Eat less. Exercise more.
Eat less. Exercise more. Eat less. Exercise more.

Eat less. Exercise more. Eat less. Exercise more.
Eat less. Exercise more. Eat less. Exercise more.
Eat less. Exercise more. Eat less. Exercise more.
Eat less. Exercise more. Eat less. Exercise more.
Eat less. Exercise more. Eat less. Exercise more.
Eat less. Exercise more. Eat less. Exercise more.
Eat less. Exercise more. Eat less. Exercise more.
Eat less. Exercise more. Eat less. Exercise more.
Eat less. Exercise more. Eat less. Exercise more.
Eat less. Exercise more. Eat less. Exercise more.
Eat less. Exercise more. Eat less. Exercise more.
Eat less. Exercise more. Eat less. Exercise more.
Eat less. Exercise more. Eat less. Exercise more.
Eat less. Exercise more. Eat less. Exercise more.
Eat less. Exercise more. Eat less. Exercise more.
Eat less. Exercise more. Eat less. Exercise more.
Eat less. Exercise more. Eat less. Exercise more.
Eat less. Exercise more. Eat less. Exercise more.
Eat less. Exercise more. Eat less. Exercise more.
Eat less. Exercise more. Eat less. Exercise more.
Eat less. Exercise more. Eat less. Exercise more.
Eat less. Exercise more. Eat less. Exercise more.
Eat less. Exercise more. Eat less. Exercise more.
Eat less. Exercise more. Eat less. Exercise more.
Eat less. Exercise more. Eat less. Exercise more.
Eat less. Exercise more. Eat less. Exercise more.
Eat less. Exercise more. Eat less. Exercise more.
Eat less. Exercise more. Eat less. Exercise more.
Eat less. Exercise more. Eat less. Exercise more.
Eat less. Exercise more. Eat less. Exercise more.
Eat less. Exercise more. Eat less. Exercise more.
Eat less. Exercise more. Eat less. Exercise more.
Eat less. Exercise more. Eat less. Exercise more.

Eat less. Exercise more. Eat less. Exercise more.
Eat less. Exercise more. Eat less. Exercise more.
Eat less. Exercise more. Eat less. Exercise more.
Eat less. Exercise more. Eat less. Exercise more.
Eat less. Exercise more. Eat less. Exercise more.
Eat less. Exercise more. Eat less. Exercise more.
Eat less. Exercise more. Eat less. Exercise more.
Eat less. Exercise more. Eat less. Exercise more.
Eat less. Exercise more. Eat less. Exercise more.
Eat less. Exercise more. Eat less. Exercise more.
Eat less. Exercise more. Eat less. Exercise more.
Eat less. Exercise more. Eat less. Exercise more.
Eat less. Exercise more. Eat less. Exercise more.
Eat less. Exercise more. Eat less. Exercise more.
Eat less. Exercise more. Eat less. Exercise more.
Eat less. Exercise more. Eat less. Exercise more.
Eat less. Exercise more. Eat less. Exercise more.
Eat less. Exercise more. Eat less. Exercise more.
Eat less. Exercise more. Eat less. Exercise more.
Eat less. Exercise more. Eat less. Exercise more.
Eat less. Exercise more. Eat less. Exercise more.
Eat less. Exercise more. Eat less. Exercise more.
Eat less. Exercise more. Eat less. Exercise more.
Eat less. Exercise more. Eat less. Exercise more.
Eat less. Exercise more. Eat less. Exercise more.
Eat less. Exercise more. Eat less. Exercise more.
Eat less. Exercise more. Eat less. Exercise more.
Eat less. Exercise more. Eat less. Exercise more.
Eat less. Exercise more. Eat less. Exercise more.
Eat less. Exercise more. Eat less. Exercise more.
Eat less. Exercise more. Eat less. Exercise more.
Eat less. Exercise more. Eat less. Exercise more.
Eat less. Exercise more. Eat less. Exercise more.
Eat less. Exercise more. Eat less. Exercise more.

Eat less. Exercise more. Eat less. Exercise more.
Eat less. Exercise more. Eat less. Exercise more.
Eat less. Exercise more. Eat less. Exercise more.
Eat less. Exercise more. Eat less. Exercise more.
Eat less. Exercise more. Eat less. Exercise more.
Eat less. Exercise more. Eat less. Exercise more.
Eat less. Exercise more. Eat less. Exercise more.
Eat less. Exercise more. Eat less. Exercise more.
Eat less. Exercise more. Eat less. Exercise more.
Eat less. Exercise more. Eat less. Exercise more.
Eat less. Exercise more. Eat less. Exercise more.
Eat less. Exercise more. Eat less. Exercise more.
Eat less. Exercise more. Eat less. Exercise more.
Eat less. Exercise more. Eat less. Exercise more.
Eat less. Exercise more. Eat less. Exercise more.
Eat less. Exercise more. Eat less. Exercise more.
Eat less. Exercise more. Eat less. Exercise more.
Eat less. Exercise more. Eat less. Exercise more.
Eat less. Exercise more. Eat less. Exercise more.
Eat less. Exercise more. Eat less. Exercise more.
Eat less. Exercise more. Eat less. Exercise more.
Eat less. Exercise more. Eat less. Exercise more.
Eat less. Exercise more. Eat less. Exercise more.
Eat less. Exercise more. Eat less. Exercise more.
Eat less. Exercise more. Eat less. Exercise more.
Eat less. Exercise more. Eat less. Exercise more.
Eat less. Exercise more. Eat less. Exercise more.
Eat less. Exercise more. Eat less. Exercise more.
Eat less. Exercise more. Eat less. Exercise more.
Eat less. Exercise more. Eat less. Exercise more.
Eat less. Exercise more. Eat less. Exercise more.
Eat less. Exercise more. Eat less. Exercise more.
Eat less. Exercise more. Eat less. Exercise more.
Eat less. Exercise more. Eat less. Exercise more.
Eat less. Exercise more. Eat less. Exercise more.

Eat less. Exercise more. Eat less. Exercise more.
Eat less. Exercise more. Eat less. Exercise more.
Eat less. Exercise more. Eat less. Exercise more.
Eat less. Exercise more. Eat less. Exercise more.
Eat less. Exercise more. Eat less. Exercise more.
Eat less. Exercise more. Eat less. Exercise more.
Eat less. Exercise more. Eat less. Exercise more.
Eat less. Exercise more. Eat less. Exercise more.
Eat less. Exercise more. Eat less. Exercise more.
Eat less. Exercise more. Eat less. Exercise more.
Eat less. Exercise more. Eat less. Exercise more.
Eat less. Exercise more. Eat less. Exercise more.
Eat less. Exercise more. Eat less. Exercise more.
Eat less. Exercise more. Eat less. Exercise more.
Eat less. Exercise more. Eat less. Exercise more.
Eat less. Exercise more. Eat less. Exercise more.
Eat less. Exercise more. Eat less. Exercise more.
Eat less. Exercise more. Eat less. Exercise more.
Eat less. Exercise more. Eat less. Exercise more.
Eat less. Exercise more. Eat less. Exercise more.
Eat less. Exercise more. Eat less. Exercise more.
Eat less. Exercise more. Eat less. Exercise more.
Eat less. Exercise more. Eat less. Exercise more.
Eat less. Exercise more. Eat less. Exercise more.
Eat less. Exercise more. Eat less. Exercise more.
Eat less. Exercise more. Eat less. Exercise more.
Eat less. Exercise more. Eat less. Exercise more.
Eat less. Exercise more. Eat less. Exercise more.
Eat less. Exercise more. Eat less. Exercise more.
Eat less. Exercise more. Eat less. Exercise more.
Eat less. Exercise more. Eat less. Exercise more.
Eat less. Exercise more. Eat less. Exercise more.
Eat less. Exercise more. Eat less. Exercise more.
Eat less. Exercise more. Eat less. Exercise more.
Eat less. Exercise more. Eat less. Exercise more.
Eat less. Exercise more. Eat less. Exercise more.

Eat less. Exercise more. Eat less. Exercise more.
Eat less. Exercise more. Eat less. Exercise more.
Eat less. Exercise more. Eat less. Exercise more.
Eat less. Exercise more. Eat less. Exercise more.
Eat less. Exercise more. Eat less. Exercise more.
Eat less. Exercise more. Eat less. Exercise more.
Eat less. Exercise more. Eat less. Exercise more.
Eat less. Exercise more. Eat less. Exercise more.
Eat less. Exercise more. Eat less. Exercise more.
Eat less. Exercise more. Eat less. Exercise more.
Eat less. Exercise more. Eat less. Exercise more.
Eat less. Exercise more. Eat less. Exercise more.
Eat less. Exercise more. Eat less. Exercise more.
Eat less. Exercise more. Eat less. Exercise more.
Eat less. Exercise more. Eat less. Exercise more.
Eat less. Exercise more. Eat less. Exercise more.
Eat less. Exercise more. Eat less. Exercise more.
Eat less. Exercise more. Eat less. Exercise more.
Eat less. Exercise more. Eat less. Exercise more.
Eat less. Exercise more. Eat less. Exercise more.
Eat less. Exercise more. Eat less. Exercise more.
Eat less. Exercise more. Eat less. Exercise more.
Eat less. Exercise more. Eat less. Exercise more.
Eat less. Exercise more. Eat less. Exercise more.
Eat less. Exercise more. Eat less. Exercise more.
Eat less. Exercise more. Eat less. Exercise more.
Eat less. Exercise more. Eat less. Exercise more.
Eat less. Exercise more. Eat less. Exercise more.
Eat less. Exercise more. Eat less. Exercise more.
Eat less. Exercise more. Eat less. Exercise more.
Eat less. Exercise more. Eat less. Exercise more.
Eat less. Exercise more. Eat less. Exercise more.
Eat less. Exercise more. Eat less. Exercise more.

Eat less. Exercise more. Eat less. Exercise more.
Eat less. Exercise more. Eat less. Exercise more.
Eat less. Exercise more. Eat less. Exercise more.
Eat less. Exercise more. Eat less. Exercise more.
Eat less. Exercise more. Eat less. Exercise more.
Eat less. Exercise more. Eat less. Exercise more.
Eat less. Exercise more. Eat less. Exercise more.
Eat less. Exercise more. Eat less. Exercise more.
Eat less. Exercise more. Eat less. Exercise more.
Eat less. Exercise more. Eat less. Exercise more.
Eat less. Exercise more. Eat less. Exercise more.
Eat less. Exercise more. Eat less. Exercise more.
Eat less. Exercise more. Eat less. Exercise more.
Eat less. Exercise more. Eat less. Exercise more.
Eat less. Exercise more. Eat less. Exercise more.
Eat less. Exercise more. Eat less. Exercise more.
Eat less. Exercise more. Eat less. Exercise more.
Eat less. Exercise more. Eat less. Exercise more.
Eat less. Exercise more. Eat less. Exercise more.
Eat less. Exercise more. Eat less. Exercise more.
Eat less. Exercise more. Eat less. Exercise more.
Eat less. Exercise more. Eat less. Exercise more.
Eat less. Exercise more. Eat less. Exercise more.
Eat less. Exercise more. Eat less. Exercise more.
Eat less. Exercise more. Eat less. Exercise more.
Eat less. Exercise more. Eat less. Exercise more.
Eat less. Exercise more. Eat less. Exercise more.
Eat less. Exercise more. Eat less. Exercise more.
Eat less. Exercise more. Eat less. Exercise more.
Eat less. Exercise more. Eat less. Exercise more.
Eat less. Exercise more. Eat less. Exercise more.
Eat less. Exercise more. Eat less. Exercise more.
Eat less. Exercise more. Eat less. Exercise more.
Eat less. Exercise more. Eat less. Exercise more.

Eat less. Exercise more. Eat less. Exercise more.
Eat less. Exercise more. Eat less. Exercise more.
Eat less. Exercise more. Eat less. Exercise more.
Eat less. Exercise more. Eat less. Exercise more.
Eat less. Exercise more. Eat less. Exercise more.
Eat less. Exercise more. Eat less. Exercise more.
Eat less. Exercise more. Eat less. Exercise more.
Eat less. Exercise more. Eat less. Exercise more.
Eat less. Exercise more. Eat less. Exercise more.
Eat less. Exercise more. Eat less. Exercise more.
Eat less. Exercise more. Eat less. Exercise more.
Eat less. Exercise more. Eat less. Exercise more.
Eat less. Exercise more. Eat less. Exercise more.
Eat less. Exercise more. Eat less. Exercise more.
Eat less. Exercise more. Eat less. Exercise more.
Eat less. Exercise more. Eat less. Exercise more.
Eat less. Exercise more. Eat less. Exercise more.
Eat less. Exercise more. Eat less. Exercise more.
Eat less. Exercise more. Eat less. Exercise more.
Eat less. Exercise more. Eat less. Exercise more.
Eat less. Exercise more. Eat less. Exercise more.
Eat less. Exercise more. Eat less. Exercise more.
Eat less. Exercise more. Eat less. Exercise more.
Eat less. Exercise more. Eat less. Exercise more.
Eat less. Exercise more. Eat less. Exercise more.
Eat less. Exercise more. Eat less. Exercise more.
Eat less. Exercise more. Eat less. Exercise more.
Eat less. Exercise more. Eat less. Exercise more.
Eat less. Exercise more. Eat less. Exercise more.
Eat less. Exercise more. Eat less. Exercise more.
Eat less. Exercise more. Eat less. Exercise more.
Eat less. Exercise more. Eat less. Exercise more.
Eat less. Exercise more. Eat less. Exercise more.
Eat less. Exercise more. Eat less. Exercise more.

Eat less. Exercise more. Eat less. Exercise more.
Eat less. Exercise more. Eat less. Exercise more.
Eat less. Exercise more. Eat less. Exercise more.
Eat less. Exercise more. Eat less. Exercise more.
Eat less. Exercise more. Eat less. Exercise more.
Eat less. Exercise more. Eat less. Exercise more.
Eat less. Exercise more. Eat less. Exercise more.
Eat less. Exercise more. Eat less. Exercise more.
Eat less. Exercise more. Eat less. Exercise more.
Eat less. Exercise more. Eat less. Exercise more.
Eat less. Exercise more. Eat less. Exercise more.
Eat less. Exercise more. Eat less. Exercise more.
Eat less. Exercise more. Eat less. Exercise more.
Eat less. Exercise more. Eat less. Exercise more.
Eat less. Exercise more. Eat less. Exercise more.
Eat less. Exercise more. Eat less. Exercise more.
Eat less. Exercise more. Eat less. Exercise more.
Eat less. Exercise more. Eat less. Exercise more.
Eat less. Exercise more. Eat less. Exercise more.
Eat less. Exercise more. Eat less. Exercise more.
Eat less. Exercise more. Eat less. Exercise more.
Eat less. Exercise more. Eat less. Exercise more.
Eat less. Exercise more. Eat less. Exercise more.
Eat less. Exercise more. Eat less. Exercise more.
Eat less. Exercise more. Eat less. Exercise more.
Eat less. Exercise more. Eat less. Exercise more.
Eat less. Exercise more. Eat less. Exercise more.
Eat less. Exercise more. Eat less. Exercise more.
Eat less. Exercise more. Eat less. Exercise more.
Eat less. Exercise more. Eat less. Exercise more.
Eat less. Exercise more. Eat less. Exercise more.
Eat less. Exercise more. Eat less. Exercise more.
Eat less. Exercise more. Eat less. Exercise more.
Eat less. Exercise more. Eat less. Exercise more.

Eat less. Exercise more. Eat less. Exercise more.
Eat less. Exercise more. Eat less. Exercise more.
Eat less. Exercise more. Eat less. Exercise more.
Eat less. Exercise more. Eat less. Exercise more.
Eat less. Exercise more. Eat less. Exercise more.
Eat less. Exercise more. Eat less. Exercise more.
Eat less. Exercise more. Eat less. Exercise more.
Eat less. Exercise more. Eat less. Exercise more.
Eat less. Exercise more. Eat less. Exercise more.
Eat less. Exercise more. Eat less. Exercise more.
Eat less. Exercise more. Eat less. Exercise more.
Eat less. Exercise more. Eat less. Exercise more.
Eat less. Exercise more. Eat less. Exercise more.
Eat less. Exercise more. Eat less. Exercise more.
Eat less. Exercise more. Eat less. Exercise more.
Eat less. Exercise more. Eat less. Exercise more.
Eat less. Exercise more. Eat less. Exercise more.
Eat less. Exercise more. Eat less. Exercise more.
Eat less. Exercise more. Eat less. Exercise more.
Eat less. Exercise more. Eat less. Exercise more.
Eat less. Exercise more. Eat less. Exercise more.
Eat less. Exercise more. Eat less. Exercise more.
Eat less. Exercise more. Eat less. Exercise more.
Eat less. Exercise more. Eat less. Exercise more.
Eat less. Exercise more. Eat less. Exercise more.
Eat less. Exercise more. Eat less. Exercise more.
Eat less. Exercise more. Eat less. Exercise more.
Eat less. Exercise more. Eat less. Exercise more.
Eat less. Exercise more. Eat less. Exercise more.
Eat less. Exercise more. Eat less. Exercise more.
Eat less. Exercise more. Eat less. Exercise more.
Eat less. Exercise more. Eat less. Exercise more.
Eat less. Exercise more. Eat less. Exercise more.
Eat less. Exercise more. Eat less. Exercise more.

Eat less. Exercise more. Eat less. Exercise more.
Eat less. Exercise more. Eat less. Exercise more.
Eat less. Exercise more. Eat less. Exercise more.
Eat less. Exercise more. Eat less. Exercise more.
Eat less. Exercise more. Eat less. Exercise more.
Eat less. Exercise more. Eat less. Exercise more.
Eat less. Exercise more. Eat less. Exercise more.
Eat less. Exercise more. Eat less. Exercise more.
Eat less. Exercise more. Eat less. Exercise more.
Eat less. Exercise more. Eat less. Exercise more.
Eat less. Exercise more. Eat less. Exercise more.
Eat less. Exercise more. Eat less. Exercise more.
Eat less. Exercise more. Eat less. Exercise more.
Eat less. Exercise more. Eat less. Exercise more.
Eat less. Exercise more. Eat less. Exercise more.
Eat less. Exercise more. Eat less. Exercise more.
Eat less. Exercise more. Eat less. Exercise more.
Eat less. Exercise more. Eat less. Exercise more.
Eat less. Exercise more. Eat less. Exercise more.
Eat less. Exercise more. Eat less. Exercise more.
Eat less. Exercise more. Eat less. Exercise more.
Eat less. Exercise more. Eat less. Exercise more.
Eat less. Exercise more. Eat less. Exercise more.
Eat less. Exercise more. Eat less. Exercise more.
Eat less. Exercise more. Eat less. Exercise more.
Eat less. Exercise more. Eat less. Exercise more.
Eat less. Exercise more. Eat less. Exercise more.
Eat less. Exercise more. Eat less. Exercise more.
Eat less. Exercise more. Eat less. Exercise more.
Eat less. Exercise more. Eat less. Exercise more.
Eat less. Exercise more. Eat less. Exercise more.
Eat less. Exercise more. Eat less. Exercise more.
Eat less. Exercise more. Eat less. Exercise more.

Eat less. Exercise more. Eat less. Exercise more.
Eat less. Exercise more. Eat less. Exercise more.
Eat less. Exercise more. Eat less. Exercise more.
Eat less. Exercise more. Eat less. Exercise more.
Eat less. Exercise more. Eat less. Exercise more.
Eat less. Exercise more. Eat less. Exercise more.
Eat less. Exercise more. Eat less. Exercise more.
Eat less. Exercise more. Eat less. Exercise more.
Eat less. Exercise more. Eat less. Exercise more.
Eat less. Exercise more. Eat less. Exercise more.
Eat less. Exercise more. Eat less. Exercise more.
Eat less. Exercise more. Eat less. Exercise more.
Eat less. Exercise more. Eat less. Exercise more.
Eat less. Exercise more. Eat less. Exercise more.
Eat less. Exercise more. Eat less. Exercise more.
Eat less. Exercise more. Eat less. Exercise more.
Eat less. Exercise more. Eat less. Exercise more.
Eat less. Exercise more. Eat less. Exercise more.
Eat less. Exercise more. Eat less. Exercise more.
Eat less. Exercise more. Eat less. Exercise more.
Eat less. Exercise more. Eat less. Exercise more.
Eat less. Exercise more. Eat less. Exercise more.
Eat less. Exercise more. Eat less. Exercise more.
Eat less. Exercise more. Eat less. Exercise more.
Eat less. Exercise more. Eat less. Exercise more.
Eat less. Exercise more. Eat less. Exercise more.
Eat less. Exercise more. Eat less. Exercise more.
Eat less. Exercise more. Eat less. Exercise more.
Eat less. Exercise more. Eat less. Exercise more.
Eat less. Exercise more. Eat less. Exercise more.
Eat less. Exercise more. Eat less. Exercise more.
Eat less. Exercise more. Eat less. Exercise more.
Eat less. Exercise more. Eat less. Exercise more.

Eat less. Exercise more. Eat less. Exercise more.
Eat less. Exercise more. Eat less. Exercise more.
Eat less. Exercise more. Eat less. Exercise more.
Eat less. Exercise more. Eat less. Exercise more.
Eat less. Exercise more. Eat less. Exercise more.
Eat less. Exercise more. Eat less. Exercise more.
Eat less. Exercise more. Eat less. Exercise more.
Eat less. Exercise more. Eat less. Exercise more.
Eat less. Exercise more. Eat less. Exercise more.
Eat less. Exercise more. Eat less. Exercise more.
Eat less. Exercise more. Eat less. Exercise more.
Eat less. Exercise more. Eat less. Exercise more.
Eat less. Exercise more. Eat less. Exercise more.
Eat less. Exercise more. Eat less. Exercise more.
Eat less. Exercise more. Eat less. Exercise more.
Eat less. Exercise more. Eat less. Exercise more.
Eat less. Exercise more. Eat less. Exercise more.
Eat less. Exercise more. Eat less. Exercise more.
Eat less. Exercise more. Eat less. Exercise more.
Eat less. Exercise more. Eat less. Exercise more.
Eat less. Exercise more. Eat less. Exercise more.
Eat less. Exercise more. Eat less. Exercise more.
Eat less. Exercise more. Eat less. Exercise more.
Eat less. Exercise more. Eat less. Exercise more.
Eat less. Exercise more. Eat less. Exercise more.
Eat less. Exercise more. Eat less. Exercise more.
Eat less. Exercise more. Eat less. Exercise more.
Eat less. Exercise more. Eat less. Exercise more.
Eat less. Exercise more. Eat less. Exercise more.
Eat less. Exercise more. Eat less. Exercise more.
Eat less. Exercise more. Eat less. Exercise more.
Eat less. Exercise more. Eat less. Exercise more.
Eat less. Exercise more. Eat less. Exercise more.
Eat less. Exercise more. Eat less. Exercise more.
Eat less. Exercise more. Eat less. Exercise more.

Eat less. Exercise more. Eat less. Exercise more.
Eat less. Exercise more. Eat less. Exercise more.
Eat less. Exercise more. Eat less. Exercise more.
Eat less. Exercise more. Eat less. Exercise more.
Eat less. Exercise more. Eat less. Exercise more.
Eat less. Exercise more. Eat less. Exercise more.
Eat less. Exercise more. Eat less. Exercise more.
Eat less. Exercise more. Eat less. Exercise more.
Eat less. Exercise more. Eat less. Exercise more.
Eat less. Exercise more. Eat less. Exercise more.
Eat less. Exercise more. Eat less. Exercise more.
Eat less. Exercise more. Eat less. Exercise more.
Eat less. Exercise more. Eat less. Exercise more.
Eat less. Exercise more. Eat less. Exercise more.
Eat less. Exercise more. Eat less. Exercise more.
Eat less. Exercise more. Eat less. Exercise more.
Eat less. Exercise more. Eat less. Exercise more.
Eat less. Exercise more. Eat less. Exercise more.
Eat less. Exercise more. Eat less. Exercise more.
Eat less. Exercise more. Eat less. Exercise more.
Eat less. Exercise more. Eat less. Exercise more.
Eat less. Exercise more. Eat less. Exercise more.
Eat less. Exercise more. Eat less. Exercise more.
Eat less. Exercise more. Eat less. Exercise more.
Eat less. Exercise more. Eat less. Exercise more.
Eat less. Exercise more. Eat less. Exercise more.
Eat less. Exercise more. Eat less. Exercise more.
Eat less. Exercise more. Eat less. Exercise more.
Eat less. Exercise more. Eat less. Exercise more.
Eat less. Exercise more. Eat less. Exercise more.
Eat less. Exercise more. Eat less. Exercise more.
Eat less. Exercise more. Eat less. Exercise more.
Eat less. Exercise more. Eat less. Exercise more.

Eat less. Exercise more. Eat less. Exercise more.
Eat less. Exercise more. Eat less. Exercise more.
Eat less. Exercise more. Eat less. Exercise more.
Eat less. Exercise more. Eat less. Exercise more.
Eat less. Exercise more. Eat less. Exercise more.
Eat less. Exercise more. Eat less. Exercise more.
Eat less. Exercise more. Eat less. Exercise more.
Eat less. Exercise more. Eat less. Exercise more.
Eat less. Exercise more. Eat less. Exercise more.
Eat less. Exercise more. Eat less. Exercise more.
Eat less. Exercise more. Eat less. Exercise more.
Eat less. Exercise more. Eat less. Exercise more.
Eat less. Exercise more. Eat less. Exercise more.
Eat less. Exercise more. Eat less. Exercise more.
Eat less. Exercise more. Eat less. Exercise more.
Eat less. Exercise more. Eat less. Exercise more.
Eat less. Exercise more. Eat less. Exercise more.
Eat less. Exercise more. Eat less. Exercise more.
Eat less. Exercise more. Eat less. Exercise more.
Eat less. Exercise more. Eat less. Exercise more.
Eat less. Exercise more. Eat less. Exercise more.
Eat less. Exercise more. Eat less. Exercise more.
Eat less. Exercise more. Eat less. Exercise more.
Eat less. Exercise more. Eat less. Exercise more.
Eat less. Exercise more. Eat less. Exercise more.
Eat less. Exercise more. Eat less. Exercise more.
Eat less. Exercise more. Eat less. Exercise more.
Eat less. Exercise more. Eat less. Exercise more.
Eat less. Exercise more. Eat less. Exercise more.
Eat less. Exercise more. Eat less. Exercise more.
Eat less. Exercise more. Eat less. Exercise more.
Eat less. Exercise more. Eat less. Exercise more.
Eat less. Exercise more. Eat less. Exercise more.
Eat less. Exercise more. Eat less. Exercise more.

Eat less. Exercise more. Eat less. Exercise more.
Eat less. Exercise more. Eat less. Exercise more.
Eat less. Exercise more. Eat less. Exercise more.
Eat less. Exercise more. Eat less. Exercise more.
Eat less. Exercise more. Eat less. Exercise more.
Eat less. Exercise more. Eat less. Exercise more.
Eat less. Exercise more. Eat less. Exercise more.
Eat less. Exercise more. Eat less. Exercise more.
Eat less. Exercise more. Eat less. Exercise more.
Eat less. Exercise more. Eat less. Exercise more.
Eat less. Exercise more. Eat less. Exercise more.
Eat less. Exercise more. Eat less. Exercise more.
Eat less. Exercise more. Eat less. Exercise more.
Eat less. Exercise more. Eat less. Exercise more.
Eat less. Exercise more. Eat less. Exercise more.
Eat less. Exercise more. Eat less. Exercise more.
Eat less. Exercise more. Eat less. Exercise more.
Eat less. Exercise more. Eat less. Exercise more.
Eat less. Exercise more. Eat less. Exercise more.
Eat less. Exercise more. Eat less. Exercise more.
Eat less. Exercise more. Eat less. Exercise more.
Eat less. Exercise more. Eat less. Exercise more.
Eat less. Exercise more. Eat less. Exercise more.
Eat less. Exercise more. Eat less. Exercise more.
Eat less. Exercise more. Eat less. Exercise more.
Eat less. Exercise more. Eat less. Exercise more.
Eat less. Exercise more. Eat less. Exercise more.
Eat less. Exercise more. Eat less. Exercise more.
Eat less. Exercise more. Eat less. Exercise more.
Eat less. Exercise more. Eat less. Exercise more.
Eat less. Exercise more. Eat less. Exercise more.
Eat less. Exercise more. Eat less. Exercise more.
Eat less. Exercise more. Eat less. Exercise more.
Eat less. Exercise more. Eat less. Exercise more.

Eat less. Exercise more. Eat less. Exercise more.
Eat less. Exercise more. Eat less. Exercise more.
Eat less. Exercise more. Eat less. Exercise more.
Eat less. Exercise more. Eat less. Exercise more.
Eat less. Exercise more. Eat less. Exercise more.
Eat less. Exercise more. Eat less. Exercise more.
Eat less. Exercise more. Eat less. Exercise more.
Eat less. Exercise more. Eat less. Exercise more.
Eat less. Exercise more. Eat less. Exercise more.
Eat less. Exercise more. Eat less. Exercise more.
Eat less. Exercise more. Eat less. Exercise more.
Eat less. Exercise more. Eat less. Exercise more.
Eat less. Exercise more. Eat less. Exercise more.
Eat less. Exercise more. Eat less. Exercise more.
Eat less. Exercise more. Eat less. Exercise more.
Eat less. Exercise more. Eat less. Exercise more.
Eat less. Exercise more. Eat less. Exercise more.
Eat less. Exercise more. Eat less. Exercise more.
Eat less. Exercise more. Eat less. Exercise more.
Eat less. Exercise more. Eat less. Exercise more.
Eat less. Exercise more. Eat less. Exercise more.
Eat less. Exercise more. Eat less. Exercise more.
Eat less. Exercise more. Eat less. Exercise more.
Eat less. Exercise more. Eat less. Exercise more.
Eat less. Exercise more. Eat less. Exercise more.
Eat less. Exercise more. Eat less. Exercise more.
Eat less. Exercise more. Eat less. Exercise more.
Eat less. Exercise more. Eat less. Exercise more.
Eat less. Exercise more. Eat less. Exercise more.
Eat less. Exercise more. Eat less. Exercise more.
Eat less. Exercise more. Eat less. Exercise more.
Eat less. Exercise more. Eat less. Exercise more.
Eat less. Exercise more. Eat less. Exercise more.
Eat less. Exercise more. Eat less. Exercise more.

Eat less. Exercise more. Eat less. Exercise more.
Eat less. Exercise more. Eat less. Exercise more.
Eat less. Exercise more. Eat less. Exercise more.
Eat less. Exercise more. Eat less. Exercise more.
Eat less. Exercise more. Eat less. Exercise more.
Eat less. Exercise more. Eat less. Exercise more.
Eat less. Exercise more. Eat less. Exercise more.
Eat less. Exercise more. Eat less. Exercise more.
Eat less. Exercise more. Eat less. Exercise more.
Eat less. Exercise more. Eat less. Exercise more.
Eat less. Exercise more. Eat less. Exercise more.
Eat less. Exercise more. Eat less. Exercise more.
Eat less. Exercise more. Eat less. Exercise more.
Eat less. Exercise more. Eat less. Exercise more.
Eat less. Exercise more. Eat less. Exercise more.
Eat less. Exercise more. Eat less. Exercise more.
Eat less. Exercise more. Eat less. Exercise more.
Eat less. Exercise more. Eat less. Exercise more.
Eat less. Exercise more. Eat less. Exercise more.
Eat less. Exercise more. Eat less. Exercise more.
Eat less. Exercise more. Eat less. Exercise more.
Eat less. Exercise more. Eat less. Exercise more.
Eat less. Exercise more. Eat less. Exercise more.
Eat less. Exercise more. Eat less. Exercise more.
Eat less. Exercise more. Eat less. Exercise more.
Eat less. Exercise more. Eat less. Exercise more.
Eat less. Exercise more. Eat less. Exercise more.
Eat less. Exercise more. Eat less. Exercise more.
Eat less. Exercise more. Eat less. Exercise more.
Eat less. Exercise more. Eat less. Exercise more.
Eat less. Exercise more. Eat less. Exercise more.
Eat less. Exercise more. Eat less. Exercise more.
Eat less. Exercise more. Eat less. Exercise more.
Eat less. Exercise more. Eat less. Exercise more.

Eat less. Exercise more. Eat less. Exercise more.
Eat less. Exercise more. Eat less. Exercise more.
Eat less. Exercise more. Eat less. Exercise more.
Eat less. Exercise more. Eat less. Exercise more.
Eat less. Exercise more. Eat less. Exercise more.
Eat less. Exercise more. Eat less. Exercise more.
Eat less. Exercise more. Eat less. Exercise more.
Eat less. Exercise more. Eat less. Exercise more.
Eat less. Exercise more. Eat less. Exercise more.
Eat less. Exercise more. Eat less. Exercise more.
Eat less. Exercise more. Eat less. Exercise more.
Eat less. Exercise more. Eat less. Exercise more.
Eat less. Exercise more. Eat less. Exercise more.
Eat less. Exercise more. Eat less. Exercise more.
Eat less. Exercise more. Eat less. Exercise more.
Eat less. Exercise more. Eat less. Exercise more.
Eat less. Exercise more. Eat less. Exercise more.
Eat less. Exercise more. Eat less. Exercise more.
Eat less. Exercise more. Eat less. Exercise more.
Eat less. Exercise more. Eat less. Exercise more.
Eat less. Exercise more. Eat less. Exercise more.
Eat less. Exercise more. Eat less. Exercise more.
Eat less. Exercise more. Eat less. Exercise more.
Eat less. Exercise more. Eat less. Exercise more.
Eat less. Exercise more. Eat less. Exercise more.
Eat less. Exercise more. Eat less. Exercise more.
Eat less. Exercise more. Eat less. Exercise more.
Eat less. Exercise more. Eat less. Exercise more.
Eat less. Exercise more. Eat less. Exercise more.
Eat less. Exercise more. Eat less. Exercise more.
Eat less. Exercise more. Eat less. Exercise more.
Eat less. Exercise more. Eat less. Exercise more.
Eat less. Exercise more. Eat less. Exercise more.
Eat less. Exercise more. Eat less. Exercise more.
Eat less. Exercise more. Eat less. Exercise more.

Eat less. Exercise more. Eat less. Exercise more.
Eat less. Exercise more. Eat less. Exercise more.
Eat less. Exercise more. Eat less. Exercise more.
Eat less. Exercise more. Eat less. Exercise more.
Eat less. Exercise more. Eat less. Exercise more.
Eat less. Exercise more. Eat less. Exercise more.
Eat less. Exercise more. Eat less. Exercise more.
Eat less. Exercise more. Eat less. Exercise more.
Eat less. Exercise more. Eat less. Exercise more.
Eat less. Exercise more. Eat less. Exercise more.
Eat less. Exercise more. Eat less. Exercise more.
Eat less. Exercise more. Eat less. Exercise more.
Eat less. Exercise more. Eat less. Exercise more.
Eat less. Exercise more. Eat less. Exercise more.
Eat less. Exercise more. Eat less. Exercise more.
Eat less. Exercise more. Eat less. Exercise more.
Eat less. Exercise more. Eat less. Exercise more.
Eat less. Exercise more. Eat less. Exercise more.
Eat less. Exercise more. Eat less. Exercise more.
Eat less. Exercise more. Eat less. Exercise more.
Eat less. Exercise more. Eat less. Exercise more.
Eat less. Exercise more. Eat less. Exercise more.
Eat less. Exercise more. Eat less. Exercise more.
Eat less. Exercise more. Eat less. Exercise more.
Eat less. Exercise more. Eat less. Exercise more.
Eat less. Exercise more. Eat less. Exercise more.
Eat less. Exercise more. Eat less. Exercise more.
Eat less. Exercise more. Eat less. Exercise more.
Eat less. Exercise more. Eat less. Exercise more.
Eat less. Exercise more. Eat less. Exercise more.
Eat less. Exercise more. Eat less. Exercise more.
Eat less. Exercise more. Eat less. Exercise more.
Eat less. Exercise more. Eat less. Exercise more.

Eat less. Exercise more. Eat less. Exercise more.
Eat less. Exercise more. Eat less. Exercise more.
Eat less. Exercise more. Eat less. Exercise more.
Eat less. Exercise more. Eat less. Exercise more.
Eat less. Exercise more. Eat less. Exercise more.
Eat less. Exercise more. Eat less. Exercise more.
Eat less. Exercise more. Eat less. Exercise more.
Eat less. Exercise more. Eat less. Exercise more.
Eat less. Exercise more. Eat less. Exercise more.
Eat less. Exercise more. Eat less. Exercise more.
Eat less. Exercise more. Eat less. Exercise more.
Eat less. Exercise more. Eat less. Exercise more.
Eat less. Exercise more. Eat less. Exercise more.
Eat less. Exercise more. Eat less. Exercise more.
Eat less. Exercise more. Eat less. Exercise more.
Eat less. Exercise more. Eat less. Exercise more.
Eat less. Exercise more. Eat less. Exercise more.
Eat less. Exercise more. Eat less. Exercise more.
Eat less. Exercise more. Eat less. Exercise more.
Eat less. Exercise more. Eat less. Exercise more.
Eat less. Exercise more. Eat less. Exercise more.
Eat less. Exercise more. Eat less. Exercise more.
Eat less. Exercise more. Eat less. Exercise more.
Eat less. Exercise more. Eat less. Exercise more.
Eat less. Exercise more. Eat less. Exercise more.
Eat less. Exercise more. Eat less. Exercise more.
Eat less. Exercise more. Eat less. Exercise more.
Eat less. Exercise more. Eat less. Exercise more.
Eat less. Exercise more. Eat less. Exercise more.
Eat less. Exercise more. Eat less. Exercise more.
Eat less. Exercise more. Eat less. Exercise more.
Eat less. Exercise more. Eat less. Exercise more.
Eat less. Exercise more. Eat less. Exercise more.
Eat less. Exercise more. Eat less. Exercise more.
Eat less. Exercise more. Eat less. Exercise more.

Eat less. Exercise more. Eat less. Exercise more.
Eat less. Exercise more. Eat less. Exercise more.
Eat less. Exercise more. Eat less. Exercise more.
Eat less. Exercise more. Eat less. Exercise more.
Eat less. Exercise more. Eat less. Exercise more.
Eat less. Exercise more. Eat less. Exercise more.
Eat less. Exercise more. Eat less. Exercise more.
Eat less. Exercise more. Eat less. Exercise more.
Eat less. Exercise more. Eat less. Exercise more.
Eat less. Exercise more. Eat less. Exercise more.
Eat less. Exercise more. Eat less. Exercise more.
Eat less. Exercise more. Eat less. Exercise more.
Eat less. Exercise more. Eat less. Exercise more.
Eat less. Exercise more. Eat less. Exercise more.
Eat less. Exercise more. Eat less. Exercise more.
Eat less. Exercise more. Eat less. Exercise more.
Eat less. Exercise more. Eat less. Exercise more.
Eat less. Exercise more. Eat less. Exercise more.
Eat less. Exercise more. Eat less. Exercise more.
Eat less. Exercise more. Eat less. Exercise more.
Eat less. Exercise more. Eat less. Exercise more.
Eat less. Exercise more. Eat less. Exercise more.
Eat less. Exercise more. Eat less. Exercise more.
Eat less. Exercise more. Eat less. Exercise more.
Eat less. Exercise more. Eat less. Exercise more.
Eat less. Exercise more. Eat less. Exercise more.
Eat less. Exercise more. Eat less. Exercise more.
Eat less. Exercise more. Eat less. Exercise more.
Eat less. Exercise more. Eat less. Exercise more.
Eat less. Exercise more. Eat less. Exercise more.
Eat less. Exercise more. Eat less. Exercise more.
Eat less. Exercise more. Eat less. Exercise more.
Eat less. Exercise more. Eat less. Exercise more.
Eat less. Exercise more. Eat less. Exercise more.

Eat less. Exercise more. Eat less. Exercise more.
Eat less. Exercise more. Eat less. Exercise more.
Eat less. Exercise more. Eat less. Exercise more.
Eat less. Exercise more. Eat less. Exercise more.
Eat less. Exercise more. Eat less. Exercise more.
Eat less. Exercise more. Eat less. Exercise more.
Eat less. Exercise more. Eat less. Exercise more.
Eat less. Exercise more. Eat less. Exercise more.
Eat less. Exercise more. Eat less. Exercise more.
Eat less. Exercise more. Eat less. Exercise more.
Eat less. Exercise more. Eat less. Exercise more.
Eat less. Exercise more. Eat less. Exercise more.
Eat less. Exercise more. Eat less. Exercise more.
Eat less. Exercise more. Eat less. Exercise more.
Eat less. Exercise more. Eat less. Exercise more.
Eat less. Exercise more. Eat less. Exercise more.
Eat less. Exercise more. Eat less. Exercise more.
Eat less. Exercise more. Eat less. Exercise more.
Eat less. Exercise more. Eat less. Exercise more.
Eat less. Exercise more. Eat less. Exercise more.
Eat less. Exercise more. Eat less. Exercise more.
Eat less. Exercise more. Eat less. Exercise more.
Eat less. Exercise more. Eat less. Exercise more.
Eat less. Exercise more. Eat less. Exercise more.
Eat less. Exercise more. Eat less. Exercise more.
Eat less. Exercise more. Eat less. Exercise more.
Eat less. Exercise more. Eat less. Exercise more.
Eat less. Exercise more. Eat less. Exercise more.
Eat less. Exercise more. Eat less. Exercise more.
Eat less. Exercise more. Eat less. Exercise more.
Eat less. Exercise more. Eat less. Exercise more.
Eat less. Exercise more. Eat less. Exercise more.
Eat less. Exercise more. Eat less. Exercise more.
Eat less. Exercise more. Eat less. Exercise more.
Eat less. Exercise more. Eat less. Exercise more.

Eat less. Exercise more. Eat less. Exercise more.
Eat less. Exercise more. Eat less. Exercise more.
Eat less. Exercise more. Eat less. Exercise more.
Eat less. Exercise more. Eat less. Exercise more.
Eat less. Exercise more. Eat less. Exercise more.
Eat less. Exercise more. Eat less. Exercise more.
Eat less. Exercise more. Eat less. Exercise more.
Eat less. Exercise more. Eat less. Exercise more.
Eat less. Exercise more. Eat less. Exercise more.
Eat less. Exercise more. Eat less. Exercise more.
Eat less. Exercise more. Eat less. Exercise more.
Eat less. Exercise more. Eat less. Exercise more.
Eat less. Exercise more. Eat less. Exercise more.
Eat less. Exercise more. Eat less. Exercise more.
Eat less. Exercise more. Eat less. Exercise more.
Eat less. Exercise more. Eat less. Exercise more.
Eat less. Exercise more. Eat less. Exercise more.
Eat less. Exercise more. Eat less. Exercise more.
Eat less. Exercise more. Eat less. Exercise more.
Eat less. Exercise more. Eat less. Exercise more.
Eat less. Exercise more. Eat less. Exercise more.
Eat less. Exercise more. Eat less. Exercise more.
Eat less. Exercise more. Eat less. Exercise more.
Eat less. Exercise more. Eat less. Exercise more.
Eat less. Exercise more. Eat less. Exercise more.
Eat less. Exercise more. Eat less. Exercise more.
Eat less. Exercise more. Eat less. Exercise more.
Eat less. Exercise more. Eat less. Exercise more.
Eat less. Exercise more. Eat less. Exercise more.
Eat less. Exercise more. Eat less. Exercise more.
Eat less. Exercise more. Eat less. Exercise more.
Eat less. Exercise more. Eat less. Exercise more.
Eat less. Exercise more. Eat less. Exercise more.

Eat less. Exercise more. Eat less. Exercise more.
Eat less. Exercise more. Eat less. Exercise more.
Eat less. Exercise more. Eat less. Exercise more.
Eat less. Exercise more. Eat less. Exercise more.
Eat less. Exercise more. Eat less. Exercise more.
Eat less. Exercise more. Eat less. Exercise more.
Eat less. Exercise more. Eat less. Exercise more.
Eat less. Exercise more. Eat less. Exercise more.
Eat less. Exercise more. Eat less. Exercise more.
Eat less. Exercise more. Eat less. Exercise more.
Eat less. Exercise more. Eat less. Exercise more.
Eat less. Exercise more. Eat less. Exercise more.
Eat less. Exercise more. Eat less. Exercise more.
Eat less. Exercise more. Eat less. Exercise more.
Eat less. Exercise more. Eat less. Exercise more.
Eat less. Exercise more. Eat less. Exercise more.
Eat less. Exercise more. Eat less. Exercise more.
Eat less. Exercise more. Eat less. Exercise more.
Eat less. Exercise more. Eat less. Exercise more.
Eat less. Exercise more. Eat less. Exercise more.
Eat less. Exercise more. Eat less. Exercise more.
Eat less. Exercise more. Eat less. Exercise more.
Eat less. Exercise more. Eat less. Exercise more.
Eat less. Exercise more. Eat less. Exercise more.
Eat less. Exercise more. Eat less. Exercise more.
Eat less. Exercise more. Eat less. Exercise more.
Eat less. Exercise more. Eat less. Exercise more.
Eat less. Exercise more. Eat less. Exercise more.
Eat less. Exercise more. Eat less. Exercise more.
Eat less. Exercise more. Eat less. Exercise more.
Eat less. Exercise more. Eat less. Exercise more.
Eat less. Exercise more. Eat less. Exercise more.
Eat less. Exercise more. Eat less. Exercise more.
Eat less. Exercise more. Eat less. Exercise more.
Eat less. Exercise more. Eat less. Exercise more.
Eat less. Exercise more. Eat less. Exercise more.

Eat less. Exercise more. Eat less. Exercise more.
Eat less. Exercise more. Eat less. Exercise more.
Eat less. Exercise more. Eat less. Exercise more.
Eat less. Exercise more. Eat less. Exercise more.
Eat less. Exercise more. Eat less. Exercise more.
Eat less. Exercise more. Eat less. Exercise more.
Eat less. Exercise more. Eat less. Exercise more.
Eat less. Exercise more. Eat less. Exercise more.
Eat less. Exercise more. Eat less. Exercise more.
Eat less. Exercise more. Eat less. Exercise more.
Eat less. Exercise more. Eat less. Exercise more.
Eat less. Exercise more. Eat less. Exercise more.
Eat less. Exercise more. Eat less. Exercise more.
Eat less. Exercise more. Eat less. Exercise more.
Eat less. Exercise more. Eat less. Exercise more.
Eat less. Exercise more. Eat less. Exercise more.
Eat less. Exercise more. Eat less. Exercise more.
Eat less. Exercise more. Eat less. Exercise more.
Eat less. Exercise more. Eat less. Exercise more.
Eat less. Exercise more. Eat less. Exercise more.
Eat less. Exercise more. Eat less. Exercise more.
Eat less. Exercise more. Eat less. Exercise more.
Eat less. Exercise more. Eat less. Exercise more.
Eat less. Exercise more. Eat less. Exercise more.
Eat less. Exercise more. Eat less. Exercise more.
Eat less. Exercise more. Eat less. Exercise more.
Eat less. Exercise more. Eat less. Exercise more.
Eat less. Exercise more. Eat less. Exercise more.
Eat less. Exercise more. Eat less. Exercise more.
Eat less. Exercise more. Eat less. Exercise more.
Eat less. Exercise more. Eat less. Exercise more.
Eat less. Exercise more. Eat less. Exercise more.
Eat less. Exercise more. Eat less. Exercise more.
Eat less. Exercise more. Eat less. Exercise more.

Eat less. Exercise more. Eat less. Exercise more.
Eat less. Exercise more. Eat less. Exercise more.
Eat less. Exercise more. Eat less. Exercise more.
Eat less. Exercise more. Eat less. Exercise more.
Eat less. Exercise more. Eat less. Exercise more.
Eat less. Exercise more. Eat less. Exercise more.
Eat less. Exercise more. Eat less. Exercise more.
Eat less. Exercise more. Eat less. Exercise more.
Eat less. Exercise more. Eat less. Exercise more.
Eat less. Exercise more. Eat less. Exercise more.
Eat less. Exercise more. Eat less. Exercise more.
Eat less. Exercise more. Eat less. Exercise more.
Eat less. Exercise more. Eat less. Exercise more.
Eat less. Exercise more. Eat less. Exercise more.
Eat less. Exercise more. Eat less. Exercise more.
Eat less. Exercise more. Eat less. Exercise more.
Eat less. Exercise more. Eat less. Exercise more.
Eat less. Exercise more. Eat less. Exercise more.
Eat less. Exercise more. Eat less. Exercise more.
Eat less. Exercise more. Eat less. Exercise more.
Eat less. Exercise more. Eat less. Exercise more.
Eat less. Exercise more. Eat less. Exercise more.
Eat less. Exercise more. Eat less. Exercise more.
Eat less. Exercise more. Eat less. Exercise more.
Eat less. Exercise more. Eat less. Exercise more.
Eat less. Exercise more. Eat less. Exercise more.
Eat less. Exercise more. Eat less. Exercise more.
Eat less. Exercise more. Eat less. Exercise more.
Eat less. Exercise more. Eat less. Exercise more.
Eat less. Exercise more. Eat less. Exercise more.
Eat less. Exercise more. Eat less. Exercise more.
Eat less. Exercise more. Eat less. Exercise more.
Eat less. Exercise more. Eat less. Exercise more.
Eat less. Exercise more. Eat less. Exercise more.

Eat less. Exercise more. Eat less. Exercise more.
Eat less. Exercise more. Eat less. Exercise more.
Eat less. Exercise more. Eat less. Exercise more.
Eat less. Exercise more. Eat less. Exercise more.
Eat less. Exercise more. Eat less. Exercise more.
Eat less. Exercise more. Eat less. Exercise more.
Eat less. Exercise more. Eat less. Exercise more.
Eat less. Exercise more. Eat less. Exercise more.
Eat less. Exercise more. Eat less. Exercise more.
Eat less. Exercise more. Eat less. Exercise more.
Eat less. Exercise more. Eat less. Exercise more.
Eat less. Exercise more. Eat less. Exercise more.
Eat less. Exercise more. Eat less. Exercise more.
Eat less. Exercise more. Eat less. Exercise more.
Eat less. Exercise more. Eat less. Exercise more.
Eat less. Exercise more. Eat less. Exercise more.
Eat less. Exercise more. Eat less. Exercise more.
Eat less. Exercise more. Eat less. Exercise more.
Eat less. Exercise more. Eat less. Exercise more.
Eat less. Exercise more. Eat less. Exercise more.
Eat less. Exercise more. Eat less. Exercise more.
Eat less. Exercise more. Eat less. Exercise more.
Eat less. Exercise more. Eat less. Exercise more.
Eat less. Exercise more. Eat less. Exercise more.
Eat less. Exercise more. Eat less. Exercise more.
Eat less. Exercise more. Eat less. Exercise more.
Eat less. Exercise more. Eat less. Exercise more.
Eat less. Exercise more. Eat less. Exercise more.
Eat less. Exercise more. Eat less. Exercise more.
Eat less. Exercise more. Eat less. Exercise more.
Eat less. Exercise more. Eat less. Exercise more.
Eat less. Exercise more. Eat less. Exercise more.
Eat less. Exercise more. Eat less. Exercise more.
Eat less. Exercise more. Eat less. Exercise more.

OTHER
MERCK PROFESSIONAL HANDBOOKS

THE MERCK INDEX
First Edition, 1889

THE MERCK VETERINARY MANUAL
First Edition, 1955

THE MERCK MANUAL OF GERIATRICS
First Edition, 1990

Merck Professional Handbooks
are published on a nonprofit basis
as a service to the scientific community.

THE

MERCK
MANUAL

SIXTEENTH EDITION

1st Edition – 1899	9th Edition – 1956
2nd Edition – 1901	10th Edition – 1961
3rd Edition – 1905	11th Edition – 1966
4th Edition – 1911	12th Edition – 1972
5th Edition – 1923	13th Edition – 1977
6th Edition – 1934	14th Edition – 1982
7th Edition – 1940	15th Edition – 1987
8th Edition – 1950	16th Edition – 1992

VOLUME II

SPECIALTIES

SIXTEENTH EDITION

THE
MERCK
MANUAL
OF

DIAGNOSIS AND THERAPY

VOLUME II

SPECIALTIES

GYNECOLOGY PSYCHIATRY
OBSTETRICS PHARMACOLOGY
PEDIATRICS OTHER SPECIALTIES

Robert Berkow, M.D., EDITOR-IN-CHIEF

Andrew J. Fletcher, M.B., B.Chir., ASSISTANT EDITOR

Editorial Board

Philip K. Bondy, M.D.
Preston V. Dilts, Jr., M.D.
R. Gordon Douglas, Jr., M.D.
Douglas A. Drossman, M.D.
L. Jack Faling, M.D.
Eugene P. Frenkel, M.D.

Robert A. Hoekelman, M.D.
Fred Plum, M.D.
John Romano, M.D.
G. Victor Rossi, Ph.D.
Paul H. Tanser, M.D.

Published by

MERCK RESEARCH LABORATORIES

Division of
MERCK & Co., INC.
Rahway, N.J.

1992

MERCK & CO., INC.
Rahway, N.J.
U.S.A.

MERCK HUMAN HEALTH DIVISION
Rahway, N.J.
U.S. HUMAN HEALTH
West Point, Pa.

MERCK RESEARCH LABORATORIES
Rahway, N.J.
West Point, Pa.

MERCK VACCINE DIVISION
Rahway, N.J.

MERCK AGVET DIVISION
Woodbridge, N.J.

HUBBARD FARMS, INC.
Walpole, N.H.

MERCK CONSUMER HEALTHCARE GROUP
Woodbridge, N.J.

MERCK MANUFACTURING DIVISION
Rahway, N.J.

CALGON CORPORATION
WATER MANAGEMENT DIVISION
Pittsburgh, Pa.
CALGON VESTAL LABORATORIES
St. Louis, Mo.

KELCO DIVISION
San Diego, Calif.

Library of Congress Catalog Card Number 1–31760
ISBN Number 0911910–15–8
ISSN Number 0076–6526

First Printing—August 1992

Printed in the U.S.A.

FOREWORD TO VOLUMES I AND II

These two volumes together contain all of the 16th Edition of THE MERCK MANUAL with the text rearranged to solve a problem most often encountered by medical students and house officers, to whom these volumes are specifically dedicated. THE MANUAL—probably the most widely used medical text in the world—has steadily grown in size and become too large to be carried conveniently in a jacket pocket or small medical bag. Dividing the book into two smaller volumes provides greater portability for those users who are constantly confronted with a variety of complex problems and need instant access to a pocket-sized reference text.

The objectives of THE MERCK MANUAL have always been ambitious. It attempts to provide clinically useful information that might be required by a family practitioner working anywhere in the world. THE MANUAL covers not only disorders of interest to general internists but also clinical pharmacology, psychiatry, ophthalmology, otorhinolaryngology, dermatology, dental disorders, special subjects (eg, clinical procedures, laboratory medicine, radiation reactions and injuries, and dental emergencies), obstetrics, gynecology, and pediatrics. Since the book is used worldwide, more subjects are covered than would be required for a purely domestic text. Furthermore, THE MANUAL is not just a brief outline or simple cookbook presentation of diseases. Rather, disease discussions include relevant data about incidence, epidemiology, etiol-

ogy, pathophysiology, symptoms and signs, and laboratory data, as well as differential diagnosis and treatment. Review of the physical examination, the analysis of symptoms and signs, and the approach to patients with various types of disorders, as well as basic information about major technologic advances, is presented in detail. Despite this extraordinary coverage, the size of the book has been well controlled. Nevertheless, achieving a pocket size required a different approach.

Rather than sacrifice coverage by abridging THE MANUAL, we offer our readers more choices. The 16th Edition is available in a single volume with a hard cover, as in the past. Additionally, the book is divided into these two smaller volumes: Volume I covers general internal medicine, while Volume II covers the specialties and special subjects noted above. Some subjects (eg, tables of laboratory values, weights and measures, and certain disease discussions) are reproduced in both volumes for the convenience of the user.

Abbreviations and symbols, used liberally as essential space savers, are listed on pages xxix and xxx.

The basic quality of the text, which relates to the excellence of our Editorial Board and distinguished authors as well as to extensive review procedures, remains the same in the two smaller volumes as in the single, larger text. We hope you will find these smaller volumes to be of value.

Robert Berkow, M.D.

NOTICE

Volume I: GENERAL MEDICINE

covers the following subjects:

INFECTIOUS DISEASE

IMMUNOLOGY; ALLERGIC DISORDERS

CARDIOVASCULAR DISORDERS

PULMONARY DISORDERS

GASTROINTESTINAL DISORDERS

HEPATIC AND BILIARY DISORDERS

NUTRITIONAL AND METABOLIC DISORDERS

ENDOCRINE DISORDERS

HEMATOLOGY AND ONCOLOGY

MUSCULOSKELETAL AND CONNECTIVE TISSUE DISORDERS

NEUROLOGIC DISORDERS

GENITOURINARY DISORDERS

LABORATORY AND REFERENCE GUIDES

Volume II: SPECIALTIES

FOREWORD TO EDITION 16

It has been 93 years since THE MERCK MANUAL first appeared in 1899 as a slender 262-page text titled MERCK'S MANUAL OF THE MATERIA MEDICA. It was expressly designed to meet the needs of general practitioners in selecting medications, noting that "memory is treacherous" and that even the most thoroughly informed physician needs a reminder "to make him at once master of the situation and enable him to prescribe exactly what his judgment tells him is needed for the occasion." It was well received and, by the 6th Edition (1934), THE MERCK MANUAL had become highly valued by medical students and house staff as well; by the end of World War II the pocket-sized manual was an established favorite ready-reference book. Today THE MANUAL is the most widely used medical text in the world. While the book has grown to about 2800 pages, its primary purpose remains the same—to provide useful clinical information to practicing physicians, medical students, interns, residents, and other health care professionals.

Fewer physicians now attempt to manage the whole range of medical disorders that can occur in infants, children, and adults, but those who do must have available a broad spectrum of current and accurate information. Specialists require precise information about subjects outside their areas of expertise. All physicians need more and more information for study and examination purposes, as well as for patient care. Keeping up with the rapid and extraordinary advances in cellular and molecular biology, molecular genetics, and medical technology is more challenging than ever, but THE MERCK MANUAL continues to try to meet these needs, excluding only details of surgical procedures.

Precisely how do we attempt to meet these needs? First, from a disease orientation, THE MANUAL covers all but the most obscure disorders of mankind, not only those that a general internist might expect to encounter but also problems associated with pregnancy and delivery; common and serious disorders of neonates, infants, and children; and many special situations. Disorders are organized mainly according to the organ systems primarily affected, on the basis of their etiology (as with most of the infectious diseases and disorders due to physical agents), or on the basis of disciplines (eg, gynecology, obstetrics, pediatrics, genetics, psychiatry). In addition, THE MANUAL contains information for special circum-stances, such as radiation reactions and injuries; problems encountered in deep-sea diving, and dental emergencies. The entire book is updated for each new edition, and new subjects are added, such as discussions of genetic evaluation and counseling, human immunodeficiency virus (HIV) infection in children, sports medicine, hospice medicine, cross-cultural issues in medicine, anabolic steroid abuse, and special considerations in performing cardiopulmonary resuscitation on infants and children. This edition has 140 more pages of text (approximately 5%) than the preceding edition. We therefore urge you to check the Index whenever you need information, even on unusual subjects or those not commonly found in other texts.

A completely disease-oriented compendium, however, would have serious limitations. Since patients usually present with complaints or concerns that must be meticulously described, sorted, and deciphered, many chapters are devoted to discussions of symptoms and signs and of how to elicit the historical and physical data required for diagnosis. Common clinical procedures and laboratory tests used as diagnostic and management aids are described, with emphasis on their indications, contraindications, and possible complications. New and sophisticated laboratory and technologic procedures are also described, with comments on their uses, interpretations, and limitations.

Current therapy is presented for each disorder and supplemented with a separate section on clinical pharmacology that describes general principles, new advances (eg, the role of drug receptors, plasma concentration monitoring), and details of pharmacologic groups and specific agents; it even discusses the use of placebos. The use of complex equipment (eg, respirators) is also described. Prophylaxis is emphasized wherever possible. Finally, reference guides are provided for checking normal values, for calculating dosages, and for converting weights, measures, and volumes to metric equivalents.

Can so many subjects be covered adequately in a single book? You, the reader, must be the ultimate judge, but we believe the answer is in the affirmative. This edition required a concerted effort by many people, beginning with an internal analysis and critique of the previous edition, even though it enjoyed highly favorable reviews and outstanding reader acceptance. Sections of that book were then sent to outside experts who had had nothing to do with its preparation, to solicit their most candid criticism. Published reviews and letters from readers were analyzed. Next, the Editorial Board met to compare reviews and critiques and to plan this 16th Edition. Distinguished special consultants were enlisted to provide additional expertise. Then, 290 authors with outstanding qualifications, experience, and knowledge were engaged. Their manuscripts were painstakingly edited by our in-house staff to retain every valuable morsel of knowledge while eliminating sometimes elegant but unneeded words. Each manuscript was then reviewed by a member of the Editorial Board or a consultant. In many cases, additional special reviewers were invited to comment. Every mention of a drug and its dosage was reviewed by still another outside consultant. The objective of all these reviews was to ensure accuracy, adequate and relevant coverage of each subject, and simple and clean exposition. The authors then reworked, modified, and polished their manuscripts. Almost all of the manuscripts were revised at least 6 times; 15 to 20 revisions were not uncommon. We believe that no other medical text undergoes as many reviews and revisions as THE MERCK MANUAL does.

Owing to the extensive subject matter covered and to a successful tradition, the style and organization of THE MANUAL have some unique characteristics. Readers are urged to spend a few minutes reviewing the Table of Contents (p. ix) and the Index (p. 1179). Scrutiny of the arrangement of subject headings within each section, of internal headings within a subject discussion, and of boldfaced terms in the text will reveal a pattern of outlining intended to aid study of the text.

The foregoing description is a simplified review of the complex and arduous but rewarding 5-year enterprise that culminated in the presentation of this 16th Edition of THE MERCK MANUAL. The members of the Editorial Board, special consultants, contributing authors, and in-house staff and their affiliations are listed on the pages that follow. They deserve a degree of gratitude that cannot be adequately expressed here, but we know they will feel sufficiently rewarded if their efforts serve your needs.

We hope this edition of THE MERCK MANUAL will be a welcome aid to you, our readers—compatible with your needs and worthy of frequent use. Suggestions for improvements will be warmly welcomed and carefully considered.

Robert Berkow, M.D., *Editor-in-Chief*
MERCK RESEARCH LABORATORIES
West Point, Pa. 19486

CONTENTS

Volume II

SPECIALTIES

§1. GYNECOLOGY AND OBSTETRICS

§3.   PEDIATRICS AND GENETICS (Cont'd)

§3.   PEDIATRICS AND GENETICS (*Cont'd*)

§3.   PEDIATRICS AND GENETICS (*Cont'd*)

§7. DERMATOLOGIC DISORDERS (*Cont'd*)

§9.   DISORDERS DUE TO PHYSICAL AGENTS

§10.   SPECIAL SUBJECTS

§11.   CLINICAL PHARMACOLOGY

ABBREVIATIONS AND SYMBOLS

The following abbreviations are used throughout the text; other abbreviations are expanded at first mention in the chapter or subchapter.

ACTH	adrenocorticotropic hormone	GI	gastrointestinal
ADH	antidiuretic hormone	gm	gram
ADP	adenosine diphosphate	G6PD	glucose-6-phosphate dehydrogenase
AIDS	acquired immunodeficiency syndrome	GU	genitourinary
ALT	alanine aminotransferase (formerly SGPT)	h	hour
		Hb	hemoglobin
AST	aspartate aminotransferase (formerly SGOT)	HCl	hydrochloric acid; hydrochloride
		HCO₃	bicarbonate
ATP	adenosine triphosphate	Hct	hematocrit
bid	2 times a day	Hg	mercury
BMR	basal metabolic rate	HI	hemagglutination inhibition, inhibiting
BP	blood pressure		
BSA	body surface area	HIV	human immunodeficiency virus
BUN	blood urea nitrogen	HLA	human leukocyte group A
C	Celsius; centigrade; complement	Hz	hertz (cycles/second)
		ICF	intracellular fluid
Ca	calcium	IgA, etc	immunoglobulin A, etc
CBC	complete blood count	IM	intramuscular(ly)
CF	complement fixation, fixating	IPPB	intermittent positive pressure breathing
Ch.	chapter		
Ci	curie	IU	international unit
CK	creatine kinase	IV	intravenous(ly)
Cl	chloride; chlorine	IVU	intravenous urography
cm	centimeter	K	potassium
CNS	central nervous system	kcal	kilocalorie (food calorie)
CO₂	carbon dioxide	kg	kilogram
CPR	cardiopulmonary resuscitation	17-KS	17-ketosteroids
CSF	cerebrospinal fluid	L	liter
CT	computed tomography	lb	pound
cu	cubic	LDH	lactic dehydrogenase
D & C	dilation and curettage	LE	lupus erythematosus
dL	deciliter (= 100 mL)	M	molar
DNA	deoxyribonucleic acid	m	meter
DTP	diphtheria-tetanus-pertussis (toxoids/vaccine)	m²	square meter
		MCH	mean corpuscular hemoglobin
D/W	dextrose in water	MCHC	mean corpuscular hemoglobin concentration
ECF	extracellular fluid		
ECG	electrocardiogram	mCi	millicurie
EEG	electroencephalogram	MCV	mean corpuscular volume
ENT	ear, nose, and throat	mEq	milliequivalent
ESR	erythrocyte sedimentation rate	Mg	magnesium
F	Fahrenheit	mg	milligram
FDA	U.S. Food and Drug Administration	MI	myocardial infarction
		MIC	minimum inhibitory concentration
ft	foot; feet (measure)		
FUO	fever of unknown origin	min	minute
GFR	glomerular filtration rate	mIU	milli-international unit

mL	milliliter		RF	rheumatic fever; rheumatoid factor
mm	millimeter		RNA	ribonucleic acid
mmol	millimole		Sa_{O_2}	arterial oxygen saturation
mo	month		SBE	subacute bacterial endocarditis
mol wt	molecular weight		s.c.	subcutaneous(ly)
mOsm	milliosmole		sec	second
MRC	Medical Research Council (units)		SI	International System of Units
MRI	magnetic resonance imaging		SLE	systemic lupus erythematosus
N	nitrogen; normal (strength of solution)		soln	solution
			sp gr	specific gravity
Na	sodium		sq	square
NaCl	sodium chloride		STS	serologic test(s) for syphilis
ng	nanogram (= millimicrogram)		TB	tuberculosis
nm	nanometer (= millimicron)		tid	3 times a day
NSAID	nonsteroidal anti-inflammatory drug		u.	unit
			URI	upper respiratory infection
17-OHCS	17-hydroxycorticosteroid		USPHS	United States Public Health Service
OTC	over-the-counter (pharmaceuticals)		UTI	urinary tract infection
oz	ounce		WBC	white blood cell
P	phosphorus; pressure		WHO	World Health Organization
Pa_{CO_2}	arterial carbon dioxide pressure		wk	week
PA_{O_2}	alveolar oxygen pressure		wt	weight
Pa_{O_2}	arterial oxygen pressure		yr	year
P_{CO_2}	carbon dioxide pressure (or tension)		μ	micro-; micron
			μCi	microcurie
pg	picogram (= micromicrogram)		μg	microgram
pH	hydrogen ion concentration		μL	microliter
PMN	polymorphonuclear leukocyte		μm	micrometer (= micron)
po	orally		μmol	micromole
P_{O_2}	oxygen pressure (or tension)		μOsm	micro-osmole
PPD	purified protein derivative (tuberculin)		$m\mu$	millimicron (= nanometer)
			/	per
ppm	parts per million		<	less than
prn	as needed		>	more than
psi	pounds per square inch		≤	equal to or less than
q	every		≥	equal to or more than
q 4 h, etc	every 4 hours, etc		≅	approximately equal to
qid	4 times a day		±	plus or minus
RA	rheumatoid arthritis		§	section
RBC	red blood cell			

CONSULTANTS

CONTRIBUTORS TO EDITION 16

Hagop S. Akiskal, M.D.

Senior Science Advisor on Affective and Related Disorders, National Institute of Mental Health

Mood Disorders

Philip O. Alderson, M.D.

Professor and Chairman, Department of Radiology, Columbia-Presbyterian Medical Center

Radionuclide Imaging of the Heart

James K. Alexander, M.D.

Professor of Medicine (Cardiology), Baylor College of Medicine

Pulmonary Embolism

Chloe G. Alexson, M.D.

Professor of Pediatrics, University of Rochester

Congenital Heart Disease; Heart Failure (Pediatric)

James R. Allen, M.D.

Director, National AIDS Program Office, Public Health Service

Nosocomial Infection in the Newborn; Human Immunodeficiency Virus Infection in Children

Terry D. Allen, M.D.

Professor of Urology, University of Texas Southwestern Medical Center at Dallas

Intersex States

Roy D. Altman, M.D.

Professor of Medicine, University of Miami; Chief, Arthritis Division, VA Medical Center, Miami

Paget's Disease of Bone

Michael C. Appleton, M.D.

Associate Professor of Internal Medicine, College of Osteopathic Medicine of the Pacific, Pomona; Medical Director, The Visiting Nurse Association of Los Angeles, Hospice in the Home

Hospice Medicine

Jacob V. Aranda, M.D., Ph.D.

Professor of Pediatrics and of Pharmacology and Therapeutics, McGill University; Director, Apnea Treatment and Research Center, and Developmental Pharmacology and Perinatal Research Unit, Montreal Children's Hospital (Canada)

Special Considerations of Drug Treatment in Neonates, Infants, and Children

Hervy E. Averette, M.D.

Professor and Director, Division of Gynecologic Oncology, University of Miami

Gynecologic Neoplasms

Richard F. Bakemeier, M.D.

Professor of Medicine, Director of Cancer Education, and Associate Dean for Continuing Medical Education, University of Colorado

Tumor Immunology

Zuhair K. Ballas, M.D.

Associate Professor of Internal Medicine, University of Iowa; VA Medical Center, Iowa City

Biology of the Immune System

Mark Ballow, M.D.

Professor of Pediatrics, State University of New York at Buffalo; Chief, Division of Allergy/Immunology, Children's Hospital of Buffalo

Immunologic Status of the Fetus and Newborn

Peter A. Banks, M.D.

Professor of Medicine, Tufts University; Chief of Gastroenterology, St. Elizabeth's Hospital of Boston

Pancreatitis

John G. Bartlett, M.D.

Chief, Division of Infectious Diseases, Johns Hopkins University

Pneumonia; Lung Abscess

Peter Beighton, M.D., Ph.D.

Professor of Human Genetics, University of Cape Town (South Africa)

Arthrogryposis Multiplex Congenita; Inherited Disorders of Connective Tissue; The Osteochondrodysplasias; The Osteopetroses; The Osteochondroses

Robert Berkow, M.D.

Editor-in-Chief, THE MERCK MANUAL; Clinical Professor of Medicine and of Psychiatry, Hahnemann University

Psychiatry in Medicine

Richard W. Besdine, M.D.

Travelers Professor of Geriatrics and Gerontology, and Professor of Medicine, University of Connecticut; Director, Travelers Center on Aging

Geriatric Medicine

Don C. Bienfang, M.D.

Assistant Professor of Ophthalmology, Harvard University

Optic Nerve, Visual Pathways

Jacob D. Bitran, M.D.

Professor of Medicine, University of Chicago

Oncology

John H. Bland, M.D.

Professor of Medicine and Rheumatology (Emeritus), University of Vermont

Osteoarthritis

Harvey Blank, M.D.

Professor of Dermatology and Cutaneous Surgery (Emeritus), University of Miami

Herpes Gestationis; Pruritic Urticarial Papules and Plaques of Pregnancy; Impetigo, Ecthyma; Dermatologic Disorders; Reactions to Sunlight

M. Donald Blaufox, M.D., Ph.D.

Professor and Chairman, Department of Nuclear Medicine, and Professor of Medicine and Radiology, Albert Einstein College of Medicine

Radiation Reactions and Injuries; Nuclear Medicine

Rodney Bluestone, M.B., F.R.C.P.

Clinical Professor of Medicine, University of California, Los Angeles

Vasculitis; Polyarteritis Nodosa; Wegener's Granulomatosis

Philip K. Bondy, M.D.

Professor of Medicine (Emeritus), Yale University; Chief of Staff (Retired), VA Medical Center, West Haven

Adrenal Cortical Hypofunction; Addison's Disease; Adrenal Cortical Hyperfunction; Nonfunctional Adrenal Masses; Polyglandular Deficiency Syndromes; Congenital Adrenal Hyperplasia

William K. Bottomley, D.D.S.

Professor of Histopathology, Howard University

Disorders of the Lips, Mouth, and Tongue; Dental Caries and Its Complications; Periodontal Disease; Preneoplastic and Neoplastic Lesions

Glenn D. Braunstein, M.D.

Professor of Medicine, University of California, Los Angeles; Chairman, Department of Medicine, Cedars-Sinai Medical Center

The Testes

Peter C. Brazy, M.D.

Associate Professor of Medicine and Head, Nephrology Section, University of Wisconsin, Madison

Renal Disease Associated with Systemic and Metabolic Syndromes; Anomalies in Kidney Transport (Pediatric)

James L. Breeling, M.D.

Instructor in Medicine, Harvard University; Associate Physician, Brigham and Women's Hospital

Bacteroides and Mixed Anaerobic Infections

Dick D. Briggs, Jr., M.D.

Professor and Vice-Chairman, Department of Medicine, Eminent Professor of Pulmonary Diseases and Director, Division of Pulmonary and Critical Care Medicine, University of Alabama at Birmingham; President, University of Alabama Health Services Foundation

Special Procedures (Pulmonary)

John G. Brooks, M.D.

Professor of Pediatrics and Director, Pediatric Pulmonary Medicine, University of Rochester

Sudden Infant Death Syndrome

Marilyn R. Brown, M.D.

Associate Professor of Pediatrics, Chief of Pediatric GI/Nutrition Unit, and Co-Medical Director of Nutritional Support Service, University of Rochester

Obesity (Pediatric)

Felix E. Bruckner, M.B., F.R.C.P.

Director, Department of Rheumatology, St. George's Hospital; Senior Lecturer, University of London (England)

Neuropathic Disorders

Michael F. Bryson, M.D.

Clinical Associate Professor of Pediatrics, University of Rochester

Growth and Development from Birth Through Childhood

Roger J. Bulger, M.D.

President and Chief Executive Officer, Association of Academic Health Centers; Clinical Professor of Medicine, Georgetown University

Rat-Bite Fever

John F. Burke, M.D.

Helen Andrus Benedict Professor of Surgery (Emeritus), Harvard University; Visiting Surgeon, Trauma Services, Massachusetts General Hospital

Burns

Benjamin Burrows, M.D.

Chalfant-Moore Professor of Internal Medicine and Director, Division of Respiratory Sciences, University of Arizona

Acute Bronchitis; Chronic Airways Obstructive Disorders

James R. Campbell, M.D.

Fellow, General Academic Pediatrics, University of Rochester

Hemorrhagic Shock and Encephalopathy

Ronald W. F. Campbell, M.B., Ch.B., F.R.C.P.

British Heart Foundation Professor of Cardiology, Freeman Hospital; Honorary Consultant Cardiologist, University of Newcastle upon Tyne (England)

Cardiac Arrhythmias

Jesse M. Cedarbaum, M.D.

Clinical Associate Professor of Neurology, Cornell University; Program Director, Clinical Research, Regeneron Pharmaceuticals, Inc.

Disorders of Movement: Extrapyramidal and Cerebellar Disorders

Mary C. Ciotti, M.D.

Assistant Professor of Obstetrics and Gynecology, Michigan State University

Common Gynecologic Problems

Fredric L. Coe, M.D.

Professor of Medicine and Physiology, and Head, Nephrology Program, University of Chicago

Urinary Calculi

Alan S. Cohen, M.D.

Conrad Wesselhoeft Professor of Medicine, Boston University; Chief of Medicine and Director, Thorndike Memorial Laboratory and Boston City Hospital

Amyloidosis

Sidney Cohen, M.D.

Richard Laylord Evans Professor of Medicine and Chairman, Department of Internal Medicine, Temple University

Disorders of the Esophagus

Florence Comite, M.D.

Assistant Professor of Medicine (Endocrinology), Pediatrics, and Obstetrics and Gynecology, Yale University

Precocious Puberty

Jules Constant, M.D.

Clinical Associate Professor of Medicine, State University of New York, Buffalo

Valvular Heart Disease

Eugene L. Coodley, M.D.
Professor of Medicine, University of California, Irvine; Chief of General Internal Medicine, VA Medical Center, Long Beach
Laboratory Medicine

Mary Ann Cooper, M.D.
Residency Research Director, Emergency Medicine Program, University of Illinois
Electric Shock

John K. Crane, M.D.
Assistant Professor of Medicine and Pharmacology, University of Texas at Houston
Enterobacteriaceae Infections; Salmonella Infections; Shigellosis; Hemophilus Infections; Brucellosis; Tularemia; Bartonellosis

Drew C. Cutler, M.D.
Assistant Professor of Pediatrics, Loma Linda University
Inherited and Congenital Disorders; Autosomal Recessive (Childhood) Polycystic Kidney Disease

Ralph E. Cutler, M.D.
Professor of Medicine and Pharmacology, and Chief, Clinical Pharmacology, Loma Linda University; Chief, Nephrology Section, Jerry L. Pettis Memorial VA Hospital, Loma Linda
Clinical Evaluation of Genitourinary Disorders; Renal Failure; The Glomerular Diseases; Tubulointerstitial Disease; Infections of the Kidney, Urinary Tract, and Male Genital Tract; Vascular Disease

Ron Dagan, M.D.
Associate Professor of Pediatrics and Director, Pediatric Infectious Diseases Unit, Ben-Gurion University of the Negev, Beer Sheva, Israel
Acute Infectious Neonatal Diarrhea

David C. Dale, M.D.
Professor of Medicine, University of Washington
Infections in the Compromised Host; Leukopenia, Neutropenia

Patricia A. Daly, M.D.
Instructor in Endocrinology, Harvard University
Multiple Endocrine Neoplasia Syndromes

Ronald G. Davidson, M.D.
Professor of Pediatrics and Director (Retired), Program in Human Genetics, McMaster University (Canada)
General Principles of Medical Genetics

Anne L. Davis, M.D.
Associate Professor of Clinical Medicine, New York University; Assistant Director, Chest Service, Bellevue Hospital
Bronchiectasis; Atelectasis

Dwight Davis, M.D.
Associate Professor of Medicine, Director of Cardiac Catheterization Laboratory, Cardiology Director of Cardiac Transplantation Program, Pennsylvania State University, Milton S. Hershey Medical Center
Calcium Antagonists

W. Howard Davis, D.D.S.
Clinical Professor of Oral Surgery, University of Southern California; Associate Professor, Loma Linda University
Dental Emergencies

Norman L. Dean, M.D.
Associate Clinical Professor of Medicine, Yale University
Near-Drowning

Ronald Dee, M.D.
Associate Clinical Professor of Surgery, Albert Einstein College of Medicine; Associate Attending Surgeon, St. Joseph's Hospital, Stamford
Varicose Veins

Roman W. DeSanctis, M.D.
Professor of Medicine, Harvard University; Director of Clinical Cardiology, Massachusetts General Hospital
Diseases of the Aorta and Its Branches

Paul Dieppe, M.D.
Professor of Rheumatology, University of Bristol (England)
Introduction (Musculoskeletal and Connective Tissue Disorders)

Preston V. Dilts, Jr., M.D.

Bates Professor of Diseases of Women and Children, and Chairman, Department of Obstetrics and Gynecology, University of Michigan

Gynecologic Practice and Approach to the Patient; Conception, Implantation, Placentation, and Embryology; Normal Pregnancy, Labor, and Delivery; Abnormalities and Complications of Pregnancy; Abnormalities and Complications of Labor and Delivery; Postpartum Care

Eugene P. DiMagno, M.D.

Professor of Medicine, Mayo Medical School; Consultant in Gastroenterology and Internal Medicine, and Director of GI Diagnostic Unit, Mayo Clinic

Cancer of the Pancreas

R. Gordon Douglas, Jr., M.D.

President, Merck Vaccine Division, Merck & Co., Inc.; Clinical Professor of Medicine, Cornell University; Attending Physician, New York Hospital

The Nature of Infectious Disease

George E. Downs, Pharm.D.

Professor of Clinical Pharmacy, Philadelphia College of Pharmacy and Science

Some Trade Names of Generic (Nonproprietary) Drugs

Douglas A. Drossman, M.D.

Professor of Medicine and Psychiatry, University of North Carolina, Chapel Hill

Diagnostic and Therapeutic Gastrointestinal Procedures; Functional Dyspepsia and Other Nonspecific Gastrointestinal Complaints

Bruce H. Drukker, M.D.

Professor and Chairperson, Department of Obstetrics, Gynecology, and Reproductive Biology, Michigan State University

Common Gynecologic Problems

Felton J. Earls, M.D.

Professor of Child Psychiatry and of Human Behavior and Development, Harvard University

Childhood Psychosis; Affective Disorders (Pediatric)

Sherman Elias, M.D.

Professor of Obstetrics and Gynecology, and Director, Division of Reproductive Genetics, University of Tennessee, Memphis

Genetic Evaluation and Counseling

Elliot F. Ellis, M.D.

Pulmonary/Allergy/Immunology Division, Nemours Children's Clinic, Jacksonville

Asthma

Kent Ellis, M.D.

Professor of Radiology, Columbia University; Attending Radiologist, Columbia-Presbyterian Medical Center

Plain Chest Radiography; Cardiac Fluoroscopy; Positron Emission Tomography; Magnetic Resonance Imaging

W. Edmund Farrar, M.D.

Professor of Medicine and Microbiology, Medical University of South Carolina

Leptospirosis

Harvey Feigenbaum, M.D.

Distinguished Professor of Medicine, Krannert Institute of Cardiology, Indiana University

Echocardiography

Robert Fekety, M.D.

Professor of Internal Medicine and Head, Division of Infectious Diseases, University of Michigan

Bacterial Diseases Caused by Gram-Positive Cocci; Rheumatic Fever; Sydenham's Chorea

Daniel Finkelstein, M.D.

Associate Professor, The Wilmer Institute, Johns Hopkins University

Retina

Andrew J. Fletcher, M.B., B.Chir.

Assistant Editor, THE MERCK MANUAL; Adjunct Professor of Pharmaceutical Health Care, Temple University

Gas; Osteoporosis

Kathleen M. Foley, M.D.
Professor of Neurology, Neuroscience, and Clinical Pharmacology, Cornell University; Chief, Pain Service, Memorial Sloan-Kettering Cancer Center

Pain

Michael R. Foley, M.D.
Assistant Director, Maternal-Fetal Medicine, and Director, Obstetric Intensive Care, Phoenix Perinatal Associates, Good Samaritan Medical Center

Drugs in Pregnancy

Noble O. Fowler, M.D.
Professor of Medicine (Emeritus) and of Pharmacology and Cell Biophysics (Emeritus), University of Cincinnati

Pericardial Disease

Howard R. Foye, Jr., M.D.
Clinical Associate Professor of Pediatrics, University of Rochester

Behavioral Problems

Irwin N. Frank, M.D.
Professor of Urology and of Health Services, and Senior Associate Dean for Clinical Affairs, University of Rochester

Obstructive Uropathies; Myoneurogenic Disorders; Urinary Incontinence; Male Genital Lesions; Genitourinary Trauma; Neoplasms (Genitourinary); Congenital Abnormalities— Renal and Genitourinary Defects; Wilms' Tumor; Neuroblastoma

Eugene P. Frenkel, M.D.
Professor of Internal Medicine and Radiology, Patsy R. & Raymond D. Nasher Distinguished Chair in Cancer Research, and Director, Division of Hematology-Medical Oncology, University of Texas Southwestern Medical Center at Dallas

Anemias; Eosinophilic Disorders

Gerald Friedman, M.D., Ph.D.
Clinical Professor of Medicine, Mount Sinai School of Medicine

Irritable Bowel Syndrome

Peter L. Frommer, M.D.
Deputy Director, National Heart, Lung, and Blood Institute

Sudden Cardiac Death

William A. Frosch, M.D.
Professor and Vice Chairman, Department of Psychiatry, Cornell University; Medical Director, Payne Whitney Clinic, New York Hospital

Psychiatric Emergencies

Steven M. Fruchtman, M.D.
Assistant Professor of Medicine, Mount Sinai School of Medicine; Director, Bone Marrow Transplantation, Mount Sinai Hospital

Myeloproliferative Disorders

Robert H. Gelber, M.D.
Clinical Professor of Epidemiology and Biostatistics, University of California, San Francisco; Medical Director, San Francisco Regional Hansen's Disease Center and National Ambulatory Hansen's Disease Program

Leprosy

Michael C. Gelfand, M.D.
Clinical Associate Professor of Medicine and Pediatrics, Georgetown University

Immunologically Mediated Renal Diseases

Michael A. Gerber, M.D.
Associate Professor of Pediatrics, University of Connecticut

Neonatal Hepatitis B Virus Infection

Ray W. Gifford, Jr., M.D.
Vice Chairman, Division of Medicine, and Senior Physician, Department of Hypertension and Nephrology, Cleveland Clinic Foundation

Hypertension

Robert Ginsburg, M.D.
Clinical Assistant Professor of Medicine, Stanford University

Peripheral Vascular Disorders

Stephen E. Goldfinger, M.D.
Associate Professor of Medicine and Faculty Dean for Continuing Education, Harvard University

Familial Mediterranean Fever

Frederick J. Goldstein, Ph.D.
Professor of Pharmacology and Toxicology,
Philadelphia College of Pharmacy and Science

Pharmacodynamics; Pharmacogenetics

M. Jay Goodkind, M.D.
Clinical Associate Professor of Medicine, University of Pennsylvania; Chief of Cardiology,
Mercer Medical Center, Trenton

Syphilis of the Cardiovascular System; Cardiac Tumors

Richard L. Guerrant, M.D.
Professor of Medicine and Head, Division of
Geographic Medicine, University of Virginia

Enterobacteriaceae Infections; Salmonella Infections; Shigellosis; Hemophilus Infections; Brucellosis; Tularemia; Bartonellosis

Laurence B. Guttmacher, M.D.
Associate Professor of Clinical Psychiatry, University of Rochester

Antianxiety Drugs; Antipsychotic Drugs

G. Peter Halberg, M.D.
Professor of Clinical Ophthalmology, New York
Medical College; Chief of Glaucoma Service and
of Contact Lens Service, St. Vincent's Hospital
and Medical Center of New York

Congenital Glaucoma; Glaucoma; Contact Lenses

Caroline B. Hall, M.D.
Professor of Pediatrics and Medicine, University
of Rochester

Acute Epiglottitis; Croup; Bronchiolitis

Robert W. Hamilton, M.D.
Professor of Medicine and Chief of Nephrology,
Medical College of Ohio

Dialysis and Filtration Procedures

Margaret R. Hammerschlag, M.D.
Professor of Pediatrics and of Medicine, State
University of New York, Brooklyn

Neonatal Conjunctivitis

Paul G. St. J. Hammond, M.B., D.Phil., F.R.C.P.(C)
Associate Professor of Medicine, Loma Linda
University; Assistant Chief, Nephrology Section,
Jerry L. Pettis Memorial VA Hospital, Loma
Linda

The Glomerular Diseases

James P. Harnisch, M.D.
Clinical Professor of Medicine, University of
Washington

Diphtheria

William R. Harrison, M.A.
Research Specialist, University of Arizona

Cross-Cultural Issues in Medicine

Donald H. Harter, M.D.
Clinical Professor of Neurology, George Washington University; Senior Scientific Officer and
Director, HHMI-NIH Research Scholars Program, Howard Hughes Medical Institute

Slow Virus Infections; Subacute Sclerosing Panencephalitis; Progressive Rubella Panencephalitis

Daniel H. Hechtman, M.D.
Clinical/Research Fellow in Surgery, Harvard
University, Brigham and Women's Hospital

Invasive Cardiovascular Procedures

Herbert B. Hechtman, M.D.
Professor of Surgery, Harvard University; Surgeon, Brigham and Women's Hospital

Invasive Cardiovascular Procedures

I. Craig Henderson, M.D.
Associate Professor of Medicine, Harvard University; Medical Coordinator, Breast Evaluation
Center, Dana-Farber Cancer Institute

Breast Disorders

Jan V. Hirschmann, M.D.
Professor of Medicine, University of Washington; Assistant Chief of Medicine, VA Medical
Center, Seattle

*Antimicrobial Chemoprophylaxis; Superficial
Infections; Abscesses; Osteomyelitis*

Basil I. Hirschowitz, M.D.
Professor of Medicine and Physiology, University of Alabama at Birmingham

*Disorders of the Stomach and Duodenum;
Childhood Peptic Ulcer*

Jack Hirsh, M.D.
Professor of Medicine, McMaster University; Director, Hamilton Civic Hospitals Research Centre (Canada)

Arteriosclerosis, Atherosclerosis

Christopher H. Hodgman, M.D.
Associate Professor of Psychiatry and Pediatrics, and Director, Division of Child and Adolescent Psychiatry, University of Rochester

Adolescent Psychiatric Conditions; Suicide in Children and Adolescents

Robert A. Hoekelman, M.D.
Professor and Chairman, Department of Pediatrics, University of Rochester

Introduction (Pediatrics and Genetics); Health Supervision of the Well Child; Pinworm Infestation

Paul D. Hoeprich, M.D.
Professor of Medicine (Emeritus), University of California, Davis

Erysipelothricosis; Listeriosis

Dorothy R. Hollingsworth, M.D.
Professor of Reproductive Medicine and of Medicine (Emeritus), University of California, San Diego

Pregnancy Complicated by Disease—Diabetes Mellitus, Thyroid Disease

Charles S. Houston, M.D.
Professor of Environmental Health and of Medicine (Emeritus), University of Vermont

Heat Disorders; Cold Injury; High-Altitude Illness

Douglas M. Huestis, M.D.
Professor of Pathology and Chief, Transfusion Medicine, University of Arizona

Transfusion Medicine

Graham R. Hughes, M.D., F.R.C.P.
Consultant Physician, Rheumatology Department, and Head of Lupus-Arthritis Research Laboratories (Rayne Institute), St. Thomas' Hospital, London, England

Discoid Lupus Erythematosus; Systemic Lupus Erythematosus

Daniel A. Hussar, Ph.D.
Remington Professor of Pharmacy, Philadelphia College of Pharmacy and Science

Drug Interactions

Harold L. Israel, M.D.
Professor of Medicine (Emeritus), Thomas Jefferson University

Sarcoidosis

Michael Jacewicz, M.D.
Assistant Professor of Neurology and Neuroscience, Cornell University

Approach to the Patient (Neurologic); Disorders of Smell and Taste; Vision and Eye Movement Disorders; Hearing Loss, Vertigo, Dizziness; Motor Weakness; Nutritional Neurologic Disorders; CNS Infections

George Gee Jackson, M.D.
Professor of Medicine (Emeritus), University of Illinois, Chicago; Clinical Professor of Medicine, University of Utah

Respiratory Viral Diseases; Respiratory Syncytial Virus

Harry S. Jacob, M.D.
Professor and Vice Chairman of Medicine, and Head, Division of Hematology, University of Minnesota

The Spleen

William R. Jarvis, M.D.
Chief, Epidemiology Branch, Hospital Infections Program, Center for Infectious Diseases, Centers for Disease Control

Nosocomial Infections in the Newborn

Dennis M. Jensen, M.D.
Professor of Medicine, University of California, Los Angeles

Gastrointestinal Bleeding

R. Joe Jopling, M.D.
Associate Clinical Professor, University of Utah

Anabolic Steroid Abuse

Attallah Kappas, M.D.
Sherman Fairchild Professor, Vice President, and Physician-in-Chief, Rockefeller University Hospital, New York

Anomalies in Pigment Metabolism

Karl D. Kappus, Ph.D.
Epidemiologist, Center for Infectious Diseases, Centers for Disease Control
Rabies

Dennis L. Kasper, M.D.
William Ellery Channing Professor of Medicine, Harvard University; Director, Division of Infectious Disease, Beth Israel Hospital
Bacteroides and Mixed Anaerobic Infections

Stephen I. Katz, M.D., Ph.D.
Chief, Dermatology Branch, National Cancer Institute
Herpes Gestationis; Pruritic Urticarial Papules and Plaques of Pregnancy; Impetigo, Ecthyma; Dermatologic Disorders; Reactions to Sunlight

Donald Kaye, M.D.
Professor and Chairman, Department of Medicine, Medical College of Pennsylvania
Antimicrobial Chemotherapy

Thomas Killip, M.D.
Professor of Medicine, Mount Sinai School of Medicine; Executive Vice President, Beth Israel Medical Center
Myocardial Ischemic Disorders

Eric P. Kindwall, M.D.
Associate Professor of Hyperbaric Medicine, Department of Plastic and Reconstructive Surgery, Medical College of Wisconsin, Milwaukee
Hyperbaric Oxygen Therapy

James R. Klinenberg, M.D.
Professor of Medicine, University of California, Los Angeles; Senior Vice President, Office of Academic Affairs, Cedars-Sinai Medical Center
Progressive Systemic Sclerosis; Polymyositis/ Dermatomyositis

Arthur E. Kopelman, M.D.
Director of Neonatology, East Carolina University
Perinatal Physiology; Parent-Infant Bonding: The Sick Neonate; Gestational Age and Birth Weight; Asphyxia and Resuscitation; Respiratory Disorders; Hematologic Problems; Metabolic Problems in the Newborn; Neonatal Pneumonia; Necrotizing Enterocolitis; Gastrointestinal Defects

Douglas R. Labar, M.D., Ph.D.
Director, Comprehensive Epilepsy Center, New York Hospital-Cornell Medical Center
Seizure Disorders

Gary L. Lage, Ph.D.
Principal, Environ Corp., Princeton
Drug Toxicity

Lewis Landsberg, M.D.
Cutter Professor and Chairman, Department of Medicine, Northwestern University
Multiple Endocrine Neoplasia Syndromes

Edward H. Lanphier, M.D.
Senior Scientist, Department of Preventive Medicine, and Assistant Director for Biomedical Research, The Biotron, University of Wisconsin, Madison
Medical Aspects of Diving and Work in Compressed Air

Louis Lasagna, M.D.
Dean, Sackler School of Graduate Biomedical Sciences, and Dean for Academic Affairs of the School of Medicine, Tufts University
Placebos

Daniel M. Laskin, D.D.S.
Professor and Chairman, Department of Oral and Maxillofacial Surgery, and Director, Temporomandibular Joint and Facial Pain Research Center, Medical College of Virginia
Temporomandibular Joint Disorders

Ruth A. Lawrence, M.D.
Professor of Pediatrics and of Obstetrics and Gynecology, University of Rochester
Management of the Normal Newborn—Initial Care, Complete Physical Examination, The First Few Days, Feeding, Hospital Accommodations; Infant Nutrition; Poisoning (Pediatrics)

Chinh Trung Lê, M.D.
Infectious Disease Consultant, Kaiser Permanente Medical Center, Santa Rosa; Clinical Faculty, University of California, San Francisco
Antimicrobial Therapy for Newborns; Neonatal Listeriosis; Perinatal Tuberculosis

James B. Lee, M.D.
Professor of Medicine, State University of New York, Buffalo; Director, Hypertension Program, Erie County Medical Center

Prostaglandins, Thromboxanes, and Leukotrienes

Harvey Lemont, D.P.M.
Professor and Chairman, Department of Medicine, Pennsylvania College of Podiatric Medicine; Director, Laboratory of Podiatric Pathology, Philadelphia

Common Foot Disorders

Roland A. Levandowski, M.D.
Center for Biologics Evaluation and Research, National Institutes of Health

Respiratory Viral Diseases; Respiratory Syncytial Virus

Gerald S. Levey, M.D.
Senior Vice President, Medical and Scientific Affairs, Merck Human Health Division, Merck & Co., Inc.

Thyroid; Congenital Goiters; Hypothyroidism; Hyperthyroidism (Pediatric)

Daniel Levinson, M.D.
Associate Professor, Department of Family and Community Medicine, University of Arizona

Medical Aspects of Air and Foreign Travel

David E. Levy, M.D.
Clinical Associate Professor of Neurology and Neuroscience, Cornell University; Associate Attending Neurologist, New York Hospital

Cerebrovascular Disease

Robert I. Levy, M.D.
President, Sandoz Research Institute; Adjunct Professor of Medicine, Columbia University

Anomalies in Lipid Metabolism

Edward B. Lewin, M.D.
Associate Clinical Professor of Pediatrics and Communicable Diseases, University of Michigan; Head, Division of Pediatric Infectious Diseases, Henry Ford Hospital

Neonatal Sepsis; Neonatal Meningitis; Fever of Unknown Origin in Children

Harold I. Lief, M.D.
Professor of Psychiatry (Emeritus), University of Pennsylvania; Psychiatrist (Emeritus) to the Pennsylvania Hospital

Psychosocial Issues; Disorders of Sexual Function; The Medical Examination of the Rape Victim; Gender Identity Disorders of Childhood

Gregory S. Liptak, M.D.
Associate Professor, University of Rochester

Management of Chronic Disability (Pediatric)

James H. Liu, M.D.
Associate Professor and Director, Division of Reproductive Endocrinology and Infertility, University of Cincinnati

Hypothalamic-Pituitary Relationships; Pituitary Disorders; Infertility; Endometriosis; Pituitary Dwarfism

Elliot M. Livstone, M.D.
Sarasota, Florida

Neoplasms of the Bowel

Henry S. Loeb, M.D.
Professor of Medicine, Loyola University, Chicago; Program Director in Cardiology, VA Hospital, Hines

Shock (Cardiovascular)

Earl G. Long, Ph.D.
Enteric Diseases Branch, Division of Bacterial and Mycotic Diseases, Center for Infectious Diseases, Centers for Disease Control

Parasitic Infections

Mortimer Lorber, D.M.D., M.D.
Associate Professor of Physiology and Biophysics, Georgetown University

Dentistry in Medicine; Examination of the Oral Region

Robert G. Loudon, M.B., Ch.B.
Professor of Medicine and Director, Pulmonary and Critical Care Medicine, University of Cincinnati

Approach to the Pulmonary Patient

Robert F. Mahler, M.B., F.R.C.P.
Consultant in Diabetes, Clinical Research Centre, Northwick Park Hospital, Harrow, Middlesex, England

Genetic Abnormalities of Carbohydrate Metabolism

Lois A. Maiman, Ph.D.
Head, Section on Prevention Research, National Institute of Child Health and Human Development

Special Considerations of Drug Treatment in Neonates, Infants, and Children—Compliance

Stephen E. Malawista, M.D.
Professor of Medicine, Section of Rheumatology, Department of Internal Medicine, Yale University

Lyme Disease

Gerald L. Mandell, M.D.
Professor of Medicine and Owen R. Cheatham Professor of Sciences, University of Virginia

Biology of Infectious Disease

Frank E. Manson, B.S.
Senior Staff Editor, THE MERCK MANUAL (Retired)

Ready Reference Guides

John J. Marini, M.D.
Professor of Medicine, University of Minnesota; Director, Pulmonary and Critical Care Medicine, St. Paul-Ramsey Medical Center

Respiratory Failure

Michael A. Martin, M.D.
Assistant Professor, Infectious Diseases, Oregon Health Sciences University

Hospital Infection Control

Alfonse T. Masi, M.D., Dr.P.H.
Professor of Medicine and Epidemiology, University of Illinois, Peoria

Nonarticular Rheumatism

Richard G. Masson, M.D.
Associate Professor of Medicine, Boston University; Chief, Pulmonary Medicine, and Medical Director, Intensive Care Unit, Framingham Union Hospital

Pulmonary Function Tests

Alvin M. Mauer, M.D.
Professor of Medicine and Chief, Medical Oncology and Hematology, University of Tennessee, Memphis

The Leukemias

Elizabeth R. McAnarney, M.D.
Professor of Pediatrics and Chief, Division of Adolescent Medicine, University of Rochester

Physical Conditions in Adolescence—Developmental Conditions; Teenage Pregnancy and Contraception

Carol A. McCarthy, M.D.
Assistant Professor of Pediatrics, University of Chicago

Congenital Rubella; Congenital and Perinatal Cytomegalovirus Infection; Congenital Toxoplasmosis

Daniel J. McCarty, M.D.
Will and Cava Ross Professor of Medicine and Director, Arthritis Institute, Medical College of Wisconsin

Crystal-Induced Conditions

J. Allen McCutchan, M.D.
Professor of Medicine, University of California, San Diego

Human Immunodeficiency Virus Infection; Sexually Transmitted Diseases; Congenital Syphilis

Donald S. McLaren, M.D., Ph.D., F.R.C.P.
Department of Preventive Ophthalmology, Institute of Ophthalmology, London (England)

Nutrition: General Considerations; Undernutrition; Vitamin Deficiency, Toxicity, and Dependency; Element Deficiency and Toxicity—Phosphate Depletion, Iodine, Fluorine, Zinc, Other Trace Elements; Nutritional Disorders (Pediatric)

Carole M. Meyers, M.D.
Fellow, Division of Reproductive Genetics, and Instructor, Obstetrics and Gynecology, University of Tennessee, Memphis

Genetic Evaluation and Counseling

Marco K. Michelson, M.D.
Parasitic Diseases Branch, Centers for Disease Control

Parasitic Infections

Gabe Mirkin, M.D.
Associate Clinical Professor, Georgetown University
Sports Medicine

Daniel R. Mishell, Jr., M.D.
Professor and Chairman, Department of Obstetrics and Gynecology, University of Southern California
Family Planning

John P. Morgan, M.D.
Professor of Pharmacology, City University of New York; Associate Professor of Pharmacology and Medicine, Mount Sinai School of Medicine
Drug Dependence

W. K. C. Morgan, M.D.
Professor of Medicine, University of Western Ontario; Director, Chest Diseases Service, University Hospital, London, Ontario, Canada
Occupational Lung Disease

José L. Muñoz, M.D.
Associate Professor of Pediatrics, New York University
Urinary Tract Infection in Children

Gary J. Myers, M.D.
Professor of Neurology, University of Rochester
Birth Trauma; Seizure Disorders in the Newborn; Congenital Abnormalities—General Considerations, Musculoskeletal Defects, Neurologic Defects; Common Foot and Leg Problems in Children and Adolescents

Nancy M. Nealon, M.D.
Assistant Professor, Cornell University; Assistant Attending Neurologist, New York Hospital
Craniocervical Junction Abnormalities; Spinal Cord Disorders; Disorders of the Peripheral Nervous System; Muscular Dystrophies and Other Myopathies

John C. Nemiah, M.D.
Professor of Psychiatry, Dartmouth Medical School; Professor of Psychiatry (Emeritus), Harvard University
The Neuroses

Robert A. Nozik, M.D.
Clinical Professor of Ophthalmology, Proctor Foundation, University of California, San Francisco
Uveal Tract

Raymond F. Orzechowski, Ph.D.
Professor of Pharmacology, Philadelphia College of Pharmacy and Science
Pharmacodynamics; Pharmacogenetics

Stephen E. Oshrin, Ph.D.
Professor and Chair of Speech and Hearing Sciences, University of Southern Mississippi
Clinical Measurement of Hearing in Children; Congenital Sensorineural Hearing Loss

Bosco A. Paes, M.B., B.Ch., F.R.C.P.(I), F.R.C.P.(C)
Director of Nurseries, St. Joseph's Hospital; Associate Professor of Pediatrics (Neonatal Division), Children's Hospital at Chedoke-McMaster, Hamilton, Ontario, Canada
Cardiopulmonary Resuscitation (Pediatric)

Lawrence L. Pelletier, Jr., M.D.
Professor and Vice Chairman of Internal Medicine, University of Kansas, Wichita; Chief, Medical Service, Wichita VA Medical Center
Endocarditis

Peter L. Perine, M.D.
Professor and Director, Tropical Public Health, and Joint Professor of Medicine, Uniformed Services University of the Health Sciences
Endemic Treponematoses; Relapsing Fever

Steve Perkins, M.D.
Assistant Professor of Medicine, University of Texas Southwestern Medical Center at Dallas
Eosinophilic Disorders

Hart deC. Peterson, M.D.
Clinical Professor of Neurology and of Neurology in Pediatrics, Cornell University
Cerebral Palsy Syndromes

Marjorie C. Pfaudler, R.N., M.A.
Associate Professor of Nursing (Emeritus), The Daisy Marquis Jones Rehabilitation Center, University of Rochester
Aids for the Disabled Patient

Dale L. Phelps, M.D.

Professor of Pediatrics and Ophthalmology, University of Rochester

Retinopathy of Prematurity

Sidney F. Phillips, M.D.

Professor of Medicine, Mayo Medical School; Director, Gastroenterology Unit, Mayo Clinic

Diarrhea and Constipation

Michael E. Pichichero, M.D.

Clinical Professor of Pediatrics, University of Rochester

Immunization Procedures Throughout Childhood

Nathaniel F. Pierce, M.D.

Professor of Medicine, Johns Hopkins University

Cholera

Fred Plum, M.D.

Anne Parrish Titzell Professor of Neurology and Neuroscience, Cornell University; Neurologist-in-Chief, New York Hospital

Disorders of the Cerebral Hemispheres and Higher Brain Functions; Headache; Hiccup; Sleep Disorders; Trauma of the Head and Spine; Poliomyelitis

Russell K. Portenoy, M.D.

Associate Professor of Neurology, Cornell University; Director of Analgesic Studies, Pain Service, and Associate Attending Neurologist, Memorial Sloan-Kettering Cancer Center

Pain

Keith R. Powell, M.D.

George Washington Goler Professor and Associate Chairman for Clinical Affairs, Department of Pediatrics, and Chief, Division of Infectious Diseases, University of Rochester

Occult Bacteremia; Periorbital and Orbital Cellulitis

Douglas J. Pritchard, M.D.

Professor of Orthopedic Surgery and of Oncology, Mayo Medical School

Neoplasms of Bones and Joints

Charles E. Rackley, M.D.

Anton and Margaret Fuisz Professor of Medicine, Georgetown University

Heart Failure

Steven B. Raffin, M.D.

Associate Clinical Professor of Medicine, University of California, San Francisco

Bezoars and Foreign Bodies

Samuel I. Rapaport, M.D.

Professor of Medicine and Pathology, University of California, San Diego

Hemorrhagic Disorders

C. George Ray, M.D.

Professor of Pathology and Pediatrics, University of Arizona

Antiviral Drugs; Viral Diseases—Introduction; Herpesviruses; Pertussis; Measles; Rubella; Roseola Infantum; Erythema Infectiosum; Chickenpox; Enteroviral Diseases; Mumps; Reye's Syndrome; Kawasaki Syndrome

Robert W. Rebar, M.D.

George B. Riley Professor and Chairman, Department of Obstetrics and Gynecology, University of Cincinnati

Hypothalamic-Pituitary Relationships; Pituitary Disorders; Reproductive Endocrinology; Infertility; Amenorrhea and Abnormal Genital Bleeding; Endometriosis; Pituitary Dwarfism

John D. Reid, M.D.

Professor of Pathology, Northeastern Ohio Universities; Pathologist (Honorary), Robinson Memorial Hospital, Ravenna

Carcinoid Syndrome

James C. Reynolds, M.D.

Associate Professor of Medicine, University of Pittsburgh

Disorders of the Esophagus

Hal B. Richerson, M.D.

Professor of Internal Medicine and Director, Allergy/Immunology Division, University of Iowa

Hypersensitivity Diseases of the Lungs

Jean E. Rinaldo, M.D.

Associate Professor of Medicine, Vanderbilt University; Chief, Pulmonary Critical Care, Nashville VA Medical Center

Adult Respiratory Distress Syndrome

Melvin I. Roat, M.D.

Assistant Professor of Ophthalmology, The Eye and Ear Institute, University of Pittsburgh

Congenital Cataract; Ophthalmologic Disorders (Pediatric); Clinical Examination (Ophthalmologic); Ocular Symptoms and Signs; Eye Injuries; Orbit; Lacrimal Apparatus; Eyelids; Conjunctiva; Cornea; Cataract

Kenneth B. Roberts, M.D.

Professor of Pediatrics, University of Massachusetts

Fluid and Electrolyte Disorders in Infants and Children

William O. Robertson, M.D.

Professor of Pediatrics, University of Washington; Director, Washington Poison Network

Poisoning

Robert M. Rogers, M.D.

Professor of Medicine and Anesthesiology, and Chief, Pulmonary Medicine, University of Pittsburgh

Cardiac Arrest and Cardiopulmonary Resuscitation; Pulmonary Alveolar Proteinosis

John Romano, M.D.

Distinguished University Professor of Psychiatry (Emeritus), University of Rochester

Introduction (Psychiatric Disorders); Schizophrenic Disorders; Delusional (Paranoid) Disorders

Beryl J. Rosenstein, M.D.

Professor of Pediatrics, Johns Hopkins University; Director, Cystic Fibrosis Center, Johns Hopkins Hospital

Pulmonary Disorders (Pediatric)

David Y. Rosenzweig, M.D.

Associate Professor of Medicine, Medical College of Wisconsin, Milwaukee

Other Mycobacterial Infections Resembling Tuberculosis

Fred H. Rubin, M.D.

Clinical Assistant Professor of Medicine, University of Pittsburgh; Chief, Division of Geriatric Medicine, Shadyside Hospital

Immunization Procedures for Adults

Trenton K. Ruebush, II, M.D.

Medical Officer, US Public Health Service

Parasitic Infections

Findlay E. Russell, M.D., Ph.D.

Professor of Pharmacology and Toxicology, University of Arizona; Adjunct Professor of Neurology, University of Southern California

Venomous Bites and Stings

Paul S. Russell, M.D.

John Homans Professor of Surgery, Harvard University; Visiting Surgeon and former Chief, Transplantation Unit, Massachusetts General Hospital

Transplantation

Edwin A. Rutsky, M.D.

Professor of Medicine and Director, Medical Dialysis Facilities, University of Alabama at Birmingham

Water, Electrolyte, Mineral, and Acid-Base Metabolism

David B. Sachar, M.D.

Professor of Medicine, Mount Sinai School of Medicine; Director, Division of Gastroenterology, Mount Sinai Hospital

Chronic Inflammatory Diseases of the Bowel; Antibiotic-Associated Colitis

Olle Jane Z. Sahler, M.D.

Associate Professor of Pediatrics, Psychiatry, Medical Humanities, and Medical Informatics, University of Rochester

Failure to Thrive; Recurrent Abdominal Pain

Jay P. Sanford, M.D.

Dallas, Texas; Dean (Emeritus), Uniformed Services University of the Health Sciences

Plague; Melioidosis; Cat-Scratch Disease; Chlamydial Diseases; Arbovirus and Arenavirus Diseases

Mathuram Santosham, M.D.
Associate Professor of International Health, Johns Hopkins University

Acute Infectious Gastroenteritis

Shigeru Sassa, M.D., Ph.D.
Associate Professor and Physician, Rockefeller University, New York

Anomalies in Pigment Metabolism

James W. Sayre, M.D.
Associate Clinical Professor of Pediatrics, University of Rochester

Screening Procedures for Infants and Children; Common Feeding and Gastrointestinal Problems; Child Abuse and Neglect

Dennis R. Schaberg, M.D.
Professor of Medicine, University of Michigan

Pseudomonas Infections; Campylobacter and Noncholera Vibrio Infections

Peter M. Schantz, V.M.D., Ph.D.
Epidemiologist, Center for Infectious Diseases, Centers for Disease Control

Parasitic Infections

Kurt Schapira, M.D., F.R.C.P., F.R.C.Psych.
Consultant Psychiatrist (Emeritus), Royal Victoria Infirmary; Lately Senior Lecturer, University of Newcastle upon Tyne (England)

Suicidal Behavior

I. Herbert Scheinberg, M.D.
Professor and Head, Division of Genetic Medicine, Albert Einstein College of Medicine

Disturbances in Copper Metabolism

Albert P. Scheiner, M.D.
Professor of Pediatrics, Division of Behavioral and Developmental Pediatrics, University of Massachusetts

Mental Retardation

Robert T. Schooley, M.D.
Professor of Medicine, University of Colorado

Infectious Mononucleosis

George E. Schreiner, M.D., F.R.C.P.
Distinguished Professor of Medicine, Georgetown University

Nephrotoxic Disorders

H. Ralph Schumacher, Jr., M.D.
Professor of Medicine, University of Pennsylvania; Director, Arthritis-Immunology Center, VA Medical Center, Philadelphia

Approach to the Patient with Joint Disease; Rheumatoid Arthritis; Juvenile Rheumatoid Arthritis

Cindy L. Schwartz, M.D.
Assistant Professor of Pediatrics, University of Rochester

Retinoblastoma

Ira K. Schwartz, M.D.
Associate Professor of Community and Preventive Medicine, Emory University; Medical Epidemiologist, Centers for Disease Control

Parasitic Infections—Malaria

Ronald W. Schworm, Ph.D.
Educational Consultant, The Reading and Learning Disorders Center, Rochester; Adjunct Professor, University of Rochester and Rochester Institute of Technology

Learning Disorders

Charles H. Scoggin, M.D.
President and Chief Executive Officer, Somatogen, Boulder

Tumors of the Lung

David W. Seldin, M.D.
Lecturer, Harvard University; Section Head, Nuclear Medicine, Lahey Clinic

Radionuclide Imaging of the Heart

Eldon A. Shaffer, M.D., F.R.C.P.(C)
Professor and Head, Department of Medicine, University of Calgary; Director, Department of Medicine, Foothills Provincial General Hospital, Calgary, Alberta, Canada

Laboratory and Radiologic Evaluation of the Liver and Biliary System; Fatty Liver; Liver Disease due to Alcohol; Fibrosis and Cirrhosis; Chronic Liver Diseases; Vascular Lesions of the Liver

William R. Shapiro, M.D.
Chairman, Division of Neurology, Barrow Neurological Institute, Phoenix

CNS Neoplasms; Demyelinating Diseases

Gordon C. Sharp, M.D.
Professor of Medicine and Pathology, and Director, Division of Immunology and Rheumatology and the Multipurpose Arthritis Center, University of Missouri, Columbia

Mixed Connective Tissue Disease

Martin A. Shearn, M.D.
Clinical Professor of Medicine (Emeritus), University of California, San Francisco

Sjögren's Syndrome

Ziad M. Shehab, M.D.
Clinical Associate Professor of Pediatrics, University of Arizona

Antiviral Drugs; Viral Diseases—Introduction; Herpesviruses; Pertussis; Measles; Rubella; Roseola Infantum; Erythema Infectiosum; Chickenpox; Enteroviral Diseases; Mumps; Reye's Syndrome; Kawasaki Syndrome

Roger C. Sider, M.D.
Professor of Psychiatry, Michigan State University; Medical Director, Pine Rest Christian Hospital

The Psychiatric Interview

Jerome B. Simon, M.D., F.R.C.P(C)
Professor of Medicine, Queen's University, Kingston, Ontario, Canada

Introduction (Hepatic and Biliary Disorders); Clinical Features of Liver Disease; Hepatitis; Drugs and the Liver; Postoperative Liver Disorders; Hepatic Granulomas; Neoplasms of the Liver; Pregnancy Complicated by Disease—Hepatic Disorders

Arthur T. Skarin, M.D.
Associate Professor of Medicine, Harvard University; Attending Physician, Dana-Farber Cancer Institute

Lymphomas

Charles B. Smith, M.D.
Associate Dean and Professor, Department of Medicine, University of Washington; Chief of Staff, VA Medical Center, Seattle

Behçet's Syndrome; Relapsing Polychondritis; Reiter's Syndrome; Infectious Arthritis

Celia A. Snavely, M.S.W.
Senior Nephrology Social Worker, Piedmont Dialysis Center, Inc., Winston-Salem

Psychosocial Aspects of Chronic Dialysis

Gordon L. Snider, M.D.
Maurice B. Strauss Professor of Medicine, Boston University; Chief, Medical Service, VA Medical Center, Boston

Pleural Disorders

James B. Snow, Jr., M.D.
Director, National Institute on Deafness and Other Communication Disorders

Adenoid Hypertrophy; Retropharyngeal Abscess; Nose and Throat Disorders (Pediatric); Otolaryngology; Motion Sickness

Selma E. Snyderman, M.D.
Professor of Pediatrics, New York University; Director, Metabolic Disease Center, New York University Medical Center

Anomalies in Amino Acid Metabolism

Norman Sohn, M.D.
Clinical Assistant Professor of Surgery, New York University; Associate Attending Surgeon, Lenox Hill Hospital

Anorectal Disorders

P. Frederick Sparling, M.D.
Professor and Chairman, Department of Medicine, University of North Carolina, Chapel Hill

Neisseria

Gabriel Spergel, M.D.
Clinical Associate Professor of Medicine, State University of New York, Brooklyn; Chief of Endocrinology, Lutheran Medical Center; Senior Staff Endocrinologist, Brookdale Hospital Medical Center

Pheochromocytoma

Harry Spiera, M.D.
Clinical Professor of Medicine and Chief, Division of Rheumatology, Mount Sinai Hospital

Polymyalgia Rheumatica and Temporal Arteritis

William W. Stead, M.D.
Professor of Medicine, University of Arkansas; Director, Tuberculosis Program, Arkansas Department of Health
Tuberculosis

E. Richard Stiehm, M.D.
Professor of Pediatrics and Head, Division of Immunology, University of California, Los Angeles
Immunodeficiency Diseases

Bradford G. Stone, M.D.
Assistant Professor of Medicine, University of Minnesota; VA Medical Center, Minneapolis
Extrahepatic Biliary Disorders

Marvin J. Stone, M.D.
Clinical Professor of Internal Medicine, University of Texas Southwestern Medical Center at Dallas; Chief of Oncology, Baylor University Medical Center
Plasma Cell Dyscrasias

Albert J. Stunkard, M.D.
Professor of Psychiatry, University of Pennsylvania
Obesity; Anorexia Nervosa; Bulimia Nervosa

Michael W. Sue, M.D.
Chief of Gastroenterology, White Memorial Medical Center, Los Angeles
Gastrointestinal Bleeding

Michael J. Sullivan, M.D., F.R.C.P.
Associate Clinical Professor of Medicine, McMaster University; Staff Cardiologist, St. Joseph's Hospital, Hamilton, Ontario, Canada
Cardiopulmonary Resuscitation (Pediatric)

Jan Peter Szidon, M.D.
Professor of Medicine, Rush University
Cor Pulmonale; Goodpasture's Syndrome; Idiopathic Infiltrative Diseases of the Lung

Paul H. Tanser, M.D., F.R.C.P.(C)
Professor of Medicine, McMaster University; Chief of Medicine, St. Joseph's Hospital, Hamilton, Ontario, Canada
An Approach to the Cardiac Patient; Cardiomyopathy

Robert V. Tauxe, M.D.
Chief, Epidemiology Section, Enteric Diseases Branch, Division of Bacterial and Mycotic Diseases, Center for Infectious Diseases, Centers for Disease Control
Gastroenteritis: Infective and Toxic

J. Richard Thistlethwaite, Jr., M.D., Ph.D.
Associate Professor of Surgery, University of Chicago
Transplantation

Ronald G. Tompkins, M.D., Sc.D.
Associate Professor of Surgery, Harvard University; Associate Visiting Surgeon, Massachusetts General Hospital
Abdominal Pain; Intestinal Obstruction; Appendicitis; Peritonitis; Colorectal Diverticular Disease; Meckel's Diverticulum; Burns

Thomas N. Tozer, Pharm.D., Ph.D.
Professor of Pharmacy and Pharmaceutical Chemistry, University of California, San Francisco
Drug Input and Disposition; Kinetic Principles of Drug Administration; Monitoring Drug Treatment

Allan R. Tunkel, M.D., Ph.D.
Assistant Professor of Medicine, Medical College of Pennsylvania
Biology of Infectious Disease

John E. Ultmann, M.D.
Professor of Medicine and Director of Cancer Research Center, University of Chicago
Oncology

John P. Utz, M.D.
Professor of Medicine, Georgetown University
Nocardiosis; Actinomycosis; Systemic Fungal Diseases

George E. Vaillant, M.D.
Raymond Sobel Professor of Psychiatry, Dartmouth Medical School
Personality Disorders

Paul P. VanArsdel, Jr., M.D.
Professor of Medicine and Head, Allergy Section, University of Washington
Disorders due to Hypersensitivity

Elise W. van der Jagt, M.D.
Associate Professor of Pediatrics, University of
Rochester; Director, Strong Children's Critical
Care Center
Injuries (Pediatric)

Jack A. Vennes, M.D.
Professor of Medicine, University of Minnesota;
VA Medical Center, Minneapolis
Extrahepatic Biliary Disorders

Wolfgang H. Vogel, Ph.D.
Professor and Acting Chairman of Pharmacology, Professor of Psychiatry and Human Behavior, Thomas Jefferson University
Neurotransmission

Jacob S. Walfish, M.D.
Clinical Assistant Professor, Mount Sinai School
of Medicine
*Chronic Inflammatory Diseases of the Bowel;
Antibiotic-Associated Colitis*

Louis R. Wasserman, M.D.
Distinguished Service Professor (Emeritus) and
Albert A. and Vera G. List Professor (Emeritus)
of Medicine (Hematology), Mount Sinai School
of Medicine
Myeloproliferative Disorders

William C. Watson, M.D., Ph.D.
Professor of Medicine, Victoria Hospital, Lon-
don, Ontario, Canada
Malabsorption Syndromes

Max Harry Weil, M.D., Ph.D.
Distinguished Professor of Medicine, Physiology, and Biophysics, University of Health Sciences, Chicago Medical School; President, Institute of Critical Care Medicine
Bacteremia and Septic Shock

John M. Weiler, M.D.
Professor of Internal Medicine, University of
Iowa; VA Medical Center, Iowa City
Biology of the Immune System

Allan B. Weingold, M.D.
Chairman, Department of Obstetrics and Gyne-
cology, George Washington University
*High-Risk Pregnancy; Pregnancy Complicated
by Disease—Cardiac Disease, Thromboembolic
Disease, Hypertension, Renal Disease, Urinary
Tract Infection, Infectious Disease, Anemia,
Asthma, Autoimmune Diseases, Malignancy,
Disorders Requiring Surgery*

Michael Weintraub, M.D.
Associate Professor of Community and Preventive Medicine and of Pharmacology and Medicine, University of Rochester
Patient Compliance

Claude E. Welch, M.D.
Clinical Professor of Surgery (Emeritus), Harvard University; Senior Surgeon, Massachusetts
General Hospital
*Abdominal Pain; Intestinal Obstruction; Appen-
dicitis; Peritonitis; Colorectal Diverticular Disease; Meckel's Diverticulum*

Nanette K. Wenger, M.D.
Professor of Medicine (Cardiology), Emory University; Director, Cardiac Clinics, Grady Memorial Hospital
*Syncope; Orthostatic Hypotension; Exercise
and the Heart*

Richard J. Whitley, M.D.
Professor of Pediatrics, Microbiology, and Medi-
cine, University of Alabama at Birmingham
Neonatal Herpes Simplex Virus Infection

Albert I. Winegrad, M.D.
Professor of Medicine and Director, Cox Insti-
tute, University of Pennsylvania
Disorders of Carbohydrate Metabolism

Walter S. Wood, M.D.
Professor of Medicine (Emeritus), Loyola Uni-
versity, Chicago
Anthrax; Clostridial Infections

Theodore E. Woodward, M.D.
Professor of Medicine (Emeritus), University of
Maryland; Distinguished Physician, VA Medical
Center, Baltimore
Rickettsial Diseases

Verna Wright, M.D., F.R.C.P.
Professor of Rheumatology, University of Leeds (England)

Ankylosing Spondylitis; Psoriatic Arthritis; Miscellaneous Disorders (Musculoskeletal and Connective Tissue)

Robert Zelis, M.D.
Professor of Medicine and Physiology, and Director, Cardiovascular Research, Pennsylvania State University

Calcium Antagonists

EDITORIAL AND BUSINESS STAFF

Shirley Claypool, EXECUTIVE EDITOR

Arlene Elisabeth Dahlbeck, SENIOR STAFF EDITOR

Keryn A.G. Lane, SENIOR STAFF EDITOR

Frank E. Manson, SENIOR STAFF EDITOR

Catherine J. Humber, TEXTBOOK PRODUCTION COORDINATOR/COPY EDITOR

Diane C. Zenker, SECRETARY

Gary Zelko, PUBLISHER

Pamela J. Barnes, ADVERTISING AND PROMOTION ADMINISTRATOR

Lynn Foulk, BOOK DESIGNER (VOLUMES I AND II)

§1. GYNECOLOGY AND OBSTETRICS

1. GYNECOLOGIC PRACTICE AND APPROACH TO THE PATIENT

A young woman's first visit with a physician is often for contraception or pregnancy. This first visit is of major importance, as it may affect her attitude and actions toward future care needs; as wife-mother, she will likely select health care providers for her family.

A patient's personal expectations, interpretations, and response to symptoms and therapy, as well as disease patterns, are influenced by her culture and socioeconomic status. Modesty may make the physical, particularly the pelvic, examination an ordeal. The patient may be ignorant of generative and sexual functions. Religious and cultural backgrounds influence attitudes about pregnancy, contraception, and abortion. Visual exploration of any portion of the genital tract may be proscribed. For some, an absolute or highly desirable requirement may be virginity at marriage, frequently equated with the size of the hymenal orifice; thus, an examination may be limited or impossible. On the other hand, premarital sexual activity with multiple partners is common in young people and leads to infection, cervical neoplasia, and unplanned pregnancy. Taboos and attitudes toward menstruation vary markedly; eg, menses were traditionally associated with soiling, shame, and "sickness"; or the menstrual flow was thought of as "cleansing," so that a heavy flow might be welcomed as feminine and a light flow or longer interval interpreted as unhealthy.

Gynecologic and obstetric problems account for 20% of office visits by women. Many women have physical examinations only because of need for contraception, pregnancy detection and subsequent care, or sexual counseling, or they postpone examinations until an urgent problem arises. Important symptoms might be considered too minor or embarrassing to mention (eg, annoying discharge, dyspareunia, urinary incontinence, or pelvic pressure) and are elicited only by tactful interviewing and thorough examination. Patients may or may not be aware of psychologic stress that could be augmenting or causing their symptoms. Some patients use minor symptoms as a pretense when they actually wish to explore other problems, such as fear of cancer or venereal disease, pregnancy, need for counseling in sexual or reproductive functions, or effects of menopause.

Increasingly, women are becoming better educated, working outside the home, having fewer children, changing residences, being divorced or separated, rearing children alone, and outliving their mates. The pressures of these changes may affect a woman's health, needs, and ability to handle problems. An affluent, better-educated woman who has easy access to health care generally is more likely to practice preventive care and seek attention early for symptoms. However, health practices vary widely, and each patient's attitudes must be assessed individually.

Venereal disease, pregnancy, and sexual dysfunction are occurring in epidemic proportions in adolescents, who make up about 40% of obstetric and gynecologic patients. Physicians have a unique opportunity to establish continuing relationships, teach about body function and health care maintenance, and counsel. This contact must be nonjudgmental, because an adolescent will perceive insensitivity regarding her physical and emotional feelings. Her vulnerability emphasizes the effect the physician has on her attitude toward and feelings about future medical care. Confidentiality must be observed and affirmed to adult and adolescent patients. The rights of minors who do not want parents informed of medical problems, especially those associated with sexual activities, should be respected. Many states have laws "emancipating" minors for visits concerning pregnancy, contraception, abortion, sexually transmitted diseases, or marriage. Women now expect to be involved in decisions affecting their health care. Therefore, patients must receive support and counsel as well as sufficient information to understand their problem, the nature of therapy, and available alternatives.

The Gynecologic History

Rapport begins with the physician's courtesy, attention, and friendly, unhurried manner while compiling the medical history. A nonjudgmental approach in questions, gestures, and attitudes avoids moralizing or expressing dogmatic opinion and encourages an accurate history. Since the physician's attitude toward women may differ from that of the patient, care must be exercised to avoid making the patient feel embarrassed, helpless, or dependent. An appropriate response recognizes her worth and encourages realization of her independence.

The patient's **primary complaint** should be identified and explored in detail. **Background data** reveal the patient as an individual. **Menstrual history** includes the age of menarche of the patient (and other family members); frequency, regularity, duration, amount of flow, and pain or other symptoms with or before menses; abnormal bleeding; and dates of last 2 menses. **Sexual activity,** orientation, and possible problems can influence further questioning. A **history of venereal disease,** including herpes and condyloma, should be noted. The possibility of pregnancy should be explored, along with attitudes, knowledge, and experience with contraceptives. **History of pregnancy** includes the number of pregnancies, their dates and outcomes, and problems in becoming pregnant. **Pain,** if present, should be described: when and where it occurs, its severity, its tendency to radiate, what exacerbates it or gives relief, and how it relates to GI or urinary functions. **Fever** should be noted.

A review of **past illnesses** follows, including hospitalization and surgery, with details of abdominal or pelvic surgery. Any **history of radiation therapy** for benign disease—eg, mastitis, enlarged thymus, menorrhagia, or skin disorders—should be elicited, as well as reports of possible exposure to diethylstilbestrol (**DES**) by mothers who were pregnant or by daughters born during the years of its use (1947 to 1971). The patient's **general health** should be reviewed, including her **psychologic status,** with particular attention to depression, anxiety, or drug abuse. Any history of **weight change,** bulimia, or anorexia nervosa should be investigated. **Drug intake** should be noted, with reference to allergies and especially to drugs affecting the present condition, since they may conflict with proposed treatment or be contraindicated in pregnancy. Reference to use or abuse of tobacco, alcohol, or other drugs must be explored.

Since the **urinary tract** is frequently involved in gynecologic disease, the patient should be questioned about urinary frequency, nocturia, dysuria, involuntary loss of urine, and vaginal protrusion. Similarly, **GI symptoms** should be reviewed: change of bowel habit, stool color, anorexia, nausea, vomiting, abdominal pain, food intolerance, and possible symptoms (past or present) of liver disorder.

Breast problems, including pain or growth, should be noted. A review of general **endocrine status** includes abnormal hair growth or lactation and symptoms of other endocrine dysfunction. A history of **bleeding abnormalities,** anemias, phlebitis, or other abnormal clotting may give clues to the cause of abnormal menses or preclude hormone medication. The **cardiac status**; history of cardiac disease, hypertension, or smoking; or cholesterol or triglyceride abnormality may also influence therapy. A history of migraine headache or seizures may affect treatment; drugs used to control migraine or seizures may be detrimental in pregnancy. A **family history** may disclose hereditary disease—especially pertinent are ovarian, uterine, and breast cancer; diabetes; bowel polyps or cancer; and genetic abnormalities.

The Gynecologic Examination

The bladder must be emptied before pelvic examination; the urine specimen should be examined for sugar, albumin, and bacteria. Measurements of Hb or Hct should be done as indicated (eg, by heavy menses, tiredness, pallor, or previous anemia). Laboratory assessments may include CBC, urinalysis, and cholesterol and lipid levels.

The **physical examination** includes height, weight, BP, and a check of heart, lungs, and lymph nodes. Abnormal body hair texture or distribution should be noted. The thyroid gland may be enlarged, nodular, or tender.

A thorough **breast examination** (see Ch. 9) in both seated and supine positions notes maturation, tenderness, symmetry, retraction of skin or nipples, and masses. Gentleness and warm hands are appreciated. During this procedure, the physician may instruct the patient in breast self-examination.

Abdominal examination always begins away from an area of pain. Using a flat hand, the physician should systematically probe (not poke) each quadrant of the abdomen for masses and tenderness. The following findings should be noted: presence of a mass and its size, location, mobility, and tenderness; scars or distention; and ascites or suggestion of other abdominal fluids. Liver size and possible tenderness and palpability of the kidneys, liver, and spleen should also be noted. If the patient has an abdominal complaint, bowel sounds should be checked. If tenderness is present, its severity, location, and any accompanying rigidity of the abdominal wall should be noted. Referral of tenderness elsewhere in the abdomen or rebound tenderness indicates peritoneal irritation.

The **pelvic examination** is usually deferred until last. The physician's unhurried explanations and sensitive and gentle but matter-of-fact attitude help the patient to relax, ensuring a more thorough examination. Having emptied her bladder, the patient should assume the lithotomy position (in which the hips and knees are flexed with the buttocks at the edge of the table and the legs supported by heel or knee stirrups). **Inspection** of the genital area shows hair distribution, clitoral size, vulvar lesions, discoloration, discharge, inflammation, and hymenal orifice patency. A gentle touch on the inner thigh just before touching the genitalia reduces the startle reflex. The labia should be spread with the fingers of one hand. To expose the cervix and avoid pressure on the urethra, a warmed, water-lubricated speculum should be inserted into the upper vagina and then opened. (Lubricating jelly should not be used, since it may interfere with the Papanicolaou test.)

The **Papanicolaou (Pap) test** examines exfoliated cells to detect preinvasive lesions (eg, dysplasia, carcinoma in situ) as well as invasive lesions. The Pap test should detect 80 to 85% of cervical malignancies and premalignant states. The patient should have refrained from douching or using vaginal medication for 24 h. An inadequate sample or an infected malignant lesion may produce false-negative results. Only 50% of tests are positive in patients who have endometrial malignancies. Viral and other infections may be diagnosed, and the estrogen level may be obtained.

An endocervical sample should be taken with a saline-moistened, cotton-tipped applicator or a brush that is rotated or rolled thinly on a slide. The visible cervix should then be firmly scraped circumflexually with an Ayre spatula; a sample from the posterior fornix (vaginal pool) may be included. These specimens may be placed on the same slide as the endocervical smear or on a separate slide, at the discretion of the cytologist. DES-exposed women should also have vaginal wall scrapings examined. The sample should be fixed immediately with an alcohol solution or spray.

With the speculum in place, gross lesions may be noted; specimens should be taken if discharge or other symptoms warrant. The vaginal walls should be inspected as the patient bears down and the speculum is gradually withdrawn.

Bimanual palpation of the uterus is done with the index and middle finger of one hand in the vagina and the fingers of the other hand on the abdomen. The uterus is normally felt as a pear-shaped, smooth muscular organ; the fingers, shifting from anterior to posterior fornix, ascertain its position, size, consistency, surface contour, mobility, and tenderness. A retroflexed uterus is more difficult to outline and may seem larger than its actual size. **Enlargements** may be due to pregnancy, myoma, adenomyosis, simple hypertrophy, malignancy, or inflammation. **Softening** may be due to pregnancy, malignancy, degenerating myoma or sarcoma, or low estrogen levels—as with immaturity or postmenopause. **Irregularities** may be due to myomas, varying in size from several millimeters to many centimeters; anomalies of the uterus, usually felt as an indentation of the fundus; malignancies; or adhesions of other pelvic structures, such as between ovary and uterus. **Adnexal structures** should be palpated by approximating the fingers of the 2 hands, the painful side last. The normal adult ovary, 3 by 2 by 2 cm, may be difficult to palpate, especially if the abdominal wall is thick or tense; but performing this examination is important because early diagnosis of malignant lesions depends upon early findings in an asymptomatic patient. Enlargements of ovary or adnexal mass, including tubes, should be noted, as well as abnormalities similar to those mentioned above in palpation of the uterus. On the right, the position of **the cecum** may be differentiated by its mobility and the presence of gas. The cul-de-sac area behind the uterus should be palpated at this time and again in the rectal examination. The vagina should be palpated for vaginal cysts or nodules. **Pelvic support** may be evaluated with 2 fingers held gently against the posterior vaginal wall; the physician should check for descensus of the uterus and evidence of cystocele, rectocele, and enterocele by noting support both before and after the patient bears down. Protrusion of the anterior wall is termed **cystocele.** Posteriorly, the levator ani muscles offer support, with weakness and protrusion of the posterior wall termed **rectocele.** Herniation near the apex of the vagina between the major supporting uterosacral ligaments is termed **enterocele.** This can also occur after a hysterectomy, when the apex of the vagina may descend to varying degrees.

Rectovaginal examination should be done last, with the index finger in the vagina and the second finger in the rectum to confirm the findings. The physician should palpate uterosacral ligaments, the back of the uterus and cervix, and the contents of the cul-de-sac (pouch of Douglas) and parametria to search for masses, tenderness, or induration. This part of the examination is especially important with a retroflexed uterus. **Rectal lesions** within the range of the examining finger (eg, hemorrhoids, fissures, polyps, masses) or the presence of blood should be noted.

The upper posterior vagina between the uterosacral ligaments, the thinnest layer of the abdominal wall, is a common site for needle aspiration of fluid contents of the peritoneum (**culdocentesis**).

Following the examination, the physician, using diagrams or pictures as indicated, should discuss the findings with the patient so that she understands her condition and the alternatives of therapy.

2. REPRODUCTIVE ENDOCRINOLOGY

Normal human reproductive function requires the complex interplay of endocrine and target organs (see FIG. 2–1). **Gonadotropin-releasing hormone (GnRH)**, also known as luteinizing hormone–releasing hormone (**LHRH, LRH**), is a small peptide (secreted by the hypothalamus) that regulates release of the pituitary gonadotropins **luteinizing hormone (LH)** and **follicle-stimulating hormone (FSH)** from the anterior pituitary gland. LH and FSH, termed gonadotropins, are important in stimulating secretion of hormones by the gonads and also play an essential role in inducing maturation of germ cells. Androgens from the testes in men and estrogens from the ovaries in women in turn stimulate the target organs of the reproductive tract (ie, breasts, uterus, and vagina in women and accessory reproductive organs in men) and exert feedback effects on the CNS-hypothalamic-pituitary unit to influence its hormone secretion.

Steroids are polycyclic compounds derived from cholesterol with carbon atoms arranged in 4 rings. They circulate in the bloodstream, bound almost entirely to various plasma proteins. Only free or unbound steroids appear to be biologically active. Steroid hormones can exert both **negative** and **positive feedback** effects on gonadotropin secretion. Negative feedback occurs when steroids *inhibit* release of LH and FSH; positive feedback occurs when steroids *stimulate* gonadotropin secretion.

Inhibin, a peptide hormone secreted by the granulosa cells of the ovary and by the Sertoli cells of the testis, specifically inhibits FSH secretion. It is made up of an α chain and one of 2 β chains, termed A and B. If 2 β chains combine, the peptide, termed activin, stimulates FSH secretion in vitro, but any physiologic significance remains to be determined.

Virtually all hormones are released in short bursts or pulses at intervals of 1 to 3 h. Constant levels are not observed in the circulation. The patterns described are therefore merely idealized representations on which the minute-to-minute fluctuations must be superimposed. Such factors must be considered in interpreting single hormonal values obtained for clinical purposes.

Infancy, Childhood, and Puberty

Both LH and FSH are elevated at birth but fall to low levels within a few months and remain low through the prepubertal years (see FIG. 2–2). Serum FSH levels are generally slightly higher than LH levels in children, when expressed in terms of milli-international units (**mIU**)/mL. The hypothalamic-pituitary unit appears to be exquisitely sensitive to extremely low levels of circulating steroids, and negative feedback influences predominate. Early in puberty there is a decrease in the sensitivity of the hypothalamus to gonadal steroids, resulting in increased secretion of pituitary gonadotropins, stimulation of gonadal steroid production, and development of secondary sexual characteristics. Increased secretion of both LH and FSH first occurs only during sleep and is associated with increased gonadal steroid secretion. Later, secretion of LH and FSH increases throughout the 24-h period. The patterns of increase in basal LH and FSH levels differ between boys and girls, but in both, the increases in basal LH levels exceed those of FSH.

The adrenal androgens, dehydroepiandrosterone (**DHEA**) and its sulfate (**DHEAS**), begin to increase several years prior to puberty in both sexes. It is possible that the increase in adrenal androgens may play a role in activating other pubertal events and may be important in initiating pubic and axillary hair growth (ie, adrenarche). Since ACTH and cortisol do not increase with these androgens, it has been suggested that another as yet unidentified pituitary peptide initiates adrenal androgen secretion.

The mechanisms responsible for initiating puberty are not understood; there must be some "CNS program." In addition to decreased sensi-

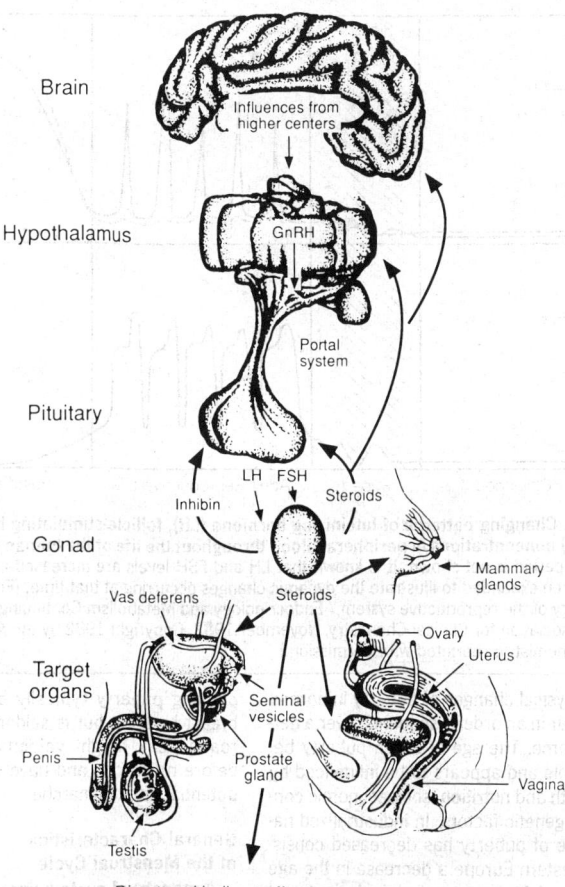

Brain

Influences from
higher centers

Hypothalamus

GnRH

Portal
system

Pituitary

LH FSH

Inhibin   Steroids

Gonad

Vas deferens   Steroids

Mammary
glands

Target
organs

Ovary

Uterus

Penis

Seminal
vesicles

Prostate
gland

Vagina

Testis

Direct and indirect effects on other
tissues (bone, skin, muscle, etc.)

FIG. 2–1. The CNS-hypothalamic-pituitary-gonadal-target organ axis in men and women. FSH = follicle-stimulating hormone, GnRH = gonadotropin-releasing hormone, LH = luteinizing hormone. (Modified from Rebar RW: "Normal physiology of the reproductive system," Endocrinology and Metabolism Continuing Education Program, American Association of Clinical Chemistry, November 1982. Copyright 1982 by the American Association for Clinical Chemistry; reprinted with permission.)

tivity to the inhibitory feedback effects of circulating gonadal steroids, maturation of a positive stimulating feedback response to estrogen must occur in girls in order to result in the midcycle LH surge preceding ovulation. Data in monkeys demonstrate that puberty can be initiated precociously simply by giving GnRH in a pulsatile fashion. Thus, a central "clock" that matures and initiates pulsatile GnRH release may be an early

and critical event in pubertal development. Central inhibitory influences may diminish pulsatile GnRH secretion in childhood.

Puberty: *The sequence of maturational events by which a child is transformed into an adult.* Puberty occurs during **adolescence**, the period during which complete growth and sexual maturity are achieved. Regardless of the mecha-

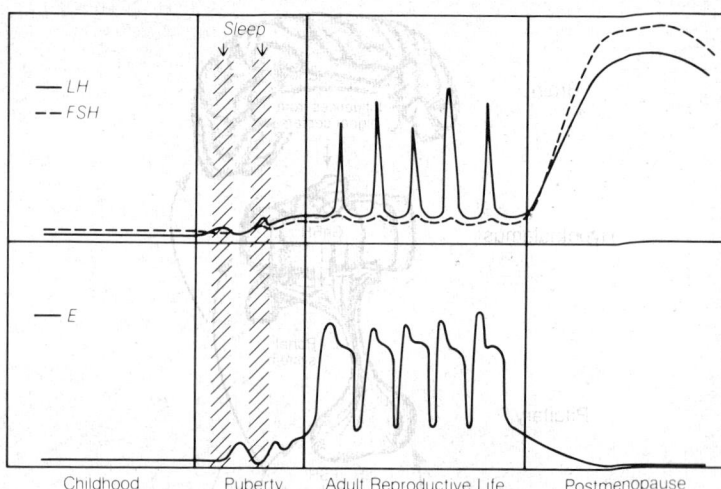

FIG. 2–2. Changing patterns of luteinizing hormone (LH), follicle-stimulating hormone (FSH), and estradiol (E₂) concentrations in peripheral blood throughout the life of the human female. The immediate neonatal period is not shown. It is known that LH and FSH levels are increased at birth. The pubertal period has been expanded to illustrate the dynamic changes occurring at that time. (From Rebar RW: "Normal physiology of the reproductive system," Endocrinology and Metabolism Continuing Education Program, American Association for Clinical Chemistry, November 1982. Copyright 1982 by the American Association for Clinical Chemistry; reprinted with permission.)

nism, the physical changes of puberty in normal children occur in an orderly sequence over a definite time frame. The age at which puberty begins is variable and appears to be influenced by general health and nutrition, socioeconomic conditions, and genetic factors. In industrialized nations the age of puberty has decreased consistently: In Western Europe a decrease in the age of menarche of 4 mo for each decade occurred between 1850 and 1950. Moderate obesity for age is associated with earlier menarche, while delayed menarche is common in severely underweight and malnourished girls. Such observations have led to the theory that a critical body weight of 48 kg (106 lb) must be attained before menarche occurs. Earlier pubertal development also occurs in girls living in urban areas, in blind girls, and in those whose mothers noted early sexual maturation.

Breast budding in girls is usually the first pubertal change, followed closely by the first appearance of pubic and axillary hair (see FIG. 2–3). The interval from breast budding to menarche is generally about 2 yr. Habitus in girls changes as well, and the percentage of body fat increases. The adolescent growth spurt accompanying puberty typically begins even before breast budding but is seldom recognized. Girls reach peak height velocity early in puberty before menarche and have only limited growth potential after menarche.

General Characteristics of the Menstrual Cycle

A **menstrual cycle** *begins with the first day of genital bleeding (day 1) and ends just before the next menstrual period*. **Menarche** refers to *the onset of menses*, **menopause** to *the cessation of menses*. Although the median menstrual cycle length is 28 days, only 10 to 15% of normal cycles are exactly 28 days in length; the range is about 18 to 40 days. Maximal variation with the longest intermenstrual intervals generally occurs in the years following menarche and those preceding menopause, when anovulatory cycles are more common.

Hormonal events during the menstrual cycle: On the basis of known endocrine events, the menstrual cycle can be divided into 3 distinct phases (see FIG. 2–4). The **preovulatory** or **follicular phase** varies in length, beginning with the first day of bleeding and extending to the day

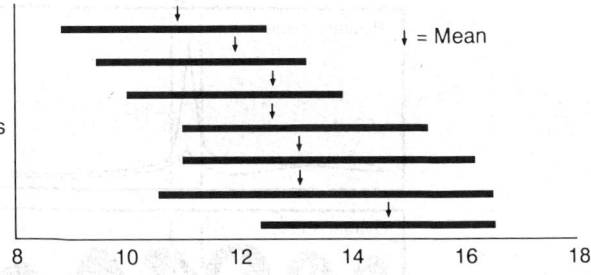

FIG. 2–3. **Puberty—age of development of female sexual characteristics.** The bars indicate normal ranges.

before the preovulatory LH surge. During the first half of the follicular phase, slightly increased FSH secretion from the anterior pituitary gland initiates growth and development of a cohort of 3 to 30 follicles, consisting of oocytes and their surrounding cells. One of these follicles will ovulate; all the others will undergo degeneration (**atresia**). In the absence of appropriate increase in FSH, follicular development will not be normal. Circulating LH levels rise slowly during this time, beginning 1 to 2 days after the FSH rise. Steroid hormone estrogen and progesterone secretion by the ovaries is relatively constant and remains low during this period.

About 7 to 8 days before the preovulatory surge, estrogen (particularly **estradiol, E₂**) secretion from the ovaries begins to increase slowly, but then accelerates and generally peaks during the day of the LH surge. This rise in estrogen is accompanied by a slow but steady increase in LH and a fall in FSH levels. The divergence in LH and FSH levels may be due to the preferential inhibitory action of estrogens on FSH, compared to LH release, and of inhibin. Just before the LH surge, **progesterone** levels also begin to increase significantly.

In the **ovulatory phase**, a series of complex endocrine events culminates in the massive release (ie, preovulatory surge) of LH by the pituitary gland. The mechanism for the process of ovulation itself is unclear, but this LH surge is necessary to cause release of the ovum from the mature preovulatory (ie, graafian) follicle, generally 16 to 32 h after onset of the surge. (In this discussion of endocrine changes during the menstrual cycle, the day of maximal LH release is referred to as day 0. Hormonal events are centered around this surge, with days before the LH surge numbered negatively from 0 and days after the

surge numbered positively.) Although ovulation may result, the subsequent luteal phase may be short and inadequate and preclude pregnancy.

The ovulatory release of LH occurs partly as a result of positive estrogen feedback and leads to final maturation of the follicle and ovulation. Although there is a smaller simultaneous increase in FSH secretion, its significance is not understood. With rising LH levels, estradiol levels fall but progesterone concentrations continue to increase. The LH surge typically lasts 36 to 48 h and consists of multiple large bursts of LH released in a pulsatile fashion.

The **postovulatory** or **luteal phase** is the most constant half of the cycle, averaging 14 days in length in the absence of pregnancy and ending with the onset of menstruation. The name and length of this phase come from the functional lifespan of the **corpus luteum** (ie, yellow body) of the ovary, which supports the released ovum by secreting progesterone. After ovulation the granulosa and theca cells that make up the follicle reorganize to form the corpus luteum. The corpus luteum secretes increasing quantities of progesterone, peaking with secretion of about 25 mg during each 24-h period 6 to 8 days after the LH surge. Circulating LH and FSH levels decline and are low throughout most of the luteal phase but begin to increase again with menstruation.

Cyclic Changes in the Ovary

By the 6th wk of gestation, primordial germ cells, now called **oogonia**, have migrated by ameboid movement from their site of origin in the yolk sac to the genital ridges (ie, presumptive ovaries) of the fetus. Their number markedly increases by mitosis through the 20th wk of fetal age. The germ cells then undergo meiosis so that

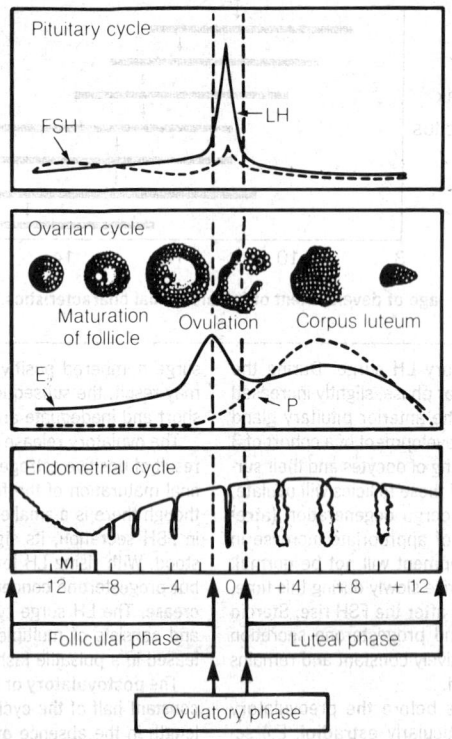

FIG. 2–4. The idealized cyclic changes observed in pituitary gonadotropins, estradiol (E2), progesterone (P), ovarian follicles, and uterine endometrium during the normal menstrual cycle. The data are centered about the day of the LH surge (day 0). Days of menstrual bleeding are indicated by M. FSH = follicle-stimulating hormone, LH = luteinizing hormone. (From Rebar RW: "Normal physiology of the reproductive system," Endocrinology and Metabolism Continuing Education Program, American Association for Clinical Chemistry, November 1982. Copyright 1982 by the American Association for Clinical Chemistry; reprinted with permission.)

all germ cells are arrested in the diplotene stage of meiotic prophase by the 7th mo of gestation and can be called **oocytes**. Between 7 and 9 mo of gestation, the fetal ovary becomes organized and each oocyte becomes a part of a **primordial follicle**, consisting of a basement membrane, a single layer of squamous epithelial granulosa cells, and an oocyte arrested in meiosis. These primordial follicles represent the pool of nongrowing follicles from which all mature follicles develop. Thus, the human female is born with a limited number of germ cells (ova). These are eliminated from the ovary by atresia, which accounts for elimination of 99.9% of all germ cells, and by ovulation. The estimated number in the

ovaries throughout life is cited in TABLE 2–1. Each viable oocyte remains arrested in meiotic prophase until after the midcycle LH surge of the cycle in which it is ovulated, making it one of the longest lived cells in the body (from embryo up to about 50 yr). The long life span of oocytes may account for the increased incidence of genetically abnormal pregnancies as mothers increase in age.

Follicular growth involves the transformation of a small primordial follicle 50 μm in diameter into a mature graafian follicle 1 to 2.5 cm in diameter (see FIG. 2–5). Follicular growth begins with the oocyte increasing in diameter from 15 to 150 μm. This larger oocyte becomes surrounded

TABLE 2–1. THE ESTIMATED POTENTIAL OF HUMAN OVARIES

Parameter	Approximate Number
Maximum number of oocytes in both fetal ovaries	7–20 million
Oocytes present at birth	2 million
Oocytes present at menarche	200–400,000
Oocytes undergoing some development during reproductive life	8000
Number of ovulatory menstrual cycles during reproductive life	300–400
Number of follicles beginning to develop each cycle	3–30
Number of ova normally shed at each ovulation	1 (rarely 2)

Modified from Rebar RW: "Normal physiology of the reproductive system," Endocrinology and Metabolism Continuing Education Program, American Association for Clinical Chemistry, November 1982. Copyright 1982 by the American Association for Clinical Chemistry; used with permission.

by a **zona pellucida,** a translucent "shell" of gly-coproteins. The fully grown oocyte surrounded by a single layer of granulosa cells is termed a **primary follicle.** Development into a **secondary follicle** occurs with mitosis of granulosa cells so that the oocyte becomes surrounded by 2 or more cell layers. The initiation of oocyte and follicular growth is not controlled by gonadotropins and is not understood.

Although the oocyte itself fully differentiates early in follicular development, it cannot be extruded from the ovary until the follicular unit develops into a mature graafian follicle capable of responding to the midcycle LH surge. This phase of follicular maturation is completely dependent upon gonadotropin and steroid hormones and is controlled by changes in the type and number of hormone receptor sites on the granulosa and theca cells of the follicle.

FSH induces the appearance of FSH receptors on granulosa cells, necessary to stimulate the aromatase enzyme needed to convert androgens to estrogens. Specific steroid receptors for estradiol and testosterone appear in granulosa cells with the appearance of the FSH receptors. The estrogen-receptor interaction stimulates multiplication of granulosa cells and thus follicular growth, while androgen-receptor interaction has been implicated in follicular atresia. In addition, many factors, especially insulin-like growth factor I **(IGF-I),** also known as somatomedin-C, appear to be important in follicular growth and atresia.

Theca interstitial cells begin to develop around the basement membrane surrounding the granulosa cells shortly after the oocyte completes its growth. The theca develop specific receptors for LH but not FSH. LH stimulates the theca to synthesize androgens, mainly androstenedione

and testosterone. The androgens produced in the theca diffuse across the basement membrane into the granulosa cells where they are converted into estradiol, which then diffuses into the systemic circulation to feed back on the hypothalamic-pituitary unit (see under Neuroendocrine Regulation of the Menstrual Cycle, below).

The mature tertiary, preovulatory, **graafian follicle** contains an antrum or fluid-filled cavity, created by proliferating granulosa cells, which secrete fluid and mucopolysaccharides. The tertiary follicle grows from 200 μm to 1 to 2.5 cm in diameter, primarily because of accumulation of follicular fluid under the control of FSH, which also induces the appearance of specific LH receptors on granulosa cells. These LH receptors are responsible for the stimulation of progesterone secretion prior to ovulation and for continued production of progesterone in the luteal phase. Granulosa cells also develop specific membrane receptors for prolactin in early tertiary follicles, but these decrease as the follicles mature, and their physiologic role is unclear. About 2 wk are required for the presumptive preovulatory follicle to complete its growth and expel a mature oocyte. The mechanism of preovulatory selection from the cohort of developing follicles is unknown, but intraovarian factors must be important. This is also apparent because the fully grown oocyte is inhibited from resuming meiotic maturation by granulosa-oocyte interactions until after ovulation. If the oocyte is removed from the follicle, meiotic division begins. Increases in the size of preovulatory follicles clinically can be monitored by ultrasonography, which is useful when ovulation is induced in anovulatory patients.

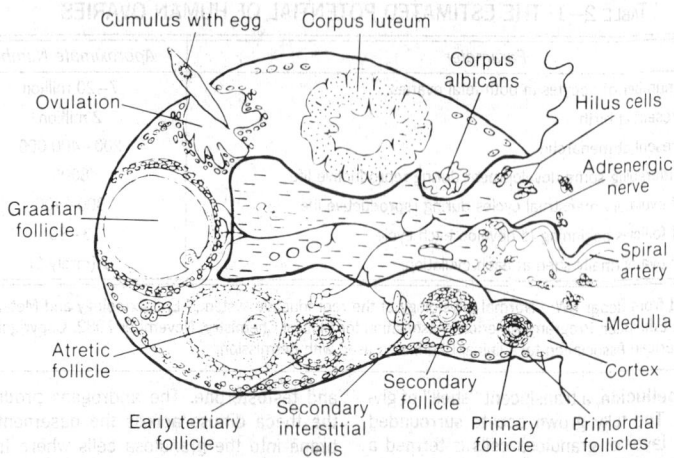

Fig. 2-5. **Morphologic and histologic depiction of a human ovary.** The follicles, corpora lutea, and secondary interstitial cells are embedded in the outer cortex, while the hilus cells, autonomic nerves, and spiral arteries are found in the medulla. (From Erickson GF in *Gynecology and Obstetrics,* edited by JD Sciarra. Philadelphia, JB Lippincott Company, 1984; used with permission.)

Within 36 h of the LH/FSH surge, the oocyte completes the first meiotic division, when each cell receives only 23 chromosomes of the original 46 and the first polar body is extruded. The 2nd meiotic division, when each chromosome divides longitudinally with identical pairs, is not completed and the 2nd polar body not extruded unless the egg is penetrated by a spermatozoon. During the LH surge, the preovulatory follicle swells and bulges above the ovarian epithelium. A **stigma** or avascular spot appears on the follicle surface. A small vesicle forms on the stigma, the vesicle breaks, and the oocyte and some granulosa cells surrounding the oocyte (forming the **cumulus** mass) are extruded. Proteolytic enzymes in the granulosa cells and in the epithelial cells overlying the preovulatory follicle appear to play an important role in rupturing the follicle. Prostaglandin production by the follicle itself, perhaps under the regulation of LH and/or FSH, also appears essential for the ovulatory process.

The corpus luteum produces progesterone and estradiol for about 14 days and then degenerates unless fertilization occurs. Because progesterone is also thermogenic, basal body temperature increases by at least 0.33° C (0.6° F) in the luteal phase and remains elevated until menstruation. Prostaglandins and IGF-I may play a role in regulating the life span of the corpus luteum; however, this is as yet poorly under-stood. If fertilization occurs, **human chorionic gonadotropin (HCG)** from the fertilized ovum supports the corpus luteum until the feto-placental unit can support itself endocrinologically. HCG is structurally and functionally similar to LH; however, pregnancy tests typically use antibodies specific to the β subunit of HCG and have little if any cross-reactivity with LH.

Cyclic Changes in the Other Target Organs of the Reproductive Tract

During the menstrual cycle, the **endometrium** undergoes remarkable histologic and cytologic changes that culminate with menstrual bleeding. The endometrium consists of 3 layers: (1) the nonfunctioning **basal layer,** which is not lost during menses and serves to regenerate the other 2 layers during the menstrual cycle; (2) the **superficial layer** of compact epithelial cells that line the uterine cavity; and (3) the intermediate **spongiosa layer.** The latter 2 layers are functioning, show the greatest changes during the menstrual cycle, and are shed with menstruation. Following menstruation in the early follicular phase, the endometrium, which is made up of glands and stroma, is thin. The endometrial glands are narrow and straight with low columnar epithelium, and the endometrial stroma is dense. With rising levels of estradiol during the late follicular phase, the endometrium undergoes progressive proliferation and extensive mitoses (ie, regeneration from the basal layer), the mucosa thickens, and the tubular glands lengthen but remain straight. In the luteal phase, under the influence of progesterone, the glands become coiled, sawtoothed, and secretory, with increased vascularity of the stroma. As both estradiol and progesterone decline in the late luteal phase, the stroma becomes increasingly edematous, endometrial and blood vessel necrosis occurs, and endometrial bleeding ensues. Because the histologic changes during the menstrual cycle are characteristic, endometrial biopsies may be used to accurately date the stage of the cycle and to assess the tissue response to gonadal steroids. Although the mechanism for the onset of menstruation is not understood, prostaglandins have been implicated in causing the initial vasoconstriction and subsequent tissue anoxia and necrosis. Since prostaglandin release may also explain the uterine contractions accompanying menstrual flow, the use of prostaglandin inhibitors to treat dysmenorrhea is logical and should be effective (see under PRIMARY DYSMENORRHEA in Ch. 5). The average duration of menstrual bleeding is 5 (± 2) days, with blood loss averaging 130 mL (range 13 to 300 mL). A saturated pad or tampon absorbs 20 to 30 mL. Menstrual blood does not usually clot (unless bleeding is very heavy), probably because fibrinolysin and other factors inhibiting clotting are present.

Cyclic changes in the diameter of the external cervical os, dimensions of the cervical canal, quantity and biophysical properties of cervical mucus, and tissue vascularity are also observed during the menstrual cycle. During the follicular phase, there is a progressive increase in cervical vascularity, congestion and edema, and secretion of cervical mucus. The external cervical os opens to a diameter of 3 mm at ovulation and then decreases to 1 mm. Under the influence of increasing levels of estrogen, there is a ten- to thirty-fold increase in the quantity of cervical mucus. The elasticity or **spinnbarkeit** increases. "Palm leaf" arborization or **ferning** becomes prominent when cervical mucus obtained just prior to ovulation is allowed to dry on a glass slide and examined microscopically. This ferning is a result of increased NaCl in cervical mucus from estrogenic stimulation. Under the influence of progesterone in the luteal phase, cervical mucus thickens, becomes less watery, and loses its elasticity and ability to fern. The characteristics of cervical mucus are clinically useful in evaluat-

ing the stage of the cycle and the hormonal status of the individual.

Proliferation and maturation of the vaginal epithelium are also influenced by estrogen and progesterone. When ovarian estrogen secretion is low in the early follicular phase, vaginal epithelium is thin and pale. As estrogen levels increase in the follicular phase, the vaginal epithelium thickens and the squamous cells mature and become cornified. During the luteal phase, the number of precornified intermediate cells increases, and there are increased numbers of leukocytes and debris as the mature squamous cells are shed. Changes in the vaginal epithelium can be quantitated histologically and can be used as a qualitative index of estrogenic stimulation. The vagina and cervix are the most sensitive indicators of estrogenic stimulation in the body.

Neuroendocrine Regulation of the Menstrual Cycle

The release of both LH and FSH appears to be dependent on the secretion of GnRH from the hypothalamus. No separate releasing hormone for FSH has been identified. Since strong evidence suggests that LH and FSH are sometimes found in the same cells, differential release of LH and FSH must be dependent upon interactions of various inputs (eg, GnRH, estradiol, and inhibin) and the different disappearance rates of LH (half-life, 20 to 30 min) and FSH (half-life, 2 to 3 h) from the circulation. Like virtually all hormones, both LH and FSH are secreted in an episodic or pulsatile fashion. The frequency and amplitude of the pulses are modulated by ovarian steroids and vary throughout the menstrual cycle. GnRH also appears to be secreted in a pulsatile fashion and is responsible for the pulsatile gonadotropin secretion.

Of the ovarian steroids, 17β-estradiol is the most potent *inhibitor* of gonadotropin secretion, acting on both the hypothalamus and the pituitary gland. Only small increases in estradiol levels are needed to initiate negative feedback action. Inhibin, produced by ovarian granulosa cells, also appears to play a role in suppressing FSH release. Surgical removal of the ovaries leads to rapid increases in LH and FSH, and administration of estradiol to hypoestrogenic women leads to a prompt decline in circulating gonadotropin levels. For ovulation to occur, estradiol must also exert a *positive* effect on gonadotropin secretion. The feedback effects of estradiol appear to be both time and dose dependent. High physiologic concentrations of estrogen stimulate synthesis and storage of gonadotropin and also augment the effect of GnRH in stimulating gonadotropin release. In the normal menstrual cycle, the positive feedback action of estradiol leading to the midcycle LH/FSH surge is preceded by a period when lower estradiol levels are present with their negative feedback effects.

Thus, the secretion of LH and FSH is determined by the direct input of GnRH modulated by the feedback effects of gonadal steroids. Early in the follicular phase, the gonadotropes in the anterior pituitary gland have relatively small amounts of LH and FSH available for release. Increasing estradiol augments synthesis of LH and FSH but inhibits their secretion. As estradiol increases further to midcycle, it finally induces the midcycle release of LH and FSH, aided by the low but increasing quantities of circulating progesterone. Whether pulsatile release of GnRH is also increased at midcycle is unknown. The onset of the midcycle surge could represent merely a rapid increase in the number of GnRH receptors (stimulated by estrogen) on the gonadotropes.

Menopause
(See also MENOPAUSE in Ch. 5)

The time at which cyclic ovarian function as manifested by menstruation ceases. Menopause generally occurs at 51 yr of age but may occur normally in women as young as 40 yr. Symptoms and signs of the **menopausal syndrome** are related primarily to decreased concentrations of circulating estrogen.

Symptoms include hot flushes, insomnia, paresthesias, palpitations, cold hands and feet, headache, vertigo, anxiety, irritability, nervousness, depression, fatigue, forgetfulness, inability to concentrate, and weight gain. The hot flush has been characterized most thoroughly. The woman feels warm or hot and may perspire, sometimes profusely; the hot flush or "flash" lasts from a few seconds to 3 to 5 min. The skin, especially of the head and neck, becomes red and warm. The flush may be followed by chills. Hot flushes occur in > 75% of all women at menopause and may occur in 25% for > 5 yr.

The vasomotor symptoms of the hot flush occur coincidently with the onset of LH pulses, but not every rise in LH is associated with a hot flush, suggesting that anterior hypothalamic centers independently control both flushes and pulsatile release of LH. Since hot flushes occur following pituitary ablation in women who do not secrete LH and FSH, the 2 events must be independent.

A number of other objective changes occur at menopause. Most apparent is the cessation of menstrual flow. Any genital bleeding in a woman who has not bled for $\geq$ 6 mo demands investigation. Severe osteoporosis occurs in about 25% of menopausal women, especially among those who are thin and white. The vulvar skin and vaginal epithelium become thin, and the labia minora, clitoris, uterus, and ovaries decrease in size.

Many hormonal changes occur in the perimenopausal period (see FIG. 2–2). Regular menstrual cycles may continue up to the menopause. However, the cycles may become shorter, owing to a shortened follicular phase, with increased FSH and decreased estradiol and progesterone levels in comparison with normal ovulatory cycles. Cycles may become quite variable in length, with some being ovulatory and others being anovulatory. Such changes must be due to decreasing ovarian follicular activity, but a few viable appearing oocytes have been observed in the ovaries of postmenopausal women.

Circulating LH and FSH levels are greatly increased in postmenopausal women, with the ratio of FSH to LH typically being > 1 (in terms of mIU/mL) because of decreased negative feedback by estradiol. Obviously, estrogen levels are markedly reduced. Androgen levels are also decreased, but only slightly, because the stroma of the postmenopausal ovary (as well as the adrenal) continues to secrete substantial amounts of androgen. These androgens are converted to estrogens in the periphery, especially in fat cells and skin. This peripheral conversion of androgens accounts for most circulating estrogen found in postmenopausal women.

3.   INFERTILITY

Failure by a couple to conceive after 1 yr of unprotected intercourse.

Infertility affects an estimated 1 in 5 couples in the USA. This growing incidence partly reflects

deferment of marriage and of first birth within marriage. Diagnosis and treatment require a thorough assessment of both partners, the extent and time course of which should be individualized (eg, more rapid if the woman is > 35 yr).

Major etiologic factors include male sperm factors (40%), ovulatory dysfunction (20%), abnormal tubal function (30%), and cervical factors (5%) and are unidentified in 10%.

MALE FACTORS

Spermatogenesis

Spermatogenesis is continuous and requires about 72 to 74 days for germ cell maturation from spermatogonia to spermatozoa. It is most efficient at 34° C (93.2° F), so that exposure to excessive heat or a prolonged fever within 2 to 3 mo of evaluation can adversely affect sperm count, motility, and morphology. Within the seminiferous tubules, Sertoli's cells sustain and regulate maturation, and Leydig's cells produce testosterone required for maintenance of spermatogenesis. The endocrine regulation of the testes is discussed in greater detail under THE TESTES in Ch. 40. Azoospermia is associated with obstruction, congenital absence of the vas deferens, or a primary testicular disorder. The presence of fructose, which is normally secreted by the seminal vesicles, will indicate patency of the ejaculatory ducts.

A **varicocele** is the most common anatomic abnormality found in the infertile male (25%, vs. 10 to 15% in the general population), resulting from abnormal dilation of the veins within the pampiniform plexus draining the testes. The varicocele is more commonly left-sided, where the spermatic vein empties into the left renal vein. In theory, a varicocele causes insufficient drainage of blood from the testes, resulting in excessive pooling of blood and higher intrascrotal temperatures.

Occasionally, **retrograde ejaculation** into the bladder can occur, especially with diabetes mellitus, prior retroperitoneal dissection for Hodgkin's disease, prostatectomy, and neurologic dysfunction.

Diagnosis

Following a history and physical examination to search for causes of infertility, **semen analysis** is the major screening test for the evaluation of the male partner. It should be performed after 2 to 3 days of sexual abstinence. At least 2 to 3 ejaculates should be examined because of sperm count variability, each being obtained by masturbation into a clean glass jar, preferably at the laboratory site. For men who have difficulty, special

Silastic condoms devoid of lubricants and chemicals toxic to sperm can be used.

After liquefaction at room temperature for 20 to 30 min, the following parameters should be evaluated: ejaculate volume (normal, 2 to 6 mL), viscosity (normally liquefies within 1 h), gross and microscopic appearance (normally opaque, cream colored, 1 to 3 WBC/hpf), pH (normal, 7 to 8), sperm count (normal, > 20 million/mL), sperm motility at 1 and 3 h (normal, > 50%), and sperm morphology (normal, > 60%). Additional computer-assisted measures of sperm motility (ie, linear sperm velocity) are now available; however, clinical correlation of velocity with fertility remains unclear.

An abnormal semen analysis should be repeated because of normal variability. The history in men should exclude mumps orchitis, cryptorchidism, testicular injury, exposure to industrial or environmental toxins, excessive heat exposure, acute illness or prolonged fever within the previous 3 mo, recreational drug use, alcohol intake, exposure to diethylstilbestrol or anabolic steroids, inadequate length of abstinence prior to analysis, and failure to deposit the entire semen sample in the collection vessel.

Physical examination should focus on anatomic abnormalities; eg, decreased testicular volume (normal, 20 to 25 mL), prostatitis, hypospadias, or a varicocele. A testicular biopsy may be required to assess the functional capacity of the seminiferous tubules.

Endocrine disorders that can be associated with defective spermatogenesis are uncommon but include hyperprolactinemia, hypothyroidism, adrenal disorders, Klinefelter's syndrome, gonadal dysgenesis, abnormalities of the hypothalamic-pituitary-gonadal axis, and hypogonadism (see under THE TESTES in Ch. 40 and Ch. 48).

Specialized tests of sperm function and quality are now available at major infertility centers and may be appropriate prior to in vitro fertilization **(IVF)** or gamete intrafallopian tube transfer **(GIFT—described under ASSISTED REPRODUCTIVE TECHNOLOGIES, below).** The most commonly used test for detection of antisperm antibodies uses small beads coated with antibodies that bind to the IgG and IgA that may be present on the sperm head, midpiece, or tail **(immunobead test).** The **hypo-osmolar swelling test,** which measures the structural integrity of the sperm plasma membranes, is performed by placing sperm in a hypo-osmolar culture medium. Normally, excess extracellular water shifts into the sperm head, causing it to swell.

Two tests determine the ability of sperm to fertilize the egg in vitro. The **hemizona assay** evaluates sperm binding to protein receptors on the surface of the isolated shell (zona pellucida) of human oocytes. The **sperm penetration assay** evaluates sperm penetration of hamster eggs after the zona pellucida has been removed.

Treatment

There is no good evidence that treatment of men with reduced sperm counts who do not have endocrine disturbances is associated with an increased likelihood of pregnancy.

Varicoceles are generally treated. In *un*controlled studies, ligation of the internal spermatic vein results in a 30 to 50% pregnancy rate, but controlled, randomized studies are needed to confirm this.

In the absence of obvious endocrine defects, moderate oligospermia (10 to 20 million/mL) may be improved with clomiphene citrate (25 to 50 mg/day for 25 days monthly for 3 to 4 mo). Unfortunately, sperm motility and morphology do not seem to be significantly improved, and there are no controlled studies indicating increased fertility.

Artificial insemination (AI): Use of this technique has focused on sperm selection. Most studies suggest that AI of whole sperm ejaculates, using a cervical cup, does not enhance pregnancy rates. AI using a split ejaculate (the first portion, with the greatest sperm density and motility) may slightly enhance pregnancy rates when ejaculate volumes are large. More recently, intrauterine insemination with washed semen samples has been used to treat infertility associated with low sperm counts, decreased motility, antisperm antibodies, or abnormal cervical mucus. The ejaculate is washed several times with tissue culture medium; the motile sperm "swim up" from the sperm pellet and are selected for insemination. This approach appears most successful in men with low sperm counts and normal motility or in couples with cervical factors; most pregnancies will be achieved by the 6th treatment cycle. In azoospermia, therapeutic insemination with donor sperm is an option. Timing by monitoring of ovulation is critical, eg, by measuring basal body temperature or determining the day of urinary luteinizing hormone (LH) rise (see OVULATION FACTORS, below). Because sexually transmitted disease, including AIDS, is a concern, fresh donor semen samples should no longer be used.

Frozen sperm specimens can be obtained from reputable sperm banks. Oligospermia, decreased sperm motility, and antisperm antibodies also can be treated with either the IVF or GIFT procedures (see ASSISTED REPRODUCTIVE TECHNOLOGIES, below).

OVULATION FACTORS

Women with regular menses (26 to 35 days) accompanied by premenstrual molimina (*breast tenderness, lower abdominal bloating, moodiness*) are usually ovulatory. For those with irregular menses or amenorrhea, a cause should be established before ovulatory treatment. A discussion of the physiology of the menstrual cycle is found in Ch. 2 and of the evaluation of amenorrhea in Ch. 6.

Ovulation Monitoring

Daily measurements of basal body temperature **(BBT)** have been used to monitor ovulation. A nadir in BBT suggests impending ovulation, while a rise $\geq 0.5°$ C is characteristic of the postovulatory period. However, the BBT is not reliable or accurate. At best, it can predict ovulation only within 2 days. Much more reliable are pelvic ultrasound monitoring of ovarian follicle diameter and ovulation predictor kits designed to detect an increase in the urinary luteinizing hormone **(LH)** excretion 24 to 36 h prior to ovulation.

Several other biochemical parameters can be used to determine if ovulation occurred in a given cycle; eg, an elevation in serum progesterone (≥ 4 ng/mL) or in its urinary metabolite pregnanediol glucuronide. The quality of ovulation can be evaluated by endometrial biopsy during the late luteal phase (10 to 12 days after ovulation). Endometrial histologic findings of a > 2-day lag in development (compared with subsequent menstrual period onset) are suggestive of inadequate luteal phase production or action of progesterone (luteal phase deficiency—**LPD**). To establish the diagnosis of LPD, delay should be present in 2 menstrual cycles.

Treatment

The selection of ovulation-inducing agents must be tailored to the defect; eg, in patients who are anovulatory or oligo-ovulatory secondary to **hyperprolactinemia**, bromocriptine is the drug of choice.

In patients with **polycystic ovary syndrome** or **chronic anovulation**, clomiphene citrate (an oral antiestrogen derived from diethylstilbestrol) is the most appropriate initial agent. Uterine bleeding should first be induced with medroxyprogesterone acetate 5 to 10 mg once/day for 5 to 10 days. Starting on the 5th day of either spontaneous or withdrawal bleeding, clomiphene 50 mg/day is given for 5 days. Ovulation will generally take place 5 to 10 days (mean, 7 days) after the last day of clomiphene administration; in ovulatory cycles, menses will occur within 35 days.

For those who remain **amenorrheic after clomiphene treatment**, a pregnancy test and pelvic examination should be performed. In the absence of significant ovarian enlargement, withdrawal bleeding is induced as described above and clomiphene restarted atthe 50-mg dose. If ovulation is not achieved after 2 cycles, the dosage is increased to 100 mg/day and further increased at 50-mg increments every 2 cycles until a maximum of 200 mg/day for 5 days is reached (although clomiphene is approved for use at ≤ 100 mg/day, numerous studies have documented the efficacy and safety of these larger dosages). Once a threshold dose for ovulation is determined, treatment should be continued for at least 6 cycles. The conception rate is maximal by the 6th ovulatory cycle.

Side effects of clomiphene citrate include vasomotor flushes (10%), abdominal distention (6%), breast tenderness (2%), nausea (3%), visual symptoms (1 to 2%), and headaches (1 to 2%). The incidence of multiple pregnancy (primarily twins) and ovarian hyperstimulation (see below) is about 5%.

For those who fail to ovulate or to conceive during clomiphene therapy, human *menopausal* gonadotropins **(HMG)**, extracted from urine of postmenopausal women, can be used. Two forms are available. Menotropins (Pergonal®) contains 75 IU/ampul of LH and 75 IU/ampul of follicle-stimulating hormone **(FSH)**. Urofollitropin (Metrodin®) contains only 75 IU/ampul of FSH. The medications are used in a similar fashion. They are quite expensive and have significant side effects; therefore, male and tubal factors must be adequately evaluated prior to initiating treatment, and treatment cycles must be closely supervised by a physician experienced in their use. HMG is given daily IM, beginning on the 2nd day after withdrawal bleeding or spontaneous menses. Because of variability in ovarian responses, daily doses (1 to 4 ampuls) are individualized. The goal is to stimulate follicular growth and maturation of 2 to 4 ovarian follicles within a 7- to 14-day period, monitored by serum estradiol levels and pelvic ultrasonography. After follicular maturation is achieved, human chorionic gonadotropin **(HCG)** 10,000 to 20,000 u. is given IM to trigger ovulation. The major risks of HMG therapy are the **ovarian hyperstimulation syndrome** (10 to 20%) and multiple pregnancy (10 to 30%). *The hyperstimulation syndrome can be life-threatening,* associated with massively enlarged ovaries and a shift of the intravascular fluid volume into the peritoneal space, resulting in hypovolemia, oliguria, hemoconcentration, and massive ascites. It can usually be avoided with close monitoring and the withholding of HCG if ovarian response becomes excessive.

For treatment of **hypothalamic amenorrhea**, gonadorelin acetate, a synthetic gonadotropin-releasing hormone **(GnRH)** for pulsatile IV infusion, recently has become available as an ovulation-inducing agent. GnRH is given either 5 μg/pulse IV or 20 μg/pulse s.c. q 90 min, using a computerized peristaltic pump. This stimulates pituitary release of LH and FSH in a physiologic manner; therefore, usually only one dominant follicle is stimulated to ovulate during a 14-day treatment period. Because the risk of ovarian hyperstimulation is low, extensive monitoring is unnecessary. After ovulation, GnRH can be continued during the luteal phase or HCG can be given as a single dose of 1500 u. IM q 3 days 4 times.

In ovulatory disorders (eg, polycystic ovary syndrome), GnRH agonists have been increasingly used to abolish endogenous gonadotropin secretion and increase the efficacy of subsequent HMG and pulsatile GnRH treatment. This approach awaits validation.

Inadequate luteal phase (luteal insufficiency, luteal phase defect) can be treated with clomiphene citrate 50 to 100 mg/day for 5 days beginning on day 2 or 3 of the menstrual cycle or with progesterone suppositories (not available in the USA and requiring preparation by a pharmacist) 25 mg bid for 14 days beginning 2 days after ovulation. If conception occurs during a treatment cycle, progesterone support is continued uninterrupted until the 10th wk of gestation.

TUBAL FACTORS

Abnormal tubal function is found in about 30% of infertile couples. There may be a history of pelvic inflammatory disease, intrauterine device use, ruptured appendix, lower abdominal surgery, or ectopic pregnancy. To determine tubal patency, a hysterosalpingogram (HSG) should be performed under fluoroscopy 2 to 5 days after cessation of menstrual flow. HSG can demonstrate intrauterine anomalies, uterine filling defects or adhesions (Asherman's syndrome), tubal patency, and potential pelvic adhesions. Because fertility appears to be enhanced slightly following a normal HSG, additional diagnostic tests of tubal function can be delayed for several cycles.

If the HSG indicates an intrauterine abnormality, such as Asherman's syndrome (intrauterine adhesions), a hysteroscopic evaluation can be performed. Hysteroscopic lysis of adhesions is very effective in improving the chances of pregnancy. A diagnostic laparoscopy can further evaluate tubal function and, in some cases, allow simultaneous fulguration or laser ablation of pelvic endometriosis or lysis of pelvic adhesions.

CERVICAL FACTORS

Cervical mucus serves as a biologic filter, preventing the influx of vaginal bacterial flora and enhancing sperm survival. During the follicular phase of the menstrual cycle, rising concentrations of estradiol stimulate increased production of clear, stretchable mucus. The postcoital test provides a measure of mucus receptivity and ability of sperm to survive and access the upper reproductive tract. Although this test is commonly performed, its value has been questioned because some studies have found no correlation between the presence or absence of viable sperm in the mucus and subsequent fertility. The test should be done at midcycle when estradiol levels are highest. A specimen of endocervical mucus is obtained with nasal polyp forceps or a tuberculin syringe between 2 and 8 h after intercourse. In a normal test, the mucus is clear, stretchable for 8 to 10 cm (spinnbarkeit), exhibits a ferning pattern, and contains $\geq$ 5 motile sperm/hpf. Agglutination of sperm, increased cervical mucus viscosity, or absence of sperm may suggest the presence of sperm antibodies, improper timing of the test, or improper coital technique. Treatment must be individualized and can include intrauterine insemination or use of mucolytic agents.

ASSISTED REPRODUCTIVE TECHNOLOGIES

In vitro fertilization (IVF) has been used increasingly, eg, in tubal disease, endometriosis, oligospermia, presence of sperm antibody, and unexplained infertility. This procedure involves ovarian hyperstimulation, oocyte retrieval, fertilization and embryo culture, and embryo transfer. Ovarian hyperstimulation matures multiple oocytes (3 to 10) by using a combination of clomiphene citrate and HMG, HMG alone, or a GnRH agonist and HMG. After appropriate follicular growth is achieved, HCG is given to induce final follicular maturation. About 34 h after HCG administration, the oocytes are retrieved by direct needle puncture of the follicle, either transvaginally by ultrasound guidance or by laparoscopy. The oocytes are then fertilized in vitro with washed sperm and the embryos cultured for about 40 h, after which 3 to 4 embryos are transferred into the uterine cavity. Additional embryos can be frozen in liquid nitrogen for transfer in a subsequent natural cycle. Despite the transfer of multiple embryos, the average term pregnancy rate for a couple starting each IVF cycle is about 8 to 10%.

For women who have unexplained infertility, endometriosis, and normal tubal function, gamete intrafallopian tube transfer (GIFT) also can be used. In GIFT, multiple oocytes and sperm are obtained as in IVF but are subsequently transferred to the distal fallopian tubes, either transabdominally by laparoscopy or vaginally through the uterine-tubal junction by ultrasound guidance, where fertilization occurs. Success rates are about 20 to 30% at most experienced centers. Several variations of the IVF and GIFT procedures include zygote intrafallopian tube transfer (ZIFT), use of donor oocytes, and transfer of frozen embryos to a surrogate mother. These techniques raise additional moral and ethical issues, eg, disposition of stored embryos (especially in cases of death or divorce), legal parentage in surrogate motherhood, and selective reduction of implanted embryos in multiple pregnancy.

PSYCHOLOGIC ASPECTS

Failure to conceive often generates frustration, emotional stress, feelings of inadequacy, anger, guilt, and resentment. The financial burden and time commitment for diagnostic and therapeutic infertility procedures can cause marital strife. Provision of counseling and psychologic support is an important adjunct to treatment. Support groups for infertile couples (eg, Resolve)

have been organized at local and national levels. Despite all efforts, some couples will fail to achieve pregnancy. They should be counseled on when to stop treatments and when to consider adoption.

4. FAMILY PLANNING

One or both members of a couple can use **contraception** to avoid pregnancy temporarily or **sterilization** to prevent pregnancy permanently. **Induced abortion** (elective termination of pregnancy) can be used to correct failures of contraception. The couple's decision to begin, prevent, or interrupt a pregnancy may be influenced by **prenatal diagnosis** or **genetic counseling** (see Chs. 13 and 48). **Infertility** is discussed in Ch. 3.

CONTRACEPTION

The contraceptive methods most commonly used in the USA are (in order of popularity) oral steroid pills, condoms, spermicides, withdrawal, diaphragms, periodic abstinence, and intrauterine devices (**IUDs**). A new modality, polysiloxone capsules containing levonorgestrel that are implanted subcutaneously, was initially marketed in 1991. The advantages and disadvantages of each technique should be explained so that the woman can choose the one most suitable for herself and her partner. Many factors affect rates of contraceptive failure. Age, level of education, and degree of motivation are inversely related to contraceptive failure rates. In general, methods used at the time of coitus (eg, diaphragm, condom, foam, sponge, withdrawal) are more effective in theory than in practice. Overall effectiveness is greater with methods unrelated to coitus (eg, oral contraceptives, IUDs) because patient involvement is simpler. Over a period of several years, pregnancy:use rates are < 1%/yr for oral contraceptives, IUDs, and subdermal implants and about 5%/yr for coitus-related methods.

Diaphragm and Cervical Cap

The **diaphragm**, a dome-shaped rubber cup with a flexible rim that fits over the cervix, acts as a barrier to sperm. The diaphragm must be carefully fitted by the health provider, and the woman must know how to insert it so that the cervix is covered. Contraceptive cream or jelly should always be used with the diaphragm to

improve contraceptive effectiveness in case the diaphragm is displaced during coitus. The diaphragm should cause no discomfort, and neither partner should be aware of its presence. It should be inserted prior to coitus and remain in place for 8 h after the last coitus. Additional spermicide should be added before each coital act to improve effectiveness. When the diaphragm is properly used, the pregnancy rate is about 3%/yr and the overall failure rate about 14%.

The **cervical cap** is similar to the diaphragm, comes in several sizes, and must be fitted by a clinician. It can be left in place for 48 h. Failure rates are similar to those with the diaphragm.

Vaginal Foam, Cream, Suppository, and Sponge

These agents must be placed into the vagina before each coital act. They contain a spermicide, usually nonoxynol 9, that immobilizes or kills sperm on contact; they also provide a mechanical barrier to sperm. No single type of foam or suppository seems to be more effective than another, but the contraceptive sponge has the advantage of remaining effective for 24 h. Its failure rate is about the same as that of the diaphragm. Efficacy with all these agents increases greatly as the woman's age increases; in women > 30 yr, it is similar to that of the IUD.

Natural Family Planning (Periodic Abstinence)

This method depends on abstaining from sexual intercourse during the fertile period. Ovulation most often occurs about 14 days before onset of the next menstrual period. Although the human ovum may be fertile for only about 24 h, motile sperm have been identified up to 7 days after coitus; fertilization has occurred following coitus 3 days before ovulation. The **calendar rhythm method** is the least effective technique of natural family planning, even for women who have regular menstrual cycles. To determine the period of abstention with this method, 18 days should be subtracted from the length of the shortest of the previous 12 cycles and 11 days from the longest. Thus, if the woman's cycles vary between 26 and 29 days, the couple must abstain from coitus from day 8 through day 18 of each cycle. With greater variance in cycle length, longer periods of abstinence are required. Other, more effective techniques require a high degree of motivation as well as training. One such method is based on measuring the woman's **basal body temperature** each morning before arising. Basal body temperature rises about 0.6° F, from a relatively lower level before ovulation to a somewhat higher level, usually > 98° F (37° C), after ovulation. The couple abstains from intercourse until at least 48 to 72 h after the temperature rise. Detection of an increased amount of **cervical mucus** (usually near the time of ovulation) has been used to more accurately determine the fertile time. Intercourse is permitted every other day after menses ends until cervical mucus secretion is detected. Abstinence is then required until 4 days after the peak amount of mucus is observed. The **sympto-thermal method** combines the cervical mucus changes with temperature changes and other symptoms associated with ovulation. It is the most effective method for determining duration of periodic abstinence. However, even with these adjuvants, the use:failure rate is about 10%/yr after training is completed.

Condom

Condom use, the 3rd most common contraceptive method in the USA (after male/female sterilization and oral contraceptives) is the only reversible effective male method other than coitus interruptus (withdrawal). If used properly, the condom also provides considerable protection against sexually transmitted diseases and may possibly prevent premalignant changes of the cervix. The condom should not be applied tightly (the tip should overlap about 1/2 in. to collect the ejaculate) and must be removed carefully so that none of the contents is spilled. The failure rate with careful use is 3 to 4%. Adding a spermicidal agent, either in the lubricant or by insertion into the vagina, may further lower this rate.

Oral Contraceptive (OC)

There are 2 major categories of OCs: **combination** and **progestogen only**. Combination types contain both a synthetic estrogen and a synthetic progestogen and are given continuously for 3 wk. No medication is given in the 4th

wk, to allow for withdrawal bleeding. With progestogen alone, a small dose of a synthetic progestogen is given every day; this regimen, associated with a relatively high incidence of irregular bleeding episodes and a pregnancy rate of 2 to 8%/yr, is recommended only when estrogen is contraindicated—eg, when breast-feeding.

Effectiveness does not differ significantly among the various combination formulations; if no tablets are omitted, the pregnancy rate is < 0.2% at the end of 1 yr. However, formulations with 50 μg or more of estrogen have a higher incidence of adverse effects and, in general, should not be prescribed. Low-dose formulations with 30 to 35 μg of ethinyl estradiol should be given to new users of OCs. These formulations are as effective as higher dose formulations, but the incidence of breakthrough bleeding may be somewhat higher in the first few months of use.

The benefits of OCs must be weighed against risks for the individual patient. Not taking OCs may result in an unwanted pregnancy, and the risk of death associated with normal pregnancy as well as with elective abortion is greater than that associated with OCs.

Starting OC treatment: All women receiving OCs should be examined initially, 3 mo later (to determine if BP has changed), and at least annually thereafter. When a personal or family history suggests increased risk of diabetes mellitus or arteriosclerotic cardiovascular disease, a 2-h postprandial blood glucose level should be obtained, along with a serum lipid profile that includes HDL and LDL cholesterol, total cholesterol, and triglyceride levels. If the glucose or lipids are abnormal, low-dose OCs can be used, but these metabolic values should be assessed to be sure they have not been adversely altered. At each visit, breast and pelvic examinations should be performed and the liver carefully palpated. BP and weight should be measured annually and a cervical cytologic examination performed.

OC use following pregnancy: The woman who has had a term delivery differs from one who has had an abortion in the interval between resumption of ovulation and recurrence of menstruation. The first episode of menstrual bleeding following an abortion is usually preceded by ovulation, which generally occurs between 2 and 4 wk. The first menstruation following a term delivery in a nonnursing mother is usually anovulatory, but occasionally ovulation occurs 4 to 5 wk after delivery. Nursing mothers usually do not ovulate until 10 to 12 wk after delivery, but they may ovulate before the first menses. After spontaneous or induced abortion of a fetus of < 12 wk gestation, OCs should be started immediately. After termination of pregnancy between 12 and 28 wk, the start of OCs should be delayed 1 wk. Since the risk of thromboembolism normally increases postpartum and may be enhanced by OCs, patients who have a delivery after 28 wk gestation and are not nursing should delay taking OCs until 2 wk after delivery. During lactation, OCs diminish the amount of milk produced and reduce the concentrations of protein and fat in the milk; also, measurable amounts of the hormonal compounds can be found in the milk. Therefore, combination OCs are *not* advised for nursing mothers; progestogen-only formulations should be used. **Galactorrhea** is an uncommon side effect.

No benefits of intermittently stopping therapy have been documented. Thus, OCs need not be stopped for any interval (unless the woman wishes to conceive), as long as she does not develop adverse effects or other contraindications to their use. Healthy women who do not smoke can take low-dose OCs continuously until menopause or age 50. *However, in women **over age 35** who smoke cigarettes or have other cardiovascular risk factors (eg, untreated hypertension or hypercholesterolemia) and use OCs with ≥ 50 μg of estrogen, an increased risk of death has been reported from circulatory diseases, including stroke and myocardial infarction.*

Physiology: Because OCs provide negative feedback to the hypothalamus, inhibiting gonadotropin-releasing hormone, the pituitary does not secrete gonadotropins at midcycle to stimulate ovulation. The endometrium of the uterus becomes thin, and the cervical mucus becomes thick and impervious to sperm.

Side effects and contraindications: Women who develop breakthrough bleeding while taking OCs should be given a combination with a higher ratio of estrogen; ie, a more estrogenic formulation. For women who develop amenorrhea, the progestogenic component should be decreased. Many side effects, such as nausea, breast tenderness, fluid retention, higher BP, and depression, are related to the dose of estrogen. Progestogens produce anabolic effects, such as weight gain, acne, and a sensation perceived by some women as nervousness. Levonorgestrel is 10 to 20 times as potent per unit weight as the other 3 progestogens used in OCs—norethindrone, norethindrone acetate, and ethynodiol diacetate, which are about equal in potency.

In addition to affecting the female genital tract, the metabolic activities of synthetic hormonal components of OCs affect nearly every other organ system. Serious complications, however, are relatively rare. **Absolute contraindications** to OCs besides smoking after age 35 include pregnancy, active liver disease, hyperlipidemia, uncontrolled hypertension, diabetes mellitus with vascular changes, prolonged immobilization of a lower extremity, and a history of thromboembolic phenomena, thrombophlebitis, coronary artery disease, stroke, sickle cell disease, estrogen-dependent cancer, liver adenoma, and cholestatic jaundice of pregnancy. **Relative contraindications** include depression, migraine headache, oligomenorrhea, undiagnosed amenorrhea, and heavy cigarette smoking under age 35.

Inhibition of ovulation persists in a few women after they stop taking the tablets, but OCs do not cause permanent sterility or affect the outcome of pregnancies conceived any time after their discontinuance. OCs taken early in pregnancy do not adversely affect the fetus.

Most **serum protein changes** that occur during OC therapy do not represent medical hazards, but *results of some clinical laboratory tests are altered.* Serum copper and iron levels increase, while tests of thyroid function are altered to the same extent as in pregnancy; eg, thyroxin-binding globulin capacity increases, while free thyroxine remains normal. There is no evidence that OCs alter thyroid function itself. However, increased levels of the globulins involved in the clotting process, particularly factors VII and X, result in a hypercoagulable state.

The incidence of **deep vein thrombophlebitis** and **thromboembolism** in OC users is estimated to be 3 to 4 times higher than in nonusers in healthy women using 50-μg or higher estrogen formulations. Thrombus formation appears to be related to increases in blood-clotting factors (and, possibly, increased platelet adhesion) produced by the estrogenic component. The incidence of thromboembolic disorders has steadily decreased as amounts of estrogen in the formulations have been lowered. There is no evidence that the incidence of thromboembolism is increased in women with varicosities of the leg veins. If a woman develops signs of deep vein thrombophlebitis or pulmonary embolism while receiving OCs, she should discontinue them and further diagnostic studies should be done. Because of the increased risk of thromboembolic disease, OCs should be discontinued 1 mo before elective surgery and not restarted until 1 mo after surgery.

CNS effects of OCs include nausea and vomiting, headache, and depression. The risk of stroke was previously estimated to be greater in OC users, but recent epidemiologic studies, in which formulations with lower doses of estrogen were used, have shown the incidence to be no different in healthy OC users than in healthy nonusers of similar age. Women who have headaches more frequently or develop any peripheral neurologic symptoms, fainting, or aphasia while taking OCs should discontinue them, since these symptoms may be prodromes of a stroke. Depression and sleep disturbances are noted in 1 to 2% of OC users.

Estrogen increases production of angiotensin, which causes some OC users to develop **increased BP**; the incidence is lower with lower-dose estrogen formulations. BP should be monitored in all women before and during treatment with OCs. If BP increases, OCs should be discontinued, and usually it will return to normal.

Alterations in glucose metabolism, both impairment of glucose tolerance and increase in plasma insulin levels due to peripheral insulin resistance, have been associated with the progestogen component of OCs. These changes are usually reversible and rarely occur with low progestogen dose formulations. OCs can be prescribed for patients who previously had an elevated blood glucose test but are not currently diabetic. A 2-h postprandial blood glucose test should be performed annually in all women using OCs who are likely to develop diabetes mellitus; eg, those who have a family history, whose infants were large at birth, or who have a history of unexplained fetal deaths. If this test is abnormal, a glucose tolerance test should be performed and, if abnormal, the OCs should be stopped. OCs are not recommended for insulin-dependent diabetics with vascular changes, because their use may increase the risk of cardiovascular disease.

Estrogens may cause **sodium retention**; some users develop **edema** and may gain 3 to 5 lb in weight. Progestogens are anabolic, and some women gain weight because of increased appetite. Thus, if a woman gains > 10 lb/yr, an OC containing a less potent progestogen should be used or, if the woman has tried unsuccessfully to lose weight, OCs should be discontinued.

Serum levels of some vitamins, trace elements, and lipids may be altered by OCs. Levels of pyridoxine, folic acid, and most other B vitamins, as well as ascorbic acid, calcium, manganese, and zinc, are decreased, while vitamin A levels are increased. These changes have no known clinical significance, and women taking OCs do not need vitamin supplements. Serum lipid levels may be slightly altered with high progestogen dose formulations but not with lower-dose formulations.

Drug interactions: Although synthetic sex steroids can retard biotransformation of certain drugs such as antipyrine and meperidine because of substrate competition, such interference is not important clinically. OC use has not been shown to inhibit the actions of other drugs. However, certain drugs (barbiturates, sulfonamides, cyclophosphamide, and rifampin) can interfere with the action of OCs by inducing liver enzymes that accelerate biotransformation of the steroids to more polar and less biologically active metabolites. A relatively high incidence of OC failure has been reported in women taking rifampin, and the 2 agents should not be given concurrently. Data concerning OC failure in users of other antibiotics (eg, penicillin, ampicillin, and sulfonamides) and other agents (eg, phenytoin and phenobarbital) are based on anecdotal reports and are less clear. However, when therapeutic doses of antibiotics are also prescribed, use of a barrier method may be suggested in addition to the OCs. Epileptic patients who take phenobarbital daily should use a 50-µg estrogen formulation, since they have an increased incidence of abnormal bleeding with lower estrogen dose formulations.

The incidence of **cholelithiasis** in OC users increases during the first few years of use and then declines. Thus, OCs accelerate gallstone formation but do not cause new stones to form. Women who develop **idiopathic recurrent jaundice of pregnancy** (cholestasis of pregnancy) may also become jaundiced when treated with OCs and should not use them. **Active liver disease** is another contraindication to hormonal contraceptive therapy, but hepatitis followed by complete recovery is not an absolute contraindication. Women with a history of liver disease should have normal liver function before taking OCs. Rarely, **benign liver adenomas** develop in OC users and may rupture spontaneously. The incidence, which is related to duration of use and dose of the formulation, is estimated to be about1/30,000 to 500,000 users. The adenomas usually regress spontaneously after therapy is stopped. **Hepatic vein thrombosis** with Budd-Chiari syndrome has occurred in OC users, but a causal relationship has not been established.

Melasma, similar to that which develops in pregnancy, occurs in some patients receiving OCs. This change is accentuated by exposure to sunlight and disappears slowly after stopping the OCs. Since treatment is difficult (see HYPERPIG-MENTATION in Ch. 101), OCs should be stopped as soon as melasma becomes apparent.

The risk of **breast cancer** is not increased in OC users overall nor in high-risk subgroups such as those with a family history of breast cancer. After 30 yr of OC use in humans, vast amounts of epidemiologic data have been amassed regarding the neoplastic effects of OCs. Although some studies show an increased risk of breast cancer in certain groups of OC users, other studies do not confirm such an association. Because of the conflicting results of studies, an FDA advisory committee recently stated that there should be no change in OC use or prescribing. Several other epidemiologic studies show that **cervical neoplasia** is increased in OC users, particularly those who have used OCs for > 5 yr. A causal relationship has not been established, but such women need to have cytologic screening performed at least annually. A number of studies have shown that OC use decreases the risk of the lethal endometrial and ovarian cancers by about 50%, and this reduced risk persists after OC use is stopped. Other documented noncontraceptive health benefits of OC use include decreased incidences of menorrhagia, dysmenorrhea, premenstrual tension, iron-deficiency anemia, benign breast disease, and functional ovarian cysts; reduced incidences of ectopic pregnancy and salpingitis associated with their use should decrease infertility. These benefits result in an estimated reduction of 50,000 hospitalizations/year in the USA.

Subdermal Implant

Polysiloxone capsules containing levonorgestrel are inserted subcutaneously in the upper arm; when released, the drug inhibits ovulation and prevents sperm from penetrating the thick cervical mucus. A small incision is made under local anesthesia in an outpatient setting. Then 6 capsules are inserted through a 10-gauge trocar in a fan-shaped pattern to obtain sufficiently high circulating levels of levonorgestrel for effective contraception. The incision is closed without sutures. The capsules remain in place and are effective for 5 yr, with a cumulative pregnancy rate of $< 2\%$.

The major side effects are irregular uterine bleeding and amenorrhea. Headache and weight gain may also prompt premature removal of the capsules. With proper counseling, many women choose to continue using this method of contraception after 5 yr, but because the capsules are not biodegradable, they need to be removed and replaced. Removal is similar to insertion but more difficult because fibrosis develops around the capsules. Normal ovarian activity and return of fertility resume immediately after removal.

Intrauterine Device (IUD)

Only about 1 million women in the USA use IUDs for contraception, even though they are very effective. IUDs have some advantages over OCs: their effects are limited to the female genital tract, and insertion requires only one decision by the patient. Only 2 types of IUDs are currently marketed in the USA; the progesterone-releasing IUD needs to be inserted annually, while the copper-bearing T380A is effective for at least 6 yr. Pregnancy rates at the end of 6 yr of use with this device are $< 2\%$. Although it had been advised that the IUD be inserted during menstruation, the device can be inserted at any time in the cycle, provided the woman is not pregnant. A high fundal insertion must be obtained for the device to be effective.

Discontinuance rates for the T380A are higher in the first year than in subsequent years, but only about 10 to 15% of patients who receive proper counseling discontinue use in the first year. There is no need to change a plastic unmedicated IUD unless the patient develops increased bleeding after it has been in place for > 1 yr. The roughness of calcium salts deposited on the plastic over time, however, can cause ulceration and bleeding of the endometrium. If increased bleeding develops after 1 yr or more, the old IUD should be removed and a new one inserted.

Physiology: A sterile tissue reaction in the endometrial cavity is generally accepted as the main cause of the contraceptive effect. Bacterial contamination is present for 24 h after insertion of an IUD, and although the endometrial cavity rapidly becomes sterile, inflammation persists after the bacterial infection disappears. Breakdown products of intrauterine neutrophils are toxic to the sperm and blastocyst; this is the major means by which IUDs prevent fertilization. The inflammatory foreign body reaction ceases when the IUD is removed. The monthly incidence of conception in the first year after removal of an

IUD is the same as after stopping the use of condoms or diaphragms; at the end of 1 yr, 90% of women who wish to conceive have done so.

Side effects and complications: Bleeding and pain are the major medical reasons for removing an IUD; these problems account for > 50% of all discontinuances and occur in about 15% of patients during the first year and 7% during the second year of use. Insertion during menses is usually less painful than at other times in the menstrual cycle.

The **expulsion rate** for most devices is greatest during the first year (about 10%) and occurs most frequently in the first few months after insertion. The expulsion rate is higher in younger women and in nulligravidas. If another IUD is inserted, there is a good chance it will be retained. *About 20% of expulsions are unnoticed and can be followed by an unwanted pregnancy;* therefore, a plastic string should be attached to the IUD so that the user can check periodically, especially after menses, to see that the device has not been expelled.

Perforation of the uterus is a potentially serious but uncommon problem; for devices in current use it occurs in about 1/1000 insertions. Perforation occurs during insertion. Sometimes only the distal portion of the IUD penetrates the uterine muscle during insertion; then uterine contractions during the next few months force the IUD into the peritoneal cavity. Perforation should always be suspected if a patient states she cannot feel the string but did not notice that the device was expelled. If the device or the tail is not visible after pelvic examination, the uterine cavity should be probed (unless pregnancy is suspected). If the IUD cannot be felt with a uterine sound or biopsy instrument, a sonogram or a lateral x-ray with contrast medium inside the uterine cavity should be obtained (an IUD located in the cul-de-sac can be missed on an ordinary anteroposterior film). All intraperitoneal IUDs should be removed, as they may cause bowel adhesions. Extrauterine IUDs containing copper can cause severe intraperitoneal reactions and should be removed promptly, usually via laparoscopy.

Bacterial contamination of the endometrial cavity occurs at the time of insertion and clears after 24 h. IUD appendages do not provide continuous access for bacteria to enter the endometrial cavity. However, an IUD should not be inserted in a patient with clinical evidence of salpingitis, since additional bacteria would be introduced. Most infections occurring after an IUD has been in place for ≥ 30 days are sexually transmitted and are not caused by the IUD; they can be treated without removing it, unless the infection is severe or the patient is pregnant. Although IUD users have a three-fold greater incidence of clinical salpingitis than nonusers, the increased risk with copper IUDs occurs during only the first 4 mo after insertion and probably is related to bacteria introduced during insertion. Prophylactic systemic antibiotic use following insertion is not cost-effective. An IUD should not be inserted if there is clinical evidence of cervicitis. Since the shield type of IUD with its multifilament tail string has been associated with increased risk of salpingitis, all IUDs of this type should be removed. Individuals at high risk for developing salpingitis, including those with a prior history of pelvic inflammatory disease, nulliparous women < 25 yr of age, and women with multiple sexual partners, should not use IUDs.

The incidence of congenital defects in babies born to mothers with an IUD in place is no greater than that of the general population; nor is the incidence of fetal death increased, but the incidence of **spontaneous abortion** is significantly higher (about 55%). If a woman who becomes pregnant with an IUD in place wishes to continue the pregnancy and the appendage is visible, the IUD should be removed, since the abortion rate is lower after removal of the device. The IUD will not be located in the amniotic sac, since implantation does not occur immediately adjacent to the device. If the appendage is not visible, the uterus should not be probed in an attempt to remove the IUD. A number of serious and even fatal **systemic infections** have been reported in women who became pregnant with the IUD (particularly the shield type with its multifilament tail) in place; thus, it is recommended that the IUD be removed if pregnancy occurs and the string is visible. If the string is not visible, removal will result in abortion. *Therefore, if the patient refuses removal and wants to retain the pregnancy, she must be warned of the possibility of sepsis and should report symptoms of infection promptly.* If uterine infection during pregnancy occurs with an IUD in place, appropriate antibiotics should be given and the endometrial cavity should be evacuated.

Pregnancies overall are effectively prevented by IUDs; however, a woman who becomes pregnant with an IUD in place has about a ten-fold greater than normal (or 3 to 9%) chance of having an **ectopic pregnancy.** After an induced abortion for an IUD failure, the uterine contents should be examined histologically to ensure that the gestation was intrauterine.

Several long-term studies have shown no clinical evidence that IUDs cause adenocarcinoma of the endometrium or carcinoma of the cervix.

STERILIZATION

One partner is sterilized in about 1/3 of all married couples in the USA who use some method of family planning. Sterilization is the most popular contraceptive method for couples in whom the wife is over age 30. *Sterilization should always be considered permanent.* Both partners should be counseled regarding the risks and irreversibility of the procedures. The reconstructive operation (reanastomosis) is much more difficult following vasectomy than tubal ligation. Pregnancy rates are 45 to 60% following reanastomosis of the vas, 50 to 80% following oviduct reanastomosis.

Sterilization in men is by vasectomy, an outpatient procedure of about 20 min that requires only local anesthesia. The vas deferens is isolated and cut, the ends of the vas are closed by either ligation or fulguration and then replaced in the scrotal sac, and the incision is closed. About 15 to 20 ejaculations are usually required after the operation before sterility is achieved. Semen analysis should be performed after the procedure, and *the man is not considered sterile until 2 sperm-free ejaculates have been produced.* Complications of vasectomy include hematoma (incidence ≤ 5%), sperm granulomas (inflammatory responses to sperm leakage), and spontaneous reanastomosis, which usually occurs shortly after the procedure.

Female sterilization is by tubal ligation, a more complicated procedure requiring an intraperitoneal incision and general or local anesthesia. Ligation can be performed through a small infraumbilical incision either immediately after delivery in the operating room or the following day without prolonging the hospital stay. The same operative techniques can be used for female sterilization at other times (interval sterilization). The oviducts can usually be easily and rapidly ligated through an abdominal incision or through a colpotomy incision. If a small, 2-cm suprapubic incision is made (minilaparotomy), the patient may be cared for in an ambulatory surgery setting, as with laparoscopy (see below). The minilaparotomy is usually performed under general anesthesia, but it can also be done under local anesthesia. The same technique can be

used as is used with laparoscopy—eg, fulguration; occluding the tubes with bands or clips; or ligation/partial excision, such as the Pomeroy method.

Laparoscopy has become a popular gynecologic operative technique. Working through the laparoscope, the physician fulgurates the oviducts and cuts through 1 or 2 small intraperitoneal punctures. Although general anesthesia is usually used for laparoscopic sterilization, the patient does not have to be hospitalized overnight. The failure rate following laparoscopic fulguration is reported to be only 1/1000 procedures, but a high percentage of such pregnancies are ectopic. The incidence of complications following laparoscopic fulguration ranges from 1 to 6%; major complications, such as hemorrhage or puncture or burns of the bowel, occur at a rate of 0.6%. Because the rate of bowel injury is lower with bipolar than with unipolar coagulation operations, the former should always be used for fulguration.

Various mechanical devices (Silastic bands and spring-loaded clips) are currently being used to occlude the tubes instead of fulgurating or cutting them, thereby avoiding problems associated with electric current. Because these devices cause less tissue damage, such sterilization is potentially more reversible, but even with microsurgical techniques, reversibility rates are only about 75%.

Elective vaginal hysterectomy is accepted for sterilization alone in some communities. If other chronic problems with the uterus exist (such as menorrhagia, cervical dysplasia, or severe dysmenorrhea), abdominal or vaginal hysterectomy may be the preferred method of sterilization. Although the morbidity, blood loss, and hospital stay are greater after hysterectomy than after tubal sterilization, there are long-term benefits, such as 100% effectiveness, the absence of menstrual disorders, and the prevention of possible development of leiomyomas or cancer.

INDUCED ABORTION

Throughout history, women have used abortion to terminate unwanted pregnancies. Its legal status worldwide varies from complete prohibition to elective procedures on request. Legal abortion is available to about 2/3 of the women in the world; about 1/12 of all women are in countries with strictly enforced abortion prohibitions. In the USA, abortion is permitted on request in the first trimester; after that, abortion is regulated by each state in ways reasonably related to maternal health.

The number of reported abortions in the USA has progressively increased, especially since 1974, when the laws were liberalized. In 1963, the *rate* of abortions was 0.13/1000 women in childbearing years (ages 15 to 44); in 1984, the rate was 26.9/1000. Therefore, $\approx$ 3% of women aged 15 to 44 have abortions in a year. The ratio of abortions to live births increased more markedly, from 13/1000 in 1963 to 287/1000 in 1985. Thus, in 1985, 30% of all pregnancies in the USA were terminated by abortion. Abortion is one of the most common surgical procedures in the USA; > 1.5 million abortions were reported in 1985. About 27% of women having abortions were under age 20, 35% were 20 to 24, and the remaining 38% were 25 or older; 19% of the women were married. In 1983, > 90% of abortions were in the first trimester (12 wk or less), with > 50% of these at 8 wk or less. About 97% were performed by curettage; 3% by saline, prostaglandin, or urea instillation; and < 0.1% by other methods, including major surgical procedures.

Abortion methods currently used are (1) instrumental evacuation through the vagina; (2) medical induction, with stimulation of uterine contractions; and (3) uterine surgery (hysterotomy or hysterectomy). The procedure varies with the length of gestation. Weeks of gestation are calculated from the *last menstrual period*, with the assumption that ovulation occurred at about day 14 of the cycle. **Instrumental evacuation** is used in 97% of abortions. In pregnancies < 12 wk, curettage is virtually the only procedure used. **Suction curettage** at 4 to 6 wk of gestation (sometimes called "menstrual extraction," a term from earlier days when sensitive early pregnancy tests were not readily available) requires little or no dilatation of the cervix. The curet most commonly used is a small, flexible cannula (4, 5, or 6 mm in diameter); rigid, 6-mm plastic curets are also used, as well as metal endometrial aspiration biopsy curets. The cannula, attached to a vacuum source (usually a machine suction pump, but hand pumps and occasionally vacuum syringes are also used), is inserted through the cervix. The uterine cavity is gently and thoroughly curetted. Failure to terminate the pregnancy occurs more frequently in these early weeks than later.

After 7 wk of gestation, the cervix usually requires dilatation in order to use the larger-diameter suction curets needed to evacuate the larger amount of products of conception. The cervix may be gently dilated by using tapered dilators of progressively increased sizes until the diameter of the desired cannula is reached. The size of the disposable cannula generally correlates with gestational age—eg, 8 mm for 8 wk of gestation, up to a maximum of 10 mm for 12 wk. To reduce potential injury to the cervix by mechanical dilatation, *Laminaria* (dried seaweed stems) or other osmotic dilators are frequently used. They are inserted into the cervical canal through the internal os and left for 4 to 5 h, usually overnight; expansion of the *Laminaria* and/or stimulation of prostaglandin release dilates the cervix.

In pregnancies of > 12 wk, dilatation and evacuation (**D & E**) is the method most commonly used; it is increasingly replacing medical methods of termination because its rate of serious complications is lower. Before 1979, patients with gestations of 13 to 15 wk had to wait until 16 wk, when medical induction could be effectively performed. Currently, D & E is most often used for termination at 13 to 15 wk and has replaced amniotic instillation as the method most commonly used at 16 to 20 wk. In this procedure (after 12 wk), the cervix is dilated (usually with multiple *Laminaria* or other osmotic dilators); forceps are used to dismember and remove the fetus; and a 14- to 16-mm suction cannula is used to aspirate the amniotic fluid, placenta, and fetal debris. In more advanced pregnancies, multiple *Laminaria* may be used to gently dilate the cervix to 3 to 4 cm to make the evacuation easier and safer. D & E requires more skill than does suction curettage.

Although D & E has been shown to have lower rates of minor morbidity than medical induction through 20 wk, medical induction is still used—especially after 18 wk—because D & E has a greater risk of major morbidity (including bowel injury and uterine injury requiring hysterectomy).

First trimester abortion has been performed without **anesthesia**. However, since the procedure usually produces considerable pain, anesthesia should be used for humane reasons and also because the operator is more likely to remove all of the tissue if the patient is not in acute discomfort. In the first trimester, local anesthesia is more commonly used, with paracervical block the preferred method. Local anesthetic is injected into the paracervical tissue at 4 and 8 o'clock and into the anterior cervix; after a 6- to

8-min wait, good anesthesia is usually obtained. Local or general anesthesia is used for D & E.

Abortion may be initiated by **medical induction** of uterine contractions, especially in the 2nd trimester. In the USA, the most common procedure involves instilling hypertonic saline solution via a needle through the abdominal wall and uterus into the amniotic sac. Commonly, 50 to 200 mL of amniotic fluid is removed, and 200 mL of hypertonic (20%) saline is carefully injected into the sac. Labor usually starts within 24 h; fetus and placenta are delivered about 36 h after instillation. To expedite the abortion, augmenting agents such as *Laminaria,* oxytocin, or prostaglandins are usually used. Complications include hypernatremia, coagulopathy, hemorrhage, infection, and cervical injuries.

Prostaglandins (see also Ch. 142) stimulate uterine contractions. Either vaginal prostaglandin E_2 (dinoprostone) suppositories or IM injections of 15-methylprostaglandin $F_{2\alpha}$ (dinoprost tromethamine) can be used. This method has a shorter installation-to-abortion time but an increased incidence of retained placenta and is more likely to result in abortion of a live fetus. Using IV oxytocins accelerates the process but increases the risk of lower uterine tears and hypernatremia. The suppositories are more commonly used to supplement other methods, especially when membranes rupture without active contractions occurring. Using *Laminaria* or other osmotic dilators singly or multiply in the 2nd trimester prior to medical induction usually shortens labor and decreases the incidence of cervicovaginal lacerations. Side effects of prostaglandins include nausea, vomiting, diarrhea, hyperthermia, facial flushing, vasovagal symptoms, and bronchospasm. Prostaglandins may precipitate bronchial asthma in susceptible patients; in those with severe kidney and liver disease, activation of the drug may be decreased; patients with epilepsy may develop seizures.

Mifepristone (RU 486), a progesterone-receptor blocker, when combined with a prostaglandin is very effective in terminating pregnancy of < 7 wk. Currently, this drug is available only in France.

One major surgical procedure, **hysterotomy**—in essence a cesarean section—is rarely indicated. The uterine scar increases the risk of uterine rupture in a subsequent pregnancy. **Hysterectomy** should be reserved for women who have had a previous indication for this procedure and who recognize that permanent sterilization

follows. The mortality of these procedures is 44 times that of a first-trimester curettage.

Complications

Complication rates are directly related to the gestational age and to the method used. They increase with advancing gestational age. If any doubt exists about the gestational age, an ultrasound examination should be done. Bleeding after conception may be misconstrued as the "last menstrual period"; the retroflexed uterus as well as the uterus of an obese patient may be difficult to assess. Serious early complications include perforation of the uterus (0.1%) by one of the instruments used for abortion (sometimes the intestine or other organs are also injured); major hemorrhage (0.06%) may occur secondary to trauma or atonic uterus; late hemorrhage may be due to retained placenta or infection. Laceration of the cervix (0.1 to 1%) ranges from superficial tenaculum tears to cervicovaginal fistula (associated with an instillation procedure in the 2nd trimester). Untoward effects of general or local anesthesia may occur. Additional complications of medical inductions have been noted previously.

The most frequent delayed complications include postabortion bleeding due to retention of placenta fragments; infection (0.1 to 2%), ranging from mild endometritis to severe pelvic inflammation, peritonitis, and septicemia; and thrombophlebitis. Sterility may occur secondary to pelvic infection or from synechiae in the endometrial cavity. Rh sensitization may occur in susceptible Rh-negative women if Rh immune globulin is not used. The effect of elective abortion on subsequent pregnancies continues to be disputed. Recent extensive studies report no significantly increased risk. Forceful dilatation of the cervix in more advanced pregnancies may predispose to incompetent cervix. Complication rates, including mortality, have progressively decreased, especially since 1972. The safest method is suction curettage, followed by D & C, D & E, prostaglandin instillation, saline instillation, hysterotomy, and hysterectomy.

In general, contraception has a much lower complication rate than abortion, especially for young women. The serious complication rate for abortion is < 1% and the mortality rate is < 1 death/100,000 cases. Morbidity in permanent sterilization with tubal ligation is ≈ 5%; mortality is < 4/100,000 cases. Maternal mortality in 1982 was 8.9/100,000 live births; the rate for nonwhite women was 3 times the rate for white women, and the rate for women > 35 was 3 times the rate for younger women. Therefore, contraception or sterilization should be used to *prevent* unwanted pregnancy, and abortion should be used when safer techniques fail.

Psychologic Aspects

For most women, abortion is not a threat to mental well-being and has no adverse psychologic sequelae. Before abortion was easily and legally obtainable, psychologic difficulties may have been related more to the problems and stress desperate women encountered in obtaining the procedure. The women more prone to psychologic sequelae are those who had psychiatric symptoms before pregnancy, who terminated a desired pregnancy for medical reasons (maternal or fetal), who have considerable ambivalence, who are young adolescents, or who had an abortion at late gestational age.

5. COMMON GYNECOLOGIC PROBLEMS
(See also Chs. 6 and 7)

PELVIC PAIN

Pelvic pain is a common complaint. Its nature and intensity may fluctuate, and its cause is often obscure. Pelvic pain may originate in genital or extragenital organs; in some cases no disease can be shown. Causes include intense muscular contractions or cramps, inflammation or direct irritation of nerves, and psychogenic factors. Both smooth and skeletal muscles can produce pain by strong or sustained contractions resulting from overdistention or obstruction of a hollow viscus, ischemia, or tetany. Nerves can be irritated by acute or chronic trauma, fibrosis, pressure, or intraperitoneal inflammation. Psychogenic factors can cause pain or aggravate minor aches. Often pelvic pain has multiple causes.

In evaluating acute lower abdominal pain, prompt decisions must be made about which conditions are surgical emergencies; ie, twisted ovarian cyst, ectopic pregnancy, ruptured tuboovarian abscess, appendicitis, and bowel perforation. A ruptured corpus luteum cyst and pelvic inflammation are usually treated medically.

The cause of pelvic pain can often be established by a thorough history, with special attention to type of discomfort; distribution and radiation of pain; time and suddenness of onset; circumstances at onset; duration of pain; associated symptoms; relation to various activities such as movement or defecation; frequency of recurrence; and relationship to the menstrual cycle, sleep, coitus, eating, and micturition. Physical and laboratory findings aid the diagnosis.

Differential Diagnosis

Colicky pain is caused by contraction of an obstructed hollow viscus (eg, intestine, ureter, gallbladder, appendix). **Sudden onset of pain** usually results from ischemia (eg, twisted ovarian cyst) or sudden perforation and spillage into the peritoneal cavity. A more insidious onset over several hours occurs with inflammation or obstruction (eg, salpingitis, appendicitis, intestinal obstruction). **Localized pain** may represent a localized inflammation or a problem with one adnexum or part of the uterus. **Pain involving the entire abdomen** suggests a generalized reaction (eg, flooding of the peritoneum with blood, pus, or intestinal contents). Pain from intraperitoneal irritation usually increases with abdominal, general body, or bowel or bladder movement or with examination. A **tender adnexal mass** suggests an ectopic pregnancy, ovarian cyst, or inflammatory mass. **Vomiting** occurs early with acute appendicitis or cholecystitis and may or may not accompany salpingitis or pyelonephritis; it occurs later with bowel obstruction.

Pain of genital origin: Sudden, severe pelvic pain associated with a pelvic mass is usually not difficult to diagnose. Less severe and especially chronic pain makes the diagnosis less obvious unless a mass is present. However, the mass may not be the cause of the pain. **Acute salpingitis,** usually bilateral, causes severe lower abdominal pain and tenderness, especially on movement of the cervix. The pain is often accompanied by low- to high-grade fever, leukocytosis, and a purulent discharge from the cervical canal. Generally, few findings are related to the GI tract, and no mass is present during the first few days of symptoms. If salpingitis persists for several days, a pelvic abscess may develop, most often pointing toward the vagina or rectum. A sudden easing of symptoms may mean that the abscess has ruptured intra-abdominally and immediate laparotomy is required.

Ectopic pregnancy is most commonly signaled by pelvic pain, menstrual irregularity, and an adnexal mass (see Ch. 15). In pregnant women, sudden pelvic pain also may be caused by an associated torsion of an ovarian cyst, acute degeneration of a uterine myoma, placental abruption, rupture of the uterus, or if fever is present, parametritis.

Ovarian cysts, including malignant tumors, are frequently asymptomatic, but the pressure of an abdominal mass may cause discomfort, aching, or heaviness. Sudden or sharp pain may indicate rupture, hemorrhage, or torsion; varying degrees of tenderness, fever, leukocytosis, or signs of shock may be present. Hemorrhage into a cyst is common and produces pain. Follicular or corpus luteum cysts with thin walls usually bleed very little when ruptured and are treated conservatively. Cysts with thicker walls rarely rupture. Severe peritonitis can follow a catastrophic intra-abdominal event (eg, ruptured dermoid cyst, perforated endometrioma), producing intra-abdominal hemorrhage. A twisted ovarian cyst produces intermittent colicky pain; the cyst should be removed without untwisting the pedicle, which might risk an embolism. Malposition of the uterus rarely causes pelvic pain unless it is retrodisplaced and fixed by adhesions or scar tissue. An invasive neoplasm may cause pain as a result of invasion of pelvic tissue or pelvic nerve roots.

Endometriosis may cause pain and tenderness by acting directly on nerve endings or by interfering with functions of involved or adjacent organs. Characteristically, the pain is worse a few days before menstruation and during the early period of flow. Occasionally a patient has severe pain for a few hours during midcycle (mittelschmerz) from ovarian bleeding following ovulation; this pain may be mistakenly diagnosed as appendicitis.

Pelvic congestion, occurring most commonly between ages 30 and 50, may cause discomfort 7 to 10 days before menses. Pelvic pain present on sitting or standing but relieved by lying down is frequently accompanied by low back and leg aches, increased vaginal discharge, and dyspareunia. The condition may worsen with stress or anxiety that accompanies premenstrual symptoms of fatigue, headache, and insomnia. The uterus is usually tender and may be retroverted. The condition may result from chronic pelvic hyperemia and vascular congestion or psychosomatic factors.

Pain with intercourse (dyspareunia) is discussed in Ch. 55.

Pain of extragenital origin: Most pelvic pain of extragenital origin is related to the urologic or GI systems, skeletal and supporting tissues, or psychologic factors. Pain of urologic origin is frequently associated with urinary symptoms such as frequency, dysuria, burning, fever, chills, hematuria, and ureteral colic. Occasionally, the only finding is tenderness in the suprapubic or bladder trigone area. Urinalysis, cystoscopy, urography, and urodynamic studies are usually helpful in diagnosis.

Pain of musculoskeletal origin from the spine or pelvis may occur at the site of involvement or may be referred. Pain that radiates down the legs or is aggravated by the motion of the involved part rather than by vaginoabdominal or rectovaginal examination suggests a skeletal cause, as does pain or hyperesthesia in other pelvic areas, such as the skin or abdominal wall. Various disturbances in the pelvic supporting tissues (eg, cystocele, rectocele, and uterine descensus) can produce symptoms of pressure, pelvic heaviness, and insecurity ("as if the organs will drop out"). Pelvic tumors and threatened abortion may produce a similar discomfort. The slow progression of symptom severity makes some patients irritable, while others adapt and are not even aware of the symptoms until surgical correction relieves the anatomic displacements. Backache is common but seldom due to gynecologic disorder except in cases of advanced tumors. Backache may be caused by poor posture, lack of exercise, strain or other trauma, or a primary disease of the skeletal system (eg, osteoporosis, herniated nucleus pulposus, osteoarthritis, or bone tumor). In some women, pelvic joints are loosened so much during pregnancy that motion is painful; this diagnosis can be confirmed (and symptoms relieved) by tightening a belt around the pelvic girdle to stabilize the bony pelvis.

Pain originating from the GI tract or its appendages, especially appendicitis or diverticulitis, is often confused with pain of gynecologic origin. In GI disorders, tenderness and accompanying muscle spasm usually are more intense away from the uterine and adnexal area, while nausea, vomiting, and disturbance of bowel motility (diarrhea or constipation) are more pronounced. Peritonitis from pelvic infection is difficult to differentiate from that with a bowel origin. During pregnancy, the pain of appendicitis tends to be less severe and more variable in intensity; after the first trimester, it may occur higher in the abdomen. If pelvic pain is predominantly left-sided and recurrent, the possibility of diverticulitis should be considered. Functional bowel disease (irritable or spastic colon) is often diagnosed in patients complaining of pelvic pain. The pain is not directly related to eating. The colon may be palpable and tender; rolling the examining fingers across the colon usually reproduces the pain. Whenever the diagnosis is not clear but the findings do not require immediate surgery and GI symptoms predominate, further search for the cause is indicated. Surgical emergencies must be ruled out, but if the pain is not progressive and if fever and leukocytosis are not present, endoscopy and radiologic studies of the gallbladder and bowel usually can be deferred until after the acute episode. However, ultrasound studies during the episode can reveal the presence of stones in the gallbladder or GU tract. If any doubt exists that acute surgical conditions can be ruled out, surgery usually is indicated without undue delay.

In **psychogenic pain**, extensive laboratory studies may be needed to rule out other disorders. WBC counts help to establish the presence or absence of infection, and other hematologic studies rule out porphyria and blood dyscrasias. Radiologic and ultrasound studies rule out gallbladder and GI or urinary tract disease. Endoscopic examination and psychiatric or orthopedic evaluation may be indicated. Surgery, except for diagnostic endoscopy, is seldom indicated unless there is unmistakable evidence that it will correct the cause of the pain; exploratory laparotomy should rarely be needed for diagnosis. Diagnostic laparoscopy for pelvic examination may be useful, especially for early diagnosis of ectopic pregnancy, differential diagnosis of appendicitis vs. pelvic inflammation, and endometriosis.

Treatment

Treatment of pelvic pain should be directed at the specific cause but may be only symptomatic. Hypnosis by experienced persons has been useful in relieving pelvic pain due to functional causes that are not amenable to surgery. Presacral and sacrouterine neurectomy can be helpful in selected patients, especially those with endometriosis. Nerve block or transection may be helpful in inoperable malignancies, but usually the disease has spread beyond the area that can be included in the nerve block.

VULVOVAGINITIS

Infectious diseases and other inflammatory conditions affecting the vaginal mucosa and often secondarily involving the vulva; vaginal discharge is common.

Etiology

Most vulvovaginitis and symptomatic vaginal discharges are caused by bacteria, usually *Gardnerella vaginalis* in combination with various anaerobes. Protozoa (*Trichomonas vaginalis*) cause $1/3$ of all cases, *Candida* is a frequent cause in pregnant women and diabetics, and occasionally oral contraceptives increase susceptibility. Another major cause is the human papillomavirus (**HPV**), which has many types. Type 6 is most commonly associated with vaginal infection, as are types 11, 16, and 18 to a lesser degree (the latter 2 with cervical dysplasia and malignancy). Less commonly encountered are types 31, 33, 35, 39, 41, 42, 43, 44, 51, 52, and 56. Other less common causes are other bacteria (eg, *Neisseria gonorrhoeae*, members of the *Chlamydia* and *Mycoplasma* groups, streptococci, *Escherichia coli*, and staphylococci), foreign bodies, viral infections (herpes simplex), pinworms (*Enterobius vermicularis*), fistulas, radiation, and tumors of the genital tract. Extensive vaginal and cervical adenosis, as found in some women exposed to diethylstilbestrol (**DES**), may produce excessive discharge. Frequent douching, especially with chemicals, may disturb normal vaginal milieu. Deodorant sprays, laundry soaps and fabric softeners, and bath water additives may cause vulvar irritation. Tight, nonporous, nonabsorbent underclothing, as well as poor hygiene, may foster fungal and bacterial growth. Occasionally, sensitivity to spermicides, coital lubricants, or latex in a diaphragm or condom causes irritation.

Age groups must also be considered in determining etiology because of differences in estrogen and sexual activity. In the reproductive years, when estrogen is present, vulvitis is usually secondary to vaginal infection, whereas in premenarchal and postmenopausal years, vulvitis alone is common.

Newborns may have a sterile mucoid discharge secondary to the maternal estrogen effect that subsides in < 2 wk; a small amount of bleeding may occur from this "estrogen withdrawal" effect.

In **children,** *E. coli* is most commonly found with vulvitis; streptococci, staphylococci, and *Candida* are found less often. Occasionally, pinworms or *N. gonorrhoeae* cause infection. Bubble baths or soaps may cause irritation. When discharge is present, especially with blood, a foreign body must be considered, as well as a DES-related tumor. Immature anatomy and poor hygiene contribute to infection; premenarchal girls have small labia minora, thin vaginal mucosa, and little cervical secretion. Discharge is scant and usually alkaline in pH, with few bacteria. The amount of discharge increases when estrogen production increases, up to a year or more before menarche.

In **females of reproductive age,** a milky-white, watery or mucoid discharge arises primarily from the cervix or as a result of desquamation of vaginal cells. The amount and type of discharge vary with phase of the menstrual cycle and sexual stimulation and from transudation of vaginal fluid and Bartholin's gland secretion. Bacteria, chiefly lactobacilli and corynebacteria, and small numbers of fungi usually are present. The vaginal pH is normally 3.5 to 4.5; acidity tends to be decreased by menstrual blood, infected cervical mucus, vaginal transudate, or semen. The glycogen content is high, the vaginal mucosa is thick, and the labia are well developed. Elevated hormonal levels, as in pregnancy and oral contraceptive use, can change vaginal metabolism. Vaginal discharges due to infections are discussed below.

In **postmenopausal women,** bacteria and fungi are the most common infecting agents, and *Trichomonas* is less common. Menopausal estrogen depletion due to aging, ovariectomy, or radiation of the pelvis, or temporarily low estrogen levels (similar to those during lactation) cause vulvar structures to regress and vaginal mucosa to thin. Discharge becomes scant, and the pH rises to 4.5 to 5.5. The atrophic vaginal and vulvar epithelium is more easily traumatized and infected. Dystrophies and tumors, symptomatic and asymptomatic, become increasingly common with aging. Folliculitis and other dermatologic disorders can affect the skin of the vulva. Foreign bodies, especially forgotten pessaries, can also cause discharge.

Symptoms, Signs, and Diagnosis

The most common complaint is of vaginal discharge, with or without vulvar irritation. Vaginal discharge is abnormal when the odor is offen-

sive; when pruritus, irritation, or pain occurs; or when the amount distresses the patient.

The initial visit should include a complete physical examination and history, with attention to details of the discharge (color, consistency, presence of odor, duration, and symptoms). The type of discharge may suggest the cause, or it may be misleading. The patient should be asked to describe when the discharge occurs in the menstrual cycle; whether it is recurrent; how it responded to previous therapy; whether vulvar itching, burning, pain, or lesion is present; and what aspect of the problem is most troublesome. Questions should also concern sexual activity; contraceptive use; whether the sexual partner has had urethral discharge, pruritus, penile lesions, postcoital irritation, or therapy for infection; use of chemicals on the vulva or vagina; recent change in laundry products; any present or past venereal disease or parasitic infection; and whether anyone in the household has pubic itching.

After the general physical examination, the vulva is examined for redness, edema, excoriation, and abnormal lesions. A biopsy of discrete vulvar lesions should be performed; if much of the vulva is white and thickened (as in lichen sclerosus) or otherwise appears abnormal, a site may be selected by staining with toluidine blue 1%, then decolorizing with acetic acid 2 to 3% (vinegar diluted 1:1 with water), and targeting the biopsy at a persistent stain. Examination should include searching for parasites, palpating enlarged nodes, culturing ulcers for viruses, and noting urethral and Bartholin's gland discharge. In **children,** a culture may be obtained from the vulva or fourchette; if discharge is present, a vaginal culture should be done. The child should be checked for a foreign body and for pinworms.

Physiologic discharge is annoying because of the feeling of wetness and soiled clothing it produces, but it is not malodorous nor does it produce vulvitis.

Bacterial vaginosis tends to produce a white, gray, or yellowish turbid discharge with a foul or "fishy" odor that becomes stronger when the discharge becomes alkaline (eg, after coitus or washing with soap). Vulvar pruritus or irritation may be present, but redness or edema is not usually marked.

Candida infection (see also Genital Candidiasis in Ch. 21) is suggested by moderate to severe vulvar itching and burning, with redness and possibly excoriation. The thick, cheesy discharge that may be present tends to cling to the vaginal walls. Symptoms usually increase in the week before menses. Infection tends to recur in poorly controlled diabetics and patients routinely using tetracycline for acne.

Trichomonas infection is marked by a white, grayish-green, or yellowish discharge that may be frothy. It often appears shortly after menses and may be malodorous owing to coexisting anaerobic organisms. Itching is severe. Acute inflammation of the vagina with small "strawberry" spots may be found.

A watery discharge, especially if bloody, may suggest **malignancy** of the vagina or upper genital tract. **Cervical polyps** or **vaginal endometriosis** may also produce this type of discharge, with bleeding after coitus.

A discharge may be related to **atrophic vaginitis, radiation vaginitis,** or a **foreign body.** The atrophic vagina is fragile, and bleeding sites may be identified. An acutely painful vulvar lesion suggests **herpes infection** or **local abscess.** Chronic itching or vulvar discomfort suggests **lichen sclerosus** or **carcinoma in situ.** In chronic vulvitis, atypical dystrophies and malignancy should be ruled out by biopsy.

Using a water-lubricated speculum, the physician inspects the vagina, checks the pH, and obtains a specimen with a cotton-tipped applicator. The specimen is diluted on 2 slides—one with 0.9% sodium chloride, the other with 10% potassium hydroxide; at the same time, the latter specimen is checked for released odor. On microscopic examination, *T. vaginalis* can be seen as motile, unicellular flagellated organisms. White cells and "clue" cells (epithelial cells with a granular appearance) with large numbers of bacteria suggest bacterial vaginosis. In the potassium hydroxide preparation, mycelia and/or spores of *Candida* may be seen. Cultures for *Chlamydia trachomatis* and *N. gonorrhoeae* may be indicated; cultures for other organisms are not helpful.

The cervix is inspected, a Papanicolaou **(Pap)** smear taken, and the remainder of the bimanual examination performed.

Treatment

Physiologic discharge requires only reassurance of normalcy. Occasionally, douching with water may reduce the amount of secretion and thus the discharge. Prepubertal girls should be instructed about perineal hygiene. Foreign bodies should be removed.

Specific causes of discharge require specific therapy. Topical anti-inflammatory agents such as hydrocortisone 0.5% tid can be used until specific therapy is instituted after culture results have been obtained. If labial adhesions have occurred secondary to previous inflammation of the labia, application of vaginal estrogen cream daily for 7 to 10 days usually opens the labia. Povidone iodine douche 15 to 30 mL/L (2 tbsp/qt) of water may give relief until specific therapy is effective and may reduce recurrences of *Candida.*

Candida is treated topically with miconazole 2% or clotrimazole 1% cream, vaginal tablets, or suppositories for 3 to 7 days. Ketoconazole is rarely indicated—only in recurrent, recalcitrant disease. *Trichomonas* is treated with metronidazole 250 mg tid or 500 mg bid orally for 5 days; 2 gm in a single daily dose may be used. Ideally, the sexual partner should also be treated. *Gardnerella* or **anaerobic infections** are treated similarly to *Trichomonas,* with metronidazole. About 25% of patients have recurrences and require re-treatment in 2 to 3 mo. Lowering vaginal pH with propionic acid jelly may help. **Chlamydial infections** are treated with doxycycline 100 mg bid or erythromycin 500 mg qid orally for 7 days. *Mycoplasma* is treated with doxycycline 100 mg bid orally for 10 days. For any of these infections, sexual partners should be treated simultaneously, if possible.

Acute vulvitis: The cause should be treated as discussed above, and measures should be taken to reduce acute inflammation; eg, wearing loose, absorbent clothing that allows air circulation and keeping the vulva clean (soaps should be avoided). Intermittent use of ice packs reduces soreness and pruritus; sometimes warm sitz baths or compresses help. Topical steroids are useful, and oral antihistamines may be helpful, especially at night when a sedative effect may be welcome. Oral acyclovir may reduce symptoms and shorten the course of a herpes infection. Symptomatic treatment with pain relievers and anesthetic ointments may be helpful.

Atrophic vaginitis is treated with estrogen replacement; many patients respond to oral estrogen (eg, conjugated estrogen 0.625 mg, ethinyl estradiol 0.05 mg, or estradiol 1 mg) given daily for $\geq$ 25 days. If estrogen is used regularly, medroxyprogesterone acetate is needed to prevent endometrial hyperplasia. Symptoms will recur if the drug is stopped. Some patients prefer estrogen vaginal cream ($^1/_2$ applicator [2.0 gm] every night for 1 mo, then $^1/_4$ applicator 2 or 3 times a week) to maintain a healthy, cornified vaginal epithelium. In some situations, the vaginal mucosa will respond to ½ these dosages.

Chronic vulvitis often leads to chronic inflammation. Occasionally it is due to poor hygiene, especially in elderly patients who are incontinent and bedridden; cleanliness improves the condition. Skin conditions that can cause chronic vulvitis (eg, psoriasis or tinea versicolor) should be treated appropriately, and infection is treated with specific antibiotics. All substances that may cause chronic irritation should be removed.

Vulvar dystrophies can occur at any age but usually are seen in postmenopausal patients. Atrophic vulvar dystrophy has been called lichen sclerosus et atrophicus, kraurosis vulvae, and atrophic vulvitis. Testosterone propionate 2% in petrolatum applied in small amounts bid is often beneficial. Hyperplastic dystrophy usually produces a white or reddish area on the surface of the vulva. Initial treatment with fluorinated topical steroids relieves pruritus. For long-term use, hydrocortisone cream 0.5% prevents vulvar atrophy and contraction. Surgical excision usually is not indicated. Follow-up examinations with constant search for progressive change and possible malignancy are essential. Atypical dystrophies should be removed. Biopsies should be performed on all dystrophies before treatment is begun.

SALPINGITIS
(Pelvic Inflammatory Disease [PID])

Infection of the fallopian tubes. Although the term **pelvic inflammatory disease (PID)** is used by some to include infection of the cervix (cervicitis), the uterus (endometritis), or the ovaries (oophoritis), it should not be used as a catchall for pelvic pain of unknown origin.

Etiology and Pathogenesis

Salpingitis occurs predominantly in women under age 35 who are sexually active and results from microorganisms transmitted most commonly by intercourse, less often by childbirth (puerperal fever) or abortion. Patients with intrauterine devices (IUDs) are especially vulnerable, probably because the transcervical appendage assists pathogen transport. Salpingitis rarely occurs before the menarche, after the menopause, or during pregnancy. The cause may be a single organism or several organisms. *Chlamydia trachomatis* has replaced *Neisseria gonorrhoeae* as the most common cause of PID, but numerous other aerobic and anaerobic organisms can also be present. *C. trachomatis* may affect the lower or upper genital tract; often upper genital tract infections have a deceptively benign onset and seem quite mild. Chlamydial organisms may remain in tubal mucosa for many months before manifestations of acute disease appear. *N. gonorrhoeae* usually produces more acute, typical pelvic inflammation, with rapid onset and development of pelvic pain shortly after the start of a menstrual period.

Salpingitis due to actinomycosis, schistosomiasis, leprosy, oxyuriasis, sarcoidosis, and foreign bodies (eg, x-ray contrast media) has been reported.

Infection begins intravaginally in most cases. The endocervical glands provide an optimal environment for organisms such as *C. trachomatis* and *N. gonorrhoeae* to flourish before spreading upward to produce a superficial endometritis and endosalpingitis. Although symptoms and signs may predominate on one side, both tubes are probably affected. The tubal infection produces a profuse exudate, leading to agglutination of mucosal folds, adhesions, and tubal occlusion. Peritonitis, from spread of the exudate to the pelvic peritoneum, is common; the ovaries tend to resist infection but may also be invaded.

Symptoms and Signs

Acute salpingitis: Onset is usually shortly after menses. Lower abdominal pain becomes progressively more severe, with guarding, rebound tenderness, and discomfort that increases with cervical motion. Unless related to an IUD, involvement is usually bilateral. Vomiting may occur; bowel sounds are normal early, although paralytic ileus may ensue. High fever, leukocytosis, and copious purulent cervical discharge have commonly been associated with PID, but low-grade fever, mild to moderate abdominal pain, irregular bleeding, and vaginal discharge may also signal the disease.

Chronic salpingitis may follow an acute attack with subsequent tubal and pelvic scarring and adhesions, chronic pain, menstrual irregularities, and, possibly, infertility. An obstructed tube may distend with fluid (hydrosalpinx). In **chronic interstitial salpingitis,** the tube is enlarged as a result of a thickened wall. Exacerbations may occur, commonly from organisms other than gonococcus.

Abscesses may develop in the tubes, ovaries, or pelvis during the acute or subacute stage. A small perforation may seal off the abscess and still allow response to antibiotics; those that do not respond require surgical removal. Massive perforation of an adnexal abscess is a **surgical emergency,** rapidly progressing in a characteristic pattern of severe low abdominal pain, generalized peritonitis, nausea, vomiting, and shock secondary to peritonitis and endotoxemia. **Pyosalpinx,** in which one or both fallopian tubes are filled with pus, may be sterile but almost always is associated with symptoms of inflammation. The ovary, if involved, becomes incorporated into the tubal inflammatory mass, producing a **tubo-ovarian abscess. Hydrosalpinx** occurs with late or incomplete therapy, resulting from closure of the fimbriated end of the fallopian tube. It may be present without symptoms for years. As a result of the mucosal destruction and tubal occlusion, **infertility** is a common sequela of salpingitis.

Diagnosis

The history may disclose recent coitus, insertion of an IUD, childbirth, or abortion. Temperature and WBC count may be elevated. The ESR is usually elevated. On pelvic examination, the most striking finding is that moving the cervix or palpating the adnexa produces severe pain. Peritoneal irritation frequently produces marked abdominal, referred, and rebound tenderness (therefore, gentle palpation is important if a pelvic mass is to be identified). Surgical emergencies must be ruled out, especially appendicitis and ectopic pregnancy. Specimens for cultures and smear for Gram stain should be obtained from the cervical, urethral, and rectal areas and from the pharynx. Culdocentesis, with examination of the fluid, may help in differential diagnosis as well as in identifying organisms. Laparoscopy should be performed if the clinical diagnosis is questioned for any reason; it also aids in differential diagnosis.

Treatment

Acute salpingitis requires immediate and vigorous treatment to stop the infection and prevent infertility. Antibiotics should be started as soon as specimens have been obtained for culture and sensitivity tests, without waiting for the results of these studies. If a patient can be treated as an outpatient (ie, findings are minimal), appropriate therapy includes single doses of cefoxitin 2 gm IM plus probenecid 1 gm orally followed by doxycycline 100 mg orally bid for 10 days. Alternatively, a single dose of ceftriaxone 250 mg IM plus probenecid 1 gm orally followed by doxy-cycline 100 mg orally bid for 10 days may be given. Patients should be followed up within 48 h; if no improvement is noted, they should be hospitalized.

Current optimal inpatient therapy consists of combinations of antibiotics to control infection as quickly and completely as possible, since infertility increases with degree of inflammation. The Centers for Disease Control recommend 2 regimens: One is cefoxitin 2 gm IV qid plus doxycycline 100 mg IV bid for 4 days or until 48 h after defervescence, followed by doxycycline 100 mg orally bid to complete 10 days. The other regimen is clindamycin 600 mg IV qid plus gentamicin 2 mg/kg IV once, followed by gentamicin 1.5 mg/kg IV q 8 h for 4 days or until 48 h after defervescence, followed by clindamycin 450 mg orally qid to complete 10 to 14 days.

Adequate treatment of women with acute salpingitis must include examination and treatment of sexual contacts, many of whom may be found to have nonsymptomatic urethritis.

PREMENSTRUAL SYNDROME (PMS)
(Premenstrual Tension)

A condition characterized by nervousness, irritability, emotional instability, depression, and possibly headaches, edema, and mastalgia; it occurs during the 7 to 10 days before menstruation and disappears a few hours after onset of menstrual flow.

Etiology

The syndrome seems to be related to fluctuations in estrogen and progesterone. Estrogen exerts fluid-retaining action; transitory increases in fluid in different body tissues seem to explain symptoms such as weight gain, edema, breast tenderness, and possibly, bloating. However, many symptoms do not correlate in intensity with fluid retention and weight gain; eg, diuretics promote sodium and water excretion but do not relieve all of the symptoms and may have no effect on the symptom complex.

Estrogen-progesterone imbalance, excessive aldosterone or ADH, carbohydrate metabolism changes, hypoglycemia, hyperprolactinemia, allergy to progesterone, retention of sodium and water by the kidneys, and psychogenic factors have all been implicated.

Symptoms and Signs

Most women experience some symptoms referable to the menstrual cycle; in many women, the symptoms are significant but of short duration and not disabling. Other women have one or more of a broad range of symptoms that temporarily disturb normal functioning. Symptoms last from a few hours to 10 to 12 or more days and usually cease with onset of menses; however, in perimenopausal women, symptoms may persist through and after menses. Type and intensity of symptoms vary in the general population and may also vary in individuals.

With onset of menses, PMS is replaced by **dysmenorrhea** in many women. Significant dysmenorrhea is more common in the teens and tends to diminish with maturity. Conversely, PMS may begin in the 20s and increase with age.

The most common complaints are **mood alteration and psychologic effects:** irritability, nervousness, lack of control, agitation, anger, insomnia, difficulty in concentrating, lethargy, depression, and severe fatigue. Symptoms related to **fluid retention** are edema, transient weight gain, oliguria, and breast fullness and pain. **Neurologic and vascular symptoms** include headache, vertigo, syncope, paresthesias of extremities, easy bruising, and cardiac palpitation. Epilepsy may be aggravated. **GI symptoms** include bloating, constipation, nausea, vomiting, and changes in appetite. **Pelvic heaviness or pressure** and **backache** may occur. **Skin problems** of acne, neurodermatitis, and aggravation of other skin disorders may also occur. **Respiratory problems** (allergies and infection) and **eye complaints** (visual disturbance and conjunctivitis) may be worse premenstrually.

Treatment

Treatment involves symptomatic relief and, when possible, correcting the cause. **Fluid retention** may be relieved by reducing sodium intake and using a diuretic (eg, hydrochlorothiazide 50 to 100 mg/day orally), starting just before the time symptoms are usually noted. **Counseling** about the symptoms can increase understanding and lead to modification of activities for **stress reduction.** Because of the normal variation of the disorder, having the patient record symptoms and therapies helps to determine the effectiveness of the treatment. **Partner involvement,** directly or indirectly, may help both to cope with the PMS. **Hormonal manipulation** is effective for some women. Possible regimens include (1) oral contraceptives, (2) natural progesterone by vaginal suppository (200 to 400 mg/day) or injection (progesterone in oil 5 to 10 mg IM) for 10 to 12 days premenstrually, or (3) long-acting progestin (eg, medroxyprogesterone acetate 200 mg IM every 2 to 3 mo) to eliminate cyclic changes. **Tranquilizers** (eg, alprazolam 0.25 mg/day orally at bedtime) may be used in patients with irritability, nervousness, and lack of control, especially if they are unable to change their stressful environments. **Dietary changes,** increasing protein and decreasing sugars as well as supplementing with vitamin B complex (especially pyridoxine and/or magnesium), may be helpful for some women. Other regimens, using spironolactone, bromocriptine, or monoamine oxidase **(MAO)** inhibitors, do not show clear benefits.

PRIMARY DYSMENORRHEA
(Functional Dysmenorrhea)

Cyclic pain associated with menses during ovulatory cycles but without demonstrable lesions affecting the reproductive structures.

Etiology and Incidence

The pain is thought to result from uterine contractions and ischemia, probably mediated by the effect of prostaglandins produced in secretory endometrium; therefore, primary dysmenorrhea is almost always associated with ovulatory cycles. The passage of tissue through the cervix, a narrow cervical os, malposition of the uterus, lack of exercise, and anxiety about menses may be contributing factors. This common disability usually appears during adolescence, causes significant absence from school or work, and tends to decrease with age and after pregnancy.

Symptoms and Signs

Low abdominal pain is usually crampy or colicky but may be a dull constant ache and may radiate to the lower back or legs. It may start before or with menses, tends to peak after 24 h, and usually subsides after 2 days. Sometimes endometrial casts **(membranous dysmenorrhea)** or clots are expelled. Headache, nausea, constipation or diarrhea, and urinary frequency are often present; vomiting occurs occasionally. Premenstrual syndrome symptoms (see above) of irritability, nervousness, depression, and abdominal distention may persist during part or all of the menses.

Treatment

Assurance that her reproductive organs are normal will give a woman psychologic support. The most effective drugs are the prostaglandin synthetase inhibitors; ibuprofen, naproxen, and mefenamic acid are helpful. Effectiveness may be increased if the drug is started 24 to 48 h before menses and continued through 1 or 2 days of the cycle. If pain continues to interfere with normal activity, suppression of ovulation with low-dose estrogen-progesterone oral contraceptives is advisable. Although antiemetics may be used, nausea and vomiting usually disappear as cramps subside. Adequate rest and sleep and regular exercise may be beneficial.

SECONDARY DYSMENORRHEA
(Acquired Dysmenorrhea)

Pain with menses caused by demonstrable pathology.

Etiology

One of the most common causes is endometriosis; adenomyosis also causes dysmenorrhea. A few women have an extremely tight cervical os, secondary to conization or to cryo- or thermal cautery, that results in pain when the uterus attempts to expel tissue. Cramping pain occurs occasionally when a pedunculated submucosal fibroid or an endometrial polyp is being extruded from the uterus (although it may be painless).

Chronic pelvic inflammatory disease (PID) and adhesions may cause diffuse low abdominal pain that is vague and continuous. Patients with both acute and chronic PID tend to have increased pain with menses. Acute pain may be associated with acute pelvic inflammation, fever, and diffuse abdominal symptoms during or just after menses.

Treatment

Secondary dysmenorrhea can be relieved symptomatically or by correction of the underlying abnormality. Dilation of a narrow cervical canal may give 3 to 6 mo of relief (and also permits diagnostic curettage). Interruption of uterine nerves by presacral neurectomy and division of the sacrouterine ligaments may help selected patients; hypnosis has also been useful.

MENOPAUSE

The physiologic cessation of menses as a result of decreasing ovarian function. It is usually a retrospective diagnosis, made when menses have not occurred for a year. Menopause may be natural, artificial, or premature.

Etiology

Natural menopause occurs at an average age of 50 to 51 yr. As ovaries age, response to pituitary-produced gonadotropins (follicle-stimulating and luteinizing hormones) decreases, initially with shorter follicular phases (hence, shorter cycles), fewer ovulations, decreased progesterone production, and more cycle irregularity. Eventually, the follicle fails to respond and, without feedback of estrogen, the circulating gonadotropins rise substantially. Circulating levels of estrogens and progesterone are markedly reduced; androgen (androstenedione) is reduced by half, but testosterone decreases only slightly. This transitional phase beginning before menopause and continuing after it, during which a woman passes from her reproductive stage, is properly referred to as the climacteric, although most people refer to it also as menopause. Premature menopause refers to ovarian failure of unknown cause that occurs before age 40. Smoking is associated with early menopause. Radiation exposure, chemotherapeutic drugs, and surgery that impairs ovarian blood supply can also hasten menopause. Artificial menopause follows ovariectomy or radiation of the pelvis, including the ovaries.

Symptoms and Signs

Menopausal women may be asymptomatic, or they may have severe symptoms. Hot flushes and sweating secondary to vasomotor instability affect 75% of women. Most have hot flushes for > 1 yr and 25 to 50% for > 5 yr. Psychologic and emotional symptoms of fatigue, irritability, insomnia, and nervousness may be related to both estrogen deprivation and the stress of aging and changing roles. Lack of sleep due to disturbance by recurrent hot flushes contributes to fatigue and irritability. Intermittent dizziness, paresthesias, and cardiac symptoms of palpitations and tachycardia may occur; the incidence of heart disease increases. Dyspareunia, increasing pelvic relaxation, urinary incontinence, cystitis, and vaginitis tend to occur. Nausea, flatulence, constipation, diarrhea, arthralgia, and myalgia are common complaints.

Osteoporosis is the major health hazard. Those at highest risk are slender, white women who smoke, take corticosteroids, or have little physical activity. Bone mass losses average 1 to 2%/yr after menopause and result in numerous fractures. Primary sites are the vertebrae, which show anterior collapse, leading to stooping and backache; hip (200,000/yr in the USA); and wrist. These fractures may occur with little trauma, and in the elderly, with no trauma.

Diagnosis

Menopause is usually obvious. In younger patients, the diagnosis is substantiated by elevated levels of follicle-stimulating hormone. Endocrine disorders such as thyroid disease or diabetes mellitus should be ruled out. Patients with symptomatic osteoporosis should be evaluated for causes other than menopause (eg, hyperparathyroidism).

Treatment

Counseling about the physiologic causes and the concerns, fears, and stresses related to this phase of life is important. When psychic factors dominate, psychotherapy is indicated and, if necessary, antidepressants, minor tranquilizers, and mild sedatives can be used as adjunctive therapy for depression, anxiety and irritability, and insomnia, respectively.

Estrogen replacement is the only consistent and satisfactory therapy to sustain systems dependent on ovarian hormone secretion and to relieve **hot flushes.** Patient selection, determination of risk/benefit ratio, and observation during therapy are necessary. When hot flushes and subsequent insomnia and fatigue from night-awakening decrease, the feeling of well-being usually returns. When estrogens are contraindicated, treatments for reducing discomfort due to hot flushes include sedative-hypnotics (eg, barbiturates or benzodiazepines), progestin (medroxyprogesterone acetate 10 mg/day orally or 100 to 150 mg/mo IM, megestrol acetate 40 mg/day orally), or clonidine (0.1 mg transdermally).

Symptomatic **vaginal atrophy and vaginitis** and **atrophic changes of the lower urinary tract** (especially of the urethra and trigone of the bladder), with urinary frequency, dysuria, and sometimes incontinence, are reversible with estrogen therapy.

Preventing **osteoporosis** requires extended estrogen replacement. Adequate nutrition, including elemental calcium (1000 mg/day for pre-menopausal and estrogen-treated women, 1500 mg/day for untreated postmenopausal women), and weight-bearing exercise are also necessary. For those who have inadequate daily exposure to sunlight, vitamin D supplementation (600 u. bid) is indicated. The efficacy and safety of other modalities have not been established (eg, sodium fluoride, calcitriol, calcitonin, weak androgenic anabolic steroids, thiazides, diphosphonates, and 1-34 parathyroid hormone). To prevent falls, side effects of other drugs need to be considered and home hazards should be minimized.

The therapeutic effects of estrogen replacement on **cardiovascular disease** in postmenopausal women are becoming more clearly delineated. Documented improvement in morbidity and mortality suggests that cardiovascular mortality is $1/3$ lower in estrogen users than in nonusers, largely as a result of estrogen-induced increases in high density lipoprotein. Although BP increases have been reported in some women receiving estrogen replacement therapy, this has not been associated with an increased risk for cerebrovascular accident.

Estrogen administration usually is cyclic. If the patient has a uterus, a progestin is added to the cycle. Estrogen (conjugated estrogen 0.3 to 1.25 mg/day or ethinyl estradiol 0.02 to 0.05 mg/day) is taken orally once a day from the first through the 25th day each month. Progestins (eg, medroxyprogesterone acetate 5 or 10 mg or norethindrone acetate 2.5 to 5 mg orally) are given from the 15th through the 25th day of the cycle. Bleeding, if it occurs, should happen only during the hormone withdrawal period; if bleeding occurs at other times, an endometrial biopsy should be performed. (Some physicians advocate an endometrial biopsy before therapy and at yearly intervals thereafter; others recommend it only if symptoms warrant, as it is an uncomfortable procedure, increases expense, and has a low yield in asymptomatic women.) Estrogen can be increased or decreased, according to the symptoms. If hot flushes occur during the end of the cycle, the days without estrogen can be decreased by 1 day each month until symptoms are relieved. Alternative regimens include conjugated estrogen 0.3 to 0.625 mg/day or ethinyl estradiol 0.02 to 0.05 mg/day plus medroxyprogesterone acetate 2.5 mg/day continuously (spotting is minimal or eliminated after a few months with this regimen), or transdermal estrogen twice weekly with daily or cyclic oral progestin. If the uterus has been removed, only estrogens need to be given.

Topical estrogen (eg, conjugated, natural or synthetic estrogen cream) may be used for atrophic vaginal changes and dyspareunia; 1 applicator/night for 5 nights, then ¹/₂ applicator/night for 1 mo, followed by ¹/₄ applicator 2 to 3 times/wk will correct atrophic changes and maintain a healthy, cornified vaginal epithelium. The estrogen is readily absorbed systemically from the vaginal mucosa. Injectable estrogen (estradiol valerate 10 to 20 mg IM q 4 wk) is rarely indicated, except immediately after oophorectomy.

Contraindications to estrogen therapy include a history of estrogen-dependent neoplasia of the endometrium or breast, a history of thrombophlebitis or thromboembolism, and the presence or a history of severe liver disease. There are also relative contraindications.

Mammography should be routine in postmenopausal women and is particularly pertinent as a screen and to provide a baseline in those receiving estrogen treatment. Most evidence indicates that estrogen therapy does not increase risk for breast cancer.

6.   AMENORRHEA AND ABNORMAL GENITAL BLEEDING

AMENORRHEA

Absence of menstruation, ie, either lack of menarche or cessation of menses.

Normal menstruation: By definition, the first day of menstrual flow is day 1 of the cycle. The interval is 28 ($\pm$ 3) days for 65% of women, with a range of 18 to 40 days; once a menstrual pattern has been established, the variation does not normally exceed 5 days. The average duration of menstrual flow is 5 ($\pm$ 2) days with a blood loss averaging 130 mL (range, 13 to 300 mL), usually heavier on the 2nd day.

Amenorrhea indicates failure of hypothalamic-pituitary-gonadal interaction to produce cyclic changes in the endometrium resulting in menses, and thus may indicate an abnormality at any level of the reproductive tract. It is important to remember that amenorrhea is merely a sign, potentially of any of a large number of disorders involving several organ systems. Amenorrhea is **physiologic** *when it occurs in the prepubertal girl, during pregnancy and early lactation, and after the menopause.* At any other time it should be considered **pathologic.** Amenorrhea is traditionally categorized as **primary** (*the absence of menarche by age 16*) or **secondary** (*the absence of menstruation for $\geq$ 3 mo in women with past menses*). However, such categorization may lead to diagnostic omissions and should not be considered in the evaluation of the amenorrheic woman.

Menarche may be delayed physiologically until the age of 16 yr. **Physiologic delay** must always be a diagnosis of exclusion. Evaluation is indicated in girls with no evidence of puberty by age 13, in girls with absence of menarche by age 16, and in those in whom $\geq$ 5 yr pass from the onset of pubertal development without menarche. Girls in whom evaluation as outlined below is normal should be reassured and followed at 3- to 6-mo intervals for pubertal progression. Although some physicians suggest use of exogenous progestins and/or estrogens to induce cyclic bleeding, this is unnecessary once normalcy of the outflow genital tract is established. Additionally, continued administration of sex steroids can obscure both initiation of menses and pathologic processes.

Clinical Evaluation

Even subtle hormonal alterations may be manifested by symptoms and signs. Central to the diagnostic evaluation is the history and physical examination with regard to the influence of altered hormonal secretion on the pubertal process and secondary sexual characteristics. Patients should be questioned for evidence of psychologic disturbances, dietary and exercise habits, life-style, environmental stresses, a family history of genetic anomalies, and abnormal growth and development. Patients should also be asked about any signs of increased androgen secretion (**hyperandrogenism**), especially **hirsutism**, which may be defined as *an increase in sexually stimulated hair.* **Virilization** refers to *an increase in masculine secondary sexual characteristics* (**masculinization**), including hirsutism, temporal balding, voice deepening, increased muscle mass, clitoromegaly, and increased libido; and to a decrease in feminine secondary sexual characteristics (**defeminization**), including decreased breast size and vaginal atrophy. In addition, any history of **galactorrhea,**

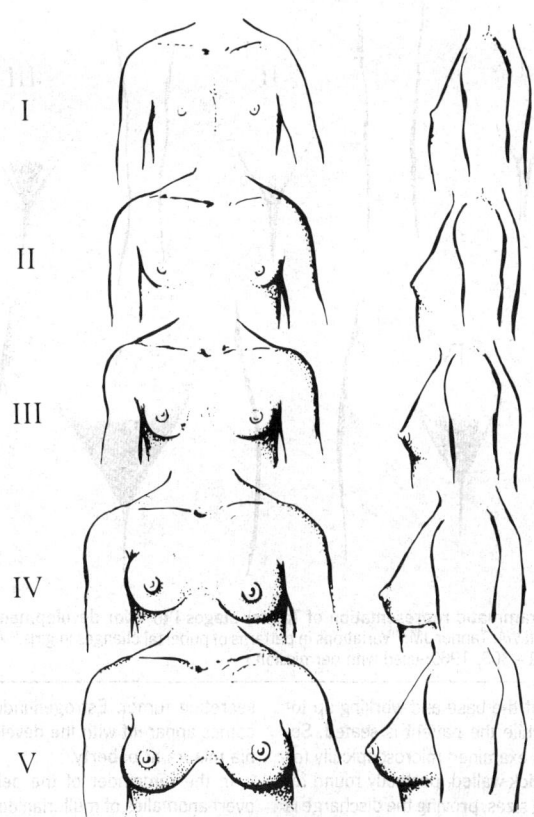

FIG. 6–1. Diagrammatic representation of Tanner stages I to V of human breast maturation. (From Marshall WA, Tanner JM: "Variations in patterns of pubertal changes in girls." *Archives of Disease in Childhood* 44:291–303, 1969; used with permission.)

defined as *nonpuerperal secretion of milk or lactation,* should be sought.

Although the entire physical examination is important, special emphasis should be placed on evaluating (1) body dimensions and habitus, (2) the extent and distribution of body hair, (3) breast development and secretions, and (4) the genitalia. In normal individuals the arm span is similar to the height, whereas in hypogonadal individuals the span is typically > 2 in. (5 cm) greater than the height. The distribution and quantity of hair should be considered in light of the family history. **Hypertrichosis,** *the excessive growth of hair on the extremities, head, and back,* must not be mistaken for true hirsut-

ism and virilization. Some hypertrichosis is not uncommon in women ,of Mediterranean descent, whereas any facial hair growth in the relatively hairless and androgen-insensitive Oriental woman may require thorough evaluation. The extent of hirsutism should be recorded, preferably by photographs. It is most practical to grade only facial hirsutism (since this is generally the reason the patient seeks aid) from 0 to 4 +, giving 1 + each for excess chin, upper lip, or sideburn hair, and 4 + for a full beard.

The breasts should be inspected and development noted according to the method of Tanner (see FIG. 6–1). Any breast secretion should be elicited by applying pressure to all sections of the

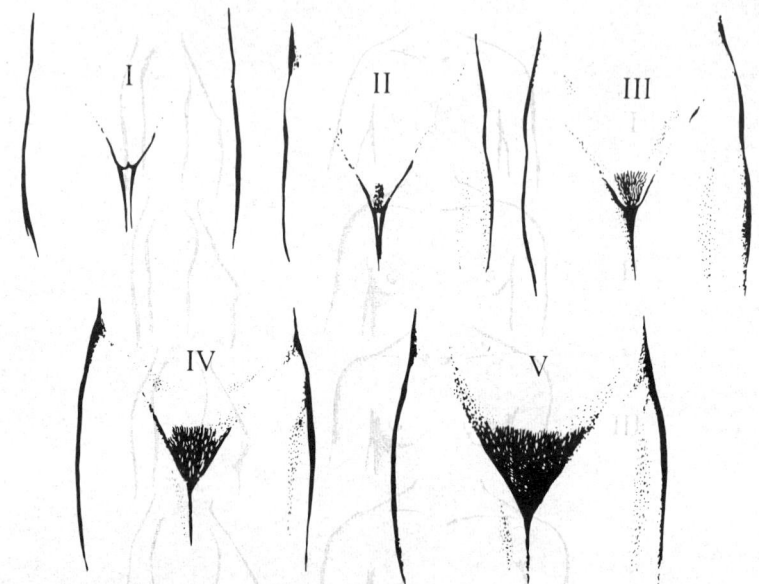

Fig. 6–2. Diagrammatic representation of Tanner stages I to V for development of pubic hair in girls. (From Marshall WA, Tanner JM: "Variations in patterns of pubertal changes in girls." *Archives of Disease in Childhood* 44:291–303, 1969; used with permission.)

breast beginning at the base and working up toward the nipple while the patient is seated. Secretions should be examined microscopically for the presence of thick-walled, perfectly round fat globules of varying sizes, proving the discharge is milk.

Lastly, the genitalia should be examined carefully because they are sensitive indicators of hormonal milieu. Stages of pubic hair development should be noted (see Fig. 6–2). Since the sensitivity of the genitalia to androgens decreases in time from the early stages of fetal development to adulthood, the extent of any virilization is important. The most marked changes, fusion of the labia and enlargement of the clitoris (with or without formation of a penile urethra), are observed in women exposed to androgens during the first 3 mo of their fetal development and in patients with congenital adrenal hyperplasia, hermaphroditism, and drug-induced virilization (see CONGENITAL ADRENAL HYPERPLASIA in Ch. 40). Significant development of clitoromegaly postnatally requires marked hormonal stimulation and, without a history of intake of exogenous steroids, strongly implicates an androgen-

secreting tumor. Estrogen-induced change becomes apparent with the development of the labia minora at puberty.

In the remainder of the pelvic examination, overt anomalies of müllerian duct derivatives, including imperforate hymen, vaginal and uterine aplasia, and vaginal septa, should be sought. Any obstruction to the escape of menstrual blood may lead to the collection of blood in the vagina (hematocolpos) and distention of the uterus (hematometra). A bulging vagina and a pelvic mass are typically felt on abdominal and rectal examinations, but establishing whether the cause is vaginal agenesis, a vaginal septum, or an imperforate hymen may prove difficult. In such circumstances the development of the external genitalia and other secondary sex characteristics is normal (because of normal ovarian function), but the presence of associated urinary tract and skeletal abnormalities is frequent (about 15 to 40%) in the first 2 instances. The external genitalia also appear normal in testicular feminization, but pubic and axillary hair is decreased, breast development is incomplete, and the vagina is of variable length with no identifi-

TABLE 6–1. CLINICAL CATEGORIZATION OF AMENORRHEA

Physiologic causes
  Prepuberty
  Pregnancy
  Postmenopause

Chronic anovulation or premature ovarian failure
  Due to CNS-hypothalamic-pituitary dysfunction
  Due to inappropriate feedback (eg, polycystic ovary syndrome)
  Due to thyroid and adrenal disorders
  Premature ovarian failure

Pathologic end-organ disease
  Gestational trophoblastic disease
  Asherman's syndrome

Disorders of sexual differentiation
  Müllerian agenesis and dysgenesis
  Gonadal dysgenesis
  Male pseudohermaphroditism

able cervix or uterus. Bimanual palpation can also document the existence of pelvic pathology, including tumors. Visual inspection of the quality of the vaginal mucosa and the cervical mucus is important because of their exquisite sensitivity to estrogen. Under the influence of estrogen, the vaginal mucosa progresses during sexual maturation from a tissue with a shiny, bright-red appearance with sparse, thin secretions to a dull, gray-pink rugated surface with copious, thick secretions.

The history and physical examination should permit classification of patients into the categories listed in TABLE 6–1. The various disorders of sexual differentiation and the physiologic and pathologic end-organ causes are often apparent on inspection. The stigmas of **Turner's syndrome**, for example, including short stature of < 63 in., shield-like chest, webbed neck, short 4th metacarpals and metatarsals, hypoplastic nails, multiple pigmented nevi, and congenital heart disease, generally make the diagnosis, which may be confirmed by karyotype, 45,X (see GONADAL DYSGENESIS under SYNDROMES ASSOCIATED WITH SEX CHROMOSOME ABERRATIONS in Ch. 48). In male pseudohermaphrodites and in women with müllerian duct abnormalities, the abnormal genitalia should raise suspicions. In individuals with suspected intersex disorders, a karyotype should be obtained (see INTERSEX STATES in Ch. 28). In amenorrheic individuals, pregnancy and gestational trophoblastic disease may be suspected and confirmed by measuring human chorionic gonadotropin (HCG). In women with amenorrhea developing after curettage or acute endome-

tritis, the possibility of intrauterine adhesions or synechiae **(Asherman's syndrome)** must be entertained. Without laboratory studies it may be impossible to distinguish individuals with chronic anovulation from those with ovarian failure.

A **progestational challenge** can help to assess the competence of the outflow tract and the level of endogenous estrogens. Medroxyprogesterone acetate 5 to 10 mg/day orally for 5 days or, alternatively, progesterone in oil 100 to 200 mg IM is given. Within 10 days after conclusion of progestational medication, the patient will or will not bleed. Any bleeding excludes the possibility of Asherman's syndrome in most patients and suggests strongly, but does not confirm, the diagnosis of anovulation. It also confirms the presence of sufficient estrogen to have stimulated growth of endometrium. If bleeding does not occur, orally active estrogen, such as conjugated estrogens 2.5 mg/day for 21 days, with the addition of 5 to 10 mg oral medroxyprogesterone acetate for the last 5 of those days, will produce bleeding in the absence of a uterine abnormality. TB affecting the endometrium and Asherman's syndrome may preclude bleeding, although hysterosalpingography and hysteroscopy may be required for definitive diagnosis, because some patients continue to have cyclic bleeding.

Laboratory Studies

If possible, **basal levels of serum follicle-stimulating hormone (FSH) and prolactin (PRL) should be obtained in all women with amenorrhea to rule out ovarian failure and**

hyperprolactinemia. Thyroid function studies are also indicated to rule out thyroid disorders as the cause of the amenorrhea (or oligomenorrhea). Simultaneous measurement of luteinizing hormone **(LH)** may assist in making a definitive diagnosis. LH and FSH levels will show 1 of 4 patterns:

1. **A hypogonadotropic pattern** (LH and FSH both < 10 mIU/mL of the 2nd International Reference Preparation of Human Menopausal Gonadotropin) is found in patients with panhypopituitarism, isolated gonadotropin deficiency (who may also present with anosmia, color blindness, cleft lip or other midline defects as Kallmann's syndrome), anorexia nervosa, amenorrhea-galactorrhea, and severe hypothalamic chronic anovulation.

2. **A normogonadotropic pattern** (LH and FSH both 7 to 20 mIU/mL with at least one ≥ 10 mIU/mL) includes women with hypothalamic chronic anovulation and, less frequently, inappropriate steroid feedback (ie, polycystic ovary syndrome).

3. **An inappropriate increase in the LH:FSH ratio** to > 2 with LH generally > 20 mIU/mL includes women with chronic anovulation due to inappropriate feedback (a typical finding in polycystic ovary syndrome) and rarely testicular feminization. Such levels may also be seen at the time of the midcycle LH surge (in which case menses will occur 2 wk later), in pregnant women, and sometimes in those with trophoblastic disease (because immunoassay determinations of LH cross-react with those of HCG).

4. **A hypergonadotropic pattern** (LH > 20 and FSH > 40 mIU/mL) is suggestive of ovarian "failure." As discussed subsequently, ovarian failure may be reversible in some instances. Elevated FSH levels in a young amenorrheic woman indicate the need for a karyotype.

Basal PRL levels are elevated in perhaps $^1/_3$ of women who have amenorrhea (normal, 2 to 15 ng/mL). Because PRL levels are increased by nonspecific stressful stimuli, sleep, food ingestion, and breast examination, an elevated value (generally > 20 to 30 ng/mL, depending on the laboratory) should be repeated before more extensive testing. PRL is typically increased by a number of pharmacologic agents as well, including phenothiazines, L-dopa, reserpine, and oral contraceptives. If either galactorrhea or persistent hyperprolactinemia is present, primary hypothyroidism must be ruled out, with elevated thyroid-stimulating hormone **(TSH)** levels being diagnostic. In primary hypothyroidism, increased secretion of thyrotropin-releasing hormone **(TRH)** stimulates increased PRL as well as increased TSH release.

X-rays of the sella turcica are indicated in euthyroid women with hyperprolactinemia to rule out pituitary tumors. Sellar x-rays should not be obtained in hypothyroid women with mild hyperprolactinemia and amenorrhea-galactorrhea, because any enlargement of the sella turcica will return to normal following appropriate thyroid hormone replacement. Views of the sella turcica are also indicated whenever gonadotropin concentrations are low, regardless of the PRL level, to rule out a pituitary neoplasm.

Pituitary testing, especially of adrenal and thyroid function, is warranted whenever panhypopituitarism is suspected or a large tumor is present. CT or MRI of the sella will determine if the patient has any suprasellar extension of a pituitary neoplasm or if she suffers from the **empty sella syndrome,** in which the sella turcica is enlarged but has been largely replaced by CSF. Formal visual field testing is indicated whenever a pituitary neoplasm is ≥ 10 mm in diameter on x-ray or there is evidence of suprasellar extension.

Anovulatory women with masculinization (hyperandrogenic women) should be evaluated to exclude serious disorders. In most cases, this can be done easily at the bedside and confirmed with the aid of laboratory tests. Inappropriate gonadotropin secretion with elevated LH and low to normal FSH levels are common, but both may be in the normal range. Total circulating androgen levels may be elevated but need not be because of altered metabolic clearance and decreased levels of sex-hormone–binding globulin **(SHBG),** which binds androgens in plasma. **Hirsutism** may also result because of increased sensitivity of the pilosebaceous unit (ie, hair follicle) to normal quantities of androgen. It is now recognized that "idiopathic" hirsutism results from increased conversion of testosterone to dihydrotestosterone **(DHT)** within the hair follicle.

Initial laboratory evaluation of hirsute women should include measurement of serum testosterone **(T)** and dehydroepiandrosterone sulfate **(DHEAS).** T levels > 200 ng/dL should lead to investigation for an androgen-producing tumor, most commonly of ovarian origin. DHEAS levels twice as high as the upper limit of the normal range for the laboratory should lead to evaluation for an adrenal neoplasm. There is no need for extensive testing if T or DHEAS is not markedly elevated, because the possibility of a serious cause has been eliminated. Likewise, the presence of hirsutism obviates the need to measure biologically free T. The measurement of 3-androstanediol glucuronide has been suggested to detect increased metabolic activity within the pilosebaceous unit in response to the circulating androgens; however, 3-androstanediol glucuronide is elevated in all hirsute women. Consequently, its measurement adds little to the physical examination and is not recommended.

If T and DHEAS measurements are obtainable, there is no need to measure urinary 17-ketosteroids **(17-KS)** and 17-hydroxycorticosteroid **(17-OHCS)** excretion. It is difficult to obtain complete 24-h urine collections, and results are inconclusive. 17-KS secretion is not a reliable indicator of testosterone secretion and a poor indicator of ovarian androgen production. Major sources of urinary 17-KS are secreted by the adrenal gland and, if 17-KS excretion is > 20 mg/24 h, the source of excess androgens is probably adrenal. Measurement of 17-OHCS excretion is of no value in the diagnosis of androgen excess, although it is elevated in most cases of Cushing's syndrome (ie, adrenocortical hyperfunction). Likewise, the use of dexamethasone suppression and of stimulation with ACTH and HCG is not of consistent value in evaluating the hirsute woman. Individuals with suspected Cushing's syndrome should be screened for cortisol excess.

Hirsute women with a history and examination suggestive of **congenital adrenal hyperplasia (CAH)**, most commonly due to 21-hydroxylase deficiency, can have the diagnosis confirmed by the presence of elevated levels of 17-hydroxyprogesterone **(17-OHP)** in the serum or pregnanetriol in the urine (see CONGENITAL ADRENAL HYPERPLASIA in Ch. 40). Patients with severe hirsutism beginning during adolescence, high levels of T and/or DHEAS, a strong family history of hirsutism, or hypertension are candidates for the measurement of 17-OHP to rule out nonclassic 21-hydroxylase deficiency. (Girls with classic 21-hydroxylase deficiency generally present with heterosexual precocity and short stature with a masculinized habitus and failure to develop female secondary sexual characteristics and menstrual periods—see in Ch. 40.) Basal levels of 17-OHP > 3 ng/mL but < 8 ng/mL require ACTH stimulation testing to make a distinction between CAH and other disorders such as polycystic ovary syndrome (see under CHRONIC ANOVULATION DUE TO INAPPROPRIATE FEEDBACK SIGNALS, below). Levels > 8 ng/mL are virtually diagnostic of CAH. Many protocols for ACTH testing have been used; the most common involves measuring serum levels of 17-OHP 30 min after injection of synthetic ACTH 250 μmg IV. Patients with classic 21-hydroxylase deficiency have levels > 3000 ng/dL; those with nonclassic 21-hydroxylase deficiency typically achieve levels ≥ 1500 ng/dL; whereas heterozygotic carriers achieve levels ≤ 100 ng/dL. A plasma level of 17-OHP > 3 ng/mL 15 min after IV administration of exogenous ACTH at a dose of 10 μg/m^2 BSA in a patient suppressed with dexamethasone (2 mg orally at midnight before morning testing) is also diagnostic of 21-hydroxylase deficiency. Some clinicians recommend ACTH stimulation in all women with hirsutism to diagnose nonclassic forms of CAH. The frequency of this disorder varies according to population, but in most geographic areas is probably too low to justify such extensive testing.

Ultrasonography, CT, and selective adrenal and ovarian vein angiography with androgen measurement are useful in attempting to localize any androgen-producing neoplasm prior to surgical excision. Selective adrenal and ovarian vein sampling should be performed only in specialized centers familiar with this procedure. The neoplasms should be biopsied during surgery to assess malignant potential.

CHRONIC ANOVULATORY DISORDERS

Chronic anovulation may be viewed as a steady state in which the monthly rhythm manifested by menses is no longer operational. The term chronic anovulation further implies that functional ovarian follicles remain and that cyclic ovulation can be induced or reinitiated with appropriate management. Chronic anovulation is the most frequent form of amenorrhea when there are no anatomic abnormalities of the target organs precluding menstruation (see TABLE 6–2). Selected syndromes are discussed in this chapter. Rational and appropriate management can be instituted only after the cause of the anovulation has been determined. Unfortunately, until the mechanisms for the several forms of chronic anovulation are better understood, the anovulation can be interrupted only by transient and nonspecific ovulation induction in a large percentage of affected women.

TABLE 6–2. CLASSIFICATION OF CHRONIC ANOVULATION

Chronic anovulation of suprapituitary origin
  Hypothalamic chronic anovulation (HCA)
    Psychogenic
    Exercise-associated
    Associated with malnutrition
    Of mixed or unknown etiology
  Anorexia nervosa
  Pseudocyesis (ie, false pregnancy)
  Forms of isolated gonadotropin deficiency

Chronic anovulation of pituitary origin
  Hypopituitarism
  Pituitary tumors
  Forms of isolated gonadotropin deficiency

Chronic anovulation due to inappropriate feedback (eg, polycystic ovary syndrome)
  Excessive extraglandular estrogen production (eg, obesity)
  Abnormal buffering involving sex-hormone–binding globulin (including liver disease)
  Functional androgen excess (adrenal or ovarian)
  Neoplasms producing androgens or estrogens
  Neoplasms producing human chorionic gonadotropin

Chronic anovulation due to other endocrine or metabolic dysfunctions
  Adrenal hyperfunction
    Cushing's syndrome and disease
    Congenital adrenal hyperplasia (female pseudohermaphroditism)
  Thyroid dysfunction
    Hyperthyroidism
    Hypothyroidism
  Prolactin and/or growth hormone excess
    Hypothalamic dysfunction
    Pituitary dysfunction (micro- and macroadenomas)
    Drug-induced
    Malnutrition

Modified from Rebar RW: "The reproductive age: Chronic anovulation," in *The Ovary*, edited by GB Serra. New York, Raven Press, 1983; used with permission.

HYPOTHALAMIC CHRONIC ANOVULATION (HCA)

Evidence suggests that HCA is a heterogeneous group of disorders with similar manifestations. Emotional and physical stresses, diet, body composition, exercise, environment, and other unrecognized factors contribute in varying proportions to the anovulation. (Anorexia nervosa is a related but distinct entity discussed under EATING DISORDERS in Ch. 47.) These disorders are characterized by low to normal levels of gonadotropins and relative hypoestrogenism. Psychologic counseling and/or a change in the life-style of the patient is often effective in inducing ovulation. Ovulation may also be induced with clomiphene citrate. If these measures are ineffective, then treatment with human menopausal gonadotropin and human chorionic gonadotropin (HMG-HCG) or with gonadotropin-releasing hor-

mone (GnRH) given in a pulsatile fashion may be required. Most authorities now advocate the use of exogenous estrogens supplemented cyclically with an oral progestin to prevent osteoporosis in women with low concentrations of circulating estrogen who do not desire pregnancy. An oral daily regimen of 0.625 to 1.25 mg conjugated estrogens, 1.25 to 2.5 mg estrone sulfate, 20 μg ethinyl estradiol, or 0.5 to 1.0 mg micronized estradiol-17β, with oral medroxyprogesterone acetate 5 to 10 mg administered for the first 12 to 14 days of each month, can be used. Alternatively, oral contraceptives can be administered to affected women who are sexually active.

CHRONIC ANOVULATION DUE TO PITUITARY DYSFUNCTION

Following appropriate therapy for the pituitary dysfunction, ovulation can be induced if pregnancy is desired. Gonadal stimulation with

HMG-HCG is required if the pituitary no longer produces gonadotropins.

CHRONIC ANOVULATION DUE TO INAPPROPRIATE FEEDBACK SIGNALS

A heterogeneous group of disorders with great clinical and biochemical variability in which chronic anovulation, because of inappropriate feedback signals to the hypothalamic-pituitary unit, appears to be the common denominator. The most prominent example is the **polycystic ovary syndrome (PCO; Stein-Leventhal syndrome)**, which is characterized by LH-dependent hyperandrogenism but not necessarily hirsutism. Included are such disorders as Cushing's syndrome, mild congenital adrenal hyperplasia, virilizing tumors of adrenal or ovarian origin, hyper- and hypothyroidism, and obesity.

Symptoms and Signs

Typically, patients present with amenorrhea, hirsutism, and obesity, but they may instead complain of irregular, profuse uterine bleeding (because of endometrial hyperplasia that results from unopposed estrogenic stimulation—see under ABNORMAL GENITAL BLEEDING, below), have no hirsutism, and be of normal weight. Evidence indicates that the hypothalamic-pituitary unit is intact, but that a functional derangement resulting in abnormal gonadotropin secretion is present. Excess androgen from any source or increased extraglandular conversion of androgens to estrogens can lead to the constellation of findings observed. In all these disorders, the ovaries may be enlarged, with smooth and thickened capsules, or they may be normal in size. Typically, the ovaries contain many 2- to 6-mm follicular cysts, and thecal hyperplasia surrounds the granulosa cells. Large cysts containing atretic cells may be present.

Diagnosis

In PCO, the irregular menses, mild obesity, and hirsutism usually begin in the pubertal years and generally worsen with time. Although patients may present with either primary or secondary amenorrhea (as well as uterine bleeding), all patients are clinically well estrogenized with abundant cervical mucus on examination. LH levels are typically elevated, with relatively low and constant FSH levels, but both may be in the normal range. Generally, levels of most circulating androgens tend to be mildly elevated. Hirsutism should be evaluated as described under AMENORRHEA, above. The aim of the diagnostic evaluation is to discover a cause (eg, a neoplasm) that can be treated definitively. PCO is a benign disorder.

Treatment

No ideal therapy for either PCO or hirsutism exists. Patients may require therapy to induce ovulation if pregnancy is desired and to prevent estrogen-induced endometrial hyperplasia. Treatment must be individualized to the needs and desires of the patient.

In the anovulatory woman who is not hirsute and does not desire pregnancy, intermittent progestin (eg, medroxyprogesterone acetate 5 to 10 mg/day orally for 10 to 14 days q 1 to 2 mo) or oral contraceptives (if she is premenopausal, does not smoke, and has no other significant risk factors [see Oral Contraceptives in Ch. 4]) should be given to reduce the increased risks of endometrial hyperplasia and carcinoma present because of unopposed estrogen. An endometrial biopsy should be obtained before initiating medical therapy in any woman with a prolonged history of anovulatory bleeding and in all affected women > 35 yr. Women using intermittent progestins should be cautioned about the need for contraception because of the possible (although unproven) association of these agents with birth defects if taken during early pregnancy.

In the anovulatory woman who is hirsute and does not desire pregnancy, treatment differs but is similar to that offered to the ovulatory hirsute woman. The use of physical treatment modalities (including bleaching, electrolysis, plucking, waxing, and depilation) should be encouraged. No pharmacologic modality is ideal or completely effective, and the various agents have not been compared directly in controlled studies. **Oral contraceptive agents** are the first line of therapy for patients with mild hirsutism. These drugs suppress gonadotropin and steroid secretion and increase production of sex-hormone–binding globulin (**SHBG**), thus reducing biologically active free testosterone levels. Unfortunately, several months are required to observe any effect, and that effect is often slight. All preparations seem to be equally efficacious. For the patient for whom oral contraceptives are undesired or contraindicated, continuous suppression with oral progestin (medroxyprogesterone acetate 5 to 20 mg/day) can be used. Side effects of progestin include mastodynia, bloating, and depression.

Cyproterone acetate, a potent progestational agent and an antiandrogen, appears to control hirsutism in 50 to 75% of affected women. It is used to treat hirsute women throughout the world except in the USA, where it has not been approved because of its propensity to cause breast cancer in beagles and fetal anomalies in pregnant rats. Cyproterone is generally used in a cyclic manner with ethinyl estradiol so that periodic withdrawal bleeding occurs. Contraception should be used. Significant side effects include decreased libido and depression.

Spironolactone, a mild diuretic that also inhibits the biosynthesis of androgen and competes with androgens for the androgen receptor in target tissues such as the hair follicle, has been used effectively to treat hirsutism at doses of 100 to 200 mg/day orally. Side effects include initial diuresis and postural changes (including syncope and hypotension), mastodynia, and irregular uterine bleeding. Spironolactone has not been approved for such use in the USA, and effects on a developing fetus are unknown. Thus, contraception should be used. Furthermore, the long-term effects of this agent remain unknown.

Glucocorticoids, used to achieve adrenal suppression, are not indicated in most hirsute women because no advantage of adrenal over ovarian suppression has been demonstrated and because the source of excess androgen in most hirsute women is largely ovarian. The potential hazards of adrenal steroids would seem to militate against their use except in patients with documented adrenal hyperfunction or enzyme defects in the steroidogenic pathway.

In the future, both GnRH agonists and antagonists have potential in the treatment of hirsutism. These agents suppress gonadotropins and thus gonadal steroid secretion and produce what has been called a medical oophorectomy. Effective topical antiandrogens also are being sought.

In women with PCO who desire pregnancy, clomiphene citrate 50 to 100 mg/day for 5 days remains the first choice with which to induce ovulation because of its simplicity and high success rate (75% ovulation rate, 35 to 40% pregnancy rate). Previous failure to induce ovulation with clomiphene should not contraindicate its use in the future. Other methods of ovulation induction include use of HMG-HCG, human purified FSH, pulsatile administration of GnRH, and ovarian wedge resection. **Wedge resection** should be reserved for patients in whom all other methods fail, in whom there is a question of an ovarian tumor because of ovarian size or circulating androgen levels, and/or in whom fertility is not an issue (because pelvic adhesions can form after the surgery). Ablation of ovarian cysts by laser or electrocautery is advocated by some but must be regarded as experimental. It is likely that these procedures will cause pelvic adhesions as well, and medical therapy is very effective in inducing ovulation.

PREMATURE OVARIAN FAILURE
(Premature Menopause)

Several disorders in which women < 40 yr present with symptoms and signs due to estrogen deficiency and have elevated circulating levels of gonadotropins (especially FSH) and low levels of estradiol. See TABLE 6–3 for the disorders presenting as ovarian failure.

Although high levels of gonadotropin as observed in castrates and postmenopausal women are usually associated with the absence of oocytes in the ovaries, there are several rare circumstances in which high gonadotropin levels are found in women whose ovaries still contain viable follicles. Rare pregnancies have been reported in sexually active women with hypergonadotropic hypogonadism during and after treatment with estrogens. Other patients have resumed regular menses and conceived after several years of hypergonadotropic amenorrhea.

All patients < 30 yr in whom the diagnosis of ovarian failure has been made on the basis of elevated gonadotropins should have a karyotype determination. The presence of a Y chromosome requires laparotomy and excision of gonadal tissue to prevent the 25% incidence of malignant tumor formation occurring in such patients. Genetic evaluation is unnecessary in women > 35 yr presenting with elevated gonadotropin levels, because gonadal neoplasms have not been reported in these older women. They should be presumed to have premature menopause.

A number of cases of ovarian failure occur in association with other autoimmune disorders, including thyroiditis, hypoparathyroidism, hypoadrenalism, diabetes mellitus, rheumatoid arthritis, myasthenia gravis, and pernicious anemia. Some patients have circulating antibodies to ovarian tissue (presumably to ovarian receptors for FSH). Therefore, in young women desiring pregnancy, blood tests to evaluate the possibility of an autoimmune disorder are indicated. Such tests may also indicate which patients may develop other endocrine disorders

TABLE 6-3. CAUSES OF ELEVATED LEVELS OF FSH

Menopause

Physical causes
Surgical extirpation of the gonads
Irradiation of the gonads
Viral agents
Chemotherapeutic agents

Gonadotropin-producing neoplasms (rare)

Chromosomal abnormalities
Gonadal dysgenesis
With stigmas of Turner's syndrome (45,XO)
Pure (46,XX or 46,XY)
Mixed
Trisomy X with or without chromosomal mosaicism

Gonadotropin gonadal receptor and/or postreceptor defects (resistant ovary or Savage syndrome)

Defects in gonadotropin secretion
Secretion of biologically inactive forms
Defects in α or β subunits

Enzymatic defects
17 α-Hydroxylase deficiency
Galactosemia

Autoimmune disorders
Polyglandular disorders involving ovarian failure and any combination of thyroiditis, hypoadrenalism, hypoparathyroidism, diabetes mellitus, pernicious anemia, myasthenia gravis, vitiligo, and mucocutaneous candidiasis
Isolated ovarian failure

Congenital thymic aplasia

Idiopathic premature ovarian failure

FSH = follicle-stimulating hormone.

with time. These tests should include measurements of serum calcium and phosphorus to rule out hypoparathyroidism, thyroid function and antibodies to rule out thyroiditis, and at least an AM cortisol to rule out hypoadrenalism. Also indicated are a CBC and tests for sedimentation rate, total protein, albumin/globulin ratio, rheumatoid factor, and antinuclear antibodies. Serum gonadotropin and estradiol levels can be determined weekly on 2 to 4 occasions. If LH levels are ever greater than FSH levels or if estradiol is ever > 50 pg/mL, then ovarian follicles should be present.

Ovulation induction with gonadotropins can be offered empirically, but any patient electing treatment must recognize that the possibility of pregnancy is very low. Pregnancy can be achieved in these women by use of oocyte donation, with artificial cycles stimulated with exogenous estrogen and progesterone so that the embryos fertilized in vitro can be transferred to appropriately stimulated endometrium.

ABNORMAL GENITAL BLEEDING

*Abnormal uterine bleeding includes (1) excessive duration (**menorrhagia**) or amount (**hypermenorrhea**) of menstruation or both; (2) too frequent menstruation (**polymenorrhea**); (3) nonmenstrual or intermenstrual bleeding (**metrorrhagia**); and (4) **postmenopausal bleeding**, which denotes any bleeding occurring ≥ 6 mo after the last normal menstrual period at the menopause.*

Abnormal genital bleeding is due to organic causes in about 25% of patients; in the remainder there is a functional abnormality of the hypothalamic-pituitary-ovarian axis (**dysfunctional uterine bleeding**). In considering the individual patient, age is the most important factor. Dysfunctional bleeding is much more common during the early reproductive years, whereas organic causes, including neoplasias of the genital tract, become more frequent with advancing age (see below).

Infancy and Childhood

Newborn girls may have some spotting for a few days because of stimulation of the endometrium in utero by placental estrogens. Any other bleeding from the reproductive tract is rare in childhood and warrants investigation. Accidental traumatic lesions of the vulva and vagina are most common. Vaginitis (often as a result of a foreign body), prolapse of the urethral meatus, and tumors of the genital tract can also present with bleeding. Ovarian tumors generally do not bleed unless they are endocrinologically active.

Precocious puberty (see also in Ch. 47) must always be considered in the differential diagnosis of childhood bleeding and can be recognized in most cases by the development of secondary sexual characteristics. The cause for precocious development remains unknown in many cases but may be due to drug ingestion, CNS lesions, hypothyroidism, or adrenal or ovarian neoplasms.

Bleeding and vaginal discharge are the presenting symptoms in > 80% of cases of **vaginal adenosis** and **clear cell adenocarcinoma of the vagina and cervix.** These lesions have been linked to diethylstilbestrol **(DES)** exposure in utero and are diagnosed by cytologic smear and colposcopically directed biopsy of suspicious areas. In the absence of malignancy, most lesions do not require treatment and patients can be followed with periodic examinations.

Women of Reproductive Age

Hematologic disorders with abnormal clotting, whether primary (eg, idiopathic thrombocytopenia purpura, leukemia, bone marrow aplasia, hemolytic anemia) or secondary to systemic causes (eg, uremia, liver disease, anticoagulant therapy), can lead to abnormal bleeding throughout the reproductive years. Hematologic evaluation is indicated in adolescents and in others with a history suggestive of clotting disorders. Von Willebrand's disease most commonly presents as dysfunctional uterine bleeding.

Complications of pregnancy are the most frequent organic causes of abnormal bleeding in women of reproductive age. Patients with symptoms of pregnancy or with a confirmed early pregnancy and uterine bleeding spontaneously abort the pregnancy in perhaps half the cases. Ectopic pregnancy and gestational trophoblastic

disease are the most important entities to be considered in the differential diagnosis. These topics are discussed in Chs. 10 and 15. Endometritis and infected retained products of conception usually cause bleeding shortly after delivery or abortion but occasionally may present ≥ 2 wk later (see Ch. 19).

Endometriosis (see Ch. 7) causes dysfunctional uterine bleeding by unknown mechanisms in 20 to 88% of affected women.

Vulvar bleeding in the reproductive years is almost always due to trauma.

Vaginal lesions vary greatly and may cause bleeding during this time of life. Vaginitis causes bleeding more commonly in children and postmenopausal women because their vaginal mucosa is thinner, but spotting may occur in severe cases during the reproductive years. Granulomatous tissue formed after surgery (especially hysterectomy) may also cause bleeding. Biopsy may be necessary to rule out malignancy. Although cauterization with silver nitrate or cryotherapy is sufficient to stop bleeding in most cases, surgical resection may be required for large lesions. Vaginal adenosis, which frequently presents with bleeding, was discussed above as a cause of bleeding in children. Malignant lesions of the vagina, which may also cause bleeding, are discussed in Ch. 10.

Cervical cancer (see Ch. 10) and several **benign cervical lesions** are associated with bleeding. Cervicitis only rarely causes bleeding, except in association with **ectropion of the cervix** (extension of columnar epithelium to the exposed portion of the cervix). Patients may complain of postcoital spotting, but the usual complaint is a vaginal discharge tinged with blood. Diagnosis and treatment are discussed in Ch. 5. Women with cervical polyps may present with intermenstrual or postcoital bleeding. Most polyps are easily removed by merely twisting them off at the pedicle. Endometrial polyps and submucosal myomas should be considered in the differential diagnosis. Condylomata acuminata of the cervix can cause bleeding and are treated with cryotherapy, surgical resection, or laser therapy as discussed in Ch. 21.

Endometrial hyperplasia, a common cause of uterine bleeding, is discussed under DYSFUNCTIONAL UTERINE BLEEDING, below.

Adenomyosis, *the benign invasion of endometrium into the myometrium,* is a common disorder that causes symptoms in only a small percentage of affected patients, most commonly late in the reproductive years. Menorrhagia and intermenstrual bleeding are the most common complaints, followed by nonspecific pelvic pain and bladder and rectal pressure. On pelvic examination, the uterus may feel enlarged, globular, and softer than normal; and there may be associated leiomyomas. Hysterectomy may be indicated for symptomatic relief in some patients.

Leiomyomas are present in the uterus of as many as 40% of women by age 40, but in only a few women are they symptomatic. Any kind of bleeding abnormality can be caused by myomas. Hysterectomy is indicated for symptomatic women in whom fertility is not an issue, those with a uterus > 12 to 14 wk gestation in size, those in whom the uterus is increasing rapidly in size, and those with significant bleeding not controlled medically. Myomectomy is an option for symptomatic women who wish to preserve reproductive potential. The use of GnRH analogs before surgery to decrease the size of the fibroids may make myomectomy more simple, but it is not always possible to preserve the uterus if there are many large fibroids.

Functional ovarian cysts are relatively common, and > 50% of patients present with some form of menstrual irregularity, ranging from amenorrhea to menorrhagia. In young women cystic adnexal masses may disappear spontaneously. Adnexal masses of > 5 cm that persist for > 1 mo require surgical exploration to exclude a neoplasm. Although any ovarian tumor may cause abnormal uterine bleeding, it is common only in endocrinologically active neoplasms. Treatment of these neoplasms is discussed in Ch. 10.

Contraceptives, including birth control pills, IUDs, and progestins, may cause abnormal bleeding. It is unclear if tubal ligation is followed by an increased incidence of menstrual irregularities. These issues are discussed in Ch. 4.

Thyroid dysfunction may also be associated with menstrual irregularity. Although oligomenorrhea and amenorrhea are more common, menorrhagia can result.

Postmenopausal Bleeding

Gynecologic malignancies must be ruled out in any postmenopausal woman with genital bleeding (see Ch. 10). Of the benign conditions associated with postmenopausal bleeding, the most frequent are atrophic vaginitis (see Ch. 5), an atrophic endometrium, endometrial polyps, and endometrial hyperplasia. Why a patient with atrophic endometrium bleeds is not clear. Endometrial polyps need no further treatment after

diagnostic curettage but need to be observed for possible recurrence. Hyperplastic endometrial changes should generally be treated by hysterectomy in older women (see below).

DYSFUNCTIONAL UTERINE BLEEDING (DUB)
(Functional Uterine Bleeding)

Abnormal uterine bleeding not associated with tumor, inflammation, or pregnancy.

DUB, the most common cause of abnormal uterine bleeding, must be a diagnosis of exclusion. It occurs most commonly at the extremes of reproductive life; > 50% of the cases of DUB occur in women > 45 yr, and 20% are seen in adolescents. Although DUB may occur with either ovulatory or anovulatory cycles, > 70% of episodes are associated with anovulation. Thus, DUB is common in women with polycystic ovary syndrome **(PCO)**. The bleeding in anovulatory women is generally the result of stimulation of the endometrium with unopposed estrogen and may result in **endometrial hyperplasia**. The endometrium, thickened by the estrogen, then sloughs incompletely and irregularly, and bleeding becomes irregular, prolonged, and sometimes profuse. Abnormal bleeding may also occur in women taking some form of exogenous estrogen. In ovulatory cycles the abnormal bleeding is generally due to luteal phase abnormalities.

History and physical examination cannot distinguish patients with abnormal uterine bleeding who have endometrial hyperplasia from those who do not. Women ≥ 35 yr, those with PCO and/or a prolonged history of anovulatory bleeding, and obese and nulliparous women should have an endometrial biopsy before initiation of medical therapy, because they are at increased risk for endometrial carcinoma (see Ch. 10). A Hct and Hb should be done on each patient presenting with abnormal bleeding to evaluate the chronicity and severity of the bleeding.

Treatment

Treatment varies with the age of the patient, the extent of the bleeding, pathologic assessment of the endometrium, and the patient's wishes. Even acute episodes of profuse bleeding in anovulatory women can generally be treated by giving 1 combination oral contraceptive agent q 6 h for 5 to 7 days. Bleeding should stop in 12 to 24 h, but patients will have heavy bleeding, often with cramping, 2 to 4 days after stopping therapy. Recurrence is prevented by giving combination oral contraceptive agents cyclically for at least 3 mo. If spontaneous cyclic menses do not resume and pregnancy is not desired, or if use of oral contraceptives is contraindicated for some reason, the patient can be treated with progestin (medroxyprogesterone acetate 5 to 10 mg/day orally for 10 to 14 days each month). Uterine curettage is indicated in patients failing to respond to hormonal therapy (as indicated in a subsequent biopsy) and in those in whom irregular bleeding persists. If pregnancy is desired, then ovulation can be induced as discussed in treatment of PCO, above.

An alternative approach to the treatment of an acute episode of anovulatory bleeding is the administration of conjugated estrogens 25 mg IV q 4 h up to 3 doses until bleeding abates. Progestin therapy (medroxyprogesterone acetate 5 to 10 mg/day orally for 10 days) should be started simultaneously. Following cessation of therapy, withdrawal bleeding will result. The patient can then be treated with oral contraceptives for at least 3 cycles.

For women with anovulatory bleeding without a profuse bleeding episode, treatment with cyclic oral contraceptives or progestin can be offered if pregnancy is not desired. Ovulation induction with clomiphene citrate can be offered to those desiring pregnancy. Similarly, clomiphene citrate can be used to treat luteal dysfunction. HCG 2500 to 5000 IU IM q 2nd or 3rd day beginning with the midcycle increase in basal body temperature and progesterone 12.5 mg/day IM in oil or 25 mg bid as rectal or vaginal suppositories have also been used to treat luteal dysfunction.

Treatment of women with endometrial hyperplasia must be individualized, based on the pathologic findings, the age of the patient, and the patient's reproductive desires. Women with atypical adenomatous hyperplasia are most easily treated with hysterectomy regardless of age because of the risk of subsequent adenocarcinoma of the uterus. A fractional D & C should be performed prior to any therapy in any woman with atypical hyperplasia on biopsy to rule out coexisting carcinoma. In women who are poor surgical risks and in those who wish to preserve future fertility, medroxyprogesterone acetate 20 to 40 mg/day orally can be given for 3 to 6 mo. Patients can then undergo a repeat endometrial biopsy. If the biopsy indicates resolution of the hyperplasia, patients may be treated with cyclic medroxyprogesterone acetate (5 to 10 mg/day orally for 10 to 14 days each month) or with clomiphene citrate to induce ovulation if pregnancy is desired. Women with more benign cystic hyperplasia or adenomatous hyperplasia can generally be treated cyclically with medroxyprogesterone acetate, but again should undergo a repeat biopsy in about 3 mo.

7. ENDOMETRIOSIS

A benign disease in which functioning endometrial tissue is present in sites outside the uterine cavity.

Endometriosis is usually confined to the peritoneal or serosal surfaces of intra-abdominal organs, commonly the ovaries, posterior broad ligament, posterior cul-de-sac, and the uterosacral ligaments. Less common sites include the serosal surfaces of the small and large bowel, ureters, bladder, vagina, surgical scars, and pleural cavity.

Etiology and Epidemiology

The most widely accepted hypothesis is that endometrial cells are transported from the uterine cavity to implant at ectopic sites. Retrograde flow of menstrual tissue through the fallopian tubes could cause intra-abdominal endometriosis, while the lymphatic or circulatory systems could spread endometriosis to distant sites (eg, the pleural cavity). Another possible explanation is the transformation of coelomic epithelium into endometrium-like glands (ie, coelomic metaplasia).

There is evidence of a familial inheritance pattern, with the occurrence of endometriosis increased by 6% in first-degree relatives of women with endometriosis. Additional factors associated with an increased incidence include delay in childbearing, Oriental race, and müllerian duct anomalies.

Although the reported incidence varies, endometriosis is commonly found in 10 to 15% of women between the ages of 25 and 44 yr who are actively menstruating. Increased use of diagnostic laparoscopy has also detected endometriosis in teenagers. It has been estimated that 25 to 50% of infertile women have endometriosis. In patients with severe endometriosis and distor-

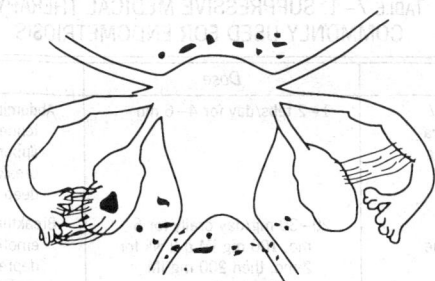

FIG. 7–1. Stage III (moderate) endometriosis. Filmy adhesions are present on the right fallopian tube and ovary; dense adhesions are found on the left fallopian tube and ovary. The latter also has deep endometrial implants; superficial implants are noted on the peritoneum. (Adapted from "Revised American Fertility Society Classification of Endometriosis." *Fertility and Sterility* 43:351, 1985; reproduced with permission of the publisher, The American Fertility Society.)

tion of normal pelvic anatomy, the incidence of infertility is high because of impaired ovum pickup and tubal transport mechanisms. However, some patients with minimal endometriosis and normal pelvic anatomy are also infertile and may have an increased incidence of luteal phase dysfunction, luteinized unruptured ovarian follicle syndrome ("trapped oocyte"), increased peritoneal prostaglandin production, and/or increased peritoneal macrophage activity to account for their decreased fertility.

Symptoms and Signs

The clinical manifestations are pelvic pain, pelvic mass, alterations of menses, and infertility. Some women with severe endometriosis may be asymptomatic, while others with minimal disease may have incapacitating pain. Dyspareunia and midline pelvic pain pre- or perimenstrually, particularly beginning after several years of pain-free menses, may occur. Such dysmenorrhea is an important diagnostic clue. Lesions on the large bowel or bladder may cause pain with defecation, abdominal bloating, rectal bleeding with menses, or suprapubic pain during urination. Endometriotic implants on the ovary or adnexal structures can form an endometrioma (ie, a cystic mass of endometriosis localized to an ovary) or adnexal adhesions, giving rise to a pelvic mass. Occasionally, rupture or leakage from an endometrioma may be associated with acute abdominal pain.

Diagnosis

The diagnosis is suspected on the basis of the symptoms described above and/or physical findings (see FIG. 7–1). Pelvic examination may be normal or may reveal visible lesions on the vulva or cervix, in the vagina, the umbilicus, and in surgical scars. There may be a retroverted and fixed uterus, enlarged ovaries, or uterosacral nodularity.

The diagnosis can be established only by visualizing lesions, usually by endoscopy of the pelvis. In the absence of visible lesions on physical examination, the primary diagnostic modality is direct visualization and/or biopsy of lesions by laparoscopy. Diagnosis could also be made during laparotomy or on sigmoidoscopy or cystoscopy. Microscopically, endometriotic implants consist of endometrial glands and stroma, structurally identical to endometrium (most implants can bleed during menstruation). *By definition, both glands and stroma must be present to diagnose endometriosis.* These tissues contain estrogen and progesterone receptors that allow for growth and differentiation in response to the sequential changes in ovarian steroids during the menstrual cycle. Thus, the macroscopic appearance (clear, red, brown, black) and size of these implants vary. When confined to the peritoneal cavity, bleeding from these lesions is thought to initiate an inflammatory process followed by fibrin deposition and adhesion formation, which eventually leads to distortion of peritoneal surfaces and of normal pelvic anatomy. Other diagnostic procedures (eg, ultrasonography, barium enema, IV urogram, CT, or MRI) may be useful for demonstrating the extent of disease and following its course but are not specific or adequate for diagnosis. Investigational serum markers for endometriosis (eg, CA-125 and antiendometrial

TABLE 7-1. SUPPRESSIVE MEDICAL THERAPY
COMMONLY USED FOR ENDOMETRIOSIS

Drugs	Dose	Side Effects
Combination estrogen/ progestin oral contraceptives* (30–35 μg ethinyl estradiol)	1–2 tabs/day for 4–6 mo	Abdominal swelling, breast tenderness, increased appetite, edema, nausea, breakthrough bleeding, deep venous thrombosis
Progestogens (medroxyprogesterone acetate)	20–30 mg/day orally for 6 mo; 100 mg IM q 2 wk for 2 mo; then 200 mg IM monthly for 4 mo	Breakthrough bleeding, emotional lability, depression, atrophic vaginitis
Danazol	400–800 mg/day orally for 4–6 mo	Weight gain, acne, lowering voice, hirsutism, hot flushes, atrophic vaginitis, edema, muscle cramps, breakthrough bleeding, decreased breast size, emotional lability, liver dysfunction, carpal tunnel syndrome, adverse effects on lipids
GnRH agonists Nafarelin	400–800 mg/day intranasally	Hot flushes, vaginal dryness, bone demineralization, emotional lability
Leuprolide	1 mg/day s.c.	
Leuprolide depot	3.75 mg IM q 30 days	

GnRH = gonadotropin-releasing hormone.
* Monophasic.

antibody levels) may help monitor the disease but will require further refinement. Infertility studies may be indicated (see Ch. 3).

Staging the disease as minimal, mild, moderate, or severe is important to formulate a treatment strategy and evaluate response to therapy. The revised staging criteria of the American Fertility Society are based on the location of implants, presence of superficial or deep endometriosis, and presence of filmy or dense adhesions. This classification scheme divides the degree of endometriosis into minimal, mild, moderate, or severe categories. Shown in FIG. 7–1 is an example of stage III (moderate) endometriosis.

Treatment

Treatment must be individualized to the patient's age, symptoms, desire for pregnancy, and extent of disease. In general, treatment modalities include medically suppressing ovarian function to arrest the growth and activity of the endometrial implants, conservative surgical resection of as much of the endometriosis as possible, a combination of the 2 therapies, and extirpative

surgery (total abdominal hysterectomy with or without unilateral or bilateral salpingo-oophorectomy).

Various drugs are available that suppress ovarian function and/or growth of the endometrial tissue. These are listed in TABLE 7–1 with examples of dosages and side effects. Continuous oral contraceptives are less commonly used because other agents, such as danazol (an antigonadotropin that blocks ovulation) and gonadotropin-releasing hormone (GnRH) agonists (which produce a state of relative and reversible hypoestrogenemia), have become available. Pregnancy rates with medical therapy range from 40 to 60%. It is not clear that fertility rates are improved by treatment of mild or minimal endometriosis. It must be emphasized that suppressive medical therapy or conservative surgery does not effectively cure endometriosis, and recurrence is observed in most patients. *Only total ablation of ovarian function will prevent recurrence of endometriosis.* Cyclic oral contraceptives given following medical therapy and/or conservative surgery may slow progression of the disease and are warranted in women wishing to delay childbearing.

Moderate to severe cases are treated most effectively by excision of as many implants as possible, while preserving reproductive potential. Indications for surgery include the presence of endometriomas ($>$ 2 to 3 cm), significant pelvic adhesions, fallopian tube obstruction, and intractable and incapacitating pelvic pain not responsive to medical therapy. Care must be taken to prevent adhesion formation during surgery by using microsurgical techniques. With the newer operative laparoscopic approach, it is possible in some cases to electrocauterize peritoneal or ovarian lesions or to vaporize or excise them with a CO_2, argon, or neodymium:yttrium-aluminum-garnet (Nd:YAG) laser. Pregnancy rates following this conservative surgical approach are about proportional to the severity of the endometriosis

and range from 40 to 70%. In patients with midline pelvic pain, laparoscopic resection of the uterosacral ligaments with electrocautery or laser therapy may reduce the degree of pain. For patients who undergo conservative surgery with incomplete resection of disease, adjunctive suppressive medical treatment may enhance fertility rates.

Extirpative surgery should be reserved for patients with intractable pelvic pain who have completed childbearing. Following removal of the uterus and ovaries, replacement estrogen therapy can be started postoperatively or may be delayed for 4 to 6 mo if significant disease is left in situ. Adjunctive suppressive medical therapy may be necessary in this interval. In the younger patient, one should consider preserving ovarian function, although recurrence rates of 3.5 to 85% have been reported.

8.   TOXIC SHOCK SYNDROME (TSS)

A syndrome characterized by high fever, vomiting, diarrhea, confusion, and skin rash that may rapidly progress to severe and intractable shock. This syndrome was first described in children (8 to 17 yr old) in 1978. In 1980, a large number of cases began to be recognized, predominantly in young women (age 13 to 52 yr), almost always associated with menstruation and the use of vaginal tampons. The incidence is not known, but estimates made from small series have suggested about 3 cases/100,000 menstruating women. Overall, about 700 cases were reported in the USA in 1980. By 1981, after widespread publicity, as well as withdrawal of some vaginal tampons from the market, the incidence in women dropped precipitously, but cases are still reported in women who do not use tampons and in postoperative and postpartum women. About 15% of cases occur in men, usually postoperatively. Cases have also been reported in association with influenza. Less severe instances of the syndrome that may lack some of the manifestations are fairly common.

Etiology and Pathogenesis

The exact cause of TSS is unknown, but almost all patients have been found to be infected with exotoxin-producing strains of phage-group 1 *Staphylococcus aureus*. These infections appear to be caused by the same toxin, now called the **toxic shock syndrome toxin-1 (TSST-1)**. The organism has been found in mucosal (nasophar-

ynx, vagina, trachea) or sequestered (empyema, abscess) sites. In menstruating women it has been found in the vagina, and in almost every case the affected women used vaginal tampons for their menses. (Tampon manufacturers had modified the absorbent material to increase absorbency and more completely obstruct outflow from the vagina.) Presumably, women most at risk are those with preexisting *S. aureus* colonization of the vagina who also use tampons regularly for their menses. Conceivably, mechanical or chemical factors related to tampon use result in production of the bacterial exotoxin, which enters the bloodstream through a mucosal break or via the uterus to the peritoneal cavity. TSS may also occur as a complication of a postoperative staphylococcal wound infection that is often minor, deep, and difficult to detect.

Symptoms and Signs

The onset is sudden, with fever (temperature 39 to 40.5° C [102 to 105° F] that remains elevated) associated with headache, sore throat, nonpurulent conjunctivitis, profound lethargy, intermittent confusion without focal neurologic signs, vomiting, profuse watery diarrhea, and a diffuse sunburnlike erythroderma. The syndrome may progress rapidly (within 48 h) to orthostatic hypotension, syncope, and shock. Between the 3rd and 7th days after onset, desquamation of the skin occurs that may lead to epidermal sloughing, particularly of the palms and soles.

Other organ systems are usually involved, resulting in mild nonhemolytic anemia, moderate leukocytosis with a predominance of immature granulocytes, and early thrombocytopenia followed by thrombocytosis. Although clinically important bleeding phenomena are rare, the prothrombin time and partial thromboplastin time tend to be prolonged. In children particularly, impaired perfusion of the extremities may be associated with profound hypotension. Renal dysfunction, characterized by diminished urine output and increases in BUN and creatinine levels, is almost universal. Laboratory evidence of hepatocellular dysfunction (hepatitis) and skeletal myolysis are common during the first week of illness. Cardiopulmonary involvement occurs, manifested by peripheral and pulmonary edema (despite abnormally low central venous pressures, suggesting adult respiratory distress syndrome).

Mortality rates range between 8 and 15% but may not reflect the true incidence, since these figures are probably based on recognition of only the more severe cases. Recurrence is common in women who continue to use tampons during the first 4 mo following an episode of TSS, although there is evidence that this pattern does not apply to women treated with antibiotics to eradicate S. aureus.

Diagnosis

TSS resembles Kawasaki syndrome (mucocutaneous lymph node syndrome—see also in Ch. 32) but can usually be differentiated on clinical grounds. Shock usually is not seen in Kawasaki syndrome; the skin rash is maculopapular in Kawasaki syndrome but a diffuse erythema in TSS; azotemia and thrombocytopenia are rarely seen in Kawasaki syndrome but are common in TSS. Though the cause of Kawasaki syndrome is uncertain, it generally occurs in children < 5 yr of age, and the staphylococcal exotoxin implicated in Kawasaki syndrome by some investigators is different from that in TSS. Other disorders to be considered in differential diagnosis are scarlet fever, Reye's syndrome, the staphylococcal scalded skin syndrome, meningococcemia, Rocky Mountain spotted fever, leptospirosis, and viral exanthematous diseases. These are ruled out by specific differences in the clinical picture and by appropriate cultures and serologic studies.

Treatment

Patients suspected of having TSS should be hospitalized immediately and treated intensively. Tampons, diaphragms, or any other foreign bodies should be removed at once when the diagnosis is suspected. Immediate consideration must be given to supportive care, particularly adequate fluid and electrolyte replacement to prevent or treat hypovolemia, hypotension, or shock. Since shock may be profound and resistant, large quantities of fluid and electrolyte replacement are sometimes required. Specimens for Gram stain and culture should be obtained from mucosal surfaces and blood; then treatment with a β-lactamase–resistant penicillin or a cephalosporin may be started. Whether antibiotics modify the acute course of the illness is unclear, but eradicating staphylococcal foci appears to protect against recurrences.

Other than eradicating S. aureus, precise recommendations for prevention (primary or secondary) cannot be made with certainty. However, it seems prudent to advise women to avoid constant use of tampons throughout the menstrual period and to intermittently use napkins or other hygienic measures. Additionally, avoiding newer types of tampons designed for maximum absorbency may be advisable.

9.   BREAST DISORDERS

Incidence and Epidemiology

Breast cancer is the most common cancer in women, and symptoms suggesting this disease are even more common. About 15 million women in the USA seek medical attention every year because of concern about breast cancer, and >140,000 new cases are diagnosed annually. For every woman diagnosed with the disease, another 5 to 10 undergo biopsies that prove benign, and another 10 present with a breast mass causing them anxiety. In addition, many women present with mastalgia, either associated with an underlying cyst or unrelated to any findings within the breast, and some with nipple discharge, usually unrelated to cancer.

Screening and Diagnostic Techniques

Breast examination by patient or physician begins with visual inspection for asymmetry in breast size, nipple inversion, bulging, or dimpling. FIG. 9–1 A and B shows the usual positions for such inspection. An underlying cancer is

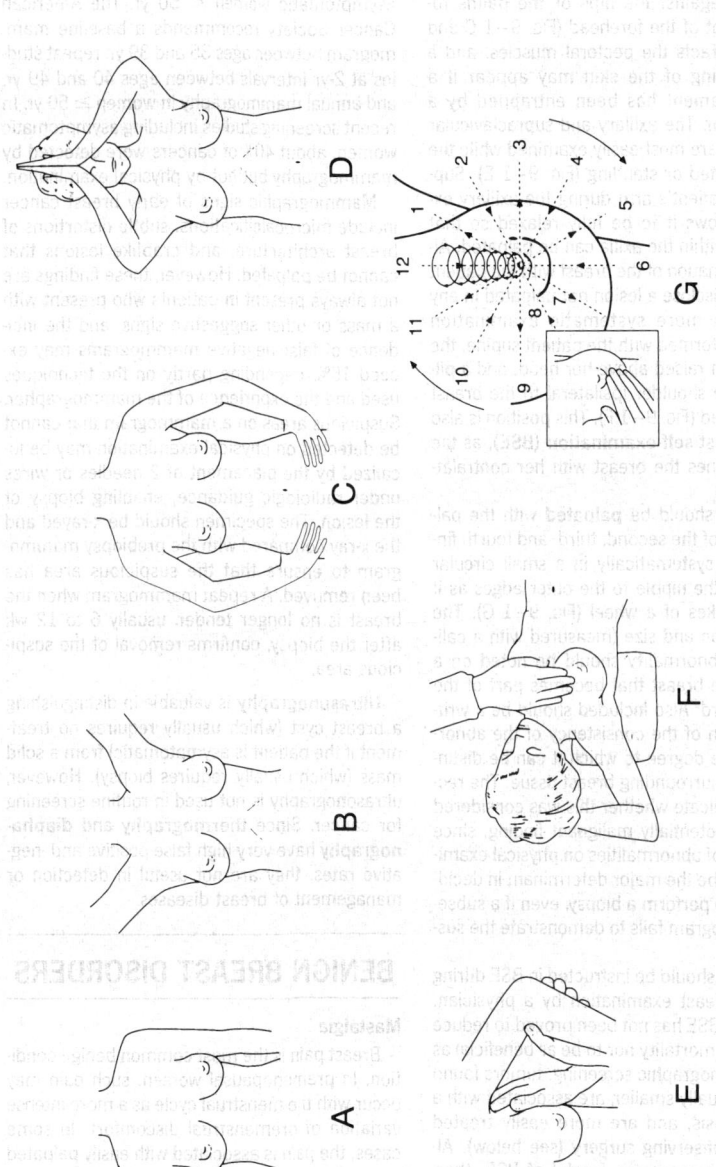

Fig. 9–1. Positions for breast examination. Patient seated or standing: (A) Arms at side. (B) Arms raised over head, elevating pectoral fascia and breasts. (C) Hands pressed firmly against hips, or (D) palms pressed together in front of forehead, contracting pectoral muscles. (E) Palpation of axilla; arm supported as shown, relaxing pectoral muscles. Patient supine: (F) Pillow under shoulder and arm raised above head on side being examined. (G) Palpation of breast in circular pattern from nipple outward.

sometimes detected by having the patient press both hands against the hips or the palms together in front of the forehead (FIG. 9–1 C and D). This contracts the pectoral muscles, and a subtle dimpling of the skin may appear if a Cooper's ligament has been entrapped by a growing tumor. The axillary and supraclavicular lymph nodes are most easily examined while the patient is seated or standing (FIG. 9–1 E). Supporting the patient's arm during the axillary examination allows it to be fully relaxed so that nodes deep within the axilla can be palpated. Although examination of the breast with the patient seated may disclose a lesion not palpated in any other way, a more systematic examination should be performed with the patient supine, the ipsilateral arm raised above her head, and a pillow under the shoulder ipsilateral to the breast being examined (FIG. 9–1 F). This position is also used for **breast self-examination (BSE)**, as the patient examines the breast with her contralateral hand.

The breast should be **palpated** with the palmar surfaces of the second, third, and fourth fingers, moving systematically in a small circular pattern from the nipple to the outer edges as if along the spokes of a wheel (FIG. 9–1 G). The precise location and size (measured with a caliper) of any abnormality should be noted on a drawing of the breast that becomes part of the patient's record. Also included should be a written description of the consistency of the abnormality and the degree to which it can be distinguished from surrounding breast tissue. The record should indicate whether this was considered a benign or potentially malignant finding, since the presence of abnormalities on physical examination should be the major determinant in deciding whether to perform a biopsy, even if a subsequent mammogram fails to demonstrate the suspicious area.

The patient should be instructed in BSE during her annual breast examination by a physician. While routine BSE has not been proved to reduce breast cancer mortality nor to be as beneficial as routine mammographic screening, tumors found on BSE are usually smaller, are associated with a better prognosis, and are more easily treated with breast-conserving surgery (see below). Although many women are fearful of BSE, thorough instruction by a nurse or other specialist can alleviate much anxiety.

Routine mammography reduces breast cancer mortality by 25 to 35% in asymptomatic women ≥ 50 yr of age and by a lesser degree in asymptomatic women < 50 yr. The American Cancer Society recommends a baseline mammogram between ages 35 and 39 yr, repeat studies at 2-yr intervals between ages 40 and 49 yr, and annual mammography in women ≥ 50 yr. In recent screening studies including asymptomatic women, about 40% of cancers were detected by mammography but not by physical examination.

Mammographic signs of early breast cancer include microcalcifications, subtle distortions of breast architecture, and crablike lesions that cannot be palpated. However, these findings are not always present in patients who present with a mass or other suggestive signs, and the incidence of false-negative mammograms may exceed 15%, depending partly on the techniques used and the experience of the mammographer. Suspicious areas on a mammogram that cannot be detected on physical examination may be localized by the placement of 2 needles or wires under radiologic guidance, enabling biopsy of the lesion. The specimen should be x-rayed and the x-ray compared with the prebiopsy mammogram to ensure that the suspicious area has been removed. A repeat mammogram when the breast is no longer tender, usually 6 to 12 wk after the biopsy, confirms removal of the suspicious area.

Ultrasonography is valuable in distinguishing a breast cyst (which usually requires no treatment if the patient is asymptomatic) from a solid mass (which usually requires biopsy). However, ultrasonography is not used in routine screening for cancer. Since **thermography** and **diaphanography** have very high false-positive and -negative rates, they are not useful in detection or management of breast diseases.

BENIGN BREAST DISORDERS

Mastalgia

Breast pain is the most common benign condition. In premenopausal women, such pain may occur with the menstrual cycle as a more intense variation of premenstrual discomfort. In some cases, the pain is associated with easily palpated **cysts** and can be relieved by aspirating the cyst with a fine-gauge needle. The aspirated fluid need not be examined cytologically, but the color and volume should be recorded, and whether the cyst disappeared after aspiration should be noted. Cancer in the wall of a cyst, although extremely rare, can be suspected if the fluid is bloody or reaccumulates rapidly (within 12 wk) following aspiration. Under these circumstances, the entire cyst should be excised.

Other causes of mastalgia are thought to be primarily hormonal. Methylxanthines have been proposed, but controlled trials have failed to demonstrate that restricting intake of methylxanthine-containing substances (eg, coffee) is more beneficial than a placebo. In most patients, mastalgia remits spontaneously after months or years, thus complicating the evaluation of potential therapeutic modalities. Danazol, an attenuated androgen with low androgenic side effects, given 100 to 400 mg/day orally for 3 to 6 mo, and tamoxifen, an antiestrogen with almost no side effects, given 10 mg bid orally for 3 to 6 mo, have been shown to relieve mastalgia. Since the long-term side effects of these drugs are not yet known, their use should be limited to a short course in patients with unusually severe symptoms, though tamoxifen can probably be given safely, especially in older women, for up to 5 yr.

Most women have areas of relatively indistinct lumpiness in the breast, usually in the upper outer quadrant. Mastalgia, breast cysts, and nondescript lumpiness are common conditions and often occur together. The combination is frequently described under the catchall term **fibrocystic disease**, a condition important primarily because of its possible relation to subsequent risk of developing breast cancer (see below). However, none of these conditions should in itself be considered abnormal. There is no evidence that treatment of these conditions will reduce the risk of developing breast cancer.

Fibroadenomas

These benign tumors usually appear in young women, often in teenagers, and may be easily mistaken for cancer. However, they tend to be more circumscribed and mobile and may feel like a small, slippery marble under the examining fingers. Fibroadenomas can usually be excised under local anesthesia but frequently recur. Often, after several such tumors have been established as benign, the patient feels comfortable in leaving a fibroadenoma intact rather than having it excised. Other benign, solid breast masses include **fat necrosis** and **sclerosing adenosis**, which can be diagnosed only by biopsy.

Nipple Discharge

This is not necessarily abnormal, even in postmenopausal women. Cancer is an underlying cause in < 10% of patients with nipple discharge (see Paget's disease under OTHER CANCEROUS BREAST DISORDERS, below). While the gross appearance of the discharge is of little help in diagnosing an underlying cancer, a guaiac-positive secretion was identified with breast cancer in one study. The most common cause of a bloody discharge is an underlying **intraductal papilloma**. In some cases, the cancer or benign tumor causing the discharge can be palpated. In other cases, routine or contrast ductographic mammography is helpful in locating the lesion. If breast cancer is not apparent on these evaluations, the cause of the discharge is probably benign, and a nipple-flap duct resection, usually performed as an outpatient procedure under local anesthesia, can eradicate the symptom and relieve the patient's anxiety. A milky discharge, or galactorrhea, in a woman who is not postpartum should prompt an endocrine evaluation.

Infections

These are extremely rare except as a puerperal event or following trauma. Infection occurring under other circumstances should prompt consideration of other underlying disorders, such as cancer.

Gynecomastia

Enlargement of the male breast is normal and usually transient during puberty. Similar changes may occur in senescence; with various diseases, especially of the liver; following drug treatment (eg, with estrogens, reserpine, digitalis, isoniazid, spironolactone, calcium channel blockers, ketoconazole, theophylline, cimetidine, metronidazole, methadone, and antineoplastic drugs); or with marijuana use. Endocrine disorders are less commonly the cause of gynecomastia. Ultrasonography of the testis is valuable in detecting estrogen-secreting testicular tumors, and CT or MRI of the abdomen is useful in detecting estrogen-secreting tumors of the adrenals.

Gynecomastia may be unilateral or bilateral, and most of the enlargement is usually due to proliferation of stroma rather than breast ducts. The patient may experience some tenderness; generally this is associated with benign causes. In most cases, no specific treatment is needed, since gynecomastia will spontaneously remit or disappear after treatment of the underlying cause. Reports of benefit from various endocrine

TABLE 9–1. BREAST CANCER RISKS IN WHITE FEMALES

Age	Risk of Developing Breast Cancer (%)	Risk of Developing Invasive Breast Cancer (%)	Risk of Dying from Breast Cancer (%)
Birth–110	10.2	9.8	3.6
20–30	0.04	0.04	0.00
20–40	0.49	0.42	0.09
20–110	10.34	9.94	3.05
35–45	0.88	0.83	0.14
35–55	2.53	2.37	0.56
35–110	10.27	9.82	3.56
50–60	1.95	1.86	0.33
50–70	4.67	4.48	1.04
50–110	8.96	8.66	2.75
65–75	3.17	3.08	0.43
65–85	5.48	5.29	1.01
65–110	6.53	6.29	1.53

From Seldman H, et al. Surveillance, Epidemiology, and End Results (SEER): "Breast cancer: Current trends in diagnosis and treatment." *CA—A Cancer Journal for Clinicians*, 1985, p 186; used with permission.

treatments are contradictory; surgical removal of the excess breast tissue remains the only reproducibly effective treatment. Recently, suction lipectomy, alone or with cosmetic surgery, has been used with increasing success.

BREAST CANCER

Risk Factors

In the USA, the cumulative risk of developing breast cancer is 10.2%, but that of dying from the disease is only about 3.6%. Much of this risk is after age 75 (see TABLE 9–1). For example, the oft-cited 10% lifetime risk of developing breast cancer is based on an actuarial analysis and calculated from birth to age 110. The cumulative risk for the disease in any 20-yr period is considerably lower; cumulative risks > 40% are rare for even the highest risk groups.

A family history of breast cancer in a first-degree relative (parent, sibling, child) increases two- to threefold an individual's chance of developing the disease, but a history in more distant relatives increases the risk only slightly. Some studies have shown that relatives of women with bilateral breast cancer or in whom the cancer was diagnosed prior to menopause are at higher risk for the disease, but other studies have failed to confirm these observations. Thus, it is unlikely that any family history profile is associated with a > 30% probability of developing breast cancer before age 75.

The women at highest risk of developing breast cancer are those with a history of in situ or invasive breast cancer. The risk of developing cancer in the contralateral breast following mastectomy is about 0.5 to 1.0%/yr of follow-up.

Women with early menarche, late menopause, and late first pregnancy are at increased risk. Women with a first pregnancy after age 30 may be at higher risk than those who are nulliparous. Although a history of fibrocystic disease has been shown to increase the risk, this is an imprecise histologic diagnosis often assigned to a breast biopsy that reveals normal breast tissue or very minimal proliferation and a few cysts; therefore, it has little meaning. Among women who have had a biopsy for a benign breast condition, the increased risk appears to be limited to those with a histologic picture of ductal proliferation, and even then the risk is moderate except in women with atypical hyperplasia or a positive family history. Women with multiple breast lumps but no histologic confirmation of a high-risk pattern should not be considered at high risk; lumpy breasts is a normal condition.

Most studies have failed to demonstrate an association between the use of oral contraceptives and subsequent development of breast cancer, but prolonged use (ie, > 4 yr) before the first pregnancy may increase the risk. Similarly, the use of postmenopausal estrogen replacement therapy appears to increase the risk modestly but only after 10 to 20 yr of exposure. Whether use of a cyclic estrogen-progestin regimen has an effect on risk is not known.

Evidence indicates that environmental factors, such as diet, play a role in causing or promoting the growth of breast cancers, but there is no conclusive evidence that a particular diet (eg, one high in fats) is more likely to be associated with the disease. Obese postmenopausal women are at increased risk, but no evidence shows that dietary modification decreases this risk. Radiation exposure before age 30 also increases risk.

Symptoms, Signs, and Diagnosis

More than 80% of breast cancers are discovered as a lump found by the patient herself. Less commonly, patients present with a history of pain and no mass, with breast enlargement, or with a nondescript thickening in the breast. A typical finding on physical examination is a dominant mass—a lump distinctly different from the surrounding breast tissue. Diffuse fibrotic changes in a quadrant of the breast, usually the upper outer quadrant, are more characteristic of benign disorders, but a slightly firmer thickening not noted in the contralateral breast may be a sign of cancer. More advanced, usually inoperable, breast cancers are characterized by fixation of the mass to the chest wall or the overlying skin, by the presence of satellite nodules or ulcers in the skin, or by exaggeration of the usual skin markings resulting from lymphedema (peau d'orange). Matted or fixed axillary lymph nodes and supra- or infraclavicular lymphadenopathy are also considered inoperable. Inflammatory breast cancer is particularly virulent, characterized by a diffuse inflammation and enlargement of the breast, often without a mass.

If cancer is suspected on physical examination, biopsy should be planned. A prebiopsy mammogram may help delineate other areas of the breast on which biopsies also should be performed and serves as a baseline for future reference. However, the results of the mammogram should not dissuade the physician from performing the biopsy. Fine-needle aspiration and cytologic evaluation may be sufficient to confirm cancer but should be used only by those experienced in the technique. If aspirate from a suspicious lesion is negative, a more definitive procedure should be performed: a needle or incisional biopsy or an excisional one if the tumor is small. For most lesions, including those requiring mammographically guided needle localization

(see under Screening and Diagnostic Techniques, above), biopsy can be performed under local anesthesia. The excised specimen may be placed in India ink before sectioning, so normal tissue margins surrounding the tumor mass can be defined more precisely.

A part of the biopsy specimen should routinely undergo estrogen- and progesterone-receptor analysis. These cytoplasmic proteins can be measured by either a steroid-binding assay, which requires about 1 gm fresh tumor pulverized to form a crude tumor cell homogenate, or by immunochemical assay (ER-ICA), which requires smaller amounts of fresh tissue. The ER-ICA can also be performed with fixed tissue sections, but the results are less reliable. About $2/3$ of patients have an estrogen-receptor positive (ER+) tumor; the incidence of positive tumors is greater among post- than premenopausal women. Patients with receptors have a somewhat better prognosis and are more likely to benefit from endocrine therapy. A tumor progesterone receptor is thought to reflect a functional estrogen receptor, and the presence of both receptors predicts a higher likelihood of response than the presence of estrogen receptor alone and a much greater likelihood of response than might be expected if neither receptor is present. Knowledge of receptor status at the time of diagnosis may be useful in the selection of both adjuvant therapy (after mastectomy or radiation therapy) and palliative therapy if the patient later develops metastatic disease.

Tumor tissue specimens may also be evaluated for ploidy and S-phase fraction of cells. The prognosis is worse if aneuploid tumors and those with a high percentage of cells in S phase are found. Even though these tests can be performed at many commercial laboratories, no standardized values have been established to identify the patient with a poor prognosis, nor have quality control programs been instituted to ensure the comparability of results obtained in different laboratories. Eventually, these tests may help determine prognosis in patients whose breast cancer has no histologic involvement of axillary lymph nodes.

In situ carcinoma, once fairly uncommon, now accounts for > 10% of all breast cancers diagnosed in the USA. Lobular carcinoma in situ (LCIS), or lobular neoplasia, occurs predominantly in premenopausal women and is usually found incidentally, since it does not form a palpable mass. Between 25 and 35% of patients with LCIS subsequently develop an invasive breast cancer after a latency of up to 40 yr. These invasive cancers occur with equal frequency bilaterally. Many specialists link LCIS with atypical hyperplasia, considering it an indication of propensity for breast cancer rather than a true precursor.

Ductal carcinoma in situ (DCIS) occurs in both pre- and postmenopausal women, forms a palpable mass, and is more frequently localized to one quadrant of a breast. DCIS is frequently the cause of microcalcifications seen in mammograms. Patients are likely to develop an invasive cancer following biopsy if no further treatment is undertaken. However, DCIS is still considered a precursor of invasive cancer, and because it is localized, it can be totally removed surgically.

Invasive ductal and lobular tumors are the most common histologic types, accounting for about 90% of all breast cancers. Patients with less common histologic types, eg, medullary and tubular lesions, have a somewhat better prognosis.

Most patients choose to delay initiation of treatment for one to several weeks after biopsy. During this time, a thorough evaluation should be performed to rule out metastatic disease. Minimally, this should include a physical examination for lymphadenopathy, skin metastases, and hepatomegaly; a chest x-ray; liver function studies; and a CBC. Baseline measurements of carcinoembryonic antigen (CEA) and CA 15-3 might also be obtained, since these tumor markers are elevated in > 50% of patients with metastatic disease. A bone scan should be obtained routinely for patients with larger tumors or lymphadenopathy. Although bone scans rarely are positive in patients without lymphadenopathy whose tumors are < 2 cm in diameter, they can provide a valuable baseline for comparison with future scans if signs of metastatic disease (eg, musculoskeletal pain) develop. Liver scans rarely are positive in patients with normal liver function studies, a normal CEA, and no evidence of hepatomegaly on physical examination.

Primary Treatment

Survival rates in patients treated with **mastectomy** compared with those treated with **breast-conserving surgery** (lumpectomy, tylectomy, wide excision, partial mastectomy, or quadrantectomy) **plus radiotherapy** appear to be identical, at least for the first 20 yr. The choice of treatment depends primarily on patient preference. The major advantage of breast-conserving sur-

gery and radiotherapy is cosmetic and its resulting sense of body integrity. However, this advantage may not be achieved if the tumor is large in relation to the breast, since total removal of the tumor mass along with a tumor-free margin of normal tissue is necessary for long-term control of breast cancer. In about 15% of patients treated with breast-conserving surgery and radiotherapy, it may be difficult to determine which breast was treated. More often, however, some shrinkage occurs in the treated breast and possibly some thickening or disruption of contour in the area of the wide excision. These changes can be minimized by attention to cosmetic detail during initial biopsy and during reexcision if that becomes necessary. Other adverse effects of radiotherapy are usually transient and mild; they include erythema or painless blistering of the skin during therapy, mild pneumonitis 3 to 6 mo after completion of radiotherapy in about 10 to 20% of patients, and asymptomatic rib fractures in < 5% of patients.

Although most invasive tumors have one or more small areas of intraductal (or in situ) cancer, some studies have shown that tumors characterized by an extensive (> 25%) intraductal component (EIC+) *both within the invasive tumor area and in nearby tissue* have a high recurrence rate *within* the breast following breast-conserving surgery and radiotherapy. However, there is no difference in the distant recurrence rate or survival rates of EIC+ and EIC− tumors treated by breast-conserving surgery. Local control of EIC+ tumors is best achieved by either mastectomy or a reexcision of the original tumorous area to rule out multiple foci of remaining tumor.

The Halsted **radical mastectomy** has been almost universally superseded by a **modified radical mastectomy**, which removes all breast tissue but preserves the greater pectoral muscle and eliminates the need for skin graft. **Radiotherapy** administered as an adjuvant after mastectomy significantly reduces the incidence of local recurrence on the chest wall and in the regional lymph nodes but does not improve overall survival. Consequently, adjuvant radiotherapy is being used less often. Length of survival following modified radical mastectomy is equivalent to that following a radical mastectomy, and **breast reconstruction** is considerably easier. Techniques for reconstruction include simple placement of a submuscular (or less commonly, subcutaneous) silicone implant, the use of a tissue expander with delayed implantation of a silicone prosthesis, the transference of muscle and blood supply from either the latissimus dorsi or the lower rectus abdominis muscles, or the creation of a free flap by anastomosing the gluteus maximus muscle to the internal mammary vessels. The choice of procedure depends on the extent of previous surgery or radiotherapy, the experience of the plastic surgeon, and the patient's willingness to undergo more extensive surgical procedures. Patients may elect to undergo reconstruction immediately following mastectomy, but this requires prolonged anesthesia and coordination between the general and plastic surgeons.

A **lymph node dissection** or **node sampling** can be performed as part of a modified radical mastectomy or as a separate axillary incision during breast-conserving surgery. Considerably less morbidity is associated with the procedure if node dissection is limited to the areas medial and inferior to the subclavian muscle. More extensive procedures are probably not justified, since the main value of lymph node removal is diagnostic, not therapeutic. No other prognostic factor is as well correlated with disease-free and overall survival as is nodal status. In most studies, the 10-yr disease-free survival rate exceeds 70%, and overall survival exceeds 80% for node-negative patients. In contrast, the rates are about 25 and 40%, respectively, for node-positive patients. The prognosis is worse with each additional positive lymph node found, but 3 nodal group classifications have traditionally been used: node-negative, 1 to 3 positive nodes, and ≥ 4 positive nodes. The 10-yr disease-free and overall survival rates for the last group are about 15 and 25%. Larger lesions are more likely to be node-positive, but size has independent prognostic value (ie, each 1-cm increase in size worsens prognosis). Some authorities believe that a tumor < 1 cm indicates an excellent prognosis, and no adjuvant therapy is required; others believe that a tumor > 5 cm calls for adjuvant systemic therapy before mastectomy or breast-conserving surgery. Although patients with poorly differentiated tumors have a worse prognosis than those whose tumors are well differentiated, precision in making this assessment is not good; different pathologists examining the same slides tend to judge them differently.

In situ carcinoma: LCIS is treated with either close observation after diagnosis or bilateral mastectomy. Most patients with DCIS are cured by simple mastectomy, which has been standard treatment for this type of cancer. However, increasing numbers of patients are being treated with wide excision alone, especially if the lesion is < 2.5 cm and the type of DCIS is histologically favorable, or with wide excision plus radiotherapy when size and histologic characteristics are less favorable. Wide excision, alone or with radiotherapy, is being evaluated for both groups of patients in randomized trials.

Inflammatory cancers are treated initially with systemic therapy, usually chemotherapy, followed by radiotherapy. Although about $2/3$ of inflammatory breast cancers are ER +, the role of hormone therapy, alone or with chemotherapy, is not well defined in these tumors.

Adjuvant Systemic Therapy

Chemotherapy or endocrine therapy, begun soon after the completion of primary therapy and continued for months or years, delays recurrence in almost all patients and prolongs survival in some. No evidence shows that these therapies will cure patients who have not been cured by mastectomy or radiotherapy.

Adjuvant chemotherapy increases survival rates by 25 to 35% in premenopausal women during the first 10 yr of follow-up. Studies with longer follow-up suggest that the difference in median length of survival between premenopausal, node-positive patients treated with adjuvant chemotherapy and those treated with mastectomy alone may exceed 5 yr. Chemotherapy combination regimens, such as cyclophosphamide, methotrexate, and 5-fluorouracil **(CMF)**, are more effective than a single drug, but use of a regimen for 6 to 24 mo is no more effective than that for 4 to 6 mo. Although adjuvant chemotherapy prolongs disease-free survival in postmenopausal women, it does not significantly prolong overall survival. Acute side effects depend on the regimen used but usually include nausea, infrequent vomiting, mucositis, easy fatigability, mild to severe alopecia, myelosuppression, and thrombocytopenia. No long-term side effects have been noted with most regimens, and death from infection or bleeding is rare (< 0.2%). However, L-phenylalanine mustard has been reported to increase more than tenfold the incidence of acute leukemia, and there may be an increased incidence of other tumor types after longer follow-up of patients treated with other drugs.

Adjuvant tamoxifen therapy increases survival rates about 20% in women ≥ 50 yr of age in the first 5 yr following diagnosis. In one study of postmenopausal women, the difference in median survival time between patients treated with mastectomy plus 5 yr of tamoxifen therapy and those treated with mastectomy alone was 2 yr. Although adjuvant tamoxifen delays recurrence in premenopausal women, it does not prolong overall survival. The optimal duration of adjuvant therapy with tamoxifen is not known, but treatment for > 5 yr is not recommended until evidence shows that prolonged courses offer additional benefits without additional toxicity. While tamoxifen has almost no acute side effects, especially in postmenopausal women, its antiestrogenic effects on breast tissue are balanced by estrogenic effects in other parts of the body. Thus, tamoxifen decreases the incidence of contralateral breast cancer (an antiestrogenic effect) while also decreasing serum cholesterol (an estrogenic effect). Tamoxifen therapy may reduce cardiovascular mortality and osteoporosis but may simultaneously increase the risk of developing subsequent uterine cancer.

Until recently, patients whose axillary lymph nodes show no histologic involvement have not been treated with adjuvant therapy, because most of them are cured by local therapy. Adjuvant chemotherapy and adjuvant tamoxifen significantly delay recurrence in these patients, but no proof exists that overall survival is substantially or significantly improved.

Some form of adjuvant chemotherapy, such as CMF for 6 mo, should be given routinely after mastectomy or lumpectomy plus radiotherapy to all premenopausal, node-positive patients. Adjuvant tamoxifen should be routinely given after local therapy for at least 2 yr but not > 5 yr to postmenopausal women who are node-positive and have ER+ tumors. Since use of these therapies in other patients remains controversial, they should be used only with full disclosure of the uncertainty regarding benefits and long-term side effects.

Treatment of Metastatic Disease

Breast cancer may metastasize to almost any organ in the body. Those most commonly involved include the lung, liver, bone, lymph nodes, and skin. Because metastases frequently appear in breast cancer patients years or decades after initial diagnosis and treatment, symptoms should prompt an immediate physical examination followed by appropriate blood and radiologic studies. Breast cancer is a common cause of metastases to the CNS. About 10% of patients with metastases to bone eventually develop hypercalcemia. Although most metastases to skin occur in the region of the breast surgery, metastases frequently appear on the scalp as well.

Treatment of metastases only marginally affects survival, but appropriately used, even relatively toxic therapies (eg, chemotherapy) palliate symptoms and improve quality of life. The choice of one therapy over another depends on (1) the estrogen- and/or progesterone-receptor determination of the primary tumor or biopsy of a metastatic lesion; (2) the interval from diagnosis to presentation of metastases (the disease-free interval); (3) the number of sites of metastases and organs involved; and (4) the patient's menopausal status. Patients with one focus of metastases always have others, even if they are not immediately apparent on initial relapse. Thus, most patients with metastatic disease are treated with systemic therapy, either endocrine or chemotherapy. However, there are exceptions. Patients with a long disease-free interval (eg, ≥ 2 yr) and a single site of metastasis may not have evidence of additional metastases for months or years; in such patients, radiotherapy alone might be used to treat isolated, symptomatic bone lesions or local skin recurrences not amenable to surgical resection. Radiotherapy is the most effective treatment for brain metastases, occasionally achieving long-term control. Patients with multiple sites of metastases outside the CNS should initially be given systemic therapy; radiotherapy is usually withheld until evidence shows that a site cannot be adequately palliated with systemic treatment. Since there is no proof that treatment of patients with asymptomatic metastases substantially increases survival, therapy, especially toxic, may be withheld until either the patient has symptoms or evidence of rapid progression appears.

Endocrine therapy is preferred over chemotherapy in patients with estrogen receptor−positive (ER+) tumors, a disease-free interval > 2 yr, or disease that is not life-threatening. Endocrine therapies are especially effective in premenopausal women in their 40s and postmenopausal women > 5 yr past their last menstrual period. However, none of these factors should be the sole criterion for choosing endocrine therapy over chemotherapy. For example, a 70-yr-old woman with an estrogen receptor−negative (ER−) tumor and a disease-free interval of > 5 yr and whose metastatic disease is limited to several bones might reasonably be treated with endocrine therapy. Conversely, a 35-yr-old premenopausal woman with an ER+ tumor and a disease-free interval of 6 mo and who has extensive liver involvement might be a candidate for chemotherapy.

Tamoxifen is usually the first endocrine therapy used because of its relative lack of toxicity. In premenopausal women, ovarian ablation by surgery or radiation is a reasonable alternative. Patients who initially respond to endocrine therapy but whose disease progresses months or years later should be treated with additional forms of endocrine therapy until no further response is seen. The progestins, either medroxyprogesterone acetate or megestrol acetate, are almost as nontoxic as tamoxifen and are often used as a secondary endocrine treatment. **Aminoglutethimide,** an aromatase inhibitor that decreases the availability of estrogen needed to maintain tumor growth, may also be used as either 2nd- or 3rd-line endocrine therapy in postmenopausal women. This drug should be administered with hydrocortisone replacement because of its suppressive effects on the adrenal gland. It is especially effective in patients with painful bone metastases. Although **estrogens** and **androgens** are also effective, they are not used frequently because they produce more side effects than other forms of endocrine therapy. For the same reason, adrenalectomy and hypophysectomy are rarely used.

The most effective **cytotoxic drugs** for the treatment of metastatic breast cancer are cyclophosphamide, doxorubicin, and mitomycin-C. The response rate to a combination of drugs is higher than that to a single agent, and most patients requiring palliative treatment with a chemotherapy combination are initially given either cyclophosphamide, methotrexate, and 5-fluorouracil **(CMF)** or cyclophosphamide, doxorubicin, and 5-fluorouracil **(CAF).** Response rates to regimens containing doxorubicin are higher than those to CMF regimens. However, combinations containing doxorubicin provide little additional survival benefit and are associated with more severe alopecia and cardiotoxicity. The administration of prednisone with CMF increases the response rate and decreases myelosuppression and GI toxicity, but prednisone increases the incidence of secondary infection and thromboembolic phenomena. Patients refractory to cyclophosphamide and doxorubicin are sometimes successfully palliated with either mitomycin-C or vinblastine. However, prolonged remissions are rarely achieved in these patients with other agents, including experimental programs.

The use of new drugs and treatment strategies, such as **biological response modifiers,** must be considered early in the course of disease, before extensive chemotherapy has been given, if it is to have any benefit. The biological response modifiers, including interferons, interleukin-2, lymphocyte-activated killer cells, tumor necrosis factors, and monoclonal antibodies, do not yet have an established role in breast cancer therapy.

OTHER CANCEROUS BREAST DISORDERS

Paget's disease of the nipple presents as a crusting, scaling erosion or as a discharge, usually so benign it is ignored by the patient and diagnosis is delayed for a year or more. Definitive diagnosis is made by biopsy of the nipple, but a cytologic smear of the nipple discharge often yields the diagnosis. Somewhat more than half these patients have a palpable mass at diagnosis. The underlying cancer may be invasive or in situ. Standard treatment is identical to that for other forms of breast cancer, and the prognosis depends on the invasiveness of the tumor, the size of the mass, and the presence or absence of histologically involved lymph nodes. Rarely, patients may be treated successfully with a limited excision of the nipple and some surrounding normal tissue.

Cystosarcoma phyllodes has many of the clinical characteristics of a fibroadenoma but generally should be treated as a sarcoma. The usual treatment is wide excision, but a simple mastectomy may be more appropriate if the mass is large in relation to the breast. Between 20 and 35% of these tumors recur locally, and distant metastases occur in 10 to 20% of patients.

Breast cancer in men occurs with 1% of the frequency seen in women. Although these cancers more often progress to an advanced stage because the diagnosis is seldom suspected by patient or physician, the prognosis for men is identical to that for women in the same stage. The treatment is also nearly identical, although breast-conserving surgery is rarely used and no firm data are available on the value of adjuvant therapy. Metastatic tumors respond to all of the endocrine therapies used to treat female breast cancer and to orchiectomy. Men with metastatic disease refractory to endocrine therapy may be successfully palliated with combination chemotherapy.

10.   GYNECOLOGIC NEOPLASMS

ENDOMETRIAL CARCINOMA
(Adenocarcinoma of the Uterus)

Of the malignancies affecting women, endometrial carcinoma ranks 4th in frequency, after breast, colorectal, and lung cancers. This adenocarcinoma is an epithelial lesion of the endometrium and is usually postmenopausal, with peak incidence between ages 50 and 60.

Etiology and Pathology

Endometrial carcinoma is more frequent in women with estrogen-producing ovarian tumors; with prolonged, and especially atypical, adenomatous endometrial hyperplasia; with delayed menopause; or with an abnormal menstrual history and infertility. Obesity, hypertension, diabetes mellitus, breast cancer, conditions that predispose to unopposed estrogen (ie, absence of ovulation and therefore no periodic progesterone), and a family history of breast or ovarian cancer are possible predisposing factors.

Endometrial carcinoma spreads (1) down the surface of the uterine cavity into the cervical canal; (2) through the myometrium to the serosa and into the peritoneal cavity; (3) by transplantation via the lumen of the fallopian tube to the ovary, broad ligament, and peritoneal surfaces; (4) via the bloodstream, leading to distant metastases; or (5) via the lymphatics. Downward spread may lead to cervical stenosis and pyometra. Vaginal metastases may cause a mucosanguineous discharge that, upon examination, leads to diagnosis of the metastases in advanced stages.

Symptoms, Signs, and Diagnosis

The cardinal symptom is inappropriate uterine bleeding, such as any postmenopausal bleeding or recurrent metrorrhagia in the premenopausal patient; *as many as ¹/₃ of all cases of postmenopausal bleeding are due to endometrial carcinoma.* The presence of myomas should not lead to complacency regarding abnormal bleeding, especially in susceptible women (see Etiology, above). A mucoid or watery discharge may precede bleeding by several weeks or months.

In **diagnosis**, the **Papanicolaou test (Pap test**—see below under CERVICAL CARCINOMA) is helpful but undependable, since 30 to 40% of smears yield false-negative results. Obtaining cellular material by aspiration of the endocervix may increase the rate of detection by Pap test to 70%. Vaginal douching should be avoided for at least 24 h before the examination. **Endometrial biopsy** has a 92% rate for detecting carcinoma. However, if cancer is not diagnosed by biopsy and surgical staging is not performed, the diagnostic procedure of choice is **fractional curettage** (endocervical curettement, sounding of the uterus, dilation of the cervical canal, and curettement of the endometrium). This procedure permits histologic confirmation and grading of the tumor, including determination of extension into the cervix, which may be important in planning therapy. Care should be taken in biopsy performance, sounding of the uterus, or curettement, since perforation may occur with these procedures.

IVU, cystoscopy, proctosigmoidoscopy, barium enema, and chest x-ray should be performed before initiating therapy. Other studies (eg, mammography, bone and liver scans, arteriography, lymphangiography) may be considered and performed when appropriate but are not a routine part of staging.

The staging system developed by the International Federation of Gynecology and Obstetrics (**FIGO**) for endometrial carcinoma recently changed from a clinical to a surgical classification and is outlined in TABLE 10–1.

Treatment and Prognosis

In the USA, the surgical approach includes extrafascial total abdominal hysterectomy with a wide vaginal cuff, combined with bilateral salpingo-oophorectomy and retroperitoneal lymph node sampling in the pelvic and para-aortic areas. Radical hysterectomy with retroperitoneal lymph node dissection is not warranted unless the cervix is clearly involved.

Progesterone therapy in patients with advanced or recurrent disease has led to regression in 35 to 40% of cases. Continuous, large doses of nonestrogenic progesterone derivatives (hydroxyprogesterone caproate 1 gm/wk IM or medroxyprogesterone acetate 500 mg/wk IM) or megestrol acetate 20 to 40 mg qid orally may be given. Treatment continues indefinitely if a favorable response is noted. Progesterone therapy also has produced regression of pulmonary, vaginal, and mediastinal metastases; difficulties with sodium and water retention are rarely en-

TABLE 10-1. STAGING OF ENDOMETRIAL CARCINOMA
AS A GUIDE TO TREATMENT AND PROGNOSIS*

Stage		Definition
IA	(G1,2,3)†	Tumor limited to endometrium
IB	(G1,2,3)	Invasion to $< 1/2$ myometrium
IC	(G1,2,3)	Invasion to $> 1/2$ myometrium
IIA	(G1,2,3)	Tumor involves only endocervical glands
IIB	(G1,2,3)	Invasion to cervical stroma
IIIA	(G1,2,3)	Tumor has invaded serosa and/or adnexa and/or peritoneal cytologic results are positive
IIIB	(G1,2,3)	Metastases to vagina
IIIC	(G1,2,3)	Metastases to pelvic and/or para-aortic lymph nodes
IVA	(G1,2,3)	Tumor has invaded bladder and/or bowel mucosa
IVB		Distant metastases, including intra-abdominal and/or inguinal lymph nodes

* Staging as described by the International Federation of Gynecology and Obstetrics (FIGO), 1988. Since uterine corpus cancer is now surgically staged, procedures previously used for differentiation of stages are no longer applicable. However, since there may be a small number of patients who will be treated primarily with radiation therapy, the clinical staging adopted by FIGO in 1971 still applies in these cases, but designation of that staging system should be noted. Ideally, in current staging, width of the myometrium should be measured along with the width of tumor invasion.

† G1 = ≤ 5% of a nonsquamous or nonmorular solid growth pattern; G2 = 6–50% of a nonsquamous or nonmorular solid growth pattern; G3 = 50% of a nonsquamous or nonmorular solid growth pattern. Notable nuclear atypia, inappropriate for the architectural grade, raises the grade of a grade 1 or 2 tumor by 1. In serous adenocarcinomas, clear cell adenocarcinomas, and squamous cell carcinomas, nuclear grading takes precedence. Adenocarcinomas with squamous differentiation are graded according to the nuclear grade of the glandular component.

countered. Remissions last 2 to 3 yr or occasionally longer.

Recently, cytotoxic chemotherapy has been used with progestins for metastatic cancer. Monthly chemotherapy combining cyclophosphamide 500 mg/m², doxorubicin 50 mg/m², and cisplatin 50 mg/m², given IV, plus megestrol acetate 120 mg/day orally has improved the overall response in 60% of patients. Frequent monitoring and complete knowledge of potential toxicity are essential with this regimen.

Prognosis is influenced by the histologic appearance and grading of the tumor, age of the patient (older women have a poorer prognosis), and spread of the tumor before therapy. The overall 5-yr survival rates for endometrial carcinoma are encouraging. Almost 63% of patients are alive without evidence of disease ≥ 5 yr after treatment; 28% succumb within 5 yr of treatment; 9% are alive with disease still present. In stage I disease, the reported 5-yr survival rate is between 70 and 89%.

Rarely, malignancies originate from other histologic components of the uterus, eg, sarcomas, carcinosarcomas, and mixed mesodermal tumors. Results of therapy in these cases are uniformly poor. Degenerating myomas rarely become sarcomatous, but when they do, cure rates with hysterectomy approach 80% if the lesion has remained within the myoma.

CERVICAL CARCINOMA

Carcinoma of the uterine cervix, the 2nd most common malignancy of the female reproductive tract, usually affects women aged 40 to 55 yr. The incidence is higher among women from lower socioeconomic groups and those with a history of early, frequent coitus and multiple sexual partners. Recently, venereal transmission of human papillomavirus (**HPV**)—especially subtypes 16, 18, 31, 33, and 35—has been implicated in the etiology of cervical neoplasia.

Pathology

The earliest histologic change in what is considered a continuum from normal to invasive cancer is **minimal cervical dysplasia**, in which abnormal cell proliferation occurs in the lower 1/3 of the epithelium. Most minimal dysplasias are self-limiting and regress to normal, but most **severe dysplasias** (2/3 of the epithelium showing abnormal proliferation) progress to **carcinoma**

TABLE 10-2. THE BETHESDA SYSTEM FOR REPORTING CERVICAL
AND VAGINAL CYTOLOGIC DIAGNOSES

Category	Description
Group 1	Findings within normal limits
Group 2	Infections
Group 3	Reactive and reparative changes
Group 4	Squamous cell abnormalities
	Squamous atypia
	Low-grade squamous intraepithelial lesion, including HPV or mild dysplasia
	High-grade squamous intraepithelial lesion, including moderate dysplasia (CIN 2), severe dysplasia, and carcinoma in situ (CIN 3)
	Squamous cell carcinoma
Group 5	Glandular cell abnormalities
	Atypia of undetermined significance
	Adenocarcinoma
Group 6	Nonepithelial malignant neoplasm

HPV = human papillomavirus; CIN = cervical intraepithelial neoplasia.

in situ, in which a full thickness of epithelium contains abnormal cells. When cancer cells penetrate the basement membrane and invade the stroma (invasive carcinoma), they can spread to adjacent pelvic organs by direct extension or by lymphatic permeation and dissemination.

Some 85 to 90% of cervical carcinomas are squamous cell carcinomas. These vary from well-differentiated cells with keratinization to highly anaplastic spindle cells. Adenocarcinomas account for 10 to 15% of cervical tumors. Sarcoma is rare.

Diagnosis

Early, asymptomatic cervical neoplasia can be detected preclinically by cytologic examination of cervical smears obtained during routine annual pelvic examinations. The Papanicolaou (Pap) test can detect ≥ 90% of early cervical neoplasias, and its use has reduced deaths from cervical cancer by > 50% through recognition and treatment of preinvasive neoplasia. Cervical cancer could be eliminated as a cause of death if all women had an annual Pap test; unfortunately, < 40% of women do so. (See directions for taking Pap test specimens in Ch. 1.)

Pap test results have been described in a system of cellular classification. However, most cytopathologists and many clinicians now prefer to report findings descriptively (eg, smear is consistent with infection, dysplasia, etc) rather than by class. The Bethesda System groups findings into 6 categories, listed in TABLE 10-2.

Biopsy is mandatory if a suspicious lesion (a friable mass or an ulcer) is seen. Dysplasia or carcinoma detected on Pap smear can be investigated with the colposcope. Colposcopy may reveal the biopsy site (and avoid the need for cone biopsy) in 85% of cases. If colposcopy is not available, biopsy sites may be identified by staining the cervix with an iodine solution, such as Lugol's (strong iodine) or Schiller's (potassium iodide 2 gm, iodine 1 gm, and water 300 mL). Nonstaining areas may be malignant, dysplastic, atypical, or glandular areas on the cervix. Outpatient cervical punch biopsy and endocervical curettage (to identify lesions higher in the cervical canal) diagnose invasion in 90% of cases with abnormal smears. Cold knife (noncautery) cone biopsy or laser cone biopsy with fractional D & C performed under local or general anesthesia is used only when simple biopsy fails to establish the presence or absence of invasion or when colposcopic examination is inconclusive or unsatisfactory.

Clinical staging of cervical carcinoma by physical examination of the pelvis is the basis for estimating prognosis and planning therapy (see TABLE 10-3). In addition, a metastatic survey, including cystoscopy and sigmoidoscopy (with biopsies as needed in each), IVU, and chest x-rays, is always done.

Treatment

Carcinoma in situ: Localized preinvasive lesions may be totally excised by cold knife or laser conization with diligent follow-up or by total hysterectomy. The choice depends upon the patient's desire to remain reproductive and her reliability in follow-up. If conization is chosen, Pap tests should be repeated every 3 mo for the first year and every 6 mo thereafter to ensure that all

TABLE 10–3. CLINICAL STAGING OF CERVICAL CARCINOMA
AS A GUIDE TO TREATMENT AND PROGNOSIS*

Stage	Description
0	Carcinoma in situ, intraepithelial carcinoma
I	Carcinoma strictly confined to the cervix (extension to the corpus should be disregarded)
IA	Preclinical carcinoma (diagnosed only by microscopy)
IA1	Minimal microscopically evident stromal invasion
IA2	Lesions detected microscopically that can be measured (depth of invasion ≤ 5 mm from base of epithelium; horizontal spread of ≤ 7 mm)
IB	Lesions of greater dimension than stage IA2; preformed space involvement should be recorded for determination of future treatment decisions
II	Carcinoma extends beyond the cervix but not onto the pelvic wall; carcinoma involves the vagina but not the lower $1/3$
IIA	No obvious parametrial involvement
IIB	Obvious parametrial involvement
III	Carcinoma extends to the pelvic wall; on rectal examination there is no cancer-free space between the tumor and the pelvic wall; tumor involves the lower $1/3$ of the vagina; includes all cases with hydronephrosis or nonfunctioning kidney
IIIA	Extension onto the pelvic wall
IIIB	Extension onto the pelvic wall and hydronephrosis or nonfunctioning kidney or both
IV	Carcinoma extends beyond the true pelvis or clinically involves the mucosa of the bladder or rectum (bullous edema as such does not permit a case to be allotted to stage IV)
IVA	Spread of the growth to adjacent organs
IVB	Spread to distant organs

* Staging as described by the International Federation of Gynecology and Obstetrics (FIGO), 1987.

of the lesion has been removed and that it does not recur. Cryotherapy and occasionally laser therapy are being used as outpatient treatment in carefully selected patients when colposcopy and biopsy have clearly defined the lesion and invasive cancer has been ruled out.

Invasive squamous cell carcinoma remains well localized for a considerable time, with distant metastases occurring only late in its course. Since the tumor spreads by contiguity and via the lymphatics, effective treatment must include affected nodes as well as the primary tumor but without excessively or irreversibly damaging surrounding normal body tissues. Radiotherapy and surgery, used alone or together, are nearly equally effective.

Radiotherapy: A common, effective technique consists of 2 cesium applications to the cervix (17,000 to 20,000 rads) for about 35 h each, followed by external radiation therapy encompassing the lymphatics along the pelvic wall. The cesium applications are sufficient to destroy the primary tumor, and external therapy raises irradiation to tumor-destroying levels in critical node regions. To shrink bulky or very advanced disease, external therapy may precede cesium applications. Major complications of radiother-

apy include radiation proctitis and cystitis and occasionally recto- and vesicovaginal fistula formation. With primary radiotherapy for invasive squamous cell carcinoma, the overall 5-yr survival rate is about 55%. In stages I and II, 5-yr cure rates are 75 to 90%.

Surgery: Primary surgical treatment is limited to patients in whom ovarian function can be preserved, lesions show limited local spread, and para-aortic lymph node biopsy is negative. Young women with stages IB and IIA lesions are preferred candidates. Surgery involves radical hysterectomy, including all of the parametria, and bilateral retroperitoneal lymph node dissection ending just above the bifurcation of the aorta. Five-year cure rates of 85 to 90% for women with stages IB and IIA lesions have been reported following radical hysterectomy. The major complication of radical surgery, uretero- and vesicovaginal fistula formation, occurs in about 1 to 2% of operations. If para-aortic node biopsy is positive or if the disease extends outside the pelvis, surgery is generally contraindicated. If tumors are restricted to the pelvis but involve the rectum or bladder, exenteration (excision of all pelvic organs) may be performed in physically and psychologically appropriate patients. Exenteration usually is the treatment of choice for recurrent or persistent cancer confined to the central pelvis following conventional radiotherapy; occasionally it is used as primary therapy for advanced disease. It is successful in 25 to 45% of cases.

Chemotherapy: Systemic treatment usually provides only temporary pain relief. When radiation therapy has failed, distant metastases appear to respond better to chemotherapy than the primary tumor. Many cytotoxic agents are being investigated, but they have achieved objective regression in only 25 to 30% of tumors.

Cervical carcinoma in pregnancy: About 1% of all cervical carcinomas are complicated by pregnancy or occur in recently pregnant women. With carcinoma in situ, treatment is delayed until after delivery, which may occur vaginally. Invasive disease is treated as in nonpregnant women: in the first trimester, radical hysterectomy or therapeutic irradiation will terminate the pregnancy; in the 2nd trimester, the uterus is emptied by hysterotomy, followed by radiation therapy or surgical excision for early lesions; in the 3rd trimester, a short delay is encouraged to achieve fetal viability. Vaginal delivery is contraindicated in invasive cervical disease because it lowers the cure rate, regardless of treatment.

OVARIAN CARCINOMA

Ovarian cancers account for 18% of all gynecologic neoplasms, most commonly occurring in women in their 50s. Since an ovarian neoplasm usually remains occult until it enlarges or extends enough to produce symptoms, early detection is difficult; in 70 to 80% of patients, the disease is not diagnosed until it has become extensive within or beyond the pelvis. Thus, if routine pelvic examination reveals an ovary enlarged > 5 cm in diameter, close follow-up is required. In the young woman, detection of functional cysts is common; reexamination after 6 wk will show whether spontaneous resolution has occurred. Tumor size may be the only criterion for surgery, and 1 in 4 ovarian tumors removed surgically is malignant. This ratio increases with patient age. Ovaries in postmenopausal women are small and normally not palpable. *Thus, any enlargement of the ovary in a postmenopausal woman should signify a malignancy that requires prompt surgical excision.* Serous cystadenocarcinoma is the most common type (found in 50% of cases) and occurs bilaterally in 30 to 50% of patients.

Pathology

About 80% of malignant ovarian tumors arise from the ovarian epithelium and are classified histologically as (1) serous cystadenocarcinomas, (2) mucinous cystadenocarcinomas, (3) endometrioid tumors (similar to adenocarcinoma of the endometrium), (4) celioblastomas (Brenner tumors), (5) clear cell carcinomas, and (6) unclassified carcinomas. Tumors arising from germ cells or stroma that do not fall into this classification include granulosa-theca cell tumors, Sertoli-Leydig cell tumors, dysgerminomas, and malignant teratomas.

Ovarian cancer tends to spread by both direct extension and lymphatics to regional nodes in the pelvis and paraaortic region. With lymphatic involvement, dissemination to the abdominal and pelvic peritoneum usually occurs. With abdominal involvement, hematogenous dissemination can lead to liver and pulmonary inclusion.

Symptoms, Signs, and Diagnosis

An ovary may grow to considerable size before clinical symptoms appear. The earliest symptoms are vague lower abdominal discomfort and mild digestive complaints. Inappropriate endometrial bleeding is uncommon, presumably resulting from hormone secretion by the tumor. Abdominal swelling due to ovarian enlargement or accumulation of ascitic fluid, pelvic pain, anemia, and cachexia appear late in the course of disease. Additional physical signs include functional tumor effects (eg, hyperthyroidism, feminization, virilization) or, more commonly, a lobulated, fixed solid mass associated with nodular implants in the cul-de-sac. A cervical smear of the vaginal pool or pleural or peritoneal fluids may contain cells diagnostic of ovarian malignancy. X-rays may show distant metastases to lung and bone.

Although a pelvic mass and ascites usually signify a malignant ovarian tumor, a benign ovarian fibroma is rarely associated with ascites and right hydrothorax (**Meigs' syndrome**).

Clinical staging for ovarian carcinoma is outlined in TABLE 10–4.

Treatment and Prognosis

Standard therapeutic approaches are hindered by the variety of histologic types of tumors, by late discovery, and by the prevalence of widespread metastases, bilateral involvement, and extension to the uterus and contigu-

TABLE 10-4. CLINICAL STAGING OF OVARIAN CARCINOMA
AS A GUIDE TO TREATMENT AND PROGNOSIS*

Stage	Description
I	Growth limited to the ovaries
IA	Growth limited to one ovary; no ascites. No tumor on the external surface; capsule intact
IB	Growth limited to both ovaries; no ascites. No tumor on the external surface; capsules intact
IC	Tumor either stage IA or IB, present on the surface of one or both ovaries, or capsule ruptured, or with ascites present containing malignant cells, or with positive peritoneal washings†
II	Growth involving one or both ovaries, with pelvic extension
IIA	Extension and/or metastases to the uterus and/or tubes
IIB	Extension to other pelvic tissues
IIC	Tumor either stage IIA or IIB, present on the surface of one or both ovaries, or capsule ruptured, or with ascites present containing malignant cells, or with positive peritoneal washings†
III	Growth involving one or both ovaries with peritoneal implants outside the pelvis and/or positive retroperitoneal or inguinal nodes. Tumor limited to the true pelvis with histologically proven malignant extension to small bowel or omentum
IIIA	Tumor grossly limited to the true pelvis with negative nodes but with histologically confirmed microscopic seeding of abdominal peritoneal surfaces
IIIB	Tumor of one or both ovaries with histologically confirmed implants of abdominal peritoneal surfaces, < 2 cm in diameter; nodes negative
IIIC	Abdominal implants > 2 cm in diameter and/or positive retroperitoneal or inguinal nodes
IV	Growth involving one or both ovaries with distant metastases. If pleural effusion is present, there must be positive cytologic test results to allot a case to stage IV. Parenchymal liver metastasis equals stage IV
Special category	Unexplored cases that are thought to be ovarian carcinoma

* Staging as described by the International Federation of Gynecology and Obstetrics (FIGO), 1987.
† To evaluate impact on prognosis for cases allotted to stages IC and IIC, it would be of value to know if rupture of the capsule was spontaneous or caused by the surgeon and if source of malignant cells detected was peritoneal washings or ascites.

ous structures. Not all lesions require extensive or radical therapy. In a young patient with a histologically low-grade unilateral lesion (such as a mucinous tumor), reproductive capability can be preserved by excising only the involved ovary and tube. In advanced disease, total abdominal hysterectomy and bilateral salpingo-oophorectomy with omentectomy are applied for excisable tumors, but each case involves considerable latitude. Thorough surgical staging should be performed, including biopsy of the diaphragm, parietal peritoneum, and retroperitoneal lymph nodes. Radical surgery with node dissections and exenterations is ineffective, but radiotherapy and especially chemotherapy are becoming increasingly useful and are under continuous reevaluation. When tumor involvement precludes a realistic expectation of total excision, the initial laparotomy is performed to diagnose, grade, and remove as much tumor as possible; chemotherapy or abdominal radiotherapy follows.

Widespread disease and stage IV tumors are treated with chemotherapy after adequate surgical excision. Most oncologists agree that in patients with advanced stages III and IV tumors, combination therapy with ≥ 2 cytotoxic agents is preferable to single-agent treatment. (See drugs and dosage recommendations above for cytotoxic chemotherapy of endometrial cancer.)

For patients with common epithelial tumors, the overall 5-yr survival rate without evidence of recurrence is 15 to 45%. Prognosis for the rare germ cell and stromal tumors varies considerably, depending upon the stage at diagnosis. For recurrent disease, the factor most strongly correlated with survival is the time between diagnosis and start of multiagent therapy. With aggressive tumor-reductive surgery and combination chemotherapy, the long-term survival rate for all ovarian cancer patients is improving (67% with stage III tumors in one series). However, the death rate from ovarian cancer surpasses that from cervical and corpus cancer combined and ranks 5th in cancer fatalities in women.

VULVAR CARCINOMA

Malignancy of the vulva accounts for about 3 to 4% of all gynecologic neoplasms and usually occurs after menopause. Though patients can readily visualize and palpate these malignancies, they may not seek treatment for up to 3 yr because of embarrassment or fear. Also, the physician may delay treatment by striving to provide symptomatic relief of the accompanying pruritus rather than obtaining an immediate biopsy.

Pathology

About 90% of cases are squamous cell carcinomas and about 4% are basal cell carcinomas; the remainder include intraepithelial carcinomas, such as Paget's disease, adenocarcinoma of Bartholin's gland, fibrosarcoma, and melanoma. Often, the intraepithelial lesions have multifocal origins. Growth is initially superficial, but later the tumors extend into the vagina, the urethra, or the anus. The superficial inguinal and femoral nodes are involved in up to 50% of cases. Squamous cell carcinoma may be well differentiated or anaplastic.

Symptoms and Signs

Epithelial alterations, such as typical and atypical hyperplastic dystrophy, coexist in 40% of patients, and foci of lichen sclerosus may be associated with the cancer but are not necessarily considered precancerous. **Kraurosis vulvae,** a gross clinical diagnosis characterized by shrinkage and constriction of the vaginal outlet, is histopathologically identical to lichen sclerosus. Until the lesion reaches 1 to 2 cm or more in diameter, it is often asymptomatic, although carcinoma in situ tends to be pruritic. When the tumor becomes necrotic and infected, symptoms resemble those of an ulcer with bleeding and/or watery discharge.

Diagnosis

Diagnosis usually is made by simple biopsy. Sites can be delineated by staining the vulva with toluidine blue (1%), allowing the dye to be absorbed for 3 to 5 min, and then decolorizing with dilute (2 to 3%) acetic acid. Abnormal areas retain the blue dye. Differential diagnosis must include the various venereal diseases (granuloma inguinale, chancroid, lymphogranuloma venereum,

syphilis); basal cell carcinoma (rodent ulcer); intraepithelial (in situ) cancers characterized by small red, white, or pigmented friable papules; Paget's disease, manifested by red, moist, elevated patches; and bowenoid papulosis, usually small elevated lesions considered a carcinoma in situ. Melanomas frequently appear as bluish-black, pigmented, or papillary lesions; they metastasize via the lymphatics, the bloodstream, or both. Prognosis depends on the depth of involvement into the underlying epidermis.

Treatment

Since **squamous cell carcinoma** of the vulva spreads by local extension as well as by lymphatic embolization, all existing and potential tumor sites in this region should be removed. The tumors drain to the inguinal lymph nodes; however, those extending deep into the vagina drain into the retroperitoneal nodes. A correlation between tumor size and lymph node involvement has been noted.

The treatment of choice is radical vulvectomy and bilateral superficial inguinal and femoral node dissection. Recent reports show the importance of individualization in specific instances (eg, unilateral lesions with minimal invasion). Retroperitoneal lymph node dissection is warranted only if the superficial nodes are affected or the tumor extends deeply into the vagina. Nevertheless, with deep pelvic nodal involvement, few (if any) 5-yr survivors are reported, and irradiation should be considered. Up to $\frac{1}{3}$ of the distal urethra may be excised without producing urinary incontinence. Lymphedema is common for a year or so, until collateral lymph channels have been established.

Preoperative external radiotherapy can be used to sterilize or decrease the size of large tumors. Radium needle implants may be used for inoperable tumors and metastases.

The treatment of **basal cell carcinoma** is local excision. Paget's disease requires total vulvectomy, since the presence of an underlying malignancy must be ruled out. The treatment of in situ carcinoma should be individualized, since $\geq$ 40% of cases are found in patients < 40 yr old, in whom vulvectomy is rarely indicated.

VAGINAL CARCINOMA

About 1% of gynecologic malignancies are vaginal carcinomas; the peak incidence is from age 45 to 65.

Etiology and Pathology

Except for clear cell carcinoma, in which tumor development has been linked to intrauterine exposure to diethylstilbestrol **(DES)**, the etiology is unknown. Current evidence suggests that, as with cervical neoplasia, exposure to human papillomavirus **(HPV)** may be important.

Of malignancies arising primarily in the vagina, 95% are squamous cell carcinomas. The rest include primary and secondary adenocarcinomas, secondary squamous cell carcinomas in older women, clear cell adenocarcinomas in younger women, and botryoid sarcomas (embryonal rhabdomyosarcomas) in infants and children. Extension to the bladder and rectum is common.

Symptoms, Signs, and Diagnosis

Bleeding occurs after coitus or examination. Ulceration of the tumor may cause bleeding and infection. Watery discharge, dyspareunia, and (when the bladder or rectum is involved) urinary frequency or urgency or painful defecation occur. The tumor is most commonly found in the upper $1/3$ of the vagina on the posterior wall.

In clinically unsuspected lesions, a Papanicolaou test may disclose carcinomatous cells, and a Schiller's test may outline the biopsy site. Extension is usually superficial and toward the cervix, following the lymphatics. Every girl who has been or may have been exposed prenatally to DES should be examined at menarche, regardless of symptoms, and at regular intervals (at least yearly) thereafter.

Treatment and Prognosis

Treatment depends partly on the location and extent of the disease (it is complicated by extension to the bladder or rectum) and partly on the age and physical condition of the patient. A tumor localized in the upper $1/3$ of the vagina is treated either by radical hysterectomy with upper vaginectomy and pelvic lymph node dissection or with radium and external radiotherapy. Treatment of primary and secondary carcinomas is usually combined and may be either radiotherapy or radical surgery. The 5-yr survival rate without recurrence is about 30%.

FALLOPIAN TUBE CARCINOMA

Primary carcinoma of the oviduct is rare, the peak incidence being from age 50 to 60. Chronic salpingitis and TB have been considered possible etiologic factors but probably are unimportant. Infertility is common.

Pathology, Symptoms, Signs, and Diagnosis

These tumors spread either directly or by the lymphatics. Lymphatic spread is chiefly to the iliac, lumbar, and preaortic nodes. The tumors are usually unilateral and located in the distal $1/3$ of the tube. Symptoms, as with any enlarging pelvic mass, are usually related to a vague feeling of discomfort due to pressure on the bladder or rectum. Occasionally, a watery or blood-tinged vaginal discharge occurs. Physical findings may include enlargement of the abdomen secondary to a large pelvic mass or to ascites, so the usual preoperative diagnosis is ovarian carcinoma. The tumor may close the fimbriated end of the tube, simulating the gross appearance of a hydrosalpinx.

Treatment

The 5-yr survival rate without evidence of recurrence varies from 5 to 48%. The treatment of choice, like that of the more common ovarian cancers, is total abdominal hysterectomy and bilateral salpingo-oophorectomy with omentectomy, followed by combination chemotherapy. Radiotherapy (confined to the pelvis) may be useful in earlier disease.

TROPHOBLASTIC DISEASE

Neoplasms of trophoblastic origin that can follow intra- or extrauterine pregnancy.

A **hydatidiform mole** is the end stage of a degenerating pregnancy in which the villi have become hydropic and the trophoblastic elements have proliferated. **Persistent trophoblastic disease (PTD, chorioadenoma destruens, or invasive mole)** is a local invasion of the myometrium by the villi of the hydatidiform mole. In contrast, **metastatic trophoblastic disease (MTD, choriocarcinoma, or chorioepithelioma)** is an invasive—usually widely metastatic—tumor composed of syncytiotrophoblastic and cytotrophoblastic elements only.

A mole is more common in older patients. Molar pregnancies occur in about 1/2000 gestations in the USA; however, for unknown reasons, the incidence in Asiatic countries approaches 1/200. Over 80% of hydatidiform moles are benign. However, 15% lead to local invasion characteristic of PTD; 2 to 3% are followed by MTD. The locally invasive variant may cause uterine perforation, hemorrhage, and sepsis. A mole always precedes PTD but precedes only 50% of MTDs. MTD occurs in about 1/25,000 to 1/45,000 pregnancies.

Symptoms, Signs, and Diagnosis

Hydatidiform mole often manifests itself shortly after conception by a rapid increase in the size of the uterus, often causing it to be larger than it should be by dates. Vaginal bleeding, lack of fetal movement, lack of fetal heart tones at the appropriate time (12 wk with Doppler ultrasonography), and severe nausea and vomiting should arouse clinical suspicion. Passage of typical grapelike molar tissue suggests the diagnosis, and histologic examination confirms it. Without such proof, the diagnosis may be difficult to differentiate from other pregnancy complications involving a possibly normal fetus. Ultrasonography, the diagnostic modality of choice, is not infallible but usually demonstrates absence of an amniotic sac with a fetus in it.

Human chorionic gonadotropin (HCG) is produced by the proliferating trophoblastic tissue, and high levels of HCG found on radioimmunoassay are valuable in evaluating treatment. Serum and urinary HCG levels are elevated during the first 100 days of gestation (even more so with multiple pregnancy); therefore, the value of the test early in pregnancy is diminished. Radioimmunoassay for the β subunit of HCG is used for diagnosis and management of trophoblastic disease.

Complications of a mole include intrauterine infection and septicemia, hemorrhage, toxemia of pregnancy (the only condition in which true toxemia is seen in the first half of pregnancy), and development of MTD. PTD, because it is intramural, tends to cause bleeding; it may infiltrate adjacent tissue and occasionally metastasize to distant sites. MTD metastasizes early and widely via the venous and lymphatic systems and is highly malignant.

Treatment

Evacuation of **hydatidiform mole** is essential. The treatment of choice is suction curettage, followed by oxytocin stimulation and curettage of the uterus. Hysterotomy is no longer used for evacuation. Hysterectomy may be selected, based on the age, parity, and future pregnancy plans of the patient. After evacuation, serial chest x-rays should be taken and serum β-HCG titers should be determined. The titer should progressively fall to a normal level in 8 wk. If it fails to fall or if it rises after once falling, studies for malignant progression should be performed. The patient should use contraception for a year, since detection of malignant change is compromised by pregnancy.

Patients with persistent or rising HCG levels may have either **PTD** (invasive mole) or **MTD** and should receive chemotherapy with methotrexate, dactinomycin, or a combination of drugs, depending on the organs involved, β-HCG titers, and postevacuation duration. Chemotherapy has largely replaced hysterectomy in both conditions; results are good, reproductive capacity is preserved, and major surgery is avoided. However, hysterectomy may be considered in patients > 40 yr or those desiring sterilization and may be required for those with infection, uncontrolled bleeding, or invasion of disease through the uterine wall. For patients with trophoblastic malignancy, the overall remission rate is 75 to 85%.

11.   MEDICAL EXAMINATION OF THE RAPE VICTIM

Rape is the *illegal sexual penetration of any body orifice*. While the definition does not include touching without penetration, in some jurisdictions it may include penetration of body orifices by inanimate objects. Except when a child is seduced by offers of affection or bribes, rape is usually a sexual act committed by threat or use of force against an unwilling person. Reported cases of female victims in the USA total 75,000/yr; estimates of unreported rape range from 2 to 10 times that number. Approximately 90% of rapists attack victims of the same race; 50% are known to their victims and are often members of the extended family. This is particularly important for preteen and teenage victims and has implications for follow-up and child abuse prevention (see also Ch. 31). Most rapes are planned (not the result of sudden impulse), and over half the attacks involve a weapon, usually a knife. About 50% of female rape victims show signs of physical trauma; over 10% require emergency treatment.

Although rape is usually thought of in the context of the female victim, a growing number of rape victims are males who are not necessarily part of a prison or homosexual community. The male victim is more likely to have physical trauma than the female, to have been victimized by several assailants, and to be more unwilling to report the crime. For both males and females, however, the assault is the sexual expression of aggression, anger, or need for power. It is a violent, even more than a sexual, act (see also Ch. 54). A few cases of female rapes of males have been reported in the last several years.

Evaluation Procedures

Although provision of medical care and psychologic support for the rape victim is the first concern, the patient is a victim of a crime, and forensic medicine requires certain special details of medical evaluation and record-keeping. TABLE 11–1 may serve as a guide for examination procedures and the medical record, to be adapted according to local requirements. Such a record is sometimes admissible in court and aids recall if testimony is required later. Unless subpoenaed, the record should never be released without written consent of the patient.

Whenever possible, the patient should be treated in a rape treatment center, which should be separate from the emergency room and staffed by trained, concerned support personnel.

History and physical examination: A brief account of the attack by the patient will indicate areas for medical investigation and treatment. However, recounting the events is often frightening for the patient, and a complete history may have to be deferred until more immediate needs have been met. The reasons for the questions asked and for the examination procedure are not always clear to patients; eg, the female patient may need to be told that knowledge of the last menstrual period or the use of a contraceptive will help determine the risk of pregnancy, or that information concerning the time of the last previous coitus is important in establishing validity of sperm testing.

Since these patients have been through an experience to which they did not consent, enlisting their cooperation and requesting permission for the examination are important. Details of the pelvic examination should be described and explained as it proceeds, and the results should be reviewed with the patient. Since rape victims may feel anxiety at being examined by a physician of the opposite sex, a nurse or volunteer of the victim's sex should be present to lend support and to corroborate the procedures.

The evidence collected during the examination and all laboratory specimens should be placed in individual packages and carefully labeled, dated, and sealed. Receipts should be obtained upon delivery to the laboratory or police. Samples for DNA genetic determinations to identify the attacker are not routinely collected. Accurate testing is difficult, and some authorities believe it can be done properly only by the Federal Bureau of Investigation **(FBI)**. However, the FBI does not investigate all rape cases. Additionally, the legal use of the results of such determinations is controversial.

Psychologic assessment: Rape presents both psychologic and social problems for the victims, who must handle their own feelings as well as face the often negative reactions (eg, judgmental, derisive) of friends, family, and officials. Patients should be viewed as undergoing a **posttraumatic stress disorder** that typically has an *acute phase* lasting a few days to a few weeks, followed by a *long-term process* of reorganization and recovery.

Acute phase reactions are fear and anger, although patients' outward responses range from talkativeness, tenseness, crying, and trembling to shock and disbelief, with dispassion, quiescence, and smiling. The latter responses are rarely an indication that the patient is unconcerned; they may be avoidance reactions or may occur in patients who have coping styles that require control of emotion or who are physically exhausted. Patients are usually severely frightened and embarrassed and feel degraded. The anger felt by many victims may be displaced onto hospital personnel, who should be aware of this and not troubled by it.

Long-range effects of rape include reexperiencing the assault, aversion to sex, anxiety, phobias, suspiciousness, depression, nightmares and sleep disorders, somatic symptoms, and social withdrawal. Guilt and shame occur when patients feel, generally irrationally, that somehow they provoked or should have prevented the attack or that the attack was a punishment for some wrongdoing.

The physician's report may include a brief account of the attack in the patient's words and a statement of the physician's clinical determination as to injuries and sexual activity. It is not necessary to state whether rape occurred since that is a legal determination, but one should record a diagnosis including all probable or possible physical and psychologic problems.

TABLE 11–1. EXAMINATION FOR ALLEGED RAPE

Name of patient: Date of examination:
   Address: Time:
   Phone: Location:
   Age:
   Sex:
Name of guardian, if patient is under age:
   Address:
   Phone:
Name of person accompanying patient to hospital:
   Address:
   Phone:
Name of police officer, badge number, and department:

HISTORY
  Circumstances of attack
    Date and time:
    Location (familiar to patient?):
    Assailant(s):
     Number:
     Name(s), if known:
     Description(s):
     Weapon:
    Type of sexual contact (vaginal, oral, rectal):
    Condom used?
    Activities of patient after attack
     Douche: Medication:
     Bath: Other:
     Clothing change:
    Last menstrual period:
    Date of previous coitus and time, if recent:
    Contraceptive history (oral, IUD, etc):

PHYSICAL EXAMINATION
  General trauma (extragenital)
    Head: Chest:
    Face: Abdomen:
    Throat: Back:
  Genital trauma
    Perineum: Vulva:
    Hymen: Vagina:
                 Cervix:
                 Anus:
  Foreign material on body (stains, hair, dirt, twigs, etc):
  Evidence of alcohol or other drugs:
  Evidence of existing pregnancy:

PSYCHOLOGIC ASSESSMENT
  Patient's emotional or mental state:

LABORATORY FINDINGS
  Clothing: Note condition (damaged, stained, foreign material adhering)
               Provide small samples, including unstained sample, or give clothing to police or
               laboratory
  Hair samples: Loose hairs adhering to patient or clothing
               Semen-encrusted pubic hair
               Clipped pubic hair of victim—at least 10 (for comparison)

(Continued)

TABLE 11—1. EXAMINATION FOR ALLEGED RAPE *(Cont'd)*

LABORATORY FINDINGS *(Cont'd)*

Other specimens, as indicated by the history or physical examination:

	Tests	From	To determine
Semen	Papanicolaou	Vagina	Sperm motility, nonmotility
	Saline suspension*	Cervix	Sperm morphology
	Acid phosphatase†	Rectum	Presence of A, B, or H blood
	Other (eg, bacterial cultures)	Mouth	group substances‡
	Baseline VDRL and gonorrhea cultures	Thighs	Gonorrhea
Blood (including dried samples on patient's		Other	Blood group
body and clothing)			Presence of drugs, alcohol
			Pregnancy
Urine			Presence of drugs, alcohol
			Pregnancy

TREATMENT

REFERRAL

PHYSICIAN'S CLINICAL COMMENTS
    Signed: MD State License No:

WITNESS TO EXAMINATION
    Signed:

DISPOSITION OF EVIDENCE
    Delivered by: Date: Time:
    Received by: Date: Time:

---

* Should be performed by examining physician if time factor permits discovery of motile sperm.

† A useful test, since no sperm will be found if the assailant had a vasectomy, is oligospermic, or used a condom. If test cannot be performed immediately, specimen should be placed in a freezer.

‡ In 80% of cases, blood group substances are found in semen.

Adapted from Root I, Ogden W, Scott W: "The medical examination of alleged rape." *The Western Journal of Medicine* 120(4):329–333, 1974; used with permission of *The Western Journal of Medicine.*

Treatment

Most physical trauma is minor and treated conservatively, but severe injuries can occur and may require surgical repair. Overall, the psychosocial aspects are the most potentially damaging and require sophisticated management. It is very important to treat patients with respect, to see that they are not left alone, to assure them that they are safe, to demonstrate understanding and empathy, and to explain in detail how the evaluation will proceed.

Psychologic trauma: An unhurried, nonjudgmental, willing-to-listen attitude by the examiner is therapeutic. Since patients are in a traumatic state and many details may be embarrassing, they often omit important data. Therefore, specific details of the attacker's aggression, threats, violent behavior, and of the sex acts committed must be elicited with careful questioning. Empathy can be shown by acknowledging that the questions may be embarrassing or may exacerbate the patient's fears. Properly done, such a potentially distressing interview may begin the therapeutic process. *The full psychologic impact*

cannot be ascertained at the first examination, and follow-up visits must be scheduled. At the first visit, the patient should be given an explanation of the possible psychologic and social sequelae, and arrangements should be made for introduction to someone trained in rape crisis intervention. If the patient's acute stress reactions do not subside or if long-range psychologic problems seem likely, psychiatric referral is indicated. NOTE: Some patients appear to adjust quickly by unconsciously denying the rape and rapidly returning to normal activities but later manifest the symptoms and signs of posttraumatic stress disorder.

Support network: The physician often has to deal with the intense reactions of family and friends, who can be sources of support or of additional stress. In the immediate situation, the physician should try to decrease their strong feelings of anxiety, anger, or guilt, for these usually increase the intensity of the patient's emotional reactions. Instead, family and friends must be shown how to listen to the patient in a supportive fashion, and they can do this only if they can control their feelings when they are with the patient.

A support network of health workers, friends, and family is a vital ingredient of long-term care.

Prophylaxis for sexually transmitted disease (STD): Since the risk of becoming infected with an STD (eg, gonorrhea, chlamydia, syphilis) is almost always a concern, preventive measures should be taken. In most rape centers, the patient is questioned about hypersensitivity to penicillin, and ceftriaxone 250 mg IM is given in a single dose to prevent gonorrhea. Tetracycline 0.5 gm orally qid is recommended for 7 to 14 days to prevent chlamydia or for 15 days to prevent syphilis. Some clinicans prefer doxycycline 200 mg/day orally (100 mg q 12 h) for 7 to 10 days to prevent chlamydia or for 15 days to prevent syphilis.

Transmission of the human immunodeficiency virus **(HIV)** is always a concern, despite the odds against its occurring in a single encounter. Health care personnel should suggest that blood samples for HIV testing be drawn at the time of the examination and 30 and 60 days afterward. If any test is positive, treatment with zidovudine should be instituted immediately, following the guidelines for accidental needlesticks.

Pregnancy: Factors determining the possibility of a pregnancy include the patient's menstrual cycle phase and whether or not contraceptives were used. Tests for human chorionic gonadotropin make such determinations easier.

Rape-induced pregnancy is very rare, but if it seems possible, an oral contraceptive such as 0.5 mg norgestrel/0.05 mg ethinyl estradiol may be given. Two tablets orally immediately plus 2 tablets 12 h later will induce menses (99% effective) if given within 72 h of rape. Antiemetic medication such as oral hydroxyzine will counter nausea and vomiting. If there is a possibility that the patient was pregnant at the time of the rape, estrogens should not be given until this situation is evaluated. The patient's attitude toward abortion should be explored.

Additional considerations include (1) provision of privacy for examination and consultation; (2) provision of cleansing facilities and toilet (many patients will want to wash—some will have been urinated on or have been raped out of doors—some will want to use a mouthwash); and (3) provision of money or transportation to get home. Also, if a rape crisis team operates in the area, referral can provide helpful medical, psychologic, and legal support to the victim.

Follow-up should include tests for HIV, as described above, and for gonorrhea, chlamydia, syphilis, and pregnancy within 6 wk. If pregnancy occurs, consideration should be given to its termination. A further test for syphilis should be done at 6 mo. (See also discussion of follow-up under psychologic trauma, above.)

12. CONCEPTION, IMPLANTATION, PLACENTATION, AND EMBRYOLOGY

CONCEPTION

Ovulation and conception occur about 14 days before a menstrual period. If the periods are irregular, the time of conception and thus the due date of the pregnancy and due date may be difficult to determine.

At the time of ovulation, the cervical mucus becomes less viscid, facilitating rapid transit of sperm from the vagina to the endometrial cavity. Under experimental conditions, sperm have migrated from the vagina to the fimbriated end of the uterine tube in 5 min. Before ovulation, sperm may be stored in the cervix for at least a few days.

Conception, or fertilization, occurs in the uterine tube, usually near the fimbriated end. The tubal epithelium must function properly for the sperm and

ovum to unite and for continued division and development of the zygote during its transit down the tube to the endometrial cavity. The zygote moves from the fimbriated end of the tube to the endometrial cavity in 3 to 5 days and to the site of implantation in 1 to 2 more days. During this time the conceptus is dividing; at the time of implantation it has formed a blastocyst, a single layer of cells surrounding a central cavity. On one wall of the blastocyst is a thickening 3 to 4 cell layers deep. This is the embryonic pole of the blastocyst; it soon becomes recognizable as an embryo.

IMPLANTATION

Implantation usually occurs in the front or back wall of the endometrial cavity near the fundus. Trophoblast cells proliferate from the surface of the blastocyst, invading and penetrating the endometrium so that the blastocyst burrows into the central layer of endometrium. This process begins between days 5 and 8 and is completed by day 9 or 10.

By day 10 both syncytial and cytotrophoblast cells are identifiable. Beginning about this time, fluorescent staining shows chorionic gonadotropin in syncytial cells. Presumably all the other trophic hormones produced by the placenta appear in the syncytial cells relatively shortly thereafter. The blastocyst wall changes into the chorion and becomes the outer layer of the membranes surrounding the fetus and amniotic fluid.

The amniotic sac develops about day 10 to 12 as a split in the embryonic ectodermal layer; the sac fills with fluid and expands to cover the embryo and line the inner wall of the future chorionic membrane. The old blastocyst cavity disappears.

The embryo continues to grow, but the pregnancy is confined within one wall of the uterine cavity until the 12th wk. At that time the endometrium or decidua overlying the embryo comes in such close contact with the decidua of the opposite wall of the uterus that they fuse and obliterate the endometrial cavity. After that time, the only cavity in the uterus is the amniotic cavity, containing amniotic fluid and the fetus.

PLACENTATION

The first evidence of placental formation is development of the trophoblast cells at day 10. Invasion of these cells into maternal blood vessels causes blood to leak into the space between cells, forming lakes or lacunae, which will become the intervillous space. Meanwhile, the fetus derives its nourishment from the lacunae. Initially the placenta surrounds the entire blastocyst, transmitting nutrients and discharging wastes directly across cell membranes. From the time vessels appear within the placenta at day 19, the villous pattern of transfer from maternal blood to fetal blood begins. Villi begin to form on the chorionic surface as early as day 11 or 12 and bud out around the entire surface of the chorion; they branch and rebranch in a complicated treelike arrangement.

Beginning at about 12 wk and apparently influenced by the location of the major source of the maternal blood supply, the true, or discoid, placenta begins to demarcate at the old embryonic

pole of the blastocyst; it is attached by anchoring villi to the decidua directly overlying maternal spiral arterioles. These arterioles empty into the intervillous space so that the maternal blood circulates around and through the latticework of villi, draining out through 2 or 3 venous sinuses associated with each spiral arteriole. The villi are divided into groups called cotyledons, each supplied by 1 or 2 spiral arterioles. A placenta at term contains between 10 and 20 cotyledons. Nutrients are transferred from maternal blood in the intervillous space, across the trophoblast cells, through the fibrous core of the villus, and through the endothelial cells of the fetal capillaries to the fetal blood itself. Wastes move in the opposite direction. This arrangement is called a hemochorial placenta, since maternal blood is in apposition to fetal chorionic, or trophoblast, tissue.

The discoid placenta reaches its final form at 18 to 20 wk of pregnancy. At 12 wk, the remaining villous structures covering the chorionic sac begin to atrophy; they disappear entirely by 16 to 18 wk. The placenta grows throughout pregnancy until it reaches its final size of about 500 gm (1 lb) at delivery.

EMBRYOLOGY

The conceptus first becomes recognizable as an embryo about 10 days after fertilization, when the future ectoderm splits to form the amniotic sac. All 3 germ layers (ectoderm, mesoderm, endoderm) are present and can usually be distinguished. The primitive streak, or future neural tube, begins to develop thereafter; around day 16 or 17, the mesoderm thickens near the cephalic end, forming a central channel that ultimately becomes the heart and great vessels. The heart begins to pump plasma through the vessels on day 20, and on day 21 fetal RBCs appear. At this time they are very immature forms; however, nucleated RBCs soon disappear and reappear only in erythroblastosis. Fetal vessels develop throughout the body shortly thereafter. Some arise within the body stalk, which connects the allantoic sac to the fetal abdomen at the umbilicus and contains blood vessels and the extension of the urachus through which urine drains from the bladder into the allantoic sac.

The allantoic sac atrophies rapidly, and the body stalk becomes the umbilical cord connected to vessels within the placenta. Umbilical vessels carry blood to and from the placenta. Organ formation is complete by the 12th wk of pregnancy (70 days from conception) except in the CNS, which continues to develop throughout pregnancy. Most malformations occur during the first 12 wk, when outside teratogenic influences such as the rubella virus are most destructive. All medications and immunizations should be avoided until after the 12th wk of pregnancy, unless they are essential to protect the mother's health; great care should be taken to avoid a teratogenic drug.

13.   GENETIC EVALUATION AND COUNSELING

(See also Ch. 48)

GENETIC SCREENING

An accurate **family history** should routinely be obtained and summarized as a pedigree (commonly used symbols are described in Ch. 48). Minimum information for an uncomplicated family history should include 3 generations, with all first-degree relatives (parents, siblings, offspring) and second-degree relatives (aunts and uncles, grandparents) of the proband, and their state of health. Complicated family histories require extended pedigrees. Ethnic background, as well as any consanguineous matings, should routinely be sought. Review of medical records is necessary whenever genetic diagnoses are suggested.

Many genetic diagnoses are based on **physical signs (phenotype)** rather than symptoms. A detailed description of physical findings is therefore vital, particularly in stillborns or infants dying soon after birth. Photographs and full-body x-rays should be taken as part of the permanent record and can be invaluable for future counseling. Cryopreservation of fetal tissues (fibroblasts, liver) for future DNA or enzymatic studies is also recommended.

Carrier screening generally refers to *identification of heterozygotes (carriers) for autosomal or X-linked recessive disorders.* The most common indication for carrier screening in obstetrics is to provide prospective parents with reproductive alternatives, eg, prenatal diagnosis with possible termination or treatment of affected fetuses, artificial insemination, or deferral of childbearing.

Screening of all individuals for even the most common disorders would be impossible and is usually based on such criteria as availability of a simple, accurate, inexpensive carrier test; an ethnic, racial, or geographic heritage of increased risk for a specific genetic disorder; and the availability of treatment or reproductive options for identified carriers. In the USA, 3 disorders currently meet these criteria: Tay-Sachs disease, sickle cell anemia, and the thalassemias. For other diseases, screening based on family history may be possible (eg, for hemophilia, cystic fibrosis, or Huntington's disease). **Molecular techniques** (see also Ch. 48) can often substantially alter theoretic risk, sometimes obviating the need for invasive prenatal diagnostic procedures. For example, a pregnant women who has a brother with hemophilia theoretically has a 50% risk of carrying the hemophilia gene; if she is found not to be a carrier, the risk becomes essentially zero. Participation of multiple family members (including affected individuals) is usually required for the most accurate risk assessment.

Sickle cell anemia (see also Ch. 35), the most common mendelian disorder in American blacks (about 1/400), is autosomal recessive. Individuals with sickle cell *disease* are homozygous for the mutant gene, while the *trait* is autosomal dominant (ie, heterozygous individuals express both the normal and sickle genes). A single nucleotide substitution (GAG to GTG) in the 6th codon of the β-globin gene leads to the transcription of the amino acid valine (rather than glutamic acid), which results in an abnormal Hb molecule. About 10% of sickle cell anemia patients born in the USA die by the age of 10 yr. **Carrier screening** is available by several tests, with confirmation by using Hb electrophoresis. **Prenatal diagnosis** is available through the direct analysis of DNA obtained from chorionic villi or amniotic fluid cells (see under PRENATAL DIAGNOSTIC TECHNIQUES, below). **Newborn screening** for sickle cell disease is recommended because prophylactic antibiotics can decrease the incidence of infection, often an inciting event in the sickle crisis.

Tay-Sachs disease (GM_2 gangliosidosis—see also under OTHER LIPIDOSES in Ch. 40) occurs in about 1/3600 infants of Ashkenazi Jewish and French Canadian parents as an autosomal recessive disorder. The biochemical abnormality is the absence of hexosaminidase A, which is involved in the metabolism of gangliosides (a class of nervous system lipids). **Carrier detection** is possible by demonstrating *intermediate* reduction of hexosaminidase A activity in serum. However, hexosaminidase A activity in serum normally decreases during pregnancy relative to total hexosaminidase and may produce a false-positive result. Leukocyte hexosaminidase assays are not altered during pregnancy and thus are recommended whenever pregnant women are screened. Similarly, many noncarrier women taking oral contraceptives may have reduced serum hexosaminidase A (in the inconclusive or heterozygous range), and leukocyte assays are again recommended for screening. **Prenatal diagnosis** is available by assay of hexosaminidase A activity in cells from chorionic villi or amniotic fluid.

The **thalassemias** (see also THALASSEMIAS in Ch. 35) are a heterogeneous group of hereditary anemias that share a diminished synthesis of Hb. The α-thalassemias involve mutations with deletion of from 1 to 4 genes, present at 2 different loci, which code for the 2 α chains in the Hb molecule, and are most common in individuals from Southeast Asia.

The β-thalassemias fall into 2 general groups with defective β-chain synthesis. In the β^+ group, reduced amounts of mRNA are due to incomplete suppression of the β gene. In the β^o group, mRNA for the β chain is absent or nonfunctional. β-Thalassemia is present in all populations but is more common in Mediterranean countries, the Middle East, and parts of India and Pakistan.

Screening for carriers of both α- and β-thalassemia is possible by evaluation of RBC indexes. A mean corpuscular Hb value of 20 to 22 pg and MCV values of 50 to 70 fL suggest the diagnosis of thalassemia minor. Confirmation is by demonstration of elevated levels of Hb A_2 by electrophoresis. **Prenatal diagnosis** for both α- and β-thalassemia is possible by molecular techniques. However, accurate characterization of the Hb defect is essential.

INDICATIONS FOR PRENATAL DIAGNOSIS

CHROMOSOME ABNORMALITIES

Chromosome abnormalities occur in about 0.5% of all live births. Down syndrome is the most common and best known chromosome disorder, but many others exist. All are prenatally diagnosable, but invasive prenatal tests are not appropriate for every couple, as the risks may outweigh the benefits. Prenatal diagnosis should be offered to all individuals at increased risk for chromosome abnormalities.

Advanced maternal age is the most common indication for prenatal cytogenetic studies. Chromosome abnormalities occur in offspring of mothers at all ages, but the frequency of trisomic offspring increases with age, rising exponentially after age 30. No biologic explanation is known. TABLE 13–1 lists the risk of having a liveborn child with a chromosome abnormality by 1-yr maternal age intervals. At 16 to 18 wk gestation, the prevalence of chromosome abnormalities is 30% higher than that for liveborn infants because of a high spontaneous loss rate in such pregnancies.

Prenatal diagnosis should be offered to all women who will be ≥ 35 yr at delivery. The age threshold is largely arbitrary, and prenatal diagnosis may be considered in younger women.

Low maternal serum α-fetoprotein (MSAFP): Amniocentesis (see under PRENATAL DIAGNOSTIC TECHNIQUES, below) may be considered for women identified by MSAFP screening to be at increased risk for carrying a Down syndrome fetus.

Family history of anomalous child: Counseling should reflect the recurrence risk for any confirmed disorder. When a definitive diagnosis has not been made, risk assessment must be empiric, based on the most likely diagnosis.

Known chromosome abnormalities: After a couple has had a liveborn child with trisomy 21, their risk of having another chromosomally abnormal child is about 1% for women < 30 yr at delivery. For women > 30 yr, the risk is the same as the background maternal age risk (see TABLE 13–1). These figures assume the parents do not carry a robertsonian translocation (see below). Information is limited for other trisomies, but the recurrence risk seems to be increased to about 1% for another chromosomally abnormal offspring. Prenatal diagnosis should be offered to all such couples. Even when risk is not increased, parental anxiety alone may warrant prenatal diagnosis.

Unknown chromosomal status of a previous anomalous infant, liveborn or stillborn: Chromosome abnormalities are more frequent in anomalous infants as well as in phenotypically normal

TABLE 13−1. RISK OF HAVING A LIVEBORN CHILD WITH DOWN SYNDROME
OR OTHER CHROMOSOME ABNORMALITY

Maternal Age	Risk of Down Syndrome	Total Risk for Chromosome Abnormalities*
20	1/1667	1/526
21	1/1667	1/526
22	1/1429	1/500
23	1/1429	1/500
24	1/1250	1/476
25	1/1250	1/476
26	1/1176	1/476
27	1/1111	1/455
28	1/1053	1/435
29	1/1000	1/417
30	1/952	1/384
31	1/909	1/384
32	1/769	1/323
33	1/625	1/286
34	1/500	1/238
35	1/385	1/192
36	1/294	1/156
37	1/227	1/127
38	1/175	1/102
39	1/137	1/83
40	1/106	1/66
41	1/82	1/53
42	1/64	1/42
43	1/50	1/33
44	1/38	1/26
45	1/30	1/21
46	1/23	1/16
47	1/18	1/13
48	1/14	1/10
49	1/11	1/8

* 47,XXX excluded for ages 20−32 (data not available).

Data from Hook EB: "Rates of chromosome abnormalities at different maternal ages." *Obstetrics and Gynecology* 58:282−285, 1981; and Hook EB, Cross PK, Schreinemachers DM: "Chromosomal abnormality rates at amniocentesis and in live-born infants." *Journal of the American Medical Association* 249:2034−2038, 1983.

stillborns (5%). Prenatal diagnostic evaluation may be indicated if the previous anomalies were due to a chromosome abnormality, increasing the risk in future pregnancies.

Parental chromosome abnormality: Carriers of a chromosome abnormality may be phenotypically normal, yet at increased risk of producing a chromosomally abnormal offspring. Balanced parental rearrangements include **translocations (robertsonian** or **reciprocal)** and **inversion (paracentric** or **pericentric).** These individuals should be referred for genetic counseling and consideration of prenatal diagnosis.

Parental **aneuploidy** for an autosome is unusual. Trisomy for a sex chromosome (eg,

47,XXX) is more common, although it is frequently associated with reduced fertility. Theoretically, 50% of offspring of an aneuploid parent should also be aneuploid. However, for women with trisomy 21, $\frac{1}{3}$ of their offspring are trisomic. Men with trisomy 21 are sterile. For parents with sex chromosome trisomies, very few offspring are aneuploid. Prenatal diagnostic study should be offered to any parent carrying an aneuploid or mosaic chromosome complement. Parental chromosome abnormalities are most often diagnosed during evaluation for recurrent miscarriage or abnormal offspring.

Multiple spontaneous abortions: At least 50% of early spontaneous abortions have chromosome abnormalities, about $\frac{1}{2}$ of which are trisomies. If the initial loss is aneuploid, subsequent losses are also likely to be aneuploid, although not necessarily for the same chromosome. A trisomy in one pregnancy may be lethal and result in miscarriage (eg, trisomy 16), but subsequent pregnancies may result in a chromosome abnormality compatible with an abnormal liveborn (eg, trisomy 18). A previous aneuploid *liveborn* increases the risk in subsequent pregnancies of another aneuploid liveborn (see above). However, it is not clear whether aneuploidy in a *spontaneous abortus* increases the risk for future liveborn offspring with aneuploidy. Some geneticists accept recurrent spontaneous abortions as an indication for prenatal diagnosis. Recurrent spontaneous abortion is an indication to study the parental chromosomes for rearrangements; if any are identified, prenatal diagnosis is offered.

Mendelian disorders: Not all are detectable prenatally, but the number is increasing rapidly. The incidence and inheritance of common mendelian disorders and availability of prenatal diagnosis are summarized in TABLE 13-2. The methods used for DNA analysis are reviewed in Ch. 48. In patients at increased risk, prenatal diagnosis is often available by chorionic villus sampling, amniocentesis, fetal skin or blood sampling, or ultrasound (US) examination.

Prenatal screening of selective ethnic, racial, or geographic populations may identify carriers of specific mendelian disorders, such as Tay-Sachs disease, sickle cell disease, and the thalassemias. **Newborn screening** will identify additional couples as carriers for certain metabolic disorders; in these cases, family history is usually negative. For other couples, **family history** will be positive, particularly for those with autosomal dominant or X-linked recessive inheritance. **Physical examination** of the couple may reveal a mendelian disorder, eg, achondroplasia.

Risk assessment in any of these situations is dependent upon several factors. Type of inheritance (ie, autosomal recessive or dominant, X-linked recessive or dominant) is the major factor in assessing risk (see also Ch. 48). Frequency of the disorder in the general population may be important (the more common the disorder, the more likely an unselected individual will carry the gene). Detection of carrier status can change theoretic to actual risk assessment.

POLYGENIC DISORDERS

The incidence of **neural tube defects (NTDs)** in the USA is 1 to 2:1000 births. Most NTDs (either spina bifida or anencephaly) are inherited as polygenic/multifactorial disorders. A few are consequences of single gene disorders, chromosome abnormalities, or teratogens (eg, valproic acid), and recurrence risks are based on the underlying etiology. When the proband has an NTD, the risk for offspring of first-degree relatives (sibling, parent, offspring) is 1 to 2%. For offspring of second-degree relatives (aunt, uncle, niece, nephew), it is about 1%. When the proband is a first cousin, the risk remains slightly increased over that of the general population. Couples who have 2 children with NTDs have a 5% risk. Recurrence risks are also related to the incidence of NTDs in the general population; in the United Kingdom, both the incidence and the recurrence risks are higher than in the USA. Amniocentesis is recommended for couples at $\geq$ 1% risk. Only about 5% of NTDs occur in families with a previously affected offspring, but amniocentesis is indicated for such patients who desire prenatal diagnosis. Counseling should be individualized for lower risks.

PRENATAL SCREENING TECHNIQUES

MATERNAL SERUM α-FETOPROTEIN (MSAFP)

MSAFP screening for neural tube defects **(NTDs)** and other fetal abnormalities (eg, Down syndrome) should be offered to all eligible pregnant women. MSAFP programs were developed to determine those pregnant women with sufficient risk to justify amniocentesis (about 1 to 2% of those screened). However, MSAFP does not detect every fetus with NTD; about 80% with open spina bifida and 90% with anencephaly will be detected (see below). Accurate gestational age assessment at the time the sample is obtained is essential. If ultrasound **(US)** assessment of gestational age is done prior to MSAFP sampling, fewer false-positives will be identified. To maximize accuracy of screening, the initial sample should be obtained between 16 and 18 wk gestation. Median values for the test are available from 15 to 20 wk; outside this range, the test is uninterpretable. Corrections for maternal weight and diabetes mellitus are necessary, and most programs also adjust for race.

First screen: Prior to screening, the couple should be informed as to the voluntary nature,

TABLE 13–2. SELECTED MENDELIAN DISORDERS FOR WHICH PRENATAL DIAGNOSIS IS AVAILABLE*

Disorder	Incidence	Inheritance	Prenatal Diagnosis
Cystic fibrosis	1/1500 in white population	Autosomal recessive	Molecular techniques on AFC or CV; microvillar intestinal enzyme (amniotic fluid)
Congenital adrenal hyperplasia	1/10,000	Autosomal recessive	Molecular techniques on AFC or CV; prenatal therapy available
Duchenne type muscular dystrophy	1/3300 male births	X-linked recessive	Molecular techniques on AFC or CV
Hemophilia A	1/8500 male births	X-linked recessive	Molecular techniques on AFC or CV; rarely, fetal blood sampling
Homozygous α- and β-thalassemia	Varies widely but present in most populations	Autosomal recessive	Molecular techniques on AFC or CV
Huntington's disease	4–7/100,000	Autosomal dominant	Molecular techniques on CV or AFC
Polycystic kidney disease (adult type)	1/3000 by clinical diagnosis	Autosomal dominant	Molecular techniques on CV or AFC
Sickle cell anemia	1/400 in blacks in USA	Autosomal recessive	Direct DNA analysis on AFC or CV
Tay-Sachs disease (GM₂ gangliosidosis)	1/3600 Ashkenazic Jews and French Canadians; 1/400,000 other populations	Autosomal recessive	Hexosaminidase A levels in cultured AFC or CV

AFC = amniotic fluid cells; CV = chorionic villi.

* Absence of a disorder in this table does not imply that prenatal diagnosis is not available for that condition.

Adapted from Simpson JL, Elias S: "Prenatal diagnosis of genetic disorders," in *Maternal-Fetal Medicine: Principles and Practice*, ed. 2, edited by RK Creasy and R Resnick. Philadelphia, *WB Saunders Company*, 1989, pp 99–102; used with permission.

limitations, and implications of the test, as well as a possible need for further testing. Programs defining elevated values as the 95th to 98th percentile, or 2 to 2½ multiples of the median (MoM), will identify about 5 to 7% of those screened as being at increased risk. The lower the cutoff, the higher the sensitivity but the lower the specificity and therefore the greater the need for amniocentesis.

Second screen: Some programs recommend that patients with an elevated MSAFP level be retested. The 2nd sample must be drawn ≥ 7 days after the initial sample. About 4% of the originally screened population will have serially elevated MSAFP levels and require further evaluation.

With an **elevated MSAFP,** the pregnancy is at increased risk for NTD. US examination is the next step in evaluation. Other reasons for elevated MSAFP demonstrable by US include underestimation of gestational age (20 to 30%), multiple gestation (5 to 15%), threatened abortion (10%), fetal demise, and other rare congenital abnormalities. High resolution US may give further information.

In about 2% of the originally screened population, US cannot identify a cause for the elevated MSAFP, and **amniocentesis** is indicated. Indeed, unless the diagnosis by US is certain, **amniotic fluid α-fetoprotein (AFAFP)** remains the standard method for detection of NTDs. Contamination by fetal blood may result in a falsely elevated AFAFP. The presence of acetylcholinesterase (AChE) supports the diagnosis of NTD or other fetal abnormality. Virtually all cases of anencephaly and 90 to 95% of spina bifida will have elevated AFAFP and positive AChE. About 5 to 10% of spina bifida lesions are covered with skin and will not be detected by amniotic fluid studies. When fetal blood is present but AChE is absent, elevated α-fetoprotein (AFP) is due to the blood contamination or a defect other than NTD.

Many abnormalities other than NTDs may be associated with elevated AFAFP (eg, omphalocele, congenital nephrosis, cystic hygroma, gastroschisis, upper GI atresias). In these disorders, elevations of AChE may or may not occur. High-resolution US should be used to identify other abnormalities; however, a negative US study does not exclude abnormality. If AFP is elevated and AChE is present, a fetal abnormality is likely, regardless of the US findings.

Women with unexplained MSAFP elevations whose fetus does not have an NTD may still be at increased risk for other obstetric complications,

intrauterine growth retardation, placental abruption, and fetal demise.

Low MSAFP is associated with Down syndrome, overestimation of gestational age, fetal demise (found with both low and high MSAFP), or presence of a hydatidiform mole. If US is insufficient for diagnosis, amniocentesis should be offered. Repeating low MSAFP values is not recommended and will only decrease the prenatal detection of Down syndrome.

Risk of Down syndrome can be estimated using MSAFP level and maternal age. For example, the risk in a 25-yr-old woman based on age alone is 1:890. However, if her MSAFP level is 0.36 MoM at 16 wk gestation, her risk is 1:182. Using such a protocol in women under age 35, $^1/_4$ to $^1/_3$ of fetuses with Down syndrome can be identified by doing amniocentesis in 2 to 4% of women. Physicians should consult their local genetic diagnostic service concerning MSAFP screening and interpretation of low results. Until further data become available, offering of prenatal diagnosis for the detection of chromosome abnormalities should be as discussed under INDICATIONS FOR PRENATAL DIAGNOSIS, above, irrespective of the MSAFP value. In addition to low MSAFP levels, other maternal serum markers proposed to aid in the screening for fetal Down syndrome include elevated levels of human chorionic gonadotropin (HCG) and low levels of unconjugated estriol. However, use of these new markers must be regarded as investigational at present.

Other congenital anomalies, including congenital heart disease, cleft lip and palate, pyloric stenosis, and congenital hip dislocation, show risks of recurrence consistent with polygenic/multifactorial inheritance. Prenatal diagnosis may be available in some cases, particularly with high resolution US (see below), allowing optimal antepartum management and immediate neonatal care. Confirmation of the diagnosis to rule out a multiple malformation syndrome is essential.

PRENATAL DIAGNOSTIC TECHNIQUES

AMNIOCENTESIS

The most commonly performed technique for prenatal diagnosis is midtrimester amniocentesis. This is best performed from 15 to 17 wk gestation (menstrual age). Amniocentesis earlier in pregnancy is technically possible but of unknown risk.

Real-time US examination for fetal cardiac motion, gestational age assessment, placental position, amniotic fluid location, and fetal number should be done immediately prior to amniocentesis (see below). The abdomen is cleansed with an antiseptic solution. Under US guidance, a 20- or 22-gauge spinal needle is passed transabdominally into the amniotic fluid. An initial aspirate of 1 to 2 mL of fluid should be discarded to decrease the chances of maternal cell contamination. A total of 20 to 30 mL of fluid is aspirated and the needle removed. Fetal heart motion should be documented immediately after the procedure. $Rh_o(D)$ immune globulin 300 μg should be given to Rh-negative, unsensitized patients after the procedure to decrease the likelihood of sensitization.

Bloody amniotic fluid is obtained in about 2% of amniocenteses. The blood does not usually affect amniotic cell growth and is usually maternal in origin; however, it may falsely elevate AFAFP (see above). Conversely, dark red or brown fluid is indicative of previous intra-amniotic bleeding and is associated with an increased frequency of adverse pregnancy outcome. Green fluid does not appear to be associated with poor pregnancy outcome.

Amniocentesis carries risks for both mother and fetus. Significant maternal morbidity (eg, symptomatic amnionitis) is rare. Transient vaginal spotting or amniotic fluid leakage occurs in aggregate in 1 to 2% of all cases and is usually self-limited.

Several collaborative studies in the USA and Europe have assessed fetal loss from amniocentesis. Some studies have shown no increased loss. However, the probable risk is about 0.5%. Needle injuries to the fetus have been reported very rarely. Inability to obtain amniotic fluid, culture failure, and maternal cell contamination are unusual.

Amniocentesis in twin pregnancies is usually possible. Amniotic fluid is aspirated from the first sac. Prior to removal of the needle, 2 to 3 mL of indigotindisulfonate sodium (indigo carmine), diluted 1:10 in bacteriostatic water, is injected into the first sac. Amniocentesis is then done on the second sac, at a location selected after visualization of the separating membrane. Aspiration of clear fluid confirms that the second sac has been sampled. In experienced hands, amniocentesis is possible in > 95% of twin pregnancies. Amniocentesis may also be possible with triplet or higher pregnancies, injecting indigo carmine after aspiration of each sac.

CHORIONIC VILLUS SAMPLING (CVS)

CVS is a more recently developed technique used for first trimester prenatal diagnosis. Indications for CVS are the same as for amniocentesis, with one exception. Testing that requires amniotic fluid rather than amniotic fluid cells (eg, AFAFP levels for NTD screening—see above) cannot be performed by CVS.

CVS can be performed in an ambulatory surgery unit that provides a sterile environment and is equipped to handle immediate obstetric complications. Prior to the procedure, fetal viability and gestational age are confirmed by US. CVS is currently done from 9 to 12 wk gestation. Rh sensitization is an absolute contraindication to any CVS procedure because it may exacerbate the condition; however, midtrimester amniocentesis remains an option in such cases.

The primary advantage of CVS over amniocentesis is that results are available much earlier in pregnancy, allowing simpler, safer methods of pregnancy termination in cases with abnormal results. If normal, the earlier results decrease parental anxiety. Early diagnosis may also be required for prenatal treatment; eg, prevention of female virilization in a fetus affected with 21-hydroxylase deficiency by administration of dexamethasone to the mother.

There are 2 CVS approaches: transcervical and transabdominal. In the USA, a Portex® catheter or similar device (1.5 mm diameter) is most commonly used for transcervical CVS. This catheter consists of a plastic cannula encasing a metal obturator that extends just beyond the tip of the cannula. A new catheter must be used for each sampling. The patient is placed in the lithotomy position and the vagina cleansed with povidone-iodine. Gentle traction on a tenaculum placed on the anterior cervical lip helps stabilize the cervix and straighten an angulated canal. Under US guidance, the catheter is passed through the cervix into the placenta, parallel to the long axis, away from the decidua or gestational sac (see FIG. 13–1). The obturator is removed. A 20- or 30-cc syringe containing 5 cc of culture media with heparin is connected to the cannula. Villi are aspirated by intermittent negative pressure on the syringe plunger; the cannula is then removed while applying continuous negative pressure. Contraindications to transcervical CVS include active infections (eg, genital herpes

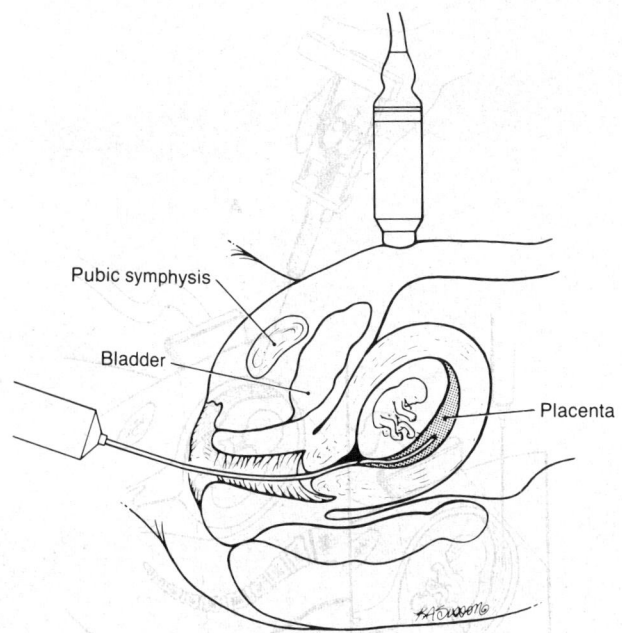

FIG. 13–1. **Transcervical chorionic villus sampling (CVS) procedure with cannula in a posterior placenta.** (From Elias S, Simpson JL: "Chorionic villus sampling," in *Diagnostic Ultrasound, Applied to Obstetrics and Gynecology,* ed. 2, edited by RE Sabbagha. Philadelphia, JB Lippincott Company, 1987; used with permission.)

or gonorrhea, chronic cervicitis) or cervical pathology.

Alternatively, CVS may be done **transabdominally.** After determining the insertion site by US, the skin is infiltrated with local anesthetic, then cleansed with povidone-iodine. An 18-gauge spinal needle with stylet is passed lengthwise into the long axis of the placenta (see FIG. 13–2). The remainder is similar to the transcervical procedure (see above). Contraindications to transabdominal CVS include interference of the needle path by bowel or bladder or active infection of the skin in the area of needle insertion.

Placental location is the primary determinant in the selection of approach for CVS. Low-lying or posterior placentas are usually more easily sampled by the transcervical approach. Fundal placentas or those located anteriorly in a slightly anteflexed uterus are most amenable to the transabdominal approach, as are women with cervical leiomyomas or long, angulated endocervical canals. Transabdominal CVS may also be useful later in pregnancy for rapid karyotyp-

ing. In rare patients with a severely retroflexed uterus and posterior placenta, a **transvaginal approach** through the posterior cul-de-sac has been used. Some patients will not be candidates for CVS, because of either of an inaccessible placenta or another contraindication to the procedure. Amniocentesis may be offered as an alternative.

Following CVS, fetal heart rate is verified by US. $Rh_0(D)$ immune globulin 300 µg is given to unsensitized Rh-negative women. Adequacy of all samples is assessed immediately under a dissecting microscope. A minimum of 5 mg of villi is necessary for analysis; 10 to 25 mg is optimal. Cytotrophoblast cells are harvested directly for cytogenetic analysis after an overnight incubation. In situ cultures of mesenchymal core cells are harvested in 5 to 8 days. Most centers do both methods of analysis. Later, between 15 and 18 wk, MSAFP is obtained to screen for neural tube defects (see above).

Risks of transcervical CVS compared with risks of amniocentesis have been assessed in

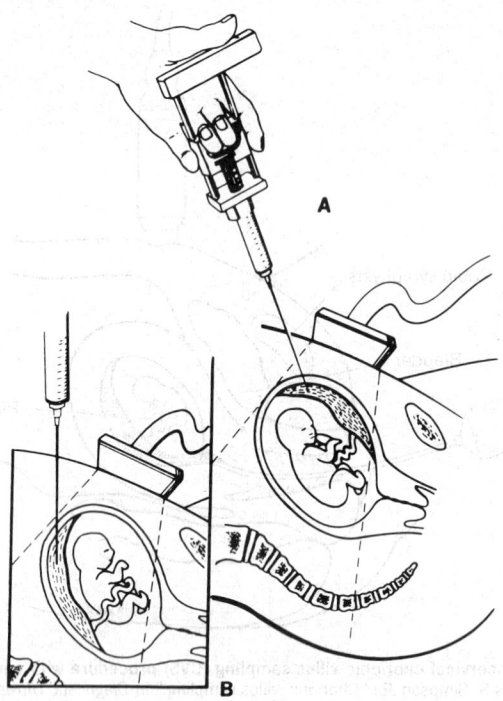

FIG. 13–2. **Transabdominal chorionic villus sampling (CVS) procedure.** Approach used with anterior placenta **(A)** and with posterior placenta **(B)**. From Elias S, Simpson JL, Shulman LP, et al: "Transabdominal chorionic villus sampling for first-trimester prenatal diagnosis." *American Journal of Obstetrics and Gynecology* 160(4):879–886, 1989; used with permission.)

several collaborative studies. In one, the CVS group had a 0.6% higher total loss rate (including spontaneous and induced abortions and losses after 20 wk), which was not statistically significant. In another study, the excess loss rate in the CVS group was 0.8%, which was again not statistically significant. From a practical standpoint, the risks of miscarriage from amniocentesis and from CVS are comparable. Higher loss rates were experienced in patients requiring > 1 catheter pass. Later complications in pregnancy were no more frequent in CVS patients.

An error in diagnosis arising from maternal cell contamination is a potential problem with CVS but occurs rarely with good laboratory techniques. With CVS, detection of certain chromosome abnormalities (ie, tetraploidy, lethal trisomies, monosomy X) may not reflect the true fetal status but rather a localized placental abnormality. In cases in which the diagnosis is unclear, am-

niocentesis may be necessary to reach a definitive diagnosis. In general, however, the accuracy of CVS is considered comparable to that of amniotic fluid analysis.

ULTRASONOGRAPHY (US)

US during pregnancy has become widely used. There are no known risks to either mother or fetus. A National Institutes of Health task force concluded in 1984 that there was no benefit in perinatal outcome from routine US screening of all pregnant women; however, this remains controversial. There are many obstetric indications for US throughout pregnancy. A basic examination in the first trimester should include fetal number, documentation of fetal viability, placental localization, gestational dating, amniotic fluid volume, and evaluation for any maternal pelvic masses. A basic examination in the 2nd or 3rd trimester should also include fetal presentation and a survey for gross malformations. Patients should be informed of the indication for US, as well as the information to be obtained, prior to the examination. Consistency in the content of the evaluation within a specific center is important.

Many of the indications for prenatal diagnosis dictate a targeted US for fetal anomalies; eg, elevated MSAFP or family history of congenital anomalies. Targeted US examination should include evaluation of intracranial structures (specifically ventricles and cerebellum) and of spine in both longitudinal and sagittal views; 4-chamber view of the fetal heart; and visualization of the fetal bladder, kidneys, stomach, umbilical cord insertion site, and long bones. Determination of the fetal gender is usually possible in the late 2nd trimester but usually is not essential except for accurate counseling of some genetic disorders. Experienced ultrasonographers should readily diagnose major anomalies (anencephaly), but few centers can state their sensitivity and specificity for detection of specific anomalies. Patients must be aware that anomalies cannot be detected with 100% accuracy, and a normal US result does not guarantee a phenotypically normal infant.

PERCUTANEOUS UMBILICAL BLOOD SAMPLING (PUBS)
(Funipuncture)

Fetal blood samples can now be obtained by PUBS, without the use of a fetoscope. Under US guidance, a 25- or 23-gauge needle is usually directed into the umbilical cord vein near the site of cord insertion into the placenta. Originally developed for the evaluation and treatment of erythroblastosis, PUBS may be useful for the detection of genetic disorders. Loss rates from PUBS are not established. Therefore, PUBS should not be used if the same information can be obtained from amniocentesis.

Until recently, fetal blood was necessary for the prenatal diagnosis of many common genetic disorders, eg, hemoglobinopathies, thalassemias, hemophilia. The rapid progress in molecular diagnosis of these disorders has now made prenatal diagnosis possible on specimens obtained by CVS or amniocentesis. Fetal blood is still necessary for prenatal diagnosis of a few rare genetic disorders, eg, chronic granulomatous disease, hereditary congenital neutropenia, and severe combined immunodeficiency dis-

ease. As more disorders are diagnosable by molecular studies, this list will continue to decrease.

PUBS is particularly useful for rapid chromosome analysis, particularly late in the 3rd trimester when fetal anomalies are present. Obstetric management may be influenced by a chromosome abnormality incompatible with life. Short-term lymphocyte cultures can establish the fetal chromosome complement in 48 to 72 h. More recently, rapid techniques have made cytogenetic results available within 24 h.

FETAL SKIN SAMPLING

Prenatal diagnosis is available for several severe, hereditary skin disorders (genodermatoses). Biopsy of fetal skin is the only method for prenatal diagnosis of some disorders, eg, harlequin ichthyosis, **epidermolysis bullosa letalis** (junctional type), epidermolytic hyperkeratosis. Fetal skin samples may be obtained after direct visualization with a fetoscope, followed by biopsy performed through the fetoscopic sleeve. More recently, biopsies have been obtained without direct fetoscopic visualization. Biopsy forceps are passed through a 14-gauge sleeve under concurrent ultrasonographic visualization. The fetal back is the preferred biopsy site. Loss rates after fetal skin sampling are perhaps 2 to 3% above background.

PRINCIPLES OF COUNSELING

In genetic counseling, one should use readily comprehensible terms, yet avoid a patronizing attitude. It may be useful briefly to recount major causes of genetic disorders: cytogenetic, single gene (mendelian), polygenic/multifactorial (can be labeled "complex"), and environmental. It helps to write out unfamiliar words or use diagrams to reinforce important concepts. Repetition is essential. Time should be allowed not only for couples to ask questions but also to talk privately to formulate their concerns and decisions.

In prenatal diagnosis counseling, some patients believe pregnancy termination is required if an abnormality is identified, and this misconception should be addressed. For patients in whom pregnancy termination is not an option, valid indications for prenatal diagnosis still exist. Many couples use prenatal diagnosis for reassurance that their fetus is not affected with a particular disorder. Without the availability of this reassurance, a significant number of couples would decide against pregnancy, and many would choose abortion upon becoming pregnant. For those with abnormal pregnancies, realistic expectations for the outcome of the pregnancy can be discussed prior to delivery, ie, anticipated anomalies and expected neonatal course. Appropriate referrals can be instituted prior to delivery and will optimize pregnancy and neonatal management.

In complex cases, letters provide a permanent record, allay misunderstanding, and help individuals communicate with relatives. For more common problems (eg, advanced maternal age, repetitive spontaneous abortions, previous offspring with neural tube defects, previous

trisomic offspring), brochures or preprinted forms emphasize that a couple's problem is not unique.

A counselor should attempt to provide objective information but not direct toward a particular decision. However, completely nondirective counseling is probably a myth. For example, a counselor's unwitting facial expression or vocal inflection will invariably be interpreted by the patient. Merely offering antenatal diagnostic services implies approval. In fact, many couples believe prenatal diagnosis is required, and this misconception should be addressed.

14. NORMAL PREGNANCY, LABOR, AND DELIVERY

DIAGNOSIS OF PREGNANCY

The first sign of pregnancy and the first reason most pregnant women see a physician is absence of an expected menstrual period. If a patient's periods are usually regular, absence of menses for $\geq$ 1 wk is presumptive evidence of pregnancy. Breast engorgement and nausea with occasional vomiting may also be noted. The engorgement is caused by increased levels of estrogen (primarily) and progesterone and is an extension of premenstrual breast engorgement. Nausea and vomiting may be caused by human chorionic gonadotropin (HCG) and estrogen, which the syncytial cells of the placenta begin to produce in increasing amounts 10 days after fertilization. HCG stimulates the corpus luteum in the ovary to continue secreting high levels of estrogen and progesterone in order to maintain the integrity of the pregnancy. Many women become fatigued at this time, and an occasional patient notices abdominal enlargement (bloating) very early in her pregnancy.

Pregnancies are usually dated in weeks, starting from the first day of the last menstrual period. Thus, if the patient's menses were regular and if ovulation did occur on day 14 of the cycle, obstetric dates are about 2 wk longer than embryologic dates. If the patient's periods are irregular, the difference is greater or less than 2 wk. Usually, 2 wk after missing a period, the patient is considered to be 6 wk pregnant and the uterus is correspondingly enlarged.

By the time a patient whose periods were regular has missed a period for 2 wk, she is usually certain she is pregnant. Pelvic examination shows uterine enlargement compatible with

pregnancy. The cervix is softer, and the uterus is irregularly softened and enlarged. The vagina and cervix usually become bluish to purple, apparently because they are engorged with blood.

A blood or urine test is usually positive. The recently developed enzyme-linked immunosorbent assay (ELISA) for HCG allows quick and easy determination of the presence of even small quantities of this hormone in the urine. Some of the most sensitive pregnancy tests developed with this method (eg, ICON, TestPack) can provide positive results in about $^1/_2$ h with HCG levels as low as 50 mIU (First International Reference Preparation standard)/mL of urine (levels often found several days before the missed menstrual period). With radioimmunoassays (RIAs) using specific antibodies to the β subunit of HCG (β-HCG), lower levels of HCG can be detected. Because the minimum detection level of HCG for most RIAs is about 0.05 mIU/mL of serum, pregnancy can be diagnosed even several days after conception.

During the first 60 days of normal single gestation, HCG levels double about every 2 days, demonstrating an exponential rise. Although in normal pregnancies HCG levels correlate with gestational age, the use of different standards for measuring HCG, interassay variation, and inherent biologic variation preclude the designation of one quantitative HCG value for the diagnosis of a normally growing fetus. The best approach is comparison of 2 quantitative serum HCG values, obtained 48 h apart, and performed by the same laboratory; a doubling in the HCG value is highly predictive of a normally growing fetus. In abnormal pregnancy, such as spontaneous abortion, blighted ovum, and ectopic pregnancy, HCG levels fall off the normal curve and do not double in 2 days.

The uterus at 6 wk of pregnancy sometimes can be easily flexed on the markedly softened isthmus. At 12 wk, the uterus is larger than the pelvic cavity and rises out of the true pelvis into the abdomen; it can be palpated above the symphysis pubis. At 20 wk, the upper pole of the uterus is at the level of the umbilicus (and about 20 cm from symphysis to top of uterus by tape measurement); at 36 wk, it is near the xiphoid process.

Positive proof of pregnancy is delivery of a fetus. Traditionally, 3 other signs have been accepted as positive: (1) fetal heart tones heard by a physician or recorded via phonocardiography or a Doppler ultrasound instrument (fetal heart tones can ordinarily be detected with a stethoscope at 18 to 20 wk, and as early as 10 to 12 wk with a Doppler ultrasound device if the uterus is accessible abdominally); (2) fetal movements felt or heard by the examining physician; and (3) identification of a fetal skeleton on x-ray, usually after 16 wk. Today, however, positive proof can be obtained by noting a doubling of HCG levels and by ultrasound detection of an intrauterine sac and a fetus with cardiac motion. The presence within the uterus of a cavity compatible with pregnancy can be diagnosed at about 6 wk (4 wk after ovulation) with ultrasound scanning. Fetal cardiac motion may also be seen at about 6 wk with real-time ultrasound scanning and is detectable at 8 wk in > 95% of cases. The patient ordinarily begins to detect fetal motion between 16 and 20 wk.

Pregnancy is considered to last 266 days from the time of conception or 280 days from the first day of the last menstrual period if menses are regular at 28 days. **Nägele's rule** calculates the estimated date of confinement **(EDC)** by subtracting 3 mo from the first day of the last menstrual period and adding 7 days. This calculation is only approximate; ≤ 10% of patients deliver on the calculated day, but 50% deliver within 1 wk and 74 to 88% within 2 wk. Patients should be told that the EDC is ± 2 wk and that delivery up to 2 wk earlier or later is normal.

A pregnant woman is described as a **gravida**. Each pregnancy (twins are one pregnancy) increases gravidity, so that a patient with 2 pregnancies is a gravida 2. Parity describes outcome and may be recorded in 2 ways. Each delivery past 20 wk is recorded as para 1, 2, or 3 (twins are together 1 para). Each loss prior to 20 wk is recorded as abortus 1, 2, or 3. The sum of para and abortus equals gravidity. A newer, more widely used and more informative system records para in 4 numbers: The first indicates the number of deliveries past 20 wk; the 2nd, the number of abortuses; the 3rd, the number of premature deliveries; and the 4th, the number of living children. Thus, a woman pregnant for the 3rd time with 1 set of twins born at 32 wk and 1 abortion would be recorded as gravida 3, para 1-1-1-2.

PHYSIOLOGY

Pregnancy causes physiologic changes in all organ systems, most of which revert to normal after delivery.

Cardiovascular Physiology

Cardiac output (CO) rises 30 to 50%, beginning by 6 wk of pregnancy and peaking between 16 and 28 wk (usually at about 24 wk). CO remains elevated until after 30 wk, then may decrease slightly because the enlarging uterus obstructs the vena cava. During labor, CO increases another 30%. After delivery, the uterus contracts and CO drops markedly to about 15 to 25% above normal, then slowly declines over the next 3 to 4 wk until, at about 6 wk postpartum, it reaches the prepregnancy level. Increased CO is accompanied by an increase in heart rate from the normal 70 beats/min to 80 or 90 beats/min and by proportional stroke volume increases. BP usually drops (with a widening pulse pressure) as the uteroplacental circulation expands during the 2nd trimester but may return to normal in the 3rd trimester.

The rise in CO is probably due to changes in uteroplacental circulation. As the placenta and fetus develop, the uterus requires greater blood flow. At term, blood flow to the uterus is about 1 L/min or 20% of normal CO. Since the volume of the uteroplacental circulation also increases markedly, more blood is needed. In addition, the circulation within the intervillous space acts partly as an arteriovenous shunt to further increase requirements for blood volume and CO.

Exercise increases CO, heart rate, O_2 consumption, and respiratory volume/min more during pregnancy than postpartum. The hyperdynamic circulation of pregnancy increases the frequency of functional murmurs and accentuates heart sounds. X-ray or ECG examination may show the heart displaced into a horizontal position, rotating to the left, with increased transverse diameter. Premature atrial and ventricular beats are common during pregnancy. All these changes should be recognized as normal and should not be erroneously diagnosed as heart disease; they usually can be managed with reassurance alone. However, paroxysms of atrial tachycardia occur more frequently in pregnant women and may require prophylactic digitalization.

Blood volume increases proportionally with CO, but the increase in plasma volume is greater (close to 50%) than that in RBC mass (about 25%), and the Hb may be lowered by dilution, from 13.3 to 12.1 gm.

The **WBC count** (from 5000 to 7000) increases slightly to 9,000 to 12,000. The total mass of WBCs must also increase to fill the increased blood volume. The reason for this increase in WBCs is unknown. A marked leukocytosis ($\geq$ 20,000) occurs during labor and the first few days postpartum.

Iron requirements increase to about 1 gm during pregnancy. The fetus and placenta use about 300 mg of iron, and the increased maternal RBC mass requires an additional 500 mg. Excretion accounts for 200 mg. Supplemental iron therapy is needed, since the average woman has iron stores of only 0.3 to 0.5 gm. The amount absorbed from diet, with that absorbed from stores, is usually insufficient to meet the demands of pregnancy. Iron requirements become great during the 2nd half of pregnancy—6 to 7 mg/day. Supplemental iron is therefore valuable during pregnancy. Iron salts providing 30 mg of iron/day should be used, or 60 to 90 mg/day if anemia is present.

Renal Physiology

Changes in kidney function parallel those in cardiac function. GFR increases 30 to 50%, peaks between 16 and 24 wk of pregnancy, and remains at that level until nearly term, when it may decrease slightly because of positional stasis due to pressure on the vena cava. Renal plasma flow rises correspondingly. Backup, due to pressure from the pregnant uterus on the ureters and hormonal influences (predominantly progesterone), markedly dilates the ureters. These increases in kidney function cause the BUN to drop, usually to < 10 mg/dL, and creatinine levels correspondingly drop to 0.7 mg/dL.

Kidney function, like cardiac function, is very responsive to posture during pregnancy. Normally, kidney function increases in the supine po-

sition and decreases in upright positions; this difference is accentuated in pregnancy. In addition, kidney and cardiac function also markedly increase in the lateral position, because in the supine position, the heavy pregnant uterus resting on the great vessels causes stasis in the lower extremities. This increase is one reason a pregnant woman feels a need to urinate frequently when trying to sleep.

Pulmonary Physiology

Changes in lung function during pregnancy are due partly to the hormonal stimulus of progesterone and partly to positional problems caused by the enlarging uterus. Tidal and minute volume, respiratory rate, and plasma pH and O_2 consumption increase, while inspiratory and expiratory reserve, residual volume and capacity, and plasma P_{CO_2} decrease. Vital capacity and plasma P_{O_2} do not change. Thoracic circumference increases about 10 cm. Considerable hyperemia and edema of the respiratory tract occur, as do occasional symptomatic nasopharyngeal obstruction and nasal stuffiness, transient blockage of eustachian tubes, and changes in tone and quality of voice. Mild dyspnea on exertion is consistently noted, and deep respirations become more frequent.

Gastrointestinal and Hepatobiliary Physiology

As pregnancy progresses, the enlarging uterus pressing against the rectum and lower portion of the colon may cause constipation. In addition, GI motility decreases because elevated progesterone levels relax smooth muscle. Heartburn and belching are common, possibly because of the delay in gastric emptying time and relaxation of the sphincter at the junction of the esophagus and stomach, with reflux of gastric fluids; relaxation of the diaphragmatic hiatus adds to this complaint. However, peptic ulcer disease is uncommon in pregnancy, and preexisting ulcers often improve; HCl production decreases. The incidence of gallbladder disease is somewhat increased; women who have been pregnant have more gallbladder problems than women who have not. Physiologic changes in the liver are discussed in Ch. 17.

Endocrine Physiology

Pregnancy alters the function of most endocrine glands, partly because most hormones are circulated in protein-bound forms and protein binding increases in pregnancy. **Thyroid func-**

tion changes markedly. Thyroid tests indicate an increase in function that mimics hyperthyroidism, and the symptoms and signs of this condition—tachycardia, palpitations, excessive perspiration, emotional instability, and an enlarged thyroid gland—are frequently present. However, true hyperthyroidism occurs in only 0.08% of pregnancies. Adrenal hormone levels increase, probably causing the pink skin striae known as stretch marks and contributing to edema.

Increased levels of glucocorticoids, estrogens, and progesterone modify glucose metabolism and increase the need for insulin, as does the stress of pregnancy and possibly the increased level of human placental lactogen. Also, insulinase manufactured by the placenta may affect insulin requirements, so that patients with prediabetes frequently develop more overt forms of the disease. Diabetes mellitus and pregnancy is discussed in Ch. 17.

The trophic hormones manufactured by the placenta include HCG, which functions much like follicle-stimulating and luteinizing hormones from the anterior pituitary gland in maintaining the corpus luteum, thereby preventing ovulation. The placenta also manufactures a hormone (similar to thyroid-stimulating hormone) that changes thyroid function, and a melanocyte-stimulating hormone that increases skin pigmentation. The placenta may also produce a variety of ACTH that increases adrenal gland function.

Skin

Melasma (mask of pregnancy), a blotchy, brownish pigment, occurs over the forehead and malar eminences. Increased pigment of the mammary areolae and a dark line down the midabdomen commonly occur. Incidence of spider angiomas (usually only above waist level) and thin-walled, dilated capillaries (especially in the lower legs) also increases.

PRENATAL CARE

Ideally, all patients should be seen and examined before conception to allow the physician to screen for medical disease; counsel against use of tobacco, drugs, alcohol, and other substances; and verify physical normality. Health promotion measures such as diet, exercise, and spacing of pregnancies should be discussed, and appropriate agency referral should be made. Any identified social or medical problems should receive specific attention. All patients should be exam-

ined between 6 and 8 wk of pregnancy (ie, when a menstrual period is 2 to 4 wk late) so that duration of pregnancy can be estimated early and the estimated date of confinement (EDC) can be determined more accurately.

The first examination should include a complete physical examination, including weight, height, and BP measurements; palpation of the neck and thyroid gland; auscultation of heart and lungs; examination of the breasts, abdomen, and extremities; and ideally, a funduscopic examination of the eyes. Laboratory tests should include a CBC; STS; serum test for hepatitis B virus; culture for gonorrhea and chlamydia; blood typing for the major blood groups and Rh factor and screening for antibodies; a rubella antibody titer (unless a previous titer was positive); a complete urinalysis and screening test for bacteria in the urine; and a Papanicolaou test of the cervix. Black patients should be tested for sickle cell trait or disease. Genetic studies should be recommended for those in higher risk categories (see Chs. 13 and 48). Women from Asia or south of the US border should have skin tests for TB. A chest x-ray is needed only when the patient has a history of heart or lung disorder; otherwise, x-ray exposure should be avoided during pregnancy, especially during the first 3 mo. If an x-ray is required, the fetus should be shielded.

At 15 to 16 wk, an α-fetoprotein (AFP) test (see also Diagnostic and Screening Procedures under Prevention of Genetic Disorders in Ch. 48) should be offered. Elevated AFP levels may indicate neural tube defect, multiple pregnancy, or miscalculation of dates. An abnormally low AFP may be associated with chromosomal abnormalities.

Screening for abnormal carbohydrate metabolism should be done early in the 2nd trimester in women with a history of large infants or unexplained fetal losses, persistent glucosuria, or a strong family history of diabetes. At 28 wk, all women should be screened: the patient consumes 50 gm glucose in water or soda at a random time (without fasting) and blood glucose concentration is measured 1 h later. Patients with blood glucose levels $\geq$ 135 mg/dL should be given a standard 100-gm, 3-h glucose tolerance test.

The first examination should also include a full pelvic examination with cytologic smear of the cervix and bimanual and rectovaginal examinations to determine the size and configuration of the uterus and normality of adnexa. Pelvic capacity can be determined by attempting to touch the sacral promontory with the middle finger in the vagina; if the distance to the sacral promontory is > 11.5 cm from the underside of the symphysis, the pelvic inlet is almost certainly adequate. The distance between the ischial spines should also be estimated; ≥ 9 cm is considered normal. The length of the sacrospinous ligaments should be estimated so the depth of the pelvis can be judged; 4 to 5 cm or more is considered normal. The subpubic arch in a woman is normally 90° or wider. X-ray pelvimetry is rarely indicated. The combination of adequate pelvic examination for size and configuration, ultrasound examination for position and abnormality, and trial of labor for dilatation and descent usually suffices for either vertex or breech presentation.

Ultrasonography is the imaging method of choice in obstetrics. Many obstetricians believe at least one ultrasonic examination should be performed in each pregnancy to ensure that progress is satisfactory. Since the equipment is portable, it can be used in the office or labor room. The fluid-filled uterus improves ultrasonic visualization of the fetus and the placenta, while the rounded contour of the pregnant abdomen makes scanning more effective. Before examination, especially in early pregnancy, the patient must drink water, since a full bladder pushes the uterus out of the pelvis and improves visualization of its contents. Evidence of pregnancy can be visualized as early as the 4th or 5th wk, and fetal growth can be followed until delivery. Ultrasonography performed with a vaginal transducer eliminates the need for a full bladder and frequently detects a gestational sac earlier than abdominal scanning does. With establishment of a nomogram based on ultrasonic measurements of either fetal biparietal or chest diameters or both, fetal growth can be estimated in terms of weight. This enables the physician to detect sudden changes in fetal growth, check fetal size with predicted delivery dates, and determine fetal growth if early delivery is indicated for the mother's health. A biophysical profile has been devised for a fetus suspected of being in distress; it includes measurement of amniotic fluid, fetal tone, movement, and breathing pattern. Doppler monitoring of the fetal heart or monitoring of fetal respiratory movement has been advocated to detect a high-risk pregnancy.

Ultrasonography also is used to determine multiple pregnancy, hydatidiform mole, polyhydramnios, placenta previa, placental location, fetal position and size, ectopic pregnancy, needle guidance for amniocentesis or fetal transfusion, and

the reason a uterus is too large or too small for given dates of gestation.

Techniques for diagnosing in utero fetal structural abnormalities (eg, anencephaly, hydrocephaly, spina bifida, meningomyelocele, congenital heart defects, bowel or urinary tract obstruction, and polycystic kidney disease) are steadily improving. Real-time scanning allows direct observation of fetal and heart movements. In most hospitals, ultrasonography is used routinely for needle guidance during amniocentesis and fetal transfusion.

Follow-up visits should occur at 4-wk intervals until 32 wk of pregnancy, at 2-wk intervals until 36 wk, and then weekly until delivery. At each examination, the patient's weight and BP should be noted, and the size and shape of the uterus should be measured to determine whether growth and advancement are normal for gestational age. The urine should be tested for albumin and glucose. Fetal heart tones may be heard at 10 to 12 wk with Doppler ultrasonography. Beginning at 18 wk, fetal heart tones may be listened for with a specially designed (DeLee-Hillis) stethoscope and recorded at each visit. The patient's ankles should be examined for edema. The Hct should be measured in each trimester. The patient at high risk for gonorrhea or chlamydia should have culture specimens drawn at the first visit and again at 36 wk. If the patient is Rh-negative, an Rh antibody titer should be repeated at 26 to 27 wk; if she is Rh-negative and the father of the baby is known *with certainty* not to be Rh-negative, the patient should be given $Rh_0(D)$ immune globulin 300 μg at 28 wk. A similar dose should also be given if amniocentesis is performed or whenever significant bleeding occurs. Titers should not be done thereafter. A weakly positive direct Coombs' test may be found in fetal cord blood, but it is not significant. If the infant is $Rh_0(D)$-positive, the mother should receive more $Rh_0(D)$ immune globulin.

These follow-up examinations can be performed by a physician's assistant or nurse and do not require the presence of a physician unless abnormalities are detected. If the EDC is uncertain, the pregnancy should be dated by ultrasound scanning. Dating is most accurate within the first 12 wk. Dating accuracy has a range of ± 4 days at 8 wk, ± 10 days at 13 wk, and ± 3 wk in the 3rd trimester. If normal uterine growth does not occur, fetal growth can be evaluated by ultrasonography. This can be done as early as 18 wk and is most accurate between 28 and 32 wk. At each examination, some time should be spent answering questions and preparing the woman for labor and delivery; she and her husband or other support person should be encouraged to attend childbirth education classes. The combination of early first-trimester pelvic examination, ultrasonography in the first or early 2nd trimester, and auscultation of heart tones at 18 wk (weekly until heard) is accurate for dating in normal pregnancies and should be done in all pregnancies. Late in pregnancy, decisions concerning repeated cesarean section, premature rupture of membranes, or preterm labor can be made with certainty on the basis of these data.

Weight gain during pregnancy for an average-size woman should be about 11.2 to 13.5 kg (25 to 30 lb) or 0.9 to 1.4 kg (2 to 3 lb)/mo of pregnancy. Weight gain beyond 13.5 to 15.8 kg (30 to 35 lb) is excessive and represents fat on both the fetus and the mother. The patient should be warned that controlling weight gain late in pregnancy is more difficult, and she should not gain most of the total weight during the first months; however, failure to gain weight is an ominous sign, especially if weight gain is < 4.5 kg (10 lb). Fluid retention due to stasis in the legs occasionally causes weight gain but can be relieved by having the patient lie on her side (preferably her left side) for 30 to 45 min tid or qid.

About 250 kcal should be added to the patient's daily **diet** to provide for fetal nutrition. Although protein should supply most of these calories, the diet should be well balanced, including fresh fruits and vegetables. High-fiber, sugar-free cereals should be encouraged. Salt (preferably iodized) may be used in moderation, but foods that are excessively salty or have added preservatives should be avoided. Dieting during pregnancy is not recommended, even for a grossly obese patient; some weight gain is essential for proper fetal development, and dieting reduces the supply of nutrients to the fetus. Although the fetus has first choice of nutrients, the choice must involve something worth having. The value of a nutritious, well-balanced diet should be emphasized throughout pregnancy.

Drugs, including vitamins and aspirin, should be discouraged. No drugs should be prescribed unless specifically indicated (see also DRUGS IN PREGNANCY, below). Most women need an iron supplement, and ferrous sulfate 300 mg orally bid usually suffices. Ferrous gluconate 450 mg orally bid may be better tolerated. If the diet is adequate, no other vitamin or supplement is needed.

For **nausea and vomiting,** dietary management should precede medication. The patient should be advised to drink or eat only small amounts frequently, avoid hunger, and limit her intake to bland foods such as bouillon, consommé, rice, pasta, and similar foods. Soda crackers and a soft drink often relieve the nausea. Eating before rising may be helpful. No drugs for morning sickness have been approved by the FDA. If nausea and vomiting are so intense or persistent that the patient becomes dehydrated, develops ketosis, or loses weight, she may need to be hospitalized and given IV fluids.

Edema, especially of the legs, is common. **Varicosities** of the legs and vulva are also common and may give discomfort. Clothing should be nonconstrictive at the waist and legs. Edema usually decreases with use of elastic support hose or increased rest with the legs elevated or, preferably, lying on the side. **Hemorrhoids** are common; if symptomatic, they should be treated with stool softeners, topically applied anesthetics, and warm soaks. **Backache** in varying degrees is common; eliminating excessive strain and wearing a lightweight maternity girdle may be helpful. **Pain at the symphysis pubis** occurs occasionally. **Heartburn,** usually caused by reflux of gastric contents into the lower esophagus, is common. Treatment includes eating smaller meals, avoiding bending or lying flat for several hours after eating, and using antacid preparations (except sodium bicarbonate). **Fatigue** is common, especially in the first trimester and again in late pregnancy. Pregnant women frequently develop increased **vaginal discharge,** which is usually nonpathologic. Vaginal trichomoniasis and candidiasis are common but probably should be treated only if symptomatic. **Pica,** a bizarre craving for strange foods or, at times, inedible materials (eg, starch or clay) may occur. Occasionally, profuse salivation, **ptyalism,** may cause distress.

Normal activities and **customary exercises** may be continued throughout pregnancy. Swimming and other mildly strenuous sports are permissible. There is no reason a pregnant woman should not ride horseback or engage in similar vigorous activity if she is accomplished at it and is cautious. Many women find that their sexual desire increases or decreases during pregnancy. Sexual intercourse is permissible throughout pregnancy but should be prohibited if any vaginal bleeding, pain, or leakage of amniotic fluid is present and especially if uterine contractions occur. Several maternal deaths have been reported from blowing air into the vagina during cunnilingus.

Any of the following warning symptoms should be reported promptly: persistent headaches, persistent nausea and vomiting, dizziness, visual disturbances, pain or cramps in the lower abdomen, contractions, vaginal bleeding, rupture of membranes, swelling of hands or feet, diminished urinary output, or any illness or infection. The patient should also be encouraged to consult her physician about any problems that puzzle her.

Finally, the **signs of beginning labor** should be reviewed with the patient. The principal signal is the onset of back pain or lower abdominal contractions that recur at regular intervals. A multipara with a history of rapid labors should notify the physician even earlier. Toward the end of pregnancy, after 36 wk, many doctors prefer to examine the patient vaginally to try to predict when labor will occur. This procedure is *contraindicated* if the head is floating above the inlet, because of the possibility of placenta previa, unless the placenta has been localized in normal position by a previous ultrasound examination.

FETAL MONITORING

Several methods of fetal monitoring are available that are technically more sophisticated than the traditional method of intermittent auscultation, and electronic external fetal heart rate monitoring is routinely used in all labors by many obstetricians. However, a growing body of evidence shows that patients monitored electronically have a higher rate of cesarean section than those monitored by auscultation. The addition of fetal scalp pH determination to decide the need for cesarean section may help reduce the rate, but this procedure requires sophisticated equipment and readily available, experienced technicians. Thus, for monitoring low-risk patients in normal labor, auscultation with a fetoscope q 15 min in the 1st stage and q 3 min or after each contraction in the 2nd stage is reliable. This intermittent auscultation is associated with a lower false-positive rate and incidence of intervention than continuous electronic monitoring, and it provides opportunities for greater personal contact with the woman in labor. Electronic fetal monitoring can be reserved for high-risk patients or those in whom auscultation is difficult or indicates a possibly abnormal heart rate.

Electronic fetal heart rate monitoring with external devices applied to the maternal abdomen detects and records fetal heart tones and uterine contractions. Leads may also be placed internally, with an electrode attached to the fetal scalp and a catheter through the cervix into the uterus to measure amniotic fluid pressure. The external devices are generally used for normal pregnancies; the internal methods are reserved for high-risk or problem pregnancies.

External fetal monitoring can also be used as a **nonstress test (NST)** or as a **contraction stress test (CST)**, sometimes called the **oxytocin challenge test (OCT)**. In these tests, fetal heart rate is recorded and compared with fetal movement (NST) or with contractions induced by oxytocin (OCT) or those occurring spontaneously or secondary to breast stimulation. These tests are frequently used to monitor problem pregnancies.

If a problem has been previously identified or is detected by auscultation or external monitoring, internal monitoring is used to provide more reliable information about fetal heart rate and uterine contraction patterns. When a problem is discovered on electronic monitoring or on auscultation verified by electronic monitoring, **fetal scalp blood sampling for pH** may be used to confirm the need for intervention. A value of ≥ 7.25 is reassuring; 7.0 to 7.24 is worrisome, indicating that scalp sampling for pH should be repeated after O_2 and IV fluids have been given and maternal position has been changed; < 7.0 indicates that prompt delivery is needed.

DRUGS IN PREGNANCY

Most pregnant women take drugs. A recent study from the Centers for Disease Control showed that 90% of 492 women surveyed took either prescription or OTC medications representing 48 classes of drugs. Those taken most commonly include antiemetics, antacids, antihistamines, analgesics, antimicrobials, tranquilizers, hypnotics, diuretics, and social or illicit drugs. Yet, drug-induced teratology accounts for only 2 to 3% of all fetal congenital malformations; most result from genetic, environmental, or unknown causes.

Drug use in pregnancy is complicated by the changing biochemical dynamics of the mother and the fetus. Drugs circulate between mother and fetus by the same pathway that provides the fetus substrates for growth and development and removes waste products. The exchange takes place primarily in the placenta, where maternal arterial blood spurts into sinuses (the intervillous space) and then drains into the maternal uterine veins to be returned to the maternal systemic circulation. Maternal and fetal blood do not merge; exchange of solutes takes place across fetal capillaries contained in villi protruding into the intervillous space. Solutes must cross the epithelial cells of the villi and the endothelium of the fetal capillaries; they are then carried to the fetus by fetal placental veins, which converge into the umbilical vein.

Drugs given during pregnancy can affect the fetus by (1) acting directly on the embryo to produce a lethal, toxic, or teratogenic effect; (2) altering placental function (constricting vessels), affecting gas and nutrition exchange between fetus and mother; (3) changing the myometrial activity (producing severe uterine hypertonia resulting in fetal anoxic injury); or (4) altering the biochemical dynamics of the mother, indirectly affecting the fetus.

The magnitude and seriousness of a drug effect on fetal development or reactivity is determined largely by **fetal age, drug potency,** and **dosage.** Drugs given during the embryonic or zygotic stage (before the 20th day after conception) may have an all-or-nothing effect, either killing the embryo or not affecting it at all. The fetus is highly resistant to teratogenesis during this stage. The period of organogenesis (between the 3rd and 8th conceptual wk) is critical for teratogenesis. Drugs reaching the embryo at this stage may produce (1) no measurable effect, (2) abortion, (3) a sublethal gross anatomic defect (true teratogenic effect), or (4) a permanent subtle metabolic or functional defect that might manifest itself later in life (covert embryopathy). Drugs given after organogenesis (ie, in the 2nd and 3rd trimesters) are unlikely to be teratogenic, but they may alter the growth and the physiologic and biochemical functions of normally formed fetal organs and tissues.

The characteristics of drug diffusion across the placental barrier are similar to those of passage across other epithelial barriers (see DRUG ABSORPTION in Ch. 133). After a drug is administered to a pregnant woman, its concentration is higher in cord venous plasma than in cord arterial plasma. Equilibration between maternal blood and fetal tissues takes at least 40 min. To avoid producing a toxic effect, drugs that pass through the placenta, such as those commonly used during labor (ie, local anesthetics, narcotics), should be given cautiously within the hour before delivery; after the cord is cut, the newborn (whose metabolic and excretory processes are still immature) must assume the task of clearing the transferred drug from its body.

The FDA rates drugs in 5 categories of safety for use in pregnancy. In **category A,** controlled human studies have demonstrated no fetal risks (these are the safest drugs). In **category B,** animal studies indicate no risk to the fetus and no controlled human studies have been done, or animal studies show a risk to the fetus but well-controlled human studies do not. In **category C,** no adequate studies, either animal or human, have been done, or adverse fetal effects have been shown in animals but no human data are available. In **category D,** positive evidence of human fetal risk exists, but benefits in certain situations (eg, life-threatening situations or serious diseases for which safer drugs cannot be used or are ineffective) may outweigh the risks. In **category X,** proven fetal risks exist that outweigh any possible benefit. These labeling definitions are universally accepted and are often helpful in directing the risk-benefit decision making encountered when prescribing drugs during pregnancy.

Specific drugs or classes of drugs and their potential adverse effects on the fetus are discussed below.

Teratogens

Antineoplastic agents are foremost among the teratogens. Since embryonic tissues undergo rapid growth characterized by a high DNA turnover rate, they resemble neoplastic tissues and are very susceptible to antineoplastic agents. Aminopterin was the first drug shown to be teratogenic in humans. Many antimetabolites and alkylating agents (including methotrexate, 6-mercaptopurine, cyclophosphamide, chlorambucil, and busulfan) can cause fetal abnormalities such as intrauterine growth retardation, mandibular hypoplasia, cleft palate, cranial dysostosis, ear defects, and club foot. Colchicine, vinblastine, vincristine, and actinomycin D are teratogenic in animals but have not proved to be so in man. Colchicine has been shown to increase abnormal chromosomes in lymphocyte cultures, raising concerns about increasing the risk of Down syndrome in offspring.

Thalidomide, another known teratogenic agent, was introduced in 1956 as a remedy for influenza and was also recommended as a sedative. In the early 1960s, a thalidomide embryopathy was described that included bilateral fetal limb reduction as well as GI and cardiovascular malformations in fetuses of women who took the drug during organogenesis.

Isotretinoin is also a significant human teratogen. More than 17 cases of birth defects and 20 incidences of spontaneous abortion have been reported in women taking isotretinoin early in pregnancy. The most significant anomalies reported include cardiac defects, microtia (small ears), and hydrocephalus. The actual risk of anomalies in exposed fetuses is estimated to be 25%. **Etretinate**, another synthetic retinoid, has been implicated as an animal and human teratogen. After oral administration, the drug is stored in subcutaneous fat and slowly released; its metabolite etretin produces teratogenic effects for up to 6 mo after the drug is discontinued.

Other potential teratogens include **androgenic hormones** and synthetic **progestins** given during the first 12 wk of gestation, which produce masculinization of the external genitalia in female fetuses. A relationship has been reported between adenocarcinoma of the vagina in adolescent girls and their mothers' use during pregnancy of **diethylstilbestrol (DES)**, a synthetic nonsteroidal estrogen. Aside from the rare occurrence of clear cell adenocarcinoma in females exposed in utero to DES, the following abnormalities have been observed: poor preovulatory mucus, abnormal endometrial cavity, menstrual dysfunction, spontaneous abortion, incompetent cervix, increased rate of ectopic pregnancy, and an increase in preterm labor and perinatal mortality. In males exposed to DES, meatal stenosis and hypospadias have been observed. Other human tumors have appeared many years after exposure to carcinogens (thymus radiation, aniline, etc), but the DES effect is the first implication of transplacental carcinogenesis in humans. **Meclizine**, an agent frequently prescribed for motion sickness, nausea, and vomiting, is teratogenic in rodents, but this effect has not been documented in humans.

An association of fetal abnormalities with **anticonvulsants** is strengthened by increasing reports of cleft palate, cardiac abnormalities, craniofacial anomalies, nail and digit hypoplasia, visceral defects, and mental subnormality in the children of epileptic mothers taking anticonvulsant drugs. Additionally, risk factors for teratogenesis in these women may include the frequency and severity of epileptic seizures. The anticonvulsants **trimethadione** and **valproic acid** have been clearly shown to be strongly teratogenic and are contraindicated in almost all circumstances. The previous association of the **fetal hydantoin syndrome** (craniofacial anomalies, deficient growth, mental retardation, and limb defects) with phenytoin is now disputed because studies have shown similar defects in babies born to untreated epileptic mothers. During the first day of life, newborns exposed to phenytoin and phenobarbital in utero are at increased risk for bleeding due to drug-induced vitamin K deficiency. This complication can be prevented by daily oral vitamin K administration to the mother 1 mo before delivery or an IM injection to the newborn after birth. Recently, carbamazepine has also been implicated as a potential teratogen. However, to minimize the complications resulting from frequent seizures during pregnancy, epilepsy should be treated with phenytoin, carbamazepine, phenobarbital, or a combination of these, using the smallest effective dose under close supervision.

Immunization with a **live virus** should be avoided when pregnancy is suspected; eg, giving rubella vaccine risks viral placental and fetal infection. Vaccinations for cholera, hepatitis A and B, measles or mumps, influenza, plague, poliomyelitis, rabies, tetanus-diphtheria, typhoid, varicella, and yellow fever may be given during pregnancy if a substantial risk of infection exists.

Thyroid drugs: Radioactive iodine (^{131}I), when used to treat thyroid disease, can cross the placenta and destroy the thyroid gland of the fetus or produce severe hypothyroidism. Triiodothyronine, propylthiouracil, and methimazole also cross the placenta and can cause fetal goiter. Methimazole has been associated with scalp defects (aplasia cutis) in newborns. Thus, propylthiouracil is the drug of choice for treating hyperthyroidism during pregnancy.

Oral hypoglycemics given chronically to diabetic mothers may result in inadequate control of diabetes and profound hypoglycemia in newborns.

Narcotics, sedatives, and analgesics (see also discussions on pregnancy and opioid addiction in Ch. 53 and on medications for mood disorders in Ch. 57): Narcotics, barbiturates, and salicylates cross the placental barrier and attain significant levels in the fetus. Neonates born to narcotic addicts may show withdrawal symptoms 6 h to 8 days after birth. Maternal phenobarbital ingestion alters the usual course of physiologic jaundice in the neonate, perhaps due to induction of the neonatal hepatic conjugating enzymes. Salicylates compete with bilirubin for albumin binding sites and may produce fetal kernicterus. Large doses of aspirin may result in delayed onset of labor, premature closure of the fetal ductus arteriosus, a maternal bleeding diathesis during the intrapartum or postpartum period, or neonatal bleeding.

The **fetal alcohol syndrome** is seen in babies born to mothers who drink alcohol. The syndrome consists of prenatal growth retardation, microcephaly, shortened palpebral fissures, borderline mental deficiency, and less frequently, joint anomalies, cardiovascular defects, perinatal mortality, and postnatal failure to thrive. The critical volume of ingested alcohol that results in fetal alcohol syndrome is unknown. In one study, an increased frequency of abnormalities was not found until 45 mL of alcohol (equivalent to 3 drinks per day) was exceeded.

Tranquilizers and antidepressants: Phenothiazines have been used during pregnancy as antiemetics and psychotropics. They readily pass the placental barrier and, as a group, appear to present an insignificant fetal risk. However, when examined individually, certain drugs have shown an association with fetal abnormalities (eg, chlorpromazine may be associated with an increased risk of fetal malformation).

Studies of fetal exposure to meprobamate and chlordiazepoxide showed no evidence of increased malformations or fetal deaths. Mental and motor tests of these children at age 8 mo and intelligence tests at 4 yr did not document brain damage. Because of reports that some fetal abnormalities have been associated with intake of tranquilizers, the FDA requires that tranquilizer labels warn about the increased risk of congenital malformation when administered during the first trimester of pregnancy.

Tricyclic antidepressants have not been conclusively associated with congenital malformations. Isolated reports note that neonates born to mothers who received tricyclics just before delivery may show tachycardia, respiratory distress, and urinary retention. Lithium carbonate given in the first trimester also has been associated with fetal congenital malformations; eg, a report from the International Register of Lithium Babies concluded that when lithium was given during the first trimester, up to 11.5% of the fetuses were malformed. Cardiovascular abnormalities, including Ebstein's anomaly, were most common. Perinatal effects of lithium have also been reported, including lethargy, hypotonia, poor feeding, goiter, and nephrogenic diabetes insipidus in the newborn.

Antibacterials: Tetracyclines pass the placenta and are concentrated and deposited in fetal bones and teeth, where they combine with calcium; the period of risk is from the middle to the end of pregnancy. Permanent yellowish discoloration of the teeth, enamel hypoplasia, and decreased resistance to caries have been observed in children of mothers given tetracyclines during pregnancy. Bone growth may be retarded. Because several safe alternatives are available, tetracyclines should be avoided during pregnancy.

Streptomycin, gentamicin, kanamycin, and other ototoxic drugs should be avoided in pregnancy, since they cross the placenta and may damage the fetal labyrinth. However, their benefits in treating penicillin- or cephalosporin-resistant organisms may outweigh the risks. Chloramphenicol, even when given to the mother in large doses, does not produce adverse effects in the fetus. The neonate, though, cannot adequately metabolize chloramphenicol, and the resulting high blood levels may lead to circulatory collapse **(the gray baby syndrome)**. Penicillins appear to be safe in pregnancy, but sensitization may occur in utero.

Long-acting sulfonamides also pass the placenta; since they are highly protein-bound, they can displace bilirubin from binding sites. If the sulfonamides are given well before the perinatal period, the placenta efficiently excretes the bilirubin, minimizing fetal risk. When sulfonamides are given near or during the late perinatal period, the neonate may develop severe jaundice and kernicterus because of its inability to clear the bilirubin, owing to its deficient conjugation system. Sulfasalazine is a notable exception in that the active fetal metabolite, sulfapyridine, has weak bilirubin-displacing activity, presenting minimal risk to the fetus.

Anticoagulants: Coumarins given during pregnancy can pass to the fetus, which is highly sensitive to them. The **fetal warfarin syndrome** may occur in up to 25% of fetuses exposed during the first trimester; abnormalities including nasal hypoplasia, bone stippling on x-ray examination, bilateral optic atrophy, and various degrees of mental retardation have been described. Optic atrophy, cataracts, mental retardation, microcephaly, and microphthalmia have been described with 2nd- or 3rd-trimester warfarin exposure. Fetal and maternal hemorrhage has also been seen in pregnant women during warfarin therapy. Heparin, a large, highly charged molecule that has little appreciable transplacental access, is the anticoagulant of choice for use in pregnancy. Protracted use during pregnancy, however, may result in maternal osteoporosis or thrombocytopenia.

Cardiovascular drugs: Cardiac glycosides cross the placenta, but neonates (and children) are relatively resistant to their toxicity. Of a dose of ^{14}C-digitoxin injected into the mother, only 1% appears in the fetus as unchanged digitoxin and 3% as metabolites. Higher concentrations of digitoxin have been seen in fetuses, mostly in the first trimester. Neonates born to mothers using digoxin have a plasma concentration approximating that of the mother, with no indication of ill effects on the fetus. Mothers of children with congenital heart defects have a high incidence of amphetamine use, suggesting a possible teratogenic association.

Antihypertensive drugs frequently taken by mothers with preeclampsia or eclampsia also cross the placenta and can adversely affect the neonate. Magnesium sulfate causes respiratory depression. Ganglionic blockers may produce autonomic effects such as hypotension and paralytic ileus. Propranolol passes the placental barrier and can cause bradycardia and hypoglycemia; it may also be responsible for varying degrees of intrauterine growth retardation. Thiazide diuretics should be avoided in pregnancy. Thiazide contracts the mother's plasma volume and can compromise fetal oxygenation and nutrition. It can also cause hyponatremia, hypokalemia, and thrombocytopenia in the neonate.

Oxidant drugs such as primaquine, nitrofurantoin, naphthalene, vitamin K, sulfonamides, and chloramphenicol may cause hemolysis in mothers and fetuses with a genetic G6PD deficiency.

Drugs commonly used during labor and delivery: Placental transfer of local anesthetics (mepivacaine, lidocaine, prilocaine) from various sites of administration (epidural, caudal, paracervical) has been associated with fetal CNS depression and bradycardia. Catecholamines and oxytocin given to the mother may affect her fetus by causing vasoconstriction or increased myometrial activity, possibly resulting in anoxia or asphyxia. Narcotics, scopolamine, barbiturates, ketamine, and analgesics all pass the placental barrier. Thiopental, which is commonly used during cesarean delivery under general anesthesia, is concentrated in the fetal liver, shielding the CNS from high concentrations. Large doses of IV diazepam given to mothers before delivery have been reported to produce hypotonia, hypothermia, low Apgar scores, impaired metabolic response to cold stress, and neurologic depression in their babies.

Social and Illicit Drugs

Cigarette smoking: The mean birth weight of infants born to mothers who smoke during pregnancy is 6 oz less than that of infants born to nonsmoking mothers. The incidence of spontaneous abortion, stillbirth, preterm birth, and sudden infant death syndrome may also be increased in pregnant women who smoke.

Caffeine: Several studies have suggested that drinking > 7 to 8 cups of coffee per day is associated with an increased incidence of stillbirths, preterm births, low-birth-weight infants, and spontaneous abortions. These studies, however, did not control the use of tobacco and alcohol. A recent controlled study of women who took small doses of caffeine showed no evidence of a teratogenic effect. However, evidence is conflicting as to whether heavy ingestion of caffeine is associated with increased perinatal complications. Decaffeinated beverages, however, theoretically pose little risk to the developing fetus.

Alcohol is described above as being responsible for an increased incidence in perinatal morbidity. **Cocaine** use during pregnancy has been associated with an increased miscarriage rate, abruptio placentae, fetal CNS and GU malformations, and a depression of interactive behavior in newborns. **Marijuana** use during pregnancy is more common. Though no specific evidence shows that marijuana is teratogenic or associated with adverse fetal growth and development, studies do suggest that heavy use is associated with neurobehavioral abnormalities in newborns.

MANAGEMENT OF NORMAL LABOR

Labor consists of a series of rhythmic, progressive contractions of the uterus that cause effacement and dilation of the uterine cervix. The stimulus for labor is unknown. Circulating oxytocin secreted by the posterior pituitary gland may initiate labor, but no direct evidence supports this thesis. Labor usually begins within 2 wk (before or after) of the estimated date of confinement. In a first pregnancy, labor usually lasts a maximum of 12 to 14 h; succeeding labors are shorter, averaging 6 to 8 h.

During labor, contractions increase in duration, intensity, and frequency. A latent phase, with irregular contractions of varying intensity that apparently ripen or soften the cervix, usually precedes actual labor. This latent phase may be intermittent over several days or may last only a few hours. Bloody show (a small amount of blood with mucous discharge from the cervix) may precede the onset of labor by as much as 72 h.

Occasionally, the amniotic and chorionic sac (the membranes) ruptures before labor begins, and amniotic fluid leaks through the cervix and vagina. When a patient's membranes rupture, she should contact her physician immediately. About 80 to 90% of patients with ruptured membranes go into labor spontaneously within 24 h. If the patient does not and if the fetus is at term, labor is usually induced because of risk of infection.

Upon admission, the patient's BP, heart and respiratory rates, temperature, and weight should be recorded and the presence or absence of edema noted. A urine specimen should be collected for protein and glucose analysis, and blood should be drawn for a CBC and blood type, if not known. A physical examination should be performed. Examination of the abdomen includes estimating the size, position, and presentation of the fetus and noting the presence or absence of fetal heart tones. Preliminary estimates of the quality of contractions and their duration and frequency should also be recorded.

Vaginal examination should be performed with a clean glove after the patient's vulva is washed. Such examination is *contraindicated* if any bleeding is present; it may also be contraindicated if the membranes are ruptured, unless they were ruptured by the physician. If membranes are ruptured, the presence of fetal meconium (producing greenish discoloration) should be noted, as it may be a sign of fetal distress. The degrees of **dilation and effacement of the cervix** and of descent **(station)** of the fetus within the pelvic cavity should be recorded, and the presentation and position should be noted. **Presentation** describes the lowermost part of the fetus, such as breech, vertex, or shoulder. **Position** describes the relationship of the presenting part to the pelvis, such as occiput left anterior **(OLA)** or sacrum right posterior **(SRP)**. Dilation is recorded in centimeters as the diameter of a circle. Effacement is estimated in percentages, progressing from zero (no effacement) to 100% (complete taking up of the cervix). Station is determined in centimeters above or below the level of the ischial spines. At this time, the physician should determine whether or not the membranes

are intact. A brief description of the **powers** (labor quality, rate, and duration), **passage** (pelvic measurements), and **passenger** (fetal size, position, heart rate pattern, etc) should be noted in the labor record.

The patient should be admitted to the labor suite for observation until delivery. An enema is not necessary; no evidence shows that it stimulates labor, but it does contaminate the vulva and perineum throughout labor and delivery. Shaving (or clipping) vulvar hair is also not indicated, since shaving is irritating and may lead to infection. An IV infusion of Ringer's solution may be started, using a large-bore indwelling catheter inserted in a vein in the hand or forearm. During a normal labor of 6 to 10 h, the patient should receive 500 to 1000 mL of solution. This infusion prevents dehydration during labor and subsequent hemoconcentration, while providing an adequate circulating blood volume. It also provides immediate access for drugs or blood in an emergency or if drugs are needed to stimulate contraction of the uterus. Fluid preloading is also of value if conduction anesthesia is to be used.

The patient should be observed frequently during labor. She should receive little by mouth, to prevent possible vomiting and aspiration during delivery. An antacid should be given orally on admission and q 3 h to neutralize gastric acidity. Maternal heart rate and BP and fetal heart rate should be checked q 15 min during the 1st stage of labor. In the 2nd stage, the patient should be attended constantly, and fetal heart tones should be checked after every contraction or q 3 min, whichever is closer together. In many institutions, the fetal heart rate and uterine contractions are electronically monitored for all deliveries, since 30 to 50% of babies who develop fetal distress or die during delivery show no antecedent signs that would call for intense observation. Electronic fetal monitoring may save the life of such a baby (see also FETAL MONITORING under PRENATAL CARE, above).

Analgesia may be provided during labor as necessary, but as little drug as possible should be given because of the depressant effects on the fetus. Better preparation and education for childbirth lessen anxiety, so the need for an analgesic is markedly decreased. Meperidine (up to 50 mg) or morphine sulfate (up to 5 mg) given IV q 60 to 90 min is most commonly used and provides good analgesia with only a small total amount of drug. Although both narcotics cross the placenta and affect the fetus, naloxone 0.01 mg/kg can be given IM, IV, or s.c. to the newborn as a specific antagonist, if necessary. "Synergistic" drugs (eg, promethazine) are popular but are not ideal, since no antidote is available if an overdose is given or a problem arises. These drugs are more additive than synergistic; thus, if more analgesia is needed, additional meperidine or morphine is better, or epidural analgesia may be used (see under MANAGEMENT OF NORMAL DELIVERY, below).

The 1st stage of labor, *from onset of labor to full dilation of the cervix* (about 10 cm), can be divided into several phases. In the **latent phase**, the contractions become progressively better co-ordinated, discomfort is minimal, and the cervix effaces but has minimal dilation. The duration of this phase varies but averages $8^1/_2$ h in nulliparas and 5 h in multiparas. The **active phase**, during which the cervix dilates from 2 to 3 cm to full dilation and the presenting part descends well into the midpelvis, lasts about 5 h in nulliparas and 2 h in multiparas. The patient may begin to feel the urge to bear down as the presenting part descends in the pelvis. However, discouraging the patient from pushing until the cervix is fully dilated prevents tearing the cervix and wasting her energy before it is useful.

The 2nd stage of labor, *the time from complete cervical dilation to delivery of the fetus*, lasts about 60 min in nulliparas and 15 min in multiparas. In addition to contractions of the uterus, expulsive bearing-down efforts are required of the patient for spontaneous delivery.

Various abnormalities of both 1st and 2nd stages of labor (problems of fetal distress, abnormal presentations, disproportions between fetus and maternal pelvis, bleeding disorders, infection, or premature labor) require special investigation; correction of the problems if feasible; and possible use of forceps, vacuum extractor, or cesarean section delivery (see Ch. 18).

MANAGEMENT OF NORMAL DELIVERY

Ideally, when delivery is imminent, the patient is taken to the delivery room with the IV infusion of Ringer's solution still running. The father or other support persons should be offered the opportunity to accompany her. In the delivery room, the patient is washed and draped and delivery is accomplished.

Methods of **anesthesia** for delivery include pudendal block, regional anesthesia, and general anesthesia. In all cases, skill and experience in administration are required for safe, effective anesthesia. **Pudendal block** involves injecting a local anesthetic through the wall of the vagina so that the pudendal nerve is flooded with anesthetic as it swings around the ischial spine. The nerve pathways are such that anesthesia is provided for the lower part of the vagina, the perineum, and the posterior portion of the vulva; the anterior vulva is innervated by lumbar dermatomes and is not anesthetized. Pudendal block is useful for uncomplicated deliveries in which the patient wishes to push and there are no contraindications. **Paracervical block** is no longer recommended because it is associated with a high incidence ($> 15\%$) of fetal bradycardia. Infiltration of the perineum is also commonly used, although anesthesia is not as effective as with well-administered pudendal block.

Several **methods of regional analgesia** may be used; that most frequently used for labor and delivery is lumbar epidural injection of local anesthetic. Narcotics (eg, fentanyl and sufentanil) may be given by continuous infusion in the epidural space. Caudal injection is rarely used today. Spinal anesthesia may be used for cesarean section but has a risk of spinal headache afterwards, so it is used less often. Constant attendance and frequent (q 5 min) vital sign checks are necessary to detect and treat possible hypotension.

General anesthesia with potent inhalation agents such as isoflurane can be very depressing to both mother and fetus and therefore is not recommended for routine delivery. Analgesia by 40% nitrous oxide may be used as long as verbal contact with the patient is maintained. Greater interest in prepared childbirth has lessened the use of such agents except for breech or twin delivery or cesarean section. Considerable experience is required to use them safely.

A vaginal examination is performed to determine the position and station of the head. The patient is instructed to bear down and strain with each contraction to move the head down through the pelvis and progressively dilate the vaginal introitus so that more and more of the head will appear. When about 3 or 4 cm of the head is visible in a primipara during a contraction (somewhat earlier in a multipara), the following maneuvers can facilitate delivery and reduce the possibility of perineal laceration: The physician (if right-handed) places the left palm over the baby's head during a contraction to control and, if necessary, slightly retard its progress, while placing the curved fingers of the right hand against the dilating perineum through which the baby's brow or chin is felt. Applying pressure against the brow or chin with the curved fingers helps to advance the head. The physician controls advancement or retardation of the head to effect slow and controlled delivery.

Use of forceps for delivery is often an arbitrary decision. If an epidural anesthetic that precludes vigorous straining is used, forceps may be required and are safe. However, if a local anesthetic that allows bearing-down efforts is used, forceps usually are not needed unless complications interfere. If the 2nd stage of labor is likely to be prolonged because the patient is having difficulty straining, forceps should be used.

An **episiotomy**, *surgical incision of the perineum,* should be performed for patients in whom the perineum does not stretch readily and is obstructing delivery. This procedure substitutes a surgical incision for excessive stretching and possible tearing of the perineal tissues. The incision is easier to repair properly than a tear and may decrease anterior tears. The most common episiotomy is a midline incision made with scissors from the midpoint of the posterior fourchette directly backward toward the rectum. This type risks extension into the rectal sphincter or rectum itself, but if recognized promptly, the extension can be repaired successfully and will heal well. Episioproctotomy (intentionally cutting into the rectum) is not recommended because the incidence of recto-vaginal fistula is unacceptably high. Tears or extensions into the rectum can usually be prevented by keeping the baby's head well flexed until the occipital prominence passes beyond the subpubic arch. Another type of episiotomy is a mediolateral incision made with scissors from the midpoint of the posterior fourchette at a 45° angle laterally on either side. Although this type usually does not extend into the sphincter or rectum, postoperative pain and healing time are increased. Thus, unless problems are expected, the midline episiotomy is recommended.

Following delivery of the head, the baby's body rotates so that the shoulders are in an anteroposterior position; *gentle* downward pressure on the head delivers the anterior shoulder under the symphysis. The head is *gently* lifted, the posterior shoulder slides over the perineum, and the rest of the baby's body follows without difficulty. The baby's nose, mouth, and pharynx are aspirated with a bulb syringe to remove obstructions (mucus and fluids) and help establish respirations. The cord should be double-clamped and cut between the clamps, and a plastic clip should be applied. The baby is then placed in a warmed resuscitation bassinet or on the mother's abdomen. Care of the newborn is described in Ch. 23.

The 3rd stage of labor *begins after delivery of the infant and ends with delivery of the placenta.* After delivery, the physician places a hand gently on the uterine fundus to detect contractions; placental separation usually occurs during the 1st or 2nd contraction, often with a gush of blood from behind the separating placenta. The mother can usually push out the placenta. If not, and if significant bleeding occurs, the placenta can usually be expressed by firm, downward pressure on the uterus. If this is not effective, the umbilical cord is held taut while the uterus is pushed *upward,* away from the placenta. (Manual removal by inserting the entire hand into the uterine cavity, separating the placenta from its attachment, then extracting the placenta may be necessary.) The placenta should be examined for completeness, as fragments left in the uterus can cause delayed hemorrhage. If the placenta is incomplete, the uterine cavity should be explored manually. Some obstetricians routinely explore the uterus after each delivery. Immediately after delivery of the placenta, an oxytocic drug should be given (oxytocin 10 IU IM or, if the IV infusion is running, in the IV fluid) to aid in firm contraction of the uterus. Oxytocin should *not* be given as a single large IV dose, since cardiac arrhythmia may occur.

After inspection to rule out or repair lacerations in the cervix or vagina and to make sure the uterus is contracting, and after repair of the episiotomy, the patient may be taken to the recovery room. If all is well, the infant can be presented to the mother so that they can be taken there together. Many mothers wish to begin breast-feeding soon after delivery, and this should be encouraged. Mother, infant, and father should remain together in a warm, private area for an hour or more, as this may increase parent-infant emotional attachment (bonding). The baby may then be taken to the nursery (see Ch. 23). The mother should be observed for about 1 h for bleeding, BP problems, and general well-being. The time from delivery of the placenta to 4 h postpartum is frequently called the **4th stage of labor**; most complications, especially hemorrhage, occur at this time, and frequent observation is mandatory.

PSYCHOLOGIC ASPECTS

For many women, the father's presence during labor is helpful and should be encouraged. His moral support, encouragement, and expressions of affection decrease the need for analgesia and make the process of labor less frightening and unpleasant. Childbirth education classes are available to prepare both the father and mother for a normal labor and delivery. Sharing the stresses of labor, the sight of their own child, and the sound of its crying constitute a dramatic episode that tends to create strong bonds between parents and with the child. The couple should be fully informed regarding any complications.

HOME DELIVERY

Although home delivery has been advocated by some, it is not recommended because of the incidence of unexpected complications during labor and delivery, such as sudden abruption (premature separation) of the placenta, fetal distress during labor, unexpected multiple pregnancy, or unexpected postpartum complications (eg, neonatal depression or abnormality or maternal hemorrhage). Hospitals are responding to patients' desires by providing homelike birthing room facilities with fewer formalities and rigid regulations but with the availability of emergency equipment and personnel.

15. ABNORMALITIES AND COMPLICATIONS OF PREGNANCY

SPONTANEOUS ABORTION
(Miscarriage)

Abortion generally is defined as *delivery or loss of the products of conception before the 20th wk of pregnancy*, but definitions vary. For this discussion, 20 wk of gestation, which corresponds to a fetal weight of about 500 gm, is used as the limit for abortion. *Delivery between 20 and 38 wk is considered preterm birth.*

Incidence and Etiology

About 20 to 30% of women bleed or have cramping sometime during the first 20 wk of pregnancy; 10 to 15% actually spontaneously abort. Since in 60% of spontaneous abortions the fetus is either absent or grossly malformed, and in 25 to 60% it has chromosomal abnormalities incompatible with life, spontaneous abortion may be a natural rejection of a maldeveloping fetus.

About 85% of spontaneous abortions occur in the first trimester and tend to be related to fetal causes; those occurring in the 2nd trimester usually have maternal causes. Maternal factors that have been suggested as causes of spontaneous abortion include an incompetent, amputated, or lacerated cervix; congenital or acquired anomalies of the uterine cavity; hypothyroidism; diabetes mellitus; chronic nephritis; acute infection; use of cocaine, especially crack; and severe emotional shock. Many viruses, most notably cytomegalo-, herpes-, and rubella viruses, have

been implicated as causes. The importance of uterine fibroids or retroversion and impaired corpus luteum function appears to have been overestimated. A relationship to physical trauma has not been substantiated.

Classification

An abortion is termed either **early** (before 12 wk of pregnancy) or **late** (between 12 and 20 wk). This distinction is made because more difficulties are encountered in treating late abortions. After 12 wk of pregnancy, the uterine cavity is obliterated and instrumentation is more likely to cause perforation. Since a definitive placenta has begun to form with a more organized and larger blood supply, bleeding is more likely. Fetal bones have also begun to form, and the long bones of the limbs may perforate the uterus during evacuation. Further, the size of a fetus at > 12 wk of pregnancy makes it difficult to dilate the cervix enough to pass the fetus.

Abortions may be spontaneous or induced. **Spontaneous abortions** occur without any instrumentation. **Induced abortions**, those done for medical or elective reasons, are discussed in Ch. 169. Abortions performed to save the pregnant woman's life or health are referred to as **therapeutic.**

Spontaneous abortions may be threatened, inevitable, incomplete, or complete. **Threatened abortion** is any bleeding or cramping of the uterus in the first 20 wk of pregnancy. **Inevitable abortion** is intolerable pain or bleeding that threatens the woman's well-being. If part of the products of conception is passed or if the membranes are ruptured, the abortion is **incomplete.** If all of the products of conception are passed, the uterus has contracted toward normal size, and the cervix has closed, the abortion is **complete.**

The occurrence of 3 or more consecutive spontaneous abortions is termed **habitual abortion** and requires extensive diagnostic investigation. Genetic and chromosomal studies should be performed. Among the endocrinopathies and metabolic diseases to be ruled out are hypo- and hyperthyroidism, diabetes mellitus, and chronic renal disease. Immunologic causes such as the lupus anticoagulant should be investigated. Defective corpus luteum function is always suspected. Anatomic abnormalities of the uterus (eg, polyps, fibroids, congenital defects) should be evaluated by hysterography, D & C, or hysteroscopy. Specific treatment, such as unification of a double uterus, excision of septum, or myomectomy, may be needed.

Missed abortion occurs when the fetus has died but has been retained in utero 4 wk or longer. After 6 wk, the **dead fetus syndrome** may develop, with disseminated intravascular coagulation and progressive hypofibrinogenemia and possible massive bleeding when delivery finally occurs. The dead fetus syndrome usually occurs only when the loss is in the 2nd trimester or later. Missed abortion should be suspected when the uterus fails to grow, when the fetal heart is not heard at the appropriate time with Doppler ultrasonography, or when a previously present fetal heart sound is absent. A serum or urine test for the β subunit of HCG becomes negative earlier than expected, and ultrasonography fails to show cardiac activity. The diagnosis can be confirmed with ultrasound imaging, and treatment can be started much earlier.

Septic abortion develops when the contents of the uterus become infected before, during, or after an abortion. The patient is acutely ill, with symptoms and signs of infection and threatened or incomplete abortion—chills, high temperature, septicemia, and peritonitis. Leukocytosis (WBC count 16,000 to 22,000) is present. Critically ill patients may evidence bacterial shock (**septic** or **endotoxic shock**) with vasomotor collapse, hypothermia, hypotension, oliguria or anuria, and respiratory distress. Causative organisms include *Escherichia coli, Enterobacter aerogenes, Proteus vulgaris,* hemolytic streptococci, staphylococci, and some anaerobic organisms, such as *Clostridium perfringens.* If septi-

cemia develops with the latter, anuria, anemia, jaundice, and thrombocytopenia with ecchymoses may result. In the USA before legalization of abortion, septic abortions were often associated with induced abortions performed by untrained persons using nonsterile techniques and were commonly called **criminal abortions.** The incidence of septic abortion in the USA has fallen dramatically.

Treatment

Treatment of **threatened abortion** is conservative; bed rest should be suggested, since it seems to lessen the amount of bleeding and cramping. The diagnosis should be confirmed with ultrasonography. If an empty sac is found or if cardiac activity has disappeared, evacuation of the uterus is indicated. Intercourse should be avoided; although no evidence shows that it is harmful, guilt feelings associated with abortion immediately after intercourse may be great enough to warrant abstention. The patient should be encouraged not to work and to stay off her feet at home. No evidence has been found that hormones save pregnancies except in very few instances, but they may cause fetal congenital anomalies, particularly transposition of the great vessels of the heart. Also, vaginal cancer or other genital abnormality in female offspring has been associated with the use of estrogen for threatened abortions. **Inevitable** and **incomplete abortions** must be completed, usually by D & C or suction curettage. Many physicians consider curettage mandatory to prove that a spontaneous abortion is complete; others prefer to watch the patient for a few days and, if no further bleeding occurs, avoid curettage.

In spontaneous abortions due to incompetence of the internal cervical os, the cervix seems unable to resist the progressive pressure of the enlarging components of pregnancy, and thus begins to dilate. Weakness of the cervical connective tissue may be congenital (including from the effects of DES exposure in utero) or secondary to deep cervical lacerations or previous excessive operative dilation. Cervical cerclage may enable the pregnancy to continue to term.

Missed abortion should be completed by physician intervention as soon as the diagnosis is certain; with ultrasound examination, the death of a fetus in utero can be diagnosed earlier than was previously possible. Up to a gestational age of 28 wk, missed abortion or retained dead fetus is frequently managed by inserting a 20-mg dinoprostone (E_2 prostaglandin) suppository into the vagina q 3 or 4 h as necessary to achieve contractions. Pretreatment of the cervix with *Laminaria* decreases complications. This drug is not approved for use after the 28-wk gestational age limit. Vigorous antibiotic management and early emptying of the uterus are mandatory to save the patient's life in cases of **septic abortion.**

Late spontaneous abortion may be completed with a dilute IV infusion of oxytocin, which causes contraction of the uterus and delivery of the products of conception. After the uterus has contracted following delivery of the fetus, curettage may be needed to remove fragments of the placenta. Suction curettage is used in up to 18 wk of pregnancy.

Psychologic problems may develop in the woman who has a spontaneous abortion with her first pregnancy or who is having a second or third consecutive spontaneous abortion. Some psychologic upset probably occurs in every patient who has an abortion, whether it is spontaneous, therapeutic, or induced. Usually a couple can be reassured and their difficulties diminished with sympathetic discussion and counseling. Many communities have active support groups.

ECTOPIC PREGNANCY

Pregnancy in which implantation occurs outside the endometrium and endometrial cavity; ie, in the cervix, uterine tube, ovary, or the abdominal or pelvic cavity. The incidence, 1/100 to 1/200 diagnosed pregnancies, is rising and is higher in nonwhites. Its likelihood increases with previous tubal disease, ectopic pregnancy (10 to 25%), exposure to DES, or induced abortion. Intrauterine devices do not prevent ectopic pregnancies.

The most common site of ectopic implantation is somewhere in a uterine tube. In many cases (50%), tubal implantation is caused by a previous tubal infection. Cervical, ovarian, and abdominal pregnancies are rare and are not discussed here.

The death rate for ectopic pregnancy has been falling, but much less rapidly than for maternal mortality in general. In the USA, it is estimated at 1/826. Untreated ectopic pregnancy is usually fatal.

Symptoms, Signs, and Diagnosis

In ectopic pregnancy, spotting and cramping pain usually begin shortly after the first missed menstrual period. The symptoms are similar to those of threatened abortion. Gradual hemorrhage from the tube causes pain and pressure, but rapid hemorrhage results in hypotension or shock. Often, uterine bleeding precedes these events as HCG levels decrease. Physical examination shows signs of hemorrhage, shock, and lower abdominal peritoneal irritation that may be lateralized. On pelvic examination, the uterus is enlarged (but smaller than anticipated from dates), the cervix is tender to motion, and a tender mass may be palpated in one adnexum. The cul-de-sac may bulge. If the serum or urine test for the β subunit of HCG is positive and ectopic pregnancy is suspected, ultrasound scanning should be performed. Serial titers of β subunit HCG are helpful in questionable cases. In normal pregnancy, the titer doubles about q 48 h; in ectopic pregnancy, the HCG titer may be lower than expected for the gestation time and usually does not show normal doubling time. Also, when the HCG titer is 6500 mIU/mL, a gestational sac in the uterus is normally found on transvaginal or abdominal ultrasound examination. An empty uterus strongly suggests ectopic pregnancy. If, in addition, a mass is detected in the adnexum, the diagnosis is confirmed. Culdocentesis may be helpful; blood aspirated from the cul-de-sac does not usually clot. Ultrasonography (either transvaginal or abdominal) can be helpful in diagnosis, and laparoscopy can be very helpful. At about 6 to 8 wk of pregnancy, marked sudden lower abdominal pain may occur, followed by fainting. This usually indicates rupture of the tube with intra-abdominal hemorrhage.

Interstitial (cornual) pregnancies have a somewhat longer course, since the uterine wall provides support and delays rupture. In these cases, the uterus is usually asymmetric and somewhat tender on examination. The usual signs include cramping and spotting. Cornual pregnancies rupture between 12 and 16 wk, and the rupture is catastrophic.

Treatment

Even if a tubal pregnancy is diagnosed before rupture, treatment is surgical. However, every effort should be made to conserve the tube by salpingotomy and evacuation of the products of pregnancy, with repair of the tube. Laparoscopy with cautery or laser may allow successful salpingostomy without laparotomy. If a damaged portion of the tube must be resected, as much tube as possible should be left behind. Future tubal reconstructive surgery may allow a subsequent pregnancy. After cornual pregnancy, the tube and ovary involved can usually be resected and the uterus repaired; rarely, repair is impossible and hysterectomy must be performed.

ANEMIA

Anemia during pregnancy is defined as *a Hb concentration < 10 gm/dL* and may be found in as many as 80% of some gravid populations. However, any patient with a Hb level < 11 to 11.5 gm/dL at onset of pregnancy must be treated as anemic, since the hemodilution that occurs as pregnancy advances will bring the Hb level into the anemic range.

Etiology

Most anemia during pregnancy is due to dietary iron deficiency (especially in teenage girls), to the normal loss of iron in blood with menses (which approximates the amount normally ingested each month, so iron stores are never built up), or to previous pregnancy. Rarely, anemia during pregnancy is caused by folic acid deficiency. This condition is sometimes called megaloblastic anemia because in extreme cases early forms of RBCs are found in the peripheral circulation. In certain populations, both sickle cell trait and anemia may be found, as well as thalassemia minor and major. Other hemoglobinopathies are occasionally diagnosed. All present special problems in pregnancy and are discussed more fully in Ch. 35.

Diagnosis

Iron-deficiency anemia is diagnosed from the CBC and by finding characteristic hypochromic microcytic RBCs in the peripheral blood smear. It can be confirmed by RBC indexes and by serum iron and iron-binding capacity measurements. If the anemia does not respond to therapy for iron deficiency, folic acid deficiency should be suspected.

Treatment

Iron-deficiency anemia is treated with supplemental iron, preferably as ferrous sulfate 300 mg given not more often than bid. The side effects of the iron (gastric upset and constipation) are increased if > 2 tablets/day are given. Also, if > 2 tablets are taken daily, one dose blocks absorption of the succeeding doses, thereby reducing total intake. **Megaloblastic anemia** due to folic acid deficiency is treated with folic acid 1 mg bid. True megaloblastic anemia may require hospitalization for bone marrow examination and further treatment. These anemias can be profound enough (Hb ≤ 6 gm/dL) to necessitate transfusion. Resistant iron-deficiency anemia or megaloblastic anemia warrants consultation for definitive treatment. "Shotgun" vitamin therapy (treatment with multiple vitamins) or administration of iron by injection is occasionally warranted.

There is conflicting evidence that routine supplemental iron therapy is necessary in pregnancy. However, most pregnant patients should be given supplemental iron (ferrous sulfate 300 to 600 mg/ day), even though the Hb level is normal at the beginning of the pregnancy. This prophylactic measure prevents depletion of reserves and the anemia that may ensue with any abnormal bleeding or with a subsequent pregnancy.

Treatment of **sickle cell anemia** is more controversial. Exchange transfusion for the mother is recommended by some but disputed by others. No evidence confirms any treatment other than supportive care.

HYPEREMESIS GRAVIDARUM

Malignant nausea and vomiting to the extent that the pregnant woman becomes dehydrated and acidotic. Ordinary morning sickness with nausea and vomiting is discussed under PRENATAL CARE in Ch. 14; this discussion refers to women in whom starvation, dehydration, and acidosis are superimposed on the vomiting syndrome.

Pathology

Persistent hyperemesis gravidarum may be associated with serious liver damage. Autopsies in such cases usually show severe necrosis in the central portion of the lobules or widespread fatty degeneration similar to that seen in starvation. Hemorrhagic retinitis is a serious complication and indicates a grave prognosis: the mortality rate in such patients is 50%.

Symptoms, Signs, and Diagnosis

Patients do not gain weight; they usually lose weight. Weight loss, dehydration, and ketosis confirm that the vomiting is extensive. Many pregnant women with morning sickness feel as though they are vomiting everything they ingest, but if they continue to gain weight and are not dehydrated, the condition is not hyperemesis gravidarum. Psychologic factors are prominent in this syndrome but do not lessen the danger. Patients should be evaluated for unsuspected liver disease, kidney infection, pancreatitis, intestinal obstruction, GI tract lesions, and intracranial lesions, since these conditions can cause vomiting.

Treatment

The acidosis and dehydration are corrected with IV infusion of water, glucose, and electrolytes. The patient should be kept in bed in a hospital and given nothing by mouth for 24 h. Antiemetics and sedatives should be used as necessary. Occasionally, IV vitamin therapy is required. After the dehydration and acute vomiting are corrected, bland oral feedings in small amounts at frequent intervals may be started and increased as tolerated. Usually vomiting ceases within a few days, but sometimes the regimen of fasting, IV fluids, and small meals has to be repeated once or twice.

Repeated ophthalmoscopic examinations are imperative, and if hemorrhagic retinitis appears, the pregnancy should be terminated at once. Even in the absence of a developing retinitis, termination of the pregnancy should be considered in the rare cases that do not respond to therapy (as evidenced by continued weight loss, jaundice, and increasing pulse rate).

PREECLAMPSIA AND ECLAMPSIA

Preeclampsia: *Development of hypertension with albuminuria or edema between the 20th wk of pregnancy and the end of the first week postpartum.* **Eclampsia:** *Coma and/or convulsive seizures in the same time period, without other etiology.* The etiology of preeclampsia and eclampsia is unknown. Preeclampsia develops in 5% of pregnant women, usually in primigravidas and women with preexisting hypertension or vascular disease. If untreated, preeclampsia characteristically smolders for a variable length of time and suddenly progresses to eclampsia. Eclampsia develops in 1/200 preeclamptic patients and is usually fatal if untreated. A major complication of preeclampsia is abruptio placentae (see below under THIRD TRIMESTER BLEEDING), apparently caused by the vascular disease. Low-dose aspirin therapy has been tried as a preventive measure in high-risk patients; however, the data on results are mixed, and this therapy should probably be considered experimental.

Symptoms, Signs, and Diagnosis

Any pregnant woman who develops a BP of 140/90 mm Hg, edema of the face or hands, or albuminuria of $\geq 1+$ or whose BP rises by 30 mm Hg systolic or 15 mm Hg diastolic (even though it does not reach levels above 140/90) must be considered to have preeclampsia. Mild preeclampsia develops as borderline hypertension, unresponsive edema, or albuminuria. Patients with a BP of 150/110 or with marked edema or albuminuria are considered to have severe preeclampsia. All routine laboratory tests (CBC, urinalysis, electrolyte levels, uric acid concentration, prothrombin time, and partial thromboplastin time) should be obtained and any abnormalities corrected. BUN and creatinine levels should also be obtained to rule out unsuspected kidney disease.

Treatment

Treatment is aimed at preserving the life and health of the mother; the fetus usually also survives. A patient with **mild preeclampsia** occasionally may be treated as an outpatient requiring bed rest, but she should be seen by her physician every 2 days. If her condition does not immediately improve, she should be hospitalized. *The primary treatment of preeclampsia and eclampsia is delivery.* No data indicate that delay in delivery enhances neonatal survival, except in the patient with unusually mild and immediately responsive preeclampsia. Therefore, any patient with preeclampsia that is nonresponsive or more severe than very mild should be stabilized and delivered.

Diuretics have no place in the treatment of preeclampsia, since they further disturb the already deranged electrolyte balance and reduce both renal and uteroplacental perfusion. A low-salt diet is also of no value. The patient needs a normal salt intake and an increased intake of water. Keeping the patient in bed and encouraging her to lie on her left side will promptly increase her urinary output and lessen the intravascular dehydration and hemoconcentration. Since etiology is unknown, the treatment prior to delivery is to lessen symptoms, and the principal agent is magnesium sulfate **(MgSO₄)**, as described below.

In **severe preeclampsia**, more vigorous therapy is indicated. Upon admission, an IV infusion of a balanced salt solution (eg, Ringer's solution) is started through a large-bore catheter. Then 4 gm of MgSO₄ is given slowly IV over 15 min until the hyperreflexia that usually accompanies this disorder diminishes, thereby decreasing the risk of convulsions. Concomitant lowering of BP usually occurs. With infusion of 3 or 4 L of balanced salt solution in a 24-h period, a rise in urinary output and lessening in edema also occur. $MgSO_4$ should be given continuously via an IV infusion pump at about 1 to 3 gm/h with supplemental doses as necessary. Usually within 4 to 6 h, BP stabilizes at a lower level and hyperreflexia is dampened. At that time, delivery can be accomplished. If BP does not respond to $MgSO_4$ therapy, an IV infusion of hydralazine (40 mg/1000 mL) may be started, with the rate of infusion titrated to BP levels. BP should never be lowered to < 130/80 in cases of severe preeclampsia or eclampsia, because perfusion of the uterus would be decreased so markedly that the fetus would be jeopardized. Calcium gluconate 1 gm IV is a specific antidote for excess $MgSO_4$. If urinary output does not increase, addition of furosemide 10 to 20 mg IV will produce diuresis; diuretics are not used otherwise. Sedatives should not be used because of effects on the fetus. Stabilization can be accomplished in 6 to 8 h, and delivery at that time is indicated. Once the decision to treat preeclampsia with other than bed rest has been made, delivery should be the objective.

The patient admitted with **established eclampsia** should be treated in the same fashion. Early administration of $MgSO_4$ usually controls the seizures. If not, diazepam in doses of 5 mg IV may be added until the seizures are controlled. Constant monitoring and attendance are required; BP, pulse, respirations, and reflexes should be recorded every 15 min, and urinary output and IV intake should be recorded hourly. Observation for complications such as blurring of vision, confusion, pain, vaginal bleeding, or loss of fetal heart tones must be made and recorded every 15 min. Again, the condition should be stabilized in 4 to 6 h, and delivery accomplished at that time. The **HELLP syndrome** (Hemolysis, Elevated Liver enzymes, and Low Platelet count) is a major complication. Treatment is similar to that described above, but delay in treatment is frequently associated with this syndrome.

Delivery should be accomplished by the most efficient method. If the cervix is ripe and vaginal delivery seems probable, amniotomy should be performed and a dilute infusion of oxytocin started to induce labor. If the cervix is unfavorable and vaginal delivery is unlikely, cesarean section should be performed.

After delivery the patient must be monitored as carefully and frequently as during labor; 25% of eclampsia occurs in the postpartum period, usually in the first 2 to 4 days. As the patient gradually improves, a mild sedative such as phenobarbital 30 to 60 mg tid orally may be added and ambulation allowed. Hospitalization may be prolonged, and medication may be necessary after discharge. The patient should be seen every 2 wk or more often during the postpartum period. Her BP may remain elevated for 6 to 8 wk, but if it is still elevated after this time, a possible diagnosis of hypertension must be considered. Throughout this time, determinations of CBC, urinalysis, BUN, and creatinine must be obtained regularly.

THIRD TRIMESTER BLEEDING

ABRUPTIO PLACENTAE

Premature separation of a normally implanted placenta from the uterus. All degrees of placental separation, from a few millimeters to complete detachment, may occur. The cause is unknown. Abruptio placentae develops in 0.4 to 3.5% of all deliveries. It is associated with the various hypertensive, cardiovascular, and rheumatoid diseases in pregnancy and especially with use of cocaine in any form.

Symptoms, Signs, and Diagnosis

Retroplacental bleeding occurs, and the blood may pass behind the membranes and through the cervix (**external hemorrhage**) or may be retained behind the placenta (**concealed hemorrhage**). Symptoms and signs depend on the degree of separation and blood loss. In severe cases, they include vaginal bleeding, a tender and tightly contracted uterus, evidence of fetal cardiac distress or death, and maternal shock. Abruptio placentae may be confused with placenta previa (see below). The diagnosis can usually be established with abdominal ultrasonography. Serious complications, particularly with preexisting toxemia, include hypofibrinogenemia with disseminated intravascular coagulation (**DIC**), acute renal failure, and uteroplacental apoplexy (**Couvelaire uterus**).

Treatment

If the patient's bleeding is not life-threatening, if the fetal heart tones are normal, and if the pregnancy is not near term, bed rest is advised and may lessen the bleeding. If the condition improves, the patient may be allowed to ambulate and may even be discharged if no further bleeding occurs and she has easy access to the hospital. If the bleeding continues or worsens, delivery is indicated in both fetal and maternal interests. Once the decision to deliver promptly has been made, a vaginal examination should be performed. If the cervix is dilated, the membranes should be ruptured, as this seems to lessen the incidence of DIC. However, unless vaginal delivery is imminent, cesarean section should be performed. Vigorous and active treatment markedly lessens maternal and fetal or neonatal morbidity and mortality.

PLACENTA PREVIA

Implantation of the placenta over or near the internal os of the cervix. The placenta may cover the internal os completely (total previa) or partially (partial previa), or it may encroach on the internal os (low implantation or marginal previa). Placenta previa occurs in 1/200 deliveries, usually in multiparas or in patients with abnormalities of the uterus, such as fibroids, that inhibit normal implantation.

Symptoms, Signs, and Diagnosis

Sudden, painless vaginal bleeding begins late in pregnancy when the lower uterine segment begins to thin and lengthen and is followed by painless, massive, bright red bleeding. Placenta previa frequently cannot be distinguished from abruptio placentae (see above) by clinical findings. Vaginal examination is contraindicated until the diagnosis of abruptio placentae has been firmly established, since inadvertent vaginal examination in the presence of placenta previa will precipitate greater hemorrhage. The best way to differentiate the 2 diagnoses is with abdominal ultrasound examination.

Treatment

If bleeding is minor and the patient is not near term, bed rest is advised. If the bleeding stops, ambulation is allowed. The patient may be discharged from the hospital if bleeding does not resume, transportation is good, and distance to the hospital is short.

Once the decision for delivery has been reached, cesarean section almost always is preferable; very rarely, with a marginal or low-lying placenta previa on the anterior wall of the uterus, vaginal delivery may be allowed if the head effectively compresses the placenta. Blood must be available for replacement as needed.

ERYTHROBLASTOSIS FETALIS

Hemolytic anemia of the fetus or neonate, caused by transplacental transmission of maternal antibody, usually evoked by maternal and fetal blood group incompatibility.

Etiology and Pathophysiology

Rh incompatibility may develop when an Rh-negative woman is impregnated by an Rh-positive man and an Rh-positive fetus is conceived. RBCs from the fetus cross the placenta and enter the woman's circulation throughout pregnancy (the greatest transfer is at delivery), stimulating maternal antibody production against the Rh factor. The antibodies reach the fetus via the placenta and cause lysis or destruction of the fetal RBCs. The resulting anemia may be so profound that the fetus may die in utero. To overcome the anemia, the fetal bone marrow releases immature RBCs, or erythroblasts, into the fetal peripheral circulation.

The Hb from the lysed RBCs breaks down to bilirubin, which is cleared from the fetus in utero by crossing the placenta into the woman's blood. After birth, however, bilirubin builds up in the newborn's circulation; high levels can be deposited in the basal ganglia of the brain, resulting in kernicterus, *a clinical syndrome of poor feeding, flaccidity, opisthotonus, seizures, apnea, and neonatal death.* Survivors may have choreoathetosis, mental retardation, and hearing loss.

Incidence

The incidence and severity of isoimmunization and the reaction are influenced by (1) the variable potencies of different antigens (producing variable antibody responses), (2) the distribution of the antigen in the population (affecting the probability of parents' having antigenically dissimilar RBCs), and (3) the zygosity of the father—if he is homozygous, all of his offspring will have the antigen; if heterozygous, 50% of his offspring will have the antigen. In the USA, 85% of whites are Rh-positive, and about 13% of marriages among whites result in pairing of an Rh-positive man and an Rh-negative woman. Only 1/27 children born to these couples will have erythroblastosis.

A first pregnancy is rarely affected, unless the woman was previously sensitized by transfusion. The risks of sensitization increase with each subsequent pregnancy. In women who have developed Rh sensitization, the second pregnancy often produces a mildly affected infant, although $1/3$ of infants who die do so in the first sensitized

TABLE 15-1. LEVEL OF BILIRUBIN IN AMNIOTIC FLUID

Clinical Interpretation	Net Spectrophotometric Absorptivity	Total Bilirubin (mg/dL)
Normal or possibly affected	< 0.20	< 0.28
Affected but not in jeopardy	0.20–0.34	0.28–0.46
Distressed and probably in failure	0.35–0.70	0.47–0.95
Impending fetal death	> 0.70	> 0.95

pregnancy. Succeeding pregnancies produce more seriously affected infants until, at the third, fourth, or fifth pregnancy, the fetus dies in utero.

Feto-maternal **incompatibilities of the ABO blood types** leading to neonatal erythroblastosis are less severe but more common. In these cases, production of maternal anti-A or anti-B antibodies is sensitized by fetal RBCs carrying these antigens. The most frequent pairing resulting in sensitivity is maternal blood group O and fetal blood group A. Neonatal jaundice rarely reaches serious levels, and a Coombs' test of the newborn's blood may be negative or only weakly positive.

Prevention and Treatment

Since antibody production does not usually begin in a previously unsensitized mother until after delivery, erythroblastosis can be prevented by injecting a high-titer anti-Rh γ-globulin preparation within 72 h after delivery. The preparation must be given after each pregnancy—whether it ends in delivery, ectopic pregnancy, or abortion. The anti-Rh antibody destroys fetal cells that crossed the placenta before they could stimulate the maternal immune system endogenous antibodies. If a massive fetal-maternal hemorrhage has occurred, additional injections of anti-Rh antibody may be necessary. This technique has a failure rate of about 1 to 2%, apparently because of the mother's sensitization during pregnancy rather than at delivery. Therefore, all Rh-negative mothers with no apparent sensitization (as indicated by antibody titer—see below) should be treated with a standard 300-μg dose of anti-Rh antibody at about 28 wk of pregnancy. These exogenous antibodies are gradually destroyed over the next 3 to 6 mo, and the mother remains unsensitized.

At the first prenatal visit, all patients should be screened for blood and Rh type. If the patient is Rh-negative, the father's blood type and zygosity should also be investigated. If he is Rh-positive and the woman's Rh antibody titer is negative, maternal Rh antibody titers should be repeated antepartum at 26 to 27 wk. While titers are of limited value in patients who are already sensi-

tized, they are very useful in patients at risk but not yet affected.

If the titers are > 1:32, **amniocentesis** and spectrophotometric determinations of bilirubin concentration in amniotic fluid should be done at 2-wk intervals beginning at 28 wk. Patients already sensitized to the Rh factor are candidates for amniocentesis at 26 to 30 wk, depending on the estimated severity of the disease. High-resolution spectrophotometric determination of bilirubin levels in amniotic fluid (see TABLE 15-1) is useful in the antepartum assessment of erythroblastosis fetalis.

If bilirubin levels in amniotic fluid remain normal, the pregnancy can be allowed to continue to term and spontaneous labor. If bilirubin levels are elevated, indicating impending intrauterine death, the fetus can be given **intrauterine transfusions** at 10-day to 2-wk intervals, generally until 32 to 34 wk gestation, at which time delivery should be performed. Intrauterine transfusion is performed by inserting a needle through the maternal abdominal and uterine walls and the fetal abdominal wall into the fetal abdominal cavity. RBCs from blood transfused into the fetal abdominal cavity are absorbed intact into the fetal circulation. Percutaneous umbilical blood sampling or blood transfusion may also be useful. These procedures must be performed in an institution equipped for care of high-risk pregnancies.

Delivery should be as nontraumatic as possible. The placenta should not be removed manually. An infant born with erythroblastosis should be attended to immediately by a pediatrician who is prepared to do an **exchange transfusion** at once if required (see HEMATOLOGIC PROBLEMS in Ch. 27).

HERPES GESTATIONIS

A polymorphous, vesiculobullous, nonviral-related eruption occurring during pregnancy or puerperium. The term herpes is a misnomer—the eruption is not associated with herpes or any other type of virus.

Etiology

The disease is uncommon, usually beginning in the 2nd or 3rd trimester or immediately postpartum. It is thought to have an autoimmune etiology, since complement and immunoglobulins are localized to the skin basement membrane zone, the site of earliest histopathologic change, where the vesicle forms.

Symptoms, Signs, and Diagnosis

The eruption is very pruritic and may be polymorphic; vesicles and bullae are usually present. Lesions often start on the patient's abdomen and become widespread; they may be annular, with vesicles on the outer border. In addition, the lesions may be grouped as in herpes zoster or simplex. Exacerbation of the eruption in the immediate postpartum period is common. The eruption usually remits within a few weeks to a few months postpartum but often recurs with subsequent pregnancies or with oral contraceptive use. The infant may be born with erythematous plaques or vesicles that resolve in a few weeks without therapy.

Herpes gestationis may be confused clinically with several other pruritic eruptions of pregnancy, particularly with pruritic urticarial papules and plaques of pregnancy (PUPPP), discussed below. Herpes gestationis can be diagnosed with certainty by direct immunofluorescence examination of perilesional skin: The third component of complement (C3) and occasionally IgG are deposited linearly at the epidermal basement membrane zone.

Treatment

Treatment aims at suppressing eruption of new lesions and relieving the intense pruritus. Some patients with mild disease require only frequent applications (5 to 6 times/day) of 0.1% triamcinolone acetonide cream. Others, with more widespread disease, require prednisone 40 mg every morning or, if this does not control the itching, 10 mg qid for several days, then tapered to a level at which only an occasional lesion erupts. At parturition, the dosage may have to be increased because of severe exacerbations of itching and lesions. Systemic corticosteroids given late in pregnancy do not seem to harm the fetus.

PRURITIC URTICARIAL PAPULES AND PLAQUES OF PREGNANCY (PUPPP)

A common pruritic eruption of pregnancy of unknown etiology.

Symptoms, Signs, and Diagnosis

Intensely pruritic, erythematous, urticaria-like papules and plaques, at times with minute vesicles in the center, begin on the abdomen (frequently on the striae distensae) and spread to involve the thighs, buttocks, and occasionally the arms. Often halos of blanching surround the papular lesions. The eruption most frequently begins in the last 2 to 3 wk of pregnancy (occasionally in the last few days) but may begin at any time during the 3rd trimester. Most patients have hundreds of lesions. Although the eruption is itchy enough to keep the patient awake, excoriated lesions are rare. The eruption usually resolves promptly after delivery and does not usually recur in subsequent pregnancies.

PUPPP must be differentiated from other pruritic eruptions of pregnancy. There is no specific diagnostic test for PUPPP as there is for herpes gestationis, and clinical differentiation is sometimes difficult.

Treatment

Symptoms and lesions may resolve within 2 to 4 days with frequent (5 to 6 times/day) applications of 0.1% triamcinolone acetonide cream. At times, the intensity of symptoms and lack of response to topical corticosteroids necessitate use of oral prednisone, which should be given in divided daily doses totaling 30 to 40 mg. The dosage can be tapered by 5 mg q 3 to 4 days. Systemic corticosteroids, especially late in pregnancy, do not seem to harm the fetus.

16. HIGH—RISK PREGNANCY

Pregnancy in which the mother, fetus, or newborn is or will be at increased risk for morbidity or mortality before or after delivery.

All pregnancies should be evaluated to determine whether there are or will be risk factors.

Classifying pregnancies as high risk is an effective way to ensure extra attention to patients who need medical care the most. The incidence of high-risk pregnancy varies according to population. Many factors are involved; to weight each factor as a risk increment requires the use of a systematic review and scoring system. TABLE 16–1 illustrates one such system that identifies and assigns relative weights to various ante- and intrapartum events, making risk assessment quantifiable.

Besides immediately identifying patients likely to have an unfavorable perinatal course, a risk assessment program offers other advantages. Most important, it enables referral of high-risk patients to a perinatal center before delivery, thereby significantly decreasing neonatal morbidity and mortality rates, compared with those for neonates of similar gestational age and weight who are transported to such centers after birth. (The perinatal center is usually associated with an obstetric service and neonatal intensive care unit that have the physical resources and personnel to provide the highest level of care to the obstetric patient, fetus, and newborn.) Referred patients may be identified as high risk during the antepartum period or during labor because of acute events that change risk status. The most common reason for referral is the risk of preterm delivery often associated with premature rupture of the membranes (see in Ch. 18).

Maternal mortality occurs in 6/100,000 births in the USA. The leading cause is motor vehicle accidents, followed by thromboembolic disease, complications of anesthesia, hemorrhage, infection, and complications of hypertension.

Perinatal mortality in the USA occurs in 17/1000 deliveries. Slightly > 50% of these deaths are stillbirths and the remainder occur in neonates up to the 28th day of life. Most perinatal deaths not directly due to congenital anomalies are associated with prematurity often accompanied by abnormal presentation, abruptio placentae, multiple pregnancy, preeclampsia and eclampsia, placenta previa, or polyhydramnios.

Risk factors can be categorized as inherent, or present before conception, and antepartum, or occurring after conception.

INHERENT RISK FACTORS

Demographics

Maternal age: Patients age 16 or younger are at increased risk for preeclampsia and eclampsia and for delivering low-birth-weight or nutritionally deficient infants. Patients age 35 or older are at increased risk for associated chronic or superimposed pregnancy-induced hypertension, ges-

tational diabetes, uterine myomas, and dystocia. Risk of fetal chromosomal abnormalities increases from 0.9% at age 35 to 7.8% at age 43. Chorionic villus sampling or amniocentesis for chromosome analysis should be offered to patients in this age group.

Nutritional status: Women who weigh < 100 lb when not pregnant have an increased risk of delivering a small-for-gestational-age (SGA) infant. When inadequate weight gain (< 15 lb) is added to the initial low-weight risk, the incidence of SGA babies approaches 30%. Conversely, maternal obesity is a risk factor for fetal macrosomia, gestational diabetes, and hypertension.

Stature: Women < 5 ft tall are at increased risk for fetal-pelvic disproportion, preterm labor, and intrauterine growth retardation.

Obstetric History

Habitual abortion: The risk of recurrent abortion after 3 consecutive early pregnancy losses is about 35%. Habitual abortion also is associated with 2nd trimester and early 3rd trimester stillbirth and preterm labor. Parental balanced chromosomal translocations, uterine and cervical anomalies, infections, connective tissue diseases, and hormonal abnormalities should be ruled out before pregnancy is reattempted.

Previous stillbirth or neonatal death: A history of perinatal loss may suggest fetal or parental cytogenetic abnormality, maternal diabetes, chronic renal vascular disease, hypertension, connective tissue disease, or drug abuse.

Previous preterm or growth-retarded infant: The greater the number of previous preterm deliveries, the greater the risk in the current pregnancy. A woman whose sole obstetric experience has resulted in delivering a baby weighing ≤ 1500 gm has a 50% chance of a preterm delivery in her next pregnancy. A woman who has had a previous growth-retarded infant should be evaluated for hypertension, renal disease, inadequate weight gain, infection, cigarette smoking, or alcohol abuse.

Previous large infant: A previous delivery of a macrosomic infant (> 4500 gm) suggests maternal diabetes. Patients with this suspected diagnosis should be screened with 1-h, 50-gm glucose tests at 20 and 28 wk of pregnancy; abnormal glucose levels should be corroborated by a 3-h glucose tolerance test.

Multiparity: Women who have had 6 or more previous pregnancies are at increased risk for

TABLE 16-1. PREGNANCY RISK ASSESSMENT

Risk Factors	Score*
Antepartum	
Cardiovascular and renal	
Moderate to severe toxemia	10
Chronic hypertension	10
Moderate to severe renal disease	10
Severe heart disease (class II–IV, New York Heart Association classification)	10
History of eclampsia	5
History of pyelitis	5
Class I heart disease (New York Heart Association classification)	5
Mild toxemia	5
Acute pyelonephritis	5
History of cystitis	1
Acute cystitis	1
History of toxemia	1
Metabolic	
Insulin-dependent diabetes	10
Previous endocrine ablation	10
Thyroid disease	5
Prediabetes (diet-controlled gestational diabetes)	5
Family history of diabetes	1
Pregnancy histories	
Previous fetal exchange transfusion for Rh	10
Previous stillbirth	10
Post-term > 42 wk	10
Previous preterm infant	10
Previous small-for-gestational-age infant	10
Previous neonatal death	10
Previous cesarean section	5
Habitual abortion	5
Infant > 10 lb	5
Multiparity > 5	5
Epilepsy or cerebral palsy	5
Fetal anomalies	1
Anatomic abnormalities	
Uterine malformation	10
Incompetent cervix	10
Abnormal fetal position	10
Polyhydramnios	10
Small pelvis	5
Miscellaneous	
Abnormal cervical cytologic findings	10
Multiple pregnancy	10
Sickle cell disease	10
Age ≥ 35 or ≤ 15 yr	5
Viral disease	5
Rh sensitization only	5
Positive serologic results	5
Severe anemia (Hb < 9 gm/dL)	5
Excessive use of drugs	5
History of TB or PPD injection site induration ≥ 10 mm	5
Weight < 100 or > 200 lb	5
Pulmonary disease	5
Flu syndrome (severe)	5
Vaginal spotting	5

(Continued)

TABLE 16-1. PREGNANCY RISK ASSESSMENT *(Cont'd)*

Risk Factors	Score*
Miscellaneous *(Cont'd)*	
Mild anemia (Hb 9.0–10.9 gm/dL)	1
Smoking ≥ 1 pack/day	1
Alcohol (moderate)	1
Emotional problem	1
Intrapartum	
Maternal	
Moderate to severe toxemia	10
Hydramnios or oligohydramnios	10
Amnionitis	10
Uterine rupture	10
Mild toxemia	5
Premature rupture of membranes > 12 h	5
Preterm labor	5
Primary dysfunctional labor	5
Secondary arrest of dilation	5
Meperidine > 300 mg	5
Magnesium sulfate > 25 gm	5
Labor > 20 h	5
Second stage > 2.5 h	5
Clinical small pelvis	5
Medical induction	5
Precipitous labor < 3 h	5
Primary cesarean section	5
Repeat cesarean section	5
Elective induction	1
Prolonged latent phase	1
Uterine tetany	1
Oxytocin augmentation	1
Placental	
Placenta previa	10
Abruptio placentae	10
Post-term > 42 wk	10
Meconium-stained amniotic fluid (dark)	10
Meconium-stained amniotic fluid (light)	5
Marginal separation	1
Fetal	
Abnormal presentation	10
Multiple pregnancy	10
Fetal bradycardia > 30 min	10
Breech delivery total extraction	10
Prolapsed cord	10
Fetal weight < 2500 gm	10
Fetal acidosis pH ≤ 7.25 (stage I)	10
Fetal tachycardia > 30 min	10
Operative forceps or vacuum extraction	5
Breech delivery spontaneous or assisted	5
General anesthesia	5
Outlet forceps	1
Shoulder dystocia	1

* A score of 10 or more indicates a high risk.

uterine inertia during labor and for postpartum hemorrhage due to uterine atony. Multiparas may also have precipitate labor, with increased risk of hemorrhage and amniotic fluid embolism. Placenta previa is more common in the grand multiparous patient.

Previous infant with isoimmunization: A history of significant hemolytic newborn disease calls for blood typing of both parents and blood group antibody screening as early as possible. Clear, effective protocols exist for the management of pregnancy complicated by atypical maternal antibodies.

Previous preeclampsia and eclampsia: A history of these complications increases the risk for hypertension in a future pregnancy, particularly if an identifiable underlying chronic hypertensive vascular disease is present.

Previous infant with genetic disorder or congenital anomaly: Tests should be performed to determine the presence of congenital defects that are likely to recur; these procedures include ultrasonography, chorionic villus sampling or amniocentesis, and DNA analysis.

Previous birth injury: A history of difficult delivery or neonatal intensive care suggests the presence of shoulder dystocia or prolonged labor and an increased risk for mid-pelvic operative delivery.

Reproductive System Disorders

Genital tract abnormalities: Hysteroscopy or hysterosalpingography may be indicated to diagnose septate or bicornuate uterus and may be useful to confirm an impression of cervical incompetency.

Uterine leiomyomas: These lesions occur more frequently in older women and may be associated with an increased risk of preterm labor, dystocia, malpresentation, placenta previa, recurrent pregnancy loss, and carneous degeneration.

Bacterial cervicovaginitis: Bacterial infections during pregnancy may lead to preterm labor or premature rupture of the membranes. Offending organisms include Group B streptococcus, chlamydia, mycoplasma, and *Ureaplasma*. Appropriate antibiotic therapy reduces the frequency of recurrent premature rupture of membranes and arrests early preterm labor.

Medical Conditions

While pregnancy may enhance medical disorders, specific diseases may adversely affect the outcome of pregnancy for both mother and infant. The most important medical complications of pregnancy are chronic hypertension, renal disease, diabetes mellitus, cyanotic heart disease, hemoglobinopathy, thyroid disorder, connective tissue disorder, and coagulopathy. These are discussed in detail in Ch. 17.

Family History

Any occurrences of mental retardation, twins, or familial diseases in a patient's family increases the risk of these events; thus, a detailed family history should be obtained.

ANTEPARTUM RISK FACTORS

A pregnant patient may initially be classified as low risk after reviewing the preceding areas of potential maternal complications, but later that patient may have a change in condition that significantly affects risk status. Such changes include teratogenic exposure and medical or pregnancy complications.

Exposure to Teratogens

Drugs known to have teratogenic effects include alcohol, phenytoin, folic acid antagonists, lithium, streptomycin, tetracycline, thalidomide, and warfarin (see also DRUGS IN PREGNANCY in Ch. 14). Infections that may be teratogenic include herpes simplex, viral hepatitis, influenza, mumps, rubella, varicella, syphilis, listeriosis, toxoplasmosis, and those caused by coxsackie- and cytomegalovirus. A detailed history of drug ingestion and infectious disease exposure should be taken for each pregnant patient as early as possible.

Of particular concern in current obstetric practice is the impact of cigarette smoking, alcohol intake, and substance abuse on the fetus and on subsequent development.

Cigarette smoking is probably the most common addiction among pregnant women in the USA. Despite increasing publicity regarding the health hazards of smoking, the overall proportion of adult women who smoke has dropped only slightly over the past 20 yr, and the percentage of female heavy smokers has actually increased. Smoking among teenage girls has increased substantially and exceeds that among teenage boys. Although smoking is detrimental not only to the mother but also to the fetus, only about 20% of smokers who become pregnant quit during pregnancy. The most consistently observed effect of smoking is the reduction in birth weight among infants of smokers. This effect is directly related to degree of smoking. It appears to be more pronounced with older smokers, who are more likely to deliver babies who weigh less and are shorter. Pregnant smokers have a higher incidence of abruptio placentae, placenta previa, and premature rupture of the membranes and amnionitis. Anencephaly, congenital heart defects, and orofacial clefts are reported more frequently in infants of smokers than in those of control subjects. Several studies have reported a positive association between maternal smoking and sudden infant death syndrome, and evidence shows that children of smoking mothers have slight but measurable deficiencies in physical growth, intellectual development, and behavior. These effects are thought to be mediated through both carbon monoxide, which may cause chronic tissue hypoxia, and nicotine, which stimulates the release of catecholamines producing uteroplacental vasoconstrictions.

Alcohol is now recognized as the leading known teratogen. The incidence of fetal alcohol syndrome **(FAS)**, one of the major consequences of drinking during pregnancy, is about 2.2/1000 live births. Alcohol can produce a wide spectrum of defects, ranging from spontaneous abortion to severe behavioral effects in the absence of physical anomalies. FAS includes growth retardation before or after birth; facial anomalies; and CNS dysfunction including microcephaly, varying degrees of mental retardation, and abnormal neurobehavioral development (see also FETAL ALCOHOL SYNDROME under METABOLIC PROBLEMS IN THE NEWBORN in Ch. 27).

The risk for spontaneous abortion increases about twofold with maternal drinking during pregnancy, particularly heavy drinking. Decreased birth weight is the most reliable indicator of prenatal alcohol exposure, with the average birth weight of such children estimated to be about 2000 gm; the median birth weight for all infants is about 3300 gm. FAS is the leading known cause of mental retardation, which has an incidence exceeding that of Down syndrome and cerebral palsy. In general, the extent of mental retardation is positively related to the severity of dysmorphogenesis. Microcephaly, a common feature of FAS, is probably a result of the overall decrease in brain growth.

Drug addiction and substance abuse during pregnancy continue to escalate. Besides women with chronic **heroin** dependence, a large number of adolescents experiment with a variety of stimulants, sedatives, and mood-altering drugs, producing a complex polydrug-abuse syndrome. The use of cocaine and cocaine derivatives (eg, crack) has become endemic in recent years, spreading across all social classes. About 25% of the adult population is estimated to have used marijuana or cocaine at least once and > 5 million people are reported to be regular users— many of them, women of childbearing age.

While menstrual abnormalities are found in 60 to 90% of women dependent on heroin, these irregularities are not drug-specific; rather, they are related to associated malnutrition, hepatitis, pelvic infection, and distress stemming from the unstable social, economic, and emotional environment in which the women exist. Use of amphetamines, diazepam, and cocaine has little effect on the menstrual cycle, leading to numerous pregnancies being associated with concurrent drug use.

Thin-layer chromatography is a practical, economic, and sensitive method for detecting in urine such drugs as heroin, morphine, amphetamines, barbiturates, codeine, cocaine, methadone, methaqualone, and phenothiazines. Once IV drug addiction has been diagnosed, its extensive impact on both the woman and her child in utero must be considered. For instance, IV substance abusers are at greater risk for anemia, bacteremia, endocarditis, cellulitis, acute and chronic hepatitis, phlebitis, pneumonia, tetanus, venereal disease, and AIDS. Some 75% of infants and children who acquire AIDS are born to women at risk for the disease through either IV drug use or heterosexual transmission via prostitution. Babies of these women are also at risk for hepatitis, intrauterine growth retardation, other venereal diseases, prematurity, and sepsis.

About 14% of all pregnant women use **marijuana** to some degree. Since Δ-9 tetrahydrocannabinol **(THC)** is able to cross the placenta, the potential exists for damage to the conceptus. However, few documented human studies have confirmed an increased risk of congenital anomaly, growth retardation, or postnatal neurobehavioral effects resulting from marijuana use.

In contrast, **cocaine** abuse during pregnancy is associated with various maternal and fetal problems. Cocaine, a CNS stimulant, has both local anesthetic and vasoconstrictive effects. In the isolated human placenta, cocaine causes intense vasoconstriction, potentiating a bradykinin-induced pressure response. This suggests that cocaine produces episodes of significantly decreased blood flow to the fetus, resulting in periods of hypoxia. In addition, fetal exposure to other chemical substances, normally innocuous but rendered dangerous because of rebound vasodilation, may be increased. Since many cocaine users are polydrug users, such increased exposure is of special concern. In women who use cocaine throughout pregnancy, a preterm delivery rate of 31% has been reported, along with a 19% incidence of growth retardation and a 15% incidence of abruptio placentae. In women who stop using cocaine after the first trimester, the incidences of preterm delivery and abruptio placentae are still increased, but fetal growth appears normal.

A pregnant woman who has acute nonproteinuric hypertension, signs of abruptio placentae, or an unexplained stillbirth should be routinely evaluated for the presence of cocaine in the urine. This symptom complex is frequently seen in hospitals serving rural and suburban areas as well as in urban tertiary care centers. In women who used cocaine regularly during pregnancy, a number of anomalies have been reported, particularly clustering in areas where circulatory compromise affects organ growth. Thus, skeletal defects and isolated atresias in the infants are particularly prominent. Finally, evidence shows that infants exposed to chronic maternal cocaine intake during pregnancy have disturbances in neurobehavioral activity exemplified by hyperactivity, tremulousness, and significant learning deficits that may last through the 4th and 5th yr of life.

Medical Complications

Hypertension: When hypertension is diagnosed for the first time during pregnancy, the specific cause should be determined if possible. The need for treatment of mild to moderate hypertension is uncertain. Management is discussed in Ch. 17.

Pyelonephritis: In patients with a history of UTIs, a midstream urine specimen should be collected for culture early in pregnancy. Patients with bacteriuria should be given antibiotics to minimize the risk of pyelonephritis associated with preterm labor and premature rupture of the membranes.

Fever: Temperature $> 39.5°$ C (103° F) in the first trimester has been associated with both pregnancy loss and increased risk of CNS anomaly. Similar temperatures in late pregnancy are associated with preterm labor.

Acute surgical problems: Any acute surgical intervention in pregnancy is associated with a risk of preterm labor. Since a specific disorder (eg, appendicitis, cholecystitis, intestinal obstruction) is difficult to diagnose because of the physiologic changes of pregnancy, the condition is often more advanced when the diagnosis is finally established, increasing the risk of maternal morbidity and mortality.

Pregnancy Complications

Isoimmunization: The most common type of sensitization is to the $Rh_o(D)$ antigen. If the patient's blood is Rh-negative, her antibody status should be assessed. The nonsensitized patient should be given $Rh_o(D)$ immune globulin after any episode of bleeding, after amniocentesis or chorionic villus sampling, at the 28th wk of pregnancy, and in the puerperal period.

Third trimester bleeding: The most common causes of 3rd trimester bleeding are placenta previa, abruptio placentae, and lower genital tract disease. All patients who bleed in the 3rd trimester should be considered at risk and should have a full evaluation, including sonography, inspection of the cervical area, and cytologic studies of the cervix.

Polyhydramnios and oligohydramnios: Polyhydramnios can lead to severe maternal dyspnea and preterm labor. It is associated with uncontrolled maternal diabetes, fetal anomalies (esophageal atresia, anencephaly, spina bifida), multiple gestation, and isoimmunization. In about $1/2$ of the cases, the cause remains occult. Oligohydramnios is associated with congenital anomaly of the fetal urinary tract, severe intrauterine growth retardation, and fetal demise. Potter's syndrome, marked by pulmonary hypoplasia and surface compression abnormalities, is a common sequela.

Preterm labor: Uterine anomalies, incompetent cervix, previous uterine surgery, maternal stress, multiple gestation, and antepartum bleeding are associated with preterm labor. Maternal infections (pneumonia, asymptomatic bacteriuria, appendicitis) also can cause preterm labor. In some 30% of patients who have preterm labor, amnionitis exists with intact membranes; the role of antibiotic therapy in such cases is unclear.

Multiple gestation: The incidence of preterm labor, fetal malformation, and complications of labor and delivery increases in all forms of multiple gestation.

Post-term pregnancy: A pregnancy that continues beyond 42 wk is considered prolonged. The neonatal mortality and stillbirth rates in this situation increase threefold. Nonstress testing and biophysical profile obtained by sonography can identify the fetus at risk.

17. PREGNANCY COMPLICATED BY DISEASE

CARDIAC DISEASE

Cardiac disease in pregnancy is becoming uncommon in the USA, mainly because of the marked decline in rheumatic heart disease (even though better diagnosis and treatment of other types of cardiac disease are allowing more patients with those diseases to achieve pregnancy and delivery). Cardiac disorders in pregnancy are predominantly congenital diseases that frequently have been corrected surgically.

The physiology of the cardiovascular system in pregnancy (discussed in Ch. 14) is the basis for the symptoms and treatment of heart disease in pregnancy, since pregnancy imposes predictable burdens on the cardiovascular system. Knowing that the patient has a history of heart disease is helpful, because primary diagnosis of cardiac lesions during pregnancy is complicated by frequent systolic functional murmurs, venous distention, tachycardia, and chest x-ray distortions that are related to pregnancy and not to disease. On the other hand, the unexpected finding of a diastolic or presystolic murmur during pregnancy demands investigation. In about 25% of patients with mitral stenosis, symptoms first appear during pregnancy.

The New York Heart Association's functional status classification is helpful in managing patients with heart disease and assessing their prognosis in pregnancy. Almost all deaths from heart failure during pregnancy are in class III and IV patients. Class I and II patients with mitral stenosis sometimes advance rapidly to higher-risk classifications. Class III patients need digitalis as well as bed rest beginning in the 20th wk of pregnancy. Class IV patients may be considered candidates for early therapeutic abortion.

In women with preexisting heart disease, pregnancy is associated with a maternal mortality of about 1%, but these deaths account for about 10% of all maternal mortality. Successful pregnancy does not shorten life or permanently impair the functional capacity of mothers with heart disease. Congenital heart disease is more common among the children of mothers with congenital heart disease. Patients in class I or II have no increased risk of death during pregnancy, even when their predominant lesion is mitral stenosis. Patients in class III or IV, who are symptomatic after limited activity or at rest, have an increased risk of maternal and fetal death and should not conceive until they have been thoroughly evaluated and have shown maximum improvement following medical and surgical therapy.

In patients with rheumatic heart disease (RHD), the murmurs of mitral and aortic stenosis are amplified, while those associated with mitral and aortic insufficiency are diminished. Patients with **mitral or aortic insufficiency** who are asymptomatic or only mildly symptomatic usually tolerate pregnancy without difficulty; those with severe symptoms should be advised to have valve replacement before becoming pregnant. Relatively little information about **aortic stenosis** and pregnancy is available, but reported maternal and fetal mortality rates are high, and patients with severe stenosis should be advised to have surgical correction before becoming pregnant. **Mitral stenosis** is especially dangerous because the tachycardia, increased blood volume, and increased cardiac output of pregnancy interact with this lesion to elevate pulmonary capillary pressure; atrial fibrillation also is common. Together, these factors increase the risk of pulmonary edema, the most lethal complication of mitral stenosis. Mitral stenosis often leads to pulmonary capillary hypertension before the menopause, but left ventricular failure secondary to mitral regurgitation or aortic valve disease is unusual during childbearing years. Mitral valvotomy can be performed during pregnancy, but open heart surgery increases the risks of abortion and fetal damage.

Maximum improvement of RHD should be achieved by surgical and medical means before conception. Prophylactic antibiotic therapy should be continued during pregnancy. Medical management is based on limitation of physical activity, fatigue, and anxiety; prevention or prompt treatment of anemia; and prompt treatment of infection. In all patients with mitral stenosis, digoxin 0.25 mg/day orally is used prophylactically if atrial fibrillation develops. Labor and delivery are best tolerated at full term, and close attention to analgesia and relief of anxiety is essential. Occasionally, sudden postpartum episodes of pulmonary congestion occur, but generally the most hazardous time is at peak cardiac output (20 to 34 wk). Antibiotics should always be used in the immediate postpartum period as well as when risk of infection is increased—eg, with premature rupture of the membranes (PROM).

Most asymptomatic patients with **congenital heart disease** are not at increased risk during pregnancy. Patients with **Eisenmenger syndrome** and **primary pulmonary hypertension** (and perhaps isolated pulmonary stenosis) are liable to sudden collapse and death during labor or the postpartum period; this danger also exists following abortion later than the 20th wk of pregnancy. The cause of death in these patients is unclear, but the hazard is great enough to make pregnancy inadvisable. If pregnancy occurs, delivery should be accomplished under the best available conditions, with close attention to anesthesia, availability of cardiac resuscitation, and prevention of right-to-left shunting by maintaining peripheral vascular resistance and minimizing pulmonary vascular resistance. Venous return must be maintained. Patients with **Marfan's syndrome** are at increased risk for aortic dissection and rupture of aortic aneurysms during pregnancy; childbearing is not advised.

Mitral valve prolapse occurs more frequently in younger women and tends to be familial. It is usually an isolated abnormality but may be associated with Marfan's syndrome or atrial septal defect secundum. Women with mitral valve prolapse generally tolerate pregnancy well. The relative increase in ventricular size diminishes the discrepancy between the disproportionately large mitral valve and the ventricle. Asymptomatic patients require no treatment other than antibiotic prophylaxis during delivery, when bacterial endocarditis is a possible complication. In patients with recurrent arrhythmias, β-adrenergic blocking agents are indicated, and in the rare pregnant patients who develop systemic or pulmonary emboli, anticoagulation is required. Since the course of mitral valve prolapse in pregnancy is generally benign, patients should be reassured that this minor developmental anomaly is not cause for undue concern.

Occasionally, cardiomyopathy begins near term or in the postpartum period. This syndrome, called **peripartum cardiomyopathy,** is especially liable to affect women over age 30, multiparas, those carry-ing twins, and those whose pregnancy is complicated by toxemia. The syndrome is associated with a 50% mortality within 5 yr and a high probability of recurrence in subsequent pregnancies, which are therefore contraindicated.

In pregnancy, the cardiac patient's status may deteriorate despite the precautions of frequent visits to her physician, ample rest, elimination of stress or anemia, prophylactic penicillin, and weight restriction. Any arrhythmia or evidence of pulmonary congestion requires hospitalization and bed rest. Periods of special concern, when digitalization may be required, occur between 28 and 34 wk, during labor, and immediately postpartum, when the heart experiences maximum physiologic loads.

The fetus shares the increased risk from maternal cardiac disease. The fetus may die during an episode of maternal heart failure, or the neonate may succumb to prematurity.

Labor and delivery are threatening to a cardiac patient, since the work of labor, straining in the 2nd stage, and the increased amount of venous blood returning to the heart from the contracting uterus markedly alter cardiac hemodynamics. Cardiac output increases about 20% during each uterine contraction. A skilled anesthesiologist should be in attendance during labor. Conduction anesthesia is preferred for patients with mitral valve disease. Since patients with aortic valve disease cannot tolerate the stasis and occasional drops in BP that occur with conduction anesthesia, they should have local anesthesia, or if necessary, general anesthesia. No straining should be allowed in the 2nd stage of labor, because this effort halts all oxygenation, and the patient can become anoxic within seconds. Forceps delivery should be performed if feasible, or a cesarean section, if indicated (see Ch. 18). Forceps delivery is preferred, since it poses less threat to the patient than does a cesarean section.

In the **postpartum period,** the patient should be closely monitored, because mobilization of fluid produces wide swings in cardiac function. Diuretic therapy must be administered cautiously, and appropriate digitalis therapy should be continued. These patients are not out of danger for several weeks.

THROMBOEMBOLIC DISEASE

Thromboembolism is the leading cause of maternal mortality due to medical complications in the USA, having surpassed hemorrhage, infection, and hypertensive disease during the past 10 yr. This increased incidence is related to the higher rate of cesarean sections being performed and to improved diagnosis. During pregnancy, the risk for thrombosis is significantly greater because of increased venous capacitance and elevated venous pressure in the lower extremities, resulting in decreased flow (stasis). Though the pregnant patient's blood is hypercoagulable, most thromboembolic episodes occur in the postpartum period as a result of vascular trauma during delivery. In pregnancy, the symptoms of thrombophlebitis correlate poorly with severity of disease and risk of embolization; the lower extremities are often edematous, and calf cramping and tenderness (a physiologic process of pregnancy) may be misinterpreted as Homans' sign.

Diagnosis is complicated by concern over the hazards of radiation associated with venography. Doppler ultrasonography and plethysmography of the lower extremities are noninvasive, nonradiologic means of establishing the presence of venous occlusion. However, venography should be performed when the diagnosis is in doubt or when prolonged anticoagulation therapy increases maternal and fetal risk. In the puerperal period, CT scanning with contrast material is useful in diagnosing iliac, ovarian, and other pelvic venous thromboses.

Warfarin therapy in pregnancy has been associated with fetal death and anomaly, and low mol wt dextran and the NSAIDs have not been proved safe; thus, the anticoagulant of choice is **heparin**. Because of its molecular size, heparin does not cross the placenta. In patients with confirmed deep venous thrombosis **(DVT)** or pulmonary embolism **(PE)**, treatment with heparin is instituted promptly.

When patients have a documented history of DVT or PE in a previous pregnancy or preceding pregnancy, strong consideration should be given to **prophylactic anticoagulation** toward the end of pregnancy when the risk of recurrence is highest. The venous system should be assessed by Doppler ultrasonography at 20 and 28 wk. If impediment of venous flow is noted, prophylactic therapy with s.c. heparin 5000 u. q 12 h is begun without delay. Without signs of venous impediment, and unless the patient is thought to be at risk for preterm delivery, prophylactic therapy can be delayed until 34 wk of pregnancy and continued until the patient is fully ambulatory in the postpartum period.

If PE is suspected, a ventilation-perfusion scan may be performed safely, since the radiation dose to the fetus is $< .002$ rads. Perfusion defects are seen in 20% of postpartum patients, probably resulting from trophoblastic embolization during delivery. When the diagnosis of PE is uncertain, pulmonary angiography is required. Acute treatment, besides IV heparin, includes enzymatic dissolution with urokinase or tissue plasminogen activator **(tPA)**. Recurrent embolization despite what appears to be effective anticoagulation requires surgical therapy, best accomplished by percutaneous insertion of a Greenfield umbrella at the level of the renal vessels.

HYPERTENSION

The management of **chronic hypertension** in pregnancy is one of the most controversial areas of therapy in obstetric practice, despite the relative frequency of the condition (1.5 to 2.0%). Association between chronic hypertension and increased risk for morbidity and mortality to both mother and fetus is undisputed: cerebral, cardiac, and renal complications occur frequently in the mother; stillbirth, placental abruption, intrauterine growth retardation, and hypoxic effects of superimposed pregnancy-induced hypertension are common in the fetus. The controversy centers largely on the issue of whether treatment of mild to moderate disease reduces the incidence and severity of these complications and, if so, whether the fetus is at risk from direct or indirect pharmacologic actions of the drugs used for treatment.

While the maintenance of BP at normal levels for pregnancy ultimately depends on the interplay between cardiac output and systemic vascular resistance, each is significantly altered. Cardiac output increases gradually by 40%, resulting from an increase in both pulse rate and stroke volume. Although circulating angiotensin and renin increase significantly in the 2nd trimester, BP tends to fall, indicating a reduction in systemic vascular resistance. This is due to decreases in blood viscosity and vascular sensitivity to angiotensin caused mainly by the vasodilator prostaglandins.

Evaluation of new hypertension noted before the 28th wk of pregnancy and not associated with multiple pregnancy or trophoblastic disease should include studies to rule out renal artery stenosis, coarctation of aorta, Cushing's syndrome, SLE, and pheochromo-cytoma.

Since most patients have mild hypertension and the prognosis for mother and fetus is generally quite good, hypertension is not a contraindication to pregnancy. However, mortality may be increased in those in the first trimester whose BP is > 180/110 mm Hg or who have a creatinine clearance < 60 mL/min or a plasma creatinine level > 2 mg/dL or both. Death is due to hypertensive encephalopathy or cerebrovascular accident secondary to severe superimposed pregnancy-induced hypertension with eclampsia, renal failure, left ventricular failure, or microangiopathic hemolytic-uremic syndrome. About 45% of eclamptic mortality occurs in older multiparas with preexisting hypertension, although > 80% of eclampsia occurs in young primigravidas.

Fetal outcome in chronic hypertensive women is directly related to the reduced effective blood flow to the uteroplacental circuit. Fetal death is usually due to hypoxia, often acute and secondary to placental abruption or vasospasm, and is generally preceded by intrauterine growth retardation.

Antihypertensive drugs that are effective and appropriate in a nonpregnant patient may directly or indirectly harm the fetus in a pregnant patient. Since the placental circulation is in a maximally dilated state and incapable of autoregulation, reducing maternal pressure to the point of hypotension may immediately jeopardize the fetus. Diuretics reduce the mother's effective circulating blood volume, but since fetal growth is directly related to plasma volume, consistent reduction in this volume increases fetal risk.

The first-line drugs for hypertension during pregnancy are methyldopa 0.75 to 3.0 gm/day and hydralazine 100 to 200 mg/day. Second-line drugs include combined α- and β-blocking agents, which appear to be effective as adjuncts to the first-line therapy while reducing many adverse effects associated with high-dose treatment.

Patients with mild hypertension (140/90 to 150/100 mm Hg) should discontinue drug therapy before conception or as soon as pregnancy is confirmed. Restricted salt intake and drastically reduced physical activity appear to benefit fetal growth. Most patients do not require reinstitution of antihypertensive therapy because of decreased systemic vascular resistance. In these patients, perinatal outcome is generally similar to that for nonhypertensive patients. The 15% incidence of superimposed pregnancy-induced hypertension can and should be treated aggressively. A BP that does not decrease in the 2nd trimester is an ominous sign.

In patients with preexisting moderate hypertension (150/90 to 180/110 mm Hg), diuretics should be discontinued and methyldopa therapy initiated. The dosage can be increased to 2 gm/day or more if the patient is observed for excessive somnolence or symptomatic orthostatic hypotension. Hydralazine is added when necessary to increase antihypertensive effect. These patients must be taught self-monitoring of BP and serum protein levels, and they should have monthly renal function tests and ultrasound evaluation to monitor fetal growth. Early maturational studies should be performed on the fetus, which should be delivered at the 38th wk or earlier.

Patients with severe hypertension (≥ 180/110 mm Hg) require an immediate evaluation of maternal status. Values should be obtained for BUN, creatinine, creatinine clearance, and total urinary protein, and retinal photography should be performed as a basis for patient counseling. Both maternal and fetal prognoses are poor. If continuation of pregnancy is appropriate and desired, a second-level antihypertensive α- and β-blocking agent is often required. These labile patients with fragile fetuses must be hospitalized for much of the latter part of pregnancy. Further adverse change in maternal condition mandates termination of the pregnancy.

RENAL DISEASE

Occasional pregnancies are complicated by a significant decrease in renal function due to congenital anomalies or acquired renal disease. As a rule, a patient with significant dysfunction (serum creatinine > 3 mg/dL or BUN > 30 mg/dL) before pregnancy cannot carry to term. Nevertheless, some women with more severe renal disease have borne viable infants. Similar success has occasionally occurred in women on maintenance dialysis or who have had renal transplantation. Pregnancy seems to have no significant effect on the occurrence of noninfectious renal disease as long as hypertension is absent or controlled.

Treatment requires close consultation with a nephrologist. Frequent office visits are needed to monitor kidney function. BUN and creatinine levels plus creatinine clearance should be measured at least monthly; BP and weight should be recorded at 2-wk intervals. Sodium restriction is indicated, and diuretics are given only to control BP or excessive edema; in some instances, other drugs may be needed to control BP. The incidence of preeclampsia is high. Hospitalization after 28 wk of pregnancy should be considered, since delivery before term may be necessary to save the infant. An oxytocin challenge test (OCT) and nonstress test (NST) should be performed (see in FETAL MONITORING under PRENATAL CARE in Ch. 14); if results are normal, the pregnancy can continue. The lecithin/sphingomyelin (L/S) ratio should be determined. If it is > 2:1, especially with a falling creatinine clearance or abnormal OCT or NST results, delivery should be accomplished. If the cervix is ripe and vaginal delivery appears easy, this route may be chosen, but cesarean section is usually necessary.

URINARY TRACT INFECTION

Urinary tract infection (UTI) is common in pregnancy, apparently because hormonal dilation and ureteral hypoperistalsis as well as pressure of the pregnant uterus against the ureters cause urinary stasis. Asymptomatic bacteriuria occurs in about 15% of pregnancies and sometimes progresses to symptomatic cystitis or pyelonephritis. Frank UTI is not always preceded by asymptomatic bacteriuria. Diagnosis and treatment of UTI in pregnant patients are as in nonpregnant patients, except for avoidance of drugs that may harm the fetus.

Both asymptomatic bacteriuria and pyelonephritis are associated with an increased incidence of preterm labor and premature rupture of the membranes (PROM). In patients with a history of PROM or preterm delivery, urine should be cultured monthly and treatment should be based on sensitivity studies. Proof-of-cure cultures are required; reinfection is best managed by long-term suppressive therapy. Any patient who has had pyelonephritis during pregnancy should be given suppressive therapy for the remainder of pregnancy.

DIABETES MELLITUS (DM)

DM is a genetically and clinically heterogeneous group of disorders that have carbohydrate intolerance in common. In pregnant women, the syndrome should be defined and classified as accurately as possible, because the complex metabolic alterations of normal gestation complicate diabetic control and may place the fetus in jeopardy. Thus, management of women with different types of DM

should be individualized. In contemporary perinatal and neonatal centers, with preconception counseling and early prenatal care, the risks for diabetic mothers and their infants no longer exceed those for nondiabetic women. A successful diabetic pregnancy requires (1) preconception counseling and optimal diabetic control before, during, and after the pregnancy as well as meticulous management by a diabetes team or an obstetrician, internist, or family physician well versed in DM in pregnancy and by a pediatrician; (2) prompt diagnosis and treatment of both trivial and serious complications of pregnancy; (3) careful timing and appropriate mode of delivery; (4) attendance at delivery of a pediatrician knowledgeable in assessing and caring for infants of diabetic mothers; and (5) proximity of a neonatal intensive care nursery.

Classification

Nomenclature based on that adopted by the National Diabetes Data Group and WHO is presented in TABLE 17–1. The previous classification of DM in pregnancy was based on age at onset, duration, and complications of the disease. **Gestational diabetes (GDM)** is *carbohydrate intolerance of variable severity with onset or first recognition during the present pregnancy.* All pregnant women should be screened for GDM because unrecognized or untreated gestational carbohydrate intolerance is associated with increased fetal and neonatal loss and higher neonatal and maternal morbidity (see also PRENATAL CARE in Ch. 14). GDM occurs in 1 to 3% of all pregnancies, although the figure may be much higher in selected populations (eg, Mexican-Americans, American Indians, Orientals, Indians, Pacific Islanders). Pregnancy is a metabolic stress test for DM; women who fail the test and develop GDM may be obese, hyperinsulinemic, and insulin-resistant or thin and relatively insulin-deficient. Thus, GDM is also a heterogeneous syndrome.

Management of Diabetic Pregnancies

Good control of DM at conception and throughout gestation is important for an optimal maternal and infant outcome. Most diabetes centers use a team approach that combines the skills of physicians, nurses, nutritionists, and social workers. In addition, regional perinatal centers have experts in ophthalmology, renal disease, neurology, cardiology, anesthesiology, perinatology, and neonatology readily available.

Preconception counseling and diabetes control are important because congenital malformations in pregnancy complicated by DM may be

TABLE 17–1. CLASSIFICATION OF GLUCOSE INTOLERANCE IN PREGNANT WOMEN

Nomenclature	Former Names	Clinical Characteristics During Pregnancy
Type I, insulin-dependent diabetes mellitus (IDDM)	Juvenile diabetes (JD) Juvenile-onset diabetes (JOD) Ketosis-prone diabetes Brittle diabetes	Ketosis-prone. Insulin-deficient because of islet cell loss. Often associated with specific HLA types with predisposition to viral insulitis or autoimmune (*islet cell antibody*) phenomena. Occurs at any age. Common in youth. These women are usually of normal weight but may be obese
Type II, non–insulin-dependent diabetes mellitus (NIDDM) Nonobese Obese Maturity-onset diabetes of youth (MODY)	Adult-onset diabetes (AOD) Maturity-onset diabetes (MOD) Ketosis-resistant diabetes Stable diabetes	Ketosis-resistant. More frequent in adults but occurs at any age. Majority are overweight. May be seen in family aggregates as an autosomal dominant genetic trait. *Always require insulin for hyperglycemia during pregnancy.* Previous history of "borderline diabetes," impaired glucose tolerance, or treatment with oral hypoglycemic agents. Hb A_{1c} elevated $\leq$ 20 wk gestation*
Type III, gestational carbohydrate intolerance (GCI)[†] Nonobese Obese	Gestational diabetes mellitus (GDM)	Screening tests: All pregnant women. 50-gm oral glucose load given randomly (need not be fasting) at 24–28 wk gestation. A plasma glucose value 1 h later $\geq$ 140 mg/dL (7.8 mmol/L) is an indication for a 3-h oral glucose tolerance test (OGTT) with 100 gm glucose
Type IV, secondary diabetes	Conditions and syndromes associated with impaired glucose tolerance	Cystic fibrosis; endocrine disorders— eg, acromegaly, hyperprolactinemia, Cushing's syndrome; drugs or chemical agents; renal dialysis; organ transplantations; certain genetic syndromes

* Laboratory methods and normal values vary. Women with gestational carbohydrate intolerance have normal Hb A_{1c} concentrations during the first half of pregnancy.

† All pregnant women at higher risk for gestational carbohydrate intolerance should be screened at the first prenatal visit. Risk factors are glycosuria, family history of diabetes in a first-degree relative, history of an unexplained fetal demise or stillbirth in a previous pregnancy, a previous heavy-for-date baby, obesity (body mass index [kg $\div$ m^2] > 30), maternal age > 35 yr, or parity of 5 or more.

Diagnosis of GDM based on National Diabetes Data Group criteria (with a 100-gm glucose load) that 2 or more of the following plasma glucose values be met or exceeded: Fasting, 105 mg/dL (5.8 mmol/L); 1-h, 190 mg/dL (10.5 mmol/L); 2-h, 165 mg/dL (9.1 mmol/L); 3-h, 145 mg/dL (8.0 mmol/L).

Diagnosis of GDM based on 1985 WHO criteria (for pregnant and nonpregnant women) for impaired glucose tolerance following a 75-gm glucose challenge: Venous plasma glucose levels—fasting, < 140 mg/dL (7.8 mmol/L); 2-h, 140–200 mg/dL (7.8–11.1 mmol/L). For diabetes: venous plasma glucose levels—fasting, $\geq$ 140 mg/dL (7.8 mmol/L); 2-h, $\geq$ 200 mg/dL (11.1 mmol/L).

Modified from *Pregnancy, Diabetes, and Birth*, ed. 2, by DR Hollingsworth. Baltimore, Williams & Wilkins, 1992; used with permission.

linked to disturbances in maternal metabolism during the period of embryogenesis, and organogenesis is completed by the 6th or 7th wk of gestation.

TABLE 17-2 is a simple guide for managing pregnant women with type I (insulin-dependent diabetes mellitus [IDDM]), type II (non-insulin-dependent diabetes mellitus [NIDDM], but always **insulin-requiring** during gestation), and gestational carbohydrate intolerance (GCI) disorders. Details of treatment vary from one center to another, and patient care must be individualized.

In type I patients, **overinsulinization** is a risk of tight metabolic control regardless of the route of administration. In some type I patients, hypoglycemia does not trigger the normal release of counterregulatory hormones (catecholamines, glucagon, cortisol, and growth hormone). In these individuals, hypoglycemic coma may occur *with no premonitory symptoms.* All such patients should have glucagon kits and should be instructed (as should their families) in giving subcutaneous injection of glucagon for severe hypoglycemia (unconsciousness, confusion, or plasma glucose levels < 40 mg/dL). In pregnancy, good diabetic control consists of *absence* of wide glucose excursions with marked hyper- or hypoglycemia, Hb A_{1c} concentration of < 8%, and quantitative urinary glucose loss of < 1 gm/day. During pregnancy, normal fasting blood glucose levels are about 76 mg/dL (4.2 mmol/L), and 2-h postprandial values are ≤ 120 mg/dL (6.6 mmol/L). Purified pork and human insulin (as opposed to beef) are recommended during pregnancy to minimize antibody formation. Insulin antibodies cross the placenta, but their effect (if any) on the fetus is unknown.

Complications of Diabetic Pregnancies

Medical and obstetric complications such as infection, diabetic ketoacidosis, preterm labor, and pregnancy-induced hypertension are managed by current perinatal principles. No differences have been found in prevalence or severity of retinopathy, nephropathy, or neuropathy in diabetic women who have or have not experienced pregnancy. Diabetic retinopathy and nephropathy are not contraindications for conception or reasons for terminating pregnancy, but they require preconception counseling and close management before and during gestation. Initial and monthly ophthalmologic examinations are recommended. When proliferative retinopathy is noted at the first prenatal visit, the patient should receive photocoagulation treatment as soon as possible to prevent progressive deterioration. Women who have background retinopathy are followed expectantly.

No evidence indicates that diabetic renal disease worsens because of pregnancy, and renal complications during pregnancy are rare. Women with chronic renal failure who are undergoing hemodialysis rarely have a successful pregnancy, but surviving infants have been reported. One of 50 women who have functional renal transplants becomes pregnant. Pregnancy-induced hypertension occurs in 25% of such pregnancies, and other complications are common. The incidence of preterm births is related to maternal renal function and time interval from transplantation; the best prognosis for term deliveries of normal-birth-weight infants is ≥ 2 yr after transplantation.

In type I or II diabetic pregnancies, the major cause of neonatal mortality is congenital malformation incompatible with life. Therefore, a maternal serum α-fetoprotein determination is recommended at 16 to 18 wk gestation and a thorough ultrasound examination at 20 to 22 wk (with measurement of amniotic fluid α-fetoprotein level if the maternal serum value was abnormal). Abnormal maternal serum and amniotic fluid tests or an abnormal ultrasound examination suggests neural tube or other developmental defects. Fetal echocardiography should be performed if the Hb A_{1c} value was abnormally high in the first trimester or at the first prenatal visit. Congenital malformations of major organs have been positively correlated with elevated Hb A_{1c} concentrations at conception and during embryogenesis (the first 8 wk). In women with type II DM, use of oral hypoglycemic agents in the first trimester has been associated with cardiac defects, ear malformations, and the VATER anomaly.

Labor and Delivery

During the 3rd trimester, the 3 major aspects of care for diabetic women are control of maternal plasma glucose concentration, assessment of fetal well-being, and determination of fetal pulmonary maturation.

Most women with **GDM** have spontaneous onset of labor at term and are delivered vaginally. When induction of labor is necessary, it is initiated with IV oxytocin and amniotomy. If these pregnancies are permitted to go beyond term (> 42 wk), the fetus is at risk for death in utero. Even when maternal glucose levels in GDM have been normal or nearly so throughout pregnancy, infants are at risk for macrosomia. Thus, cesar-

Table 17-2. MANAGEMENT OF DIABETES MELLITUS IN PREGNANCY

Type	Care Before Conception	Prenatal Care	Labor and Delivery
I*	Regulate diabetes Hb A1c concentration should be ≤ 8% at conception† Check for renal, retinal, and cardiac complications	Start care after missed period Recommend prenatal clinic visits each week Individualize diet following 1979 ADA guidelines and coordinate with insulin administration Recommend 3 meals and 3 snacks/day; emphasize consistent timing Individualize amount and type of insulin. In AM, 2/3 total dosage (60% NPH, 40% regular); in PM, 1/3 (50% NPH, 50% regular)‡ Instruct in home blood-glucose monitoring Check Hb A1c level every 4–6 wk Caution about dangers of hypoglycemia during exercise and at night Instruct patient and family in glucagon administration Perform fetal monitoring with nonstress tests, biophysical profiles, and kick counts from 35 wk to term (or earlier if indicated)	Deliver vaginally at term if patient has well-documented dating criteria and good diabetic control; amniocentesis may not be required. Deliver by cesarean section if perinatal complications are present, dating criteria are poor; prenatal care is inadequate, or diabetic control is poor; perform amniocentesis for mature lecithin/sphingomyelin ratio (≥ 2) and phosphatidylglycerol (≥ 3%) Deliver with constant low-dose insulin infusion, or alternatively, give usual PM NPH insulin dose and withhold insulin on AM of labor induction. Administer regular insulin s.c. as needed during labor and delivery Arrange for transitional and postpartum diabetes care
II*	Encourage weight loss if patient is obese (BMI > 27) Control hyperglycemia§ Hb A1c concentration should be ≤ 8% at conception† Recommend diet low in fat, relatively high in complex carbohydrates, high in dietary fiber Encourage exercise	Individualize amount and type of insulin. For obese patients: Prescribe regular insulin before each meal. For normal-weight patients: In AM, 2/3 of total dosage (60% NPH, 40% regular); in PM, 1/3 (50% NPH, 50% regular). Use highly purified pork or human insulin Individualize daily caloric intake to avoid excessive weight gain (> 9 kg, or > 20 lb) in obese patients Discourage daytime snacks for obese patients Recommend moderate walking exercise after meals Instruct in home blood-glucose monitoring Monitor weekly at clinic visits: 2-h postbreakfast plasma glucose level Check Hb A1c level every 4–6 wk	Same as for type I

		Deliver at term; avoid prolonged gestation (> 42 wk)
Gestational	Modify diet: Eliminate concentrated sweets, monitor caloric intake to prevent excessive weight gain (> 9 kg, or > 20 lb) Discourage daytime snacks for obese patients Recommend moderate exercise after meals Prescribe small doses of purified pork or human short-acting insulin before meals if postprandial plasma glucose levels are > 120 mg/dL Monitor weekly at clinic visits: 2-h postbreakfast plasma glucose level	
	No special care unless patient has a history of GDM, then try to achieve normal weight, encourage modest exercise, check FBG and Hb A1c	

ADA = American Diabetes Association; NPH = neutral protamine Hagedorn; BMI = body mass index; GDM = gestational diabetes mellitus; FBG = fasting blood glucose.
* Suggested guidelines only; marked individual variations require appropriate adjustments.
† Normal values may differ, depending on laboratory methods used.
‡ Some hospital programs recommend up to 4 daily insulin injections. Continuous s.c. insulin infusion (CSII) given in medical research settings is a possible alternative. This is labor-intensive and should be used only in special circumstances and at a diabetes center.
§ Women taking oral hypoglycemics should discontinue them and control plasma glucose levels with insulin; possible adverse effects on fetal development due to oral agents cannot be excluded.

TABLE 17-3. MANAGEMENT OF DIABETES DURING LABOR AND DELIVERY*

One day before induction of labor
Give usual insulin dose and diet to maintain euglycemia

Morning of induction†
Withhold insulin and breakfast
Measure baseline fasting blood glucose
Initiate labor and delivery flow sheet
Start IV infusion of 5% dextrose in 0.5% sodium chloride at 125 mL/h, using an infusion pump

During labor
Measure blood glucose hourly with meter at bedside‡
For glucose level > 110 mg/dL (6.1 mmol/L), add 10 U regular insulin to 1000 mL 5% dextrose in 0.5% sodium chloride and continue infusion rate of 125 mL/h (1.25 U insulin/h); *keep infusion rate constant*
Adjust insulin hourly, if necessary, by doubling or halving the insulin concentration to maintain blood glucose at 70–120 mg/dL (3.8–6.6 mmol/L)

* This protocol for women with insulin-dependent and non–insulin-dependent diabetes mellitus is adapted from Coustan (1988).
† For spontaneous labor, follow the same procedure. Insulin requirement will be less if the patient has taken intermediate-acting insulin in the previous 12 h. Patients with fever or infection will require higher doses (see TABLE 17-4).
‡ Obese patients with non–insulin-dependent diabetes mellitus who have required > 100 U of insulin/day prepartum, and patients with fever, infection, or other complications, will require higher insulin doses.
Modified from *Pregnancy, Diabetes, and Birth*, ed. 2, by DR Hollingsworth. Baltimore, Williams & Wilkins, 1992; used with permission.

ean section may be necessary in case of dysfunctional labor or cephalopelvic disproportion or to avoid shoulder dystocia and injury to the infant and the birth canal.

In DM types I and II, the obstetrician should assess fetal well-being at 35 wk by external fetal heart rate monitoring (nonstress tests) and biophysical profiles. In addition, the patient should be instructed to count fetal movements for 30 min daily; a sudden decrease should be reported immediately to the obstetrician. Nonstress tests may begin earlier in women with complications such as hypertension, hydramnios, premature rupture of membranes, intrauterine growth retardation, preterm labor, infection, or developmental defects.

Most diabetologists and perinatologists do not measure maternal serum or urinary estriol levels, since these expensive assays are not the most practical or useful tests for assessing fetal well-being.

Amniocentesis is not routinely performed to assess fetal lung maturity in women whose DM is well controlled and who have well-documented dating criteria. In these patients, spontaneous vaginal delivery at term is more common. Vaginal delivery is planned unless labor fails to progress, marked fetal macrosomia is present, or the patient has had a previous cesarean section and a trial labor is considered undesirable or unwanted by the patient.

However, in women with obstetric complications, inadequate prenatal care, or poor diabetic control, amniocentesis is often necessary to assess fetal lung maturity. In these patients, the rate of cesarean sections is ≥ 50%.

Control of plasma glucose levels during labor and delivery is easier when insulin is administered as a continuous, low-dose infusion during the intrapartum period (see TABLES 17-3 and 17-4). The patient is hospitalized one day before delivery and given her usual diet and insulin dose. The following morning, breakfast and insulin are withheld and an IV infusion of 5% dextrose in 0.5% sodium chloride is started at 125 mL/h, using an infusion pump. Plasma glucose values are checked hourly, and the insulin dose is closely monitored to maintain normal glucose levels (70 to 120 mg/dL [3.8 to 6.6 mmol/L]). A pediatrician should attend the delivery to assess and care for the infant.

Postpartum Care

An immediate decrease in insulin requirement after delivery is related to the abrupt loss of the placenta, which has synthesized high levels of peptide and steroid hormones throughout pregnancy. In the immediate postpartum period, women with GDM and many of those with type II DM require no insulin. In type I patients, insulin

TABLE 17-4. GUIDELINES FOR INSULIN AND GLUCOSE INFUSION
DURING LABOR AND DELIVERY*

Fluids Given by Infusion Pump	Capillary Glucose Level mg/dL	mmol/L	Insulin U/h
5% dextrose in 0.5% sodium chloride at constant rate: 125 mL/h	< 80	4.4	0.0
	80-100	4.4-5.5	0.5
	101-140	5.6-7.7	1.0
	141-180	7.8-10.0	1.5
	181-220	10.1-12.2	2.0
	> 220	> 12.2	2.5

* These guidelines for women with insulin-dependent and non-insulin-dependent diabetes mellitus should be adjusted for each patient.
Modified from *Pregnancy, Diabetes, and Birth*, ed. 2, by DR Hollingsworth. Baltimore, Williams & Wilkins, 1992; used with permission.

requirements decline dramatically but gradually increase after about 72 h.

During the first 6 wk postpartum, women with types I and II DM require careful readjustment of their insulin regimens to obtain close control. They should check blood glucose levels before meals and at bedtime. Breast-feeding is not contraindicated but may be associated with hypoglycemia in women with IDDM. In women with NIDDM, continuation of insulin therapy rather than oral hypoglycemic agents is recommended during lactation.

Women who have had GDM should have a 2-h oral glucose tolerance test with 75 gm of glucose at 6 to 12 wk postpartum to determine whether they are normal, clearly diabetic, or have impaired glucose tolerance (based on WHO criteria).

Infants of diabetic mothers require thorough neonatal assessment. These infants are at risk for respiratory distress, hypoglycemia, hypocalcemia, hyperbilirubinemia, polycythemia, and hyperviscosity.

THYROID DISEASE

Thyroid problems are common during pregnancy. Symptoms of hypo- and hyperthyroidism in pregnant patients do not differ from those in nonpregnant patients. Normal values of thyroid function tests vary with different laboratories, but generally serum T_4 values are increased 2 to 4 μg/dL and T_3 values are increased 20 to 50 ng/dL during pregnancy, while free T_4 and thyroid-stimulating hormone (TSH) values are normal. Oral contraceptives may produce the same changes in test values. Women with mild to moderate hypothyroidism may become pregnant, since affected women frequently have normal menstrual cycles. If the diagnosis was established before pregnancy, the usual replacement dose of L-thyroxine is continued. Modest increases or decreases in L-thyroxine may be necessary as pregnancy progresses. When hypothyroidism is first diagnosed during gestation, oral replacement therapy with L-thyroxine 0.1 mg/day is started as soon as the diagnosis is confirmed. Response to therapy is monitored by repeating serum T_4 and sensitive TSH determinations after several weeks and adjusting medication accordingly.

Treatment of **Graves' disease** during pregnancy varies in different medical centers. In general, the lowest possible dose of oral propylthiouracil (50 to 100 mg q 8 h) is the treatment of choice. *Caution is exercised,* as this drug crosses the placenta and may cause fetal goiter and hypothyroidism. The therapeutic response occurs gradually over 3 to 4 wk, and usually the dose does not need to be adjusted at shorter intervals. Simultaneous administration of L-thyroxine or L-triiodothyronine is *contraindicated,* since these hormones may mask the maternal effects of excessive doses of propylthiouracil and cause fetal hypothyroidism. Maternal thyroid status is monitored by physical examination and by serum T_4 and/or free T_4 determinations. Amelioration of Graves' disease in the 3rd trimester is common, and often propylthiouracil may be reduced to 25 to 50 mg/day or discontinued. In centers where experienced thyroid surgeons are available, a 2nd-trimester thyroidectomy may be considered when the mother is euthyroid. If this treatment is selected, the mother should receive a full replacement dose of L-thyroxine (0.15 to 0.2 mg/day) beginning 24 h after surgery. Radioactive iodine (diagnostic or therapeutic) and iodide solutions are *contraindicated* during pregnancy because of adverse effects on the fetal thyroid. β-Blocking agents (eg, propranolol) are *not* recommended (unless drug reactions to propylthiouracil or the similar blocking agent methimazole are encountered) because of neonatal side effects such as possible intrauterine growth retardation, bradycardia, floppiness, and severe hypoglycemia.

In Graves' disease, maternal thyroid status does *not* correlate with fetal thyroid function. Women with Graves' disease or a history of the disorder can be clinically euthyroid, hyperthyroid, or hypothyroid; whichever condition prevails, their thyroid-stimulating immunoglobulins (TSIs) cross the placenta and may be associated with **fetal hyperthyroidism** in utero. Thyroid-blocking antibodies, if present, also cross the placenta; fetal thyroid status reflects the relative titers of the stimulatory or blocking immunoglobulins received. TSI measurements can be performed in commercial laboratories and should be requested for pregnant women with Graves' disease or a history of the disorder, regardless of current clinical status. In infants at risk for in utero hyperthyroidism, fetal tachycardia (> 160 beats/min) and intrauterine growth retardation documented by ultrasonography may indicate fetal hypermetabolism. In infants of women receiving propylthiouracil, congenital Graves' disease may not become apparent until 7 to 10 days after birth, when the effect of the drug subsides. Mothers and infants should be followed closely postpartum to monitor their metabolic status.

Hashimoto's thyroiditis and previous treatment for Graves' disease are the most common causes of hypothyroidism. Maternal immune suppression associated with pregnancy often ameliorates the course of chronic thyroiditis. In some women, however, hypo- or hyperthyroidism occurs and may require treatment to maintain a maternal euthyroid status.

Acute (subacute) thyroiditis, a common problem during pregnancy, often is misdiagnosed as Graves' disease. A tender goiter is noted along with or following a respiratory infection. *Transient* symptoms of hyperthyroidism are associated with serum T4 levels above normal pregnancy values. Usually, no treatment is necessary.

Postpartum maternal thyroid dysfunction has been reported in 4 to 7% of women in the first 6 mo after delivery. Pregnant women with goiters, Hashimoto's thyroiditis, a strong family history of autoimmune thyroid disease, or type I

(insulin-dependent) diabetes mellitus are particularly prone to this dysfunction. During the first trimester, their thyroid microsomal autoantibodies (MSA) should be measured. Women with hemagglutination titers for MSA of ≤ 1:100 rarely develop postpartum thyroid dysfunction, but those with titers of ≥ 1:6400 more commonly do. With intermediate titers, the outcome is uncertain. Postpartum hypo- or hyperthyroidism is usually transient but may require treatment. In women with Graves' disease, a recurrence of hyperthyroidism after delivery may be either transient or persistent.

Painless thyroiditis with transient hyperthyroidism, a newly recognized postpartum entity, is probably an autoimmune disorder. It develops abruptly in the first few weeks after delivery, is associated with a low radioactive iodine uptake, and is characterized histologically by lymphocytic infiltration. In contrast to subacute thyroiditis, this disorder may be persistent or progressive, and recurrent transient episodes of hyperthyroidism are described.

HEPATIC DISORDERS

Normal pregnancy subtly affects hepatic function, especially bile transport, but routine function test values are normal. Alkaline phosphatase values rise progressively during the 3rd trimester and may reach 2 to 3 times normal at term; this is due to placental production rather than hepatic dysfunction. Jaundice results from usual hepatic disorders or from conditions unique to pregnancy.

Not Unique to Pregnancy

Jaundice may be caused by **drugs** prescribed for morning sickness or intercurrent illnesses during pregnancy. Acute cholecystitis and biliary obstruction from **gallstones** appear to be more common during pregnancy, probably because of increased lithogenicity of bile and impaired gallbladder contractility.

Viral hepatitis is the most common cause of jaundice during pregnancy. The course generally is unremarkable, but among patients in underdeveloped countries, the epidemic form of non-A, non-B hepatitis particularly may be unusually severe, possibly as a result of malnutrition. There is no clear evidence that hepatitis is teratogenic in the first trimester. Hepatitis B virus (HBV) may be transmitted to the infant at parturition or, less often, transplacentally. Transmission is particularly likely if the mother is e-antigen positive and either is a chronic carrier of hepatitis B surface antigen (**HBsAg**) or has contracted hepatitis during the 3rd trimester. Affected babies often become carriers of HBV and have subclinical liver dysfunction, but they only occasionally develop frank neonatal hepatitis. To help minimize such vertical transmission, routine testing of all pregnant women for HBsAg is increasingly being performed. Prophylaxis prenatally with immune globulin and vaccination for HBV-exposed infants are discussed under NEONATAL INFECTIONS in Ch. 27.

Unique to Pregnancy

Minor nonspecific hepatic dysfunction may develop in **hyperemesis gravidarum**. Jaundice occurring in **septic abortion** is multifactorial, resulting from septic hepatocellular injury, hemolysis, and hypoxia.

Severe **preeclampsia** may be associated with hepatic fibrin deposition, necrosis, and hemorrhage and may be manifested by abdominal pain, nausea and vomiting, and mild jaundice. **Spontaneous rupture of the liver** from subcapsular hematoma with intra-abdominal hemorrhage is a rare but life-threatening event associated with pregnancy; the pathogenesis is unknown, but it is usually associated with preeclampsia and may represent an extreme vascular complication of the disorder. Occasionally, women with otherwise relatively mild preeclampsia develop an obscure syndrome of **He**molysis, **E**levated **L**iver enzyme values, and **L**ow **P**latelet counts (**HELLP syndrome**), with variable abdominal and systemic symptoms; the cause is unknown. Recent evidence suggests that preeclampsia may also be associated with fatty liver of pregnancy (see below).

Cholestasis (pruritus) of pregnancy is a relatively common disorder, apparently caused by an idiosyncratic exaggeration of normal hormonal effects on bile transport. Intense pruritus, the earliest manifestation of cholestasis, develops in the 2nd or 3rd trimester; dark urine and jaundice sometimes follow. Hepatic inflammation is not present, and there are no systemic symptoms. The condition is benign, disappearing after delivery; however, it tends to recur with each pregnancy, and affected women often develop the same syndrome when given oral contraceptives (see Ch. 70). When pruritus is severe, oral cholestyramine 8 to 12 gm daily in 2 or 3 divided doses usually relieves the itching. Bleed-

ing from hypoprothrombinemia occasionally develops but is readily reversed by vitamin K therapy (phytonadione 5 to 10 mg/day IM for 2 to 3 days).

Fatty liver of pregnancy (obstetric yellow atrophy) is a rare and poorly understood illness that occurs near term, sometimes with preeclampsia. It presents with acute nausea and vomiting, abdominal discomfort, and jaundice, often followed by rapidly progressive hepatocellular failure. Clinical and laboratory findings mimic fulminant viral hepatitis, though aminotransferase levels < 500 u./L and hyperuricemia are clues to the disorder. The cause is unknown. Mortality for both mother and fetus is high in full-blown cases, although less severe cases are increasingly being recognized. Whether immediate termination of pregnancy alters the outcome is debatable, though this is usually advised. Liver biopsy shows diffuse small droplets of fat in the hepatocytes, usually with minimal apparent necrosis, though in some cases the features overlap with those of viral hepatitis. Recovery is complete if the patient survives, and the disorder does not recur in subsequent pregnancies. A seemingly identical illness may develop at any stage of pregnancy if tetracyclines are given IV in high doses.

Chronic Liver Disease and Pregnancy

In women with chronic active hepatitis and especially with cirrhosis, fertility is often decreased; with severe liver disease, pregnancy is relatively uncommon. When it does occur, fetal losses are high because of spontaneous abortion and prematurity; successful outcome of the pregnancy is unpredictable. In contrast, prognosis for the mother is generally favorable, as maternal mortality is not substantially increased. Although pregnancy may temporarily worsen cholestasis in primary biliary cirrhosis and other cholestatic disorders, pregnancy per se is not detrimental to patients with underlying chronic liver disease. Increased plasma volume in the 3rd trimester enhances the risk of variceal hemorrhage in cirrhotic patients, but this is a relatively uncommon event. Most patients can tolerate cesarean section.

Corticosteroids given for chronic active hepatitis need not be stopped during pregnancy, since fetal hazard has not been proved. Need for azathioprine and other immunosuppressive drugs must be balanced against potential hazards.

INFECTIOUS DISEASE

Infectious diseases other than UTIs and common viral infections rarely complicate pregnancy and usually are not a problem. However, certain viral diseases can have specific effects on the fetus. These diseases are discussed very briefly here in relation to pregnancy.

Rubella is a major cause of congenital anomalies, particularly of the cardiovascular system and inner ear. Cytomegalovirus infection can cross the placenta and damage the fetal liver. Toxoplasmosis can affect the fetal brain. Patients should avoid contact with cats during pregnancy unless the cats are strictly confined to the house and are not exposed to street cats. Infectious hepatitis (see HEPATIC DISORDERS, above) follows a clinical course like that in the nonpregnant patient, but it can be particularly devastating during pregnancy, especially in malnourished women. The fetus may be infected in the latter part of pregnancy, and the incidence of preterm delivery increases.

SEXUALLY TRANSMITTED DISEASE
(See also §2)

Chlamydial infection during pregnancy may be associated with premature rupture of the membranes and preterm labor. The presence of mucopurulent cervicitis or recurrent culture-negative urethritis mandates testing for *Chlamydia*. Culture and sensitivity testing, though complex and expensive, is the best means of establishing the diagnosis in high-risk populations. The treatment agent of choice is erythromycin.

Human immunodeficiency virus (HIV) infection during pregnancy is a major obstetric problem, as heterosexual transmission of the disease along with IV drug abuse is significantly increasing its incidence in women. Vertical transmission to the fetus occurs in nearly half the patients, resulting in an aggressive, shortened disease course in the child that usually ends in death before the age of 2 yr. Evidence that early treatment with pentamidine and/or zidovudine may delay the onset of clinical AIDS in patients who are HIV-positive and asymptomatic suggests that a widespread program of prenatal testing for this virus may be useful. Pregnancy does not seem to accelerate the process of the HIV infection. Because of the high risk of fetal transmission, termination of pregnancy generally is advocated once the diagnosis is confirmed. In most urban hospitals, HIV transmission precautions are mandatory for all obstetric staff because of the risk of exposure to blood and body fluids.

Herpesvirus infection during pregnancy has major perinatal implications through fetal inoculation during delivery. Pregnant patients and their partners should be specifically questioned about recurrent herpes infections. Serial cultures of asymptomatic patients taken in the antepartum period to identify mothers at risk for transmitting herpes to the newborn are of no value. The risk of fetal transmission of herpes in patients with recurrent infections who have no visible lesions is extremely low. Without herpetic lesions or prodrome, the patient should not require cesarean section delivery unless traditional obstetric indications are present. An exception may be mothers who acquire a primary first episode of herpes during the late 3rd trimester and are known to continue excreting herpesvirus from the cervix at term. Patients with active lesions or a clear prodrome at term should be offered the option of cesarean section regardless of how long the membranes have been ruptured. When the patient is known to have recurrent herpes infections but presents in labor without lesions or a prodrome, vaginal delivery may be performed. Culture specimens should be obtained from the mother and infant in case such information is relevant to caring for the infant in the first weeks of life. In patients with recurrent herpes infection during pregnancy, delivery should be arranged during a risk-free interval at term. This may involve induction of labor.

ANEMIA

The Hct value in nonpregnant women normally ranges from 38 to 45%, but in pregnant women normal values can be much lower (eg, 34% in a single and 30% in a multiple pregnancy), even with adequate stores of iron, folic acid, and vitamin B_{12}. This lower range represents "the physiologic hydremia of pregnancy" and does not indicate a decrease in O_2-carrying capacity or true anemia. Normally, a pregnant patient has erythroid hyperplasia of the marrow and a measurable increase in red cell mass. However, a disproportionate rise in plasma volume results in the "hydremia." Unless excessive blood loss occurs at delivery, the Hct generally rises in the immediate postpartum period. In late pregnancy, the absence of this dilutional effect suggests inadequate blood volume expansion, which has been associated with growth retardation, pregnancy-induced hypertension, and intrauterine fetal death.

Since pregnancy represents a state of negative iron balance, **iron deficiency** is responsible for 95% of anemia in pregnancy. Unless normal nutritional intake is supplemented during pregnancy, pregnant women at term will have deficits in iron stores. Diagnostic indexes for iron-deficiency anemia include a Hct of $\leq$ 33%, an MCV of $<$ 79 μm^3, or serum iron level of $<$ 60 $\mu g/dL$. Iron deficiency during pregancy can be successfully treated with oral iron preparations totaling 180 mg/day. One 325-mg ferrous sulfate tablet taken at midmorning, another at midafternoon, and a multivitamin (pregnancy formula) with citrus juice at bedtime provide adequate dosage. About 20% of pregnant women fail to ingest or absorb adequate iron and may require parenteral therapy. Iron dextran is given IM in divided doses every other day for a total of $\geq$ 1000 mg over 3 wk. Prompt response, denoted by an elevation in the reticulocyte count, is usually apparent.

Because of the preferential transport of iron across the placenta, the neonatal Hct is generally normal despite maternal anemia. However, total iron stores in these infants are usually reduced, indicating a need for early dietary iron supplementation.

Folate deficiency with severe anemia, megaloblastic marrow changes, and glossitis is relatively uncommon, but laboratory evidence of folic acid deficiency is found in 0.5 to 1.5% of pregnant women. The earliest evidence of folic acid deficiency in pregnancy is the finding of macrocytes in the peripheral blood. The diagnosis is confirmed by low serum or erythrocyte folate levels.

Folate deficiencies are likely to occur with hemolytic complications of pregnancy, such as the hemoglobinopathies; absorptive defects in chronic granulomatous bowel disease or following jejunoileal bypass surgery; the increased demand of multiple pregnancy; and the ingestion of drugs (eg, alcohol and phenytoin) interfering with folate absorption. Folic acid deficiency has been implicated in fetal alcohol syndrome and in the syndrome associated with anticonvulsant therapy based on phenytoin (fetal hydantoin syndrome). Daily prophylaxis with 1 mg folic acid is recommended in all pregnancies.

HEMOGLOBINOPATHIES

Hemoglobinopathies complicating pregnancy, particularly **SS disease (sickle cell disease)**, SC disease (Hb S-C disease), sickle cell—thalassemia, and **α-thalassemia**, significantly affect maternal morbidity and perinatal morbidity and mortality. Routine antenatal testing for Hb status is recommended for all women at risk on the basis of racial or geographic origin and family history. All of these hemoglobinopathies can be diagnosed by restriction endonuclease analysis of the DNA present in uncultured placental cells, by chorionic villus sampling, or by amniocentesis.

The pregnant patient with **SS disease** is especially susceptible to infection; pneumonia, UTIs, and endometritis are most common. Anemia almost invariably becomes more severe as pregnancy progresses. About $^1/_3$ of these patients have pregnancy-induced hypertension. Sickle cell crisis occurs commonly, as do heart failure and pulmonary infarction. The more complicated the history before pregnancy, the higher the risk of morbidity and mortality. Fetal wastage is markedly increased, with perinatal mortality rates of $\leq$ 25%. Intrauterine growth retardation and intrauterine death account for most of this increase, although severe maternal debility and the high rate of preeclampsia contribute.

Treatment of SS disease during pregnancy is currently under reassessment. Prophylactic exchange transfusions designed to keep Hb A at $\geq$ 60% are successful in reducing the frequency of hemolytic crises and pulmonary complications. However, these benefits must be weighed against the risks of transfusion reaction, hepatitis, HIV transmission, and blood group isoimmunization.

SC disease often first manifests itself during pregnancy in otherwise asymptomatic patients. While less common than SS disease, it may be associated with a higher incidence of pulmonary infarction secondary to bony spicule embolization. Obstetric management involves aggressively treating the painful crisis with IV fluids, O_2 supplementation, and analgesics. **Sickle cell—thalassemia** is relatively uncommon and more benign. Though **α-thalassemia** is not associated with maternal morbidity, in its homozygous state it is lethal for the fetus; intrauterine death secondary to hydrops occurs during the 2nd or early 3rd trimester.

ASTHMA

The incidence of asthma in pregnancy is 1% and that of severe asthmatic attacks and status asthmaticus is $< ^1/_{10}$ of the patients at risk. Pregnancy has no consistent effect on asthma, although deterioration is more common than improvement. Similarly, asthma has no consistent effect on pregnancy, although it is associated with preterm delivery and intrauterine growth retardation. Treatment of asthma during pregnancy is based on severity and chronicity of attacks. Therapy for mild episodes is nebulized isoproterenol 1:200 q 3 h. More severe attacks require IV aminophylline, and status asthmaticus requires aggressive hydration and IV corticosteroids. Antibiotics should be used when infectious components are present. For maintenance therapy after control of an acute attack, anhydrous theophylline sustained action tablets 300 mg bid is recommended, with monitoring of theophylline levels. Increased dosage may be required during pregnancy to achieve therapeutic levels of ≥ 10 µg/mL. Nebulized bronchodilators and corticosteroid inhalants (eg, beclomethasone dipropionate) have been widely used and are both effective and safe.

AUTOIMMUNE DISEASES

Autoimmune diseases are 5 times more frequent in women than in men and tend to reach a peak incidence during reproductive years. Thus, association with pregnancy is common.

Systemic lupus erythematosus (SLE) may first appear during pregnancy or may have an increased risk of activity if it was present before pregnancy. If the disease is active at the time of conception, remission during pregnancy is less likely. Preexisting significant renal or cardiac disease is associated with major maternal morbidity and risk of mortality. The course of SLE during a particular pregnancy cannot be predicted on the basis of events in previous pregnancies or on duration of remission. The most likely time for exacerbation is the immediate puerperal period.

The effect of SLE on pregnancy is noted before the clinical onset of disease. Recurrent abortion, 2nd-trimester stillbirth, intrauterine growth retardation, and preterm delivery occur frequently in the obstetric history of women whose diagnosis of SLE is subsequently confirmed. A further increase in perinatal mortality is associated with diffuse nephritis, hypertension, or the presence of circulating antiphospholipid antibodies. The first line of treatment is prednisone; immunosuppressants are reserved for refractory clinical situations. Peripartal corticosteroid prophylaxis reduces the incidence of puerperal exacerbation. The neonate may test positive for antinuclear antibodies and may show thrombocytopenia, hemolytic anemia, or leukopenia. These serologic stigmas of SLE are transitory, resulting from passive immunization by transplacental passage of IgG. A specific effect of SLE is congenital heart block produced by direct involvement of the septal conduction system with an antibody to tissue ribonucleoproteins.

The lupus anticoagulant, present in about 5 to 15% of patients, is associated with significant increased risk of abortion, stillbirth, and maternal thromboembolic disease. The anticoagulant reacts with platelet membrane phospholipid, reducing the production of prostacyclin; it also has an apparent direct effect on the vascular endothelium, leading to thrombosis in the placenta and in maternal organs. High-dose corticosteroids (50 mg/day prednisone) and low-dose aspirin (80 mg/day), which affects platelet thromboxane synthesis, can suppress the lupus anticoagulant.

Rheumatoid arthritis may have its onset in pregnancy, particularly in the postpartum period. Its clinical course is generally improved during pregnancy, perhaps in response to increased circulating levels of free cortisol. The fetus is not specifically affected, but delivery may be difficult because of maternal hip joint or lumbar spine involvement.

Myasthenia gravis has a variable course during pregnancy. Frequent acute myasthenic episodes may require increasing doses of anticholinesterase agents (eg, neostigmine), risking cholinergic signs of overdosage (eg, abdominal pain, diarrhea, and vomiting), which may require atropine. In some patients, the myasthenia becomes refractory to standard therapy, requiring corticosteroids or immunosuppressants to control symptoms. During labor, these patients may require assisted ventilation; they are extremely sensitive to sedatives, analgesics, narcotics, and magnesium sulfate. Because of the transplacental passage of IgG, neonatal myasthenia may occur in 20% of infants; it may occur with even greater frequency if the mother has not had a prior thymectomy.

Immune thrombocytopenic purpura (ITP) generally has its onset before age 30 and has a female predominance of 3:1. Untreated in pregnancy, ITP tends to be more severe and is associated with increased maternal morbidity. Of particular concern is the passage of the antiplatelet antibody to the fetus, leading to intrauterine and neonatal thrombocytopenia. Fetal intracranial bleeding during labor and delivery is a risk, resulting in increased neonatal mortality and long-term morbidity. Sampling of maternal plasma for direct or indirect antiplatelet antibody is not predictive of fetal involvement, nor is the absence of maternal thrombocytopenia as a result of corticosteroid therapy or previous splenectomy. Recently, the availability of percutaneous umbilical blood sampling has allowed identification of affected fetuses and subsequent selection of cesarean section delivery to prevent intracranial bleeding. Unaffected fetuses can be delivered vaginally.

Corticosteroids produce transient remission in most patients with ITP but sustained improvement in only 50%. Immunosuppression and plasmapheresis further reduce IgG antibody titer. A recent addition to treatment is the infusion of high-dose IgG, which produces short-term but significant increases in platelets, allowing planned induction of labor and vaginal delivery. Platelet transfusions are indicated only when delivery by cesarean section is required for obstetric reasons and maternal platelet counts are < 50,000/μL. Rarely, splenectomy is required for refractory clinical situations; it is best performed in the 2nd trimester, when it produces sustained remission in some 80% of patients.

MALIGNANCY

Malignancy of any kind is generally treated as if the patient were not pregnant. Malignancies of the upper abdomen, lung, or extremities are uncommon in pregnancy and should be treated as usual. (See also MALIGNANT MELANOMA in Ch. 104.) Breast cancer is a major problem because the breast engorgement that occurs during pregnancy makes recognizing a new lump difficult. Any solid or cystic breast mass should be investigated. This can usually be done by ultrasound-guided needle aspiration or biopsy. Excisional biopsy is rarely indicated. Delay may be fatal for the patient. Malignancy of the lower abdomen, excluding the genital tract, should be treated as in nonpregnant women. However, for rectal cancers, hysterectomy may be needed to ensure complete removal of the malignancy. Delay should not be allowed, and after 28 wk of pregnancy, cesarean section should be performed in an attempt to save the infant. Before 28 wk, the

fetus should be sacrificed, unless the patient refuses.

Malignancy of the genital tract is somewhat different. Ovarian cancer should be treated by bilateral oophorectomy as soon as it is recognized. Before the 12th wk of pregnancy, the ovaries are usually easily palpable, but after that time they rise out of the pelvis with the uterus, and the cancer may be missed. Survival rates for these patients are very low. Endometrial and tubal carcinomas rarely occur during pregnancy.

Carcinoma of the cervix is becoming less common, since cytologic smears allow early diagnosis of the preinvasive form. However, cancer of the cervix can develop during pregnancy, and an abnormal Pap smear should not be attributed to pregnancy but must be followed up with colposcopically directed biopsies. Conization usually can be avoided. If biopsy shows mild forms of dysplasia, the patient can be allowed to deliver normally, and appropriate follow-up by cytologic smear and biopsy can start at the 6-wk checkup. Severe dysplasia or carcinoma in situ (CIS) warrants further investigation during pregnancy. A very superficial conization of the cervix may be necessary for complete diagnosis to rule out invasion, although colposcopy is usually accurate. If true severe dysplasia or CIS is found, hysterectomy may be suggested at the time of delivery. However, some authorities believe that hysterectomy may not be indicated at all for cervical intraepithelial neoplasia III (CIN III), that risk for hysterectomy at time of delivery is much higher, and that recuperation will interfere with infant care. Therefore, further investigation can be delayed until the 6-wk checkup, when appropriate treatment can be instituted. If invasive cancer of the cervix is diagnosed in the first 20 wk of pregnancy, either hysterotomy and radical hysterectomy with lymph node dissection or whole pelvis irradiation followed by intravaginal radium treatment is required. Evidence is accumulating that radical surgery is more successful than irradiation during pregnancy. Treatment for microinvasive cancer may be deferred until after delivery, as more conservative surgery may be possible. If the cancer is diagnosed after 20 wk, some patients prefer to wait for treatment until 32 wk, when the fetus has some chance of surviving; but if abortion is acceptable, treatment should be begun. Near term, cesarean section combined with radical hysterectomy and lymph node dissection is preferred.

Leukemia and **Hodgkin's disease** are uncommon in pregnancy. If they are diagnosed early in the pregnancy, they should be treated appropriately with assistance and guidance by a hematologist or oncologist. Many infants have developed normally while the mothers were treated with antileukemic drugs, but use of such drugs also has been associated with loss of the pregnancy and fetal anomalies. Since leukemias rapidly become fatal, no attempt should be made to save the pregnancy, and the disease must be treated promptly. Hodgkin's disease is not so rapidly fatal, and cure is possible. If Hodgkin's disease is confined above the diaphragm, a pregnant patient may receive appropriate irradiation therapy with shielding of the abdomen. If the disease is below the diaphragm, abortion may be required for adequate treatment.

DISORDERS REQUIRING SURGERY

Most of these disorders in young women are confined to the abdomen and may cause problems during pregnancy, since pregnancy may obscure the diagnosis and affect necessary surgical procedures. When surgery must be performed, mother and fetus tolerate it well if the supportive care before and during surgery is good and if anesthetics are administered carefully so that hypotension and hypoxia do not occur. Certain conditions present particular diagnostic problems during pregnancy.

Appendicitis mimics the general cramping pain that patients may experience during pregnancy, and the WBC count of pregnant patients is normally somewhat elevated. In addition, since the appendix rises in the abdomen as pregnancy progresses, pain in the right lower quadrant does not reliably establish this diagnosis. If appendicitis is suspected, laparotomy should be performed *without delay* (the death rate from a ruptured appendix during pregnancy is high) or in the immediate puerperium (when appendicitis is more common).

Benign ovarian cysts can develop during pregnancy. Unless the cyst is obviously malignant, operative intervention should be delayed during the first trimester, since the cyst may be a corpus luteum. The operation should be delayed, if possible, until after 12 wk of pregnancy; however, if the cyst continues to enlarge or if there is tenderness, exploration is necessary. After 12 wk of pregnancy, ovarian tumors are difficult to diagnose because the ovaries rise out of the pelvis with the uterus and are difficult to find. Torsion or infarction can mimic appendicitis and will be discovered at laparotomy.

Gallbladder disease occurs occasionally and, if possible, should be treated expectantly; if the patient does not improve, immediate surgery is needed. **Bowel obstruction** can be devastating during pregnancy. Loss of pregnancy can occur if gangrene of the bowel with accompanying peritonitis develops. Prompt exploration is warranted in a patient with symptoms and signs of small or large bowel obstruction and a history of previous surgical intervention or intra-abdominal infection that might predispose to intestinal obstruction.

---

18. ABNORMALITIES AND COMPLICATIONS OF LABOR AND DELIVERY

INDUCTION OR STIMULATION OF LABOR

Elective induction of labor is rare and usually used only with patients who live long distances from the hospital or would have difficulty getting there in adequate time for delivery. Some of these patients should be hospitalized when they are near term. Dating must be accurate, and amniocentesis for lecithin/sphingomyelin (L/S) ratio may be advisable.

When induction of labor is indicated in obstetric or medical disease, the disease process should be under control; reasons for the induction should be precise and should be recorded. The most successful and safest method for induction is giving dilute oxytocin IV, using an infusion pump for precise control. Labor usually starts at a flow of 0.5 to 2 mU/min; if contractions are inadequate, the dose is increased at 20- to 30-min intervals. External fetal monitoring is essential. Internal monitoring should be performed as soon as the membranes can be safely ruptured. A total of 40 mU/min should not be exceeded, since at that point water retention becomes a hazard. Rarely is 10 to 12 mU/min exceeded.

Stimulation or augmentation of labor with oxytocin is indicated when the patient has developed contractions with an unsatisfactory pattern; before stimulation is attempted, the diagnosis must be reasonably precise. If the patient is in the latent phase of labor—ie, has little effacement, minimal dilation, and irregular contractions—then rest, walking, or support is better treatment than oxytocin. After true labor has begun (4-cm dilation with nearly completed effacement), progress should be > 1-cm dilation/h. If true labor does not occur, the patient is considered to have **hypotonic uterine dysfunction.** The best treatment is dilute oxytocin stimulation until a more normal pattern of contractions is achieved.

An occasional patient has **hypertonic dysfunctional labor,** in which contractions are too strong, too close together, or both. This contraction pattern is difficult to control. Administration of any oxytocic agent should be discontinued promptly. Repositioning the patient and administering analgesia may help. A tocolytic agent, such as ritodrine, may be effective.

PRETERM LABOR

Onset of labor with effacement and dilation of the cervix before 37 wk of gestation.

Preterm labor associated with vaginal bleeding or rupture of the membranes is difficult to stop. Bed rest helps occasionally, but if dilation and effacement of the cervix begin, labor usually progresses to delivery. Preterm labor not associated with bleeding or leaking amniotic fluid can be stopped in 50% of patients by bed rest and hydration. Ethyl alcohol and barbiturates should not be used because of maternal and fetal side effects. **Ritodrine,** a β-adrenergic sympathomimetic agent, has a 70 to 80% success rate; however, side effects include maternal tachycardia and hypotension, as well as fetal tachycardia. If ritodrine is not tolerated, magnesium sulfate infusion (similar to that used for preeclampsia—see in Ch. 15) may also be effective. Terbutaline has been used with a success rate similar to that of ritodrine. If preterm labor is arrested, treating the mother with dexamethasone 5 mg IM q 12 h for 4 doses (betamethasone sodium phosphate and betamethasone acetate suspension 12 mg IM q 24 h for 2 doses/wk is also used) before delivery appears to accelerate maturation of the fetal lungs and decreases the incidence of neonatal respiratory distress syndrome (see under RESPIRATORY DISORDERS in Ch. 27). The problems to which preterm infants are predisposed are discussed in GESTATIONAL AGE AND BIRTH WEIGHT in Ch. 27.

PREMATURE RUPTURE OF MEMBRANES (PROM)

Rupture of the membranes 1 h or more before onset of labor. Previous practice was to have these patients delivered promptly because of risk of neonatal infection, but this no longer is done. Patients with PROM should *not* have a digital examination of the cervix. Rather, examination with a clean speculum is performed to verify rupture, estimate dilation, and collect fluid for maturity studies. Firm diagnosis of rupture of membranes is made when fluid is seen escaping from the cervix or the presence of fetal vernix or meconium is observed; other less reliable tests are determination of pH with nitrazine paper (amniotic fluid is alkaline, turning it blue) and microscopic fern pattern of fluid dried on a glass slide. If the amniotic fluid indicates by L/S ratio or other tests that the fetal lungs are not mature, an attempt should be made to delay delivery until maturity. Bed rest is effective in some patients; ritodrine may be needed in many. If no digital examination is performed and speculum examination is not repeated, the risk of infection is minimal. The patient should be kept on bed rest, and her temperature and pulse should be recorded at least twice daily. Delivery should be accomplished if infection is suspected or when amniotic fluid studies indicate maturity.

PROLAPSE OF THE UMBILICAL CORD

This rare complication can be occult or overt. **Occult prolapse** occurs with intact membranes when the cord is expelled ahead of the presenting part or is trapped in front of a shoulder. A specific pattern on the electronic fetal monitoring tracing is generally diagnostic. **Treatment** is changing the patient's position or elevating the fetus to relieve pressure on the cord. Occasionally, cesarean section is necessary.

Overt prolapse occurs with ruptured membranes when the cord presents in front of the presenting part. This most commonly occurs spontaneously with breech presentation. It also occurs with vertex presentation, particularly when membranes are ruptured with the presenting part not engaged. The cause may be iatrogenic, which is one reason why membranes should not be artificially ruptured unless the head is well engaged in the pelvis. **Treatment** is immediate delivery, usually by cesarean section, to avoid fetal damage. An attendant or the obstetrician must hold the presenting part up off the prolapsed cord to prevent further and prolonged compression of the cord.

AMNIOTIC FLUID EMBOLISM

This extremely rare event can occur at any gestational age, usually with tumultuous labor and ruptured membranes. Amniotic fluid is embolized into the pulmonary circulation, and the patient responds as though a blood clot had embolized to the lungs, with collapse, shock, tachycardia, cardiac irregularity and arrest, and death. Autopsy reveals fetal squamous cells and hair in the pulmonary circulation. If the patient survives, disseminated intravascular coagulation is a common complication.

POSTDATISM AND POSTMATURITY

Postdatism: *Pregnancy continuing after 42 wk.* **Postmaturity:** *An uncommon syndrome of failing placental function and fetal jeopardy that occurs after 42 wk.*

Since calculation of the estimated date of confinement is subject to error, the diagnosis of **postdatism** may be uncertain. If the mother's menstrual cycles were 35 days or longer, delivery may be late by definition although the infant is really only at term. The **signs of postmaturity** are lessening in uterine size and decrease in fetal motion in a pregnancy that is > 42 wk gestation by dates. Postmaturity can be confirmed by a yellow finding on amniocentesis, secondary to meconium staining of the amniotic fluid. Frequently, however, the amount of amniotic fluid is markedly decreased in postmature pregnancies, and amniocentesis may be difficult.

Postdatism can be treated expectantly, as long as no signs of postmaturity occur. Accurate dates should be established as early as possible in pregnancy. If this cannot be done because of an irregular or unobtainable menstrual history, ultrasound examination should be performed early in pregnancy to determine the length of gestation. Later in pregnancy, prior to 32 wk, serial ultrasound examinations for biparietal diameter

of the fetal head can help confirm the date. After 32 wk, dating by ultrasound is ±3 wk. If the pregnancy continues past 42 wk, a nonstress test or a contraction stress test should be performed to help evaluate the condition of the fetus. Some physicians recommend starting testing at 41 wk and including a biophysical profile (eg, amount of amniotic fluid, fetal movement, respiratory status, head:abdomen ratio). If results are abnormal, delivery should be accomplished. If the cervix is not ripe, cesarean section should be performed. Problems associated with postmaturity are discussed under GESTATIONAL AGE AND BIRTH WEIGHT in Ch. 27.

PROBLEMS IN LABOR AND DELIVERY

FIRST AND SECOND STAGES OF LABOR

Most of the problems that occur during delivery can and should be anticipated. Signs of danger during the 1st stage of labor include **vaginal bleeding** (see THIRD TRIMESTER BLEEDING in Ch. 15) or **abnormal fetal heart rate**. Other problems include **abnormal fetal presentation and position**. All of these problems must be accurately diagnosed early in the 1st stage of labor so that appropriate treatment can be started at the proper time. Failure to diagnose potential problems at the initial examination threatens both mother and infant.

Occasionally, for various reasons, an infant is born apneic although no problems existed before delivery. Appropriate resuscitative measures must be started immediately (see ASPHYXIA AND RESUSCITATION in Ch. 27). Thus, in addition to the obstetrician, individuals trained in resuscitation, who can be freed from providing anesthesia or tending to maternal problems, should be present during delivery if possible.

The primary event of the 2nd stage of labor is descent of the presenting part into the pelvis. In general, both cervical dilation and descent of the head into the pelvis should proceed by at least 1 cm/h; if they do not, **fetopelvic disproportion** is likely and appropriate treatment should be instituted. If disproportion is not present and labor does not progress normally with good descent of the infant, oxytocin infusion (see INDUCTION OR STIMULATION OF LABOR, above) should be tried. If that is unsuccessful, a cesarean section should be performed. Fetal heart tones must be monitored; any significant abnormality of heart rate requires immediate delivery by forceps or cesarean section (see below).

In fetopelvic disproportion, forceps delivery or cesarean section is required. When an attempt at forceps delivery proves too difficult, the obstetrician should realize that the pull is too hard to be safe and should perform a cesarean section.

Abnormal Presentations

When the **fetal occiput is posterior** in the pelvis rather than anterior (the most frequent abnormal presentation), the fetal neck is usually deflexed to some extent and a larger diameter of the head is presented for passage through the maternal pelvis. Any degree of disproportion may prolong labor and make delivery difficult. The obstetrician must evaluate this problem and decide between forceps delivery and cesarean section (see below). In **face presentation**, the head is hyperextended, and the chin presents; if the chin is posterior and remains so, vaginal delivery is not possible. **Brow presentation** rarely persists; vaginal delivery is not possible.

In **breech presentation**, the next most common abnormality, the fetal buttocks present rather than the head. The perinatal death rate for breech presentation is 4 times that for cephalic presentations; prematurity is a major contributing factor. Complications can be prevented only by diagnosing the problem before delivery (eg, the fetus can be moved to vertex presentation by external version prior to labor, usually at 37 or 38 wk). There are several varieties of breech presentation: In a **frank breech presentation**, the fetal hips are flexed but the knees are extended. In a **complete breech presentation**, the infant seems to be sitting with hips and knees flexed. Single or double **footling presentation** occurs when one or both legs are completely extended and present before the breech. *The primary problem with breech presentation is that the soft parts of the lower portion of the body and trunk can mold to fit through the pelvis, but the head has no chance to undergo molding.* Thus, disproportion is not discovered until the body has been delivered and the head is caught. Consequently, the infant may die. The incidence of nerve damage due to stretching the brachial plexus or spinal cord and brain damage due to anoxia is increased in breech presentation. When the infant's umbilicus is visible at the introitus, the cord is being compressed by the fetal head against the inlet of the pelvis so that little exchange of O$_2$ takes place, resulting in anoxia. These problems are compounded in primigravidas because the pelvic tissues have not been softened by previous deliveries. Many obstetricians advocate cesarean section for most breech presentations in primigravidas and all preterm breech presentations.

Other abnormal presentations may occur. Occasionally an infant presents shoulder-first with a transverse lie in which the long axis is oblique or perpendicular rather than parallel to the mother's long axis. These infants, except second twins, should be delivered by cesarean section.

Twins occur in 1/70 to 1/80 deliveries and can be diagnosed before delivery by ultrasonography, x-ray, or the recording of 2 distinct heart-rate patterns on the fetal ECG. **Complications of twin presentations:** Twins are usually small and premature because an overdistended uterus tends to go into labor before term. They present in various ways, and abnormal presentations may complicate delivery. Because the uterus contracts after delivery of the first twin and tends to shear away the placenta of the second twin, morbidity and mortality are higher for second twins. In some cases, the overdistended uterus does not contract well after delivery, causing maternal hemorrhage. The obstetrician should decide whether to deliver vaginally or by cesarean section.

Shoulder Dystocia

An uncommon occurrence in which the anterior shoulder in vertex presentation impinges on the symphysis pubis. The head, following delivery, appears to be pulled back tightly against the vulva. The crisis in this event is that the baby is unable to breathe because the chest is compressed by the vaginal canal and the mouth is kept shut by pressure against the vulva, preventing the obstetrician from inserting any kind of tube. Oxygen deficit occurs within 4 to 5 min. This condition occurs most commonly with large infants, but the only consistent predictor is the need to perform midforceps delivery. Large babies cannot be accurately predicted and do not always have shoulder dystocia.

When this situation occurs, the first step is to apply suprapubic pressure in combination with fundal pressure to disengage the shoulder and allow the baby to descend farther into the pelvis. Hyperflexing the mother's hips may be helpful by flattening the lower spine and causing the birth canal to be straighter. If this fails, a hand should be inserted into the posterior part of the vagina and pressure placed on either the anterior or posterior part of the posterior shoulder to rotate the baby in whichever direction it will go easily. With rotation, the anterior shoulder should disengage.

If neither attempt works, the posterior shoulder is pushed up into the hollow of the sacrum, the obstetrician's hand is inserted to the fetal elbow, the fetal elbow is flexed, and the fetal hand is grasped and pulled outside to deliver the entire fetal arm. The arm is then used (like a crank for an old automobile) to turn the entire baby and disengage the anterior shoulder. When all maneuvers fail, the baby's head is flexed and pushed back into the vagina; the baby is then delivered by cesarean section.

Forceps Delivery

Forceps delivery is **elective** when used to ease delivery or to provide greater control of the head; it is **indicated** in problems of fetal distress or fetal position or to shorten the 2nd stage of labor when no complications are present but lengthy vaginal delivery is anticipated. The 2nd stage occasionally fails to progress when use of conduction anesthesia prevents the patient from bearing down adequately. The decision to use forceps must be made by an obstetrician, since cesarean section may be a better alternative in each of these situations.

Contraindications to vaginal (forceps) delivery include cephalopelvic disproportion, incomplete dilation of the cervix, failure of engagement, indeterminate presentation or position, and insufficient skill of the operator. An alternative to forceps delivery is vacuum extraction; its application requires specific and sufficient training in the use of a vacuum extractor.

Major complications that occur with use of either forceps or vacuum extraction are injury to the fetus and to the mother. Only specific training, skillful use, and experience will prevent these complications.

Cesarean Section

Cesarean section (*surgical delivery by incision in the body of the uterus*) should be performed whenever it is safer for the mother or baby than vaginal delivery. About 20% of deliveries are done by cesarean section. The decision and procedure require an obstetrician, and management of anesthesia and resuscitation of newborns require an anesthesiologist and neonatologist or someone skilled in neonatal resuscitation. The procedure is safe because of current-day anesthesia, IV therapy, antibiotics, blood transfusions, and early ambulation.

Two types of uterine incision are used: classic and lower segment. A classic incision is longitudinal in the anterior wall of the uterus, starting at the top or fundus. This incision is usually reserved for patients with placenta previa or a transverse lie of the fetus. The uterine wall is more vascular in this area, blood loss is greater than with a lower segment incision, and the scar is not as strong in subsequent pregnancies. A lower segment incision is made in the thinned, elongated lower portion of the uterine body behind the bladder reflection; it may be either transverse or longitudinal. A longitudinal incision should be used for most abnormalities of presentation and for excessively large infants to avoid lateral extension of a transverse incision into the uterine arteries. Blood loss is lessened and, since the incision is covered by bladder and peritoneum, adhesions are reduced. Vaginal birth after cesarean section has a success rate approaching 75% and should be offered to all pregnant patients who previously had a cesarean section with a lower segment incision. The best treatment for repeated cesarean section is correct management of the previous labor.

THIRD STAGE OF LABOR
(Delivery of the Placenta)

Maternal hemorrhage must be prevented during the 3rd stage. Ordinarily, 400 to 500 mL of blood is lost during delivery; if the loss is greater, the reasons must be sought. Possible sources of bleeding include uterine atony, vaginal or cervical lacerations, or retained portions of the placenta. If the uterus does not contract, hemorrhage will occur, since the primary mechanism for hemostasis within the uterus is contraction of myometrium. When the placenta has dropped into the lower uterine segment and presents at the cervix, the corpus may be depressed toward the pelvis to help push the placenta into the vagina. However, the uterus can be inverted if this procedure is done incorrectly, especially if traction is applied on the cord before the placenta is completely separated. Exploration of the uterine cavity and birth canal for lacerations or retained placental fragments is discussed in Ch. 14. During this time, the patient must be observed by a trained individual, preferably an anesthesiologist; BP, heart rate, respirations, and alertness must be monitored.

19. POSTPARTUM CARE

THE NORMAL PUERPERIUM

The clinical manifestations of the **puerperium,** *the 6-wk period following delivery,* are numerous and variable. They generally reflect reversal of the physiologic changes that occurred in pregnancy, are mild and temporary, and should not be confused with more serious conditions. Within the first 24 h, the mother's pulse rate drops and her temperature may be slightly elevated. Since WBCs increase during labor, marked leukocytosis (to 20,000) occurs in the first 24 h postpartum. Vaginal discharge is grossly bloody **(lochia rubra)** for 3 or 4 days but changes over the next 10 to 12 days to pale brown **(lochia serosa)** and finally to yellowish white **(lochia alba).** The total volume is about 250 mL; intravaginal tampons (changed frequently) or external pads may be used to absorb it. Urine temporarily increases in volume and may contain protein and sugar. Loss of fluid elevates the Hct and ESR for a few days. The uterus involutes progressively; after 5 to 7 days, it is firm and nontender, extending midway between symphysis and umbilicus. By 2 wk, it is no longer palpable abdominally. Contractions of the involuting uterus are often painful and may require analgesics.

Management in the Hospital

The possibility of maternal infection, hemorrhage, and pain must be minimized. Observation, periodic uterine massage, and dilute oxytocin drip administration (or IM injection of 10 u. of oxytocin) are required for 1 h immediately after delivery of the placenta to ensure that the uterus contracts and remains contracted to prevent excess bleeding. If general anesthesia was used during delivery, additional supervision (preferably in a recovery room equipped with suction devices), O_2 administration, a ready source of blood tested for compatibility or type O-negative, and IV fluids must be available for 2 to 3 h after delivery.

After the first 24 h, postpartum recovery is rapid. Regular diet should be offered as soon as the patient requests food, sometimes shortly after delivery. Full ambulation is encouraged as soon as possible. Exercises to strengthen abdominal muscles may be started after 1 day. Sit-ups done lying in bed with the knees elevated tighten only the abdominal muscles and will not cause a backache. The perineum should be washed with

warm water 2 or 3 times daily. Shower baths can be encouraged, but vaginal douching is prohibited during the early puerperium. Pain from an uncomfortable or painful episiotomy can be relieved with hot sitz baths several times daily as long as necessary; codeine 30 mg and aspirin 650 mg q 4 h may be required (if the woman is breast-feeding, use acetaminophen 650 mg without codeine instead of aspirin).

Bladder care is important. Urine retention, bladder overdistention, and catheterization should be avoided if possible. Rapid diuresis may occur, especially when oxytocins are discontinued. Ambulation, encouragement to void, and surveillance to prevent asymptomatic bladder overfilling are essential. The patient should be encouraged to defecate before leaving the hospital, although with early discharge, patients often leave before a bowel movement has occurred. Laxatives may be needed if constipation exists. If a bowel movement has not occurred within 3 days, a mild cathartic can be given. Hemorrhoids can be prevented by maintaining good bowel function and can be treated with hot sitz baths.

A CBC should be done before discharge to verify that the mother is not anemic. Seronegative women should be immunized against rubella on the day of discharge. If the mother is Rh-negative, is not sensitized, and has an Rh-positive infant, she should be given 300 μg of γ globulin with a high titer of anti-Rh within 72 h of delivery to prevent sensitization.

Breast engorgement may become very painful during early lactation, when the amount of milk is beginning to increase. Managing engorgement in the nursing mother is discussed under MANAGEMENT OF THE NORMAL NEWBORN in Ch. 23. If the mother is not going to breast-feed, lactation can be suppressed by giving bromocriptine mesylate 2.5 mg bid with meals for 14 days. Rebound symptoms are common. Firm support of the breasts is needed, since drooping stimulates the let-down reflex and encourages milk flow. Many women find that tight binding of the breasts, oral fluid intake, and aspirin prn followed by firm support work well, with symptoms lasting only 3 to 5 days.

Postpartum depression ("blues") usually appears within 24 h of delivery, is usually limited to 72 h, and is common. If this depression lasts longer than 72 h or is associated with lack of interest in the infant, suicidal or homicidal thoughts, hallucinations, or psychotic behavior, it is pathologic. True psychosis is probably the emergence of preexisting mental illness in response to the physical and psychic stress of pregnancy and delivery; psychotherapy is needed.

Management at Home

The mother and child can be discharged as early as 24 h postpartum if both are normal. Medication may be offered for sleep and pain as necessary but should be limited in the nursing mother, since most drugs are secreted in breast milk (see under DRUGS IN LACTATING MOTHERS in Ch. 23). Normal activities may be resumed at will. Many family-centered obstetric units discharge patients as early as 6 h postpartum if major anesthesia was not used and no complications occurred. Major problems are rare, but a home visit or close follow-up regimen is necessary.

Intercourse may be resumed as soon as desired and comfortable; however, contraceptive measures are required, since pregnancy is possible. Oral contraceptives should be started after the first menstrual period but only in women who are not breast-feeding. Some authorities advocate starting oral contraceptives within the first postpartum week in non-nursing mothers. A diaphragm should be fitted only after complete involution of the uterus at 6 to 8 wk. In the meantime, foams, jellies, and condoms should be used. In nonlactating women, earliest ovulation is about 6 wk postpartum, usually following the first menses. However, conception has been reported as early as 2 wk postpartum, so ovulation can occur earlier. Nursing mothers tend to ovulate, then menstruate, usually at 10 to 12 wk postpartum. An occasional nursing mother ovulates and menstruates (and becomes pregnant) as quickly as a nonlactating woman. Prevention of pregnancy for several months to allow complete recovery is in the woman's best interest. Rubella immunization mandates a delay of 3 mo before a woman should become pregnant.

PUERPERAL INFECTION

Puerperal infection is presumed when the mother's temperature rises to 38° C (100.4° F) or above on any 2 successive days after the first 24 h postpartum and other causes are not apparent. Infections directly related to delivery commonly involve the genital tract; they occur in the vagina, uterus, or parametria. Renal infections also commonly occur early after delivery. Other causes of fever, such as femoral thrombophlebitis and breast infection, tend to occur after the 3rd postpartum day.

Etiology

Febrile amnionitis during labor may be followed by a secondary endometritis, myometritis, parametritis, or puerperal pyrexia. Certain conditions predispose normal vaginal bacteria (such as anaerobic streptococci and staphylococci) to become pathogenic in the puerperium; these include anemia, preeclampsia, prolonged rupture of the membranes, prolonged labor, traumatic delivery, repeated examination, retention of placental fragments within the uterus, and postpartum hemorrhage. The same factors enable exogenously introduced contaminants (Escherichia coli, β- hemolytic streptococci, Streptococcus faecalis, anaerobic organisms, and even Clostridium perfringens) to multiply in the uterus and vagina.

Symptoms, Signs, and Diagnosis

Even in the first 12 h, a significant fever must be evaluated by examining the lungs and uterus and obtaining cultures of the urinary tract and lochia. After 2 or 3 days of low-grade fever, higher temperatures occur. The most common cause of fever in early puerperium is dehydration, but puerperal infection typically begins with evidence of uterine infection.

Chills, headache, malaise, and anorexia are common. Pallor, tachycardia, and leukocytosis are the rule. The uterus is soft, large, and tender. Lochia may be diminished or profuse and malodorous; the prognosis is more ominous when uterine drainage is reduced. When the parametria are involved, pain and pyrexia are severe; the large, tender uterus is fixed by painful induration at the base of the broad ligaments and extending to the pelvic walls. Peritonitis and/or pelvic thrombophlebitis (with risk of pulmonary embolization) may complicate the illness. Endotoxemia, endotoxic shock, and renal tubular or cortical necrosis may follow virulent puerperal sepsis due to aerobic streptococci or other anaerobes and E. coli and may be fatal.

Treatment

Preventing or decreasing the predisposing factors is primary. Although vaginal delivery cannot be made sterile, postpartum infections are uncommon today because of better aseptic techniques. The most commonly found organism is E. coli; coagulase-negative staphylococci, enterococci, anaerobic cocci, and *Bacteroides* have also been isolated frequently.

An initial antibiotic (eg, ampicillin/sulbactam 1.5 to 3.0 gm q 6 h or ticarcillin/clavulanate potassium 3.1 gm q 6 h) should be given IV until the patient is afebrile for 48 h. Oral treatment is not necessary.

PYELONEPHRITIS

Pyelonephritis may occur postpartum, the result of bacteria ascending from the bladder. The infection may begin as asymptomatic bacteriuria during pregnancy and is sometimes associated with catheterization of the bladder to relieve urinary distention during and after labor. The symptoms include high fever, flank pain, general malaise, constipation, and occasionally, painful urination. The causative organism is usually coliform, and **treatment** is cefazolin 1 gm q 8 h IV until the patient is afebrile for 48 h. Sensitivities should be checked and appropriate treatment continued for 2 wk after discharge. High intake of liquids should be encouraged to maintain good kidney function. A urine culture should be repeated 6 to 8 wk after delivery to verify cure.

OTHER PUERPERAL INFECTIONS

A fever between days 4 and 10 postpartum may indicate a developing femoral thrombophlebitis; it should be treated by standard methods. Latent pulmonary TB may be activated by lowering the diaphragm following delivery and should also be treated by standard methods. Febrile reactions late in the puerperium are frequently due to mastitis, although cystitis is also common. Breast abscesses are exceedingly rare and are treated with antibiotics aimed at *Staphylococcus aureus*. Breast-feeding need not be stopped if the infection improves. If an abscess occurs, incision and drainage is necessary.

POSTPARTUM HEMORRHAGE

Blood loss of > 500 mL during or after the 3rd stage of labor. After infection, postpartum hemorrhage is the major cause of maternal mortality. The causes vary, and most are avoidable. They include hemorrhage from the placental site (associated with an atonic uterus resulting from overdistention, prolonged or dysfunctional labor, grand multiparity, or relaxant anesthesia) and from lacerations, retained products of conception, or hypofibrinogenemia. Serious blood loss

usually occurs early but may appear as late as 1 mo after delivery.

Treatment, as for infection, begins with prevention. Antepartum correction of anemia, recognition of hydramnios or multiple gestation, and discovery of an unusual blood type or history of puerperal hemorrhage are helpful. Careful, unhurried delivery, with a minimum of intervention, is always wise. After placental separation, oxytocin 10 u. IM or dilute oxytocin drip (10 u./1000 mL) generally ensures uterine contraction and reduces the inevitable blood loss. The placenta must be examined thoroughly for completeness. If it is incomplete, the uterus must be explored manually and missing fragments recovered. If the placenta does not separate spontaneously within 30 min after delivery, manual removal is advised. Rarely, curettage is required to remove infected placental fragments and decidua. Uterine contraction and the amount of vaginal bleeding must be observed for 1 h after completion of the 3rd stage of labor.

If hemorrhage occurs, bimanual uterine massage and IV oxytocin drip are required. If bleeding persists, blood should be replaced and the uterus explored for lacerations or retained secundines. The cervix and the vagina are also examined. Injection of prostaglandin $F_{2\alpha}$ directly into the myometrium has been used with success. If contractions cannot be stimulated in a refractory atonic uterus, hypogastric artery ligation or hysterectomy may be required.

INVERTED UTERUS

A crisis that occurs when the corpus turns inside out, emerging through the cervix into the vagina or out beyond the introitus. It most commonly occurs with too much fundal pressure by an inexperienced operator or with too much traction on the cord of an adherent placenta.

The easiest and simplest way to reinvert the uterus is to push the corpus up into the vaginal canal, then pass a catheter into the vagina and occlude the introitus with the hand. Saline is flushed by hydraulic pressure (the saline is held 3 to 4 ft above the patient's abdomen) so that it inflates the vagina and reinverts the uterus.

Manual attempts to reinvert the uterus may result in its inadvertent puncture by the examiner's fingers. Rarely, surgical exploration is necessary. The constricting ring between the uterosacral ligaments is incised, and the uterus is reinverted.

§2. SEXUALLY TRANSMITTED DISEASES

20. HUMAN IMMUNODEFICIENCY VIRUS (HIV) INFECTION

Infection caused by one of several related retroviruses that become incorporated into host cell DNA and result in a wide range of clinical presentations varying from asymptomatic carrier states to severely debilitating and fatal disorders. **Acquired immunodeficiency syndrome (AIDS)** *is a secondary immunodeficiency syndrome resulting from HIV infection and characterized by opportunistic infections, malignancies, neurologic dysfunction, and a variety of other syndromes.*

Etiology and Pathogenesis

A transmissible retrovirus that was isolated by 3 different laboratories and named human T-cell lymphotropic virus type III (**HTLV-III**), lymphadenopathy-associated virus (**LAV**), and AIDS-associated retrovirus (**ARV**) has been renamed the **human immunodeficiency virus (HIV)**. Two closely related viruses, **HIV-1** and **HIV-2**, have been identified as causing AIDS in different geographic regions. HIV-1 causes most cases of AIDS in the Western Hemisphere, Europe, and Central, South, and East Africa; HIV-2, which appears less virulent than HIV-1, is the principal agent of AIDS in West Africa. In certain areas of West Africa, both organisms are prevalent.

All retroviruses contain an enzyme called reverse transcriptase that converts viral RNA into a proviral DNA copy that becomes integrated into the host cell DNA. These integrated proviruses are duplicated with normal cellular genes during each cell division. Thus, all progeny of the originally infected cell will contain the retroviral DNA. In addition, multiple copies of the infectious virus may be produced, causing other cells to become infected.

Retroviruses cause both malignant and nonmalignant diseases. Expression of the viral genes of some retroviruses may be oncogenic, converting the cell into a cancer, or may have other pathologic effects that may alter normal cell function or produce cell death. The same virus may cause different diseases in different animals; eg, bovine leukemia virus causes a B cell lymphoma in cows, a T cell lymphoma in sheep, and an immunodeficiency disorder similar to AIDS in rabbits and subhuman primates. Of the retroviruses known to infect humans, HTLV types I and II are associated with lymphoid neoplasms

and neurologic disease but not with severe immunosuppression, while HIV causes immunosuppression but does not appear to cause neoplasms directly.

HIV infects a major subset of T cells defined phenotypically by the T4 or CD4 transmembrane glycoprotein and functionally as helper/inducer cells. HIV also infects nonlymphoid cells, such as pulmonary macrophages, microglial cells of the brain, and dendritic cells in the skin and lymph nodes. As a result, the numbers and functions of T cells, B cells, natural killer cells, and monocytes-macrophages are disturbed. Despite abnormalities of other than CD4+ lymphocytes, much of the immunologic dysfunction in AIDS appears to be explained by loss of these critically important helper lymphocytes.

The best single predictor of onset of the serious opportunistic infections that define AIDS (see TABLE 20–1) has been the total circulating number of **CD4+ lymphocytes**. This number is the product of (1) the WBC count, (2) the percentage of lymphocytes in the WBCs, and (3) the percentage of lymphocytes that bear the CD4+ marker. Vulnerability to opportunistic infections increases markedly when CD4+ lymphocyte levels are < 200 to 300/μL. Other evidence of decreased cell-mediated (lymphocyte-macrophage) immunity is loss of delayed hypersensitivity to intradermally injected antigens such as the PPD skin test for TB.

The pattern of loss of CD4+ lymphocytes proceeds in 3 phases and at rates varying from patient to patient. Within months of infection, circulating CD4+ cell numbers drop rapidly by 40 to 50%, from 1000 to 1300/μL to 600 to 800/μL. Then a prolonged period of slower decline is followed by another rapid decline in the 1- to 2-yr period before AIDS develops. The reason lymphocyte depletion rates vary over time and between individuals is unclear, and the mechanisms underlying their destruction are unknown.

Humoral immunity is also defective. Hyperplasia of B (antibody-producing) lymphocytes in lymph nodes causes lymphadenopathy and increased secretion of antibodies, leading to hyperglobulinemia. Production of antibodies to previously encountered antigens persists, providing adults with partial protection against a vari-

TABLE 20−1. REVISED SURVEILLANCE CASE DEFINITION FOR AIDS IN ADULTS*

Diseases diagnosed definitively without laboratory evidence of HIV infection or immunosuppressive drugs or other causes of immunodeficiency

Candidiasis of esophagus, trachea, bronchi, or lungs
Cryptococcosis outside the lung
Cryptosporidial diarrhea for > 1 mo
Cytomegalovirus infection exclusive of liver, spleen, or lymph nodes
Herpes simplex causing skin ulcers for > 1 mo or pneumonia, bronchitis, or esophagitis
Kaposi's sarcoma in patients < 60 yr
Lymphoma of the brain in patients < 60 yr
Lymphoid interstitial pneumonitis
Disseminated *Mycobacterium avium* complex infection
Pneumocystis carinii pneumonia
Progressive multifocal leukoencephalopathy or parvovirus encephalitis
Toxoplasmic encephalitis

Diseases diagnosed definitively with laboratory evidence of HIV infection

Multiple or recurrent bacterial infections
Disseminated coccidioidomycosis
HIV encephalopathy
Disseminated histoplasmosis
Isosporal diarrhea for > 1 mo
Kaposi's sarcoma at any age
Lymphoma of brain at any age
Non-Hodgkin's lymphoma of B cell or unknown phenotype
Disseminated mycobacterial infections
Recurrent salmonella (nontyphoidal) septicemia
Severe wasting or slim disease

* Centers for Disease Control, 1987.

ety of pathogens such as encapsulated bacteria. However, response to new antigens is defective, if not totally absent. Thus, total antibody levels (especially IgG and IgA) may be elevated and titers of antibodies to specific agents (eg, cytomegalovirus) may be unusually high, but response to immunizations is usually suboptimal.

Epidemiology

HIV is not transmitted by casual contact or even the close, nonsexual contact that normally occurs at work, in school, or at home. Transmission requires **contact with body fluids** containing infected cells or plasma. HIV may be present in any fluid or exudate that contains plasma or lymphocytes, specifically blood, semen, vaginal secretions, breast milk, or saliva. However, transmission by saliva or droplet nuclei produced by coughing or sneezing has not been documented.

Infected cells can reach target cells in a new host via blood transfusion, accidental injection, or after mucous membrane exposure. The role of mucous membrane inflammation is illustrated by the enhancing effect of other sexually transmitted diseases **(STDs)** on susceptibility to HIV infection. Epidemiologic studies suggest that sexual transmission of HIV is more likely in the presence of herpes, syphilis, and other STDs. Nevertheless, female chimpanzees have been infected experimentally via vaginal exposure without trauma or coexisting infection.

Transmission by **accidental needlestick**, estimated at about 1/200 accidents, is much more difficult and much less frequent than transmission of hepatitis B, presumably because of the relatively low number of HIV virions in blood. Risk of transmission may be increased by deep injections or injection of blood.

The extremely low risk of transmission by casual contact deserves emphasis. In one study, nonsexual household contacts (68 children, 33 adults) of patients with AIDS or AIDS-related complex with oral candidiasis were evaluated. The contacts had lived in the same household with a patient for ≥ 3 mo and had shared household items and facilities with the patient for a median of 22 mo. Close personal interactions (eg, assisting the patient with bathing, dressing, and eating) were common. The only contact found to have HIV infection was a 5-yr-old daughter of 2 IV drug abusers; the daughter had most likely been infected perinatally, rather than horizontally.

Since AIDS was first recognized in 1981, when cases of *Pneumocystis carinii* pneumonia and Kaposi's sarcoma were reported in homosexual men in California and New York, it has reached epidemic proportions; > 100,000 deaths were reported through 1990. Two epidemiologic patterns of HIV transmission are recognized. In the USA and Europe (pattern 1), epidemiologic characteristics of persons with AIDS remained remarkably similar throughout the first decade (1980–1990) of the epidemic. Some 90% of patients were 20 to 49 yr old, 93% were men, and 94% could be placed in groups that suggest a possible means of acquiring the disease (eg, homosexual or bisexual men, IV drug users, heterosexual sex partners of infected persons, and recipients of transfused blood or blood components). Of those unassigned to a high-risk group, many could not be fully investigated. The proportions in these risk groups remained relatively stable. While heterosexual spread of AIDS has been much less rapid than the spread among homosexual men in Western countries, experts predict it will increase on the basis of experience in Central Africa and other tropical areas, as well as certain trends. In the USA, > 10% of AIDS cases have occurred in women, and new diagnoses of AIDS in women are increasing at a more rapid rate than those in men.

Among persons with hemophilia, AIDS has become the leading cause of death. Before 1985, the risk of HIV infection among hemophiliacs correlated with large requirements for Factor VIII concentrates and the origin of plasma products used in the USA. The widespread use of commercial plasma products for hemophiliacs resulted in a high rate of HIV infection, even in areas not affected by the epidemic until after 1985. In most of Europe, where clotting factor material was collected from populations with lower risk of HIV infection, fewer hemophiliacs were infected. However, routine heat treatment of plasma products in the USA has subsequently eliminated the risk of infection.

In Africa, the Caribbean Basin, and Southeast Asia, the epidemiologic pattern (pattern 2) is very different from that in the USA and Europe. Transmission is primarily heterosexual, the sexes are equally affected, and homosexuality is not a common risk factor. Mixtures of patterns 1 and 2 are found in some Latin American countries (eg, Brazil).

Infection of large numbers of women of childbearing age has led to a substantial number of pediatric cases of AIDS (see HUMAN IMMUNODEFI-

CIENCY VIRUS INFECTION IN CHILDREN under VIRAL INFECTIONS in Ch. 32). HIV can be transmitted transplacentally or perinatally. The virus has been demonstrated in breast milk, and breast-feeding has also been implicated, although rarely, in transmission. In addition, several major epidemics of HIV infection among neonates have resulted from contamination of inadequately sterilized needles. The continuing spread of HIV in developing countries with minimal resources to manage the epidemic is an ominous pattern with grave implications.

AIDS is the most severe manifestation of a spectrum of HIV-related conditions (see Symptoms and Signs, below). The risk that a person infected with HIV will develop AIDS is estimated to be 1 to 2%/yr in the first several years after infection and about 5%/yr thereafter. The cumulative risk is 35 to 45% after the first 8 to 10 yr. Because of the limited (1 decade) experience with HIV, the pattern of progression to AIDS after the first decade is not known, but the possibility remains that almost all HIV-infected persons will develop AIDS. Furthermore, some of the long-term sequelae of HIV infection (eg, other malignancies and chronic neurologic diseases) may not yet have been elucidated, because they will appear only after more prolonged carriage.

Symptoms and Signs

A broad spectrum of sequential clinical problems may occur after infection with HIV. Immediately after infection and for a prolonged period (several years in a small number of persons), there may be an antibody-negative asymptomatic carrier state. During this time, the virus may be truly latent or reproducing so slowly that it is not recognized by the immune system. However, highly sensitive techniques for amplifying HIV nucleic acids (the polymerase chain reaction) can detect the infection, even when no antibody to HIV is detectable. Within 2 to 4 wk after infection, a minority of patients have a 3- to 14-day acute mononucleosis-like syndrome (primary HIV infection) with fever, malaise, rash, arthralgias, and generalized lymphadenopathy, usually followed in 1 to 3 mo by seroconversion for antibody to HIV. Subsequently, these manifestations disappear (although lymphadenopathy usually persists) and the patients may become antibody-positive asymptomatic carriers. During the asymptomatic, seropositive stage, most patients have reduced numbers of CD4+ lymphocytes. Some of these patients develop mild, remittent symptoms and signs that do not meet the definition of AIDS or AIDS-related complex (eg, persistent generalized lymphadenopathy).

The AIDS-related complex (ARC) is a constellation of chronic symptoms and signs manifested by HIV-infected persons who have not had the opportunistic infections or tumors that define AIDS. These symptoms, signs, and laboratory abnormalities include generalized lymphadenopathy, weight loss, intermittent fever, malaise, fatigue, chronic diarrhea, leukopenia, anemia, immune-mediated thrombocytopenia, oral hairy leukoplakia, and oral thrush (candidiasis). A severe manifestation of ARC is the wasting syndrome (called slim disease in Africa), which is characterized by progressive weight loss $\geq$ 15% body wt.

AIDS is defined by the development of opportunistic infections and/or certain secondary cancers known to be associated with HIV infection, such as Kaposi's sarcoma and non-Hodgkin's lymphoma, especially primary lymphoma of the brain (see TABLE 20–1). Many patients are first seen with a life-threatening opportunistic infection or malignancy without the preceding symptoms of ARC.

Neurologic symptoms often are the first manifestation of AIDS and commonly occur during its course. Neurologic disorders include acute and chronic aseptic meningitis (see Ch. 32), peripheral neuropathies with weakness and paresthesias, and encephalopathy with seizures, with focal motor, sensory, or gait deficits, and with progressive dementia. Infections, neoplasms, vascular complications, aseptic meningitis, and neuropathy are among the more prominent sequelae.

CNS infections: The most common treatable neurologic illness is toxoplasmic encephalitis. Headache, lethargy, confusion, seizures, and focal signs evolve over days to weeks. CT findings include ring-enhancing lesions with a predilection for basal ganglia. Serologic tests for IgG antitoxoplasmal antibodies reflecting previous infection are almost always positive but do not always provide conclusive proof that the lesion is caused by Toxoplasma organisms. The CSF shows a mild to moderate pleocytosis and elevated protein content. Brain biopsy can be diagnostic. Treatment is with pyrimethamine and sulfadiazine (or clindamycin if the patient is allergic to sulfa). Prognosis is at best guarded, since recurrence is possible and other complications of AIDS are likely. Cryptococcal and tuberculous meningitides (Mycobacterium avium-intracellulare) also occur in AIDS. Progressive multifocal

leukoencephalopathy and infections with Candida, Aspergillus, and gram-negative organisms occur less frequently.

A serious neurologic complication is a subacute encephalitis caused by either HIV or cytomegalovirus. The gray matter exhibits nodular collections of microglial cells without other inflammatory infiltrates. Intranuclear and intracytoplasmic inclusions have been observed within the nodules. Small, poorly defined foci of perivenular demyelination are found in white matter. Memory loss, confusion, psychomotor retardation, myoclonus, seizures, and dementia progressing to coma are typical findings spanning weeks to months prior to death. Cortical atrophy on CT, CSF pleocytosis and elevated protein level, and a diffusely abnormal EEG are often, albeit inconsistently, found but are nonspecific.

Neoplasms: Primary CNS lymphoma is a frequent intracranial mass lesion in AIDS. It may be clinically silent or may produce focal signs consistent with its anatomic location. CT usually shows a contrast-enhancing mass that cannot always be distinguished from abscess or other lesions; in these cases, MRI may be more discriminating.

Systemic lymphomas in AIDS may involve the CNS. Kaposi's sarcoma rarely involves the CNS.

Vascular complications: Nonbacterial endocarditis, usually with neoplasm or severe infection, can produce transient ischemic attacks and focal ischemic stroke. Cerebral hemorrhage can occur in thrombocytopenic states (eg, lymphoma, idiopathic thrombocytopenic purpura).

Aseptic meningitis: Rapid onset of headache, fever, stiff neck, and photophobia may be associated with a CSF mononuclear pleocytosis, elevated proteins, slightly depressed glucose, and consistently negative cytologic studies and cultures. The episodes are transient but can be recurrent.

Peripheral neuropathy: Painful dysesthesias, moderate distal sensory loss (stocking-and-glove), depressed ankle reflexes, distal weakness, and atrophy can occur in varying degrees and can coincide with rapid weight loss from poor nutrition; no metabolic cause has been identified. A Guillain-Barré type of neuropathy has been reported. Myopathy similar to polymyositis may complicate AIDS or zidovudine therapy.

Treatment of neurologic disorders: Most CNS complications of AIDS respond poorly or not at all to treatment, since the primary immune defect remains uncorrected. The prognosis is poor; responses to retrovirals have been well documented only for cognitive dysfunction.

A few patients present with **renal insufficiency or nephrotic syndrome** (see in Ch. 41), with **symptomatic anemia**, or with **immune-mediated thrombocytopenia.** HIV-associated thrombocytopenia occurs throughout the full spectrum of HIV infections, usually responds to the same interventions (corticosteroids, splenectomy, IV immune globulin) as idiopathic thrombocytopenic purpura, and seldom leads to bleeding.

Patterns of specific opportunists vary both geographically and between risk groups. In the USA and Europe, > 90% of AIDS patients with Kaposi's syndrome (**KS**) were homosexual or bisexual men, possibly because of an unidentified, sexually transmissible cofactor. Recently the incidence of KS has been diminishing. Most AIDS cases in the USA and Europe (about 60%) present with *Pneumocystis carinii* pneumonia, which is reported less frequently in Africa. Toxoplasmosis and TB are more common in tropical areas where the prevalence of latent infections with *Toxoplasma gondii* and *Mycobacterium tuberculosis* in the general population is high. Even in developed countries where background levels of TB are low, HIV infections have caused increased rates and atypical presentations of TB.

The clinical presentation and course of HIV infection in women has not been as well defined as that in men and children. HIV prevalence appears to be greater in women with some sexually transmitted diseases (**STDs**) and with chronic refractory vaginal candidiasis. Some of these STDs may be clinically atypical, more aggressive, and resistant to treatment. While these issues need further study, cervical neoplasia and pelvic inflammatory disease are of particular concern. Meanwhile, it seems prudent to recommend HIV testing to women with recurrent, aggressive, or unusually resistant STDs. In HIV-infected women, careful attention to evaluation of genital organs is recommended; eg, annual or perhaps semiannual Pap tests and a rigorous approach to colposcopic evaluation and biopsy when Pap tests are abnormal.

Laboratory Findings and Diagnosis

Clinical suspicion of HIV infection should be high for persons with potential exposure to HIV and any of the clinical manifestations described above. The isolation of HIV or detection of HIV antigen in blood provides the most specific diag-

nosis of HIV infection, but the former is expensive, cumbersome, and not widely available and the latter is insensitive. The demonstration of antibodies to HIV is sensitive and specific at most stages of infection, inexpensive, and widely available.

Two tests for detecting antibody to HIV are widely used. The first is an enzyme-linked immunosorbent assay (**ELISA**), which detects antibodies to HIV proteins. Newer generations of ELISA are both highly sensitive and specific in most situations. However, most positive ELISA tests in asymptomatic persons who do not belong to a high-risk group (eg, those that occur during blood screening) are false-positives. When an ELISA is positive in low-risk patients, *the test should be repeated on the same sample.* If it is positive a second time, the recommendation is to confirm the ELISA with a test that is more specific; ie, the **Western blot.** The Western blot is an immunoelectrophoretic procedure for identifying antibodies to specific viral proteins separated by their molecular weight. Patients with repeatedly positive ELISA and confirming test (eg, Western blot) results should be considered infected and contagious. Use of ELISA to screen blood donors can vastly reduce the risk of acquiring HIV by transfusion.

Individuals in the early stages of HIV infection, who have not yet mounted an antibody response, may have negative ELISA and Western blot results (**false-negatives**). A few persons have been reported to remain antibody-negative while yielding positive results for viral nucleic acids by the highly sensitive polymerase chain reaction (**PCR**) for several years. These persons may account for the very low, but continuing, risk of transfusion-associated HIV infection (estimated at between 1/10,000 and 1/100,000 per unit transfused). Levels of antibody to HIV may decrease in advanced stages of AIDS, but this usually does not represent a diagnostic problem.

ELISAs that directly measure viral antigens (eg, p24) rather than antiviral antibodies are commercially available but are relatively insensitive. They are useful for prognosis and for measuring the antiviral effect of drugs.

The immunologic abnormalities in AIDS include anergy (demonstrated by lack of delayed hypersensitivity responses to intradermal injection of common antigens; eg, tetanus, mumps, *Candida albicans*), poor T cell proliferative responses to mitogens (phytohemagglutinin, concanavalin A) and antigens, polyclonal hypergammaglobulinemia, elevated immune complex levels, diminished antibody responses to both recall and new antigens, decreased natural killer function, and increased levels of α_1-thymosin, acid-labile interferon, neopterin, and β_2-microglobulin. The T cell deficiency is due to decreased numbers and function of CD4 + lymphocytes. Suppressor/cytotoxic CD8 + lymphocytes, which are functionally normal and increased in number, may contribute further to immunosuppression. This leads to reduction of the normal CD4:CD8 ratio (about 2:1) to < 1. Decreased CD4:CD8 ratios are not diagnostic of AIDS, since a variety of viral infections (eg, cytomegalovirus, Epstein-Barr virus, influenza, and hepatitis B) may produce transient reductions. In patients with AIDS who develop opportunistic infections, circulating CD4 + lymphocytes are usually < 200/µL.

The risk for an HIV-infected person of developing AIDS within 2 to 3 yr can be estimated by combining several measures, such as CD4 + lymphocyte count, levels of B2-microglobulin or neopterin, and the presence of detectable p24 antigen. These estimates may also be used to determine indications for beginning antiretroviral therapy or prophylaxis against opportunistic infections.

Prognosis

Although there have been no complete recoveries from AIDS, a few patients are long-term (> 5 yr) survivors; eg, patients with KS who do not have severe immune defects or opportunistic infections. In one large study conducted before use of zidovudine (ZDU, formerly called azidothymidine [AZT]), the median survival varied with the initial clinical manifestation: For patients with KS alone, it was 125 wk; with P. carinii pneumonia alone, 35 wk; and with any other opportunistic infection, 18 wk. While about 85% of these patients survived their initial hospitalization, their quality of life was markedly compromised and about 1/2 spent 30 to 50% of their remaining lifetime in the hospital. ZDU has increased severalfold the median survival for patients diagnosed with P. carinii pneumonia (80% survive for 1 yr). Despite these advances, opportunistic infections are the cause of death in > 95% of AIDS patients. However, advances in prophylaxis for Pneumocystis and in management of other opportunistic infections have decreased their incidence as well as their morbidity and mortality.

Prevention

A number of strategies are being developed to induce protective immunity in persons not infected with HIV. Immunogens include whole killed virus, genetically-engineered viral proteins and peptides (eg, from the viral envelope), and vaccinia virus genetically modified to express HIV viral proteins. These efforts are hampered by the lack of a defined marker of protective immunity such as broadly cross-reactive, neutralizing antibody or a convenient animal model. Nevertheless, some of these vaccines seem likely to be field-tested for protective efficacy within the next few years.

Most infections occur as a result of repeated and close contact with a carrier of HIV, specifically mucous membrane contact with blood or body fluids. Sexual relationships are the major source of such contacts, and people must be educated to avoid unsafe sexual practices by reducing the number and frequency of sexual contacts, avoiding high-risk practices (eg, anal intercourse), and using barrier protection such as condoms. Consistent use of condoms reduces transmission of HIV by preventing exposure to semen and genital sores. Whether symptomatic or not, HIV carriers should be counseled to avoid unsafe sexual practices with uninfected persons. Because people tend to not change sexual practices readily, most homosexual men in the USA had to have some personal experience with AIDS before decreasing dangerous sexual practices and thus diminishing transmission. Although transmission among older homosexual men has been dramatically reduced, transmission and high rates of infection among younger homosexual men continue.

Since HIV may be transmitted in utero, intrapartum, or postpartum, women at risk for infection should be tested for antibody to HIV; HIV-positive women should be advised to defer pregnancy. The risk of transmission from infected women to their babies is estimated to be 30 to 50%. Use of ZDU to prevent intrapartum infection is under study, but failures have been observed. For many HIV-infected women, given the risk of transmission and the uncertainty of their own health, termination of pregnancy is the more acceptable alternative.

Parenteral drug users need to be educated and counseled with regard to the risk of sharing needles with other drug users. Ideally, this effort should be combined with rehabilitation and treatment of drug dependence.

Testing for antibody to HIV should be offered on a confidential basis to anyone requesting it but only in conjunction with pre- and posttest counseling by someone familiar with its significance. HIV carriers and persons belonging to a high-risk group—*even those with negative HIV antibody test results*—should not donate blood or organs for transplantation.

Medical and dental professionals should wear gloves when examining *all* patients if contact with mucous membranes or other wet surfaces may occur. Body fluids and tissue samples should be handled in the same manner as those from patients with hepatitis B. Accidental needle-sticks of health care personnel are remarkably common, and special emphasis must be placed on teaching all health care students and professionals how to avoid these potentially dangerous accidents. While the risk of HIV transmission appears to be much lower than that of hepatitis B transmission, the potential consequences are much worse.

Hospitalized patients with HIV infection generally need not be isolated, except when their complicating infections (eg, suspected or proven TB) require that other patients and hospital personnel be protected. Surfaces contaminated by blood or other body fluids should be cleaned and disinfected. HIV is readily inactivated by heat and commonly used disinfecting agents, including peroxide, alcohols, phenolics, and hypochlorite. Although AIDS patients are ordinarily not infectious to hospital personnel or other patients, their body fluids and blood are and should be handled with extreme care.

Use of ZDU or dideoxyinosine (DDI) for post-exposure prophylaxis following penetrating injuries involving HIV-infected blood (needlesticks) or heavy mucous membrane contamination is controversial. Because of the low risk of infection for most injuries, controlled studies of effectiveness have not proved to be practical. The potential carcinogenic or teratogenic effects of brief exposures to ZDU are unknown. Some women in early pregnancy will be offered postexposure ZDU before their pregnancy tests are positive; therefore, special caution must be used with this group, despite the perceived (but unproved) need for administration of ZDU immediately after exposure. Additional problems arise when the source or HIV status of blood is unknown.

Patients with CD4+ lymphocyte counts < 200/μL should be encouraged to begin primary prophylaxis for *P. carinii* pneumonia with trimethoprim/sulfamethoxazole, dapsone, or aerosolized pentamidine. The relative efficacy of these regimens is under study. Because the sulfonamides and sulfones appear to provoke adverse effects (eg, fever, neutropenia, skin rashes) in these patients more frequently than in persons with normal immunity, many of these patients must rely on aerosolized pentamidine.

Adequate primary prophylaxis for fungal, mycobacterial, and toxoplasmal infections is desirable but has not yet been developed. Secondary prophylaxis is indicated to prevent relapses of *P. carinii* pneumonia, cryptococcal infections, toxoplasmic encephalitis, herpes simplex, and thrush.

Treatment

As of late 1991, both **ZDU and DDI** were licensed for treatment of HIV infection. A modified form of the nucleoside thymidine, ZDU appears to slow viral replication through inhibition of reverse transcriptase, which is necessary for establishing infection in uninfected cells. As noted above, ZDU prolongs survival and reduces incidence and severity of opportunistic infections in both AIDS and ARC patients. In asymptomatic patients with CD4+ lymphocyte counts between 200 and 500/μL, ZDU appears to reduce the rate of progression to AIDS. Although evidence for the beneficial effects of DDI is less complete, DDI probably has activity similar to that of ZDU in slowing progression of infection.

The development of resistance to ZDU in isolates from AIDS patients taking the drug for more than a year raises the possibility that for some patients, ZDU will provide only a limited period of effective treatment. Fortunately, ZDU resistance does not appear to induce cross-resistance to other nucleosides. Most experts believe that persons with CD4+ counts < 500/μL should be encouraged to start ZDU therapy because they are at significant risk for progression to AIDS in several years if untreated. Treatment has been approved for all patients with CD4+ counts < 500/μL. An alternative to beginning treatment in these patients is semiannual or quarterly monitoring of those with counts > 350/μL; those whose counts drop below this level are strongly encouraged to begin treatment. Longer follow-up of treated, asymptomatic patients will probably clarify which of these strategies is more effective in the long run. Patients with HIV-related dementia, thrombocytopenia, and other HIV-related syndromes may also benefit from ZDU therapy, regardless of CD4+ count.

The toxicity of ZDU is primarily hematologic (anemia and granulocytopenia), appears to be dose-related but not necessarily cumulative, and is partially reversible. The anemia is macrocytic ($MCV > 100$ in most patients receiving the drug) but unresponsive to folate or vitamin B_{12}. Less frequently, nausea or headache may be limiting. Mild symptoms are common initially but decrease or disappear with continued use.

Hematologic toxicity may be managed by dose reduction, by erythrocyte transfusions, or by stimulation of bone marrow with cytokines such as erythropoietin or granulocyte− or granulocyte-macrophage−colony-stimulating factor (G-CSF, GM-CSF). The long-term utility and immunologic effects of these cytokines have not yet been established.

The optimal dose of ZDU has not been established, but comparative studies of 500 to 600 and 1000 to 1200 mg/day indicate equivalent benefit and less toxicity at the lower dose. The lowest effective dose of ZDU (eg, 300 mg/day) is not known, nor have optimal dosing intervals (eg, q 4 h vs. q 8 h) been established. Most patients are initially given 100 mg q 4 h with the option of missing a dose during sleep (500 to 600 mg/day).

The toxicities of DDI are primarily peripheral neuropathy and pancreatitis.

Resistance to ZDU appears to result from at least 3 nucleic acid substitutions in the reverse transcriptase enzyme of HIV. Prolonged administration (6 to 18 mo) may be necessary to select for this resistance. The clinical significance of ZDU resistance in HIV-1 is unclear, but it may help to explain the loss of both clinical and an-

tiviral effects in most patients after 1 to 2 yr. Patients taking ZDU often have a decrease in serum p24 antigen; slight increase in CD4+ lymphocyte counts; and increases in weight, energy, and well-being for many months, after which deterioration resumes.

Another nucleoside, dideoxycytidine (DDC), with excellent in vitro antiviral activity and with toxicities differing from those of ZDU, is undergoing clinical trial. DDC has similar toxicity to DDI in peripheral nerves but not in the pancreas. Alternating combinations of ZDU with DDC and DDI is being investigated; the goal of combination therapy is to achieve continuous antiviral effect with reduced toxicity and resistance.

Alternative approaches to HIV-1 treatment under study include (1) use of soluble forms of CD4; (2) inhibition of glycosylation reactions necessary for attachment of sugar molecules to viral glycoproteins; (3) inhibition of HIV protease, an enzyme necessary to cleave functional proteins from large protein precursors; and (4) immunization of infected persons to boost their protective immunologic responses. Other approaches will emerge from the intense effort aimed at improving the limited benefit provided by ZDU.

The prospect for a cure of HIV infection through conventional chemotherapy alone now seems remote. However, the goals of sustained inhibition of viral reproduction and arrest of immunodeficiency progression through chronic chemotherapy appear realizable in the near future. Restoration of immune function to normal has not yet been achieved and is the next important goal of treatment.

21.   OTHER SEXUALLY TRANSMITTED DISEASES (STDs)

(See also in Ch. 17 and Ch. 20)

The incidence of STDs, among the most common communicable diseases in the world, steadily increased from the 1950s to the 1970s but generally stabilized in the 1980s. Some diseases (eg, HIV infection, syphilis, gonorrhea) increased in incidence at the end of the 1980s in the USA and elsewhere. Diseases such as nonspecific urethritis, trichomoniasis, chlamydial infections, genital candidiasis, genital and anorectal herpes and warts (all discussed in this chapter), vulvovaginitis (see in Ch. 5), proctitis, scabies, pediculosis pubis, and molluscum contagiosum (see

Chs. 93 and 94) probably are more prevalent than the 5 historically defined venereal diseases—syphilis, gonorrhea, chancroid, lymphogranuloma venereum, and granuloma inguinale. However, because the former group is not consistently reported, incidence rates are not available. For gonorrhea, > 250 million persons worldwide and close to 3 million in the USA are estimated to be infected annually. For syphilis, annual worldwide incidence is estimated at 50 million persons, with 400,000 in the USA annually needing treatment. Other infections, including salmonellosis, giardiasis, amebiasis, shigellosis, campylobacteriosis, hepatitis A and B, and cytomegalovirus infection, sometimes are sexually transmitted. Strong associations between cervical cancer (see Ch. 10) and herpesviruses and papillomaviruses have been discovered. Since 1978, the epidemic of acquired immunodeficiency syndrome (AIDS) has spread rapidly in certain groups of homosexual men and IV drug abusers in Western countries and among heterosexuals in Africa and increasingly in developed nations (see Ch. 20).

STD incidence has risen despite advances in diagnosis and treatment that rapidly render patients with many STDs noninfectious and cure the majority. While changes in sexual behavior and access to medical care underlie the epidemic of STDs, a number of more specific causes can be delineated. Both physicians and patients have been reticent to deal openly and candidly with sexual issues. Changing sexual mores and oral contraceptives have relaxed traditional sexual restraints, especially for women. Before the AIDS epidemic, homosexual men had very high rates of STDs, which have plummeted in most American cities affected by AIDS. Additionally, reemergence of rare (eg, chancroid-producing bacillus) or evolution of drug-resistant (eg, penicillinase-producing gonococci) agents reflects highly mobile populations that import organisms from abroad. This has been most dramatically illustrated by the rapid distribution of the AIDS virus (HIV-1) in Europe and North America.

STD control depends on having good facilities for diagnosis and treatment; tracing and treating all sexual contacts of the patients; continuing to observe those who received treatment to ensure that they have been cured; educating doctors, nurses, and the public; counseling patients about responsible sexual behavior; and developing methods for producing artificial immunity against infection.

GONORRHEA

An acute infectious disease of the epithelium of the urethra, cervix, rectum, pharynx, or eyes that may lead to bacteremia and result in metastatic complications.

Etiology and Epidemiology

The causative organism, *Neisseria gonorrhoeae*, can be identified in discharges (by direct smear or after culture) as pairs or clumps of gram-negative, kidney-shaped diplococci, often intracellular and with their adjacent surfaces slightly concave.

The disease usually spreads by sexual contact. Women are frequently asymptomatic carriers of the organisms for weeks or months and often are identified when sexual contacts are traced. Symptomless infection is also common in the oropharynx and rectum in homosexual men and is occasionally found in the urethra in heterosexual men in some geographic regions.

Gonorrhea occurring in the vagina of prepubertal girls is usually caused by adults, through either sexual abuse or, rarely, fomites.

Symptoms and Signs

In men, the incubation period is from 2 to 14 days. Onset is usually marked by mild discomfort in the urethra, followed a few hours later by dysuria and a purulent discharge. Frequency and urgency of micturition develop as the disease spreads to the posterior urethra. Examination shows a purulent, yellowish-green urethral discharge; the lips of the meatus may be red and swollen.

In women, symptoms usually begin within 7 to 21 days after infection. Though symptoms generally are mild, in a few women the onset may be severe, with dysuria, frequency, and vaginal discharge. The cervix and deeper reproductive organs are the sites most frequently infected, followed by the urethra, rectum, Skene's ducts, and Bartholin's glands. The cervix may be reddened and friable, with a mucopurulent or purulent discharge. Pus may be expressed from the urethra on pressure against the symphysis pubis or from Skene's ducts or Bartholin's glands. Salpingitis is a common complication (see Ch. 5).

In women or homosexual men, rectal gonorrhea is common. It usually is symptomless in women, but perianal discomfort and a rectal discharge may occur. Severe rectal infection is more common in homosexual men. Patients may note a coating of mucopus on stools, perianal excoriation may be present, and proctoscopy may show mucopus on the rectal wall. Gonococcal pharyngitis from orogenital contact is being recognized more frequently. Although symptoms and signs often are absent, some patients may complain of a sore throat and discomfort on swallowing; the pharynx and tonsillar area may be red, sometimes with a mucopurulent exudate and occasionally with edema of the uvula and faucial pillars.

In female infants and prepubertal girls, irritation, erythema, and edema of the vulva with a purulent vaginal discharge may be accompanied by proctitis. The child may complain of soreness or dysuria, and the parents may notice staining of the underclothes.

Diagnosis

A gram-stained smear of urethral discharge allows rapid identification of the gonococcus in most (> 90%) men. However, the cervical Gram stain is only about 60% sensitive in women. Identification of the gonococcus by culture of genital exudate should always be made for women and for men with negative or equivocal urethral Gram stains. When symptoms of rectal or pharyngeal infection are present, cultures should be performed in both sexes, since Gram stains are unreliable (insensitive and nonspecific). Exudates from the urethra, cervix, rectum, and other infected sites are inoculated onto a suitable medium (eg, modified Thayer-Martin medium) and incubated at 35 to 36° C for 48 h in an atmosphere containing 3 to 10% CO_2 (a candle jar may be used). Some colonies become visible after 24 h, but most appear after 48 h. The colonies are small, circular, transparent, and usually 1 to 4 mm in diameter. Complete identification depends on characteristic appearance on Gram stain; on the oxidase test, in which positive colonies turn purple and later black on exposure to 1% di- or tetramethyl-p-phenylenediamine HCl; and on fermentation reactions. All Neisseria are oxidase-positive. N. gonorrhoeae ferments dextrose (glucose) but not maltose or sucrose. The meningococcus (N. meningitidis) ferments dextrose and maltose but not sucrose. Nonpathogenic Neisseria spp ferment either ≥ 3 carbohydrates or none and are usually inhibited by antibiotics (eg, colistin, vancomycin, nystatin) in selective media.

If adequate laboratory facilities are not immediately available, the specimen may be inoculated onto a transport medium for transfer to a laboratory. Containers with suitable media and a self-contained CO_2 supply are commercially available. For successful growth of gonococci, the specimens must be subcultured within 48 h, preferably within 24 h. Reliable serologic or rapid nonculture diagnostic tests for gonococci are not yet available for routine clinical use.

Complications

In men treated early, postgonococcal urethritis is the most common sequela. Often it results from the presence of other organisms (eg, Chlamydia trachomatis) that were acquired simultaneously with N. gonorrhoeae but have longer incubation periods and do not respond to penicillin. Less dramatic discharge or dysuria recurs 7 to 14 days after penicillin treatment for gonorrhea. Epididymitis, another important complication, is usually unilateral; if it is bilateral, sterility may result. Infection descends from the posterior urethra along the vas deferens to the lower pole of the epididymis. The testicle is painful, and the epididymis and spermatic cord become hot, tender, and swollen. A secondary hydrocele may follow. Abscesses of Tyson's and Littre's glands, periurethral abscesses, infection of Cowper's glands and the prostate, urethral stricture, and infection of the seminal vesicles are less common complications.

In women, salpingitis is the most important clinical problem (see Ch. 5).

In either sex, disseminated gonococcal infection (DGI) with bacteremia may occur, but it is more common in women. In the arthritis-dermatitis syndrome, the patient presents with a mild febrile illness, malaise, migratory polyarthralgias or polyarthritis, or a few pustular skin lesions, often on the periphery of the limbs (each symptom is present in about $2/3$ of the patients). The genital infection is often symptomless, but bacteriologic tests of the genital secretions may show gonococci. In about $1/2$ of the cases, the organism can be grown from the bloodstream (blood cultures are most often positive in the first week) or joint fluid. The gonococcus can sometimes be demonstrated in pus from skin lesions by using immunofluorescence techniques. Any potential source of bacteremia should be cultured. Patients with DGI almost never have positive blood and synovial fluid cultures simultaneously. Bacteremia has serious potential sequelae; pericarditis, endocarditis, meningitis, and perihepatitis occasionally occur and rarely are fatal.

Gonococcal arthritis, a more focal form of DGI, may or may not be preceded by symptomatic bacteremia. The onset is acute, with fever, severe pain, and limitation of movement (usually in one or a few joints, as opposed to DGI, which involves multiple joints). The joint is swollen and tender, and the overlying skin is hot and red. Synovial fluid is increased, and aspiration produces purulent fluid (WBCs > 25,000) from which gonococci can be visulized on Gram stain and cultured. Analysis should be performed and treatment started immediately, before destruction of the articular surfaces of the joint occurs.

Any purulent joint effusion should be considered septic and treated until proved otherwise.

Ocular infections may occur in newborns (see under NEONATAL INFECTIONS in Ch. 27) and adults (see Ch. 79).

Treatment

Blood specimens for STS should always be obtained before treatment is started, and the patient should be thoroughly examined to exclude other STDs. STS should be repeated in 3 mo.

The infectious nature of gonorrhea should be explained to the patient, who should abstain from sexual activity until cure is confirmed. Men should also be advised not to squeeze the penis in a search for urethral discharges. All sexual contacts of the patient should be traced, examined, and treated.

The emergence of penicillin- and tetracycline-resistant gonococci has shifted treatment from previously recommended penicillin-, ampicillin-, and tetracycline-based regimens. However, co-existing chlamydial infections are sufficiently common to require presumptive treatment with a prolonged course of an oral tetracycline.

The Centers for Disease Control now recommend a single dose of ceftriaxone 250 mg IM plus doxycycline 100 mg orally bid for 7 days as initial therapy for urethral, endocervical, pharyngeal, and rectal infections. Alternatives to ceftriaxone are spectinomycin 2 gm IM once, ciprofloxacin 500 mg orally once, norfloxacin 800 mg orally once, cefuroxime 1 gm orally once with probenecid 1 gm, cefotaxime 1 gm IM once, and ceftizoxime 500 mg IM once. All regimens should be accompanied by doxycycline 100 mg orally bid for 7 days, except in pregnant women, for whom erythromycin base 500 mg orally qid for 7 days should be substituted. In patients known to harbor penicillin-sensitive gonococci, amoxicillin 3 gm orally once may be used instead of ceftriaxone.

For **DGI**, ceftriaxone 1 gm IM or IV daily, ceftizoxime 1 gm IV q 8 h, cefotaxime 1 gm IV q 8 h, and spectinomycin 2 gm IM q 12 h are considered equivalent. For known penicillin-sensitive infections, ampicillin 1 gm orally q 6 h is adequate. Duration of treatment for DGI is not well defined, but regimens ranging from 3 to 10 days appear equally successful. Repeated cultures of joint fluid may be advisable for slowly responsive arthritis.

In **gonococcal arthritis**, in which sterile joint effusions may persist for 7 to 14 days, addition of an anti-inflammatory drug seems beneficial. Repeated drainage is usually unnecessary, but initially the joint is kept immobilized in an optimal functional position. Passive range-of-motion exercises should be started as soon as possible, as should quadriceps-setting exercises, if the knee is involved. As soon as the pain subsides, more active exercises, with stretching, active range of motion, and muscle strengthening, should be done at least twice daily. Over 95% of patients treated for gonococcal arthritis recover complete joint function.

One week after treatment, to confirm that the patient is cured and no longer infectious, specimens from accessible infected sites (except joints) should be cultured. Ideally, a second test for cure should be performed 2 wk later and STS should be carried out 3 mo after treatment, but most incubating syphilis is cured by the treatment for gonorrhea. Many recurrent infections are reinfections.

SEXUALLY TRANSMITTED CHLAMYDIAL AND UREAPLASMAL INFECTIONS

(Nongonococcal Urethritis [NGU]; Nonspecific Urethritis [NSU]; Mucopurulent Cervicitis; Nonspecific Genital Infections)

Etiology and Incidence

The sexually transmitted organisms causing most cases of cervicitis and urethritis in women, urethritis in men, and proctitis and pharyngitis in both sexes have been identified. Terms previously used to describe the nongonococcal forms of these infections, **nonspecific urethritis (NSU)** or **nongonococcal urethritis (NGU)**, are inexact. This group of sexually transmitted infections, although not reportable, may be the most common STDs in the USA. The causal agents include *Chlamydia trachomatis* (responsible for about 50% of cases of NGU and most cases of nongonococcal mucopurulent cervicitis) and *Ureaplasma urealyticum*, but some cases remain unexplained.

Symptoms and Signs

In **men**, symptoms of urethritis generally appear between 7 and 28 days after intercourse, usually with mild dysuria and discomfort in the urethra and a clear-to-mucopurulent discharge. Although the discharge may be slight and the symptoms mild, they are frequently more marked early in the morning when the lips of the meatus often are stuck together with dried secretions. On examination, the meatus may be red, with evidence of the dried secretions on underclothes. Occasionally the onset is more acute, with dysuria, frequency, and a copious purulent discharge.

Proctitis and pharyngitis may develop after rectal and orogenital contact.

Most **women** are asymptomatic, although vaginal discharge, dysuria, frequency, pelvic pain, and dyspareunia, as well as symptoms of proctitis and pharyngitis, may occur. Cervicitis with characteristic yellow, mucopurulent secretion may be seen.

Diagnosis

Diagnosis is based on bacteriologic examination to exclude gonorrhea in men and other causes of discharge in women, including herpes, trichomoniasis, and candidiasis. In **men**, gram-stained slides of the urethral discharge show many polymorphonuclear leukocytes **(PMNs)** and some epithelial cells but no pathogenic organisms. In mild cases, evidence of urethritis may require examination of urine, which shows $\geq$ 5 PMNs/1000 × (oil) field. If the diagnosis is in doubt, examination is made on first-voided, morning urine. If infection is present, urethral swabbing usually produces enough material for laboratory examination to confirm the diagnosis. *C. trachomatis* can be grown on culture in nearly half the cases but requires inoculation of tissue cultures. The introduction of specific monoclonal antibodies and fluorescent staining to identify *Chlamydia* in genital secretions allows most laboratories to diagnose *C. trachomatis*. In **women**, Gram stain of a purulent cervical discharge often shows many leukocytes but no gonococci.

Complications

In **men**, local complications include epididymitis (especially chlamydial infections in men < 35 yr) and urethral stricture; in **women**, bartholinitis, cysts of Bartholin's glands, salpingitis, and Fitz-Hugh–Curtis syndrome (perihepatitis). Infection of the perihepatic peritoneum by either *Chlamydia* or, less commonly, the gonococcus may simulate cholecystitis or acute right upper quadrant peritonitis of other causes. Chlamydial salpingitis is increasingly recognized as an important source of morbidity and has focused attention on the diagnosis and treatment of chlamydial infections in women. A serious systemic complication occurring more commonly in

men than in women is Reiter's syndrome, consisting of nonspecific urethritis, polyarthritis, and conjunctivitis or uveitis.

Chlamydial ophthalmia neonatorum is increasingly recognized in infants born to women with chlamydial cervicitis (see NEONATAL CONJUNCTIVITIS under NEONATAL INFECTIONS in Ch. 27).

Treatment

Uncomplicated infections are treated with tetracycline 500 mg orally q 6 h or doxycycline 100 mg orally bid for 7 days. Patients who relapse or develop complications require longer courses (tetracycline 500 mg q 6 h or doxycycline 100 mg bid orally for 21 to 28 days). In **pregnant women**, erythromycin (500 mg orally q 6 h for at least 7 days) should be substituted for tetracycline; if this schedule cannot be tolerated, a lower dosage can be used for a longer interval. Infected Bartholin's glands may require aspiration, drainage, or surgical removal. About 20% of patients have one or more relapses on follow-up and require re-treatment. They may become anxious and should be assured that they will be cured eventually. Chlamydial infections coexist with gonorrhea so frequently that presumptive therapy with doxycycline is now standard practice (see Treatment under GONORRHEA, above).

If appropriate treatment is not given, the symptoms and signs subside within 4 wk in about 60 to 70% of patients but may persist in women, resulting in chronic pelvic infection and its sequelae—pain, infertility, or ectopic pregnancy.

Patients should be advised to abstain from sexual intercourse until treatment is completed and symptoms subside. Sex partners should be examined and treated. Treated persons should be followed for 3 mo with regular clinical examinations. STS should be performed before treatment and after 3 mo.

SYPHILIS
(Lues)

A contagious systemic disease caused by the spirochete Treponema pallidum, *characterized by sequential clinical stages and by years of symptomless latency.* It can affect any tissue or vascular organ of the body and can be passed from mother to fetus (**congenital syphilis**—see under NEONATAL INFECTIONS in Ch. 27).

Classification of both acquired and congenital syphilis is shown in TABLE 21–1.

TABLE 21–1. CLASSIFICATION OF SYPHILIS

Acquired	Congenital*
Early infectious syphilis	**Early congenital syphilis**
Primary stage: chancre; regional lymphadenopathy	(symptomatic): the overt disease
Secondary stage (immediately follows primary stage): varied	seen in infants up to age 2
dermatologic lesions that mimic several disorders—eg, skin	**Late congenital syphilis**
rashes, erosions of mucous membranes, alopecia	(symptomatic): the stigmas seen in
Latent stage (asymptomatic; may persist indefinitely or be	later life—eg, Hutchinson's teeth,
followed by late stage, below)	scars of interstitial keratitis, bony
Early latent syphilis (infection < 2 yr† duration; infectious	abnormalities
lesions may recur)	
Late latent syphilis (infection > 2 yr† duration)	
Late or **tertiary** stage (symptomatic; not contagious)	
Benign tertiary (late benign) syphilis	
Cardiovascular syphilis	
Neurosyphilis	

* Congenital syphilis can also exist in a permanently latent, or asymptomatic, state.
† For reporting purposes, the division is sometimes made on a 4-yr rather than a 2-yr basis.

ACQUIRED SYPHILIS

Etiology and Pathology

T. pallidum is a delicate spiral organism about 0.25 μm wide and from 5 to 20 μm long. It can be identified by morphologic characteristics and motility, using a darkfield microscope or fluorescence techniques (see under Diagnosis, below). It does not grow on artificial media and cannot survive for long outside the human body but remains viable for several days in tissue culture.

In acquired syphilis, *T. pallidum* enters the body through the mucous membranes or skin. Within hours the organisms reach the regional lymph nodes and rapidly disseminate throughout the body. Host reaction includes perivascular infiltration of lymphocytes, plasma cells, and later, fibroblasts. The resulting swelling and proliferation of the endothelium of the smaller blood vessels leads to **endarteritis obliterans.** Healing occurs with scar tissue formation. In late syphilis, hypersensitivity to *T. pallidum* leads to gummatous ulcerations and necrosis. Inflammatory changes may subside despite progressive damage, especially in the cardiovascular and central nervous systems.

The CNS is invaded early in the infection; during the secondary stage of the disease > 30% of patients have an abnormal CSF. During the first 5 to 10 yr after infection, the disease involves principally the meninges and blood vessels, resulting in **meningovascular neurosyphilis;** later the pa-

renchyma of the brain and spinal cord are damaged, leading to **parenchymatous neurosyphilis.** Involvement of the cerebral cortex and overlying meninges results in **general paresis.** Destruction of the posterior columns and root ganglia of the spinal cord results in **tabes dorsalis.**

Epidemiology

Infection is usually transmitted by sexual contact, including orogenital and anorectal, and occasionally by kissing or close bodily contact. Highly active homosexual men had been at greatest risk in the USA, but during the 1980s this pattern changed as a result of the AIDS epidemic. Untreated patients with primary or secondary syphilis who have skin lesions are the most infectious. Early latent syphilis is potentially infectious during mucocutaneous relapses, but late latent syphilis is not. Tertiary syphilis is not contagious. Infection with syphilis does not confer lasting immunity against subsequent reinfection, particularly if treatment is given early in the course of the disease.

Symptoms, Signs, and Course

The incubation period of primary syphilis can vary from 1 to 13 wk but is usually from 3 to 4 wk. The disease may appear in any stage, without a history of prior stages and remote from the time of initial infection. Because the disease has diverse clinical manifestations and is now relatively rare in the USA, clinicians there may find it difficult to recognize. The clinical course of syphilis may be accelerated by coexisting HIV infection, but experience is insufficient to determine how frequently this occurs.

Primary syphilis: The primary lesion or **chancre** generally evolves and heals within 4 to 8 wk in untreated patients. At the inoculation site, a red papule develops and soon erodes to form a painless ulcer. It is usually single, occasionally multiple, with an indurated base. It does not bleed, but when abraded, it exudes a clear serum containing numerous *T. pallidum* organisms. A red areola may surround it. The regional lymph nodes usually enlarge painlessly and are firm, discrete, and nontender. Primary chancres occur on the penis, anus, and rectum in men and on the vulva, cervix, and perineum in women. Chancres may be found on the anogenital skin or mucous membranes as well as the lips, tongue, buccal mucosa, tonsils, or fingers, and rarely on other parts of the body, often producing such minimal symptoms that they are ignored.

Secondary syphilis: Cutaneous rashes usually appear within 6 to 12 wk after infection and are most florid after 3 to 4 mo. About 25% of patients have a healing primary chancre. The lesions may be transitory or may persist for months. In untreated patients they frequently heal, but fresh ones may appear within weeks or months. Over 80% of patients have mucocutaneous lesions; 50% have generalized enlargement of the lymph nodes; and about 10% have lesions of the eyes (uveitis), bones (periostitis) and joints, meninges, kidney (glomerulitis), liver, and spleen. Mild constitutional symptoms of malaise, headache, anorexia, nausea, aching pains in the bones, and fatigability are often present, as well as fever, anemia, jaundice, albuminuria, and neck stiffness. At this stage, a small number of patients develop acute syphilitic meningitis, with headache, neck stiffness, cranial nerve lesions, deafness, and occasionally, papilledema.

Syphilitic skin rashes may simulate a variety of dermatologic conditions (see Diagnosis, below). Usually they are symmetric and more marked on the flexor and volar surfaces of the body, especially the palms and soles. The rashes generally occur in crops as macules, papules, pustules, or squamous lesions. The individual spots are pigmented in black persons and pinkish or pale red in whites; they are round, tend to become confluent and indurated, and generally do not itch. They eventually heal, usually without leaving a scar but with areas of residual hyper- or depigmentation in some patients.

The surface of the mucous membranes frequently becomes eroded, forming mucous patches that are circular and often grayish-white with a red areola. These patches occur mostly in the mouth, on the palate, pharynx, or larynx; on the glans penis or vulva; or in the anal canal and rectum. Papules developing at the mucocutaneous junctions and in moist areas of the skin become hypertrophic, flattened, and dull pink or gray; they are called **condyloma lata** and are extremely infectious. The hair often falls out in patches, leaving a moth-eaten appearance (alopecia areata).

Frequently, a generalized, nontender, firm, discrete enlargement of the lymph nodes affects the cervical, suboccipital, epitrochlear, axillary, and inguinal groups, and the liver and spleen may be palpable.

Latent syphilis: In the early latent period (< 2 yr after infection), infectious mucocutaneous relapses may occur, but after 2 yr contagious lesions rarely develop, and the patient appears normal. The latent stage may resolve spontaneously in a few years or last for the rest of the patient's life. About $^1/3$ of untreated persons develop late or tertiary syphilis, though perhaps not until many years after the initial infection.

Late or **tertiary syphilis:** The lesions of late syphilis may be clinically described as (1) benign tertiary syphilis of the skin, bone, and viscera, (2) cardiovascular syphilis, or (3) neurosyphilis.

Lesions of benign tertiary syphilis usually develop within 3 to 10 yr of infection and have almost vanished in the antibiotic era. The typical lesion is a **gumma**, a chronic granulomatous reaction that leads to necrosis and fibrosis. It is frequently localized but may diffusely infiltrate an organ or tissue. With localized lesions, an area of central necrosis is surrounded by granulation tissue. Gummas are indolent, increase slowly in size, heal gradually, and leave scars. Gummatous lesions may develop in the skin, where they result in nodular, ulcerative, or squamous skin eruptions. If they are subcutaneous, they result in punched-out ulcers with sloughing, washed-leather-appearing bases that leave typical tissue-paper scars on healing. Often they occur in submucous tissue (especially of the palate, nasal septum, pharynx, and larynx) and lead to tissue destruction with perforation of the palate or septum. Though they are most common on the leg just below the knee, the upper trunk, the face, and the scalp, they may occur almost anywhere in the body, including the stomach, lung, liver, testicle, and choroid of the eye.

Diffuse gummatous infiltration affects the tongue and leads to chronic interstitial glossitis with leukoplakia and deep fissure formation. Carcinoma is a common sequela.

Benign tertiary syphilis of the bones results in either periostitis with bone formation or osteitis with destructive lesions. The patient complains of a deep, boring pain, characteristically worse at night. A lump or swelling may be noticed if the area involved is superficial.

Cardiovascular syphilis produces a dilated aneurysm of the ascending aorta, narrowing of the coronary ostia, or aortic valvular insufficiency that usually appears 10 to 25 yr after the initial infection.

Symptomatic neurosyphilis produces various clinical syndromes that develop in about 5% of untreated syphilitics. **Asymptomatic neurosyphilis** generally precedes symptomatic neurosyphilis and is found in about 15% of those originally diagnosed as having latent syphilis, in 12% of those with cardiovascular syphilis, and in 5% of those with benign tertiary syphilis. In asymptomatic neurosyphilis, abnormalities may be present in the CSF (see Diagnosis, below).

Meningovascular neurosyphilis: When the brain is principally involved, headache, dizziness, poor concentration, lassitude, insomnia, neck stiffness, and blurred vision occur. Mental confusion, epileptiform attacks, papilledema, aphasia, and mono- or hemiplegia may also be present. Cranial nerve palsies and pupillary abnormalities occur with basilar meningitis. The **Argyll Robertson pupil**, which occurs almost exclusively in neurosyphilis, is a small irregular pupil that reacts normally to accommodation but not to light.

When the spinal cord is involved, there may be bulbar symptoms, weakness and wasting of shoulder girdle and arm muscles, a slowly progressive spastic paraplegia with bladder symptoms, and in rare cases, a transverse myelitis with sudden flaccid paraplegia and loss of sphincter control.

Parenchymatous neurosyphilis: General paresis or **dementia paralytica** generally affects patients in their 40s or 50s. The onset usually is insidious and manifested by behavior changes. Convulsions, aphasia, or transient hemiparesis may be present, but irritability, difficulty in concentrating, deterioration of memory, defective judgment, headaches, insomnia, or fatigue and lethargy are more common. The patient's hygiene and grooming deteriorate. Emotional instability, asthenia, depression, and delusions of grandeur with lack of insight may occur.

Physical signs include tremors of the mouth, tongue, outstretched hands, and whole body; pupillary abnormalities; dysarthria; brisk tendon reflexes; and in some cases, extensor plantar responses. Handwriting usually is shaky and illegible. The posterior column lesions of **tabes dorsalis (locomotor ataxia)** result in pain, ataxia, sensory changes, and loss of tendon reflexes. Onset is slow and insidious. The first and most characteristic symptom usually is an intense, stabbing pain (lightning pain) in the legs that recurs in irregular episodes. Later, unsteadiness of gait develops that is worse in the dark. The patient may walk on a broad base with the feet wide apart. There may be a feeling of walking on foam rubber, with hyperesthesia and paresthesia. Loss of bladder sensation leads to urine retention, incontinence, and recurrent infections. Impotence is common.

Most patients with tabes dorsalis are thin and have characteristic sad-looking, tabetic facies. Argyll Robertson pupils usually are present, and there may be primary optic atrophy. Examination of the legs discloses hypotonia, diminished or absent tendon reflexes, impaired vibratory and joint position sense, ataxia in the heel-shin test, and absence of deep pain sensation. **Romberg's sign** is positive, and ataxia occurs on walking. The bladder is frequently palpably enlarged.

Visceral crises appear as paroxysms of pain in various organs, the most common being gastric crises with vomiting. Rectal, bladder, and laryngeal crises also occur. **Trophic lesions,** secondary to hypoesthesia of the skin or periarticular tissues, may develop in the later stages of the disease. Trophic ulcers may develop on the soles of the feet, penetrate deeply, and involve the underlying bone. **Charcot's arthropathy,** a painless joint degeneration with bony swelling and an abnormal range of movement, is a common manifestation.

Diagnosis

Diagnostic studies for syphilis should include a clinical history, physical examination, serologic tests, darkfield examination of fluids from lesions, CSF tests, radiologic examination, and investigations of sexual contacts.

Darkfield examination: In darkfield microscopy, light is directed obliquely through the slide so that rays striking any organisms cause them to appear as bright objects against a dark background. The external morphologic characteristics and motility of spirochetes present in exudates and tissue fluids from primary and secondary lesions may thus be observed and identified. Experience and skill are needed in collecting the specimens and identifying the organism by its regular coils, corkscrew rotation, and bending. The organism should be distinguished from nonpathogenic spirochetes, which may be part of the normal flora.

Serologic tests for syphilis (STS): Two principal classes of STS aid in diagnosing syphilis and other treponemal diseases: (1) screening, nontreponemal tests using lipoid antigens detect syphilitic reagin, and (2) specific treponemal tests detect antitreponemal antibodies.

The screening tests most frequently used are the Venereal Disease Research Laboratory (VDRL) and the rapid plasma reagin (RPR) tests. Specific treponemal tests include the fluorescent treponemal antibody absorption (FTA-ABS) test, microhemagglutination assay for antibodies to T. pallidum (MHA-TP), and the hemagglutination treponemal tests for syphilis (HATTS).

The VDRL test is a flocculation test for syphilis in which reagin antibody (not to be confused with the reaginic antibodies that mediate allergy) in the patient's serum reacts visibly with cardiolipin, the antigen. A number of conditions (eg, acute hepatitis) can increase serum reagin and produce a reactive VDRL test. Results are reported as reactive, weakly reactive, borderline, or nonreactive. Reactive and weakly reactive sera are considered positive for syphilitic antibodies. All reactive and weakly reactive VDRL tests should be confirmed by one of the more specific treponemal tests.

The screening tests are easy to perform and inexpensive, but they lack the specificity of the treponemal tests and sometimes give biologic false-positive (BFP) results. A BFP reaction (defined as a reactive reagin test but a nonreactive treponemal test) may be a clue to the presence of autoimmune or collagen-vascular disorders, viral infection, or various conditions with altered immunoglobulins. Quantitative reagin titers decline following treatment, becoming negative by 1 yr in primary and by 2 yr in secondary syphilis. Reagin tests do not become positive until 3 to 6 wk after the initial infection. Since the chancre usually develops before this, an early negative STS cannot rule out syphilis. In patients with undiagnosed genital lesions, the reagin tests should be repeated at 2-wk intervals for the first 6 wk before the diagnosis of syphilis can be excluded. The treponemal tests usually become positive after infection has been established 3 to 4 wk and remain so for many years, despite effective treatment.

CSF examination: Before treatment is given in all but the early ($<$ 1 yr) infectious cases, examination of the CSF is recommended to exclude neurosyphilis. The cell count and differential, total protein, and VDRL or other nonspecific (reagin) serologic tests are usually performed. The value of treponemal tests of CSF is unclear.

Immediate diagnosis of primary syphilis depends on demonstrating T. pallidum in exudates taken from the chancre by darkfield microscopy. If initial results are negative, the examinations should be repeated and serologic tests ordered. Aspirates from lymph node punctures may be needed to demonstrate T. pallidum in some cases, especially if topical antiseptics or antibiotics have reduced organisms in the chancre to below detectable levels.

Differential diagnosis of genital ulceration includes herpes genitalis, chancroid, lymphogranuloma venereum, scabies, mucous patches of secondary syphilis, erosive balanitis, Behçet's disease, gummatous ulceration, epithelioma, granuloma inguinale, tuberculous ulceration, and trauma; dual infections with 2 pathogens (eg, herpes simplex and treponema) are not rare. All genital ulcers should be considered syphilitic until proved otherwise. Because physicians frequently overlook the possibility of syphilis, extragenital chancres are often misdiagnosed.

Diagnosis of secondary syphilis: Because syphilis can mimic most skin diseases, any undiagnosed cutaneous eruption or mucosal lesion should be considered syphilitic, especially if it is associated with generalized lymphadenopathy or occurs in patients at risk for syphilis. The diagnosis is established by demonstrating T. pallidum on darkfield examination or by positive STS. These tests are reactive in virtually all cases, often with a high titer of reagin antibody. Common errors include misdiagnosing secondary syphilis as a drug eruption, pityriasis rosea, rubella, infectious mononucleosis, erythema multiforme, pityriasis rubra pilaris, or fungal infection. Condyloma lata may be mistaken for warts, hemorrhoids, or pemphigus vegetans; scalp lesions for ringworm or alopecia areata; and mucous patches for various other conditions.

Diagnosis of latent syphilis is made by excluding the other forms of syphilis in patients with persistently positive reagin and treponemal STS but without clinical evidence of active syphilitic lesions. The CSF is normal, as are the heart and aorta on clinical and radiologic examination. Latent acquired syphilis must be differentiated from latent congenital syphilis (see under NEONATAL INFECTIONS in Ch. 27), latent yaws and other treponemal diseases found in patients from tropical areas, and BFP reactions. Since many patients give no history of primary or secondary manifestations, one must presume that they were asymptomatic during the early stages, the manifestations were trivial or ignored, or the diagnosis was missed.

Diagnosis of tertiary syphilis: In **benign tertiary syphilis**, STS is positive in most cases, but differentiation from coincidental granulomatous conditions may be difficult without biopsy. In **cardiovascular syphilis**, symptoms and signs are sometimes so typical that a clinical diagnosis can easily be made. The diagnosis may be confirmed by echocardiographic and radiologic examination, ECG, and STS. The CSF should be examined, as neurosyphilis and cardiovascular syphilis often occur concurrently. In **asymptomatic neurosyphilis**, the CSF usually shows an elevated cell count, increased protein level, and positive reagin test. In **paresis**, the treponemal test in serum is positive and the CSF is always abnormal, usually with an elevated cell count of 7 to 100 lymphocytes, increased protein level, and positive reagin test. In **tabes dorsalis**, the serum treponemal tests are usually positive, but the reagin screening tests may be negative. The CSF usually shows an increased cell count, a raised protein level, and weakly positive STS. In many advanced cases, the CSF may be normal.

Treatment

In **primary and secondary syphilis**, all the implications should be explained to the patient. All sexual contacts of the past 3 mo (in cases of primary syphilis) and those of up to 1 yr (in cases of secondary syphilis) should be examined, treated, and informed that they may be contagious. They should not have any form of sexual relations until they and their partners have been examined and completed treatment.

Penicillin is the antibiotic of choice for all stages of syphilis. A serum level of 0.03 IU/mL for 6 to 8 days is required to cure early infectious syphilis. Benzathine penicillin G 2.4 million u. IM produces a satisfactory blood level for 2 wk (usu-

ally, 1.2 million u. is given in each buttock). Two additional injections of 2.4 million u. q 7 days should be given for secondary syphilis because of treponemal persistence in the CSF of some patients after single-dose regimens. Alternatively, aqueous procaine penicillin G 600,000 u./day IM for 10 days may be given but offers no advantage. For penicillin-allergic patients, erythromycin 500 mg orally q 6 h for 15 days or tetracycline (at the same dosage) may be used. Because the latter regimens require the patient's compliance, they should be monitored closely.

Patients with **early and late latent syphilis** should be treated with penicillin to prevent subsequent development of tertiary manifestations. Benzathine penicillin G at a total dose of 7.2 million u. may be given as single injections of 2.4 million u. IM once/wk for 3 wk. Alternatively, aqueous procaine penicillin G 600,000 u./day IM for 14 days may be given. Those intolerant of penicillin may be treated with erythromycin 500 mg q 6 h for 15 days. **Benign tertiary syphilis** is treated in the same way as latent syphilis, above; however, for those who cannot tolerate penicillin and are treated with erythromycin, a second course of erythromycin at the same dosage 3 mo later is advisable.

Because of apparently increased rates of complications, patients with **coexistent HIV infection** should be routinely investigated for evidence of neurosyphilis and ocular syphilis, and treatment regimens should be adjusted accordingly.

Cardiovascular syphilis: Treatment is the same as for latent syphilis, above, but procaine penicillin G usually is given for a total of 21 days.

Neurosyphilis: Penicillin is given as in latent syphilis, above, but procaine penicillin G, if used, should be given for a total of 21 days. Treatment of asymptomatic neurosyphilis prevents development of symptomatic neurosyphilis but usually does not reverse established symptoms. Chlorpromazine 25 or 50 mg orally or IM is effective in controlling restless patients with paresis; analgesics should be used freely for tabetic patients with lightning pains. Carbamazepine 200 mg orally tid or qid is sometimes effective in controlling the pains.

Over 50% of the patients with early infectious syphilis, especially those with secondary syphilis, have a **Jarisch-Herxheimer reaction** within 6 to 12 h after the initial treatment. The reaction—manifested by general malaise, fever, headache, sweating, rigors, and a temporary exacerbation of the syphilitic lesions—usually subsides within 24 h and poses no danger other than the anxiety it may produce. However, patients with general paresis or a high CSF cell count are likely to develop a Herxheimer reaction that occasionally causes serious disorders, such as seizures, hemiplegia, or monoplegia. The Herxheimer reaction should be explained to the patient before treatment is started. Herxheimer reactions may be confused with penicillin allergy and may provide a clue to coexistent syphilis in persons treated for other conditions.

Posttreatment Surveillance

The importance of repeated tests to confirm a permanent cure should be explained to the patient before treatment. Examinations and quantitative reagin tests should be performed at 1, 3, 6, and 12 mo or until no reaction is found, whichever period is longer. Following successful treatment, lesions heal rapidly, serologic titers fall, and the reagin tests usually become negative within 9 to 12 mo. The treponemal tests, such as the FTA-ABS and the MHA-TP, usually remain positive for years or even for the rest of the patient's life. The CSF should be examined after 1 yr of surveillance. If the VDRL test remains positive for > 1 yr or if the titer starts to rise, more intensive re-treatment should be considered. Serologic or clinical relapse is uncommon but occasionally occurs about the 6th to 9th mo, most commonly affecting the nervous system. Relapse requires re-treatment with a more intensive regimen of antibiotics, but the possibility of reinfection should also be considered and investigated. If all the clinical and serologic examinations remain satisfactory for 2 yr after treatment, the patient can be reassured that cure is complete and permanent and that no further follow-up is needed.

All patients with syphilis should be encouraged to undergo testing for HIV, and those found to be negative should be retested at 6 mo to detect infection acquired simultaneously with syphilis. Those with positive tests should undergo CSF examination.

Patients with latent syphilis should be kept under surveillance and tested at 3, 6, 12, 18, and 24 mo; those with persistently positive serologic tests should be seen annually indefinitely. The prognosis is excellent. Patients with benign tertiary syphilis should be examined at regular intervals after treatment, and those with cardiovascular syphilis should be followed for the rest of their lives.

In asymptomatic neurosyphilis, the CSF should be examined q 6 mo until it has been normal for 2 yr; abnormal CSF should be examined q 3 mo until it is normal, and then annually for another 2 yr. Tabes dorsalis tends to progress despite treatment. A close watch should be kept for UTIs.

TRICHOMONIASIS

Etiology

Trichomonas vaginalis, a flagellated protozoan found in the GU tract of either sex, is a common cause of vaginitis. The organism is usually pear-shaped, with average dimensions of 7 × 10 μm but occasionally as long as 25 μm. It has 4 anterior flagella and a fifth flagellum embedded in an undulating membrane. The organism is more common in women, affecting about 20% of them during the reproductive years and causing vaginitis, urethritis, and possibly cystitis. *T. vaginalis* is more difficult to detect in men; probably causes urethritis, prostatitis, and cystitis; and may account for 5 to 10% of all cases of male urethritis in some areas. Most infected men are asymptomatic carriers but can infect their sex partners.

Symptoms and Signs

In women, onset typically is accompanied by a copious, greenish-yellow, frothy vaginal discharge associated with irritation and soreness of the vulva, perineum, and thighs and with dyspareunia and dysuria. Some women have only a slight discharge, and many are asymptomatic carriers for long periods, although symptoms may develop at any time. The infection frequently coexists with gonorrhea. In severe cases, the vulva and perineum may be inflamed, with edema of the labia. The vaginal walls and surface of the cervix frequently are normal but may show punctate, red strawberry spots, or they may have a small amount of discharge in the vaginal fornices. Complications, including bartholinitis, skenitis, and cystitis, are rare.

Men generally are asymptomatic. Some may have a transient, frothy, or purulent urethral discharge with dysuria and frequency, usually early in the morning; mild urethral irritation and occasionally moisture at the urethral meatus; and discomfort in the perineum or deeper in the pelvis. A subpreputial discharge may appear in uncircumcised men. Epididymitis and prostatitis are the only known complications.

Diagnosis

In women, the diagnosis can usually be made immediately by examining a sample of vaginal secretion taken from the posterior fornix under either a darkfield, phase-contrast, or ordinary light microscope. The lashing movements of the flagella and striking motility of the oval-shaped organisms are readily observed. The organism can be cultured on a suitable medium. Trichomoniasis is also commonly diagnosed on a Papanicolaou smear. Tests should be done to exclude gonorrhea and other STDs.

In men, if examination is done early in the morning before urinating, a slight mucoid discharge may be present, and some fine threads may be found in the 2-glass urine test. A wet film of the urethral secretions in men should be examined microscopically for trichomonads and cultures inoculated. Examining the centrifuged sediment of urine and prostatic secretions may also be helpful.

Treatment

Metronidazole 2 gm orally in a single dose cures up to 95% of women submitting to initial treatment if sex partners are treated simultaneously. Because the effectiveness of single-dose regimens in men is unclear, men should be treated with 500 mg bid for 7 days. Metronidazole may cause leukopenia, disulfiram-like adverse interactions with alcohol, or candidal superinfections; it is relatively contraindicated in pregnancy, although human data suggest it is not dangerous to the fetus after the first trimester. Povidone-iodine should also be avoided. All sex partners should be examined and treated, and patients should abstain from intercourse until a cure is established.

GENITAL CANDIDIASIS

Etiology

Yeast infections of the genital tract caused by *Candida albicans* are increasing in frequency, especially in women. Uncommonly transmitted sexually, the infection usually spreads from the patient's normal skin or intestinal flora. The increased incidence is primarily due to widespread use of broad-spectrum antibiotics and the large number of women taking oral contraceptives, although better diagnostic methods may also contribute. Other predisposing factors include pregnancy, menstruation, diabetes mellitus, constrictive undergarments, and use of immunosuppressive drugs and corticosteroids. *Systemic candidiasis is evidence of severe underlying disease or immunologic abnormality; it is rarely a complication of genital infection.*

Symptoms and Signs

Women usually develop vulval irritation and vaginal discharge. Frequently the irritation is severe and the discharge scanty. The vulva may be reddish and swollen, with excoriation and fissures. The vaginal wall may be covered with a white, cheesy material or may appear normal. **Men** often are symptomless but may complain of irritation and soreness of the glans penis and prepuce, especially after intercourse. Occasionally, they may notice a slight urethral discharge. The glans penis and prepuce are reddish on examination, and vesicles or erosions may be present. White, cheesy material may adhere to the surface. In severe cases, the prepuce may be edematous, causing phimosis (constriction of the foreskin).

Diagnosis

An immediate diagnosis can be made by taking smears from the vagina, glans penis, or prepuce and examining them microscopically for *C. albicans* by Gram stain with potassium hydroxide (the organisms are gram-positive, oval, budding, yeastlike cells having typical elongated, filamentous pseudohyphae). Culture media should also be inoculated, as this increases the number of positive findings by 25% and confirms the presence of *C. albicans*. Since candidiasis is rarely transmitted sexually, tests for coexisting STDs should be performed only if clinically or epidemiologically indicated.

Treatment

Once the diagnosis and the underlying cause have been identified, predisposing conditions such as antibiotic therapy should be controlled to avoid recurrences.

Vaginal candidiasis can be treated locally with (1) clotrimazole one 100-mg vaginal tablet/day for 6 days or 200 mg/day for 3 days, (2) miconazole 200 mg/day intravaginally for 3 days, (3) butaconazole 2% cream 5 gm/day intravaginally for 3 days, or (4) terconazole one 80-mg suppository/day for 3 days or 0.4% cream 5 gm/day for 7 days. All of these agents are given once daily at bedtime. An oral regimen of ketoconazole 200 mg bid for 6 days also has produced satisfactory results.

Candidal balanoposthitis is treated by carefully washing the genitalia with soap and water, drying with a clean towel, and applying nystatin cream bid for 7 to 10 days. Urethritis may be treated with daily irrigations of a 100,000-u./mL nystatin suspension, but usually it is secondary to balanitis and does not require additional treatment.

Relapse is common in either sex and may be due to reinfection by the sex partner or, more commonly, from the normal flora in combination with a provoking condition. Occasionally, oral contraceptives must be discontinued for several months during treatment. Women who require antibiotics recurrently or for prolonged periods or have other unavoidable predispositions may require prophylaxis with any of the treatment regimens.

BALANOPOSTHITIS; BALANITIS

Inflammation of the glans penis and the prepuce.

Etiology

Balanoposthitis (balanitis in the circumcised) may be caused by complications of gonorrhea, trichomoniasis, candidiasis, herpes simplex, and primary or secondary syphilis. Other noninfectious causes include Reiter's syndrome, fixed drug eruptions, contact dermatitis, psoriasis, lichen planus, seborrheic dermatitis, lichen sclerosus et atrophicus, and erythroplasia of Queyrat. In many cases, no cause can be found. Balanoposthitis is often associated with a tight prepuce. The subpreputial secretions become infected with anaerobic bacteria, resulting in inflammation and tissue destruction. Diabetes mellitus predisposes to balanoposthitis.

Symptoms and Signs

Soreness, irritation, and a subpreputial discharge often occur 2 or 3 days after sexual intercourse. Phimosis (constriction of the foreskin) due to surface edema of the glans penis and prepuce may be present. Both may be eroded with superficial ulcerations. The inguinal lymph nodes may be tender and enlarged.

Diagnosis and Treatment

Common STDs should be excluded by smears and cultures of material from the inflamed surface, STS performed, and the urine tested for glucose.

Appropriate treatment should be given if a specific cause is found. Saline washes should be carried out several times daily if no cause can be found. Subpreputial irrigations should be given for true phimosis. Oral sulfonamides, which will not mask incubating syphilis, should be given for significant secondary infection. Circumcision should be considered in patients with persistent phimosis once the inflammation has resolved.

CHANCROID

An acute, localized, contagious disease characterized by painful genital ulcers and suppuration of the inguinal lymph nodes.

Etiology

The causative agent is *Hemophilus ducreyi*, a short, slender, gram-negative bacillus with rounded ends that is usually found in chains or groups. It grows slowly on nutritionally enriched culture media containing hemin and albumin, but many laboratories do not have such capabilities. The reemergence of chancroid in North America and its association with increased risk of HIV transmission have heightened interest in this previously exotic infection.

Symptoms and Signs

The incubation period is 3 to 7 days. Small, painful papules rapidly break down to become shallow ulcers with ragged, undermined edges. Each ulcer is shallow, nonindurated, painful, and surrounded by a reddish border. Ulcers vary in size and often coalesce. Phagedenic erosion occasionally leads to marked tissue destruction. The inguinal lymph nodes become tender, enlarged, and matted together, forming a fluctuant abscess (bubo) in the groin. The skin over the abscess may become red and shiny and may break down to form a sinus. Autoinoculation may result in new lesions. Complications include phimosis, urethral stricture, urethral fistula, and severe tissue destruction. Chancroid may coexist with other causes of genital ulcers.

Diagnosis

Diagnosis usually has been based on clinical findings, since culture of the organism is difficult and the polymicrobial flora of ulcers makes microscopic identification uncertain. However, attempts should be made to identify *H. ducreyi* in material taken from the edge of the ulcers or in pus from a bubo. Cultures should also be attempted on media containing fresh defibrinated rabbit blood or the patient's own serum. Biopsy of a specimen from an ulcer edge may be helpful, but the changes are often nonspecific. Tests to exclude other STDs should be performed—especially STS and culture for herpes, if available.

Treatment

Ceftriaxone 250 mg IM once or erythromycin 500 mg q 6 h for at least 7 days is recommended. Increasing resistance to sulfonamides alone and tetracycline have rendered these drugs less effective. Buboes should be aspirated, not incised. All sexual contacts should be examined and the patient kept under surveillance for 3 mo, with STS performed regularly.

LYMPHOGRANULOMA VENEREUM (LGV)
(Lymphopathia Venereum; Lymphogranuloma Inguinale)

A sexually transmitted chlamydial disease having a transitory primary lesion followed by suppurative lymphangitis and serious local complications.

Etiology

LGV is caused by a limited number of immunotypes of *Chlamydia trachomatis* distinct from the agents causing trachoma, inclusion conjunctivitis, urethritis, and cervicitis. The disease is found mostly in tropical and subtropical areas but occurs uncommonly in the USA.

Symptoms and Signs

After an incubation period of 3 to ≥ 12 days, a small, transient, nonindurated vesicular lesion is formed that ulcerates rapidly, heals quickly, and may pass unnoticed. Usually, the first symptom is unilateral, tender enlargement of the inguinal lymph nodes, which progresses to form a large, tender, fluctuant mass that adheres to the deep tissues and inflames the overlying skin. Multiple sinuses may develop and discharge purulent or bloodstained material. Healing eventually occurs with scar formation, but the sinuses can persist or recur.

The patient may complain of fever, malaise, headaches, joint pains, anorexia, and vomiting. Backache is common in women, in whom the ini-

tial lesions may be on the cervix or upper vagina, resulting in enlargement and suppuration of perirectal and pelvic lymphatics. Involvement of the rectal wall in women or homosexual men may result in an ulcerative proctitis with bloodstained purulent rectal discharges.

Chronic inflammation obstructs the lymphatic vessels, leading to edema, ulcerations, and fistula formation. Large polypoid masses develop, and gross swellings may eventually result in genital elephantiasis. Rectal strictures may be found in females and male homosexuals.

Diagnosis

Clinical diagnosis can be confirmed by a CF test in which a rising titer of antibody may be demonstrated. A microimmunofluorescence (micro-IF) test measures type-specific antibody and distinguishes various serotypes of antibody. Cross-reactions, however, are common. Isolation in cell culture is available in relatively few laboratories. Commercially available immunofluorescence kits using monoclonal antibodies for staining of *Chlamydia* in pus has increased the availability of specific tests. If micro-IF and cell culture tests are not available, diagnosis can be made by a thorough history, clinical examination, and the presence of high or rising titers of complement-fixing antibodies.

Treatment

Doxycycline 100 mg orally bid, erythromycin 500 mg orally qid, or tetracycline 500 mg orally qid, each for 21 days, is the treatment of choice, producing rapid healing of early lesions. Fluctuant buboes should be aspirated, not incised. Abscesses and fistulas usually require surgery, but rectal strictures can usually be dilated. Elephantiasis is treated by plastic surgery. All sexual contacts should be examined, and the patient should be kept under observation for 6 mo after apparently successful treatment.

GRANULOMA INGUINALE

A chronic granulomatous condition usually involving the genitalia and probably spread by sexual contact.

Etiology

Granuloma inguinale is rare in temperate climates but common in some tropical and subtropical areas. It is believed to be caused by a gram-negative, intracellular bacillus found in mononuclear cells and known as *Calymmatobacterium granulomatis* (formerly *Donovania granulomatis*).

Symptoms and Signs

The incubation period varies from about 1 to 12 wk. The initial lesion is a painless, beefy-red nodule that slowly develops into a rounded, elevated, velvety, granulomatous mass. Sites of infection are the penis, scrotum, groin, and thighs in men; the vulva, vagina, and perineum in women; the anus and buttocks in homosexual men; and the face in both sexes. There is no lymphadenopathy, and the disease spreads by continuity and autoinoculation. Progress is slow, but eventually the lesions may cover the genitalia. Healing also is slow and scar tissue forms. Secondary infection is common and can cause gross tissue destruction. Anemia, cachexia, and death may follow in neglected cases, and hematogenous dissemination to bones, joints, or liver occurs occasionally.

Diagnosis

Bright, beefy-red, granulomatous lesions are characteristic. Confirmation of the diagnosis is made microscopically by demonstrating Donovan bodies (intracytoplasmic bacilli in macrophages stained by Giemsa or Wright's stain) in smears taken from edge scrapings of the lesions. Biopsy specimens from such scrapings contain many plasma cells but few mononuclear cells.

Treatment

Streptomycin, tetracycline, erythromycin, chloramphenicol, and trimethoprim/sulfamethoxazole produce satisfactory healing of the lesions. Streptomycin does not mask incubating syphilis, is given 1 gm IM q 12 h for 21 days, and remains effective in some areas. Tetracycline is given 500 mg orally q 6 h for 10 to 14 days. Treatment should result in a response in 7 days but should be continued for 3 wk or until lesions have been healed to minimize relapses. The patient's sexual contacts should be located and thoroughly examined. Surveillance after apparently successful treatment should continue for 6 mo and should include STS.

GENITAL HERPES

Infection of the genital or perirectal area skin by herpes simplex.

Etiology

Infection of the genital and anorectal skin and mucosa, usually with herpes simplex virus type 2 (HSV-2), but also (in ≈ 5%) type 1 (HSV-1), is the most common cause of genital ulceration in developed countries. It is moderately contagious and usually spreads by sexual contact. Lesions frequently develop 4 to 7 days after contact, and the condition tends to recur because the virus establishes latent infection of the sacral sensory nerve ganglia, from which it reactivates and reinfects the skin.

Symptoms and Signs

Primary lesions are more painful, prolonged, and widespread than those of recurrent outbreaks. Itching and soreness usually precede a small patch of erythema on the skin or mucous membranes. A small group of painful vesicles develop; they erode and form several superficial, circular ulcers with a red areola, which may coalesce. The ulcers, usually painful, become crusted after a few days and generally heal in about 10 days, with scarring. The inguinal lymph nodes are usually slightly enlarged and tender.

Lesions may occur on the prepuce, glans penis, and penile shaft in men, and on the labia, clitoris, perineum, vagina, and cervix in women. They may occur around the anus and in the rectum in homosexual men or rectally exposed women. In addition to pain in primary infections, the patient may experience generalized malaise, fever, and difficulty with micturition (because of bladder paresis or dysuria) or with walking.

In patients with depressed cell-mediated immunity from HIV infections or other causes, prolonged or progressive lesions may persist for weeks or longer. Failure to heal requires that HIV infection be investigated.

Diagnosis

Clinical diagnosis is confirmed by taking material from the base of ulcerated lesions on a cotton-tipped swab (or by aspiration from a vesicle), placing it in a suitable virus transport medium, and inoculating it into tissue cultures. A characteristic cytopathic effect is produced within 24 to 48 h. Paired serum samples, taken at 10- to 14-day intervals, may show a rise in antibody titer in primary infections. Immediate diagnosis can be made by finding characteristic multinucleated giant cells in Wright-Giemsa stained smears of cells from lesions (Tzanck preparation).

Complications

Genital herpes may be complicated by aseptic meningitis, transverse myelitis, or autonomic nervous system dysfunction involving the sacral regions. Aseptic meningitis presents with fever, headache, vomiting, photophobia, and nuchal rigidity 3 to 12 days after onset of primary or recurrent genital lesions. WBCs range from 10 to > 1000, predominantly lymphocytes, and the CSF protein may be slightly elevated. The disease almost always resolves spontaneously in a few days without sequelae. Symptoms of autonomic dysfunction, including inability to urinate, constipation, and impotence in men, frequently complicate primary infection. Less commonly, the syndrome of transverse myelitis affecting the legs complicates primary infections.

Hematogenous dissemination of virus to the skin, joints, liver, or lung occasionally occurs in apparently immunologically normal patients but is more common in immunosuppressed or pregnant patients.

Extragenital lesions, usually involving the buttock, groin, or thigh, may occur in primary or recurrent disease by neuronal spread or direct inoculation. The latter mechanism accounts for occasional infections of the fingers or eye. Extension into the genitals or urinary system is extremely rare. Bacterial superinfection of herpetic ulcers is uncommon, although herpes may coexist with *Treponema pallidum*, *Hemophilus ducreyi*, or *Candida albicans*.

By far the most common complication of genital herpes is recurrent disease, usually confined to one side of the body, milder than the initial attack, and associated with prodromal symptoms that may be severe. The likelihood and rate of recurrence are greater with HSV-2 (80%) than HSV-1 (50%). Recurrences vary greatly in their courses but may be frequent and prolonged over many years. Reinfection with different strains of HSV-2 can also occur.

Treatment

Acyclovir, available in IV, topical, and oral forms, effectively treats primary herpetic infections of the mouth, genitalia, and rectum. It (1) reduces viral shedding and symptoms in severe primary infections, (2) marginally reduces shedding and symptoms in recurrent disease, (3) cures chronic infections in immunocompromised patients, and (4) reduces rates of recurrence when used prophylactically. However, even early treatment of primary infections does not abort latent infections or prevent recurrences. Oral acyclovir seems likely to become standard outpatient therapy for most of the indications listed above. Patients with severe primary disease or immunocompromised patients with chronic progressive lesions (eg, AIDS) should receive acyclovir 200 mg orally 5 times/day or 800 mg bid for 5 days or, if necessary, 5 mg/kg IV q 8 h. Prophylaxis for severe recurrent disease with acyclovir 200 mg orally 2 to 5 times/day or 400 mg bid dramatically reduces the rate and severity of recurrences.

GENITAL WARTS
(Condylomata Acuminata;
Moist or Venereal Warts)

Etiology and Incidence

Genital warts are caused by papillomaviruses (human papillomavirus [HPV] types 1, 2, 6, 11, 16, and 18) and usually are transmitted sexually. They have an incubation period of 1 to 6 mo and occur most commonly on warm, moist surfaces in the subpreputial area, the coronal sulcus, within the urethral meatus, and on the penile shaft in men; and on the vulva, the vaginal wall, the cervix, and the perineum in women. They are particularly common in the perianal region and rectum in homosexual men.

Genital wart infections in the USA have increased in the past 10 yr at twice the rate of genital herpes and are medically important, especially in association with cancer.

Symptoms and Signs

Genital warts usually appear as soft, moist, minute, pink or red swellings that grow rapidly and may become pedunculated. Usually several of them are found in the same area, resembling cauliflower; occasionally they are solitary. In pregnant patients or in those with immunosuppression or maceration of the skin, they may grow more rapidly.

Diagnosis

Genital warts usually can be identified by their appearance but must be differentiated from the flat-topped condyloma lata of secondary syphilis. Biopsies should be performed on atypical or persistent warts to exclude carcinoma. Women with cervical warts should not be treated until Papanicolaou smear results are available to guide therapy.

Treatment

No treatment is completely satisfactory.

Genital warts may be removed by electrocauterization, laser, cryotherapy, or surgical excision under local or general anesthesia. Topical applications of podophyllin or trichloroacetic acid are widely used, usually require multiple applications over weeks to months, and frequently fail. For **urethral lesions**, thiotepa has been effective. Topical 5-fluorouracil applied 2 to 3 times a day by the patient is highly effective in the urethra in men, but the patient should be watched for acute (though rare) urethral obstruction. Removal with a resectoscope under general anesthesia may be the most satisfactory treatment. Circumcision may prevent recurrence.

Sexual contacts should be examined and STS performed initially and after 3 mo. Relapse is frequent and requires re-treatment.

Need for follow-up of patients and their sex partners with genital warts (types 6, 11, 16, and 18) has radically changed with the knowledge that many women with endocervical warts may develop dysplastic changes or invasive carcinoma of the cervix. Finding HPV type 16 or 18 in bowenoid papulosis and in bladder cancers is also cause for regular follow-up examinations. The fact that type 16 integrates with the host's cell DNA rather than remaining as an episome, as with other types of wart virus, may account for its greater invasiveness and its possibly lesser susceptibility to interferon treatment. Cervical cytologic or colposcopic examination of women at yearly or shorter intervals is necessary to detect and treat dysplasia, which is sometimes premalignant.

Interferon-α, intralesionally or IM, has cleared intractable lesions of skin and genitals. Its optimal administration and long-term results are under study in several countries. However, caution is suggested by reports of patients with bowenoid papulosis of the genitals (type 16), in whom the lesions initially disappeared after treatment with interferon-β but reappeared as invasive cancers.

SEXUALLY TRANSMITTED ENTERIC INFECTIONS

Various bacterial (*Shigella, Campylobacter,* or *Salmonella*), viral (hepatitis A), or parasitic (*Giardia* or ameba) pathogens are transmitted by sexual practices that promote anal-oral contamination. Although the bacterial pathogens may coexist with or cause proctitis, they usually produce symptoms (diarrhea, fever, bloating, nausea, and abdominal pain) suggesting disease more proximal in the GI tract. Multiple infections are frequent, especially in homosexual men with many sex partners. Asymptomatic infections also occur with all these pathogens and are the rule with *Entamoeba histolytica*, which is usually of a nonpathogenic type in homosexual men in Western countries.

§3. PEDIATRICS AND GENETICS

22. INTRODUCTION

In recent years, pediatrics has enlarged its scope to include perinatology and adolescent medicine; has placed increasing emphasis on health promotion and on the prevention and early recognition of disease through appropriate periodic screening; and has acknowledged the importance and interdependency of the organic, functional, behavioral, sociologic, economic, and political aspects of child health care. Most of these changes have been prompted by societal changes that have generated disruptions in our homes, schools, and communities. For many, this has led to poor child rearing, poor individual prospects for success and happiness, and increased stress, self-depreciation, substance abuse, violence, depression, and self-destructive behaviors.

Because this section of THE MANUAL discusses medical care of the newborn, infant, child, and adolescent, it is helpful to define those age groups as they are used here: ie, **the neonate (newborn)**—birth to 1 mo; **the infant**—1 mo to 1 yr; **early childhood**—1 yr through 5 yr; **late childhood**—6 yr through 12 yr; **adolescence**—13 yr through 17 yr. The term "child" may be used in a general way from birth on, as in discussions of the number of children in a family. Specifically, "child" refers to ages 1 through 12.

Prenatal diagnosis and genetic counseling are discussed in Chs. 13 and 48. Diseases and disorders occurring in the pediatric age group that are also prevalent in adults are covered more fully elsewhere in THE MANUAL.

23. HEALTH MANAGEMENT IN NORMAL NEONATES, INFANTS, AND CHILDREN

Most pediatricians in developed countries, especially the USA and Canada, are primary care practitioners who direct their efforts to keeping neonates, infants, and children well. This is done through illness prevention, early detection and treatment of diseases, and provision of guidance and support to parents in their child-rearing practices. Health management as described below accounts for 35 to 50% of visits to pediatricians' offices and 55 to 60% of pediatricians' practice time. Except for providing care to normal newborns, little of the primary care pediatrician's time is spent in hospital. Most childhood diseases do not require hospitalization, and those that do most often are managed by pediatric subspecialists practicing in tertiary care hospitals.

MANAGEMENT OF THE NORMAL NEWBORN

PERINATAL PHYSIOLOGY

The successful transition of the term fetus, immersed in amniotic fluid and totally dependent on the placenta for gas exchange, nutrition, and

excretion, to a squalling air-breathing neonate is a source of wonder. A number of neonatal disorders can now be seen as failures to accomplish this transition successfully. Several specific areas of perinatal physiology will be reviewed briefly.

Ventilation and Lung Function

The placenta provides gas exchange for the fetus. Fetal lungs develop anatomically throughout gestation, and fairly well developed alveoli are present by the 25th wk. The fetal lungs continually produce fluid, a transudate from pulmonary capillaries plus some pulmonary surfactant secreted by type II pneumonocytes. Fetal breathing movements occur intermittently, usually during rapid eye movement (REM) sleep that is present about 1/3 of the time in the fetus. During these breathing movements, lung fluid moves up through the tracheobronchial tree and contributes to amniotic fluid. Fetal breathing movements appear to be essential for development of neuromuscular control of breathing, which the neonate will require to survive.

Surface tension is not involved in fetal breathing movements, since fetal lung alveoli are fluid-filled. Following the first breath after delivery, however, the air spaces contain air, and air-fluid interfaces exist, since a layer of water lines the alveolar surface. Pulmonary surfactants must be present in this layer of water; otherwise, excessively high surface tension would cause alveolar collapse **(atelectasis)**, greatly increasing the work of breathing. **Pulmonary surfactant** (a complex mixture of phospholipids, including phosphatidyl choline, phosphatidyl glycerol, phosphatidyl inositol, and 3 lipoproteins) is largely stored in lamellar inclusions in the type II pneumonocytes or alveolar lining cells during fetal life. At the first breath, surfactant is secreted into the alveolar-lining water layer. By 35 wk gestation, there is usually sufficient surfactant to prevent diffuse atelectasis, the primary defect in respiratory distress syndrome **(RDS)**, which may complicate more premature birth (see in Ch. 27).

For normal respirations to occur, pulmonary interstitial and alveolar fluid must be cleared promptly at birth. There are 2 mechanisms to accomplish this: (1) During vaginal delivery, the fetal thorax is compressed, expelling some lung fluid. As the thorax is delivered, elastic recoil of the ribs draws some air into the pulmonary tree. The first strong inspiratory efforts further fill the alveoli with air. (2) Fetal epinephrine and norepinephrine levels resulting from the stress of labor increase the absorption of sodium and water across the respiratory epithelium, which leads to a markedly increased pulmonary lymph flow. Neonatal **wet lung syndrome (transient tachypnea of the newborn**—see RESPIRATORY DISORDERS in Ch. 27) is believed to be caused by delayed resorption of fetal lung fluid.

Changes in the Circulation at Birth

A profound change in the circulation coincides with the first breath of air. Pulmonary arteriolar resistance is very high in the fetal circulation; as a result, there is little blood flow to the fetal lungs (only 5 to 10% of cardiac output). In contrast, there is low resistance to blood flow in the systemic circulation, largely because of low resistance to blood flow through the placenta. Low fetal systemic Pa_{O_2} (about 25 mm Hg) along with locally produced prostaglandins, keeps the fetal ductus arteriosus dilated. Blood ejected by the right ventricle preferentially flows from right to left, from the pulmonary artery into the aorta, through the ductus arteriosus because of the high pulmonary resistance. Another right-to-left shunt occurs through the foramen ovale. Left atrial pressure is low in the fetus because little blood is returned from the lungs, while right atrial pressure is relatively high because of the large volume of blood returning from the placenta. The difference in atrial pressures keeps the flap of the foramen ovale open and permits blood to shunt from right to left atrium.

The first breaths of air enhance pulmonary blood flow and closure of the foramen ovale. Pulmonary arteriolar resistance drops acutely, the result of vasodilation caused by expansion of the lungs, by increased Pa_{O_2}, and by reduction in Pa_{CO_2}. Air breathing also creates alveolar air-fluid interfaces that exert force toward alveolar collapse, which is counteracted by the elastic forces of the ribs and chest wall. As a result, pulmonary interstitial pressure drops, reducing tissue pressure on the pulmonary capillaries and further enhancing pulmonary blood flow.

As pulmonary blood flow is established, venous return from the lungs increases and left atrial pressure is raised. When air breathing begins, the umbilical arteries contract in response to an increased Pa_{O_2}. Placental blood flow is reduced or ceases, and blood return to the right atrium is reduced. Right atrial pressure falls, while left atrial pressure increases; the foramen ovale therefore closes as air breathing begins and pulmonary blood flow increases.

Soon after birth, systemic resistance becomes higher than pulmonary resistance, a reversal of the fetal state. Therefore, the direction of blood flow through the patent ductus arteriosus reverses, creating left-to-right shunting of blood. This state of circulation in which pulmonary blood flow has been established, placental circulation has been removed, and blood flows from left to right through the ductus arteriosus is called the **transitional circulation**. It lasts from moments after birth (when the pulmonary blood flow and functional closure of the foramen ovale occur) until about 24 h of age when the ductus arteriosus closes. Blood entering the ductus and its vasa vasorum from the aorta has a high P_{O_2}, which, along with alterations in prostaglandin metabolism, leads to constriction and closure of the ductus arteriosus. Once the ductus arteriosus has closed, an adult-type circulation exists. The 2 ventricles now pump in series, and there are no major shunts between the pulmonary and systemic circulations.

During the first days following delivery, a stressed newborn may revert to a fetal-type circulation. Asphyxia with hypoxia and hypercarbia causes the pulmonary arterioles to constrict and the ductus arteriosus to dilate, reversing the processes described above, resulting in right-to-left shunting through the now patent ductus arteriosus and the reopened foramen ovale. As a consequence, the newborn becomes severely hypoxemic. This condition is called **persistent pulmonary hypertension** or **persistent fetal circulation** (of course, there is no umbilical circulation). The goal of treatment is to reverse the conditions that produced pulmonary vasoconstriction; ie, to ventilate with 100% O_2.

Bilirubin Excretion
(See also METABOLIC PROBLEMS IN THE NEWBORN in Ch. 27)

In the fetus, bilirubin is cleared from the circulation by placental transfer into the mother's plasma following the concentration gradient. The maternal liver then conjugates and excretes the fetal bilirubin.

At birth, the placenta is lost and the neonatal liver must then take up, conjugate, and excrete bilirubin into bile so it can be eliminated when the infant passes stools. These steps required for neonatal bilirubin elimination apparently function, at least in part, during fetal life. Fetal hepatocytes contain Y- and Z-binding proteins, which take up free bilirubin from blood in the hepatic sinusoids. The bilirubin is then diglucuronidated and secreted into bile, which makes its way into meconium but cannot be eliminated from the body, since the fetus does not normally pass stools. The enzyme β-glucuronidase, present in the fetus' small intestinal luminal brush border, is released into the intestinal lumen, where it breaks the bilirubin glucuronide bonds; free (unconjugated) bilirubin is then reabsorbed from the intestinal tract and reenters the circulation. The **fetal enterohepatic circulation of bilirubin** "anticipates" the steps in bilirubin metabolism and excretion that will be required in the newborn. However, fetal bilirubin is still cleared by the placenta. Following delivery, feedings produce the gastrocolic reflex and bilirubin is excreted in the stools before it can be deconjugated and reabsorbed.

Delay in initiating feedings and circumstances that prevent enteral feedings (eg, intestinal atresia) are often complicated by unconjugated hyperbilirubinemia. One reason appears to be that β-glucuronidase still present in the neonate's GI tract results in a continuing enterohepatic circulation of bilirubin when GI transit time is prolonged (see also HYPERBILIRUBINEMIA under METABOLIC PROBLEMS IN THE NEWBORN in Ch. 27).

Fetal Hemoglobin

Because of its high affinity for O_2, fetal Hb is especially suited to extract O_2 from maternal Hb across the placenta. This increased O_2 affinity is less useful following delivery, because fetal Hb less readily gives up O_2 to tissues; this may be deleterious if severe pulmonary or cardiac disease with hypoxemia exists. The transition from fetal to adult Hb begins before delivery.

The abrupt increase in Pao_2 from about 25 to 30 mm Hg in the fetus to 90 to 95 mm Hg in the normal newborn results in a drop in serum erythropoietin, which accounts for a shutdown of RBC production that normally occurs at birth and persists for 6 to 8 wk. This bone marrow shutdown results in **physiologic anemia,** particularly in premature newborns whose body mass and blood volume are now increasing rapidly. However, the falling Hb eventually results in reduced tissue O_2 tension and an appropriate increase in erythropoietin release, which stimulates the bone marrow to produce new RBCs. Recently, it has been shown that erythropoietin given to anemic preterm infants produces a normal bone marrow response; this may prove to be an effective therapy for **physiologic anemia of the premature** (not to be confused with iron-deficiency anemia, which is not usually seen until age 4 to 6 mo).

IMMUNOLOGIC STATUS OF THE FETUS AND NEWBORN

Individual host defense factors develop at different rates in the fetus. At birth, the function of most immune mechanisms is proportional to gestational age, but even in term infants is lower than in adults. Thus the newborn and young infant (especially between ages 3 and 12 mo) have a significant transient immunodeficiency involving all limbs of the immune system, putting the neonate at risk of overwhelming infection. The risk can be enhanced by prematurity, traumatic delivery, maternal illness, neonatal stress, and some medications. (Immunization procedures are discussed below under IMMUNIZATION PROCEDURES THROUGHOUT CHILDHOOD.)

Phagocytic System

Phagocytic cells, first seen at the yolk sac stage of development, are critical for the inflammatory response that combats bacterial and fungal infection. Granulocytes and monocytes can be identified in the 2nd and 4th mo of gestation, respectively. In general, their level of function increases with gestational age but is still low at term. The newborn's decreased inflammatory response contributes to increased susceptibility to infections and may help explain the absence of localized clinical signs (eg, fever or meningismus) that are seen in older children with infections.

Ultrastructure of newborn neutrophils is normal, but membrane deformability and adherence are decreased, possibly influencing cell functions such as chemotaxis and phagocytosis. In most neonates, neutrophil and monocyte **chemotaxis** is decreased because of an intrinsic abnormality of cellular locomotion and adherence to surfaces. The latter can be attributed to failure to up-regulate the surface expression of adhesion glycoproteins (LFA, CR3) and to decreased fibronectin. The serum of neonates also has a decreased ability to generate chemotactic factors (*substances that attract phagocytes to sites of microbial invasion*). Decreased chemotaxis of newborn monocytes may contribute to their cutaneous anergy. Chemotaxis does not reach adult levels until several years of age. Neutrophil and monocyte **phagocytosis** and microbial killing usually are normal in healthy infants after 12 h of age, but are decreased in low-birth-weight or stressed term newborns.

Opsonization is necessary for efficient phagocytosis of many microorganisms. Serum opsonic factors include IgG and (heat-stable) IgM antibody **(Ab)** and (heat-labile) complement. IgM opsonizes gram-negative bacteria more efficiently than does IgG, but complement is needed for optimal serum opsonic activity. Unlike IgG, IgM and complement components do not cross the placenta. Levels of IgM production are low at birth unless stimulated by intrauterine infection. Synthesis of complement components begins as early as $5^{1}/_{2}$ wk gestation, but levels of most classical and alternative pathway components reach only 50 to 75% of adult levels by term. Therefore, normal newborns have very low serum levels of IgM and complement components. WBCs in newborns have normal Fc and C3 receptors for both groups of opsonins, but the C3 receptors fail to undergo increased expression on the cell surface after stimulation. Serum opsonic activity varies with gestational age, being decreased in low-birth-weight infants for all organisms tested and in term infants usually for some organisms, particularly gram-negative bacteria.

The circulating monocyte is the precursor of the fixed tissue macrophage, which is capable of phagocytosis in utero and has low-to-normal microbicidal activity at term. Pulmonary alveolar macrophages migrate into position at or near birth and help clear the alveoli of amniotic fluid debris as well as microorganisms. These and other tissue macrophages, including those in the spleen, have diminished phagocytic capacity. Decreased efficiency of the reticuloendothelial system of the newborn is, at least in part, due to decreased serum opsonic activity.

Cellular (T Cell) Immunity

In man, the thymus anlage is generated from the epithelium of the 3rd and 4th pharyngeal pouches at about the 6th wk of gestation; by the 12th wk it can participate in the immune response. The thymus is most active during fetal development and in early postnatal life. It grows rapidly in utero and is readily noted on chest x-ray in the normal neonate, and then involutes gradually over many years. The thymus is considered the mediator of tolerance to "self" antigens **(Ags)** during the fetal and perinatal periods and is essential to the development and maturation of peripheral lymphoid tissue. The epithelial elements in the thymus produce humoral substances that are important in T cell differentiation and maturation.

At birth, delayed hypersensitivity skin test responses are markedly diminished, and skin graft rejection is impaired. These functions improve during the first few months of life. In contrast, T cell numbers, T cell subsets (helpers and suppressors), and T cell proliferative responses to mitogens and allogeneic cells are normal or increased. Some lymphokines (interleukin [IL]-1, IL-2, IL-6, tumor necrosis factor [TNF], interferon [IFN]-α), but not all (IL-4, IFN-γ), are produced in near-normal quantities by lymphocytes in the newborn. Cytotoxic activity, including natural killer, Ab-dependent, and cytotoxic T cell killing is considerably lower than in adult lymphocytes. Also, T cell suppressor activity is considerably increased in the neonate, which may account for abnormalities of immunoregulation and decreased Ab production. The net effect is a partial T cell immunodeficiency, which may cause increased susceptibility to infection and, under rare circumstances, engraftment of transfused or maternal lymphocytes. A number of factors such as viral infections, hyperbilirubinemia, drugs taken by the mother late in pregnancy (eg, corticosteroids or antimetabolites) may depress T cell function in the neonate.

Antibody (B Cell) Immunity

B cells are found in fetal bone marrow, blood, liver, and spleen by 12 wk of gestation. Trace amounts of IgM and IgG synthesis occur by 20 wk and IgA synthesis by 30 wk. However, since the fetus is normally in an Ag-free environment, only small amounts of immunoglobulin (predominantly IgM) are produced in utero. Elevated levels of cord serum IgM (> 20 mg/dL) indicate in utero Ag challenge, usually from congenital infection. Almost all IgG is acquired from the mother via the placenta. At term birth, the infant has IgG levels comparable to or greater than adult levels (110% of maternal level). IgG levels at birth in premature infants are decreased in proportion to gestational age. After birth, catabolism of the transplacental IgG with a half-life of about 25 days results in a "physiologic hypogammaglobulinemia" by age 2 to 6 mo, which begins to resolve after 6 mo as the infant's rate of IgG synthesis begins to exceed catabolism of maternal Ab. Premature infants, in particular, may become profoundly hypogammaglobulinemic during the first 6 mo of life. By 1 yr of age the IgG level is about 70% of average adult values. IgA, IgM, IgD, and IgE do not cross the placenta. Their levels increase slowly from very low to about 30% of adult levels by 1 yr of age. Adult immunoglobulin levels are achieved approximately as follows: IgM, 1 yr; IgG, 8 yr; and IgA, 11 yr.

The newborn has deficient Ab responses to a number of Ags, including vaccine Ags. Ab responses to polysaccharide Ags such as hemophilus and pneumococcal polysaccharides are particularly poor in the first 2 yr of life, unless conjugated to diphtheria toxoid. When an Ab response occurs, usually there is a prolonged IgM response and a diminished IgG response. Immunization of an infant too early may result in a decreased Ab response to subsequent challenge with the same Ag.

Passive transfer of maternal immunity as transplacental IgG Ab and immune factors in breast milk helps compensate for the newborn's immature immune system and gives immunity to many serious bacterial (eg, pneumococcus, hemophilus, meningococcus) and viral pathogens (eg, measles, varicella). However, occasionally, passively acquired IgG can also inhibit the newborn's response to immunization against agents such as measles or rubella. Breast milk contains many antimicrobial factors (eg, IgG, secretory IgA, WBCs, complement proteins, lysozyme, and lactoferrin) that coat the GI and upper respiratory tracts and help prevent invasion of mucous membranes by respiratory and enteric pathogens. Breastfeeding is particularly important where the water supply may be contaminated.

The morbidity and mortality due to neonatal infections remain significant despite appropriate antibiotic therapy. Attempts have been made to augment the neonate's immature immune system in the prevention and treatment of infection. Recent studies suggest a possible role for immune or hyperimmune globulin in some kinds of neonatal infection (eg, Group B streptococcal disease). Data on the efficacy of exchange and leukocyte transfusions are conflicting, and the advisability of their routine use awaits the results of controlled trials.

INITIAL CARE

At birth, the normal newborn breathes spontaneously once his airway is cleared of mucus and debris by gentle bulb suction. The cord is clamped and cut after the first breath; one vein and 2 arteries should be visible on the fresh-cut surface. The newborn is dried gently and placed on a sterile, dry receiving blanket on a warm table; maintaining body temperature is critical.

Initial delivery-room inspection is limited to identifying any life-threatening or major abnormalities, such as gross deformities (omphalocele, myelomeningocele, cleft lip and palate) and orthopedic anomalies (clubfoot, an abnormal number of digits on hands or feet). Other abnormalities to be noted include a scaphoid abdomen, as seen in diaphragmatic hernia, and asymmetry or increased anteroposterior diameter of the chest, as seen in both diaphragmatic hernia and spontaneous pneumothorax. General condition is noted using the Apgar score (see ASPHYXIA AND RESUSCITATION in Ch. 27). Generalized cyanosis indicates significant heart or lung disease or major CNS depression; differential cyanosis indicates specific cardiac lesions. Many normal newborns have transient cyanosis that clears by the 5-min Apgar score. The heart and lungs are auscultated and the abdomen palpated. Gestational age is estimated (see method in FIG. 23–1) in order to plan special care for any neonate < 37 wk or > 42 wk gestation, or whose weight is inappropriate for his estimated gestational age (see GESTATIONAL AGE AND BIRTH WEIGHT in Ch. 27).

Except in resuscitation efforts, a tube should not be passed to check the esophagus and stom-

NEUROMUSCULAR MATURITY

Score	−1	0	1	2	3	4	5
Posture							
Square Window (wrist)	>90°	90°	60°	45°	30°	0°	
Arm Recoil		180°	140°–180°	110°–140°	90°–110°	<90°	
Popliteal Angle	180°	160°	140°	120°	100°	90°	<90°
Scarf Sign							
Heel to Ear							

PHYSICAL MATURITY

Skin	Sticky, friable, transparent	Gelatinous, red, translucent	Smooth, pink; visible veins	Superficial peeling and/or rash; few veins	Cracking, pale areas; rare veins	Parchment, deep cracking; no vessels	Leathery, cracked, wrinkled
Lanugo	None	Sparse	Abundant	Thinning	Bald areas	Mostly bald	
Plantar Surface	Heel-toe 40–50 mm: −1 <40 mm: −2	>50 mm, no crease	Faint red marks	Anterior transverse crease only	Creases anterior 2/3	Creases over entire sole	
Breast	Imperceptible	Barely perceptible	Flat areola, no bud	Stippled areola, 1–2 mm bud	Raised areola, 3–4 mm bud	Full areola, 5–10 mm bud	
Eye/Ear	Lids fused loosely: −1 tightly: −2	Lids open; pinna flat; stays folded	Slightly curved pinna; soft; slow recoil	Well-curved pinna; soft but ready recoil	Formed and firm, instant recoil	Thick cartilage, ear stiff	
Genitals (male)	Scrotum flat, smooth	Scrotum empty, faint rugae	Testes in upper canal, rare rugae	Testes descending, few rugae	Testes down, good rugae	Testes pendulous, deep rugae	
Genitals (female)	Clitoris prominent, labia flat	Clitoris prominent, small labia minora	Clitoris prominent, enlarging minora	Majora and minora equally prominent	Majora large, minora small	Majora cover clitoris and minora	

MATURITY RATING

Score	Weeks
−10	20
−5	22
0	24
5	26
10	28
15	30
20	32
25	34
30	36
35	38
40	40
45	42
50	44

FIG. 23–1. Assessment of gestational age—new Ballard score. (Modified from Ballard JL, Khoury JC, Wedig K, et al: "New Ballard score, expanded to include extremely premature infants." *The Journal of Pediatrics* 119(3):417–423, 1991; used with permission of the CV Mosby Company.)

ach until the newborn is stable (a minimum of 5 to 10 min after birth), since this maneuver may produce severe vasovagal reflex apnea in an otherwise normal infant. After 10 min of life, a tube is passed to check patency of the nares and esophagus in newborns born to mothers with polyhydramnios or diabetes, in those born in the breech position or by cesarean section delivery, and in *any* newborn with increased secretions, in order to rule out tracheoesophageal fistula and other anomalies of the esophagus and stomach. The stomach, if reached, is aspirated, and the volume of its contents measured. Neonates delivered in the vertex position may have little fluid left in the stomach, but this does not rule out obstruction. In premature newborns, the normal stomach volume is as follows:

Birth Weight	Fluid Volume
2.5 kg	12–15 mL
2.0 kg	10 mL
1.5 kg	7–8 mL
1.0 kg	5 mL

As soon as possible, the newborn is swaddled to maintain body temperature, being sure to cover the head, a large surface area capable of losing considerable heat. Two drops of 1% silver nitrate solution, or an antibiotic ointment such as erythromycin, are instilled in each eye. Before leaving the delivery area, or in the first hour of life, the newborn may be held by the mother and put to breast if she wishes (see FEEDING, below). *Good hand-washing technique must be used by all personnel, since the newborn's defense mechanisms against infection are not fully developed* (see IMMUNOLOGIC STATUS OF THE FETUS AND NEWBORN, above).

On arrival in the nursery, if the newborn's temperature is < 35.5° C (96° F), an infant warmer is required. Normally, the crib is left flat and the newborn is placed on his side to facilitate mucus drainage. Phytonadione (vitamin K_1) 1 mg IM is given to prevent hypoprothrombinemia, which causes hemorrhagic disease of the newborn. Triple Dye® may be applied with a swab to the fresh-cut cord and periumbilical area to prevent infection; one application is sufficient.

The admission bath is not given for 6 h or until the temperature has been stabilized at 37° C (98.6° F) for 2 h. The bath should not remove all the **vernix caseosa** (*a whitish, greasy material that covers most of the body at birth*), as it provides some antibacterial protection. A mild soap such as castile may be used with thorough rinsing. Oils, powders, and ointments should not be routinely used.

Initial Parent-Infant Interactions

Although pregnancy allows a woman to prepare herself psychologically for the new baby and to share that preparation with the father, there are important events that enhance parenting during and following birth. The physiologic aspects of birth include adaptations of the woman's body to the movement of the fetus from the uterus to the outside world. Participation in the birth by a prepared, knowledgeable woman and her spouse makes the new role of parenting go more smoothly. An optimal environment that helps the couple to be secure and confident also helps the mother relax and work with her body during labor and delivery.

Parental feelings at the first moments of their newborn's life vary from ecstasy to disappointment; for some, these moments are totally forgotten because of concurrent events requiring priority, such as resuscitation of the infant or obstetric complications in the mother. (Parent-infant bonding with a sick neonate is discussed in Ch. 24.) It has been suggested that early physical contact with the infant, looking eye to eye, establishes an early bond essential to a lasting parental love and relationship. In humans, however, such a "critical period" may not exist. Unquestionably, mothers can relate well to their infants even when the first hours are not spent enraptured with each other.

Immediately following a normal birth, the mother should be helped to hold and cuddle her baby while warmth and stabilization are provided for the newborn. The mother should be offered an opportunity to put the newborn to breast for the first suckling (see FEEDING, below), and the father should have the opportunity to share these moments. This may require providing appropriate garb for the father and some staff support if he is uncomfortable or insecure.

The first few days after birth are ideal times to provide the parents with additional information about breastfeeding, bathing, dressing, and understanding the newborn. When the neonate spends the entire days at his mother's bedside, where the parents can become familiar with his activities and sounds, the transition to the home is smoother. (See also HOSPITAL ACCOMMODATIONS, below.)

COMPLETE PHYSICAL EXAMINATION

This examination of the newborn should be done within the first 12 h of life and should include a more precise determination of the gestational age, utilizing both physical and neuromuscular findings (see Fig. 23–1).

Measurements: Body length is measured from crown to heel. Head circumference (largest measurement above the ears) should be about half the body length + 10 cm. Fig. 27–1 shows the relationship between birth weight and gestational age classifications. The average weight for term babies is 7 lb (3.2 kg). Measured against gestational age, the newborn's size may provide important clues to several conditions. For example, if the infant is small for gestational age, an intrauterine infection or a chromosomal abnormality may be the cause. An infant may be large for gestational age because of maternal diabetes mellitus or hyperinsulinism, as in Beckwith's syndrome; cyanotic congenital heart disease due to transposition of the great vessels; maternal obesity; or familial predisposition, as in Crow and Cheyenne Indians in Montana.

Skin: The skin is usually ruddy, and acrocyanosis is common in the first few hours. Dryness and peeling often occur in a few days, especially at wrist and ankle creases. Petechiae may be seen over the scalp and face because of pressure exerted during delivery but are not normally present below the umbilicus. Vernix caseosa covers most of the body after 24 wk of gestation.

Head: In a vertex delivery the head will be molded, with overriding of the cranial bones at the sutures and some swelling and/or ecchymosis of the scalp (**caput succedaneum**). In breech deliveries the head is usually unmolded, with swelling and ecchymosis occurring in the presenting part (ie, buttocks, genitalia, or feet). The fontanelles may vary in diameter from a fingertip breadth to several centimeters. A **cephalhematoma** is an accumulation of blood between the periosteum and the bone, producing a swelling that does not cross suture lines. It may present over one or both parietal bones and occasionally over the occiput. Cephalhematomas gradually disappear over several months and should not be aspirated.

Asymmetry of the face may be present because of in utero positioning. Facial nerve palsy should be suspected when there is asymmetry of the nasolabial folds and the creases around the eyes when the baby cries. The **eyes** should open symmetrically. Pupils should be equal and react to light, and the fundi should be visualized. If a red reflex is obtained on ophthalmoscopic examination, opacities may be excluded. Scleral hemorrhages are common. The **ears** are inspected for gestational age determination and positioning; low-set ears often signal a renal or genetic abnormality. The ear canals should be patent and the tympanic membranes visible. Although inexpensive portable devices are available to test the newborn's hearing, their reliability and validity have not been demonstrated except for gross screening purposes. Auditory evoked response testing (see in Ch. 64) may be available for high-risk patients, who should be identified by careful history of family deafness, fetal rubella, neonatal jaundice, or maternal or neonatal treatment with aminoglycosides.

The **mouth** should be inspected for an intact palate and uvula, gum cysts, and a congenitally short frenulum (**tongue-tie**). Small pearl-like elevations (**Epstein's pearls**) and small ulcerations (**Bednar's aphthae**) on the hard palate are normal. The infant's ability to suck should also be evaluated.

Cardiorespiratory system: Respirations are normally abdominal and range between 40 and 50/min. Breath sounds are harsh but should be heard equally throughout the chest. Heart sounds are audible by stethoscope, most prominently beneath the sternum. The heart rate is 100 to 150/min (average, 120). There may be marked sinus arrhythmia. Heart murmurs are frequently heard, but only about 10% are associated with congenital heart disease (see Ch. 28).

Severe congenital heart diseases, such as aortic atresia or hypoplasia of the right or left ventricle, may present with cyanosis or heart failure in the newborn period. Femoral pulses are palpable and their strength should be checked and compared; if the pulses are weak, aortic coarctation or left ventricular abnormalities may be present. Weak pulses should be confirmed with a flush or Doppler BP taken in all extremities. **Flush BP** is a technique in which blood is removed from a limb by elevating it until the skin pales. A previously applied BP cuff is pumped up as in taking regular BP; then, with the limb at the patient's side, pressure is gradually dropped and a reading is taken when color returns to the limb. **Doppler BP** (eg, using a Doptone® device) uses a transducer in the inflatable cuff to transmit and receive ultrasound waves. The technique detects vessel turbulence and so determines systolic and diastolic pressures with accuracy.

Abdomen: The abdominal examination is very important, as 10% of all newborns have anomalies or findings that require careful monitoring during the first few days of life, including abnormal shape, size, or position of the kidneys or other organs. (See also RENAL AND GENITOURINARY DEFECTS in Ch. 28.) Normally, the liver is felt 1 to 2 cm below the costal margin, and the spleen tip is easily palpated. Both kidneys are ordinarily palpable, the left more easily than the right; if they cannot be palpated, agenesis or hypoplasia may be suspected. Large kidneys may be caused by obstruction, tumor, or cystic disease. Failure of the male infant to void may indicate posterior urethral valves. An umbilical hernia, due to a weakness of the umbilical ring musculature, is common but rarely causes symptoms or needs therapy.

Genitalia: In the full-term male, the testes should be present in the scrotum. Hydroceles and inguinal hernias are often encountered in the newborn. A firm, discolored scrotal mass may represent **testicular torsion**, particularly in breech deliveries. Although rare and apparently not painful in the neonate, *torsion represents a surgical emergency.* Torsion can be distinguished from simple bruising by the distribution of the ecchymoses and the firmness of the testes if torsion is present. The mass will transilluminate if it is a hydrocele. In females, the labia are prominent. Mucoid and occasionally serosanguineous secretions (pseudomenses) may occur and are transient and nonirritating. A small tag of tissue at the posterior fourchette, believed to be due to maternal hormonal stimulation, will disappear over the first few weeks.

Neuromuscular system: The extremities should be symmetrically placed and actively mobile. Completely abducting the thighs to the surface of the examining table, while the infant is supine with the hips and knees flexed, should be possible; limited abduction and a palpable "clunk" as the femoral head slides into the hip socket are the cardinal signs of **congenital hip dislocation.** (See also MUSCULOSKELETAL DEFECTS in Ch. 28.) Female infants and those delivered in the breech position are particularly prone to have a dislocated hip. If hip mobility is in question, an ultrasound should be obtained and an orthopedic specialist consulted. With minimal congenital dysplasia of the hip joint, using double or triple diapers may be adequate treatment. In

more severe cases, an orthopedist should apply an abduction splint, but only after the ultrasound is reviewed. If a specialist is not available immediately, triple diapers should be used 24 h/day until a splint can be applied. If **clubfoot** or any other significant orthopedic abnormality is present, therapy should begin immediately. (See MUSCULOSKELETAL DEFECTS in Ch. 28.)

The **neurologic examination** should include elicitation of the Moro, sucking, and rooting reflexes. The deep tendon reflexes should be present and equal. (Neurologic congenital abnormalities are discussed in Ch. 28.)

THE FIRST FEW DAYS

Weight: Loss of 5 to 10% of birth weight in the first few days of life is considered normal and is common for most newborns. Passage of meconium, loss of vernix caseosa, and drying of the umbilical cord account for some weight loss, but most is due to urinary and insensible water losses. **Umbilical cord:** The plastic cord clamp should be removed in 24 h to avoid undue tension on the drying stump. Daily application of 70% alcohol to the stump hastens drying and reduces infection. The cord should be observed daily for redness or drainage, since it is an excellent portal of entry for infection (see also INITIAL CARE, above). It is the first area to colonize with bacteria and usually is the site cultured in infection control programs. **Circumcision,** if indicated, generally is performed within the first few days of life but should be delayed indefinitely if there is any displacement of the urethral meatus, hypospadias, or any other abnormality of the glans or penis, since the prepuce may be used later in plastic repair. Circumcision usually is requested by the parents and is rarely indicated medically. An increase in incidence of UTI among uncircumcised males is cited as an indication by some. It should not be done if a family history of hemophilia or other bleeding disorders exists, or if the mother is taking medication associated with coagulation disturbances, such as anticoagulants or aspirin.

Voiding: The first urine voided is concentrated and often contains urates, which turn the diaper pink. Failure to void within the first 24 h of life must be investigated thoroughly. Delayed voiding is more common in males and may be associated with a tight foreskin, or edema and swelling of the penis in the recently circumcised infant. **Defecating** (stooling): **Meconium** is *a sticky green-black substance that contains lanugo and* squamous epithelial cells from swallowed amniotic fluid and intestinal secretions. Every infant should pass meconium by age 24 h. The infant who is meconium-stained at birth may delay defecating, but in this case it is evident that the anus is patent. Delayed defecation is most commonly the result of a plug of inspissated meconium (see under GASTROINTESTINAL DEFECTS in Ch. 28).

Skin: Erythema toxicum, a benign self-limited rash, is the most common lesion and may occur at any time during the first week but most often on the second day. Usually found where clothing rubs the arms, legs, and back, and rarely on the face, the rash appears as a blotchy erythematous wheal with a central papule that may become quite prominent. A Wright-stained smear of the papule contents reveals eosinophils. A family history of allergy should be sought in severe cases; if found, use of lotions, powders, perfumed soaps, and plastic pants should be avoided. Subcutaneous fat necrosis may occur over any bony prominence subjected to trauma or pressure, especially the head, cheek, and neck where forceps are applied. Lesions are indurated, isolated, and well demarcated. A lesion may rupture through to the skin surface, releasing a clear yellow, sterile fluid that should disappear spontaneously or with use of a "pressure doughnut" dressing.

Slight jaundice may occur in normal newborns but is of concern if it appears before 24 h of age, and if the serum bilirubin is > 12 mg/dL in a term newborn (concern is greater at lower levels in a premature neonate and under other circumstances—see HYPERBILIRUBINEMIA under METABOLIC PROBLEMS IN THE NEWBORN in Ch. 27 for a full discussion).

Screening tests for metabolic and hematologic disorders should be undertaken (see SCREENING PROCEDURES FOR INFANTS AND CHILDREN, below).

FEEDING

(See also INFANT NUTRITION, below)

The normal newborn has active rooting and sucking reflexes and can receive oral feedings immediately. Ordinarily, these should not be delayed > 4 h.

Spitting and regurgitating mucus are common during the first day, but if they persist the stomach should be emptied by gentle aspiration through a feeding tube and washed out with 5% D/W until the returns are clear of mucus. If vomiting continues in a newborn who is bottle fed, a hypoallergenic milk formula should be tried, and, if unsuccessful, a more comprehensive diagnostic assessment should be done. A breastfed newborn who continues to vomit should have a full diagnostic assessment for obstruction, since babies are not allergic to human milk.

Bottle Feeding

The first offering tests whether or not the newborn can coordinate suck, swallow, and gag reflexes. Sterile distilled water is given, since even 5% D/W may irritate the newborn lung if aspirated. If this is not regurgitated, the next feeding can be a milk formula. Full-term newborns are usually fed on a 4-h schedule for the sake of hospital efficiency.

Prepackaged formulas are available in sterile 4-oz bottles providing 13 or 20 kcal/oz with adequate vitamins for the normal newborn. Full-term neonates can tolerate 20 kcal/oz immediately. The mother should be told not to overfeed the newborn simply because 4 oz of formula are available. Feedings should be increased gradually during the first week of life from 1 or 2 oz to 3 or 4 oz given 6 times/day. This supplies about 120 kcal/kg (55 kcal/lb) at age 1 wk.

The newborn should be offered water between feedings, particularly in hot weather or in a hot, dry environment. Newborns should retain at least 65 mL of fluid/kg the first 24 h, 75 mL/kg the second 24 h, and up to 100 mL/kg the third 24 h. Those who fall appreciably behind these amounts are given 5% glucose in 0.25% sodium chloride by IV drip to make up the deficit. A cause for the poor feeding pattern should be sought.

Breastfeeding

Over 50% of mothers breastfeed their infants today and the number is increasing, primarily in higher socioeconomic groups. Given adequate support and encouragement, most women can nurse their infants successfully. Physicians should discuss infant feeding with the mother, prenatally presenting the benefits of breastfeeding (nutritional, immunologic, including protection against infection, and psychologic—see also INFANT NUTRITION, below, and IMMUNOLOGIC STATUS OF THE FETUS AND NEWBORN, above) and other points to be aware of (see DRUGS IN LACTATING MOTHERS, below), so that each mother can make an informed choice. The chief contraindication is the mother's lack of desire and interest.

When breastfeeding is planned, the technique should be familiar before delivery. Physicians who counsel nursing mothers should be conversant with the better literature on this subject before they recommend any reading to their patients. The physician should discuss the physiology of lactation with the mother and answer her questions. It is often helpful if the mother talks to a woman who has nursed successfully and even observes the process. Preparation of the nipple before delivery is not necessary, nor is manual expression of the breast, which at this time may lead to mastitis or early labor. Nature prepares the areola and nipple for the suckling by secreting a lubricant from Montgomery's glands to protect the surface. This lubricant should not be buffed away with a towel or elaborate nipple exercises.

At delivery, if the mother has had little medication and a normal delivery and the newborn is alert and active, he may be put to breast immediately for a few minutes on each side. He will receive a small amount of **colostrum**, a high-caloric, high-protein, thin yellow fluid present in the breast before birth and for the first few days thereafter, which contains antibodies, lymphocytes, and macrophages as well as nutrients. Colostrum also stimulates the passage of meconium.

Whether or not the newborn is nursed in the delivery room, he can be taken to the mother for nursing within the first 4 h of age. The mother should assume a comfortable, relaxed position, such as lying almost flat and turning from one side to the other to offer each breast. The newborn should be placed so he faces the mother, ventral surface to ventral surface. The mother should support her breast with thumb on top and fingers below to ensure that it is centered in the baby's mouth, minimizing any soreness. The corner of the newborn's mouth should be stimulated with the nipple so that he will root and grasp the breast. Suction should be broken before removing the newborn from the breast. Feedings are started on alternate sides, initially at least 2 min at each breast to allow time for the let-down reflex to act. Although there should not be stopwatch timing, excessive suckling should be avoided initially, as sore nipples are easier to prevent than to cure. On the other hand, milk production is dependent on adequate suckling time. Nursing times are gradually increased until the "milk is in." Ten minutes at the first breast and a time sufficient to satisfy the newborn at the second are usually appropriate. In primiparas, lactation is established in 72 to 96 h; less time is required in multiparas. If the mother is especially

fatigued, the 2 AM feeding may be replaced with water until full milk secretion begins, but with never > 6 h between breastfeedings during the first few days. Feeding should be on demand rather than by the clock, and feeding duration should also reflect newborn needs.

Breast engorgement, which occurs during early lactation, may be minimized by early frequent feeding. Engorgement can be alleviated if the mother wears a comfortable nursing brassiere 24 h/day for support. Manually expressing milk during a warm shower may provide considerable comfort. The mother may have to express her milk manually just before nursing to allow the newborn to get the swollen areola into his mouth, but excessive expression between feedings encourages continued engorgement and should be done only to relieve discomfort. Should sore nipples occur, positioning of the baby should be checked as noted above. Sometimes the newborn will draw in his lower lip and suck the lip, which is irritating to the nipple. The mother can ease the lip out with her thumb. Between feedings, she can use a hairdryer set on low to warm and dry her nipples for 15 min, letting the milk dry on the nipples. Plastic brassiere liners should be avoided.

Special dietary increases during lactation include 600 extra kcal, of which 20 gm are protein. The major nutrient a mother must add is 400 mg extra calcium (dairy products are an excellent source). If milk products are not tolerated, nuts and green vegetables should be increased, or calcium gluconate supplements by capsule may be used. Vitamin supplementation is not necessary if the diet is well balanced and includes vitamin C and animal protein for B_6 and B_{12} (the average US diet is low in B_6, and vegetarian diets may be low in B_{12}). A daily vitamin supplement such as those used prenatally may be used but usually are not necessary.

All newborns, especially breastfeeding ones, should be seen by the physician at 10 days to 2 wk of age to evaluate progress and answer any questions the mother may have before they become problems. This is especially urgent if the mother is a primipara. A normal newborn wets 6 to 8 diapers a day or more, stools daily, and has a vigorous cry, good skin turgor, and a good suck reflex. Weight gain is also a good test of adequate feeding. Although sleeping long periods of time between feedings may be a sign of a good milk supply, it can be associated with inadequate supply and starvation; thus all newborns should be checked early.

DRUGS IN LACTATING MOTHERS

Drugs pass into the breast milk of lactating mothers differentially, depending on the drug's lipid solubility, pK_a, and protein-binding capacity, and on the pH of the milk. The concentration gradient is the primary determinant of drug transfer between plasma and milk.

The pH of milk is slightly lower than plasma pH; hence weak bases tend to have a higher milk-to-plasma ratio than do weak acids. Lincomycin, erythromycin, antihistamines, alkaloids, isoniazid, antipsychotics, antidepressants, lithium, quinine, thiouracil, and metronidazole—all weak bases—have concentrations in milk equal to or higher than in plasma. Barbiturates, phenytoins, sulfonamides, diuretics, and penicillins—weak acids—have concentrations in milk equal to or lower than in plasma.

Almost all drugs pass to some extent into breast milk, but the clinical significance of this depends on (1) the degree of drug passage into milk, (2) the amount of milk ingested by the infant at the feeding, (3) whether the amount ingested at each feeding is the same, (4) the frequency of feeding, (5) whether the drug is absorbed by the infant, and (6) whether the infant is affected by the drug.

There are problems in determining what drugs are contraindicated in lactating mothers because of very limited human studies. Data often are taken from casereports, human studies with very small numbers of subjects, or anecdotal reports of adverse effects in nursing infants associated with drug medication of the mother. Animal data are inappropriately projected to humans on a theoretic basis. The concentrations of drugs in milk are generally expressed relative to the mother's plasma concentration. A milk:plasma ratio of ≥ 1 creates a false alarm for potential adverse effects in the nursing infant, not considering that milk concentration does not equate with plasma concentration in relation to target sites of action. A clear example is isoniazid. Given at therapeutic dosage, the plasma concentration achieved is 6 $\mu g/mL$. Assuming that the milk:plasma ratio is 1, an infant consuming 8 oz of milk will ingest only 1.4 mg/feeding. The therapeutic dose of isoniazid for children is 10 to 20 mg/kg. Considering absorption, distribution, metabolism, and excretion processes of the drug, one would expect an insignificant plasma concentration in the infant. Unless a drug is highly potent and toxic even in very low concentrations or has cumulative effects in infants because of the infant's immature drug metabolism and excretion, drug excretion in milk would not be a hazard to infants. As more studies are reported on drugs and lactation, fewer drugs are considered **absolute contraindications** to nursing infants. These are the anticancer drugs, radiopharmaceuticals, ergot and its derivatives (methysergide, etc), lithium, chloramphenicol, phenylbutazone, atropine, thiouracil, iodides, and mercurials.

Over-the-counter medications are important to consider because of their availability to consumers and the increasing trend in self-diagnosis and treatment of self-limited minor illnesses. The nonprescription drugs include (1) analgesics—aspirin, ibuprofen, and acetaminophen; (2) antihistamines in cold, sinus, cough and antivertigo remedies, and sleeping aids; (3) sympathomimetics like ephedrine, pseudoephedrine, phenylephrine, and phenylpropanolamine, which are selectively utilized for anticongestant, anorexiant, and antiasthmatic medications; (4) antacids, laxatives, and cathartics; (5) topical medications (skin, rectal, and vaginal), which include corticosteroids, local anesthetics, astringents like zinc and bismuth, and antihistamines. In general, all the above medications *are safe* for nursing mothers, when taken short-term and in doses prescribed on the labels. Over-the-counter drugs are formulated using the least toxic class of drugs at the lowest effective therapeutic doses.

Some controversies exist over the significance in breast milk of propylthiouracil, methimazole, warfarin, dicumarol, morphine, codeine, methadone, neuroleptics and antidepressants, sedatives and tranquilizers, contraceptives, alcohol, nicotine, and metronidazole. Although some studies have shown that these drugs have been given to nursing mothers without ill effects in their nursing infants, experts advise that these drugs should be used only when critically indicated. When they are prescribed, close observation of the infant is required because of potential toxicity with prolonged medication in specific conditions.

Analgesics: Salicylates are excreted into the breast milk in moderate amounts. With larger doses and chronic medication, nursing neonates may achieve plasma concentrations that can cause greater risk from hyperbilirubinemia (salicylates compete for albumin-binding sites), hemorrhagic problems, and hemolysis in G6PD-deficient babies. **Acetaminophen** appears safe when taken in therapeutic doses. There are no data for ibuprofen. **Narcotic analgesics** (eg, codeine, morphine, meperidine, or methadone) in therapeutic doses are excreted in the milk at very low concentrations that minimally affect nursing infants in single doses. However, in narcotic addicts using high doses of drugs, significant amounts are excreted in milk, affecting the nursing infant and causing withdrawal symptoms when feeding is missed (see also Ch. 53 and METABOLIC PROBLEMS IN THE NEWBORN in Ch. 27).

Antibiotics generally can be prescribed to nursing mothers without significant hazards to their infants. However, because almost all antibiotics are excreted in milk, infants may develop hypersensitivity, diarrhea, and candidiasis. Levels of **penicillin** are detectable in breast milk as early as 1 h and as long as 9 h after IM injection. **Tetracycline** is significantly excreted in milk, but because it is precipitated by calcium in the milk, absorption by nursing infants could be too insignificant to cause adverse effects. However, the tetracyclines (eg, minocycline, which is 100% absorbed orally and not affected by food) *should be avoided by nursing mothers.* **Metronidazole,** a useful antiprotozoal and antibacterial for giardiasis, trichomoniasis, and hemophilus vaginitis, and a radiosensitizer in the treatment of various tumors, is significantly excreted in breast milk. The agent is carcinogenic in rodents and mutagenic in bacteria. When metronidazole is inevitably indicated, a single-dose regimen of 2 gm should be given and breastfeeding should be suspended for 24 h, pumping and discarding the milk. **Nalidixic acid, sulfonamides,** and **other oxidant drugs** can cause hemolysis in G6PD-deficient infants. The orally nonabsorbable antibiotics like **streptomycin, kanamycin,** and **gentamicin** pose no systemic problems in infants, but their continuous ingestion may alter the infant's intestinal flora and consequently affect some immune mechanisms.

Antihypertensives, diuretic drugs, digoxin, and β **blockers** can be continuously prescribed without significant adverse effects in nursing infants. Drug choice should be based on minimal levels in milk. **Hormones** that are orally absorbed, when given to nursing mothers in large doses, can attain high concentrations in milk. **Oral contraceptives** often are prescribed postpartum to prevent pregnancy. The hormones ethinyl estradiol and mestranol are excreted into breast milk; they can reduce milk production and also reduce pyridoxine (vitamin B_6) in the milk. Breast enlargement was observed in one male infant. Newer low-dose and single-hormone contraceptive pills are preferable. **Corticosteroids,** when given to the mother in large doses for extended periods, can attain high concentrations in milk and pose the danger of suppressing growth and interfering with endogenous corticosteroid production in the infant. **Barbiturates** and **phenytoin** can induce microsomal oxidizing enzymes in infants, enhancing the degradation of endogenous steroids, but in small doses are usually considered safe. **Diazepam** is excreted in breast milk and causes lethargy, drowsiness, and loss of weight in breastfed infants. Evidence indicates that metabolism of diazepam by nursing infants of mothers on moderate diazepam dosage (≥ 30 mg/day) is slow. Since diazepam is metabolized by glucuronide conjugation, competition with bilirubin for glucuronic acid may predispose neonates under 1 mo of age to kernicterus. The **antipsychotics** and **tricyclic antidepressants** pass into the milk but are not likely to produce any significant adverse reactions in the infant, since low plasma concentration is achieved as a result of poor absorption from the GI tract. **Warfarin** and **dicumarol** can be given cautiously to nursing mothers, but the synthetic anticoagulants can cause kernicterus. **Heparin** does not pass into milk.

Tetrahydrocannabinol (9-THC), the most psychoactive component of marijuana, is highly bound to lipoproteins after oral absorption, and excretion into breast milk is very low in animals. Since the plasma half-life in man may be as long as 2 days, it is wise for nursing mothers to avoid marijuana. **Cocaine** cannot be safely used while breastfeeding, as it persists in the milk for up to 24 h.

Drugs taken by nursing mothers that are not generally considered hazardous to the infant include insulin, epinephrine, alcohol, nicotine, and caffeine. However, *large doses of alcohol, caffeine, and theophylline can adversely affect the infant,* eg, hyperirritability from caffeine and theophylline.

Drugs to be avoided in the absence of studies on their excretion in breast milk are those with long half-lives; those that are potent toxins to the bone marrow; those given in high doses chronically; insecticides, pollutants, and other toxins; and vaccines.

The following drugs can **suppress or inhibit lactation** in nursing mothers: bromocriptine, bendroflumethiazide, estradiol, large-dose oral contraceptives, levodopa, and the antidepressant trazodone.

HOSPITAL ACCOMMODATIONS

Rooming-in is an arrangement that permits the infant to remain with the mother in her hospital room all or part of each day. Properly done, it facilitates establishment of the critically important mother-child relationship. The primipara can learn about her baby with professional help available, while the experienced mother is reassured that her baby is being managed her way. The plan provides a flexible feeding and sleeping routine and may reduce the risk of cross infection. This service is more an applied attitude to neonatal care than provision of a physical facility and can be offered in any hospital with sympathetic medical and nursing personnel. Alternatively, **nursery care** generally allows the mother more rest and permits more direct continual supervision of the infant by nursery personnel when these considerations are paramount.

Early discharge from the hospital (under 48 h) should be accompanied by a plan to supervise home management closely with home or office visits.

HEALTH SUPERVISION OF THE WELL CHILD

Periodic health supervision visits intended to promote the optimal health of infants and children.

The objectives are (1) prevention of disease through routine immunizations (see IMMUNIZATION PROCEDURES THROUGHOUT CHILDHOOD, below) and through education (parental instruction on nutrition, accident prevention [see Ch. 30], sanitation, etc); (2) early detection of disease through interview, physical examination, and screening procedures (discussed separately below); (3) early treatment of disease; and (4) provision of guidance in child rearing to afford optimal conditions for normal emotional and intellectual development. To meet these objectives, child and parent are seen at regular intervals throughout the early years of life (see TABLE 23–1). The frequency and content of these visits are determined by the child's age, the population served, and the physician's and parents' opinion of their value.

Inquiries as to the child's intellectual and psychosocial development are essential in preventive health care. Personal adaptive development (social, language, gross motor, fine motor) can be estimated by using the Denver Developmental

Screening Test (DDST). Routine testing should be started at age 4 to 6 mo and can be repeated periodically into early childhood.

Assessing the parents' perception of their child and the interactions between parents and child cannot be accomplished easily by any convenient, standardized method; rather it requires skillful interviewing and observation, beginning with discussions at the first contact in the hospital. Some parents and physicians prefer to meet prior to the baby's delivery, usually early in the 3rd trimester, to discuss parental expectations for their newborn and plans for care during infancy and childhood. Subsequently, parental attitudes may be identified tactfully by determining how the parents feel they are being affected by caring for a new infant, how they handle difficult situations, and how easily they can obtain help when feeling tired or short-tempered. In helping to establish good parent-child interactions, the physician is fulfilling an ongoing, integral responsibility that requires individualized attention.

The American Academy of Pediatrics (**AAP**) has recommended preventive health care schedules (see TABLE 23–1) for children who have not manifested any important health problems and who are growing and developing satisfactorily. More frequent and sophisticated visits are recommended for children who do not meet these criteria. If a child comes under care for the first time at a late point on the schedule, or if any items are not accomplished at the suggested age, the schedule should be brought up to date as rapidly as possible. The recommended schedule is based upon the opinion of the AAP membership; there is no scientific evidence that adherence to these recommendations (except for those on immunization) has any positive overall effect on childhood mortality or morbidity, or exerts any significant influence on developmental and social functioning outcomes.

SCREENING PROCEDURES FOR INFANTS AND CHILDREN

Screening procedures are a part of preventive health care in infants and children, often detecting disorders before frank symptoms of disease exist. To be useful, screening must show that early detection of a disorder can improve an infant's health through therapeutic intervention or that genetic counseling may be provided to aid the family. The number of cases detected by screening tests varies greatly with each disorder but, in general, is low, and false positives may be anticipated. Some patients need retesting, re-evaluation, or referral to an appropriate specialist before a clear, definitive diagnosis can be reached.

Testing in the Newborn Period

Screening of the neonate is important for identifying a number of physical anomalies and diseases, such as hip dislocation, renal masses, or cataracts. A complete physical examination should be performed (see under MANAGEMENT OF THE NORMAL NEWBORN, above), and each parent's family history and the mother's pregnancy history should be reviewed. Screening for metabolic and hematologic disorders also should be undertaken, especially for the following conditions.

Metabolic diseases (recognition markers for certain diseases are discussed in Ch. 13 and under PREVENTION OF GENETIC DISORDERS in Ch. 48): At the time of hospital discharge, the newborn should have capillary blood specimens taken to screen for a number of diseases (eg, phenylketonuria **[PKU]**, hypothyroidism, tyrosinosis, homocystinuria, maple syrup urine disease, galactosemia). Many metabolic disorders (eg, PKU) are proving to be amenable to dietary management. **Galactosemia** (see GENETIC ABNORMALITIES OF CARBOHYDRATE METABOLISM in Ch. 40) may be reliably diagnosed and treated before affected infants must risk the consequences of high blood galactose levels (liver disease, cataracts, brain damage due to hypoglycemia, or death). **Hypothyroidism** diagnosed and treated before age 3 mo has a greatly improved prognosis. (Hypothyroidism in children is discussed in Ch. 40.)

Sickle cell screening: Case finding of sickle cell disease using Hb electrophoresis is advisable in the newborn because early prophylaxis with penicillin reduces the risks of pneumococcal disease. Because of cost and technical limitations of Hb electrophoresis, newborn testing is not done routinely in all US states. However, the physician may want to do this test on an individual basis. (Prenatal testing for sickle cell disease is discussed in Ch. 13 and under PREVENTION OF GENETIC DISORDERS in Ch. 48.)

Anemia: Blood loss during birth or in the neonatal observation period (when extensive studies may require multiple blood samples) may cause anemia. Determining the Hct or Hb level at the time of discharge provides a baseline value for tests undertaken later in infancy.

Urinary screening for drugs: Recent studies suggest that many pregnant women use cocaine and opioids. Because of toxic effects on newborns of such prenatal drug use and the high risk for child abuse and neglect when mothers continue drug use after the infant is born, urinary screening of newborns has been advised when indicated by (1) a maternal history of drug abuse, < 5 prenatal visits, hepatitis B, syphilis, gonorrhea, HIV infection, unexplained placental abruption, or unexplained premature labor; or (2) the infant exhibits unexplained neurologic disease, evidence of drug withdrawal, or unexplained intrauterine growth retardation.

Newborns of mothers whose blood type is O and/or Rh-negative should be typed and a Coombs' test performed. Those with a positive indirect Coombs' test should be watched for jaundice. Many recommend a total bilirubin determination upon discharge as a routine procedure.

G6PD deficiency: About 10% of black American males suffer from a mild form of this disorder and only occasionally have symptoms in early infancy; Orientals and some groups of Mediterranean origin develop a more severe form, with hemolytic anemia and hyperbilirubinemia. Sensitivity of RBCs to various drugs occurs later. These select groups should be screened during the neonatal period.

Procedures After the Newborn Period

Growth and development: Length (crown-heel), weight, and head circumference should be measured at each visit or health examination during the first year of life. Continued systematic plotting of the infant's measurements on a growth curve with percentiles facilitates growth-rate monitoring. The infant's developmental level and performance should be assessed at each visit. (See also TABLE 23-1 and the discussion below in GROWTH AND DEVELOPMENT FROM BIRTH THROUGH CHILDHOOD.)

Hips, legs, and feet: When unstable or dislocated hips are (occasionally) undetected in the newborn, later signs provide clues, eg, unequal leg length or adductor tightness. Internal tibial torsion is common and may need orthopedic evaluation. Forefoot adduction usually is not apparent at birth and should be sought at each infant examination. It is easily corrected at a young age. (See also COMMON FOOT AND LEG PROBLEMS IN CHILDREN AND ADOLESCENTS in Ch. 42.)

Cardiac auscultation should be performed to identify the presence of murmurs, and femoral

TABLE 23–1. RECOMMENDATIONS FOR PREVENTIVE PEDIATRIC HEALTH CARE*

	Infancy							Early Childhood					Late Childhood					Adolescence²			
Age³	2–3 days¹	By 1 mo	2 mo	4 mo	6 mo	9 mo	12 mo	15 mo	18 mo	24 mo	3 yr	4 yr	5 yr	6 yr	8 yr	10 yr	12 yr	14 yr	16 yr	18 yr	20+ yr
History Initial/interval	•	•	•	•	•	•	•	•	•	•	•	•	•	•	•	•	•	•	•	•	•
Measurements																					
Height and weight	•	•	•	•	•	•	•	•	•	•	•	•	•	•	•	•	•	•	•	•	•
Head circumference	•	•	•	•	•	•	•	•	•	•											
Blood pressure											•	•	•	•	•	•	•	•	•	•	•
Sensory screening																					
Vision	S	S	S	S	S	S	S	S	S	S	S	S	O	O	O	O	O	O	O	O	O
Hearing	S	S	S	S	S	S	S	S	S	S	S	S	O	O	S⁴	S⁴	O	S	O	O	S
Development/behavioral assessment⁵	•	•	•	•	•	•	•	•	•	•	•	•	•	•	•	•	•	•	•	•	•
Physical examination⁶	•	•	•	•	•	•	•	•	•	•	•	•	•	•	•	•	•	•	•	•	•
Procedures⁷																					
Hereditary/metabolic screening⁸	•																				
Immunization⁹		•	•	•	•		•	•				•	•								
Tuberculin test¹⁰							•														
Hct or Hb¹¹					•																
Urinalysis¹²							•														
Anticipatory guidance¹³	•	•	•	•	•	•	•	•	•	•	•	•	•	•	•	•	•	•	•	•	•
Initial dental referral¹⁴											•										

● = to be performed; S = subjective, by history; O = objective, by a standard testing method; arrows = once within that period.

* Recommended by the American Academy of Pediatrics' Committee on Practice and Ambulatory Medicine. Reprinted with permission from *AAP News*, July 1991. Copyright 1991 American Academy of Pediatrics.

1. For newborns discharged ≤ 24 h after delivery.
2. Adolescence-related issues (eg, psychosocial, emotional, substance use, and reproductive health) may necessitate more frequent health supervision.
3. If a child comes under care for the first time at any point on the schedule, or if any items are not accomplished at the suggested age, the schedule should be brought up to date at the earliest possible time.
4. At these points, history may suffice; if a problem is suggested, a standard testing method should be used.
5. By history and appropriate physical examination; if suspicious, by specific objective developmental testing.
6. At each visit, a complete physical examination is essential, with infant totally unclothed, older child undressed and suitably draped.
7. These may be modified, depending on entry point into schedule and individual need.
8. Metabolic screening (eg, thyroid, phenylketonuria [PKU], galactosemia) should be done according to state law.
9. Schedule(s) per *Report of Committee on Infectious Diseases*, 1991 Red Book, and current AAP Committee statements.
10. For high-risk groups, the Committee on Infectious Diseases recommends annual TB skin testing.
11. Present medical evidence suggests the need for reevaluation of the frequency and timing of Hb or Hct tests. One determination is therefore suggested during each time period. Performance of additional tests is left to the individual practice experience.
12. Present medical evidence suggests the need for reevaluation of the frequency and timing of urinalysis. One determination is therefore suggested during each time period. Performance of additional tests is left to the individual practice experience.
13. Appropriate discussion and counseling should be an integral part of each visit for care.
14. Subsequent examinations as prescribed by dentist.

NOTE: Special chemical, immunologic, and endocrine tests are usually carried out upon specific indications. Other screening tests (eg, for sickle cell disease and lead poisoning) are discretionary with the physician.

pulses should be palpated at each health examination.

Abdominal palpation also should be repeated at every visit, because many masses, particularly Wilms' tumor and neuroblastoma, may be apparent only as the infant grows.

Hearing (see also CLINICAL MEASUREMENT OF HEARING IN CHILDREN, below): About 1/600 neonates has a congenital hearing loss, and many more acquire hearing loss owing to conditions encountered during the neonatal period. Detecting this problem in infancy depends on understanding high-risk conditions as well as behaviors and responses that suggest a hearing loss. **High-risk factors** include birth weight < 1500 gm; Apgar score ≤ 5 at 5 min; serum bilirubin > 22 mg/dL in a neonate whose birth weight is > 2000 gm, or > 17 mg/dL in a newborn < 2000 gm; anoxia; neonatal sepsis or meningitis; neonatal hyperbilirubinemia; seizures or apneic spells; congenital intrauterine infection, such as rubella, cytomegalovirus, or toxoplasmosis; use of aminoglycoside drugs; or a history of early hearing loss in a parent or close relative.

In about 1/3 of infants deaf from birth, a hereditary recessive etiology that is not present in either parent is assumed. These children must be identified by **observations that the parents can learn to make.** By age 3 mo, an infant can be expected to startle to a nearby loud sound, stir or awaken from sleep when someone talks or makes a noise, and be soothed by the mother's voice. By age 6 mo, an infant should look toward an interesting sound, turn when his name is called, make sounds such as "moo," "ma," "da," and "di" to toys or objects, and coo when listening to music. By age 10 mo, the infant should make sounds on his own, imitate some sounds made by others, and understand "no" and "bye-bye." By age 18 mo, the appropriate use of a few single words, the understanding of many single words or commands, and babbling in sentence-like patterns is expected. Infants who do not pass these minimal performance standards or whose parents suspect that there is a hearing loss at any age should be referred for hearing testing.

Ear infections, middle ear serous fluid accumulations, or frequent respiratory infections may cause enough hearing loss in infants and children to seriously affect development of language skills. Prompt audiologic referral may be indicated.

Vision: While sight cannot be tested easily or very satisfactorily at < 3 yr of age, attention to the infant's and young child's eyes should start early in life. The premature infant of < 32 wk gestation must be repeatedly examined for evidence of **retinopathy of prematurity** (see under PREMATURE INFANT in Ch. 27). This is best done by an ophthalmologist. Such infants also commonly develop refractive errors as they grow.

In the first 2 to 4 wk of life, an eye examination by the primary physician should note abnormalities of the globe (globe size in particular, because congenital glaucoma causes enlargement of the globe), color of the iris, pupillary size and asymmetry, character of the red reflex, and whether choroidal vessels can be visualized by direct ophthalmoscopy. A cataract may be seen, or merely suspected, when the red reflex is missing or distorted. Untreated cataracts may cause amblyopia (visual loss) if not detected early. By age 6 wk, the infant should begin to fix the parent with his eyes. Strabismus that is demonstrated at any age may cause loss of visual acuity, and an ophthalmologist should be consulted. Other conditions that obscure vision are ptosis and eyelid hemangioma.

In the growing child, alignment of the eyes should be examined repeatedly. Esotropia (inward deviation or convergent strabismus) accounts for much of childhood amblyopia. A cover test is of value. By 3 or 4 yr of age, vision testing by Snellen charts or newer testing machines can be done routinely. The E charts are better than pictures. Visual acuity of $< 20/30$ should be checked by an ophthalmologist.

Further laboratory studies: (1) Newborn screening tests for PKU are discussed under ANOMALIES IN AMINO ACID METABOLISM in Ch. 40. (2) Hct or Hb should be determined at age 8 to 9 mo for full-term infants and at age 5 to 6 mo for premature infants. (3) Sickledex® test for Hb S can be done at age 6 to 9 mo (diagnosis of sickle cell disease is discussed in Ch. 35). (4) Periodic blood testing for lead exposure should begin at age 1 yr *in all children* and be repeated yearly thereafter. Those living in substandard or old housing should be tested more frequently. The Centers for Disease Control (CDC) has determined that blood lead levels > 10 µg/dL constitute a risk for neurobiologic damage (see also LEAD POISONING in Ch. 30).

After the age of 3 yr, children should be routinely checked as follows. **Blood pressure** measured with an appropriate-sized cuff, depending on arm size, should be done routinely (see FIG. 23–2). The inflatable rubber bag portion of the BP cuff should be long enough to encircle the up-

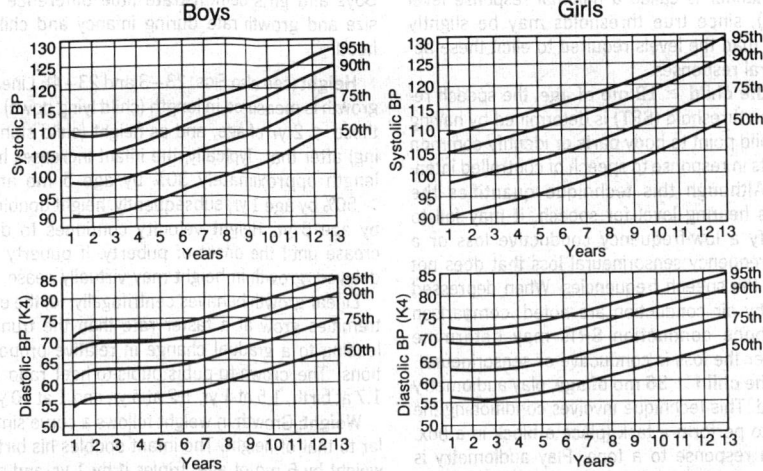

FIG. 23–2. **Age-specific percentiles of BP measurements in boys and girls aged 1 to 13.** K4 = Korotkoff phase IV sound (low-pitched and muffled). Normal BP was defined as *systolic and diastolic BPs < 90th percentile for age and sex*; high-normal BP as *average systolic and/or average diastolic BPs between the 90th and 95th percentiles for age and sex*. (From the Second Task Force on Blood Pressure Control in Children; National Heart, Lung, and Blood Institute. *Pediatrics* 79(Suppl): 1–25, 1987; reproduced by permission of *Pediatrics*.)

per arm completely (with or without overlap) and should be wide enough to cover approximately 75% of the upper arm. **Scoliosis** can quickly be checked for, along with evaluation of posture. Shoulder tip and scapular symmetry, torso list, and spine position and rotation on forward bending are useful tests. **Urinalysis** for screening purposes should be performed once during infancy, early childhood, late childhood, and adolescence.

CLINICAL MEASUREMENT OF HEARING IN CHILDREN

(See also CLINICAL MEASUREMENT OF HEARING in Ch. 64)

Early identification and correction of hearing loss is essential for normal development of communication skills. If risk factors are identified in the history, audiometry should be done by age 3 mo. Parents may suspect profound hearing loss if their infant does not seem to respond to a spoken voice or ordinary household sounds. Parents' observations are very important, and questions they raise about a child's hearing should be investigated. Risk factors and simple tests of hearing are discussed in SCREENING PROCEDURES FOR INFANTS AND CHILDREN, above.

Special audiometric techniques, usually performed by an audiologist, can assess hearing ability starting at birth. These tests use reflexive, behavioral, and physiologic responses to auditory stimuli of controlled intensity.

In the infant from birth to age 6 mo, the audiometric test battery includes both electrophysiologic and behavioral tests. Electrophysiologic tests (most often, Auditory Brainstem Response [ABR] audiometry) provide a reliable estimate of overall hearing threshold but cannot provide frequency-specific thresholds. ABR testing can be conducted within 1 to 2 days of birth and is often used to screen high-risk infants. When sensorineural hearing loss is suspected, behavioral tests must be done to provide information necessary for the fitting of hearing aids. Behavioral audiometric techniques depend on the age of the child.

In the child age 6 mo to 2 yr, localization responses to tones and speech are evaluated. In Conditioned Orientation Response (COR) audiometry, sometimes called Visual Response Audiometry (VRA), a lighted toy mounted on a loudspeaker is flashed after presentation of the test tone. After a brief conditioning period, the child localizes toward the tone, if audible, in anticipation of the flashing toy. A threshold recorded in this manner is called a minimal response level (MRL), since true thresholds may be slightly lower than the levels required to elicit these behavioral responses.

In the child ≥ 12 mo of age, the speech reception threshold (SRT) is determined by having the child point to body parts or identify common objects in response to speech of controlled intensity. Although this technique quantifies the child's hearing level for speech, it may fail to identify a low-frequency conductive loss or a high-frequency sensorineural loss that does not affect the speech frequencies. When depressed SRTs by air conduction are noted, comparison with bone conduction SRTs may determine whether the loss is conductive or sensorineural.

In the child > 36 mo of age, play audiometry is used. This technique involves conditioning the child to perform a task (place a block in a box, etc) in response to a tone. Play audiometry is usually used until age 4 or 5, when the child can respond by raising his hand.

Tympanometry and acoustic reflex measurements can be used with a child of any age and are useful in determining abnormal middle ear function. Abnormal tympanograms often denote eustachian tube dysfunction and/or the presence of middle ear fluid that cannot be visualized by otoscopic examination.

GROWTH AND DEVELOPMENT FROM BIRTH THROUGH CHILDHOOD

PHYSICAL DEVELOPMENT

A multifaceted process involving genetic, nutritional, and environmental (physical and psychologic) factors. Disturbances in any of these may alter growth. Optimal growth requires optimal health.

Growth from birth to adolescence occurs in 2 distinct patterns. The 1st (from birth to about age 2 yr) is one of rapid but decelerating growth. The 2nd (from about 2 yr to the onset of puberty) shows more consistent and steady annual increments. A child's position relative to his peers tends to remain the same. An exception may occur during the 1st yr of life, when some children grow faster or slower than their peers before establishing their ultimate pattern, which is primarily genetic in origin. This early growth variation is due in part to maternal factors (eg, uterine size).

Boys and girls demonstrate little difference in size and growth rate during infancy and childhood.

Height (see also FIGS. 23–3 and 23–4): Linear growth is measured in length (child lying down) in those < 2 yr of age, and as height (child standing) after that. Typically, the infant increases his length approximately 30% by age 5 mo and > 50% by age 1 yr; subsequently, height doubles by age 5 yr. Height velocity continues to decrease until the onset of puberty. If puberty is delayed, growth in height may virtually cease.

Linear growth behaves centrifugally; ie, the extremities grow at a faster rate than the trunk, leading to a gradual change in relative proportions. The crown-to-pubis:pubis-to-heel ratio is 1.7 at birth, 1.5 at 1 yr, 1.2 at 5 yr, and 1 at 10 yr.

Weight: Growth in weight follows a curve similar to that of height. The infant doubles his birth weight by 5 mo of age, triples it by 1 yr, and almost quadruples it by 2 yr. Between ages 2 and 5 the annual increments are fairly similar. Subsequently, yearly increments increase slowly until the onset of puberty.

Organ systems: Three organ systems do not follow the general pattern of growth seen with height and weight. The lymphoid system grows fairly constantly and rapidly throughout childhood, so that at the onset of puberty a child has almost twice the lymphoid tissue that an adult has. Thereafter, the size recedes. The reproductive system, except for a brief time in the immediate postnatal period, shows little growth until later childhood and puberty. Growth of the central nervous system (CNS) occurs almost exclusively during the early years of life. At birth, the brain is 25% of adult size. By the child's 1st birthday, the brain has completed half its postnatal growth and is 75% of adult size. Gradually decelerating in growth rate, it reaches 80% of adult size by age 3 yr, and 90% by age 7 yr.

Functional development of organs, independent of organ size, occurs primarily during the early growth period. The most notable changes occur in renal, immune (see above, IMMUNOLOGIC STATUS OF THE FETUS AND NEWBORN), and CNS functions. At birth, renal function is generally reduced. Shortly afterward, however, renal acidifying and concentrating abilities are functionally similar to those of adults. By age 1 yr, glomerular filtration rate, urea clearance, and maximum tubular clearances have reached adult levels. CNS functional changes occur largely and most rapidly during the first 4 to 5 yr of life and are best

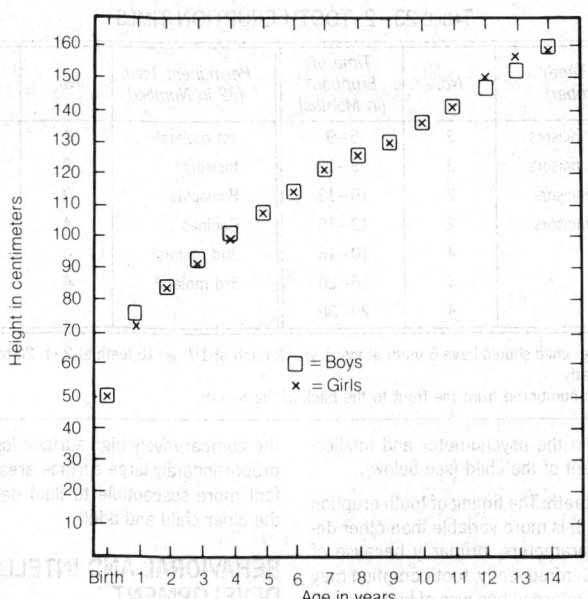

FIG. 23-3. Height and age equivalents in boys and girls.

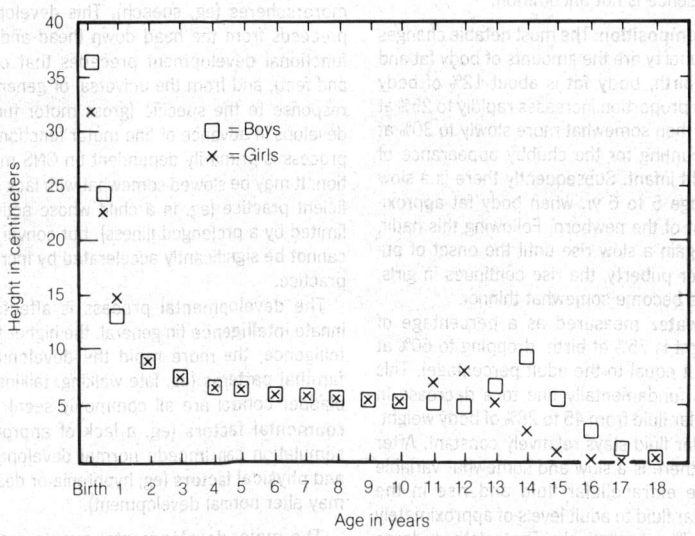

FIG. 23-4. Velocity of linear growth (height) in boys and girls in cm/yr.

TABLE 23-2. TOOTH ERUPTION TIMES

Deciduous Teeth* (20 in Number)	No.	Time of Eruption† (in Months)	Permanent Teeth (32 in Number)	No.	Time of Eruption† (in Years)
Lower central incisors	2	5-9	1st molars‡	4	5-7
Upper central incisors	2	8-12	Incisors	8	6-8
Upper lateral incisors	2	10-12	Bicuspids	8	9-12
Lower lateral incisors	2	12-15	Canines	4	10-13
1st molars‡	4	10-16	2nd molars‡	4	11-13
Canines	4	16-20	3rd molars‡	4	17-25
2nd molars‡	4	20-30			

* The average child should have 6 teeth at age 1 yr, 12 teeth at 1½ yr, 16 teeth at 2 yr, 20 teeth at 2½ yr.
† Varies greatly.
‡ Molars are numbered from the front to the back of the mouth.

demonstrated in the psychomotor and intellectual development of the child (see below).

Deciduous teeth: The timing of tooth eruption (see TABLE 23-2) is more variable than other developmental parameters, primarily because of familial factors. Infrequently, tooth eruption may be significantly retarded because of hypothyroidism. Eruption of deciduous teeth is similar in both sexes; permanent teeth tend to appear earlier in girls. Deciduous teeth generally are smaller than their permanent counterparts. The presence of supernumerary teeth or their congenital absence is not uncommon.

Body composition: The most notable changes prior to puberty are the amounts of body fat and water. At birth, **body fat** is about 12% of body weight. Its proportion increases rapidly to 25% at 6 mo and then somewhat more slowly to 30% at 1 yr, accounting for the chubby appearance of the 1-yr-old infant. Subsequently there is a slow fall until age 5 to 6 yr, when body fat approximates that of the newborn. Following this nadir, there is again a slow rise until the onset of puberty. After puberty, the rise continues in girls, while boys become somewhat thinner.

Body water measured as a percentage of body weight is 75% at birth, dropping to 60% at 1 yr (about equal to the adult percentage). This change is fundamentally due to a decrease in extracellular fluid from 45 to 28% of body weight. Intracellular fluid stays relatively constant. After age 1 yr, there is a slow and somewhat variable fall in the extracellular fluid and rise in the intracellular fluid to adult levels of approximately 16 and 47%, respectively. The relatively large amount of body water, its high turnover rate, and the comparatively high surface losses (due to a proportionately large surface area) make the infant more susceptible to fluid deprivation than the older child and adult.

BEHAVIORAL AND INTELLECTUAL DEVELOPMENT

Behavioral and intellectual development is a continuous process that occurs in the same sequence in all children. The rate of development, however, varies from child to child; even in a specific child, temporary pauses may occur in 1 or more spheres (eg, speech). This development proceeds from the head down (head and hand functional development precedes that of legs and feet), and from the universal or generalized response to the specific (gross motor function develops in advance of fine motor function). The process is primarily dependent on CNS maturation. It may be slowed somewhat with lack of sufficient practice (eg, in a child whose activity is limited by a prolonged illness), but conversely it cannot be significantly accelerated by increased practice.

The developmental process is affected by innate **intelligence** (in general, the higher the intelligence, the more rapid the development); **familial patterns** (eg, late walking, talking, and bladder control are all commonly seen); **environmental factors** (eg, a lack of appropriate stimulation can impede normal development); and **physical factors** (eg, hypotonia or deafness may alter normal development).

The major developmental events are summarized below.

Birth: The newborn sleeps most of the time. He can eat, clean his airway, and respond with crying to discomforts and intrusions. **Six weeks:** The infant regards objects in the line of vision, begins to smile when spoken to, lies flat on his abdomen, and has head lag when pulled to a sitting position. **Three months:** Smiles spontaneously, vocalizes, and follows a moving object with his eyes. His head is steady on sitting, and objects are grasped when placed in his hand. **Six months:** Sits with support and rolls over, supports himself in a standing position, transfers an object from hand to hand, and babbles to toys. **Nine months:** Sits well, crawls, and pulls himself to a standing position; says "mama" and "dada"; plays pat-a-cake; waves bye-bye; and holds his bottle. **One year:** Walks with his hand held, speaks several words, and helps to dress himself. **Eighteen months:** Walks well, can climb stairs holding on, turns several book pages at a time, speaks about 10 words, pulls toys on strings, and partially feeds himself. **Two years:** Runs well, climbs up and down stairs alone, turns single book pages, puts on simple clothing, makes 2- or 3-word sentences, and verbalizes toilet needs. **Three years:** Rides a tricycle, dresses well except for buttons and laces, counts to 10 and uses plurals, questions constantly, and feeds himself well. **Four years:** Alternates feet going up and down stairs, throws a ball overhand, hops on one foot, copies a cross, knows at least one color, washes hands and face, and takes care of toilet needs. **Five years:** Skips, catches a bounced ball, copies a triangle, knows 4 colors, and dresses and undresses without assistance.

IMMUNIZATION PROCEDURES THROUGHOUT CHILDHOOD

ACTIVE IMMUNIZATION

GENERAL RECOMMENDATIONS

The recommended schedule for **routine active immunization** of healthy infants and children in the USA is given in TABLE 23−3. Immunization requirements may differ in other parts of the world. Parents should give written consent for their children to be immunized and should be informed about the antigens to be given, the reasons these antigens are used, and associated reactions that might occur. They should be encouraged to tell the physician about any severe or unusual response, which in turn should be

thoroughly evaluated and reported to local or state health officials.

In the USA, the National Childhood Vaccine Injury Act requires that health care providers report selected events that occur after routine immunization (eg, events described in the vaccine package inserts as contraindications to receiving additional doses of vaccine and vaccine-associated events that are compensable) to the US Department of Health and Human Services. Forms and instructions have been developed by the Vaccine Adverse Event Reporting System **(VAERS)** and distributed to physicians. The forms and information on reporting requirements can be obtained by calling 800-822-7967.

Age at which immunization is begun: Routine immunization of normal infants is usually begun at 6 to 8 wk. The first vaccines given are diphtheria and tetanus toxoids combined with pertussis vaccine **(DTP)**, trivalent oral poliovirus vaccine **(OPV)**, and *Hemophilus* b conjugate vaccine **(HbCV)**.

Dosage and administration techniques: Depot antigens should be injected deep into the muscle, preferably into the midlateral aspect of the thigh or the deltoid muscle. The manufacturer's package insert should be consulted for dosage recommendations.

General precautions and contraindications: An acute febrile illness may necessitate delaying immunization until a subsequent visit or until the infection is controlled. A minor infection such as the common cold (even if associated with low-grade fever) is not a contraindication to immunization. Some vaccines are produced in cell culture systems and may contain trace amounts of cell culture materials. However, no adverse reactions have been reported from administration of these vaccines to individuals able to eat products containing the foreign antigen (eg, egg-sensitive persons who are able to eat bread or cookies).

Interruption of schedule: A delay between doses does not interfere with the final immunity achieved, nor does it necessitate restarting an immunization series, regardless of the time elapsed.

Immunization records: Parents should maintain a written history of each child's immunizations.

Combined vaccines and simultaneous administration: Simultaneous administration of various live virus vaccines offers obvious advantages, particularly if the child may be inaccessi-

TABLE 23–3. RECOMMENDED SCHEDULE FOR ACTIVE IMMUNIZATION OF HEALTHY INFANTS AND CHILDREN*

Recommended Age†	Vaccines	Comments
2 mo	DTP, OPV, HbCV (HbOC or PRP-OMP)	DTP and OPV can be initiated as early as 4 wk after birth in areas of high endemicity or during epidemics. Either a 3-dose series of HbOC or a 2-dose series of PRP-OMP may be started at 2 mo, with subsequent doses at 2-mo intervals; the same vaccine product should be used for subsequent (booster) doses in children < 15 mo
4 mo	DTP, OPV, HbCV (HbOC or PRP-OMP)	2-mo interval (minimum of 6 wk) desired for OPV to avoid interference from previous dose
6 mo	DTP, HbCV (HbOC)	3rd dose of OPV is not indicated in USA but is desirable in areas where polio is endemic; 3rd dose of HbOC should be given
12 mo	HbCV (PRP-OMP)	Booster dose of PRP-OMP should be given
15 mo	Measles-mumps-rubella, HbCV (HbOC)	Measles-mumps-rubella vaccine may be given at 12 mo in areas with recurrent measles transmission; booster dose of HbOC should be given. Tuberculin testing may be done at the same visit
15–18 mo	DTP, OPV	DTP should be given 6 to 12 mo after the 3rd dose; may be given simultaneously with measles-mumps-rubella vaccine at 15 mo. OPV may be given at 15 mo, simultaneously with measles-mumps-rubella vaccine and HbCV, or at any time between 12 and 24 mo. *Priority should be given to administering measles-mumps-rubella vaccine at the recommended age*
4–6 yr	DTP, OPV	At or before school entry; DTP may be given up to the 7th birthday. In some public health jurisdictions, a 2nd dose of measles-mumps-rubella vaccine is required
11–12 yr	Measles-mumps-rubella	At entry to middle or junior high school unless 2nd dose was given previously
14–16 yr	Td	Repeat q 10 yr for lifetime

DTP = diphtheria and tetanus toxoids with pertussis vaccine; OPV = oral poliovirus vaccine containing attenuated poliovirus types 1, 2, and 3; HbCV = *Hemophilus* b conjugate vaccine; HbOC = oligosaccharide-CRM_{197} conjugate vaccine; PRP-OMP = outer membrane *Neisseria meningitidis* protein conjugate vaccine; Td = adult tetanus toxoid (full dose) and diphtheria toxoid (reduced dose) for adult use.

* For all products used, consult manufacturer's package insert for instructions on storage, handling, dosage, and administration. Biologics prepared by different manufacturers may vary, package inserts from the same manufacturer may change from time to time. Therefore, physicians should be aware of the contents of the current package insert.

† These ages should not be construed as absolute; eg, 2 mo can be 6 to 10 wk. However, measles-mumps-rubella vaccine usually should not be given to children < 12 mo. (If measles vaccination is indicated, monovalent measles vaccine is recommended, and measles-mumps-rubella vaccine should be given subsequently, at 15 mo.)

Modified and reprinted with permission from *Report of the Committee on Infectious Diseases.* Copyright © 1991 American Academy of Pediatrics.

ble for further immunization. In addition, the licensed combination vaccines DTP, trivalent OPV, and measles-mumps-rubella may be administered simultaneously with HbCV, using separate sites and syringes for the injectable products.

SPECIFIC IMMUNIZATIONS

Diphtheria-tetanus-pertussis (DTP) vaccine: Diphtheria and tetanus vaccines are toxoids prepared from *Corynebacterium diphtheriae* and *Clostridium tetani*, respectively. The whole-cell pertussis vaccine currently available is composed of formaldehyde-treated bacterial cell wall fragments from *Bordetella pertussis*. Acellular pertussis vaccines consisting of semipurified or purified components of the pertussis bacteria (eg, pertussis toxin, filamentous hemagglutinin, agglutinogens, and 69-kd protein) have been used in Japan and recently were licensed in the USA for use as booster vaccines (4th and 5th doses) at 15 to 20 mo and 4 to 6 yr.

All children should receive active immunization with DTP, starting at age 6 to 8 wk, unless a specific contraindication precludes administration of the vaccine (eg, a moderate or severe illness with or without fever or hypersensitivity to a vaccine component). Adverse events after immunization that usually contraindicate further administration of pertussis vaccine include encephalopathy within 7 days; a convulsion, with or without fever, within 3 days; persistent, severe, inconsolable screaming or crying for $\geq$ 3 h or an unusual, distinctive, high-pitched cry within 48 h; collapse or a shock-like state within 48 h; temperature of $\geq$ 40.5° C ($\geq$ 104.9° F), unexplained by another cause, within 48 h; and immediate severe or anaphylactic reaction to the vaccine. The initial series of 3 doses is followed by a booster at age 18 mo and another when the child reaches school age. Subsequent routine tetanus boosters (indicated for all children and adults) q 10 yr should maintain protection; use of adult-type tetanus and diphtheria toxoids, adsorbed **(Td)** is preferred for these. More frequent boosters are unwarranted, since adverse reactions to toxoid may occur. At any interval after basic immunization, immunity can be reestablished by a single booster dose; however, after an interval of $>$ 10 yr from the last injection of tetanus toxoid, the rate of antibody rise to the booster response may be somewhat slower.

Hemophilus b conjugate vaccines: Vaccines prepared from the purified capsule of *Hemophilus influenzae* type b **(Hib)**—polyribosylribitol phosphate **(PRP)**, conjugated to protein carriers: diphtheria toxoid **(PRP-D)**, *Neisseria meningitidis* outer membrane protein **(PRP-OMP)**, tetanus toxoid **(PRP-T)**, and diphtheria mutant carrier protein CRM_{197} **(HbOC)**— have been developed and are effective in preventing Hib disease in children. The administration schedule for primary immunization of infants varies with the product: PRP-OMP is administered in 2 primary doses at ages 2 and 4 mo, with a booster at 12 mo; HbOC and PRP-T are administered in 3 primary doses at ages 2, 4, and 6 mo, with a

booster at 15 mo. PRP-D is not recommended for children $<$ 15 mo of age.

Poliomyelitis vaccine (see also POLIOMYELITIS under VIRAL INFECTIONS in Ch. 32): A primary series of 3 adequately spaced doses of trivalent oral polio vaccine **(OPV)**, consisting of a mixture of attenuated poliovirus types 1, 2, and 3, produces immunity in about 95% of recipients. Infection of the GI tract with OPV is a prerequisite to the establishment of immunity. Since a subclinical or ongoing wild enterovirus infection may interfere with this process, several doses of poliovirus vaccine at spaced intervals are recommended. The only known side effect of trivalent OPV is the very rare development of polio vaccine—induced paralysis, which occurs in 0.06/1,000,000 doses. Nevertheless, concern over OPV-induced paralysis combined with the development of improved inactivated polio vaccine **(IPV)** has led to consideration of introducing a combined OPV-IPV schedule. Use of IPV is recommended in immunodeficient patients, including HIV-infected infants.

Measles (rubeola) vaccine (see also MEASLES under VIRAL INFECTIONS in Ch. 32): Measles vaccine is a live, attenuated strain of measles virus. Antibodies are induced in 95% of children vaccinated at about 15 mo of age; antibody titers confer protection, which is durable. Because replication of the vaccine virus may be inhibited by preexisting serum antibody, immunization in infants preferably should be delayed until after the disappearance of passively acquired maternal antibody. There is some controversy as to when maternal antibody wanes sufficiently for measles vaccination to be efficacious. The current recommendation is for vaccination at about 15 mo of age. However, in an epidemic, children $\geq$ 6 mo old should be vaccinated and then revaccinated after 15 mo of age. Children initially immunized at age 15 mo should be revaccinated at age 11 to 12 yr (or in some localities, at age 4 to 6 yr, at school entry) to boost immunity or to induce immunity in those who were initial nonresponders. Measles vaccine produces a mild, noncommunicable infection in 15% of recipients. Symptoms occur 7 to 10 days after immunization and may include fever, malaise, and a measleslike exanthem.

Subacute sclerosing panencephalitis **(SSPE)** is a slow virus infection of the CNS associated with measles virus (see also SUBACUTE SCLEROSING PANENCEPHALITIS under VIRAL INFECTIONS in Ch. 32). About 6 to 22 cases of SSPE result per 1,000,000 cases of natural measles infection, while vaccination with live, attenuated measles virus is associated with development of SSPE in 1/1,000,000 cases.

Rubella vaccine (see also CONGENITAL RUBELLA under NEONATAL INFECTIONS in Ch. 27 and RUBELLA under VIRAL INFECTIONS in Ch. 32): This live, attenuated vaccine was developed to prevent congenital rubella; it produces antibodies in 95% of the recipients, and immunity is sustained. Current recommendations for routine immunization are to administer rubella vaccine in combination with measles and mumps vaccine. Joint pain, usually in the small peripheral joints, is the most common side effect, usually occurring 2 to 8 wk after immunization in about 5 to 10% of recipients. A rash, lymphadenopathy, or both occasionally occur. Live rubella virus vaccine should not be given to pregnant women because of the theoretic risk to the developing fetus. However, inadvertent administration during pregnancy does not routinely mandate a therapeutic abortion, since reports indicate that the real risk to the fetus may be nil.

Mumps vaccine (see also MUMPS under VIRAL INFECTIONS in Ch. 32): Mumps occurring in postpubertal males may result in orchitis, with subsequent sterility. Live mumps vaccine produces protective antibodies in 95% of those vaccinated; immunity is durable. Rarely, side effects of mumps vaccination have been reported, including encephalitis, seizures, nerve deafness, parotitis, purpura, rash, and pruritus.

Other vaccines: Immunization recommendations for pneumococcal pneumonia, meningococcal disease, TB, influenza, rabies, hepatitis B, and other infections are discussed under the specific diseases.

SPECIAL CIRCUMSTANCES

Children not immunized in infancy: For children who have not been immunized according to the schedule outlined in TABLE 23–3, alternative recommendations have been developed by the American Academy of Pediatrics (AAP) and are shown in TABLE 23–4). In brief, the recommendations state that children < 7 yr of age may be immunized with DTP, using 3 doses IM at intervals of 4 to 8 wk. For children ≥ 7 yr old, use of adult-type tetanus and diphtheria toxoids, adsorbed (Td) is preferred. Pertussis vaccine is not recommended at this age, but it may be used in special circumstances (eg, when an outbreak occurs in closed populations such as a day-care center, hospital, or residential facility). Live, attenuated measles, mumps, rubella vaccines may be used in persons of any age if no contraindication exists. Similarly, live poliovirus vaccines may be used in older children and adolescents.

Preterm infants: Since transplacental antibody acquisition is terminated at birth and the newborn has the capacity to produce immunoglobulin in response to antigenic stimulation, immunization can be started at 6 to 8 wk of age, regardless of gestational age at birth. If the infant is still hospitalized, OPV should not be given because of the risk of spreading a live vaccine virus to other babies.

Children with neurologic disease: Children with fluctuating or progressive neurologic disease should not be immunized until their condition has been stabilized for at least 1 yr because of the risk of cerebral irritation. Deferring or withholding routine immunizations in infants and children with static neurologic disorders is not necessary.

Immunodeficient or immunosuppressed children: *Children with known or suspected immunodeficiency disease should not receive any live virus vaccines,* since they could initiate a severe or fatal infection. Asplenic children are at increased risk for overwhelming bacteremia, usually due to *Streptococcus pneumoniae, N. meningitidis,* or *H. influenzae* type b. These children should be given pneumococcal and *Hemophilus* b conjugate vaccines at the earliest age at which efficacy can be expected. Children receiving immunosuppressive agents (corticosteroids, antimetabolites, alkylating compounds, radiation) may have aberrant responses to active immunization procedures. Immunizations for patients on short-term therapy should be deferred until treatment is discontinued. Children on long-term therapy should not be given live vaccines but may receive inactivated vaccines such as DTP; ≥ 3 mo after therapy is discontinued, they should be given an additional dose of inactivated vaccine, and then live vaccines may be started. Children who have undergone bone marrow transplantation should be considered unimmunized; they should be reimmunized according to the schedule in TABLE 23–3 or according to the AAP recommendations for older children.

Children who have recently received blood, plasma, or γ globulin: Immunization with live, attenuated virus vaccines should be delayed for

TABLE 23–4. RECOMMENDED IMMUNIZATION SCHEDULES FOR CHILDREN NOT IMMUNIZED IN FIRST YEAR OF LIFE

Recommended Time/Age	Vaccines	Comments
< 7 yr		
First visit	DTP, OPV, measles-mumps-rubella HbCV	Measles-mumps-rubella vaccine if child ≥ 15 mo old; tuberculin testing may be done at same visit For children aged 15–59 mo, can be given simultaneously with DTP and other vaccines (using separate sites and syringes)*
Interval after first visit		
2 mo	DTP, OPV (HbCV)	2nd dose of HbCV is indicated only in children whose first dose was received when younger than 15 mo
4 mo	DTP	3rd dose of OPV is not indicated in the USA but is desirable in other areas where polio is endemic
10–16 mo	DTP, OPV	OPV is not given if 3rd dose was given earlier
4–6 yr (at or before school entry)	DTP, OPV	DTP is not necessary if 4th dose was given after the 4th birthday; OPV is not necessary if 3rd dose was given after the 4th birthday
11–12 yr	Measles-mumps-rubella	At entry to middle school or junior high
10 yr later	Td	Repeat q 10 yr throughout life
≥ 7 yr		
First visit	Td, OPV, measles-mumps-rubella	If a person is ≥ 18 yr old, routine poliovirus vaccination is not indicated in the USA; minimum interval between doses of measles-mumps-rubella vaccine is 1 mo
Interval after first visit		
2 mo	Td, OPV	
8–14 mo	Td, OPV	
11–12 yr	Measles-mumps-rubella	At entry to middle school or junior high
10 yr later	Td	Repeat q 10 yr throughout life

DTP = diphtheria and tetanus toxoids with pertussis vaccine; OPV = oral poliovirus vaccine containing attenuated poliovirus types 1, 2, and 3; HbCV = Hemophilus b conjugate vaccine; Td = adult tetanus toxoid (full dose) and diphtheria toxoid (reduced dose) for adult use.

* The initial 3 doses of DTP can be given at 1- to 2-mo intervals; hence, for the child in whom immunization is initiated at age ≥ 15 mo, one visit could be eliminated by giving DTP, OPV, and measles-mumps-rubella vaccine at the first visit; DTP and HbCV at the 2nd visit (1 mo later); and DTP and OPV at the 3rd visit (2 mo after the first visit). Subsequent doses of DTP and OPV 10 to 16 mo after the first visit are still indicated. HbCV, measles-mumps-rubella, DTP, and OPV can be given simultaneously at separate sites if failure to return for future immunizations is a concern.

Modified and reprinted with permission from *Report of the Committee on Infectious Diseases.* Copyright © 1991 American Academy of Pediatrics.

at least 1 mo (preferably 3 mo) after administration of blood, plasma, or immune globulin, because these products may inhibit the desired antibody response.

Children with HIV infection: Live virus and bacterial vaccines (eg, measles-mumps-rubella, OPV, BCG) usually should not be given to children with symptomatic AIDS; generally, immunization with inactivated vaccines (eg, DTP, IPV, and Hemophilus b conjugate) is recommended. How-

ever, an exception can be made for measles-mumps-rubella vaccine. The occurrence of severe, often fatal, measles following wild virus infection in symptomatic HIV-infected children and the lack of reported complications from measles-mumps-rubella vaccine have led to the recommendation for immunization with the vaccine. Children with positive serologic tests for HIV infection, but without clinical manifestations of infection, should be immunized according to routine recommendations, except that IPV should be substituted for OPV.

PASSIVE IMMUNIZATION

Passive immunization provides temporary immunity when vaccines for active immunization are unavailable or have not been given before exposure to an infection.

Immune Globulin (IG)

Human IG is an antibody-rich fraction of pooled plasma obtained from normal healthy donors. Commonly referred to as γ globulin, it consists primarily of IgG, though trace amounts of IgA, IgM, and other serum proteins may be present. IG is a concentrated antibody solution that does not contain transmissible viruses (eg, hepatitis or HIV) and is stable for many months if stored at 4° C. Since maximal serum antibody levels may not be achieved until about 48 h after IM injection, IG must be given as soon after exposure as possible. The half-life of IG in the circulation is about 3 wk.

Disadvantages of IG include (1) only a temporary protective effect, (2) variation in the antibody content against specific agents by as much as tenfold between preparations, (3) painful administration, and (4) anaphylaxis from inadvertent IV injections as a result of complement activation by immunoglobulin aggregates.

IG may be used for prophylaxis in hepatitis A, measles, immunoglobulin deficiency, varicella (in immunocompromised patients when varicella-zoster immune globulin is unavailable), and rubella exposure in the first trimester of pregnancy.

Other Immune Globulins

Hyperimmune globulin is prepared from the plasma of individuals who have high titers of antibody against a specific organism or antigen. It is derived from artificially hyperimmunized donors or from persons convalescing from natural infections. Specific immune globulins available include those for hepatitis B, rabies, tetanus, and varicella-zoster.

IV immune globulin (IVIG) was developed to provide larger and repeated doses of γ globulin. Administration is painless (once IV access has been established), and side effects are uncommon, although fever, chills, headache, faintness, nausea, vomiting, hypersensitivity, anaphylactic reactions, and cardiovascular manifestations have been reported. IVIG is the product of choice in the treatment and prophylaxis of severe bacterial and viral infections such as septicemia in preterm and low-birth-weight infants, bacterial meningitis, Kawasaki syndrome, and AIDS in children. Other indications are under study.

INFANT NUTRITION

Measurement of diet adequacy cannot be precise. Increases in the infant's weight and length only grossly reflect nutritional progress. The daily requirements for adequate nutrition are especially significant for the growing child compared with the adult (see TABLES 23-5, 39-1, and 39-2). Protein is one constituent of the diet that varies with the rate of growth as well as the state of health. Because of a deceleration in growth rate as compared with body weight, the caloric needs of the child calculated as a function of body weight gradually decrease as the child grows older, so that at < 6 mo, the requirement is 50 to 55 kcal/lb/day (110 to 120 kcal/kg); at 1 yr, 45 kcal/lb/day (95 to 100 kcal/kg); and at age 15 yr, 20 kcal/lb/day (44 kcal/kg). When protein and calories are provided by human milk, the requirements between 3 and 9 mo of age may actually be lower than those stated. The relative need for protein, vitamins, and minerals remains constant and is greater than that of adults. Requirements for various vitamins depend on the intake of calories, protein, fat, carbohydrate, and specific amino acids.

Nutritional deficiency diseases are unusual in our culture today unless associated with another disease that alters intake, absorption, or metabolism; therefore, personal opinion regarding nutrition often is applied more than scientific data. Since the stomach is not very discriminating, babies may be satisfied on nearly any diet, but the retention of a formula does not necessarily make it adequate for optimal growth and development.

For infants, drinking and eating are intense experiences, comprise most of their socializing, and are integral parts of their developmental progress. Thus, the act of feeding provides emotional and psychologic benefits, as well as an opportunity to gratify both sucking and nutritional needs. Problems caused by failure to satisfy these needs are discussed under COMMON FEEDING AND GASTROINTESTINAL PROBLEMS, below.

Breastfeeding

Management of breastfeeding in the hospital is discussed under FEEDING in MANAGEMENT OF THE

TABLE 23–5. RANGE OF AVERAGE WATER REQUIREMENTS OF CHILDREN
AT DIFFERENT AGES UNDER ORDINARY CONDITIONS

Age	Average Body Wt in Kg	Total Water in 24 h, mL	Water/Kg Body Wt in 24 h, mL
3 days	3.0	250–300	80–100
10 days	3.2	400–500	125–150
3 mo	5.4	750–850	140–160
6 mo	7.3	950–1100	130–155
9 mo	8.6	1100–1250	125–145
1 yr	9.5	1150–1300	120–135
2 yr	11.8	1350–1500	115–125
4 yr	16.2	1600–1800	100–110
6 yr	20.0	1800–2000	90–100
10 yr	28.7	2000–2500	70–85
14 yr	45.0	2200–2700	50–60
18 yr	54.0	2200–2700	40–50

From Barness LA: "Nutrition and nutritional disorders," in *Nelson Textbook of Pediatrics*, ed. 13, edited by RE Behrman, VC Vaughan III, and WE Nelson (Senior Editor). Philadelphia, WB Saunders Company, 1987, p 115; used with permission.

NORMAL NEWBORN, above. Once the mother and baby are discharged, nursing usually settles into a routine pattern. A modified ad lib schedule that allows the infant to sleep as long as possible at night is usually best. Infants generally should not be put to breast more often than q 2 h. Some infants, however, have a regular fussy period daily, and more frequent feeding may be temporarily necessary.

The mother's diet should be well balanced, and she should avoid foods that may cause colic, such as garlic, onions, legumes, cabbage, chocolate, and excessive amounts of exotic or seasonal fruits (melons, rhubarb, peaches), unless trial shows that they are tolerated by the baby. Maternal fatigue and emotional stress more often result in failure to satisfy the infant than do any other factors. **Breast engorgement,** which occurs during early lactation, is discussed above under FEEDING.

Human milk contains nutritional substances ideal in quantity and quality for optimal growth and development of the human infant. For example, breast milk contains a predominance of monounsaturated fatty acids, which are easily absorbed and do not combine with calcium to make unabsorbable soaps; it also contains lipase, which facilitates the digestion of fat; it has the highest lactose content of the mammalian milks, providing a readily available energy source compatible with neonatal enzymes; it

contains large amounts of vitamin E, which may be related to preventing anemia and is an important antioxidant in fat metabolism; and it has a calcium:phosphorus ratio of 2:1, preventing calcium-deficiency tetany (the ratio in cow's milk is almost reversed). In addition to its nutritional value, breast milk favorably changes the pH of stools and the intestinal flora, thus protecting against bacterial diarrheas. Because of the protective quality of these factors, all infectious diseases are less frequent in infants who are breastfed rather than bottle fed.

If the mother's diet is adequate, no supplement is needed by the breastfed infant. The American Academy of Pediatrics no longer recommends fluoride supplementation unless the water supply in the region is deficient. In areas with little sunshine, infants, especially those with dark skins, may require 400 u. of vitamin D daily, especially in the winter.

Drugs in lactating mothers are discussed above under FEEDING in MANAGEMENT OF THE NORMAL NEWBORN.

Weaning should be related to the individualized needs and desires of both mother and infant. Nursing at least 6 mo, until solid foods are added to the diet, is considered by many as an ideal minimum. Gradual weaning over weeks or months is easiest. One breastfeeding/day should be replaced by a bottle or cup of fruit juice, modified formula, or fresh cow's milk when the infant is about 7 mo old. Weaning to a cup can be completed by age 10 mo; some infants will cling to 1 or 2 nursings daily, often until age 18 to 24 mo. Some infants are nursed even longer but should also receive solid foods and fluids by cup.

Bottle Feeding

By the time the infant leaves the hospital, he has adapted to the bottle and usually takes 2 to 3 oz/feeding approximately q 4 h. A modified ad lib schedule is satisfactory for most infants. If more volume is needed, water may suffice, especially in warm weather. A baby should be held and cuddled for all feedings; *the bottle should never be propped.*

Nutritional requirements: Commercial infant formulas have made formula-making at home rare. They are generally available as powder, concentrated liquid, and prediluted liquid, and are generally preferable to cow's milk. Preparing 20 kcal/oz of prepared formula requires 1 tbsp powder to 2 oz water, 1 oz liquid concentrate to 1 oz water, and no adjustment in the prediluted form. Each type contains the minimum daily requirement of vitamins and is available with iron 10 to 12 mg/qt, a maintenance dose. The American Academy of Pediatrics now recommends that all infants who are bottle fed receive a formula containing iron. Special hypoallergenic or carbohydrate-free formulas are available, as are predigested formulas with triglycerides, amino acids, and monosaccharides, and simulated breast milk; each has a different vitamin content and preparation procedure. If a **nonproprietary formula** is desired, the most reliable, easily made, and flexible formula is made from 13 oz evaporated milk, 1 to 3 tbsp sugar (for additional calories), and 19 oz water. This will provide 21 kcal/oz of formula. Each infant should receive 50 to 55 kcal/lb/day (110 to 120 kcal/kg) and 2 to 2½ oz of fluid/lb/day (130 to 160 mL/kg).

Nutritionally, milk is a well-balanced food for an infant except that it lacks iron. An infant not receiving a proprietary formula with iron may require an iron supplement, such as ferrous sulfate drops 15 mg/day, for maintenance after neonatal stores begin to deplete, at age 4½ to 6 mo. When an evaporated, skim, or whole milk formula is used, the infant should also receive supplemental vitamins A, C, and D daily for the first year of life and the second winter in cold climates. Fluoride is provided by using fluoridated water to prepare the formula or by giving fluoride drops (0.25 mg/day orally) when fluoridated water is not available or when prediluted liquid formula that does not contain fluoride is used.

Initiating Solid Foods

The time to start solid foods depends on the infant's needs and readiness, but infants do not need solids before age 6 mo. The infant must develop a new movement for tongue and mouth. Neurologic development has progressed sufficiently for this to occur at about 3 to 4 mo in full-term infants. Infants can swallow solids at a younger age if the food is placed on the back of the tongue, but refusal is normal. Some parents coax the infant to take large amounts of solid food in an effort to get the baby to sleep through the night; no sound evidence supports this practice. Some infants who are force-fed early rebel and develop feeding problems later.

Many infants take solids *after* being bottle fed, which satisfies the need to suck and more rapidly appeases hunger. Solids should be offered by spoon and introduced individually to determine tolerance. Many commercial baby foods, especially desserts and soup mixtures, are high in starch, which has no vitamins or minerals and is high in calories, and cellulose, which is poorly digested by infants. Some commercial baby foods have a high sodium content (over 200 mg/jar); they can be identified by reading labels carefully and should be avoided. (The daily infant sodium requirement is 17.6 mg/kg.) Pureed home foods are adequate. Meat should be introduced in preference to foods that are high in carbohydrates; but because many infants tend to reject meat, it should be introduced with care and attention so that it is accepted well. Wheat, eggs, and chocolate should be avoided until the child is 1 yr of age to prevent unnecessary food sensitivities.

COMMON FEEDING AND GASTROINTESTINAL PROBLEMS

Most common feeding and GI problems are not serious medically, and many can be handled by explanation and reassurance with a minimum of medication and formula manipulation. However, such problems may be of major concern to parents, and careful appraisal of the infant is always indicated. Evaluation should also include observing the parent-child interaction in the office and checking the infant's length and weight. If growth rate is normal when plotted on a standard growth chart, and the parent's complaints appear out of proportion to the findings, this overconcern may be a clue to deeper anxieties or problems in the parent-child relationship requiring further exploration.

A number of disorders mentioned in this chapter are detailed elsewhere in THE MANUAL. Eating problems of older children are discussed under BEHAVIORAL PROBLEMS in Ch. 29 and under EATING DISORDERS in Ch. 47.

Regurgitation and Vomiting

Infants commonly bring up small amounts (seldom > 5 to 10 mL) of milk during or soon after feedings, often when being burped. Feeding too fast and swallowing air may be related to this; using bottles with firmer nipples and smaller holes and burping the baby more often may help. Study of this problem is seldom indicated, and a formula change usually is valueless. Excessive regurgitation may be due to overfeeding (see below). However, **vomiting** may signal a more serious condition. Repeated projectile vomiting of increasing amounts may indicate **pyloric stenosis** or **gastroesophageal reflux. Upper small bowel obstruction** from duodenal bands, duodenal stenosis, or volvulus causes bile-stained vomitus. **Metabolic disorders** (eg, adrenogenital syndrome and galactosemia) may present with vomiting. Vomiting with fever and/or lethargy may signal **infection** (eg, sepsis or meningitis).

Underfeeding

Adequately fed infants usually become quiet or sleep soon after a feeding. The underfed infant often remains restless, almost seems to look around for more to eat, and awakens 1 to 2 h after being fed, appearing hungry. Such clear signs of underfeeding are not always present or may not be fully appreciated by a parent. Weight gain < 200 to 250 gm/wk (6 to 8 oz) in infants under age 4 mo is inadequate. A detailed feeding history must be taken to determine whether the difficulty is underfeeding or a more serious metabolic or systemic problem. Constituents and proportions of the formula should be reviewed. Underfeeding also may be a sign of parental inadequacy (eg, lack of concern or neglect). Breastfed infants who do not show adequate weight gain may be weighed before and after several feedings to determine milk intake more accurately. The breastfed infant's diet may be supplemented with an appropriate milk formula and cereal; treatment of the formula-fed infant may include a change of the formula constituents and an increase in total quantity of formula offered. Parents should be instructed in how much and how often the baby should be fed. Follow-up weight checks should be arranged.

Overfeeding

Monitoring the infant's weight by serial recording on a standard growth chart readily shows too-rapid weight gain. Other signs of overfeeding include crying and excessive regurgitation. Since problems of obesity may begin with excessive eating in infancy, attempts to control rate of weight gain may be of value, particularly if the infant has 2 obese parents and, therefore, an 80% chance of becoming obese. The overweight infant's daily intake should be reviewed, and the parents should be encouraged to reduce the amounts offered. Dietary supplements of solids must be introduced at appropriate times and in modest amounts.

Diarrhea

Frequent loose bowel movements (4 to 6/day) may occur in the normal infant; they are of no concern unless anorexia, vomiting, weight loss, failure to gain weight, or passage of blood also occurs. Breastfed infants tend to have frequent, frothy bowel movements, especially if they are not receiving solid baby foods.

Sudden onset of diarrhea with vomiting, bloody stools, fever, anorexia, or listlessness may be due to **infection.** A low-grade diarrhea persisting for weeks or months may result from several conditions. (1) **Gluten-induced enteropathy (celiac disease):** The gluten fraction of wheat protein causes a malabsorption of dietary fats, resulting in malnutrition, anorexia, and bulky, foul-smelling stools. Removing gluten from the diet by excluding all wheat products corrects the condition. (2) **Cystic fibrosis:** Pancreatic insufficiency results in trypsin and lipase deficits, causing high fecal losses of protein and fats with consequent malnutrition and growth retardation. The stool is large in quantity and often foul-smelling. Pancreatic extract may be given orally to improve this problem. (3) **Sugar malabsorption:** Intestinal mucosal enzymes, such as lactase, which splits lactose to galactose and glucose, may be congenitally absent or temporarily deficient secondary to GI infection. Improvement after eliminating carbohydrates from the diet or after substituting a lactose-free formula strongly suggests such a malabsorption state. (4) **Allergic gastroenteropathy:** Milk protein may cause diarrhea, especially when associated with vomiting and the presence of blood in the stools, but intolerance to the carbohydrate fraction of the ingested food should be suspected also. Symptoms often abate promptly on substitution with a soybean formula and return with a challenge feeding of cow's milk. Those infants intolerant of cow's milk commonly are soy-intolerant, so there may be a need to use one of several special elemental noncarbohydrate-based formulas available. Spontaneous improvement usually occurs toward the end of the first year of life, regardless of alterations in the content of the formula offered to the infant.

Constipation

The infant's bowel movements vary so much in frequency that it is difficult to define constipation. The same infant who has a bowel movement 4 times/day may, at other times, have one every 2 days. Most infants pass a hard, large stool with minimal discomfort, while some cry when passing a soft one. Infants < 2 to 3 mo commonly have a minor degree of anal stenosis that causes persistent straining and passage of small-caliber stools. A gentle digital examination of the anus easily identifies this condition, revealing a tight band-like circumanal constriction. Anal dilation once or twice provides relief of symptoms. A large bowel movement may cause an **anal fissure,** which presents with pain on defecation and the occasional passage of a small amount of bright red blood. The fissure can be identified by inspecting the anal canal with an anoscope or an otoscope, using a large speculum. In infants, most fissures clear quickly without intervention, but a mild stool softener, such as dioctyl sodium sulfosuccinate 3 to 5 mg/kg/day divided into 2 to 3 doses, may be used for 7 to 10 days to allow the fissure to heal; the value of locally applied corticosteroid cream has not been proved. Persistent constipation, particularly if it begins before age 1 mo, may be a symptom of **congenital megacolon** (see DISTAL SMALL BOWEL AND LARGE BOWEL OBSTRUCTION under GASTROINTESTINAL DEFECTS in Ch. 28).

COLIC

A symptom complex of early infancy that is characterized by paroxysms of crying, apparent abdominal pain, and irritability.

Etiology, Symptoms, and Signs

Colic may begin shortly after a baby comes home from the hospital, but often begins some weeks later, and may persist until age 3 or 4 mo. The term "colic" is descriptive, suggesting a cause of intestinal origin, but the specific mechanisms of infantile colic are unknown. Typically, the colicky infant eats and gains weight well, may seem excessively hungry, and often will suck vigorously on almost anything available, but paroxysms of crying may transform a peaceful home into chaos and strain family tempers. Colic often occurs at a predictable time of day or night, but a few infants cry almost incessantly. Excessive crying causes aerophagia, which results in flatulence and abdominal distention. Such crying *may* be an early manifestation of an insistent, impatient personality style, which may have counterpart behavior patterns in the older child. Parents are apt to assume that the infant is irritable because of the way they handle him; some explanation of the infant's individuality is justified to overcome any such guilt feelings.

Diagnosis

Before colic is diagnosed, other reasons for similar behavior must be ruled out. A hungry baby may cry incessantly, but shows an inadequate weight gain. An over-attended infant may not get sufficient sleep. Sickness, such as a fever, a cold, or an ear infection, may cause irritability. A physical examination may reassure both physician and parents; a blood count, urinalysis, or other study may be indicated. Careful questioning may reveal that crying is not the chief concern, but a symptom that the parents have used to justify their visiting the doctor to present another problem—eg, concern over the death of a previous child or over their feelings of inability to cope with a new infant.

Treatment

The infant who cries for short periods may respond to being held, rocked, or patted gently. An infant with a strong sucking urge who fusses soon after a feeding may need more sucking. If a bottle feeding takes < 20 min, new nipples with smaller holes should be tried; a pacifier also may quiet the infant. A very active, restless infant may respond, paradoxically, to being swaddled rather tightly with a small sheet and placed on his stomach. A short trial of a milk substitute formula is useful to ascertain whether a form of milk intolerance may exist. In exceptional circumstances, the judicious use of a sedative such as phenobarbital (in liquid form) 2 mg/kg/day orally in 2 divided doses may help when given 1 h before the anticipated fussy period. Parents should be assured that the colicky infant is basically healthy, that this behavior will cease in a few weeks, and that too much crying is not harmful.

24. SPECIAL CONSIDERATIONS IN CARING FOR SICK CHILDREN AND THEIR FAMILIES

PARENT–INFANT BONDING: THE SICK NEONATE

Strong psychologic attachments between parents and their newborn that begin to develop in the first hours and days following birth. The process is influenced by the parents' own experiences as they were reared by their parents, by their cultural and social attitudes toward child rearing, by their personality development, by their desire to have a child, and by the psychologic planning for the arrival of the newborn, which progresses through the pregnancy. Parent-infant bonding establishes the intense emotional ties that normally exist between parents and their children. It ensures the necessary parental support of the child during his developmental years, and it supports the development of the child's personality (see also INITIAL CARE in Ch. 23).

When the neonate is sick or premature, the situation is much more difficult, and special care must be taken to be realistically encouraging to the parents and to help them understand the newborn's problems. Parents should be encouraged to visit their newborn early and frequently and to participate in his care as much as possible. Supportive attention to the parents helps minimize their anxiety and promotes the bonding process.

Particular difficulties arise when a critically ill newborn must be transferred to an **intensive care nursery**. The parents may be separated from their infant for many days or weeks, and the development of normal attachments may not be possible. In the past, parental visiting and contact with premature or very ill neonates were either impossible or extremely limited, and in many such cases parental neglect or abuse of these children developed. In the modern intensive care nursery, parents and close relatives are encouraged to visit the newborn frequently and as soon after birth as possible. After appropriate hand washing and gowning, they should be helped to touch or hold the newborn as his condition allows. *No newborn, even if on a respirator, can be considered too ill for the parents to see and touch.* Parent-newborn bonds are strengthened if the parents can feed, bathe, and change their newborn, and if the mother can provide breast milk for her sick baby, even if he must initially be fed by tube. (See also MANAGEMENT OF CHRONIC DISABILITY, below.)

Malformed newborns: When a newborn has a birth defect, the parents should see him together as soon after birth as possible, regardless of his medical condition. In the past, parents sometimes were discouraged from seeing their malformed or critically sick newborn, but this often led them to imagine his appearance and condition to be much worse than was actually the case. Intensive parental support is essential, with as many counseling sessions as are needed for questions and concerns to be answered and to achieve understanding and then acceptance of their newborn's condition. It is important to emphasize what is normal about the child and what potential he has, and not to dwell totally on the abnormalities.

When an infant dies, parents who have never seen or touched him may feel as though they had never had a baby. Such parents have reported exaggerated feelings of emptiness; prolonged pathologic depression may result because the parents could not grieve for the loss of a "real infant." The process of mourning will then be incomplete. In most situations, parents who have not been able to see or hold their infant will be helped if allowed to do so after the infant has died. In all cases, follow-up visits with the physician and a social worker are helpful to review the circumstances of the infant's illness and death, to answer questions that often arise later, and to assess and alleviate inappropriate guilt feelings. This also gives the physician an opportunity to recommend genetic counseling and/or counseling with a perinatologist regarding possible future pregnancies. The physician can evaluate the parents' grieving process, and if it is pathologic, he can provide appropriate guidance or make a referral for more extensive support.

MANAGEMENT OF CHRONIC DISABILITY

Chronic disabilities are defined as *physical conditions that affect daily functioning for > 3 mo/yr, cause cumulative hospitalization of > 1 mo/yr, or are likely to;* eg, asthma, cerebral palsy, cystic fibrosis, congenital heart disease, diabetes mellitus, meningomyelocele, inflammatory bowel disease, renal failure, epilepsy, cancer, juvenile arthritis, hemophilia, and sickle cell disease. Although each is uncommon, together they affect about 10% of all children and constitute an important part of medical practice.

Despite many differences, these children share pain and discomfort, restricted growth and development, frequent hospitalizations and outpatient visits, painful and embarrassing treatments, inability to participate in peer activities, significant daily burden of care, and an unpredictable course. For the family, the chronic disability leads to loss of the "ideal child," neglected siblings, major expense and time commitment, confusing systems of health and other care (eg, third-party payers), lost opportunities (eg, the mother who cannot return to work), and social isolation. Such stress may cause family breakup, especially when other marital and intrafamily problems exist. For the community, the common issues include poor understanding (for many people, their only exposure is during telethons designed to raise sympathy), inconsistent policies and funding, inadequate facilities (including barriers to access), and poor communication and coordination within and between the health care and other systems (eg, education).

Understanding Child Development

Conditions that affect the physical appearance of an infant, eg, cleft lip and palate or hydrocephalus, can affect the bonding between child and family or caretakers. Once the diagnosis of abnormality is made, parents may grieve for the lost "normal child" with shock, denial, anger, sadness or depression, guilt, and anxiety. This may occur at any time in the child's development, and each parent may be at a different stage, making communication between them difficult. They may express their anger at the health care provider, or their denial may cause them to seek multiple opinions.

The demands placed on the family, and sympathy for the child, may make discipline inconsistent and can lead to behavior problems. One parent (often the mother) may become overinvolved with the child, thus blurring normal family boundaries. The working father may become isolated (the office hours of most health care providers preclude him from attending health care visits).

The paucity of disabled adult role models (eg, television stars) makes it more difficult for these children to establish identities. Physical differences may lead to social rejection by peers and decreased motivation. The disability may also interfere with the child's ability to achieve goals (eg, a sense of autonomy in the child who cannot physically walk away from his parents to show independence) and may interact with the child's temperament, leading to poor adaptation (eg, the child who is distractible by nature and is also deaf).

Case Management

Children with chronic disabilities have complex needs, the medical system is fragmented, and communication between it and other systems is often inadequate.

Maximal functioning for child and family requires attention to many factors (case management) to ensure coordination of care. Without it, care will be crisis-oriented; some services will be duplicated, while others will be neglected. Case management includes (1) **needs assessment** (medical, educational, social, and psychologic) of the child and family; (2) **comprehensive care planning** for medical and nonmedical services (communication between the primary care physician and consultants should clearly define the roles and responsibilities of each provider); (3) **facilitation and coordination of services** (including the training of community providers); (4) **follow-up** (monitoring services and patient and family progress, after which the goals of the treatment plan should be reviewed and modified as needed); and (5) **empowerment** (counseling, education, training, and supporting the child and family), which can include volunteer parent groups, respite care, and direct intervention such as with schools or third-party payers. Case management requires knowledge about the child's condition, the family, and the community in which he functions.

Any professional who provides care for the child must ensure that *someone* is providing case management. Ideally, this should be the child's parents. However, the systems that must be understood and negotiated are often so complex that even the most capable parents need assistance. Other possible case managers include the primary care physician, the specialty program staff, the community health nurse, and third-party payer (insurance and government)

staff members. Regardless of who assists, the family and child must be partners in the process.

The care of children with chronic disability rarely leads to dramatic cures. Physicians' understanding of their own attitudes is important to successful management.

25. SPECIAL CONSIDERATIONS OF DRUG TREATMENT IN NEONATES, INFANTS, AND CHILDREN
(See also appropriate chapters in §11 and Drugs in Lactating Mothers in Ch. 23)

Effective and safe drug therapy in neonates, infants, and children requires an understanding of maturational changes that affect drug action, metabolism, and disposition. Virtually all pharmacokinetic parameters change with age. Pediatric drug dosage regimens must be adjusted for the kinetic characteristics of individual drugs, age (the major determinant), disease states, sex, and individual needs. Otherwise, ineffective treatment or toxicity may result.

Drug absorption: GI drug absorption may be slower than in adults, especially in the newborn with prolonged gastric emptying time and in children with celiac disease. Absorption of some drugs given IM (eg, digoxin, kanamycin) may be erratic in neonates. Dermal and subcutaneous absorption of drugs is remarkably enhanced in newborns and young infants; eg, topically administered epinephrine may cause systemic hypertension, and dermal absorption of dyes and antibacterials (hexachlorophene) may result in poisoning. Theophylline administered subcutaneously to premature newborns with apnea is well absorbed and maintains therapeutic plasma concentrations.

Changes in **drug distribution** during growth parallel changes in body composition. Total body water is greater in neonates (ranging from 86% of body weight in premature newborns to about 70% at full term) than in adults (55%). Therefore, to maintain equivalent drug plasma concentrations, water-soluble drugs are given in decreasing doses (per kilogram of body weight) with advancing postnatal age. Interestingly, this decline in total body water continues into old age.

Plasma **protein binding** of drugs is less in newborns than in adults but approaches adult capacity a few months after birth. This decreased protein binding could be due to qualitative and quantitative differences in neonatal plasma protein and also to the presence of exogenous and

endogenous substrates in the plasma. Decreased protein binding may alter pharmacologic responses and drug clearance but is seldom considered in older children. The increased sensitivity of newborns to certain drugs, eg, theophylline, has been attributed in part to decreased protein binding, resulting in more available drug at the receptor site and leading to a more intense pharmacologic effect. Thus, adverse reactions may occur at much lower plasma drug concentrations, considered safe in the adult population.

Drug metabolism and elimination: The maintenance dosage of a drug is largely a function of body clearance, which depends mainly on rates of metabolism and elimination. These processes tend to be very slow in the newborn, increase progressively during the first few months of life, and exceed adult rates by the first few years of life. Drug elimination slows during adolescence and probably attains adult rates by late puberty.

Changes in drug metabolism and disposition as a function of age are extremely variable and depend also on the substrate or drug. Carbamazepine is excreted by neonates at rates similar to those in adults (plasma half-life ranges from 8 to 28 h in neonates and from 21 to 36 h in adults). Most drugs (phenytoin, barbiturates, analgesics, cardiac glycosides) have plasma half-lives 2 to 3 times longer in newborns than in adults. Other drugs are eliminated exceedingly slowly in newborns and young infants; eg, the mean plasma half-life of theophylline is 30 h in the neonate and 6 h in the adult. Whereas adult rates of elimination for some drugs (barbiturates, phenytoin) may be achieved 2 to 4 wk postnatally, others (theophylline) require months.

Metabolism and drug elimination show marked interpatient variability and vulnerability to pathophysiologic states. Moreover, activation of alternative biotransformation pathways occurs in the newborn (eg, conversion of theophylline to caffeine). These observations have been adapted in dosage regimens for infants and children. The principles are illustrated in Fig. 25–1 by theophylline, a bronchodilator and CNS stimulant. This drug, used commonly in pediatrics, is eliminated very slowly in the neonate, reaches adult rates within months, and by age 1 to 2 yr exceeds them. Thus, in order to maintain drug plasma concentrations in therapeutic ranges, the dose/body wt is extremely low during the neonatal period but increases and exceeds adult dosages within 6 mo to 4 yr of age.

Renal drug elimination is the primary route for antimicrobial agents, which are the most commonly used drugs in newborns and young children. Renal elimination is dependent on glomerular filtration and tubular secretion. Both functions are deficient in the newborn and undergo active maturational changes during the first 2 yr of life. Neonatal glomerular filtration rate is about 30% of the adult rate and is greatly influenced by gestational age at birth. Effective renal blood flow (RBF) affects the rate at which drugs are presented to and eliminated by the kidneys. The effective RBF is low during the first 2 days of life (34 to 99 mL/min/1.73 m²), increasing to 54 to 166 mL/min/1.73 m² by 14 to 21 days, and further increasing to adult values of about 600 mL/min/1.73 m² by age 1 to 2 yr. Plasma clearances of drugs are significantly increased in early childhood beyond the first year of life. This is partly due to increased renal and hepatic elimination of drugs in early childhood relative to adults, especially the elderly. Dose regimens of aminoglycosides and other antimicrobials are adjusted accordingly.

Pediatric Drug Dosages

No rules are adequate to guarantee efficacy and safety of drugs in the pediatric patient, especially the newborn. Dosages based on pharmacokinetic data for a given age group, adjusted to the desired response and each individual's drug handling capability, offer the most rational approach.

Many drugs currently used in pediatric practice have not been studied adequately or at all in a pediatric population. Many formulas have been suggested for calculating the pediatric dose from the adult dose (eg, Clark's, Cowling's, and Young's rules), assuming *incorrectly* that the adult dose is always right and that the child is a miniature adult. As shown in Fig. 25–1, dosage requirements constantly change as a function of age. Dosage based on body weight is practical but not ideal. Infants receive an underdosage if given mg/kg doses that are satisfactory for adults. The body surface area (BSA) method of calculating drug dosages (BSA [m²] divided by 1.73 and multiplied by the adult dose) approximates the pediatric dose and is more consistent throughout all age groups, *but does not apply to the premature and full-term newborn.*

Pharmacokinetic considerations and therapeutic monitoring: Knowledge of a drug's kinetic profile allows manipulation of the dose to achieve and maintain a given plasma concentration. Many drugs exhibit a biexponential plasma disappearance curve in the neonate and older pediatric patient; ie, the log of the plasma drug concentration decreases linearly as a function of time, with a brief but fast distributive (α) phase and a slower elimination (β) phase. This exemplifies a 2-compartment model and first-order kinetics, in which a certain fraction (not amount) of the drug remaining in the body is eliminated per unit time; and, after the distribution phase, the plasma concentration is proportional to the concentration of drug in other portions of the body. This model is applicable to a wide variety of drugs used in newborns and older children, although some drugs (eg, gentamicin, diazepam, digoxin) may fit a multicompartmental model; others (eg, salicylates) exhibit saturation kinetics (ie, a certain amount—not a fraction—of the drug is eliminated per unit of time). In the young toddler and prepubertal child, the α phase may be very short relative to the β phase, and its contribution to overall elimination and to dosage computations may not be significant. Similarly, drugs given to the newborn usually have an extremely prolonged β phase relative to the α phase. Thus, the entire body during the newborn period could be considered as if it were a single compartment for purposes of dose calculations.

For the majority of drugs, which follow first-order kinetics, dose adjustments can be based on plasma drug concentration, which at steady state is proportional to dose. For example, if phenobarbital plasma concentration is only 5 mg/L at 10 mg/kg/day, doubling the dose to 20 mg/kg/day should also double the plasma drug concentration to 10 mg/L.

Administering a loading dose (mg/kg) may be useful to achieve a given plasma concentration quickly when rapid onset of drug action is required. For many drugs, loading doses (mg/kg) are generally greater in neonates and young infants than in older children or adults. However,

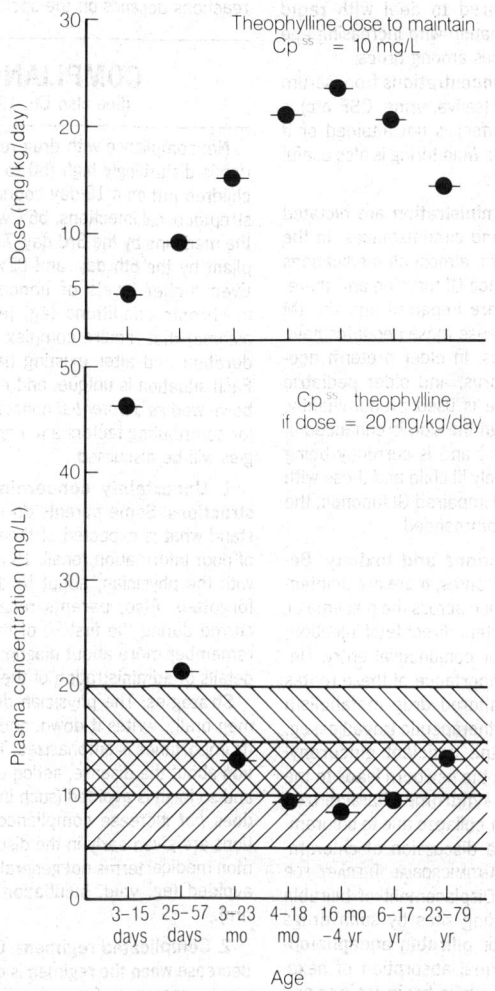

FIG. 25–1. **Theophylline dose requirements and plasma concentrations.** *Top panel*: Estimated dose requirements of theophylline (mg/kg/day) to maintain a plasma concentration of 10 mg/L. *Lower panel*: Estimated plasma concentrations of theophylline at steady state if dose is kept at 20 mg/kg/day. Shaded areas indicate tentative therapeutic level for bronchodilatation and anti-apneic activity. Cp^{ss} = Plasma concentration at steady state. (From Aranda JV: "Maturational changes in theophylline and caffeine metabolism and disposition: Clinical implications," in *Proceedings of the Second World Conference on Clinical Pharmacology and Therapeutics*, July 31–August 5, 1983, edited by L Lemberger and MM Reidenberg. Copyright by the American Society for Pharmacology and Experimental Therapeutics, Bethesda, 1984, p 870; used with permission.)

the prolonged elimination of drugs in the first few weeks of postnatal life warrants substantially lower maintenance doses given at longer intervals to prevent toxicity. Adjustment of maintenance doses is required to deal with rapid changes in drug elimination with increasing age and also with differences among drugs.

Monitoring drug concentrations from serum or other biologic fluids (saliva, urine, CSF, etc) is useful if the desired effect is not attained or if adverse reactions occur. Monitoring is also useful in assessing compliance.

Routes of drug administration are dictated by the clinical needs and circumstances. In the sick premature newborn, almost all medications are administered IV, since GI function and therefore drug absorption are impaired and the IM route is precluded because these neonates have very poor muscle mass. In older preterm neonates, full-term newborns, and older pediatric patients, the oral route is used predominantly. Drug absorption through the skin is enhanced in the neonate (see above) and is currently being evaluated. For the acutely ill child and those with vomiting, diarrhea, and impaired GI function, the parenteral route is recommended.

Adverse drug reactions and toxicity: Besides the usual desired routes, there are unintentional ones; eg, absorption across the placenta or via breast milk; inadvertent direct fetal injection; and pulmonary, skin, or conjunctival entry. Underestimation of the importance of these routes and unawareness of altered drug metabolism and disposition lead to therapeutic tragedies; eg, failure to recognize the deficient glucuronyl transferase activities in the newborn leads to the **gray baby or toddler syndrome** characterized by acute cardiovascular collapse due to chloramphenicol toxicity (for a discussion of chloramphenicol, see under ANTIMICROBIAL THERAPY FOR NEWBORNS in Ch. 27). Displacement of bilirubin from the albumin-binding sites by sulfa drugs leads to **kernicterus** or **bilirubin encephalopathy** in neonates. Dermal absorption of hexachlorophene produces **cystic brain lesions** and **neuropathologic abnormalities** in young infants. Boric acid and aniline dye poisoning occurs from unexpected absorption of these agents from diapers.

Drug toxicities (as in overdosage) usually are exaggerations of the known pharmacologic effects of a drug (eg, cardiac arrhythmias with overdosage of cardiac glycosides). However, host factors such as **hypersensitivity** or **genetic** abnormalities (eg, G6PD deficiency) may also predispose to adverse drug reactions (see Ch. 138). Drug withdrawal generally reverses the adverse reaction. Management of persistent toxic reactions depends on the specific drug.

COMPLIANCE
(See also Ch. 139)

Noncompliance with drug regimens in pediatrics is disturbingly high (50 to 75%); eg, among children put on a 10-day course of penicillin for streptococcal infections, 56% were not receiving the medicine by the 3rd day, 71% were noncompliant by the 6th day, and 82% by the 9th day. Even higher levels of noncompliance occur in chronic conditions (eg, juvenile diabetes, asthma) that require complex regimens of long duration and alter existing behavior patterns. Each situation is unique, and *every* parent must be viewed as a *potential* noncomplier. Some major contributing factors and improvement strategies will be discussed.

1. Uncertainty concerning physician instructions. Some parents do not clearly understand what is expected of them, partly because of poor information recall: 15 min after meeting with the physician, about $1/2$ the information is forgotten. Also, parents recall best what occurred during the first $1/3$ of the discussion and remember more about diagnosis than about the details of administration of therapy.

Strategies: The physician describes the regimen orally, writes it down, and reviews it again. Its importance is emphasized. Technical information about the disease, action of the medication, and so forth is avoided (such information usually does *not* increase compliance). These instructions are given early in the discussion, and common medical terms not generally understood are avoided (eg, void, incubation period, workup, prn).

2. Complicated regimens. Compliance levels decrease when the regimen is complex, inconvenient, expensive, of long duration, or requires alterations in life-style.

Strategies: The regimen is kept as simple as possible by reducing the number of medications, doses, and variations in scheduling. If clinically appropriate, larger, less frequent doses and preparations that combine several drugs or provide more sustained action are used; doses are synchronized when more than one medication is required. Routine prescribing of additional nonessential medications (eg, over-the-counter [OTC] cough and cold preparations, decongestants, vitamins) is avoided, and critical aspects of the treatment plan are emphasized (eg, giving the antibiotic regularly for the full course of the regimen). Unavoidably complex regimens might be divided into less complex stages implemented sequentially (eg, gradually increasing frequency of urine testing for diabetes patients). Matching the regimen schedule to the parent's/patient's regular daily activities minimizes inconvenience and forgetfulness.

Scheduling follow-up visits or phone calls in quick succession (eg, 3 to 4 days) can identify progress or problems, offers an illusion of short-term therapy, and provides motivation for adherence and opportunity for suggestions to overcome difficulties or concerns. If life-style must be modified (eg, changes in diet or exercise), changes should be introduced singly over several visits. Realistic goals should be set (eg, if the child should lose 30 lb, a target is set to lose 2 lb by a 2-wk follow-up visit). Good compliance should be reinforced with praise, and only then should the next objective be added. The cost of the regimen may be reduced by prescribing generic drugs and by avoiding unnecessary and OTC prescribing.

3. **Obstructive health beliefs** and attitudes (see also Ch. 132), often based on misinformation about, or experience with, the illness or regimen, cause the parent not to follow some or all of the physician's recommendations.

Strategies: Beliefs must be elicited by specific questions and often can be altered. The physician should ask if the parent (1) agrees with the diagnosis, (2) perceives the condition (or its sequelae) as serious, (3) feels the recommended treatment will work, (4) fears regimen side effects, and (5) believes the regimen will be difficult to follow.

The parent may possess powerful, well-defined (although erroneous) health beliefs that conflict with the assessment and diagnosis ("My child can't have the flu because he's had it before and you don't get that twice—it's like measles"). Such beliefs have multiple origins, including cultural standards, handed-down family beliefs, prior illness experience, misinterpretation of factual information, and acceptance of erroneous information from nonmedical sources.

The physician should encourage parents to discuss concerns about diagnosis or treatment. If certain beliefs appear to be contributing to noncompliance, corrective information is provided. Persuasion may require appeals to feelings of responsibility or support from a more credible source to the parent (eg, other parents whose children were successfully treated with the same regimen).

4. **Troubled physician-parent interaction.** Parental dissatisfaction with the amount of information and emotional support obtained from the physician, inability to express concerns, difficulty in understanding responses to questions, and unfulfilled expectations for the visit are associated with negative outcomes for children (eg, failure to keep follow-up appointments, lack of problem resolution, and noncompliance).

Strategies: Correction of these problems requires that they be recognized; ie, privacy and adequate time must be provided for discussion, and the physician must be secure and sensitive enough to encourage parents to express their expectations, concerns, misconceptions, and complaints. Compliance will improve when the parent perceives that sincere concern and sympathy have been shown and when responsive information about the condition and progress is provided.

Other strategies: Although physicians are becoming aware that noncompliance is a significant problem, surprisingly little supervision of the patient or **monitoring of regimen adherence** is performed (eg, reminder calls from the physician or staff about the regimen or follow-up visit; requests that medication bottles be brought to the next visit or that a record be kept of what dosage was taken each day and when; urine testing with antibiotics). Poor adherence should always be considered a possible cause of therapeutic failure and should be ruled out before starting other diagnostic or treatment efforts. **Utilizing other health care providers** can be beneficial. **Nurses** and **pharmacists** can execute most of the strategies described above. They can provide verbal and written reinforcement of regimen information; send telephone or mailed reminders before the medication would be running out; issue written instructions concerning special precautions; and maintain a patient medication profile to avoid overdose, allergic reactions, and adverse drug interactions and also to help monitor compliance.

26.   FLUID AND ELECTROLYTE DISORDERS IN INFANTS AND CHILDREN

Dehydration, usually due to diarrhea, remains a major cause of morbidity and mortality in infants and children worldwide. Too much fluid and electrolyte may be as devastating as too little in seriously ill pediatric patients who have cerebral edema, impairment of renal or circulatory function, or immature organ systems (eg, premature infants). In general, the younger the child, the more careful the calculations of fluid and electrolyte requirements must be.

The young infant is compromised by being unable to communicate thirst or seek fluid, and has a relatively large obligatory evaporative fluid loss, which is partly due to the high ratio of body surface area (BSA) to volume. The infant's metabolic rate is 2 to 3 times that of the adult when expressed per unit of body weight. Heat generated by metabolic activity must be dissipated (largely through evaporation), and solutes must be excreted (largely in the urine). The net result is a more rapid turnover of body fluids in the infant than in the adult and less margin for error in calculating fluid and electrolyte needs.

In the clinical management of infants and children with fluid and electrolyte disorders, complete precision is impossible; nevertheless, sufficient accuracy can usually be attained to restore and maintain normal balance and avoid serious complications. Attention to basic principles, a commitment to monitor progress carefully, and experience are required. Situations that demand particular attention to detail are those in which organ function (especially skin, heart, brain, or kidney) is critically compromised.

Fluid and electrolyte problems are most easily approached by considering separately the deficit, maintenance, and ongoing losses—see TABLE 26–1—and by calculating first the amount of fluid required, then its composition (electro-

lytes), and, finally, the rate of replacement. In this way, even complex problems can be dissected and are not as overwhelming as they first may appear. The examples in this chapter focus on the IV administration of fluid and electrolyte therapy, but the concepts and principles apply to oral rehydration therapy as well (see under ACUTE INFECTIOUS GASTROENTERITIS in Ch. 32).

Deficit

Deficit refers to the losses incurred prior to beginning corrective measures.

The amount can best be determined directly from changes in body weight when such information is available. An acceptable presumption is that a short-term weight loss in excess of 1% body weight/day represents a fluid deficit. When the child's prior weight is unknown, a clinical estimate of fluid loss must be made, although there are shortcomings and pitfalls in this method (see TABLE 26–2).

The composition of fluid required to replace a deficit depends on (1) the duration of the loss, (2) the nature of fluid lost, and (3) current serum electrolyte concentrations. If the loss is hyperacute, ie, minutes to a few hours, the composition is essentially that of serum. Usually, however, dehydration develops over 2 to 3 days, and there is more time for equilibration between extracellular fluid (ECF) and intracellular fluid (ICF); thus, less Na and more K are required. TABLE 26–3 presents approximate concentrations of electrolytes to replace deficit losses in the most frequently encountered clinical situations leading to dehydration.

The patient's current serum electrolyte concentrations (in particular the Na concentration) guide the selection of fluid composition after initial resuscitation of the circulation. Abnormalities

TABLE 26–1. APPROACH TO FLUID AND ELECTROLYTE PROBLEMS

Problem	Amount (Fluid)	Composition (Electrolyte)
Deficit	Short-term weight change Clinical estimate (TABLE 26–2)	TABLE 26–3
Maintenance	Calculate by either surface area method or caloric methods	TABLE 26–6
Ongoing loss	Measure	TABLE 26–7 or measure

TABLE 26-2. CLINICAL ESTIMATE OF THE SEVERITY OF DEHYDRATION

Infant EWL mL/kg		Adolescent EWL mL/kg		Severity of Dehydration	Clinical Data	Problems in Assessment
5%	50	3%	30	Mild	Dry mucous membranes Oliguria	Oral mucosa may be dry in chronic mouth-breathers Frequency of urination may be unknown in cases of infantile diarrhea, especially in girls
10%	100	5%	50	Moderate	Marked oliguria Poor skin turgor Sunken fontanelle Tachycardia	As for oliguria, above Affected by serum Na concentration ([Na])* Infants only Affected by fever, [Na],* underlying disease
15%	150	7%	70	Severe	Hypotension Poor perfusion	Affected by [Na],* underlying disease Affected by [Na],* underlying disease

EWL = estimated weight loss; [Na] = serum Na concentration.
* [Na] > 150 mEq/L gives falsely low estimate of severity; [Na] < 130 mEq/L exaggerates clinical estimate of severity.

of serum Na concentration also affect the clinical estimation of the severity of dehydration (see TABLE 26-2).

The rate at which the deficit is replaced depends on the severity of dehydration and the rate of fluid loss. In general, when signs of circulatory compromise exist, 20 mL/kg of ECF-like fluid (eg, lactated Ringer's or 0.9% sodium chloride solution) is infused IV over 30 to 60 min to restore adequate perfusion—the "resuscitative phase." If the circulation does not improve satisfactorily, more ECF-like fluid or 10 mL/kg of a colloid (eg, plasma, human plasma protein fraction, blood) is infused rapidly; the need for this additional resuscitative measure must alert the physician to anticipate the many possible complications and sequelae of acute shock. The remainder of the deficit can be replaced over 8, 12, 24, or 48 h, depending on the patient's apparent need for

volume and on practical considerations. If serum electrolyte concentrations were abnormal initially, the postresuscitative phase of the deficit replacement must be tailored accordingly.

Maintenance

Fluids are required to maintain homeostasis, to dissipate the heat generated by metabolic activity, and to excrete the solute products of cellular metabolism. Evaporative losses from the skin and respiratory tract (in a ratio of 2:1) account for about 50% of maintenance fluid needs. The other 50% is provided for urine formation, to permit excretion of solute in urine that is neither concentrated nor dilute (ie, 300 mOsm/L, sp gr about 1.010).

The amount of maintenance fluid required depends on metabolic rate and thus bears a complex relationship to weight: the younger the child,

TABLE 26-3. USUAL DEFICITS OF ELECTROLYTES BY CAUSE OF DEHYDRATION

Cause	Sodium (mEq/L)	Potassium (mEq/L)
Fasting and thirsting	50	10
Diarrhea		
Isotonic dehydration	80	80
Hypotonic dehydration	100	80
Hypertonic dehydration	20	10
Pyloric stenosis	80	100
Diabetic ketoacidosis	80	50

TABLE 26−4. STANDARD BASAL METABOLIC RATES

Weight (kg)	Kcal/24 h		
	Male	Both Sexes	Female
3		140	
5		270	
7		400	
9		500	
11		600	
13		650	
15		710	
17		780	
19		830	
21		880	
25	1020		960
29	1120		1040
33	1210		1120
37	1300		1190
41	1350		1260
45	1410		1320
49	1470		1380
53	1530		1440
57	1590		1500
61	1640		1560

Increments or decrements:
1. Add or subtract 12% of above for each degree C (8% for each degree F) above or below rectal temperature of 37.8° C (100° F).
2. Add 0−30% increments for usual activity; hypo- or hypermetabolic states require greater adjustments.

the greater the metabolic activity/kg body wt (50 kcal/kg for newborn, 26 to 28 kcal/kg for adult). Thus, the amount of fluid for maintenance needs cannot be determined directly from body weight with the same ease as deficit needs.

Three systems for estimating the amount of maintenance fluid required are widely used: One is based on BSA, the others on caloric expenditure. Surface area, like metabolic rate, is not a linear function of weight and requires the use of a table or nomogram (see FIG. 26−1). The advantage of this system is the convenience of a single number to remember: Maintenance needs for individuals of all ages are about 1500 to 2000 mL/m²/day.

Basal calorie method: Caloric expenditure can be estimated by referring to a table of basal calories and applying appropriate situation-specific modifications for activity and alterations in body temperature (see TABLE 26−4). Alternatively, estimating caloric expenditure based on the **Holliday-Segar formula** eliminates the need for tables (see FIG. 26−2). This formula includes an allowance for activity (as does the surface area system); it presumes the very young hospitalized infant to be at normal or near-normal activity, but the older child to be more restricted.

For both of the systems based on caloric expenditure, calories can reasonably be translated to milliliters of fluid (see TABLE 26−5).

Each system can be used successfully; however, the systems do not give exactly the same estimate. The basal calorie method yields the lowest recommended fluid volume and, therefore, is the safest when activity is reduced or when fluid overload is a concern. However, since the Holliday-Segar formula requires no tables, it is the easiest to use. Becoming thoroughly familiar with one of the systems is advised.

Determining the amount of maintenance fluid often appears complex to the inexperienced; deciding the **composition** of the fluid is more straightforward. Virtually all the electrolyte loss occurs in the urine (see TABLE 26−6), so the anuric patient requires no electrolyte replacement; the patient with normal renal function is well maintained by fluids containing 32 mEq/L of Na and 24 mEq/L of K, approximated by the commercially available solution of 5% dextrose and 0.2% sodium chloride with added K.

By convention, when maintenance fluids are given parenterally, the amount is distributed evenly over 24 h. This is not the case in normal individuals meeting their maintenance fluid re-

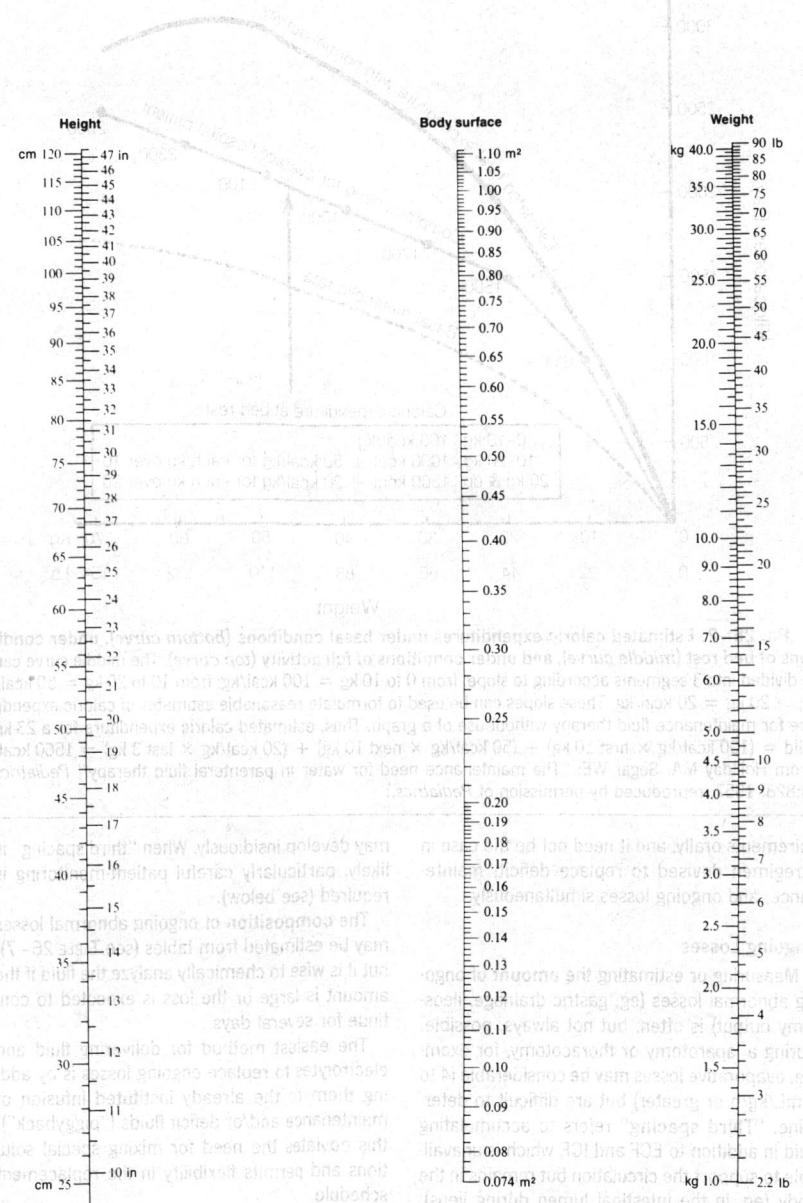

FIG. 26-1. Nomogram for calculating the body surface area of children. (Adapted from *Geigy Scientific Tables*, ed. 8, Vol. 1, edited by C Lentner. Basle, Switzerland, Ciba-Geigy Ltd, 1981, pp 226-227; used with permission.)

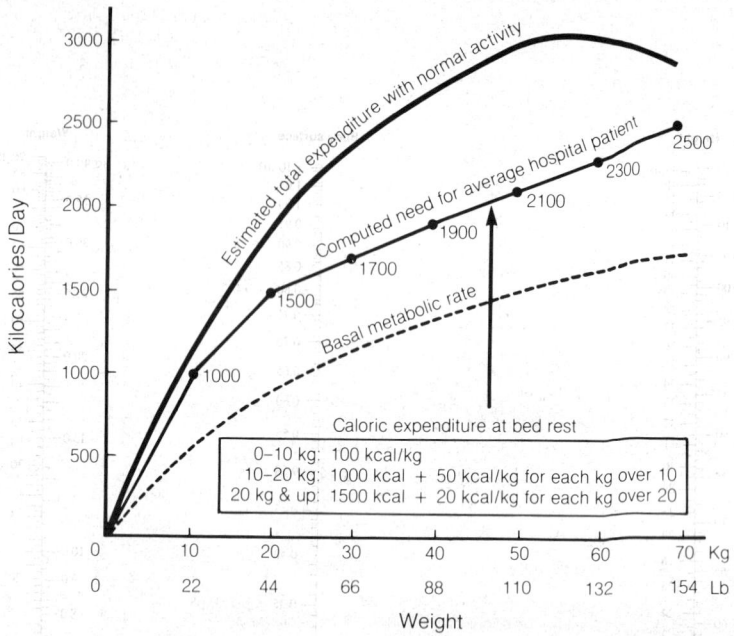

FIG. 26–2. Estimated caloric expenditures under basal conditions (*bottom curve*), under conditions of bed rest (*middle curve*), and under conditions of full activity (*top curve*). The middle curve can be divided into 3 segments according to slope: from 0 to 10 kg = 100 kcal/kg; from 10 to 20 kg = 50 kcal/kg; > 20 kg = 20 kcal/kg. These slopes can be used to formulate reasonable estimates of caloric expenditure for maintenance fluid therapy without use of a graph. Thus, estimated caloric expenditure for a 23-kg child = (100 kcal/kg × first 10 kg) + (50 kcal/kg × next 10 kg) + (20 kcal/kg × last 3 kg) = 1560 kcal. (From Holliday MA, Segar WE: "The maintenance need for water in parenteral fluid therapy." *Pediatrics* 19:823, 1957; reproduced by permission of *Pediatrics*.)

quirements orally, and it need not be the case in a regimen devised to replace deficit, maintenance, and ongoing losses simultaneously.

Ongoing Losses

Measuring or estimating the **amount** of ongoing abnormal losses (eg, gastric drainage, ileostomy output) is often, but not always, possible. During a laparotomy or thoracotomy, for example, evaporative losses may be considerable (4 to 6 mL/kg/h or greater) but are difficult to determine. "**Third spacing**" refers to accumulating fluid in addition to ECF and ICF, which is unavailable to support the circulation but remains in the body (eg, in the intestinal lumen during ileus). This situation is particularly difficult to manage clinically, since no external losses are seen as an alerting sign, and body weight does not decrease as the ECF is depleted; thus, severe dehydration

may develop insidiously. When "third spacing" is likely, particularly careful patient-monitoring is required (see below).

The **composition** of ongoing abnormal losses may be estimated from tables (see TABLE 26–7), but it is wise to chemically analyze the fluid if the amount is large or the loss is expected to continue for several days.

The easiest method for delivering fluid and electrolytes to replace ongoing losses is by adding them to the already instituted infusion of maintenance and/or deficit fluids ("piggyback"); this obviates the need for mixing special solutions and permits flexibility in the replacement schedule.

Gains

Not all fluid and electrolyte problems are those of deficits and losses; some result from

TABLE 26-5. RELATIONSHIP BETWEEN CALORIC EXPENDITURE
AND MAINTENANCE FLUID REQUIREMENTS

Source of Water Loss	Usual Losses (mL H_2O/100 kcal metabolized)
Lungs	15–20
Skin	30–40
Stool	5
Urine	55–65
Total	115
Water generated Metabolism ($CH_2O + O_2 \rightarrow H_2O + CO_2$)	–15
Net	100

overhydration (particularly when there is disordered renal or cardiac function), excessive electrolyte administration, or both. It is important to be alert to additional sources of fluid and electrolytes, such as the diluent used to reconstitute medications, eg, sterile water vs. sodium chloride for injection.

The principles used for restoring homeostasis in dehydration can be applied, with some modification, to problems of excess: Fluid amounts and compositions are estimated, and the appropriate restrictions on intake are applied.

Monitoring

All of the guidelines discussed are approximations and in no way obviate the need for careful monitoring of the patient. Unfortunately, there is no single, simple sign or test that infallibly reflects fluid and electrolyte balance; TABLE 26-8 lists 10 measures in rough order of practical value, considering degree of ease, availability, invasiveness, time to perform, and cost. Frequency of monitoring must be individualized, depending on the present severity of the disorder and the potential rate of change. Once daily is rarely sufficient.

Practical Example

An infant has diarrhea for 3 days with weight loss of 1 kg (from 10 kg to 9 kg). Clinical findings support the estimate of 10% fluid deficit—dry mucous membranes, poor skin turgor, markedly decreased urine output, and tachycardia, but BP is normal and adequate peripheral perfusion is shown by compression-release of the nail beds. Serum Na is 136 mEq/L; K, 4 mEq/L; Cl, 104 mEq/L; and HCO_3, 20 mEq/L.

Calculations

Deficit

Amount (from TABLE 26-2): 1 L

Composition (electrolyte losses from TABLE 26-3: diarrhea-isotonic): 80 mEq of Na, 80 mEq of K

Maintenance

Amount:

Surface area method (FIG. 26-1): 0.47 m^2 × 1500 to 2000 mL/m^2/day = 705 to 940 mL/day

Basal calorie method (TABLE 26-4): 550 basal kcal + 20% (110 kcal) for activity = 660 kcal ~ 660 mL/day

TABLE 26-6. APPROXIMATE, PROPORTIONATE SOURCES
OF FLUID AND ELECTROLYTE LOSSES

Source of Loss	Water (mL)	Sodium (mEq/L)	Potassium (mEq/L)
Lungs	150	0	0
Skin	300	1	2
Stool	50	1	2
Urine	500	30	20
Total	1000	32	24

TABLE 26–7. APPROXIMATE COMPOSITION OF EXTERNAL ABNORMAL LOSSES

Fluid	Sodium (mEq/L)	Potassium (mEq/L)	Chloride (mEq/L)
Gastric	20–80	5–20	100–150
Pancreatic	120–140	5–15	40–80
Small intestinal	100–140	5–15	90–130
Bile	120–140	5–15	80–120
From ileostomy	45–135	3–15	20–115
Diarrheal	10–90	10–80	10–110
Sweat			
Normal	10–30	3–10	10–35
Cystic fibrosis	50–130	5–25	50–110
From burns (see Ch. 114)	140	5	110

TABLE 26–8. SIGNS AND TESTS FOR MONITORING STATE OF HYDRATION

Sign or Test	Problem
1. Physical signs of dehydration (see TABLE 26–2)	May be deceiving if [Na] abnormal; may be influenced by fever (especially pulse), etc (see TABLE 26–2)
2. Body weight	Can be fooled by "third spacing"
3. Urine volume	Low output may represent SIADH, dehydration, or renal failure
4. Urine specific gravity	Concentrating ability of infant kidney limited; high sp gr may indicate dehydration, SIADH, or renal failure; low sp gr may indicate good hydration, pyelonephritis, or acute tubular necrosis
5. Intake and output with direct measure of all losses (and gains)	Must estimate maintenance; cannot measure "third space" loss
6. Urea nitrogen (SUN, BUN)	GFR severely reduced before urea nitrogen rises; elevated by blood in GI tract; infant level normally lower than adult; need creatinine to differentiate dehydration from renal disease
7. Hematocrit	Useful serially but not as single value; much less helpful if patient is actively bleeding
8. TSS (total serum solids) or TSP (total serum protein)	Good serially in same patient but not as single value
9. Concurrent serum and urine osmolalities	Good for detecting SIADH problem
10. Serum electrolyte concentrations	By themselves, say little about state of hydration

[Na] = serum Na concentration; SIADH = syndrome of inappropriate antidiuretic hormone; SUN = serum urea nitrogen.

Holliday-Segar formula: 100 kcal/kg × 10 kg = 1000 kcal ~ 1000 mL/day

Composition: 5% dextrose and 0.2% sodium chloride + 20 mEq/L of potassium acetate or potassium chloride

Ongoing losses

Amount: To be determined as course progresses

Procedure

Resuscitative portion of deficit

Lactated Ringer's solution at 20 mL/kg × 1 h

Amount: 20 mL/kg × 10 kg = 200 mL

Composition: 130 mEq/L of Na; 4 mEq/L of K

Remainder of deficit

Amount: 1000 mL (total deficit) − 200 mL (already given) = 800 mL

Composition of Na: 80 mEq (deficit) − 26 mEq (given in the Ringer's solution) = 54 mEq. The 54 mEq in 800 mL is a concentration of 68 mEq/L and approximates the Na content of commercially used 5% dextrose and 0.45% sodium chloride (77 mEq/L).

Rate: Arbitrary; let us choose 100 mL/h × 8 h

Maintenance

Amount: 660 to 1000 mL

Composition of Na: 5% dextrose and 0.2% sodium chloride

Rate: If begun after deficit replacement, then the first day requirements must be given over 15 rather than 24 h

$$\left(rate = \frac{660 \text{ to } 1000}{15} = 50 \text{ to } 60 \text{ mL/h} \right)$$

After the first day, the maintenance fluids can be distributed evenly over the full 24-h period

$$\left(rate = \frac{660 \text{ to } 1000}{24} = 30 \text{ to } 40 \text{ mL/h} \right)$$

Ongoing losses

As occur

Summary:

Lactated Ringer's solution, 200 mL/h × 1 h

5% dextrose and 0.45% sodium chloride, 100 mL/h × 8 h

5% dextrose and 0.2% sodium chloride, 50 to 60 mL/h × 15 h

5% dextrose and 0.2% sodium chloride, 30 to 40 mL/h thereafter

Notes

1. Only Na needs are calculated in this example: The amount and rate of K administered are governed by the need for safety, and full replacement is not achieved acutely. Once urine output is assured and it is thus considered safe to administer K, 20 to 40 mEq/L is added to the replacement solutions.

2. Sequential replacement of deficit and maintenance fluids is demonstrated in the example; the method is convenient and illustrates the approach presented in the text. Many clinicians prefer to combine deficit and maintenance replacement and to proceed more slowly; that method is equally acceptable and is preferred in hypernatremic dehydration (see below).

3. If the child is accepting fluids by mouth, oral fluid therapy should be considered unless prohibited by vomiting; it is effective, safe, convenient, and inexpensive compared with IV therapy. The oral *rehydration* solution used to replace the calculated deficit should contain complex carbohydrate or 2% glucose and 50 to 90 mEq/L of Na (see under Acute Infectious Gastroenteritis in Ch. 32). Once the deficit has been replaced, an oral *maintenance* solution, containing less Na, should be used.

HYPERNATREMIA IN INFANTS AND CHILDREN

(See also Hypernatremia in Ch. 27)

A serum sodium (Na) concentration > 150 mEq/L. Hypernatremia results from water loss in excess of solute loss (**hypernatremic dehydration**), solute overload (**salt poisoning**), or both. Water loss in excess of solute loss occurs commonly in disorders such as diarrhea, but hypernatremic dehydration develops only when fluid intake is insufficient to offset the loss. Clinical situations of particular concern include those in which intake is compromised and/or the fluid loss is underestimated or overlooked.

Salt poisoning most commonly results from errors in infant formula preparation or from the administration of hyperosmolar solutions and appears less frequently nowadays, presumably owing to the introduction of partially and fully preprepared formulas.

As hypernatremia develops, the "extra" Na does not diffuse into the cell but remains an obligatory extracellular ion; water then leaves the cell and enters the extracellular space in an attempt to reduce the osmolarity of the ECF. This serves to bolster the intravascular volume—but at the expense of cellular size and function. Intracranial hemorrhage and acute renal tubular necrosis are the major complications.

Because the intravascular volume is preserved, the physical examination underestimates the degree of dehydration. A doughy feel to the skin and subcutaneous tissue is a suggestive physical sign, as is a dissociation between the severe degree of dehydration (as judged by weight loss and by the state of the mucous membranes) and the relatively mild degree of circulatory compromise. **Diagnosis** is established by measuring the serum Na concentration. Additional laboratory findings may include an increase in the BUN, a modest increase in blood glucose, and if serum K is low, a depression in the level of serum Ca.

Treatment is designed to avoid a rapid fall in serum osmolality, since the osmotic gradient favoring movement of water into cells may cause cerebral edema. Correction of hypernatremia should be extended over 2 to 3 days (48 to 72 h). The fluid *volume* administered is the sum of the estimated deficit and 2 to 3 days of maintenance

requirements; this total amount is divided by 48 to 72 to determine the hourly volume and is given at a constant *rate* over the 48 to 72 h of correction. The *composition* of the fluid is 5% dextrose with approximately 70 mEq/L of cation. Initially the cation is Na; once adequate urine output is demonstrated, the cation should be Na and K in approximately equal amounts. Extreme hypernatremia (Na > 200 mEq/L) caused by salt poisoning should be treated by peritoneal dialysis.

Prophylaxis requires attention to the volume and composition of unusual fluid losses and of solutions used to maintain homeostasis. In newborns and young infants, who are unable to signal thirst effectively and to replace losses voluntarily, the opportunity for dehydration is greatest; factors that increase radiant heat loss (including warmers and phototherapy lights) raise the risk of hypernatremia. The composition of feedings whenever mixing is involved (eg, some infant formulas, concentrated preparations for tube feeding) requires particular attention, especially when the potential for developing dehydration is high, such as during episodes of diarrhea, poor fluid intake, vomiting, or high fever.

27.   DISTURBANCES IN NEWBORNS AND INFANTS

GESTATIONAL AGE AND BIRTH WEIGHT

CLASSIFICATION

Each newborn is classified as premature, full-term, or postmature. Rapid, accurate determination of gestational age can be done in the first days after birth using the new Ballard score (see Fig. 23–1). This permits anticipation of clinical problems, since the level of organ system maturation is determined primarily by gestational age. Each infant's intrauterine growth status should be determined at birth as small, appropriate, or large for gestational age, by plotting his weight (see Fig. 27–1) and by plotting his length and head circumference (see Fig. 27–2). The fetal growth rate may be altered by genetic factors and by abnormal intrauterine states, which can also predispose the infant to perinatal problems. This assessment also helps to predict growth and development potential.

PREMATURE INFANT

Any infant born before 37 wk gestation. Previously, any infant weighing < 2.5 kg (5.5 lb) was termed premature; this definition was inappropriate, since many newborns weighing < 2.5 kg are actually mature or postmature but small for gestational age (**SGA**) and have a different appearance and different problems than do premature infants.

Etiology and Prevention

In most cases, the cause of premature labor or premature rupture of the membranes followed by premature labor is unknown. However, the maternal histories commonly show low socioeconomic status, inadequate prenatal medical care, poor nutrition, poor education, unwed state, and intercurrent, untreated illness or infection.

The risk of preterm delivery, which is the greatest cause of neonatal morbidity and mortality, can be reduced by ensuring that all women, especially those in "high-risk groups," have access to early and appropriate prenatal care. The

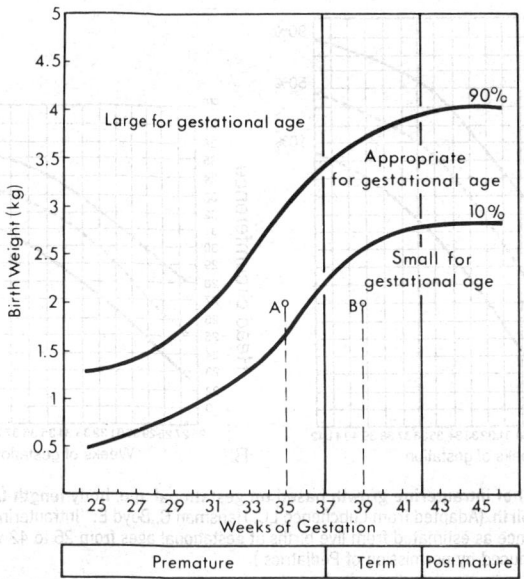

Fig. 27-1. **Level of intrauterine growth based on birth weight and gestational age of liveborn, single, white infants.** Point A represents a premature infant, while point B indicates an infant of similar birth weight, who is mature but small for gestational age. The growth curves are representative of the 10th and 90th percentiles for all of the newborns in the sampling. (Adapted from Sweet AY: "Classification of the low-birth-weight infant," in Care of the High-Risk Neonate, ed. 3, edited by MH Klaus and AA Fanaroff. Philadelphia, WB Saunders Company, 1986; used with permission.)

use of tocolytics to arrest premature labor and to hasten maturation of the fetal lungs if premature delivery is likely is discussed in Ch. 18.

Signs

The premature infant is small, usually weighs < 2.5 kg, and tends to have thin, shiny, pink skin through which the underlying veins are easily seen. Little subcutaneous fat, hair, or external ear cartilage exists. Spontaneous activity and tone are reduced, and extremities are not held in a flexed position. In males the scrotum may have few rugae, and the testes may be undescended. In females the labia majora do not yet cover the labia minora.

Problems

Most problems of premature infants relate to the immature functioning of organ systems.

Lungs: In many premature infants, surfactant production is not adequate to prevent alveolar collapse and atelectasis, which results in the re-

spiratory distress syndrome (**RDS**—see under RESPIRATORY DISORDERS, below).

CNS: Inadequate coordination of sucking and swallowing reflexes in the infant born before 34 wk gestation may require that the infant be fed IV or by gavage. Immaturity of the respiratory center in the brainstem results in apneic spells (**central apnea**—see APNEA OF PREMATURITY under RESPIRATORY DISORDERS, below). Apnea may also result from nasopharyngeal and soft palate obstruction (**obstructive apnea**). In preterm infants, the periventricular germinal matrix (see under BIRTH TRAUMA, below) is prone to hemorrhage, which may extend into the cerebral ventricles (**intraventricular hemorrhage**). Hemorrhagic or nonhemorrhagic infarction of the periventricular white matter (**periventricular leukomalacia**) may also occur, but the reasons for this are not understood. Hypotension, inadequate or erratic brain perfusion, and BP peaks (as when fluid or colloid is given rapidly IV) may all contribute to cerebral infarction or hemorrhage.

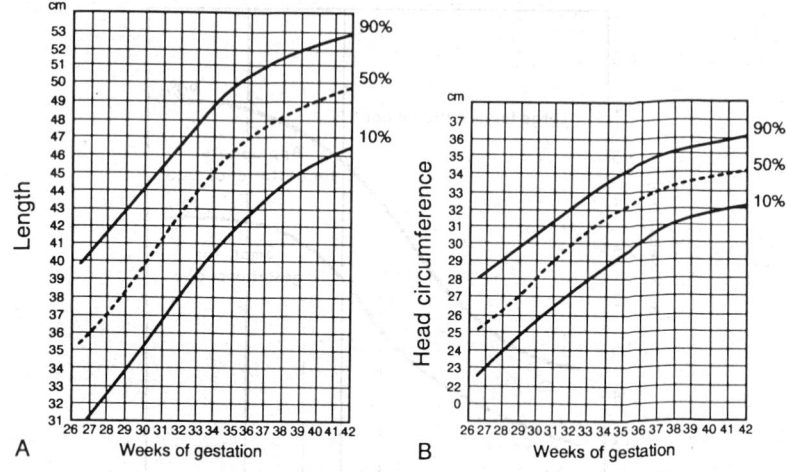

FIG. 27–2. Level of intrauterine growth based on gestational age, body length (A), and head circumference (B) at birth. (Adapted from Lubchenco LC, Hansman C, Boyd E: "Intrauterine growth in length and head circumference as estimated from live births at gestational ages from 26 to 42 weeks." *Pediatrics* 37:403, 1966; reproduced by permission of Pediatrics.)

Infection: The risk of developing sepsis or meningitis is about 4 times greater in the premature infant than in the full-term newborn. This increased susceptibility to infection is due to the need for indwelling intravascular catheters and endotracheal tubes and to the markedly reduced serum immunoglobulin levels in preterm infants. (See NEONATAL INFECTIONS, below; and IMMUNOLOGIC STATUS OF THE FETUS AND NEWBORN in Ch. 23.)

Temperature regulation: Premature infants have an exceptionally large body surface area to body mass ratio; therefore, when exposed to temperatures below the neutral thermal environment, they lose heat quickly and have difficulty maintaining their body temperature. (See METABOLIC PROBLEMS IN THE NEWBORN, below.)

GI tract: The small stomach capacity of the premature infant, coupled with immature sucking and swallowing reflexes, hinders adequate oral or nasogastric tube feedings and creates a risk of aspiration. Most premature infants tolerate human breast milk, proprietary milk formulas containing 20 kcal/oz, or specially prepared formulas that contain 24 kcal/oz. Small premature infants have been successfully tube-fed with their own mother's milk, which provides immunologic and nutritional factors that are absent in altered cow's milk formulas. However, human milk will not provide sufficient calcium, phosphorus, and protein for very-low-birth-weight in-

fants (< 1.5 kg, or 3.3 lb), for whom it should be mixed with one of several available breast milk fortifiers. In the first days, if adequate fluids and calories cannot be given by mouth or nasogastric or nasoduodenal tube, solutions with 10% glucose and maintenance electrolytes may be given IV to prevent dehydration and malnutrition, especially in the infant weighing < 1.5 kg. Continuous breast milk or formula feeding via nasoduodenal or gastric tube is a satisfactory method of maintaining caloric intake in small, sick, premature infants, especially if respiratory distress or recurrent apneic spells are present. Feedings are begun with small amounts of half-strength formula; if tolerated, the volume and concentration of feedings are slowly increased over 7 to 10 days. In very tiny or critically sick infants, adequate nutrition may be provided by total parenteral hyperalimentation via peripheral IV or a percutaneously or surgically placed central catheter.

Necrotizing enterocolitis: Preterm infants are uniquely susceptible (see NECROTIZING ENTEROCOLITIS, below).

Hyperbilirubinemia (see also METABOLIC PROBLEMS IN THE NEWBORN, below): Premature infants develop hyperbilirubinemia more often than do full-term newborns, and kernicterus may occur at serum bilirubin levels as low as 10 mg/dL in small, sick, premature neonates. Delayed clamping of the umbilical cord increases the risk of significant hyperbilirubinemia by allowing the transfusion of a large RBC mass; as a result, RBC breakdown and bilirubin production are increased. The higher bilirubin levels in premature infants may be partially due to inadequately developed hepatic excretion mechanisms, including deficiencies in bilirubin uptake from the serum, in its hepatic conjugation to bilirubin diglucuronide, and in its excretion into the biliary tree. In addition, decreased bowel motility enables more bilirubin diglucuronide to be deconjugated within the intestinal lumen by the enzyme β-glucuronidase, permitting increased reabsorption of free bilirubin (enterohepatic circulation of bilirubin). Early feedings can significantly decrease the incidence and severity of physiologic jaundice by increasing bowel motility, thus interrupting the enterohepatic circulation of bilirubin as the bilirubin is more rapidly excreted in the stools.

Hypo- and hyperglycemia: See METABOLIC PROBLEMS IN THE NEWBORN, below.

Kidney: Renal function is immature, so that concentration or dilution of urine is less effective than in the full-term infant. The inability of the immature kidney to excrete fixed acids, which accumulate with high-protein formula feedings and as a result of bone growth, may cause metabolic acidosis **(late metabolic acidosis of the premature)** and resultant growth failure. Late metabolic acidosis is easily treated with oral sodium bicarbonate; and although the amount given depends on the severity of acidosis, 1 to 2 mEq/kg/day in 4 to 6 divided doses is often adequate and may need to be continued for several days. Reduction of the protein content of the formula may also be necessary.

RETINOPATHY OF PREMATURITY (ROP)
(Retrolental Fibroplasia)

A bilateral ocular disorder of premature infants, occuring mainly in those of lowest birth weight, with outcomes ranging from normal vision to blindness.

Etiology and Pathogenesis

The blood vessels supplying the inner retina begin to grow about halfway through pregnancy and have fully vascularized the retina by full term. Thus, they are incomplete when an infant is born prematurely. ROP results if these vessels continue their growth in an abnormal pattern. In infants < 1 kg at birth, > 80% develop ROP and more often when there are many medical complications. Administration of excessive (especially prolonged) O_2 without adjustment to need increases the risk of ROP, but a threshold safe level or duration of elevated Pa_{O2} is not known. Significant degrees of ROP are rare in appropriately treated infants > 1500 gm birth weight, and alternative diagnoses should be considered (eg, familial exudative retinopathy or **Norrie's disease**).

Clinical Course

Susceptibility to ROP is variable but correlates with the extent of retina that remains avascular at birth. An abnormal ridge of vascular tissue forms between the vascularized and nonvascularized peripheral retina. In severe ROP, these new vessels invade the vitreous, and sometimes the entire vasculature of the eye becomes engorged (**"plus disease"**). The abnormal vessel growth often subsides spontaneously but, in about 4% of survivors < 1 kg birth weight, may progress to retinal detachments and vision loss in the 2 to 12 mo after birth. Children with healed ROP have a higher incidence of myopia, strabismus, and amblyopia. A few children with moderate, healed ROP are left with cicatricial scars (eg, dragged retina or retinal folds) but no initial retinal detachments and carry a risk of retinal detachments later in life.

Prevention and Treatment

The most important preventive action is to provide prenatal care to reduce the incidence of prematurity. After a preterm birth, optimal stabilization is most important, including use of O_2 only in amounts sufficient to avoid hypoxia. The prophylactic use of vitamin E as an antioxidant and the restriction of light exposure (a pro-oxidant) are areas of active research.

In severe ROP, cryotherapy to ablate the avascular retina can halve the incidence of severe retinal damage. Therefore, all high-risk infants should have their eyes examined by 6 wk after birth. The progress of retinal vascularization must be closely followed at 1- to 2-wk intervals until the vessels have matured without reaching the preconditions for cryotherapy. If retinal detachments occur, scleral buckling surgery or vitrectomy with lensectomy may be considered, but these procedures are investigational.

Infants with residual scarring from ROP should be followed at least annually for life; scars and retinal holes that lead to late retinal detachments can often be treated effectively if detected before progression. Treatment of amblyopia and refractive errors in the first year will optimize residual vision. Infants with total retinal detachments should be monitored for possible complications of secondary glaucoma and phthisis, and referred to appropriate early intervention programs for the visually impaired.

Complete prevention of ROP has not been achieved, and intensive investigation continues worldwide.

POSTMATURE INFANT

Any infant born after 42 wk gestation.

Etiology

The cause of postmature delivery generally is unknown. Very rarely, abnormalities of the fetal pituitary-adrenal axis (eg, anencephaly or adrenal agenesis) can result in postmaturity.

Signs

Postmature infants are alert and appear mature, but there is a decreased amount of soft tissue mass, particularly subcutaneous fat; the skin may hang loosely on the extremities and is often dry and peeling. The finger- and toenails are long. The nails and umbilical cord may be stained with meconium passed in utero.

Problems

The main clinical problem is that past term the placenta involutes, and multiple infarcts and villous degeneration produce the **placental insufficiency syndrome**. The fetus may receive inadequate nutrients from the mother, resulting in fetal soft tissue wasting. Postmature infants are prone to develop (1) **asphyxia** during labor secondary to placental insufficiency (see ASPHYXIA AND RESUSCITATION, below); (2) the **meconium aspiration syndrome** (see under RESPIRATORY DISORDERS, below), which may be unusually severe since, past term, amniotic fluid volume is decreased and the aspirated meconium is less diluted; and (3) neonatal **hypoglycemia** because of insufficient glycogen stores at birth. Hypoglycemia is exaggerated if perinatal asphyxia has occurred, during which anaerobic metabolism rapidly utilizes the last of the glycogen stores (see METABOLIC PROBLEMS IN THE NEWBORN, below).

SMALL−FOR−GESTATIONAL−AGE (SGA) INFANT
(Dysmaturity; Intrauterine Growth Retardation)

Any infant whose weight is below the 10th percentile for gestational age, whether premature, full-term, or postmature. Despite his small size, a full-term SGA infant does not have the problems related to organ system immaturity that the premature infant has.

Causes

An infant may be small at birth because of genetic factors (short parents or a genetic disorder associated with short stature) or from other factors that can retard intrauterine growth. These intrauterine (nongenetic) factors usually are not operative before 32 to 34 wk gestation, and include placental insufficiency that often results from maternal disease involving the small blood vessels (as in preeclampsia, primary hypertension, renal disease, or long-standing diabetes); placental involution accompanying postmaturity; or infectious agents such as cytomegalovirus, rubella virus, or *Toxoplasma gondii.* An infant may be SGA if the mother is a narcotic or cocaine addict or a heavy user of alcohol and, to a lesser degree, if she smokes cigarettes during pregnancy.

Signs

Despite their small size, SGA infants have physical characteristics and behavior similar to those of normal-sized infants of like gestational age. Thus, a 1.4-kg infant born between 37 and 42 wk gestation may have the skin, external ear cartilage, sole creases, genital development, and the neurologic development, alertness, spontaneous activity, and zest for feeding of a full-term infant. If the intrauterine growth retardation has been caused by chronic malnutrition, SGA infants may demonstrate remarkable "catch-up" growth following delivery if they maintain an adequate caloric intake.

Problems

Birth asphyxia: If intrauterine growth retardation is due to placental insufficiency (with marginally adequate placental perfusion), the infant will be at risk of asphyxia during labor, since each uterine contraction slows or stops maternal placental perfusion by compressing the spiral arteries. Therefore, when placental insufficiency is suspected, the fetal state should be assessed before labor and the fetal heart rate monitored during labor. If fetal asphyxia is imminent, rapid delivery, often by cesarean section, is indicated. The SGA infant with asphyxia is likely to have low Apgar scores and mixed acidosis at birth (see ASPHYXIA AND RESUSCITATION, below). Perinatal asphyxia is the greatest problem for these infants, and if it can be avoided, their neurologic prognosis appears to be quite good. Infants who are SGA because of genetic factors, congenital infection, or maternal drug use may not have such a good prognosis.

Meconium aspiration: During birth asphyxia, SGA infants, especially those who are post-term (see POSTMATURE INFANT, above), may pass meconium into the amniotic sac and begin deep gasping movements. The consequent aspiration of meconium is likely to result in meconium aspiration syndrome after delivery (often most severe in the growth-retarded or postmature infant, as the meconium is contained in a smaller volume of amniotic fluid; see under RESPIRATORY DISORDERS, below).

Hypoglycemia: The SGA infant is very prone to hypoglycemia in the first hours and days of life because of lack of adequate glycogen stores (see METABOLIC PROBLEMS IN THE NEWBORN, below.)

LARGE−FOR−GESTATIONAL−AGE (LGA) INFANT

Any infant whose weight is above the 90th percentile for gestational age, whether premature, full-term, or postmature.

Etiology

Other than genetically determined size, the major cause of an infant's being large for gestational age is **maternal diabetes mellitus.** Macrosomia results from exposure to excessive blood glucose and insulin levels during gestation. The less well controlled the mother's diabetes during pregnancy, the more severe will be the fetal macrosomia and early neonatal hypoglycemia.

Signs

The infant of a diabetic mother is generally large, obese, and plethoric; is often listless and limp; and may feed poorly.

Problems

Delivery: Because of the infant's large size, vaginal delivery is often difficult and may be traumatic. Shoulder dystocia, fractures of the clavicles or limbs, and birth asphyxia may occur. Therefore, cesarean section delivery should always be considered when the fetus is thought to be LGA, especially if the mother's pelvic measurements are not adequate.

Hypoglycemia: The infant of a diabetic mother is very likely to become hypoglycemic in the first 1 to 2 h following delivery because of his state of hyperinsulinism and the sudden termination of a glucose infusion from the mother when

the umbilical cord is cut. This can be prevented by close prenatal control of the mother's diabetes and by prophylactic use of 10% glucose in water IV in the infant until early frequent feedings can be instituted to provide calories and glucose. The blood glucose should be closely monitored during the transition period. Glucose oxidase reagent strips are often used to screen for low blood glucose in neonates. However, these strips are not precise at low glucose levels, and treatment should not be based on the reagent strip alone. Any questionably low values should be verified by laboratory determination of serum glucose. (See also METABOLIC PROBLEMS IN THE NEWBORN, below.)

Hyperbilirubinemia (see also METABOLIC PROBLEMS IN THE NEWBORN): Infants of diabetic mothers frequently develop hyperbilirubinemia because of their intolerance for oral feedings in the first days of life (increased enterohepatic circulation of bilirubin), because of their relatively high Hct (one manifestation of macrosomia), and probably because of other, unknown factors.

Lungs: In infants of diabetic women, pulmonary maturation with production of surfactant may be delayed until late in gestation; therefore, these infants may develop respiratory distress syndrome even if delivered only a few weeks prematurely. Following amniocentesis, the lecithin/sphingomyelin ratio and especially the presence of phosphatidyl glycerol **(PG)** in the amniotic fluid can be determined to evaluate fetal lung maturity, and so determine the optimal time for safe delivery. Indeed, lung maturity can be assumed *only* if PG is present.

ASPHYXIA AND RESUSCITATION
(Asphyxia Neonatorum)
(See also CARDIOPULMONARY RESUSCITATION in Ch. 30)

A newborn who does not breathe spontaneously or is in shock requires immediate resuscitation to sustain life and minimize the possibility of brain damage. Although instituting ventilation usually is the main concern, rapid correction of hypovolemia to support circulation may be equally critical.

Etiology and Pathophysiology

High-risk pregnancies account for only 70% of cases in which resuscitation will be needed, so that personnel at *every* delivery should have re-

TABLE 27-1. THE APGAR SCORE

Criteria	Score		
	0	1	2
Color	Blue, pale	Body pink, extremities blue	All pink
Heart rate	Absent	< 100	> 100
Respiration	Absent	Irregular, slow	Good, crying
Reflex response to nose catheter	None	Grimace	Sneeze, cough
Muscle tone	Limp	Some flexion of extremities	Active

suscitation skills. Newborns are likely to require resuscitation in situations such as premature birth, multiple births, prolapsed umbilical cord, severe maternal bleeding, maternal hypotension, toxemia, or intrauterine growth retardation. During an otherwise apparently uncomplicated labor, the appearance of thick meconium in the amniotic fluid, abnormalities of the fetal heart rate pattern, or a drop in the fetal scalp blood pH to < 7.25 may indicate fetal distress, especially when more than one finding is present.

Perinatal asphyxia may be due to placental or neonatal pulmonary dysfunction. The infant may become asphyxiated before or during labor and may already be in a critical state at the moment of delivery, or may become asphyxiated after delivery unless effective spontaneous breathing begins. Asphyxia in utero may result from severe uteroplacental insufficiency, abruptio placentae, umbilical cord compression, uterine tetany, maternal hypotension, or fetal exsanguination. The newborn may not breathe spontaneously because of prior asphyxiation, placental passage of maternal analgesics and anesthetics, or malformations (eg, choanal atresia, diaphragmatic hernia, or hypoplastic lungs). A premature infant with immature lungs and surfactant deficiency may be unable to breathe adequately at birth because of low lung compliance.

Asphyxia produces both hypoxemia and hypercapnia. Respiratory acidosis results from CO_2 retention; superimposed metabolic acidosis occurs as tissues are deprived of adequate O_2 and lactic acid accumulates. Secondary effects include a fall in cardiac output (CO) with a drop in pulse rate and BP, hypovolemia from pooling of blood in central veins or escape of fluid from the capillary bed damaged by hypoxemia, and CNS depression. Anaerobic glycolysis causes increased use of glycogen stores; therefore, asphyxiated infants, particularly those small for

gestational age, are prone to early hypoglycemia.

Clinical Evaluation

The Apgar scoring system (see TABLE 27-1) estimates the severity of respiratory and neurologic depression at birth by rating certain physical signs. Every infant should be rated at exactly 1 and 5 min after birth, and both scores should be recorded. The maximum score of 10 is rare; the lower the score, the more severely depressed is the infant (≤ 5 indicates severe depression). Low scores, particularly at 5 min or later, are more likely to be associated with residual neurologic damage or neonatal death, although most of these infants will survive and be normal.

A low score may be caused by either perinatal asphyxia or respiratory and neurologic depression from transplacental passage of anesthetics given to the mother. An infant with low scores due to asphyxia will appear cyanotic or pale and have a slow heart rate and low BP, while an infant depressed by anesthetics is likely to have normal color, heart rate, and BP. Thus a low Apgar score by itself is not evidence of perinatal asphyxia. A cord-blood pH < 7.2 is a more direct measure of perinatal asphyxia. Premature infants often have low scores because they are hypotonic, have depressed reflexes, and may not establish respirations because of stiff lungs. Thus, low Apgar scores may be considered "normal" for a premature infant—these infants often require immediate positive pressure ventilation at delivery.

Preparations for Effective Resuscitation

Delivery room personnel must be skilled in resuscitation, as the apneic infant cannot wait for a consultant. In high-risk situations, preparations should be made in advance, with trained personnel present at delivery. All personnel must be familiar with the following equipment, which should be simple, dependable, and in working order: sources of O_2 and suction, suction catheters of various sizes, infant airways, an infant resuscitation bag and mask, a laryngoscope with newborn- and premature-size blades (sizes 1 and 0), endotracheal tubes (sizes 2.5, 3, and 3.5 mm), an endotracheal tube stylet, and umbilical catheters (sizes 5 and 8 French). Fluids (eg, 5 or 10% D/W and 5% human serum albumin) should be on hand, as should sodium bicarbonate (see step 4, below). Basic equipment and drugs (in common doses and dilutions) can be displayed clearly on a pegboard in the delivery room (see TABLES 30−7 and 30−8). To maintain the infant's body temperature during evaluation and resuscitation, a radiant heater is essential.

Treatment

Step 1. Airway: The airway must be quickly cleared of secretions, fluid, or blood by gently suctioning the pharynx and nostrils with a soft catheter. Suctioning is limited to 5 to 10 sec, since prolonged vigorous suctioning of the posterior pharynx may cause apnea or bradycardia (by stimulating the vagal reflex).

The well-oxygenated infant who is depressed by anesthetics may be stimulated repeatedly (eg, by gently slapping the feet) before other efforts at resuscitation are begun. However, if central cyanosis or bradycardia develops, positive pressure ventilation (see step 2, below) must begin immediately.

For a neonate who is covered with meconium and depressed, it is essential to intubate the trachea at once; endotracheal suctioning is repeated until the airway is clear of aspirated meconium. An endotracheal tube with the largest possible diameter should be used (a 3.5- or 4-mm tube can usually be used for full-term infants, a 3-mm tube for infants < 1.5 kg, and a 2.5-mm tube for infants < 1 kg), so that the largest possible size suction catheter can be inserted. Mechanical suction must be available at all deliveries; *risk of HIV transmission proscribes endotracheal suctioning by mouth.* To prevent severe anoxia, these procedures should be done quickly, followed by positive pressure O_2 ventilation with a bag and an endotracheal tube.

Step 2. Ventilation: Positive pressure ventilation (with 100% O_2) can usually be effectively and safely provided with bag and mask resuscitation, by placing the infant's head in the neutral position and raising the jaw slightly to ensure an unobstructed airway. So that valuable time is not lost or errors made, only experienced personnel should perform endotracheal intubation. Ventilation rate should be started at about 40/min; its effectiveness is judged by watching chest wall movement (since hearing transmitted breath sounds is not always a reliable indicator of adequate ventilation in a small infant).

Step 3. Circulation: If the infant does not rapidly become pink with effective positive pressure ventilation, the circulation may be inadequate. If the heart rate is < 80/min and not increasing, with thready pulses and poor capillary refill (> 2 sec), cardiac massage is immediately begun by placing the thumbs over the midsternum with both hands encircling the chest or placing 2 fingers over the lower $1/3$ of the sternum in the midline and compressing the chest about 120 times/min about $1/2$ to $3/4$ in. After 3 or 4 chest compressions, one positive pressure ventilation is given to maintain a respiratory rate of about 40/min. This sequence is repeated smoothly and requires 2 experienced persons. If the heart rate remains low with thready pulses and poor skin perfusion, epinephrine 0.1 to 0.2 mL/kg of a 1:10,000 solution IV is given. In emergency situations, if IV access is not immediately available, 0.2 mL/kg of a 1:10,000 dilution of epinephrine can be given endotracheally. Following severe asphyxia, dopamine or dobutamine may be required as a continuous IV infusion to maintain CO and perfusion.

Step 4. Fluid and glucose: For the severely asphyxiated infant with a poor CO, rapid infusion of fluid using a plasma expander (eg, 10 mL/kg of either 5% human serum albumin or fresh frozen plasma) will improve circulation and facilitate the distribution and buffering of fixed acids. In emergencies, infusions and sampling of blood are most quickly accomplished through an umbilical vein catheter. Sodium bicarbonate may be needed to correct metabolic acidosis. Whenever possible, the acid-base status should be determined first; otherwise, the infant may be given sodium bicarbonate 2 mEq/kg IV. Sodium bicarbonate comes as a hypertonic solution (44.5 mEq/50 mL) and should be diluted three- to fourfold with sterile water and then infused over 5 to 10 min while positive pressure ventilation is continued. Since asphyxiated infants are prone to hypoglycemia, the blood glucose levels should be monitored and 10% D/W should be given IV, starting shortly after delivery.

Step 5. Depression secondary to narcotics: If the infant's respiratory depression may be due to narcotics given to the mother, naloxone (a narcotic antagonist) 0.1 mg/kg IV is given. The recommended pediatric dosage form of naloxone hydrochloride comes as 0.4 mg/mL, so up to 1 mL can be given safely to any infant. This may need to be repeated several times at 5- to 20-min intervals if the initial response is good, since naloxone has a short half-life compared with those of narcotics. Naloxone is not indicated for any other type of drug or anesthetic depression in the neonate, as it is an antidote only for narcotics. Naloxone should not be given to the infant of a known drug addict, as it may result in seizures.

Step 6. Temperature: Maintaining the infant's temperature during resuscitation is essential. Cooling may double or triple the infant's BMR, thus increasing O_2 requirements. In the face of O_2 lack, severe O_2 debt can ensue rapidly and result in neurologic damage or death. After the infant is dried thoroughly, radiant heating (rather than blankets) is recommended to permit continuous observation of the infant's color and activity.

Sequelae

Infants with significant asphyxia at birth require close observation for evidence of sequelae. Cerebral hypoxia may produce **hypotonia** and **lethargy** or **coma** initially, as well as **convulsions** that may not occur for 1 or 2 days. The premature infant with cerebral hypoxia is more likely to develop (1) **germinal matrix hemorrhages** that can rupture into the lateral ventricles, resulting in **intraventricular hemorrhage** of varying severity, or (2) periventricular leukomalacia (*softening of the white matter*) from infarction of periventricular white matter. (See also BIRTH TRAUMA, below.) Following asphyxia, fluid intake should be restricted initially (eg, 10% D/W 60 mL/kg/day IV), with electrolytes added at 24 h of life; weight, urine output, and serum electrolytes should be monitored closely since **inappropriate ADH secretion** may develop. Severe renal hypoxia and hypoperfusion can result in **acute tubular necrosis**, also resulting in fluid retention and hyponatremia. Ischemia of the bowel wall, particularly in premature infants, may damage the mucosa and its ability to secrete mucus, which protects against enteric bacterial invasion. Several days later, after milk feedings are begun, **necrotizing enterocolitis**, possibly associated with peritonitis or sepsis, may occur. For this reason, feedings may be delayed for several days in such infants, during which total parenteral nutrition is instituted. Meconium-stained, asphyxiated infants may develop **meco-**nium aspiration syndrome with respiratory distress, pneumomediastinum, and tension pneumothorax.

All organ systems, except the CNS, usually will recover from even the most severe hypoxic insults. Asphyxiated infants with documented fetal distress and metabolic acidosis who remain severely neurologically depressed (coma, poor responsiveness, inability to feed orally, seizures) for several days to a week are likely to suffer residual CNS damage. If the infant's neurologic state returns to normal rapidly, the probability of normal development is strong. The infant with severe asphyxia at birth and abnormal neurologic examination for many days after delivery is at risk for long-term residual CNS damage including mental retardation, cerebral palsy, and seizure disorder. Unless damage is proved, reasonably optimistic and supportive but honest assessments will help parents relate positively to their infant. Most infants who have sustained perinatal asphyxia will be normal. Parental attachment is essential for developing the warm, loving, and stimulating home environment that will in large measure ultimately determine the child's mental development.

RESPIRATORY DISORDERS

Respiratory disorders due to altered RBC mass and blood volume are discussed under HEMATOLOGIC PROBLEMS, and neonatal pneumonia is discussed under NEONATAL INFECTIONS, in this chapter below.

RESPIRATORY DISTRESS SYNDROME (RDS)
(Hyaline Membrane Disease)

A disorder primarily of prematurity, manifested clinically by respiratory distress and pathologically by pulmonary hyaline membranes and atelectasis.

Etiology

RDS is due to diffuse atelectasis that develops when pulmonary surfactants are deficient at birth. The air-fluid interfaces of the film of water lining the alveoli exert large forces that cause the alveoli to collapse if surfactants are lacking. Pulmonary surfactant, a mixture of phospholipids and 3 surfactant apoproteins, is manufactured in the type II alveolar cells (see PERINATAL PHYSIOLOGY in Ch. 23).

RDS almost always occurs in infants born before 37 wk gestation; the more premature the infant, the greater the chance of developing RDS. RDS is also more likely to develop in infants of diabetic mothers, but is less likely at any gestational age in infants with signs of fetal growth retardation or when the mother has toxemia or hypertension. Prolonged rupture of the membranes also seems to afford some protection against RDS.

Fetal lung maturity with regard to surfactant production may be assessed before delivery by measuring surfactants in amniotic fluid obtained by amniocentesis or collected from the vagina (if the membranes have ruptured). Fetal lung maturity is shown if the lecithin/sphingomyelin ratio (L/S ratio) is > 2 and phosphatidyl glycerol is present. Use of this information to choose the optimal time for delivery in a variety of maternal disorders as well as for repeat cesarean section has reduced the incidence of RDS (see Chs. 17 and 18). Also systemic administration of betamethasone for at least 24 h to the woman who must be delivered when the fetal lung profile is immature may induce fetal surfactant production and thus reduce the risk of RDS or decrease its severity.

Symptoms and Signs

The infant with RDS is almost always premature. A diagnosis of RDS in an infant of ≥ 37 wk gestational age is unusual and should make one suspect that the mother may have had unrecognized diabetes mellitus or that the diagnosis is incorrect (eg, early-onset Group B streptococcal pneumonia and sepsis can mimic RDS clinically and on x-ray).

The infant will usually develop rapid, labored respirations immediately or within a few hours after delivery. There will be supra- and substernal retractions, flaring of nasal alae, and grunting respirations. Both the extent of atelectasis and the severity of respiratory failure will increase with time. The lack of surfactant causes lung compliance to be very low, and the work of inflating the stiff lungs is increased. The premature infant is further handicapped because his ribs are more easily deformed; respiratory effort is wasted in deforming the ribs (sternal retractions). In severe disease, the diaphragms and intercostal muscles fatigue and CO_2 retention and respiratory acidosis develop. Additionally, there is shunting of blood through the atelectatic portions of lung, so that oxygenation does not occur

and the infant becomes hypoxemic. Unless adequate O_2 is delivered to the body tissues, metabolic acidosis will supervene. Ultimately, if untreated, severe hypoxemia will result in multiple organ failure and death. However, if respirations can be mechanically supported and lung expansion effected, surfactant production will begin and the RDS will resolve in about 4 to 5 days.

Not all infants with RDS will present with signs of respiratory distress; tiny infants with very low birth weight (eg, < 1000 gm) may be unable to initiate respirations at birth because their lungs are so stiff and will present with primary apnea in the delivery room. All such infants must be immediately intubated and given positive pressure ventilation.

Premature infants with RDS are at greater risk of intraventricular hemorrhage (**IVH**) and neonatal death. Intracranial pathology (from ischemia and IVH) has been associated with hypoxemia, hypercarbia, hypotension, swings in arterial BP, and low cerebral perfusion. Tension pneumothorax, a potential complication of RDS, produces sudden hypotension and also may result in reduced cerebral blood flow (see INTRACRANIAL HEMORRHAGE under BIRTH TRAUMA and HEMORRHAGIC SHOCK AND ENCEPHALOPATHY, below).

Diagnosis

The diagnosis is based on the history (eg, premature labor, maternal diabetes, assessment of fetal lung maturity [see above]), physical examination (eg, respiratory distress, cyanosis), and laboratory assessment. Arterial blood gases (**ABGs**) show variable degrees of hypoxemia and hypercarbia. Chest x-ray shows diffuse atelectasis and roughly correlates with the clinical severity of the RDS; **grade I RDS**: reticulogranular pattern of the lung parenchyma with aerated areas (black dots) exceeding atelectatic areas (white dots); **grade II RDS**: reticulogranular areas of lung parenchyma with atelectatic lung areas in excess of aerated lung; **grade III RDS**: same as grade II plus prominent air bronchograms; and **grade IV RDS**: almost total loss of heart borders because of severe diffuse atelectasis.

Once the infant is placed on a respirator, positive pressure inflation of the lung may reduce the extent of the atelectasis as seen on x-ray. Early-onset Group B streptococcal pneumonia can masquerade as RDS radiologically as well as clinically.

Treatment and Prognosis

Monitoring: It is important to monitor respiratory and circulatory status closely, so that treatment is proportional to the clinical severity of the disease. An umbilical artery catheter (**UAC**) is usually placed in infants with moderate-to-severe respiratory disease; ie, those who require the flow of inspired O_2 (**FIO_2**) to be $\geq 40\%$. If a UAC cannot be inserted, a percutaneous radial artery catheter can be used for continuous BP monitoring and for sampling ABGs.

Devices that can continuously and noninvasively monitor both O_2 and CO_2 tension transcutaneously (**tcPO_2** and **tcPCO_2**) reduce the need for frequent blood samples. After transcutaneous values have been correlated with simultaneously obtained arterial samples, they can be used to follow trends in ABGs and ABG responses to changes in ventilator settings. Intermittent blood gas sampling (eg, radial artery punctures or heel sticks) has the disadvantage of causing pain and may yield results different (usually worse) from the true values that are present at rest. A pulse oximeter placed on a finger or toe can provide accurate information regarding Hb saturation with O_2.

Acceptable PaO_2 in preterm infants is 50 to 70 mm Hg; these O_2 tensions provide almost full saturation of Hb with O_2 because these infants have fetal Hb, which has a higher affinity for O_2 and is almost fully saturated at these values. Higher PaO_2 may increase the risk of **retinopathy of prematurity**, while delivering very little additional O_2 to tissues. As in adults, normal $PaCO_2$ is 35 to 45 mm Hg.

Specific treatment is individualized. Infants with mild RDS may do well with supplemental O_2 given by hood; more severe RDS will respond to continuous positive airway pressure (**CPAP**) with the infant breathing spontaneously; the sickest infants will require ventilator support.

Treatment with **pulmonary surfactants** instilled intratracheally have been shown to reduce the severity of RDS as measured by improvement in ABGs, by the ability to reduce ventilator support rapidly, and by improvement in the chest x-ray. Multi-hospital trials showed that infants treated with these surfactants have a significantly improved rate of survival as well as a reduced risk of developing pulmonary air leaks (eg, tension pneumothorax, pulmonary interstitial emphysema). Some (but not all) trials have also shown a reduced incidence of bronchopulmonary dysplasia developing in infants treated with surfactants as compared with matched controls.

Exosurf Neonatal® (colfosceril palmitate, cetyl alcohol, tyloxapol), a synthetic protein-free surfactant, is approved for use in infants in the USA. It is instilled intratracheally via a sideport of a specially designed endotracheal tube adapter while the infant is on a respirator. The manufacturer recommends its use in 3 situations: (1) *prophylaxis* for infants weighing < 1350 gm who are at risk for developing RDS; (2) *prophylaxis* for infants weighing > 1350 gm who have evidence of fetal lung immaturity; and (3) rescue treatment for infants who have developed moderate or severe RDS.

Each dose is 5 mL/kg. When given for prophylaxis, the first dose is given within several minutes after delivery as quickly as the infant can be stabilized on a ventilator, and 2 additional doses are given q 12 h. Rescue treatment is indicated for an infant with a clinical and x-ray diagnosis of at least moderate RDS, defined as having a PaO_2 to PAO_2 ratio (a/A ratio) of < 0.22 as determined from an ABG sample. A second dose is given 12 h later.

The infant needs to be monitored closely during and after surfactant therapy to be sure that the treatment is tolerated and that changes in oxygenation, ventilation, or systemic BP are quickly corrected. After instillation of the surfactant, pulmonary compliance may improve rapidly; in that case ventilator pressure may need to be reduced rapidly to lower the risk of pulmonary air leak. Other ventilator parameters (eg, FIO_2, rate) may also be reduced. Professionals can prepare themselves to give surfactant by reviewing the manufacturer's videotape. Until now its use has been limited to tertiary neonatal centers. It is appropriate for physicians at community hospitals to discuss with their tertiary centers the advisability and risks of giving surfactant to infants with RDS who are to be transferred to tertiary centers. Surfactant administration does not eliminate the risk of complications or ensure a good outcome; treated infants still should be referred to regional centers.

The most serious side effect to date has been an increased incidence of pulmonary hemorrhage, especially in tiny infants, and most often in those who have a patent ductus arteriosus. The incidence is about 10% in the highest risk population, infants weighing < 700 gm, as compared with 2% in untreated infants. There have been a few reports of plugging of the endotracheal tube after Exosurf® administration.

Another surfactant product (Survanta®, produced from purified bovine lung extract supplemented with lecithin) has also proved to be effective in clinical trials for prophylaxis or treatment of premature infants with RDS. The indications, timing, and mode of delivery are somewhat different. Survanta® is currently available to be given according to an investigational new drug protocol (IND) by the FDA. The natural surfactant (Survanta®) and the artificial surfactant (Exosurf®) have not been directly compared regarding efficacy or safety.

As RDS resolves, usually in 4 to 5 days, the type of support is reduced proportionally: The infant may be weaned from a ventilator, to CPAP, to an O₂ hood.

O₂ hood: O₂ must be mixed with air using a blender; the O₂ percentage being delivered must be measured with an O₂ analyzer and recorded. O₂ delivery should never be measured as L/min, since the flow rate tells nothing about how much O₂ the infant is actually inspiring. The O₂ should be warmed (36 to 37° C) and humidified to prevent cooling. Cool O₂ or air can also induce bronchospasm.

Continuous positive airway pressure (CPAP) is indicated for a spontaneously breathing infant who requires an $FI_{O_2} \geq 40\%$ to maintain a normal Pa_{O_2} (50 to 70 mm Hg). It may be started earlier if an infant with RDS is worsening rapidly. CPAP can deliver an O₂ mixture, usually under positive pressure of 5 to 8 cm of H_2O, via nasal prongs, nasopharyngeal tube, or endotracheal tube. The positive pressure holds alveoli open throughout the respiratory cycle and improves oxygenation by reducing the amount of blood shunted through atelectatic areas (see PERINATAL PHYSIOLOGY in Ch. 23). Once the Pa_{O_2} improves, it is usually possible to reduce the FI_{O_2}.

Ventilator support is required if the infant has respiratory failure with a $Pa_{CO_2} > 50$ mm Hg, has apnea, or cannot be oxygenated with CPAP. Clinical judgment plays a large role: Infants who are at risk of severe RDS and IVH (eg, infants weighing < 1250 gm at birth) and infants whose RDS is worsening rapidly may do better if started on a ventilator without waiting for respiratory failure or hypoxemia to develop, and then they can be weaned as tolerated.

The infant is intubated with an endotracheal tube (the smallest is a 2.5-mm-diameter tube for infants < 1250 gm; a 3-mm tube is usually appropriate for infants of 1250 to 2500 gm; and a 3.5-mm tube is used for those > 2500 gm). Intubation is safer if O₂ is insufflated into the airways during the procedure.

This text does not describe all details of ventilator therapy for neonates. Ventilators can deliver gas at either a predetermined pressure or volume; each type has advantages and indications. Many neonatal ICUs find the pressure-limited, time-cycled continuous-flow ventilators easy to use in tiny infants. The FI_{O_2}, inspiratory time **(IT)**, expiratory time **(ET)**, peak inspiratory pressure **(PIP)**, and positive end expiratory pressure **(PEEP)** are set independently.

Initial ventilator settings are estimates based upon past experience and judgment of the severity of the lung disease. Typical settings for an infant with moderate RDS follow: $FI_{O_2} = 40\%$; $IT = 0.5$ sec; $ET = 1.0$ sec, rate = 40 breaths/min, $PIP = 25$ cm H_2O, $PEEP = 5$ cm H_2O. The infant's oxygenation, chest wall movements, breath sounds, and respiratory efforts should be observed; the first ventilator settings are quickly adjusted, depending on the clinical response. Readjustments are based on ABGs or transcutaneous monitoring. Pa_{CO_2} is lowered by increasing the minute ventilation by the following maneuvers: increase tidal volume (increase PIP or decrease PEEP) or increase rate (while decreasing ET). The Pa_{O_2} will be increased by either increasing the FI_{O_2} or increasing the mean airway pressure (increase PIP, increase PEEP, or prolong IT).

Any sudden deterioration in the infant's condition, including changes in oxygenation, ABGs, BP, or perfusion, should lead one to check the endotracheal tube immediately for its position and patency. The tip of the tube is properly placed when it can be palpated through the tracheal wall just at the sternal notch. If there is any doubt, the tube should be removed and the infant supported by bag and mask ventilation until a new tube is inserted.

Tension pneumothorax, *an emergency that must be treated at once,* is another common cause of sudden clinical deterioration occurring in up to ¼ of premature infants with RDS who are on respirators. It may be detected by clinical signs (loss of breath sounds and shift of the heart away from the affected side, positive transillumination) and by x-ray. The free air may be drained with a scalp vein needle and syringe until a chest tube can be inserted. The chest tube should be attached to water seal with 10 to 15 cm of continuous suction. Free air rises to the highest point in the hemithorax; thus it is important to position the chest tube with the tip lying anterior in the chest (and the infant supine).

As the infant's respiratory status improves, he can be weaned from intermittent mandatory ventilation (IMV) by lowering the FIO_2, inspiratory pressure, and rate (by prolonging the ET). Continuous-flow positive pressure ventilators permit the infant to breathe spontaneously against a PEEP while the ventilator rate is progressively slowed. This permits a gradual transition; after the IMV rate has been reduced to 10 breaths/min, the infant will usually tolerate extubation. The final steps involve extubation and support with nasal (or nasopharyngeal) CPAP, and then use of a hood to provide humidified O_2 or air. Some infants with very low birth weight may be weaned earlier if they are begun on aminophylline (loading dose of 8 mg/kg IV and maintenance of 1.5 mg/kg IV q 8 h, adjusted as needed to maintain a blood level of 7 to 14 μg/mL). The same dose of theophylline may be given orally or by gastric tube. Aminophylline and other xanthines are CNS-mediated respiratory stimulants that increase ventilatory efforts and may prevent apneic and bradycardic episodes that may interfere with successful weaning from the ventilation.

TRANSIENT TACHYPNEA OF THE NEWBORN (TTNB)
(Neonatal Wet Lung Syndrome)

Respiratory distress with rapid respirations and hypoxemia requiring O_2 supplementation, a condition caused by delayed resorption of fetal lung fluid.

Infants with TTNB are usually born at or close to term. They are likely to have been delivered by cesarean section and may have had perinatal distress. Rapid respirations, grunting, and retractions begin soon after delivery, and cyanosis may develop. Chest x-ray shows hyperinfiltrated lungs with heavy perihilar markings, giving the appearance of a shaggy heart border. Fluid is often present in the fissures. The lung periphery remains clear. The mechanism for resorption of fetal lung fluid is described under PERINATAL PHYSIOLOGY in Ch. 23.

Treatment involves giving O_2 by hood and monitoring blood gases by arterial sampling or by transcutaneous monitoring and pulse oximetry. Some infants may require support with CPAP and rarely may require IMV. TTNB may occur along with RDS in the more preterm infant. Recovery within 2 to 3 days is the rule.

APNEA OF PREMATURITY

Many infants of ≤ 34 wk gestation will have apneic spells, often beginning after the first 2 to 3 days. The incidence is highest at the lowest gestational ages. These infants often have periodic breathing (rapid respirations with brief pauses), which is attributed to immaturity of medullary respiratory center control. If the respiratory pauses last > 20 sec (apnea), they may be associated with hypoxemia and bradycardia, and active intervention to stimulate breathing may be required. Hypoxemia briefly stimulates respiratory efforts in the newborn but, after a few seconds, acts to suppress respirations.

Central apnea may occur and is due to a lack of sufficient neural impulses from the respiratory center in the medulla to the respiratory muscles; the infant is flaccid and makes no respiratory efforts. Other apneic spells are due to upper airways obstruction (obstructive apnea) in which apposition of the posterior pharyngeal wall with the tongue occludes the nasopharynx; the infant makes respiratory efforts but cannot inhale air into the lungs and becomes hypoxemic and bradycardic. Because chest wall movements are present, obstructive apnea will not be detected by an impedance type of apnea monitor. Thus, infants with low birth weight at risk for apnea should be on a heart rate monitor as well; they must be observed closely to detect color change and to confirm the presence of apnea or bradycardia.

Treatment

While it is common for well infants with low birth weight to have spells of "premature apnea," apnea is also a common sign of neonatal disorders (eg, hypoglycemia, sepsis, and intracranial hemorrhage). Therefore, it is important to evaluate each premature infant who develops apnea to avoid missing these underlying, treatable conditions.

The infant should lie with the head in the midline and the neck in the neutral position or slightly extended to prevent upper airways obstruction (obstructive apnea). Lowering the environmental temperature slightly (eg, to lower the skin temperature from 36.5° C [97.7° F] to 36.2° C [97.2° F]) may reduce the frequency of apnea in some infants. If apneic spells continue, especially if they are associated with cyanosis or bradycardia, the infant can be treated with aminophylline (for dosage, see under Treatment of RDS, above). If the infant is taking enteral feedings, theophylline may be given orally or via gastric tube at the same dose.

If apnea continues despite treatment with aminophylline or another xanthine, the infant may be treated with continuous positive airway pressure

(CPAP); it can be started by nasal prongs or nasopharyngeal tube at 5 cm H_2O pressure. Intractable apneic spells require ventilator support (see RESPIRATORY DISTRESS SYNDROME, above).

Aminophylline treatment is stopped after the infant has been apnea-free for about 7 days. The infant may be sent home after another 10 days if apnea does not recur after theophylline treatment has been discontinued. Most premature infants will stop having apneic spells by the time they reach about 37 wk gestational age. Those who continue to experience apnea or bradycardia, including those who have intracranial hemorrhage or periventricular leukomalacia, may be considered candidates for home monitoring to avoid sudden infant death syndrome. A 24-h pneumogram may help with this evaluation. After the parents are thoroughly taught (including CPR instruction and plans for ongoing evaluation and parental support), an infant at risk of life-threatening apnea at home is discharged on aminophylline and home monitoring.

PERSISTENT PULMONARY HYPERTENSION (PPH)
(Persistent Fetal Circulation)

A life-threatening disorder in which there is a return to the fetal condition with the pulmonary arterioles vasoconstricted and the effective pulmonary blood flow reduced to a fraction of normal. As in the fetus, in PPH blood is shunted from the right to the left circulatory system, either through the foramen ovale or through a persistent patent ductus arteriosus. (For a description of the perinatal circulation and the development of PPH, see PERINATAL PHYSIOLOGY in Ch. 23.) The right-to-left shunting leads to profound hypoxemia, even when the infant is breathing 100% O_2.

Etiology, Symptoms, and Signs

In many infants who have died with PPH, examination of lung pathology has shown abnormal muscular hypertrophy of the walls of the small pulmonary arterioles, possibly the result of chronic hypoxemia in utero. PPH occurs most commonly in term or post-term infants and in infants with fetal growth retardation secondary to placental insufficiency (eg, preeclampsia and maternal hypertension). Commonly, an episode of perinatal or postdelivery asphyxia seems to trigger the persistence or recurrence of pulmonary arteriolar constriction. If postmature, these infants are also very prone to meconium aspiration syndrome (see below). PPH has also been observed after treating the mother with large

doses of prostaglandin synthetase inhibitors (eg, aspirin or indomethacin); presumably these drugs may have produced constriction of the fetal ductus arteriosus in utero, leading to an abnormally increased pulmonary blood flow with a secondary "protective" hypertrophy of the pulmonary arteriolar walls. Congenital diaphragmatic hernia **(CDH)** is also often associated with muscular hypertrophy of the pulmonary arterioles in both lungs, also presumed secondary to an abnormally increased pulmonary blood flow in utero (the left lung is usually severely hypoplastic and most of the pulmonary blood flow must go through the right lung). PPH often complicates the course of infants with CDH, accounting for its high mortality rate.

Diagnosis

The diagnosis usually is based on history, physical findings, and x-ray and laboratory data. The infant with PPH will be near term or post term, and will remain hypoxemic even when breathing unassisted or being ventilated with 100% O_2. The lungs may be entirely clear on chest x-ray, but parenchymal lung disease (eg, meconium aspiration syndrome or neonatal pneumonia) or congenital diaphragmatic hernia may be present. Occasionally, it may be difficult to exclude the possibility of cyanotic congenital heart disease with right-to-left shunting. A cardiac assessment with echocardiogram will resolve most of these questions. In PPH the echocardiogram may show a prolonged right ventricular pre-ejection phase reflecting pulmonary hypertension. Occasionally, cardiac catheterization may be needed to rule out cyanotic congenital heart disease.

The increased pulmonary vascular resistance that leads to pulmonary hypertension and right-to-left shunting is worsened by hypoxemia and hypercarbia. Therefore, PPH should be suspected in any near-term infant with arterial hypoxemia; treatment should begin as quickly as possible to prevent progression of the pulmonary hypertension.

Treatment

Treatment primarily involves positive pressure ventilation of the infant with 100% O_2, since O_2 is the most potent pulmonary vasodilator. Alkalinization also helps to dilate the pulmonary arterioles. Alkalinization may be achieved by giving a slow IV infusion of sodium bicarbonate. The dosage is adjusted to keep the pH $\geq$ 7.5. Rapid bag and mask ventilation with 100% O_2 for 10 to 15 min may also be helpful because mechanical expansion of the alveoli also causes vasodilation.

Until recently, hyperventilation with a respirator was used to maintain a marked respiratory alkalosis. Now many believe that the high ventilator rates and pressures required to achieve this caused severe barotrauma that in turn led to lung injury and the death of some infants. Therefore, the goal of ventilation is to maintain blood gases near the normal range; the Pa_{O_2} as low as 40 mm Hg and the Pa_{CO_2} as high as 50 mm Hg may be acceptable.

The use of muscle paralysis (eg, pancuronium bromide 0.1 mg/kg IV repeated prn to prevent movements) may help to stabilize some infants, but it should be used selectively; paralyzed infants often need greater support from a respirator, which can lead to increased barotrauma.

Since some of these infants will have a large right-to-left shunt via a patent ductus arteriosus, the Pa_{O_2} may be significantly higher in the right radial artery than in the descending aorta; thus, it is advisable to obtain at least 1 ABG measurement from the right radial artery. Pulse oximeters simultaneously placed on the right hand and on a lower extremity will also detect a right-to-left shunt at the level of an existing ductus arteriosus.

Tolazoline, an α-adrenergic blocker, may be tried to see if it helps cause pulmonary vasodilation and hence improves oxygenation. Tolazoline is given in a loading dose of 1 to 2 mg/kg IV over 5 to 10 min, then 1 to 2 mg/kg/h IV. Since tolazoline may also induce systemic vasodilation and hypotension, it should be given by a route that will provide maximum delivery to the pulmonary circuit; in PPH with a right-to-left shunt at the atrial level, this is done by giving it into a vein in the upper part of the body (upper extremity or scalp vein) or directly into a catheter placed in the pulmonary artery. Systemic hypotension should be treated immediately because it will increase the right-to-left shunting. Initially, a volume expander can be used (eg, 5% human albumin 10 mL/kg over 10 min). If BP or perfusion remains decreased, the infant is treated with dopamine 2 to 20 μg/kg/min IV (*maximum dose 40 μg/kg/min; never given through an arterial line*) and/or dobutamine 2.5 to 20 μg/kg/min IV (*never given through an arterial line*). Tolazoline causes histamine release, and upper GI bleeding has been associated with its use; antacids may be given prophylactically.

Careful attention also must be paid to maintenance of fluid, electrolyte, glucose, and Ca homeostasis. Infants should be kept at the neutral thermal environment and treated with antibiotics for possible sepsis. Once Pa_{O_2} has been stabilized at $\geq$ 100 mm Hg, weaning is begun, first by reducing the FI_{O_2} in very small decrements of 2 to 3%. Later, FI_{O_2} and ventilator pressures can be reduced alternately. The goal is to avoid large changes, since a sudden drop in the Pa_{O_2} can lead to a recurrence of pulmonary vasoconstriction.

Despite medical management, a number of these infants cannot be oxygenated and will not survive. It has become feasible to maintain oxygenation (in these and other term infants with respiratory failure) with **extracorporeal membrane oxygenation (ECMO)** used from a few days up to 1 wk until the underlying pulmonary disease resolves to the point where they will survive. This technique requires transfer to neonatal intensive care centers in which ECMO therapy is available. *EMCO cannot be used for preterm infants because heparinized blood, which must be used, causes intraventricular hemorrhage in them.*

One cannula is surgically placed in the right common carotid artery and another in the right internal jugular vein, requiring sacrifice of both vessels. Blood is diverted from the jugular vein through the membrane oxygenator, which serves as an artificial lung to remove CO_2 and add O_2 to the blood. Oxygenated blood is then returned to the arterial system. On ECMO it is possible to maintain the Pa_{O_2} and Pa_{CO_2} at any desired levels even without respiratory efforts.

ECMO can save the lives of some larger neonates (eg, those with PPH, congenital diaphragmatic hernia, overwhelming pneumonia), and many survive without neurologic sequelae. However, there is still considerable controversy about the indications for instituting an invasive procedure with real risks (including the risk of transporting the critically sick neonate to an ECMO center). In the past, ECMO was intended for infants whose risk of mortality with medical management could be predicted to be at least 80%; recent improvements in medical management have led to uncertainty about when that criterion is met. Each ECMO center develops criteria for instituting this procedure in term infants with respiratory failure based on local experience regarding the prospects of survival with conventional management. To optimize patient selection, some infants will need to be transported to ECMO centers who in the final analysis will not require ECMO.

MECONIUM ASPIRATION SYNDROME (MAS)

Aspiration of meconium that has entered the amniotic sac, leading to a chemical pneumonitis and mechanical obstruction of bronchi. Complete bronchial obstruction results in atelectasis, while partial blockage leads to air-trapping on expiration, causing hyperinflation of the lungs and pulmonary air leaks (eg, pneumomediastinum or pneumothorax).

MAS occurs in the setting of fetal distress that may be associated with placental insufficiency (eg, in maternal preeclampsia, hypertension, or postmaturity). In response to stress, the fetus passes meconium stools and gasps forcefully, aspirating meconium mixed with amniotic fluid into the tracheobronchial tree. MAS is often most severe in post-term infants who have a reduced amniotic fluid volume, because the less dilute, thicker meconium is more likely to cause airways obstruction.

Diagnosis

The infant with MAS will have mild to extremely severe respiratory distress. Air-trapping caused by partial bronchial obstruction with meconium, or a secondary tension pneumothorax, may in turn cause an increased anteroposterior chest diameter, giving a barrel-chested appearance. The infant may appear dysmature or postmature, and there may be meconium staining of the umbilical cord and nails.

Chest x-rays show patchy atelectasis and intervening areas of emphysematous hyperinflation. Progressive air-trapping may lead to pulmonary interstitial emphysema or cysts, pneumomediastinum, or pneumothorax. Occasionally, fluid is seen in the major fissures or pleural spaces.

Treatment

Attempts to prevent MAS begin in the delivery room. The delivering physician should immediately aspirate the mouth and nasopharynx using a DeLee suction apparatus as soon as the infant's head is delivered. This is the most important step to prevent MAS.

Until recently it was believed that all infants should then be immediately intubated to allow suctioning of meconium from the trachea in deliveries in which there was meconium in the amniotic fluid. Newer recommendations are that intubation and tracheal suctioning need be done only in infants who are depressed at birth, but not for those who are vigorous. This point is still somewhat controversial.

In any case, skilled personnel should be immediately available to intubate and begin tracheal suctioning of at least all depressed infants when meconium is present. Suctioning is most effective if it is done before the infant breathes and cries, which distributes meconium through the pulmonary tree. A 3.5- or 4.0-mm endotracheal tube is first used to suction the trachea. Several types of meconium aspirators attach directly to the endotracheal tube, which then serves as the suction catheter. An 8 or 10 (French scale) suction catheter is then passed through the endotracheal tube to complete the aspiration of meconium from the tracheobronchial tree. Oral suctioning of the endotracheal tube is proscribed because of the possibility of HIV transmission to the resuscitator. After suctioning is completed, positive pressure ventilation is provided through the endotracheal tube. If no meconium has been obtained and if the infant appears vigorous, he may then be extubated. If significant MAS is suspected, the infant is admitted to the neonatal ICU.

After admission to the nursery, intermittent chest physiotherapy, suctioning, and administration of humidified air or O_2 may also help to loosen and remove meconium from the airway.

Respiratory support is provided according to the severity of the pneumonitis; it varies from supportive care and chest physiotherapy to providing supplemental O_2 by hood or positive pressure ventilation. Infants with MAS, especially those who are post term, are susceptible to developing persistent pulmonary hypertension **(PPH).** It is essential to anticipate this life-threatening complication and to initiate treatment for it at once (see PERSISTENT PULMONARY HYPERTENSION, above). If the infant's blood gases are only marginally satisfactory in an O_2 hood or are worsening over time, it may be safest to initiate positive pressure ventilation to avoid hypoxemia or hypercarbia, which may trigger the chain of events leading to PPH.

Infants with MAS trap air beyond bronchi that are partially blocked with aspirated meconium. During the first few days they are prone to develop air-leak syndrome (pneumomediastinum and pneumothorax). Regular evaluations by auscultation of breath sounds, transillumination of the chest, and chest x-rays are important to detect these complications. Evaluation and treatment for tension pneumothorax or for an endotracheal tube plugged by meconium should be instituted at once if the infant's BP, perfusion, or ABG values suddenly worsen (see PULMONARY AIR-BLOCK SYNDROME, below).

Since meconium may enhance bacterial growth and it is difficult to rule out bacterial pneumonia on x-ray, it is customary to obtain cultures of blood and tracheal aspirate and to begin antibiotics (ampicillin and an aminoglycoside).

ASPIRATION OF OTHER SUBSTANCES

During delivery infants may also aspirate vernix caseosa, amniotic fluid, and maternal or fetal blood. They will have respiratory distress and signs of aspiration pneumonia on chest x-ray. As in meconium aspiration, treatment is supportive; if bacterial infection is suspected, cultures are taken and antibiotics are begun.

PULMONARY AIR–BLOCK SYNDROME

(Pulmonary Interstitial Emphysema [PIE];
Pneumomediastinum; Pneumothorax;
Pneumopericardium)

Dissection of air (air leaks) out of the normal pulmonary air spaces.

Air leak has been described following delivery in 1 to 2% of normal infants, probably as a result of the large negative intrathoracic forces created by the first breaths of air. Many of these infants are asymptomatic or have only tachypnea.

However, pulmonary air leaks usually occur in infants with serious lung diseases (eg, RDS or MAS—see above) who are predisposed because of poor lung compliance and the need for high distending pressures (eg, an infant with RDS on a respirator) or because of increased airways resistance (eg, meconium partially obstructing bronchi in MAS).

Pulmonary Interstitial Emphysema (PIE)

PIE occurs if *air dissects from the alveoli into the pulmonary interstitium, lymphatics, or subpleural space.* This often occurs in infants with poor lung compliance who are being treated with positive pressure ventilation, but it may occur spontaneously. The location of PIE is highly variable: It may involve one or both lungs and may be focal or generalized within each lung. The infant's respiratory status may worsen (raised $Paco_2$, lowered pH, lowered Pao_2) if there is diffuse dissection of air, as lung compliance is suddenly reduced.

Chest x-ray shows several or many cystic or linear lucencies in the lung fields that are too large or too peripheral to represent bronchi. Some lucencies are elongated; others appear as enlarged subpleural cysts and may be several centimeters in diameter.

The course of PIE is highly variable. It may resolve dramatically over 1 or 2 days or persist on x-ray for weeks or months. Some infants with severe respiratory disease will develop bronchopulmonary dysplasia (BPD)—see below, and the cystic changes of PIE then merge into the x-ray picture of BPD.

Treatment: The goal is to lower the ventilator inspiratory pressure as much as possible to allow the lung to heal. It is reasonable to achieve adequate oxygenation in the presence of PIE by increasing the Fio_2 while lowering the inspiratory pressure as much as possible, but this may be difficult or impossible if the lungs with diffuse PIE become very noncompliant.

If PIE is very severe in one lung and mild or absent in the other lung, differential bronchial intubation may be attempted. An endotracheal tube is advanced into the mainstem bronchus on the normal or less involved side; this may be facilitated by advancing the endotracheal tube while turning the head and neck to the side opposite the bronchus to be intubated. If lung auscultation is done during this maneuver, breath sounds will be lost over the lung with PIE when differential bronchial intubation has been achieved. Position is confirmed on x-ray, which will soon show total atelectasis of the lung with PIE. Since only one lung is now being ventilated, ventilator settings and Fio_2 may need to be increased at once. After 24 to 48 h, the endotracheal tube is pulled back into the trachea, in hopes that the PIE has resolved. There has been some success in treating severe PIE and other chronic forms of pulmonary air leak with high-frequency ventilators, which can provide ventilation without high peak inspiratory pressures, thus allowing the air leaks to heal.

Pneumomediastinum (PM)

PM results if *pulmonary interstitial emphysema dissects into the loose connective tissue of the mediastinum.* Usually, the infant will not develop additional signs of respiratory distress, but the chest may transilluminate positively and, on x-ray, air in the mediastinum will be seen lifting the lobes of the thymus away from the cardiac silhouette. This may best be seen on a lateral x-ray. Air may dissect further into the subcutaneous tissues of the neck and scalp; subcutaneous air is also asymptomatic and will resolve spontaneously.

Specific treatment is not needed. However, since PM indicates that an air leak has occurred, it may be advantageous to try to lower ventilator pressures, as PM may progress to pneumothorax.

Pneumothorax

Pneumothorax develops *when air dissects into the pleural space from a pneumomediastinum or from the rupture of a subpleural bleb (as in PIE).* Although sometimes asymptomatic, pneumothorax is often life-threatening, especially in an infant with severe parenchymal lung disease (eg, RDS, MAS) on positive pressure ventilation.

Clinical signs of a **tension pneumothorax** may include a sudden increase or more commonly a fall in BP, poor skin perfusion, poor pulses, and reduced or absent breath sounds on the affected side. Heart sounds may be muffled if the pneumothorax is on the left side. Positive transillumination with a fiberoptic light source strongly suggests that there is free air in the thorax. If the infant's condition permits before treatment is initiated, a chest x-ray will confirm the diagnosis.

Treatment: Immediate evacuation of a pneumothorax is required in the infant with lung disease or on positive pressure ventilation. In an emergency, a scalp vein needle and syringe can be used temporarily to evacuate free air. Definitive treatment is by insertion of a 5 or 8 French chest tube. Chest tubes should be inserted with a curved hemostat after a small incision is made in the skin. (NOTE: Insertion of a chest tube with a trocar is more likely to result in lung laceration.) The tube should be positioned with the tip anterior in the chest, since free air will collect in the most superior space (anterior when the infant is supine). The chest tube should be connected to a water trap at 10 to 15 cm of negative H_2O pressure suction. Follow-up auscultation, transillumination, and x-ray will confirm that the tube is functioning properly.

In an infant free of underlying lung disease, a pneumothorax may produce only mild tachypnea or may even be asymptomatic. In this situation, one can simply wait for spontaneous resolution while closely observing the infant.

Other Air Leaks

In an infant on positive pressure ventilation, air may dissect into the pericardial sac and cause pneumopericardium, resulting in **cardiac tamponade** with reduced cardiac output and BP. X-ray will show air surrounding the heart within the pericardial sac. Rapid evacuation of the air using a scalp vein needle, followed by surgical insertion of a pericardial tube, may be lifesaving.

Occasionally a pulmonary air leak may result in free air dissecting retroperitoneally and then into the peritoneal cavity, producing a **pneumoperitoneum.** This will resolve spontaneously, but it needs to be distinguished from pneumoperitoneum due to a ruptured abdominal viscus, which is a surgical emergency.

BRONCHOPULMONARY DYSPLASIA (BPD)

A chronic lung disorder in infants who have been treated for respiratory distress with intermittent mandatory ventilation. At 28 days of age, they will have respiratory distress, characteristic x-ray changes, and an ongoing need for O_2.

Etiology

Lung injury may be associated with barotrauma from positive pressure ventilation, high inspired O_2 concentrations, and endotracheal intubation; it is more common among infants of low gestational age. It is often a sequela of RDS and its treatment and is more likely to develop during the occurrence of pulmonary interstitial emphysema (see PULMONARY AIR-BLOCK SYNDROME, above). The transition from RDS to BPD is gradual; often the infant simply fails to wean from O_2 and intermittent mandatory ventilation (**IMV**) at the age of 5 to 6 days (when RDS should have resolved).

Since BPD is at least in part caused by ventilator use, it is important to wean infants from ventilator support as soon as possible. In an infant with RDS who fails to wean from IMV at an appropriate time, possible underlying problems (eg, patent ductus arteriosus and nursery-acquired pneumonia) should be sought and treated if present. Early use of aminophylline as a respiratory stimulant may rapidly help to wean preterm infants from IMV.

Symptoms and Signs

In the early stages of BPD there is inflammation and exudate. The alveolar epithelium may slough, and macrophages may be found in the tracheal aspirate. At this time the chest x-ray may show only a diffuse haziness of the lung fields. Later, scarring and breakdown of alveolar walls occur. Alternating areas of emphysema with hyperaeration and pulmonary scarring and atelectasis lead to a "hobnail appearance" pathologically and to a multicystic appearance with many coarse streaks and hyperinflation on chest x-ray. Pathologically, there is also muscular hypertrophy of the peribronchial and arteriolar smooth muscle and squamous metaplasia of the bronchial epithelium.

Prognosis and Treatment

BPD may require weeks or months of additional ventilator support and/or supplemental O_2. Ventilator pressures and FIO_2 should be reduced as tolerated, but the infant should not be allowed to become hypoxemic, because low PaO_2 will cause pulmonary vascular constriction and may result in pulmonary hypertension, cor pulmonale, and right heart failure. Pulmonary hypertension can be evaluated by echocardiography and will be manifested by a prolonged right ventricular pre-ejection time. Arterial oxygenation may be continuously monitored with a pulse oximeter and should be maintained at or above 90% saturation.

Infants with chronic lung disease may have a compensated respiratory acidosis while breathing spontaneously. It is therefore appropriate to let the PCO_2 rise above normal while weaning from the ventilator as long as the pH remains normal (pH > 7.30) and the infant's respiratory distress is not too great.

Good nutrition is essential in these chronically ill infants, who often have increased caloric needs because of the increased work of breathing. Depending on the infant's condition, nutrition may be provided by IV alimentation or by nasoduodenal or orogastric tube feedings. Infants with BPD may be very susceptible to developing pulmonary congestion or edema if challenged with excessive fluids. It is often necessary to restrict the daily fluid intake to 100 to 120 mL/kg/day; this may present a challenge to provide adequate calories (eg, by adding glucose polymers or medium chain triglyceride oil to supplement enteral feedings).

Chronic diuretic therapy is customarily used to treat these infants, because of their tendency to develop pulmonary congestion with decreased lung compliance. Furosemide (1 mg/kg given IV or IM, or 2 mg/kg given orally) once daily to tid may be used for short periods, but prolonged use causes hypercalciuria with resultant osteoporosis, fractures, and renal stones. Chronic diuretic therapy can be more safely provided with the combination of chlorothiazide 10 to 20 mg/kg/day and spironolactone 1 to 2 mg/kg/day both given orally bid. The state of hydration and serum electrolytes should be closely monitored.

After the infant with BPD is weaned from a ventilator, supplemental O_2 may be required for an additional period of several weeks. O_2 may be given by nasal cannula with gradual reduction in the percentage of O_2 or the O_2 flow rate. Oxygenation can be monitored with a pulse oximeter.

The parents will require a great deal of emotional support because the course of resolution of BPD may be both slow and unpredictable, and some infants may die even after many months of care. Surviving infants' respiratory distress gradually resolves, although reduced lung compliance and increased airways resistance may persist for several years. These infants are at increased risk of lower respiratory tract infections, especially viral infections, in the first years, and may quickly develop respiratory decompensation if pulmonary infection supervenes. The infant will likely require rehospitalization if signs of a respiratory infection develop or there is increased respiratory distress.

BIRTH TRAUMA

The incidence of neonatal injury from a difficult or traumatic delivery is decreasing. Improved prenatal diagnosis and monitoring during labor have helped to prevent neurologic injury. In addition, cesarean section, which presents fewer risks to the mother than previously, often replaces attempts at difficult versions, vacuum extractions, or mid- or high-forceps deliveries.

A traumatic delivery is anticipated when the mother has small pelvic measurements, when the infant seems large for gestational age (often the case with diabetic mothers), or when there is a breech or other abnormal presentation, especially in a primipara. In such situations, both the labor and the fetal condition should be monitored closely. If fetal distress is detected, the mother should be positioned on her side and given O_2. If fetal distress persists, an immediate cesarean section should be performed.

INJURIES TO THE CENTRAL AND PERIPHERAL NERVOUS SYSTEMS

(See also CEREBRAL PALSY SYNDROMES in Ch. 43)

The mechanics of labor and delivery are such that physical injury to the infant can easily occur. The strength of these forces is apparent from the head molding that follows vertex deliveries, but even severe molding usually does not cause problems or require treatment.

Head trauma varies in degrees: **Caput succedaneum,** *edema of the presenting portion of the scalp,* results from mild trauma as this area is forced against the uterine cervix. **Subgaleal hemorrhage** results from greater trauma and is characterized by a boggy feeling over the entire scalp, including the temporal regions. **Cephalhematoma,** or hemorrhage beneath the periosteum, can be differentiated from more superficial bleeding because it is sharply limited to the area overlying a single bone, the periosteum being adherent at the sutures. Cephalhematomas are commonly unilateral and parietal. A small percentage have an associated **linear fracture** in the bone underlying them. Cephalhematomas do not require treatment, but anemia or hyperbilirubinemia may rarely result from the volume of subperiosteal bleeding. **Depressed skull fractures** are uncommon. Most result from forceps pressure; rarely, they are caused by resting of the head against a bony prominence in utero. They can be seen and felt as depressions and must be differentiated from the depressions secondary to an elevated periosteal rim seen with cephalhematomas. X-rays will confirm the diagnosis. Depressed fractures may require neurosurgical elevation. Depressed skull fractures or other head trauma may be associated with subdural bleeding, subarachnoid hemorrhage, or even contusion or laceration of the brain itself (see INTRACRANIAL HEMORRHAGE, below).

Trauma to cranial nerves primarily involves the **facial nerve.** Involvement of other cranial nerves is uncommon and not usually due to birth injuries. Although frequently attributed to forceps pressure, most such injuries probably occur from pressure on the nerve in utero. This may be due to fetal positioning (eg, from the lying of the head against the shoulder) or to pressure against the nerve by the sacral promontory or a uterine fibroid.

Facial nerve injury is usually peripheral, and the face appears asymmetric. In complete peripheral 7th nerve injuries, movement of facial muscles on the entire involved side is absent. Injury also occurs in individual branches of the 7th nerve, most often the mandibular. Intrauterine pressure on the mandible can also lead to facial asymmetry, but the muscle innervation is intact. Comparison of the maxillary and mandibular occlusal surfaces, which should be parallel, differentiates this from a true 7th nerve injury. No test or treatment is needed for peripheral facial nerve injuries, which usually resolve by age 2 to 3 mo.

Injuries to nerve roots and peripheral nerves may result from difficult deliveries and are usually seen in the upper extremities. **Brachial plexus injuries** follow stretching caused by shoulder dystocia, breech extraction, or hyperabduction of the neck in cephalic presentations. The injury can be due to simple stretching, hemorrhage within a nerve, tearing of the nerve or root, or avulsion of the roots with associated cervical cord injury. Associated traumatic injuries (eg, fractures of the clavicle or humerus or subluxations of the shoulder or cervical spine) may occur.

The site and type of nerve root injury determine the prognosis. Injuries of the upper brachial plexus (C5, 6) affect muscles about the shoulder and elbow, while lesions of the lower plexus (C7, 8; and T1) primarily affect muscles of the forearm and hand. **Erb's palsy** is an upper brachial plexus injury causing adduction and internal rotation of the shoulder with pronation of the forearm; ipsilateral paralysis of the diaphragm is common. Treatment includes protecting the arm through immobilization across the upper abdomen and preventing contractures by daily passive gentle range of motion exercises to involved joints starting at 1 wk of age. **Klumpke's palsy** is a lower plexus injury resulting in paralysis of the hand and wrist, often with ipsilateral Horner's syndrome (miosis, ptosis, anhidrosis). Passive range of motion is the only treatment indicated. Neither of these brachial plexus injuries is usually associated with demonstrable sensory loss. Improvement in both is usually rapid. If a significant deficit persists > 3 mo, surgical exploration and repair should be considered.

When the entire brachial plexus is injured, there is no movement of the involved upper extremity, and sensory loss is often present. Ipsilateral pyramidal signs indicate associated spinal cord trauma. Passive range of motion is used to prevent contractures, and surgical exploration should be considered. The prognosis for recovery is poor. Subsequent growth of the involved extremity may be impaired.

Injuries to other peripheral nerves (eg, the radial, sciatic, and obturator) are rare in the newborn and are not ordinarily related to the birth process. They are usually secondary to a local traumatic event (eg, an injection in or near the sciatic nerve or fat necrosis over the radial nerve). The muscles antagonistic to those paralyzed should be placed at rest until recovery occurs. In most peripheral nerve injuries recovery is complete. Neurosurgical exploration of the nerve is seldom indicated.

Trauma to the spinal cord is rare. It is usually seen in breech deliveries and follows excessive longitudinal traction to the spine. Sometimes a click or snap is heard at delivery. It can also follow hyperextension of the fetal neck in utero (the "flying fetus"). The trauma usually occurs in the lower cervical region (C5, 6, 7), since higher lesions generally are fatal. The injury may consist of varying degrees of spinal cord disruption, often with hemorrhage. Initially there is spinal shock with flaccidity below the level of injury. Spasticity develops within days or weeks. Breathing is diaphragmatic, since the phrenic nerve arises higher (C3, 4, 5). There is paralysis of intercostal and abdominal muscles, and voluntary control of rectal and bladder sphincters cannot develop. Sensation and sweating are lost below the involved level and can result in fluctuations of body temperature with environmental changes. The CSF usually is bloody. X-rays of the neck are normal. An MRI, CT, or myelogram of the cervical cord may demonstrate the lesion and will exclude surgically treatable lesions. The usual causes of death are progressive loss of renal function (making evaluation of the urinary tract essential) and recurring pneumonia. Some infants survive for many years. Treatment of spinal cord injury consists of nursing care to prevent skin ulcerations, prompt treatment of urinary and respiratory infections, and regular evaluations to identify obstructive uropathy early.

INTRACRANIAL HEMORRHAGE

Hemorrhage in or around the brain is a major problem in the newborn infant, especially when premature. Hypoxia, pressures exerted on the infant's head during labor, and the presence of the germinal matrix in premature infants are 3 major reasons. Small hemorrhages frequently are found at autopsy in the subarachnoid space, falx, and tentorium. Larger hemorrhages are less common but usually more serious. About 40% of premature infants < 1500 gm have intracranial hemorrhage. Cranial ultrasound (US) and CT studies can detect blood and are useful in diagnosis. Hemorrhage can occur into several spaces related to the CNS. Bleeding into the subarachnoid space probably is the most common in full-term infants and may account for the RBCs so often seen in the newborn's CSF. The diagnosis, made by CSF examination and CT scan, should be suspected in any infant with apnea, seizures, lethargy, or an abnormal neurologic examination. The associated meningeal inflammation may lead to a communicating hydrocephalus as the baby grows. Bleeding into the subdural space, which occurs less often as obstetric techniques have improved, results from tears in the falx, the tentorium, or the bridging veins. Such tears are most common in infants of primiparas, in large infants, or after difficult deliveries. All these conditions can produce unusual pressures on the skull. The presenting finding may be seizures, a rapidly enlarging head, an abnormal neurologic examination with hypotonia, a poor Moro reflex, retinal hemorrhages, or a positive transillumination of the skull.

Hemorrhages within the ventricles or parenchyma are the most serious type of intracranial bleeding. They occur in about 40% of premature infants, generally during the first 3 days of life. Most are asymptomatic, but there can be apnea, cyanosis, or even a sudden collapse. Hemorrhage in premature infants is frequently bilateral and usually arises in the germinal matrix (a mass of embryonic cells lying over the caudate nucleus, and present only in the fetus) on the lateral wall of the lateral ventricles. Most bleeding episodes are subependymal or have a small amount of blood in the ventricles. In severe ones, there may be casts of the ventricular system and large amounts of blood in the cisterna magna and basal cisterns. Hypoxia, particularly in premature infants, often precedes intraventricular and subarachnoid bleeding. Hypoxia damages the capillary endothelium, impairs cranial vascular autoregulation, and increases cerebral blood flow and venous pressure, all of which make hemorrhage more likely.

Suspected intracranial hemorrhage requires careful evaluation for skin petechiae or hemorrhage from other sites, signs that suggest a systemic hematologic or vascular disorder (eg, vitamin K deficiency, hemophilia, or disseminated intravascular coagulation).

Laboratory evaluation of an infant with suspected intracranial hemorrhage should begin with a lumbar puncture. The CSF should be examined for RBCs and usually contains gross blood. A CBC (especially Hct and platelet count) and metabolic studies to identify other causes of neurologic dysfunction (hypoglycemia, hypocalcemia, electrolyte imbalance) should be done. Clotting studies may also be needed. Cranial US or CT scan can readily identify blood within the ventricles or brain substance, but thin layers of subarachnoid or subdural blood lying over the hemispheres may be missed. An EEG may help establish the prognosis if the infant survives the acute bleeding episode.

Treatment of most intracranial hemorrhages is supportive unless a hematologic abnormality has contributed to the bleeding. The infant should receive vitamin K if it was not previously given. Platelets should be given if they are deficient. Subdural hematomas should be treated with daily bilateral subdural taps if the infant is symptomatic or the head is enlarging rapidly. *Only 10 to 15 mL of subdural fluid should be removed from each side at one time, as removing larger amounts may precipitate shock.* If symptoms persist after 2 wk of daily drainage, then a subdural shunting procedure should be considered.

The prognosis for infants with large intraventricular hemorrhages is poor, especially if the hemorrhage extends into the parenchyma. Most infants with smaller hemorrhages survive the acute bleeding episode and do well. A few may be left with variable degrees of neurologic deficit. The prognosis is much better if the hemorrhage is subarachnoid. The outlook for infants with subdural hematomas is guarded, but some infants do well.

FRACTURES

Midclavicular fracture, the most common fracture during birth, usually occurs with shoulder dystocia or when the obstetrician must fracture the clavicle to facilitate a difficult breech delivery. The infant is first noted to be irritable and does not move the arm on the involved side either spontaneously or when the Moro reflex is elicited. Most clavicular fractures are greenstick and heal rapidly and uneventfully. A large callus forms at the fracture site within a week, and remodeling is completed within a month. The major significance of clavicular fractures is their association with brachial plexus injury and with pneumothorax from perforation of the apical pleura.

The humerus and the femur may be fractured in difficult deliveries. Most of these are greenstick, mid-shaft fractures, and excellent remodeling of the bone usually follows, even if there is an initial moderate degree of angulation. A long bone may be fractured through its epiphysis, but even here the prognosis for newborns is excellent.

SOFT TISSUE INJURIES

Any soft tissues are susceptible to injury with subsequent edema and hemorrhage if they have been the presenting part or the fulcrum for the forces of uterine contraction. Edema and ecchymosis of the periorbital and facial tissues commonly occur in face presentations, while the scrotum or labia are traumatized during breech deliveries. Breakdown of blood within the tissues and conversion of heme to bilirubin result whenever a hematoma develops in any injury. This added burden of bilirubin in borderline cases may produce sufficient neonatal jaundice to require exchange transfusion (see HYPERBILIRUBINEMIA under METABOLIC PROBLEMS IN THE NEWBORN, below). No other treatment is needed.

HEMATOLOGIC PROBLEMS

To evaluate anemias in the newborn during the first week of life, blood should be obtained by venipuncture or from a central catheter; Hcts obtained by heel prick may be as much as 15% higher owing to sludging of blood in skin capillaries.

ACUTE BLOOD–LOSS ANEMIA

Massive perinatal blood loss may result from abnormal placental separation (abruptio placentae) or placenta previa; from a traumatic tear of the umbilical cord or of a torn vessel if there is velamentous insertion of the cord into the placenta; or from incision into an anterior-lying placenta during cesarean section delivery. If the umbilical cord is wrapped tightly around the infant's neck or body, arterial blood from the infant may be pumped into the placenta, while compression of the cord prevents blood from returning via the umbilical vein to the infant; clamping the cord immediately upon or during delivery may then result in significant acute occult blood loss (into the placenta).

In such cases, shock and severe asphyxia may occur before delivery or at birth. The infant is hypotensive and extremely pale, has weak or absent pulses, makes poor respiratory efforts, and does not respond well to CPR. A normal Hct at birth does not rule out acute massive blood loss, because it may not have had time to equilibrate downward.

Acute blood loss with hypovolemic shock should be corrected by immediate transfusion of whole blood via an umbilical vein catheter; 15 mL/kg over 5 to 10 min are given, followed by repeated aliquots until adequate circulation is restored. If blood is not immediately available, circulation may be supported initially by infusing the same volume of colloid (5% human albumin or fresh frozen plasma). If shock persists, repeated infusions of blood or colloid should be given. Central venous pressure may be monitored via an umbilical vein catheter (after the catheter tip is confirmed on x-ray as being above the diaphragm) to help determine when the blood deficit has been replaced.

A **twin-to-twin transfusion** may occur in identical twins who have an anastomotic vessel between their portions of a shared placenta. A chronic transfusion from one twin into the other results. The donor is usually small for gestational age and anemic; the recipient is significantly larger and plethoric. The donor may need an exchange transfusion or a simple transfusion to raise the Hct rapidly to a safe level, while the recipient, who may suffer from polycythemia (see below), may require partial exchange transfusion with plasma to lower the Hct to a safe level ($< 65\%$).

HEMOLYTIC ANEMIAS OF THE NEWBORN
(See also ERYTHROBLASTOSIS FETALIS in Ch. 15)

RHESUS (RH) INCOMPATIBILITY

Rh incompatibility may occur when an Rh-negative woman carries an Rh-positive fetus. Isoimmunization of the mother occurs after some (incompatible) fetal RBCs cross the placenta and induce an immunologic response of maternal antibodies **(Abs)** that subsequently cross the placenta into the fetus and lead to hemolysis. The severity of the hemolytic process can be evaluated by doing sequential amniocenteses to measure the amount of bilirubin present in the amniotic fluid (see TABLE 15–1). These bilirubin levels are measured as the optical density at 450 nm (OD 450) and are corrected for gestational age.

The first immunization may occur with a miscarriage or in a pregnancy with an Rh-positive fetus. The severity of isoimmunization usually increases in subsequent pregnancies, and each subsequent infant is more likely to be affected. Rh incompatibility usually indicates that Ab to group D RBC surface antigen is present, although C and E factor incompatibilities of the Rh system may also occur. Rh isoimmunization can usually be prevented by proper administration of Rh₀(D) immune globulin to the unsensitized Rh-negative woman at 28 wk gestation and again following delivery or at the time of amniocentesis or miscarriage. Rh-negative immune globulin does not have to be given if the father is also known with certainty to be Rh-negative, as the fetus will also have Rh-negative antigen on its RBCs. (See also ERYTHROBLASTOSIS FETALIS in Ch. 15.)

Symptoms and Signs

The most severely affected fetuses develop profound anemia in utero with intrauterine fetal death or are delivered with **hydrops fetalis**, which may be diagnosed before delivery on fetal ultrasound **(US)** examination, which shows scalp edema, cardiomegaly, hepatomegaly, pleural effusions, and ascites. Polyhydramnios may also be present. These newborns are extremely pale and may have severe generalized edema, including pleural effusions and ascites. The liver and spleen are enlarged because of extramedullary hematopoiesis. Heart failure may occur. Because of anemia and prematurity, asphyxia is more likely during labor and delivery, and cesarean section is indicated. Prematurity and asphyxia, along with hypoproteinemia, predispose these infants to respiratory distress syndrome **(RDS)**, the signs of which may be difficult to distinguish from those of heart failure. Less severely affected neonates may be anemic but do not have edema or other signs of hydrops; mildly affected infants may have little or no anemia at birth. Affected infants usually develop severe hyperbilirubinemia soon after delivery because of the continuing hemolytic effect of Rh Abs that have crossed the placenta; kernicterus may develop if this is not treated (see HYPERBILIRUBINEMIA, below).

Treatment

Severely affected immature fetuses may be treated with intraperitoneal transfusion of type O Rh-negative RBCs, which should first be irradiated to kill lymphocytes that might otherwise cause graft-vs.-host disease. It is possible to sample fetal blood (for analysis of Hct, blood type, and direct Coombs' test) and to give transfusions of packed RBCs to the severely affected fetus by means of a needle inserted into an umbilical vessel near the placental insertion of the umbilical cord. This procedure is done with US guidance at a perinatal center.

A newborn infant with hydrops fetalis or severe erythroblastosis fetalis without hydrops is critically ill and should be delivered at a perinatal intensive care facility. Fetal heart rate should be monitored during labor; if signs of fetal distress occur or if the infant is severely affected, cesarean delivery is indicated.

The mainstay of treatment is exchange transfusion using Rh-negative RBCs. An exchange transfusion using twice the infant's calculated blood volume (a 2-volume transfusion) removes 85% of the infant's blood, including circulating Abs, sensitized RBCs, and accumulated bilirubin.

In hydrops fetalis, profound anemia should be treated at once by doing a partial (1-volume) exchange transfusion using packed Rh-negative RBCs (Hct 70%). After the infant's condition stabilizes, a 2-volume exchange transfusion should be done with Rh-negative blood. In addition, digoxin and diuretics for heart failure, alkali therapy for metabolic acidosis, and respiratory support for RDS may be required.

When an Rh-negative, sensitized woman delivers, the cord blood should be examined immediately to determine the infant's blood type, and the direct Coombs' test should be done. If the infant is Rh-positive and the direct Coombs' test is positive, the infant's Hct and reticulocyte count should be determined, and a blood smear should be obtained to check for reticulocytes and nucleated RBCs. The bilirubin level in cord blood should be determined also. A cord-blood Hct < 40% and a cord-blood bilirubin > 5 mg/dL are indicators of severe hemolysis.

Laboratory and clinical evaluations of some infants suggest such a severe rate of hemolysis that exchange transfusion will almost certainly be required in the future. If the infant's condition is stable, an early exchange transfusion will remove sensitized RBCs and Abs before hemolysis produces large amounts of bilirubin and may avert the need for multiple exchange transfusions at a later time. **Criteria suggesting the need for an early, but not emergency, exchange transfusion include** a Hct < 40%, reticulocytes > 15%, and a bilirubin concentration > 5 mg/dL at birth; the most useful information

is obtained by observing the rate at which serum bilirubin rises over several hours. If the level rises ≥ 1 mg/dL/h, the infant will likely come to need exchange transfusion, although treatment with phototherapy may slow the rise in bilirubin and may avoid the need for exchange transfusion in some infants.

If an exchange transfusion is not indicated immediately, the infant can be followed by clinical evaluation and by serial determinations of both serum bilirubin and Hct. If bilirubin levels become dangerously elevated (see hyperbilirubinemia under PREMATURE INFANT, above, and under METABOLIC PROBLEMS IN THE NEWBORN, below) or significant anemia develops, exchange transfusion is indicated.

Many affected Rh-positive infants will not require an exchange transfusion in the newborn period; however, the Hct must be followed serially *for several months,* as severe anemia may develop because of slow, ongoing hemolysis. Such infants will require a simple transfusion with packed type-specific Rh-negative RBCs.

ABO BLOOD GROUP INCOMPATIBILITY

In almost all cases of ABO incompatibility, the mother's blood type is O and the infant's is either A or B. (See also ERYTHROBLASTOSIS FETALIS in Ch. 15.) Anti-A sensitization is more common, but anti-B sensitization is likely to produce more severe hemolytic disease when it occurs. Although the infant may develop anemia in utero, it is almost never severe enough to cause hydrops fetalis or intrauterine death. The major clinical problem is the development of significant hyperbilirubinemia following birth.

The required laboratory studies are similar to those for Rh disease. The direct Coombs' test is usually weakly positive but may occasionally be negative; this does not rule out ABO incompatibility if other diagnostic criteria are met. Usually anti-A or anti-B Abs can be found in the infant's serum (positive indirect Coombs' test) or following Ab elution from the infant's RBCs. Also, numerous microspherocytes in the infant's blood and reticulocytosis suggest ABO incompatibility. Principles of surveillance and treatment of these infants are identical to those for Rh incompatibility.

RARE BLOOD GROUP INCOMPATIBILITIES

Many rare blood group incompatibilities have been documented (eg, Kell, Duffy). Although infrequent, they may be severe; and because hemolysis is involved, they produce anemia and hyperbilirubinemia, as does Rh or ABO incompatibility. Treatment is similar to that for Rh incompatibility; blood used for exchange transfusion must lack the sensitizing antigen. Since diagnosis of these incompatibilities may take a considerable amount of time, many advise routine screening of the mother's blood for rare or atypical antibodies during pregnancy.

ANEMIA DUE TO CONGENITAL SPHEROCYTOSIS

(See also ANEMIAS DUE TO ALTERATIONS OF RED CELL MEMBRANE in Ch. 35)

Hemolysis in infants born with congenital spherocytosis often causes significant hyperbilirubinemia. Anemia may develop as well. Significant splenomegaly usually does not occur in neonates. Spherocytes are seen on the blood smear, and the RBCs have increased osmotic fragility. This disorder may be inherited as a dominant trait, so a family history of one parent with hemolytic anemia or splenectomy may help in making the diagnosis. However, in many cases the family history is negative for spherocytosis. Early hyperbilirubinemia, if severe, is treated by exchange transfusion. Splenectomy may be required at a later age to control chronic hemolytic anemia.

NONSPHEROCYTIC HEMOLYTIC ANEMIAS

Occasionally neonates develop hemolytic anemia secondary to RBC enzymatic defects, such as pyruvate kinase deficiency or G6PD deficiency (see ANEMIAS DUE TO ALTERATIONS OF RED CELL MEMBRANE in Ch. 35). If a Heinz body preparation is positive in an infant with hemolytic anemia, these disorders are suspected and specific tests for enzyme activity can be done. A definitive diagnosis in the neonate may be difficult. The course of the hemolytic anemia should be observed over time; if the hemolytic process continues, amounts of blood large enough to diagnose specific RBC enzymatic defects will be easier to obtain when the infant is older.

HEMOLYTIC ANEMIA DUE TO INFECTIONS

Hemolysis is found in many congenital infections (eg, toxoplasmosis, rubella, cytomegalovirus disease, herpes simplex, and syphilis) and in infections due to hemolytic bacteria (eg, Escherichia coli or β-hemolytic streptococci). Jaundice, which is often present also, should suggest the possibility of an infectious process, particu-

larly if the direct serum bilirubin is elevated (> 1.5 mg/dL).

HEMOGLOBINOPATHIES

(See also ANEMIAS DUE TO DEFECTIVE HEMOGLOBIN SYNTHESIS in Ch. 35)

Most clinical hemoglobinopathies involve abnormalities of the β-chain of Hb (sickle cell disease, β-thalassemia). Since the newborn has a large amount of fetal Hb (α-2, γ-2), these disorders are not clinically evident at birth, but most are gradually manifested later, in the first 6 mo of life. However, the rare disorder α-thalassemia results in hydrops fetalis with either fetal or early neonatal death due to profound intractable anemia. Micromethods available to screen for various hemoglobinopathies in the newborn are done routinely in many states as part of screening for metabolic disorders.

POLYCYTHEMIA AND HYPERVISCOSITY

Increased viscosity due to a high Hct (usually 70% or more), which may result in stasis of blood within vessels, pulmonary congestion, cardiomegaly, and, possibly, vascular thrombosis. The affected newborn may appear plethoric or can present with neurologic signs (eg, seizures, lethargy, poor feeding) or with cardiorespiratory distress (eg, tachypnea, tachycardia, cyanosis). Symptomatic newborns with a central venous Hct > 65% should receive a partial exchange transfusion in which aliquots of blood are removed and replaced by equal volumes of plasma to reduce the Hct to safe levels; simple phlebotomy alone should not be used, because hypovolemia results and the symptoms may worsen. A possible association between neonatal polycythemia and subsequent developmental delay has been suggested but remains unproved.

METABOLIC PROBLEMS IN THE NEWBORN

HYPOTHERMIA

An abnormally low body temperature. Newborns are prone to becoming hypothermic in a cool environment. Hypothermia is a serious hazard that can result in hypoglycemia, metabolic acidosis, and death. Since the O_2 requirement (metabolic rate) increases with cold stress, hypothermia may also result in tissue hypoxia and neurologic damage in neonates with respiratory insufficiency (eg, the preterm neonate with respiratory distress syndrome). Prolonged unrecognized cold stress may divert calories to heat production and impair growth.

Newborns respond to cooling by a sympathetic nerve discharge of norepinephrine to the "brown fat." This specialized organ of the newborn, located in the nape of the neck, between the scapulae, and around the kidneys and adrenals, responds by lipolysis followed by oxidation or reesterification of the fatty acids that are released. These reactions produce heat locally, and a rich blood supply to the brown fat helps to transfer this heat to the rest of the newborn's body. This reaction may increase the metabolic rate and O_2 utilization two- to threefold above baseline.

Nevertheless, the low-birth-weight neonate may become hypothermic because he has a high ratio of surface area to body weight and rapidly loses heat by radiation. Evaporative heat loss (eg, a newborn wet with amniotic fluid in the delivery room) and conductive and convective heat losses can also be significant. The newborn's thermal environment is affected by relative humidity, air flow, and the proximity of cold surfaces (to which heat is lost by radiation) as well as by the ambient air temperature.

Hypothermia can be prevented by rapidly drying the newborn in the delivery room (to avoid evaporative heat loss) and then swaddling him (including his head) in a warm blanket. The neonate who is exposed for resuscitation or closer observation, or to provide skin-to-skin contact with the mother, should be warmed under a radiant warmer.

Sick newborns should be maintained in a **neutral thermal environment**—the environmental conditions under which the metabolic rate is minimal while maintaining a normal core temperature (37° C or 98.6° F). This can be approximated by setting the isolette temperature indicated in TABLE 27–2 according to the newborn's birth weight and postnatal age. An alternative approach to achieving a neutral thermal environment is to provide heat using an isolette or radiant warmer with a servo-control mechanism set to maintain the skin temperature at 36.5° C (97.7° F).

TABLE 27–2. NEUTRAL THERMAL ENVIRONMENTAL TEMPERATURES*

Age and Weight	Starting Temperature (°C)	Range of Temperature (°C)
0–6 h		
< 1200 gm	35.0	34.0–35.4
1200–1500 gm	34.1	33.9–34.4
1501–2500 gm	33.4	32.8–33.8
> 2500 gm (and > 36 wk)	32.9	32.0–33.8
6–12 h		
< 1200 gm	35.0	34.0–35.4
1200–1500 gm	34.0	33.5–34.4
1501–2500 gm	33.1	32.2–33.8
> 2500 gm (and > 36 wk)	32.8	31.4–33.8
12–24 h		
< 1200 gm	34.0	34.0–35.4
1200–1500 gm	33.8	33.3–34.3
1501–2500 gm	32.8	31.8–33.8
> 2500 gm (and > 36 wk)	32.4	31.0–33.7
24–36 h		
< 1200 gm	34.0	34.0–35.0
1200–1500 gm	33.6	33.1–34.2
1501–2500 gm	32.6	31.6–33.6
> 2500 gm (and > 36 wk)	32.1	30.7–33.5
36–48 h		
< 1200 gm	34.0	34.0–35.0
1200–1500 gm	33.5	33.1–34.1
1501–2500 gm	32.5	31.4–33.5
> 2500 gm (and > 36 wk)	31.9	30.5–33.3

(Continued)

TABLE 27–2. NEUTRAL THERMAL ENVIRONMENTAL TEMPERATURES* (Cont'd)

Age and Weight	Starting Temperature (°C)	Range of Temperature (°C)
48–72 h		
< 1200 gm	34.0	34.0–35.0
1200–1500 gm	33.5	33.0–34.0
1501–2500 gm	32.3	31.2–33.4
> 2500 gm (and > 36 wk)	31.7	30.1–33.2
72–96 h		
< 1200 gm	34.0	34.0–35.0
1200–1500 gm	33.5	33.0–34.0
1501–2500 gm	32.2	31.1–33.2
> 2500 gm (and > 36 wk)	31.3	29.8–32.8
4–12 days		
< 1500 gm	33.5	33.0–34.0
1501–2500 gm	32.1	31.0–33.2
> 2500 gm (and > 36 wk)		
4–5 days	31.0	29.5–32.6
5–6 days	30.9	29.4–32.3
6–8 days	30.6	29.0–32.2
8–10 days	30.3	29.0–31.8
10–12 days	30.1	29.0–31.4
12–14 days		
< 1500 gm	33.5	32.6–34.0
1501–2500 gm	32.1	31.0–33.2
> 2500 gm (and > 36 wk)	29.8	29.0–30.8
2–3 wk		
< 1500 gm	33.1	32.2–34.0
1501–2500 gm	31.7	30.0–33.0
3–4 wk		
< 1500 gm	32.6	31.6–33.6
1501–2500 gm	31.4	30.0–32.7
4–5 wk		
< 1500 gm	32.0	31.2–33.0
1501–2500 gm	30.9	29.5–32.3
5–6 wk		
< 1500 gm	31.4	30.6–32.3
1501–2500 gm	30.4	29.0–31.8

* These are appropriate isolette temperatures if the room is warm and the isolette wall temperature is within a degree of the air temperature in the isolette. In a cool room, add 1° C to the isolette temperature given in the table for every 7° C that the room is below the isolette temperature.

Modified from Klaus MH, Fanaroff AA: "The physical environment," in Care of the High-Risk Neonate, ed. 3, edited by MH Klaus and AA Fanaroff. Philadelphia, WB Saunders Company, 1986; used with permission.

HYPOGLYCEMIA
(See also Ch. 40)

A blood glucose < 40 mg/dL in the full-term neonate, or < 30 mg/dL in the premature neonate. The correlation between symptoms and low blood glucose levels is inexact, as is the correlation between hypoglycemia and subsequent neurologic damage. However, since neurologic damage can occur, it is important to prevent neonatal hypoglycemia or to treat it promptly when it develops.

Etiology
Hypoglycemia usually occurs because of deficient glycogen stores at birth or secondary to hyperinsulinism. Since glycogen stores may be deficient in very-low-birth-weight (VLBW) preterm infants, these newborns are prone to

hypoglycemia unless they receive a sustained input of exogenous glucose. Glycogen stores are also depleted in newborns who experience intrauterine malnutrition because of placental insufficiency (small-for-gestational-age neonates). If they also sustained perinatal asphyxia with hypoxia, any glucose stores (as glycogen) will have been rapidly consumed during anaerobic glycolysis. Glycogen-deficient neonates may become hypoglycemic at any time in the first few days, especially if there is a prolonged interval between feedings or if nutritional intake is poor.

Hyperinsulinism is seen in newborns of diabetic mothers (inversely related to the degree of diabetic control), in severe erythroblastosis fetalis, and in **Beckwith-Wiedemann syndrome** (macroglossia, umbilical hernia, and hypoglycemia). Elevated insulin levels characteristically result in a rapid fall in the blood glucose in the first 1 to 2 h after birth when the continuous supply of glucose from the placenta is interrupted. Hypoglycemia may also occur in these infants if an IV infusion of glucose in water is abruptly interrupted.

Symptoms, Signs, and Diagnosis

Although many newborns remain asymptomatic, listlessness, poor feeding, hypotonia, jitteriness, apneic spells, tachypnea, and seizures may occur. These signs are nonspecific and may be seen as well in infants who have been asphyxiated, have hypocalcemia, or are experiencing drug withdrawal (eg, "cocaine babies"—see Cocaine Abuse and Withdrawal, below).

Prophylaxis and Treatment

Newborns in the following categories are at risk for developing hypoglycemia: newborn infants of diabetic mothers, premature newborns, small-for-gestational-age newborns, newborns with severe isoimmune hemolytic disease, newborns with Beckwith-Wiedemann syndrome, and newborns who have experienced perinatal asphyxia. Neonates at risk who are sick, extremely premature, or have respiratory distress should receive their maintenance fluids as 10% glucose IV. Because they frequently develop early hypoglycemia and often feed poorly, newborns of insulin-dependent diabetic women should also be started on an IV 10% glucose infusion at birth. Newborns at risk who are not sick should be started on early, frequent formula feedings to provide a source of carbohydrate and other nutrients. In addition, all such newborns should have their blood glucose checked at frequent in-

tervals. This can be screened at the bedside using diagnostic glucose test strips (eg, Chemstrip bG®). However, the determination of capillary blood glucose in neonates using glucose oxidase test strips is inexact. Any values that are marginally low, or any infant with symptoms suggestive of hypoglycemia, should have a laboratory-determination of true blood glucose.

The newborn who develops hypoglycemia should be treated at once by an IV infusion of 10% glucose in water, 5 mL/kg over 10 min. The infusion should then be continued at a rate that provides 4 to 8 mg/kg/min of glucose (ie, 10% glucose in water at about 60 to 120 mL/kg/day). Blood glucose values must be monitored to guide adjustments in the infusion rate. Once the newborn's condition has improved, enteral feedings can gradually replace the IV infusion while the blood glucose is monitored. The IV glucose infusion should always be tapered gradually, as sudden discontinuation may result in hypoglycemia.

If there is difficulty in starting an IV infusion promptly in a hypoglycemic neonate, giving **glucagon** 300 µg/kg IM usually will raise the blood glucose rapidly, an effect lasting 2 to 3 h, except in neonates with depleted glycogen stores. Hypoglycemia that is refractory to high rates of glucose infusion may be treated with **hydrocortisone** 5 mg/kg/day IM in 2 divided doses. If hypoglycemia is refractory to treatment, an endocrine evaluation and search for other etiologies (eg, sepsis) should be considered.

HYPERGLYCEMIA

An abnormal increase of the blood glucose above 120 mg/dL in newborns. This condition occurs less frequently than hypoglycemia. However, VLBW newborns (< 1.5 kg) may not tolerate rapid IV infusions of glucose during the first few days of life and may become significantly hyperglycemic. Very severely stressed or septic newborns may also develop hyperglycemia. **Transient neonatal diabetes mellitus** is a rare entity that usually occurs in small-for-gestational-age neonates. Until this resolves spontaneously, usually within a few weeks, glucose homeostasis and hydration should be carefully maintained.

Hyperglycemia may cause glycosuria with osmotic diuresis and dehydration, and severe hyperglycemia with marked serum hyperosmolarity may cause neurologic damage.

Treatment includes reducing the glucose infusion rate (either by changing the concentration from 10% to 5% glucose or by slowing the rate). Fluid and electrolyte losses resulting from diuresis are replaced IV. Hyperglycemia persisting at low glucose infusion rates (eg, 4 mg/kg/min) may indicate relative insulin deficiency or insulin resistance. Human insulin may be added to the IV 10% glucose infusion at a uniform rate of 0.01 to 0.1 u./kg/h. It is convenient to add the insulin to a separate IV of 10% glucose in water and "piggyback" it into the maintenance 10% glucose IV so the insulin rate can be adjusted without changing the total IV infusion rate. The response to insulin therapy is unpredictable in the newborn, and it is extremely important to monitor the blood glucose frequently.

HYPOCALCEMIA

A serum calcium (Ca) concentration < 8 mg/dL. Neonatal hypocalcemia occurs fairly frequently in the intensive care nursery. High-risk groups include premature newborns, newborns of diabetic mothers, small-for-gestational-age newborns, and newborns who have had perinatal asphyxia.

Etiology

The etiology of **early-onset hypocalcemia** is not well understood. Some preterm or sick newborns appear to have a transient period of relative hypoparathyroidism following birth; when the constant infusion of ionized Ca from the placenta is interrupted, their serum Ca falls. This may be exaggerated in newborns of diabetic mothers, as these women have higher-than-normal ionized Ca levels during pregnancy, and therefore at birth the neonatal parathyroid glands do not function as well to maintain a normal serum Ca level. Hypocalcemia may also be seen for the same reason in newborns of women with hyperparathyroidism. In other neonates there appears to be a lack of the normal phosphaturic renal response to parathyroid hormone. Perinatal asphyxia may cause increased serum calcitonin, which inhibits Ca release from bone and results in hypocalcemia.

After 3 days of age, newborns with **late hypocalcemia** may present with tetany or seizures. Now rare, it is caused by infant feedings of cow's milk or formula preparations with too high a phosphate (PO₄) load; elevated serum PO₄ leads to hypocalcemia.

Symptoms and Signs

Newborns with hypocalcemia are often asymptomatic, but may present with hypotonia, apnea, poor feeding, jitteriness, or seizures. Similar symptoms may occur with hypoglycemia or

drug withdrawal. Prolongation of the corrected QT interval (QT$_c$) on the ECG is suggestive of hypocalcemia. Signs of hypocalcemia rarely occur unless the total serum Ca is < 7 mg/dL.

Treatment

Early-onset hypocalcemia ordinarily resolves in a few days, and asymptomatic infants usually do not need treatment. Neonates with serum Ca levels > 7 mg/dL rarely require treatment. Those with levels < 7 mg/dL should be treated with 10% calcium gluconate solution, 200 mg/kg of calcium gluconate (2 mL/kg) by slow IV infusion over 5 to 10 min. Ten percent calcium gluconate solution contains 100 mg calcium gluconate/mL and 9 mg elemental calcium/mL. Too rapid an infusion can cause bradycardia, and the heart rate should be monitored during the infusion. The IV site should also be watched closely, as tissue infiltration by Ca solution is very irritating and may cause local tissue damage.

After acute correction of hypocalcemia, calcium gluconate may be mixed in the IV fluids and given continuously. Starting with 400 mg/kg/day of calcium gluconate, the dose may be increased gradually to 800 mg/kg/day, if needed, to prevent recurrence of hypocalcemia. When oral feedings are begun, they may be supplemented with the same daily dose of calcium gluconate by adding the 10% calcium gluconate solution into the day's formula.

The goal of treatment in late-onset hypocalcemia is to add sufficient Ca to the formula to provide a 4:1 molar ratio of Ca to PO₄. This will precipitate calcium phosphate in the GI tract, thus preventing PO₄ absorption and enhancing Ca absorption from the GI tract.

HYPERNATREMIA
(See also Ch. 26)

Serum sodium (Na) > 150 mEq/L. Extreme neonatal hypernatremia has been associated with seizures, intracranial hemorrhage, and later neurologic impairment.

Excessive loss of free water **(hypertonic dehydration)** frequently occurs in VLBW neonates via cutaneous evaporation of water (insensible water losses) in association with immature renal function and reduced ability to produce a concentrated urine. The skin of VLBW neonates of 24 to 28 wk gestation lacks a stratum corneum and is extremely permeable to water. Skin blood flow and insensible water loss are also much increased if the newborn is nursed under a radiant warmer or is under bili-lites; these newborns may require 200 to 250 mL/kg/day of water IV in the first few days, after which insensible water loss decreases. Body weight, serum electrolytes, urine volume, and sp gr must be checked at least every 12 h in these tiny newborns, so fluid administration can be adjusted appropriately. This type of hypernatremia is treated by replacing water losses using 5 or 10% glucose in water IV.

Hypernatremia may also occur if Na in isotonic or hypertonic fluids is administered in excess of renal losses. Daily Na maintenance for low-birth-weight newborns is 2 to 4 mEq/kg/day. It is important to remember that fresh frozen plasma and human serum albumin are isotonic Na solutions. Even catheter flushes of isotonic saline may provide a significant amount of Na to VLBW infants. Sodium bicarbonate is a hypertonic solution and should be diluted 1:3 with water before administration. The neonate with this type of hypernatremia often will be edematous and will have high urine Na excretion unless there is cardiac or renal insufficiency. **Treatment** is best addressed by stopping the administration of Na and maintaining the administration of water as 5 or 10% glucose IV until the serum Na concentration returns to normal.

In the past, errors in preparing evaporated milk formulas by adding excess sodium chloride resulted in neurologic damage or death of some newborns. Formulas should not be mixed at home nor should proprietary formulas be altered by the addition of salt.

HYPERBILIRUBINEMIA

Normal Route of Bilirubin Excretion

Old or damaged RBCs are removed from the circulation by reticuloendothelial cells, which then metabolize the heme to bilirubin. The breakdown of 1 gm of Hb yields 34 mg of bilirubin. The bilirubin (unconjugated), bound to serum albumin, is carried to the liver and transferred to binding proteins (Y and Z proteins) in the hepatocytes. Glucuronyl transferase then conjugates the bilirubin with uridine diphosphoglucuronic acid (UDPGA) to bilirubin diglucuronide (conjugated, direct-reacting bilirubin), which is secreted actively into the bile ducts and enters the GI tract. The newborn lacks proper intestinal bacteria for oxidizing bilirubin to urobilinogen in the gut; consequently, unaltered bilirubin is excreted in the stools, giving them a typical bright-yellow color. However, the newborn's (and fetus') GI tract contains β-glucuronidase, which deconjugates some of the bilirubin so that unconju-

gated bilirubin can be reabsorbed and returned to the circulation from the intestinal lumen (**enterohepatic circulation of bilirubin**). In the fetus, the circulating reabsorbed bilirubin can be excreted by the placenta, but it persists in the newborn and may contribute to **physiologic jaundice.**

The exact cause of physiologic hyperbilirubinemia is not known; limiting rates in the binding of bilirubin in the hepatocytes, in the conjugation of bilirubin with glucuronic acid, and in bile secretion have all been implicated, as well as the enterohepatic circulation of bilirubin. Physiologic jaundice appears after 24 h in about 50% of full-term newborns and in a higher percentage of premature newborns. It usually is not accompanied by constitutional symptoms or signs and resolves within 1 wk. However, excess bilirubin accumulation from any cause can produce kernicterus (see below), especially in the preterm or sick neonate.

Etiology of Hyperbilirubinemia

An **increased production** of bilirubin (eg, from elevated Hb from hypertransfusion, hemolytic diseases, hematomas), a **decreased excretion** of bilirubin (eg, from decreased glucuronyl transferase in the preterm neonate, hepatitis, biliary atresia), or both will result in neonatal hyperbilirubinemia. Therefore, the appearance of jaundice can signal a variety of disorders. Known causes of neonatal hyperbilirubinemia are listed in TABLE 27–3.

Neonatal hyperbilirubinemia is most often of the unconjugated (indirect-reacting) type. Conjugated hyperbilirubinemia is seen fairly often owing to cholestasis as a complication of parenteral alimentation. Other causes of direct hyperbilirubinemia are listed in TABLE 27–3. The specific etiology must always be sought and treated; eg, extrahepatic biliary atresia may progress to irreversible cirrhosis if not diagnosed and surgically corrected in the first 4 to 6 wk.

Evaluation of Neonatal Hyperbilirubinemia

Jaundice appearing on the first day in any newborn and a bilirubin concentration > 10 mg/dL in premature infants or > 15 mg/dL in full-term infants warrant investigation. When the blood level of bilirubin is about 4 to 5 mg/dL, jaundice becomes apparent. With increasing bilirubin levels, visible jaundice advances in a head-to-foot direction.

In addition to a complete history and physical examination, evaluation should include determi-

TABLE 27–3. CAUSES OF NEONATAL HYPERBILIRUBINEMIA

Overproduction	Undersecretion	Mixed
Fetal-maternal blood group incompatibility—Rh, ABO, others	Metabolic-endocrine Familial nonhemolytic jaundice types 1 and 2 (Crigler-Najjar syndrome)	Sepsis
Hereditary spherocytosis (elliptocytosis, somatocytosis)	Gilbert's disease Hypothyroidism	Intrauterine infections Toxoplasmosis Rubella Cytomegalovirus
Nonspherocytic hemolytic anemias G6PD deficiency and drugs Pyruvate kinase deficiency	Tyrosinosis Hypermethioninemia Drugs and hormones Novobiocin	inclusion disease Herpes simplex Syphilis
Other red-cell enzyme deficiency α Thalassemia β-δ Thalassemia	Pregnanediol Lucey-Driscoll syndrome	Hepatitis Respiratory distress syndrome
Acquired hemolysis due to vitamin K₃, nitrofurantoin, sulfonamides, antimalarials, penicillin, oxytocin?, bupivacaine, or infection	Diabetic mother Prematurity Hypopituitarism and anencephaly	Asphyxia Infant of diabetic mother
Extravascular blood—petechiae; hematomas; pulmonary, cerebral, or occult hemorrhage	Obstructive disorders Biliary atresia* Dubin-Johnson and Rotor's syndromes*	Severe erythroblastosis fetalis
Polycythemia Maternal-fetal or feto-fetal transfusion Delayed umbilical cord clamping	Choledochal cyst* Cystic fibrosis* (inspissated bile) Tumor or band* (extrinsic obstruction)	
Increased enterohepatic circulation Pyloric stenosis* Intestinal atresia or stenosis, including annular pancreas Hirschsprung's disease Meconium ileus or meconium plug syndrome Fasting or other cause for hypoperistalsis Drug-induced paralytic ileus (hexamethonium) Swallowed blood	α₁-Antitrypsin deficiency* Parenteral nutrition	

* Jaundice may not be seen in the neonatal period.
Adapted from Poland RL, Ostrea EM Jr: "Neonatal hyperbilirubinemia," in *Care of the High-Risk Neonate*, ed. 3, edited by MH Klaus and AA Fanaroff. Philadelphia, WB Saunders Company, 1986; used with permission.

nation of both total and direct serum bilirubin concentration, direct Coombs' test, Hct, blood smear, reticulocyte count, and the determination of blood type and Rh group of both newborn and mother. Other studies, such as blood, urine, and CSF cultures, or determination of RBC enzyme levels, may be indicated by the history, physical examination, or initial laboratory findings.

Breast milk jaundice is diagnosed by exclusion. Therefore, it is important for the physician to evaluate the newborn for other possible causes of the hyperbilirubinemia that may require specific treatment (see also PREMATURE INFANT under GESTATIONAL AGE AND BIRTH WEIGHT, above). The mechanism of breast milk jaundice is not understood. Occasional term newborns who are breast fed will develop progressive unconjugated hyperbilirubinemia during the first week; the problem tends to recur in subsequent pregnancies. If the bilirubin level continues to increase to 17 or 18 mg/dL, a change from breast milk to formula feedings is required; phototherapy may also be indicated. Discontinuation of breast-feeding will only be necessary for 1 or 2 days, and the mother should be encouraged to continue to express breast milk regularly so that she can resume nursing as soon as the infant's bilirubin level is < 15 mg/dL. She should also be assured that the hyperbilirubinemia has not caused any harm and that she may safely resume breast-feeding.

Kernicterus

Brain damage due to deposition of bilirubin in the basal ganglia and brainstem nuclei.

Early symptoms of kernicterus in term infants are lethargy, poor feeding, and vomiting. Opisthotonos, oculogyric crisis, seizures, and death may follow. In preterm infants, kernicterus may not be associated with recognizable clinical signs. During childhood, late signs of kernicterus may be manifested as mental retardation, choreoathetoid cerebral palsy, sensorineural hearing loss, and paralysis of upward gaze. It is not known if minor degrees of bilirubin encephalopathy can result in less severe neurologic impairment (eg, perceptual-motor handicaps and learning disorders in school).

There is no clinically proven test that indicates the risk of kernicterus in a particular newborn. Bilirubin is firmly bound to serum albumin and is not free to cross the blood-brain barrier and cause kernicterus as long as there are unused bilirubin binding sites on serum albumin. The risk of kernicterus is therefore greater in newborns who have a markedly elevated serum bilirubin concentration, a low albumin concentration, or substances in their serum that compete for bilirubin binding sites on albumin. Such substances include free fatty acids, hydrogen ion, and certain drugs such as sulfisoxazole, ceftriaxone, and aspirin. Serum albumin concentrations are lower in preterm newborns, putting them at greater risk. Competing molecules (eg, free fatty acids and hydrogen ions) are likely to be elevated in the serum of newborns who undergo fasting, are septic, or have respiratory or metabolic acidosis. These clinical conditions would therefore place a newborn at increased risk of kernicterus at any particular serum bilirubin concentration.

Treatment

Early, frequent feedings of newborns will reduce the incidence and severity of hyperbilirubinemia by increasing GI motility and frequency of stools, thereby minimizing the enterohepatic circulation of bilirubin. The type of feedings does not appear important in increasing bilirubin excretion.

Phototherapy: Exchange transfusion remains the definitive treatment for hyperbilirubinemia that has reached the level at which kernicterus may occur. However, phototherapy has proved to be a safe and effective method to treat hyperbilirubinemia, and it has greatly reduced the need for exchange transfusion. A maximal effect is obtained by exposing the infant to visible light in the blue range. However, if blue lights are used, cyanosis cannot be detected; therefore, phototherapy using broad-spectrum white light is often preferred. Since there are many biologic effects of exposure to bright light, phototherapy should be used only when specifically indicated. Temporary intestinal lactose intolerance occurs during phototherapy, but the resultant diarrhea is not usually significant.

Phototherapy produces configurational photoisomers of bilirubin in the skin and subcutaneous tissues; these more water-soluble configurations can be excreted rapidly by the liver without the need for prior glucuronidation. Phototherapy is not indicated if there is biliary or intestinal obstruction, since the photoisomers then cannot be excreted. Brownish discoloration of the serum and skin has occurred in such circumstances (**bronze baby syndrome**), but it is not known if this condition is hazardous to the newborn.

All possible etiologies for hyperbilirubinemia should be considered before starting phototherapy; otherwise the symptom of "jaundice" may be treated without making the correct diagnosis. Phototherapy can be started when the serum bilirubin reaches within 3 or 4 mg/dL of the serum concentration at which exchange transfusion would be performed (see discussion of exchange transfusion, below).

A Plexiglas shield should be placed between the phototherapy lights and the infant to screen out ultraviolet radiation, and the infant should be blindfolded during phototherapy to prevent eye damage. Care must be taken to avoid nasal obstruction by the blindfold. Since visible jaundice may disappear during phototherapy while the serum bilirubin remains elevated, skin color should not be trusted to evaluate the severity of jaundice. The light should be turned off and the blindfold removed during feedings; blood taken for bilirubin determinations should also be protected from light, since bilirubin in the collection tubes may photo-oxidize rapidly.

Exchange transfusion: Traditionally, dangerous levels of bilirubin are treated by exchange blood transfusion via an umbilical vein catheter. Overall mortality is < 1% for this procedure when done by experienced personnel, and it should be much less when the procedure is done on otherwise healthy full-term newborns.

Since there is no exact test to determine the risk of kernicterus and hence the level at which exchange transfusion is necessary, the following has proved useful as a rough guide. The bilirubin level (in mg/dL) used for exchange transfusion is the newborn's weight in grams divided by 100. Thus, a 1000-gm newborn would receive an exchange transfusion at a bilirubin level of 10 mg/dL, and a 2000-gm newborn at 20 mg/dL. It is rarely necessary to do an exchange transfusion if the total serum bilirubin is < 10 mg/dL. Traditionally, in term newborns exchange transfusion has been done if the total serum bilirubin reaches 20 mg/dL. Although clinical correlations are not available, in the absence of hemolytic disease the bilirubin may safely be allowed to rise slightly above 20 mg/dL if the newborn is not sick. In addition to the determination of exchange transfusion bilirubin level based upon weight, it is customary to lower the level by 1 to 2 mg/dL if the newborn has clinical factors that would increase the risk of kernicterus (eg, fasting, sepsis, acidosis). Only unconjugated hyperbilirubinemia can cause kernicterus; if the conjugated bilirubin is significantly elevated, only the level of unconjugated bilirubin is used to calculate the need for exchange transfusion.

INBORN ERRORS OF METABOLISM

Many inherited biochemical disorders may be detected at or soon after birth. In the USA, many states require that newborns be screened routinely for the more common inborn errors of metabolism, including congenital hypothyroidism, galactosemia, hemo globinopathies, and phenylketonuria. Inborn errors of metabolism are discussed elsewhere in THE MANUAL.

FETAL ALCOHOL SYNDROME (FAS)
(See also Ch. 16)

Maternal alcohol abuse during pregnancy is the most common cause of drug-induced teratogenesis. The most serious consequence is severe mental retardation due to impaired brain development. Affected neonates have growth retardation and are microcephalic. Multiple malformations may occur—microphthalmia, short palpebral fissures, midfacial hypoplasia, abnormal palmar creases, cardiac defects, and joint contractures; no single finding is pathognomonic and only partial expression of FAS may occur, making diagnosis of mild cases difficult. The mental retardation is thought to be part of ethanol teratogenesis, since infants of alcoholic women are often retarded even if raised in foster homes.

FAS has been diagnosed in neonates born to chronic alcoholics who drank heavily throughout pregnancy. Lesser degrees of alcohol abuse result in less severe manifestations of FAS. Because it is not known when during pregnancy ethanol is most likely to harm the fetus, or whether there is a lower limit of ethanol use that can be considered safe, pregnant women should be advised to avoid all alcohol intake. When a child is affected, the mother's other children should be examined for subtle manifestations of FAS.

COCAINE ABUSE AND WITHDRAWAL
(See also Chs. 16 and 53)

Cocaine inhibits reuptake of neurotransmitters such as norepinephrine and epinephrine. In addition to producing a feeling of euphoria, it also causes strong sympathomimetic effects including vasoconstriction and hypertension. Cocaine crosses the placenta, and the same physiologic effects are believed to occur in the fetus. Cocaine abuse in pregnancy is associated with a higher rate of spontaneous abortion and fetal death. There is also a well-documented increased risk of placental abruption, which may lead to intrauterine fetal demise or to neurologic damage if the infant survives. Abruption may be caused by reduced maternal blood flow to the placental vascular bed. Infants born to addicted mothers have low birth weight, reduced body length and head circumference, and lower Apgar scores.

Several anomalies have been associated with cocaine use early in pregnancy, and all are reported to be the result of vascular disruption, presumably secondary to the intense vasoconstriction of fetal arteries produced by cocaine. These malformations include limb reduction malformations, GU malformations including prune-belly syndrome, and intestinal atresia or necrosis. Some infants with cerebral infarcts noted at birth may have had their blood supply to the brain impaired secondary to cocaine effects in utero. Prognosis for infants born to cocaine-addicted mothers in terms of future growth and development is unknown.

Infants may show withdrawal symptoms if the mother has been using cocaine up until the day of delivery. Signs of withdrawal and treatment are the same as for opioid withdrawal (see below).

OTHER DRUG WITHDRAWAL SYNDROMES

The infant of a woman addicted to opioids (eg, heroin, morphine, methadone) should be observed for the development of withdrawal symptoms within 72 h after delivery. Newborns rarely die from drug withdrawal, but long-term effects have not been studied. Characteristic signs include irritability, jitteriness, hypertonicity, vomiting, diarrhea, sweating, convulsions, and hyperventilation that produces respiratory alkalosis. Mild withdrawal symptoms are treated by swaddling and frequent feedings to reduce restlessness. Severe symptoms can be controlled by diluting tincture of opium, which contains 10 mg morphine/mL, 25-fold with water and giving 2 drops/kg orally q 4 to 6 h as needed. Phenobarbital 5 to 7 mg/kg/day given orally or IM in 3 divided doses may also control withdrawal symptoms. Treatment is tapered and stopped over several days or weeks as symptoms subside.

Most crucial in the management of infants born to mothers addicted to opioids or cocaine is evaluation of the home situation to determine if the infant will be safely cared for following hospital discharge. The supportive help of relatives, friends, and visiting nurses may enable the mother to care for her infant. Otherwise, foster home care or an alternative care plan may be in the best interests of the child. The incidence of **sudden infant death syndrome** is greater in infants born to narcotic addicts, but still is less than 10/1000 infants, so routine use of home cardiorespiratory monitors is not recommended for all such infants.

Prolonged maternal abuse of **barbiturates** may cause neonatal drug withdrawal with jitteriness, irritability, and fussing that often does not develop until 7 to 10 days postpartum when the neonate has been discharged from the nursery. Sedation with phenobarbital 5 to 7 mg/kg/day given orally or IM in 3 divided doses may be required and then tapered over a few days or weeks, depending upon the duration of symptoms.

SEIZURE DISORDERS IN THE NEWBORN

(See also Ch. 43)

General Considerations

Seizures, *abnormal involuntary electrical discharges from the CNS usually manifested by stereotyped muscular activity or autonomic changes,* are a frequent, serious neonatal problem. They may occur with any disorder that directly or indirectly affects the CNS and require immediate evaluation to determine their cause and treatment.

They are usually focal *and may be difficult to recognize.* Migratory clonic jerks of extremities, alternating hemiseizures, or primitive subcortical seizures (respiratory arrest, chewing movements, persistent deviations of the eyes, episodic changes in tone) are common. A typical grand mal seizure is infrequent. The focal nature of neonatal seizures may be due to the lack of myelination, the primarily inhibitory nature of the newborn cortex, or incomplete formation of dendrites and synapses in the brain at this age.

It is important to separate the clonic activity seen with hypertonicity and jitteriness from true seizure activity. Jitteriness produces clonus with stimulation, and holding the extremity will stop it. Seizures occur spontaneously, and their motor activity can be felt to continue when the limb is held.

Seizures can arise only from an abnormal CNS discharge, but this may be from a primary intracranial process (meningitis, tumor, encephalitis, intracranial hemorrhage) or secondary to a systemic or metabolic problem (anoxia, hypoglycemia, hypocalcemia, hyponatremia, etc). The type of seizure seen in the newborn does *not* help distinguish focal CNS lesions from metabolic problems.

Etiology

Since specific treatment for many causes of neonatal seizures is known, the etiology must be pursued. **Hypoglycemia** is common in infants born to diabetic mothers, infants small for gestational age, and those with a hypoxic insult or other stress. In full-term infants, blood glucose levels < 30 mg/dL are considered hypoglycemic; in low-birth-weight infants, < 20 mg/dL. Not all infants have symptoms at hypoglycemic levels. Whether asymptomatic hypoglycemia leads to neurologic damage is unknown, but the possibility exists. **Hypocalcemia,** defined as a serum Ca level < 7.5 mg/dL, is usually accompanied by a serum P level of > 3 mg/dL and, like hypoglycemia, can be asymptomatic. It is often associated with prematurity or difficult births. **Hypomagnesemia** is uncommon, but can produce seizures when the serum Mg level is < 1.4 mEq/L. Hypomagnesemia is often associated with hypocalcemia and should be considered in a hypocalcemic infant when the seizures continue after adequate Ca therapy. Either hyper- or **hyponatremia** may cause seizures. Hypernatremia can result from accidental oral or IV NaCl overloading. Hyponatremia can be dilutional when too much water is given orally or IV or may follow

Na loss in stool or urine. **Inborn errors of metabolism** and **drug withdrawal** may also present as neonatal seizures.

Seizures are frequent with **meningitis.** They also occur in **sepsis** but generally are not a presenting sign. Gram-negative organisms often cause intracranial and systemic infections. Cytomegalovirus, herpes simplex virus, rubella virus, *Treponema pallidum,* and *Toxoplasma gondii* should also be considered. **Pyridoxine deficiency** or dependency is rare but readily treated. Other causes of seizures in newborns that are more difficult to diagnose and to treat include the sequelae of **hypoxia, intraventricular hemorrhage, birth trauma,** and **CNS malformations.**

Diagnosis

The evaluation of neonatal seizures should begin with blood glucose, Ca, Mg, and electrolyte determinations. Commercially available test strips provide a rapid blood glucose determination, but a concomitant true blood glucose should also be obtained. Next, infection is sought through cultures from peripheral sites, blood, and CSF. The CSF should also be examined for abnormal numbers of RBCs or WBCs, and for the glucose and protein content. The need for further metabolic tests (eg, arterial pH, blood gases, serum bilirubin, or urine amino acids) depends on the clinical situation. X-rays of the skull may reveal intracranial calcifications, and long-bone films may show changes due to congenital infections (eg, rubella and syphilis). An EEG is useful to document and follow the seizures; it is especially helpful if there is difficulty in deciding whether or not the infant is having seizures. The presence of a normal EEG or one with focal abnormalities during a seizure has been shown clinically to be a good prognostic sign, while an EEG with diffuse abnormalities is a poor one. Cranial ultrasound or CT scans can document intracranial hemorrhage. If no cause is found, the mother should also be studied for evidence of addiction to drugs.

Prognosis and Treatment

Although conditions causing neonatal seizures have a high mortality and are often associated with permanent neurologic damage, nearly 50% of neonates who have seizures and survive will be normal at age 5 yr. Early onset of seizures is associated with the highest morbidity and mortality. The longer seizure activity continues, the more likely the infant is to have later neurologic impairment (eg, cerebral palsy, mental retardation).

Therapy should be directed primarily at the underlying pathology and secondarily at the seizure. Except for seizures presenting as apnea, it is usually unnecessary to stop seizures in progress, since they generally are self-limited and rarely compromise vital function in a newborn. If blood glucose is low, 10% dextrose 2 mL/kg IV is given. If hypocalcemia is present, 5% calcium gluconate 4 mL/kg IV (50 mg/mL) can be given. *Calcium gluconate should be given no faster than 1 mL/kg/min and with continuous cardiac monitoring.* Extravasation should be avoided, since sloughing of the skin can result. If Mg deficiency is diagnosed, 0.2 mL/kg of a 20% magnesium sulfate solution is given IM. Infections should be treated with antibiotics.

Symptomatic treatment of the seizure itself should begin immediately after completing the initial efforts to identify its cause. Phenobarbital is the drug of choice and should be given in a loading dose of 20 mg/kg IV. If seizures continue, then 5 mg/kg can be given q 15 min until seizures cease or a maximum of 40 mg/kg has been given. Maintenance therapy, consisting of 5 mg/kg/day in 2 divided doses, should be started 12 h later. Phenobarbital should be given IV, especially if seizures are frequent or prolonged. When the seizures are controlled, the oral route can be used. If a second drug is needed, then phenytoin in a loading dose of 20 mg/kg should be used. In neonates, it is effective only IV and should be given slowly in two 10 mg/kg increments to avoid hypotension or arrhythmias. Signs of phenytoin toxicity may be difficult to detect in newborns, and prolonged high levels may be harmful. If blood levels can be monitored, the risk is smaller. Therapeutic blood levels for phenobarbital are 15 to 40 μg/mL; for phenytoin, 10 to 20 μg/mL. Infants taking anticonvulsant drugs need to be closely observed; *overmedication with resulting respiratory depression and even arrest may be more dangerous than the seizures.* Medication should be continued until the seizures have been controlled and the risk of further seizures is small.

CONGENITAL SENSORINEURAL HEARING LOSS

In the past, epidemics of rubella resulted in the birth of large numbers of children with congenital deafness. Particularly during the first trimester of pregnancy, the rubella virus may invade the developing inner ear (viral **endolymphatic labyrinthitis**), producing much destruction and a profound sensorineural hearing loss. Other causes of profound congenital sensorineural hearing loss are anoxia during birth, bleeding into the inner ear from trauma to the base of the skull during delivery (particularly in preterm infants), ototoxic drugs given to the mother, erythroblastosis fetalis, congenital toxoplasmosis, neonatal herpes simplex infection, persistent fetal circulation, and numerous hereditary conditions including Waardenburg syndrome, albinism, and Hurler's syndrome.

Diagnosis and Treatment

If severe bilateral sensorineural hearing loss is present at birth, parents may note within the first week or so that the newborn does not respond to their voices or environmental sounds. When parents suspect hearing loss, it is almost always present. (See also CLINICAL MEASUREMENT OF HEARING IN CHILDREN in Ch. 23.)

If a child does not develop speech normally, a differential diagnosis of deafness, mental retardation, aphasia, and autism must be considered.

Since children must hear language to learn it, deaf children do not develop language without special training. They require special education, beginning as soon as the hearing loss is identified. Because there is an optimum time for acquisition of language, early diagnosis of deafness in infants is essential.

Amplification with a **hearing aid** should be started as early as possible after diagnosis (even as early as 6 mo of age). In bilateral sensorineural hearing loss, binaural amplification using postauricular or in-the-ear aids is indicated to maximize hearing and permit development of auditory localization. For information on various types of hearing aids, see Ch. 67.

NEONATAL INFECTIONS

ANTIMICROBIAL THERAPY FOR NEWBORNS

Rapid physiologic changes during the neonatal period significantly affect the pharmacokinetic and toxicologic properties of antimicrobial agents. Absorption, distribution, metabolism, and excretion of drugs vary in neonates according to body weight, surface area, and gestational and chronologic ages (see below and the appropriate chapters in §11). These changes necessi-

tate complex dosing and frequency interval selections based on data derived from studies of antimicrobials in newborns (see TABLE 27–4).

Pharmacologic Principles
(See also Ch. 25)

Antibiotic distribution: The ECF compartment comprises up to 45% of total body weight in neonates. This increases the volume of distribution of certain drugs (eg, aminoglycosides) and requires larger doses relative to weight than those used in adults. Lower serum albumin concentrations in premature infants may affect antibiotic protein binding. Drugs that displace bilirubin from albumin (eg, sulfonamides, ceftriaxone) may increase the risk of kernicterus.

Antibiotic metabolism and excretion: Absence or deficiency of certain enzymes during early neonatal life may prolong the half-life of certain drugs and increase the risk of toxicity. For example, immaturity of hepatic glucuronyl transferase activity in neonates diminishes conjugation of chloramphenicol to the inactive form, resulting in prolonged and elevated blood levels. This can cause cardiovascular collapse and death, the **gray baby syndrome**, in infants treated with excessive chloramphenicol. Diminished GFR and renal tubular secretion in neonates increases the half-life values of penicillins and aminoglycosides. With changing renal function during the first month of life, dosage and frequency of administration of these antibiotics must be readjusted.

When using antibiotics that have unpredictable pharmacokinetics or a narrow therapeutic index (eg, chloramphenicol, vancomycin, and aminoglycosides), plasma drug levels should be measured at appropriate intervals to ensure sufficient but not excessive levels. Chloramphenicol levels should be measured, especially when the newborn is given concurrent treatment with rifampin, phenobarbital, or acetaminophen, because of interference with hepatic metabolism. The measurement can usually be done in the USA in reference or university laboratories.

Route of administration: Vasomotor instability of newborns with serious bacterial infection results in unpredictable drug absorption when drugs are given s.c. or IM. Therefore, antibiotics for severe infections should preferentially be given IV. Oral antibiotics can be used for outpatients who are not seriously ill (see TABLE 27–5).

Antibiotic therapy in pregnant or lactating women: Most commonly used antimicrobial agents cross the placenta and are excreted in

TABLE 27–4. DOSAGE RECOMMENDATIONS FOR SELECTED PARENTERAL ANTIMICROBIAL AGENTS FOR NEWBORNS

Antimicrobial Agent	Route of Administration	Individual Dose	Infant Weight < 2000 gm		Infant Weight ≥ 2000 gm		Comments
			Age 0–7 days	≥ 8 days	Age 0–7 days	≥ 8 days	
Aqueous penicillin G							Maximum for Group B streptococcal meningitis, 250,000 u./kg/day
Meningitis	IV	50,000 u./kg	q 12 h	q 8 h	q 8 h	q 6 h	
Other diseases	IV, IM	25,000 u./kg	q 12 h	q 8 h	q 8 h	q 6 h	
Penicillin G							CAUTION: sterile abscess and procaine toxicity
Procaine	IM	50,000 u./kg	q 24 h	q 24 h	q 24 h	q 24 h	
Ampicillin							IV as 15- to 30-min infusion
Meningitis	IV	50 mg/kg	q 12 h	q 8 h	q 8 h	q 6 h	
Other diseases	IM, IV	25 mg/kg	q 12 h	q 8 h	q 8 h	q 6 h	
Ticarcillin	IM, IV	75 mg/kg	q 12 h	q 8 h	q 8 h	q 6 h	No primary indication. Use in combination with aminoglycoside against *Pseudomonas aeruginosa.* Potential bleeding with renal failure
Mezlocillin	IM, IV	75 mg/kg	q 12 h	q 8 h	q 8 h	q 6 h	Limited data
Methicillin, nafcillin, oxacillin							Monitor renal function when using methicillin. Monitor CBC, liver function when using nafcillin
Meningitis	IV	50 mg/kg	q 12 h	q 8 h	q 8 h	q 6 h	
Other diseases	IM, IV	25 mg/kg	q 12 h	q 8 h	q 8 h	q 6 h	
Cefazolin*	IM, IV	20 mg/kg	q 12 h	q 12 h	q 12 h	q 8 h	No primary indication. Limited data. Do not use for initial therapy of sepsis or meningitis
Cefotaxime	IM, IV	50 mg/kg	q 12 h	q 8 h	q 12 h	q 6–8 h	For very-low-birth-weight newborns (< 1000 gm), use 50 mg/kg q 24 h
Ceftazidime	IV, IM	30 mg/kg	q 12 h	q 8 h	q 8 h	q 8 h	
Ceftriaxone	IM, IV						Limited data. May cause biliary pseudolithiasis. May increase risk of bilirubin encephalopathy in jaundiced premature newborns
Meningitis		50–75 mg/kg	q 12 h	q 12 h	q 12 h	q 12 h	
Other diseases		50 mg/kg	q 24 h	q 24 h	q 24 h	q 24 h	
Aztreonam	IV, IM	30 mg/kg	q 12 h	q 12 h	q 12 h	q 8 h	Limited data. For gram-negative bacilli only

Drug	Route	Dose						Comments
Clindamycin	IV, IM	5 mg/kg	q 12 h	q 8 h	q 8 h	q 8 h	q 6 h	For anaerobes and gram-positive cocci (not enterococci)
Kanamycin[†], amikacin[†]	IM, IV	10 mg/kg	—	q 8 h	q 8 h	q 8 h	q 8 h	Monitor serum peak drug levels (kanamycin or amikacin = 15–25 µg/mL; gentamicin or tobramycin = 5–10 µg/mL; trough = < 10 µg/mL). Reduce dose for impaired renal function. Reduce frequency in very small premature infants (q 18–24 h)
Gentamicin[†]	IM, IV	7.5 mg/kg	q 12 h	q 12 h	q 8 h	q 8 h	q 8 h	
Tobramycin[†], netilmicin[†]	IM, IV	2 mg/kg	q 12 h	q 12 h	q 12 h	q 12 h	q 8 h	
Chloramphenicol	IV	25 mg/kg	q 24 h	q 24 h	q 24 h	q 12 h	q 8 h	Adjust doses by monitoring serum drug levels (peak = 15–25 µg/mL) and hematologic parameters
Vancomycin	IV	15 mg/kg loading dose; then 10 mg/kg	q 12 h	q 8 h	q 8 h	q 8 h	q 8 h	Limited data. Give by slow IV infusion, no less than 60 min. Monitor serum levels (peak = 25–40 µg/mL; trough = < 10 µg/mL); adjust doses in renal failure. For premature infants < 1000 gm, give 15–20 mg/kg q 24–36 h
Metronidazole	IV	7.5 mg/kg	q 12 h	q 12 h	q 12 h	q 12 h	q 12 h	Limited data. Give loading dose of 15 mg/kg. Followed 48 h later in preterm and 24 h later in full-term infants, then q 12 h
		15 mg/kg	q 12 h	—	—	—	—	
Trimethoprim/ sulfamethoxazole (TMP/SMX)[‡]	IV	2 mg/kg TMP, 10 mg/kg SMX loading dose; then 0.6 mg/kg TMP, 3 mg/kg SMX	q 12 h	q 12 h	q 12 h	q 12 h	q 12 h	Limited data. Monitor bilirubin and hematologic and renal parameters. Safety not established in premature infants or those < 2 mo old; use only under extraordinary circumstances
Imipenem	IV	20 mg	q 12 h	q 12 h	q 8 h	q 8 h	—	Limited data.
		25 mg	—	—	—	q 8 h	q 6 h	
Amphotericin B	IV	0.25–1 mg/kg						Dilute in 5% D/W (do not use saline solution) Limited data. Start at 0.25 mg/kg single daily dose over 3-h infusion. After patient improves, give dose every other day. Increase by 0.25 mg/kg every other day, up to 1 mg/kg/day. Total dose over a 4- to 6-wk period, about 30–35 mg/kg. Monitor hematologic and renal functions

* Does not cross the blood-brain barrier.
† Sample to be obtained after end of IV infusion or 60 min after IM injection.
‡ In shigellosis, 2 mg/kg TMP and 10 mg/kg SMX loading dose followed by 0.6 mg/kg TMP and 3 mg/kg SMX q 12 h. In gram-negative meningitis and *Pneumocystis carinii* pneumonitis, use higher doses. Measure TMP levels on the 3rd day of therapy (desirable peak of TMP is 5 to 6 µg/mL).

TABLE 27-5. DOSAGE RECOMMENDATIONS FOR SELECTED
ORAL ANTIMICROBIAL AGENTS FOR NEWBORNS

Antimicrobial Agent	Dosage (mg/kg/dose)	Interval	Comments
Amoxicillin	15	q 8 h	Limited data. Cefaclor is associated with serum sickness
Cefaclor			
Erythromycin estolate	10	q 8-12 h	For chlamydial infections or pertussis
Erythromycin ethyl succinate	10	q 6 h	
Neomycin	30-35	q 8 h	For gastroenteritis caused by enteropathogenic strains of *Escherichia coli*, and for prophylaxis of neonates at high risk for necrotizing enterocolitis, for 5 days. May be systemically absorbed in the presence of significant diarrhea. Unproven efficacy and safety
Colistin	3-5	q 8 h	
Rifampin*	10	q 24 h	For tuberculosis
	5	q 12 h	For meningococcus prophylaxis for 2 days
	10	q 24 h	For *Hemophilus influenzae* prophylaxis for 4 days
Flucytosine	25	q 6 h	Limited data. Use only in combination with amphotericin B, to retard emergence of resistance
Chloramphenicol†	25	q 12 h	Monitor blood levels and CBC
Clindamycin	5	q 6-8 h	Limited data

* Serum levels in preterm infants should be monitored with rifampin therapy.
† Chloramphenicol should be administered q 24 h for those 0-14 days; q 24 h for those ≤ 2000 gm or 15-30 days; q 12 h for those > 2000 gm.

breast milk. Sulfonamides, chloramphenicol, and tetracyclines should particularly be avoided in pregnant and nursing mothers (see DRUGS IN PREGNANCY in Ch. 14 and DRUGS IN LACTATING MOTHERS in Ch. 23).

Choice of antimicrobial regimen: Specific therapy should be tailored according to the results of cultures and antimicrobial susceptibility tests. Empiric treatment, usually a combination of ampicillin plus an aminoglycoside, or a broad-spectrum cephalosporin with good CSF penetration, is often started pending these results (see also under NEONATAL SEPSIS in this chapter, below). Knowing the prevalence of antibiotic-resistant organisms in a particular nursery is helpful in choosing the first-line antibiotic regimens. If skin lesions are present or nosocomial infections are suspected, additional antistaphylococcal coverage is recommended.

Physicians should be cautious when using potent broad-spectrum antimicrobial agents such as the newer cephalosporins; these agents can induce drastic changes in bowel flora, bleeding disorders, emergence of resistant organisms, and superinfections with yeasts or enterococci.

TABLES 27-4 and 27-5 recommend dosages for selected antimicrobial agents for newborns. Pharmacologic data and safety and efficacy data are limited for many drugs; however, as new, safer agents become available, older drugs (such as chloramphenicol) with known toxic effects and unpredictable pharmacokinetics will no longer be used routinely. Other drugs, although less commonly used in the newborn, that do have specific therapeutic values are vancomycin for infections caused by methicillin-resistant staphylococci; metronidazole for anaerobic infections; ceftazidine for *Pseudomonas aeruginosa*; trimethoprim-sulfamethoxazole for shigellosis, salmonellosis, *Pneumocystis carinii*, and rare cases of gram-negative bacillary meningitis refractory to other regimens; and rifampin for TB and prophylaxis for meningococcal and *Hemophilus influenzae* diseases.

NOSOCOMIAL INFECTION IN THE NEWBORN

Infections not present or incubating at the time of birth. This includes infections acquired from the mother during delivery (maternally acquired infections) and those acquired after admission to the nursery (hospital-acquired infections). This definition eliminates subjective assessment of whether an infection such as early-onset Group B streptococcal disease was acquired at delivery or after birth. Obviously, not all nosocomial infections are preventable.

Nosocomial infection rates vary by type of nursery and infant birth weight. Well-baby nursery infection rates are usually < 1%, while those reported in neonatal intensive care units range from 5.9 to 30.4% (mean, 22.5%). Bloodstream infections and pneumonia are most common. Mortality rates from nosocomial infections in infants are about 33%: for those with a birth weight < 1000 gm, 18 to 45%; and those with a birth weight > 2000 gm, 2 to 12%.

Most infants at birth move from a sterile intrauterine environment to one teeming with microorganisms. Colonization with bacteria and other organisms is inevitable, but exposure to more virulent organisms before a balanced and inhibitory normal flora is established can result in illness. Preterm or ill infants do not have fully functional defenses (see IMMUNOLOGIC STATUS OF THE FETUS AND NEWBORN under MANAGEMENT OF THE NORMAL NEWBORN in Ch. 23) and are likely to undergo multiple invasive diagnostic, therapeutic, and monitoring procedures that breach barriers to infection.

Term Nurseries

Skin infection due to methicillin-sensitive *Staphylococcus aureus* acquired in the nursery is the most frequent nosocomial infection in term infants. However, methicillin-resistant *S. aureus* infections have also recently been reported in term infants. Other types of infection include meningitis or sepsis resulting from Group B streptococci, *Citrobacter,* or *Listeria monocytogenes;* diarrhea caused by enterotoxigenic or enteropathogenic *Escherichia coli, Salmonella,* or rotaviruses; disease from HIV, herpes simplex virus, enteroviruses, or respiratory syncytial virus; ophthalmitis or complicated infection due to *Neisseria gonorrhoeae;* or conjunctivitis or pneumonitis caused by *Chlamydia trachomatis.* Most of these infections are transmitted from mother to infant during the perinatal period, although transmission among infants in the nursery is possible if appropriate infection control measures are not followed. Sepsis from *E. coli* or other gram-negative pathogens is uncommon in healthy term infants, but clusters of infection caused by virulent strains occur. Except for Group A streptococcal infection, most postpartum maternal genital infections are not likely to be transmitted to the newborn. Consequently, a febrile postpartum woman who feels well enough and has no infection that endangers her infant may be allowed to handle and feed her newborn if she washes her hands thoroughly, wears a clean hospital gown, and prevents the baby from touching any contaminated items.

Staphylococcus aureus **disease and skin care regimens:** Pustular skin lesions in the periumbilical or diaper area are the most frequent manifestations, although complicated and disseminated infections (including osteomyelitis, pneumonia, and meningitis) occur. **Staphylococcal scalded skin syndrome,** ranging in severity from scarlatiniform erythema to bullous lesions to generalized exfoliative disease **(Ritter's disease),** is caused by *S. aureus* that produces exfoliative toxin. Clinical onset of *S. aureus* infection varies from a few days to several months of age but usually occurs at 2 to 3 wk. *S. aureus* resistant to penicillinase-resistant penicillin (eg, methicillin, oxacillin, nafcillin), gentamicin, and other antibiotics is becoming more common in nurseries.

Colonization of infants in the nursery with *S. aureus* ranges from < 10 to 70% or more. Since different strains vary markedly in virulence, the probability of disease occurring in colonized infants also varies greatly, and a high colonization rate per se is not an indication for instituting specific control measures. In fact, colonization by a noninvasive strain may interfere with colonization by disease-producing strains. Therefore, culturing for surveillance should be undertaken only if the nursery is experiencing an outbreak of disease (ie, a rate significantly greater than the baseline rate) due to *S. aureus.* Since most such infections appear after the infant has left the nursery, a surveillance system to assess infections occurring within the first month of life should be established with the community's infant health care providers.

Although nursery personnel who are *S. aureus* nasal carriers and disseminators are potential sources of infection for infants, colonized infants in the nursery are usually the reservoir; **transmission** is from infant to infant via the transiently colonized hands of personnel. The umbilical stump and groin are most frequently colonized during the first few days of life, while the nares are more frequently colonized later.

Skin care for newborns may affect colonization patterns. Bathing infants with 3% hexachlorophene decreases frequency of *S. aureus* colonization, but *routine* use of this product is inadvisable because of its potential neurotoxicity, particularly in low-birth-weight infants. The American Academy of Pediatrics recommends dry skin care for infants, but in some hospitals this has resulted in high rates of colonization with *S. aureus* and epidemics of disease. During disease outbreaks, application of Triple Dye® to the cord area or bacitracin or mupirocin ointment to the cord and/or nares and circumcision site helps reduce colonization. Hospitals troubled with *S. aureus* disease may temporarily institute daily bathing of the diaper area of each term infant with 3% hexachlorophene emulsion, which should then be rinsed off. Routine cultures of either personnel or the environment are not recommended.

Special-Care Nurseries

Infants in special-care nurseries often are sick, preterm, and of low birth weight. They require numerous supportive invasive procedures and frequently receive antimicrobial therapy. Because of the widespread use of antimicrobial agents in these nurseries, the bacterial flora colonizing the preterm and sick infants tends to be the predominantly gram-negative organisms prevalent there (eg, *Klebsiella, Enterobacter, Pseudomonas*, and *Proteus*), which frequently are resistant to multiple antibiotics.

Organisms are transmitted via the hands of personnel and material used in the multiple invasive procedures these infants undergo; eg, long-term arterial and venous catheterization for intravascular pressure monitoring, parenteral nutrition, or access for fluids, medicine, or blood sampling; endotracheal intubation with ventilatory assistance or continuous airway pressure; and nasogastric or nasojejunal feeding tubes for alimentation. All these procedures have been implicated as causes of epidemic or endemic nosocomial infections. **Prevention** of colonization and infection requires provision of sufficient space (80 to 100 sq ft/infant in intensive care, 50 sq ft/infant in intermediate care, 6 ft between incubators or warmers, edge-to-edge in each direction) and personnel (nurse:patient ratio 1:1 to 2 in intensive care, 1:3 to 4 in intermediate care); knowledge of recommended methods for patient care (including techniques for placement and care of invasive devices); and meticulous cleaning and disinfection or sterilization of equipment after each use between infants. Active surveillance for infection (not colonization) and monitoring of procedure methods are essential.

Since **nosocomial infection rates** vary markedly by birth weight, calculation of birth-weight–specific rates (ie, rates of infection for birth-weight groups ≤ 1000 gm, 1001 to 1500 gm, 1501 to 2500 gm, and > 2500 gm) is a useful monitoring tool. The length of stay in special-care nurseries often is a good predictor of infection; the number of infant-days in the unit rather than the number of infants admitted or discharged can be used as the denominator in calculating infection rates (ie, number of infections/1000 infant-days in the unit). Since many infections result from invasive procedures, calculation of procedure-specific rates (eg, bloodstream infection rate/1000 intravascular-line–days or pneumonia rate/1000 ventilator-days) may facilitate comparison of infection rates over time and identification of areas in which more intensive investigation or prevention efforts are needed.

While establishing a strict cohort of infected or colonized babies may be necessary during outbreaks, it is impractical as a routine measure in most special-care nurseries. However, many infected infants can be cared for in these units if personnel follow appropriate **isolation technique,** including the use of gowns (to prevent contamination of uniforms and forearms) and gloves (when touching lesions or handling items potentially contaminated with infectious secretions or excretions). With the increased concern in recent years about blood-borne infections (eg, hepatitis B virus, HIV), the concept of universal blood and body fluid precautions has become widely accepted. With **universal precautions,** the blood and certain body fluids of *all* patients are considered potentially infectious, and appropriate precautions are used. Body fluids are those that may contain a blood-borne infectious agent or may be contaminated with blood, eg, cerebrospinal, synovial, pleural, peritoneal, pericardial, or amniotic fluid; semen; and vaginal secretions. Forced-air incubators provide limited protective isolation but should not be relied upon to prevent transmission from an infected infant; the exteriors and interiors of the units rapidly become heavily contaminated, and personnel are likely to contaminate their hands and forearms while working with the infants in the incubators.

Prophylaxis: Although frequently used, nonspecific antibiotic prophylactic therapy is *not* effective, hastens development of resistant bacteria in the nursery, alters the balance of normal flora in the infant, and predisposes the infant to colonization with more resistant strains. Routine prophylactic antimicrobial therapy is recommended only for prevention of gonorrheal ophthalmia neonatorum (see NEONATAL CONJUNCTIVITIS, below) or complicated gonococcal infection in exposed infants. Antibiotics against specific pathogens may be considered under special circumstances; eg, penicillin G for prophylaxis against Group A streptococcal infection or oral colistin or neomycin for prophylaxis against enterotoxigenic or enteropathogenic *E. coli* during a confirmed nursery epidemic. Prophylaxis for neonatal hepatitis B virus is discussed below, under NEONATAL HEPATITIS B VIRUS INFECTION.

An infant who remains in the hospital > 2 mo should be immunized against diphtheria, tetanus, and pertussis according to the routine schedule for adjusted age (see IMMUNIZATION PROCEDURES THROUGHOUT CHILDHOOD in Ch. 23). To avoid cross infection with other infants in the nursery, oral (live virus) polio vaccine should not be given in the hospital.

Screening blood prior to transfusions is now routinely done to detect units that may be contaminated with HIV (see HUMAN IMMUNODEFICIENCY VIRUS INFECTION IN CHILDREN in Ch. 32). Infants born to cytomegalovirus (**CMV**)-seronegative mothers are at risk for serious infection or death if transfused with CMV-positive blood; every effort should be made to transfuse infants with only CMV-negative blood or components (see CONGENITAL AND PERINATAL CYTOMEGALOVIRUS INFECTION, below).

Routine practices for nursery personnel include active surveillance for infections; knowledge of disease transmission; provision of sufficient space (in the term nursery, 30 sq ft of floor space/bassinet, and in the admission-observation nursery, 40 sq ft/bassinet, with a minimum of 3 ft between bassinets, edge-to-edge in each direction) and personnel (1 nurse/6 to 8 term infants requiring routine care); and thorough handwashing between infant contacts. Providing each infant with its own supplies and equipment (eg, stethoscope) in a separate bassinet reduces the risk for cross-contamination. Since airborne transmission of disease in a nursery is relatively uncommon, infants with various infections may be cared for in a general nursery if personnel are meticulous in techniques to avoid transmission between infants, as described above. The environs of infants with diarrhea or draining skin lesions may be heavily contaminated; a separate room for these infants is desirable. Similarly, a separate room or establishment of a strict cohort is desirable for infants with many types of congenital infection (CMV, rubella, syphilis) or those with potentially serious and transmissible viral infections (herpes simplex, respiratory syncytial, adeno- or enterovirus infection).

Nursery personnel should wear short-sleeved scrub clothes provided and laundered by the hospital, but long-sleeved gowns are recommended for handling infants outside incubators and bassinets. Caps, beard bags, and masks are recommended, and sterile gloves are essential only during invasive procedures, such as inserting an umbilical catheter. *Handwashing is the keystone to infection control in the nursery.* At the start of a shift, personnel should scrub hands and forearms to the elbows. Between handling infants, a vigorous 15-sec wash with an antiseptic agent is recommended (vigorous washing is more important than the antiseptic agent chosen). Disposable gloves may limit hand contamination when working with infected infants or contaminated items. Jewelry should not be worn on duty.

Personnel with respiratory tract infections (including pharyngitis), furuncles, draining skin lesions, diarrhea, or fever should not work with infants. Those with *active* nasolabial herpes preferably should not work with infants, but the risk of compromising patient care by excluding essential personnel must be weighed against that of infecting an infant. Personnel with chronic dermatitis on their hands should be individually evaluated. Serologic tests for rubella should be performed on all personnel; susceptible women should be counseled about the risk of infection and offered rubella vaccine or the option of working in another area during pregnancy. No evidence of increased risk of cytomegalovirus transmission for nursery personnel has been reported.

Encouraging mothers to room-in with their infants and establishing alternative birth centers as part of the delivery facility can enhance the birth experience without increasing the risk of infection to mother or infant, when instituted with care. Having sufficient personnel is important (1 nurse/3 mother-infant pairs for rooming-in). The presence of siblings at the birth and liberal visiting policies with the mother (eg, in a family lounge or private room) should be encouraged; only visitors with active infectious illness should be excluded.

In an epidemic, establishing cohorts of diseased or colonized infants and assigning them a separate nursing staff is useful; unexposed infants may be discharged early or may room-in with their mothers rather than be admitted to the nursery. Continuing surveillance of infants for 1 mo after discharge is necessary for assessing the adequacy of controls instituted to abort an epidemic.

NEONATAL CONJUNCTIVITIS
(Conjunctivitis Neonatorum; Ophthalmia Neonatorum)

Purulent ocular drainage is common during the neonatal period. The major causes are, in decreasing order, chemical injury, chlamydial infection, and bacterial infection. Chemical conjunctivitis is generally secondary to the instillation of silver nitrate drops for ocular prophylaxis. *Chlamydia trachomatis,* the most common infectious cause of neonatal conjunctivitis, accounts for the disease in 2 to 4% of live births. Chlamydial inclusion conjunctivitis (inclusion blennorrhea), acquired by the infant during parturition, may account for 30 to 50% of all cases of conjunctivitis seen in infants < 4 wk of age. The prevalence of maternal chlamydial infection ranges from 2 to 20%. About 33% of infants born to affected women develop conjunctivitis and 10% develop pneumonia. Other bacteria, including *Streptococcus pneumoniae* and *Hemophilus influenzae,* account for another 15% of all cases of neonatal conjunctivitis. The incidence of ophthalmia neonatorum in the USA due to *Neisseria gonorrhoeae* is 2 to 3/10,000 live births. Isolation of bacteria other than *H. influenzae* and *N. gonorrhoeae,* including *Staphylococcus aureus,* usually represents colonization rather than infection. The major viral agent that causes neonatal conjunctivitis is herpes simplex virus (HSV) types 1 and 2.

Clinical Presentation

The different types of neonatal conjunctivitis are difficult to distinguish on clinical grounds alone, because they overlap in both presentation and onset. Chemical conjunctivitis secondary to silver nitrate usually appears within 6 to 8 h after instillation and disappears spontaneously within 24 to 48 h. Gonorrheal ophthalmia produces an acute purulent conjunctivitis that appears 2 to 5 days after birth or earlier if there has been premature rupture of membranes. The infant has severe eyelid edema followed by chemosis and a profuse purulent exudate that may spurt out of the lids when they are separated. If treatment is delayed, corneal ulcerations may occur. Inclusion conjunctivitis due to C. trachomatis usually occurs 5 to 14 days after birth. It may range from mild conjunctivitis with minimal mucopurulent discharge to severe edema of the eyelids with copious drainage and pseudomembrane formation. Follicles are not present in the conjunctiva in neonates with this infection, as they are in older children and adults. The onset of conjunctivitis following infection with other bacteria is extremely variable, ranging from 4 days to 3 wk. Keratoconjunctivitis due to HSV can occur as an isolated infection or with disseminated or CNS infection. Herpetic conjunctivitis can be mistaken for bacterial or chemical conjunctivitis, but the presence of dendritic keratitis is pathognomonic.

Diagnosis

The first diagnostic procedure should be a culture and Gram stain of a conjunctival specimen. *Gonococcal infection must be ruled out.* The presence of intracellular gram-negative, coffee-bean–shaped diplococci suggests gonococcal infection. Cultures should be placed on appropriate media (eg, Thayer-Martin) for isolating *N. gonorrhoeae.* Examining the Gram stain also helps to suggest other bacterial pathogens. In chlamydial infection, a smear of the conjunctiva should show a predominantly mononuclear reaction with no organisms.

The most sensitive means of diagnosing chlamydial ophthalmia is isolation of *C. trachomatis* in tissue culture. Cultures of the conjunctiva can be obtained by firmly stroking the everted lower eyelid with a cotton or Dacron swab. Two types of nonculture diagnostic tests are commercially available: direct monoclonal antibody tests, which detect chlamydiae in smears of purulent exudate, and enzyme-linked immunoassays. Both appear to be very sensitive and specific for detecting chlamydiae in conjunctival specimens.

The diagnosis of herpetic conjunctivitis can best be confirmed by isolating the virus, detecting specific HSV-1 or HSV-2 antigen by immunofluorescence in conjunctival scrapings, or identifying HSV particles by electron microscopic evaluation.

Prophylaxis

Routine use of 1% silver nitrate, erythromycin, or tetracycline ophthalmic ointments or drops instilled into each eye after delivery is recommended by the Centers for Disease Control for prevention of neonatal **gonococcal conjunctivitis**. Although it had been suggested that ocular prophylaxis with erythromycin ointment would also prevent chlamydial conjunctivitis, recent studies have not confirmed this. Neither erythromycin nor tetracycline nor silver nitrate will prevent neonatal **chlamydial conjunctivitis**. Since infants born to mothers with untreated gonorrhea are at increased risk for infections at other sites, full-term exposed infants should be treated prophylactically with a single injection IM or IV of ceftriaxone 50 mg/kg, up to 125 mg. Penicillin is no longer the first-line drug for treatment of gonococcal infections, because high rates of penicillinase-producing *N. gonorrhoeae* are found in many areas.

Treatment

For **gonorrheal ophthalmia**, the infant should be hospitalized and given ceftriaxone 125 mg IM as a single dose. Frequent irrigation of the eye with saline prevents secretions from adhering. Topical antimicrobial preparations alone are not sufficient and are not required if appropriate systemic antibiotic therapy is given. Conjunctivitis due to other bacteria usually responds to topical ointments containing polymyxin plus bacitracin, erythromycin, or tetracycline. Since at least $1/2$ of the infants with **chlamydial conjunctivitis** also have nasopharyngeal infection and some develop chlamydial pneumonia, systemic therapy is preferable to topical therapy. Erythromycin ethylsuccinate 50 mg/kg/day orally in divided doses q 6 or 8 h for 10 days to 2 wk is recommended. **HSV conjunctivitis** should be treated (*in association with an ophthalmologist*) with trifluridine ophthalmic drops or ointment q 2 to 3 h while the infant is awake and in combination with idoxuridine ointment at bedtime, until 3 to 5 days after healing appears to be complete. If there is no response within 7 to 8 days, therapy with systemic acyclovir should be considered. Specific diagnosis is important. Since ointments containing steroids may seriously exacerbate eye infections due to *C. trachomatis* and HSV, they should be avoided in neonates.

ACUTE INFECTIOUS NEONATAL DIARRHEA

(See also ACUTE INFECTIOUS GASTROENTERITIS under BACTERIAL INFECTIONS in Ch. 32)

A syndrome characterized by passage of unformed stool with increased frequency; it is often associated with vomiting and usually caused by bacteria or viruses. Although these manifestations are common to many disorders, including a variety of noninfectious causes (eg, anatomic, metabolic and enzymatic, inflammatory), infection is by far the most common cause during the neonatal period.

Etiology and Epidemiology

Newborns are relatively protected from acute infectious diarrhea since they are usually cared for with better hygienic practices than are older infants and children. However, where poor hygiene prevails, or in poor and crowded families, diarrhea can be found more frequently. Nosocomial outbreaks may occur, especially in overcrowded nurseries. The transmission is almost exclusively fecal-oral. Newborns are mostly infected by pathogens ingested during passage through a contaminated birth canal or acquired from the contaminated hands of patients, parents, siblings, or nursery personnel. Other less common sources are fomites and contaminated formulas. Occasionally, airborne infection is suspected, especially when viral outbreaks occur.

The incidence and relative frequency of the various pathogens causing neonatal infectious diarrhea have not been determined, but any infectious organism causing diarrhea in older infants and children may also cause diarrhea in neonates. The most commonly reported associated organisms derive from nursery outbreaks and include bacteria (eg, *Escherichia coli, Salmonella* spp, and *Campylobacter jejuni*) and viruses, especially rotaviruses. Less commonly reported agents are bacteria such as *Shigella* spp, *Yersinia enterocolitica, Klebsiella* spp, Pseudomonas spp, and *Proteus* spp and viruses such as enteric adeno-, entero-, and coronaviruses. The role of Norwalk-like agents and astro- and caliciviruses in neonatal diarrhea is not established.

It is important to note that although rotaviruses are important pathogens in newborns, they are often found in asymptomatic neonates. Parasites (eg, *Giardia lamblia, Entamoeba histolytica*) are rare in neonates. Although *Clostridium difficile* and its toxin may often be isolated from infants during the first weeks of life, the organism is only rarely associated with postantibiotic diarrhea (pseudomembranous enterocolitis) in neonates.

Symptoms, Signs, and Complications

GI infections, clinically presenting as diarrhea, often accompanied by vomiting, can cause a rapidly progressive serious illness in newborns. Normal stools of breast-fed newborns are similar to those that occur with diarrhea. **Common complications** that should be of concern in every neonate with infectious diarrhea are (1) dehydration, (2) electrolyte imbalance, and (3) bacteremia or septicemia.

Mild dehydration ($\leq 5\%$) may be manifested by dry oral mucous membranes only. When **moderate dehydration** occurs (7 to 10%), decreased skin turgor and sunken eyes and fontanelles may be found. **Severe dehydration** ($> 10\%$) is usually accompanied by hemodynamic changes consistent with hypovolemic shock. Oliguria usually does not appear until a late phase of dehydration, since mechanisms of renal concentration in neonates are immature. **Electrolyte imbalance and metabolic acidosis** often accompany dehydration in neonates and young infants. Dehydration with electrolyte imbalance may cause alterations in the infant's behavior (lethargy or irritability) or other more rare complications (eg, arrhythmia, intracranial hemorrhage, renal vein thrombosis).

The macroscopic appearance of the stool suggests the nature of the causative organisms but is not diagnostic. Bloody stools and mucus suggest colitis, usually caused by enteroinvasive *E. coli* **(EIEC)**, *Salmonella* spp, *Shigella* spp, or *C. jejuni*. In contrast, watery and voluminous stools that continue to be passed even while the infant is fasting suggest secretory diarrhea caused by enterotoxigenic bacteria (eg, enterotoxigenic *E. coli* **[ETEC]**) or by viruses (eg, rotavirus). Watery diarrhea that remits with fasting suggests secondary lactase deficiency. Bacteremia secondary to gastroenteritis caused either by enteric pathogens (eg, *Salmonella* spp, *Shigella* spp, or *Campylobacter*) or by normal enteric inhabitants may occur and may cause septicemia or focal infections. Symptoms of septicemia are often subtle and nonspecific (see Neonatal Sepsis, below). Necrotizing enterocolitis may also occur as a complication of bacterial or viral gastroenteritis (see below).

Laboratory Diagnosis

Microscopic examination of fresh stool specimens is useful; to prepare a slide for microscopic examination, one usually mixes fresh mucus from stool with a drop of normal saline and methylene blue. Evidence of fecal WBCs provides information that may suggest the nature and extent of the mucosal inflammation and the type of pathogen. Fecal WBCs are produced in response to bacteria that invade the colonic mucosa (eg, *Shigella*, *Salmonella*, EIEC, *Campylobacter*, or *Y. enterocolitica*); *G. lamblia* cysts or trophozoites may also be seen.

In nursery outbreaks, **stool cultures** are important, especially since knowledge of the causative organism and its antibiotic sensitivity may help in early treatment and prevention of new cases. Cultures should also be taken from the medical personnel and other contacts, including parents. Seriously ill neonates should be evaluated for systemic infections, and therefore **CSF, blood, and urine cultures** should be obtained.

Reducing substances and stool pH should be tested in freshly passed watery stool; pH of < 6 and the presence of reducing substances may help to diagnose sugar malabsorption due to mucosal damage or, very rarely, primary lactase deficiency. However, conditions such as breast-feeding and antibiotic therapy may result in decreased pH or positive reducing substances in stool.

Microscopic examination and standard stool culture provide the diagnosis in a minority of cases. Other more specific tests extend the diagnosis of enteric pathogens. **Special cultures** are useful for isolating *Y. enterocolitica*, *Vibrio cholerae*, *C. difficile*, *Aeromonas*, and others; **immunoassays** (eg, ELISA, latex agglutination) may provide a variety of diagnoses (eg, rotavirus, other viral antigens, and enterotoxins); and **serotyping** of *E. coli* may help to characterize ETEC, EIEC, enteropathogenic *E. coli* (*EPEC*), enterohemorrhagic *E. coli* (*EHEC*), etc. (Suckling mouse assay, gene probe hybridization assay, rabbit ileal loop assay for invasiveness, cell culture cytotoxicity, electron microscopy, and others help to characterize various enteropathogens and enterotoxins. Unfortunately most of these tests are still performed only in research laboratories.) **Proctosigmoidoscopy** may help to diagnose pseudomembranous enterocolitis.

The WBC count and differential are important, because they may suggest an invading process, but are of little help in differentiating between the various enteric pathogens. **Serum electrolytes,**

BUN, and creatinine are important as guidelines for fluid and electrolyte therapy.

Treatment

Fluid and electrolyte therapy is the primary and most urgent step. Infants who look toxic or have profuse diarrhea and persistent vomiting, refuse to drink, have unreliable parents or caretakers, or have underlying illness must be hospitalized and often require parenteral fluids. Emergency fluid replacement may be given in some cases through bone marrow or peritoneum when peripheral or central IV access is impossible. Unless the infant has one or more of the severe problems mentioned above, oral fluid replacement and maintenance are indicated. Oral therapy should consist of rapid rehydration with replacement of ongoing losses during the first day or two with a glucose-electrolyte or oral rehydration solution **(ORS)** that can be given in the hospital or at home. Commercially available ORSs are preferable to those prepared at home.

The **World Health Organization solution (WHO-ORS)** contains 90 mEq/L of sodium, 20 mEq/L of potassium, and 2% glucose concentration. Other commercial ORSs (eg, Pedialyte®, Lytren®, Infalyte®, and others) usually contain less sodium than the WHO-ORS but equivalent amounts of potassium and carbohydrate, and therefore have decreased osmolarity. Such solutions may be preferable for newborns, especially during the first 2 wk of life, since the kidneys of newborns are deficient in sodium regulation. Breast-feeding may be continued while giving ORS. When moderate-to-severe dehydration exists, or in neonates with initially abnormal serum electrolytes, the serum pH, electrolytes, and BUN should be monitored q 12 to 24 h during the rehydration phase. Special attention should be paid to development of hypernatremia.

Diet: Early restoration of feeding is important to prevent acute malnutrition. Breast-feeding should be resumed as soon as possible. The non-breast-fed infant should be offered a lactose-free formula immediately after initial rehydration and stabilization with either IV solution or ORS. Milk or formula can be resumed gradually a few days later, but if diarrhea recurs, the lactose-free formula should be readministered for several weeks. If protracted diarrhea (lasting > 2 wk) occurs, elemental or casein-hydrolysate formulas, and sometimes the addition of IV alimentation, are often required. In parallel, a search for primary or secondary causes of noninfectious prolonged diarrhea (eg, cystic fibrosis, allergic enteropathy, protein intolerance) must be undertaken.

Antimicrobials are not usually needed in acute bacterial gastroenteritis, since the disease is often self-limited. However, in neonates, preventing systemic spread of enteric pathogens and secondary invasion of normal enteric inhabitants is an important goal. Drug susceptibility of enteric pathogens varies among different geographic regions and even during different periods in the same area.

Shigella infections should be treated with parenteral ampicillin 50 to 100 mg/kg/day for 5 to 7 days. If an ampicillin-resistant strain is isolated or prevails in the community and a drug is to be given before sensitivity is known, trimethoprim/sulfamethoxazole **(TMP/SMX)** 10/50 mg/kg/day orally or IV should be given in 2 divided doses. During the very first days of life, sulfa drugs may be contraindicated because of their ability to increase jaundice. Unfortunately, many worldwide reports indicate resistance of *Shigella* to both TMP/SMX and ampicillin. In such cases, newborns should initially be given a 3rd-generation cephalosporin (eg, cefotaxime, ceftriaxone). In very ill infants, in whom sepsis is suspected, parenteral 3rd-generation cephalosporins are indicated.

Antibiotics usually are not helpful in *Salmonella* **gastroenteritis.** However, since *Salmonella* tends to cause bacteremia, owing to its invasive properties, all neonates with *Salmonella* gastroenteritis should receive antibiotic treatment. Ampicillin 50 to 100 mg/kg/day can be used to treat susceptible strains. Chloramphenicol should be avoided in neonates unless serum level monitoring is available. Most *Salmonella* strains are sensitive to 3rd-generation cephalosporins, and these drugs are effective against systemic *Salmonella* infections. The treatment for gastroenteritis is 5 to 7 days. For **systemic infections,** a more prolonged treatment (10 to 14 days) is needed. Many neonates will become asymptomatic carriers after successful treatment. There is no need to treat such patients. However, enteric precautions (see below) should be carried out throughout the hospitalization.

Campylobacter **gastroenteritis** usually responds to oral erythromycin estolate 30 to 40 mg/kg/day in 3 divided doses for 5 days but only if given during the early phase of illness. When bacteremia is suspected, addition of parenteral gentamicin 5 to 7.5 mg/kg/day is recommended. No data are available for the efficacy of antibiotic therapy of other invasive bacteria (eg, *Yersinia* or

EIEC) in neonates. However, these organisms are usually sensitive to aminoglycosides and 3rd-generation cephalosporins, and neonates with such invasive enteric infections should receive parenteral antibiotics. In **noninvasive bacterial diarrhea**, such as caused by EPEC or ETEC, oral colistin 15 mg/kg/day in 3 divided doses or oral gentamicin 10 to 20 mg/kg/day in 3 divided doses may be given. This is especially important in nursery outbreaks for reducing spread of enteropathogens.

Any attempt to alter the course of neonatal gastroenteritis with antiperistaltic or antidiarrheal agents is contraindicated. Impairment of bowel motility not only potentiates persistent colonization of the host with enteropathogens, but also permits significant sequestration of fluid in the bowel, masking the seriousness of dehydration by decreasing the number of stools and preventing accurate monitoring of weight.

Enteric precautions must be very carefully kept, particularly handwashing and establishing cohorts of contacts. These precautions should be followed even for culture-negative cases, since a minority of pathogens are identified by routine laboratory procedures. Epidemiologic investigation must be initiated in the event of a nursery outbreak.

NEONATAL SEPSIS
(Sepsis Neonatorum)

Invasive bacterial infection occurring in the first 4 wk of life. Bacterial infection, the primary cause in up to 30% of neonatal deaths, occurs 5 times more often in low-birth-weight **(LBW)** newborns than in full-term newborns.

Neonatal sepsis occurs in from 0.5 to 8.0/1000 live births; the highest rates occur in LBW newborns, those with depressed respiratory function at birth, and those with maternal perinatal risk factors. The risk is greater in males (2:1) and in neonates with congenital malformations, particularly of the GU tract.

A newborn may be predisposed to neonatal sepsis by obstetric complications, eg, premature rupture of the membranes **(PROM)** occurring 12 to ≥ 24 h before birth (or as little as 6 h before, if accompanied by active labor), maternal bleeding (placenta previa, abruptio placentae), toxemia, precipitous delivery, or maternal infection (particularly of the urinary tract or endometrium, most commonly manifested as maternal fever shortly before or during parturition). **Early-onset neonatal sepsis** is clinically apparent within 6 h of birth in > 50% of cases; the great majority

present within the first 72 h of life. **Late-onset neonatal sepsis** usually presents after 4 days of age and includes nosocomially acquired infections.

Until recently, advances in antimicrobial therapy and supportive care have not significantly altered the overall mortality rate of either early-onset (15 to 50%) or late-onset (10 to 20%) neonatal sepsis. The fatality rate is twice as high in LBW as in full-term neonates.

Etiology

Before 1940, Group A β-hemolytic streptococcus was the major cause of neonatal sepsis; it was subsequently replaced by gram-negative enteric bacilli. Coagulase-positive staphylococci caused nursery epidemics in the late 1950s. During the 1960s, coliforms returned to prominence (perhaps in part because of the routine use of hexachlorophene in bathing), with *Escherichia coli* (predominantly those containing the K1 polysaccharide capsule) being the most common cause of neonatal sepsis. In the 1970s, Group B streptococcus **(GBS, Streptococcus agalactiae)** emerged as the most common cause of early-onset neonatal sepsis. In the 1980s, both GBS and gram-negative enteric organisms were the most common pathogens, accounting for 70% of early-onset sepsis.

Other gram-negative enteric bacilli (eg, *Klebsiella* spp) and gram-positive organisms—*Listeria monocytogenes,* Group D streptococci (enterococci, eg, *Enterococcus faecalis* and *E. faecium,* and nonenterococci, eg, *S. bovis* and *S. mitis*) and more recently, α-hemolytic streptococci of respiratory origin—account for most other invasive bacterial infections leading to sepsis. *S. pneumoniae, Hemophilus influenzae* (both nontypeable and type b), and less commonly, *Neisseria meningitidis* have been isolated more frequently in such cases in recent years. *N. gonorrhoeae* should be considered in evaluating a septic neonate, since asymptomatic gonorrhea occurs in 5 to 10% of pregnancies. Because an infected newborn is at risk for both ophthalmia neonatorum and disseminated gonococcal disease, endocervical cultures should be performed routinely during pregnancy and at delivery to identify mothers and infants requiring therapy.

The role of anaerobes (particularly *Bacteroides fragilis,* which requires special culture media for identification) in neonatal sepsis remains unclear, although neonatal deaths have been attributed to *Bacteroides* bacteremia. Anaerobes may account for some culture-negative cases, in which autopsy findings indicate sepsis, and should be suspected when foul-smelling amniotic fluid is present at birth.

The above-mentioned pathogens predominate in early-onset sepsis occurring in nurseries in North America. In other areas of the world, different pathogens (*L. monocytogenes* in Spain and *Salmonella* spp in Latin America) may be much more prominent.

Early-onset **GBS infection** may present in a fulminating, primarily bacteremic and pulmonic form caused by serotypes Ia, Ib, Ic, II, and III. The incidence of associated obstetric complications (particularly prematurity, prolonged rupture of the membranes, and chorioamnionitis) is high. In > 50% of infants, GBS infection presents within 6 h of birth; 45% have an Apgar score of < 5. The mortality rate for these infants is 50 to 85%. Meningitis is frequently absent. Late-onset GBS infection occurs at 1 to 12 wk (occasionally later) and is usually caused by serotype III. It is commonly associated with meningitis and has a mortality rate of about 20%. This form is generally not associated with perinatal risk factors nor with demonstrable maternal cervical colonization; even when the mother is colonized, it may not be with the same serotype as that affecting the baby. Thus, postnatal acquisition of the organism may be responsible for many of these cases.

Neonatal sepsis due to *L. monocytogenes* also may occur in an early- or late-onset form. In the early-onset form, infants present with respiratory distress and shock, with a fulminant course within the first several days of life. This form primarily involves the lungs but may disseminate, with granuloma formation in the liver (granulomatosis infantiseptica). The late-onset form, as with that of GBS infection, is frequently associated with meningitis and has a better prognosis.

E. coli is the most common **gram-negative enteric organism** causing early-onset neonatal sepsis; 40% of these pathogens causing septicemia and 80% of those causing meningitis possess the K1 capsular antigen, a virulence factor for *E. coli*.

The organisms derived from the environment that cause late-onset sepsis have a distinct bacteriologic profile. The nosocomial infection rate for newborns hospitalized for ≥ 48 h in a regional newborn intensive care unit may be as high as 25%. *Staphylococcus aureus* and gram-negative enteric bacilli (particularly *Klebsiella* spp, *E. coli*, *Proteus* spp, and *Pseudomonas aeruginosa*), as well as enterococci and *Candida* spp, had until recently been the predominant pathogens. However, *S. epidermidis* now accounts for up to 30% of late-onset cases and is most frequently associated with indwelling plastic intravascular devices (eg, umbilical artery or vein catheters, Broviac catheters). Usually, nosocomial infections are sporadic, but epidemics do occur and may be due to multiply resistant organisms (eg, *K. pneumoniae*, *Enterobacter cloacae*, *S. aureus*). The isolation of *E. cloacae* or *E. sakazakii* from blood or CSF should suggest contaminated feedings. Contaminated respiratory equipment should be suspected in nosocomial *P. aeruginosa* pneumonia or sepsis. Late-onset neonatal sepsis or meningitis due to *Flavobacterium meningosepticum* suggests colonization of objects containing, or in regular contact with, water.

In addition, certain **viral infections** (eg, disseminated herpes simplex, entero-, adeno-, and respiratory syncytial virus) may present as either early- or late-onset neonatal sepsis, with symptoms and signs indistinguishable from those produced by bacterial sepsis.

Pathogenesis

The clustering of neonatal bacterial infections in the perinatal period suggests that pathogens are usually acquired in utero during labor or delivery. Hematogenous and transplacental dissemination of maternal infection occurs in the transmission of viral (eg, rubella, cytomegalovirus, HIV), protozoal (eg, *Toxoplasma gondii*), and treponemal (eg, *Treponema pallidum*) agents. A few bacterial pathogens (eg, *L. monocytogenes*, *Mycobacterium tuberculosis*) may reach the fetus transplacentally, but most are acquired by the ascending route in utero or as the fetus passes through the colonized birth canal.

The intensity of maternal colonization is directly related to risk for invasive disease in the newborn. However, a significant number of mothers with low-density colonization give birth to infants with high-intensity colonization who are therefore at risk. The facilitated growth of GBS and *E. coli* in amniotic fluid contaminated with meconium or vernix, allowing the small number of organisms in the vaginal vault to rapidly proliferate as PROM proceeds, may contribute to this paradox. Organisms may invade the fetal circulation by contaminating superficial chorionic vessels, but more commonly they reach the bloodstream by fetal aspiration or swallowing of contaminated amniotic fluid and subsequent bacteremia. The ascending route of infection helps to explain such phenomena as the high incidence of PROM in neonatal infections, the significance of adnexal inflammation (amnionitis is more commonly associated with neonatal sepsis than is central placentitis), the increased risk of infection to the twin closer to the birth canal, and the bacteriologic characteristics of neonatal sepsis, which reflect the flora of the maternal vaginal vault.

Foci of infection, which become established in the paranasal sinuses, middle ear, lungs, or GI tract, may be disseminated to meninges, kidneys, bones, joints, peritoneum, and skin. Pneumonia is the most common invasive bacterial infection in the neonate.

Newborns (particularly those of LBW) are immunologically immature and are ill-suited to defend against the polymicrobial flora to which they are exposed during and after parturition. The role of passively acquired IgG antibody in protecting the fetus is vividly demonstrated by GBS infections. Virtually every infant with GBS infection has low levels of transplacentally acquired, type-specific IgG antibodies because its mother lacks those antibodies. Certain bacterial virulence factors (eg, GBS serotype III polysaccharide and the K1 antigen of *E. coli*) seem to play a role, particularly in producing meningitis. Most important, perhaps, are certain deficiencies in neonatal host defense related to birth weight; ie, birth weight is directly related to both heat-stable (type-specific antibodies) and heat-labile (complement) opsonins, producing a defect in opsonization efficiency. Further, neonatal polymorphonuclear leukocytes (PMNs) demonstrate decreased chemotaxis, opsonization, phagocytosis, deformability, and intracellular bacterial killing as well as depressed oxidative responses; neonatal monocytes have decreased chemotaxis and cytotoxic function. (See also IMMUNOLOGIC STATUS OF THE FETUS AND NEWBORN in Ch. 23.)

Risk factors for nosocomial infection include associated illnesses (which may be only a marker for the use of invasive supportive techniques), exposure to antimicrobial agents (which "selects" resistant bacterial strains), prolonged hospitalization, contaminated laboratory support equipment, IV or enteral solutions, and most important, prolonged use of intravascular plastic catheters. The gram-positive organisms (eg, *S. epidermidis* and *S. aureus*) may be introduced from the environment or the patient's skin. Gram-negative enteric bacteria are almost always derived from the patient's endogenous flora, which may have been altered by antecedent antibiotic therapy or populated by resistant organisms transferred from the hands of personnel or contaminated equipment. The major means of spread in the newborn nursery for all of these organisms is via the hands of nursery personnel. Therefore, situations that increase exposure of the neonate to these bacteria (eg, crowding, high nurse:newborn ratios, and inadequate handwashing) result in higher nosocomial infection rates in the newborn nursery.

Symptoms and Signs

Because the newborn can respond to perinatal insults in only a few ways, the early signs of neonatal sepsis are frequently nonspecific and subtle. Diminished spontaneous activity, less vigorous sucking, apnea, bradycardia, and temperature instability (hypo- or hyperthermia) are particularly common. Other symptoms and signs include respiratory distress, neurologic findings (eg, seizures, jitteriness), jaundice (especially occurring within the first 24 h of life without Rh or ABO blood group incompatibility and with a higher than expected direct bilirubin concentration), vomiting, diarrhea, and abdominal distention.

Specific signs of an infected organ may pinpoint the primary source or a metastatic site. Most infants with early-onset GBS infection present with respiratory distress that is difficult to distinguish from hyaline membrane disease. Examination of the ears, preferably with pneumatic otoscopy, may identify otitis media (frequently underdiagnosed in the newborn). The maxillary and anterior ethmoid sinuses may also be clinically infected in newborns. Periumbilical erythema, discharge, or bleeding in a newborn without a hemorrhagic diathesis suggests omphalitis (infection prevents obliteration of the umbilical vessels). Coma, seizures, opisthotonos, or a bulging fontanelle signals severe CNS dysfunction and suggests meningitis or brain abscess. Decreased spontaneous movement of one extremity and/or swelling, warmth, erythema, or tenderness over a joint indicate osteomyelitis or pyogenic arthritis. Unexplained abdominal distention may indicate peritonitis or necrotizing enterocolitis (particularly when accompanied by bloody diarrhea and fecal leukocytes). Cutaneous vesicles, mouth ulcers, and/or hepatosplenomegaly (particularly with disseminated intravascular coagulation—DIC) could identify disseminated herpes simplex.

Diagnosis

Early diagnosis is important and requires awareness of risk factors (particularly in LBW newborns) and a high index of suspicion when any newborn deviates from the norm in the first few weeks of life. Remarks by nurses or parents that the newborn is "not doing well" or any overt or subtle signs of sepsis should prompt investigation. The following laboratory tests can provide helpful diagnostic information.

WBC count, differential, and smear: The normal WBC count in the newborn varies, but values < 4,000 or > 25,000 are abnormal. The absolute band count is not sensitive enough to be a useful predictor of neonatal sepsis. A ratio of immature:total PMNs of < 0.2 accurately predicts the absence of bacterial sepsis. A precipitous fall in a known absolute eosinophil count, as well as morphologic changes in neutrophils (toxic granulation, Döhle bodies, and intracytoplasmic vacuolization in noncitrated blood or EDTA), may suggest sepsis.

Platelet count: The platelet count may fall hours to days before the onset of clinical sepsis but more often remains elevated until a day or so after the infant manifests illness. This is sometimes accompanied by other findings of DIC (eg, increased fibrin degradation products, decreased fibrinogen, prolonged prothrombin time).

Buffy coat examination: Because of the large numbers of circulating bacteria in the septic neonate, organisms can frequently be seen in or associated with PMNs by applying Gram stain, methylene blue, or acridine orange to the buffy coat.

Lumbar puncture should be performed in any neonate suspected of having sepsis. Because GBS pneumonia presenting in the first day of life can be confused with hyaline membrane disease, lumbar punctures are often performed routinely on infants suspected of having these diseases. However, the procedure can be difficult to perform and creates the risk of increasing hypoxia in an already hypoxemic infant. Further, when respiratory distress is the major reason to suspect sepsis, the CSF culture is not likely to be positive. Therefore, routine lumbar punctures in these infants should be discouraged. For a discussion of this procedure and CSF interpretation, see NEONATAL MENINGITIS, below.

Blood cultures: Since umbilical vessels are frequently contaminated by organisms on the umbilical stump, they yield unreliable cultures. Therefore, blood for culture should be obtained by venipuncture, preferably at 2 peripheral sites, each meticulously prepared by first applying an iodine-containing liquid, then 95% alcohol, and finally allowing it to dry. Blood should be cultured for both aerobic and anaerobic organisms. If catheter-associated sepsis is suspected, a culture should be obtained through the catheter as well as peripherally. In > 90% of positive bacterial blood cultures, growth is seen within 48 h of incubation; 50% of positive blood cultures contain > 50 colony-forming units (CFU)/mL, but only those with > 1000 CFU/mL indicate risk of developing meningitis. Because of this high-density bacteremia, a small amount of blood (eg, 1 mL) is usually sufficient for detecting organisms. Data on capillary blood culture are insufficient to recommend its use.

If fungi (eg, Candida) are suspected, a special culture medium should be used. Fungal blood cultures may require 4 to 5 days of incubation before becoming positive and may be negative even in demonstrably disseminated disease.

Urinalysis and culture: Urine should be obtained by suprapubic aspiration, not by urine collection bags. A finding of > 5 WBC/high-power field in the spun urine or any organisms in a fresh unspun gram-stained sample is presumptive evidence of a UTI, which in the newborn suggests antecedent bacteremia (neonatal sepsis). Absence of pyuria does not rule out UTI.

Counterimmunoelectrophoresis and latex agglutination tests: These tests detect antigen in body fluids (eg, CSF, concentrated urine). They can contribute additional information by detecting capsular polysaccharide antigen of GBS, E. coli K1, S. pneumoniae, and H. influenzae type b.

Acute phase reactants: These proteins are produced by the liver under the influence of interleukin-1 when inflammation from any cause is present; as such, they lack specificity. Generally, however, they are sensitive and can be useful in signaling the presence of inflammation and as indicators of resolution. The most valuable of these is the quantitative C-reactive protein. A concentration of 1 mg/dL (measured by nephelometry) has both a false-positive and false-negative rate of about 10%. Elevated levels occur within a day, peak at 2 to 3 days, and fall to normal within 5 to 10 days in infants who become clinically well. The micro-ESR correlates well with the standard Wintrobe method but has a high false-negative rate (especially early in the course and with DIC) and a slow return to normal, well beyond the time of clinical cure. Therefore, it has limited value as a diagnostic aid and as an adjunct in terminating therapy.

External ear canal fluid: Gram-stain examination and culture of this fluid may indicate the infecting organism. The presence of ≥ 3 PMNs/high-power field predicts a positive blood culture (with the same organism being cultured from the external canal).

Gastric fluid: Only 1/30 neonates having ≥ 5 PMNs/high-power field in the gastric aspirate after the first 24 h of life develops sepsis within 72 h of birth, but that 1 infant is rarely missed when this method for predicting positive blood-culture results is used.

Screening panels: Several investigators recommend using a combination of some of the above tests to identify the newborn with sepsis and thereby determine need for therapy. In general, the immature:total PMN ratio (> 0.2 being abnormal) along with culture of blood, CSF, and urine is as useful as other multiple combinations; negative results accurately identify 97% of *uninfected* newborns.

Treatment

Newborns with **early-onset sepsis** should receive ampicillin or penicillin G plus an aminoglycoside. In some nurseries, this regimen is used for infants at risk of developing sepsis, but cefotaxime is substituted for an aminoglycoside if the infant is sick and thought to be septic (eg, findings include hypotension, poor temperature control, lethargy, decreased platelets, and decreased granulocytes). Overuse of 3rd-generation cephalosporins in a closed unit such as a neonatal intensive care unit may result in cephalosporinase production by gram-negative enteric organisms and selection of these now resistant strains. Therefore, 3rd-generation cephalosporins should not be used routinely in infants with a low index of suspicion for sepsis. Once an organism is identified, antibiotic therapy is adjusted according to sensitivities and the site of infection. If foul-smelling amniotic fluid is present at birth, therapy for anaerobes (eg, clindamycin) should be considered in the initial antibiotic coverage. Chloramphenicol may also be used, but only if serum levels of the drug can be closely monitored.

The choice of which aminoglycoside to use for early-onset sepsis is dictated by the antibiotic sensitivity pattern for the nursery of each hospital. When 10% of isolated *E. coli* strains are resistant to a particular aminoglycoside, that drug should not be used for at least 6 mo and another

should be used in its place (eg, amikacin may be substituted for gentamicin). Subsequently, if resistance drops to < 10%, use of the original aminoglycoside may be resumed with continued surveillance of resistance rates, since reemergence of resistance is common.

Initial therapy of patients with **late-onset sepsis** should include nafcillin plus an aminoglycoside (or a 3rd-generation cephalosporin, as discussed above). If *P. aeruginosa* is prevalent in a particular nursery, ceftazidime may be used instead of an aminoglycoside. Newborns previously treated with an aminoglycoside who need re-treatment should receive a different aminoglycoside or a 3rd-generation cephalosporin.

If *S. epidermidis* is suspected (ie, an indwelling catheter has been in place for > 72 h) or is isolated from blood or other normally sterile fluid and considered a pathogen, initial therapy for late-onset sepsis should include vancomycin instead of nafcillin, since about 35% of *S. epidermidis* isolates are resistant to semisynthetic penicillins (eg, nafcillin). However, if the organism is found to be sensitive to this class of antibiotics, vancomycin should be discontinued and replaced with nafcillin. Removal of the presumptive source of the organism (usually an indwelling intravascular catheter) is frequently necessary to cure the infection, since *S. epidermidis* may be protected by a covering slime (glycocalyx) that encourages adherence of organisms to the plastic catheter.

Candida spp have become increasingly important as causative agents of late-onset sepsis, occurring in 2 to 4% of very LBW infants. Risk factors include prolonged (> 10 days) placement of indwelling central IV catheters, hyperalimentation, use of antecedent antibiotics, necrotizing enterocolitis, and previous surgery. Since *Candida* may take 2 to 5 days to grow in blood culture, initiation of amphotericin B therapy without positive blood or CSF cultures and removal of the infected catheter may be necessary to save the infant's life. Proof of colonization (in mouth or stool or on skin) should be sought, and indirect ophthalmoscopy with dilation of the pupils to look for retinal lesions consistent with disseminated candidiasis should be undertaken. Renal ultrasonography should be performed to look for renal mycetoma.

Since neonatal sepsis may present with nonspecific clinical signs and its effects may be devastating, an early, aggressive diagnostic assessment and rapid institution of therapy are recommended. The value of this practice is reflected in a treated:proved ratio of 15:1 and 8:1 in community and inner-city hospitals, respectively. Depending on the laboratory, culture methods, and rapidity of reporting, almost all bacterial cultures are positive within 72 h. If negative cultures of body fluids are consistent with the clinical course, clinicians may discontinue antimicrobial therapy after 72 h. Antibiotics should be used judiciously, since most newborns at risk for sepsis will continue to be under close surveillance for a time and since these drugs are detrimental to the flora of individual infants and the nursery; such use includes willingly discontinuing them when they are no longer indicated.

Vaginal or rectal cultures of women at term may show GBS colonization rates of up to 30%; at least 50% of their newborns will also become colonized. The density of infant colonization is a risk factor for the development of invasive disease (the risk is 40 times higher with heavy colonization). While only 1/100 of those colonized will develop invasive disease due to GBS, > 50% of those infants will present within the first 6 h of life. Therefore, any strategy to reduce such invasive disease must take into account this very early onset. Courses of antimicrobial therapy given before delivery do not eradicate maternal colonization nor reduce the incidence of neonatal colonization or invasive disease. Postnatal culture results of newborns and even rapid diagnosis may be available too late for treatment to be effective. Several studies have indicated that **intrapartum therapy** may reduce colonization and invasive disease in mother and newborn, respectively. When positive cervical cultures for GBS obtained at about 36 wk gestation are combined with certain perinatal risk factors—eg, preterm labor at < 37 wk gestation, PROM (> 12 h), or intrapartum fever (> 37.5° C [99.5° F] orally)—selective maternal intrapartum chemoprophylaxis with ampicillin or penicillin is recommended.

Exchange transfusions have been used for sick (particularly hypotensive and metabolically acidotic) newborns; their purported value is to increase the levels of circulating immunoglobulins, decrease circulating endotoxin, increase Hb levels (with higher 2,3-diphosphoglycerate levels), and improve perfusion. However, no controlled prospective studies of their use have been conducted. In addition, fresh whole blood must be used and prescreened to rule out the presence of hepatitis B surface antigen (**HBsAg**) and antibodies to cytomegalovirus (**CMV**) and HIV; such blood may not be readily available. There is

also a risk of developing non-A, non-B hepatitis (particularly hepatitis C). The administration of **fresh frozen plasma** may be helpful in reversing the heat-stable and heat-labile opsonin deficiencies seen in LBW infants, but controlled studies of its use are also unavailable and transfusion-associated risks must be considered.

Several uncontrolled studies have suggested that **IV immunoglobulin (IVIG)** when given at birth may be useful in preventing neonatal sepsis in certain high-risk LBW infants. Its use in prevention and in treatment of established infection in these patients is the subject of several well-controlled prospective studies that are currently under way in the USA. Until results of these investigations are available, use of IVIG should be considered experimental.

Newborns who are both septic and granulocytopenic are less likely to survive, particularly if their bone marrow neutrophil storage pool (**NSP**) is depleted to < 7% of total nucleated cells (mortality, 90%). Since NSP levels may not be readily available, the peripheral blood immature:total (**I:T**) neutrophil ratio can be used to approximate bone marrow NSP levels. I:T ratios of > 0.80 correlate with NSP depletion and death. Therefore, this ratio may help identify patients who might benefit from **granulocyte transfusion.** Granulocytes are generally collected by intermittent flow centrifugation leukapheresis using hydroxyethyl starch and are obtained from adults who are negative for antibodies to HBsAg, CMV, and HIV, and whose RBC antigens are compatible with the neonatal recipient. To prevent graft-vs.-host disease, each granulocyte pack must be treated with 1500 rads before transfusion. Transfusions of 15 mL/kg of a suspension containing 0.2 to 1.0×10^9 granulocytes/15 mL of the suspension with < 10% lymphocytes should be administered. Infusions are given once or twice daily for up to 5 days.

NEONATAL PNEUMONIA

Neonatal pneumonia, like sepsis, may be of early or late onset.

EARLY-ONSET PNEUMONIA

Pneumonia as part of generalized sepsis can present at or within hours of birth.

Etiology

Early-onset pneumonia often occurs in association with amnionitis, following prolonged rupture of the amniotic membranes. The fetus is surrounded by infected amniotic fluid, and respiratory efforts result in aspirating into the lungs organisms that cause pneumonia and sepsis. Neonatal pneumonia has been associated with low Apgar scores and perinatal complications; eg, premature labor, placental abruption, and difficult forceps delivery.

Group B streptococcus is the most common cause of early-onset sepsis and pneumonia, but occasionally *Listeria monocytogenes, Hemophilus influenzae, Escherichia coli, Klebsiella,* and other gram-positive and gram-negative organisms are responsible.

Symptoms, Signs, and Diagnosis

The infant's appearance depends on the severity of the sepsis and pneumonia, ranging from tachypnea to respiratory failure and septic shock from the time of birth. The delivery history (eg, amnionitis) may suggest the diagnosis, but bacterial pneumonia cannot be distinguished clinically or radiographically from other causes of neonatal respiratory distress, such as respiratory distress syndrome (RDS), transient tachypnea of the newborn (TTNB), meconium aspiration, or persistent pulmonary hypertension. X-rays of neonatal pneumonia may show patchy infiltrates, interstitial fluid, or rarely, lobar consolidations, or they may mimic those of RDS, TTNB, or meconium aspiration.

Evaluation for suspected pneumonia is the same as for sepsis (see NEONATAL SEPSIS, above). Cultures of blood, tracheal aspirate, and CSF are most important. A CBC with platelet count and a urine latex agglutination test for Group B streptococcus are useful.

Treatment of both early- and late-onset pneumonia is the same as that for NEONATAL SEPSIS, above.

LATE-ONSET PNEUMONIA

Pneumonia usually seen after 7 days of age, most commonly in neonatal intensive care units in infants who require prolonged endotracheal intubation because of chronic lung disease.

Symptoms, Signs, and Diagnosis

Onset of nursery-acquired pneumonia may be gradual, with increased secretions being suctioned from the endotracheal tube and need for higher ventilator settings. In other cases, infants may be acutely ill, with temperature instability and neutropenia. New infiltrates may be visible

on chest x-ray but may be difficult to recognize if the infant has severe bronchopulmonary dysplasia.

Evaluation includes cultures of blood and tracheal aspirate. Coagulase-negative staphylococcus, resistant to oxacillin, has been a common cause of nursery-acquired sepsis and pneumonia in recent years. Vancomycin is the drug of choice, but a less nephrotoxic antibiotic may be substituted after sensitivity results are available. In infants likely to have received a variety of broad-spectrum antibiotics, a wide spectrum of pathogens may be found in addition to coagulase-negative staphylococcus, including coagulase-positive staphylococcus, *E. coli, Klebsiella, Pseudomonas, Proteus,* and *Serratia,* as well as *Candida albicans* and other fungi (see NEONATAL SEPSIS, above). For treatment, see NEONATAL SEPSIS, above.

Perinatal contamination with *Chlamydia* organisms during delivery may result in development of chlamydial pneumonia at 2 to 6 wk. The infants are tachypneic but usually not critically ill and may have an associated conjunctivitis caused by the same organism. Eosinophilia may be present, and x-rays show interstitial infiltrates. Treatment with erythromycin leads to rapid resolution.

NEONATAL MENINGITIS

Inflammation of the meninges due to bacterial invasion in the first 4 wk of life. It occurs in 2/10,000 full-term and 2/1,000 low-birthweight infants; there is a male predominance. It is a frequent concomitant to neonatal sepsis (see above), occurring in about 25% of those cases.

Etiology

Group B streptococcus (GBS—predominantly type III), *Escherichia coli* (particularly those strains containing the K1 polysaccharide), and *Listeria monocytogenes* account for 75% of meningitis in the newborn. Meningitis due to GBS may be present in the first week of life, when it accompanies early-onset neonatal sepsis and frequently presents as a pneumonic illness. Usually, however, it occurs after this period (up to 3 mo of age) as an isolated illness characterized by absence of antecedent obstetric or perinatal complications, predominance of serotype III, presence of more specific signs of meningitis (eg, fever, lethargy, seizures), and a mortality rate significantly lower than that of early-onset neonatal sepsis.

Enterococci, nonenterococcal Group D streptococci, α-hemolytic streptococci, and other gram-negative enteric organisms (eg, *Klebsiella* spp, *Enterobacter* spp, and *Citrobacter diversus*) are also important pathogens. In addition, *Hemophilus influenzae* type b, *Neisseria meningitidis*, and *Streptococcus pneumoniae* have been increasingly reported as causes of neonatal bacterial meningitis. (In fact, the age-specific attack rate for *H. influenzae* type b in infants < 1 mo of age is twice as high as that for children 3 to 4 yr of age.) Organisms that cause meningitis with an associated severe vasculitis, particularly *C. diversus* and *Enterobacter sakazakii*, are likely to produce cysts and abscesses. *Pseudomonas aeruginosa* and *Serratia* spp also may cause brain abscesses in newborns.

Neonatal meningitis most frequently results from an antecedent bacteremia associated with neonatal sepsis. Blood cultures are positive in 70% of infants with neonatal meningitis; the higher the colony count (bacterial density) in the blood culture, the higher the risk for meningitis. Meningitis may also result from skin lesions of the scalp (eg, from diploic thrombophlebitis) that, along with developmental defects, lead to communication of the skin surface with the subarachnoid space. Direct extension to the CNS from a contiguous otic focus may also occur (eg, otitis media), emphasizing the importance of middle ear examination in the newborn.

Symptoms, Signs, and Diagnosis

Newborns with meningitis frequently manifest only those findings associated with neonatal sepsis (eg, temperature instability, respiratory distress, jaundice, apnea). **CNS signs** (eg, lethargy, seizures [particularly focal], vomiting, irritability) more specifically suggest meningitis. A bulging or full fontanelle occurs in about 25% and nuchal rigidity in only 15%; the absence of these signs, therefore, does not exclude the diagnosis of neonatal meningitis. Cranial nerve abnormalities (particularly those involving the 3rd, 6th, and 7th nerves) may also be seen. An early clinical sign of brain abscess is increased intracranial pressure, commonly manifested by vomiting, a bulging fontanelle, and an enlarging head size. Deterioration in an otherwise stable infant with meningitis suggests rupture of an abscess into the ventricular system.

The **definitive diagnosis** of meningitis is made by CSF examination. Lumbar puncture **(LP)** should be performed in any neonate suspected of having sepsis. LP can be difficult to perform in a newborn and may put the infant at risk for hypoxia; poor clinical condition (eg, respiratory distress, shock, thrombocytopenia) establishes excessive risk for the procedure. If LP is delayed, the infant should be treated as though meningitis were present. Even when the clinical condition improves, the presence of inflammatory cells in CSF and abnormal chemistries days after the onset of illness can still provide valuable information on the presence or absence of meningitis.

A needle with a trocar should be used for LP to avoid introducing epithelial rests and subsequent development of epitheliomas. The CSF, even if bloody or acellular, should be cultured. About 15% of infants with negative blood cultures may have positive CSF cultures.

Normal values for CSF in newborns are controversial and age-related. In general, for low-birth-weight infants up to 4 wk of age, 20 WBCs (1/2 of which may be polymorphonuclear leukocytes **[PMNs]**), a protein level of 160 mg/dL, and a glucose level of 50 mg/dL may be considered the upper limits of normal. For term infants, these limits are 10 WBCs (with 1/2 PMNs), a protein level of 80 mg/dL, and a glucose level of 50 mg/dL. Since the concentration of CSF glucose depends largely on that of serum glucose and may normally be as low as 20 to 30 mg/dL, a serum glucose value should be obtained before the LP is performed so CSF glucose level can be determined as a percentage of serum glucose (< 50% is abnormal). The median level of CSF WBCs found in GBS meningitis is ≅ 100, while that found in gram-negative meningitis is ≅ 2000.

Ventriculitis is a frequent concomitant of neonatal meningitis, particularly when caused by gram-negative enteric bacilli. It should be suspected in any newborn not responding appropriately to antimicrobial therapy. The diagnosis is made when a ventricular puncture yields a WBC count > 100/μL, Gram stain and/or culture is positive, ventricular pressure is increased, and ventricles are dilated. When the infant is not responding to therapy and ventriculitis or brain abscess is suspected, ultrasonography and CT may be helpful diagnostically.

LP should be repeated at 36 h for gram-positive and at 72 h for gram-negative organisms to ensure sterilization. It should not be routinely repeated at the end of therapy in an infant who is doing well.

Prognosis

Prognosis is determined by birth weight, etiology, and clinical presentation. Before antibiotics were introduced, the mortality rate from neonatal sepsis approached 100%. Even with modern, sophisticated support for the sick neonate, the mortality rate for gram-negative neonatal meningitis is 20 to 30% and for gram-positive (eg, GBS), 10 to 20%. For organisms that produce necrotizing meningitis and brain abscess, the mortality rate approaches 75%. Neurologic sequelae (eg, hydrocephalus, hearing loss, mental retardation) develop in 20 to 50% of infants who survive neonatal meningitis, with a poorer prognosis when gram-negative enteric bacilli are the cause.

Prognosis depends partly on the number of organisms present in CSF at the time of diagnosis, determined either by colony count or, more commonly, by amount of free antigen (eg, $E. coli$ K1). The duration of positive CSF cultures correlates directly with the incidence of complications. In general, CSF cultures from infants with GBS are usually sterilized within the first 24 h of antimicrobial therapy; those from infants with gram-negative bacillary meningitis remain positive for an average of $3^{1}/_{2}$ days.

Treatment

The major goal of antimicrobial therapy is to achieve rapid sterilization of the CSF. The rate of bacterial disappearance correlates with bactericidal titers in the CSF against the infecting organism; titers of 10 times the minimum bactericidal concentration (MBC) are required to achieve sterilization. The percentages of the CSF levels to concomitant serum concentration for antimicrobials commonly used in treating neonatal meningitis are penicillin G, 2 to 5%; ampicillin, 15 to 20%; cefotaxime, 27 to 63%; nafcillin, 10 to 15%; vancomycin, 10 to 15%. Data for tobramycin and amikacin are insufficient.

Treatment of GBS meningitis is still somewhat controversial. A number of cases of relapse or recurrence or both have been reported for early- and late-onset GBS infections; most have been attributed to a relatively low dose of penicillin or ampicillin. Additionally, about 4% of GBS isolates demonstrate penicillin tolerance (MBC > 32 × minimum inhibitory concentration [MIC]), but the clinical significance of this phenomenon has not been clearly demonstrated. In vitro and in vivo animal studies have demonstrated synergistic bactericidal activity when ampicillin and gentamicin are used in combination, but again, the clinical significance of this observation has not been indisputably established in the human infant. The recommended initial treatment of meningitis in which GBS is suspected is penicillin G 500,000 u./kg/day or ampicillin 300 to 400 mg/kg/day plus gentamicin 7.5 mg/kg/day. If CSF sterilization has been achieved by 36 h and the organism is shown not to be tolerant, gentamicin may be discontinued and the above dosages adjusted according to the MBC. If MBCs are not available, the higher dosages are continued.

In both early- and late-onset meningitis due to enterococci or L. monocytogenes, treatment should include the combination of ampicillin and gentamicin.

Therapy for gram-negative bacillary meningitis is difficult. The typical regimen of ampicillin plus an aminoglycoside results in a 20 to 30% mortality rate with a poor prognosis for survivors. Efforts to treat both the meningitis and the frequently accompanying ventriculitis by barbotage of aminoglycoside into the lumbar subarachnoid space, or by IV aminoglycosides, have not shown a significant advantage over systemic therapy alone. The excellent activity of 3rd-generation cephalosporins against most gram-negative bacilli (low MBC) and their substantial penetration of the CSF (providing impressive peak CSF bactericidal titers) have raised hopes that these antibiotics may be useful in lowering morbidity and mortality. However, the only controlled study of a 3rd-generation cephalosporin (moxalactam vs. ampicillin and amikacin) failed to show an advantage in either rapidity of CSF sterilization (positive CSF culture for 3 days in both groups) or ultimate outcome. Nevertheless, the use of moxalactam (no longer used in the newborn) did demonstrate that a 3rd-generation cephalosporin is at least as effective as ampicillin and an aminoglycoside. Therefore, because of its predictable pharmacokinetics, low toxicity, excellent activity, and good penetrability, a 3rd-generation cephalosporin (eg, cefotaxime) should be considered in treating infants with proven gram-negative meningitis (or sepsis) or those convincingly septic. These agents should not be used routinely in the large number of newborns given antibiotics for less compelling reasons, since certain gram-negative organisms induce β-lactamase production with 3rd-generation cephalosporins, resulting in the rapid emergence of resistance.

Treatment may need to be altered for a specific clinical situation. For instance, in a newborn who received ampicillin and gentamicin for suspected neonatal sepsis in the first week of life and who several weeks later develops sepsis and meningitis, the infecting organism should be assumed to be either a multiply resistant gram-negative bacterium, *Staphylococcus aureus*, or *S. epidermidis*. This newborn should initially receive a combination of vancomycin and either an aminoglycoside different from the one previously used or a 3rd-generation cephalosporin (eg, cefotaxime). Once a pathogen is isolated, antibiotic regimens are tailored to in vitro sensitivities. Parenteral therapy for gram-positive meningitis is given for a minimum of 14 days; for gram-negative, a minimum of 21 days.

Since meningitis should be considered part of the continuum of neonatal sepsis, the adjunctive measures used in treating neonatal sepsis should also be used in neonatal meningitis (see NEONATAL SEPSIS, above).

Patients should be closely followed for neurologic complications during the first 2 yr of life.

NEONATAL LISTERIOSIS

Transplacental infection with *Listeria monocytogenes* can result in fetal dissemination with granuloma formation in many organs (eg, liver, adrenal glands, lymphatic tissue, lungs, and brain)—**granulomatosis infantiseptica**. Aspiration or swallowing of amniotic fluid or vaginal secretions can lead to perinatal infection. Nosocomial acquisition also has been reported.

Symptoms and Signs

Infections in pregnant women may be asymptomatic or may be characterized by a primary bacteremia presenting as a nonspecific flu-like illness. In the fetus and newborn, clinical presentation depends on the timing and route of infection. Abortion, premature delivery with amnionitis (with a characteristic murky amniotic fluid), stillbirth, or neonatal sepsis commonly occurs. Infection may be apparent within hours or days of birth, or it may be delayed up to several weeks. Infants with early-onset disease frequently are of low birth weight, have associated obstetric complications, and show evidence of sepsis with circulatory or respiratory insufficiency, or both. Those with the delayed-onset form are full-term, previously well infants presenting with meningitis

or sepsis. Neonatal mortality, ranging from 10 to 50%, is higher in infants with early-onset disease.

Diagnosis

In neonatal listeriosis, the organism can be cultured from umbilical cord or peripheral blood vessels; the infant's CSF, gastric aspirate, and meconium; the mother's lochia and exudates from cervix and vagina; and grossly diseased parts of the placenta.

Blood and cervix specimens should be obtained from any pregnant woman with a febrile disease and cultured for *L. monocytogenes* after prolonged incubation at 4° C (39° F). A sick neonate or an infant born to a mother with listeriosis during pregnancy should be evaluated for sepsis (see above). CSF examination may show a predominance of mononuclear cells. Gram-stained smears frequently are negative but may show pleomorphic, gram-variable coccobacillary forms. The clinician should be careful not to disregard them as "diphtheroid" contaminants. Serologic tests are not useful in establishing the diagnosis.

Prophylaxis

Avoidance of food products that may be contaminated by *L. monocytogenes* (eg, unpasteurized dairy products or raw vegetables exposed to cattle or sheep manure) is important, since they cause maternal and fetal infection. Pregnant women who have previously given birth to infected infants should have cervical and stool cultures performed during the 3rd trimester to identify a carrier state of *L. monocytogenes*. Such recognition may allow prophylactic treatment before delivery or intrapartum, to prevent vertical transmission to the newborn; however, the usefulness of these measures has not been established.

Treatment

Initial treatment with ampicillin and an aminoglycoside is preferred. After clinical response is observed, ampicillin alone may be given. Synergy of ampicillin or penicillin with an aminoglycoside or rifampin has been demonstrated, and trimethoprim-sulfamethoxazole and imipenem are active against *L. monocytogenes*; however, these regimens have not been well evaluated in the newborn. A 14-day course is usually satisfactory, but the optimal duration of therapy is unknown. Other adjuncts should also be given to the newborn with bacterial sepsis (see NEONATAL

SEPSIS, above). Drainage/secretion precautions should be considered for heavily infected infants.

CONGENITAL RUBELLA
(See also RUBELLA under VIRAL INFECTIONS in Ch. 32)

Etiology and Epidemiology

Rubella is caused by an RNA virus of the Togaviridae family in the genus *Rubivirus*. Congenital rubella typically results from a primary maternal infection. The introduction of rubella vaccine in 1969 markedly decreased the incidence of both rubella and congenital rubella. Nevertheless, rubella still occurs, primarily in those > 15 yr of age, and recent studies show that 10 to 20% of postpubertal individuals lack antibody to rubella. Protection against the disease in this group must be achieved before congenital rubella can be eliminated.

Pathogenesis

Rubella is believed to invade the upper respiratory tract, with subsequent viremia and dissemination of virus to different sites, including the placenta. The fetus is at highest risk for developing the abnormalities associated with congenital rubella during the first 16 wk of gestation, particularly the first 8 to 10 wk. Early in gestation, the virus is thought to establish a chronic intrauterine infection; its effects include endothelial damage to blood vessels, direct cytolysis of cells, and disruption of cellular mitosis.

Symptoms and Signs

Rubella in the pregnant woman may be asymptomatic or characterized by upper respiratory tract symptoms, fever, lymphadenopathy (especially in the suboccipital and posterior auricular areas), and a maculopapular rash. This illness may be followed by joint symptoms.

Effects on the fetus vary from fetal death in utero, to multiple anomalies, to isolated hearing loss. Infants may also be asymptomatic at birth. The most frequently seen abnormalities include intrauterine growth retardation, meningoencephalitis, cataracts, retinopathy, hearing loss, cardiac defects (patent ductus arteriosus and pulmonary arterial hypoplasia), hepatosplenomegaly, and bone radiolucency. Other manifestations are thrombocytopenia with purpura, dermal erythropoiesis resulting in bluish-red skin lesions, adenopathy, and interstitial pneumonia. These infants also require close observation for possible subsequent hearing loss, mental retardation, ab-

normal behavior, endocrinopathies, and a rare progressive encephalitis.

Diagnosis

Both serologic tests and viral culture can be useful in the diagnosis of maternal as well as congenital infection. In the adult, virus can be isolated from nasal or throat swabs. In the infant, specimens from the nasopharynx, urine, CSF, buffy coat, and conjunctiva may grow virus.

The serologic assays used to detect IgG and IgM include the hemagglutination inhibition test, immunofluorescence assay, radioimmunoassay, and enzyme-linked immunosorbent assay (ELISA). Maternal infection is suggested by a four-fold or greater rise in rubella-specific IgG levels between specimens from acute and convalescent stages. Persistence of rubella-specific IgG in the infant after 6 to 12 mo of age suggests fetal infection. Increased rubella-specific IgM antibodies can also assist in diagnosing rubella in the pregnant woman or infant. In a few centers, the fetus has been diagnosed prenatally by isolation of virus from the amniotic fluid, detection of rubella-specific IgM in fetal blood, or application of molecular biology techniques on a chorionic villus biopsy specimen.

Other laboratory procedures that may be performed in the infant with suspected congenital rubella include a CBC with differential, CSF analysis, and radiologic examination of the bones; thorough ophthalmologic and cardiac evaluation are also useful.

Prophylaxis

No specific therapy is available for maternal or congenital rubella infections. Women exposed to rubella early in pregnancy should be informed about the potential risks to the fetus, and termination of pregnancy should be considered. Some authorities recommend administration of immune globulin (0.55 mL/kg) for exposure early in pregnancy.

Unlike many other congenitally acquired infections, rubella can easily be prevented because of the availability of an effective vaccine. In the USA, it is recommended that infants receive immunization for rubella together with measles and mumps immunizations at 15 mo of age and again at entry to grade school or junior high school (see IMMUNIZATION PROCEDURES THROUGHOUT CHILDHOOD in Ch. 23). Postpubertal females who are not known to be immune to rubella should be vaccinated. *Rubella vaccination is contraindicated in immunodeficient or pregnant women.* Following immunization, women should be advised not to become pregnant for 3 mo. Efforts should also be made to screen and vaccinate members of high-risk groups such as hospital employees, military recruits, and college students.

NEONATAL HERPES SIMPLEX VIRUS (HSV) INFECTION

Neonatal HSV infection is a serious disease with high mortality and significant morbidity. The incidence is estimated to be between 1/2500 and 1/5000 live deliveries. HSV type 2 causes about 80% of cases; the remainder are caused by HSV type 1. HSV-2 is usually transmitted to the newborn during delivery by passage through an infected maternal genital tract (see also INFECTIOUS DISEASE in Ch. 17). Transplacental transmission of virus and nosocomial spread from one neonate to another by hospital personnel or family have also been implicated in about 15% of cases. Mothers of newborns with HSV infection tend to have no history or symptoms of genital infection at the time of delivery.

Clinical Manifestations

Rapid and specific diagnosis of neonatal HSV infection is essential if therapy is to be efficacious. Disease manifestations generally occur between the 1st and 2nd wk of life; however, symptoms may not appear until as late as the 4th wk. The hallmark of infection is skin vesicles, which frequently lead to progressive or more serious forms of disease within 7 to 10 days if therapy is not started. However, up to 45% of infected newborns have no skin vesicles; usually, these babies have brain infection. Other signs of infection, which can be present singly or in combination, include temperature instability, lethargy, hypotonia, respiratory difficulty (apnea or pneumonia), convulsions, hepatitis, and disseminated intravascular coagulation (DIC). They provide the basis for classifying the disease into 2 major categories: disseminated and localized disease. Newborns considered to have **disseminated disease** with visceral organ involvement have hepatitis, pneumonitis, and/or DIC with or without encephalitis or skin disease. With no therapy, the mortality rate is 85%. Newborns with **localized disease** can be subdivided into 2 groups. The first group has encephalitis manifested by neurologic findings, CSF pleocytosis, and elevated protein concentration, with or without concomitant involvement of the skin, eyes, and mouth. Without treatment, encephalitis in the newborn has a mortality rate of about 50%,

and at least 95% of the survivors have severe neurologic sequelae. The 2nd group with localized disease includes neonates having only skin, eye, and mouth involvement and no evidence of CNS or organ disease. Death is uncommon in this group, except as the result of concomitant medical problems, but about 30% develop neurologic impairment, which may not become manifest until 2 to 3 yr of age.

Morbidity in each group parallels its mortality and is directly proportional to the extent of the disease. About 90% of infants with viscerally disseminated neonatal HSV infection have subsequent sequelae. Only 5% of those with CNS infection return to normal. Neonatal herpes is, therefore, a rapacious infection in the newborn.

Diagnosis

Neonatal HSV infection can be confirmed by isolation of virus in tissue culture, using various cell lines of human or nonhuman origin. The most common site for virus retrieval is skin vesicles; the mouth, eye, and CSF are also high-yield sites. In some newborns presenting with encephalitis, virus is found only in the brain. Cytopathologic effects can usually be demonstrated in tissue culture within 24 to 48 h after inoculation. The diagnosis can also be confirmed by neutralization with appropriate high-titer antiserum; immunofluorescence of lesion scrapings, particularly using monoclonal antibodies; and electron microscopy. If no diagnostic virology facilities are available, a Papanicolaou smear of the lesion base may be obtained and may show characteristic histopathologic evidence (multinucleated giant cells and intranuclear inclusions) but is less sensitive than culture, and false-positive results occur.

Treatment

Therapy with either vidarabine or acyclovir will decrease the mortality rate by 50% and increase the number of newborns who will develop normally from 10 to 50%. Vidarabine 30 mg/kg/day in standard IV fluid is given over a period of 12 h each day for 10 to 14 days. Acyclovir 30 mg/kg/day is given q 8 h in divided doses for 10 to 14 days and is equally effective. Treatment also requires vigorous supportive therapy, including appropriate IV fluids, alimentation, respiratory support, correction of clotting abnormalities, and control of seizure disorders. The appearance of herpes keratoconjunctivitis requires topical therapy with an agent such as trifluridine (see also NEONATAL CONJUNCTIVITIS in this chapter, above).

NEONATAL HEPATITIS B VIRUS INFECTION

Of the recognized forms of viral hepatitis (hepatitis A, hepatitis B, delta hepatitis, and hepatitis C), only hepatitis B virus (HBV) is recognized as an important cause of neonatal hepatitis. The spectrum of disease manifestations is broad, with most neonates developing chronic subclinical hepatitis.

Etiology and Epidemiology

HBV is a double-shelled DNA virus. The surface antigen (HBsAg) is found on the surface of the virus and on accompanying smaller spherical and tubular forms of excess virus-coat material.

In the USA, where the HBsAg carrier rate in the general population is quite low (about 0.1%), the major source of neonatal HBV infection is from infected mothers during delivery. (Exposure to contaminated blood products has been virtually eliminated by screening blood donors for HBsAg.) Maternal acute hepatitis B during the 3rd trimester or within 2 mo of delivery is associated with a 70% risk of transmission; in contrast, the risk from mothers with acute hepatitis B during the 1st or 2nd trimester is only 5%. Risk of maternal-infant transmission of HBV is also high from asymptomatic HBsAg-positive carriers with the e antigen. Carriers without the e antigen or with anti-HBe are less likely to transmit the disease.

Maternal-infant HBV transmission results primarily from either micro–maternal-fetal transfusions during labor or infant contact with infectious maternal secretions in the birth canal. Transplacental transmission is unusual. Postpartum transmission occurs rarely through neonatal exposure to infectious maternal blood, saliva, stool, urine, or breast milk. Neonatal HBV infection may be an important viral reservoir in certain communities.

Symptoms, Signs, and Course

Most neonates infected with HBV develop chronic, subclinical hepatitis characterized by persistent HBsAg antigenemia and variably elevated transaminase activity. Histologically, this disease resembles the "chronic persistent hepatitis" seen in adults. Long-term prognosis is unknown, although there is evidence that HBsAg carriage from early in life increases the risk of subsequent liver disease (eg, chronic-active hepatitis, cirrhosis, and hepatocellular carcinoma). Infrequently, infected newborns develop acute hepatitis B, which is usually mild and self-limited, with jaundice, lethargy, failure to thrive, abdominal distention, and clay-colored stools. An occasional infant may be severely affected with hepatomegaly, ascites, and hyperbilirubinemia (primarily conjugated bilirubin); rarely the disease may be fulminant and even fatal. Fulminant disease occurs more often in infants born to mothers who are chronic carriers than in those born to mothers with acute hepatitis B. Many children born to women with acute hepatitis B during pregnancy are of low birth weight, whether or not they are infected with HBV.

Prophylaxis

All pregnant women should be tested routinely for HBsAg during an early prenatal visit in each pregnancy, and treatment to prevent hepatitis B should be given to infants born to HBsAg-positive mothers. Women not screened prenatally should be tested when admitted for delivery.

Infants born to HBsAg-positive mothers should be given one dose of 0.5 mL IM hepatitis B immune globulin (HBIG) within 12 h of birth. Recombinant hepatitis B virus vaccine (5 μg/0.5 mL) should be given IM in a series of 3 doses. The first should be given concurrently with HBIG but at a different site; however, this dose may be given within 7 days of birth. The 2nd and 3rd doses should be given at 1 mo and 6 mo, respectively, after the first. Testing for HBsAg and anti-HBs at 12 to 15 mo is recommended.

Where hepatitis B infection is highly endemic or HBsAg screening of mothers is impractical, vaccination of all newborns with hepatitis B vaccine is the most effective strategy for controlling hepatitis B.

Separating an infant from its HBsAg-positive mother is not recommended, and breast-feeding does not appear to increase the risk of postpartum HBV transmission, particularly if HBIG and hepatitis B virus vaccine have been given. However, if a mother has cracked nipples, abscesses, or other breast pathology, breast-feeding could potentially transmit HBV.

Treatment

Neonates with acute hepatitis B should receive symptomatic care and adequate nutrition; neither steroids nor HBIG has been shown to be of value. There is no specific treatment for neonates with chronic, subclinical hepatitis, but liver function tests should be monitored periodically because of the risk of developing significant disease.

CONGENITAL AND PERINATAL CYTOMEGALOVIRUS INFECTION

(See also CYTOMEGALOVIRUS INFECTION under VIRAL INFECTIONS in Ch. 32)

Cytomegalovirus (CMV) is frequently isolated from infants at birth and in the perinatal period. Although most infants shedding this virus are asymptomatic, others have life-threatening illness and devastating long-term sequelae.

Etiology and Epidemiology

CMV, a DNA virus belonging to the Herpesviridae family, acquired its name from the characteristic large cells containing intranuclear and cytoplasmic inclusions often seen in histologic specimens. Although differences among CMV isolates can be detected with the use of restriction endonuclease analysis of viral DNA, similarities in the genome of various isolates are greater; as a result, only one serotype of CMV is recognized. Like other herpesviruses, CMV is capable of latency and reactivation. CMV has been isolated from various sites including saliva, urine, breast milk, semen, cervical secretions, amniotic fluid, and buffy coat. Initial acquisition of CMV at an early age appears to be related positively to various factors; eg, low socioeconomic status, high rates of breast-feeding, and increased exposure to other young children (eg, in day-care centers). CMV is also thought to be transmitted sexually.

Congenital CMV infection, which occurs in 0.2 to 2.2% of all live births, is thought to result from transplacental acquisition of a primary or recurrent maternal infection. Clinically apparent disease in the newborn is much more likely to occur after a primary maternal exposure, particularly in the first half of pregnancy. In some higher socioeconomic groups in the USA, 50% of young women lack antibody to CMV, making them susceptible to primary infection.

Perinatal CMV is acquired by exposure to infected cervical secretions, breast milk, or blood products. Maternal antibody is thought to be protective, and most of these term infants are asymptomatic or are not affected by contact with the virus. In contrast, *preterm* infants lacking antibody to CMV who receive seropositive blood can develop significant illness.

Symptoms and Signs

Many women who become infected with CMV during pregnancy are asymptomatic, but some develop a mononucleosis-like illness.

About 10% of infants with congenital CMV infection are symptomatic at birth; manifestations include intrauterine growth retardation, prematurity, microcephaly, jaundice, petechiae, hepatosplenomegaly, periventricular calcifications, chorioretinitis, and pneumonitis. Symptomatic newborns have a mortality rate of up to 30%, and > 90% of the survivors have neurologic impairments including hearing loss, mental retardation, and visual disturbances. About 10% of asymptomatic infants also eventually develop neurologic sequelae. Since hearing defects are a particular concern, close monitoring beyond the neonatal period is necessary. Infants who acquire CMV after birth may develop pneumonia, hepatosplenomegaly, hepatitis, thrombocytopenia, and atypical lymphocytosis.

Diagnosis

Laboratory diagnosis of CMV is made by virus isolation or serologic tests. A primary infection in the mother is more frequently diagnosed by serologic tests than by culture; a positive culture may be due to reactivation of the virus. Seroconversion from a negative to a positive CMV-specific titer most strongly suggests infection. A four-fold or greater rise in CMV-specific IgG levels between specimens from acute and convalescent stages and an elevated CMV-specific IgM level in tests performed by a reliable laboratory may also indicate newly acquired infection. IgG levels can be measured by CF, immunofluorescence, indirect hemagglutination, radioimmunoassay, or enzyme-linked immunosorbent assay (ELISA). IgM levels are most reliably measured by radioimmunoassay or ELISA.

In neonates, viral culture is the primary diagnostic tool. Culture specimens should be kept refrigerated before inoculation on fibroblast cells. Congenital CMV can be diagnosed if the virus is isolated from specimens of urine or other body fluids obtained within the first 2 wk of life. After 2 wk, positive cultures may represent perinatal or congenital infection. Infants may shed CMV for several years after both types of infection.

Symptomatic congenital CMV infection must be distinguished from other congenital infections including toxoplasmosis, rubella, herpes simplex, and syphilis. Because infected infants may have thrombocytopenia, atypical lymphocytosis, hyperbilirubinemia, and elevated AST (SGOT) levels, a CBC and differential and liver function tests may be helpful. Radiologic examination of the infant's head and an ophthalmologic evaluation should also be performed.

Prophylaxis and Treatment

Many questions regarding transmission of CMV and risk to the fetus remain unanswered. For example, when a woman with primary CMV can safely conceive is not known. Women who develop primary CMV during pregnancy should be counseled on an individual basis, since risk to the fetus is difficult to assess. Many authorities do not recommend routine serologic testing for CMV before or during pregnancy in healthy women.

Although CMV is ubiquitous and reactivation is common, the nonimmune pregnant woman may be able to limit her exposure to the virus. For instance, since CMV infection is common in children attending day-care centers, pregnant women should always wash hands thoroughly after exposure to urine and respiratory secretions of such children. Development of a vaccine against CMV is under investigation, but many complex issues need to be resolved before such a vaccine will be available.

No specific therapy for congenital or perinatal CMV infections is available. Several antiviral drugs have been used to treat symptomatic infants but none have been successful. The antiviral drug ganciclovir (an acyclic nucleoside analog of guanine) is used to treat some CMV infections. However, its role in the treatment of infants with congenital CMV infection has yet to be determined.

Transfusion-associated perinatal CMV disease can be controlled by giving preterm seronegative infants blood products from CMV seronegative donors or products that have been treated to make them noninfectious.

CONGENITAL TOXOPLASMOSIS

(See also TOXOPLASMOSIS under MISCELLANEOUS INFECTIONS in Ch. 32)

An infection caused by transplacental acquisition of the coccidian protozoan Toxoplasma gondii. This parasite, found throughout the world, causes an estimated incidence of congenital infection ranging from 1/1000 to 8/1000 live births. A pregnant woman's risk for transmitting the infection to her infant is related to both current and past contact with the organism.

Etiology

T. gondii exists in 3 forms: the tachyzoite, the tissue cyst, and the oocyst. The oocyst form multiplies sexually in the intestinal epithelium of infected cats and is excreted in feces. In the proper environment, oocysts may remain viable for many months; they become infectious upon forming sporozoites that invade the host's GI mucosa. The proliferative form is the tachyzoite, found during active infection. Tachyzoites multiply asexually and disseminate throughout the body. Tissue cysts, consisting of bradyzoites, can form at various sites, particularly in striated muscle and the brain. Infection with *T. gondii* is thought to occur primarily from ingestion of inadequately cooked meat containing these cysts and ingestion of oocysts.

With rare exception, congenital toxoplasmosis is secondary to a primary maternal infection during gestation. About 50% of women infected during pregnancy will have a congenitally infected child. The rate of transmission to the infant is higher in women infected later during pregnancy. However, in infants infected early in gestation, the disease is generally more severe.

Symptoms and Signs

Pregnant women infected with *T. gondii* generally do not have clinical manifestations. Similarly, infected infants are usually asymptomatic at birth. In infants who do manifest the disease, however, clinical presentations include prematurity, intrauterine growth retardation, jaundice, hepatosplenomegaly, myocarditis, pneumonitis, and various rashes. Neurologic involvement, often prominent, includes chorioretinitis, hydrocephalus, intracranial calcifications, microcephaly, and seizures. Associated laboratory findings are thrombocytopenia, lymphocytosis, monocytosis, eosinophilia, and CSF abnormalities (xanthochromia, pleocytosis, or increased protein concentration). Outcome in these infants varies. Some have a fulminant course with early death, while others have long-term neurologic sequelae. Studies suggest that neurologic manifestations (eg, chorioretinitis, mental retardation, deafness, seizures) may develop years later in children who appeared normal at birth. Consequently, children with congenital toxoplasmosis should be closely monitored beyond the neonatal period.

Diagnosis

Serologic tests are important in diagnosing both maternal and congenital infection, but they require that the clinician be familiar with the characteristics of particular tests and the laboratory's methods of standardization. Some tests are performed only in reference laboratories.

The most reliable tests for measuring IgG antibodies to *T. gondii* include the Sabin-Feldman dye test, the indirect fluorescent antibody (IFA) test, and the direct agglutination assay. Acute maternal infection is suggested by seroconversion or a four-fold or greater rise in IgG levels between samples collected in acute and convalescent stages. Interpretation of IgG antibodies in the infant is often difficult because maternal IgG antibodies may be detectable through the first year of life. IgM antibody to *T. gondii* may be detected by the IgM indirect fluorescent antibody (IgM-IFA) test, the double-sandwich enzyme-linked immunosorbent assay (ELISA), and other immunosorbent assays. The double-sandwich ELISA is the preferred test. Recently, efforts have been made to diagnose congenital infection prenatally; fetal blood and amniotic fluid have been sampled and inoculated into mice or tissue culture to isolate the organism.

In infants suspected of having congenital toxoplasmosis, serologic tests should be performed, in addition to head x-rays, CSF analysis, and a thorough eye examination by an ophthalmologist. Inspection of the placenta for evidence of *T. gondii* infection can also be helpful.

Prophylaxis and Treatment

Education of all women of childbearing age and identification of recently infected pregnant women are the best means of preventing congenital toxoplasmosis. Women should be instructed to avoid contact with cat litter boxes and other areas contaminated with cat feces. Meat should be thoroughly cooked before consumption, and hands should be washed after handling raw meat or unwashed produce. Women at risk for primary infection should be screened during pregnancy. Those infected during the 1st or 2nd trimester should be counseled regarding available treatment methods as well as possible termination of pregnancy.

Although studies are limited, data suggest that treatment of infected women during pregnancy may be beneficial to the fetus. Spiramycin (available in the USA from the FDA) has been used to prevent transmission of maternal infection to the fetus. Pyrimethamine and sulfonamides have been used later in gestation to treat the infected fetus.

More data are needed concerning the treatment of congenitally infected infants. Consultation with an expert is advised. Infants with clinically apparent disease have been treated with pyrimethamine, sulfadiazine, spiramycin, folinic acid, and if inflammation is evident, corticosteroids. Treatment of infants with subclinical infection should be individualized.

CONGENITAL SYPHILIS
(See also SYPHILIS in Ch. 21)

A multisystem infectious disease caused by Treponema pallidum *and transmitted from mother to fetus via the placenta.* Risk of transplacental infection of the fetus (overall, about 60 to 80%) is related to the stage of the mother's infection and stage of pregnancy when she was infected; ie, untreated primary or secondary syphilis usually is transmitted, but latent and tertiary syphilis usually is not. In untreated mothers with late syphilis, a healthy child may be born between 2 others who have congenital syphilis. Nevertheless, congenital syphilis is preventable with adequate treatment of infected pregnant women. The incidence of congenital syphilis can be greatly reduced by routinely administering prenatal serologic tests for syphilis (STS—see in Ch. 21), retesting women who acquire other sexually transmitted diseases during pregnancy, and adequately treating those infected.

Symptoms and Signs

In **early congenital syphilis,** the characteristic skin lesions are bullous eruptions or a macular copper-colored rash on the palms and soles and papular lesions around the nose and mouth and in the diaper area. Generalized lymphadenopathy and hepatosplenomegaly are often present. The infant may fail to thrive and have a characteristic "old man" look, with fissured lesions around the mouth (rhagades) and a mucopurulent or blood-stained nasal discharge causing snuffles. A few infants may develop meningitis, choroiditis, hydrocephalus, or convulsions, and others may be mentally retarded. Within the first 3 mo of life, osteochondritis (chondroepiphysitis), especially of the long bones and ribs, may result in pseudoparalysis of the limbs with characteristic radiologic changes in the bones.

Many patients with congenital syphilis remain in the **latent stage** of the disease throughout their lives and never present any active manifestations. In others, **late manifestations** appear: gummatous ulcers tend to involve the nose, septum, and hard palate, while periosteal lesions result in saber shins and bossing of the frontal and parietal bones. Neurosyphilis is usually asymptomatic, but juvenile paresis and tabes may develop. Optic atrophy, sometimes leading to blindness, may occur. Interstitial keratitis is the most common eye lesion; it frequently recurs, often resulting in scarring of the cornea. Sensorineural deafness, which is often progressive, may appear at any age. **Hutchinson's incisors, Moon's molars,** and maldevelopment of the maxilla resulting in "bulldog" facies are typical, if infrequent, sequelae.

Diagnosis

Clinical suspicion of **early congenital syphilis** is confirmed when scrapings from the skin or mucosal lesions demonstrate *T. pallidum* by darkfield microscopy. If this does not yield a definitive diagnosis, STS should be performed, along with CSF analysis for cell count, protein level, and Venereal Disease Research Laboratory (VDRL) test, and long-bone x-rays should be obtained.

Since most neonates do not have signs of disease during their nursery stay, those whose mother has a history of any sexually transmitted disease before or especially during pregnancy should be tested serologically. Positive nonspecific (reagin) and specific (treponemal) serologic results may be due to passive transfer of maternal IgG across the placenta. Therefore, a positive STS in an otherwise asymptomatic infant should be interpreted with caution. The Centers for Disease Control **(CDC)** have provided guidelines for interpreting serologic and clinical signs of early congenital syphilis and classifying cases as confirmed, compatible, or unlikely (see TABLE 27–6). The value of the fluorescent treponemal antibody absorption immunoglobulin (**FTA-ABS[IgM]**) assay is controversial, but it has been used in detecting infection in the neonate.

Late congenital syphilis is diagnosed by the clinical history, distinctive physical signs, and positive serologic tests (see also the discussion on screening tests for syphilis in Ch. 21). **Hutchinson's triad** of interstitial keratitis, Hutchinson's incisors, and 8th nerve deafness is diagnostic. Sometimes the standard STS are negative and the *T. pallidum* immobilization **(TPI)** test is negative, but the FTA-ABS test is usually positive. The diagnosis should be considered in cases of unexplained deafness, progressive intellectual deterioration, or keratitis.

Prophylaxis

Adequate maternal treatment during pregnancy usually (99% of cases) cures both mother and fetus. However, in some cases, treatment late in the pregnancy eliminates the infection but not certain signs of syphilis that are apparent after birth.

When a diagnosis of congenital syphilis is made, other family members should be examined for physical and serologic evidence of infection at regular intervals. Re-treatment of the mother in subsequent pregnancies is necessary only if serologic titers remain positive. Women who remain sero-fast after adequate treatment may have been reinfected and should be re-treated. A mother without lesions who is seronegative but has had venereal exposure to a known patient with syphilis should be treated, as there is a 25 to 50% chance she acquired reactivating syphilis without yet being seropositive.

Treatment

For **pregnant women with early stages of syphilis,** benzathine penicillin G 2.4 million u. IM as a single injection (1.2 million u. may be given in each buttock) is recommended. For **later stages of syphilis** or **neurosyphilis,** the appropriate regimen for nonpregnant patients should be followed (see in Ch. 21). Occasionally, a severe **Jarisch-Herxheimer reaction** occurs after such therapy, leading to spontaneous abortion. Those allergic to penicillin may be desensitized and then treated with penicillin. Reagin tests become negative at 3 mo after adequate treatment in most patients and by 6 mo in nearly all patients. Since erythromycin therapy is inadequate for both the mother and fetus, it is not recommended. Tetracycline is *contraindicated.*

For **confirmed or compatible cases of early congenital syphilis,** the CDC recommends aqueous procaine penicillin G 50,000 u./kg IM daily for 10 days. A less intense regimen may be used for those at lower risk. Infants who have normal CSF, no other signs of active disease, and received standard penicillin therapy in utero may be given benzathine penicillin G 50,000 u./kg IM as a single or divided dose at one session if prolonged surveillance is impractical. The prognosis is usually favorable if serious damage has not already been done. The mother and other infected family members should also be treated.

In **late congenital syphilis,** the CSF should be examined before treatment is started. Because the adequacy of less intense regimens has not been established, the CDC recom-

TABLE 27–6. DIAGNOSTIC CLASSIFICATION OF CONGENITAL SYPHILIS

Confirmed/definite

Identification of *Treponema pallidum* by darkfield microscopy, fluorescent antibody, or other specific stains in specimens from lesions, autopsy material, placenta, or umbilical cord

---

Compatible (formerly "probable" or "possible")

A reactive STS in a stillborn

or

A reactive STS in an infant whose mother had syphilis during pregnancy and was not adequately treated, regardless of symptoms in the infant

or

A reactive VDRL test in CSF

or

A reactive STS in an infant with any of the following signs: snuffles, condyloma lata, osteitis, periostitis or osteochondritis, ascites, skin and mucous membrane lesions, hepatitis, hepatomegaly, spleno-megaly, nephrosis, nephritis, hemolytic anemia

or

Four-fold or greater rise in titers* of nontreponemal tests (VDRL or RPR) and a confirmed treponemal test (FTA-ABS or MHA-TP) over a 3-mo interval

or

A reactive treponemal test or nontreponemal test that does not revert to nonreactive in 6 mo

---

Unlikely

No reactive STS

or

Treponemal tests revert to nonreactive within 6 mo

or

No symptoms in live-born infants whose mothers were treated for syphilis during pregnancy and subsequently had a four-fold or greater fall in titer *provided* the infant's own STS is also four-fold or lower than the maternal titer at time of treatment

---

VDRL = Venereal Disease Research Laboratory; RPR = rapid plasma reagin; FTA-ABS = fluorescent treponemal antibody absorption; MHA-TP = microhemagglutination assay for antibody to *T. pallidum*.

* "Four-fold rise in titer," "four-fold fall in titer," and other similar phrases refer to changes in serum titers of at least 2 dilutions (2 "tubes"), eg, from 1:2 to 1:8 (and the reverse), or from 1:4 to 1:16 (and the reverse), or from 1:32 to 1:8 (and the reverse).

Adapted from "Guidelines for the Prevention and Control of Congenital Syphilis." *Morbidity and Mortality Weekly Report*, Vol. 37, No. S-1, Centers for Disease Control, U.S. Public Health Service, U.S. Department of Health and Human Services, Jan. 15, 1988.

mends that any child with congenital syphilis be treated with aqueous crystalline penicillin G 200,000 to 300,000 u./kg IV daily (up to adult doses) in divided doses for 10 days. Many patients do not revert to seronegativity but do have a four-fold decrease in titer of reagin (eg, VDRL) antibody. Interstitial keratitis is usually treated with corticosteroids and atropine drops; an ophthalmologist should be consulted. Patients with nerve deafness may benefit from combining penicillin therapy with a corticosteroid such as prednisone 0.5 mg/kg/day orally in divided doses for 1 wk, followed by 0.3 mg/kg/day for 4 wk, after which the dose is gradually reduced over a period of 2 to 3 mo. (Corticosteroids have not been critically evaluated in either of these conditions.) Family contacts should be traced, and patients should be kept under long-term surveillance.

PERINATAL TUBERCULOSIS

(See also TUBERCULOSIS IN CHILDREN under BACTERIAL INFECTIONS in Ch. 32)

Infants may acquire TB by (1) transplacental spread through the umbilical vein to the fetal liver, (2) aspiration or ingestion of infected amniotic fluid, or (3) postnatal exposure to active TB in a close contact (family or nursery personnel) via airborne inoculation. About 50% of children born to mothers with active pulmonary TB develop the disease during the first year of life if chemoprophylaxis or bacille Calmette-Guérin (BCG) vaccine is not given. Routine neonatal BCG vaccination is not indicated in developed countries but may curb the incidence of childhood TB or decrease its severity in populations at increased risk for infection.

Symptoms and Signs

The clinical presentation of neonatal TB is non-specific but is usually marked by multiple organ involvement. The infant may look acutely or chronically ill. Fever, lethargy, respiratory distress, hepatosplenomegaly, or failure to thrive should alert the physician to the possibility of TB in an infant with a history of TB exposure.

Diagnosis

Screening for TB by detailed history and skin testing is an essential part of prenatal evaluation. A pregnant woman with a positive tuberculin reaction should have a chest x-ray (with precautions against fetal exposure to radiation), and her close contacts should be screened for TB.

The result of skin testing may be difficult to interpret in the newborn infant: It may be negative in the neonate with active TB. Conversely, a false-positive test may result from transfer of tuberculin-sensitized lymphocytes to the fetus by maternal-fetal transfusion or to the neonate via ingested breast milk. Examination and culture of tracheal aspirates, urine, gastric washings, and CSF for acid-fast bacteria can be helpful. Chest x-ray usually shows miliary infiltrates. Biopsy of the liver, lymph nodes, or lung and pleura may be necessary to confirm the diagnosis.

Prophylaxis and Treatment

1. Pregnant women with a positive tuberculin test: Use of isoniazid (INH) in women who do not have acute TB can be deferred until the 3rd trimester or after delivery, because the potential hepatotoxicity of INH is increased in pregnancy. The risk of contracting TB from a mother with a positive tuberculin test is greater for the newborn during the postpartum period than for the fetus during pregnancy. *However, pregnant women with HIV infection should receive INH prophylactic therapy for 9 to 12 mo and should be evaluated for active TB.* The newborn whose mother has a positive tuberculin test but no clinical or radiologic evidence of infection does not need prophylaxis but should be given a skin test every 3 mo for 1 yr; the infant's family should also be investigated. If the reaction becomes positive, or if the family cannot be tested promptly or is noncompliant with follow-up, the infant should receive INH 5 to 10 mg/kg/day orally in a single daily dose for 9 to 12 mo and should be closely followed.

2. Pregnant women with active TB: INH, ethambutol, and rifampin used in recommended doses during pregnancy have not been shown to be teratogenic to the human fetus. If the disease is not extensive, pregnant women can be treated with a combination of INH (300 mg), pyridoxine (50 mg), and rifampin (600 mg). Ethambutol (15 to 25 mg/kg) may be added initially if INH resistance is a possibility. All these drugs can be given in single daily doses. The recommended duration of therapy is 9 mo unless the organism is drug-resistant, in which case an infectious disease consultation is recommended and therapy may need to be extended to 18 mo. Streptomycin is potentially ototoxic to the developing fetus and should not be used early in pregnancy unless rifampin is contraindicated. Other antituberculous agents should be avoided because of teratogenicity (eg, ethionamide) or lack of clinical experience during pregnancy. Breast-feeding is not contraindicated for mothers receiving therapy who are not infective.

3. Asymptomatic infants of women with active TB: The infant usually should be separated from the mother until effective treatment is under way and acid-fast stains of her sputum become negative (usually 2 to 12 wk). Family contacts should be investigated for undiagnosed TB before the infant is sent home. If compliance can be reasonably assured and the familial environment is nontuberculous, the infant should be started on a regimen of INH and may be sent home at the usual time; skin testing should be performed at ages 6 wk, 3 mo, and 6 mo. If the infant remains tuberculin-negative after that period, INH may be discontinued and the infant followed with skin tests at ages 9 mo and 12 mo.

If, on the other hand, good compliance in a nontuberculous environment *cannot* be ensured, BCG vaccine may be considered for the infant, and INH therapy should be started as soon as possible. (Although INH inhibits the multiplication of BCG organisms, the combination of BCG vaccine and INH is supported by clinical trials and anecdotal reports.) The infant is separated from the mother until she has received antituberculous therapy and her sputum becomes negative for acid-fast bacilli. The infant may then be sent home on a regimen of INH and given a tuberculin skin test at age 8 to 12 wk. If the infant's skin test is still negative, BCG vaccination should be repeated. BCG vaccination does not ensure against exposure to and development of tuberculous disease but offers the infant significant protection against serious and widespread invasion (eg, tuberculous meningitis). These infants should be followed closely for development of tuberculous illness, particularly in the first year of life. (CAUTION: *BCG vaccine is contraindicated in immunosuppressed patients and infants suspected of being infected with HIV*). However, in populations in which the risk of TB is high, the WHO recommends that asymptomatic HIV-infected infants receive BCG vaccine at birth or shortly thereafter.

4. Newborns with active TB: The newer recommendations for short-course therapy are based on experience with adults, since few data are available on experience with neonates and young children; however, it seems reasonable to assume that such therapy will be effective in infants. The regimen of INH (10 to 15 mg/kg), rifampin (10 to 20 mg/kg), and pyrazinamide (20 to 40 mg/kg) in single daily doses is given for 2 mo, followed by INH and rifampin for another 4 mo. Alternatively, a 9- to 12-mo regimen of INH and rifampin can be given, along with a third drug (pyrazinamide 20 to 30 mg/kg, streptomycin 20 to 30 mg/kg, ethambutol 15 to 25 mg/kg, or ethionamide 15 to 20 mg/kg), pending results of testing for resistance. **When the CNS is involved,** the initial therapy should include corticosteroids (prednisone 1 mg/kg/day for 4 to 8 wk, then gradually tapered), INH 20 mg/kg/day, rifampin 20 mg/kg/day, streptomycin 20 to 30 mg/kg/day, and pyrazinamide 20 to 40 mg/kg/day for 1 to 3 mo; therapy should be continued until all signs of meningitis have disappeared and cultures are negative on 2 successive lumbar punctures at least 1 wk apart. Then therapy can be continued with INH and rifampin daily or twice weekly for another 10 mo. Recent data suggest that nonmeningeal, nondisseminated extrapulmonary TB can be treated effectively with a 9-mo (total) course of therapy. The organism recovered from the infant or mother should be tested for drug sensitivity. Clinical monitoring for symptoms and signs of drug toxicity (hematologic, hepatic, and otologic) should be frequent.

NECROTIZING ENTEROCOLITIS (NEC)

An acquired disease, primarily of preterm or sick neonates. Mucosal or even deeper intestinal necrosis is present most commonly in the terminal ileum, with the colon and the proximal small bowel involved less frequently. The necrosis begins in the mucosa and may progress to involve the full thickness of the bowel wall, resulting in perforation. Associated sepsis occurs in 1/3 of infants.

Etiology and Pathogenesis

In infants who develop NEC, 3 factors are usually present in the intestine: a preceding ischemic insult, bacterial colonization, and intraluminal substrate (ie, enteral feedings).

The cause of NEC is not clear. It is believed that an ischemic insult damages the bowel lining so that mucus is not produced, leaving the bowel susceptible to bacterial invasion. Once feedings are begun, ample substrate is provided for proliferation of luminal bacteria, which can penetrate into the bowel wall; there they produce hydrogen gas that collects, producing the characteristic appearance of pneumatosis intestinalis on x-ray. Gas may also enter the portal veins, and intraportal gas may be seen over the liver on plain films of the abdomen or by ultrasound examination of the liver. Disease progression may lead to full-thickness bowel necrosis, perforation, peritonitis, sepsis, and death.

The ischemic insult may result from vasospasm of the mesenteric arteries, which can be produced by an anoxic insult triggering the primitive "diving reflex" that markedly diminishes intestinal blood flow. Ischemic intestinal insult may result as well from low blood flow states encountered during an exchange transfusion, during sepsis, or from the use of hyperosmolar formulas. Similarly, congenital heart disease with reduced systemic blood flow or arterial O_2 desaturation may lead to bowel hypoxia/ischemia and predispose to NEC. The suggestion that feeding breast milk offers protection from NEC has not been proved.

NEC may occur as clusters of cases or outbreaks in neonatal units; epidemiologic studies have identified some clusters of cases associated with specific organisms (eg, *Klebsiella, Escherichia coli,* coagulase-negative staphylococcus), but often no specific pathogen is identified. However, because some outbreaks may be infectious, it is recommended that isolation of infants with NEC and establishment of cohorts of possibly exposed neonates be considered if several cases of NEC occur within a short time.

Epidemiology and Clinical Findings

Certain neonates are at particular risk of developing NEC; 75% of NEC occurs in premature infants, particularly if prolonged rupture of the membranes with amnionitis or asphyxia occurred at birth. The incidence may also be higher in infants fed hypertonic formulas or in those who have undergone exchange transfusion. It is believed that delaying feedings for several days

TABLE 27-7. DOSAGE OF SYSTEMIC ANTIBIOTICS FOR INFANTS

Drug and Route		Age < 1 to 7 days	Age > 7 days
Ticarcillin	IV, IM	15 mg/kg/day* q 12 h	15-22.5 mg/kg/day* q 8-12 h
Mezlocillin	IV, IM	150-225 mg/kg/day* q 8-12 h	225-300 mg/kg/day* q 6-8 h
Amikacin	IM, IV	15 mg/kg/day* q 12 h	15-22.5 mg/kg/day* q 8-12 h
Gentamicin	IM, IV	5 mg/kg/day* q 12 h	7.5 mg/kg/day* q 8 h

* Given in divided doses.

to weeks in tiny or sick premature infants while providing total parenteral nutrition, and then slowly advancing the enteral feedings over a period of weeks, decreases the risk of developing NEC. Infants with NEC may present with ileus manifested by abdominal distention, bilious gastric residuals (after feedings) that may progress to bile emesis, and/or gross or microscopic blood in the stools. Screening the stools of premature infants (who are being fed) for occult blood or reducing substances may help to diagnose NEC at an early stage. Associated sepsis may be manifested by lethargy, temperature instability, increased apneic spells, and metabolic acidosis.

Early x-rays may be nonspecific and reveal only ileus. However, a fixed, dilated bowel loop that does not change on repeated x-rays indicates NEC. Specific x-ray signs diagnostic of NEC are pneumatosis intestinalis and portal venous gas. *Pneumoperitoneum indicates bowel perforation and an urgent need for surgery.*

Treatment

The treatment is **nonoperative support** in about 70% of cases. Feedings must be discontinued at once if NEC is suspected, and the bowel should be decompressed with a double-lumen nasogastric tube attached to suction. Appropriate colloid and crystalloid parenteral fluids must be given to support the circulation, as extensive bowel inflammation and/or peritonitis may lead to considerable third-space fluid losses. Total parenteral nutrition will be needed for 14 to 21 days while the bowel heals. Systemic antibiotics should be started at once with ticarcillin or mezlocillin and amikacin or gentamicin, and treatment should be continued for 10 days. (For dosage, see TABLE 27-7.) Most important, the infant with NEC requires frequent clinical reevaluation (eg, at least q 6 h), along with sequential abdominal x-rays, CBCs, platelet counts, and blood gases.

Operative intervention will be necessary in up to 1/3 of neonates with NEC. Absolute indications are intestinal perforation (pneumoperitoneum), signs of peritonitis (absent bowel sounds and diffuse guarding and tenderness or erythema of the abdominal wall), or aspiration of purulent material from the peritoneal cavity on paracentesis. In the newborn, erythema and edema of the abdominal wall is a sign of peritonitis. Serious consideration for surgery should be given in an infant with NEC whose clinical and laboratory condition worsens over time despite nonoperative support (see above). At surgery, gangrenous bowel is resected, and ostomies are created. (Primary reanastomosis may be done if the remaining bowel shows no signs of ischemia.) With resolution of sepsis and peritonitis, bowel continuity can be reestablished several weeks or months later. Rarely, infants treated nonoperatively will develop an intestinal stricture over the following weeks or months, usually at the splenic flexure of the colon. Resection of the stricture will then be required to relieve intestinal obstruction. About 2/3 of infants with NEC will survive; the outcome has been improved by aggressive support and the judicious timing of surgical intervention.

SUDDEN INFANT DEATH SYNDROME (SIDS)

The sudden death of any infant or young child that is unexpected from the history and in which a thorough postmortem examination fails to show an adequate cause of death. SIDS is the most common cause of death between 2 wk and 1 yr of age, accounting for 30% of all deaths in this age group. Distribution of SIDS is worldwide, occurring in 1.5/1000 live births in the USA. Peak incidence is between the 2nd and 4th mo of life. Incidence is increased in the cold months, in lower socioeconomic groups, in prematurely born infants, in infants who have experienced episodes of severe apnea requiring resuscitation, in subsequent siblings of SIDS victims, and in infants born to mothers who smoke during pregnancy. Many risk factors for SIDS apply to non-SIDS infant deaths as well. Almost all SIDS deaths occur when the infant is thought to be sleeping.

Etiology and Diagnosis

The cause is unknown, although it is most likely due to dysfunction of neural cardiorespiratory control mechanisms. The dysfunction that causes the death may be only intermittent or transient, and it is likely that multiple mechanisms are involved. Fewer than 5% of SIDS victims have been noted to have episodes of prolonged apnea before their death, so the overlap between the SIDS population and infants with recurrent prolonged apnea is very small.

The diagnosis, while largely one of exclusion, cannot be made without an adequate autopsy to rule out other causes of sudden, unexpected death (eg, intracranial hemorrhage, meningitis, and myocarditis).

Management

Parents who have lost a child from SIDS are grief-stricken and unprepared for the tragedy; because no definitive cause can be found for their baby's death, they usually have excessive guilt feelings. These may be aggravated by the nature of investigations conducted by police, social workers, or others who become involved because of the sudden, unexpected death. Family members require support not only during the days immediately following the infant's death, but for at least several months thereafter to help them deal with their grief and dispel their guilt reactions. This includes, whenever possible, an immediate home visit to (1) help the parents deal with their initial panic and prevent them from rushing carelessly to the hospital with their baby, endangering themselves and others; (2) observe the circumstances in which SIDS occurred; and (3) begin to inform and counsel the parents concerning the cause of death.

Autopsy should be performed quickly; as soon as the preliminary results are known (usually within 8 to 12 h), a 2nd home visit should be made to continue the earlier discussions with the family concerning SIDS. A 3rd meeting with the parents 2 to 3 days later reinforces the earlier discussions and answers many new questions raised. In a month or so, a 4th meeting should be held to give the family the final (microscopic) autopsy results and to discuss the parents' adjustment to their loss, especially their attitude toward having other children. Much of the counseling and support can be complemented by specially trained nurses or by lay persons who have themselves experienced the tragedy of and adjustment to SIDS (eg, a member of a local chapter of the National Foundation for Sudden Infant Death Syndrome or of the International Guild for Infant Survival).

HEMORRHAGIC SHOCK AND ENCEPHALOPATHY (HSES)
(Newcastle Syndrome)

Acute onset of severe shock, encephalopathy, and other symptoms in previously normal children, resulting in death or catastrophic neurologic outcome. The syndrome was first reported in 1979 in patients thought to have heatstroke.

Etiology and Pathology

The cause is unknown. It has been suggested that HSES is a form of heatstroke due to over-wrapping of infants who have febrile illness. However, HSES has rarely been seen in the newborn period, and overwrapping is not consistently reported. Additional etiologic theories have included a reaction to intestinal toxins, an environmental toxin, pancreatic release of trypsin, or an unidentified virus or bacterium. There are reports of an increase in plasma proteases and a decrease in plasma protease inhibitors. Whether the decrease is primary (a defect in synthesis or release) or secondary (due to increased utilization or deactivation) is not known.

Diffuse cerebral edema with herniation and focal hemorrhages in the cerebral cortex and other organs are consistently noted in postmortem examination. Other nonspecific findings are described, including patchy swelling and degeneration of hepatocytes but without fatty degeneration consistent with Reye's syndrome.

Symptoms, Signs, and Diagnosis

HSES occurs predominantly in infants 3 to 8 mo old (median age of 5 mo) but has been reported in a child 15 yr old. In most patients there is a prodrome of fever, upper respiratory tract symptoms, or vomiting and diarrhea. The major features are an acute onset of encephalopathy (manifested as seizures, coma, and hypotonia) and severe shock. Other common features include hyperpyrexia (up to 111° F [43.9° C] rectally), disseminated intravascular coagulopathy (DIC), cerebral edema, bloody diarrhea, metabolic acidosis, elevated liver transaminases, acute renal failure, thrombocytopenia, and a falling Hct. Primary pulmonary or myocardial involvement is unusual. Laboratory evaluation often reveals leukocytosis, hypoglycemia, hyperkalemia, and normal serum ammonia. Bacteriologic and viral cultures are negative. In all series most patients died (> 60%), and about 70% or more of survivors had severe neurologic sequelae.

Diagnosis is made by clinical and laboratory findings described above. **Differential diagnosis**

includes septic shock, Reye's syndrome, toxic shock syndrome, hemolytic-uremic syndrome, heatstroke, and viral hemorrhagic fevers. These conditions are excluded by their clinical course or laboratory findings.

Treatment

The treatment is entirely supportive. Infusions of isotonic solutions and blood products (up to 300 mL/kg) along with inotropic support (dopamine, epinephrine, etc) are necessary to maintain circulation. Increased intracranial pressure from cerebral edema requires intubation and hyperventilation. DIC often progresses despite administration of fresh frozen plasma.

28. CONGENITAL ABNORMALITIES

Structural defects present at birth.

GENERAL CONSIDERATIONS

Congenital malformations may be isolated or multiple, inherited or sporadic, apparent or hidden, gross or microscopic. They cause about 10% of neonatal deaths. A major anomaly is apparent at birth in 3 to 4% of newborns; by age 5 yr, up to 7.5% of all children manifest a congenital defect. The incidence of specific congenital anomalies varies with (1) the individual defect (common malformations such as Down syndrome occur in 1/660 births); (2) the geographic area because of factors such as differences in the genetic pool or the environment (the occurrence of spina bifida is 3 to 4/1000 births in areas of Ireland; recent studies suggest that it is about 1/1000 in the USA); (3) cultural practices (where marriages between relatives are frequent, the incidence of certain defects increases); and (4) certain ante- and perinatal problems (see Etiology, below).

Etiology

Several factors associated with pregnancy and delivery signal the increased likelihood of congenital malformation: (1) a primipara over age 35 yr (Down syndrome is a particular risk); (2) breech presentation, which is also often accompanied by birth asphyxia; and (3) poly- or oligohydramnios. Excess amniotic fluid is present when the fetus has difficulty swallowing (eg, severe CNS disorders such as anencephaly) or the fluid

cannot reach the GI tract to be absorbed (eg, esophageal atresia); decreased fluid is associated with GU anomalies that lower fetal urine output.

The specific cause of many congenital malformations is unknown. A variety of insults to the developing fetus may produce the same defect if they occur at similar times during embryogenesis when an organ system is most susceptible.

Genetic factors are responsible for many single malformations as well as syndromes. These can follow simple mendelian laws and be autosomal dominant, autosomal recessive, or sexlinked. Where the inheritance is more complex, as in spina bifida, multiple factors are probably involved. These may include a genetic predisposition or an increased susceptibility to certain environmental factors. Some syndromes result from chromosomal abnormalities and can be identified by chromosomal study; eg, Down syndrome (trisomy 21; see also Ch. 48).

Teratogenic agents include (1) drugs taken by the mother during pregnancy (see in Ch. 14); eg, thalidomide produced defects of the extremities, and recently valproic acid has been associated with spina bifida; (2) maternal illness such as diabetes mellitus and hypothyroidism; (3) various infectious agents; eg, rubella virus, cytomegalovirus, and *Toxoplasma gondii* (microcephaly, with subsequent motor and intellectual retardation, is one serious consequence); and (4) irradiation. Although irradiation can produce congenital malformations experimentally, its teratogenicity in man is less clear.

Treatment

Prenatal evaluation using ultrasonography, amniocentesis, and chorionic villus sampling (see Chs. 13 and 48) permits diagnosis of some defects during pregnancy. When a serious defect is identified, parents can then decide if they wish to continue the pregnancy or, alternatively, both physician and parents can make realistic plans for the labor, delivery, and care of the child. Prenatal therapy also becomes possible. In utero treatment has been tried for obstructive uropathy and hydrocephalus but is currently experimental.

If a congenital malformation is identified or suspected, the parents should be informed promptly even though extensive discussion may be deferred until specialists are consulted. The family should be given a realistic, honest appraisal of the severity of the condition, the medical care available, and the prognosis. Parents should be active participants in decision making. (See also PARENT-INFANT BONDING: THE SICK NEONATE and MANAGEMENT OF CHRONIC DISABILITY in Ch. 24.) When genetic factors are suspected, the parents should receive genetic counseling (see Chs. 13 and 48); if the condition is not inherited, they should be given that reassurance.

Discussions of some specific congenital defects follow.

CONGENITAL HEART DISEASE

Defects of the heart and major great vessels produced by abnormalities at various stages of fetal development and present at birth, but which may not be diagnosed until later. The incidence of such anomalies is 1/120 live births. In some instances, a specific cause may be identified. Chromosomal defects (eg, trisomy 13, trisomy 18) usually are associated with severe congenital cardiac anomalies. Other chromosomal or genetic diseases (eg, trisomy 21, Turner's syndrome [XO], Holt-Oram syndrome) are also often associated with congenital cardiac anomalies. Maternal illness (eg, diabetes mellitus, SLE), environmental exposure (eg, thalidomide), and combinations of the above may be implicated. The risk of congenital heart disease with an affected first-degree relative is generally considered to be 2 to 3%, with a higher risk in children of affected individuals.

Identification and diagnosis of congenital heart disease depend on recognition of affected cardiac function—heart murmurs representing turbulent flow, altered systemic and pulmonary blood flow, shunting in either direction, and evidences of altered work load of the cardiac chambers. Routine history, physical examination, ECG, and chest x-ray are usually adequate for specific anatomic diagnosis, with supportive and confirmatory data from echocardiography, cardiac catheterization, angiocardiography, and other laboratory data.

Normal Circulation
(See FIG. 28−1 and PERINATAL PHYSIOLOGY under MANAGEMENT OF THE NORMAL NEWBORN in Ch. 23)

In the presence of a normal heart (after the neonatal period of cardiovascular adaptation with closing of the foramen ovale and ductus arteriosus and a decrease in pulmonary vascular resistance to normal adult levels), there is complete separation of the systemic and pulmonary circuits and all right heart pressures are lower than their left heart counterparts. The consequences of congenital heart disease depend on these differences.

Pathophysiology

Many congenital cardiac defects, while clearly a result of abnormal cardiac development, produce no significant hemodynamic alteration. Defects with more significant effects on hemodynamics will show the results of ventricular volume load, ventricular pressure load, atrial emptying abnormalities, admixture of unoxygenated and oxygenated blood, or inadequate systemic cardiac output. Defects characterized by obstruction to blood flow (eg, pulmonic or aortic stenosis) do not depend on a drop in pulmonary vascular resistance and are therefore usually audible at birth, producing ejection murmurs, which have a crescendo/decrescendo quality as pressure within the ventricle rises in systole to overcome the obstruction. Ventricular hypertrophy, seen on the ECG, reflects this increased pressure work load on the heart, but because hypertrophy of ventricular muscle at moderate levels does not produce ventricular enlargement, the changes are not well seen on x-ray.

Since left-to-right shunts depend on decreasing pulmonary resistance for shunting to occur, they are not generally apparent until some time after birth—several days to a few weeks for high-pressure shunts (ie, ventricular or great vessel level) and considerably later for low-pressure atrial level shunts. Ventricular dilation, the result of left-to-right shunting, is well demonstrated by

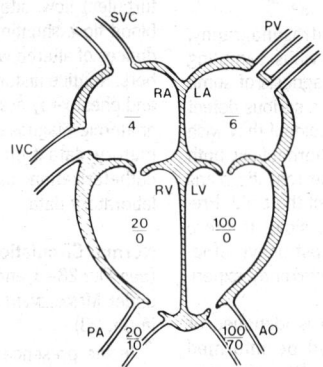

FIG. 28—1. **Normal circulation with representative right and left heart pressures.** Representative right heart saturation = 75%; representative left heart saturation = 95%. AO = aorta; IVC = inferior vena cava; LA = left atrium; LV = left ventricle; PA = pulmonary artery; PV = pulmonary veins; RA = right atrium; RV = right ventricle; SVC = superior vena cava.

cardiomegaly on x-ray but produces a less obvious ECG pattern.

Heart murmurs and thrills are the result of turbulent flow within the heart or great vessels and are transmitted to the surface at the point where they are generated, making careful localization of murmurs of great diagnostic help. Increased flow across the pulmonic valve produces a soft murmur similar to but less harsh than an aortic or pulmonic ejection murmur. Regurgitant flow from an atrioventricular valve or flow across the ventricular septum produces a pansystolic murmur, possibly obscuring the heart sounds as its intensity increases. Flow in the great vessels is continuous, and a murmur arising from aortic-pulmonary flow is continuous and uninterrupted by the heart sounds when pulmonary artery pressure is not high. The quality of the heart sounds reflects adequacy of ventricular function and arterial closing pressures. An ejection sound may be heard easily after the first sound when valve opening is restricted.

Increased pulmonary blood flow with increased pulmonary venous pressure may lead to signs of respiratory distress with tachypnea and dyspnea. Tachycardia and hepatomegaly are other consequences of heart failure. Increases in pulmonary blood flow are easily seen by chest x-ray. Cyanosis, as a presenting symptom of congenital heart disease, is seen in the neonate, but a careful search for noncardiac causes is required. Many neonatal respiratory problems are accompanied by cyanosis when there is obstruction to air flow within the bronchial tree, when large masses occupy space

otherwise occupied by lung, or when alveolar disease prevents adequate gas exchange. Recognition of cyanosis is dependent on the absolute amount of unsaturated Hb and may therefore be masked by anemia. Clubbing and polycythemia are the result of long-standing arterial unsaturation. Harlequinism, mimicking cyanosis, is not rare in the neonate or young infant. Hypothermia, hypoglycemia, hypocalcemia, sepsis, and CNS dysfunction also commonly present with cyanosis in the newborn.

Inadequate systemic perfusion presents as diminished or impalpable pulses, cold extremities, poor capillary refill and, if prolonged, evidence of organ dysfunction (eg, decreased urine output and renal failure). Evaluation of heart murmurs, adequacy of pulses, color, and the findings by ECG and x-ray will usually allow a precise cardiac diagnosis.

VENTRICULAR SEPTAL DEFECT (VSD)

One or more openings in the septum that normally separates the ventricles; such openings may undergo spontaneous closure in infancy, may lead to heart failure, may require surgical closure, or may be accompanied by pulmonary vascular disease (see FIG. 28—2).

Symptoms, Signs, and Diagnosis

VSDs are frequently heard as loud, harsh, pansystolic murmurs at the lower left sternal border in early infancy and are not accompanied by he-

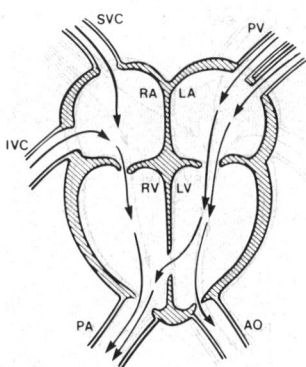

FIG. 28–2. Ventricular septal defect: increased pulmonary blood flow, increased left atrial volume, and increased left ventricular volume. (For abbreviations, see FIG. 28–1.)

modynamic abnormality. More significant VSDs are often heard somewhat later at age 2 to 3 wk as pulmonary vascular resistance decreases and left-to-right shunting increases. Heart failure (see below) may be apparent at age 6 to 8 wk as pulmonary flooding occurs. There is a long, loud, harsh systolic (pansystolic) murmur grade 3 to 4/6 at the lower left sternal border, a mid-diastolic apical murmur of mitral flow if there is a large shunt, accentuation of the pulmonic closure sound when pulmonary artery pressure is elevated, and signs of heart failure when present. X-ray findings include cardiomegaly, left atrial and left ventricular enlargement, and increased pulmonary arterial flow. ECG findings are initially those of left ventricular volume load but may include increasing right ventricular hypertrophy as right ventricular and pulmonary artery pressures increase. Cardiac catheterization and angiocardiography to determine VSD location, pulmonary vascular resistance, and the presence of associated, and sometimes masked, anomalies (eg, ductus or coarctation) are usually done before surgery.

Prognosis and Treatment

Anticongestive measures (eg, digitalis, diuresis, salt restriction) and treatment of respiratory infections may control heart failure and allow the child to maintain normal growth and development. In such children, the heart failure usually disappears in the first or second year and the defect becomes less significant and may not require surgery.

In infants who respond poorly or not at all to anticongestive measures, it may be necessary to

consider VSD closure in the first year of life. Infants with large shunts or heart failure who have not been well stabilized are at considerably higher risk for viral pneumonias (eg, respiratory syncytial virus) than are infants with smaller shunts and deserve consideration for early repair. VSDs that remain significant with cardiomegaly, growth failure, or symptoms, but without heart failure, may require closure later in childhood. All children with VSD should receive adequate protection against infective endocarditis (see antistreptococcal prophylaxis under INFECTIVE ENDOCARDITIS in Ch. 32 and RHEUMATIC FEVER in Ch. 42.)

ATRIAL SEPTAL DEFECT
(Ostium Secundum; Sinus Venosus)

Opening in the septum that normally separates the atria (see FIG. 28–3).

Symptoms, Signs, and Diagnosis

The typical murmur of atrial septal defect is usually present after age 1 yr when pulmonary blood flow has increased significantly and a grade 2 to 3/6 flow murmur is audible at the upper left sternal border in association with splitting of the second sounds throughout all phases of respiration. In the presence of a large left-to-right shunt (in which the pulmonary to systemic blood flow ratio ≥ 2:1), there may be a low-pitched diastolic murmur of tricuspid flow. By x-ray, there is dilation of the right atrium and right ventricle and an increase in pulmonary arterial flow. The ECG shows a moderate right axis, a moderate right ventricular volume load, nor-

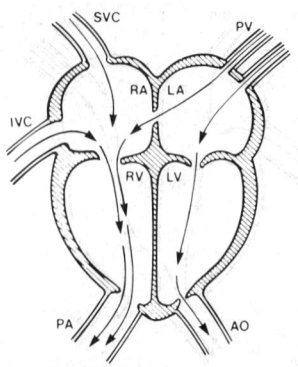

FIG. 28–3. Atrial septal defect: increased pulmonary blood flow, increased right atrial volume, and increased right ventricular volume. (For abbreviations, see FIG. 28–1.)

mal left ventricular forces, and in some patients a slightly prolonged PR and/or P wave abnormalities. Partial anomalous pulmonary venous flow is common with a sinus venosus atrial defect, and persistence of the left superior vena cava is not uncommon. The diagnosis is usually apparent on clinical grounds, and the defect is usually seen by 2-D echocardiogram. However, catheterization is often done preoperatively, not only to assess the size of the shunt and to determine the presence of anomalous systemic or pulmonary veins, but also to evaluate left ventricular function.

Treatment

Elective surgical repair is recommended at age 4 to 6 yr in children in whom the pulmonary to systemic flow ratio is > 1.5:1, although most patients undergoing atrial defect closure have a 2.5 to 3:1 ratio. Surgery may be done earlier if very large shunts are present or if atrial dysrhythmias appear. Continued medical observation is justified in children with lesser shunts if they have no cardiomegaly or symptoms and if continued medical care can be assured. Prediction of which children will develop pulmonary hypertension in adulthood is not yet possible.

PATENT DUCTUS ARTERIOSUS (PDA)

Failure of the fetal communication between the pulmonary artery and the aorta to close (see FIG. 28–4).

Symptoms, Signs, and Diagnosis

PDA in the premature infant is a frequent occurrence with increased pulmonary blood flow and further compromise of gas exchange, particularly in the infant with respiratory distress syndrome. The infant will have bounding pulses, a hyperdynamic precordium, increased pulmonary closure sound, and a pulmonic area mur-

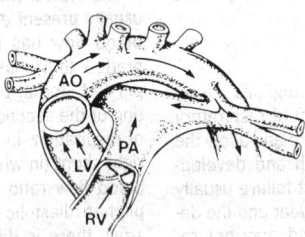

FIG. 28–4. Patent ductus arteriosus: increased pulmonary blood flow, increased left atrial and ventricular volumes, and increased ascending aorta volume. (For abbreviations, see FIG. 28–1.)

mur that may be continuous, systolic with a short diastolic component, or systolic alone. In some infants, there is no murmur, but the other findings are present. These infants will usually have normal ECGs for the degree of prematurity (ie, left ventricular prominence) but may show a left ventricular volume load. By x-ray, they will have cardiomegaly and, if the pulmonary findings of respiratory distress syndrome are not severe, an increase in pulmonary arterial flow. Echocardiography may be helpful with demonstration of left atrial size exceeding the aortic root diameter, and color-flow Doppler echocardiography usually shows reverse pulmonary artery flow in diastole.

Persistent PDA in full-term infants is usually identified after age 6 to 8 wk by a continuous murmur at the upper left sternal border. The peripheral pulses are full, with a widened pulse pressure, and the ECG may reflect left ventricular volume load. The x-ray will show prominence of left atrium, left ventricle, ascending aorta, and an increase in pulmonary blood flow if the ductus has significant flow. Care must be taken to be sure that the ductus is not compensating for pulmonary atresia and that the murmur does not represent a systemic arteriovenous fistula, branch pulmonary stenosis, or aortic-pulmonary window. Evaluation of femoral pulses and leg BP is necessary to rule out a hidden coarctation.

Prognosis and Treatment

If the respiratory status of **the premature infant** is compromised by ductal patency, attempts at closure are indicated. These include fluid restriction (90 to 100 mL/kg/day), diuresis, maintenance of good oxygenation, and consideration of pharmacologic closure with indomethacin, or surgical ligation. Indomethacin is a prostaglandin inhibitor and, in the absence of excessive jaundice (indirect bilirubin > 10 mg/dL), renal failure (creatinine > 1.4 mg/dL, BUN > 35 mg/dL), or thrombocytopenia (platelet count < 100,000/μL), usually will produce prompt ductal closure after 1 or 2 doses of 0.2 mg/kg IV 12 h apart or 0.2 mg/kg orally 3 times. Moderate fluid restriction should be maintained for 2 to 3 days with subsequent gradual and steady fluid increase. If contraindications to indomethacin exist or if indomethacin is ineffective, surgical ligation may be undertaken at little risk as long as experienced anesthesiologists and surgeons are available. While less significant ductus in premature infants will frequently undergo spontaneous closure or will close with fluid restriction alone, some will remain patent and require surgical clo-

sure at age 1½ to 2½ yr. **In full-term infants** with persistent PDA, surgical repair by ligation or transection is indicated if heart failure occurs or electively at age 6 mo to 3 yr to remove the risk of infective endarteritis.

ATRIOVENTRICULAR (A-V) CANAL DEFECTS
(Ostium Primum Atrial Septal Defect; Complete A-V Canal Defect [or Endocardial Cushion Defect])

A-V canal defects are openings in the atrial and/or ventricular septa at the level of the A-V valves and are usually accompanied by mitral and/or tricuspid valve abnormalities (see FIG. 28–5).

Symptoms, Signs, and Diagnosis

Complete A-V canal defects, often seen in infants with Down syndrome, may present with cyanosis at birth, the result of right-to-left shunting at either atrial or ventricular level, and may have systolic regurgitant murmurs of mitral and/or tricuspid insufficiency. Heart failure may be present early as the result of large volume shunts or A-V valve insufficiency or both. The diagnosis may be made from the typical ECG pattern of a superior, left axis deviation and counterclockwise loop due to congenital absence of the anterior division of the left bundle, frequent prolongation of the PR interval, and the presence of left ventricular hypertrophy and/or right ventricular hypertrophy, depending on the specific hemodynamic changes in the individual infant. The x-ray will show cardiomegaly with a typical bulge of the upper right atrial shadow, right and left ventricular dilation, prominent main pulmonary artery segment, and increased pulmonary artery flow. The diagnosis may be confirmed by 2-D echocardiography. Cardiac catheterization and left ventricular angiography usually are done before surgery, although the echocardiographic delineation of ventricular chamber size and chordal attachments provides the major information needed preoperatively.

Treatment

Surgical repair of complete A-V canal defects should be done early to prevent fixed pulmonary vascular disease, clearly before the age of 2 yr, and in many centers as early as 3 to 4 mo. The indication for surgical repair should be taken in the context of the child's overall medical state, since many children are severely retarded.

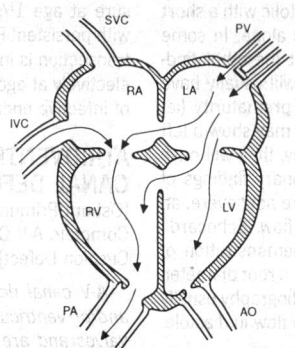

FIG. 28–5. Atrioventricular canal defect: increased blood flow; increased volumes of all chambers; often, increased pulmonary vascular resistance. (For abbreviations, see FIG. 28–1.)

CONGENITAL AORTIC VALVE STENOSIS

Congenital aortic valve abnormalities, usually a bicuspid valve, may produce severe left ventricular **(LV)** outflow tract obstruction in infancy with severe LV dysfunction, heart failure, evidence of ischemic changes by ECG, and poor systemic output. This is uncommon but requires an immediate attempt at aortic valvotomy to prevent death. Surgical results are not uniformly good, and residual aortic valve insufficiency may result. Valve replacement is usually required at a later age when the child has grown.

More commonly, bicuspid aortic valve with stenosis and sometimes with insufficiency is found later in childhood. There are usually no symptoms, and an ejection systolic murmur is heard loudest at the upper right sternal border, usually with a prominent systolic ejection click; an accentuated aortic closure sound is also heard. There may be a soft, early diastolic murmur of aortic insufficiency. The ECG shows increasing evidence of LV hypertrophy and ischemia as the severity of LV dysfunction increases but is not well correlated with the degree of obstruction. The x-ray may reflect poststenotic dilation of the ascending aorta and in long-standing obstruction may show LV hypertrophy. Complete evaluation by echocardiography, cardiac catheterization, and angiocardiography may be necessary at any age if there is evidence of severe obstruction or if symptoms occur (eg, exercise-induced chest pain or syncope), but this is usually delayed until adolescence.

A decision as to surgical palliation by aortic valvotomy is based not only on a significant LV-aortic gradient (≥ 50 mm Hg) but also on evidence of LV dysfunction and symptoms. Aortic valvotomy must be considered palliative rather than curative, and restenosis requiring aortic valve replacement is frequent. Significant aortic insufficiency following surgery may also require valve replacement.

LV outflow tract obstruction **at the subaortic level** by a fibrous ridge or by muscular hypertrophy will have essentially the same findings except that the ejection click will not be heard, the murmur may be most intense over the mid-sternum, and there will be no poststenotic dilation. **Supravalvar aortic obstruction** is not common but is frequently seen in hypercalcemia syndrome (Williams syndrome). Surgical repair, while possible, is difficult.

Congenitally bicuspid aortic valves occasionally produce severe obstruction in childhood and commonly become obstructive in adult life, at that time requiring valve replacement. Appropriate antibiotic prophylaxis against infective endocarditis/endarteritis is indicated in any patient with bicuspid aortic valves (see antistreptococcal prophylaxis under INFECTIVE ENDOCARDITIS in Ch. 32 and RHEUMATIC FEVER in Ch. 42).

PULMONIC VALVE STENOSIS

In the immediate neonatal period, pulmonic valve stenosis with severe obstruction to right ventricular **(RV)** outflow is associated with right-to-left atrial shunting and presents as an emergency, requiring immediate diagnosis: by ECG showing either diminished RV forces (when the right ventricle is hypoplastic) or RV hypertrophy; by x-ray with decreased pulmonary blood flow; by echocardiography, which may identify a severely narrowed valve with restricted movement; and by catheterization and angiography to evaluate potential RV function. Usually the right ventricle is severely hypoplastic, and immediate creation of a systemic-pulmonary anastomosis (eg, Blalock-Taussig shunt) is indicated to provide adequate pulmonary blood flow. Temporary palliation by maintaining ductal patency with prostaglandin E_1 (alprostadil) 0.05 to 0.1 μg/kg/min may be lifesaving until a systemic-pulmonary anastomosis can be done. Pulmonary valvotomy may also be indicated. These are palliative procedures; further surgery may be necessary in later childhood to provide further relief of RV outflow obstruction.

In older children, there is no cyanosis, although somewhat poor peripheral color may be the result of a prolonged circulation time and a wide arteriovenous O_2 difference. There is an ejection murmur, usually with a prominent ejection click, at the upper left sternal border with an increasingly late peak with increasing degrees of obstruction. The pulmonic component of the second sound is progressively delayed and diminished. RV hypertrophy of increasing severity is seen on the ECG. The x-ray shows a normal heart size and prominence of the main pulmonary artery segment with increasing RV hypertrophy. Cardiac catheterization to evaluate the degree of obstruction, the nature of the pulmonic valve, and RV function is indicated before treatment either by balloon valvuloplasty or surgical valvotomy. If not severe, treatment may be delayed until the immediate preschool period.

PERIPHERAL PULMONIC STENOSIS

Many neonates have soft systolic flow murmurs in the distribution of the branch pulmonary arteries without evidence of significant elevation of right heart pressures. These murmurs usually disappear by the end of the first year as growth occurs. However, in certain conditions (eg, congenital rubella, hypercalcemia syndrome [Williams syndrome]) and in some otherwise normal children, anatomic obstruction to flow to the branch pulmonary arteries occurs and may produce a continuous murmur. This is rarely amenable to surgical repair because there are multiple areas of obstruction within the lung itself and because there is usually an associated hypoplasia of the pulmonary arterial tree distal to the obstruction.

COARCTATION OF THE AORTA

Infants with aortic coarctation may have very sudden onset of heart failure, cardiovascular collapse, and severe metabolic acidosis as the ductus closes and distal perfusion is compromised. They require immediate treatment with supportive medications, intubation and ventilatory support if necessary, and may benefit from an infusion of prostaglandin (PG) E_1 at 0.05 to 0.1 μg/kg/min to reopen the ductus arteriosus. The response to PGE_1 infusion will be gradual, usually over hours, but most infants will stabilize with increased distal perfusion and improved renal blood flow and allow surgical repair of the coarctation and closure of the patent ductus.

Older children with aortic coarctation have upper extremity hypertension relative to the lower extremities and may have an absolute hypertension. A soft bruit, louder in the back, is often heard over the coarctation site. The femoral pulses, while often palpable, are clearly diminished and delayed when compared with the brachial pulses. The ECG is usually normal but may show left ventricular hypertrophy, and the x-ray shows a normal heart size with coarctation visible in a slight left anterior oblique view. Rib notching may be seen in older children. Catheterization and angiography are unnecessary unless significant associated defects (eg, aortic stenosis, aortic insufficiency, mitral valve disease, ventricular septal defect) are present or there is evidence that the narrow segment is not in the usual location just distal to the left subclavian artery or is of greater length than usual. Dilated collateral arterial vessels are usually palpable at the scapular margin. Surgical repair by resection and direct anastomosis, left subclavian artery "roofing" techniques, or grafting, if needed, is recommended at age 4 to 6 yr—or earlier with persistent upper extremity hypertension, heart failure, or other complications. Prophylaxis against endocarditis is needed (see antistreptococcal prophylaxis under Infective Endocarditis in Ch. 32 and Rheumatic Fever in Ch. 42).

TETRALOGY OF FALLOT

An anatomic abnormality with severe or total right ventricular outflow tract obstruction and a ventricular septal defect allowing right ventricular unoxygenated blood to bypass the pulmonary

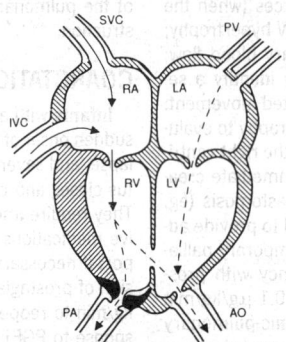

FIG. 28–6. Tetralogy of Fallot: pulmonary blood flow is decreased; right ventricle is hypertrophied; unoxygenated blood enters aorta. (For abbreviations, see FIG. 28–1.)

artery and enter the aorta directly (see FIG. 28–6).

In most instances, the upper left sternal border ejection murmur of right ventricular **(RV)** outflow tract obstruction is heard at or shortly after birth with the gradual development of cyanosis thereafter. Infants with tetralogy of Fallot with pulmonary valve atresia and ductus-dependent pulmonary blood flow, however, will present with severe cyanosis and a continuous murmur of ductal flow. Prostaglandin E_1 infusion at 0.05 to 0.1 μg/kg/min will usually maintain ductal flow until surgical palliation by a systemic-pulmonary anastomosis can be done. Prostaglandin infusion may lead to respiratory arrest, and equipment for mechanical ventilation should be available (see ASPHYXIA AND RESUSCITATION in Ch. 27 and CARDIOPULMONARY RESUSCITATION in Ch. 30). The infusion should be tapered to the lowest effective dose as quickly as possible.

Older infants will have an ejection murmur, right axis deviation, and RV hypertrophy on ECG; x-ray shows a small heart and a concave main pulmonary artery segment with diminished pulmonary blood flow. Right aortic arch is common. Intracardiac anatomy should be assessed in infancy to determine the possibility of complete intracardiac repair or the need for palliative increases in pulmonary blood flow by systemic-pulmonary anastomoses.

In some infants, tetralogy hypercyanotic "spells" with anxiety, air hunger, respiratory distress, increasing cyanosis, and altered level of consciousness may occur, usually precipitated by activity. Treatment of spells consists of supplemental O_2, knee-chest position, and morphine 0.1 to 0.2 mg/kg IM. Propranolol 0.25 to 1.0 mg/

kg orally q 6 h is useful to prevent further spells, but catheterization, angiography, and surgical palliation or repair are urgent.

TRANSPOSITION OF THE GREAT ARTERIES

An anatomic abnormality in which the aorta arises directly from the right ventricle and the pulmonary artery arises from the left ventricle, producing severe systemic hypoxemia (see FIG. 28–7).

Infants with transposition of the great arteries present with severe cyanosis immediately after birth, with rapid progression to metabolic acidosis secondary to poor tissue oxygenation and a compensatory respiratory alkalosis. They are usually otherwise healthy. Examination findings may be limited to cyanosis alone. Chest x-ray shows a narrow base as the great vessels are superimposed rather than side-by-side; there is absence of the main pulmonary artery segment in its usual location, and the overall picture is one of "an egg on its side." Pulmonary venous congestion may develop rapidly. The ECG is normal for the newborn.

Immediate confirmation of the diagnosis by echocardiography or cardiac catheterization is indicated, and palliation by balloon atrial septostomy to improve atrial mixing and decompress the left atrium is necessary. In infants with life-threatening hypoxemia, temporary palliation by giving prostaglandin E_1 will produce ductal opening, leading to an increase in pulmonary blood flow and temporary improvement in systemic oxygenation. This does not negate the need for immediate atrial septostomy. Surgical repair by re-

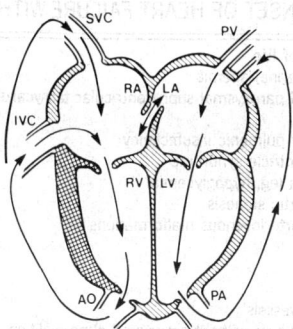

FIG. 28–7. Transposition of the great arteries: unoxygenated blood enters aorta; right ventricle is hypertrophied; foramen ovale permits minimal mixing. (For abbreviations, see FIG. 28–1.)

direction of systemic and pulmonary venous return (Mustard or Senning technique) or, in some infants, by arterial switching technique is done in early infancy.

COMPLEX CYANOTIC CONGENITAL HEART DISEASE

More complex anomalies (eg, single ventricle with or without pulmonary stenosis, tricuspid atresia with normally related or transposed great vessels, tricuspid and pulmonic atresia, mitral atresia, and truncus arteriosus) are less common. Specific anatomic diagnosis is usually possible by the usual methods of evaluation, but management is assisted by confirmatory testing (eg, angiography). Initial management of most of these infants consists of ensuring adequate pulmonary blood flow by systemic-pulmonary anastomosis or by protection of the pulmonary vascular bed and control of increased pulmonary blood flow by pulmonary artery banding. Restoration of normal blood-flow patterns and separation of oxygenated and unoxygenated blood in some of these infants are possible by the modified Fontan technique, in which blood flow is directed from the right atrium to the pulmonary artery, excluding the ventricle from the right-sided circulation. Conduit repair of truncus arteriosus is also possible for some infants.

UNDERDEVELOPED LEFT VENTRICLE SYNDROME

The abrupt appearance of severe heart failure with loss of peripheral pulses and evidence of a severe decrease in systemic perfusion in a 2- or 3-day-old infant who has been considered

healthy strongly suggest the presence of aortic and/or mitral valve atresia, with ductus-dependent systemic blood flow and cardiovascular collapse occurring as the ductus closes. Cardiomegaly, pulmonary venous congestion, and an ECG with no evidence of left ventricular forces are strongly suggestive, and echocardiography demonstrating severe hypoplasia of left heart structures is confirmatory. The prognosis for most infants with this anomaly is extremely poor, although experimental approaches (eg, the Norwood procedure or transplantation) are currently being evaluated.

LESS COMMON ANOMALIES AND ABNORMALITIES

Combinations of the more common diagnoses and other abnormalities (eg, Ebstein's malformation of the tricuspid valve), evidence of cardiac involvement with fetal disease (eg, prolonged in utero anemia, fetal dysrhythmia), severe cardiac anomalies associated with asplenia syndrome, and cardiac dysfunction secondary to noncardiac disease (eg, hypothyroidism) all require specific management guided by their manifestations in the specific infant.

Many other rare abnormalities (eg, congenital complete heart block, congenital metabolic errors usually leading to severe acidosis and secondary myocardial dysfunction, prolonged QT syndrome with risks of severe, possibly fatal dysrhythmia) and rare defects (eg, cor triatriatum) require skilled diagnostic and therapeutic intervention.

Pulmonary vascular disease **(Eisenmenger reaction)** may be a limiting factor in the care of infants and children with congenital defects (eg,

TABLE 28–1. AGE OF ONSET OF HEART FAILURE WITH COMMON CAUSES

Birth to first few hours of life
Severe chronic (intrauterine) anemia
Intrauterine or neonatal paroxysmal supraventricular tachycardia
Perinatal asphyxia
Severe tricuspid and/or pulmonic insufficiency
Underdeveloped left ventricle syndrome
Metabolic abnormalities (eg, hypoglycemia)
Critical pulmonic or aortic stenosis
Systemic or placental arteriovenous malformations

First month of life
All of the above
Transposition of great vessels
Coarctation of aorta, with or without associated abnormalities
Anomalous pulmonary vein drainage, particularly with pulmonary vein obstruction

Infancy
Ventricular septal defect, single ventricle
Truncus arteriosus
Patent ductus arteriosus
Atrioventricular canal defects
Rare metabolic diseases (eg, glycogen storage disease)

Childhood
Acute rheumatic fever with carditis
Rheumatic heart disease
Viral myocarditis
Bacterial endocarditis
Volume overload in the course of a noncardiac disease

ventricular septal defect, atrioventricular canal, truncus) in which high-pressured (ventricular, aortic-pulmonary) shunts occur and may exist alone as primary pulmonary hypertension. In these situations, pulmonary vascular resistance is maintained at a high level with medial muscular hypertrophy of the pulmonary arterioles and occlusion of the many smaller branches. As pulmonary vascular resistance approaches and equals systemic vascular resistance, left-to-right shunting is decreased and right-to-left shunting occurs, leading to systemic desaturation and visible cyanosis. Surgical repair is usually contraindicated when calculated pulmonary vascular resistance is $> 1/2$ the calculated systemic vascular resistance. Persistent and increasing right-to-left shunting leads to increasing peripheral hypoxemia and increasing polycythemia. Increased O_2-carrying capacity is provided by a Hct of up to 65% but, at higher levels, increased viscosity leads to decreasing O_2 delivery to the tissues. Cautious phlebotomy with maintenance of total blood volume may be beneficial, reducing Hct levels to about 60% when they exceed 65% and when the patient is symptomatic (eg, slurred speech, visual problems, and increased fatigue).

HEART FAILURE (HF)
(See also CONGENITAL HEART DISEASE, above)

A clinical syndrome that occurs when the heart, acting as a pump, is unable to maintain cardiac output (CO) sufficient to satisfy the metabolic demands of the body, including those necessary to support growth. A recognizable constellation of clinical and laboratory abnormalities reflects acute and chronic pulmonary and/or systemic congestion, as well as the findings of the underlying cardiac abnormality; eg, pulmonic stenosis can produce heart failure *without* pulmonary congestion.

Etiology

TABLE 28–1 gives an average age of onset of HF in infancy and childhood related to specific causes. **In utero**, HF is uncommon and is due to compromise of the pump function of the heart and its inability to maintain forward flow, rather than to shunts or obstruction. HF in utero may be produced by sustained intrauterine tachycardia chronic anemia with a subsequent volume load myocardial dysfunction secondary to myocarditis, etc. Some of these may be treated by managing the underlying abnormality; eg, maternal digitalization and diuresis may treat fetal tachycardia.

HF occurring **immediately after birth** may be the result of the above and also of perinatal asphyxia with myocardial damage, severe tricuspid and/or pulmonic insufficiency related to hypoxia, structural valve defects, or metabolic defects (eg, hypothermia, hypoglycemia, or severe metabolic acidosis from whatever cause). Critical aortic or pulmonic stenosis may be associated with early neonatal HF. Underdeveloped left ventricle syndrome is usually manifested at 48 to 72 h by abrupt HF and metabolic acidosis secondary to poor systemic perfusion.

HF occurring **in the first week of life** is the result of any of the above, complicated coarctation, various transpositions, systemic arteriovenous fistulas, or left-to-right shunts in premature infants (eg, patent ductus arteriosus **[PDA]**). Cardiac abnormalities with high-pressured left-to-right shunts (eg, ventricular septal defect, PDA, truncus arteriosus) usually show HF **by age 6 to 8 wk** as pulmonary vascular resistance decreases. More complex lesions (eg, anomalous pulmonary venous return, atrioventricular canal defects, single ventricle) may cause HF, depending on the degree of pulmonary artery flooding and pulmonary venous obstruction.

Noncardiac causes of HF include chronic anemia, upper airway obstruction, nutritional deficits, asphyxia, drug toxicity (eg, daunorubicin), and some systemic diseases such as storage diseases, Friedreich's ataxia, and iatrogenic hemodilution.

Symptoms and Signs

The onset of HF in infants may be gradual, but it is usually rapid and occasionally is extremely rapid. Tachycardia, with heart rates > 120 to 140/min and up to 200/min, is usually present. Signs of left and right heart failure usually occur together in infants. **Left ventricular failure** is manifested by respiratory difficulties. Dyspnea and tachypnea, with a respiratory rate of 60 to 100/min or more in the absence of primary lung disease, are frequently found and are due to pulmonary venous congestion, increased pulmonary capillary pressure, and transudation of fluid into alveolar, interstitial, and bronchiolar spaces. Superimposed infection may accentuate these problems. Coughing and wheezing are common. Rales and rhonchi are variable but not uncommon, while frank pulmonary edema with frothy, blood-stained sputum is rare. Fatigue from increased respiratory rate and work, as well as the increased metabolic demands to sustain the increase in respiration, leads to poor feeding, inadequate intake, and failure to thrive, although head circumference and growth in length are not usually compromised. Growth failure may be partially masked by fluid retention, decreased urine volume, and inappropriate weight gain. Other symptoms include restlessness, irritability, and excessive sweating.

Cardiomegaly is seen, except with constrictive pericarditis and severe pulmonary venous obstruction. Poor myocardial function is reflected in poor heart sounds, gallop rhythm, and signs of poor peripheral perfusion with cool extremities and decreased pulse volume and capillary filling, as well as a grayish rather than blue color. Cyanosis, an indicator of right-to-left intracardiac shunting, may also reflect inadequate alveolar gas exchange secondary to pulmonary venous congestion or a low output state with an increase in arteriovenous O_2 difference.

In **right ventricular failure**, hepatomegaly is a common and reliable sign of HF in infancy and is a sensitive guide to the effectiveness of therapy. Pain and tenderness secondary to hepatic engorgement and abnormalities of the jugular venous pulse, while useful signs in older children, are not reliable in infants. Peripheral edema occasionally is seen, particularly on the backs of hands and feet and in the periorbital area.

There are few specific laboratory findings in HF. Dilutional anemia and hyponatremia may be seen. A decrease in urine volume and albuminuria may be present. Hypoglycemia secondary to depletion of and inadequate stores of glycogen, as well as to a hypermetabolic state, is frequent, particularly in neonates. The WBC count may reflect associated infection, and prolonged systemic arterial desaturation usually results in polycythemia and later iron deficiency.

Diagnosis

HF is identified by the symptoms and signs described above. Evaluation of the infant or child in HF includes an attempt at a specific anatomic diagnosis by evaluating the history, physical examination, and basic laboratory and x-ray findings.

The precordium should be palpated for thrills, heaves, location of the maximal impulse, and sounds. Heart sounds are evaluated by listening for quality, intensity, 2 semilunar valve closures and their relative timing, and extra sounds. Heart

TABLE 28-2. PEDIATRIC DIGOXIN DOSES (ORAL OR IV)

Age	Digitalizing Dose (μg/kg)	Maintenance Dose (μg/kg/day)
Premature	20	5-8
Term, 0-1 wk	30	8-10
0-2 yr	30-50	10-12
2-5 yr	30	10-12
5+ yr	30	5-10

murmurs are identified by their location, timing, duration, intensity, and quality. Examination of the lungs for evidence of congestion or infection is required. Assessment of peripheral pulse quality and BP in all extremities is necessary. The degree of peripheral O_2 desaturation and of anemia can be determined by an examination of conjunctivae, mucous membranes, lips, and nailbeds. Liver size and fullness, as well as peripheral edema, should be noted. Fluid retention can best be determined by recording serial, carefully measured, weight increments. Frequent reevaluation of these physical findings serves as a guide to effectiveness of therapy and, as they change, as an aid to specific diagnosis.

ECG changes are of little benefit in diagnosing HF, but are of major value in making a specific anatomic diagnosis. Echocardiography, phonocardiography, vector cardiography, cardiac catheterization, and angiocardiography are required for complete anatomic diagnosis in some instances but are unnecessary in diagnosing HF. They are rarely performed before the HF and other acute problems (eg, electrolyte abnormality and infection) are controlled.

Prognosis and Treatment

Treatment is initially aimed at relieving the HF, but the prognosis is primarily influenced by the underlying disease and its treatment.

Digoxin is the most widely used drug for HF (see TABLE 28-2 for doses). The initial digitalizing dose may be given IV or orally, either in 3 divided doses, with a larger initial portion, or on a schedule of q 4, 6, or 8 h, depending on urgency. IM digoxin is rarely indicated. Digoxin maintenance divided into 2 doses daily usually provides a smoother response than 1 daily dose. Caution in digoxin prescribing is important. Digoxin concentration in the elixir for oral use is 50 μg/mL (0.05 mg), while in digoxin for IV use it is 250 μg/mL (0.25 mg). Digoxin levels in neonates and infants are not very helpful or reliable.

In very severe HF with inability to improve CO by other means, dopamine and/or dobutamine may be beneficial, beginning with 5 μg/kg/min and increasing to 15 μg/kg/min if needed. Higher doses should be *avoided* because of an adverse effect on renal blood flow. Afterload reduction with nitroprusside 0.5 to 3.0 μg/kg/min IV, hydralazine 0.5 to 5.0 mg/kg/day orally (in 3 or 4 divided doses), and captopril 0.5 to 6.0 mg/kg/day orally (in 2 to 4 divided doses) can be achieved, but the use of these drugs requires caution.

Diuresis with a rapid-acting drug (eg, furosemide or ethacrynic acid 1 mg/kg IV or 2 mg/kg orally) produces an immediate response. Either drug may be repeated in 4 to 6 h, and the dose may be doubled if an adequate response is not obtained. Chlorothiazide 20 to 40 mg/kg/day orally in 2 divided doses may be given in long-term diuretic management of infants and children. Interrupting therapy (eg, for 3 or 4 days/wk) helps to prevent electrolyte imbalance, but K supplements may be necessary. Caution must be used in prescribing diuretics if acute or chronic renal disease is present. Drugs such as amrinone should be reserved for severe HF and given only in an intensive care setting.

Therapy that may be beneficial during initial management includes humidified O_2 given by croupette, mask, or nasal prongs with adequate inspired O_2 (< 40% to prevent pulmonary epithelial damage) to prevent cyanosis and alleviate respiratory distress; sedation with morphine sulfate 0.2 mg/kg s.c. q 4 to 6 h as needed; and head elevation. While older children may benefit from a "cardiac chair" position, infants are more likely to have respiratory compromise as abdominal organs are pushed upward into the thorax. Limiting Na and, to a lesser extent, fluid intake to daily maintenance levels helps to maintain a favorable response to treatment, although care should be taken to avoid serum Na levels < 130 mEq/L. Rotating tourniquets, phlebotomy, and mechanical respiratory assistance are less commonly needed. Other general support measures (eg, attempts to increase caloric intake by formu-

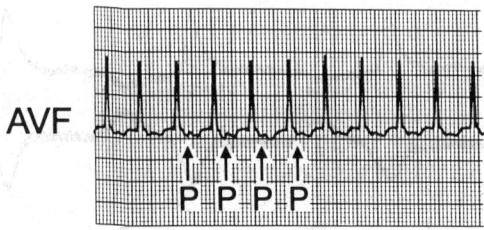

FIG. 28-8. **Narrow QRS tachycardia: orthodromic reciprocating tachycardia using an accessory pathway in a patient with Wolff-Parkinson-White syndrome.** Activation is as follows: A-V node, His-Purkinje system, ventricle, accessory pathway, atria. Note the P wave, which closely follows the QRS complex, such that PR > RP.

las of increased caloric density, rigorous fever control, treatment of anemia) are of value.

TACHYCARDIAS INVOLVING ACCESSORY PATHWAYS

Tachycardias involving accessory pathways are called **reciprocating tachycardias (RT)**. In the most common form, activation is from atria to ventricles through the normal A-V node returning via the accessory pathway to the atria. A narrow QRS tachycardia results, during which P waves are inscribed after the QRS complex (PR > RP—see FIG. 28-8). This direction of tachycardia is called **orthodromic**. Very rarely, conduction may be in the opposite direction, when a broad QRS complex **antedromic** RT results. Accessory pathways (eg, Kent bundle), which link the atria and ventricles bypassing the A-V node, are responsible for the **Wolff-Parkinson-White (WPW)** syndrome. In affected patients, a typical ECG pattern of short PR interval and slurred QRS complex (δ wave) is associated with arrhythmias (see FIG. 28-9). Antegrade conduction over the accessory pathway (see FIG. 28-10) is necessary to create the short PR interval and the δ wave, but it is retrograde conduction that is important for sustaining orthodromic RT. Thus, a concealed accessory pathway (normal PR, no δ wave in sinus rhythm) may support the arrhythmia.

In the **Lown-Ganong-Levine (LGL)/syndrome**, the accessory pathway links the atrium with His bundle tissue, bypassing the A-V node. The PR interval is short, as in the WPW syndrome, but the QRS complex is normal. Patients with the LGL syndrome have the same type of arrhythmias as do those with the WPW syndrome, and their medical management is similar (see FIGS. 28-10 and 28-11).

Symptoms and Signs

RT typically presents at 1 of 3 ages: during the 1st yr of life, in the teens and 20s, or in middle age (45 to 60 yr).

In the 1st yr of life, children may present with heart failure if the attack is protracted; otherwise episodic breathlessness, lethargy, feeding problems, or signs of rapid precordial pulsation are noticed.

RT may occur for the first time in the **teens and early 20s.** Typical attacks are of sudden onset, and many are associated with exercise. Attacks may last for only a few seconds or persist for several hours (rarely, > 12 h). In a young, otherwise fit population, RT is remarkably well tolerated and may be nearly asymptomatic. Disorganization of RT to AF is a concern, as remarkably rapid and potentially life-threatening ventricular responses may follow (> 250 beats/min).

Middle age may seem a surprising time for presentation of an arrhythmia using an accessory pathway that is congenital. Nevertheless, many patients give no prior history. Little is known of long-term changes in accessory pathway function, but more unidirectional (ventriculoatrial conduction only) pathways are seen in this age group than in symptomatic teenagers. Thus, an increased presentation rate of RT might more likely be expected with unidirectional than with bidirectional pathways. Alternatively, there may be an age-related increase in initiating atrial and ventricular premature beats.

Treatment

An established attack will frequently respond to a vagotonic maneuver (eg, the Valsalva maneuver, or ice-water facial immersion) through slowing A-V nodal conduction and destabilizing the reentry circuit.

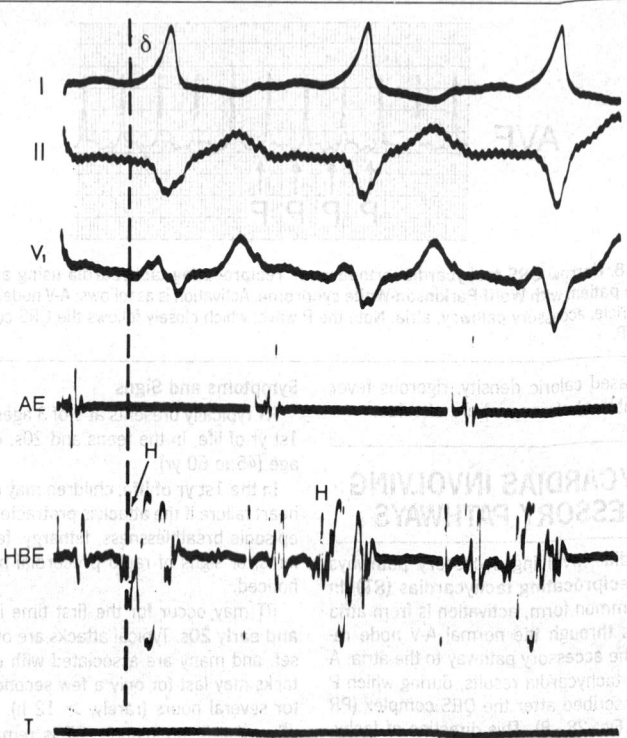

Fig. 28–9. **Wolff-Parkinson-White syndrome.** Recorded are ECG leads I, II, and V₁, an atrial electrogram (AE), a His bundle electrogram (HBE), and time marks at 10- and 100-msec intervals. Depolarization of the His bundle (HBE) occurs during inscription of the characteristic delta wave (δ). The QRS morphology represents the result of ventricular excitation via 2 independent pathways.

In infants and children (< 10 yr), AF is rare as a complication; digoxin is useful for prophylaxis but should not be continued into puberty without considering that as the child ages, digoxin may pose a risk through its facilitatory effects on the accessory pathway. *In all other circumstances, digoxin is contraindicated* as it may shorten atrial and accessory pathway refractory periods and encourage the development of VF. Established attacks may respond to vagal maneuvers, particularly if used early after symptom onset; otherwise, verapamil or adenosine will likely impose sufficient A-V nodal conduction delay to stop the reentrant activity. An alternative strategy is to slow conduction in the accessory pathway, which potentially is the weakest link in the reentrant circuit. Class Ia and Ic agents all slow accessory pathway conduction. Despite the proarrhythmic problems

seen with class Ic agents in treating ventricular arrhythmias, there is no evidence that these drugs cause similar effects in otherwise healthy individuals with accessory pathway arrhythmias. Flecainide, procainamide, and disopyramide offer efficacy and safety for acute management of attacks whether given IV or orally. In practice, on recognition of a narrow QRS tachycardia, most patients will receive IV verapamil, which will terminate the arrhythmia, not by effects on the accessory pathway but by transiently blocking or slowing conduction in the A-V node. Long-term prophylaxis requires agents with low toxicity yet exceptional efficacy. Flecainide, encainide, propafenone, and disopyramide meet these criteria. Procainamide and quinidine are rarely used in Europe, but they are widely used for chronic prophylaxis in North America. Amiodarone offers efficacy, but its

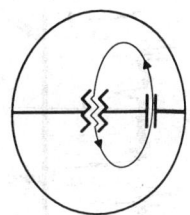

WPW syndrome
orthodromic reciprocating
tachycardia

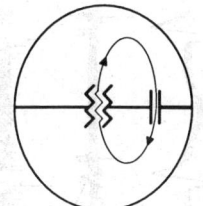

WPW syndrome
antedromic reciprocating
tachycardia

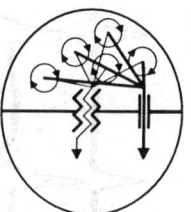

WPW syndrome
complicated by AF

|| Accessory
    pathway

§§ A-V node

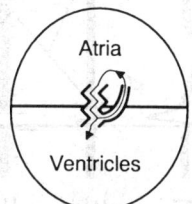

LGL syndrome
partial or complete A-V nodal
bypass inserting into the
specialized conducting tissue

FIG. 28–10. **Accessory pathways.** The anatomy of arrhythmias complicating Wolff-Parkinson-White (WPW) syndrome is shown diagrammatically, as are details of the insertion characteristics of the A-V nodal bypass in Lown-Ganong-Levine (LGL) syndrome.

substantial toxic risk requires its use only in exceptional circumstances (eg, when all else fails).

ATRIAL FIBRILLATION (AF) AND WOLFF-PARKINSON-WHITE (WPW) SYNDROME

AF is potentially serious in the setting of antegrade conduction over an accessory pathway, as the normal rate-limiting effects of the A-V node are bypassed, and excessive ventricular rates may lead to VF (see FIG. 28–12). *The situation should be considered a medical emergency.* DC cardioversion is the treatment of choice. Medical therapy must be used cautiously, since an increase in the ventricular rate may occur. The mechanism may be that drugs that block A-V nodal conduction (1) "force" conduction over the accessory pathway, (2) reduce retrograde con-

cealed penetration of the accessory pathway, and (3) thereby further enhance or release accessory pathway conduction capacity. Therefore, verapamil and other calcium antagonists are **contraindicated** in the management of AF complicating WPW. Class Ic drugs and procainamide have the best established efficacy IV but can provoke or aggravate hypotension by their negative inotropic action.

Long-Term Treatment of WPW

Chronic oral antiarrhythmic therapy can be selected empirically but, particularly for patients who have had intractable symptoms due either to RT or to AF, an electrophysiologic study is indicated to determine risk (roughly correlated with the antegrade refractory period of the accessory pathway, preferably measured after exercise or isoproterenol), to establish drug efficacy, and to locate the accessory pathway in case surgery is considered.

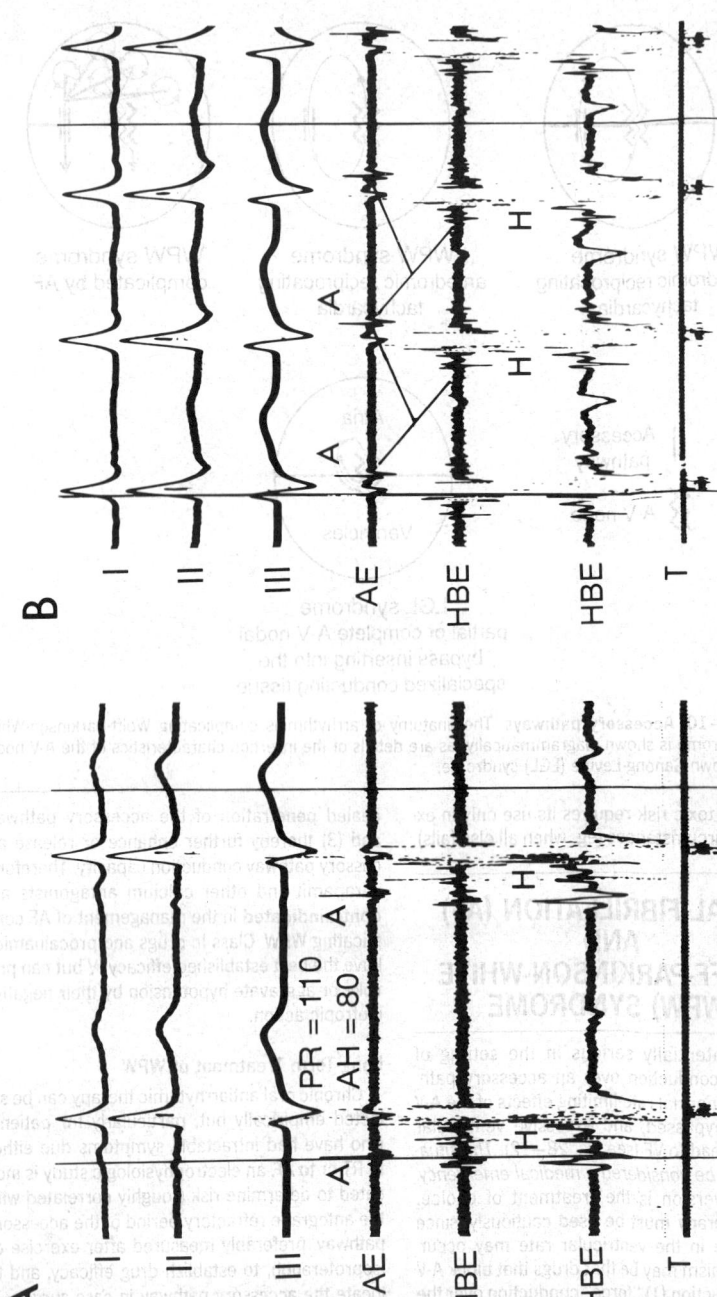

FIG. 28—11. Lown-Ganong-Levine syndrome. (A) ECG leads I, II, and III, an atrial electrogram (AE), a His bundle electrogram (HBE), and time marks at 10- and 100-msec intervals are shown during *normal sinus rhythm*. The shortened PR interval at 110 msec is a function of the short A-V nodal conduction time (AH interval, 80 msec). (B) Despite the short PR interval during sinus rhythm, prolonged A-V nodal conduction (a long AH interval) is responsible for the sustained reentrant tachycardia during *narrow tachycardia*.

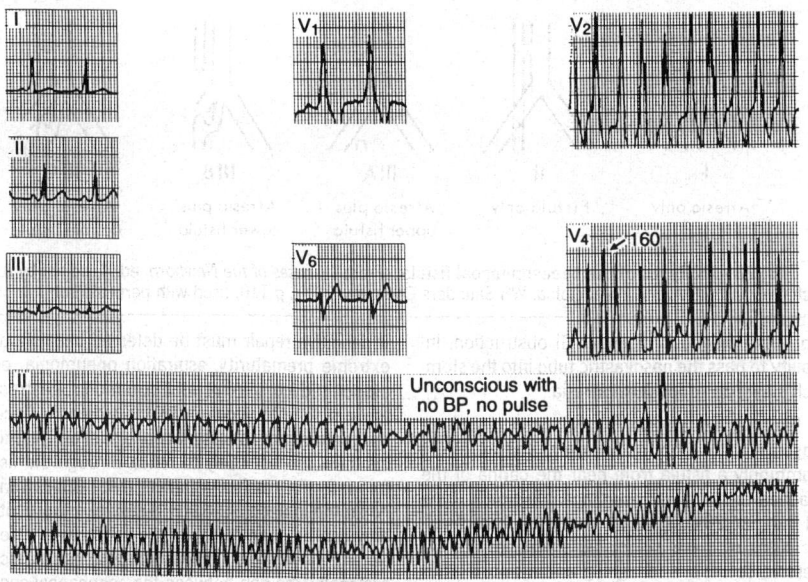

FIG. 28−12. **Wolff-Parkinson-White (WPW) syndrome.** Leads I, II, III, V₁, and V₆ (top left and center) show classic features of WPW syndrome, with a short PR interval and a δ wave. The rhythm is sinus. During the ECG recording, the patient develops atrial fibrillation (leads V₂ and V₄, at top right) with a very fast ventricular response (PR intervals as short as 160 msec are recorded). Shortly thereafter, ventricular fibrillation develops (lead II continuous rhythm strip at bottom).

Surgery and ablation: In WPW syndrome, RT and AF depend on an anatomic abnormality that is surgically removable. The accessory pathway is invisible to the naked eye but can be accurately located by electrophysiologic mapping both preoperatively by catheter mapping and intraoperatively. Accessory pathways may be anywhere in the A-V plane and are described as right lateral, left lateral, and septal. Surgical procedures have been developed to deal with all locations. Catheter ablation is a relatively new approach. It has an excellent success rate, with very low reported morbidity and mortality; however, septal variants demand considerably more technical skill than do lateral pathways.

GASTROINTESTINAL DEFECTS

In the newborn many GI anomalies with intestinal obstruction present as surgical emergencies. Immediate management includes (1) bowel decompression by continuous nasogastric suction to prevent aspiration pneumonia or further abdominal distention with respiratory embarrassment, and (2) referral within the first day to a center for neonatal surgery. Also vital are maintenance of body temperature, prevention of hypoglycemia with 10% D/W IV and electrolytes added at 24 h of age, and prevention or treatment of acidosis and infections so that the infant is in optimal condition for surgery. Since an infant with one congenital anomaly is likely to have others, the neonate should be evaluated for malformations of other organ systems, especially of the CNS, heart, and kidneys.

HIGH ALIMENTARY TRACT OBSTRUCTION

Maternal hydramnios should suggest the possibility of a high (esophageal, gastric, duodenal, jejunal) obstruction, since this disorder prevents the fetus from either swallowing or absorbing amniotic fluid. When a high obstruction is suspected, a nasogastric tube should be passed into the stomach immediately after delivery. The finding of a large volume (> 30 mL) of fluid in the stomach at birth, especially if bile-stained, sup-

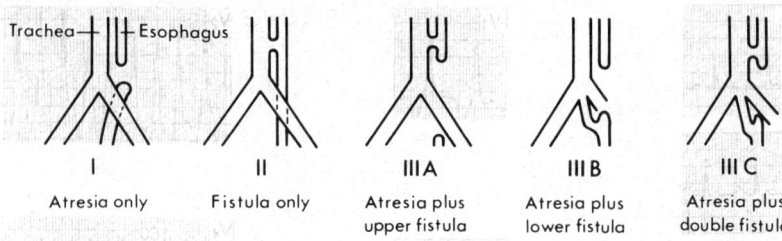

Trachea — Esophagus

I
Atresia only

II
Fistula only

III A
Atresia plus
upper fistula

III B
Atresia plus
lower fistula

III C
Atresia plus
double fistula

FIG. 28-13. Types of tracheoesophageal fistula. (From *Diseases of the Newborn*, ed. 4, edited by AJ Schaffer and ME Avery. Philadelphia, WB Saunders Company, 1977, p 110; used with permission.)

ports the diagnosis of upper GI obstruction. Inability to pass the nasogastric tube into the stomach suggests esophageal atresia.

Esophageal atresia is associated in 86% of cases with **tracheoesophageal fistula**, most commonly a fistula from near the carina of the trachea to the lower esophageal segment (type III B in FIG. 28-13). In the neonate, characteristic **signs** of these associated anomalies are excessive secretions, coughing and cyanosis after attempts at swallowing, and aspiration pneumonia. With a type III B lesion, abdominal distention develops rapidly because as the infant cries, air from the trachea is forced through the fistula into the lower esophagus and stomach.

Diagnosis of esophageal atresia can be established by inability to pass a nasogastric tube into the stomach; if a radiopaque catheter is used, its final location can be determined on x-ray. Rarely, a small amount of water-soluble radiopaque dye must be put into the upper pouch through the tube under fluoroscopy to document discontinuity of the esophagus, and then the dye should be carefully removed, since its aspiration into the infant's lungs can cause a chemical pneumonitis. This procedure should be done at the referral center where surgical treatment will occur; there is no need to determine the exact level or type of esophageal atresia that is present before referral.

Treatment: The aim of **preoperative management** is to prevent aspiration pneumonia, which makes surgical correction more hazardous. Oral feedings are withheld. A double-lumen suction catheter is inserted into the upper esophageal pouch and attached to continuous suction to prevent aspiration of swallowed saliva. The infant may be positioned prone with the head elevated 30 to 40° and with the right side down to facilitate gastric emptying and thus minimize the risk of aspirating gastric acid through the fistula.

If definitive repair must be deferred because of extreme prematurity, aspiration pneumonia, or associated congenital malformations, gastrostomy is done to decompress the stomach. Once the gastrostomy tube is placed to suction, gastric contents are not likely to reflux through the fistula into the tracheobronchial tree. **Operation:** When the infant's condition is stable, a thoracotomy can be done to repair the esophageal atresia and close the tracheoesophageal fistula. Occasionally, the gap between the esophageal segments is too great for a primary repair: Gentle stretching of the esophageal segments before later anastomosis may be beneficial, or repair by interposing a segment of colon or forming a gastric tube between the esophageal segments may be required. The most common acute complications are leakage at the site of anastomosis and stricture formation.

Prognosis: Many infants will experience feeding difficulties after a successful surgical repair because of poor motility of the distal esophageal segment and/or gastroesophageal reflux. If medical management fails, a Nissen fundoplication may be required before oral feedings can be tolerated.

Diaphragmatic hernia (*protrusion of abdominal contents into the thorax through a defect in the diaphragm*) usually occurs on the left side (90%) and in the posterolateral portion of the diaphragm (foramen of Bochdalek hernia). Loops of bowel, even most of the abdominal contents, may protrude through the defect into the hemithorax on the involved side. If the hernia is large, the lung on the affected left side is always hypoplastic. After delivery, as the newborn cries and swallows air, the loops of bowel quickly fill with air, and this rapidly enlarging mass can cause further acute respiratory embarrassment as it pushes the heart and mediastinal structures to the right, compressing the normally grown lung. After delivery, respiratory distress is immediate in severe cases and the infant is desperately ill. Besides having severe respiratory compromise, the infant will have a scaphoid abdomen (due to displacement of many of the abdominal viscera into the chest). Bowel sounds (and an absence of breath sounds) may be heard over the involved hemithorax, usually on the left side. In less severe cases, mild respiratory difficulty develops a few hours or days later as abdominal contents progressively herniate through the defect. When very small, the abnormality may appear only as a small diaphragmatic defect found on a routine chest x-ray.

X-ray reveals numerous air-filled loops of bowel in the involved hemithorax, and contralateral displacement of the heart and mediastinal structures. If the x-ray is taken immediately at birth before the infant has swallowed air, the diaphragmatic hernia may present as an opaque mass in the hemithorax. As soon as the diagnosis is made, a large double-lumen nasogastric tube should be passed into the stomach and continuous suction begun to prevent swallowed air from entering the GI tract and causing further lung compression.

Treatment: In the delivery room, the infant should be immediately intubated and ventilated. If necessary, paralysis with pancuronium may facilitate ventilation and prevent the swallowing of air. Bag and mask ventilation should *not* be used, as it further distends the bowel loops and worsens the infant's condition. Surgery is required to place the bowel in the abdomen and to close the diaphragmatic defect. The combination of one hypoplastic and one atelectatic lung often makes ventilator management extremely challenging. In infants with a hypoplastic left lung, the right lung may also have abnormally small pulmonary arteries with smooth muscle hyperplasia; this results in increased pulmonary vascular resistance with decreased pulmonary blood flow (persistent pulmonary hypertension), secondary right-to-left shunting at the level of the foramen ovale or through a patent ductus arteriosus, and severe hypoxemia. Pulmonary vessel constriction may be relieved by alkalinization (administration of sodium bicarbonate and hyperventilation with a respirator). Tolazoline can also help to reduce the increased pulmonary vascular resistance (see PERSISTENT PULMONARY HYPERTENSION under RESPIRATORY DISORDERS in Ch. 27). It is important that the empty hemithorax not be put to water-sealed drainage, as excessive negative pressure and mediastinal shift to that side may result. Re-

cently, many infants with diaphragmatic hernia and intractable pulmonary insufficiency with persistent pulmonary hypertension unresponsive to respirator support have been saved by the use of extracorporeal membrane oxygenation (ECMO—see under PERSISTENT PULMONARY HYPERTENSION in Ch. 27). Transport of a critically ill unstable infant with congenital diaphragmatic hernia and persistent pulmonary hypertension to a center for ECMO is very difficult. Thus, if the diagnosis of congenital heart disease is made by a prenatal fetal ultrasound (US) examination, it is appropriate to plan for delivery at a center that does pediatric surgery and has ECMO facilities.

Hypertrophic pyloric stenosis (*obstruction of the pyloric lumen due to pyloric muscular hypertrophy*) may cause almost complete gastric outlet obstruction. Rarely present at birth, hypertrophy develops over the first 4 to 6 wk of life, and signs of obstruction commonly do not appear until then. Forceful projectile vomiting of feedings without bile usually begins late in the first month of life. Gastric peristaltic waves may be visible, crossing the epigastrium from left to right. Delay in diagnosis may lead to repeated vomiting, dehydration, failure to gain weight, and hypochloremic metabolic alkalosis. **Diagnosis** can be made by palpation of a discrete, 2- to 3-cm, firm, movable pyloric "olive" deep in the right side of the epigastrium. If the diagnosis is uncertain, a barium-swallow x-ray will show delayed gastric emptying and the typical "string sign" of a markedly narrowed, elongated pyloric lumen. The diagnosis may also be made on abdominal US examination. The **treatment** of choice is a longitudinal pyloromyotomy, which leaves the mucosa intact and separates the incised muscle fibers. Postoperatively, the infant usually tolerates feedings well within a few days.

Duodenal obstruction has several possible causes, including atresia, stenosis, and pressure from an extraluminal mass. After the ileum, the duodenum is the most common site of primary intestinal atresia. Since the obstruction is high, there usually is a history of hydramnios, and the infant develops forceful vomiting *of bile* after the first feedings. Obstruction here is quite often found in infants with Down syndrome. Newborns with anomalies of bowel position (see under DISTAL SMALL BOWEL AND LARGE BOWEL OBSTRUCTION, below) may also have peritoneal bands that stretch across the duodenum and cause partial or complete occlusion. Choledochal cyst or annular pancreas may also cause duodenal blockage by extrinsic pressure. Infants with choledochal cyst may also present with variable degrees of obstructive jaundice.

Diagnosis: In contrast to the single large, air-filled stomach seen in pyloric obstruction, plain x-rays show the characteristic "double bubble" sign, with one large, air-filled bubble representing the stomach and a second bubble representing air in the dilated duodenum proximal to the point of blockage; no air is seen distal to the blockage. A barium swallow may identify the point of obstruction as well as extrinsic pressure from a choledochal cyst, while a barium enema will diagnose GI malrotation associated with peritoneal-band duodenal obstructions.

Treatment: When duodenal obstruction is suspected, the infant should not be fed. Continuous suction via a nasogastric tube is begun to decompress the stomach and to prevent vomiting and aspiration of vomitus. Surgical exploration is indicated to define and correct the obstruction.

DISTAL SMALL BOWEL AND LARGE BOWEL OBSTRUCTION

In most cases of distal small bowel or large intestine obstruction, no history of maternal hydramnios exists, since much of the swallowed amniotic fluid can be absorbed from the fetal bowel proximal to the obstruction. The first few feedings are usually tolerated, but late in the first day or on the second day abdominal distention appears, often accompanied by bilious or fecal vomiting. The infant may pass a small amount of meconium at first, but thereafter does not pass stools. If intestinal obstruction is suspected, a small specimen of meconium may be examined microscopically for squamous cells and lanugo hair. Since these are normally present (from swallowed amniotic fluid), they provide evidence against a complete intestinal obstruction (**Farber's test**). However, obstruction of a previously patent bowel may occur during gestation, so this finding does not absolutely rule out intestinal atresia.

The general diagnostic approach and preoperative management of distal small bowel and large bowel obstruction include the following: nothing by mouth; placement of a nasogastric suction tube to prevent further intestinal distention or possible aspiration of vomitus; correction of fluid and electrolyte disturbances; and x-ray studies, beginning with plain films followed by a contrast enema.

In **meconium plug syndrome**, thick, inspissated, rubbery meconium forms a cast of the colon and even part of the terminal ileum and can cause complete obstruction, with distention and vomiting. A contrast enema with dilute meglumine diatrizoate will demonstrate the plug, and the contrast enema or subsequent gentle enemas with 0.45% sodium chloride solution (10 to 20 mL) will usually separate the plug from the bowel wall and expel it. Although most infants will thereafter be normal, diagnostic studies may be indicated to identify the small number with underlying Hirschsprung's disease (see below) or cystic fibrosis (see also meconium ileus, below). Meconium plug is more common in infants of diabetic mothers and in toxemic mothers who have been treated with magnesium sulfate.

Meconium ileus is almost always an early manifestation of cystic fibrosis (see also Ch. 37). The abnormal meconium is thick, extremely tenacious, and stringy; it adheres to the bowel mucosa and causes obstruction at the level of the ileum. Distal to the obstruction, the colon is narrowed in diameter and contains desiccated meconium pellets. This tenacious meconium is easily distinguished from the rubbery meconium plug described above. In meconium ileus, loops of intestine can often be palpated through the abdominal wall and may have a characteristic doughy feel. Diagnosis is supported by the presence of undigested protein in the meconium. (After a meconium-and-water mixture [1:1] has been shaken and then centrifuged, 10% trichloroacetic acid is added to the supernatant. A heavy, white precipitate indicates undigested albumin.) The luminal contents may appear granular on plain films because small air bubbles are trapped in the abnormal meconium.

The loops of small bowel, distended with thick, tenacious meconium, may twist around each other to form a volvulus in utero. The bowel may then lose its vascular supply and infarct, to produce a sterile **meconium peritonitis** seen on x-ray as calcified meconium flecks lining the peritoneal surfaces and even in the scrotum. The infarcted loop may be resorbed, leaving an area or areas of bowel atresia, or it may be walled off as a large cyst.

If meconium ileus is diagnosed or strongly suspected, the obstruction may be relieved in uncomplicated cases (eg, without perforation, volvulus, or atresia) by giving one or more enemas with a dilute contrast medium (eg, a dilute solution of meglumine diatrizoate and sodium diatrizoate) under fluoroscopy. The large GI water losses that result from hypertonic contrast material must be replaced concurrently by vein in order to prevent sudden dehydration and shock. If the enema does not relieve the obstruction, laparotomy is required. A "double-barreled" ileostomy with repeated acetylcysteine lavage of both proximal and distal loops is usually required to liquefy and remove the abnormal meconium and relieve the obstruction.

Survivors with cystic fibrosis (almost 100%) have no worse pulmonary disease than other patients with cystic fibrosis. A positive sweat test is needed to make a definitive diagnosis of cystic fibrosis.

Bowel atresia occurs most frequently in the ileum, followed in order by the duodenum (see discussion of duodenal obstruction, above), jejunum, and colon. Ileal atresia usually presents late during the first day or on the second day. Abdominal distention progressively increases, the infant fails to pass stools, and finally feedings are regurgitated. The general diagnostic approach and preoperative management are similar to those for the other types of distal small bowel or large bowel obstruction (see above). At surgery, the entire bowel should be inspected for additional areas of atresia; the defect is resected, usually with a primary anastomosis. However, at times the proximal portion of the ileum is markedly dilated, while the distal, unused part is small from disuse. In some such cases, the surgeon may feel it safer to effect a double-barreled ileostomy and defer anastomosis until the distended proximal bowel has diminished in size. Prognosis is excellent.

Anomalies of bowel position (malrotation) may cause intestinal obstruction. During embryonic development, the primitive bowel protrudes from the abdominal cavity. As it returns to the abdomen, the large bowel normally rotates counterclockwise, with the cecum finally coming to rest in the right lower quadrant. If rotation is incomplete or abnormal so that the cecum ends up elsewhere (usually in the right upper quadrant or midepigastrium), bowel obstruction may result, either from retroperitoneal bands that stretch across the duodenum or from a volvulus of the small bowel that, lacking its normal peritoneal attachment, twists on its narrow stalk-like mesentery. The clinical presentation initially is the same as with other forms of bowel obstruction. The infant will soon begin to vomit bile and may appear acutely ill. Plain films of the abdomen will show a paucity of bowel gas distal to the duodenum. A barium enema will show that the cecum does not lie in the right lower quadrant. *Volvulus is an acute surgical emergency, since the involved bowel may become gangrenous if the obstruction is not immediately relieved.* Upper GI series of a patient with volvulus will show obstruction at the level of the ligament of Treitz with typical radiologic findings.

Hirschsprung's disease (congenital megacolon) is caused by congenital absence of Meissner's and Auerbach's autonomic plexuses in the bowel wall, usually limited to the colon. Peristalsis in the involved segment is absent or abnormal, resulting in continuous smooth muscle spasm and partial or complete obstruction with accumulation of intestinal contents and massive dilation of the more proximal, normally innervated bowel. Most commonly anal, the obstruction may extend proximally to involve varying portions of the colon, occasionally the entire colon, or even include the terminal ileum, but very rarely the entire GI tract. "Skip" lesions almost never occur. The infant presents with obstipation, distention, and finally vomiting. Occasionally, infants have only mild or intermittent constipation, often with intervening bouts of mild diarrhea, and Hirschsprung's disease may not be diagnosed until later in infancy. However, it is important to make the correct diagnosis as early in infancy as possible: *The longer the disease goes untreated, the greater is the chance of toxic enterocolitis, which may be fatal.* In older infants, symptoms and signs may include anorexia, lack of a physiologic urge to defecate, empty rectum on examination, palpable colon, and visible peristalsis. The child also may fail to thrive.

A barium enema shows the colon dilated proximal to the obstruction, and the narrow, distal segment, which lacks normal innervation. However, a barium enema in the newborn period may not always be diagnostic of congenital megacolon. Rectal biopsy, disclosing the absence of nerve ganglia, makes the definitive diagnosis. Neonatal Hirschsprung's disease should be treated with a colostomy at a site in the colon proximal to the aganglionic segment. Resection of the entire aganglionic portion of the colon and definitive repair with a "pull-through" procedure can then be deferred until the infant is older and the colon and anus are larger.

The obstipation of Hirschsprung's disease may lead to superimposed toxic enterocolitis, with overgrowth of bacteria in the small intestine resulting in production of bacterial toxins. The consequent *fulminant, catastrophic diarrhea* results in massive fluid loss and may rapidly lead to dehydration and death. Fluid replacement and antibiotics are important but are unlikely to prevent death unless the obstruction can be quickly relieved by colostomy. Saline lavage of the colon using a rectal tube may be helpful in the initial stages of stabilization before carrying out a colostomy.

Following a pull-through surgical procedure, the prognosis is good; most of these infants eventually achieve good bowel control.

Anal atresia is obvious on examination, since the anus is not patent. Should the diagnosis be missed on routine examination and the infant be fed, all the signs of distal bowel obstruction will, of course, soon develop. Males with anal atresia often have a fistula from the anal pouch to either the urethra or the perineum. In females, a fistula extends from the anal pouch to the vagina or, rarely, the bladder. The space between the blind anus and the skin of the perineum may be several centimeters long, or as narrow as a thin membrane of skin covering the anal opening. A cutaneous fistula generally indicates low atresia; in such cases, a definitive repair via a perineal approach is usually possible. If no perineal fistula exists, a high lesion is likely that will probably require a colostomy; definitive repair is deferred until the infant is older and the structures to be repaired are larger. The urine should be examined for the presence of meconium or bacteria. By using the lateral prone position for x-rays and fistulograms, a skilled radiologist can define the level and type of lesion. The surgical approach will depend on the findings, especially the length of the atresia.

DEFECTS IN ABDOMINAL WALL CLOSURE

An **omphalocele** is *a protrusion of variable amounts of abdominal viscera from a midline defect at the base of the umbilicus.* The herniation is covered by a thin membrane and may be small, including only a few loops of bowel, or may contain most of the abdominal viscera, including all the intestines, the stomach, and the liver. The immediate dangers are drying of the viscera, hypothermia due to heat loss through evaporation of water from the exposed viscera, and infection of the peritoneal surfaces. Immediately after delivery, the exposed viscera should be covered with sponges wet with sterile saline, and covered with an occlusive dressing to maintain sterility and to avoid hypothermia by preventing evaporation. Another useful preventive technique is to place the infant's body up to the level of the axillae in a sterile "bowel bag" containing warm sterile saline. Among infants with omphalocele, there is a higher than usual incidence of other anomalies, including bowel atresias and cardiac and renal anomalies. *After a search for associated anomalies, surgical repair of the defect is indicated as quickly as possible.*

Primary closure is performed when feasible. With a large omphalocele, the abdominal cavity may be too small to accommodate the viscera. In this case, the viscera are covered by a pouch or chimney of Silastic sheeting, which is progressively reduced in size over several days as the abdominal capacity slowly increases so that all of the viscera can finally be returned to the abdominal cavity.

In **gastroschisis**, the abdominal viscera protrude through an abdominal wall defect, usually to the right side of the umbilical cord insertion. There is no membranous covering, and the intestines are markedly edematous and appear shortened from being bathed in amniotic fluid containing fetal urine (ie, chemical peritonitis). It often takes several weeks before intestinal function recovers and oral feedings can be given. The surgical approach is similar to that for omphalocele, and immediate closure is required as there is no membrane to prevent bacterial contamination of the viscera.

Associated bowel anomalies (eg, atresia) must be looked for in infants with omphalocele or gastroschisis. Anomalies of other organ systems (eg, cardiac, renal) may accompany omphalocele but are rarely seen in infants with gastroschisis.

MISCELLANEOUS SURGICAL EMERGENCIES

Inguinal hernias develop most often in the male newborn and particularly in premature infants. Since hernias can become incarcerated, repair should be early, usually when the infant weighs about 2.27 kg (5 lb). (In contrast, **umbilical hernias** rarely become incarcerated, close spontaneously after several years, and should not ordinarily be surgically repaired.) **Intussusception,** *prolapse of one portion of the bowel into another,* although rare in neonates, is an extreme emergency because of the danger of intestinal gangrene, as is **volvulus** (see above under anomalies of bowel position). Extensive **bowel infarction** may rarely occur from mesenteric arterial occlusion due to mural thrombi or emboli following high placement of an umbilical artery catheter. Most **gastric perforations** in newborns are spontaneous and may occur because of a congenital defect in the stomach wall. The infant with gastric perforation suddenly becomes distended and has massive pneumoperitoneum on abdominal x-ray. Prognosis is usually good following surgical repair of the perforation, usually on the greater curvature of the stomach. Ileal perforation in premature infants has been reported following the use of indomethacin given to close a patent ductus arteriosus.

BILIARY ATRESIA; NEONATAL HEPATITIS

The **neonatal hepatitis** (giant cell hepatitis) syndrome is usually of unknown cause, though infection with cytomegalovirus or hepatitis B virus or a deficiency of α_1-antitrypsin is rarely responsible. **Biliary atresia** reflects total or partial agenesis of the biliary tree and usually affects extrahepatic, rather than intrahepatic, bile ducts. Recent evidence indicates that biliary atresia and neonatal hepatitis probably represent a spectrum of overlapping disorders rather than distinct entities. In most cases, biliary atresia develops several weeks after birth, probably following inflammation and scarring of the bile ducts. It is rarely found in stillborns or in the immediate neonatal period. The etiology of the inflammatory response is often unknown.

In both conditions, cholestatic jaundice with mixed hyperbilirubinemia, progressively dark urine (conjugated bilirubin), acholic stools, and hepatomegaly are usually first noted about 2 wk after birth. By age 2 to 3 mo, retarded growth, irritability from pruritus, and signs of portal hypertension may be present. Liver function tests reflect both cholestasis and hepatocellular inflammation. Appropriate investigations can usually exclude other specific causes of neonatal obstructive jaundice (eg, specific infections, α_1-antitrypsin deficiency, galactosemia, and cystic fibrosis), but differentiation between neonatal hepatitis and biliary atresia may be difficult. Direct and total bilirubin values, AST (SGOT), ALT (SGPT), alkaline phosphatase, and serum levels of bile acids often will not clearly distinguish biliary atresia from neonatal hepatitis with severe cholestasis. Ultrasound **(US)** examination of the gallbladder and extrahepatic bile ducts may be helpful. The absence of a recognizable gallbladder and of extrahepatic bile ducts on US examination is strongly suggestive of biliary atresia, while the presence of a choledochal duct cyst that is compressing and obstructing the common bile duct may be demonstrated on US examination. Placement of a nasoduodenal tube and col-

lection of a 24-h sample of duodenal fluid by gravity drainage may reveal the presence of bile (bilirubin can be measured); bile excretion is strong evidence against a diagnosis of complete bile duct atresia. Recently, liver scan using technetium Tc 99m PIPIDA has proved useful in identifying extrahepatic bile flow. Percutaneous liver biopsy is often very useful in questionable cases, and if interpreted by an experienced pathologist, it is probably the most accurate diagnostic test available, albeit the most invasive.

If the diagnosis is still uncertain, laparotomy must be done before 2 mo of age, because infants with biliary atresia will develop irreversible biliary cirrhosis if operation is deferred. At laparotomy, an intraoperative cholangiogram to delineate the state of the biliary tree and a liver biopsy for frozen section morphology are obtained. Atretic bile ducts can be successfully reanastomosed in only 5 to 10% of infants; however, a modification of the Kasai procedure (a hepatoportoenterostomy) is performed in the others and bile flow is reestablished in most. Unfortunately, many will continue to have significant chronic medical problems, including cholestasis, recurrent ascending cholangitis, and failure to thrive, with late mortality occurring in a significant number. In recent years, liver transplantation has saved the lives of some infants with liver failure. Cholestasis due to neonatal hepatitis usually resolves slowly, but permanent liver damage may ensue.

MUSCULOSKELETAL DEFECTS

Some important and common disorders of the newborn musculoskeletal system are discussed below; others are found elsewhere in THE MANUAL.

Various **craniofacial abnormalities** arise from maldevelopment of the 1st and 2nd visceral arches, which form the facial bones and ears at about the 7th wk of embryonic development. These malformations include cleft lip and cleft palate, Treacher Collins' syndrome (mandibulofacial dysostosis), Pierre Robin and Waardenburg syndromes, hypertelorism, and deformities of the external and middle ear. Most infants with craniofacial abnormalities have normal intelligence.

Cleft lips and **cleft palates** are the most common 1st arch defects and may involve the hard or soft palate or both. They occur once in 700 to

800 births. The cleft may vary from involvement of the soft palate only, to a complete cleft of the soft and hard palates, the alveolar process of the maxilla, and the lip. Cleft lips cause no disability but are cosmetically distressing, whereas a cleft palate interferes with feeding and speech development. Use of a feeder with which formula can be delivered with mild pressure (eg, a plastic bottle) often is helpful. Special cleft palate nipples and dental devices to occlude the cleft may help feeding. Plastic surgery can significantly improve either disorder. Dental, orthodontic, psychiatric, and speech therapy may be required.

Infants with defects associated with small mandibles (**Pierre Robin** and **Treacher Collins' syndromes**) cannot be fed easily and may have bouts of cyanosis because the tongue is posterior and may obstruct the pharynx. Feeding problems can be avoided by gavage. If cyanosis or respiratory problems persist, tracheostomy or surgery to fix the tongue in a forward position may be required. An otologic evaluation is indicated, since these syndromes may involve the ear.

Congenital torticollis (*head tilt present at birth*): Fractures, dislocations, or subluxations of the cervical spine (especially C-1 and C-2) or odontoid abnormalities are rare but serious causes, since permanent neurologic damage may result. Cervical x-rays can help exclude these conditions. Traumatic injury may occur before or during delivery. The most common etiology for torticollis is neck trauma during delivery, with hematoma, fibrosis, and contracture of the sternocleidomastoid (**SCM**) muscle. The torticollis is not present at birth; it appears in the first few days or weeks of life, and a nontender mass is noted in the SCM in the segment nearest the occiput. Passive SCM stretching (by rotating the head and flexing the neck laterally to the opposite side) is indicated. Other causes include abnormalities of the bony spine, such as **Klippel-Feil syndrome** (*fusion of the cervical vertebrae*), or of the atlas to the occipital bone (**atlanto-occipital fusion**). CNS tumors, bulbar palsies, and ocular dysfunction are prominent neurologic causes but rarely are present at birth.

Congenital scoliosis is rare, but **vertebral anomalies** such as hemi-, wedge-, or butterfly vertebrae are more common. Bony spinal defects should be suspected when there are posterior midline cutaneous abnormalities, bony torticollis, or congenital anomalies of the lower extremities. Since growth can lead to serious deformity, treatment with braces or body jackets should begin early. Surgery may be needed if the curvature progresses. Associated renal anomalies are common, and intravenous urography (**IVU**) is indicated.

Congenital dislocation of the hip, more common in female infants and in infants with breech presentation, a positive family history, or a hip click, has an uncertain etiology. It seems to be secondary to laxity of the ligaments about the joint or to in utero positioning. The dislocation can be uni- or bilateral. If unilateral, the involved leg is shorter and there may be asymmetric skin creases in the thigh. The major sign of subluxation or dislocation is inability to completely abduct the thigh to the surface of the examining table when the hip and knee are flexed (Ortolani's sign). This adductor spasm is often present even if the hip is not actually dislocated at the time of examination. If the hip is dislocated, abduction and external rotation of the femur may produce an audible or palpable "clunk" as the femoral head reenters the acetabulum. Minor "clicks" are more commonly found. They may disappear within a month or two but should prompt close follow-up. Partial or complete dislocation may be difficult to detect at birth; periodic testing for limitation of hip abduction during the first year of life is advised. Hip ultrasonography appears accurate in establishing early diagnosis, but hip x-rays may be difficult to interpret early and are helpful only if they confirm the clinical impression. Early treatment is critical, since the hip usually can be reduced immediately after birth, and with growth the acetabulum will then form almost normally. However, if therapy is delayed, the potential for correction declines steadily with growth. Medical treatment consists of devices (eg, splints, slings, harnesses, or large padded diapers) that hold the affected hips abducted and externally rotated, thus encouraging the acetabulum to form properly as growth occurs.

Femoral torsion or twisting, either internal (anteversion—knees pointing toward each other) or external (retroversion—knees pointing in opposite directions), is typical of newborns, in whom either condition may be striking. Spontaneous correction of even dramatic femoral torsion generally occurs when the infant stands and walks. Sleeping prone can prolong retroversion. Hip x-rays or ultrasonography for dislocation should be considered. Positioning and passive exercises may be helpful.

Knee dislocation anteriorly with hyperextension at birth is rare but requires emergency treatment. The dislocation may be related to muscle imbalance (if myelodysplasia or arthrogryposis is present) or intrauterine positioning, and it is often associated with ipsilateral hip dislocation. Immediate treatment with daily passive flexion movements and splinting in flexion frequently results in a functional knee, if the infant is otherwise normal.

Bowing and twisting (torsion) of the tibia are common at birth and are seldom pathologic. Bowing with x-ray changes of a narrow sclerotic intramedullary canal is an exception, with a high risk of fracture and pseudarthrosis; a protective orthosis is needed.

Abnormalities of the feet are common. Of the **clubfoot (talipes) deformities**, the most frequently seen is talipes equinovarus; the foot is plantar flexed, inverted, and markedly adducted. Deformities from in utero positioning can mimic clubfoot, but they can be passively corrected, whereas pathologic changes cannot. Orthopedic care beginning in the nursery with repeated cast applications to normalize the foot's position is optimal. In severe cases, surgery may be required if casting is not successful. In the **calcaneovalgus** position, the foot is flat or convex, is dorsiflexed, and can easily be approximated against the lower tibia. Early treatment with a cast to place the foot in the equinovarus position or with use of corrective shoes usually is successful. **Metatarsus adductus** (adduction of the forward part of the foot) does not require treatment. However, if the foot is also inverted and cannot be passively straightened with ease **(metatarsus varus)**, serial casts usually are required.

Congenital absence of individual muscles or groups of muscles may occur. Partial or complete agenesis of the pectoralis major is one of the most common of these defects; it can be an isolated phenomenon or it can be associated with ipsilateral hand abnormalities **(Poland's anomaly)**. One or more layers of the abdominal musculature may also be absent at birth (eg, **prune-belly syndrome**, which often is associated with severe GU abnormalities, particularly hydronephrosis). Incidence is highest in male infants, who often also have undescended testes. The prognosis is guarded, even with early relief of the urinary tract obstruction. Malformations involving the feet and rectum often accompany agenesis of the abdominal musculature.

The **chondrodystrophies** are *diseases affecting the manner in which cartilage is converted to bone.* Of these, **achondroplasia** is the best known. All are characterized by dwarfism (usually with a trunk of normal size, but with short extremities) and are often associated with abnormalities elsewhere. The osteochondrodysplasias, osteopetroses, and osteochondroses are discussed in Ch. 42. In most of the chondrodystrophies, x-rays of the long bones are needed for accurate diagnosis. Mental development usually is normal. Hypothyroidism should be ruled out. Treatment is supportive.

The **mucopolysaccharidoses (MPS—see under INHERITED DISORDERS OF CONNECTIVE TISSUE in Ch. 42)** have similarities with the chondrodystrophies, but some types also have visceral and CNS involvement with mental deficiency. Truncal shortening and limb contractures are often present. The MPS are not usually apparent in newborns.

Osteogenesis imperfecta, *abnormal fragility of bone,* is a serious disease that diffusely affects bone. Several forms have been described, but the newborn type **(congenita)** is the most severe. Infants are born with multiple fractures, which lead to shortening of the extremities. The skull is soft, has many wormian bones, and feels like a "bag of bones" when palpated. The sclerae are abnormally thin and translucent and may appear blue because a deficiency in connective tissue allows the color of the underlying vessels to show through. (Blue sclerae do not, however, always indicate osteogenesis imperfecta.) Some infants also have a hearing loss, presumably from otosclerosis due to abnormal connective tissue around the ossicles of the middle ear. Delivery trauma may lead to intracranial hemorrhage and stillbirth because of the soft skull. Infants born alive often die suddenly during the first few days or weeks of life, but some survive as deformed dwarfs. Mental development is normal unless head trauma with CNS injury occurs. Orthopedic care is indicated; there is no effective medical treatment.

Congenital hypophosphatasia is due to absence of alkaline phosphatase in the serum and results in a diffuse lack of calcium deposition in the bones. Vomiting, failure to gain weight, and enlargement of the epiphyses like that seen in rickets usually occur. Bony deformities and dwarfism, but normal mental development, are present in patients who survive infancy. There is no effective treatment.

Congenital amputations are *transverse or longitudinal limb deficiencies due to primary intrauterine growth inhibition or secondary intrauterine destruction of normal embryonic tissues.* The etiology often is unclear, but teratogenic agents (eg, thalidomide) and amniotic bands are 2 known causes. In transverse deficiencies, all elements beyond a certain level are absent, and the limb resembles an amputation stump. In longitudinal deficiencies, specific maldevelopments occur; eg, complete or partial absence of the radius, fibula, or tibia. Infants with either transverse or longitudinal limb deficiencies may also have hypoplastic or bifid bones, synostoses, duplications, dislocations, or other bony defects. One or more limbs may be affected, and defects may be of a different type in each limb. X-rays are essential in determining which bones are involved. CNS abnormalities are rare.

Treatment consists mainly of providing a prosthesis and is highly individualized. Prosthetic devices are most valuable in lower extremity deficiencies or when there is complete or nearly complete absence of an upper limb. If any activity in an arm or hand exists, no matter how great the malformation, functioning capacity must be carefully assessed before a prosthesis or operation is recommended. Therapeutic amputation of any limb or portion of a limb should be **avoided** unless essential for fitting of a prosthetic device, and it should be considered only after evaluating the functional and psychologic implications of the loss.

An upper limb prosthesis should be designed to serve as many needs as possible so that the number of devices is kept to a minimum. A child uses a prosthesis most successfully when it is fitted early and becomes an integral part of his body during the developmental years. With effective orthopedic and ancillary support, most children with congenital amputations lead normal lives.

ARTHROGRYPOSIS MULTIPLEX CONGENITA (AMC)
(Multiple Congenital Contractures)

Congenital fibrous ankylosis of multiple joints. AMC is heterogeneous (ie, consists of several similar disease entities), but the term often is loosely and incorrectly applied to some well-defined disorders in which limited joint movement is only one of several abnormalities, or in which a primary cause of joint rigidity is evident.

Etiology and Pathology

The cause is unknown but may involve impaired intrauterine fetal movement. AMC is nongenetic in most instances. Affected newborns with classic AMC have normal chromosomes, but cytogenetic abnormalities may be present in some forms that present in atypical severely affected neonates.

AMC can be **neurogenic**, with histologic and electromyographic evidence of nervous system involvement, or **myopathic**, with muscle fiber changes shown by electromyography. Neurogenic and myopathic AMC may correspond to typical and atypical clinical forms, but this is unproved.

Symptoms and Signs

In classic AMC, the joints of all limbs are fixed. The shoulders generally are adducted and internally rotated, the elbows are extended, and the wrists and digits are flexed. The hips may be dislocated and usually are slightly flexed. The knees are extended, and the feet are often in the equinovarus position.

The muscles are hypoplastic, and the limbs tend to be tubular and featureless. Soft tissue webbing is sometimes present over the ventral aspects of the flexed joints. The spine usually is uninvolved, and apart from slenderness of the long bones, the skeleton is radiographically normal. Occasional associated abnormalities in syndromic forms of AMC include cleft palate, cryptorchidism, cardiac lesions, and urinary tract malformations. Physical handicaps may be severe, but intelligence usually is unimpaired or mildly subnormal.

A relatively common, atypical form of AMC is characterized by limited joint involvement and absence of muscle wasting and associated abnormalities.

Differential Diagnosis

Congenital joint contractures may be secondary to many conditions, including spinal defects (spina bifida, sacral agenesis) and spasticity due to cerebral cortical damage. Joint rigidity also may be present in acquired disorders (juvenile RA) and several genetic conditions. Since classic AMC usually is not inherited, recognition of familial involvement or additional syndromic stigmas is diagnostically important.

Prognosis and Treatment

The deformities are at their worst at birth. AMC is not progressive; any change that occurs will be an improvement. Considerable handicap may be present, and orthopedic measures are usually required. The angle of joint ankylosis can be surgically altered, but enhanced mobility is difficult to attain. Active physiotherapy and manipulation during the first few months of life may produce considerable improvement.

NEUROLOGIC DEFECTS

Some of the most serious congenital abnormalities of the nervous system (eg, anencephaly, encephalocele, spina bifida) develop in the first 2 mo of gestation and represent *defects in neural tube formation* (**dysraphia**). Others (eg, hydranencephaly, porencephaly) occur later and appear to be secondary to destructive processes after the brain has formed. Some defects are relatively benign (eg, meningocele).

Accurate in utero detection of many malformations is now possible using amniocentesis and ultrasonography (**US**). (See also Ch. 13 and PREVENTION OF GENETIC DISORDERS in Ch. 48.) Genetic counseling for parents of a child with a major neurologic abnormality is important, since the risk of a subsequent child's having such a defect is high. These parents also need psychologic help and support. Women who have had a pregnancy resulting in an infant or fetus with a neural tube defect should be advised that folic acid supplementation (4 mg/day) before conception and during early pregnancy may substantially reduce the risk for neural tube defects in subsequent pregnancies.

Anencephaly, *absence of the cerebral hemispheres,* is incompatible with life. The absent brain is sometimes replaced by malformed cystic neural tissue, which may be exposed or covered with skin. Varying portions of the brainstem and spinal cord may be missing or malformed. No diagnostic or therapeutic efforts are helpful, and these infants either are stillborn or die within a few days.

Malformations of the cerebral hemispheres may occur: The hemispheres may be large, small, or asymmetric; the gyri may be absent, unusually large, or multiple and small; microscopic sections of normal-appearing brain may show disorganization of the normal laminar neuronal arrangement. *Decreased head size* (**microcephaly**) is often associated with these defects, and there is usually moderate to severe motor and mental retardation. Therapy consists of general support, and anticonvulsants if needed to control seizures.

Encephalocele, *a protrusion of nervous tissue and meninges through a skull defect,* is associated with incomplete closure of the cranial vault, or **cranium bifidum.** Encephalocele usually occurs in the midline and protrudes into the nasal passages or from the occiput, but can be present asymmetrically in the frontal or parietal regions. Small encephaloceles may resemble cephalhematomas, but x-rays show a bony skull defect at their base. Most encephaloceles should be repaired, since even large ones may contain mostly heterotopic nervous tissue, which can be removed without leaving major functional disability. When other serious malformations coexist, the decision to repair may be more difficult. The hydrocephalus (see below) often associated with encephalocele requires definition by CT or US scan and, if it is progressive, surgical treatment with a shunt. About ½ of affected infants have other congenital defects. The prognosis is good for many of these patients.

Porencephaly, *a cyst or cavity in a cerebral hemisphere that communicates with a ventricle,* may occur pre- or postnatally. The defect may be caused by a developmental anomaly, inflammatory disease, or a vascular accident such as intraventricular hemorrhage with parenchymal extension. The neurologic examination is usually abnormal. Cranial transillumination may be positive. Diagnosis is confirmed by CT or US scan. Progressive hydrocephalus may require a shunt procedure. Prognosis is variable; a few patients develop only minor neurologic signs and have normal intelligence.

Hydranencephaly is *an extreme form of porencephaly in which the cerebral hemispheres are almost totally absent.* Usually, the cerebellum and brainstem are formed normally and the basal ganglia are intact. The meninges, bones, and skin over the cranial vault are normal. Results of neurologic examination in the newborn period may be normal or abnormal, but the infant fails to develop normally. Externally, the head appears to be normal, but when transilluminated, light shines completely through. A CT or US scan confirms the diagnosis. Treatment is supportive, with shunting if head growth is excessive.

Dandy-Walker cysts and the Arnold-Chiari malformation are major malformations of the posterior fossa that often are associated with hydrocephalus. **Dandy-Walker cysts** are *developmental malformations in which the 4th ventricle is* cystic; hydrocephalus usually results. Diagnosis is made by observing superior displacement of the lateral sinus groove on x-ray, or by transillumination of the posterior fossa, and is confirmed by a CT or US scan. The hydrocephalus usually requires a shunt. The **Arnold-Chiari malformation** is a variable defect in the formation of the brainstem. The most extreme form consists of *elongation of the cerebellar tonsils, which protrude through the foramen magnum; beaking of the colliculi; and thickening of the upper cervical spinal cord.* Diagnosis is made by CT scan or ventriculography. Hydrocephalus may result from blockage of the 4th ventricular outlets or an associated aqueductal stenosis. Either may require a shunt procedure to relieve the obstruction. The Arnold-Chiari malformation may occur alone, but it is frequently associated with spina bifida (see below) and syringomyelia.

Spina bifida, *defective closure of the vertebral column,* is one of the most serious neural tube defects compatible with prolonged life. Its severity varies from the occult type with no findings to *a completely open spine* (**rachischisis**) with severe neurologic disability and death. In spina bifida cystica, the protruding sac can contain meninges (**meningocele**), spinal cord (**myelocele**), or both (**myelomeningocele**). US can now show bony spinal defects and soft tissue masses. Open spina bifida can be diagnosed by amniocentesis showing elevated α-fetoprotein levels. Spina bifida is most common in the lumbar, low thoracic, or sacral region, and usually extends for 3 to 6 vertebral segments. The sac in myelomeningocele usually consists of meninges with a central neural plaque. If not well covered with skin, the sac can easily rupture, increasing the risk of meningitis.

When the spinal cord or lumbosacral nerve roots are involved in the spina bifida, as is usual, varying degrees of paralysis occur below the involved level. Since this paralysis is present in the fetus, there can be orthopedic problems present at birth (eg, clubfoot, arthrogryposis, or dislocated hip—see under MUSCULOSKELETAL DEFECTS, above). The paralysis usually affects bladder and rectal functions, and the resulting GU disorder can eventually lead to severely damaged kidneys. Kyphosis, sometimes associated with spina bifida, can hinder surgical closure and prevent the patient from lying supine. Hydrocephalus occurs frequently and may be related to aqueductal stenosis or an Arnold-Chiari malformation (see above). Other congenital anomalies may be present.

Laboratory evaluation begins with x-rays of the spine, skull, hips, and, if they are malformed, lower extremities. Urinary tract evaluation is essential and includes urinalysis, urine culture, BUN and creatinine determination, IVU, and US scanning. Further testing depends on the associated defects and may include intracranial studies (CT or US scan) and CSF evaluation.

Prognosis is determined by the number and severity of abnormalities and is poorest for patients with total paralysis below the lesion, kyphosis, hydrocephalus, early hydronephrosis, and associated congenital defects. With proper care, however, many children do well.

Treatment requires a united effort by specialists from several disciplines. Initially important are neurosurgical, urologic, orthopedic, pediatric, and social service evaluations. Thorough evaluation of the infant and counseling of the family should generally precede intervention. It is important to assess the type, level, and extent of the lesion; the infant's general health status and associated deficits; the family's strengths, desires, and resources; and the community resources, including ongoing care. Following this, a decision can be made on how aggressive treatment should be.

If the defect is leaking CSF, antibiotic coverage or urgent neurosurgical evaluation and repair will reduce the risk of meningeal or ventricular infection. Hydrocephalus may require a shunt procedure. Kidney function must be carefully followed, and UTI should be treated promptly. Obstructive uropathy at either the bladder outlet or ureteral level must be treated vigorously, especially when infection is present. Loss of renal function or shunt complications are the usual causes of death in older patients with spina bifida. Orthopedic care should begin early with application of a cast for clubfoot, if present, and close observation of the hip joints, since dislocation is frequent. Other continuing orthopedic concerns are scoliosis, pathologic fractures, development of pressure sores, and muscle weakness and spasm, which may cause further deformities.

Hydrocephalus (*ventricular enlargement with excessive CSF*) is the most common cause of abnormally large heads in neonates. Obstruction is most often seen in the aqueduct of Sylvius but can also occur at the outlets of the 4th ventricle (foramina of Luschka and Magendie) or in the subarachnoid spaces around the brainstem or over the hemispheres. **Communicating hydrocephalus** is present when CSF flows freely into the subarachnoid space; **noncommunicating**

hydrocephalus indicates blockage at a site within the ventricular system or between it and the subarachnoid space. Communicating hydrocephalus usually results from meningeal inflammation, secondary either to infection or to blood in the subarachnoid space.

Laboratory evaluation includes skull x-rays and cranial US or CT scan. These may show separation of sutures, areas of thinning of the bones, or intracranial calcifications (associated with congenital infections). Plain skull films may show a "beaten-metal" appearance of the bones (common in infants with myelomeningoceles and hydrocephalus), indicating a prolonged increase in intracranial pressure. A CT scan will show the ventricular size and can also indicate the site of obstruction. US can define the degree of ventricular dilation, and serial studies can document progression of the hydrocephalus. US is especially valuable after intraventricular hemorrhage, since ventricular dilation may be transient and require only medical treatment. When congenital infection is suspected, serologic studies for *Toxoplasma gondii*, rubella virus, *Treponema pallidum,* and herpes- and cytomegalovirus are indicated. If seizures are present, an EEG may be helpful. Further studies may include subdural taps or examination of CSF.

Differential diagnosis includes intracranial space-occupying lesions (eg, subdural hematomas, porencephalic cysts, tumors). These can be identified by CT scan. *An abnormally large, usually malfunctioning brain* (megalencephaly) can also occur.

Treatment depends on etiology. Medical treatment with acetazolamide and glycerol or lumbar punctures (if the hydrocephalus is communicating) to reduce the CSF pressure can sometimes be helpful temporarily. However, progressive hydrocephalus, especially if the head circumference is growing too rapidly, requires a shunt procedure to reduce the pressure. It is important to ascertain before operation that the hydrocephalus is progressive, since some hydrocephalics arrest further progression spontaneously. The type of shunt depends on the neurosurgeon's experience and choice; ventriculoperitoneal shunts are generally preferred to ventriculoatrial shunts, since complications are fewer. After placement of the shunt, the infant's progress should be followed with attention to occipitofrontal head circumference, development, and the increased risk of related infections. Periodic, partial CT or US scans (if the anterior fontanelle is open) can be used to monitor ventricular size. Some chil-

dren cease to need the shunt as they become older, but it is difficult to determine when this occurs, and shunts are rarely removed. Fetal surgery to treat congenital hydrocephalus before birth has been unsuccessful and is experimental.

CONGENITAL EYE DEFECTS

CONGENITAL GLAUCOMA
(Infantile Glaucoma; Buphthalmos; Hydrophthalmos)

A rare condition due to a congenital defect in the region of the iridocorneal angle of the anterior chamber that obstructs the outflow of aqueous, causing a chronic increase in the intraocular pressure. The disorder is usually bilateral and is seen in infants and children. The eyeball becomes considerably enlarged; the large-diameter cornea is thinned, is sometimes milky, and may be bulging; the pupil may be large and fixed; the anterior chamber is deep. If the disease is permitted to progress, the optic nerve becomes damaged and blindness ensues. Diameter and clarity of the cornea should be carefully observed in infants. Treatment by early surgical intervention offers the only real hope of preserving useful vision (see TABLE 84–1).

CONGENITAL CATARACT

Developmental or congenital cataracts are present at birth and may result from chromosomal abnormalities, intrauterine infection (eg, rubella), metabolic disease (eg, galactosemia), or other maternal disease during pregnancy. The cataracts may be nuclear or cortical and may not be noticed unless funduscopy is performed at birth. If the cataracts are sufficiently dense to obscure the view of the optic disk and vessels, an ophthalmologist should be asked to estimate the possible effect on the infant's vision. Early surgery (within a few months of birth) is now advocated to permit development of appropriate retinal fixation and cortical visual responses. While the surgery is technically straightforward, postoperative visual correction with spectacles, contact lenses, or epikeratophakia (the suturing of a human cornea, lathed like a contact lens, onto the recipient's cornea) is difficult but necessary to achieve good vision. Extraction produces better visual results in infants with bilateral than with unilateral cataracts.

Juvenile and adult cataracts are discussed in Ch. 81.

RENAL AND GENITOURINARY DEFECTS

Congenital anomalies of the GU tract are more common than those of any other organ system. Complications include urinary obstruction and stasis with infection and stone formation, impairment of renal function, and sexual disability or infertility. Treatment of significant anatomic anomalies is usually surgical.

KIDNEY

Fusion anomalies: The most common is **horseshoe kidney,** in which *the 2 kidneys are joined at their corresponding (usually the lower) poles, generally with an isthmus of renal parenchyma across the midline at the joined poles.* Since the ureters course medially and anteriorly over this isthmus, secondary obstruction may develop. Most patients with horseshoe kidney have no difficulty; some develop hydronephrosis that requires surgery or suffer abdominal pain accentuated by hyperextension. Surgical resection of the isthmus occasionally is required and may be indicated to facilitate resection of the abdominal aorta, which lies behind the isthmus.

Other fusion anomalies include **fused pelvic kidney (pancake kidney),** in which *a single pelvic renal mass is served by 2 collecting systems and ureters* that frequently become obstructed because of anomalous position and drainage. **Crossed fused renal ectopia** also occurs, with both kidneys on one side, and usually requires no treatment unless obstruction is present.

Renal ectopia and malrotation (*displacement or failure of ascent or rotation of either or both kidneys*) may be evident on abdominal ultrasonography, CT scan, or urography even though the patient has been asymptomatic. **Pelvic kidney,** usually lying over the sacral promontory, may complicate pregnancy because of outflow obstruction. **Malrotation** of a normally positioned kidney may compromise urinary drainage and cause hydronephrosis that requires surgical correction.

Agenesis: Bilateral renal agenesis (*congenital absence of both kidneys*—Potter's syndrome) is incompatible with life. **Unilateral renal agenesis** is not uncommon and usually is accompanied by ureteral agenesis with absence of the ipsilateral trigone and ureteral orifice. The congenitally solitary kidney usually is both hyperplastic and hypertrophic, maintaining normal renal function.

Duplication anomalies: *Supernumerary collecting systems*—**accessory renal pelvis, double pelvis and ureter,** or **"duplex kidney"**—may be unilateral or bilateral and many involve the renal pelvis, calyces, ureter, and/or one or both ureteral orifices. **"Double kidney"** is a misnomer, since the single renal mass has more than one collecting system. Surgical correction is unnecessary unless renal function is compromised or complications such as hydronephrosis, infection, reflux, urinary incontinence, or obstruction develop.

Renal dysplasias (*developmental abnormalities*) with consequent compromise of renal function may result from abnormal development of the renal vasculature, the renal tubules, the collecting system, or the drainage apparatus.

Cystic hydronephrosis (*ureteral agenesis and atresia resulting in renal cystic degeneration resembling a cluster of grapes*) is due to formation of urine in the lobular segments of the fetal kidney, progressive hydrostatic atrophy, and ultimate cessation of renal function.

Renal hypoplasia (*underdevelopment of a kidney*) usually is associated with incomplete development of the main renal artery or its branches. The kidney is small, with histologically normal nephrons. Complications include ureteral abnormalities, hydronephrosis, and infection.

Polycystic kidney diseases are discussed below; **medullary sponge kidney** also is discussed below.

CYSTIC DISORDERS

The cystic disorders of the kidney represent dysplastic malformations, with single or multiple cysts varying from < 1 cm to > 10 cm in diameter. Some disorders are congenital, some are acquired, and sometimes a distinction cannot be made. The major groups are (1) polycystic disease (autosomal dominant and recessive types); (2) renal dysplasias (multicystic, focal and segmental, familial, secondary to lower urinary tract obstruction); (3) cortical cysts (simple [solitary and multiple], diffuse glomerular, and microcysts); (4) medullary cysts (medullary sponge kidney, medullary cystic disease complex); (5) cysts in hereditary disorders (Meckel syndrome, Zellweger cerebrohepatorenal syndrome, Jeune's thoracic dystrophy, tuberous sclerosis complex, Lindau's disease); and (6) miscellaneous disorders (inflammatory, neoplastic, extraparenchymal types).

Polycystic Renal Diseases

Inherited kidney disorders characterized by many bilateral cysts that increase kidney size but reduce the functioning renal tissue. Classification is by inheritance pattern. Two types are recognized: autosomal dominant polycystic kidney disease (ADPKD) and autosomal recessive polycystic kidney disease (ARPKD). The recessive type, ARPKD, may produce renal failure in childhood. Nevertheless, renal cysts in both types may be discovered even in utero. Mechanisms for the development of polycystic disease and the progressive enlargement of cysts are not well understood. The cysts are dilated portions of renal tubules and glomeruli, which maintain continuity with the remainder of the nephron.

Autosomal Recessive (Childhood) Polycystic Kidney Disease

A rare (1/10,000 births) disease involving both kidneys and liver, frequently producing renal failure in childhood. It is the most common genetically determined childhood cystic disease of the kidneys.

Symptoms, signs, and diagnosis: The clinical presentation varies with age. Generally, those first presenting in early childhood show mainly renal-related symptoms, whereas those first presenting as adolescents show mainly hepatic-related symptoms. These differences probably reflect phenotypic variation in the same genetic disorder.

Severely affected **neonates** commonly have pulmonary hypoplasia secondary to the in utero effects of renal dysfunction. These infants will often die in the first few days or weeks of life. Less severely affected neonates have a protuberant abdomen with huge, firm, smooth-surfaced, symmetric kidneys. The enlarged liver is abnormal with periportal fibrosis, bile duct proliferation, and rare cysts; the remainder of the hepatic parenchyma is normal. These pathologic findings are responsible for perisinusoidal portal hypertension with minimal or absent hepatic dysfunction. Ultrasonography is the best diagnostic tool, and in late pregnancy can allow presumptive in utero diagnosis in most cases.

Between ages 5 and 10 yr, signs of portal hypertension appear, such as esophageal and gastric varices, and hypersplenism (leukopenia, thrombocytopenia). In those individuals who first present in **adolescence**, nephromegaly is less marked. Renal insufficiency may be mild to moderate. The major symptoms are related to progressive hepatic fibrosis (portal hypertension, gastric and esophageal varices, hepatic insufficiency, and hypersplenism). Diagnosis is more difficult, especially without a positive family history. Ultrasonography may demonstrate cysts in the kidneys or liver; however, final diagnosis may require renal and liver biopsies.

Prognosis and treatment: The prognosis is limited, whether hepatic or renal dysfunction predominates. In many patients, death occurs soon after birth from pulmonary insufficiency. Infants who survive the first few years show progressive renal failure. For those with less renal involvement, progressive portal hypertension ensues. Portacaval or splenorenal shunts have been successful in reducing morbidity but not mortality. Control of hypersplenism is important, to obviate difficulty with immunosuppression if renal transplantation is attempted, although transplant experience is limited. Dialysis is used as for other children with chronic renal insufficiency.

Autosomal Dominant Polycystic Kidney Disease

The incidence of ADPKD is about 1/1000. Its penetrance is essentially complete, such that all carriers who live to 80 yr will demonstrate some signs of the disease; about 10% of patients with end-stage renal disease have ADPKD.

Symptoms and signs: Since ADPKD is slowly progressive over many years, it is often asymptomatic initially but may be discovered by ultrasonography (US) in childhood. Clinical onset is in early or middle adult life, although occasionally the disease is not discovered until autopsy. Symptoms usually are related to effects of the cysts, such as lumbar discomfort or pain, hematuria, infection, and colic due to nephrolithiasis, or may be related to a loss of renal function with uremic symptoms. Chronic infection frequently is superimposed and contributes to the progressive renal dysfunction. In about 33% of cases, cysts are present in the liver but are of no functional significance. About 10 to 22% of cases have associated intracranial aneurysms; about 15% suffer subarachnoid hemorrhage. Hypertension is found in about 50% of patients at the time of diagnosis.

Diagnosis: In advanced cases, when the kidneys are grossly enlarged and palpable, the diagnosis is obvious. The urine shows mild proteinuria and varying degrees of hematuria, but RBC casts are infrequent. Pyuria is common even in the absence of bacterial infection. Episodically, the urine is grossly bloody, apparently because of hemorrhage from a ruptured cyst or a dislodged calculus. The intravenous urogram (IVU, excretory urogram) is characteristic, with large kidneys showing irregular outlines because of the many cysts. The calyces, infundibula, and pelvis are compressed and elongated by cysts, giving a "spidery" appearance. Renal and hepatic sonograms and CT scans show a typical "moth-eaten" appearance due to the cysts that displace functional tissue; they may be diagnostic in early stages of the disease before typical IVU changes are noted. Polycystic kidney disease, with its progressive azotemia, is distinguished from solitary or multiple cysts that do not distort a sufficient portion of the renal parenchyma to cause uremia. The distinction is made on clinical grounds and by US, IVU, or radionuclide scanning.

Accurate genetic diagnosis of ADPKD may soon be available. Recombinant DNA technology has already localized one gene mutation in many ADPKD families to the short arm (p) of chromosome 16. The mutant gene, designated PKD1, shows close linkage to the genes for α globin and phosphoglycolate phosphatase (PGP). However, there appears to be genetic heterogeneity, as some ADPKD families have been identified who do not show linkage to the same chromosome 16p markers; the location of the mutant gene in these families has yet to be identified.

Prognosis and treatment: Though > 50% of patients become uremic within 10 yr of symptom onset, the course is quite variable; for many, end-stage renal failure will not occur for > 20 yr. Without dialysis or transplantation, death is usually due to uremia or the complications of hypertensive cardiovascular disease and occurs at an average age of 50. About 10% of patients die of intracranial hemorrhage from rupture of aneurysms.

Management of urinary infections and secondary hypertension may prolong life considerably. When uremia supervenes, its management is the same as in other renal diseases. With dialysis, patients with polycystic kidney disease maintain higher Hb levels than any other group of patients. Transplantation is feasible, but the use of parental and sibling donors may be impractical in view of the genetic characteristics of the disease. Genetic counseling is recommended.

Medullary Cystic Disease

A diffuse nephropathy, either genetic or congenital, characterized by the insidious onset of uremia.

The commonly described variants and their incidence are juvenile nephronophthisis, 50%; adult-onset medullary cystic disease, 20%; and renal-retinal dysplasia, 15%. A family history is common (about 85%). In a few families, the renal disease has been accompanied by pigmentary retinal degradation. The renal lesion is similar in all variants. Some authorities have noted a similarity in inheritance pattern to polycystic disease, in which the younger onset form is autosomal recessive and the adult onset form is autosomal dominant.

Symptoms, Signs, and Diagnosis

Symptoms usually begin in the first 2 decades of life, although the disease has been observed as late as the 60s. Polyuria due to a vasopressin-resistant renal concentrating defect is often the earliest symptom. Urinary Na wastage frequently is present and commonly is severe enough to require a Na intake of several hundred mEq/day to prevent extracellular volume depletion. Unexplained uremia is a good early clue in some patients. Retarded growth and evidence of bone disease are common in children. In many patients, these problems develop slowly over a period of years and are so well compensated that they are not recognized as abnormal until significant uremic symptoms appear.

Serum chemistries are similar to those in patients with chronic renal failure. Proteinuria is minimal or absent, and the urinary sediment is not remarkable. IVU demonstrates only small kidneys, but US and arteriography may reveal medullary cysts. Because cysts may be few and small, they can be missed by any or all of these imaging studies.

Prognosis and Treatment

Disease progression is variable and depends on the degree of renal dysfunction at presentation. As a rule, the disease progresses slowly but inexorably. When uremia supervenes, its management is the same as in other renal diseases. These patients may do very well with transplantation.

Medullary Sponge Kidney

Tubular ectasia or dysplasia resulting in congenital dilatation of the collecting tubules. The disorder is unrelated to medullary cystic disease (see above). The true incidence is unknown but is probably about 1/5000. Sponge kidney leads to urinary stasis and nephrocalcinosis.

Symptoms, Signs, and Diagnosis

The condition usually is asymptomatic unless the complications of calculus colic (the most common presenting complaint), hematuria, or infections supervene. Nephrocalcinosis is found in > 50% of affected kidneys. Evidence of type I (distal) renal tubular acidosis is also seen in most cases. Ultrasonography may not always be helpful because the cysts are small and located deep in the medulla. The lesion must be differentiated from renal cystic disease, papillary necrosis, pyelonephritic cysts, TB, and other conditions causing nephrocalcinosis. Diagnosis can be made by urography, which shows pyramidal cavities filled with contrast material, giving the appearance of "a bouquet of carnations." Medullary sponge kidney has been noted with increased frequency in Ehlers-Danlos syndrome, congenital hemihypertrophy, and Beckwith-Wiedemann syndrome.

Prognosis and Treatment

If uncomplicated, the condition has an excellent prognosis. Treatment is given *only* for complications. Usually, noncalcinotic forms are asymptomatic and need no therapy. Although nephrocalcinosis may be progressive, no specific medical treatment has been adequately assessed. However, thiazides (eg, hydrochlorothiazide 50 mg bid), high fluid intake, and a low Ca diet may inhibit stone formation and reduce obstructive complications. Infections are treated in the usual manner. Surgery is indicated only when obstruction occurs or if renal involvement is segmental. Extirpation of the affected tissue has proved beneficial.

HEREDITARY CHRONIC NEPHROPATHIES

Many of the genetically transmitted renal disorders produce functional or structural abnormalities, or both. Those involving mainly tubular transport defects or metabolic defects with renal involvement as in Fabry's disease (see under LIPIDOSES in Ch. 40) are discussed elsewhere. The hereditary, noncystic nephropathies discussed in this section are hereditary nephritis and the nail-patella syndrome.

Hereditary Nephritis
(Alport's Syndrome)

A heterogenous genetic disorder characterized by hematuria, renal functional impairment, frequent sensorineural deafness, and occasional ocular abnormalities.

Most evidence suggests a dominant X-linked inheritance pattern with variable penetrance, although other inheritance modes may be present in some families. There are no distinguishing histologic changes by light or immunofluorescence microscopy. Ultrastructural studies in most families show thickening and thinning of the glomerular and tubular basement membrane, with multilamination of the lamina densa in a focal or local distribution. The genetic lesion is known to affect the noncollagenous domain of type IV collagen, resulting in the production of altered collagen strands and in the loss of a common antigen on the glomerular basement membrane, which may assist in the diagnosis by monoclonal antibody techniques.

Symptoms, Signs, and Diagnosis

Disease onset may be similar to that of acute glomerulonephritis, but many patients are asymptomatic and the disease is detected by finding hematuria. The urine may contain small amounts of protein, WBCs, and casts of various types. The nephrotic syndrome occurs rarely. Females usually are asymptomatic and have little functional impairment, whereas most males develop evidence of renal insufficiency between ages 20 and 30. Sensorineural deafness frequently is present, usually affecting the higher frequencies. Some individuals with a family history may have nerve deafness alone without renal disease; such persons are capable of transmitting the renal disease to a subsequent generation. Eye lesions occur less frequently than acoustic ones; cataracts are most common, but anterior lenticonus, spherophakia, nystagmus, retinitis pigmentosa, and blindness also have been noted. Other nonrenal manifestations include polyneuropathy and thrombocytopenia.

Treatment

Treatment is indicated only when uremia occurs; its management is the same as in other renal diseases. Successful transplants have been done using kidneys from cadavers or from living, related adults. Genetic counseling is indicated.

Nail-Patella Syndrome
(Osteo-onychodysplasia; Arthro-onychodysplasia; Onycho-osteodysplasia)

A rare familial disorder of mesenchymal tissue characterized by abnormalities of bone, joints, fingernails, and kidneys.

Inheritance occurs as an autosomal dominant trait linked to the ABO blood group locus. The most common skeletal dysplasia is unilateral or bilateral hypoplasia or absence of the patella, subluxation of the radial heads at the elbows, and bilateral accessory iliac horns. The fingernails are either absent or hypoplastic, with pitting and ridges. Heterochromia of the irises may occur, but deafness is not found. Renal histologic changes by light microscopy are nonspecific, with localized thickening of the capillary wall. Focal glomerular deposits of IgM and C3 may occur. The characteristic ultrastructural changes are localized areas of rarefaction of the glomerular basement membrane, with intramembranous deposits having the appearance and periodicity of collagen.

Symptoms and Signs
Renal dysfunction occurs in about 50% of patients and is manifested by proteinuria and, rarely, hematuria. Proteinuria usually is minimal but occasionally may reach nephrotic syndrome ranges. The disease is diagnosed by the typical clinical and radiographic findings and can be further confirmed by renal biopsy. About 30% of patients with renal involvement will slowly progress to renal failure.

Treatment
Management of progressive renal failure is the same as in other renal diseases. Successful transplants have been done without evidence of disease recurrence in the renal graft. Genetic counseling is indicated.

URETER

Congenital ureteral anomalies are frequently associated with renal anomalies but may occur independently. Complications include obstruction, infection, and stone formation, as well as problems of urinary control.

Duplication anomalies (*partial or complete duplication of one or both ureters, together with duplication of the ipsilateral renal pelvis*) may occur. Duplication of only the lower ureter is rare. When complete duplication of the ureters exists, the ureter from the uppermost portion of the kidney opens at a more distal point than the orifice of the lower pole ureter. Ectopia of one or both orifices, vesicoureteral reflux into the lower or both ureters, ureterocele, or stenosis of one or both ureteral orifices is common. Surgery is unnecessary unless vesicoureteral reflux, obstruction, infection, incontinence, or compromised renal function develops. (See also ectopic orifices, below.)

Ectopia. Retrocaval ureter (*anomalous development of the ureter, usually behind a persistent right cardinal vein*) can cause obstruction. A retrocaval ureter on the left is seen only with persistence of the left cardinal vein system or complete situs inversus. Surgical treatment consisting of division of the ureter with uretero-uretero anastomosis anterior to the vena cava or iliac vessel is indicated if significant obstruction is present.

Ectopic orifices: *Displaced openings of single or duplicated ureters* may occur on the lateral bladder wall (predisposing to vesicoureteral reflux), distally along the trigone, in the bladder neck, in the female urethra distal to the sphincter (leading to incontinence), in the genital system (prostate and seminal vesicle in the male, uterus or vagina in the female), or externally. Ectopic orifices frequently lead to reflux, obstruction, incontinence, and infection. Surgical correction may be indicated.

Stricture and stenosis: Congenital stricture may occur at any portion of the ureter and frequently at the ureterovesical junction, where it is usually managed by surgical reimplantation of the ureter into the bladder. Defects in the continuity of ureteral smooth muscle may result in dysfunctional segments, disposing to proximal ureterectasis. **Megaloureter** (*congenital ureteral dilatation with no evident cause*) may be the result of a localized segmental muscular abnormality or neurogenic deficit.

Ureterocele (*bulging of the lower end of the ureter into the bladder*) may produce progressive and self-obstructing cystic dilatation, leading to ureterectasis, hydronephrosis, calculus formation, and potential loss of renal function. Diagnosis is established radiographically and cystoscopically. Treatment, when indicated, is surgical. The prognosis is good if the condition is recognized before significant renal dysfunction occurs.

VESICOURETERAL REFLUX

Reflux of urine from the bladder into the ureter is abnormal and may result in damage to the upper urinary tract by bacterial infection and by increased hydrostatic pressure.

Etiology

Vesicoureteral reflux most often is due to congenital anomalous development of the uretero-vesical junction. Incomplete development of the intramural ureteral tunnel causes a failure of the valvelike action at the ureterovesical junction and permits the reflux of bladder urine into the ureter and renal pelvis, often under the increased intravesical pressures of voiding. Other causes of vesicoureteral reflux include bladder outlet obstruction with increased intravesical pressures, lower UTI with edema and distortion of the ureteral orifice, neurogenic dysfunction of the detrusor and vesical neck mechanism, and iatrogenic reflux secondary to surgical or instrumental manipulation of the ureteral orifice.

Pathology

Intraureteral pressures are rarely greater than 10 or 12 cm of water pressure; voiding pressures may reach levels of 50 to 200 cm. Such increased pressures may be followed by progressive hydrostatic damage to the kidney when they are transmitted into the ureter and renal pelvis. Bacteria in the lower urinary tract are transmitted by reflux to the upper tract, causing persistent urinary infection with potential loss of renal function.

Symptoms, Signs, and Diagnosis

Abdominal or flank pain, persistent or recurrent urinary infection, dysuria or flank pain with voiding, frequency and urgency, or the uremic syndrome may be secondary to vesicoureteral reflux. Pyuria, hematuria, proteinuria, and bacteriuria may be present.

Intravenous urography (IVU) may show calyceal dilatation, ureteral "ribboning," and ureterectasis with dilatation of the upper collecting system. Filling and voiding cystourethrograms demonstrate vesicoureteral reflux. Cystoscopy may confirm ureteral malimplantation, with ectopia and distortion of the ureteral orifice, or bladder outlet obstruction. Reflux may also be demonstrated by isotope cystogram scan.

Prognosis and Treatment

Conservative medical management usually is adequate for mild reflux of the "high pressure" (voiding) type, with no renal damage and normal orifices, and easily controlled infection. Reflux may disappear in many such cases. Severe "low pressure" (filling) reflux secondary to malimplantation or ectopia of the ureteral orifice is best treated by vesicoureteral reimplantation. This is usually successful in eliminating reflux and may preserve renal function. Vesicoureteral reflux in association with massive hydroureter and hydronephrosis or myoneurogenic disorders may require primary urinary diversion (cutaneous ureterostomies, vesicostomy, ileal or colon segment urinary diversion). Medical management of associated urinary infection and azotemia, renal rickets, hypoproteinemia, and anemia is imperative.

BLADDER

Congenital anomalies of the urinary bladder include exstrophy, agenesis, duplication, persistent urachus, and the megacystis syndrome, which may be a primary myoneural defect.

Exstrophy of the urinary bladder is an easily detectable and serious major anomaly. The open (unroofed) bladder is seen in the suprapubic region with urine dripping from the ureteral orifices. The bladder mucosa is continuous with the abdominal skin, and the pubic bones are separated. Attempts at primary closure have been successful. Ureterosigmoidostomy, with or without proximal colostomy, and ileal or colon loop urinary diversion are the most common procedures when primary closure is not feasible or fails. Reconstruction of the genitalia is required. The prognosis for maintenance of normal renal function is relatively good.

Congenital bladder diverticula occur and predispose to urinary infection. Diverticula may be associated with reflux. Diagnosis is made by cystography and cystoscopy. Surgical removal of diverticula and reconstruction of the bladder wall may be indicated.

Contracture of the vesical outlet may occur in association with neurogenic diseases or as a primary congenital entity. Abdominal pain, weak and dribbling stream, distended urinary bladder, and persistent pyuria should suggest bladder outlet obstruction. Vesicoureteral reflux may occur. Cystography and cystoscopy establish the diagnosis. Endoscopic resection or open plastic surgical revision of the vesical orifice usually provides relief. **Congenital bladder neck obstruction** is a rare entity and an overworked diagnosis. Acquired bladder neck contracture may result from transurethral resection.

PENIS AND URETHRA

The penis in the male and the urethra in both male and female may be congenitally absent. Other anomalies include double penis, congenital penile curvature or malrotation, microphallus, and urethral stricture, stenosis, and duplication.

Hypospadias (*displaced urethral opening*): In the female, the urethra opens into the vaginal introitus. In the male, the urethral opening may be on the underside of the penile shaft, at the penoscrotal junction, between the scrotal folds, or in the perineum. **Chordee** (*ventral curvature of the penis, most apparent on erection*) usually is associated with hypospadias and is caused by a fibrous band along the usual course of the corpus spongiosum. Also present is a "dorsal hood" formed by incomplete foreskin development. The principal complications are meatal stenosis, the patient's inability to direct the urinary stream, and sexual disability in later life. Early surgical correction consists of an initial procedure to release the chordee and straighten the shaft, followed by plastic reconstruction of the urethra. One-stage surgical repairs often are performed. Prognosis for functional and cosmetic correction is good.

Epispadias: *A dorsal fusion defect of the urethra, partial or complete, the ultimate representing exstrophy of the urinary bladder.* Epispadias occurs in both males and females but is more common in males. Urinary control can be satisfactory with incomplete epispadias. Reconstruction may be effective but is often difficult and is associated with persistent incontinence.

Urethral valves: *Congenital folds of the urethra acting as valves* occur in both sexes but are much more common in the prostatic urethra of the male. Complications are due to obstruction, which may be severe and lead to massive upper tract damage. Symptoms and signs include weak and dribbling urinary stream, overflow incontinence, and urinary infection. Diagnosis is established by urography and endoscopy. Prompt surgical intervention may obviate the need for urinary diversion.

Stenosis: The most common form of congenital urethral stenosis is **meatal stricture**. Urethral meatotomy usually is successful.

Phimosis (*congenital or acquired [inflammatory] constriction of the foreskin, which cannot be retracted*) and **paraphimosis** (*inability of the retracted constricting foreskin to be reduced over the glans*). Surgical treatment by circumcision is indicated. A preliminary dorsal slit may be required. The prognosis is excellent.

TESTES AND SCROTUM

The scrotum may fail to develop unilaterally **(hemiscrotum)** or bilaterally, often associated with cryptorchidism. Congenital **hemangiomas** of the scrotum may require surgical removal, since bleeding or progressive enlargement can be anticipated. Congenital **hydrocele** communicates with the abdominal cavity through a patent processus vaginalis, a potential hernia space, but may resolve spontaneously following neonatal obliteration of the communication. **Penile-scrotal transposition** is a striking anomaly amenable to surgery.

UNDESCENDED TESTES
(Cryptorchidism)

Incomplete or improper prenatal descent of one or both testes is common. Hormonal function generally is normal. However, the undescended testis may show progressive failure of spermatogenesis if untreated. The cryptorchid testis has a higher incidence of carcinoma, which may manifest itself many years later.

In true **cryptorchidism**, the testis remains within the abdominal cavity or retroperitoneally, the result of hormonal or mechanical abnormalities. In **incomplete descent** or **maldescent of the testis**, or **arrested testis**, the testis lies within the inguinal canal but has been obstructed in its passage by mechanical factors. The **ectopic testis** lies outside the usual course of descent, suprapubically, within the perineum, or along the inner aspect of the thigh. **Hypermobile or retractile testes** may lie within the scrotum at times (eg, during a hot tub bath) but then retract into the inguinal canal.

Treatment

Human chorionic gonadotropin (HCG) 500 to 1000 IU given IM 2 or 3 times/wk for periods up to 6 wk may promote bilateral testicular descent. The usual surgical treatment is orchiopexy before 2 yr of age. Delay in surgery beyond age 5 yr may impair spermatogenesis, a critical factor when bilateral cryptorchidism occurs. Surgery generally is unnecessary for hypermobile (retractile) testes, since normal descent occurs at puberty. Orchiectomy usually is the treatment of choice when unilateral cryptorchidism is discovered in the postpubertal patient.

TESTICULAR TORSION

Twisting of the testis on its cord, spontaneously or following strenuous activity, may result from anomalous development of the tunica vaginalis and spermatic cord. Immediate **symptoms** of torsion are severe local pain, nausea, and vomiting, followed by scrotal edema and fever. Torsion must be differentiated from inflammatory conditions within the scrotum, trauma, and testicular tumor. Radioisotope scrotal scan may aid in diagnosis. **Immediate surgical intervention** is advised when torsion is suspected, since exploration within a few hours offers the only hope of testicular salvage. Fixation of the contralateral testis is performed to prevent torsion on that side. (See also under COMPLETE PHYSICAL EXAMINATION in MANAGEMENT OF THE NORMAL NEWBORN in Ch. 23.)

ANOMALIES IN KIDNEY TRANSPORT

CYSTINURIA

An inherited defect of the renal tubules in which resorption of the amino acid cystine is impaired, urinary excretion is increased, and cystine calculi often form in the urinary tract.

Cystinuria is inherited as an autosomal recessive trait. Heterozygotes may excrete increased quantities of cystine in the urine, but seldom enough to form stones.

Pathophysiology

The diminished renal tubular resorption of cystine increases its concentration in the urine. Cystine is poorly soluble in acid urine; when its urinary concentration exceeds its solubility, precipitation results, both as crystals and stones.

Resorption of dibasic amino acids (lysine, ornithine, and arginine) is also impaired, although they have an alternative transport system separate from that shared with cystine. Since they are more soluble than cystine in urine, their increased excretion does not result in precipitation. Their absorption (and that of cystine) is also decreased in the small intestine; several patterns of malabsorption have been described.

Symptoms, Signs, and Diagnosis

Radiopaque cystine stones form in the renal pelvis or bladder. Staghorn calculi are common. Symptoms usually appear between ages 10 and 30, and renal colic is the most common presenting complaint. UTI and renal failure due to obstruction may develop. In longtime survivors, end-stage renal disease is the rule.

Cystine may occur in the urine as yellow-brown hexagonal crystals. Excessive cystine in the urine may be detected by the nitroprusside cyanide test. The diagnosis is confirmed by chromatography or electrophoresis.

Treatment

The urinary concentration of cystine can be reduced by increasing urine volume. Fluid intake must be sufficient to provide a urine flow rate of up to 4 L/day. Hydration is especially important at night when urinary pH drops. Alkalinization of the urine to pH > 7.5 with sodium bicarbonate 15 to 30 gm/day orally in divided doses, and acetazolamide 5 mg/kg (up to 250 mg) orally at bedtime, will increase the solubility of cystine significantly. When high fluid intake and alkalinization do not reduce stone formation, other medications may be tried, eg, penicillamine, *although toxicity limits its usefulness.* About half of all patients treated develop some toxic manifestation, including fever, rash, arthralgias, and, less commonly, nephrotic syndrome, pancytopenia, or an SLE-like reaction.

FANCONI'S SYNDROME

An acquired or inherited disorder, often associated with cystinosis, with characteristic abnormalities of renal proximal tubular function including glucosuria, phosphaturia, aminoaciduria, and bicarbonate wasting.

Occurrence and Genetics

As an inherited trait, Fanconi's syndrome usually accompanies another genetic disorder, particularly cystinosis as an autosomal recessive disease. (See TABLE 40–10 under ANOMALIES IN AMINO ACID METABOLISM in Ch. 40.) Heterozygotes may show cystine accumulation in cells but lack other clinical and laboratory manifestations. Fanconi's syndrome may also accompany Wilson's disease, hereditary fructose intolerance, galactosemia, glycogen storage disease, Lowe's syndrome, and tyrosinemia.

Acquired Fanconi's syndrome may be caused by 6-mercaptopurine or outdated tetracycline, renal transplantation, multiple myeloma, amyloidosis, intoxication with heavy metals or other chemical agents, and vitamin D deficiency.

Pathophysiology, Symptoms, and Signs

A variety of defects of proximal tubular function occur, including impaired resorption of glucose, phosphate, amino acids, bicarbonate, uric acid, water, potassium, and sodium. The aminoaciduria is generalized, and unlike cystinuria, increased cystine excretion is only a minor component. The basic abnormality is unknown. In hereditary Fanconi's syndrome, the chief clinical features (proximal tubular acidosis, hypophosphatemic rickets, hypokalemia, polyuria, and polydipsia) usually appear in infancy.

In the **nephropathic form associated with cystinosis,** failure to thrive and growth retardation are common. The retinas show patchy depigmentation. Interstitial nephritis develops, leading to progressive renal failure that may be fatal before adolescence.

Diagnosis and Treatment

Diagnosis is made by demonstrating the abnormalities of renal function, particularly glucosuria, phosphaturia, and aminoaciduria. In cystinosis, slit-lamp examination may show cystine crystals in the cornea.

There is no specific treatment. Acidosis may be improved by giving sodium bicarbonate. **Shohl's solution** given 50 to 100 mL/day in divided doses, Bicitra®, or Polycitra-K® can be substituted for sodium bicarbonate solution and may be better tolerated. For treatment of hypophosphatemic rickets, see below. Potassium depletion may require replacement therapy. Renal transplantation has been successful in renal failure; however, when cystinosis is the underlying disease, progressive damage may continue in other organs and eventually result in death.

HYPOPHOSPHATEMIC RICKETS
(Vitamin D–Resistant Rickets)

A familial or, rarely, acquired disorder characterized by hypophosphatemia, defective intestinal absorption of calcium, and rickets or osteomalacia that is unresponsive to vitamin D.

Familial hypophosphatemic rickets is inherited as an X-linked dominant trait. Affected females have less severe bone disease than do males and may show only hypophosphatemia. Sporadic acquired cases sometimes are associated with benign mesenchymal tumors **(oncogenic rickets).**

Pathophysiology, Symptoms, and Signs

The major physiologic abnormality is decreased proximal renal tubular resorption of phosphate; decreased intestinal calcium and phosphate absorption also occurs. Parathyroid hormone and vitamin D levels are normal. Two types of hypophosphatemic rickets occur. In type I, impaired renal synthesis leads to a subnormal plasma level of 1,25-dihydroxyvitamin D_3. In type II, 1,25-dihydroxyvitamin D_3 in plasma is normal or elevated, and the disease is due to an impaired cellular response to this substance.

The disease is manifested as a spectrum of abnormalities from hypophosphatemia alone, to severe rickets or osteomalacia with bowing of the legs and other bone deformities, pseudofractures, bone pain, and short stature. Blood phosphate levels are depressed, calcium is normal, and alkaline phosphatase often is elevated. Bony outgrowth at muscle attachments may limit motion. The rickets of the spine or pelvis seen in vitamin D deficiency is rarely found. Craniostenosis and convulsions may be present in children. The age of onset is usually < 1 yr.

Hypophosphatemic rickets must be distinguished from **vitamin D–dependent rickets,** an autosomal recessive disorder with similar clinical features except that hypocalcemia is present, hypophosphatemia is mild or absent, tetany and convulsions are common, and rickets of the spine and pelvis are frequent.

Treatment

Treatment of type I hypophosphatemic rickets consists of oral phosphate 1 to 3 gm/day in divided doses, as neutral phosphate solution, plus calcitriol 0.5 to 1 μg/day in young children and 1 to 3 μg/day in older children (15 to 50 ng/kg/day). Increase in plasma phosphate concentration, decrease in alkaline phosphatase, healing of rickets, and improvement of growth rate occur. Hypercalciuria or secondary hyperparathyroidism may complicate the treatment. Type II hypophosphatemic rickets responds poorly to treatment. In adults with oncogenic rickets, dramatic improvement has followed removal of the tumor.

HARTNUP DISEASE

A rare disease due to abnormal absorption and excretion of tryptophan and other amino acids, characterized clinically by rash and CNS abnormalities.

Hartnup disease is inherited as an autosomal recessive trait. Consanguinity is common. Heterozygotes are normal. Small intestine malabsorption of tryptophan, phenylalanine, methionine, and other monoaminomonocarboxylic amino acids occurs. Accumulation of unabsorbed amino acids in the GI tract increases their metabolism by bacterial flora. Some tryptophan degradation products including indoles, kynurenine, and serotonin are absorbed by the bowel and appear in the urine. Renal amino acid resorption is also defective, causing a generalized aminoaciduria involving all neutral amino acids except proline and hydroxyproline. Conversion of tryptophan to niacinamide is also defective.

Symptoms and signs are due to niacinamide deficiency and resemble those of pellagra, particularly the rash on parts of the body exposed to the sun. Neurologic manifestations include cerebellar ataxia and psychologic abnormalities. Mental retardation, short stature, headache, and collapsing or fainting are common. Symptoms may be precipitated by sunlight, fever, drugs, or other stresses. Poor nutritional intake nearly always precedes appearance of symptoms. The eventual prognosis is good, and the frequency of attacks usually diminishes with age.

Diagnosis is made by demonstrating the characteristic amino acid excretion pattern in the urine. Indoles and other tryptophan degradation products in the urine provide supplementary evidence of the disease. **Treatment:** Attacks can be prevented by maintaining good nutrition and supplementing the diet with niacinamide or niacin.

FAMILIAL IMINOGLYCINURIA

An autosomal recessive benign defect in the renal tubular resorption of imino acids and glycine. Homozygotes excrete abnormal amounts of imino acids (proline and hydroxyproline) and glycine; heterozygotes have glycinuria only. Plasma levels of amino acids are normal. Intestinal absorption of proline may be impaired. Iminoaciduria is normal in the newborn.

INTERSEX STATES

(See also Ch. 48 and CONGENITAL ADRENAL HYPERPLASIA in Ch. 40)

Conditions in which the appearance of the external genitalia is either ambiguous or at variance with the chromosomal or gonadal sex of the individual.

Etiology and Classification

The genitalia develop during the first trimester of intrauterine life under the influence of the sex steroids. Abnormalities of sexual development may arise owing to endocrine or morphologic derangements, the latter often associated with karyotypic abnormalities. **Female pseudohermaphrodites** are normal females exposed to excessive amounts of androgenic steroids in utero. They have 46,XX karyotypes and normal internal genitalia, but ambiguous external genitalia. The offending androgen may be exogenous, eg, when the mother is given progesterone to prevent miscarriage; but more often it is endogenous, owing to accumulation of androgen caused by an enzymatic block in steroidogenesis **(adrenogenital syndrome).** True hermaphrodites have both ovarian and testicular tissue, and mixed masculine and feminine genital structures; a rare individual may be fully masculinized externally. The majority of true hermaphrodites have had 46,XX karyotypes, but the pattern can be quite variable.

Male pseudohermaphrodites have testicular tissue only and usually a 46,XY karyotype. The etiology of male pseudohermaphroditism is complex; in general, the disorder arises from (1) failure to generate adequate amounts of androgen or (2) failure to respond metabolically to the androgens produced. The former group includes some rare forms of disordered steroidogenesis as well as certain types of gonadal dysgenesis (the only type of male pseudohermaphrodite likely to have a karyotype other than 46,XY). Male pseudohermaphroditism due to an altered response to androgen includes the **testicular feminization syndrome** (a key androgen receptor is absent); **pseudovaginal perineoscrotal hypospadias** (the enzyme responsible for the conversion of testosterone to dihydrotestosterone is lacking in the tissues); and **receptor-positive defects** (nuclear binding seems to be at fault). Patients with **simple hypospadias** may have a variety of poorly defined and sometimes transient endocrinologic disturbances. In the above disorders, as with most intersex patients, the external genitalia are ambiguous. These variants are present at birth.

Patients with **mixed gonadal dysgenesis** have both testicular tissue and primitive gonadal tissue called "streaks." They usually have a 46,XY/45,XO karyotype and tend to be short of stature as adults. **Pure gonadal dysgenesis** is the name given to those with gonadal streaks bilaterally. Unlike the other intersex states in which the external genitalia are likely to exhibit some degree of ambiguity, these patients appear phenotypically to be normal females; diagnosis often is delayed until they reach puberty and fail to feminize.

Diagnosis

Patients with genital ambiguity, phenotypic females with palpable gonads, and phenotypic males with impalpable gonads should be evaluated for intersexuality. Males with hypospadias usually do not require such an evaluation if both testes are descended and appear palpably normal, but hypospadias associated with one or both testes undescended should be investigated.

Assessment of intersex patients is urgent because of pressures not only to establish a correct sex assignment, but also to identify a patient with the adrenogenital syndrome so that treatment can be started before life-threatening hyponatremia develops. Buccal smears for nuclear membrane chromatin, vaginograms to demonstrate a cervix or uterine canal, and ultrasonography to show a uterus behind the bladder are studies that can be done quickly but are somewhat nonspecific. When positive, they are suggestive but not diagnostic of the adrenogenital syndrome. Hormonal assays are more definitive. Patients with the adrenogenital syndrome characteristically show elevations of urinary 17-ketosteroids, 17-hydroxysteroids, and pregnanetriol. Even more specific is an elevated serum 17-hydroxyprogesterone. Elevated serum renin levels indicate impending hyponatremia and tendency to hyperkalemia. Karyotyping establishes the definitive diagnosis in most intersex patients, although it may be redundant in the adrenogenital syndrome, in which the diagnosis rests primarily on the biochemical data.

Patients in whom the adrenogenital syndrome can be ruled out, either because they have palpable gonads externally or because they do not exhibit the necessary biochemical abnormalities, usually require early surgical exploration and gonadal biopsy for definitive diagnosis. Sex assignment in these individuals should not be delayed beyond the first week of life, if this can be avoided.

Treatment

Assignment of sex appropriate to the individual is the most important element. Generally, female pseudohermaphrodites are sex-assigned as females. True hermaphrodites are best sex-assigned according to the ease with which their genital construction can be carried out along one sexual line or another, but most have been reconstructed as males. This may be a particularly attractive option if the individual has a normally descended testis to provide hormonal function at puberty. Male pseudohermaphrodites are sex-assigned according to their potential as determined by genital development and hormonal activity. Those with the full-blown testicular feminization syndrome must be sex-assigned as females, but for many of the other male pseudohermaphrodites, male sex assignment is reasonable and appropriate. When uncertainty exists in marginal cases, 1 or 2 courses of testosterone propionate (in oil) 25 mg IM help determine the ability of the genitalia to respond to androgen—an essential requirement in male sex assignment.

Patients with mixed gonadal dysgenesis are best sex-assigned as females, not only because of short stature, but also because of the propensity of these testes to develop tumors. Those with pure gonadal dysgenesis appear phenotypically as females and should be raised as such.

Timing of the surgical reconstruction of the genitalia is variable. Sex-assigned females other than those with the adrenogenital syndrome should have a clitoral resection as early as possible to facilitate familial acceptance in their assigned role. Those with the adrenogenital syndrome have to be deferred some months until they have been rendered endocrinologically stable by steroid therapy. Vaginal reconstruction in all of these patients is best deferred until puberty because of the high incidence of stenosis when it is done early in life. Correction of hypospadias in males usually is done at about 2 to 3 yr of age.

29. DEVELOPMENTAL PROBLEMS

FAILURE TO THRIVE (FTT)

FTT is usually defined in terms of (1) weight consistently below the 3rd percentile for age; (2) weight < 80% of ideal weight for height-age; (3) progressive fall-off in weight to below the 3rd percentile; or (4) a decrease in expected rate of growth along the child's previously defined growth curve irrespective of its relationship to the 3rd percentile.

Weight is used as the growth parameter of special interest because it is the most sensitive indicator of nutritional status; inhibition of expected height growth rate usually indicates more severe and prolonged malnutrition. A decrease in head circumference growth rate is a late finding; because of the preferential brain-sparing of protein-energy utilization, it indicates extreme or chronic malnutrition.

It is important to clarify 2 points in the above definitions: (1) by the law of normal distribution, the weight of 3% of "normal" children will fall consistently below the 3rd percentile (conversely, however, the majority of children whose weight is less than the 3rd percentile will have true growth failure); and (2) ideal weight for height-age must be adjusted for expected height (as defined by the child's previously established height growth curve) rather than current height, if there is evidence that linear growth has been impaired.

FTT is used to designate growth failure both as a symptom and as a syndrome. As a symptom, it occurs in patients with a variety of acute or chronic illnesses that are known to interfere with normal nutrient intake, absorption, metabolism, or excretion, or to result in greater-than-normal energy requirements to sustain or promote growth. In these instances, it is referred to as **organic FTT.**

When the term is used to designate a syndrome, it most commonly refers to growth failure in the infant or child who suffers from environmental neglect or stimulus deprivation. It is then designated **nonorganic FTT,** indicating the absence of a physiologic disorder sufficient to account for the observed growth deficiency.

Using the most restrictive definition, only those children who were full-term and normally grown at birth and who, by careful investigation, have no congenital or acquired illness are included in the group designated nonorganic FTT. Yet, organic FTT and nonorganic FTT are not mutually exclusive. Thus, there is a 3rd group of patients who have growth failure of **mixed etiology.** These children present the greatest challenge to the physician, who must ascertain the relative contributions of the organic entity and the deprivation syndrome to the child's abnormal growth status. This mixed etiology group includes children who were born prematurely but have evidence of disproportionate growth failure in later infancy; children who have or have had some defect that cannot sufficiently explain the current growth failure (eg, successful cleft palate

repair in the past); and children who are frustrating (eg, because of a neurologically impaired suck) or repugnant (eg, because of a deformity) to the care giver.

Etiology and Pathophysiology

In FTT of any etiology, the physiologic basis for impaired growth is inadequate nutrition to support weight gain. In organic FTT, increased metabolic needs or decreased ability to ingest, absorb, or retain foods is the primary defect; in nonorganic FTT, lack of food may be due to impoverishment, poor understanding of feeding techniques, improperly prepared formula, or inadequate supply of breast milk.

The psychologic basis for nonorganic FTT appears to be similar to that seen in **hospitalism,** a syndrome observed in infants kept in sterile enviroments who suffer from depression secondary to stimulus deprivation; ie, the unstimulated child becomes depressed, apathetic, and ultimately anorexic. In nonorganic FTT, the unavailability of the stimulating person (usually, in our society, the mother) may be secondary to that person's own depression, poor parenting skills, anxiety in or lack of fulfillment from the caregiving role, sense of hostility toward the child, or response to real or perceived external stresses (eg, demands of other children, marital dysfunction, a significant loss, or financial difficulties).

A number of recent investigators have suggested that nonorganic FTT be considered the result of a disordered interaction between mother and child in which the child's temperament, capacities, and responses help shape maternal nurturance patterns; ie, the FTT is not solely the effect of poor care giving by an inadequate or troubled mother. Thus, nonorganic FTT can be the common manifestation of a variety of interactional disorders ranging from the severely disturbed or ill child, whose care poses a major challenge to even the most competent parent, to the potentially most undemanding and compliant child being cared for by a mentally ill parent without adequate social, emotional, financial, cognitive, or physical resources. Within these extremes are maternal-child "misfits" in which the demands of the child, although not pathologic, cannot be adequately met by the mother, who might, however, do well with a child of different needs or even with the same child but under different life circumstances.

About 3 to 5% of all children admitted to tertiary care centers and 1% of all children admitted to any hospital have FTT. Approximately 50 to

80% of those who do not have an apparent growth-inhibiting disease will have nonorganic FTT (ie, failure to grow adequately for psychosocially based reasons). Children with organic FTT may present at any age depending on the underlying disorder; most children with nonorganic FTT will manifest growth failure before 1 yr of age, and in many growth failure will become evident by 6 mo of age.

Diagnosis

Initial evaluation of the child with FTT: Usually, when failure to gain weight is noted, a diet history is obtained and diet counseling is provided; the child's weight is then monitored frequently. If satisfactory weight gain does not occur, admission to the hospital, where all necessary observations and diagnostic tests can be made in the shortest time, is indicated. In the absence of a historic or physical examination finding that suggests a specific underlying pathophysiologic etiology for the growth failure, there is no single reliable clinical feature or test that distinguishes organic from nonorganic FTT. Nonorganic FTT, however, is not a diagnosis of exclusion. Accordingly, the evaluation should be designed to uncover any potential medical problem while simultaneously searching for documentation by history or observation of any personal or family characteristics that support a psychosocial etiology for the FTT. Optimally, data gathering is a multidisciplinary effort that includes a physician, nurse, nutritionist, child developmentalist, social worker, and psychiatrist or psychologist.

Engaging the parents as coinvestigators in the search for the basis of the problem and its treatment is essential and helps to foster their self-esteem. This avoids blaming those who may already feel frustrated or guilty because of an inability to perform the most basic of parental roles—adequate nurturance of their child. The family should be encouraged to visit as often and as long as possible. They should be made to feel welcome and the staff should support their attempts to feed the child, provide toys as well as ideas that promote parent-child play and other interactions, and avoid any comments that state or imply parental inadequacy, irresponsibility, or other fault as the cause of the FTT.

The history should include the following points:

1. The growth chart, including measurements obtained at birth if possible, should be examined to determine the child's trend in growth rate. Ex-

cept in severe cases where malnutrition is obvious, the diagnosis of FTT should not be based on a single measurement, because of the wide variations existing in the normal population.

2. A meticulous dietary history is essential, including techniques for preparation and feeding of formula or adequacy of breast milk supply, and feeding schedule. Observation of the primary care givers feeding the infant to evaluate their technique as well as the child's vigor of sucking should be undertaken as soon as possible. Easy fatigability may indicate underlying exercise intolerance; enthusiastic burping or rapid rocking during feeding may result in excessive spitting up or even vomiting; disinterest on the part of the care giver may be a sign of depression or apathy, indicating a psychosocial environment for the infant that is devoid of stimulation and interaction.

3. An assessment of the child's elimination pattern to determine abnormal losses through urine, stool, or emesis should be undertaken to investigate underlying renal disease, a malabsorption syndrome, pyloric stenosis, or gastroesophageal reflux.

4. Past medical history inquiries should be directed toward evidence of intrauterine growth retardation or prematurity with as-yet-uncompensated growth delay; of unusual, prolonged, or chronic infection; of neurologic, cardiac, pulmonary, or renal disease; or of possible food intolerance.

5. The family history should include information about familial growth patterns, especially in parents and siblings; the occurrence of diseases known to affect growth (eg, cystic fibrosis); or recent physical or psychiatric illness that has resulted in the infant's primary care giver being unavailable or unable to provide consistent stimulation and nurturance.

6. The social history should include attention to family composition; socioeconomic status; desire for this pregnancy and acceptance of the child; parental depression; and any stresses such as job changes, family moves, separation, divorce, deaths, or other losses. Infants in large or chaotic families or infants who are unwanted may be relatively neglected because of the demands of other children, life events, or parental apathy; financial difficulties may result in overdilution of formula to "stretch" the meager supply; breast-feeding mothers who are under stress or are poorly nourished themselves may have decreased milk production.

Physical examination should include careful observation of the child's interaction with individuals in the environment and evidence of self-stimulatory behaviors (rocking, head banging). Children with nonorganic FTT have been described as hypervigilant and wary of close contact with people, preferring interactions with inanimate objects if they are interactive at all. Although nonorganic FTT is more consistent with neglectful than abusive parenting, the child should be examined carefully for any evidence of abuse (see Ch. 31). A screening test of developmental level should be performed and followed up with a more sophisticated developmental assessment if indicated.

Laboratory findings: Extensive laboratory studies of children with FTT are nonproductive and unnecessary. In the absence of a clear indication from the history or physical examination for a particular study, most authorities recommend limiting screening tests to a CBC, an ESR, urinalysis (including ability to concentrate and acidify), BUN or serum creatinine level, urine culture, and examination of the stool for pH, reducing substances, odor, color, consistency, and fat content. Under certain circumstances other tests may be appropriate, eg, electrolyte concentrations (if there is a history of significant vomiting or diarrhea), a thyroxine level (if the patient's growth in height is more severely affected than growth in weight), and a sweat test (if there is a history of recurrent upper or lower respiratory tract disease, salty taste when kissed, ravenous appetite, foul-smelling bulky stools, hepatomegaly, or a family history of cystic fibrosis). Investigation for infectious diseases should be reserved for children with suggestive evidence of infection, eg, fever, vomiting, and diarrhea. Radiologic investigation should be reserved for children with evidence of anatomic or functional pathology, such as pyloric stenosis or gastroesophageal reflux.

Treatment

The goal of treatment is to provide sufficient health and environmental resources to promote satisfactory growth. A nutritionally appropriate diet containing adequate calories for catch-up growth (in the range of 150% "normal" kcal requirement/kg ideal wt/24 h) and individualized medical and social supports are usually required. Ability to gain weight in the hospital, however, does *not* discriminate infants with nonorganic FTT from those with organic disease; ie, all children will grow when given sufficient nutrition.

Thus, merely admitting a child to the hospital, providing adequate calories, and using weight gain as the only criterion for diagnosis of nonorganic FTT is inappropriate. Indeed, some children with nonorganic FTT will lose weight in the hospital, raising the issue of whether being cared for even by "inadequate" parents is better than being separated from them.

For children with organic or mixed FTT, the underlying physiologic disorder should be treated as quickly as possible. For children with apparent nonorganic FTT, as well as for those with FTT of mixed etiology who have both physiologic and psychologic needs, management consists of providing education and emotional support specifically designed to treat those factors that are interfering with the parent-child relationship. Because treatment frequently requires long-term social support or psychiatric treatment, it may only be possible for the evaluation team to define the family's needs, provide initial instruction and support, and institute appropriate referrals to community agencies. However, the parents should understand why the referrals are being made and should participate in decisions concerning which agencies will be involved when options are possible (eg, some families will accept and profit from community nurse intervention but refuse assistance from a social worker). If the child is hospitalized in a tertiary care center, advice should be sought from the referring physician regarding experiences with local agencies and perspectives on the level of expertise available in the community.

A predischarge planning conference involving hospital-based personnel, representatives from the various community agencies who will provide follow-up services, and the child's primary physician should be a routine part of the management process. Areas of responsibility and lines of accountability must be clearly defined, preferably in a written report distributed to everyone involved. The parents should be invited to attend a postmeeting summary session so that they can meet the community workers, ask questions, and perhaps even begin the process of entering into aftercare by arranging appointments.

In some cases, foster care placement may be necessary. If it is expected that the child will eventually be returned to the biologic parents, parenting skill training and psychologic counseling must be provided for them and monitored scrupulously while the child is in foster care. Return to the biologic parents should not be determined only by the passage of time; rather, it should be based on the parents' demonstrated ability and resources to adequately care for the child.

Prognosis

For children with nonorganic FTT, the prognosis has been disappointing. The outcome appears to be most favorable with regard to physical growth—$1/2$ to $3/4$ of children beyond infancy achieve a stable weight above the 3rd percentile. Cognitive function, especially as related to verbal skills, is below the normal range in about $1/2$ the children. General behavioral problems, as identified by teachers or mental health professionals, occur in about $1/2$ the children; problems specifically related to eating ("picky," "slow") or elimination tend to be present in a similar proportion of children, usually, but not always, those with other behavioral or personality disturbances.

These statistics, reported for patients treated in the 1960s and 1970s, emphasize the significant morbidity associated with nonorganic FTT. Although the multidisciplinary approach to diagnosis and treatment with careful follow-up that was instituted in the 1980s has not yet been fully evaluated, early indications are that this kind of care may result in more promising outcomes.

BEHAVIORAL PROBLEMS

Many behaviors that can lead to significant problems are typical of a certain stage of development (eg, the oppositional behavior of a 2-yr-old) or of a common temperamental pattern (eg, the "difficult" child who has irregular biologic functions, intense reactions, predominantly negative mood, and slowness in adapting to changes). Differentiation between difficult but normal behaviors and significant behavioral problems is often unclear. A significant problem is more likely when the behavior is frequent and chronic, when more than one problem behavior is involved, and particularly when the behavior interferes with social and cognitive functioning. A parent's or teacher's perception that a problem is significant warrants attention. Looking beyond the chief complaint often uncovers information essential for understanding a significant problem.

Prevalence figures vary according to how behavioral problems are defined and measured, but several population studies cite a rate of at least 10% for significant behavioral problems in all pediatric age groups. National surveys of office-based pediatric practice, however, show the diagnosis of behavioral problems to be < 2%.

General Principles of Dealing with Behavioral Problems

The context in which the problem evolved must be understood, including interactions between the child and care givers and the social environment surrounding those interactions. Contributing factors include characteristics of the child; eg, health (past and current), developmental status, and temperament (difficult or slow-to-warm-up). Parental factors include misinterpretations of typical stage-related behaviors, dissonance between parental expectations and child characteristics, and parental characteristics such as depression, disinterest, rejection, and overprotectiveness (to the point of stifling steps toward independence). Social environmental factors include stresses like marital discord, unemployment, and significant personal losses, particularly in the context of weak social supports.

A broad-based history is required to at least briefly survey the child and parental and environmental factors that may be contributory. Prescribing techniques to modify behavior without some understanding of the etiology merely treats symptoms. The specific behavior may be successfully modified, but if a significant underlying problem exists it is likely to manifest itself as a new symptom.

A complete, chronologic description of the child's activities in a typical day provides precise details about the problem behavior. Focus should be on the immediate context in which the problem behavior occurs and the parental response to the behavior.

Direct observation of parent-child interaction during the office visit provides valuable clues. These observations and the parent's history should be supplemented whenever possible by the observations of other relatives, teachers, nurses, etc.

Feelings of guilt and incompetence, almost universal in parents of children with behavioral problems, are difficult for parents to express. Identifying with parental frustrations and pointing out the prevalence of such problems often can allay some of the guilt and facilitate a constructive approach.

Early intervention is preferable because the longer maladaptive behaviors exist, the more difficult they are to change.

Changing behavior is a learning process for the child. **Consistency** in rules and **limit-setting** across time and among care givers facilitate this process. Parents should try to **minimize expressions of anger** when enforcing rules. Highly charged emotions may interfere with or distort the learning process.

Increasing the amount of **positive contact** between the parent and child is crucial to successful change of unacceptable behavior in the child. Mutually enjoyable interactions build the self-esteem of the parent and the child and help break vicious circle patterns (see below) that have developed.

For simple problems, parental education, reassurance, and a few specific suggestions often are sufficient; but follow-up is important to be certain that the problem is not more complex than initially assumed.

For complex or chronic problems, a more comprehensive assessment is indicated, possibly requiring multiple visits. An initially confusing history may be clarified if a detailed parental diary is kept of the timing and frequency of the problem behavior, including preceding activities and parental responses. Depending on the nature of the problem and the expertise of the clinician, referral to a psychologist, psychiatrist, neurologist, or other specialist may be indicated.

Interactional Problems in Early Infancy

The first few months of life can be a difficult adjustment period for the infant and new parents. The infant's feeding and sleeping schedules usually are unpredictable, and most infants do not sleep through the night until 2 to 3 mo of age. Many infants have periods of frequent, prolonged, intense crying in the first 3 mo (see COLIC under COMMON FEEDING AND GASTROINTESTINAL PROBLEMS in Ch. 23). Periods of alertness in the infant are still brief, providing relatively little positive feedback to the parents for their exhausting new job. A mother's ability to cope during this period may be further diminished by a difficult pregnancy or delivery, postpartum depression, or lack of adequate support from a spouse, relatives, or friends.

The quality of mother-infant interactions in the early months is related to later cognitive and social development of the infant. In extreme cases interactional failure may result in failure to thrive (see FAILURE TO THRIVE, above). Other manifestations include persistent, excessive crying, irregularity of schedules, or failure to develop positive interactive games with the infant by 3 to 4 mo.

Since a variety of factors (child, parental, or environmental) can contribute to the interactional problem, a careful history and assessment of the infant and the parent-infant interaction are indicated (see above). **Treatment** includes parental education about infant development and the temperamental characteristics of their infant in particular; reassurance if appropriate; and attempts to improve the support available to the parents (eg, emotional support, help with housework and child care, and other resources as needed).

Discipline

The noun "discipline" has several meanings, including instruction and self-control, in addition to punishment. **Positive reinforcement** for appropriate behavior is a powerful tool for molding a child's behavior, with no adverse side effects. Efforts to control a child's behavior through scolding or physical punishment may work briefly, if used sparingly, but are ineffective when frequently used and may be detrimental to the child's sense of security and self-esteem. Threats to leave or send the child away are damaging.

A good approach to altering unacceptable behavior is the use of a **"time-out" procedure.** This requires a small, portable kitchen timer, a chair in a dull place (no TV or toys, not in the bedroom, and not dark or scary), and agreement among care givers about the specific behavior that will result in time-out. Since time-outs are a learning process for the child, they are best used for one specific type of inappropriate behavior, or at most a small number of behaviors at one time. Before using time-out, the rules are explained clearly to the child, including the targeted behavior, and the procedure is demonstrated. The steps are as follows:

1. After an inappropriate behavior, it is briefly described to the child, who is calmly told to go to the time-out chair or is led there if necessary.

2. When the child is sitting in the chair, the timer is set to last 1 min for each year of age up to a maximum of 5 min.

3. If the child gets up from the chair before the bell rings, he is replaced and the timer reset. If the child gets up repeatedly, it may be necessary to hold him in the chair (not in one's lap), avoiding talking and eye contact. If it is necessary to hold him down for the entire period until the bell rings, the timer is set again.

4. If the child stays in the chair but does not quiet down before the bell rings, the timer is reset.

5. When it is time for the child to get up, he is asked the reason for the time-out; anger and nagging are avoided. If he does not recall the correct reason, he is briefly reminded.

6. Within a short period of time, praiseworthy behavior should be sought. This may be easier to achieve if the child is started in a new activity away from the scene of the inappropriate behavior.

Since most children prefer the attention they get for inappropriate behavior to no attention at all, special times for pleasant interactions with the child must occur each day. The pleasant interactions also provide an opportunity for reinforcing positive behavior.

Common Vicious Circle Patterns

Parental reaction to a child's behavior causing an adverse response from the youngster, which in turn leads to continued detrimental parental response.

In the most common vicious circle, the **aggressive-resistant child** is responded to with scolding, yelling, and spanking. This pattern may arise from parental reactions to the stage-related negativism of the 2-yr-old or back talk of the 4-yr-old, or it may evolve from parental attempts to cope with a child who has had a "difficult" temperament since birth. These children often react to stress and emotional discomfort with stubbornness, back talk, aggressiveness, and temper outbursts rather than crying.

The circular pattern may be interrupted if parents ignore behavior that does not encroach on the rights of others (tantrums, refusals to eat) and use distraction or temporary isolation to limit behavior that cannot be ignored. Friction also can be reduced and appropriate behavior reinforced by judicious use of praise. In addition, the parents and child should spend at least 15 to 20 min/day involved in a mutually pleasurable activity. If the mother is at home all day, she should be encouraged to spend some time away from the child on a regular basis.

Another circle evolves when parents react to a **fearful, clinging, or manipulating child** with overprotection and overpermissiveness. Initial complaints to the physician often are medical, but the description of a typical day reveals conflicts at mealtime, difficulties with separation, parental inability to limit behavior that encroaches on the rights of others, and a parental tendency to perform tasks that the child can do himself (eg, dressing, feeding).

Frequently, the history includes complications during the pregnancy or a serious familial illness that is believed to increase the child's vulnerability. The parents need reassurance that the child is physically well and encouragement to set reasonable limits on dependency-seeking and manipulating behavior in order to reestablish a balance of mutual respect.

When any conflicting parent-child interaction develops, the physician must provide empathetic support while the parents try to modify their response pattern. If there is no change in 3 to 4 mo, reevaluation of the problem or psychiatric consultation is indicated.

Problems Related to Eating

Not eating enough and eating the wrong foods are common complaints of parents with 2- to 8-yr-olds. At mealtime while the parents coax and threaten, the child may sit with food in his mouth or may respond to attempts at force-feeding by vomiting. The decrease in appetite usually is related to the slowing in growth rate that is normal at this time. The parents should be educated about the growth patterns of young children, reassured about the child's current height and weight status, and instructed to reduce emotions at mealtime by putting the food in front of the child and removing it in 15 or 20 min without comment about what is or is not eaten. This, along with restricting between-meal snacks, generally will restore the relationship between appetite, the amount eaten, and the child's nutritional needs. If the feeding problem is part of a pattern of overcoercion or overconcern about the child's health, a more detailed history is needed in order to determine appropriate management (see General Principles of Dealing with Behavioral Problems, above).

Sleep Problems

Normal sleep consists of cycles of **REM** sleep (rapid-eye-movement, light sleep) and **NREM** sleep (non—rapid-eye-movement, deep sleep). NREM sleep can be divided into four EEG stages, with stages 3 and 4 representing the deepest sleep. From age 2 to 3 through adulthood, individuals cycle through the stages of NREM and REM sleep about every 90 min, beginning with a sustained NREM period. About 80% of the total sleep time is spent in NREM sleep. Newborns have less well defined stages, enter sleep through active REM, and spend about half their sleep time in REM. The mature pattern gradually develops over the first 2 to 3 yr.

Nightmares are frightening dreams that occur during REM sleep. The child usually becomes fully awake and can vividly recall the details of the dream. Frightening experiences, including scary stories or television violence, can precipitate a nightmare, particularly in 3- to 4-yr-olds who cannot readily distinguish fantasy from reality. An occasional nightmare is normal, and comfort from the parent may be all that is required. Persistent or frequent nightmares, however, suggest an environmental problem that warrants evaluation.

Somnambulism (*persistent sleepwalking*) and **night terrors** are disorders of arousal that share many clinical features. They occur during arousal from deep sleep (stage 3 or 4 NREM sleep), usually in the first 1 to 3 h of sleep. Episodes last from seconds to many minutes and are characterized by sudden awakening, blank or confused stares, incomplete arousal with poor responsiveness to people, and amnesia for the episode.

Night terrors are dramatic because of the screaming and inconsolable panic of the child during the episode. They are most common between ages 3 and 8 yr. Somnambulism involves clumsy walks during which objects usually are avoided. The child appears confused but not frightened. At least one episode of sleepwalking is estimated to occur in 15% of children between 5 and 12 yr of age. Persistent sleepwalking occurs in 1 to 6% of the population, most commonly in school-aged boys. Stressful events sometimes may trigger an episode. Both disorders are almost always self-limited, though sporadic episodes may occur for years. When these disorders persist to adolescence and adulthood, an underlying psychologic disorder should be considered. A **differential diagnostic consideration** is temporal lobe epilepsy that may occur at night and is manifested by hallucinations, incomplete arousal, fear, and automatic behavior. Suspicions of seizure activity when awake, a large degree of autonomic activation, and enuresis during the episode warrant an EEG.

Treatment consists of education and assurance. Diazepam (2 to 5 mg orally before sleep) may be given for very frequent episodes.

Resistance to going to bed is a common problem, which generally peaks between 1 and 2 yr of age. The child cries when left alone in the crib or climbs out and seeks his parents. This behavior is related to separation anxiety (see below) and to increasing attempts by the child to control his environment, both of which are common at this age. Long naps late in the afternoon; rough, overstimulating play before bedtime; a disturbance in the parent-child relationship; or tension in the home also may cause the problem.

Letting the child get up, staying in the room and comforting him at length, and spanking and scolding are all ineffective. Settling the child with a brief story, offering a favorite doll or blanket, and using a night light are helpful, but sitting quietly in the hallway in sight of the child and making sure that he stays in bed may be needed to control the problem. Once the child learns that he will not be allowed out of bed or cannot entice the parent into the room for more stories or play, he will settle down and go to sleep.

Night awakening occurs in about 50% of infants between 6 and 12 mo of age and is related to the development of separation anxiety (see below). In older children, episodes often follow a move, illness, or other stressful event. Allowing the child to sleep with the parents, playing, feeding, or spanking and scolding usually prolong the problem. Returning the child to his bed with simple reassurance or sitting outside the open bedroom door until he settles down is usually more effective. Some 3-yr-olds wander around the house without waking the parents; installing a hook-and-eye lock on the outside of the child's bedroom door will solve the problem, but this procedure must be used judiciously and should not be employed indiscriminately to isolate or control the child.

Problems of Toilet Training

Most children are consistently trained for bowel control between ages 2 and 3 yr and for urinary control between 3 and 4. By age 5 the average child can go to the toilet alone, managing all aspects of dressing, undressing, and wiping. However, wide individual variations occur; eg, about 30% of normal 4-yr-olds and 10% of 6-yr-olds have not achieved regular nighttime continence.

The key to avoiding problems lies in recognizing the child's readiness to train, which is signaled when the child has dry periods lasting several hours, shows interest in sitting on a potty chair or wanting to be changed when wet, and can carry out simple verbal commands. This generally occurs between ages 18 and 24 mo.

The most common approach to toilet training is the **timing method.** After demonstrating readiness, the child is introduced to the potty chair and gradually required to briefly sit on it fully clothed and then to practice taking his pants down, sitting on the potty chair for no more than 5 or 10 min, and redressing. Simple explanations of the purpose for the exercise are given repeatedly and emphasized by placing wet or dirty diapers in the pot. The crux of this method involves the parent's anticipation of the child's need to eliminate, and then positive reinforcement for successful elimination with praise or rewards. Anger or punishment for lack of success or accidents may be counterproductive. This method works well for children with predictable elimination schedules. For the child with unpredictable schedules, however, it is difficult to provide the contingent reinforcement, and training must await the ability of the child to anticipate elimination himself.

A second training method involves **modeling** with a doll. After readiness is demonstrated, the child is taught the steps of the toileting process as the parent gives positive reinforcement to the doll for dry pants and for successful completion of each step of the process. Then the child imitates this process with the doll repeatedly, assuming the parent's role as reinforcer. Lastly the child performs the steps himself as the parent provides praise and rewards.

If the child resists sitting on the toilet, allowing him to get up and trying again after a meal is recommended. If resistance continues for days, postponing the training for several weeks is the best strategy. Behavior modification, with a reward for sitting on the toilet and producing results, has succeeded with both normal and retarded children. Once the pattern is established, rewards are given for every other success and then gradually withdrawn. In any case, *power struggles must be avoided,* since they are detrimental and may result in a strained parent-child relationship. If a repetitive pattern of pressure and resistance occurs, it should be managed as discussed under Common Vicious Circle Patterns, above.

Nocturnal Enuresis

Involuntary and repeated passage of urine while asleep, occurring at an age when voluntary control could be expected. Nocturnal enuresis is present in 30% of children at age 4 yr, 10% at age 6, 3% at age 12, and 1% at age 18. It is more common in boys than girls, appears to be familial, and is sometimes associated with sleep disorders (eg, sleepwalking and night terrors). An **organic etiology** is found in only 1 to 2% of cases, and they usually involve a UTI. Although rare,

other diagnoses to consider include congenital anomalies, sacral nerve disorders, diabetes mellitus or insipidus, or a pelvic mass. These can be excluded by a careful history, physical examination, urinalysis, and urine culture. Positive findings may indicate the need for renal ultrasound, an IV urogram, a cystourethrogram, a urologic consultation, or other evaluations. Bed-wetting occasionally is associated with moderate to severe individual or family psychopathology, indicating psychiatric referral. Bed-wetting usually represents only a delay in maturation that resolves with time. **Secondary enuresis,** in which previous bedtime control is lost, usually is due to a psychologically stressful event or condition. There is, however, a greater chance of an organic etiology (eg, UTI or diabetes mellitus) than in primary nocturnal enuresis.

Treatment: Three different modalities are commonly used, each claiming a cure rate higher than the spontaneous cure rate of 15%/yr after age 6. Even higher spontaneous cure rates before age 6 argue against imposing a treatment regimen before that age. Other factors, such as embarrassment preventing camp or overnight experiences during the school years, favor treatment after age 6.

Motivational counseling has been the most common approach, involving the following recommendations: (1) The child assumes an active role by keeping a calendar to record wet and dry nights, by talking to the physician himself, by urinating before going to bed, and by changing his clothing and bedding when wet. (2) Fluids are not consumed for 2 to 3 h before bed. (3) Punishments are discontinued and angry parental responses are avoided. (4) Positive reinforcement is given for dry nights (a star calendar or other rewards depending on the age). (5) Reassurance is given about the etiology and prognosis of enuresis, with the aim to remove blame and guilt.

Enuresis alarms have proved to be by far the most effective treatment currently available. Two studies, involving 5- to 15-yr-olds, reported a 70% cure rate with only a 10 to 15% relapse rate. These alarms are easy to set up, cost about $40, and are triggered by a few drops of urine. The disadvantage is the time required for complete success. In the first few weeks of use the child awakens after full voiding; in the next few weeks partial inhibition of urination is achieved. Eventually, the child awakens with a conditioned response to bladder contractions before urination occurs. The alarm should be used for 3 wk be-

tion or demonstration of verbal and nonverbal abilities. Specific learning disabilities are considered chronic conditions of presumed neurologic origin and distinct handicapping conditions. Learning disabilities are not due to underachievement.

Descriptions of learning disorders are diverse, and numerous syndromes have been identified. Educationally, the terms **learning disability**, **mental retardation**, and **autism** refer to learning disorders. Other labels, such as **aphasia/dysphasia**, **dysgraphia**, **dysnomia**, **dyslexia**, and **attention deficit disorder**, have been associated with learning disorders and are used to describe behavior perceived as independent and constituting specific syndromes.

Etiology and Incidence

Learning disorders are multidimensional, and affected children are heterogeneous. No single cause has been defined, but neurologic deficits are presumed. Genetic influences may be obvious, as in Down syndrome, or subtle, as in developmental reading disabilities. About 3 to 15% of the school population in the USA has been cited as needing special services; however, the actual number of students with learning disorders is undetermined. Males tend to outnumber females 5:1, suggesting familial and biologic influences.

Symptoms and Signs

Since learning disorders occur in young children who cannot express their feelings, difficulties, and symptoms well or at all, defining the characteristics of these disorders is limited to physical and behavioral signs observed by others. Although signs are manifested at early ages, mild to moderate learning disorders are not recognized until the child reaches school age and encounters the rigors of symbolic and figurative learning. Most children with learning disorders have positive neurologic findings or demonstrate lags in neurodevelopmental integrity. The neurologic factors frequently are interrelated with cognitive and behavioral liabilities, but no single sign or set of signs predicts later difficulties. Problems with visual-motor coordination, gross motor movement, and delay in paired associative learning (eg, color-naming, labeling, counting, and letter-naming) are predominant indicators of early problems with formal learning. Disturbances or delays in receptive and expressive vocabulary and comprehension of language are better predictors of academic problems beyond the preschool years. Other warning signs that are often overlooked are short attention span and distractibility, limited verbal fluency, restricted memory span, and signs related to fine motor problems (eg, poor printing and copying).

Behaviorally, difficulties with impulse control, non–goal-directed behavior and overactivity, discipline problems, withdrawal and avoidance behavior, and aggressiveness may be early indications of cognitive and communication disorders and impending school difficulties.

Cognitive disturbances: Although basic cognitive processes and learning strategies appear to be age-dependent and vary with cognitive ability (IQ), most learning disorders are related intrinsically to deficiencies in brain functions and the relationships between different functions. Problems may exist in (1) **perceptual functions**, exhibiting difficulties in personal and extrapersonal orientation, visual-spatial abilities, selective attention, pattern recognition, sound discrimination and analysis, and visual-motor integration; (2) **memory functions**, including short- and long-term information retention, memory (rehearsal) strategies, and verbal retrieval and production; and (3) **reasoning abilities**, such as conceptualizing, abstracting, generalizing, and organizing and planning information for problem solving. Subgroups of children with specific reading-learning disorders have been identified, ranging from basic language dysfunctions, dysnomia, and poor comprehension of spoken language, to visual-spatial disorders and problems in pattern recognition. Other subtypes have been noted in arithmetic disorders; eg, **anarithmia** (*disturbances in basic concept formation, and failure to acquire computation skills*) and **ageometria** (*arithmetic problems due to disturbances in spatial reasoning*). Other subtypes may exist; however, most learning disorders are complex or mixed, with problems emanating from deficiencies in more than one system.

Diagnosis

Since signs of learning disorders vary and disorders share similar and overlapping characteristics, diagnostic criteria must be comprehensive and precise. A **multidisciplinary evaluation** consisting of medical, psychologic, social, educational, speech and language, and emotional-behavioral factors is essential to establish a child's functioning levels and skill indexes, to plan treatment, and to monitor progress.

The **medical evaluation** should include detailed family history; the child's medical, developmental, and school history; a general physical examination; and a traditional and adaptive neurologic examination. Young children should be evaluated for developmental level using standardized criteria. Although causal relationships have not been firmly established, use of ototoxic drugs, maternal illnesses, and all complications during pregnancy and delivery should be noted (eg, spotting, toxemia, prolonged labor, precipitous delivery), as well as neonatal problems (eg, prematurity, low birth weight, jaundice, perinatal asphyxia, postmaturity, respiratory distress, and minor physical anomalies). Children with learning problems often have several cumulative minor physical abnormalities. Chronic and acute ear infections and insidious hearing loss, allergies, and repeated illnesses associated with autoimmune deficiencies also have been implicated.

Verbal and nonverbal intelligence testing should be done. Significant differences within and between verbal and nonverbal systems often indicate differences in ability to process information, learning preference, and learning disorders. Children with reading and generalized learning disabilities tend to have more difficulties with functions controlled by the left hemisphere than the right. Comprehensive assessment of neuropsychologic functions often is needed to test anterior and posterior brain functions of left and right hemispheres and the preferred manner in which a child processes information; eg, holistically or analytically, and visually or auditorially. These methods allow for qualitative as well as quantitative assessment and encourage comparisons of each child's development relative to his ability.

Intellectual, educational, psychologic, and language assessments are essential and must be integrated to determine the degree of discrepancy in skills, deficiencies in subskills and prerequisite skills, deficiencies in use of effective learning strategies (eg, rehearsal), and the degree of intactness of memory and reasoning. An **educational evaluation** identifies reading, writing, arithmetic, and spelling skills and deficits. **Reading evaluations** measure abilities in word decoding and recognition, passage comprehension, and passage fluency. **Arithmetic levels** should be established for computation skills, knowledge of operations, and understanding of mathematical concepts. Functional assessment to determine if the child applies all 3 of these processes to everyday experiences should be conducted. **Writing samples** should be obtained to evaluate spelling, syntax, and fluency of ideas. Dyspraxia and developmental maladroitness also should be investigated if writing problems exist.

Psychologic evaluation defines conduct disorders, poor self-esteem, and early childhood depression that frequently accompany learning disorders. Attitudes toward school, motivation, peer relationships, and self-confidence should be assessed.

Treatment

Treatment centers on effective *educational* management of the child's problem and, when necessary, the use of medical, behavioral, and psychologic therapy. No single educational program, technique, or procedure has resolved basic learning problems in children with either diverse or pervasive learning disorders or specific learning disabilities. **Direct instruction** adapted to meet a child's learning differences is advocated. Diagnostic tests, as suggested above, help determine the most effective teaching program, which may take a remedial, compensatory, or strategic (teaching the child) approach. Testing also is used for classification and educational placement decisions. When a child's learning preference and learning problem is mismatched with the instructional method implemented, the learning disorder may be aggravated.

Many children will need supplementary specialized instruction in only one area while continuing to attend regular education programs. Others will need separate and intense educational programs to accommodate their learning needs. Optimally, children with learning disorders should attend programs in the least restrictive environment compatible with the severity and extent of their learning difficulties.

Most medical, neurologic, or biochemical therapies popularly recommended for children with learning disorders (eg, eliminating food additives, prescribing large doses of vitamins, and analyzing the system for trace minerals) are *unsubstantiated* by clinical and applied research. Similarly, medication has minimal impact on academic achievement, intelligence, and general learning ability, although certain medications (eg, psychostimulants) may be effective in enhancing attention and concentration, allowing the child to respond more efficiently to instruction (see ATTENTION DEFICIT DISORDER, below). Therapies such as patterning by sensory stimulation and passive movement, sensory integrative therapy through postural exercises, and optometric training to remedy visual perceptual and sensory-motor coordination processes are controversial, and there are few positive data to encourage their use. The effectiveness of treatments such as visual and auditory perceptual and perceptual-motor training also has been difficult to substantiate through controlled investigations. Although many learning-disordered children have deficits in these processes, specific interventions designed to promote perceptual competence have not been conclusively demonstrated to improve reading and language comprehension.

ATTENTION DEFICIT DISORDER (ADD)
(Hyperactivity)

Developmentally inappropriate inattention and impulsivity, with or without hyperactivity. This definition conforms to the American Psychiatric Association's *Diagnostic and Statistical Manual, Third Edition – Revised* (DSM-III-R), shifting the focus of the disorder from excessive physical activity. Although use of the term ADD as an independent diagnosis of a specific syndrome has been challenged, no study or critique has been able to discount the constellation of signs used to describe the disorder. ADD is implicated in learning disorders and, except for moderate to profound mental retardation, can influence the behavior of children at any cognitive level. ADD is estimated to affect 5 to 10% of school-aged children, precipitating half of the childhood referrals to diagnostic clinics. ADD is seen 10 times more frequently in boys than girls.

Etiology

Etiology is unknown. Several theories advocating biochemical, sensory and motor, physiologic, and behavioral correlates and manifestations have been proposed. Less than 5% of children with ADD have evidence of neurologic damage, but CT scans and EEGs have not shown structural abnormalities. Recent research indicates neurotransmitter abnormalities, eg, decreased activity or stimulation in upper brainstem and frontal-midbrain tracts. Toxins, neurologic immaturity, and environmental problems have also been hypothesized.

Symptoms and Signs

The **primary signs of ADD** with or without hyperactivity are a child's display of inattention and impulsivity. ADD with hyperactivity is diagnosed when the signs of overactivity are obvious. Inappropriate inattention causes increased rates of activity and impersistence or reluctance to participate or respond. Although children with ADD and without hyperactivity may not manifest high activity levels, most exhibit restlessness or jitteriness, short attention span, and poor impulse control. These are qualitatively different from those seen in conduct and anxiety disorders. **Inattention** is described as *a failure to finish tasks started, easy distractibility, seeming lack of attention, and difficulty concentrating on tasks requiring sustained attention.* **Impulsivity** is described as *acting before thinking, difficulty taking turns, problems organizing work, and constant shifting from one activity to another.* Impulsive responses are especially likely when involved with uncertainty and the need to attend carefully. **Hyperactivity** is featured as *difficulty staying seated and sitting still, and running or climbing excessively.* In general, children with hyperactivity are described as "always on the go."

DSM-III-R lists 14 signs, 8 of which must be present for the diagnosis. These are (1) often fidgets with hands or feet or squirms in seat (restlessness), (2) has difficulty remaining seated when required to do so, (3) is easily distracted by extraneous stimuli, (4) has difficulty awaiting turn in games or group situations, (5) often blurts out answers before questions are completed, (6) has difficulty following through on instructions from others (not due to oppositional behavior or failure of comprehension), (7) has difficulty sustaining attention in tasks or play activities, (8) often shifts from one uncompleted task to another, (9) has difficulty playing quietly, (10) often talks excessively, (11) often interrupts or intrudes on others, (12) often does not seem to listen to what is being said, (13) often loses things necessary for tasks or activities at school or home, and (14) often engages in physically dangerous activities without considering possible consequences.

Caution is advised in interpretation. DSM-III-R does not adhere to subtypes. For example, many ADD children exhibit high degrees of inattention and low degrees of impulsivity and overactivity. Inappropriate inattention must be present for a diagnosis. Many believe that children with ADD and aggressive behavior constitute a specific subtype.

Primary signs tend to appear when the ADD child is involved in vigilance and reaction-time tasks and tasks requiring visual and perceptual search, paired associate learning, systematic listening, continuous performance, and directed attention. Inattention and impulsivity restrict development of academic skills and concepts, thinking and reasoning strategies, motivation for school, and adjustment to social demands. Behavior of

ADD children often is more resistant to treatment than that of children with other behavioral disorders.

Associated or secondary signs are frequently noted: motor incoordination, nonlocalized "soft" neurologic findings, perceptual-motor dysfunctions, EEG abnormalities, emotional lability, opposition, anxiety, aggressiveness, low frustration tolerance, and poor peer relationships.

Onset of ADD occurs typically before age 4 yr and invariably before age 7 yr. The peak age for referral has been between 8 and 10 yr. Early indicators vary, but most children diagnosed as having ADD with or without hyperactivity at school age exhibited delays in motor development, tended to have brief attention spans (eg, did not play with toys or did so in brief intervals), and usually had higher activity levels than normal during their preschool years. Children with hyperactivity often were described as hyperexcitable and were difficult to manage as toddlers and preschoolers. In school these signs persist, and difficulty with visual motor tasks such as copying and printing may become apparent. Right-left confusion and immature coordination after age 7 yr are prevalent in both types of ADD. Some children with ADD signs also have been less responsive to positive and negative reinforcement. They often seem to lack intrinsic motivation and do not consider long-term consequences of their behavior. In general, children with ADD during the school years are a more homogeneous group than those referred before age 6 yr. Many ADD signs expressed during the preschool years indicate communication disorders, anxiety, and conduct disorders. During later childhood, ADD signs usually are specific and qualitatively distinct; eg, such children often exhibit continuous movement of the lower extremities, motor impersistence such as the purposeless movement and fidgeting of hands, impulsive talking, and a seeming lack of awareness of their environment. Commonly, they are not aggressive or oppositional. Some studies have found that about 20% have learning disabilities, 40% exhibit depressed behavior by adolescence, 60% have problems such as aggressiveness, temper tantrums, and low frustration tolerance with little provocation, and 90% have academic problems.

Adolescents and adults may display residual symptoms of inattention and impulsivity such as fidgetiness, restlessness, difficulty completing assigned tasks (eg, homework), and difficulty focusing attention for extended periods of time. Although hyperactivity tends to diminish with age, residual symptoms and signs can extend well into adulthood.

Diagnosis

Diagnosis often is difficult. No particular organic signs or set of neurologic indicators are specific. Although organic factors may have a role in cause, the primary signs are behavioral, varying with situation and time. Rating scales and checklists, the predominant mode of identification, often are unable to distinguish ADD from other behavioral disorders. Such data often are based on subjective observations made by untrained personnel. In a clinical setting, most behavior is not obvious and, unless the child is excessively overactive or impulsive, diagnosis is impossible without the use of specific tasks; eg, vigilance and reaction-time tasks, tasks sampling paired associate learning, and tasks increasing response uncertainty. Also needed are behavioral recording techniques that allow the observer to document objectively the type of overactivity, inattention, and impulsivity associated with ADD. Social and medical histories and school reports are essential for diagnosis. ADD tends to occur in families. Displays of inattention, impulsivity, and overactivity are age-inappropriate and not related to behavior due to other developmental disabilities. Social and developmental immaturity is evident. ADD children with aggressive behavior have been identified as a separate subtype needing a range of interventions. Poor peer acceptance and loneliness tend to increase with age and obvious display of symptoms. Less aggressive ADD children tend to have academic problems only.

Treatment and Prognosis

No single treatment has been completely effective with all children; however, psychostimulant medications combined with behavioral and cognitive therapies (eg, self-recording, self-monitoring, modeling, and role-playing) have the greatest controlling influence on symptom expression. Used alone, medication has been effective predominantly with less aggressive ADD children coming from stable home environments. Elimination diets, megavitamin treatments, psychotherapy, and biochemical interventions (eg, the administration of neurochemicals) have had the least effect, and most studies have found minimal change in behavior and no sustained, positive long-term outcomes when such treatments have been implemented.

Methylphenidate is the drug of choice. It has proved more effective than tricyclic antidepressants (eg, imipramine), caffeine, and other psychostimulants (eg, pemoline and deanol) and has fewer side effects than does dextroamphetamine. Common side effects of methylphenidate are sleep disturbances (eg, insomnia), depression or sadness, headache, stomachache, suppression of appetite, elevated BP, and, with large continuous doses, a reduction of growth. Behavioral changes with methylphenidate are related to dosage; learning often is enhanced at lower doses (0.3 mg/kg/dose) and decreased with higher doses. Improvements in social behavior occur most often when medication levels exceed 1.0 mg/kg/dose. Dosage often is titrated, beginning at low doses and increasing to optimal levels (decrease in symptoms, improvement in task performance, and no side effects). Response to medication often is individual, and dosage is prescribed depending on the severity of the behavior and the child's ability to tolerate the substance. Methylphenidate is dispensed in 5-, 10-, and 20-mg tablets and in a 20-mg sustained-release (SR) tablet. Many children have difficulty absorbing or tolerating the SR dose and often exhibit rebound reactions as the medication dissipates. Medication often is prescribed to help the child only in school. Drug holidays are recommended; eg, the medication is not given on weekends, school holidays, or during summer vacations. Placebo conditions or periods when no medication is administered are recommended to investigate and challenge the need for medication. Challenge conditions should occur for 5 to 10 school days to ensure reliability of observations. Long-term benefits of medication have not been demonstrated conclusively. However, some research indicates that use of medication permits participation in activities previously inaccessible because of poor attention and impulsivity. Medication often interrupts the cycle of inappropriate behavior, enhancing behavioral and academic interventions.

Cognitive-behavior modification, self-monitoring techniques, environmental control of noise and visual stimulation, appropriate task length, and teacher proximity often have positive effects on the child's classroom behavior. Parents should be referred for parent training and behavior management techniques when difficulties persist at home. Children with ADD with hyperactivity and poor impulse control are often helped at home when structure, consistent parenting techniques, and well-defined limits are estab-

lished. Behavior management techniques and contingencies such as token economies and self-monitoring with reinforcement often are effective. Parents should be encouraged to seek professional assistance.

Follow-up studies have found that children identified as having ADD do not grow out of their difficulties. Later problems in adolescence and adulthood occur predominantly as academic failure, low self-esteem, and difficulty learning appropriate social behavior. Some studies have found that adolescents and adults with histories of ADD with impulsivity have a high incidence of personality trait disorders and antisocial behavior; most continue to display impulsivity, restlessness, and poor social skills. ADD individuals with hyperactivity seem to adjust better in work than in academic situations. Interpersonal and social problems often persist into adulthood; suicide attempts (not related to methylphenidate) have been reported as higher when compared with those in the normal population. Low intelligence, aggressiveness, social and interpersonal problems, and parental psychopathology are predictors of poor outcomes in adulthood.

DEVELOPMENTAL DYSLEXIA

A distinct reading problem based on specific deficiencies or deficits in phonologic processing present from birth, which affect word learning and which may also cause language disabilities. There is no universally accepted definition or precise diagnostic criterion, which raises the question whether dyslexia exists as an independent reading disorder. However, it is usually also described as *a disorder that interferes with learning to read despite average or above-average intelligence, adequate motivation and educational opportunities, socioeconomic advantage, and sensory acuity within normal limits.* Incidence is undetermined because of the lack of a universal definition. It has been estimated that 5 to 16% of children in public schools receive special education or remedial reading because of learning problems; the number of children with dyslexia included in those figures is unknown.

Phonologic processing problems are associated with deficits in sound discrimination, sound blending, memory for sounds, and sound analysis. The underlying language disorder is usually associated with the production of rather than the understanding of language and is caused presumably by auditory memory, speech production, verbal retrieval, and phonologic processing problems. Dyslexia differs from other language-related reading problems that are associated with poor comprehension of syntax and semantics. Nonlinguistic processing deficits such as visual-perceptual problems are no longer considered primary factors in dyslexia. However, many definitions of dyslexia also include the inability to learn the derivational rules of printed language (the orthography) as a factor that interferes with word learning. Individuals with this inability may have difficulty determining root words or word stems or determining which letters in words form specific sound-symbol associations such as vowel patterns, affixes, syllables, and word endings. Individuals with other reading problems may demonstrate the same word learning problems as dyslexics; however, their problems are usually associated with difficulties in oral comprehension and language usage and/or deficits in abstract reasoning.

Etiology

Dyslexia has a neurodevelopmental basis, but etiology is unknown. Most reading problems are unexplainable and are probably multidimensional, varying by degree and kind and are not age or gender related.

Dyslexia is associated predominantly with specific cortical dysfunctions stemming from congenital, neurodevelopmental deficiencies or abnormalities and is often contrasted with **alexia** (*acquired reading problems stemming from direct insults or trauma to the brain*). Lesions affecting the integration or interactions of specific brain functions are suspect. Asymmetries of left and right hemispheres, fewer neurons, and a smaller left planum temporale have also been cited. Specifically, most researchers concur that dyslexia is left hemisphere related and is associated with deficiencies or dysfunctions in the language association areas of the brain (Wernicke's area), sound and speech production areas (Broca's area), and the interconnection of Wernicke and Broca's areas via the fasciculus arcuatus. Dysfunctions or defects in the angular gyrus, the medial occipital area of the brain, and the right hemisphere have been associated with word recognition problems. Dysfunctions in or between the cerebellum and the vestibular system have also been implicated. Problems with functional vision, eye movements, and cerebral dominance have been referred to as causal; however, no clear evidence exists to substantiate these factors.

A strong genetic link has been established in dyslexia. Dyslexia tends to exist in families; more males are identified than females. Cerebrovascular accidents, prematurity, and intrauterine complications have been linked to dyslexia, often complicating a predisposition to a familial reading problem.

Symptoms and Signs

Most dyslexics are not identified until they interact with early demands of symbolic learning in kindergarten or 1st grade. However, dyslexia should be suspected in preschool children with delayed language production, speech articulation problems, and difficulties remembering the names of letters, numbers, and colors, and in children who come from families with histories of reading or learning problems. Early signs of dyslexia are associated with delays or deficiencies in phonologic or linguistic processing. Children with decoding problems often have difficulty blending sounds, rhyming words, identifying the positions of sounds in words, segmenting words into pronounceable components, and reversing the order of sounds in words. Delays or hesitations in choosing words (word finding problems), word substitutions, or naming letters and pictures are early signs of dyslexia. Short-term (working) auditory memory and auditory sequencing problems are common.

Fewer than 20% of dyslexics have difficulties with the visual demands of reading. However, many confuse letters and words with similar configurations or demonstrate difficulty visually selecting or identifying letter patterns and clusters (phoneme-graphemes) in words. Reversals and visual confusions tend to occur frequently during early elementary school years. However, most reading and writing reversals occur because of retention or retrieval problems that cause dyslexics to forget or confuse the names of letters and words that are similar in structure; subsequently, *d* becomes *b*, *m* becomes *w*, *h* becomes *n*, *was* becomes *saw*, *on* becomes *no*.

Diagnosis

Students who are not accelerating in word learning by the middle or end of 1st grade or who are not reading at the level expected for their verbal or intellectual abilities at any grade level should be evaluated. Any child with a history of delayed language acquisition or use should be monitored and referred immediately if lack of achievement occurs. Immaturity in or inappropriate use of sustained attention, visual selective attention, associate memory, and auditory analysis are often confused with a phonologic processing dysfunction. A "wait and see" attitude is not advisable if early markers and signs are apparent (see below) and a positive family history exists. Often, the best diagnostic indicator is failure of the student to respond to traditional or typical reading approaches during early 1st grade. Precise diagnosis requires sophisticated analysis of the reading problem by specially trained and equipped experts.

Since dyslexia does not simply mean "reading difficulties," students demonstrating early word learning problems need reading, psychologic, and comprehensive language and auditory processing evaluations. Language and auditory processing evaluations are essential to determine if central auditory or language processing problems exist. The objective is to identify the reading problem and assign the student to the most effective instructional approach. Ophthalmologic (refractive) and audiologic (acuity) evaluations should also be conducted. Although most pediatric and neurologic evaluations are insufficient for diagnosis, secondary features such as neurodevelopmental immaturity or soft signs are often apparent, and neurologic evaluations may rule out other disorders (eg, seizures). Psychologic evaluations are usually needed to deal with emotional concerns and rule out psychiatric disorders. The severity of a reading disorder is often increased if medical or emotional problems are present. A complete family history is needed.

Reading evaluations should be specific so that error patterns are identified. A comprehensive reading evaluation tests word recognition and word analysis skills and abilities, fluency (accuracy and rate of word recognition and passage reading), and reading or listening comprehension. **Decoding skills** are assessed by sampling the student's ability to name letter sounds and sound-symbol combinations, to segment words into pronounceable components, and to integrate sounds to form words. Evaluations of reading comprehension must also focus on the student's understanding of vocabulary, prior knowledge, thinking and reasoning skills, and metacognition, ie, the student's knowledge of the activities and strategies needed to acquire and generalize information when reading.

Language and auditory evaluations assess spoken language and phonologic processing deficiencies that are independent of intelligence and consist of deficits in sound imitation, sequencing words in sentences, and the sound elements (phonologic structures) of spoken language. Assessments of receptive and expressive language functions are also conducted. Testing cognitive abilities, eg, attention, memory, and reasoning, is also essential for a specific diagnosis.

Subgroups of dyslexics have been described recently by associating error patterns with neuropsychologic test profiles. Subgrouping is based on the assumption that students with reading disabilities can be sorted into distinct groups and that the distinctiveness of each group is due to differences in the CNS. The terms **phonologic** (word decoding), **deep** (word decoding and retrieval), **surface** (whole word learning), and **direct** (comprehension) dyslexia have been applied to distinguish subgroups. Each term has its own list of symptoms or signs. Reading disabilities have been identified also as dysphonemic-sequencing disorders, visual-spatial reading problems, and general or specific language-reading disorders. By identifying constellations or clusters of signs, errors, and characteristics, researchers hope to determine how to optimize instruction so that the strengths are emphasized and alternative approaches are developed to minimize weaknesses.

Treatment

Reading is a complex learning activity that ultimately combines word recognition with word meaning and passage comprehension. Unfortunately, many touted interventions are too simplistic and ignore or avoid the intricate interactions of phonologic, orthographic, language, and reasoning skills needed for effective reading. Therapeutic interventions are diverse and varied but can be grouped into direct instruction, indirect instruction, and indirect treatment.

Direct instruction may be explicit (eg, teaching specific phonics skills separate from other reading instruction) or implicit (eg, integrating phonics skills in reading programs as supplemental material). It has also been dichotomized as **top-down**, teaching reading from a whole word or language approach, or **bottom-up**, teaching reading by following a hierarchy of skills from the sound unit to the word to the sentence. Direct instruction for dyslexics may consist of one or more approaches to improve word decoding and reading comprehension skills and should emphasize decoding and word analysis skills following the alphabetic-phonic system. Multisensory approaches that include whole word learning and the integration of visual, auditory, and tactual procedures to teach letter names, sounds, words, and sentences are often advocated. Most programs for dyslexics are bottom-up and explicit. Typical basal reading programs are often avoided or used as supplemental material.

Indirect instruction usually consists of training to improve component skills associated with word pronunciation or reading comprehension. Teaching students to blend sounds to form words, to segment words into word parts, and to identify the positions of sounds in words are examples of component skills for word decoding. Teaching students how to identify the main idea, answer questions, isolate facts and details, and read inferentially are examples of component skills for reading comprehension.

Indirect treatments are procedures or techniques that supplant or supplement reading instruction but that usually do not include instruction in the orthography or the phonologic codes, eg, optokinetic or functional vision therapy, the use of tinted lenses, sensory integrative training, and perceptual training. **Drug therapies** have also been proposed. For instance, the use of antihistamines and motion sickness medications are recommended by one theorist to stabilize certain brain functions that may impair visual-auditory vestibular functions. Piracetam has also been investigated as treatment for reading disabilities because of its purported ability to improve certain higher cognitive functions. Most indirect treatments have not been substantiated by controlled, replicated research or have not been replicated beyond testimonials. Until the validity of these forms of treatment is established, they cannot be recommended.

Many with dyslexia may develop functional reading skills with direct instruction, although dyslexia is a lifelong problem and many dyslexic individuals never reach full literacy. Compensatory approaches such as taped texts, readers, and scribes are used to assist the dyslexic with higher-order learning. Individuals with other reading problems may overcome early weaknesses if the cause is maturational. Others may have persistent reading problems if they exhibit language impairments or cognitive deficiencies. Depending on corollary symptoms, many will have problems organizing and managing time, space, and day-to-day functions.

MENTAL RETARDATION (MR)
(Mental Handicap; Mental Subnormality)

Subaverage intellectual ability present from birth or early infancy, manifested by abnormal development and associated with difficulties in learning and social adaptation. About 3% of the total population are reported to be mentally retarded, but only about 1 to 1.5% are actually identified. The birth rate of children with IQs < 50 is 3.6/1000 live births.

Etiology

Intelligence is polygenetically and environmentally determined. Genetic and environmental predispositions to MR may be indistinguishable. The incidence of familial retardation in the offspring of 2 retarded persons is 40%; for 1, it is 20%. The percentage of retarded offspring may be altered by early intervention (see Prevention, below, and PREVENTION OF GENETIC DISORDERS in Ch. 48). In 80% of cases, the cause of MR is unknown. Etiology is more likely to be identified in the more severe cases. Factors causing MR may occur in the prenatal, perinatal, and postnatal periods.

Prenatal abnormalities causing MR may be due to genetic factors, congenital infections, teratogens (drugs and other chemical agents), radiation, or unknown conditions affecting implantation and embryogenesis.

Chromosomal abnormalities comprise the largest number of known genetic causes of MR (see also Ch. 48). The trisomies involve an additional chromosome (47 instead of the normal 46), such as trisomy 18 (Edwards' syndrome) and trisomy 13 (Patau's syndrome). The cri du chat syndrome results from a partial deletion of chromosome 5. Down syndrome is a form of trisomy 21 or (less often) a translocation from the 13-15 group to chromosome 21. Trisomy 21 is the most common trisomy, occurring in 1/600 live births. Abnormalities in sex chromosomes, such as Klinefelter's syndrome (XXY), Turner's syndrome (XO), and various mosaics, may also be associated with MR. The **fragile X syndrome** may account for a large number of persons who have been described as having mild familial MR, estimated to affect 1/1000 births (see X-LINKED MENTAL RETARDATION under CHROMOSOME ABERRATIONS in Ch. 48). Males are affected more often than females. Associated physical features include normal to increased head size, macroorchidism, a prominent jaw, and protruding ears.

Genetic metabolic disorders that cause MR include X-linked recessive defects, such as Lowe's (oculocerebrorenal syndrome), Lesch-Nyhan (hyperuricemia), and Hunter's (a mucopolysaccharidosis variant) syndromes; autosomal recessive disorders, such as phenylketonuria, galactosemia, maple syrup urine disease, and other aminoacidurias and acidemias; and autosomal recessive lysozymal defects, such as Tay-Sachs disease, Niemann-Pick disease, Gaucher's disease, and Hurler's syndrome (mucopolysaccharidosis). Screening for deficiencies in peroxisomal enzyme metabolism is important in retarded infants with idiopathic hypotonia. A positive test has important implications for genetic counseling, prognosis, and treatment.

Genetic neurologic disorders: Primary microcephaly may be caused by an autosomal recessive gene. Tuberous sclerosis, neurofibromatosis, and myotonic dystrophy are all autosomal dominant disorders that can cause MR.

Congenital infections are a major cause of MR and have been due to rubella virus, cytomegalovirus (a common cause—1/600 to 1/1000 live births), *Toxoplasma gondii,* and *Treponema pallidum.* Other viruses infecting the pregnant woman have been causally implicated but not proved.

Drugs: Children born to alcoholic mothers may have the **fetal alcohol syndrome,** which includes anomalies such as microcephaly, facial abnormalities, blepharophimosis, cardiac defects, intrauterine growth retardation, and MR (see also under METABOLIC PROBLEMS IN THE NEWBORN in Ch. 27). The **fetal hydantoin (phenytoin) syndrome** may develop in as many as 11% of children whose mothers receive hydantoin during pregnancy, and may include mental deficiency, prenatal and postnatal growth failure, microcephaly, cranial facial abnormalities, nail or distal phalangeal hypoplasia, and associated cardiac defects.

Perinatal complications related to prematurity, CNS bleeding, periventricular leukomalacia, breech or high forceps delivery, multiple births, placenta previa, preeclampsia, and asphyxia neonatorum may increase the risk of MR. Small-for-gestational-age infants have an increased incidence of MR; the intellectual impairment often is related to the cause of decreased weight. Premature infants < 32 wk gestation who weigh < 1.5 kg have a 10 to 50% chance of being retarded, depending on their gestational age, perinatal events, and the quality of care provided. Infants < 1 kg and < 28 wk gestation are at greatest risk. Infants at high risk require periodic developmental observation. The developmental outcome of infants who experience mild untoward perinatal events is often directly related to the infant's learning environment.

Postnatal factors may include viral and bacterial encephalitides (including the neuroencephalopathy associated with AIDS) and meningitides; poisoning, eg, lead and mercury; and accidents that result in severe head injuries or asphyxia.

Prenatal malnutrition in the mother or severe infant malnutrition may affect brain development, resulting in MR. This is a major concern in developing countries where famine and hunger are common. Malnutrition, coupled with environmental deprivation (lack of the physical, emotional, and cognitive support required for developmental growth and social adaptation), may be the most common cause of MR worldwide.

Diagnosis and Prognosis

Accurate diagnosis may provide developmental prognosis, suggest plans for educational and training programs, form the foundation for genetic counseling, and relieve guilt. FIG. 29-1 provides a useful general diagnostic approach when MR is suspected. Skull x-rays should be obtained when premature closure of the sutures is suspected. Cranial CT or MRI is very helpful in diagnosing cerebral malformations, cerebral atrophy, CNS hemorrhage, hydrocephalus, tumor, and intracranial calcifications associated with toxoplasmosis, cytomegalovirus infection, or tuberous sclerosis. An EEG should be performed when a seizure disorder is suspected. Urine and blood amino acid and enzyme studies are indicated when inborn errors of metabolism are suspected (see ANOMALIES IN AMINO ACID METABOLISM in Ch. 40). The major clinical manifestations of these metabolic errors may be associated with failure to thrive, lethargy, vomiting, seizures, hypotonia, hepatosplenomegaly, coarse facial features, abnormal urinary odor, or macroglossia.

Subaverage intellectual ability can be identified and measured by **standardized intelligence tests.** Such tests have a middle-class bias but are generally reasonable in appraising intellectual ability in children, particularly in the older child. Psychologic tests, such as the Bayley Scale of Infant Development (for children < age 30 mo), the Stanford-Binet (for ages 2 to adulthood), the Wechsler Preschool and Primary Scale of Intelligence (for ages 3 yr 10 mo to 6 yr 7 mo), and the Wechsler Intelligence Scale for Children—Revised (ages 6 yr to 16 yr 11 mo), should be performed by qualified psychologists. The revised Denver Developmental Screening Test (**DDST-R**) provides a gross assessment of developmental achievement for children up to age 5 yr and can be administered by the physician or his assistant.

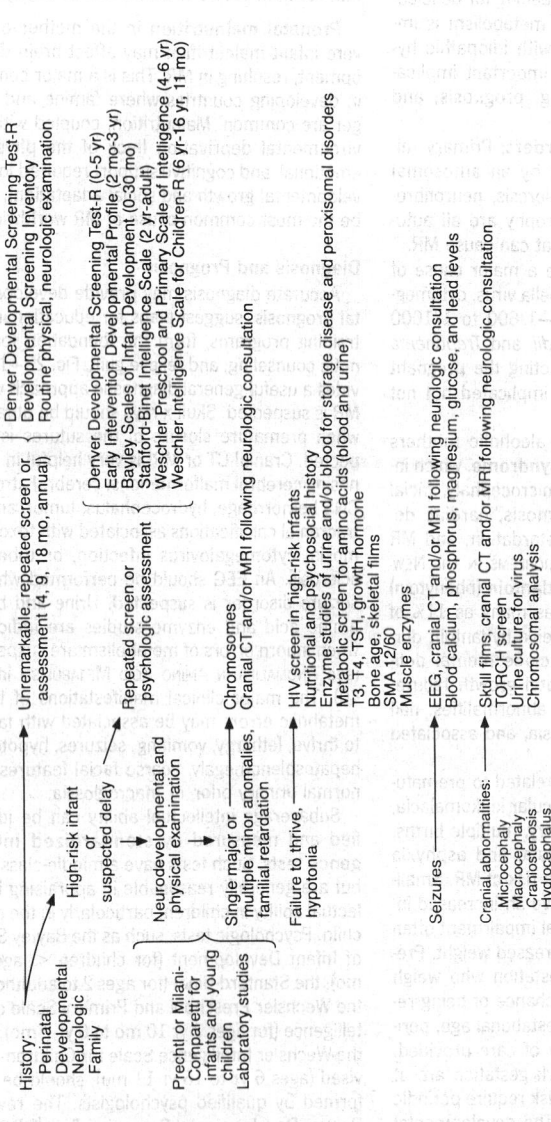

History:
- Perinatal
- Developmental
- Neurologic
- Family

Prechtl or Milani-Comparetti for infants and young children

Laboratory studies

Neurodevelopmental and physical examination

→ High-risk infant or suspected delay

→ Single major or multiple minor anomalies, familial retardation

→ Failure to thrive, hypotonia

Denver Developmental Screening Test-R
Developmental Screening Inventory
Routine physical, neurologic examination

Denver Developmental Screening Test-R (0-5 yr)
Early Intervention Developmental Profile (2 mo-3 yr)
Bayley Scales of Infant Development (0-30 mo)
Stanford-Binet Intelligence Scale (2 yr-adult)
Weschler Preschool and Primary Scale of Intelligence (4-6 yr)
Weschler Intelligence Scale for Children (6 yr-16 yr, 11 mo)

Unremarkable, repeated screen or assessment (4, 9, 18 mo, annual)

Repeated screen or psychologic assessment

Chromosomes
Cranial CT and/or MRI following neurologic consultation

HIV screen in high-risk infants
Nutritional and psychosocial history
Enzyme studies of urine and/or blood for storage disease and peroxisomal disorders
Metabolic screen for amino acids (blood and urine)
T3, T4, TSH, growth hormone
Bone age, skeletal films
SMA 12/60
Muscle enzymes

Seizures → EEG, cranial CT and/or MRI following neurologic consultation
Blood calcium, phosphorus, magnesium, glucose, and lead levels

Cranial abnormalities:
- Microcephaly
- Macrocephaly
- Craniostenosis
- Hydrocephalus

Skull films, cranial CT and/or MRI following neurologic consultation
TORCH screen
Urine culture for virus
Chromosomal analysis

ALL: Genetic counseling, visual assessment, auditory assessment, CBC, urinalysis

Fig. 29-1. The diagnostic process for mental retardation. This is meant to be a general guide. The laboratory studies should be determined by history and physical examination. TSH = thyroid-stimulating hormone; TORCH = toxoplasmosis, rubella, cytomegalovirus, herpes. References for the Prechtl and Milani-Comparetti examinations are as follows: Prechtl HFR, Beintema D: Neurological examination of full-term new born infants. Clinics of Developmental Medicine. No. 12. London, Spastic International Publications, JB Lippincott Company, 1964; and Milani-Comparetti G: Routine developmental examination in normal and retarded children. Developmental Medicine and Child Neurology 9:631-638, 1967. (From Scheiner AP, McNabb NA: "The child with mental retardation," in The Practical Management of the Developmentally Disabled Child, edited by AP Scheiner and IF Abroms. St. Louis, CV Mosby Company, 1980, p 210; used with permission.)

It should be used only for screening. Isolated delays in sitting or walking **(gross motor skills)** and in pincer grasp, drawing, or writing **(fine motor skills)** may be due to a neuromuscular disorder, while deficits in language and personal-social skills may be due to emotional problems, environmental deprivation, learning disorders, or deafness without MR. Intelligence tests are subject to error and should be questioned when they do not support clinical findings. Illness, language barriers, or cultural differences may hamper a child's test performance.

Mentally retarded children function at various levels. The child who has **borderline intelligence** or is a slow learner (IQ 84 to 69) is rarely identified before beginning school, when educational and behavioral problems become evident. About 14% of children tested in school have IQs identified as borderline retardation; however, after leaving school they usually blend into the general population without attracting attention and can support themselves if job opportunities exist that require only basic skills or manual performance.

Children with **mild retardation** (IQ 68 to 52) are educable. Those at the upper level may attain 4th- to 6th-grade reading skills and can provide for their basic self-help needs and, depending on their level of function, have varying degrees of educational achievement and social and occupational skills. They require some supervision and support, special educational and training facilities, and, frequently, a sheltered living and work situation. Usually free from gross physical defects, they may have a higher-than-normal incidence of epilepsy. Although they have difficulty reading, most mildly retarded individuals can learn the basic educational skills needed for everyday life. Socially they are often immature and unsophisticated, with a poorly developed capacity for social interaction. Because their thinking is concrete and they are often unable to generalize, adjusting to new situations is difficult, and their poor judgment, lack of foresight, and gullibility make them susceptible to delinquency. Serious offenses are uncommon, but the mildly retarded may commit impulsive crimes, often as a member of a group and sometimes to achieve peer group status. Those children at the lower mild retardation level and the **moderately retarded,** trainable child (IQ 51 to 36) have obvious language and motor delays.

Given adequate training and support, mildly and moderately retarded adults can live with varying degrees of independence within the community. Some can cope with minimal support in halfway houses, while others need greater supervision. Most will need a sheltered workshop.

The **severely retarded** child (IQ 35 to 20) is trainable but to a lesser degree. The **profoundly retarded** child (IQ 19 and below) usually cannot learn to walk and has minimal language skills (see TABLE 29–1).

Life expectancy of children with MR may be shortened, depending on the etiology and severity. In general, the more severe the retardation and the greater the immobility, the higher the mortality.

Mental illness can occur in the mentally handicapped of all levels, as it can in normal persons, and may cause sudden behavior changes. Communication difficulties may make it harder to identify thought disorders and delusions, but the relatively sudden development of a flat affect and hallucinations may suggest **schizophrenia.** When an adolescent with MR is socially rejected by the normal peer group at school, or when he realizes others see him as different and deficient, **depression** may occur. Appropriate neuroleptic and antidepressant drugs may be given in dosages similar to those used in the nonretarded. Psychotherapy and active care and training aimed at alleviating the person's sense of worthlessness or modifying unrealistic goals may also be helpful, as the use of psychotropic drugs in the absence of psychotherapy and environmental changes is *rarely* effective.

Behavior disorders are the reason for most psychiatric referrals and the most common psychiatric malady in institutionalized populations. Explosive outbursts, temper tantrums, and physically aggressive behavior are usually excessive responses to normal stresses. They are often situational, and precipitating factors usually can be found. Lack of training in socially responsible behavior, inconsistent discipline, and the reinforcement of faulty behavior are the major underlying causes of unacceptable behavior. Brain damage and impaired ability to communicate are important predisposing factors. In institutional settings, overcrowding, understaffing, and lack of occupation are important aggravating factors, and the incidence of behavioral difficulties falls dramatically when living conditions are improved and proper training and occupation are introduced.

Prevention

Genetic counseling provides parents with knowledge and understanding of the cause of re-

TABLE 29–1. OFFICIAL LEVELS OF MENTAL RETARDATION AND
SOME DEVELOPMENTAL CHARACTERISTICS*

Level and Title	IQ Range	Estimated Percentage of Total Retarded	Developmental Characteristics		
			Preschool Age 0–5 yr (Maturation and Development)	School Age 6–20 yr (Training and Education)	Adult ≥ 21 yr (Social and Vocational Adequacy)
1. Profound	< 20	5	Gross retardation; minimal capacity for functioning in sensorimotor areas; may need nursing care	Some motor development; may respond to minimum or limited training in self-help	Some motor and speech development; may achieve very limited self-care; may need nursing care
2. Severe	20–35		Poor motor development; speech is minimal; able to profit from training in self-help; few or no expressive skills	Can talk or learn to communicate; can be trained in elemental health habits; profits from systematic habit training	May contribute partially to self-maintenance under complete supervision; can develop self-protection skills to a minimal useful level in controlled environment
3. Moderate	36–51	20	Can talk or learn to communicate; poor social awareness; fair motor development; profits from training in self-help; can be managed with moderate supervision	Can profit from training in social and occupational skills; unlikely to progress beyond 2nd-grade level in academic subjects; may learn to travel alone in familiar places	May achieve self-maintenance in unskilled or semi-skilled work under sheltered conditions; needs supervision and guidance when under mild social or economic stress
4. Mild	52–68	75	Can develop social and communication skills; minimal retardation in sensorimotor areas; often not distinguished from normal until later age	Can learn academic skills up to approximately 6th-grade level by late teens; can be guided toward social conformity; "educable"	Can usually achieve social and vocational skills for adequate to minimum self-support, but may need guidance and assistance when under unusual social or economic stress

* Definition of mental retardation: significantly subaverage general intellectual functioning existing concurrently with deficits in adaptive behavior and manifest during the developmental period.
From Kenny TJ, Clemmens RL: "Mental retardation," in *Primary Pediatric Care*, edited by RA Hoekelman. St. Louis, CV Mosby Company, 1987, p 741; used with permission.

tardation and the risk of recurrence. Siblings can learn of their own risk for having a retarded child. Amniocentesis or chorionic villus biopsy may be useful in the detection of inherited metabolic and chromosomal disorders, carrier states, and the presence or absence of CNS defects such as myelodysplasia and anencephaly. Ultrasound may also identify these latter CNS defects. The serum α-fetoprotein level is a helpful screen for myelodysplasia and Down syndrome. Prenatal diagnoses permit the option of abortion and subsequent family planning. Amniocentesis is indicated in all pregnant women > 35 yr because of their increased risk for having an infant with

Down syndrome, as well as in women with a family history of mucopolysaccharidosis, galactosemia, Tay-Sachs disease, and maple syrup urine disease. (See also Ch. 13 and PREVENTION OF GENETIC DISORDERS in Ch. 48.)

The use of rubella vaccine has all but eliminated congenital rubella as a cause of MR. A vaccine is being sought for cytomegalovirus infection. Continuing improvements and availability of obstetric and neonatal care, the use of exchange transfusion and Rh₀ immunoglobulin to prevent hemolytic disease of the newborn (erythroblastosis fetalis), the regionalization of neonatal intensive care units, and improved knowledge and technology have further reduced the incidence of MR while prevalence has remained constant.

Treatment

Environmental factors can make a significant difference to the infant or child who is at high risk for developmental disabilities. Developmental vulnerability due to a perinatal insult may be overcome in a facilitating environment. Referral to an early intervention program during infancy may prevent or decrease the severity of MR.

As soon as MR is confirmed or strongly suspected, the parents should be informed, together whenever possible. Sensitive ongoing counseling is essential for family adaptation. The findings of the various consultants must be coordinated and interpreted. Parents should have ample time to discuss causes, impact, prognosis, and education and training of the child. If the family's physician cannot do this, he should refer the family to a center with a multidisciplinary team that evaluates and serves children with developmental disabilities; but the physician should plan to provide continuing medical care and advice.

A comprehensive, individualized program is developed with the help of appropriate specialists. Formal psychologic assessment may be deferred until age 3 yr unless the diagnosis is uncertain or the physician cannot assess the child's

development himself. A neurologist should investigate all cases of moderate to severe retardation, progressive disability, neuromuscular deterioration, or suspected seizure disorders. Orthopedists, physical therapists, and occupational therapists should assist in evaluating and managing retarded children with cerebral palsy or other major motor deficits. Speech pathologists and audiologists are helpful with major language delays or with a suspected hearing loss. Nutritionists, social workers, educators, ophthalmologists, psychiatrists, and dentists all can be helpful.

Family support and counseling are of major importance; however, realistic methods of caring for the child are paramount. Every effort should be made to have the child live at home or in a community-based residence. Whenever possible the retarded child should attend a normal day-care center or a regular public school. Level of social competence is as important as IQ when evaluating an individual's handicap due to retardation. IQ and social competence are highly correlated at the lower end of the IQ scale, but with higher scores other factors such as the presence of physical handicaps, personality defects, mental illness, and social abilities are increasingly important in determining effective functioning and the need for care.

Institutionalization should not be considered without extensive family discussion. While the presence of a mentally retarded child in the home can be disruptive, it is rarely the primary cause of family discord. However, the family must have psychologic support and may need help with the burdens of daily care. These can be provided by such services as day-care centers, homemakers (trained nonprofessionals who help with household chores and child care), and temporary foster homes. The retarded adult should be provided with long-term residence in apartment clusters, hostels, and nursing homes.

30. INJURIES, POISONINGS, AND RESUSCITATION

INJURIES

Injury is the most common cause of death in childhood, killing more children than cancer, congenital malformations, pneumonia, meningitis, and heart disease combined. Even the infant < 1 yr is at risk, with almost 1000 deaths/yr

occurring in this age group from falls, burns, drowning, and suffocation. Injuries are also the leading cause of disability in children. For every death from an injury, 1000 children are nonfatally injured.

Injuries are the result of a sequence of events, most of them preventable, frequently triggered by the child's curiosity. Certain factors predispose the child to sustaining injury. Injuries are more common when the child is hungry or tired (before meals or naps), is being cared for by a mother substitute, is in new surroundings (a recent family move or vacation), or has a high activity level. Injuries are likely to occur when parents are rushed and busy, or when parents do not anticipate the risks associated with each new stage of their child's development.

Safety education for parent and child is a key preventive measure. Passive protection is not enough. The child must be protected from potential hazards and taught an appropriate response to those that are unavoidable. Parents need to learn to avoid situations known to be associated with injuries. Such preventive care includes safe storage of inedible materials, use of safety caps and containers, use of safety restraints and safe car seats for children in automobiles (see below), use of bicycle helmets when riding a bicycle, and use of smoke/heat detectors in homes. Parents must set good safety examples (eg, wearing seat belts) because children will mimic their parents' actions.

Ways in which physicians can help to prevent injuries include educating parents, distributing safety information in their offices, setting good examples themselves, and anticipating potentially high-risk situations (eg, suggesting that a mother who is occupied with the care of a sick child obtain appropriate help with her other children).

Prevention of Injury in Motor Vehicle Accidents

Injury in motor vehicle accidents is a major cause of death among all age groups, claiming 4/100,000 infants < 1 yr of age, 7/100,000 children aged 1 to 14 yr, and increasing up to 40/100,000 by age 15 to 24 yr. An unrestrained child may be the only casualty of a sudden stop that results in neither property damage nor other personal injury.

To reduce the incidence and severity of injuries in a crash, all occupants should be restrained. State laws vary but most states now have child restraint laws. *It is extremely unsafe for a child to be held by a restrained adult since the adult will be unable to maintain hold on the child, who will be thrown by tremendous force even at minimal speed* (eg, restraining a 10-lb child, traveling 30 miles/h, would require the strength to lift 300 lb 1 ft off the ground). The unrestrained adult may also be thrown forward and crush the child against the interior of the car with a force equal to the adult weight × (speed)²/2.

Child restraints must be used properly to be effective. The child must be strapped into a restraint, which should be designed for his size and stage of development. The entire restraint must be secured to the car according to manufacturer's instructions, or it will serve to facilitate the trajectory path of the child in a crash. Older children in either front or back seats should be secured by seat belts. The effectiveness of car restraints in reducing trauma is undeniable; their use reduces fatalities by 40 to 50% and serious injuries by 45 to 55%.

There are a number of seats approved by the National Highway Traffic Safety Administration. Restraints that meet Federal Crash Standards are appropriately marked. A current list of approved models is available from the Academy of Pediatrics or the National Safety Council. The infant seat should face the rear of the vehicle and is appropriate up to a weight of 15 lb. Seat restraints for children from 16 to 40 lb should face forward, should be equipped with shoulder restraints and lap guards, and should provide stability for the head as well.

Head Injury

A high percentage of deaths from trauma in childhood is due to craniocerebral trauma and its complications. Serious injury to the developing nervous system often results in residual impairment of physical, cognitive, and emotional functions.

Head injury is the second most common form of trauma for which children are admitted to the hospital. The greatest incidence of head injuries occurs in children < 1 yr and > 15 yr of age. Boys exceed girls as victims, and injuries are predominantly due to falls in and around the home. Falls from a height are a major cause of preventable death in urban children. A campaign to prevent falls from windows in New York City during one year produced a 96% decrease in these injuries.

The **clinical syndrome** will depend on the location and extent of the injury. The most frequent incidents are minor trauma without loss of consciousness, concussion, contusion, and fractures. Far more serious but infrequent are subdural and epidural hematomas. The history of the event and the course of manifestations that follow are extremely important, and the details should be meticulously gathered from family and witnesses. Time, type of injury, and patient's immediate response in terms of consciousness are critical to management.

Minor head trauma without loss of consciousness and without neurologic signs may be associated with vomiting, pallor, irritability, or lethargy. However, persistence of these symptoms for > 6 mo or worsening symptoms may indicate a more severe injury, and the child should be evaluated more closely.

Concussion is *a transient and rapidly reversible state of neuronal dysfunction associated with a loss of consciousness immediately following the head injury.* Victims often have amnesia for the event and the time just prior to the event but have no neurologic signs.

Contusion is *the focal bruising or tearing of cerebral tissue accompanied by parenchymatous hemorrhage and local edema.* The neurologic signs depend on the *precise* location of the injury, but the ventral surface of the frontal lobes and inferolateral aspects of the temporal lobes are the most common sites. There may be disturbances of strength and sensation, altered sensorium, and an associated increase in intracranial pressure, particularly if the contused area is large.

Skull fractures are generally unreliable predictors of the severity of the CNS injury sustained; careful neurologic examination is more helpful. Nevertheless, the presence of a fracture is not usually consistent with a history of minor head injury, and patients with certain types of fractures may be at higher risk for intracranial problems.

In the older child, fractures across the middle meningeal artery may be associated with an epidural hematoma. Fractures through the occipital bone and the base of the skull (basilar) indicate a high-intensity impact, since these parts of the skull are thicker and more force is required to fracture them. Basilar skull fractures are usually not visible on either skull films or CT scans; however, associated signs include CSF draining from nose or ears, blood behind the tympanic membrane (or in the ear canal if the tympanic membrane has been ruptured, ecchymosis behind the ear (Battle's sign) or in the periorbital area (raccoon's eyes), or fluid noted in the frontal/maxillary sinuses. In an infant, trapping of meningeal membranes in a linear skull fracture may result in a "growing fracture." This is actually a leptomeningeal cyst, which develops over 3 to 6 wk and may be the first evidence that a linear fracture has occurred.

Depressed skull fractures require immediate evaluation, as they are more likely to be associated with injured underlying brain. Seizures are related to the associated contusion rather than to the fragment itself. Neurologic consultation should be obtained to determine if the fragment should be surgically elevated.

Epidural hematomas are collections of blood between the dura mater and the skull resulting from arterial or venous injury. Associated neurologic symptoms are usually due to compression of brain rather than direct injury. The classic symptoms in the adult (loss of consciousness, a lucid interval, and then neurologic deterioration) frequently do not occur in the child. Emergency evacuation needs to be done quickly to prevent neurologic deterioration. Ultimate prognosis is good.

Subdural hematomas are collections of blood beneath the dura mater, usually associated with a significant contusion of the brain. There is commonly associated hyperemia and cerebral edema, which results in an altered state of consciousness and signs of increased intracranial pressure. Focal deficits are also common and may be permanent. Early neurosurgical consultation is mandatory because surgical evaluation and management of increased intracranial pressure are often necessary. In addition, the incidence of seizures secondary to the contusion is high. Although most subdural hematomas occur acutely, blood may accumulate in the subdural space more gradually from small tears in the frontal and parietal cortical veins as they pass into the sagittal sinus. Symptoms of increased intracranial pressure may develop more gradually. Treatments include repeated subdural taps, surgical drainage, or shunting.

Intraventricular or subarachnoid hemorrhage is usually associated with severe head injury with considerable long-term neurologic morbidity.

Assessment: After elucidating the mechanism of injury and history of subsequent events, the physical examination is key to assessing the severity of the injury. Attention to mental status using the Glasgow Coma Scale (for children < 5 yr, the Pediatric Glasgow Coma Scale), pupillary responses, vital signs, and evidence of any associated injuries is imperative (see TABLE 30–1). A Glasgow Coma Score ≤ 12 suggests a severe head injury; a Score < 8 suggests the need for intubation and ventilation because airway protective reflexes are usually lost, and there is a high likelihood that increased intracranial pres-

TABLE 30-1. GLASGOW COMA SCALE

Eyes open	
Never	1
To pain	2
To verbal stimuli	3
Spontaneously	4
Best verbal response	
No response	1
Incomprehensible sounds	2
Inappropriate words	3
Disoriented and converses	4
Oriented and converses	5
Best motor response	
No response	1
Extension (decerebrate rigidity)	2
Flexion abnormal (decorticate rigidity)	3
Flexion withdrawal	4
Localizes pain	5
Obeys	6
Total	3-15

When carried out initially, the scale gives a rough indication of severity of brain injury. Coma grades 3 to 5 indicate potentially fatal damage, especially if accompanied by fixed pupils or absent oculovestibular responses. Conversely, admission scores of 8 or above correlate with a high chance of good recovery.

From Jennett B, Bond M: "Assessment of outcome after severe brain damage: A practical scale." *Lancet* 1:480-485, 1975; used with permission.

sure exists (hyperventilation reduces increased intracranial pressure); and a Score < 6 suggests the need for intracranial pressure monitoring. The ocular fundi should be examined carefully for the presence of retinal hemorrhages, since these provide strong evidence of child abuse (shaken infant syndrome).

Treatment: Most children with mild head trauma can be observed at home by competent parents. Children with altered consciousness at the time of examination, a history of unconsciousness for even a brief period of time, a skull fracture, and either focal or diffuse neurologic findings should be observed in the hospital. If circumstances suggest possible child abuse, these children should also be observed (see Ch. 31).

Hospitalized children must be observed closely for changes in neurologic status, including mental status, vital signs, pupillary findings, focalization or lateralization of signs, and seizures. A head CT scan should be performed in children with the following findings: alteration of consciousness, persistent vomiting, focal neurologic findings, clinical evidence of a basilar skull fracture, and seizures.

Although nothing can be done to alter the primary damage, avoidance of secondary brain dysfunction by preventing hypoxia, hypercarbia, hypotension, and elevated intracranial pressure may be accomplished by aggressive and meticulous management. Brain swelling resulting in elevated intracranial pressure requires immediate appropriate management to prevent further interference with O_2 delivery and cellular metabolism.

Management of the child with a serious head injury should be performed in a stepwise fashion. Of greatest importance initially is the adequacy of the airway, since both hypoxia and hypercarbia increase intracranial pressure by worsening cerebral hyperemia. If the Glasgow Coma Score is < 8, the child should be intubated (with appropriate medication) in a *controlled* and efficient fashion (to minimize the acute elevation in intracranial pressure seen with the intubation procedure), and mechanical ventilation should be instituted. Arterial blood gases, pulse oximetry, and end-tidal P_{CO_2} monitoring are useful in the ongoing assessment of the adequacy of oxygenation and ventilation.

Intravenous fluids consisting of 5% dextrose in 0.45% sodium chloride should be given at $2/3$ maintenance, provided there is no systemic hypotension or hypovolemic shock. Since infants and children frequently secrete an increased amount of ADH after head injury, and so are at risk for becoming overloaded with free water with subsequent worsening cerebral edema, mild fluid restriction is appropriate.

Children with a Glasgow Coma Score < 8, with or without evidence of cerebral swelling or bleeding on a head CT scan, should be mildly hyperventilated initially to keep P_{CO_2} between 25 and 30 mm Hg. Subsequently, placement of an intracranial pressure monitor should be strongly considered to determine the need for specific interventions to decrease excessively high intracranial pressure. Intracranial pressure should be kept at ≤ 15 mm Hg by using hyperventilation (to keep P_{CO_2} at 25 to 30 mm Hg or even 20 to 25 mm Hg if necessary), controlling pain, maintaining normothermia, and using muscle relaxation. The head of the bed should be elevated to 30° with the head kept in a midline position to enhance cerebral venous drainage. Judicious small doses of 20% mannitol at 0.25 to 0.5 gm/kg can be used to decrease rises in intracranial pressure or to increase the serum osmolality to 295 to 305 mOsm/kg by its dehydrating effect. Furosemide 1 mg/kg IV is also helpful in decreasing total body water, particularly when the transient hypervolemia associated with mannitol is to be avoided. In the first 24 h after a head injury, furosemide may even be preferred as a method to increase serum osmolality. Dexamethasone has not been shown to be effective in head trauma and is generally no longer used. Induced pentobarbital coma and induced hypothermia have also not been shown to be of consistent benefit and have significant risk.

Frequent evaluation of the child who has sustained a head injury is imperative. Deterioration should prompt a repeat CT scan to look for treatable lesions and/or the cause of the change in the clinical examination.

Fixed and dilated pupils, loss of oculovestibular reflexes, and decerebrate posturing are not necessarily irreversible with proper treatment. Aggressive early management directed toward maintaining adequate pulmonary gas exchange and brain perfusion can reduce the risks of increased intracranial pressure and secondary complications.

Seizures increase intracranial pressure and should be treated with phenytoin. A loading IV dose of 20 mg/kg in 2 separate 10 mg/kg boluses should be given at a maximum rate of 2 mg/kg/min (up to 50 mg/min) to prevent cardiovascular side effects (eg, hypotension, bradycardia). The maintenance IV dose is 3 to 6 mg/kg/day divided bid; duration of treatment is variable and depends on the type of injury and the results of the EEG. Seizures occur in about 5% of children > 5 yr and in 10% of those < 5 yr during the first week posttrauma. Early seizures have a more benign long-term prognosis than those that occur after 7 days.

Prognosis and rehabilitation: The degree of brain recovery depends on the age, duration of coma, and site of maximal trauma. Of the nearly 5 million children who sustain a head injury each year, 4,000 die and 15,000 require prolonged hospitalization. Of those with severe injury whose coma exceeds 24 h, 50% suffer major neurologic sequelae. Between 2 and 5% remain severely handicapped. The mortality rate in head-injured children with Glasgow Coma Scores of 5, 6, or 7 is $\leq 10\%$, with children < 5 yr (especially infants) having higher mortality rates than older children. For children who survive, functional recovery is usually quite good, but a prolonged period of rehabilitation, particularly in cognitive and emotional areas, is often required and rehabilitation services should be planned early. Common problems during recovery include retrograde amnesia, behavior changes, emotional lability, sleep disturbances, and decreased intellectual ability.

POISONING
(See also Ch. 145)

Poisoning is still the most common cause of nonfatal accidents in the home, despite the many educational programs aimed at its prevention. In a case of ingestion for which additional information is needed as to the contents of a trade name product or the appropriate therapy indicated, the nearest Poison Control Center should be consulted.

The most common serious poisonings in children (acetaminophen, aspirin, caustics, lead, iron, and hydrocarbons) are discussed here.

ACETAMINOPHEN POISONING

Acetaminophen is *not* a "harmless" alternative to aspirin. Its toxicity has been well documented in the British literature since 1960. There are > 100 products sold over the counter that contain acetaminophen. There are also many children's preparations in liquid, tablet, and capsule form. The measurement of toxicity is very different from that of aspirin, and therefore the treatment of overdose is different. Symptoms are usually mild until 48 h or later postingestion.

The cytochrome P-450–dependent enzyme system produces a potentially toxic metabolite of acetaminophen that is cleared by hepatic glutathione stores under normal circumstances. In an acute overdose, excessive levels of the metabolite deplete the glutathione stores in the liver and hepatic necrosis results.

Acetaminophen in prepubertal children is rarely fatal, even when AST (SGOT) levels reach 20,000 IU/L. The reason for this age-related difference continues to be under investigation. Children > 12 yr appear to respond as adults to the hepatic challenge of acetaminophen. An increase in symptoms and a prolongation of abnormal liver functions have been observed in adolescents.

The symptoms of acetaminophen overdose can be described in 4 stages:

Stage I (first few hours): Few if any systemic symptoms or symptoms of GI irritability occur within 12 to 24 h, even in patients with large ingestions. The patient is not perceived as ill.

Stage II (after 24 h): GI symptoms, particularly nausea and vomiting, are common, and liver function tests become abnormal. AST (SGOT) and ALT (SGPT), bilirubin, and prothrombin time are elevated in that order.

Stage III (3 to 5 days): Vomiting continues, and levels of AST, ALT, bilirubin, and prothrombin time peak. Symptoms of hepatic failure appear.

Stage IV (after 5 days): Hepatic toxic reaction resolves or death from hepatic failure occurs.

A dose of $\geq$ 140 mg/kg in a child or > 10 gm in an adult is considered toxic.

Plasma half-life is $2^{1}/_{2}$ h in normal dosage. A half-life > 4 h correlates with severe hepatocellular injury.

Treatment

At home, the stomach is immediately emptied by emesis using syrup of ipecac. In the emergency room, apomorphine 0.07 mg/kg or 0.03 mg/lb s.c. or IM may be used for emesis, since its effect can be reversed with naloxone 0.4 to 2 mg s.c., IM, or IV in adults or 0.01 mg/kg in children if vomiting persists and oral acetylcysteine cannot be retained. If the patient has ingested > 140 mg/kg of acetaminophen, acetylcysteine will probably be necessary. On arrival in an emer-

gency room, the stomach can be lavaged with water, and activated charcoal is left in the stomach. If acetylcysteine is indicated, the charcoal can be removed first, although the subsequent "interference" of charcoal with acetylcysteine is relatively negligible. At the very least, serum levels should be assessed.

At 3 to 4 h or later postingestion, a plasma assay for acetaminophen should be obtained and compared to the Rumack-Matthew nomogram (see FIG. 30–1). If the plasma level is below the possible risk zone and no toxic symptoms have developed, no specific chemical treatment is necessary. If the plasma level is above the possible risk zone ($\geq$ 15 μg/mL plasma), a loading dose of acetylcysteine 140 mg/kg should be given *orally or by stomach tube*, and the medication should be continued using 17 additional doses of 70 mg/kg at 4-h intervals; any doses vomited within 1 h should probably be repeated (some centers use less than the total dosage).

Acetylcysteine is available as a 20% solution (200 mg/mL) in vials of 4, 10, and 30 mL and should be diluted 1:4 in a carbonated beverage or fruit juice before use. A 20-kg child would need a loading dose of 140 mg/kg = 2800 mg, or 14 mL of 20% solution. This would require 56 mL of the 1:4 diluted solution. If 16 to 24 h have lapsed since ingestion, acetylcysteine is generally not used, and supportive measures are instituted appropriate to the magnitude of liver failure. If prothrombin time is 3 times normal, vitamin K_1 (phytonadione) 1 to 10 mg is given IM. Fresh plasma or clotting factor may be necessary. IV dextrose solution is given to maintain hydration. Forced diuresis may be harmful and is not helpful. Peritoneal dialysis or hemodialysis is ineffective.

Since antihistaminics, steroids, phenobarbital, and ethacrynic acid all stimulate hepatic cytochrome P-450 system activity, they should be avoided during the management of an acute acetaminophen overdose.

Residual structural and functional hepatic abnormalities do not occur following recovery from acute acetaminophen overdose in previously healthy children. The effects of chronic excessive use or repeated overdoses are still under study.

ASPIRIN AND OTHER SALICYLATE POISONING
(Salicylism)

One of the most common accidental poisonings is from ingestion of aspirin (acetylsalicylic acid). This continues to be true for children < 5

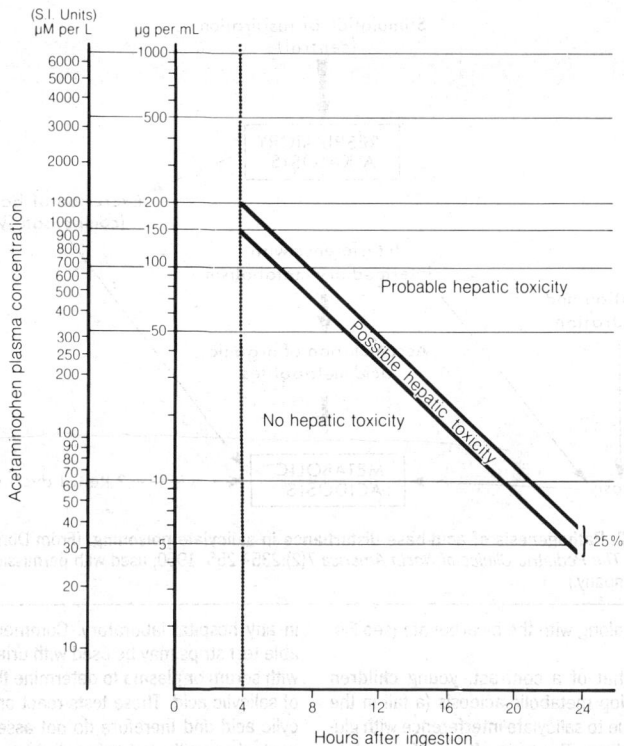

FIG. 30–1. **Rumack-Matthew nomogram for single acute acetaminophen poisoning.** Semi-logarithmic plot of plasma acetaminophen levels vs. time. *Cautions for use of this chart*: (1) The time coordinates refer to time of ingestion. (2) Serum levels drawn before 4 h may not represent peak levels. (3) The graph should be used only in relation to a single acute ingestion. (4) The lower solid line 25% below the standard nomogram is included to allow for possible errors in acetaminophen plasma assays and estimated time from ingestion of an overdose. (Adapted from Rumack BH, Matthew H: "Acetaminophen poisoning and toxicity." *Pediatrics* 55(6):871–876, 1975; reproduced by permission of *Pediatrics*.)

yr, despite safety packaging laws that limit the size of a bottle of infant aspirin to thirty-six 1¼-grain tablets and that mandate safety caps on all medications containing aspirin.

Severe intoxication is unlikely for aspirin ingestions < 200 to 300 mg/kg. Children who have been ill with a fever or who have been taking aspirin therapeutically are at greater risk. Therapeutic overdose has become a more common accident after several days of a large therapeutic dose (twice the usual dose) and is more difficult to treat.

The most toxic form of salicylate is oil of wintergreen (methyl salicylate); death has been reported from ingestion of < 1 tsp in a young child. Any exposure to methyl salicylate (found in products such as liniments and solutions used in hot vaporizers) is potentially lethal.

Clinical Course

The early symptoms of salicylism are nausea and vomiting, followed by hyperpnea, hyperactivity, hyperthermia, and even convulsions. This quickly turns to depression, with lethargy, respiratory failure, and collapse.

Hyperpnea causes a loss of CO_2 through expired air and therefore a decrease in plasma carbonic acid. In the adult especially, this tends to produce an increase in plasma pH (respiratory alkalosis), and the kidneys respond by excreting large quantities of base in the form of bicarbonate. Na, K, and large amounts of organic acids

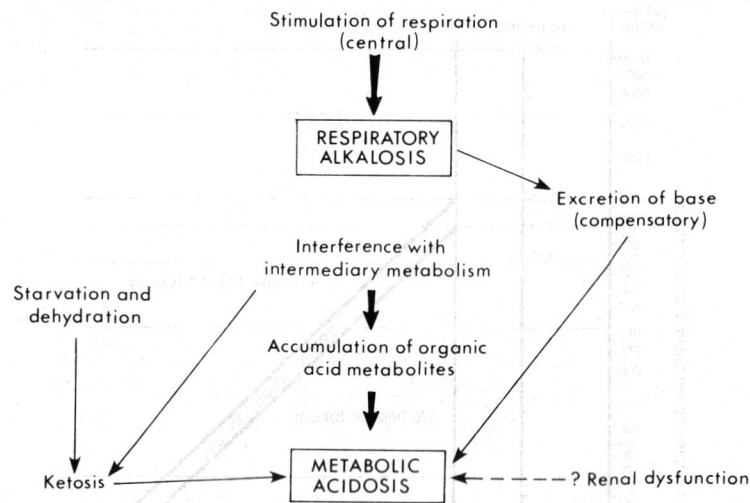

Fig. 30–2. Pathogenesis of acid-base disturbance in salicylate poisoning. (From Done AK: "Drug intoxication." *The Pediatric Clinics of North America* 7(2):235–255, 1960; used with permission of the WB Saunders Company.)

are also lost along with the bicarbonate (see Fig. 30–2).

In somewhat of a contrast, young children quickly develop metabolic acidosis (a fall in the blood pH), due to salicylate interference with glucose metabolism. The toxic effects of salicylate and the loss of buffer base interfere with metabolic processes, and ketosis develops. Because the respiratory alkalosis and metabolic acidosis occur simultaneously, a child may present with a mixed disturbance and a relatively normal pH, or with frank acidosis. The P_{CO_2} will be lower than expected. Children < 4 yr develop metabolic acidosis even more rapidly, without concurrent respiratory alkalosis. Dehydration can be a serious problem because of insensible water loss and increased renal water loss (from an increased urine solute load). Severe losses of Na and K are not uncommon.

Laboratory Findings and Diagnosis

A useful qualitative screening test for salicylic acid is performed by adding a few drops of glacial acetic acid or 0.1 N hydrochloric acid to 1 mL of urine, followed by 3 drops of 10% ferric chloride solution. A burgundy-red color appears and persists if salicylic acid is present (color may turn reddish-brown in the presence of phenothiazines). A serum salicylate level can be obtained

in any hospital laboratory. Commercially available test strips may be used with urine as well as with serum or plasma to determine the presence of salicylic acid. These tests react only with salicylic acid and therefore do not assess stomach contents or pills, but they will do so with hydrolyzed salicylate in either serum or urine.

Other laboratory tests to assist in assessment and treatment include blood pH, serum CO_2, or P_{CO_2} (any 2); serum sodium; serum potassium; BUN; blood glucose; and urine pH and sp gr. These determinations and the serum salicylate level should be followed serially during therapy.

The manifestations of salicylate toxicity are related to the peak level rather than to the level of a given moment. For single-dose ingestions of salicylate, an estimate of the relative severity of the illness can be determined by using the Done nomogram, provided the approximate time of ingestion and a single serum salicylate level are known (see Fig. 30–3).

Treatment

Early emptying of the stomach is critical and is best accomplished by giving ipecac syrup (see General Principles of Treatment in Ch. 145), unless the patient is comatose. For emphasis, with aspirin in particular the stomach should be emptied even 6 to 8 h after ingestion. As vomiting

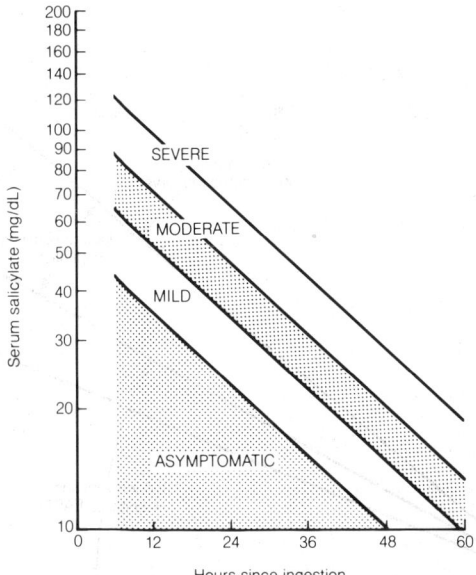

FIG. 30–3. The Done nomogram for estimating severity of salicylate poisoning at varying intervals in time, after ingestion of a single dose. (From Done AK: "Salicylate intoxication: Significance of measurement of salicylate in blood in cases of acute ingestion." *Pediatrics* 26:800–807, 1960; reproduced by permission of *Pediatrics*.)

abates, a dose of activated charcoal (15 gm in 4 oz of water) should be given orally or by stomach tube. Oral administration of sodium bicarbonate is usually not advocated, as it enhances the absorption of salicylate.

A general plan of initially treating the dehydration can be made by relating the patient's size to the dose taken and to the serum salicylate level (see FIG. 30–4). Mild cases are treated with oral fluids alone; eg, milk or fruit juice hourly, up to 50 to 100 mL/kg in the first 24 h. Potentially severe cases are treated with IV fluids immediately. A hypotonic, polyionic solution containing 1 part 0.9% sodium chloride solution and 2 parts 10% D/W can be used before the serum salicylate level is known. The initial rate of administration is rapid (20 mL/kg in the first hour) to restore hydration and establish renal blood flow. When shock is present, plasma or whole blood is also given (10 to 15 mL/kg in I h). After urinary output has been established, and if severe acidosis is present, sodium bicarbonate can be given (3 to 5 mEq/kg IV in 2 to 4 h), which is best accomplished using sodium bicarbonate as the source of Na in the polytonic solution. The real goal is to

try to alkalinize the urine and, particularly for the adult, restore K; this is best accomplished by adding potassium chloride 35 mEq/L to every liter of IV fluid administered. See TABLE 30–2 for a summary of IV fluid administration.

Fever is controlled by tepid water (not alcohol) sponging. Vitamin K_1 (phytonadione) 25 mg/day IM or IV (CAUTION: *IV use may be hazardous; refer to the package circular before prescribing*) in a single dose is given for bleeding due to hypoprothrombinemia, which is seen only rarely. Renal failure is rare; if it occurs, hemodialysis is indicated.

INGESTION OF CAUSTICS

Ingestion of strong acids and alkalies, causing burns and direct tissue damage, is not unusual. Common sources of caustics are drain and toilet bowl cleaners and electric dishwasher detergents. Formerly sold as solids, these products are now also available in the more damaging liquid form, but fortunately far fewer contain the most damaging chemicals such as sodium hydroxide or sulfuric acid. With the solid products, the burning sensation of a particle sticking to a

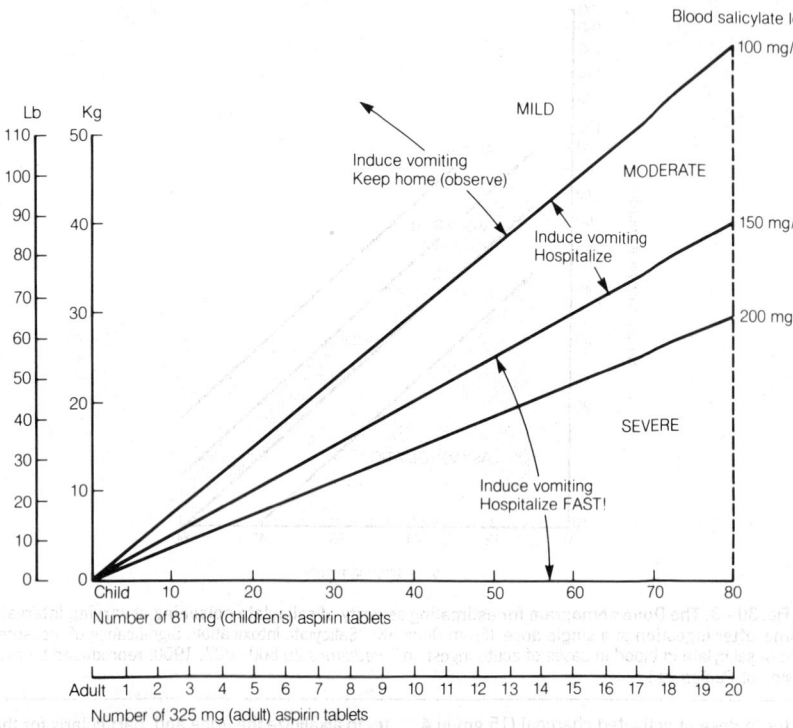

FIG. 30-4. Aspirin ingestion graph, relating severity of intoxication to the patient's size and the amount ingested. (Courtesy of the University of Rochester School of Medicine, Department of Pediatrics.)

moist surface keeps the child from consuming much. Since the liquid preparations do not stick, more is easily consumed and the entire esophagus can be affected.

Clinical Course

Pain is immediate in severe cases. The burned areas become edematous and swollen, dysphagia ensues, and secretions accumulate. Edema may obstruct the airway. The pulse is often rapid and weak. Respirations are shallow, and shock is common.

Patients who survive the initial insult may succumb to secondary infections, or the esophagus or stomach may perforate after a week or more. Perforation into the mediastinum occurs acutely, with severe chest pain. Even with a benign early course, stricture can develop weeks later. Death can result from such complications as circulatory shock, asphyxia due to pharyngeal edema, perforation of the esophagus, or pulmonary irritation.

Treatment

All patients should be seen by a physician; many will require hospitalization.

Dilution of the chemical by drinking water or milk is required immediately. Milk, a demulcent, is preferred for children. It has the advantage of coating and soothing the mucous membranes and replacing tissue protein as the target of the destruction. Contaminated clothing is removed, and the contaminated skin is washed. Emptying the stomach by emesis or lavage is *contraindicated*.

The presence or absence of mouth burns is not a reliable method of determining whether or not the esophagus is burned. Endoscopy is indicated whenever caustics are ingested to be sure that the esophagus is intact. In the presence of esophageal lesions, corticosteroid therapy is no longer considered appropriate and may even be dangerous in 3rd-degree burns. Endoscopy is an

TABLE 30-2. SCHEDULE OF IV FLUID ADMINISTRATION
FOR SALICYLATE INTOXICATION

Condition	Fluid	Rate
Initial hydration	A	2 mL/kg/h (100-200 mL/h in adults)
If shock present	Plasma or blood	10-15 mL/kg, in 1 h, then fluid as for initial hydration
After urine flow established		
Mild or no acidosis	B	8 mL/kg/24 h
Severe acidosis	C	10 mL/kg/24 h
Additional urgent buffering of profound acidosis	Sodium bicarbonate	1-1.5 mEq/kg over 10 min if pH is < 7.2
	or, if acidosis unresponsive or Na restriction desired	
	Tromethamine	3-5 mL of 0.3 M soln in 1 h
	Determine further needs by blood pH measurement (< 7.2)	

		Composition (mEq/L) and preparation of fluids			
Fluid	Na	K	Cl	HCO₃ or lactate	Preparation
A	75	0	50	25	330 mL 10% D/W 170 mL 0.9% sodium chloride 14 mL 7.5% sodium bicarbonate (44.6 mEq/mL)
B	40	35	40	20	Electrolyte 75, Electrolyte 75 with 5% dextrose
C	55	35	40	35	500 mL Fluid B 8.5 mL 7.5% sodium bicarbonate

NOTE: Sodium bicarbonate should not be added until the pH is known, especially in children.
Modified from Done AK, Temple AR: "Treatment of salicylate poisoning." *Modern Treatment* 8:528-551, Aug. 1971; used with permission.

important predictor of subsequent stricture formation and the potential need for esophageal replacement. A broad-spectrum antibiotic is given if there is fever or evidence of mediastinitis. In mild cases, oral fluids are started early; otherwise, IV therapy is instituted until oral fluids can be tolerated. A tracheostomy may be indicated to provide an airway. If strictures are not prevented, subsequent dilation therapy will be required for months or years.

LEAD POISONING
(Plumbism)

Lead poisoning is a chronic disorder, sometimes punctuated by recurrent acute symptomatic episodes, that may result in chronic irreversible effects (eg, cognitive deficits in the child and progressive renal disease in adults). "High-dose" lead sources include repetitive ingestion of chips of paint containing lead; retention of a metallic lead object (shot, curtain weight, fishing weight, bauble, etc) in the stomach or a joint, where lead is slowly dissolved; contamination of acidic foods and beverages (fruits, fruit juices, cola drinks, tomatoes, tomato juice, wine, cider) by storage in improperly lead-glazed ceramic ware; burning of lead-painted wood or battery casings in home fireplaces or stoves; folk medicines containing lead compounds; cottage industry manufactured items (lead-glazed ceramic ware, leaded glass, etc); illicit lead-contaminated whiskey or wine; inhalation of fumes of leaded gasoline; and occupational exposures without protection (respirator, ventilation, dust suppression). "Low-dose" lead sources, mainly lead-contaminated dust and soil, have been associated with asymptomatic increased lead absorption in children (see TABLE 30-3 for a classification of lead poisoning).

Symptoms, Signs, and Diagnosis

The risk of symptomatic plumbism increases with blood lead concentration (PbB) > 60 to 70 μg/dL whole blood. When PbB is > 100 μg/dL whole blood, the risk of encephalopathy is great but unpredictable. In children, sustained PbB

TABLE 30-3. CLASSIFICATION OF LEAD POISONING

Class	Risk	Laboratory Findings (Whole Blood) or Clinical Findings	Approach
I	Mild	PbB 10–19 µg/dL; FEP < 35 µg/dL	Environmental awareness; reduce exposure
		PbB 20–24 µg/dL; FEP 35–220 µg/dL: iron deficiency	Monitor PbB levels; full work-up and environmental review; remove hazards
II	Moderate	PbB 25–44 µg/dL; FEP < 35 µg/dL: minimal Pb burden; FEP 35–220 µg/dL: excess Pb burden	Complete medical examination and evaluation; consider treatment
III	High	PbB 45–69 µg/dL; FEP < 35 µg/dL: never seen; FEP 35–220 µg/dL: marked Pb burden	Mandatory treatment (see text)
IV	Urgent	Asymptomatic; PbB 70–100 µg/dL and/or FEP > 250 µg/dL: Pb toxicity	Mandatory treatment (see text)
V	Encephalopathy or impending encephalopathy	Any symptomatic patient or any patient with PbB > 100 µg/dL	Mandatory treatment (see text)

Pb = lead; PbB = whole blood lead concentration; FEP = "free" erythrocyte protoporphyrin.

> 40 to 50 µg/dL whole blood increases the risk of long-term cognitive deficits; some are convinced that these adverse effects may begin at PbB > 10 µg/dL whole blood.

In the adult, a characteristic sequence of symptoms may develop over several weeks or longer: personality changes, headache, metallic taste, anorexia, vague abdominal discomfort culminating in vomiting, constipation, and colicky abdominal pain. Encephalopathy is rare in adults. In young children, onset of clinical symptoms usually is abrupt, with the appearance over 1 to 5 days of persistent and forceful vomiting, ataxic gait, seizures, alterations in consciousness, and, finally, intractable seizures and coma. These manifestations of acute encephalopathy are primarily due to cerebral edema and may be preceded by several weeks of irritability and decreased play activity. Brain abscess, brain tumor, acute encephalitis, and meningitis should be included in the differential diagnosis. In children, chronic plumbism should be included in the differential diagnosis of mental retardation, seizure disorders, aggressive behavior disorders, developmental regression, and persistent pica. Symptoms may abate spontaneously if excessive exposure is interrupted, only to recur with renewed exposure. A hypochromic-microcytic anemia may be present in both children and adults owing to lead, concurrent iron deficiency, or both. Inhalation of tetraethyl- or tetramethyl-lead produces a different picture, with manifestations primarily of a toxic psychosis.

Definitive diagnosis requires measuring PbB. A useful screening test that reflects lead exposure is the measurement of "free" erythrocyte protoporphyrin (FEP)—see laboratory findings in TABLE 30-3. FEP is a more sensitive indicator of metabolically active lead found in soft tissue and loosely found in bone. FEP is a direct measurement of the toxic effects of lead on heme synthesis. While it is a good screening test for routine checks of at-risk children, FEP may also be elevated in Fe-deficiency states. Measurement of the total lead output in urine during the first day of chelation therapy is also highly useful. Diagnosis is confirmed if the ratio (μg Pb excreted:mg CaEDTA administered) exceeds 1. Blood and urine samples *must* be collected with lead-free equipment. To get reliable results, tests should be done by laboratories experienced in lead analysis. In acutely symptomatic cases, chelation therapy usually must be begun before blood and urine lead data are available. Presumptive diagnosis can be made on the basis of bone marrow aspirates showing basophilic stippling in > 60% of normoblasts, urinary tests for coproporphyrin and δ-aminolevulinic acid, and, in the child, positive abdominal and long-bone x-ray films. Moderate glycosuria is also suggestive.

Treatment

Succimer, also known as DMSA (meso 2,3-dimercaptosuccinic acid), is a new oral medication to treat lead poisoning. A lead chelator, it forms water-soluble chelates and, consequently, increases the urinary excretion of lead. At present, it is indicated to treat children with blood lead levels > 45 μg/dL; however, trials to date have been limited and the full range of indications has not been clarified. While the full spectrum of adverse reactions also has not yet been determined, common adverse effects include rash, GI symptoms (nausea, vomiting, diarrhea, appetite loss, metallic taste in mouth), and increases in serum transaminases. The recommended treatment course is 19 days; the safety of uninterrupted treatment for > 3 wk has not been determined, and such treatment is not recommended. Dosage and administration guidelines are given in TABLE 30–4.

In acute lead encephalopathy (class IV and V), combination treatment with dimercaprol **(BAL)** and edetate calcium disodium **(CaEDTA),** according to the dosage schedule in TABLE 30–4, is recommended and should be started as soon as urine flow is established. This is maximum dosage and should not be continued beyond 5 days to avoid depleting body stores of essential metals, particularly zinc. In asymptomatic, or very mildly symptomatic, patients with confirmed PbB in excess of 70 to 100 μg/dL whole blood (class IV), the regimen is modified as follows: Stop BAL after 48 h, but continue CaEDTA for an additional 48 to 72 h in reduced dosage of 50 to 75 mg/kg/day divided into 2 or 3 IM doses given at 8- to 12-h intervals. Patients receiving BAL should be given maintenance parenteral fluids or clear liquids orally to avoid the vomiting that BAL often causes. When PbB is 50 to 69 μg/dL whole blood (class III), CaEDTA only is suffi-

cient (TABLE 30–4). Brief courses of chelation therapy are usually associated with rebound in PbB, presumably owing to internal redistribution of lead. This rebound often can be suppressed with oral penicillamine **(PCA)** instituted after a 2-day rest period following CaEDTA treatment. Prophylactic amounts of iron, zinc, and copper probably should be given to minimize depletion of these metals during long-term treatment with PCA.

CaEDTA followed by PCA may be of some benefit in children with confirmed PbB ≥ 50 μg/dL whole blood by reducing the time that the developing brain is exposed to excess lead; reduction in exposure is critical in all cases and primarily in cases of lower PbB levels, along with attention to diet.

The use of combined BAL-CaEDTA treatment in acute lead encephalopathy is described in detail in the literature. Neurology consultation should be sought promptly, and the patient should be managed in an intensive care unit.

Precautions in the use of chelating agents: EDTA is not metabolized; it is excreted unchanged exclusively by renal glomerular filtration. CaEDTA must be withheld in anuric patients. In the combined BAL-CaEDTA regimen, CaEDTA at the dosage level in TABLE 30–4 should not exceed 5 successive days; however, in very severe, slowly responsive cases of encephalopathy, it may be given cautiously for no more than 2 additional days. The lower daily dosage of CaEDTA (50 to 75 mg/kg/day) advised for mildly symptomatic or asymptomatic cases is safer, but should not be used for more than 5 successive days with a rest period of 1 wk or more between courses. While the diagnostic CaEDTA test (75 to 100 mg/kg over 1 day only) is safe in asymptomatic persons, CaEDTA probably should not be given therapeutically in non-life-threatening situations when acute renal disease is present.

Serious reactions to CaEDTA include rising BUN, proteinuria, microscopic hematuria, shedding of renal tubular epithelial cells in urine, hypercalcemia, fever, and diarrhea. Renal toxicity, which is dose-related, is usually reversible. Side effects are probably due to depletion of zinc. **PCA** is *contraindicated* in renal disease and penicillin sensitivity. Patients on PCA must be monitored weekly for side reactions (eg, diffuse erythematous rashes, angioneurotic edema, neutropenia, and proteinuria), which are reversible if the drug is stopped promptly. **BAL** should not be given in the presence of severe hepatocellular injury, but it may be given cau-

TABLE 30–4. DOSAGE SCHEDULE FOR CHELATING AGENTS*

Combined BAL-CaEDTA

Dosage: BAL[†] 3–5 mg/kg/dose IM q 4 h; CaEDTA[‡] 25 mg/kg/dose IM

Administration: For the first dose, inject only BAL IM deep; beginning 4 h later and q 4 h thereafter for 5 to 7 days, inject BAL and CaEDTA simultaneously at separate and deep IM sites; rotate injection sites.

CaEDTA Only

Dosage: 50–75 mg/kg/dose IM divided q 12 h

Administration: IM injection simpler in children, but if IV route is preferred as in adults, infuse each dose over a 6-h period; allow 2 to 3 wk between each 3- to 5-day course of therapy.

Succimer (DMSA)[§]

Dosage: 10 mg/kg q 8 h for 5 days; then q 12 h for 2 wk

Administration: Recommended treatment course is 19 days; the continuing therapy at reduced frequency after the initial 5 days eliminates the rebound rise of blood lead levels during treatment and reduces the rebound after therapy ends. Blood lead levels should be monitored at least once weekly after therapy to determine if a repeat course is indicated. A minimum of 2 wk between courses is recommended.

Penicillamine

Dosage: Up to 20–30 mg/kg/day for long-term oral therapy; in adults, 250 mg qid not to exceed 40 mg/kg/day

Administration: Give entire daily dose on empty stomach 2 h before breakfast; contents of capsule may be mixed in a small amount of chilled fruit or fruit juice immediately prior to administration.

---

* See text for critical aspects of supportive care and precautions with chelating agents.

† BAL (dimercaprol). The dosage recommended for adults by the FDA is 2.5 mg/kg/dose q 4 h.

‡ CaEDTA. Edetate calcium disodium, available in 20% solution. For IM use, add sufficient procaine to yield a final concentration of 0.5% procaine. IM injection is more convenient in children and permits better control of IV fluids, a vital consideration in cases of encephalopathy. If given IV in combination with IM BAL, infuse the total daily dose (150 mg/kg) over 24-h period and monitor ECG continuously.

§ DMSA = meso 2,3-dimercaptosuccinic acid, also known as succimer. Approved for use in children with blood levels > 45 µg/dL.

** Penicillamine (PCA), available in 250- and 125-mg capsules. Classified as an investigational drug by the FDA when used to treat lead poisoning; see recommendation of AMA Council on Drugs.

Adapted from Chisolm Jr JJ: "Increased lead absorption and acute lead poisoning," in *Current Pediatric Therapy*, Vol. 9, edited by SS Gellis and BM Kagan. Philadelphia, WB Saunders Company, 1980; used with permission.

---

tiously early in oliguric, encephalopathic patients. BAL can induce moderate to severe acute intravascular hemolysis in patients with G6PD deficiency. Unlike CaEDTA and PCA, BAL may *not* be given concurrently with medicinal iron. Contraindications to the use of *any* chelating agent in asymptomatic persons include the concurrent presence of liver or kidney disease. In severely symptomatic cases, the risks of chelation therapy must be weighed carefully. None of these drugs should be given for prophylactic purposes to lead workers or when any patient is concurrently overexposed to lead, as they can cause a net increase in the absorption of lead present in the GI tract. *Long-term treatment requires reducing exposure to lead.*

IRON POISONING

Because of the wide distribution of iron **(Fe)** preparations, ingestion of Fe-containing products is a common but rarely lethal problem. Elemental Fe has a toxic effect on the GI, cardiovascular, and central nervous systems. The oral lethal dose of elemental Fe ranges from 200 to 250 mg/kg, but as little as 130 mg of elemental Fe has been fatal. There are > 100 commercial Fe preparations on the market; however, ferrous sulfate (20% elemental Fe), ferrous fumarate (33% elemental Fe), and ferrous gluconate (12% elemental Fe) are most widely prescribed. Moreover, Fe is compounded with multiple vitamins for both adults and children. Of note is the re-

TABLE 30–5. SERUM IRON LEVELS*

Serum Levels (µg/dL)	Toxicity
0–100	Normal
100–350	Definite poisoning; mild toxicity
350–500	Serious toxicity
500–1000	Extreme toxicity
> 1000	Potentially lethal

* 2 to 4 h postingestion.

Modified from *Medical Toxicology* by MJ Ellenhorn and P Barceloux. New York, Elsevier, 1987, p 1025. Copyright 1987 by Elsevier Science Publishing Co., Inc.

markable safety record of children's chewable vitamins containing Fe—no deaths and virtually no symptoms have been reported. On the basis of body weight, < 20 mg elemental Fe/kg is nontoxic, 20 to 60 mg elemental Fe/kg is mild to moderately toxic, and 200 to 250 mg/kg is life-threatening.

The widespread availability of measuring serum Fe concentration favors this in assessing potential toxicity (see TABLE 30–5). If the patient has already received deferoxamine, the laboratory should be notified so that the serum determination can be modified appropriately. Gastric fluid, when tested with a solution of 30% hydrogen peroxide and distilled water, will produce color if Fe is present, ranging from light-orange to dark-red depending upon the amount of Fe.

Diarrhea, vomiting, leukocytosis, and hyperglycemia are associated with serum Fe concentrations > 350 µg/dL. If any one of these findings is positive, the level will likely exceed 350. If no symptoms develop in the first 6 h, the patient is at minimal risk.

There are 4 characteristic stages of iron toxicity. In **stage I**, which occurs within 6 h, vomiting, explosive diarrhea, irritability, abdominal pain, seizures, lethargy, and coma may be present. Irritation of GI mucosa may lead to hemorrhagic gastritis. Tachypnea, tachycardia, hypotension, and metabolic acidosis may also occur when serum Fe levels are high. Shock or coma in the first 6 h is a grave prognostic sign. During **stage II** (within 10 to 14 h of ingestion), there is a latent period of up to 24 h of deceptive improvement. In **stage III** (12 to 48 h postingestion), shock, hypoperfusion, and hypoglycemia may be present. Serum Fe levels may be normal. Elevated ALT (SGPT) due to liver damage, fever, leukocytosis, bleeding disorders, inverted T waves on the ECG, disorientation, restlessness, lethargy, convulsions, coma, shock, acidosis, and death may oc-

cur. There may be a **stage IV** 2 to 5 wk later if late complications due to pyloric, antral, or intestinal obstruction, hepatic cirrhosis, or CNS damage occur.

Whenever possible, serum Fe should be determined promptly. If the serum Fe exceeds 110 µg/dL but is < 350 µg/dL, it is highly unlikely that any free Fe exists, and the patient need not be hospitalized unless symptoms are present. If the serum Fe is > 350 µg/dL or if symptoms are present, hospitalization may be necessary.

Treatment

Initially, a vigorous effort to remove the Fe from the stomach should be initiated. If the patient is awake and alert, emesis should be induced with ipecac syrup; in the hospital, apomorphine can be used IM or s.c. Gastric lavage with a large-bore tube can be carried out with 5% sodium bicarbonate as the wash solution. Activated charcoal does not absorb Fe and should not be used.

Deferoxamine therapy should be instituted in (1) any patient with a serum Fe level ≥ 350 µg/dL and evidence of GI symptoms, (2) any patient with a serum Fe level ≥ 500 µg/dL, and (3) any symptomatic patient when blood Fe levels are not available.

In a normotensive patient, the dose of deferoxamine is 1 gm IM regardless of the patient's age, followed by 1 gm q 4 to 12 h up to 6 gm/day depending on clinical signs and laboratory response to treatment. However, in the face of hypoperfusion or severe acidosis, the drug should be given IV not to exceed 15 mg/kg/h. In massive overdose this may not be adequate, as 1 gm deferoxamine chelates only 85 mg of Fe. Under such circumstances, peritoneal dialysis, hemodialysis, or exchange transfusion should be considered. Exchange transfusion is particularly effective and is important if renal shutdown develops.

Follow-up for potential sequelae should be carefully planned at 2 to 6 wk postingestion. There may be the paradox of Fe-deficiency anemia due to GI blood losses and chelation of Fe stores. The corrosive effects on the GI tract are predominantly gastric and pyloric stenosis or stricture. Radiographs, including an upper GI series, should be delayed until at least 6 wk postingestion.

Prognosis is good. Mortality is about 10% when shock and coma develop; overall it is about 1%.

HYDROCARBON POISONING

Every year the ingestion of petroleum distillates (eg, gasoline, kerosene, paint thinners) and halogenated hydrocarbons (eg, carbon tetrachloride, ethylene dichloride) is responsible for > 25,000 poisonings in children < 5 yr; but most of the deaths from acute cardiovascular arrest as a result of accidental poisonings occur in the teenage years. Viscosity and surface tension are the most important physical properties of hydrocarbon derivatives, as they determine the degree of hazard of their aspiration—small quantities can spread rapidly over large surface areas of the lung. The lower the viscosity, the higher the risk of pulmonary aspiration, with certain additives contributing to other toxic effects. Mineral seal oil (used in products such as furniture polish) is the most dangerous of the more viscous liquids in its potential for producing aspiration pneumonia.

Clinical Course

Symptoms and signs relate chiefly to the respiratory system, GI tract, and CNS. Initially, the victim coughs and chokes, even with only one small taste. Cyanosis, breath-holding, vomiting, and persistent coughing may then occur. Older children may complain of a burning sensation in the stomach and vomit spontaneously. CNS symptoms include lethargy, coma, and convulsions. These effects are usually dose-related and are most severe with lighter fluid and mineral seal oil ingestions.

In animal experiments, hydrocarbon in the respiratory tract is at least 140 times more toxic than hydrocarbon in the GI tract. If this finding were applied to humans, death of a child could occur with 350 mL in the stomach but with only 2.5 mL in the lungs. In severe cases, cardiac dilation, atrial fibrillation, and fatal ventricular fibrillation may occur. Damage to kidneys and bone marrow has been described. When death occurs from pneumonitis, it usually does so within 24 h.

Resolution of uncomplicated pneumonia takes about 1 wk except when due to mineral seal oil ingestion, when it usually takes 5 to 6 wk.

Laboratory Findings

A chest x-ray is the single most important diagnostic test and is best obtained $1\frac{1}{2}$ to 2 h postingestion unless major symptoms are present. More severe cases have visible x-ray evidence of hydrocarbon aspiration pneumonia within 2 h; 90% of all cases with pneumonia have positive films by 6 to 18 h; however, no new cases develop after 24 h. A WBC count, WBC differential, and urinalysis may help to identify secondary infection and renal involvement. Blood hydrocarbon levels have no practical value. If there are no signs or symptoms (tachypnea, tachycardia, cough or rales) of respiratory distress, the child can usually be managed at home; if the adult escapes fibrillation, the same holds true. When there is evidence of pulmonary involvement, determining arterial blood gas levels will aid both diagnosis and treatment.

Treatment

At home, once respiratory status is determined, any contaminated clothing is removed, and the skin is washed. A glass of milk may be given to dilute the ingested material and reduce stomach irritation.

Early pneumonitis is chemical in nature and does not respond to antibiotics.

Supportive therapy with IV fluids and O₂ is appropriate. Corticosteroids generally are not effective. Controlled studies of corticosteroids have not been done with a large series of life-threatening cases; however, there is some suggestion that they may negatively affect the patient's immunologic response.

When a hydrocarbon containing another poisonous substance is ingested, treatment must be directed at both poisons and at evacuation of the stomach via either emesis or lavage.

CARDIOPULMONARY RESUSCITATION (CPR)

(See also ASPHYXIA AND RESUSCITATION in Ch. 27)

Special Problems in Resuscitating Infants and Children

Pediatric CPR poses major difficulties in both basic and advanced life support. Unfortunately, survival is poor in infants and children (90 to 97%

TABLE 30–6. CAUSES OF PEDIATRIC CARDIOPULMONARY ARREST*

Motor vehicle accidents°	Smoke inhalation
Drowning°	Sudden infant death syndrome
Burns°	Airway obstruction and asphyxiation from foreign bodies
Firearms°	Infections (respiratory tract or systemic)
Poisoning°	Congenital heart disease

*Injuries (indicated by the ° symbol) cause 44% of all deaths in children between ages 1 and 14 yr.
Adapted from *Journal of the American Medical Association* 1986; 255(21):2841–3044. Copyright 1986, American Medical Association.

mortality for out-of-hospital cardiac arrests), and neurologic outcome in survivors is often severely compromised. To address the problems described on the following pages, a *standardized approach* has been developed (see A STANDARDIZED RESUSCITATION PROTOCOL, below).

Weight must be estimated accurately to allow calculation of drug doses. Weights may range from < 2 kg in a premature newborn to > 60 kg in a 16-yr-old adolescent. In critical settings, a drug dose must be calculated in *milligrams*, then converted to *milliliters* based on the specific concentration of that drug. This process often delays timely intervention and can result in serious errors. **The rate of cardiac compression** varies from 80 to 120/min, with 3 separate techniques (2 hands, 1 hand, or 2 fingers on the sternum), depending on patient size. **The ventilation rate**, while identical to the 5:1 ratio for two-person adult CPR, varies with the age-determined rate of cardiac compression. **Choosing appropriate-sized airway equipment** is complex, yet vital. Five sizes of airways, 6 sizes of masks (cuffed and uncuffed), 3 sizes of ventilation bags, 4 sizes of laryngoscope blades, 9 sizes of endotracheal tubes, and 6 sizes of suction catheters are required to meet the emergency needs of the entire pediatric population (see Airway under ADVANCED LIFE SUPPORT, below).

Major Contrasts Between Pediatric and Adult CPR

Some ½ to ⅔ of pediatric victims are < 1 yr of age, and most are < 6 mo. The **etiology** of cardiac arrests in children is very varied. The most frequent causes are listed in TABLE 30–6 and contrast markedly with those in adults (which are almost always secondary to severe diffuse coronary artery disease, most commonly with a superimposed malignant ventricular tachyarrhythmia). In children, hypoxemia and airway difficulties are major precipitants, resulting in bradyarrhythmias and asystole, while only 10% of arrhythmias are ventricular tachyar-

rhythmias. Thus a different approach is required in children, and *there is no role for routine rapid defibrillation*, as malignant ventricular arrhythmias are an unlikely cause.

Upper airway anatomy is different in children. The head is large with a small face, mandible, and external nares, and the neck is relatively short. The tongue is large relative to the mouth, and the larynx lies higher in the neck and is angled more anteriorly. The epiglottis is long, and the most narrow portion is below the vocal cords at the cricoid ring, allowing the use of uncuffed endotracheal tubes in children (unlike in adults), thereby minimizing trauma to the sensitive mucosal lining of the airway.

Children are **more susceptible to heat loss** than adults because of a larger surface area relative to body mass and less subcutaneous tissue. A "neutral external thermal environment" is crucial during CPR and may range from 36.5° C (97.7° F) in a newborn to 35° C (95° F) in a child. Hypothermia with core temperature < 35° C increases O_2 consumption and cardiac output, and adds to overall morbidity. As temperature falls, there comes a point when shivering ceases, and O_2 consumption and heart rate *decrease*.

Treatment of the precipitating disease must be considered immediately following **initial assessment**; eg, replacement of blood loss in patients with multiple trauma, removal of foreign bodies in choking patients, or aggressive management of septic shock in patients with meningococcemia.

During the entire phase of CPR, the team should be coordinated and assess the need for additional expertise or transfer to a tertiary care facility.

BASIC LIFE SUPPORT

One must establish that cardiorespiratory arrest has occurred, then rapidly assess and stabilize the airway to eliminate obstruction and provide suctioning, ventilation, and oxygenation (see

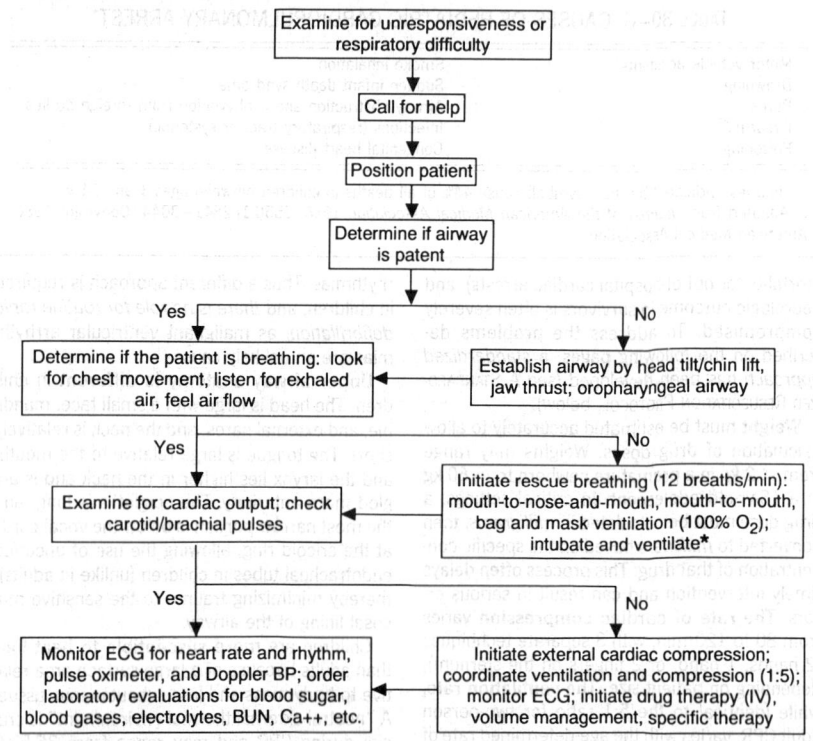

Examine for unresponsiveness or respiratory difficulty

↓

Call for help

↓

Position patient

↓

Determine if airway is patent

Yes ←→ **No**

Determine if the patient is breathing: look for chest movement, listen for exhaled air, feel air flow ← Establish airway by head tilt/chin lift, jaw thrust; oropharyngeal airway

Yes / **No**

Examine for cardiac output; check carotid/brachial pulses ← Initiate rescue breathing (12 breaths/min): mouth-to-nose-and-mouth, mouth-to-mouth, bag and mask ventilation (100% O_2); intubate and ventilate*

Yes / **No**

Monitor ECG for heart rate and rhythm, pulse oximeter, and Doppler BP; order laboratory evaluations for blood sugar, blood gases, electrolytes, BUN, Ca^{++}, etc. ← Initiate external cardiac compression; coordinate ventilation and compression (1:5); monitor ECG; initiate drug therapy (IV), volume management, specific therapy

*Disposable masks are currently being recommended for emergency ventilation instead of mouth-to-mouth resuscitation because of the risk of AIDS.

FIG. 30–5. **Management sequence for pediatric life support.** (Adapted from Ludwig S: "Life support emergencies," in *Textbook of Pediatric Emergency Medicine*, edited by G Fleisher. Baltimore, Williams & Wilkins, 1988; used with permission.)

FIG. 30–5). Obstruction may be relieved with the Heimlich maneuver, but the technique varies with patient size. If no respiratory effort is present, positive pressure breathing must be initiated, with breaths delivered over 1 to 1½ sec to provide effective ventilation while minimizing ventilatory pressure that may result in gastric distention. Next, the brachial or carotid pulse is palpated, and if absent, an appropriate external cardiac compression technique and rate is started over the lower ⅓ of the sternum (see TABLE 30–7). CPR is continued uninterrupted, except for pauses for ventilation in the unintubated child, until the patient responds or efforts are stopped. Chest compressions must always be accompanied by rescue breathing, closely observing for adequate chest excursion, adequate

pulses, pupillary reactions to light, and avoidance of gastric distention. If the latter occurs, a nasogastric tube should be inserted. The positions for chest compressions are shown in FIG. 30–6. *One must ensure that the lower ⅓ of the sternum is used, to avoid trauma to the liver.*

If there is no response to these basic measures, then advanced techniques must be instituted rapidly.

ADVANCED LIFE SUPPORT

Airway

Airway and mask must be of appropriate size (see TABLE 30–7). An oropharyngeal airway should be inserted in infants and children using a tongue depressor to hold the tongue on the floor

TABLE 30–7. GUIDE TO PEDIATRIC RESUSCITATION—MECHANICAL MEASURES

Age (yr)	Prem	Term	6–12 mo	1	2	3	4	5	6	7	8	9	10	11	12	13	14	15	16
Weight (kg)	≤2	3.5	7	10	12	14	16	18	20	22	25	28	30	35	40	45	50	55	60
Ventilation rate/min *Represents a 25% increase in rate (50% for Prem and Term) for head injury and asphyxia	40 / 60*	40 / 60*	24 / 30*	24 / 30*	24 / 30*	20 / 25*	20 / 25*	20 / 25*	20 / 25*	20 / 25*	20 / 25*	16 / 20*	16 / 20*	16 / 20*	16 / 20*	16 / 20*	16 / 20*	16 / 20*	16 / 20*
Compression rate/min	120	120	120	120	120	100	100	100	100	100	100	80	80	80	80	80	80	80	80
Compression technique	Two fingers or thumb compression, hands around chest →						→ One hand →						→ Two hands →						
Airway size (Portex) in cm	000 3.5	000 3.5	00 5	00 5	0 6	0 6	7	7	7	7	7	7	7	7	7	8	8	8	8
Masks in Laerdal sizes or use equivalent	Circular 00 0/1		Rendell-Baker type 1		Rendell-Baker type 2		→ Dome cuff mask #3 →						→ Dome cuff mask #4 →						
Ventilation bag with reservoir for 100% O₂ delivery	Infant Laerdal 240 mL →				→ Child Laerdal 500 mL →						→ Adult Laerdal 1600 mL →								
Laryngoscope blade size	Miller 0 straight blade or equivalent	1	1	1 Straight or curved blade	1	1	2	2 Curved or straight blade	2	2	3	3	3	3	3 Curved or straight blade	3	3	3	3
ETT size (Portex) in mm	2.5	3	3.5	4	4.5	4.5	5	5	5.5	5.5	6	6	6	6	6.5	6.5	6.5	6.5	7
Suction catheter — Direct oropharyngeal	10 Fr	10 Fr	Pediatric tonsil suction →						→ Adult tonsil suction →										
Suction catheter — Through ETT	6 Fr	8 Fr	8 Fr	8 Fr	→ 10 Fr →						→ 14 Fr →								
Defibrillation (watt-seconds) — Dose (2 ws/kg)	3	7	10	20	20	30	30	30	50	50	50	50	70	70†	70†	100†	100†	200†	200†
Pediatric paddles (based on HP43100A defibrillator) Frequency	If no response, give maximum dose × 2																		
Max. dose (4 ws/kg)	10	20	30	50	50	50	70	70	100	100	100	100	100	150†	150†	200†	200†	300†	300†
Cardioversion (watt-seconds) — Synchronized shock (0.2 ws/kg)	2	2	2	2	2	3	3	3	5	5	5	5	7	7†	7†	10†	10†	10†	10†
Pediatric paddles (based on HP43100A defibrillator) Frequency	Increase dose slowly at subsequent attempts, to maximum																		
Max. dose (1 ws/kg)	2	5	10	10	10	10	20	20	20	20	20	30	30	30	50†	50†	50†	50†	70†

ETT = endotracheal tube; Fr. = French; ws = watt-seconds. † Use adult paddles.

Courtesy of Dr. B Paes and Dr. M Sullivan, the Departments of Pediatrics and Medicine, St. Joseph's Hospital and McMaster University, Hamilton, Ontario, Canada.

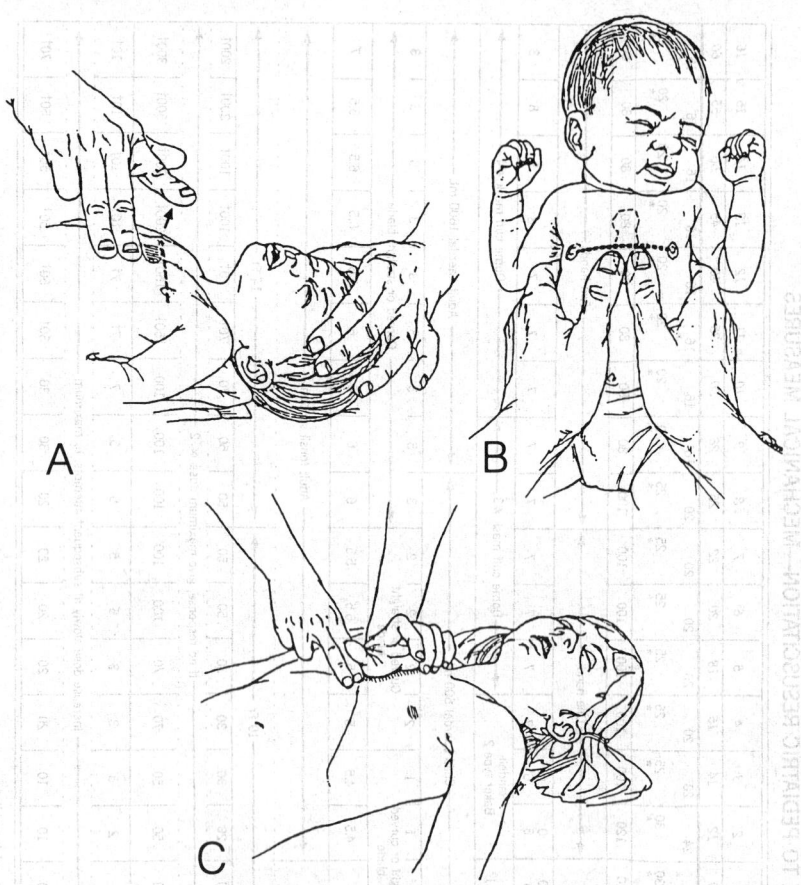

FIG. 30–6. **Chest compression techniques.** *A*, Two-finger position for neonates and infants. Note that fingers should be maintained in the upright position during compression. In premature infants, the technique shown will result in *too low a position*, ie, at or below the xiphoid; the correct position is determined at one finger's breadth above the xiphoid. *B*, Side-by-side thumb placement (preferred) in neonates and small infants whose chests can be encircled. *C*, Hand position in a child. (From American Heart Association: Standards and guidelines for CPR. *Journal of the American Medical Association* 1986; 255:2958, 2972. Copyright 1986, American Medical Association.)

of the mouth. If a depressor is not available, invert the airway on mouth insertion, using the posterior portion of the curved body as a tongue depressor; as the airway reaches the posterior oropharynx, rotate it into its proper position. Oral airways should not be used in the awake patient. Effective use of the ventilation bag requires a good seal between mask and face. Cuff masks are recommended for children > 5 yr. Early endotracheal intubation is the technique of choice to improve oxygenation, to control the airway, and to prevent aspiration. The correct size of laryngoscope blade reduces the risk of trauma to the oropharynx of young children. A straight blade in younger children is generally easier to use than a curved blade, although both are used in different centers. The endotracheal tube (which in the larger adolescent sizes should be cuffed to create a good seal) and the suction catheter should both be of correct size for direct oropharyngeal suction and to fit through the internal diameter of each endotracheal tube. (A complete range of sizes is imperative and should be immediately available.)

Vascular Access

Establishing vascular access is a priority in advanced CPR but is also difficult. It is important to acquire skill in achieving vascular access through a variety of sites, because sometimes (eg, following burns or trauma) less commonly used approaches may be necessary. Fortunately, key drugs can be given through the endotracheal tube (see Emergency Drugs, below, and TABLE 30–8). While central venous cannulation is theoretically preferable, it is difficult to achieve in inexperienced hands; therefore, femoral vein access and saphenous vein cutdown are recommended approaches. Intraosseous needle placement in the tibial bone marrow space in children < 3 yr old allows effective delivery of blood, colloid, and crystalloid infusions and of drugs such as dopamine and dobutamine. However, the safety of delivery of calcium chloride and hypertonic sodium bicarbonate by this route has yet to be established.

Emergency Drugs

After the patient has been intubated, ventilated, and oxygenated, cardiac rhythm should be determined. Ninety percent of the dysrhythmias seen in pediatric arrests are severe bradyarrhythmias and asystole (only 10% are ventricular tachyarrhythmias). Drug doses recommended during pediatric resuscitation are given (by *volume*) in TABLE 30–8. Epinephrine, atropine, naloxone, and glucose remain principal agents in CPR (when vascular access is inadequate, these drugs except glucose can be given through the endotracheal tube). Bretylium is used as a second-line drug after lidocaine for ventricular arrhythmias, although sufficient data on efficacy in children are still lacking. The use of sodium bicarbonate and calcium chloride has been de-emphasized except in clearly defined circumstances, eg, hyperkalemia, hypocalcemia, hypermagnesemia, calcium channel blocker overdose, and severe, persistent metabolic acidosis despite adequate ventilation.

It is always important to search for and treat the underlying pathophysiologic disorders that precipitated the cardiopulmonary arrest. This may include **volume replacement** with normal saline, colloid, crystalloids, or blood, eg, for trauma or burns. Fluid therapy, however, is difficult for those unaccustomed to pediatric CPR, as children have a smaller blood volume, and appropriate volume challenges must be given cautiously to avoid fluid overload.

Defibrillation and Cardioversion

Defibrillation is infrequently required, as underlying ventricular fibrillation is rare and should be documented prior to countershock. When defibrillation is used, an appropriate paddle size must be determined (neonates, infants, and young children need "pediatric" paddles; older children and adolescents should have "adult" paddles), and an appropriate "dose" of shock delivered. However, many defibrillators commonly used for pediatric CPR are standardized with large increments in the energy settings, and it is not possible to adjust the shock accurately, based on body weight. Thus, defibrillators in emergency rooms, intensive care units, or any area used to resuscitate children should be evaluated for the number and range of energy settings, and equipment upgrades should be made as appropriate.

Cardioversion, used in the treatment of symptomatic rapid supraventricular and ventricular rhythms, is very difficult in the neonate and young child, as the **"energy dose"** in watt-sec (joules)/kg is usually $1/2$ to $1/10$ the usual adult dose (see TABLE 30–7). It is probably best to start at the lowest recommended dose, with stepwise increases until the desired effect is attained.

Postarrest Assessment

Following successful CPR, subsequent care is complex and often must address the pathophysiology of multi-organ dysfunction. It is important to assess body temperature and maintain a neutral thermal environment, monitor urine output with an indwelling urinary catheter, and insert a nasogastric tube (particularly if the patient is intubated). Evaluation of neurologic function, maintenance of metabolic homeostasis, management of cardiovascular stability, and ongoing treatment of the precipitating condition are prime concerns and are best managed in a tertiary care facility.

Assessment of heart rate is mandatory. *Bradycardia in a distressed child is an ominous sign of impending cardiac arrest.* Newborns and young children tend to develop bradycardia with

TABLE 30–8. GUIDE TO PEDIATRIC RESUSCITATION—PHARMACOLOGIC MEASURES

Age (yr)	Prem	Term	6–12 mo	1	2	3	4	5	6	7	8	9	10	11	12	13	14	15	16
Weight (kg)	2	3.5	7	10	12	14	16	18	20	22	25	28	30	35	40	45	50	55	60
DRUGS FOR BRADYARRHYTHMIAS																			
Atropine (0.1 mg/mL) Dose IV/ETT mL (0.02 mg/kg)	0.5	1.0	1.5	2.0	2.5	3.0	3.0	3.5	4.0	4.5	5	5	6	7	8	9	10	10	10
Frequency	Repeat same dose q 5 min to maximum dose →																		
Max. cum. dose IV mL	5	5	5	5	10	10	10	10	15	15	15	15	20	20	20	20	20	20	20
Epinephrine 1:10,000 (0.1 mg/mL) *Loading* Dose IV/ETT mL (0.01–0.03 mg/kg)	0.5	1.0	1.5	2.0	1.0	1.5	1.5	2.0	2.0	2.5	2.5	3.0	3.0	3.5	4.0	4.5	5.0	5.5	6.0
Frequency	Repeat dose at 5-min intervals as required →																		
Infusion Final conc.	Add 10 mL (1 mg) to 90 mL 5% D/W = 10 µg/mL										Add 25 mL (2.5 mg) to 25 mL 5% D/W = 50 µg/mL								
Dose IV mL/h (0.1 µg/kg/min)	1	2	4	6	7	8	9	11	12	13	13	3	3	4	5	5	6	7	7
Frequency	Titrate to max. dose. Once achieved, increase conc. of solution to deliver smaller vol. of fluid																		
Max. dose IV mL/h (1.0 µg/kg/min)	10	20	40	60	70	80	90	110	120	130	130	30	30	40	50	50	60	70	70
Isoproterenol (1 mg/5 mL) Final conc.	Add 5 mL (1 mg) to 95 mL 5% D/W = 10 µg/mL										Add 10 mL (2 mg) to 40 mL 5% D/W = 40 µg/mL								
Dose IV mL/h (≤ 7 yr: 0–1 µg/kg/min; ≥ 8 yr: 2 µg/min)	1	2	4	6	7	8	9	11	12	13	3	3	3	3	3	3	3	3	3
Frequency	Titrate to max. dose. Once achieved, increase conc. of solution to deliver smaller vol. of fluid										Titrate to maximum dose								
Max. dose IV mL/h (≤7 yr: 1.0 µg/kg/min; ≥ 8 yr: 10 µg/min)*	10	20	40	60	70	80	90	110	120	130	15*	15*	15*	15*	15*	15*	15*	15*	15*

ELECTROLYTES

Sodium bicarbonate (4.2% + 8.4%)

Final conc.	4.2% (0.5 mmol/kg) ——— 8.4% (1 mmol/kg)
Dose IV mL (1–2 mmol/kg)	8 · 14 · 28 · 10 · 12 · 14 · 16 · 18 · 20 · 22 · 25 · 28 · 30 · 35 · 40 · 45 · 50 · 55 · 60
Frequency	Standard dose repeatable q 10 min of continued arrest
Max. cum. dose	Dependent on measured base deficit at frequent intervals

Calcium chloride (10%)

Dose IV/mL (20 mg/kg)	0.4 · 0.7 · 1.5 · 2.0 · 2.5 · 3.0 · 3.5 · 4.0 · 4.5 · 5 · 5 · 5 · 5 · 5 · 5 · 5 · 5 · 5 · 5
Frequency	Repeat × 1 in 10 min
Max. cum. dose	Based on measured calcium deficit

AGENTS FOR HYPOTENSION

Dopamine (40 mg/mL)

Final conc.	Add 1.5 mL (60 mg) to 98 mL 5% D/W = 600 µg/mL ——► Add 5 mL (200 mg) to 95 mL 5% D/W = 2000 µg/mL
Dose IV mL/h (5.0 µg/kg/min)	1 · 2 · 4 · 5 · 6 · 7 · 8 · 9 · 10 · 11 · 4 · 4 · 4 · 5 · 6 · 7 · 8 · 9
Frequency	Titrate to maximum dose
Max. dose IV mL/h (20 µg/kg/min)	4 · 7 · 14 · 20 · 24 · 28 · 32 · 36 · 40 · 44 · 15 · 17 · 18 · 21 · 24 · 27 · 30 · 33 · 36

Albumin (5% [50 mg/mL] + 25% [250 mg/mL])

Final conc.	5% [50 mg/mL] ——— 25% [250 mg/mL]
Dose IV mL (0.5 gm/kg)	20 · 35 · 70 · 20 · 24 · 28 · 32 · 36 · 40 · 44 · 50 · 56 · 60 · 70 · 80 · 90 · 100 · 110 · 120
Frequency	Repeatable depending on evidence of hypoperfusion

Blood (whole or packed cells)

Dose IV mL (10 mL/kg)	20 · 35 · 70 · 100 · 120 · 140 · 160 · 180 · 200 · 220 · 250 · 280 · 300 · 350 · 400 · 450 · 500 · 550 · 600
Frequency	Repeatable depending on evidence of hypoperfusion

Plasma (fresh frozen or stored)

Dose IV mL (10 mL/kg)	20 · 35 · 70 · 100 · 120 · 140 · 160 · 180 · 200 · 220 · 250 · 280 · 300 · 350 · 400 · 450 · 500 · 550 · 600
Frequency	Repeatable depending on evidence of hypoperfusion

0.9% NaCl

Dose IV mL (10 mL/kg)	20 · 35 · 70 · 100 · 120 · 140 · 160 · 180 · 200 · 220 · 250 · 280 · 300 · 350 · 400 · 450 · 500 · 550 · 600
Frequency	Repeatable depending on evidence of hypoperfusion

(Continued)

TABLE 30–8. GUIDE TO PEDIATRIC RESUSCITATION—PHARMACOLOGIC MEASURES (Cont'd)

Age (yr)	Prem	Term	6–12 mo	1	2	3	4	5	6	7	8	9	10	11	12	13	14	15	16
Weight (kg)	2	3.5	7	10	12	14	16	18	20	22	25	28	30	35	40	45	50	55	60
DRUGS FOR TACHYARRHYTHMIAS																			
Bretylium tosylate (50 mg/mL) — Dose IV mL (5 mg/kg)	0.2	0.4	0.7	1.0	1.0	1.5	1.5	2	2	2	2.5	2.8	3	3.5	4	4.5	5	5.5	6
Frequency	If ventricular fibrillation persists, give double above dose followed by countershock																		
Max. cum. dose IV mL (30 mg/kg)	1.2	2	4	6	7	8.5	9.5	11	12	13	15	17	18	21	24	27	30	33	36
Digoxin (0.05 mg/mL + 0.25 mg/mL) — Final conc.	← 0.05 mg/mL →			← 0.25 mg/mL →															
Load dose IV mL 10–20 µg/kg = 1/2 total dose	0.4	1.4	2.6	0.75	0.9	0.9	1.0	1.1	1.2	1.3	1.5	1.7	1.8	2.0	2.0	2.0	2.0	2.0	2.0
Frequency	Repeat 1/2 the above dose 8 h + 16 h later to complete total digitalizing dose IV																		
Maintenance dose IV	← 4–8 µg/kg/day in 2 divided doses →							← 0.125–0.25 mg/day in 2 divided doses →											
Lidocaine (20 mg/mL) — Load dose IV/ETT mL (1 mg/kg)	0.1	0.1	0.4	0.5	0.6	0.7	0.8	0.9	1.0	1.0	1.2	1.4	1.5	1.7	2.0	2.2	2.5	2.7	3.0
Final conc.	Add 5 mL (100 mg) to 45 mL of 5% D/W = 2 mg/mL										Add 25 mL (500 mg) to 25 mL of 5% D/W = 10 mg/mL								
Dose IV mL/h (20 µg/kg/min)	1	2	4	6	7	8	10	11	12	13	3	3	4	4	5	5	6	7	7
Frequency	Titrate to maximum dose																		
Max. dose IV mL/h (50 µg/kg/min)	3	5	10	15	18	21	24	27	30	33	7	8	9	10	12	13	15	16	18
Verapamil (2.5 mg/mL) (not with WPW, infants < 6 mo, or with β blockers) — Final conc.	2.5 mg/mL																		
Dose IV mL (0.1 mg/kg)	–	–	–	0.4	0.5	0.5	0.6	0.7	0.8	0.9	1	1.1	1.2	1.4	1.6	1.8	2.0	2.2	2.4
Frequency	Repeat same dose q 15 min to maximum																		
Max. cum. dose IV mL (0.3 mg/kg)	–	–	–	1.2	1.4	1.7	1.9	2.1	2.4	2.6	3	3.3	3.6	4.2	4.8	5.4	6.0	6.6	7.2

DRUGS FOR SEIZURES† (Continued)

Diazepam (Valium®) (10 mg/2 mL)

Final conc.: Add 1 mL (5 mg) to 19 mL of 0.9% NaCl = 0.25 mg/mL ——— 5 mg/mL ———

Dose in mL (0.2 mg/kg) IV mL (slow push)	1.6	2.8	6	8	10	11	13	14	16	17	1.0	1.0	1.5	1.5	2.0	2.0	2.0

Frequency: Repeat same dose q 15–30 min to maximum →

Max. cum. dose IV mL	10	15	20	20	20	30	30	40	40	2	2	3	3	4	4	4

Diazepam (Valium®) (rectal 10 mg/2 mL)

Final conc.: Add 1 mL (5 mg) to 9 mL of 0.9% NaCl = 0.5 mg/mL ——— 5 mg/mL ———

Dose in mL (0.2 mg/kg)	0.8	1.4	3	4	5	5.5	6.5	7	8	8.5	1	1	1.5	1.5	2	2	2

Frequency: Same dose repeatable q 5 min and load with long-term anticonvulsant →

Phenobarbital (30 mg/mL + 120 mg/mL)

Final conc.: —— 30 mg/mL —— ———— 120 mg/mL ————

Load dose IV mL (20 mg/kg) over 20 min	1.3	2.3	4.6	1.6	2.0	2.3	2.6	3	3.3	3.6	4.1	4.6	5	5	5	5	5	5

Maintenance dose IV: 3–5 mg/kg/day in divided doses depending on drug level →

Phenytoin (Dilantin®) (100 mg/2mL)

Final conc.: ———————— 50 mg/mL ————————

Load dose IV mL (≤7 yr: 20 mg/kg; ≥8 yr: 15 mg/kg) over 20 min	0.8	1.4	3	4	5	5.5	6.5	7	8	9	7.5	8.5	9	10.5	12	13.5	15	16.5	18

Maintenance dose IV: 4–8 mg/kg/day in divided doses depending on drug level →

(Continued)

TABLE 30–8. GUIDE TO PEDIATRIC RESUSCITATION—PHARMACOLOGIC MEASURES (Cont'd)

Age (yr)		Prem	Term	6–12 mo	1	2	3	4	5	6	7	8	9	10	11	12	13	14	15	16
Weight (kg)		2	3.5	7	10	12	14	16	18	20	22	25	28	30	35	40	45	50	55	60
MISCELLANEOUS AGENTS																				
Aminophylline (500 mg/10 mL)	*Loading* Final conc.	← 50 mg/mL →																		
	Load dose IV mL (≤7 yr: 7 mg/kg; ≥8 yr: 5–6 mg/kg) over 20 min	0.25	0.5	1.0	1.4	1.7	1.9	2.2	2.5	2.8	3.0	3.0	3.4	3.6	4.2	4.8	5.0	5.2	5.5	6.0
	Infusion Final conc.	← Add 2 mL (100 mg) to 98 mL 5% D/W = 1 mg/mL →										← Add 10 mL (500 mg) to 90 mL 5% D/W = 5 mg/mL →								
	Dose IV mL/h (≤7 yr: 1 mg/kg/h; ≥8 yr: 0.6–0.8 mg/kg/h)	–	–	7	10	12	14	16	18	20	22	4	4	5	5	6	6	6	7	7
	Max. dose IV mL/h	Dependent on theophylline level																		
Furosemide (Lasix®) (40 mg/4 mL)	Final conc.	← 10 mg/mL →																		
	Dose IV mL (1 mg/kg)	0.2	0.4	0.7	1.0	1.0	1.5	1.5	2	2	2	2.5	3	3	3.5	4	4.5	5	5.5	6
	Frequency	Repeat q 2–4 h as required																		
Hydrocortisone (100 mg/2 mL) + (250 mg/2 mL)	Final conc.	← 50 mg/mL →										← 125 mg/mL →								
	Load dose IV mL (10 mg/kg)	0.5	0.7	1.5	2	2.4	2.8	3.2	3.6	4	4.4	2	2.2	2.4	2.8	3.2	3.6	4	4.4	4.8
	Maintenance dose IV mL	As above, divided in 4 doses/day																		
Mannitol (20%)	Final conc.	← 0.2 gm/mL →																		
	Dose IV mL (0.5 gm/kg) / Rapid infusion	5	9	20	25	30	35	40	45	50	55	60	70	75	90	100	110	125	135	150
	Frequency	May be repeated as required. Consult tertiary care center.																		

Naloxone (0.4 mg/mL)															
Final conc.	0.4 mg/mL														
Dose IV/ETT mL (0.1 mg/kg)	0.5	0.8	1.7	2.5	3	3.5	4	4.5	5	5	5	5	5	5	5
Frequency	Repeat same dose q 5–10 min as required														

DRUGS FOR INHALATION

Racemic epinephrine (2.25%) (Vaponephrine®)															
Final conc.	Dose to be added to 3 mL of 0.9% NaCl for nebulization														
Dose in mL	0.1	0.1	0.5	0.5	0.5	0.5	0.5	0.5	0.5	0.5	0.5	0.5	0.5	0.5	0.5
Frequency	Repeat q 30 min as required														

Salbutamol (5 mg/mL)															
Final conc.	Dose to be added to 3 mL of 0.9% NaCl for nebulization														
Load in mL (0.02–0.03 mL/kg)	0.1	0.1	0.15	0.2	0.25	0.3	0.4	0.5	0.6	0.65	0.75	0.85	0.9	1.0	1.0
Maintenance (0.01 mL/kg)	0.1	0.1	0.1	0.1	0.1	0.15	0.2	0.2	0.25	0.25	0.3	0.34	0.34	0.34	0.34
Frequency	Repeat maintenance dose q 30 min to maximum dose														
Max. dose	0.1	0.2	0.4	0.6	0.7	0.8	0.9	1.0	1.2	1.3	1.5	1.5	1.8	2	2

ETT = endotracheal tube; WPW = Wolff-Parkinson-White syndrome.

* In severe unresponsive bradyarrhythmia, isoproterenol doses of up to 1.0 µg/kg/min may be tried.

† Intubate for respiratory depression or seizures > 30 min duration.

NOTES

1. Doses have been rounded off where necessary, to facilitate administration but avoid overdosage.
2. Loading doses may be followed by continuous infusion of the same drug if necessary.
3. Infusion rates are generally in mL/h. Drugs should be thoroughly mixed in a volume infusion burette and administered via IV pumps where available. Since rates on some infusion pumps do not exceed 99 mL/h, once a desired effect is obtained, concentration of the infused drug may be increased to allow drug delivery in a smaller volume.
4. Caution must be taken with some drugs; eg, verapamil is not recommended in WPW, in patients receiving β blockers, or in infants < 6 mo. However, treatment may be instituted following the advice and support of a tertiary care unit and under careful surveillance.
5. Drug levels should be assayed when appropriate to establish therapeutic levels and avoid overdosage.
6. Available drugs should be reviewed regularly. Medications in preloaded syringes are provided in defined volumes, set concentrations, and are graded in mL (although some are in mmol). Injecting small doses in neonatal and infant CPR may be difficult without experience and could result in drug errors.

Courtesy of Dr. B Paes and Dr. M Sullivan, Departments of Pediatrics and Medicine, St. Joseph's Hospital and McMaster University, Hamilton, Ontario, Canada.

hypoxemia, while older children tend initially to have tachycardia. In newborns, if the heart rate is < 80/min and not rising, then cardiac compression is recommended, which is a major difference from adult resuscitation (see FIG. 30–7). Tachyarrhythmias may similarly require intervention, particularly if evidence of hypoperfusion, heart failure, or CNS changes is present.

Synchronized cardioversion and/or drug therapy may be necessary to stabilize the patient. Hypoperfusion is suggested by urine output, which in the absence of renal disease should be 1 to 2 mL/kg/h but, if poor renal perfusion develops, may drop below 1 mL/kg/h. **Capillary filling deficit** suggests a reduction in cardiac output. An extremity (arm or leg) is lifted above the level of the heart and if > 3 sec are required to refill the capillary bed after blanching, then significant depression of cardiac output should be suspected and treated before changes in BP occur.

Evaluation of BP in very sick children varies significantly throughout the pediatric population. BP should be measured with an appropriate-sized cuff (see SCREENING PROCEDURES FOR INFANTS AND CHILDREN in Ch. 23). It is difficult to give an absolute normal lower limit of BP for each age group; evidence of hypoperfusion (ie, capillary refill, quality of distal pulses, urine output, level of consciousness, skin temperature) is critically important in evaluating the consequences of any level of BP. However, there are some useful guidelines for children > 2 yr of age: The lower level of normal systolic BP can be estimated as *70 plus twice the age in years.* Thus, at 6 yr systolic BP should be > 82 mm Hg. Normal systolic BP at the 50th percentile is 90 plus twice the age in years; eg, at 6 yr it would be 102 mm Hg (20 mm Hg higher than the lower norm). A drop in systolic BP of ≥ 10 mm Hg in any child, or a systolic BP < 50 mm Hg in children under 12 yr or < 80 mm Hg in children from 12 to 16 yr, is likely to represent serious hypotension requiring therapy. Even higher BP than these may represent hypotension if symptoms and signs of shock are present. Any bradyarrhythmia or tachyarrhythmia must similarly be evaluated for evidence of hypoperfusion, as this is the major factor in determining the need for volume expansion and/or pressor agents. When heart rate, perfusion, and/or BP remain unstable, vasoactive drugs (eg, epinephrine, dopamine, or dobutamine) as continuous infusions should be considered.

TECHNIQUES OF CARDIOPULMONARY RESUSCITATION (CPR)

(Techniques of CPR in neonates and children are also discussed under ASPHYXIA AND RESUSCITATION in Ch. 27)

In collapsed or unconscious persons, the state of ventilation and circulation must be determined immediately. An urgent systematic approach should ensure that only seconds elapse between recognizing arrest and intervening; speed, efficiency, and proper application of CPR directly relate to successful outcomes. While tissue anoxia for > 4 to 6 min can result in irreversible brain damage or death, wide variability in prognosis exists depending on age, cause of arrest, and clinical circumstances. Therefore, CPR must be continued until the cardiopulmonary system is stabilized, the patient is pronounced dead, or resuscitation cannot be continued (rescuer exhaustion). Following profound hypothermia or prolonged cold-water submersion, CPR should be continued until the total body core is rewarmed, since patients needing CPR for as long as 3 h have recovered.

Resuscitation efforts can be divided into basic life support **(BLS)**, which is immediately available, and advanced cardiac life support **(ACLS)**, which involves drug therapy, cardiac monitoring, and other techniques and equipment. The goal of BLS is to provide emergency ventilation and systemic perfusion. Thus, *after establishing unresponsiveness of the victim* (tap, shake, or shout), the rescuer calls for help, notes the exact time of arrest, and positions the victim horizontally on a hard surface. Then the initial 3 steps of the mnemonic A-B-C (see TABLE 30–9) that constitute BLS are carried out rapidly and in sequence. If the patient's cardiac rhythm is being monitored and VF develops, a precordial thump should be given (delivered with a clenched fist raised 10 to 30 cm [about 8 to 12 in.] above the sternum and brought down firmly). BLS and ACLS should then be immediately instituted. In an unmonitored arrest, BLS is used until ACLS is available.

A—Airway Opened

Opening the airway—A—is the first priority in respiratory inadequacy (labored, noisy breathing) and in BLS for respiratory or cardiac arrest. Sometimes A is all that is needed to restore spontaneous breathing (B) and circulation (C); in these instances, cardiac compression is not needed.

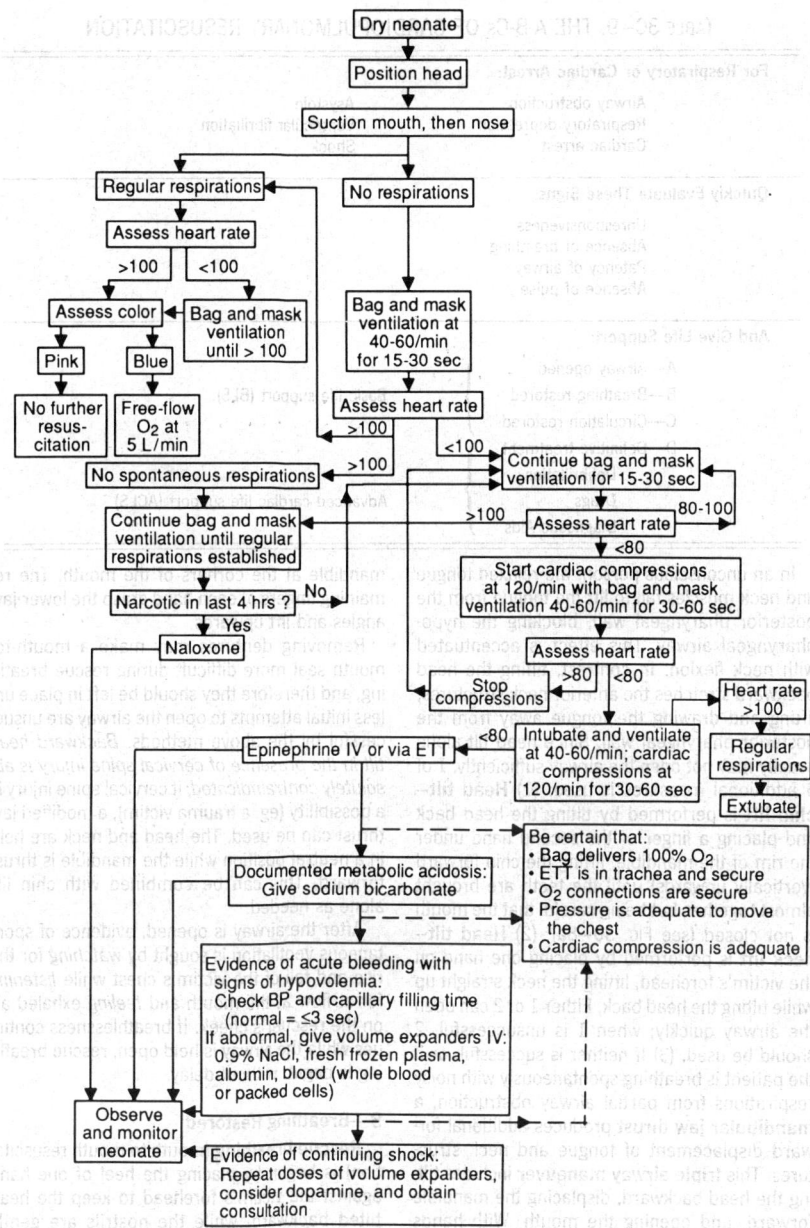

Fig. 30-7. **Management sequence for neonatal resuscitation (delivery room protocol).** ETT = endotracheal tube. (Adapted from Kattwinkel J, et al, Perinatal Continuing Education Program, University of Virginia at Charlottesville, 1991, and the Guidelines of the American Heart Association.)

TABLE 30−9. THE A-B-Cs OF CARDIOPULMONARY RESUSCITATION

For Respiratory or Cardiac Arrest:

Airway obstruction	Asystole
Respiratory depression	Ventricular fibrillation
Cardiac arrest	Shock

Quickly Evaluate These Signs:

Unresponsiveness
Absence of breathing
Patency of airway
Absence of pulse

And Give Life Support:

A—Airway opened
B—Breathing restored   } Basic life support (BLS)
C—Circulation restored
D—Definitive treatment
  Defibrillation
  Drugs   } Advanced cardiac life support (ACLS)
  Diagnostic Aids

In an unconscious person, the relaxed tongue and neck muscles fail to lift the tongue from the posterior pharyngeal wall, blocking the hypopharyngeal airway. This effect is accentuated with neck flexion. In contrast, tilting the head backward stretches the anterior neck structures, lifting and drawing the tongue away from the posterior pharyngeal wall. Since head tilt alone usually may not open the airway sufficiently, 1 of 3 additional measures is used: (1) **Head tilt–chin lift** is performed by tilting the head back and placing a finger of the second hand under the rim of the mandible, lifting the chin forward (vertically upwards) until the teeth are brought almost together, but being careful that the mouth is not closed (see Fig. 30−8a). (2) **Head tilt–neck lift** is performed by placing one hand on the victim's forehead, lifting the neck straight up while tilting the head back. Either 1 or 2 can open the airway quickly; when 1 is unsuccessful, 2 should be used. (3) If neither is successful, or if the patient is breathing spontaneously with noisy respirations from partial airway obstruction, a **mandibular jaw thrust** produces additional forward displacement of tongue and neck structures. This **triple airway maneuver** includes tilting the head backward, displacing the mandible forward, and opening the mouth. With hands placed from behind on each side of the victim's head, and the rescuer's elbows resting on the surface where the victim is lying, the head is tilted backward, while the thumbs depress the

mandible at the corners of the mouth. The remaining fingers of each hand grasp the lower-jaw angles and lift upwards.

Removing dentures may make a mouth-to-mouth seal more difficult during rescue breathing, and therefore they should be left in place unless initial attempts to open the airway are unsuccessful by the above methods. *Backward head tilt in the presence of cervical spine injury is absolutely contraindicated;* if cervical spine injury is a possibility (eg, a trauma victim), a modified jaw thrust can be used. The head and neck are held in a neutral position while the mandible is thrust forward. This can be combined with chin lift alone as needed.

After the airway is opened, evidence of spontaneous ventilation is sought by *watching* for the rise and fall of the victim's chest while *listening* for airflow at the mouth and *feeling* exhaled air on the rescuer's cheek. If breathlessness continues while the airway is held open, rescue breathing is begun without delay.

B—Breathing Restored

Rescue breathing (mouth-to-mouth resuscitation) is begun by placing the heel of one hand against the victim's forehead to keep the head tilted backward, while the nostrils are gently pinched shut with the thumb and index finger of the same hand to prevent escape of air (Fig. 30−8b). The rescuer opens his own mouth widely, takes a deep breath, places his mouth over the

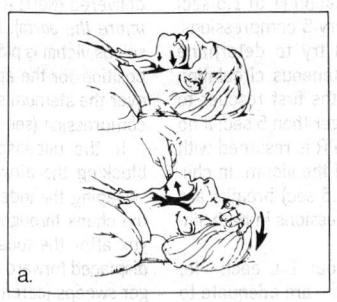

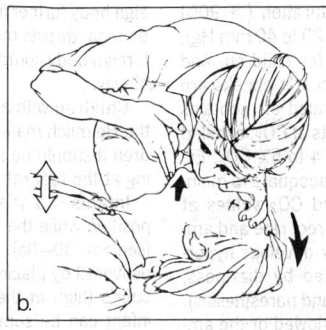

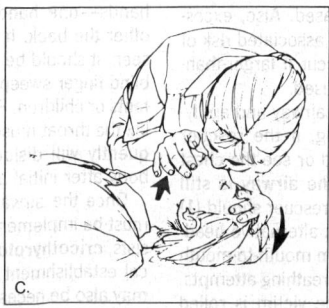

FIG. 30–8. Expired air ventilation—adult. (a) Position to open airway alone. (b) Rescue breathing: proper position of hands and patient for opening the airway and mouth-to-mouth respiration. (c) Proper positioning for mouth-to-nose respiration. (From "Standards and Guidelines for Cardiopulmonary Resuscitation [CPR] and Emergency Cardiac Care [ECC]," in *Journal of the American Medical Association* 25:2916 and 2918, June 6, 1986. Copyright 1986, American Medical Association.)

victim's (making a tight seal), and blows 2 full breaths (1 to 1.5 sec each) thereby beginning ventilation yet avoiding trapping air in the stomach. The adequacy of these ventilatory efforts is assessed by seeing the victim's chest rise and fall and by hearing and feeling his passive exhalation.

Saliva has not been implicated in HIV transmission. However, to minimize the need for emergency mouth-to-mouth resuscitation, mouthpieces, resuscitation bags, or other ventilation devices should be available in areas where the need for resuscitation is predictable.

In single-rescuer CPR, 2 breaths (about 1 to 1.5 sec each) are given to adults after each cycle of 15 cardiac compressions delivered at a rate of 80 to 100/min (see Circulation Restored, below). This totals about 12 to 15 breaths/min for adults.

In 2-rescuer CPR, one ventilation (1 to 1.5 sec) should be delivered after every 5 compressions. The second rescuer should try to determine whether restoration of spontaneous circulation has occurred by instructing the first rescuer to stop compressions for no longer than 5 sec; if no pulse is present, 2-rescuer CPR is resumed with rescuers on opposite sides of the victim. In children and infants, two (1 to 1.5 sec) breaths are delivered after each 5 compressions in both single- and 2-rescuer CPR.

For adults, breaths of about 1 L each—ie, twice the normal tidal volume—are adequate to maintain normal blood O_2 saturation ($> 90\%$) and to eliminate CO_2 ($Pa_{CO_2} = 20$ to 40 mm Hg). Smaller breaths are required for children, and only small puffs from the rescuer's cheeks are required for infants. While inhaled air contains about 21% O_2 and trace amounts of CO_2, exhaled air contains 16 to 18% O_2 and 4 to 5% CO_2. Exhaled air values are more than adequate to maintain the victim's blood O_2 and CO_2 values at close to normal levels if the correct rate and amplitude are used. If the rescuer develops hyperventilation alkalosis (manifested by dizziness, numbness, ringing in the ears, and paresthesias), the respiratory rate should be slowed or the amplitude of each breath decreased. Also, excessive gastric distention with the associated risk of subsequent aspiration may occur if larger-than-necessary volumes of air are used.

In adults, after opening the airway and applying mouth-to-mouth breathing, if the rescuer does not feel the lungs expand or see the chest rise, he should assume that the airway is still blocked. In this situation, the rescuer should (1) reposition the head and try an alternative head-tilt method, and (2) make a firm mouth-to-mouth seal again and repeat rescue breathing attempts. If the obstruction persists, the victim is rolled into the supine position and the Heimlich maneuver (*manual thrusts to the abdomen, upper abdominal thrusts*) or, in the case of pregnant or extremely obese patients, chest thrusts should be given. Six to 10 thrusts may be necessary to dislodge a foreign body. To avoid damage to chest structures and to the liver, *the hand should never be placed on the xiphoid process or over the lower rib cage.* While astride the unconscious victim (squatting above his knees), the rescuer performs the Heimlich maneuver by placing the heel of a hand in the upper abdominal area below the xiphoid process; the other hand is placed on top of the first and a firm upward thrust is

delivered (NOTE: *A straight downward thrust may injure the aorta*). For chest thrusts, the unconscious victim is placed on his back with the hand position for the application of the chest thrusts over the sternum similar to that used for cardiac compression (see Circulation Restored, below).

In the unconscious victim, a foreign body blocking the airway may also be removed by sweeping the index finger (finger sweep) along the cheek through the victim's mouth and pharynx after the tongue and lower jaw have been displaced forward (tongue-jaw lift). Additional finger sweeps (carefully so as not to dislodge a foreign body further into the airway) and manual abdominal thrusts may be required to dislodge the foreign body completely or to relieve the blocked airway.

Children with airway obstruction should have the Heimlich maneuver performed; in small children it should be performed more gently, kneeling at the feet rather than astride.

Infants < 1 yr should be held in a head-down position while the rescuer delivers 4 back blows (see FIG. 30–9a). Up to 4 chest thrusts can be delivered by placing the infant's back on the rescuer's thigh in the head-down position. Or, the infant can be supported between the rescuer's hands—one hand supports the neck and the other the back. If the obstructing object can be seen, it should be carefully removed. Otherwise, blind finger sweeps are *not* recommended in infants or children. Progressive hypoxemia may relax the throat muscles, and these maneuvers frequently will dislodge a supralaryngeal foreign body after initial attempts have failed.

Once the airway obstruction is cleared, CPR must be implemented quickly. If obstruction persists, cricothyrotomy must be performed; surgical establishment of an airway (tracheostomy) may also be necessary in the presence of severe orofacial injuries or massive inflammatory swelling of the neck and pharyngeal structures.

Mouth-to-nose resuscitation is indicated (1) when a tight seal around the victim's mouth is impossible, and (2) when the mouth cannot be opened because of muscular spasm, deformity, or severe inflammatory swelling. Backward tilt of the head in these instances is similar to mouth-to-mouth resuscitation, but with the rescuer's other hand, the lower jaw is pushed forward, closing the mouth. A tight seal is made around the victim's nose and a deep breath is delivered. The patient's mouth should be allowed to open during passive exhalation.

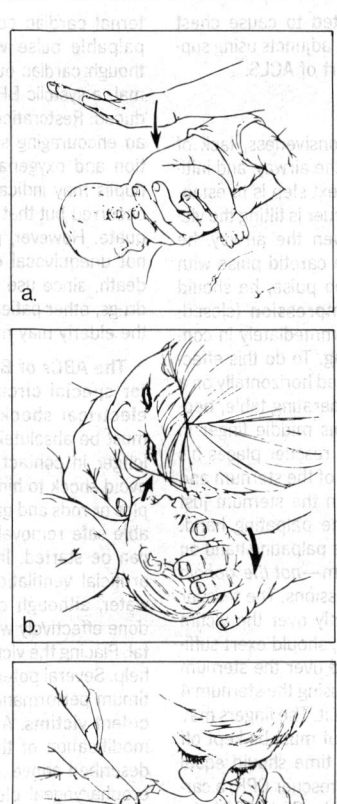

FIG. 30–9. Expired air ventilation—child. (a) Head-down position: dislodgement of foreign bodies from tracheobronchial tube. (b) Position for mouth-to-mouth respiration. (c) Combined mouth-to-nose respiration. (From "Standards and Guidelines for Cardiopulmonary Resuscitation [CPR] and Emergency Cardiac Care [ECC]," in *Journal of the American Medical Association* 255:2956 and 2959, June 6, 1986. Copyright 1986, American Medical Association.)

Combined mouth-and-nose resuscitation is used for infants and small children when a tight mouth seal cannot be maintained. The mouth of the rescuer is placed over both the mouth and nose of the victim, and the lungs are inflated with varying amounts of air according to the size of the child (see FIG. 30–9c). In general, in children ≥ 8 yr old of normal body size, adult CPR techniques can be used.

The **most common errors** in performing expired-air resuscitation are (1) delays in diagnosing respiratory or cardiac arrest; (2) failure to establish a patent airway; (3) delays in instituting BLS promptly; and (4) inadequate ventilation (eg, poor seal around mouth or nose, failure to deliver the initial 2 full breaths, inadequate amount of expired pressure generated to cause chest movements). When available, adjuncts using supplemental O_2 are used as part of ACLS.

C—Circulation Restored

After determining unresponsiveness, lack of respiratory activity, clearing the airway, and initiating rescue breathing, the next step is to establish pulselessness. As the rescuer is tilting the victim's head backward to open the airway, he should gently palpate for the carotid pulse with his other hand. If he feels no pulse, he should begin **external cardiac compression** (closed-chest cardiac compression) immediately in conjunction with rescue breathing. To do this effectively, the victim must be placed horizontally on a flat hard surface (eg, floor, operating table, bedside tray, bed-board). With his middle finger in the xiphisternal junction, the rescuer places his index finger on the lower end of the sternum and the heel of his other hand on the sternum just above the index finger of the palpating hand. Then he places the heel of the palpating hand on top of the hand on the sternum—*not the xiphoid process*—and begins compressions. The rescuer should position himself directly over the victim and, keeping his arm straight, should exert sufficient force directly downward over the sternum (to avoid rib fractures), depressing the sternum 4 to 5 cm ($1\frac{1}{2}$ to 2 in.) in the adult. The fingers may be extended or interlocked but must be kept off the chest wall. Compression time should equal release time; in both 1- and 2-rescuer CPR, a cardiac compression rate should be 80 to 100/min. The rescuer's hands should remain on the sternum during the release phase. This cycle should be repeated smoothly; jerky, bouncing, or irregular compressions increase the chance of injuries.

An infant's heart is higher in the chest, and his chest wall is more pliable. For compression, the tips of the index and middle fingers are used over the midsternum to a depth of about 1.3 to 2.5 cm ($\frac{1}{2}$ to 1 in.) at a rate of 100/min (see Fig. 30–6). In children > 1 yr but < 8 yr old, only the heel of one hand is used to perform external cardiac compression over the lower sternum, but not as low as in the adult; the depth should be increased to 2.5 to 3.8 cm (1 to $1\frac{1}{2}$ in.) at a rate of 80 to 100/min.

The effectiveness of CPR should be monitored periodically during resuscitation efforts. The carotid pulse should be palpated 1 min after beginning BLS, after the arrival of a second rescuer, and q 4 to 5 min to determine whether spontaneous circulation has returned. Ideally, external cardiac compression should produce a palpable pulse with each compression; even though cardiac output is only 30 to 40% of normal, a systolic BP > 80 mm Hg should be produced. Restoration of pupillary responsiveness is an encouraging sign of adequate brain circulation and oxygenation. Dilated, light-responsive pupils may indicate that brain damage has not occurred but that cerebral oxygenation is inadequate. However, persistently dilated pupils are not unequivocal evidence of brain damage or death, since use of high doses of cardioactive drugs, other patient medications, or cataracts in the elderly may modify pupil size and reaction.

The ABCs of BLS may need to be modified for special circumstances. When a victim of **electrical shock** is approached, the rescuer must be absolutely certain that the victim is no longer in contact with the electrical source to avoid shock to himself. Use of nonmetallic grapples or rods and grounding of the rescuer will enable safe removal of the victim, and CPR then can be started. In the case of **near-drowning**, artificial ventilation may be started in shallow water, although chest compression cannot be done effectively when the patient is not horizontal. Placing the victim on a surfboard or float may help. Several potential problems may impede optimum performance when CPR is needed in **accident victims**. A cervical spine injury requires modification of the airway-opening techniques described above. Facial injuries associated with oropharyngeal bleeding or debris may require clearing the airway before beginning ventilation. Severe facial injuries may make mouth-to-mouth resuscitation impossible without using special adjunctive devices and advanced procedures (eg, endotracheal intubation). Chest trauma, including flail chest injury or penetrating lesions of the heart or lungs, may present similar obstacles. In these situations, stabilization in the field by trained medical personnel and immediate transport to a specialized facility are indicated.

When CPR is carried out in the hospital, the adequacy of ventilation must be checked by obtaining an arterial blood sample, since peripheral cyanosis is not a reliable guide because of influence by local circulation, lighting, and Hb value.

Complications of CPR

External cardiac compression can cause injuries that are minimized if properly performed. Elevation of intrathoracic pressure by chest compression and direct cardiac compression between the sternum and spine are presumed mechanisms of blood flow during CPR, and efforts to depress the sternum further than recommended, despite an adequate pulse, are not indicated. **Laceration of the liver** is the most serious (sometimes fatal) complication and is usually caused by pressing too low on the sternum. *Do not press down on the xiphoid process!* Delayed **rupture of the spleen** after CPR has been reported, and **rupture of the stomach** can occur (particularly if gastric distention with air has occurred) following forcible abdominal thrusts. A serious complication is regurgitation followed by **aspiration of gastric contents**, producing an aspiration pneumonitis that may be fatal. Excessive **gastric distention** during artificial ventilation can be avoided by using the recommended amounts of air required for adequate ventilation, by completely opening the airway before attempting to administer rescue breathing, and by early endotracheal or nasotracheal intubation. If marked distention develops, one should recheck the airway for patency and avoid excessive airway pressure. Attempts to relieve gastric distention should wait until suction equipment is available, since regurgitation with aspiration of gastric contents may occur. If marked gastric distention interferes with ventilation and cannot be corrected by the above methods, the victim should be positioned on his side, the epigastrium compressed, and the airway cleared. **Costochondral separation** and **fractured ribs** sometimes cannot be avoided in pressing hard enough to produce a palpable pulse. **Bone marrow emboli** to the lungs have rarely been reported after external cardiac compression, but there is no clear evidence that they contribute to mortality. External cardiac compression does not cause serious **myocardial damage** unless there is a preexisting ventricular aneurysm. **Lung damage** is rare, but pneumothorax secondary to rib fracture can occur. Overall, concern for these injuries should neither deter nor modify appropriately performed CPR.

When the exact duration of cardiac arrest is uncertain, the victim should be given the benefit of the doubt, unless he is in a terminal stage of an incurable condition. Once begun, it is the physician's responsibility to decide when to end BLS.

D—Definitive Treatment

The D step of the A-B-C-D mnemonic (see TABLE 30–9) comprises advanced cardiac life support **(ACLS)** performed in conjunction with BLS. ACLS includes drug therapy, cardiac monitoring and dysrhythmia recognition (ECG diagnosis), adjunctive equipment, and special techniques for establishing and maintaining effective oxygenation and circulation.

A STANDARDIZED RESUSCITATION PROTOCOL

To reduce delays and errors, both in the calculation of drug doses and in the provision of other aspects of acute care, the protocol described earlier has been designed to standardize and streamline resuscitation maneuvers during an arrest and to standardize equipment on all CPR carts.

In summary, the sequence for resuscitation in the general pediatric age group and in newborns is shown in FIGS. 30–5 and 30–7, respectively. The protocol detailed in TABLES 30–7 and 30–8 covers all ages, from the premature infant to the 16-yr-old. Ages are listed in years, and weights are given in kilograms (the 50th percentile for the appropriate age). Dosages should be rounded down; eg, for a 2¹⁄₂-yr-old, dosages should be those for a 2-yr-old, with stepwise increments as needed but not exceeding those for a 3-yr-old.

For example, in a 5-yr-old, the recommended procedure involves the following: a ventilation rate of 20 breaths/min (25 breaths/min for a head injury); a compression rate of 100/min (1-hand technique); a size 7 airway; a size 3 dome cuff (Laerdal) mask with a child Laerdal 500-cc ventilation bag for bag-mask ventilation; a size 2 curved or straight blade for laryngoscopy; a 5-mm tracheal tube; an adult tonsil suction for direct oropharyngeal suctioning; and a size 10 French catheter passed through the endotracheal tube to suction the lower airway. Common sense must be used; eg, if even with an appropriate-sized endotracheal tube there is a leak as evidenced by an audible exhalation of gas at the glottis, then it should be replaced with a larger one once the patient is stabilized.

Drugs in TABLE 30–8 are categorized for use in bradyarrhythmias, tachyarrhythmias, and hypotension. Included also are drugs for seizures and other acute conditions, eg, respiratory disorders. Doses are given by *volume*. Higher or lower doses than those indicated may be required and must be individualized as necessary and after the patient is stabilized. Conservative fluid management can be crucial in a patient with cerebral edema, and more concentrated infusions may be necessary, but these can be recalculated once the emergency is over.

31. CHILD ABUSE AND NEGLECT

The physical or mental injury, sexual abuse, negligent treatment, or maltreatment of a child < 18 yr by a person who is responsible for the child's welfare, under circumstances that indicate the child's health or welfare is harmed or threatened thereby. Physicians are required by law to report incidents of suspected abuse or neglect in any child whom they examine or treat and are granted immunity from suit or liability for so reporting. The reports usually are made to a specifically designated agency of child protection.

Abuse and neglect of children are complicated problems of parent-child interactions that often coexist and may not be easily differentiated. Neglect probably occurs 10 to 15 times more frequently than abuse. All social classes and races contribute to these incidents, but poor children suffer neglect 12 times more frequently than others. About 25% of cases occur in children < 2 yr. Both sexes are affected equally. The incidence is difficult to determine accurately, but more than 1½ million children are involved annually. As many as 20% of physically abused children are permanently injured, and about 1200 deaths from abuse and neglect occur annually in the USA. Sexual abuse or molestation reporting has increased greatly and is thought to involve 200,000 children/yr.

Etiology

Abuse generally is caused by the breakdown of impulse control in the parent or guardian. Four contributing factors are recognized: **(1) Parental personality features:** The childhood experience of the parent may have lacked affection and warmth, often included abuse, and was not conducive to the development of adequate self-esteem or emotional maturity. Lacking an early loving environment, abusive parents may look toward their children as a source of the affection and support they never received. As a result, they may have unrealistic expectations of what their child can supply for them; they are frustrated easily and lose control, unable to give what they never experienced. Use of drugs or alcohol may provoke impulsive and uncontrolled behaviors toward the child. Less commonly a parent may be frankly psychotic. **(2) A "different" child:** Irritable, demanding, or hyperactive children may provoke parents' tempers. Handicapped children, often more dependent and needing care, are susceptible. Premature or sick infants separated from parents early in infancy, and stepchildren or those biologically unrelated, may not form adequately strong ties with their parents or guardians. Parents may have unrealistic expectations of what a child's performance should be and may punish him severely with little justification. **(3) Inadequate support:** Parents may be isolated, unprotected, and vulnerable in the absence of relatives, friends, neighbors, or peers who normally can provide physical and psychologic support in times of stress. **(4) A crisis:** Situational stress may precipitate abuse, particularly at a moment when support is not at hand.

Neglect often is seen among multiproblem families with poorly organized life-styles. Acute or chronic depression, especially maternal, is often present. Desertion by the father, himself inadequate, unable or unwilling to assert a controlling influence in the family, may precipitate neglect. Drug or alcohol abuse by one or both parents frequently results in chronic impoverishment and a distortion of priorities in family life. It is now clear that children of cocaine-using mothers are particularly at risk for desertion. Chronic medical problems of a parent may contribute.

Manifestations of Abuse

History: Features that are suggestive of abuse are (1) parental reluctance to give a history of injury; (2) an inconsistent history that may be at variance with the apparent stage of resolution of the injury and may vary depending on the source of the information; (3) history of injury that is incompatible with the developmental capability of the child; (4) an inappropriate response by the parents to the severity of the injury; and (5) delay in reporting the injury.

Physical: Skin lesions, such as ecchymoses, hematomas, burns, welts, and abrasions in various stages of development, are common (eg, round cigarette burns, arcuate bruises from extension cord whipping, symmetric scald burns of upper or lower extremities). Serious traumatic injury to the mouth, eye, internal abdominal organs, and CNS may produce permanent damage. Fractures may be single or multiple, and a skeletal survey may show bony injuries in varied stages of resolution. Metaphyseal fractures and subperiosteal elevations in long bones occur in infancy. Major diagnostic considerations in the examination are (1) multiple injuries at different stages of resolution or development; (2) cutaneous lesions specific for particular sources of injury; and (3) *repeated* injury, which is suggestive of abuse or inadequate supervision.

Emotional: Emotional manifestations of abuse are less easily defined than are physical signs. In infants, failure to thrive (see also FAILURE TO THRIVE in Ch. 29) is a common early observation. Inadequate parental stimulation and interaction with a small child often delays the development of social and language skills. Small children may be distrustful, superficial in interpersonal relationships, passive, and overly concerned with pleasing adults. The emotional impact on children usually becomes obvious at school age, when difficulties develop in forming relationships with teachers and peers. Often, emotional effects can be documented only when aberrant behaviors improve after the child is placed in another environment.

Sexual abuse or molestation: Acts of adults upon children include exposure, genital manipulation, sodomy, fellatio, and coitus. The perpetrating adult may be unknown or unrelated, in which case the abuse is considered **rape** if vaginal penetration occurred. More often, the adult is biologically related or within the close circle of family, in which case the offense is termed **incest**. When young children are involved, the offense most often is nonviolent and repetitive and may be covered over by collusive collaboration within the family. Physical signs may include difficulty in walking or sitting, genital trauma, vaginal discharge or pruritus, recurrent UTIs, or a sexually transmitted infection. However, there may be no physical indications of injury, and the behavior of the child (irritability, fearfulness, insomnia, or other behavior problems) may be the only clue. Careful interviewing of the child by a trained individual may be the only means of adding necessary details. Older children may be threatened with physical injury by the offender if they tell and, thus, may conceal repeated assaults. Sexually transmitted disease of any sort in any child < 12 to 13 yr must be viewed as the result of sexual molestation until this is ruled out.

Manifestations of Neglect

Failure to meet basic physical needs: Inadequate provision of food, clothing, or shelter, despite available supportive community resources, is common (eg, malnutrition, fatigue, lack of hygiene or appropriate clothing). Desertion or death by starvation may occur in extreme cases. As many as $1/2$ of infantile failure-to-thrive cases may be due to neglect.

Emotional deprivation: In early infancy, retardation of emotional growth may occur with blunt-

ing of affect and lack of interest in the environment. This commonly accompanies failure to thrive and is often misdiagnosed as mental retardation or physical illness. Signs in older children include poor school attendance and performance and bad relationships with peers and adults.

Failure to meet health needs: Failure to seek preventive medical or dental attention, such as immunizations and routine health supervision, and delay in seeking care for illness may be clues to inadequate family functioning.

Treatment

Providing care to involved families must be seen in long-range perspective, because the disturbed patterns of personal interaction are usually long-standing. In both abuse and neglect settings, *families should be approached in a helping rather than a punitive manner.*

A careful review of the family setting and of the parents' deficiencies and needs is essential diagnostically and is the first step in treatment. Hospitalization of the child (emergency temporary removal from the home) may be indicated, but usually it is not required and depends on how well rapport can be established with the parents. When hospitalization occurs, parents should be told that the studies to be undertaken will include discussions with them as well as the diagnostic tests on their child.

Social work consultation: Adequate understanding of the parents' backgrounds usually requires considerable review of medical records and of prior contacts with various community service agencies. If available, a social work consultant can provide valuable assistance in conducting such reviews and may help with interviews and family counseling.

Reporting to a social service or welfare department: When abuse or neglect cases are reported, a face-to-face conference should be held if possible with a child protective services representative to ensure clear understanding and to help in planning management. The parents should be told beforehand by the physician that a report is being made pursuant to the law.

Care planning: Many communities have a multidisciplinary team consisting of a social worker, psychiatrist, pediatrician, and others to provide diagnostic assistance and guidance in designing a treatment program. A source of primary medical care is fundamental and should be acceptable to both the family and the reporting physician. Periodic or ongoing social work contact usually is needed. Psychiatric assistance in understanding personality disorders and in dealing with specific conditions, such as depression, often is indicated.

Management of sexual molestation: Sex offenses may have lasting psychologic effects on the child's development and future sexual adaptations. Effects are more lasting and intense in older and teenage children. Counseling or psychotherapy of both the child and the adults concerned may prevent these effects.

Community care programs: Day-care centers for small children can relieve a mother under stress, allowing her a few hours each day for herself. Homemaker services can be arranged to give assistance. Parent aide programs, utilizing trained nonprofessional people to relate closely to abusing and neglecting parents, are being developed in some communities. "Parents Anonymous" groups also have been successful.

Temporary removal from the home: If the home setting carries a high risk to the child's health, if an abuse victim is < 1 yr of age, or if work with the family has not progressed, temporary removal may be indicated. Temporary removal on an acute basis should be strongly considered in cases of physical or sexual abuse when, after disclosure by the child, the child will be returning to a situation in which there will be contact with the suspected perpetrator, and other care givers do not support the allegations of the child. Removal requires a court petition, presented by the legal counsel of the appropriate welfare department. The procedure varies from state to state but usually entails family court testimony by a physician. When the court decides in favor of removing the child from the home, a disposition is arranged. The family's physician should participate in this disposition planning. If not, his agreement and consent to the disposition should be sought. While the child is in temporary

placement, the physician should, if possible, maintain contact with the parents and be assured that adequate efforts are being made to help them. He should also participate when the decision is made to reunite child and parents. As the dynamics of the family setting improve, it may be possible for the child to return to the parents' care. Recurrences are common.

Follow-up: The families of abused and neglected children frequently relocate, making continuity of care very difficult. Broken appointments are common; outreach and home visiting by welfare workers or a public health nurse may be needed to keep all who are concerned aware of the patient's progress.

Prevention

Knowing which settings may cause abuse and neglect of children helps to identify certain at-risk families. Parents who have been victims of abuse and/or neglect are especially apt to interact in like fashion with their children. Such parents often verbalize an anxiety about their abusive background and are amenable to assistance. Parents having their first baby and teenage mothers rebelling against their parents are also at risk. Events during pregnancy, delivery, or early infancy that risk increased morbidity can weaken parents' emotional ties to the infant (see also PARENT-INFANT BONDING: THE SICK NEONATE in Ch. 24). During such times it is important to elicit the parents' feelings about their own inadequacies and the baby's well-being. How well can they tolerate a small or sickly baby in the house? Does the father provide moral and physical support to the mother? Are there relatives or friends to help in times of need? The care provider who is alert to clues and able to give support in such settings goes a long way to prevent tragic events.

32. CHILDHOOD INFECTIONS

BACTERIAL INFECTIONS

(See also INFECTIOUS MYRINGITIS, ACUTE OTITIS MEDIA, and ACUTE MASTOIDITIS in Ch. 66)

DIPHTHERIA

An acute contagious disease caused by Corynebacterium diphtheriae, *characterized by the formation of a fibrinous pseudomembrane, usually on the respiratory mucosa, and by myocardial and neural tissue damage secondary to*

an exotoxin. **Cutaneous diphtheria** lesions are also common.

Epidemiology

Three biotypes (*mitis, intermedius,* and *gravis*) of *C. diphtheriae* exist. Only toxigenic isolates produce exotoxin. Nontoxigenic organisms may produce symptomatic diphtheria, but the clinical course is usually milder than that caused by toxigenic isolates. Spread is chiefly by the secretions of infected persons, directly or via contaminated fomites. Sporadic cases generally result from exposure to carriers who may never have had apparent disease; cases occurring during an epidemic usually can be traced.

Cutaneous diphtheria can occur when any disruption of the integument is colonized by *C. diphtheriae*. Indigent adults and native Americans living in an endemic area are particularly at risk, since poor personal and community hygiene contribute to the spread of cutaneous diphtheria. The disease is not restricted to tropical zones; large outbreaks have occurred in temperate climates.

Pathology

Ordinarily, the organisms lodge in the tonsil or nasopharynx and, as they multiply, toxigenic *C. diphtheriae* may produce exotoxins lethal to the adjacent host cells. Occasionally, the primary site is the skin or mucosa elsewhere. The exotoxin, carried by the blood, also damages cells in distant organs. Pathologic lesions are found in the respiratory passages, oropharynx, myocardium, nervous system, and kidneys.

The diphtheria bacillus first destroys a layer of superficial epithelium, usually in patches, and the resulting exudate coagulates to form a grayish pseudomembrane containing bacteria, fibrin, leukocytes, and necrotic epithelial cells. However, the areas of bacterial multiplication and toxin absorption are wider and deeper than indicated by the size of the membrane, formed in the wake of the spreading infection.

The myocardium may show fatty degeneration or fibrosis. Degenerative changes in cranial or peripheral nerves occur chiefly in the motor fibers. In severe cases, anterior horn cells and anterior and posterior nerve roots may show damage proportional to the duration of infection before antitoxin is given. The kidneys may show a reversible interstitial nephritis with extensive cellular infiltration.

Symptoms and Signs

The incubation period (1 to 4 days) and prodromal period (12 to 24 h) are among the shortest in bacterial diseases. Initially, the patient with tonsillar or faucial diphtheria has only a mild sore throat, dysphagia, a low-grade fever, increased heart rate, and rising polymorphonuclear leukocytosis. Nausea, emesis, chills, headache, and fever are more common in children.

The characteristic membrane, usually found in the tonsillar area but sometimes in other areas (eg, the nasopharynx), is dirty gray, tough, fibrinous, and may adhere firmly so that removal causes bleeding. Depending on the duration of infection, the membrane may be punctate or extensive and yellow-gray or creamy. In young children, who may show no signs of illness until the disease is well established, a membrane is often present at the first examination. In older children and adults, complaints of sore throat and fatigue may precede appearance of the membrane. Some patients never develop a membrane.

The disease may remain mild. When it progresses, dysphagia, signs of toxemia, and prostration become prominent. Pharyngeal and laryngeal edema obstructs breathing. If the larynx or the trachea and bronchi are involved, the membrane may partially obstruct the airway or suddenly detach, causing complete obstruction. The cervical lymph glands are enlarged. In severe cases, exotoxin may diffuse into the neck tissue, producing severe edema (bull neck). Nasopharyngeal involvement may produce a serosanguineous nasal discharge, often unilateral.

The lesions of **cutaneous diphtheria** are not morphologically specific. Any break in the skin can be secondarily infected with *C. diphtheriae;* lacerations, abrasions, ulcers, burns, and other wounds are potential reservoirs of the organism. The lesions generally occur on the extremities and, if untreated, may become anesthetized by exotoxin infiltration. Cutaneous diphtheritic lesions also usually harbor Group A β-hemolytic streptococci, *Staphylococcus aureus,* or both. A pseudomembrane is uncommon. Concomitant nasopharyngeal infection with the same biotype occurs in 20 to 40% of cases. Ocular infection with *C. diphtheriae* is rare and may occur with or without other cutaneous lesions.

Complications

Severe complications are likely if antitoxin is not given promptly. Myocarditis is usually evident by the 10th to 14th day but can appear any time during the 1st to 6th wk. Heart failure may follow; sudden death may occur. Insignificant ECG changes occur in 20 to 30% of patients, although atrioventricular dissociation, complete heart block, and ventricular arrhythmias are associated with a high mortality. Dysphagia and nasal regurgitation, from bulbar paralysis, may be seen in the 1st wk of illness; peripheral nerve palsies appear from the 3rd to 6th wk. Spontaneous reversal occurs slowly, over many weeks. Myocarditis and palsies are not improved by corticosteroids or delayed administration of antitoxin.

Diagnosis

The clinical appearance of the membrane suggests the diagnosis, pending confirmation by culture. Gram stain of the membrane may reveal gram-positive rods with metachromatic (beaded) staining in typical Chinese-character configuration. Loeffler's medium or tellurite agar is preferred for primary isolation of the organism, which grows well on other artificial media. The laboratory should be notified that *C. diphtheriae* is suspected. Cutaneous diphtheria should be considered when a patient develops skin lesions during an outbreak of respiratory diphtheria.

Immunization

Active immunization with DTP should be routine for all children and all susceptible contacts (see IMMUNIZATION PROCEDURES THROUGHOUT CHILDHOOD in Ch. 23). For previously immunized contacts, a booster dose of adult-type tetanus and diphtheria toxoids, adsorbed (Td), is sufficient.

Treatment

Symptomatic patients should be hospitalized in intensive care units. **Diphtheria antitoxin must be given early,** since the antitoxin neutralizes only toxin not yet bound to cells. When diphtheria is suspected, antitoxin must be given immediately upon clinical diagnosis, without waiting for culture confirmation. CAUTION: *Diphtheria antitoxin is derived from horses; hence, a skin (or conjunctival) test to rule out sensitivity should always precede administration* (see discussion of serum sickness under HYPERSENSITIVITY TO DRUGS in Ch. 34). If, after 30 min, no erythema or a flat erythematous area < 0.5 cm in diameter appears about the site of the skin-test injection, administration of antitoxin may proceed. The dose, ranging from 20,000 to 100,000 u., is determined empirically. Patients with moderately symptomatic diphtheritic pharyngitis require 20,000 to 40,000 u., while those with more severe symptoms or with complications require larger doses.

Antitoxin may be given IM or IV. Doses above 20,000 u. may be added to 200 mL of 0.9% sodium chloride solution and given slowly IV over 30 to 45 min to facilitate delivery of the large volume.

An urticarial wheal in response to the skin test indicates sensitivity and mandates **extreme caution** in giving the antitoxin. The patient must first be desensitized with dilute antitoxin, given in graduated doses, as described under HYPERSENSITIVITY TO DRUGS in Ch. 34. If untoward symptoms appear, 0.3 to 1 mL epinephrine 1:1000 should immediately be injected s.c., IM, or slowly IV. In the highly sensitive patient, IV administration of antitoxin is **contraindicated.**

Supportive treatment is important, particularly with the complications of diphtheria. Bed rest is necessary, as is intensive nursing care with emphasis on nutrition, fluid intake, oxygenation, constant observation for signs that endotracheal intubation or a tracheostomy is needed, continuous monitoring for cardiac problems, and frequent examination for CNS complications. Since the membrane can easily be dislodged, tracheostomy is the preferred emergency airway. Eradication of the organism with antibiotics is important. Adults may be given procaine penicillin G 600,000 u. IM q 12 h for 10 days or enteric-coated erythromycin 250 to 500 mg or erythromycin ethylsuccinate 400 mg orally q 6 h for 7 days. Children weighing < 25 kg should receive procaine penicillin G 300,000 u. IM q 12 h or erythromycin 50 mg/kg/day (maximum 1 gm/day) orally or IV in 4 divided doses. Ampicillin is also effective—75 mg/kg/day in 4 divided doses for children or 250 to 500 mg orally q 6 h for adults. Clindamycin and rifampin have also been used. Oral cephalosporins are not recommended.

Recovery from severe diphtheria is slow, and patients must be prevented from resuming activities too soon. Even normal physical exertion may harm the patient recovering from myocarditis.

Management of an Outbreak

1. Isolate and treat all **symptomatic patients** as described above until 2 throat (or skin, if appropriate) cultures are negative for *C. diphtheriae.* The cultures should be taken 24 and 48 h after antibiotics are discontinued. If positive cultures persist after clinical recovery, resume treatment for 10 days with erythromycin (2 gm/day orally in 4 divided doses for adults, 50 mg/kg/day for children). To avoid impaired absorption from food, use the enteric-coated base or ethylsuccinate forms. With current antibiotic regimens, tonsillectomy is no longer indicated for eradication of persistent foci.

2. Submit all isolates of *C. diphtheriae* to the local health department for biotyping and toxigenicity determination. Nontoxigenic and toxigenic biotypes may coexist in a community. Analysis of DNA restriction enzyme patterns and hybridization patterns with DNA probes of the

isolates can help characterize an outbreak epidemiologically.

3. For all close contacts of known diphtheria patients, obtain nasopharyngeal and throat cultures for *C. diphtheriae*. Examine the throat and integument; hospitalize symptomatic patients and treat as described above, pending culture reports. Confine asymptomatic contacts with positive throat cultures for *C. diphtheriae* (carriers) to their homes, without visitors, for the duration of therapy, and give erythromycin orally 250 to 500 mg q 6 h for adults (50 mg/kg/day in 4 divided doses for children). Do *not* give antitoxin to carriers. After 3 days of treatment, heads of households may resume work while taking antibiotics. *Recheck cultures after therapy.* Erythromycin treatment failures are usually due to noncompliance in taking the medicine rather than to drug-resistant organisms. Occasional resistance of *C. diphtheriae* to erythromycin has been recognized within the USA. Antimicrobial sensitivity tests should be performed on isolates from treatment failures.

4. Update diphtheria immunization in all contacts, including hospital personnel; use adult-type tetanus and diphtheria toxoids, adsorbed (Td). Protective immunity levels cannot be relied upon > 10 yr after a booster dose.

5. Presume that persons with negative cultures and full immunization are safe from both personal and public health standpoints.

PERTUSSIS
(Whooping Cough)

An acute, highly communicable bacterial disease, characterized by a paroxysmal or spasmodic cough that usually ends in a prolonged, high-pitched, crowing inspiration (the whoop).

Etiology and Epidemiology

The causative agent is *Bordetella pertussis*, a small, nonmotile, gram-negative coccobacillus. *B. parapertussis* closely resembles this organism; it causes parapertussis, which may be clinically indistinguishable from pertussis but is usually milder and less often fatal.

Transmission is by aspiration of *B. pertussis* sprayed into the air by a patient, particularly in the catarrhal and early paroxysmal stages. Transmission by contact with contaminated articles is rare. Patients usually are not infectious after the 3rd wk of the paroxysmal phase.

Pertussis is endemic throughout the world; its incidence in the USA increased in the late 1980s. In a given locality, it becomes epidemic every 2

to 4 yr. It occurs at all ages, but about $^1/_2$ of all cases occur before age 2, since infants usually have no protective antibodies. One attack does not confer natural immunity for life, but second attacks, if they occur, are usually mild and often unrecognized.

Symptoms and Signs

The incubation period averages 7 to 14 days (maximum, 3 wk). *B. pertussis* invades the mucosa of the nasopharynx, trachea, bronchi, and bronchioles, increasing the secretion of mucus, initially thin and later viscid and tenacious. The disease lasts about 6 wk and consists of 3 stages: catarrhal, paroxysmal, and convalescent. The catarrhal stage begins insidiously, generally with sneezing, lacrimation, or other signs of coryza; anorexia; listlessness; and a troublesome, hacking nocturnal cough that gradually becomes diurnal. Fever is rare.

The cough becomes paroxysmal after 10 to 14 days. There are 5 to ≥ 15 rapidly consecutive coughs followed by the whoop, a hurried, deep inspiration. After a few normal breaths, another paroxysm may begin. Copious amounts of viscid mucus may be expelled (usually swallowed by infants and children but also occurring as large bubbles via the nares) during or following the paroxysms. Vomiting subsequent to paroxysms or due to gagging on the tenacious mucus is characteristic. In infants, choking spells (with or without cyanosis) may be more common than whoops.

The convalescent stage usually begins within 4 wk; paroxysms are not so frequent or severe, vomiting decreases, and the patient looks and feels better. The average duration of illness is about 7 wk (range, 3 wk to 3 mo). Paroxysmal coughing may recur for months, usually induced by irritation from a URI.

The WBC count is usually between 15,000 and 20,000 but may be normal or as high as 60,000, usually with 60 to 80% small lymphocytes.

Diagnosis

The catarrhal stage is often difficult to distinguish from bronchitis or influenza. Adenovirus infections and TB should also be considered in the differential diagnosis, since either can mimic the pertussis syndrome. Lymphocytosis of ≥ 70% in an afebrile or slightly febrile child over age 3 with a suspicious cough often suggests pertussis but does not distinguish it from an adenoviral pertussis-like syndrome. Cultures of nasopharyngeal specimens are positive for *B. pertussis* in 80 to

90% of cases in the catarrhal and early paroxysmal stages. Best results are obtained with small sterile cotton swabs on 28-gauge, zinc-coated wire passed through the nostril to the nasopharynx. Freshly prepared Bordet-Gengou or charcoal agar medium, containing penicillin or cephalexin to inhibit overgrowth by other flora, should be used. Specific fluorescent antibody testing of nasopharyngeal smears accurately diagnoses pertussis but is not as sensitive as culture. Parapertussis is differentiated by culture or the fluorescent antibody technique.

Prognosis and Complications

Pertussis is serious in children under age 2; mortality is about 1 to 2% before age 1. The disease is troublesome but rarely serious in older children and adults, except in the aged.

The most frequent complications are respiratory, including asphyxia in infants. Bronchopneumonia and cerebral complications cause most fatalities in infants and young children. Bronchopneumonia is also a frequent complication in the aged and may be fatal at any age. Interstitial and subcutaneous emphysema and pneumothorax are infrequent consequences of the increased intrathoracic pressure during paroxysms. Bronchiectasis, particularly in debilitated children, and residual emphysema can result. Atelectasis may occur when a mucus plug occludes a bronchiole. A primary tuberculous lesion may be extended by simultaneous occurrence of pertussis. Convulsions are common in infants but rare in older children. Hemorrhage into the brain, eyes, skin, and mucous membranes can result from severe paroxysms and consequent anoxia. Cerebral hemorrhage or edema or toxic encephalitis may result in spastic paralysis, mental retardation, or other neurologic disorders. An ulcer may develop on the frenulum of tongue from lower incisor trauma during paroxysms. Umbilical hernia and rectal prolapse occasionally occur. Otitis media is frequent.

Prophylaxis

Active immunization: See IMMUNIZATION PROCEDURES THROUGHOUT CHILDHOOD in Ch. 23. **Passive immunization** is unreliable and is not recommended.

Oral erythromycin (preferably the estolate preparation) 12.5 mg/kg qid (maximum, 2 gm/day), starting during the incubation period and continuing for 14 days, may abort the infection in contacts or prevent transmission, but efficacy is not yet fully established.

Patients should be quarantined, particularly from susceptible infants, for at least 4 wk from onset of disease or until symptoms have subsided. If quarantine is uncertain or difficult, erythromycin estolate 12.5 mg/kg orally qid (maximum, 2 gm/day) for 14 days usually eradicates nasopharyngeal carriage of the organism, thus diminishing infectivity to others; however, there is no recognized therapeutic benefit after the paroxysms have begun.

Treatment

Hospitalization is recommended for seriously ill infants because expert nursing care is important. Bed rest is unnecessary for older children with mild disease. Small, frequent meals are advisable. Parenteral fluid therapy may be required to replace sodium and water losses if vomiting is severe. In infants, suction to remove excess mucus from the throat may be lifesaving, and tracheostomy or nasotracheal intubation is occasionally needed. O_2 should be given if cyanosis persists after removal of mucus. *Seriously ill infants should be kept in a darkened, quiet room and disturbed as little as possible,* since any disturbance can precipitate serious paroxysmal spells with anoxia. Close attention should be paid to the nutritional needs of the infant, since preexisting or developing malnutrition can contribute significantly to an adverse outcome.

Expectorant cough mixtures, cough suppressants, and mild sedation are of questionable value, and should be used cautiously or not at all. Adrenergic drugs such as theophylline or albuterol and corticosteroids have also been suggested for the treatment of severely ill patients; however, further controlled studies are needed to assess their effectiveness and potential hazards. Antibiotics should be used only for bacterial complications such as bronchopneumonia and otitis media.

TETANUS
(Lockjaw)

An acute infectious disease characterized by intermittent tonic spasms of voluntary muscles. Spasm of the masseters accounts for the name "lockjaw." Globally, tetanus is a preventable disease of great significance, particularly the neonatal form in developing countries.

Etiology and Pathogenesis

Tetanus is caused by an exotoxin (tetanospasmin) elaborated by *Clostridium tetani*, a slender, motile, gram-positive, anaerobic, spore-forming bacillus. Spores remain viable for years and can be found in soil and in animal feces. Tetanus may follow trivial as well as overtly contaminated wounds, depending on a suitably lowered oxidation-reduction potential in the injured tissues. In the USA, drug addicts in particular are prone to develop tetanus, as are patients with burns or surgical wounds. Infection may also develop postpartum in the uterus and in a newborn's umbilicus **(tetanus neonatorum)**. Clinical disease does not confer immunity.

The toxin may enter the CNS along the peripheral motor nerves or may be blood-borne to the nervous tissue. The tetanospasmin binds to the ganglioside membranes of nerve synapses, blocking release of the inhibitory transmitter from the nerve terminals and thereby causing a generalized tonic spasticity, usually superimposed with intermittent tonic convulsions. Once fixed, the toxin cannot be neutralized.

Symptoms and Signs

The incubation period ranges from 2 to 50 (usually 5 to 10) days. The most frequent symptom is **stiffness of the jaw**. Other symptoms include difficulty in swallowing; restlessness; irritability; stiff neck, arms, or legs; headache; fever; sore throat; chilliness; and tonic spasms. Later, the patient has difficulty opening his jaws **(trismus)**; facial muscle spasm produces a characteristic expression with a fixed smile and elevated eyebrows **(risus sardonicus)**. Rigidity or spasm of abdominal, neck, and back muscles—even opisthotonos—may be present. Sphincteral spasm causes urinary retention or constipation. Dysphagia may interfere with nutrition. Characteristic painful, generalized tonic spasms with profuse sweating are precipitated by minor disturbances such as a draft or noise or by jarring the bed. The patient's sensorium usually is clear, but coma may follow repeated spasms. During generalized spasms, the patient is unable to speak or cry out because of chest wall rigidity or glottal spasm. This also interferes with respiration, causing cyanosis or fatal asphyxia. The immediate cause of death may not be apparent.

The patient's temperature is only moderately elevated except when a complicating infection, such as pneumonia, is present. Respiratory and pulse rates are increased. Reflexes are often exaggerated. Moderate leukocytosis is usual.

Localized tetanus can occur, with spasticity of a group of muscles near the wound but without trismus. The spasticity may persist for weeks. **Cephalic tetanus**, more common in children, is associated particularly with chronic otitis media; the incidence is greatest in Africa and India. All cranial nerves can be involved, the 7th particularly. Cephalic tetanus may become generalized.

Diagnosis

A history of a wound in a patient with muscle stiffness or spasm is suggestive. A slight wound may have been overlooked. Tetanus can be confused with meningoencephalitis of other bacterial or viral origin, but the combination of an intact sensorium, normal CSF, and muscle spasms suggests tetanus. Trismus must be distinguished from signs of local causes such as a peritonsillar or retropharyngeal abscess or another local infection. The phenothiazines can induce a tetanus-like rigidity, but other signs of basal ganglia dysfunction are usually evident.

C. tetani sometimes can be cultured from the wound, but its absence does not negate the diagnosis.

Prognosis

Tetanus has a worldwide mortality rate of 50%; mortality is highest in young and old patients and in drug abusers. The prognosis is poorer if the incubation period is short and symptoms progress rapidly or if treatment is delayed. The course tends to be milder when there is no demonstrable focus of infection.

Prophylaxis

Immunization: Primary immunization against tetanus with either the fluid or adsorbed toxoid is superior to giving antitoxin at the time of injury. Immunization in a pregnant woman produces both active and passive immunity in the fetus; the former occurs at a gestational age of 5 to 6 mo with a booster at 8 mo. Passive immunity develops with maternal toxoid given before a gestational age of 6 mo. Routine DTP immunization and booster recommendations are discussed under IMMUNIZATION PROCEDURES THROUGHOUT CHILDHOOD in Ch. 23.

At the **time of injury** (see TABLE 32–1), administration of 0.5 mL of tetanus toxoid elicits a protective antibody level in a *previously immunized patient*; however, this booster dose is not necessary if the patient is known to have received a booster within the preceding 5 yr. An *inadequately immunized patient* should be given tetanus immune globulin 250 to 500 u. IM, depending on the wound potential rather than on age or body weight. At the same time, the first of three 0.5-mL doses of adsorbed tetanus toxoid should

TABLE 32–1. GUIDELINES FOR IMMUNIZING PATIENTS WHO HAVE OPEN WOUNDS

History	Susceptibility to Tetanus/Immunization Recommended		
	None	Moderate	High
Fully immunized and < 5 yr since booster	0	0	0
Fully immunized and 5–10 yr since booster	0	Td	Td
Fully immunized and > 10 yr since booster	Td	Td	Td
Incompletely immunized or uncertain	Td	Td and TIG* (250 u.)	Td and TIG† (500 u.)

Td = tetanus and diphtheria toxoids, adult type; TIG = tetanus immune globulin.
* Tetanus immune globulin not to be given if patient is known to have had 2 primary doses of toxoid.
† To be given at different sites with different syringes.

be given s.c. or IM at another injection site. The 2nd and 3rd doses of toxoid are given at monthly intervals. Tetanus antitoxin 3000 to 5000 u. IM (CAUTION: *Made from horse or bovine serum; see HYPERSENSITIVITY TO DRUGS in Ch. 34*) should be used *only* if tetanus immune globulin is not available.

Wound care: Prompt, thorough debridement—especially of deep puncture wounds—is essential, since dirt and dead tissue promote multiplication of *C. tetani*. Penicillin and the tetracyclines are effective against *C. tetani* but are not substitutes for adequate debridement.

Treatment

Therapy involves maintaining an adequate airway; ensuring early and adequate use of human immune serum globulin; neutralizing nonfixed toxin; preventing further toxin production; providing sedation; controlling muscle spasm, hypertonicity, fluid balance, and intercurrent infection; and providing continuous nursing care.

General principles: The patient should be kept in a quiet room. In moderate or severe cases, the patient should be intubated and an adequate airway maintained. Tracheotomy should be performed when intubation is expected to be prolonged—ie, 7 to 10 days. Mechanical ventilation may be necessary; it is essential when neuromuscular blockade is required to control respirations (see discussion of muscle spasm management, below). O_2 should be humidified. Gastric intubation facilitates feeding; however, IV hyperalimentation avoids the hazard of aspiration secondary to feeding by gastric tube. Since constipation is usual, stools should be kept soft; a rectal tube may help to control distention. Bladder catheterization is required if urinary retention oc-

curs. Chest physiotherapy, frequent turning, and forced coughing are essential to prevent pneumonia. Codeine is useful for pain. Patients with protracted tetanus may manifest a very labile and overactive sympathetic nervous system, including periods of hypertension, tachycardia, and myocardial irritability. Ongoing monitoring is indicated, and use of α- or β-adrenergic blockers (eg, propranolol, labetalol) or bethanidine may be indicated.

Antitoxin: The benefit of antiserum depends primarily on how much tetanospasmin is already bound to the synaptic membranes. For adults, a single IM injection of 3000 u. of tetanus immune globulin is generally recommended, with a range of 1,500 to 10,000 u., depending on wound severity. Antitoxin of animal origin is far less preferable, since the patient's serum antitoxin level is not as well maintained and there is considerable risk of serum sickness. If horse serum must be used, however, the usual dose is 50,000 u. IM or IV (CAUTION: *see HYPERSENSITIVITY TO DRUGS in Ch. 34 for necessary precautions*). Immune globulin or antitoxin can be injected directly into the wound, but this is not as important as proper wound excision and debridement.

Management of muscle spasms: The benzodiazepines, chlorpromazine, and short-acting barbiturates are all helpful in reducing the excessive neuroexcitability of tetanus. Diazepam is the drug of choice to help control seizures, counter muscle rigidity, and induce sedation. The dosage range is variable and requires meticulous titration and close observation. The most severe cases may require 10 to 20 mg q 3 h by IV push. Less severe cases can be controlled with 5 to 10 mg q 2 to 4 h orally. Dosage for children is 0.1 to 0.2 mg/kg IV or IM q 3 to 6 h; dosages as high as

10 to 15 mg/kg/day are sometimes required. Dosage for neonates (0.3 mg/kg IV or IM q 3 to 6 h) is relatively higher than that for children or adults; the usual range is 20 to 40 mg/kg/day IV. Diazepam may not preclude reflex spasms, and effective respiration may require neuromuscular blockade with a curariform agent such as pancuronium bromide or vecuronium bromide (d-tubocurarine, in contrast to pancuronium bromide, may manifest histamine release with unwanted hypotension). Use of pyridoxine in reducing spasms and possibly mortality in neonatal tetanus has been very limited but encouraging.

Antibiotics: Although the role of antibiotic therapy is minor in contrast to wound debridement and general support, either penicillin G 2 million u. IV q 6 h or tetracycline 500 mg IV q 6 h should be given for 10 days. Children are given penicillin G 200,000 u./kg/day in 6 doses or tetracycline 30 to 40 mg/kg/day. In children, as in adults, a larger amount of ischemic tissue warrants a higher dosage. Neither antibiotic is likely to prevent secondary infections (eg, pneumonia). If pneumonia develops, specimens for culture should be taken from sputum or trachea, sensitivity tests should be performed, and an appropriate antibiotic should be given if necessary. If the patient has an indwelling urethral catheter, the urine should be cultured frequently and antimicrobial therapy instituted if indicated.

Immunization: Since immunity does not follow clinical tetanus, the patient should receive a full immunizing course of toxoid after recovery.

ACUTE BACTERIAL MENINGITIS
(See also NEONATAL MENINGITIS under NEONATAL INFECTIONS in Ch. 27)

Etiology and Incidence

Although many species of bacteria can induce meningitis, 3 account for about 80% of cases: *Neisseria meningitidis* (meningococcus), *Hemophilus influenzae* type b, and *Streptococcus pneumoniae* (pneumococcus). Factors such as age, head trauma, and compromised immunity may be helpful in predicting causative agents.

Meningococcus is found in the nasopharynx of about 5% of the population; it spreads by respiratory droplets and close contact. For unknown reasons, only a small fraction of carriers develop meningitis. Meningococcal meningitis occurs most often in the first year of life. It is also apt to occur in epidemics in closed populations (eg, military barracks, boarding schools). *H. influenzae* type b accounts for most meningitis in children > 1 mo old, but not in adults unless there is a predisposing factor (eg, head trauma, immune compromise). Pneumococcus is the most common cause of adult meningitis. Especially at risk are alcoholics and persons with chronic otitis, sinusitis, mastoiditis, closed head injury, recurrent meningitis, pneumococcal pneumonia, sickle cell disease, or asplenism.

Gram-negative meningitis (most often *Escherichia coli* and *Klebsiella-Enterobacter*) is seen after CNS surgery or trauma, bacteremia (eg, genitourinary manipulations in the elderly), and nosocomial infections, and in the immune-compromised. Staphylococcal meningitis occurs after penetrating head wounds (often as part of a mixed infection), bacteremia (eg, from endocarditis), or neurosurgery. *Listeria* meningitis is found in patients with chronic renal failure and those receiving steroid therapy.

The **incidence** of meningitis is highest during the 1st mo of life with most infections due to *E. coli* and group B streptococcus. The relative incidence of meningitis for children remains high in the first 2 yr of life.

Pathophysiology

Bacteria reach the meninges by hematogenous spread, by extension from nearby infected structures (eg, sinusitis, epidural abscess), and by communication of CSF with the exterior (eg, myelomeningocele, spinal dermal sinus, penetrating traumatic injuries or neurosurgical procedures). Critical to their successful colonization (eg, of the nasopharynx by meningococci, *H. influenzae* type b, and pneumococci) and CSF seeding is the bacterial surface (eg, specialized pili permit meningococci to bind to nasopharyngeal cells for transport across the mucosal barrier). In the bloodstream, the bacterial capsule resists attack by neutrophils, cells of the reticuloendothelial system, and the classical complement pathway. Receptors for pili and other bacterial surface components in the choroid plexus, an early site of CNS inflammation, facilitate penetration into the CSF space. Due to a relative lack of antibody, complement, and WBCs in the CSF, the infection flourishes. Bacterial wall components, complement (eg, C5a), and inflammatory cytokines (eg, tumor necrosis factor and interleukin-1) draw neutrophils into the CSF space, and the growing exudate (especially dense in the basal cisterns) damages cranial nerves, obliterates the CSF pathways (causing hydrocephalus) and induces vasculitis and thrombophlebitis (causing ischemia). Arachidonic acid metabolites and cytokines generated by the exudate damage cell membranes and disrupt the blood-brain barrier to cause brain edema, which is further aggravated by ischemic brain damage and by syndrome of inappropriate antidiuretic hormone (SIADH). Intracranial pressure rises, the BP falls (septic shock), and the patient can die of systemic complications or from massive brain infarction.

Symptoms, Signs, and Complications

A prodromal respiratory illness or sore throat often precedes the fever, headache, stiff neck, and vomiting that characterize acute meningitis. Adults may become desperately ill within 24 h; the course can be even shorter in children. In older children and adults, changes in consciousness progress through irritability, confusion, drowsiness, stupor, and coma. Seizures and cranial neuropathies may be present. Dehydration is common and vascular collapse may lead to shock (Waterhouse-Friderichsen syndrome), especially in meningococcal septicemia. Hemiparesis and other focal deficits can result from cerebral infarction, but their early occurrence is relatively uncommon and should suggest brain abscess, bacterial endocarditis, or Todd's postictal paralysis.

In infants between 3 mo and 2 yr of age, symptoms and signs are less predictable. Fever, vomiting, irritability, convulsions, a high-pitched cry, and a bulging or tight fontanelle are commonly present; stiff neck may be absent. Subdural effusions may develop after several days in infants and young children; typical signs are seizures, persistent fever, or enlarging head size. Subdural taps through the coronal sutures show a high protein content in the subdural fluid. Hydrocephalus and thrombophlebitis (see in Pathophysiology, above) also may complicate meningitis.

Diagnosis

Since acute bacterial meningitis, especially meningococcal, can be lethal in hours, accurate diagnosis and treatment are urgent. Any unexplained fever in infants between 3 mo and 2 yr of age warrants a lumbar puncture (LP) if the child develops increasing irritability, poor feeding, vomiting, lethargy, seizures, or signs of meningeal irritation. When bacterial meningitis is seriously suspected, administration of antibiotics should not await the results of diagnostic tests.

The head, ears, and skin of all patients should be inspected for sources of infection. A petechial or purpuric rash can occur in generalized septicemia, but its presence with meningeal signs indicates meningococcal meningitis until proved otherwise. The skin over the entire spine should be inspected for dimples, sinuses, nevi, or tufts of hair, which may indicate a congenital anomaly communicating with the subarachnoid space. The joints, lungs, and skin may be involved in meningococcal or H. influenzae infections.

Abrupt neck flexion in the supine patient results in involuntary flexion of the hips and knees (Brudzinski's sign). Attempts to extend the knee from the flexed-thigh position are met with strong passive resistance (Kernig's sign). Both signs are thought to be due to irritation of motor nerve roots passing through inflamed meninges as they are brought under tension. Unilateral or bilateral Babinski's sign may be present. Cranial nerve abnormalities (oculomotor or facial nerve palsy and occasionally deafness) may be seen.

Laboratory findings: LP should be done immediately and the CSF cultured and examined, with the recognition that LP can precipitate acute neurologic worsening in the presence of a brain abscess or other mass lesion. If the infectious agent is not readily seen on the CSF smear, a rapid diagnosis can sometimes be made by counterimmunoelectrophoresis (CIE), latex agglutination, or other serologic detection of bacterial antigens in the CSF (in some laboratories, up to 80% of specimens are positive in meningococcal, H. influenzae type b, and pneumococcal meningitis). More recently, the polymerase chain reaction has been used successfully in the rapid, early diagnosis of meningococcal meningitis (it is also useful when cultures are negative). Search for an infectious source should also include cultures of blood, nasopharynx, respiratory secretions, urine, and any skin lesion. Disseminated intravascular coagulation commonly complicates meningitis and is characterized by elevations in the prothrombin and partial thromboplastin times, thrombocytopenia, decreased fibrinogen, and increased fibrin degradation products. Serum and urine Na and osmolarity should be monitored for presence of SIADH.

The CT scan may be normal or show small ventricles, effacement of the sulci, and contrast enhancement over the convexities. MRI with gadolinium is superior in detecting subarachnoid inflammation. Films should be scrutinized for evidence of brain abscess, sinus or mastoid infection, skull fracture, and congenital anomalies. Later, venous infarctions or communicating hydrocephalus may be seen.

Differential diagnosis: A number of infectious and noninfectious illnesses resemble bacterial meningitis. Of special importance is the need to distinguish **aseptic meningitis** (especially **viral meningitis;** see below) and **encephalitis** from bacterial infection. Diagnosis depends chiefly on the CSF findings (see ACUTE VIRAL ENCEPHALITIS AND ASEPTIC MENINGITIS under VIRAL INFECTIONS, below). Widespread use of antibiotics (eg, to treat minor respiratory infections) has made **partially treated bacterial meningitis** a diagnostic problem (see below), since infection may persist even when meningeal signs subside, the CSF reverts toward normal, and CSF cultures become negative. The slowly evolving symptoms and the CSF findings usually differentiate **subacute meningitis** from acute bacterial meningitis (see SUBACUTE AND CHRONIC MENINGITIS under MISCELLANEOUS INFECTIONS, below). **Rocky Mountain spotted fever** and other rickettsial diseases (eg, typhus) can cause fever, headache, a macular and petechial skin rash (but unlike meningococcemia, it begins in the wrists and ankles), and delirium that progresses to coma. The CSF, however, is normal or shows a modest lymphocytic pleocytosis. **Leptospirosis** causes an aseptic meningitis with fever, myalgia, headache, and meningismus followed by skin rash, and renal and liver damage. An important clue is exposure to water or soil contaminated by the urine of rats, dogs, swine, or cattle. The free-living ameba (*Naegleria*) infects swimmers in warm lakes and causes a purulent, often fatal **amebic meningoencephalitis.** Ameboid movement is detected in unspun wet mounts of the CSF, and the organism can be cultured. Combined IV and intrathecal amphotericin B (see **fungal meningitis** under SUBACUTE AND CHRONIC MENINGITIS, below, for dosage) is sometimes lifesaving. **Subacute bacterial endocarditis** (see also INFECTIVE ENDOCARDITIS, below) can produce fever, discrete skin lesions, focal embolic infarcts, and pleocytosis of the CSF. The apoplectic onset of neurologic deficits suggests embolism rather than venous infarction, whose evolution is not so abrupt. **Parameningeal infection** or **inflammation** (eg, mastoiditis, epidural abscess) can cause fever, CSF pleocytosis, and sometimes raised CSF pressure (eg, lateral sinus thrombosis secondary to phlebitis). CSF stains and cultures are negative, but treatment with antibiotics should be combined with surgical drainage of the infected structure. Young children with pneumonia or shigella infections can develop **meningismus** without any abnormality in the CSF. **Nonspecific infections in infants** may cause nonspecific symptoms (eg, lethargy, irritability) with or without fever, requiring LP to exclude meningitis.

Lead encephalopathy may mimic bacterial meningitis but onset is usually less explosive, fever is uncommon, and the CSF glucose is usually normal (see LEAD POISONING in Ch. 31). **Chemical meningitis** can occur episodically when an epidermoid tumor or craniopharyngioma leaks its keratinaceous contents into the CSF. Fever generally is absent. Intrathecal chemotherapy, spinal anesthetics, and myelographic dyes may on occasion irritate the meninges, but infection must always be ruled out. **Mollaret meningitis** is a rare, self-limiting, and often recurrent illness characterized by large endothelial cells in the CSF. PMN cells may be present, and later replaced by lymphocytes. Some cases are due to cryptic intracranial epitheliomas. **Acute cerebellar hemorrhage** or **infarction** can produce tonsillar herniation and consequent nuchal rigidity followed by obstructive hydrocephalus, stupor, coma, and death. The presence of fever may be confusing, and LP may be catastrophic. Neurologic deficits referable to the posterior fossa are diagnostic clues (see STRUCTURAL LESIONS OF THE CEREBELLUM under CEREBELLAR AND SPINOCEREBELLAR DISORDERS in Ch. 43). CT or MRI is diagnostic.

Prognosis and Prophylaxis

Antibiotics and supportive care have reduced the fatality rate of acute bacterial meningitis to < 10% in cases recognized early. However, when meningitis is diagnosed late or occurs in neonates or the elderly, it is often fatal. A low peripheral WBC count is a bad prognostic sign. Persistent leukopenia, delayed therapy, and development of the Waterhouse-Friderichsen syndrome diminish the chances of survival. Survivors occasionally show signs of cranial nerve damage, evidence of cerebral infarction, recurrent convulsions, or mental retardation.

Meningococcal vaccine is used mainly in epidemics and closed populations when epidemic spread is feared. Family members, medical personnel, and others in close contact with these patients should receive prophylaxis with rifampin over 48 h (adult, 600 mg q 12 h; children, 10 mg/kg q 12 h; infants < 1 mo old, 5 mg/kg q 12 h). Minocycline for chemoprophylaxis is less desirable because of reported vestibular side effects. A vaccine for *H. influenzae* type b has been found protective in children as young as 2 mo of age. Children and adults who have had close contact with patients with *H. influenzae* type b meningitis should receive rifampin 20 mg/kg/day (*no more than 600 mg/day*) taken orally for 4 days.

Treatment

1. **Initial therapy** should be guided by the patient's age, the clinical circumstances, suspected pathogens, and the CSF results. The Gram stain of the CSF sediment usually can discriminate between meningococcus, hemophilus, pneumococcus, staphylococcus, and gram-negative organisms. Antibiotics should be started immediately after the CSF, blood, nasopharynx, and other pertinent body fluids have been cultured; therapy should never await the results of other tests (eg, CT or MRI) when the patient is desperately ill. If the organism cannot be positively identified on smear, empiric therapy is given pending CSF culture results (see TABLE 32–2). Therapy usually includes a 3rd-generation cephalosporin (eg, ceftriaxone or cefotaxime) because of its high activity against the common meningeal pathogens in both children and adults (including hemophilus strains resistant to ampicillin and chloramphenicol, and pneumococcal strains partially resistant to penicillin). In otherwise healthy adults, bacterial meningitis is caused by pneumococci and meningococci in at least 80% of cases, and penicillin G or ampicillin remain optimal therapy. In patients > 60 yr old, pathogens (eg, gram-negative bacilli) other than hemophilus, meningococcus, and pneumococcus account for about ½ of the cases, and a 3rd-generation cephalosporin should be part of the initial treatment. The 3rd-generation cephalosporins are effective against most aerobic gram-negative bacilli but have poor activity against *Listeria* and enterococci, and variable activity against gram-positive cocci and *Pseudomonas* (ceftazidime is active against *Pseudomonas* but drug resistance may develop). Additional antibiotic coverage is necessary when these other pathogens are clinically suspected (see below).

Treatment decision problems arise when CSF pleocytosis, normal glucose content, and the absence of bacteria make it difficult to determine whether viral meningitis, partially treated bacterial infections, or early bacterial meningitis is the diagnosis. CIE and latex agglutination tests vary between laboratories, and a negative result does not exclude bacterial meningitis. Since antibiotics can cause anaphylactic reactions, drug fever, and difficulty in evaluating the response to therapy, it may be advisable, *if the patient's condition permits it*, to withhold antibiotics and examine the CSF in 8 to 12 h, or sooner if his condition deteriorates. If initial granulocyte predominance gives way to mononuclear predominance, CSF glucose remains normal, and the patient looks well, the infection is unlikely to be bacterial, and antibiotics can be withheld pending culture results. However, if the patient's condition is serious, and especially if antibiotics have been given (hindering the growth of organisms on culture), a bacterial infection must be assumed and adequate antibiotic coverage provided (see TABLE 32–2).

2. **Specific therapy:** (For dosages, see TABLE 32–2.) Once the organism is identified, penicillin G may be substituted for ampicillin in infections caused by meningococci, pneumococci, β-hemolytic streptococci, and susceptible staphylococci. Penicillinase-producing staphylococci should be treated with oxacillin or nafcillin. In hospitals where methicillin (oxacillin)-resistant *S. aureus* is endemic, vancomycin should be used as initial therapy until sensitivities are known. Because an increasing number of *H. influenzae* strains are resistant to ampicillin (and occasionally to chloramphenicol, especially outside the USA), cefotaxime or ceftriaxone should be given for the initial treatment of bacterial meningitis in children. Alternatively, chloramphenicol can be added to ampicillin. Subsequent therapy can be modified in accordance with culture results and susceptibility testing. Currently under investigation is adjuvant therapy with dexamethasone 0.15 mg/kg q 6 h for 4 days, which has been reported to reduce deafness due to *H. influenzae* meningitis.

If gram-negative bacilli are seen in the CSF, therapy should begin with cefotaxime, which covers many gram-negative organisms (but not *Pseudomonas* and *Acinetobacter*). Cefotaxime and other 3rd-generation cephalosporins appear to be as active as the aminoglycosides without their potential nephro- and ototoxicity. *Pseudomonas* coverage can be achieved by concurrent use of azlocillin, piperacillin, carbenicillin, ticarcillin, or ceftazidime with gentamicin, tobramycin, or amikacin. Amikacin should be used in hospitals where gentamicin resistance of enteric organisms is common.

The CSF should be reexamined (24 to 48 h after starting antibiotics) for sterility and conver-

TABLE 32−2. ANTIBIOTIC THERAPY FOR ACUTE BACTERIAL MENINGITIS

Organism	Antibiotic	Total Daily Dosage (Pediatric Dosage in Parentheses)	Dosing Frequency
Unknown In infants (< 1 mo old)	Ampicillin	100−150 mg/kg IV (0−7 days old) 150−200 mg/kg IV (> 7 days old)	q 8−12 h q 6−8 h
	plus Cefotaxime	200 mg/kg IV	q 6 h
	or Gentamicin	7.5 mg/kg IV (> 7 days old, 5 mg/kg)	q 8 h q 12 h
	or Tobramycin	5 mg/kg IV	q 12 h
In children (> 1 mo old)	Cefotaxime or	(dosage as above)	
	Ceftriaxone or	4 gm IV	q 12 h
	Ampicillin plus	100−200 mg/kg IV	q 3−4 h
	Chloramphenicol	50−75 m/kg IV	q 6 h
In adults	Cefotaxime or	12 gm IV	q 4−6 h
	Ceftriaxone or	(dosage as above)	q 12 h
	Chloramphenicol plus	50−100 mg/kg IV	q 6 h
	Penicillin G or	24 million u. IV	q 2−4 h
	Ampicillin	12 gm IV	q 2−4 h
Gram-negative rods in CSF (unidentified)	Cefotaxime or	(dosage as above)	q 4−6 h
	Ceftriaxone plus	(dosage as above)	q 12 h
	Gentamicin or	(dosage as above)	
	Tobramycin or	(dosage as above)	
	Amikacin*	15 mg/kg IV	q 8 h
Meningococcus	Penicillin G	24 million u. IV	q 2−4 h
Hemophilus influenzae b	Cefotaxime or	(dosage as above)	q 4−6 h
	Ceftriaxone or	2−4 gm IV	q 12 h
	Ampicillin plus	(dosage as above)	q 3−4 h
	Chloramphenicol	(dosage as above)	q 6 h
Streptococcus (pneumococcus)	Penicillin G or	(dosage as above)	q 2−4 h
	Ampicillin	(dosage as above)	q 2−4 h
Staphylococcus	Oxacillin or	12 gm IV (100−200 mg/kg IV)	q 4−6 h
	Nafcillin or	12 gm IV (100−200 mg/kg IV)	q 4 h
	Vancomycin†	2 gm IV (40 mg/kg IV)	q 6−12 h

(Continued)

TABLE 32–2. ANTIBIOTIC THERAPY FOR ACUTE BACTERIAL MENINGITIS *(Cont'd)*

Organism	Antibiotic	Total Daily Dosage (Pediatric Dosage in Parentheses)	Dosing Frequency
Listeria	Ampicillin or Penicillin G (with gentamicin)‡	(dosage as above)	
Gram-negative enterics (eg, *Escherichia coli*, *Klebsiella*, *Proteus*)	Cefotaxime or Ceftriaxone or Chloramphenicol§ with gentamicin, tobramycin, or amikacin*	(dosage as above)	
Pseudomonas	Ceftazidime with	6–8 gm IV	q 6–8 h
	Gentamicin or	(dosage as above)	
	Tobramycin or	(dosage as above)	
	Amikacin*	(dosage as above)	
	Azlocillin or	18 gm IV (225–300 mg/kg IV)	q 4 h
	Piperacillin or	18 gm IV (200–300 mg/kg IV)	q 4–6 h
	Cabenicillin	30–40 gm IV (0–7 days old, 200 mg/kg IV; infant, 300–400 mg/kg IV; child, 400–500 mg/kg IV)	q 2–4 h q 2–4 h q 2–4 h
	or Ticarcillin	200–300 mg/kg IV (0–7 days old, 150–225 mg/kg IV; > 7 days old, 225–300 mg/kg IV)	q 4 h q 8–12 h q 4–6 h

* In areas where gentamicin resistance is common. Because CSF penetration is poor, aminoglycosides may have to be given intrathecally or via an Ommaya reservoir, especially with *Pseudomonas* meningitis.
† For methicillin-resistant staphylococci or penicillin allergy.
‡ For severely ill, immunocompromised patients.
§ For patients with severe penicillin allergy.

sion to lymphocytic predominance. Antibiotics generally should be continued for at least 1 wk after fever subsides and the CSF returns toward normal (normalization of CSF, however, correlates imperfectly with success of therapy). Drug dosages should not be reduced concurrently with clinical improvement, since drug penetration in many instances will decrease as the meninges become less inflamed.

3. Supportive therapy: Fever, dehydration, and electrolyte disorders require correction (see Ch. 26). Care must be taken not to overhydrate patients with cerebral edema. Convulsions and status epilepticus are treated appropriately (see SEIZURE DISORDERS in Ch. 43 and SEIZURE DISORDERS IN THE NEWBORN in Ch. 27).

Vascular collapse and shock (Waterhouse-Friderichsen syndrome): Although attributed to adrenal insufficiency, loss of tissue fluid may be equally important, and the value of ACTH and corticosteroids remains controversial.

Cerebral edema severe enough to produce central or transtentorial herniation can be treated with controlled hyperventilation (Pa_{CO_2} 25 to 30 torr), mannitol (0.25 to 0.50 gm/kg IV), and dexamethasone (4 mg IV q 4 h).

In infants with subdural effusion, the fluid usually subsides with repeated daily subdural taps through the sutures. To avoid sudden shifts in the intracranial contents, *not more than 20 mL/day of CSF should be removed from one side*. If the effusion persists after 3 to 4 wk of taps, surgical exploration for possible excision of a subdural membrane is indicated.

Isolation: All patients with presumed bacterial meningitis (of unknown etiology) should be isolated for the first 24 h of therapy.

STREPTOCOCCAL INFECTIONS
(See also RHEUMATIC FEVER in Ch. 42)

Classification

Streptococcal infections can be classified **microbially** according to characteristics of the streptococcus and **clinically** according to the type of infection.

When grown on sheep blood agar, β-hemolytic streptococci produce zones of clear hemolysis around each colony; α-hemolytic streptococci (commonly called *Streptococcus viridans*) are surrounded by green discoloration resulting from incomplete hemolysis; and γ-hemolytic streptococci are nonhemolytic. An additional classification, based on carbohydrates present in the cell wall, divides streptococci into the Lancefield Groups A through H and K through T.

Group A β-hemolytic streptococci (*S. pyogenes*) are the most virulent species in man, causing pharyngitis, tonsillitis, wound and skin infections, septicemia, scarlet fever, pneumonia, rheumatic fever, and glomerulonephritis. **Group D** includes enterococcal (*Enterococcus faecalis, E. durans, E. faecium,* formerly *S. faecalis, S. durans,* and *S. faecium*) and nonenterococcal (*S. bovis, S. equinus*) species. Organisms formerly called enterococci have been reclassified as the genus *Enterococcus*. Most human infections caused by Group D streptococci are caused by *E. faecalis* or *S. bovis* and are distinguished from other streptococci by their ability to grow in 40% bile and to hydrolize esculin. Enterococci are identified by the PYR reaction (pyrrolidonyl-β-naphthylamide hydrolysis); these organisms also grow in 6.5% sodium chloride, but *S. bovis* does not. The latter is commonly found in the GI tract and may cause endocarditis, particularly when an intestinal neoplasm or other lesion is present. *S. bovis* is relatively susceptible to antimicrobials. Enterococci are more resistant unless exposed to a combination of a cell-wall–active drug such as penicillin, ampicillin, or vancomycin plus an aminoglycoside such as gentamicin or streptomycin. *E. faecalis* causes endocarditis, UTIs, abdominal sepsis, cellulitis, and wound infection, as well as concurrent bacteremia. Enterococci that are resistant to the bactericidal action of aminoglycosides with cell-wall–active drugs have emerged recently as an important cause of very serious and refractory infections, especially in hospitals. **Group B** streptococci may also cause infections, particularly neonatal sepsis, endocarditis, and septic arthritis. **Groups C and G** streptococci are pyogenes-like organisms and are distinguished from *S. pyogenes* in clinical laboratories by their resistance to bacitracin or by serogroup. Though often carried by animals, they colonize the human pharynx, intestinal tract, vagina, and skin. They can cause severe suppurative infections, including pharyngitis, pneumonia, cellulitis, pyoderma, erysipelas, impetigo, wound infections, puerperal sepsis, neonatal sepsis, endocarditis, septic arthritis, and poststreptococcal glomerulonephritis. Penicillin, vancomycin, the cephalosporins, and erythromycin are useful in therapy.

Extracellular Group A streptococcal antigens evoking antibody responses play important roles in the diagnostic tests described below.

Clinically, streptococcal infections can be divided into 3 broad groups: (1) the **carrier state,** in which the patient harbors streptococci without apparent infection; (2) **acute illness,** often suppurative, caused by streptococcal invasion of tissues; and (3) **delayed, nonsuppurative complications.** The nonsuppurative complications are the inflammatory states of acute rheumatic fever, chorea, and glomerulonephritis (discussed in Chs. 42, 43, and 41, respectively). They occur most commonly about 2 wk after a clinically overt streptococcal infection, but the infection may be asymptomatic and the interval may be shorter or longer than 2 wk.

Symptoms and Signs

The symptoms and signs of acute invasive streptococcal infections depend on the affected tissue, the organism, the state of the host, and the host's response.

A **carrier state** exists when streptococci can be identified in material taken from a site that shows no evidence of inflammation. Group D streptococci are normally found in the gut, α-hemolytic streptococci in the throat and respiratory tract. β-Hemolytic streptococci of Groups A, B, C, and G—the groups generally regarded as pathogenic for man—can be cultured routinely from normal-looking throats or vaginas of asymptomatic patients, and the term "carrier state" is usually reserved for such pharyngeal or vaginal discoveries. The carrier state is important as a cause of misdiagnosis in many pharyngeal or respiratory illnesses, since demonstration of bacteria does not prove that a streptococcus is responsible for the associated clinical manifestations. Throat cultures from carriers usually yield only small numbers of organisms, while those from persons with significant infections are strongly positive.

Acute streptococcal infections can be *primary*, invading normal tissue, or *secondary*, invading tissue compromised by trauma or other disease. The organism in primary invasions is usually the Group A β-hemolytic streptococcus and the site is usually the pharynx. Secondary invasions can be caused by α-hemolytic streptococci, by Group D streptococci, or by Group A organisms. Group A streptococcal erysipelas can occur in previously normal or edematous skin, or a streptococcal cellulitis can be imposed on traumatized skin or in subcutaneous tissue predisposed by venous insufficiency. A viral pneumonia or degenerative lung disease may be followed by a streptococcal pneumonia; S. viridans or Group D streptococci may cause bacterial endocarditis; Group D streptococci are frequently found in UTIs; and the endometritis of a postpartum uterus is often due to enterococci or Group A or B organisms. Group D streptococci are common causes of nosocomial wound infections. The eyes, ears, joints, bone, and gut are other sites of secondary streptococcal invasion. Infections with Group B β-hemolytic streptococci (*S. agalactiae*) are important causes of neonatal sepsis (see NEONATAL SEPSIS under NEONATAL INFECTIONS in Ch. 27). In adults, sporadic cases of bacteremia, endocarditis, UTIs, pneumonia, and meningitis are seen. In addition, Group B β-hemolytic streptococci are recovered frequently from elderly diabetic patients with cellulitis complicating severe peripheral vascular disease.

Primary or secondary infections can spread through the affected tissues and along lymphatic channels to regional lymph nodes; they can also produce bacteremia. The development of suppuration depends on the severity of infection and the susceptibility of tissue.

The most common type of streptococcal disease is **primary pharyngeal infection with Group A β-hemolytic streptococci**. Typically, the infection is manifested by sore throat, fever, a beefy red pharynx, and tonsillar exudate. About 20% of patients with Group A infections have this type of illness. The remainder are asymptomatic; have fever or mild sore throat alone, resembling viral pharyngitis; or have nonspecific symptoms such as headache, malaise, nausea, vomiting, or tachycardia. Convulsions may occur in children. The cervical and submaxillary nodes may enlarge and become tender. In children < 4 yr, rhinorrhea is common and sometimes the sole manifestation. None of these symptoms (including sore throat) and none of the signs (including pharyngeal exudate or occasional palatal petechiae) are specific for streptococcal infection; any or all of these clinical features can occur in viral infections, particularly with the adenoviruses and in infectious mononucleosis. The only sign or symptom statistically associated with serologically confirmed streptococcal disease is cervical adenitis. Cough, laryngitis, and stuffy nose are uncharacteristic of streptococcal infection, and their presence suggests that another organism is the cause or that other causative agents or complications coexist. Definitive diagnosis rests on the laboratory techniques described below.

Though formerly a common ailment, **scarlet fever** (scarlatina) is uncommon today, probably because antibiotic therapy prevents the streptococcus from progressing in individual patients or causing massive epidemics. Scarlet fever is associated with Group A streptococcal (and occasionally other) strains that produce an erythrogenic toxin, leading to a diffuse pink-red cutaneous flush that blanches on pressure. The rash, an additional feature of this illness that otherwise resembles streptococcal pharyngitis, is seen best on the abdomen, on the lateral chest, and in cutaneous folds. Among the characteristic manifestations of the rash are **circumoral pallor** surrounded by a flushed face, a **strawberry tongue** (inflamed papillae protruding through a bright red coating), and **Pastia's lines** (dark red lines in the creases of skin folds). A similar tongue can be seen in the toxic shock (see Ch. 8) and Kawasaki (see under MISCELLANEOUS INFECTIONS, below) syndromes. The upper layer of the previously reddened skin often desquamates after the fever subsides. The course and management of scarlet fever are the same as for other clinically evident Group A infections.

Streptococcal pyoderma (impetigo) is discussed below.

Laboratory Findings

Acute streptococcal inflammation is regularly associated with an elevation in both ESR (usually > 50 mm/h in the Westergren test or uncorrected Wintrobe test) and WBC count (about

12,000 to 20,000), with 75 to 90% neutrophils, many of which are young forms. The urine commonly shows no specific changes except those attributable to fever (eg, proteinuria).

The presence of streptococci can be established directly and promptly in specimens taken from the inflammatory site and examined after overnight incubation on a sheep blood agar plate or, for Group A organisms, immediate staining with fluorescent antibodies. When organisms are grown in culture, the fluorescent method obviates the need for serologic testing to differentiate Group A from other β-hemolytic streptococci, but the fluorescence often produces false-positive reactions with hemolytic staphylococci. A number of diagnostic kits for rapid identification of Group A streptococcus are also available. Though subject to false-positive and some false-negative results, they are nonetheless useful.

These direct tests can show that streptococci are *present* but *proof of infection* is obtained indirectly from streptococcal antibodies in the serum. The antistreptolysin O (ASO) titer rises in only 75 to 80% of infections; for completeness, streptococcal antihyaluronidase, antideoxyribonuclease B, antinicotinamide adenine dinucleotidase, and antistreptokinase can also be used. Penicillin given early (within the first 5 days) for symptomatic streptococcal pharyngitis may delay the appearance and decrease the magnitude of the antibody response to streptolysin O. Patients with streptococcal pyoderma usually do not have a significant ASO response.

A single value of one antibody titer is only a crude index of recent streptococcal infection. Confirmation requires comparison of sequential specimens for recent *changes* in titer, since a single value may be high as a result of slow "decay" of antibodies from a long antecedent infection. Conversely, a single value lower than the laboratory's upper limit of normal may represent an elevation for an individual patient. Serum specimens need not be taken more often than every 2 wk and may be taken every 2 mo. A significant rise (or fall) in titer should span at least 2 tube dilutions, since a 1-tube increment may be due to laboratory variation. For greatest accuracy, the sera under comparison should be saved and tested on the same day, with the same reagents, by the same technician.

Streptozyme®, an inexpensive, easily performed test for antibodies to streptolysin O, hyaluronidase, deoxyribonuclease B, and other streptococcal antigens, correlates best with an elevated ASO titer. False-positive results are seen in 3 to 5% of cases. However, 25 to 50% of patients with borderline serologic responses to specific streptococcal extracellular antigens will have false-negative agglutination with the Streptozyme® test.

Because of the time interval between serial specimens, serologic testing is not useful in managing acute invasive streptococcal infections in which diagnosis depends on clinical manifestations and results of bacteriologic tests. Serial antibody tests are particularly useful, however, in diagnosing poststreptococcal inflammatory states. Evidence of a recent Group A streptococcal infection is critical for diagnosing rheumatic fever, which can generally be ruled out if no change in titer is shown in properly performed serial tests measuring other appropriate antibodies besides ASO.

Course and Treatment

The secondarily invasive streptococcal infections can be life-threatening, particularly for a debilitated patient. Septicemias, puerperal sepsis, endocarditis, and pneumonias due to streptococci were frequent causes of death in the preantibiotic era and remain serious, especially if the infecting organism is an enterococcus. Though Group A streptococci and *S. viridans* are almost always sensitive to penicillin, enterococci are relatively resistant and require treatment with an aminoglycoside in addition to penicillin or ampicillin. In some areas, enterococci have been discovered that resist even high concentrations of gentamicin and other aminoglycosides and that show no synergism with penicillin. There is currently no reliable bactericidal therapy for these strains.

The primary pharyngeal infections, including scarlet fever, ordinarily have a finite course; the fever subsides after several days and recovery is complete within 2 wk. Antibiotics shorten the clinical illness in young children, especially those with scarlet fever, but they have little effect on the symptoms of streptococcal pharyngitis in adolescents or adults. Their value is primarily to prevent local suppurative complications such as peritonsillar abscess (quinsy), otitis media, sinusitis, and mastoiditis. Most important, they are used to thwart the nonsuppurative complications that may follow untreated Group A infections.

Penicillin is the best therapeutic agent for an established Group A streptococcal infection. A single injection of benzathine penicillin G, at a dose of 600,000 to 900,000 u. (50,000 u./kg) IM for small children and 1.2 million u. IM for adolescents or adults, will usually suffice. Since the injection is often painful, oral therapy with penicillin G or V may be preferred if the patient can be trusted to maintain the regimen. The minor differences in absorption among the diverse oral preparations of penicillin do not seem as important as an adequately high dosage and sufficient duration of the regimen. At least 200,000 u. (and preferably 400,000 u.) of penicillin G taken on an empty stomach or 125 mg (to 250 mg) of penicillin V should be taken tid or qid for at least 10 days (for children, 25 to 50 mg/kg/day in divided doses tid or qid) to achieve the effect of a single injection of benzathine penicillin G. The 10-day course *must be completed*, even if the patient becomes asymptomatic. An alternative plan for patients considered unreliable or unable to take oral medication is to give 3 injections of procaine penicillin (each usually less painful than the one large benzathine dose): 600,000 u. (for children, 50,000 u./kg) IM is given on the 1st, 4th, and 7th days.

When penicillin is contraindicated, erythromycin 250 mg qid or clindamycin 300 mg tid may be given orally for 10 days. Clindamycin (8 to 25 mg/kg/day in divided doses tid or qid) is preferred in children who have relapses of chronic tonsillitis. Sulfadiazine, which is bacteriostatic, should not be used to treat an established infection, though it is useful in preventing streptococcal infections. Tetracyclines are undesirable because a significant number of Group A streptococci are resistant to them and because they may discolor growing teeth in young children.

Antistreptococcal therapy can often be withheld for 1 or 2 days, until bacteriologic verification has been obtained, without significantly increasing the risk of suppurative or nonsuppurative complications of streptococcal pharyngitis. An effective plan is to begin oral penicillin when infection is suspected and specimens for laboratory tests have been obtained. The treatment can be stopped if laboratory tests fail to confirm the presence of streptococci. Otherwise, the oral drug is continued or replaced by an injectable agent.

Other symptoms of streptococcal infection (eg, sore throat, headache, fever) can be treated with analgesics or antipyretics. Bed rest is unnecessary unless the patient wants it. Isolation techniques are no longer warranted. Among the infected patient's close associates in family or friends, those who are symptomatic or have a history of poststreptococcal complications should be examined for streptococci, then appropriately treated with antibiotics.

OCCULT BACTEREMIA

Pathogenic bacteria in the bloodstream of young febrile children who have no apparent foci of infection and look well enough to be managed as outpatients. This disorder should be distinguished from sepsis, neonatal sepsis, and septic shock. (For a discussion of these infections in neonates, see NEONATAL SEPSIS and NEONATAL MENINGITIS under NEONATAL INFECTIONS in Ch. 27.)

Etiology and Epidemiology

Occult bacteremia is caused by *Streptococcus pneumoniae* in 65 to 75% of cases and by *Hemophilus influenzae* type b in 15 to 25%; a variety of bacteria, including *Neisseria meningitidis* and *Salmonella* spp, cause the remainder.

Occult bacteremia is detected in about 3 to 4% of febrile infants between 1 and 24 mo of age; most cases occur in infants between 6 and 24 mo of age. Children who look well enough to be managed as outpatients but who later are found to be bacteremic usually are < 24 mo of age. Incidence does not vary with sex or race.

Symptoms, Signs, and Diagnosis

Occult bacteremia is most often associated with URIs, pharyngitis, or fever alone; however, the percentage of infants with one of these complaints who are actually bacteremic is very small. It is unlikely that a child with a temperature of < 38.5° C (101.3° F) is bacteremic. The risk of bacteremia increases with higher temperatures.

Since diagnosis depends on isolating bacteria from the blood, there is no certain way to make the diagnosis when the child is first seen. Cultures usually take 24 to 48 h to become positive, and specimens often are contaminated with microorganisms from the skin. More rapid diagnostic techniques are needed since those currently available are not sensitive enough for clinical use.

Nonspecific tests may help to determine the risk of bacteremia for a particular child. In most bacteremic children, the WBC count is elevated and thus is sensitive; however, only about 10% of children with WBC counts of > 20,000 are bacteremic. Acute phase reactants add little to the WBC count. Combining risk factors—eg, 1 to 24 mo of age, temperature > 38.5° C (101.3° F), and high WBC count—helps, but at best only 10 to 25% of infants with all of these risk factors are bacteremic.

Prognosis and Treatment

Of the children who receive antibiotics before bacteremia is confirmed, > 75% improve clinically and < 10% have persistent bacteremia. In contrast, < 33% of children who do not receive antibiotics improve clinically, and nearly 33% of those with *S. pneumoniae* bacteremia and 50% of those with *H. influenzae* bacteremia are still bacteremic at the 2nd visit. The incidence of meningitis, however, is essentially the same in children who receive oral antibiotics as in those who do not.

About 50% of outpatients in whom bacteremia is suspected have treatable foci of infection—usually otitis media or pneumonia; thus, they are already receiving oral antibiotics by the time bacteremia is confirmed.

Some authorities advocate initiating treatment with IM ceftriaxone or oral amoxicillin while awaiting the results of outpatient blood cultures for infants between the ages of 3 and 24 mo who have temperatures > 40° C (104° F) and WBC counts > 15,000. Others believe treatment is not necessary if meticulous observation can be guaranteed. In either case, close observation and follow-up are essential, especially for the first 72 h.

URINARY TRACT INFECTION (UTI) IN CHILDREN

Significant bacteriuria in a child, either asymptomatic or with the manifestations of cystitis, pyelonephritis, or septicemia.

The urinary tract from the kidneys to the bladder is normally sterile, despite probable frequent contamination with colonic bacteria via the urethra. Mechanisms that maintain the tract's sterility include urine acidity and free flow, a normal emptying mechanism, intact ureteral and urethral valves, and immunologic and mucosal barriers. Abnormality in any of these mechanisms and urinary stasis are major predisposing factors to UTI.

Etiology and Incidence

In abnormal urinary tracts, many different organisms can cause infection, but in relatively normal tracts, the organisms usually are strains of *Escherichia coli* with specific attachment factors for transitional epithelium of the bladder and ureters. *E. coli* causes > 75% of UTI in all pediatric age groups. The remaining cases are due to other gram-negative enterobacteria, especially *Klebsiella, Proteus mirabalis,* and *Pseudomonas*

aeruginosa. Enterococci (Group D streptococci) and coagulase-negative staphylococci (eg, *Staphylococcus saprophyticus*) are the most frequently implicated gram-positive organisms. Fungi and mycobacteria are unusual causes of UTI. Adenoviruses are implicated in a syndrome of hemorrhagic cystitis.

One to 2% of **newborns** develop UTI, and the male:female ratio is 5:1. The infections in males often are bacteremic. Predisposing factors include malformations and obstructions of the urinary tract, prematurity, indwelling catheters, and lack of circumcision; major renal abnormalities are present in 20 to 40% of newborns with UTI.

UTIs occur in 2% of **young children beyond the newborn period** and in 5% of **school-aged children.** The female:male ratio rises with age and is > 10:1 beyond age 4 yr. Infections in females usually are ascending and not associated with bacteremia. The marked female preponderance is attributed to the shorter female urethra. Other predisposing factors in this age group include indwelling catheters, constipation, Hirschsprung's disease, and anatomic abnormalities of the urinary tract (eg, obstructions, neurogenic bladder, and ureteral duplications). Other associated risk factors include pinworms, IgA deficiency, diabetes, trauma, and, in **adolescents,** sexual intercourse. Five to 15% of school-aged children with UTI have urinary tract anomalies that will require surgery; 30 to 40% have vesicoureteral reflux that will require antibiotic prophylaxis. The incidence of reflux varies inversely with age.

Symptoms and Signs

In **newborns,** symptoms and signs are nonspecific and often mimic those of neonatal sepsis. Poor feeding, diarrhea, failure to thrive, vomiting, mild jaundice, lethargy, fever, or hypothermia can suggest UTI.

Infants and toddlers also present with poorly localizing signs. Some children are asymptomatic and diagnosed on routine screening; others have symptoms referable to the GI tract (eg, vomiting, diarrhea, or abdominal pain). In **children > 2 yr,** the more classic picture of cystitis or pyelonephritis can be seen, although, again, as many as 40% of UTIs may be asymptomatic. Symptoms of cystitis include dysuria, frequency, hematuria, urinary retention, suprapubic pain, urgency, pruritus, incontinence, foul-smelling urine, and enuresis. Symptoms of pyelonephritis include those of cystitis plus high fever, chills, costovertebral pain, and tenderness.

Diagnosis

Bladder urine is normally sterile but usually acquires some colonic and skin bacteria during passage through the urethra. The diagnosis of UTI requires demonstration of significant bacteriuria in a culture of properly collected urine.

Newborns and young children: Urine is best obtained by suprapubic aspiration or direct catheterization of the urinary bladder. Bagged specimens are reliable if negative, but a positive culture always should be confirmed with a repeat specimen, preferably suprapubic or catheterized. In **older children,** clean-voided urine specimens are acceptable, but the culture should be repeated before initiating antimicrobial therapy unless the signs are so obvious that immediate therapy is warranted. If the urine is obtained by suprapubic aspiration of the bladder, the presence of any gram-negative bacteria is significant, as are > 1000 coagulase-negative staphylococci/mL of urine. In a catheterized specimen, $> 10^3$ colonies/mL usually are significant. Clean-voided specimens from males are significant with colony counts $> 10^4$; from females, with colony counts $> 10^5$. Repeating the culture improves the diagnostic accuracy of a positive result. Occasionally UTI may be present in spite of low colony counts, possibly due to prior antibiotic therapy, very dilute urine (sp gr < 1.003), or obstruction to the flow of grossly infected urine.

Urine should be cultured as soon as possible or stored at $4°$ C if a delay of > 10 to 20 min is anticipated. Urine is best cultured in blood agar plates and incubated 24 to 48 h at $37°$ C. The urine is streaked on the plates using quantitative bacteriologic loops. When urine is from a suprapubic aspirate or is catheterized, 0.001 mL *and* 0.1 mL should be cultured. Specimens from a bag, or clean-voided, are sufficiently cultured at 0.001 mL. For office bacteriology, culturing on blood agar plates is the procedure of choice, although kit methods (eg, the dipslide or filter paper) are sensitive. Chemical tests for the presence of bacteria (eg, the nitrite test and the leukocyte esterase test) are useful for screening.

Microscopic examination of the urine is useful but not definitive. Pyuria (> 5 WBCs/high-power field in the spun urine sediment) usually indicates UTI, but is absent in 60% of culture-proven UTIs. The urine Gram stain can be a sensitive procedure for identifying UTI. The presence of one bacterium/oil immersion ($1000 \times$) field in an unspun urine, or > 100 bacteria in a spun urine sediment, correlates with the presence of $> 10^5$ bacteria/mL of urine.

Distinguishing upper from lower tract disease is not always clear-cut. When the child presents with high fever, costovertebral angle tenderness, and gross pyuria with casts, there is little doubt that the child has pyelonephritis. However, when sensitive distinguishing techniques (eg, bladder washout, concentrating ability, or the presence of antibody-coated bacteria) have been applied in research settings, many children with asymptomatic UTIs or with only symptoms of cystitis had upper tract disease. These specialized tests are not indicated in the usual clinical settings, but the physician should be aware that any child with UTI may have upper tract disease.

Treatment and Prognosis

The major goal is to preserve renal parenchymal function and to minimize acute morbidity. All children with suspected UTI should be examined for abdominal masses, enlarged kidneys, urethral abnormalities, costovertebral angle tenderness, and signs of lower spinal malformations. Force of the urinary stream may be the only clue to obstruction or neurogenic bladder. BP, height, and weight should be recorded. Hct, BUN, and creatinine should be checked in children with documented UTI.

In the newborn, blood and urine cultures should be obtained and treatment begun parenterally with ampicillin and an aminoglycoside in dosages appropriate for neonatal sepsis (see TABLE 27–4). If blood cultures are negative, clinical response is good, and repeat urine culture 48 to 72 h into therapy is negative, an appropriate oral antibiotic (eg, ampicillin, amoxicillin, or a cephalosporin) can be used to complete a 10-day course. Another urine culture should be obtained 7 to 10 days after the end of therapy. A poor response suggests either a resistant organism or an obstructive lesion and warrants urgent evaluation.

Beyond the newborn period, children with UTI can be treated with oral antibiotics unless they have high fever, prominent signs of toxicity, or are vomiting, in which case parenteral treatment is indicated. The initial antibiotics of choice are ampicillin, amoxicillin, sulfisoxazole, trimethoprim/sulfamethoxazole (TMP/SMX), or a cephalosporin (see TABLE 32–3). These agents provide adequate coverage for *E. coli*. Children hospitalized with acute pyelonephritis and signs of sepsis should receive ampicillin and an aminoglycoside parenterally. Length of treatment for UTI is 10 to 14 days, although many older chil-

TABLE 32–3. ANTIMICROBIAL DRUG DOSAGES FOR UTI IN CHILDREN

Drug	Daily Dose, Oral (mg/kg/day)	Daily Dose, Parenteral (mg/kg/day)	Dosing Interval (h)
Amikacin		15	8–12
Amoxicillin	30		8
Ampicillin	50–100	50–100	6
Carbenicillin		50–200	6
Cefadroxil	30		12
Cefamandole		50–100	6
Cefazolin		25–100	6
Cefixime	8		12–24
Cefotaxime		50–180	6
Cefoxitin		80–160	6
Ceftriaxone		50–75	12–24
Cefuroxime		50–100	8
Cefuroxime axetil	30		12
Cephalexin	25–50		6
Cephalothin		80–160	6
Cephapirin		40–80	6
Gentamicin		6–7.5	8
Kanamycin		15	8
Nitrofurantoin	5–7		6
Sulfadiazine	120–150		6
Sulfamethoxazole	50–60		12
Sulfisoxazole	120–150		6
Tetracyclines*	25–50		6
Ticarcillin		50–100	6
Tobramycin		6–7.5	8–12
Trimethoprim/ sulfamethoxazole	8/40	8/40	12

* Tetracyclines should be avoided in children < 8 yr of age.

dren with uncomplicated UTI can be successfully treated with a short course of antibiotics; eg, amikacin 7.5 mg/kg IM or gentamicin 5 mg/kg IM in a single dose may achieve a cure rate and a recurrence rate similar to 10 days of oral sulfisoxazole. Ampicillin, amoxicillin, TMP/SMX, or cefadroxil for 1 to 3 days achieves similar results in older children with uncomplicated cystitis. This approach appears promising but should not be used currently for treatment of recurrences.

Urine should be recultured 2 to 3 days after start of therapy if efficacy is not apparent and in all children with UTI 7 to 10 days after stopping antibiotics to document efficacy of treatment. Failure to sterilize the urine after 48 h of antibiotics may be due to a resistant organism, an obstructive lesion, or poor compliance.

Significant experience is accumulating with ultrasound (US) and radionuclide techniques for evaluation of the urinary tract in children. While the voiding cystourethrogram (VCUG) is the best anatomic technique for evaluation of vesicoureteral reflux, a radionuclide VCUG with tech-

netium-99m pertechnetate delivers a gonadal radiation dose 1% that of the radiographic VCUG; it is quite sensitive in detecting reflux and can be recommended as the initial test. When the radiographic or radionuclide VCUG shows no reflux, renal US can be done to rule out anatomic abnormalities; when reflux is present, the upper tract can be best evaluated with an IVU, or with a radionuclide scan with a cortical agent (eg, technetium-99m glucoheptonate), which delivers a lower radiation dose than the IVU and can be quite sensitive in detecting renal scarring. US has emerged as the procedure of choice for following renal growth in children with documented reflux.

All children with diagnosed UTI should undergo evaluation of the urinary tract with US, radionuclide scan, or IVU to search for major malformations, and a VCUG to detect significant reflux, which is found in 20 to 50% of children with UTI. Reflux of infected urine into the renal pevis or the presence of infected urine behind an obstruction can lead to chronic pyelonephritis, renal scarring, poor kidney growth, and renal failure. The IVU or US evaluation can be done at any

TABLE 32-4. KNOWN CAUSES OF GASTROENTERITIS

Bacteria		Viruses	Parasites
Enterotoxigenic	Invasive	Rotaviruses	Giardia lamblia
Vibrio cholerae 0:1	*Shigella*	Enteric adenoviruses	*Cryptosporidium*
V. cholerae, non = 0:1	*Salmonella*	Norwalk virus	*Entamoeba histolytica*
Escherichia coli	*E. coli*	Astroviruses	
Clostridium perfringens	*Staphylococcus*	Caliciviruses	
Bacillus cereus	*Yersinia enterocolitica*	Coronaviruses	
Staphylococcus aureus	*Campylobacter jejuni*		
Clostridium difficile			
Unknown mechanisms			
V. parahaemolyticus			
Aeromonas hydrophila			

time but is recommended earlier in younger infants. The VCUG is best postponed 3 to 6 wk to allow the transient reflux usually associated with cystitis to resolve and thus obtain a more accurate evaluation of the competence of the ureterovesical valves. Some physicians postpone x-ray evaluation in girls > 3 yr old until after the 2nd UTI.

Management of vesicoureteral reflux (VUR) should be based on the grade as defined by the International Reflux Study Committee. In **grade I**, only the ureters are involved; in **grade II**, the reflux reaches the calyces; in **grade III**, there is dilation of the ureter and renal pelvis; in **grade IV**, the dilation is increased and there is obliteration of the sharp angle of the fornices; in **grade V**, there is gross dilation of ureter, pelvis, and calyces, with frequent absence of papillary impressions. Children with a normal x-ray evaluation or mild, grade I VUR can be followed with periodic urine cultures. Those infants with grade II or III reflux are candidates for antibiotic prophylaxis. If grade IV or V reflux or a major renal anomaly is detected, formal urologic referral is indicated and surgery may be necessary.

Symptomatic or asymptomatic UTIs recur in about 50% of cases. The risk is increased in those with urologic abnormalities. Repeat urine cultures should be done 3 to 4 times during the first year after diagnosis, and at least twice a year during the next 2 or 3 yr (or any time the child develops UTI symptoms).

Prophylactic antibiotics are indicated for children with grade II or higher reflux to reduce recurrences and prevent kidney damage. Nitrofurantoin 2 mg/kg/day or TMP/SMX (1 mg/kg/day of the TMP) is given once daily, usually at night.

The overall prognosis for children with UTI is good. It is unusual for properly managed patients

to progress to renal failure unless they have uncorrectable urinary tract abnormalities.

ACUTE INFECTIOUS GASTROENTERITIS

(See also Acute Infectious Neonatal Diarrhea under Neonatal Infections in Ch. 27)

A syndrome of vomiting and diarrhea caused by pathogenic microorganisms that may lead to dehydration and electrolyte imbalance.

Worldwide annually about 1 billion episodes of acute gastroenteritis are estimated to occur; most happen in developing countries in children < 5 yr old. Of these episodes, 5 million are estimated to result in death because of dehydration. Most deaths can be prevented by giving fluids promptly. In addition to having a high mortality rate, infants from developing countries suffer a high morbidity from diarrhea. In many countries, infants < 2 yr old have 6 to 10 episodes annually; if they are not treated, severe nutritional consequences will ensue.

Etiology

A wide variety of organisms can cause acute gastroenteritis. Until the last few years the etiology of diarrhea was unknown in most cases. Recently (with appropriate laboratory techniques), a causative agent has been identified in 60 to 80% of cases. However, the cause remains unknown in a substantial proportion of cases. For the known bacterial, viral, and parasitic causes, see Table 32-4.

Symptoms, Signs, and Diagnosis

The epidemiology and the duration, character, and frequency of vomiting and diarrhea in relation to the child's age may indicate the cause and severity of the illness. More often than not, one

TABLE 32-5. SIGNS AND TREATMENT OF DIARRHEA

Degree of Dehydration	Signs*	Rehydration Therapy (within 4 h)	Replacement of Stool Losses	Maintenance Therapy†
Mild 5-6%	Slightly dry buccal mucous membranes, increased thirst	ORS 50 mL/kg	ORS 10 mL/kg or ½-1 cup (120-240 mL or 4-8 oz) for each diarrheal stool	Breast-feeding, half-strength lactose containing milk or formula, undiluted lactose-free formula, juices
Moderate 7-9%	Sunken eyes, sunken fontanelle, loss of skin turgor, dry buccal mucous membranes	ORS 100 mL/kg	Same as above	Same as above
Severe > 9%	Signs of moderate dehydration plus one of the following: rapid, thready pulse; cyanosis; rapid breathing; lethargy; coma	IV fluids (lactated Ringer's solution) 40 mL/kg/h until pulse and state of consciousness return to normal, then ORS 50-100 mL/kg	Same as above	Same as above

ORS = oral rehydration solution.

* If no signs of dehydration are present, rehydration therapy is not required; proceed with maintenance therapy and replacement of stool losses.

† Maintenance therapy should begin as soon as rehydration phase has been completed. Other children and adults can continue their usual diets.

From Santosham M, Greenough WB III: "Oral rehydration therapy: A global perspective." *The Journal of Pediatrics* 118(4):S44-S51, 1991; used with permission.

or more members of the patient's family or close contacts will recently have had symptoms of gastroenteritis or of a respiratory infection. Infants < 6 mo old may develop dehydration and electrolyte imbalance as early as 24 h after onset. However, severe dehydration and metabolic acidosis may develop within 24 h of onset at any age if vomiting is intractable, diarrhea is explosive, or fluid intake is drastically reduced. Physical examination should exclude any extraintestinal cause and determine the state of hydration. Lethargy, anorexia, fever, oliguria, and substantiated weight loss are signs of dehydration (see TABLE 32-5).

In older infants and overweight young children and in those with hypernatremia, some signs may not appear until dehydration is critical. These include warm, dry skin with poor tissue turgor, a sunken anterior fontanelle, sunken eyes with absent tearing (softened eyeballs are a late sign in severe dehydration), dry oral mucous membranes, weak or absent sucking, and lethargy (see TABLE 32-5).

The Hct and serum electrolytes may reflect the state of hydration and electrolyte balance.

Urinary sp gr helps assess the state of hydration, and microscopic examination of urine for bacteria determines whether or not a UTI (a common cause of symptoms similar to those of gastroenteritis) may be present. The WBC count does not usually help in the differential diagnosis or in assessing the severity of the condition, particularly when dehydration is present and the total WBC count rises owing to hemoconcentration. A shift to the left in the differential WBC count, even under these circumstances, may indicate the presence of accompanying sepsis. Stool cultures may be useful for differentiating bacterial from viral gastroenteritis, and sensitivity studies may suggest specific antibiotic therapy in the severely ill. A Wright-, Gram-, or methylene blue-stained smear of a watery stool specimen usually shows abundant polymorphonuclear leukocytes when bacterial infection is present.

Treatment

The mainstay of treatment for diarrhea, regardless of its cause, is to give appropriate fluids and electrolytes.

Assessment of dehydration: Before beginning therapy, the degree of dehydration should be clinically assessed as shown in TABLE 32–5.

Fluid therapy for infants with signs of dehydration (see TABLE 32–5): *Fluid therapy for diarrhea* should include rehydration, maintenance, and replacement of ongoing stool losses. During the rehydration phase, the estimated fluid deficit (based on clinical assessment) should be replaced. The daily individual fluid requirements should be given during the maintenance phase. During the entire period of illness, the ongoing diarrheal stool losses should be replaced.

IV fluids were formerly recommended for all patients requiring hospitalization for diarrhea. Recently an oral rehydration solution **(ORS)** has been recommended by the World Health Organization (WHO) to treat dehydration secondary to diarrhea. This solution contains (in mmol/L) sodium 90, potassium 20, chloride 80, citrate 30, and glucose 20; it is made by adding 1 L of water to the following: 3.5 gm sodium chloride, 2.5 gm sodium bicarbonate, 1.5 gm potassium chloride, and 20 gm glucose. This solution can effectively rehydrate patients with acute diarrhea regardless of age, cause, or type of electrolyte imbalance (hypo-, hyper- or isonatremia).

A solution similar in composition to the WHO-recommended ORS can be used during both rehydration and maintenance. After rehydration, the ORS intake must be supplemented by offering free water or a low-sodium fluid.

If ORS is unavailable, a sugar/salt solution can be prepared by adding 1 L of water to 15 mL (1 tbsp) of sugar and 2 mL (1/2 tsp) of salt. Although sugar/salt solution is less effective than the WHO-recommended ORS, it is adequate for treating most patients with diarrhea.

Rehydration phase: Patients who are mildly or moderately dehydrated should be given 50 and 100 mL/kg, respectively, of ORS over 4 h. If the patient is severely dehydrated, IV fluids (lactated Ringer's or similar solution) 40 mL/kg/h should be given until pulse, BP, and state of consciousness return to normal. After this occurs, the patient should be reassessed for degree of dehydration, and fluid therapy should be continued as in mild to moderate dehydration. At the end of the rehydration period (about 4 h), the patient should be reassessed. If signs of dehydration are still present, rehydration therapy should be repeated until dehydration is corrected.

Maintenance phase: Breast-fed infants should be continued on breast-feeding. In countries where lactose-free infant formulas are available and affordable, **non-breast-fed infants** should be given formula (150 mL/kg/day). In other countries, the milk normally consumed by the infant should be diluted 1:1 and given in the same volume. **Older children and adults** can take normally consumed fluids as desired.

Replacement of ongoing stool losses should proceed on a 1:1 basis with ORS. If the stool output is unknown, about 10 mL/kg or 1/2 to 1 cup (120 to 240 mL or 4 to 8 oz) of ORS should be given for each diarrheal stool.

Infants with no signs of dehydration do not need rehydration therapy. However, they should receive the same fluids recommended for patients with signs of dehydration for the maintenance phase and for ongoing stool losses. They should also be encouraged to drink fluids available at home (eg, soup, rice water, cereal-based fluids).

Antibiotics should be reserved for indications specified in TABLE 32–6. Trimethoprim/sulfamethoxazole can be used in ampicillin-resistant shigellosis. *Salmonella* gastroenteritis should *not* be treated with antibiotics because the course of the disease is not affected, fecal excretion of the organism is prolonged, and the emergence of resistant strains is enhanced. However, when *Salmonella* organisms invade the bloodstream or become localized in extra-intestinal sites, ampicillin or chloramphenicol is given in divided doses q 6 h IV dependent upon in vitro susceptibility tests. Infants < 6 mo old and T-cell–deficient children should be treated in this way, even without evidence of sepsis or extra-GI localization. *Yersinia* gastroenteritis usually subsides without antibiotic therapy. *Vibrio cholerae* gastroenteritis should be treated with tetracycline. *Campylobacter jejuni* enterocolitis severe enough to require hospitalization should be treated with erythromycin.

For discussion of infant botulism, see below.

PERIORBITAL AND ORBITAL CELLULITIS

Infections that affect primarily children, cause acute swelling and redness of the eyelid and surrounding skin (periorbital cellulitis) or of the periorbital skin and orbital contents (orbital cellulitis), progress rapidly, and can result in serious systemic or ocular complications.

TABLE 32-6. ORAL ANTIBIOTIC THERAPY
FOR ACUTE INFECTIOUS GASTROENTERITIS

Organism	Antibiotic	Dosage
Vibrio cholerae	Tetracycline TMP/SMX	50 mg/kg/day (maximum 2 gm/day) 7.5–20 mg*/kg/day for 5 days
Clostridium difficile	Vancomycin	40 mg/kg/day for 7 days (maximum 2 gm/day)
Shigella	TMP/SMX Ampicillin	7.5–20 mg/kg/day for 5 days 100 mg/kg/day for 5 days
Giardia lamblia	Furazolidone Metronidazole	6–9 mg/kg/day for 10 days 15–30 mg/kg/day for 10 days (maximum 750 mg/day)
Entamoeba histolytica	Metronidazole	50 mg/kg/day for 10 days (maximum 750 mg/day)
Campylobacter jejuni	Erythromycin	40 mg/kg/day for 7 days

NOTE: In most cases of diarrhea, antibiotic therapy is not indicated. Antibiotics may be used supportively (in addition to fluid therapy) for treating infections with the organisms listed above.

TMP/SMX = trimethoprim/sulfamethoxazole.

* Based on trimethoprim component.

Etiology and Incidence

Periorbital and orbital cellulitis can result from an external focus of infection (eg, a wound or insect bite), an internal source of infection (eg, sinusitis), or seeding from bacteremia. *Hemophilus influenzae* type b or *Streptococcus pneumoniae* can be isolated from the blood of about 33% of patients who have no evidence of trauma or another external focus of infection and have not received systemic antibiotics before blood specimens can be obtained for culture. The most common pathogens associated with external foci are *Staphylococcus aureus* and *Streptococcus pyogenes*, but these are seldom isolated from the blood. In general, a bacterial pathogen is isolated from ≤ 33% of patients with periorbital cellulitis.

Periorbital cellulitis is much more common (occurring in 85 to 90% of patients) than orbital cellulitis (10 to 15%) and occurs more frequently in children < 5 yr of age, while orbital cellulitis is more frequent in children > 5 yr.

Anatomy and Pathophysiology

The orbit is a conical cavity bounded by the paranasal sinuses. The floor of the frontal sinuses forms the roof of the orbit, the lateral walls of the ethmoid sinuses form the medial wall, and the roof of the maxillary sinus lies just below the floor of the orbit. The orbital contents are separated from the eyelids and protected anteriorly by the orbital septum. The orbital septum or palpebral fascia is a membranous extension of the periosteum, which is attached to the entire margin of the orbit and extends to the musculus levator palpebrae superioris in the upper lid and to the tarsal plate in the lower lid. The orbital septum helps prevent spread of infection from the eyelids to the orbit.

Periorbital and orbital cellulitis are most often caused by direct extension from infected ethmoid sinuses or local cutaneous infections. Spread of the infection is aided by the extensive venous network around the eye. Because these veins do not have valves, infection can spread in either direction. Local inflammation can also result in venous or lymphatic obstruction, leading to swelling in areas distant from the site of actual infection.

Symptoms and Signs

Swelling and redness of the eyelids are usually the first signs of periorbital or orbital cellulitis. Involvement is unilateral > 90% of the time. A history of trauma or signs of local infection can be found in about 33% of patients, whether or not a pathogen is isolated and regardless of what organism it is. Most children have fever; about 20% have nasal discharge and another 20% have conjunctivitis. Chemosis can be seen with periorbital cellulitis, but ophthalmoplegia, proptosis, eye pain, or decreased visual acuity indicate orbital disease.

TABLE 32–7. FINDINGS IN PERIORBITAL AND ORBITAL INFECTIONS

Infections	Lid Swelling and Erythema	Ophthalmoplegia	Proptosis	Visual Acuity
Periorbital cellulitis	+	−	−	Normal
Orbital cellulitis	+	+	+	±
Subperiosteal abscess	+	+	+	Abnormal
Orbital abscess	+	+	+	Abnormal
Cavernous sinus thrombosis	+	+	+	Abnormal

+ = present; − = absent.

Modified from Teele DW: "Management of the child with a red and swollen eye." *Pediatric Infectious Diseases* 2:258–262, 1983. © by Williams & Wilkins, 1983; used with permission.

Complications: The most common complications of orbital cellulitis are central retinal artery or retinal vein thrombosis and retinal damage secondary to ischemia caused by increased intraocular pressure. Intracranial complications, which occur when the infection is not contained within the orbit, include epidural, subdural, or cerebral abscesses, cavernous sinus or cortical vein thrombosis, or bacterial meningitis.

Diagnosis

The eye must be examined to evaluate the position of the globe, eye movement, and visual acuity. Since lid swelling frequently makes the use of lid retractors necessary for evaluation of the globe, an ophthalmologist should be consulted whenever possible. TABLE 32–7 summarizes the findings in patients with periorbital cellulitis and varying degrees of orbital involvement. The direction of proptosis may be a clue to the site of the infection; eg, extension from the frontal sinus pushes the globe down and out, and extension from the ethmoid sinus pushes the globe laterally and out. If examination of the eye fails to demonstrate proptosis, ophthalmoplegia (usually painful), or decreased visual acuity, attention should turn to seeking a local nidus of infection on the skin. If there is no evidence of local injury or infection, a sinus infection should be sought. Blood cultures yield pathogens in up to 33% of patients, but other laboratory tests are not particularly helpful. X-rays of the sinuses are useful for diagnosing sinusitis in children > 1 yr of age but generally do not differentiate preseptal from postseptal involvement. When orbital involvement is suspected, CT scanning can best assess sinus involvement, subperiosteal elevation, and intraorbital cellulitis or abscess formation and should be done as soon as specimens have been taken for culture and antibiotic therapy has begun.

Differential diagnosis of swelling and erythema of the eyelid includes trauma, insect bites, allergy, and tumor. Other inflammatory diseases (eg, hordeolum, dacryocystitis, dacryoadenitis, and conjunctivitis) can usually be distinguished by location and appearance.

Treatment

Children with periorbital or orbital cellulitis should be hospitalized and treated promptly. An ophthalmologist and otolaryngologist should be consulted early, in case surgical drainage of the orbit or a sinus is necessary. With an obvious external focus of infection, Gram stain and cultures of exudate should be obtained and an antibiotic regimen begun that treats both *S. aureus* and *S. pyogenes*. With no obvious external focus of infection, blood cultures should be obtained and therapy for *H. influenzae* type b and *S. pneumoniae* begun. In an infant < 1 yr of age with no external focus of infection, a lumbar puncture should be performed. Since the absence of an external focus of infection is usually difficult to ascertain, it is best to obtain specimens for culture and begin administering antibiotics (cefuroxime or ceftriaxone alone or chloramphenicol with nafcillin) that effectively treat *H. influenzae* type b as well as gram-positive aerobes. When CNS involvement is suspected, ceftriaxone alone or chloramphenicol with nafcillin provides adequate antibacterial coverage until culture results are known.

IMPETIGO; ECTHYMA

Impetigo (impetigo contagiosa): *A superficial vesiculopustular skin infection.* **Ecthyma:** *An ulcerative form of impetigo.*

Etiology, Symptoms, Signs, and Diagnosis

Staphylococcus aureus is the most frequent cause of pyodermas (superficial skin infections);

it is a much more common initial cause than Group A β-hemolytic streptococcus. *S. aureus* is the primary pathogen in bullous impetigo occurring anywhere on the body and in crusted impetigo of the face; its role in ecthyma varies in different parts of the world. A recent increase in furuncles and in several more serious staphylococcal infections has been observed. Purulent infections of the ears or nostrils may be the source of staphylococci, but the nose and throat seldom yield cutaneous staphylococci. Spread of untreated infection to others is often suspected, but deliberate experimental infections are difficult to induce.

The arms, legs, and face are more susceptible to impetigo and ecthyma than are unexposed areas. Both impetigo and ecthyma may follow superficial trauma with a break in the skin or may be secondary to pediculosis, scabies, fungal infections, other causes of dermatitis, or insect bites. Impetigo may occur on normal skin, especially on the legs in children. Lesions vary from a pea-sized vesicopustule to large, bizarre, circinate ringworm-like lesions. In impetigo, the lesions caused by *S. aureus* progress rapidly from maculopapules to vesicopustules or bullae to exudative and then honey-colored, crusted, circinate lesions. Ecthyma is characterized by small, purulent, shallow, punched-out ulcers with thick, brown-black crusts and surrounding erythema. Itching is common, and scratching may spread the infection. **Diagnosis** is usually based on clinical findings.

Prognosis

Neglected infection in adults can result in cellulitis, lymphangitis, or furunculosis. In children, untreated erythematous lesions may persist for months. Pigmentary changes with or without scarring may result.

Prompt recovery usually follows appropriate treatment. Acute glomerulonephritis in children, but not acute rheumatic fever, may follow cutaneous infection with a Group A β-hemolytic streptococcus; however, nephritis has become less common because nephrogenic strains of streptococci are less prevalent. Ecthyma penetrates more deeply than impetigo, resulting in ulceration with subsequent scarring.

Treatment

Until recently, systemic antibiotics were considered superior to topical antibacterials. However, application of mupirocin ointment tid has been effective in treating impetigo caused by *S.*

aureus and *Streptococcus pyogenes*, though some resistant strains have developed. Patients showing no response to mupirocin in 3 to 5 days should be treated systemically. Because most cases are caused by penicillinase-producing staphylococci, cloxacillin or a 1st-generation cephalosporin is the drug of choice. Penicillin-sensitive patients should receive cephalexin for 10 days (50 mg/kg/day divided q 6 h for children, 250 mg qid for adults) rather than erythromycin; the increased frequency of erythromycin-resistant staphylococci (10 to 40%) has decreased the effectiveness of this drug. Most streptococci are sensitive to erythromycin but rarely to tetracycline. In pure staphylococcal pyoderma, a penicillinase-resistant penicillin (eg, cloxacillin 50 mg/kg/day divided q 6 h for children or 250 mg qid for adults) should be given for 10 days.

In secondary impetigo, the underlying condition must also be treated.

ACUTE EPIGLOTTITIS
(Supraglottitis)

A severe, rapidly progressive infection of the epiglottis and surrounding tissues that may be quickly fatal because of sudden respiratory obstruction by the inflamed structures.

Etiology and Incidence

Hemophilus influenzae type b is almost always the pathogen; very rarely, streptococci may be responsible. The incidence of an *H. influenzae* type b epiglottitis is highest in children aged 2 to 5 yr; the disease is uncommon in children < 2 yr, but it may occur at any age, including in adults.

Pathophysiology

Infection, acquired through the respiratory tract, may produce initial nasopharyngitis. Subsequent downward extension produces a supraglottic cellulitis with marked inflammation of the epiglottis as well as the vallecula, the aryepiglottic folds, the arytenoids, and the ventricular bands. Bacteremia is common. The inflamed epiglottis mechanically obstructs the airway; the work of breathing increases, and CO_2 retention and hypoxia may result. Clearance of inflammatory secretions is also impaired. These combined factors may result in fatal asphyxia within a few hours.

Symptoms and Signs

Onset is usually acute and fulminating. Sore throat, hoarseness, and frequently, high fever develop abruptly in a previously well child. Dysphagia and respiratory distress characterized by drooling, dyspnea, tachypnea, and inspiratory stridor develop rapidly, often causing the child to lean forward and hyperextend the neck to enhance air exchange. On physical examination the child may appear moribund or restless and in severe respiratory distress. Deep suprasternal, supraclavicular, intercostal, and subcostal inspiratory retractions are noted. Breath sounds may be diminished bilaterally and rhonchi may be heard. The pharynx is usually inflamed.

H. influenzae type b pneumonia, occasionally with empyema, may occur concurrently with epiglottitis. Metastatic infection to the joints, meninges, pericardium, or subcutaneous tissues that results in an abscess or cellulitis may occur, though infrequently.

Diagnosis

The patient should be hospitalized immediately whenever the diagnosis is **suspected** *clinically.* Direct visualization of the epiglottis is diagnostic, but manipulation may initiate sudden, fatal airway obstruction. Visualization should be attempted *only* by designated trained personnel with equipment to establish an airway if necessary. If direct laryngoscopy confirms the diagnosis by revealing a beefy red, stiff, and edematous epiglottis, an artificial airway should be placed immediately. The type of airway may depend on the expertise of the staff, but endotracheal tube placement is generally associated with fewer complications than is tracheostomy. *H. influenzae* type b may then be cultured from the upper respiratory tract and, usually, the blood.

The major differential diagnostic concerns are acute **viral croup** (laryngotracheobronchitis) and bacterial tracheitis. Croup is usually less fulminant in onset, and its characteristic barking cough is uncommon in epiglottitis. The epiglottis in croup may be erythematous but is not markedly edematous and cherry-red as in epiglottitis. **Lateral and anteroposterior neck x-rays** differentiate the two, showing subepiglottic narrowing and a normal-sized epiglottis in croup and, in epiglottitis, an enlarged epiglottis and distention of the hypopharynx. Neck x-ray should not delay direct visualization and is preferably performed in the operating room.

Bacterial tracheitis (pseudomembranous croup), an uncommon infection affecting children of any age, needs to be differentiated from epiglottitis because of its severe, rapidly progres-

sive course. The pathogens most frequently involved are *Staphylococcus aureus*, Group A β-hemolytic streptococci, and *H. influenzae* type b. Onset is acute and is characterized by respiratory stridor, high fever, and often copious purulent secretions. The child may appear to have epiglottitis with marked toxicity and respiratory distress that may progress rapidly and may require intubation. The **diagnosis** is indicated on direct laryngoscopy by evidence of purulent secretions and inflammation in the subglottic area or by a lateral neck x-ray showing an area of subglottic narrowing with a shaggy, purulent membrane.

Diphtheria (see above) should be considered in an unimmunized patient.

Treatment

Speed is vital. A continually adequate airway must be assured and specific parenteral antibiotics given. Sudden complete airway obstruction occurs so unpredictably that an airway must be secured immediately, preferably by nasotracheal intubation. Alternatively, tracheotomy may be performed. For emergency care of children with epiglottitis, each institution should have a predetermined protocol that involves the pediatrician, otolaryngologist, and anesthesiologist. Skilled nursing care is required, since secretions can cause obstruction even after intubation or tracheostomy. The nasotracheal tube is usually required only until the patient has been stable for 24 to 48 h (usually a total intubation time < 60 h).

The inflammation is effectively controlled with parenteral antibiotics. A β-lactamase–resistant antibiotic should be used initially, since ampicillin-resistant *H. influenzae* type b organisms are common. A 3rd-generation cephalosporin or chloramphenicol 75 to 100 mg/kg/day IV may be used. Rarely, *H. influenzae* type b strains resistant to chloramphenicol have been isolated. Where this has occurred, a 3rd-generation cephalosporin should be used. If the organism is isolated and proves to be ampicillin-sensitive, ampicillin 200 mg/kg/day IV in 4 divided doses can be given. Sedatives should be *avoided*, although initial paralysis may be needed to protect the tube.

Prevention of *H. influenzae* type b epiglottitis may be possible with highly effective *Hemophilus* b conjugate vaccines now available for infants ≥ 2 mo of age.

ADENOID HYPERTROPHY

Enlargement of adenoidal tissue due to lymphoid hyperplasia.

Adenoidal lymphoid hyperplasia occurs in children and may be physiologic or secondary to infection or allergy. Consequent obstruction of the eustachian tubes may result in recurrent acute, chronic, or secretory (serous) otitis media (middle ear effusion); obstruction of the choanae may cause chronic sinusitis, mouth breathing, obstructive sleep apnea, a hyponasal voice, and purulent rhinorrhea. Chronic adenoiditis is common.

Treatment

Adenoidectomy is frequently indicated in persistent serous and chronic otitis media to reduce exacerbations of chronic otitis media and to improve the results of tympanoplasty. In recurrent acute otitis media, the decision to perform an adenoidectomy depends on the duration of the earache after antibiotic therapy is initiated, the presence of spontaneous perforation, the frequency with which myringotomy is required, and the severity of systemic symptoms. Adenoidectomy for nasal obstruction depends on the severity of the obstruction and the patient's age, since lymphoid hyperplasia reaches its maximum at puberty. Purulent rhinorrhea or sinusitis that recurs or persists despite adequate antibiotic treatment may be treated by adenoidectomy in carefully selected, otherwise healthy children.

RETROPHARYNGEAL ABSCESS

Retropharyngeal abscesses generally occur in infants or young children as complications of suppurative retropharyngeal lymph nodes to which infection (usually caused by a β-hemolytic streptococcus) has spread from the pharynx, sinuses, adenoids, nose, or middle ear. These abscesses are unusual in adults because the retropharyngeal lymph nodes diminish or disappear after childhood. Occasional causes in adults or children are TB and perforation of the posterior pharyngeal wall by foreign bodies or instrumentation.

The major manifestations are pain on swallowing, fever, cervical lymphadenopathy, and if airway obstruction occurs, stridor, dyspnea, and hyperextension of the neck. The cervical vertebrae cannot be palpated through the posterior pharyngeal wall, which is boggy and fluctuant, with a definite, usually unilateral, bulging. Widening of the prevertebral space can be seen on lateral x-rays of the neck, and abscess formation can be demonstrated on CT. **Complications** include hemorrhage; rupture of the abscess into the airway, causing asphyxia or pulmonary aspiration; laryngeal spasm; mediastinitis; and suppurative thrombophlebitis of the internal jugular veins.

Treatment includes draining the abscess through an incision in the posterior pharyngeal wall and giving penicillin G 150,000 u./kg/day IV in 6 equal doses for 3 to 4 days, then orally for a total of 14 days, unless culture and sensitivity studies of the drained abscess material indicate use of an alternative antimicrobial agent. If a β-lactamase–producing species (anaerobic gram-negative bacillus) is cultured, clindamycin 20 to 40 mg/kg/day IV in 3 or 4 equal doses or ceftizoxime 50 mg/kg IV q 6 h should be given.

TUBERCULOSIS IN CHILDREN
(See also PERINATAL TUBERCULOSIS under NEONATAL INFECTIONS in Ch. 27)

Hilar lymphadenopathy, the most common finding in children, consists of drainage from a usually obscure lesion in the well-ventilated portions of the lung (lower and middle lobes), which are most likely to harbor inhaled organisms. It has few symptoms, except for a brassy cough, but may be associated with segmental atelectasis. Further swelling of the nodes is common, even after chemotherapy is started, and may produce lobar atelectasis, which usually clears uneventfully as treatment takes effect. If treatment is not begun on the basis of suspicion and history of exposure, the infection may progress to miliary TB or tuberculous meningitis. Occasionally, if long neglected, it produces pulmonary cavitation.

Treatment: When hilar adenopathy is present (often seen only on a lateral chest x-ray), therapy with 2 drugs is usually advisable, ie, isoniazid and rifampin for 6 mo (see TABLE 32–8). When no abnormality can be detected on posterior-anterior and lateral chest x-rays and the child appears clinically well, therapy with isoniazid alone (10 to 20 mg/kg in a single daily dose for 6 mo) is adequate.

Prophylaxis

Chemoprophylaxis generally consists of isoniazid **(INH)** 300 mg/day for 6 to 9 mo for adults. For children the dosage is 10 mg/kg/day, up to 300 mg, given as a single morning dose. Chemoprophylaxis is indicated principally in persons whose tuberculin skin test converted from negative to positive within the previous 2 yr. Thus, treatment is always indicated in small children, in whom infection must be rather recent, and in older children and adults < 25 yr old, in whom infection is likely to be recent and who are in a high-risk age group for clinical TB. In the elderly, preventive treatment is indicated when conversion of the tuberculin skin test is definite (ie, an increase of at least 15 mm in size of induration over that in previous negative tests; the progression from a single negative test to an induration of 10 to 14 mm on a repeat test 1 to 6 wk later should be considered merely a booster-positive reaction, *not* a conversion). In both infected children and elderly tuberculin converters, INH therapy has been shown to be 98.5% effective in preventing development of clinical TB.

Prophylaxis is strongly indicated for any HIV-infected person whose tuberculin reaction is ≥ 5 mm, because the protective effect of T-cell immunity is lost. It is also indicated for reactors (induration of ≥ 10 mm) who show apical scarring of old TB (Simon's foci), have insulin-dependent diabetes mellitus, are on prolonged corticosteroid therapy, or have had a gastrectomy.

Chemoprophylaxis is strongly indicated in any child < 4 yr old (whether tuberculin-negative or tuberculin-positive) who is a household or close contact of a person whose sputum smear is positive for acid-fast bacilli presumed to be *M. tuberculosis.* The infection progresses so rapidly in the very young that serious disease could develop before the skin test becomes positive.

All those likely to be exposed to TB (living or working with elderly persons in a nursing home or hospital) should be tested initially with the 2-step Mantoux test in which 5 tuberculin u. of PPD are given intradermally. From 3 to 10% of persons who have no reaction to the first test will develop a significant reaction when the test is repeated 1 to 3 wk later (far too soon to have converted from a new infection). This is called a **booster-positive reaction** and has the same significance as a test that is positive the first time. Such a booster reaction may occur even on a third test, generally becoming more positive in increments rather than with a significant in-

TABLE 32–8. SUGGESTED DRUG REGIMENS FOR TUBERCULOSIS

Type of Treatment/Clinical Complication	Recommended Regimen
Initial treatment (pulmonary or extrapulmonary)	
Chemoprophylaxis (drug resistance unlikely; active disease ruled out)	INH* for 6–9 mo
Minimal disease	
1. 3 smears and culture are negative; tuberculin test, positive	INH and RMP† for 4 mo
2. 3 smears are negative, culture is positive	INH and RMP for 6 mo
Cavitary disease	INH and RMP for 9 mo or INH and RMP for 9 mo + EMB‡ for first 2 mo
Short-course intensive regimen	INH and RMP + PZA§ daily for 2 mo, followed by INH and RMP (standard doses) for total of 6 mo
Re-treatment (or probable INH resistance)	
Initiation of therapy	SM** or EMB + INH + RMP + PZA for 2 mo
Continuation of therapy (after susceptibility study reports)	
1. INH resistance confirmed	RMP + EMB + PZA
2. INH susceptibility reported	Treat as cavitary disease (see Initial treatment, above)
Multidrug-resistant *Mycobacterium tuberculosis* (not *M. avium-intracellulare*)	3 effective†† drugs; order of preference: capreomycin, PZA, ethionamide, cycloserine, kanamycin, amikacin. (No more than one aminoglycoside should be given at the same time)

(Continued)

TABLE 32-8. SUGGESTED DRUG REGIMENS FOR TUBERCULOSIS *(Cont'd)*

Type of Treatment/Clinical Complication	Recommended Regimen
Specialized treatment regimens‡‡	
Supervised twice-weekly therapy	INH + RMP daily for 1 mo, followed by INH 900 mg + RMP 600 mg twice weekly for 8 mo
Intensive short-course therapy	INH + RMP + EMB + PZA daily for 2 wk, followed by INH 15 mg/kg + RMP 10 mg/kg + EMB 50 mg/kg + PZA 50 mg/kg twice weekly to complete 6 mo of therapy
Clinical complication	
Pregnancy	Same as above, but SM and PZA should not be used
HIV infection	Same as above with additional 3 mo of therapy

INH = isoniazid; RMP = rifampin; EMB = ethambutol; PZA = pyrazinamide; SM = streptomycin.

* 300 mg/day (single dose in the morning) in adolescents and adults; 10 to 20 mg/kg (single dose) in infants and small children; 10 mg/kg, up to 300 mg/day (single dose in the morning) in children. Alternative prophylactic therapy is 15 mg/kg twice weekly in adults and children when supervision is needed.

† 600 mg/day (single dose) in adults (450 mg/day if < 40 kg [90 lb]); 10 to 15 mg/kg/day (single dose) in children.

‡ 25 mg/kg/day for 2 mo or until sputum becomes negative or while under close observation, reduced to 15 mg/kg/day for prolonged or relatively unsupervised use, in single dose, in adults; not used in younger children.

§ 25 to 30 mg/kg in single dose, usually 1.5 gm in small adults and 2.5 to 3 gm in large adults; 50 mg/kg twice weekly in adults and in children.

** 1 gm/day (single dose) 5 days/wk in adults < 60 yr old; 0.5 gm in adults > 60 yr, < 45 kg (< 100 lb), or with renal disease; 20 mg/kg (single dose) in children. Usually discontinued after 8 to 16 wk, when sputum conversion has occurred, in regimens initially using 3 drugs.

†† Effective means that the infecting microbial population is susceptible to that drug.

‡‡ To simplify treatment in children with active disease who resist taking oral medication, drugs can be given twice weekly in the same mg/kg dosages recommended for adults. Administering the drugs in applesauce rather than syrup is best for young children.

crease in size of induration after 2 negative reactions. Not using the 2-step test can result in misinterpretation of a number of booster-positive reactions as conversions and unnecessary recommendations for prophylaxis.

Vaccination with bacille Calmette-Guérin (BCG, a vaccine made from an attenuated strain of *M. bovis*) has been used in developing countries with a high prevalence and incidence of TB among young persons. It has little use in the USA, unless the index case cannot be treated satisfactorily.

Hospitalization of persons with clinical TB to protect their contacts is no longer necessary. Any risk to close contacts will already have been realized by the time the diagnosis is made and treatment started. Patients usually become noninfectious within 10 to 14 days of the start of therapy. However, good judgment should be applied; eg, an infected person should not be permitted to work in a newborn nursery until cultures are consistently negative.

LYME DISEASE (LD)
(Lyme Borreliosis)

A tick-transmitted, spirochetal, inflammatory disorder best recognized clinically by an early skin lesion, erythema chronicum migrans (ECM), that may be followed weeks to months later by neurologic, cardiac, or joint abnormalities.

Etiology, Epidemiology, and Pathophysiology

The illness is caused by a newly discovered spirochete, *Borrelia burgdorferi*, transmitted primarily by minute ticks of the *Ixodes ricinus* complex. In the USA, the white-footed mouse is the primary animal reservoir for *B. burgdorferi* and the preferred host for nymphal and larval *I. dammini* ticks. Deer are important as the preferred host for the adult ticks. Other mammals (eg, dogs) can be incidental hosts and can develop LD.

The disease was recognized in 1975 because of close geographic clustering of cases in the small community of Lyme, Connecticut. It has since appeared in 43 states in the USA, especially in foci along the northeastern coast from Massachusetts to Maryland, in Wisconsin and Minnesota, and in California and Oregon. It has become well recognized in Europe and has been reported across the USSR and in China, Japan, and Australia. Onset, usually in the summer and early fall, occurs at any age and in either sex, although most patients are children and young adults living in heavily wooded areas. For several years, LD has been the most commonly reported tick-borne illness in the USA.

B. burgdorferi has been cultured from skin (ECM) and rarely from blood (in early disease) and CSF. The spirochete enters skin at the site of a tick bite. After an incubation period of 3 to 32 days, the organism migrates outward in the skin (ECM) and may spread in lymph (regional adenopathy) or disseminate in blood to organs or other skin sites. The spirochete has been seen rarely in inflamed synovium, brain, and other tissues.

Histologically, ECM resembles an insect bite—epidermal and dermal involvement at the center (which is often indurated), dermal in the periphery. All layers of the dermis are heavily infiltrated with mononuclear cells around blood vessels and skin appendages. At the center, the papillary dermis is edematous, and the epidermis has a thickened keratin layer and intra- and extracellular edema.

Synovial membrane from affected joints of LD patients may be indistinguishable from that of RA patients. Nonspecific findings include villous hypertrophy, vascular congestion, and colonization with lymphocytes and plasma cells that may resemble early lymphoid follicles and, as in RA, are presumably capable of producing antibody locally. In addition, there may be an obliterative endarteritis and (rarely) demonstrable spirochetes. Pannus formation and erosion of cartilage and bone may occur.

LD is associated with characteristic immune findings. Over 85% of patients with subsequent arthritis have, in the prearticular (ECM) phase, serum cryoglobulins containing IgM (reflecting high serum IgM levels), compared to < 15% of patients without subsequent arthritis. Besides having prognostic value, these differences may represent different ways of responding to an im-

mune stimulus and may be determined genetically. Patients with chronic arthritis have an increased frequency of the B cell alloantigens HLA-DR4 and HLA-DR2 but not of HLA-B27 (as is found in the spondyloarthropathies).

More direct evidence for circulating immune complexes (eg, abnormal C1q-binding activity) is found in sera of most patients with ECM. These complexes tend to persist in the circulation of patients who develop neurologic or cardiac abnormalities. By the time arthritis appears, immune complexes are no longer evident in most sera but are found systematically in synovial fluid, in higher titer than in concomitant sera. T cells in fluid from affected joints and meninges respond vigorously to stimulation by *B. burgdorferi*.

Symptoms, Signs, and Course

ECM begins as a red macule or papule, usually on the proximal portion of an extremity or on the trunk (especially the thigh, buttock, or axilla), that expands, often with central clearing, to a diameter of up to 50 cm. At least 75% of patients with LD have this early lesion; of these, about 25% report having been bitten at that site by a minute tick 3 to 32 days before onset of ECM. Soon after onset, nearly $1/2$ of patients in the USA develop multiple, usually smaller, lesions without indurated centers. ECM generally lasts for a few weeks; evanescent lesions may appear during resolution. Former skin lesions may reappear faintly, sometimes before recurrent attacks of arthritis. Mucosal lesions do not occur.

The most common symptoms accompanying ECM (or preceding it by a few days) suggest a summer flu-like syndrome; they include malaise and fatigue, chills and fever, headache, stiff neck, myalgias, and arthralgias. Frank arthritis is rare at this stage. Less common are backache, nausea and vomiting, sore throat, lymphadenopathy, and splenomegaly. Symptoms are characteristically intermittent and changing, but malaise and fatigue may linger for weeks.

Frank neurologic abnormalities develop in about 15% of patients within weeks to months of ECM (often before arthritis occurs), commonly last for months, and usually resolve completely. Most common are lymphocytic meningitis (CSF pleocytosis of about 100 cells/μL) or meningoencephalitis, cranial neuritis (especially Bell's palsy, which may be bilateral), and sensory or motor radiculoneuropathies; they may occur alone or in combination. **Myocardial abnormalities** occur in about 8% of patients within weeks of ECM. They include fluctuating degrees of atrioventricular block (1st-degree, Wenckebach, or 3rd-degree) and, less commonly, myopericarditis with reduced left ventricular ejection fractions and cardiomegaly.

Arthritis occurs in about half of patients with ECM within weeks to months of its onset, although the interval has been as long as 2 yr. Intermittent swelling and pain in a few large joints, especially the knee, typically recur for several years. Affected knees commonly are much more swollen than painful, often hot, rarely red. Baker's cysts may form and rupture. Symptoms accompanying ECM, especially malaise, fatigue, and low-grade fever, also may precede or accompany recurrent attacks of arthritis. About 10% of patients develop chronic (unremittent for 6 mo or more) knee involvement. Other late findings (occurring years after onset) associated with LD include an antibiotic-responsive skin lesion—acrodermatitis chronica atrophicans—and chronic CNS abnormalities.

Laboratory and X-ray Findings

Recovery of *B. burgdorferi* from most tissues and body fluids is so far rare, difficult, and slow (requiring weeks). Specific antispirochetal antibodies in significant titer—first IgM, then IgG—appear in serum within weeks of ECM. IgG titers are higher later in the illness when arthritis is present. Titers are determined by indirect immunofluorescence or preferably by enzyme-linked immunosorbent assay (ELISA); confirmation of weak positive titers by Western blot is sometimes desirable. Elevated titers in CSF relative to serum may be helpful when neurologic disease is suspected.

Cryoprecipitates and circulating immune complexes are often seen early in the illness (see Pathophysiology, above). The ESR may be elevated when patients feel ill; the Hct and WBC and differential counts usually are normal. Rheumatoid and antinuclear factors rarely are present. The Venereal Disease Research Laboratory (VDRL) test is negative. Serum complement components are either normal or elevated during active disease (but see Pathophysiology, above). The urinalysis and serum creatinine levels usually are normal; AST (SGOT) and LDH levels may be slightly abnormal when ECM is present.

Synovial fluid findings vary but typically show a WBC count of about 25,000 (range, 500 to 110,000), mostly granulocytes; about 5 gm/dL of protein; and C3 and C4 levels usually > $^1/_3$ higher than those of serum.

Radiologic findings usually are limited to soft tissue swelling, but a few patients have had erosion of cartilage and bone.

Differential Diagnosis

In children, LD must be distinguished primarily from juvenile RA; in adults, from Reiter's syndrome and atypical RA. The distinguishing features of LD described above may occur in any combination. Important negative findings include absence (usually) of morning stiffness, subcutaneous nodules, iridocyclitis, mucosal lesions, rheumatoid factor, and antinuclear antibodies. Acute rheumatic fever is considered in the occasional patient with migratory polyarthralgias and either an increased PR interval or chorea (as a manifestation of meningoencephalitis). However, patients with LD rarely have heart murmurs or evidence of a preceding streptococcal infection. The lack of axial involvement in LD distinguishes it from spondyloarthropathies with peripheral joint involvement. LD may mimic idiopathic Bell's palsy as well as other causes of lymphocytic meningitis, peripheral neuropathies, and chronic fatigue and other CNS syndromes.

Treatment

Although all stages of LD may respond to antibiotics, early-stage treatment is generally the most successful. Optimal therapy for many aspects, including Lyme arthritis and CNS involvement associated with LD, is still evolving.

For early LD, adults (excluding pregnant women) are given oral doxycycline 100 mg bid, tetracycline 250 mg qid, or amoxicillin 500 mg (as tolerated) tid, each for 10 to 21 days, depending on the response. For uncomplicated ECM, pregnant women are given oral amoxicillin 500 mg tid for 21 days; for early disseminated LD, high-dose IV penicillin is given, as for late disease (see below). Children receive oral amoxicillin 250 mg tid or 30 to 50 mg/kg/day in divided doses (maximum 500 mg), also for 10 to 21 days. For penicillin-allergic individuals, oral erythromycin 250 mg qid or 30 to 50 mg/kg/day in divided doses (maximum 250 mg) for 10 to 21 days is almost as effective.

For early or late neurologic disease, ceftriaxone IV 2 gm/day in a single dose or penicillin G 20 million u. IV in 6 divided doses daily, each for 14 to 21 days, is recommended for adults. Children are given ceftriaxone 50 to 100 mg/kg/day (maximum 2 gm) or penicillin G 100,000 to 300,000 u./kg/day in divided doses. These regimens cure almost everyone with Lyme meningitis or peripheral neuropathies. For those allergic to both drugs, doxycycline 100 mg bid orally for 14 to 21 days or chloramphenicol 1 gm IV q 6 h for 10 to 21 days can be tried. For isolated facial (Bell's) palsy, oral regimens given for at least 21 days may suffice. For cardiac abnormalities, ceftriaxone IV 2 gm/day or penicillin G 20 million u. IV in divided doses daily, each for 14 days, is recommended, but doxycycline 100 mg orally bid or amoxicillin 500 mg orally tid, each for 14 to 21 days, may suffice.

For intermittent or chronic arthritis, any of the following regimens cures over half the patients: oral doxycycline 100 mg bid for 30 days, oral amoxicillin and probenecid 500 mg each qid for 30 days, IV penicillin G 20 million u. in 6 divided doses daily for 14 to 21 days, or IV ceftriaxone 2 gm daily for 14 to 21 days.

For symptomatic relief, aspirin (90 mg/kg/day [1.5 grains/kg/day] in children) or other NSAIDs may be used. For tense knee joints due to effusions, aspiration of fluid and the use of crutches are indicated. Patients with Lyme arthritis of the knee that persists despite antibiotic therapy may be treated successfully with arthroscopic synovectomy.

Acrodermatitis chronica atrophicans responds to oral antibiotic regimens of 3 to 4 wk.

INFECTIVE ENDOCARDITIS (IE)

(Acute Bacterial Endocarditis [ABE]; Subacute Bacterial Endocarditis [SBE])
(See also RHEUMATIC FEVER in Ch. 42)

Microbial infections of the endocardium, characterized by fever, heart murmurs, petechiae, anemia, embolic phenomena, and endocardial vegetations that may result in valvular incompetence or obstruction, myocardial abscess, or mycotic aneurysm. The course may be acute or subacute, and clinical findings vary greatly, depending on host age and susceptibility, underlying or associated disease, and the organism involved.

The overall incidence of IE has probably not changed significantly in the last 2 decades, and men continue to be affected about twice as often as women. However, epidemiologic patterns have been changing. The median age of onset has increased from about 35 yr before antibiotics were available to about age 50. There is a higher incidence of right-sided IE associated with IV drug abuse and diagnostic procedures requiring vascular lines. Cardiac surgery and other invasive procedures have led to an increase in nosocomial endocarditis (10 to 15% in recent series), and there is an increasing elderly population (almost 30%) with thickened, stiff, calcified valves. Demographic, epidemiologic, and clinical disease patterns vary greatly with setting; eg, in small, suburban private hospitals vs. large, urban medical centers.

Etiology

ABE is usually caused by *Staphylococcus aureus,* Group A hemolytic streptococcus, pneumococcus, or gonococcus but also by less virulent microorganisms.

SBE is caused usually by streptococcal species (especially viridans streptococci, microaerophilic and anaerobic streptococci, nonenterococcal Group D, and enterococci), and less commonly by *S. aureus, S. epidermidis,* and fastidious *Hemophilus* sp. SBE often develops on abnormal valves after asymptomatic bacteremias from infected gums, or GU or GI tract.

Prosthetic valvular endocarditis (PVE) develops in 2 to 3% of patients in the year following valve placement and in 0.5%/yr thereafter but is more common with aortic than mitral valve prostheses and less common with porcine (heterograft) than other prosthetic valves. **Early onset infections** (< 2 mo postsurgery) with high mortality occur mainly from antimicrobial-resistant organisms implanted during surgery (eg, *S. epidermidis,* diphtheroids, coliform bacilli, *Candida* sp, and *Aspergillus* sp). A better prognosis is associated with **later onset infections** produced by low-virulence organisms implanted at surgery, or by transient asymptomatic bacteremias often from susceptible organisms (most often *Streptococcus* sp, *S. epidermidis,* diphtheroids, and the fastidious gram-negative rods—*Hemophilus* sp, *Actinobacillus actinomycetemcomitans,* and *Cardiobacterium hominis*). (NOTE: S. epidermidis *can be susceptible or resistant and is both an early and a late pathogen.*)

Right-sided endocarditis involving the tricuspid valve and less often the pulmonary valve and artery may result from IV use of illicit drugs or from central vascular lines, which not only facilitate entry of microorganisms but may damage the endocardium. Organisms originating from the skin (eg, *S. aureus, Candida* sp, or coliform bacilli) produce septic phlebitis, fever, pleurisy, hemoptysis, septic pulmonary infarction, and tricuspid regurgitation. These infections more often respond to antimicrobial therapy and have a better prognosis than left-sided IE.

Pathology

The intravascular nidus for microorganisms within the heart and blood vessels is thought to be a sterile fibrin-platelet vegetation formed when tissue factor is released by damaged endothelial cells. Microorganisms colonizing vegetations are covered by a layer of fibrin and platelets that prevents access by neutrophils, immunoglobulin, and complement, thus permitting the pathogens to resist host defenses. *Without treatment, IE is progressive and uniformly fatal.* Death usually ensues from heart failure due to exacerbation of underlying heart disease or acute valve dysfunction, embolization of vegetations to vital organs producing infarction, rupture of a mycotic aneurysm, septic shock in ABE, renal failure, or complications of cardiac surgery.

IE occurs most often on the left side, involving the mitral, aortic, tricuspid, and pulmonic valves (in descending order of frequency). Congenital defects and rheumatic valvular disease are still major predisposing factors. Mural thrombi, arteriovenous fistulas, ventricular-septal defects, and patent ductus arteriosus sites may also become infected. Rheumatic valvular heart disease, bicuspid or calcific aortic valves, mitral valve prolapse, hypertrophic subaortic stenosis, and prosthetic valves predispose to IE. Infections treated with antimicrobial agents heal by endothelialization of vegetations.

Symptoms and Signs

SBE has an insidious onset and may mimic other systemic illnesses with low-grade fever ($< 39°$ C [102.2° F]), night sweats, fatigability, malaise, weight loss, and valvular insufficiency. Chills and arthralgias may be present. Emboli may produce stroke, myocardial infarction, flank pain and hematuria, abdominal pain, or acute arterial insufficiency in an extremity. Physical examination may be normal or show chronic illness with pallor; fever; a change in preexisting murmur or new regurgitant cardiac valvular murmur; tachycardia; petechiae over the upper trunk, conjunctiva, mucous membranes, and distal extremities; painful erythematous subcutaneous nodules about the tips of the digits (**Osler's nodes**); splinter hemorrhages under the nails; or hemorrhagic retinal lesions (particularly **Roth's spots**, *round or oval lesions with small white centers*). With prolonged infection, splenomegaly or clubbing of the fingers may also be present.

Hematuria and proteinuria may result from embolic infarction of the kidney or a diffuse glomerulonephritis due to immune complex deposi-

tion. Manifestations of CNS involvement (in about 35% of patients) may range from transient ischemic attacks and toxic encephalopathy to brain abscess, subarachnoid hemorrhage from rupture of a mycotic aneurysm, and purulent meningitis in ABE.

In **ABE**, symptoms and signs are similar to those of SBE, but the course is more rapid. ABE can develop on normal valves and is marked by the variable presence of high fever, toxic appearance, rapid valvular destruction, valve ring abscesses, septic emboli, an obvious source of infection, and septic shock.

PVE often results in valve ring abscesses, obstructing vegetations, myocardial abscesses, and mycotic aneurysms manifested by valve obstruction, dehiscence, and cardiac conduction disturbances in addition to the usual symptoms of ABE or SBE.

Diagnosis

Since symptoms and physical findings are nonspecific, highly variable, and may present insidiously, it is important to search actively for IE in high-risk patients (eg, those with a history of cardiac valvular disease or recent invasive medical procedures or dental work, drug addicts). The multitude of symptoms and signs described above may all be present, but most are being seen less frequently, perhaps because of earlier diagnosis and treatment; fever and heart murmurs are the most constant. Although up to 15% of patients with IE may not have fever or a murmur initially, almost all will have both eventually. Thus, any patient with suspected septicemia, especially with fever and a murmur, must have blood drawn for cultures as soon as possible. Because of the continuous bacteremia seen in intravascular infections, usually 3 to 5 blood cultures of 20 to 30 mL each within 24 h suffice to isolate the etiologic agent. Identification of the organism and its antimicrobial susceptibility are vital, because *bactericidal* treatment is required. Blood cultures may need 3 to 4 wk incubation, and certain infections (ie, *Aspergillus* sp) may not produce positive cultures; others (ie, *Coxiella burnetii*, *Chlamydia psittaci*) require serodiagnosis or special culture media (*Legionella pneumophila*).

Other than positive blood cultures, there are no specific laboratory findings. Patients with bacteremias from organisms known to be frequent causes of IE should be examined carefully and repeatedly for new valvular murmurs and for signs of embolic phenomena. Two-dimensional echocardiographic studies will detect vegetations in 60 to 80% of patients with IE if they have underlying valvular heart disease. In established infections, a normocytic-normochromic anemia, elevated ESR, neutrophilia, increased immunoglobulins, circulating immune complexes, and rheumatoid factor are often present.

Negative blood cultures may indicate suppression due to prior antimicrobial therapy, infection with organisms that do not grow in routine laboratory culture media, or another diagnosis (that must be established); eg, nonbacterial thrombotic endocarditis, atrial myxoma with embolic phenomenon, or one of the vasculitides.

Prognosis

Untreated, IE is always fatal. When it is treated, the mortality varies greatly, depending upon the patient's age and condition, severity of underlying diseases, site of infection, susceptibility of the microorganism to antibiotics, and complications. The expected mortality of viridans streptococcal endocarditis without major complications is < 10% but is virtually 100% with *Aspergillus* endocarditis following prosthetic valve surgery. Cardiac surgical procedures that correct acute valvular insufficiency, remove infected foreign bodies, and eliminate recalcitrant infection have significantly improved survival. A poor prognosis is associated with heart failure, extreme age, aortic or multiple valve involvement, large vegetations, polymicrobial bacteremia, antimicrobial resistance, delay in initiating therapy, prosthetic valve infections, mycotic aneurysms, valve ring abscess, and major embolic events. Following cardiac surgery, early-onset IE has a higher mortality rate than late-onset IE (as noted above), as has left-sided than right-sided IE.

Prophylaxis

(See TABLE 42–1 for prophylaxis in children)

Although effectiveness is unproved, most physicians recommend antimicrobial prophylaxis for patients with valvular or other predisposition to IE when undergoing procedures associated with bacteremias and subsequent IE. Prophylaxis is directed against viridans streptococci during oral-dental procedures, against enterococci for GI and GU tract infections, and against *S. aureus* and *S. epidermidis* during cardiac valvular surgery. Prophylaxis in the dental office consists of amoxicillin 3 gm orally 1 h before the procedure and 1.5 gm orally 6 h later, or erythromycin 1 gm orally 1 h before the procedure followed by 0.5 gm orally q 6 h for 4 to 8 doses. Prophylaxis for

enterococci consists of ampicillin 1 gm plus gentamicin 1.5 mg/kg (up to 80 mg) parenterally 30 to 60 min before the procedure, followed by 2 additional doses q 8 h. Prophylaxis during cardiac surgery usually consists of cefazolin 2 gm IV during initiation of anesthesia with 2 gm IV q 8 h for 3 to 6 doses, but other antimicrobial agents may be necessary if there are frequent postoperative infections with cefazolin-resistant organisms.

Treatment

Successful treatment requires (1) maintenance of high serum levels of an effective antibiotic, and (2) surgical management of mechanical complications and resistant organisms.

Penicillin-susceptible streptococci (penicillin G MIC ≤ 0.1 μg/mL) include most viridans streptococci, microaerophilic and anaerobic streptococci, and nonenterococcal Group D streptococci. Several regimens have equivalent results: penicillin G 10 to 20 million u./day IV in divided doses q 4 h, or procaine penicillin G 1.2 million u. IM q 6 or 12 h for 4 wk. When streptomycin 7.5 mg/kg IM (up to 500 mg) bid is administered concurrently, the length of treatment should be reduced to 2 wk, and organisms should be tested for high level (> 2000 μg/mL) streptomycin resistance, which is rare in nonenterococcal streptococci but if present, gentamicin 1 mg/kg IM (up to 80 mg) q 8 h should be used instead of streptomycin. Patients allergic to penicillin may be cautiously given cefazolin if there is no history of penicillin anaphylaxis or, alternatively, vancomycin. Oral treatment programs are less reliable and should not be used without close monitoring of serum levels to ensure adequate GI absorption.

Penicillin-resistant streptococci (penicillin G MIC > 0.1 μg/mL): Enterococcal and some other streptococcal strains (including fastidious pyridoxal-requiring viridans streptococci) are relatively resistant to penicillin G and require the synergistic activity of a penicillin or vancomycin combined with an aminoglycoside. About 40% of enterococcal strains with a high-level (> 2000 μg/mL) resistance to streptomycin do not respond to penicillin G plus streptomycin and should be treated with penicillin plus gentamicin. Penicillin G 15 to 24 million u./day IV or ampicillin 8 to 12 gm/day IV should be given concurrently with streptomycin 7.5 mg/kg IM (up to 500 mg) bid or gentamicin 1 mg/kg IV (up to 80 mg) q 8 h for 4 to 6 wk. Patients with enterococcal infections lasting > 3 mo, with large vegetations (as seen by echocardiogram), or with vegetations on prosthetic valves should be treated for 6 wk. Persons allergic to penicillin may be desensitized or treated with vancomycin 7.5 mg/kg IV (up to 500 mg) q 6 h and streptomycin or gentamicin.

Pneumococcal or Group A streptococcal endocarditis should be treated with penicillin G 10 to 20 million u./day IV for 4 wk.

S. aureus endocarditis should be treated with penicillin G 15 to 24 million u./day IV if the strain does not produce β-lactamase. Ninety percent of strains are penicillin-resistant and should be treated with a penicillinase-resistant penicillin (nafcillin or oxacillin) 1.5 to 2 gm IV q 4 h for 4 to 6 wk. Staphylococcal strains resistant to the penicillinase-resistant penicillins are also resistant to the cephalosporins, although this may be difficult to demonstrate with routine susceptibility testing. Oxacillin-nafcillin−resistant staphylococci should be treated with vancomycin 7.5 mg/kg IV q 6 h. Oxacillin-nafcillin−susceptible infections in penicillin-allergic patients may be cautiously treated with cefazolin 1 to 2 gm IV q 6 to 8 h if there is no history of penicillin anaphylaxis, or with vancomycin.

S. epidermidis endocarditis occurs most often in patients with prosthetic valves and may require surgery as well as antimicrobial agents. Penicillin- or oxacillin-susceptible strains should be treated for 6 to 8 wk as outlined above for *S. aureus.* Oxacillin-resistant strains should be treated with vancomycin 7.5 mg/kg IV q 6 h plus rifampin 300 mg orally q 8 h for 6 to 8 wk. *Hemophilus* sp should be treated with ampicillin plus gentamicin for 4 wk, using the same doses as mentioned for enterococcal infections. Coliform bacillary endocardial infections often show antimicrobial resistance and should be treated for ≥ 4 wk with a sensitivity-proven β-lactam antimicrobial agent plus an aminoglycoside.

Cardiac valve surgery (debridement and replacement of the valve) is frequently required to eradicate infection that is uncontrolled medically, particularly in early-onset prosthetic valvular endocarditis. The timing of surgical intervention requires good clinical judgment. It may be required urgently if heart failure caused by a correctable lesion is worsening (particularly when the organism is *S. aureus,* a gram-negative bacillus, or a fungus), but generally should be preceded by 24 to 72 h of an optimal antibiotic regimen.

Response to treatment: Patients with penicillin-susceptible streptococcal IE usually feel better and have a reduction in fever within 3 to 7 days of starting therapy. However, fever may persist for reasons other than continued active infection; eg, drug allergy, phlebitis, or infarction from emboli. Staphylococcal IE often responds more slowly. Sterile emboli and valve rupture may occur up to a year after successful antimicrobial therapy. Relapse after therapy usually occurs within 4 wk; the patient may respond to antibiotic re-treatment or may also require surgery. Recrudescence of IE after 6 wk in patients without prosthetic valves usually is a new infection rather than a relapse.

BOTULISM

Neuromuscular poisoning from Clostridium botulinum *toxin.* Botulism occurs in 3 forms: foodborne, wound, and infant botulism.

Etiology and Pathophysiology

The sporulating, anaerobic gram-positive bacillus *C. botulinum* elaborates 7 types of antigenically distinct toxins. Humans are usually poisoned by type A, B, E, or (rarely) F toxin. Type A and B toxins are highly poisonous proteins resistant to digestion by GI enzymes. In foodborne botulism, toxin produced in contaminated food is eaten; but in wound and infant botulism, neurotoxin is elaborated in vivo by growth of *C. botulinum* in infected tissue and in the GI tract, respectively. After absorption, the toxins interfere with release of acetylcholine at peripheral nerve endings.

C. botulinum spores are highly heat-resistant; they may survive several hours at 100° C (212° F); however, exposure to moist heat at 120° C (248° F) for 30 min will kill the spores. Toxins, on the other hand, are readily destroyed by heat, and cooking food at 80° C (176° F) for 30 min safeguards against botulism. Toxin production (especially type E) can occur at temperatures as low as 3° C (37.4° F) and does not require strict anaerobic conditions. Between 1970 and 1977 in the USA, foodborne outbreaks were caused most often by type A toxin (51%), followed by type B (21%) and type E (12%); in 16% the toxin type was not identified. Type F outbreaks are rare. Home-canned foods are the most common sources, but commercially prepared foods have been identified in about 10% of outbreaks. Vegetables, fish, fruits, and condiments are the most common vehicles, but beef, milk products, pork, poultry, and other foods have been involved. In outbreaks caused by marine products, type E accounted for about half, with types A and B causing the rest.

Botulinum toxin types are distinctively distributed in the USA: Type A is seen predominantly west of the Mississippi River, type B in the Eastern states, and type E in Alaska and the Great Lakes area.

Symptoms and Signs

In foodborne botulism, onset is abrupt, usually 18 to 36 h after ingestion of the toxin, though the incubation period may vary from 4 h to 8 days. Neurologic symptoms are characteristically bilateral and symmetric, beginning with the cranial nerves and following with descending weakness or paralysis. Common initial symptoms and signs include dry mouth, diplopia, blepharoptosis, loss of accommodation, and diminished or total loss of pupillary light reflex. Nausea, vomiting, abdominal cramps, and diarrhea frequently precede neurologic symptoms. Symptoms of bulbar paresis (dysarthria, dysphagia, nasal regurgitation) develop. Dysphagia can lead to aspiration pneumonia. Muscles of the extremities and trunk and muscles of respiration become progressively weaker in a descending pattern. There are no sensory disturbances and the sensorium usually remains clear until shortly before death. Fever is absent and the pulse remains normal or slow unless intercurrent infection develops. Routine studies of the blood, urine, and CSF are usually normal. Constipation is frequent after neurologic impairment appears. Major complications include respiratory failure due to diaphragmatic paralysis and pulmonary infections.

Wound botulism is manifested by the same symptoms of neurologic involvement as are seen in foodborne botulism, but there are no GI symptoms or epidemiologic evidence implicating food as a cause. A history of a traumatic injury or deep puncture wound in the preceding 2 wk may suggest the diagnosis. Careful search should be made for breaks in the patient's skin.

Infant botulism, seen most often in infants 2 to 3 mo old, results from the ingestion of botulinal spores and their colonization in the GI tract and toxin production in vivo; unlike foodborne botulism, infant botulism is not caused by ingestion of preformed toxin. Constipation is present initially in 2/3 of cases and is followed by neuromuscular paralysis that begins with the cranial nerves and proceeds to peripheral and respiratory musculature. Cranial nerve deficits may be

asymmetric, and a spectrum based on severity may show variation from mild lethargy and slowed feeding to severe hypotonia and respiratory insufficiency. Affected infants have characteristically been normal before the onset of illness and have usually been breastfed. However, they have generally been exposed to foods other than milk, and spores are common in the environment. Cases have been related to the ingestion of honey, dust, and soil containing C. botulinum.

Diagnosis

Foodborne botulism: The pattern of neuromuscular disturbances suggests the diagnosis of an isolated case; a likely food source provides an important clue. The simultaneous occurrence of 2 or more cases after eating the same food simplifies the diagnosis. It is confirmed by demonstrating botulinal toxin in the serum or feces of the patient or by isolating the organism from feces. Finding C. botulinum toxin in suspect food identifies the source. Pets may develop botulism from eating the same contaminated food. Botulism may be confused with the Guillain-Barré syndrome, poliomyelitis, stroke, myasthenia gravis, tick paralysis, and poisoning due to curare or belladonna alkaloids. A characteristic augmented response to rapid repetitive stimulation ($\geq$ 20 cycles/sec) makes electromyography a useful diagnostic tool for botulism, although this response may not be seen in all cases.

In wound botulism, finding toxin in serum or isolating the C. botulinum organism on anaerobic culture of the infection site confirms the diagnosis.

In infant botulism, sepsis, congenital muscular dystrophy, hypothyroidism, and benign congenital hypotonia are additional considerations. Finding C. botulinum toxin or organisms in the feces establishes the diagnosis.

Special Precautions

Since even minute amounts of botulinal toxin acquired by ingestion, inhalation, or absorption through the eye or a break in the skin can cause serious illness, all materials suspected of containing toxin require special handling. Only experienced personnel, preferably immunized with botulinal toxoid, should perform laboratory tests. Specimens should be placed in unbreakable, sterile, leakproof containers, refrigerated (preferably not frozen), and examined as soon as possible. Wound specimens are an exception and should not be refrigerated. Further details regarding specimen collection and handling can be obtained from state health department epidemiologists or the Centers for Disease Control, Atlanta, Georgia 30333.

Prophylaxis and Treatment

Proper home and commercial canning and adequate heating of home-canned food before serving are essential (see Etiology and Pathophysiology, above). Canned foods showing any evidence of spoilage should be discarded. Infants < 1 yr old should not be fed honey. Anyone known or thought to have been exposed to contaminated food must be carefully observed. To eliminate unabsorbed toxin, induction of vomiting, gastric lavage, and purgation are recommended. Toxoids can be prepared for active immunization of persons working with *C. botulinum* or its toxins.

The greatest threat to life is from respiratory impairment and its complications. All patients should be hospitalized and closely supervised with serial measurements of vital capacity. The progressive paralysis prevents patients from showing visible signs of respiratory distress while their vital capacity decreases. Respiratory impairment requires management in an ICU where intubation, tracheostomy, and mechanical ventilators are readily available. IV alimentation may be required. Improvements in such supportive care have reduced mortality to < 10%.

Trivalent antitoxin (A, B, E) is available from the Centers for Disease Control, which also stores a polyvalent antitoxin (A, B, C, D, E, F) for specific outbreaks due to C, D, or F botulism. Antitoxin will not release toxin that is already bound; therefore, preexisting neurologic impairment will not be reversed. At best it will slow or halt further progression of the disease. Antitoxin should be given as soon as possible after botulism has been diagnosed. Risks must be weighed against potential benefits. Antitoxin is unlikely to be of benefit if given > 72 h after the onset of symptoms. Since these are horse serum antitoxins, there is a risk of anaphylaxis or serum sickness. The use of antitoxin in infant botulism has not been adequately studied and at present is not generally recommended. For precautions in the use of horse serum antitoxin, see serum sickness under HYPERSENSITIVITY TO DRUGS and for treatment of reactions, see ANAPHYLAXIS under DISORDERS WITH TYPE I HYPERSENSITIVITY REACTIONS, both in Ch. 34.

VIRAL INFECTIONS
(For a condensed review of differential diagnoses of the more common exanthems, see TABLE 32–9)

MEASLES
(Rubeola; Morbilli; Nine-Day Measles)

A highly contagious, acute disease characterized by fever, cough, coryza, conjunctivitis, enanthem (Koplik's spots) on the buccal or labial mucosa, and a spreading maculopapular cutaneous rash.

Etiology and Epidemiology

Measles is caused by a paramyxovirus and is spread mainly by small droplets from the nose, throat, and mouth of a person in the prodromal or an early eruptive stage of the disease or by airborne droplet nuclei. Indirect spread by uninfected persons or by objects is unusual. The communicable period of the disease begins 2 to 4 days before the rash appears and continues during the acute stages. The virus disappears from nose and throat secretions by the time the rash clears. Persons who develop mild desquamation following the rash are no longer infectious.

Measles and chickenpox appear to be among the most readily transmitted of all infectious diseases. Before widespread immunization programs began, measles epidemics occurred every 2 or 3 yr, with small localized outbreaks during intervening years. In recent years in the USA, the epidemiology of this disease has shifted, with outbreaks now occurring in previously immunized teenagers and young adults, as well as in unimmunized preschool-aged children. An infant whose mother has had measles receives transplacental passive immunity lasting most of the first year of life; thereafter, susceptibility is high. One attack of measles confers lifelong immunity.

Symptoms and Signs

After a 7- to 14-day incubation period, typical measles begins with prodromal fever, coryza, hacking cough, and conjunctivitis. The pathognomonic Koplik's spots appear 2 to 4 days later, usually on the buccal mucosa opposite the 1st and 2nd upper molars. These spots resemble tiny grains of white sand surrounded by inflammatory areolae. If they are numerous, the entire background may be a mottled erythema. Pharyngitis and inflammation of the laryngeal and tracheobronchial mucosa develop. Characteris-

TABLE 32–9. DIFFERENTIAL DIAGNOSIS OF

Condition	Incubation (days)	Period of Communicability	Symptoms and Signs
Measles (rubeola)	7–14	From 2–4 days before appearance of rash until 2–5 days after onset	Koplik's spots, fever, coryza, cough, conjunctivitis, photophobia, usually mild pruritus
Rubella (German measles)	14–21	From shortly before onset of symptoms until rash disappears; infected newborns are usually infective for many months	Malaise, fever, headache, rhinitis, postauricular and suboccipital lymphadenopathy with tender nodes
Roseola infantum (exanthem subitum, human herpesvirus type 6)	Probably 5–15	Unknown	Characteristic disappearance of high fever and simultaneous appearance of rash in infants and preschool children, excessive risk of seizures
Erythema infectiosum (fifth disease)	4–14	From before onset of rash until a few days after	Low-grade fever, occasional arthralgias
Chickenpox (varicella)	14–21	From a few days before onset of symptoms until all crops of vesicles have crusted	Moderate fever, headache, malaise, occasional sore throat
Infectious mononucleosis	10–50	Undetermined	Malaise, headache, fever, sore throat, splenomegaly, generalized lymphadenopathy
Scarlet fever (scarlatina)	3–5 (occasionally slightly shorter or longer)	Usually from 24 h before onset of symptoms until 2–3 wk after or longer if complications occur (eg, sinusitis, otitis media)	Sore throat, chills, fever, headache, vomiting, strawberry tongue, cervical lymphadenopathy, circumoral pallor, rapid pulse
Drug rash	Variable—depends on history of recent drug use	None	Variable, including fever, malaise, arthralgia, nausea, photophobia, pruritus

tic multinucleated giant cells appear in nasal secretions, pharyngeal and buccal mucosa, and often, urinary sediment.

The characteristic rash appears 3 to 5 days after onset of symptoms, usually 1 to 2 days after

the Koplik's spots appear. It begins in front of and below the ears and on the side of the neck as irregular macules that soon become maculopapular and spread rapidly (within 24 to 48 h) to the trunk and extremities, as they begin to fade or

THE MORE COMMON EXANTHEMS

Eruption			Laboratory Findings
Site	Character	Onset; Duration	
Starts around ears, on face and neck, spreads over trunk and limbs; limbs escape in mild cases	Maculopapular, brownish-pink, and irregularly confluent in severe cases, or even petechial; discrete in mild cases	3–5 days after onset of symptoms; lasts 4–7 days	Granulocytic leukopenia; virus in blood and nasopharynx
Face, neck, and spreads to trunk and limbs	Fine pinkish macules that become confluent and often scarlatiniform or pinpoint on 2nd day	1 or 2 days after onset of symptoms; lasts 1–3 days	WBC count usually normal or slightly reduced; virus in blood and nasopharynx
Chest and abdomen, with moderate involvement of face and extremities	Diffuse macular or maculopapular	On about 4th day, rash appears as temperature drops suddenly to normal; lasts 1–2 days	Granulocytic leukopenia
Starts on cheeks, spreads to arms, legs, trunk	Maculopapular; often blotchy or reticular	Shortly after onset of symptoms; lasts 5–10 days; may recur for several weeks	Mild lymphocytosis and eosinophilia
Usually 1st on trunk, later on face, neck, extremities; infrequently on palms and soles	Lesions discrete; progress from macule to papule to vesicle to crusting; appear in crops, hence various stages are present simultaneously	Shortly after onset of symptoms; lasts a few days to 2 wk	Presence of virus in vesicle fluid; multinucleated giant cells at base of vesicle (Tzanck test)
Most prominent over trunk	Occurs in about 15% of cases as a morbilliform, scarlatiniform, or vesicular rash	5–14 days after onset of illness; lasts 3–7 days	Positive heterophil antibody test; leukocytosis with atypical enlarged lymphocytes; appearance of antibodies to Epstein-Barr virus
Face, neck, chest, abdomen, and spreads to extremities; entire body surface may be involved	Diffuse pinkish-red flush of skin, blanches on pressure, with Schultz-Charlton reaction	On 2nd day; lasts 4–10 days	Granulocytosis; throat culture positive for β-hemolytic streptococcus
Generalized; sometimes restricted to exposed surfaces	May be morbilliform, scarlatiniform, erythematous, acneiform, vesicular, bullous, purpuric, or exfoliating	Variable	Agranulocytosis possible; presence of drug in urine

the face. Petechiae or ecchymoses may be present with particularly severe rashes.

At the peak of the illness, the temperature may exceed 40° C (104° F), and periorbital edema, conjunctivitis, photophobia, a hacking cough, extensive rash, and mild itching are present; generally, the patient appears quite ill. Leukopenia with a relative lymphocytosis is usual. The constitutional symptoms and signs parallel the severity of the eruption and vary with the epidemic. In 3 to 5 days, the fever falls by lysis, the patient feels more comfortable, and the rash begins to fade rapidly, leaving a coppery-brown discoloration followed by desquamation.

Atypical measles syndrome (AMS), most common in young adults, usually occurs in individuals previously immunized with the original killed virus measles vaccines, which are no longer available. However, live, attenuated measles vaccine administration has also been known to precede development of AMS, perhaps as a result of inadvertent inactivation due to improper storage. Presumably, inactivated measles virus vaccines do not prevent wild virus infection and can sensitize patients so that disease expression is altered significantly. AMS may begin abruptly, with high fever, toxicity, headache, abdominal pain, and cough. The rash may appear 1 to 2 days later, often beginning on the extremities, and may be maculopapular, vesicular, urticarial, or purpuric. Edema of the hands and feet may occur; pneumonia and hilar adenopathy are common, and nodular densities in the lungs may persist for 12 wk or longer. Moderate to severe abnormalities in the ventilation/perfusion ratio in the lungs may result in significant hypoxemia.

Prognosis and Complications

In healthy, well-nourished children, measles has a low mortality rate unless complications ensue. Pneumonia (especially in infants), otitis media, and other bacterial infections are common. Patients with measles are highly susceptible to streptococcal infection. Measles causes transient suppression of delayed hypersensitivity, leading to a transient reversal of previously positive tuberculin and histoplasmin skin tests and sometimes to worsening of active TB or reactivation of latent mycobacterial infection. An exacerbation of fever, change in WBC count from leukopenia to leukocytosis, and development of malaise, pain, or prostration suggest a complicating bacterial infection. Immunocompromised patients may develop a severe, progressive giant cell pneumonia without a rash.

Acute thrombocytopenic purpura, at times with severe hemorrhagic manifestations, may complicate the acute phase of measles.

Encephalitis occurs about once in 1000 to 2000 cases, usually 2 days to 3 wk after onset of the exanthem, often beginning with high fever, convulsions, and coma. In most instances, the CSF lymphocyte count is between 50 and 500/μL and the protein level is increased. A normal CSF at the time of initial symptoms does not rule

out encephalitis. The course may be brief, with recovery in about a week, or may be prolonged, terminating in serious CNS impairment or death.

Measles virus is also associated with **subacute sclerosing panencephalitis (SSPE)**, which is discussed in this chapter, below. SSPE is a previously unexplained chronic brain disease of children and adolescents that occurs months to years (usually years) after an attack of measles, causing intellectual deterioration, convulsive seizures, and motor abnormalities; it is usually fatal. Measles virus has been identified in brain tissue by electron microscopy, demonstration of measles antigen through fluorescent antibody techniques, and isolation of the agent from brain biopsies.

Diagnosis

Typical measles may be suspected in a patient with coryza, photophobia, and evidence of bronchitis, but before the rash appears a definite diagnosis can be made only by identifying Koplik's spots. These, followed by high fever, malaise, and the rash with its characteristic cephalocaudal progression, establish the diagnosis in most cases. The virus can be detected in the early stage of the disease by rapid immunofluorescent staining of pharyngeal and urinary epithelial cells, or it can be grown in tissue culture. Serologic tests are also available.

Differential diagnosis of typical measles includes rubella, scarlet fever, drug rashes, serum sickness, roseola infantum, infectious mononucleosis, adenovirus, and echo- and coxsackievirus infections. Distinguishing features of rubella include its mild course with few or no constitutional symptoms, enlarged (and usually tender) postauricular and suboccipital lymph nodes, low fever, normal WBC count, usual absence of a recognizable prodrome, and short duration. Scarlet fever may be suggested at first by the pharyngitis and fever, but the leukocytosis of scarlet fever is absent in measles and the rash is morphologically distinct. Koplik's spots, the severe cough, and the characteristic rash of measles clarify what might be a difficult diagnosis. Drug rashes (eg, from phenobarbital or sulfonamides) resemble the measles eruption, but the typical prodrome, cough, and cephalocaudal progression of the rash are absent, and the palms and soles are more likely to be prominently involved. Here, even more than usual, the history is important. Roseola infantum produces a skin rash similar to that of measles but is seldom seen in children over age 3. It can usually be differentiated by its high initial temperature, absence of Koplik's spots and malaise, and appearance of the rash simultaneously with defervescence.

The differential diagnosis of AMS is similar to that of typical measles; however, the pleomorphism of the rash and the severe constitutional signs sometimes observed may suggest Rocky Mountain spotted fever, leptospirosis, hemorrhagic varicella, or meningococcal infection; other differential diagnoses include certain bacterial or viral pneumonias, appendicitis, collagen-vascular diseases such as juvenile RA, and Kawasaki syndrome (mucocutaneous lymph node syndrome). A history of measles exposure and prior administration of killed virus vaccine suggest the diagnosis, but virus isolation, serologic studies, or both may be necessary to confirm it.

Prophylaxis

A live attenuated virus vaccine is available that provides the same long-lasting immunity in vaccine respondents as does natural measles. The vaccine produces mild, or inapparent, noncommunicable infection and an antibody response similar to that of natural measles. Fever over 38° C (101° F) occurs 5 to 12 days after inoculation in < 5% of vaccinees and is often followed by a rash. CNS reactions are exceedingly rare, and simultaneous administration of measles immune globulin (MIG) or immune serum globulin with the vaccine is unnecessary and contraindicated.

Contraindications to the use of any live measles virus vaccine include generalized malignancies (eg, leukemia, lymphoma), immunodeficiency diseases, and therapy with corticosteroids, irradiation, alkylating agents, or antimetabolites. Reasons to defer vaccination include pregnancy, any acute febrile illness, active untreated TB, or administration of antibody (as whole blood, plasma, or any immune globulin) within the preceding 8 wk.

For routine immunization, see IMMUNIZATION PROCEDURES THROUGHOUT CHILDHOOD in Ch. 23.

Exposed susceptibles may be protected if the live vaccine is given within 2 days of exposure. Alternatively (eg, in pregnant patients, children < 3 yr of age, or patients with TB or an acute febrile illness), MIG or immune serum globulin 0.25 mL/kg IM is given immediately, followed by a live vaccine 8 wk later or as soon after that as health permits. An exposed susceptible patient with a condition that contraindicates use of any live measles virus vaccine (leukemia, im-

munosuppression, combined immunodeficiency, etc) is given MIG or immune serum globulin 0.5 mL/kg IM (maximum, 15 mL). If such an immunocompromised patient also has a bleeding disorder (eg, thrombocytopenia), IV γ globulin should be considered.

Treatment

Treatment is symptomatic. Patients should be protected from exposure to streptococcal infections. Secondary bacterial complications require appropriate antimicrobial drugs. In a recent study, vitamin A 400,000 IU given orally reduced morbidity and mortality in malnourished African children with severe measles. Immune serum globulin is ineffective in encephalitis; symptomatic care is the only available treatment.

SUBACUTE SCLEROSING PANENCEPHALITIS (SSPE)

A progressive, usually fatal, neurologic (brain) disorder occurring months to years (usually years) after an attack of measles and characterized by mental deterioration, myoclonic jerks, and seizures.

Etiology and Epidemiology

The mode of spread is not known. A naturally acquired altered measles virus is the probable cause. Measles virus has been demonstrated in brain tissue and isolated from brain biopsies. SSPE has been reported in children who did not have a history of natural measles but who did receive measles vaccine. Some of these cases may have resulted from unrecognized measles in the first year of life or possibly from the measles vaccination. Based on estimated nationwide measles vaccine distribution, the association of SSPE cases to measles vaccination is about one case per million vaccine doses distributed. This is far less than the association with natural measles (6 to 22 cases of SSPE per million cases of measles). Males are affected more frequently than females. The incidence has been declining in the USA and Western Europe.

Symptoms and Signs

Onset is usually before age 20. Often the first signs are diminished performance in schoolwork, forgetfulness, temper outbursts, distractibility, sleeplessness, and hallucinations. Seizures follow the mental changes and initially are myoclonic jerks—sudden flexion movements of the extremities, head, and trunk; grand mal seizures may occur. Patients show further intellectual decline; changes in speech; and abnormal involuntary movements, including athetosis, chorea, and ballistic or throwing movements. Dystonic movements and transient periods of opisthotonos are seen. Later, rigidity of the body musculature, difficulty in swallowing, cortical blindness, and optic atrophy may be noted. Focal chorioretinitis and other funduscopic abnormalities are seen in a number of patients. In the final phases, the patient becomes increasingly rigid, with intermittent signs of hypothalamic involvement (eg, hyperthermia, diaphoresis, and disturbances of pulse and BP).

The disease, almost invariably fatal within 1 to 3 yr (often as the result of terminal pneumonia), sometimes has a more protracted course, with pronounced neurologic deficits. A few patients have remissions and exacerbations.

SSPE patients have a typical EEG: paroxysmal bursts of 2 to 3 cycles/sec, high-voltage, diphasic waves occurring synchronously throughout the recording. The CT scan may show cortical atrophy or low-density lesions of the white matter. The CSF usually is under normal pressure and has a normal cell count and protein content. The CSF γ globulin is almost always markedly elevated and may constitute as much as 20 to 60% of the total spinal fluid protein. The patient's serum and CSF contain elevated levels of measles virus antibodies. Antimeasles IgG appears to increase as the disease progresses. Despite vigorous serologic responses to measles virus, SSPE patients do not develop antibodies to the M protein of the measles virion.

Diagnosis

SSPE should be considered in a child or adolescent who shows progressive mental deterioration and myoclonic jerks or seizures. The diagnosis is confirmed by the characteristic EEG, an elevated CSF γ globulin, and an excessive quantity of measles virus antibody in the serum and spinal fluid. CT abnormalities include dilatation of the lateral ventricles and atrophy of cerebral cortex, brainstem, and cerebellum.

Treatment

Antiviral agents have not proved helpful; inosiplex has been reported to retard the disease, but its effectiveness is controversial, and it has not been approved by the FDA. Generally, only symptomatic treatment with anticonvulsants and supportive measures can be offered.

RUBELLA
(German Measles; Three-Day Measles)

A contagious exanthematous disease, usually with mild constitutional symptoms, that may result in abortion, stillbirth, or congenital defects in infants born to mothers infected during the early months of pregnancy. Congenital rubella is discussed under NEONATAL INFECTIONS in Ch. 27.

Etiology and Epidemiology

The disease is caused by an RNA virus spread by airborne droplet nuclei or by close contact. A patient can transmit the disease from 1 wk before onset of the rash until 1 wk after it fades. Congenitally infected infants are potentially infectious for many months after birth. Rubella is less contagious than measles, and many persons are not infected during childhood; as a result, 10 to 15% of young adult women are susceptible. Many cases are misdiagnosed or are mild and go unnoticed. Epidemics occur at irregular intervals during the spring; major epidemics occur at about 6- to 9-yr intervals. In the USA, the number of cases of rubella and congenital rubella syndrome has increased since 1988. Immunity appears to be lifelong following natural infection.

Symptoms and Signs

After a 14- to 21-day incubation period, a 1- to 5-day prodrome, usually consisting of malaise and lymphadenopathy, occurs in children but may be minimal or absent in adolescents and adults. Tender swelling of the suboccipital, postauricular, and postcervical glands is characteristic and, with the typical rash, suggests the diagnosis.

The rash is similar to that of measles but less extensive and more evanescent. It begins on the face and neck and quickly spreads to the trunk and extremities. At the onset of the eruption, a flush simulating that of scarlet fever may appear, particularly on the face. A mild enanthem of discrete rose-colored spots is present on the palate, later coalescing into a red blush and extending over the fauces. The pharynx becomes red at the onset, but the throat is not sore. The rash usually lasts about 3 days. On the 2nd day, it often becomes more scarlatiniform (pinpoint) with a reddish flush. The slight skin discoloration that remains as the rash fades may disappear in a day.

Constitutional symptoms in children are mild—slight malaise and occasional arthralgias.

Adults characteristically have few or no complaints of constitutional symptoms, although fever, malaise, headache, stiff joints (occasionally with overt, transient arthritis), a slight feeling of lassitude, and mild rhinitis may be noted. They may become aware of the disease by noting the rash on the chest, arms, or forehead or by discovering the characteristic postauricular lymphadenopathy while washing or combing the hair. Encephalitis, a rare but occasionally fatal complication, has occurred during extensive outbreaks of rubella among young adults in the military services. Transient testicular pain is also a frequent complaint in affected men.

Diagnosis

Measles, scarlet fever, secondary syphilis, drug rashes, erythema infectiosum, and infectious mononucleosis, as well as echo-, coxsackie-, and adenovirus infections, must be considered. Rubella is clinically differentiated from measles by the milder, more evanescent rash and by the absence of Koplik's spots, coryza, photophobia, and cough. The typical patient with measles is much sicker, and the illness lasts longer. Even mild scarlet fever usually produces more constitutional symptoms than rubella, including a severely red, sore throat. The WBC count is elevated in scarlet fever but normal in rubella. Observation for a day usually establishes the diagnosis in scarlet fever.

The eruption and adenopathy of rubella can be simulated by secondary syphilis, but the adenopathy of syphilis is not tender and the skin eruption usually becomes prominent on the palms and soles. If there is doubt, a qualitative STS should be performed, and follow-up quantitative testing may be necessary. Infectious mononucleosis may also cause a rubella-like adenopathy and skin rash but can be differentiated by the initial leukopenia followed by leukocytosis, the many atypical mononuclear cells in the blood smear, the appearance of antibodies to the Epstein-Barr virus, and in many cases, an increase in the heterophil antibody titer. In addition, the pharyngeal angina of infectious mononucleosis is usually prominent, and malaise is greater and of longer duration than in rubella.

A clinical diagnosis of rubella is subject to error without laboratory confirmation, especially since enteroviral and parvovirus B19 (erythema infectiosum) exanthems closely mimic rubella. Therefore, a history of German measles is an unreliable guarantor of infection and immunity. Serum specimens from acute and convalescent stages should be obtained, if possible, for serologic testing; a four-fold or greater rise in specific antibodies is confirmatory.

Prophylaxis
(See also IMMUNIZATION PROCEDURES THROUGHOUT CHILDHOOD in Ch. 23)

Rubella immunization programs prevent some of the catastrophes associated with congenital rubella, but the most successful policy for immunization is not yet known. Routine use of live rubella virus vaccine in all susceptible mothers immediately following delivery has been suggested. Routine vaccination of children between the ages of 15 mo and puberty is recommended. The rationale is that vaccination of children will eradicate the reservoir of infection in the early age group that is presumed responsible for most adult exposures. This strategy has been largely successful in the USA. Another suggested procedure is to screen women of childbearing age for rubella antibodies (the history, whether positive or negative, is an unreliable criterion of immunity) and to immunize those who are seronegative. Such immunization, however, should not be undertaken unless conception can be prevented for at least 3 mo afterward.

Live virus vaccine prepared in human diploid fibroblast cell cultures has been shown to be effective, producing antibodies in > 95% of recipients. Transmission of vaccine virus from vaccinees to susceptible contacts rarely, if ever, occurs and is not a contraindication to immunization. Vaccine virus is transmissible to the fetus but has not been causally implicated in producing congenital rubella. In children vaccinated with live virus vaccines, solid immunity lasts ≥ 15 yr.

Fever, rash, lymphadenopathy, polyneuropathy, arthralgia, and overt arthritis are rare with vaccination in children; joint pain and swelling occasionally follow vaccination in adult women.

Vaccine should not be given to any person with a defective or altered immune mechanism (eg, with leukemia, lymphoma, other malignancy, or a febrile illness, or during prolonged corticosteroid, radiation, or chemotherapy). Data suggest that vaccine can infect a fetus during early pregnancy but has not resulted in the congenital rubella syndrome; although the risk of fetal damage is considered to be extremely low (estimated to be ≤ 3%), use of vaccine is **contraindicated** throughout pregnancy.

Treatment

Rubella requires little or no treatment. Otitis media, a rare complication, requires appropriate treatment. No specific therapy for encephalitis is available.

PROGRESSIVE RUBELLA PANENCEPHALITIS

A progressive neurologic disorder occurring in a child with the stigmas of congenital rubella and presumably due to reactivation of the rubella virus infection.

Symptoms and Signs

Children with congenital defects due to rubella virus (eg, deafness, cataracts, microcephaly, and mental retardation) develop this disease in their early teens. They show progressive spasticity, ataxia, mental deterioration, and seizures. The condition can be confused with measles-virus–related subacute sclerosing panencephalitis (SSPE), described above, but myoclonic seizure activity is more frequent in SSPE.

Diagnosis and Treatment

The diagnosis is considered when a patient with congenital rubella develops progressive neurologic deficits associated with elevated CSF cell count, total protein, and γ globulin; when elevated rubella virus antibody titers are found in CSF and serum; or when rubella virus is recovered from brain tissue. Unlike in SSPE, measles antibody titers are normal, and the EEG does not show the burst-suppression pattern typical of SSPE. CT scan may show ventricular enlargement, particularly of the 4th ventricle, due to cerebellar atrophy.

There is no specific treatment for the disorder.

ROSEOLA INFANTUM
(Exanthem Subitum; Pseudorubella)

An acute disease of infants or very young children characterized by high fever, absence of localizing symptoms or signs, and appearance of a rubelliform eruption simultaneously with, or following, defervescence.

Etiology and Epidemiology

The usual cause is the recently discovered human herpesvirus type 6 (HHV-6). The disease occurs most often in the spring and fall. Minor local epidemics have been reported.

Symptoms and Signs

The incubation period is probably 5 to 15 days. Fever of 39.5 to 40.5° C (103 to 105° F) begins abruptly and persists for 3 to 5 days without any evident cause. Convulsions are common during the early phase, particularly as the temperature rises. Despite the high fever, the child is usually clinically alert and active. Leukopenia with relative lymphocytosis is present, usually by the 3rd day. Lymphadenopathy in cervical and posterior auricular regions is often noted, and the spleen may be slightly enlarged.

The fever usually falls by crisis on the 4th day, and the macular or maculopapular eruption generally appears, profusely on the chest and abdomen and mildly on the face and extremities; it may last for a few hours to 2 days. The temperature is normal at this stage, and the child feels and acts well. The evanescent rash may be unnoticed in mild cases. In 70% of HHV-6 infections, the typical exanthem does not appear.

Diagnosis and Treatment

If roseola is known to be in the community, it should be suspected when a child aged 6 mo to 3 yr develops a persistently high temperature without apparent cause. Diagnosis is confirmed by culture and serologic tests, but these techniques are not readily available. A presumptive diagnosis usually can be made, to the relief of the parents, if pyelonephritis, otitis media, meningitis, sepsis, and bacterial pneumonia can be ruled out.

Treatment is symptomatic and includes antipyretic measures to keep the child comfortable. For treatment of convulsions, see SEIZURE DISORDERS in Ch. 43. When the temperature falls to normal and the eruption appears, the patient is so nearly well that further treatment is unnecessary.

ERYTHEMA INFECTIOSUM
(Fifth Disease; Parvovirus B19 Infection)

An acute viral disease characterized by mild constitutional symptoms and a blotchy or maculopapular rash beginning on the cheeks and spreading primarily to the exposed areas of the extremities.

Etiology and Epidemiology

The disease is caused by the recently discovered human parvovirus B19. It occurs most often during spring months, and localized outbreaks among children and adolescents are common. Parvovirus B19 is also a major cause of aplastic crisis in patients with chronic hemolytic disorders, such as sickle cell disease. Spread appears to be by the respiratory route; inapparent infection can occur.

Symptoms and Signs

The incubation period is 4 to 14 days. Symptoms and signs can vary among individuals. Typical manifestations are low-grade fever, slight malaise, and an indurated, confluent erythema over the cheeks ("slapped-cheek" appearance). Within 1 to 2 days, a symmetric eruption appears that is most prominent on the arms, legs, and trunk, usually sparing the palms and soles. The rash is maculopapular, tending toward confluence; it forms slightly raised blotchy areas and reticular or lacy patterns, usually most prominent on the exposed areas of the arms. The illness generally lasts 5 to 10 days, but the eruption may recur for several weeks afterward, exacerbated by sunlight, exercise, heat, fever, or emotional stress. Mild joint pain and swelling that may persist or recur for weeks to months is sometimes observed in adults with this disease. Immunodeficient patients can develop protracted infections with severe anemia. Like rubella, erythema infectiosum can be transmitted transplacentally during pregnancy, sometimes resulting in stillbirth or severe fetal anemia with widespread edema (hydrops fetalis). The frequency of such occurrences is unknown.

Diagnosis and Treatment

The appearance and pattern of spread of the rash are the only diagnostic features; however, diagnosis must be made with caution, since rubella and some enteroviruses have similar features. If there is any doubt, rubella infection should be ruled out by serologic testing. Parvovirus B19 viremia usually lasts 7 to 12 days and can be detected by immunoprecipitation or DNA probe techniques. The presence of IgM-specific antibody in the late acute or early convalescent phase also strongly supports the diagnosis.

Only symptomatic treatment is necessary.

CHICKENPOX
(Varicella)

An acute viral disease, usually beginning with mild constitutional symptoms that are followed shortly by an eruption appearing in crops and characterized by macules, papules, vesicles, and crusting.

Etiology and Epidemiology

Chickenpox and herpes zoster are caused by the varicella-zoster virus, chickenpox being the acute invasive phase of the virus and zoster (shingles) being the reactivation of the latent phase.

Chickenpox, like measles, is highly communicable. Epidemics occur in winter and early spring in 3- to 4-yr cycles (the period required to develop a new group of susceptibles). Susceptibility is high from birth until the disease is contracted, but some infants may have partial immunity, probably acquired transplacentally, until age 6 mo.

Chickenpox is believed to be spread by infected droplets and is most communicable during the short prodrome and early stages of the eruption. The usual incubation period is 14 to 16 days, and communicability is considered possible from 10 to 21 days after exposure. When the final lesions have crusted, the patient can no longer transmit the disease. Isolation for 6 days after the first vesicles appear is usually sufficient to control cross infection. Indirect transmission (by immune third persons) probably does not occur.

Symptoms and Signs

Mild headache, moderate fever, and malaise may be present 11 to 15 days after exposure, about 24 to 36 h before the first series of lesions appears. The prodrome, usually unrecognized in young children, is more likely to be present in children over age 10 and is usually more severe in adults.

The initial rash, a macular eruption, may be accompanied by an evanescent flush. This rash evolves within a few hours to characteristic itchy, monolocular, teardrop vesicles containing clear fluid and standing out from their red areolae; at this time, diagnosis can usually be made. The typical individual chickenpox lesions progress from macule to papule to vesicle and begin crusting within 6 to 8 h. Lesions erupt in successive crops, some macules just appearing as earlier crops are beginning to crust. The eruption may be generalized in severe cases; otherwise, the face and extremities are partially spared. When only a few lesions are present, the upper trunk is the most frequent site. Ulcerated lesions may also be present on the mucous membranes, including the oropharynx and upper respiratory tract, palpebral conjunctiva, and the rectal and vaginal mucosa. In the mouth, the vesicles rupture immediately, are indistinguishable from those of herpetic stomatitis, and often cause pain on swallowing. Laryngeal or tracheal vesicles may cause severe dyspnea. Lesions are frequently present on the scalp, resulting in tender, enlarged suboccipital and posterior cervical lymph nodes. The acute phase of illness usually lasts 4 to 7 days. New lesions usually cease to appear by the 5th day, the majority are crusted by the 6th day, and most crusts disappear in < 20 days after onset.

Chickenpox in childhood is usually benign. However, it may be severe or fatal in adults and in patients with depressed T cell immunity (eg, lymphoreticular malignancy) or in those receiving corticosteroids or chemotherapy.

Complications

Secondary streptococcal infection of the vesicles may lead to erysipelas, sepsis, acute hemorrhagic nephritis, or rarely gangrene of the skin. Staphylococci may also infect the vesicles and cause pyoderma or bullous impetigo. Pneumonia as a complication of severe chickenpox is encountered in adults, newborns, and immunocompromised patients but is unusual in young children. Myocarditis, transient arthritis or hepatitis, and hemorrhagic complications have also been reported. Hemorrhagic varicella should raise suspicion of varicella-associated thrombocytopenic purpura or secondary meningococcal sepsis.

Post-chickenpox encephalopathy is unusual, occurring in < 1/1000 cases. Like the encephalitis following measles, it tends to occur toward the end of the disease or 1 to 2 wk after its termination. One of the most common neurologic complications is acute postinfectious cerebellar ataxia. Transverse myelitis, cranial nerve palsies, and multiple-sclerosis–like clinical manifestations have also occurred. Encephalitis may be fatal, but the prognosis for complete recovery from CNS complications is generally good and is far better than in measles encephalitis. Reye's syndrome, an unusual but severe complication, may begin 3 to 8 days after onset of the rash (see REYE'S SYNDROME under MISCELLANEOUS INFECTIONS, below).

Diagnosis

Secondary syphilis, impetigo, infected eczema, insect bites and stings, drug rashes, contact dermatitis, erythropoietic porphyria (hydroa estivale), and occasionally coxsackievirus and disseminated herpes simplex virus infections must be considered in the differential diagnosis.

Immunofluorescent detection of viral antigen in lesions, culture, or serologic findings confirm the diagnosis.

Prophylaxis

Chickenpox can be prevented or modified by IM administration of zoster immune globulin (ZIG), derived from the sera of patients recovering from herpes zoster, or varicella-zoster immune globulin (VZIG), prepared from pooled plasma containing high titers of specific antibody. The recommended dose is 125 u. (about 1.25 mL/10 kg) with a maximum dose not to exceed 625 u. Such preparations should be given within 96 h after exposure to be effective; their use is primarily for exposed susceptibles with leukemia, immunodeficiency syndromes, or other severe debilitating illness. Also, newborns whose mothers developed chickenpox within 5 days before delivery or 2 days after delivery are candidates for prophylaxis. Large doses of pooled human γ globulin have also been shown to modify the disease if given IM shortly after exposure, but the quantity required is so great (0.6 to 1.2 mL/kg) that this is not generally recommended. Limited studies suggest that zoster immune plasma (ZIP) at doses ranging from 3 to 14 mL/kg IV or pooled γ globulin at doses of 4 to 6 mL/kg IV may also be useful prophylactically if given within 6 days after exposure. These preparations have no therapeutic value after the illness has begun. Live, attenuated vaccines are under study, appear to be very effective, and are expected to be available soon for use in the USA.

Treatment

Mild cases require only symptomatic treatment. Wet compresses may be applied to control itching, which may be extreme, and to prevent scratching, which may lead to widespread infection and disfigurement. Systemic antihistamines or hydroxyzine may be used in severe cases. Because of the frequency of staphylococcal or streptococcal superinfection of the vesicles, patients should be bathed often with soap and water and kept in clean underclothing; hands should be kept clean and nails clipped. Antiseptics should not be applied to individual lesions unless they become secondarily infected. Staphylococcal or β-hemolytic streptococcal infection is treated with appropriate systemic antibiotics. In severe cases with existing widespread disease, acyclovir may be given orally qid for 5 to 7 days at dosages of 20 mg/kg for 5- to 7-yr-olds, 15 mg/kg for 7- to 12-yr-olds, and 10 mg/kg for

TABLE 32-10. SYNDROMES CAUSED BY ADENOVIRUSES

Disease	Serotypes Implicated		Comments
	Common	Less Common	
Respiratory only			
Acute febrile respiratory disease of children	1, 2, 3, 5, 6	Other types	Probably the most frequent manifestation of adenoviruses; types 1, 2, and 5 endemic; type 3 occasionally epidemic; more prevalent during cold months
Acute respiratory disease (ARD)	4, 7	14, 21	Epidemic in military recruits; sporadic in adult civilians; types 4 and 7 infections rare in children
Viral pneumonia			
Infants	7	1, 3	Rare; occurs in hospital nurseries; may be fatal; similar to Goodpasture's inclusion body pneumonitis
Adults	4, 7	3, 21	Predominantly associated with ARD; cold agglutinins not developed
Ocular only			
Acute follicular conjunctivitis	3, 7	2, 4, 6, 9, 10, 21	Sporadic; affects chiefly adults; in children, usually associated with respiratory and systemic effects
Epidemic keratoconjunctivitis (EKC)	8 (classic)	3, 7, 19 (mild)	Epidemic; affects mainly adults; widespread in Japan, rare in USA
Combined respiratory and ocular			
Acute pharyngo-conjunctival fever (APC)	3, 4, 7	1, 2, 5, 6, 14, 21	Epidemic in children; sporadic in adults; summer epidemics frequently associated with swimming in pools or lakes

12- to 16-yr-olds. In patients known to be immunocompromised, acyclovir IV 1500 mg/m^2/day divided q 8 h should be given.

ADENOVIRUSES

A group of many viruses, some of which cause acute febrile disorders characterized by inflammation of the respiratory and ocular mucous membranes and hyperplasia of submucous and regional lymphoid tissue.

Etiology

Adenoviruses are DNA viruses 60 to 90 nm in size. The virion is shaped like an icosahedron. Three major antigens (hexon, penton, and fiber) are directly related to the capsid structures. The most important is the hexon, a 6-sided structure that accounts for 240 of the 252 capsid subunits. The hexon antigen has a non-type-specific CF reaction with specific antisera, thus serving as a group antigen to identify all types of ade-

noviruses. However, virus-neutralizing antibody is type-specific. The 2nd major antigen is associated with a penton, a 5-sided capsomere located at the 12 common vertices of the 20 triangles that form the icosahedron. It is a type-specific antigen that can be differentiated in neutralization or HI tests. The 3rd antigen is a fiber, related to the threadlike structure extending from the apices of the virion. Sometimes adenoviruses are accompanied by a smaller DNA virus called the **adeno-associated virus (AAV)**. It is a defective virus that must be complemented by an adenovirus to replicate. The importance of AAV in adenovirus infections is not known.

Epidemiology

About 4 to 5% of clinically recognized respiratory illnesses in civilian populations are caused by adenoviruses. Only a few of the more than 40 known serotypes have been studied adequately to determine their role in producing human disease (see TABLE 32-10). **Different serotypes** have quite different epidemiologies: Types 1, 2, and 5 cause sharp, limited outbreaks of respiratory or enteric illness during the first few months or years of life, with type 2 being somewhat more common in certain episodes. Type 3 causes a characteristic syndrome of acute pharyngoconjunctival fever (APC) in older children and adults, especially in summer camps and swimming pools. Acute respiratory disease (ARD) occurs in military camps and is caused by types 4, 7, 14, and 21. ARD epidemics also occur among civilian populations in some countries but are not identified frequently in the USA. Epidemic keratoconjunctivitis (EKC) is caused by several serotypes and is seen largely among persons in industrial plants and eye clinics. Often, adenoviruses infect primarily the intestinal tract, usually without causing symptoms, although enteritis, mesenteric adenitis, and intussusception can occur. Following infection with types 1, 2, and 5, the virus may remain latent in the tonsils and adenoids; about 80% of excised tonsils yield such virus.

The ratio of manifest disease to infection rates varies according to syndrome, serotype, and season. In winter, infection with type 4 or 7 causes recognizable illness in military recruits, with about 25% requiring hospitalization for fever and lower respiratory tract disease. In summer, APC occurs in a high proportion of type 3 infections. The ratio of illness to infection is lower with types 1, 2, 5, and some of the less-studied, higher-numbered serotypes.

Pathology

Adenoviral infections are rarely fatal; in immunocompetent hosts, they have few, if any, recognizable long-term pathologic effects. Some deaths have occurred with giant cell pneumonia associated with adenovirus types 3, 4, and 7. Autopsies have disclosed microscopically a unique, extensive inclusion body pneumonia; the intranuclear inclusions appear similar to those characteristic of adenoviral cellular invasions in tissue cultures. Biopsies of superficial lesions produced by adenoviruses in conjunctival and pharyngeal mucosa show capillary dilatation, occasional submucous hemorrhage, and mononuclear leukocyte infiltration but no intranuclear inclusions. The conjunctivitis caused by the common respiratory adenovirus types is usually benign, but sometimes it is a keratoconjunctivitis (as is caused by type 8), with corneal opacities and impaired vision.

Symptoms and Signs

Acute febrile respiratory disease is the usual manifestation of known adenoviral infection in children. Adenovirus types 1, 2, 3, 5, and 6 are most commonly isolated, though infection with these types often is not directly associated with any specific illness. Infection is airborne or water-borne (acquired by swimming); it also may be acquired by direct contact. The incubation period is up to 10 days. In a typical outbreak confined to a household or nursery, some affected children have only fever, without localizing signs; others have fever and pharyngitis; others have fever with pharyngitis, tracheitis, bronchitis, a moderately persistent nonproductive cough, and rarely, pneumonia. The cough with adenoviral pneumonia has been confused with that of pertussis in children. Pharyngeal lymphoid hypertrophy sometimes persists, leading to eustachian tube obstruction and possibly otitis media. Regional lymph nodes are frequently enlarged and sometimes tender, but they never suppurate. Laboratory findings usually are within normal limits, though a lymphocytosis is sometimes shown.

A syndrome designated ARD (acute respiratory disease) was observed in military recruits during 2 periods of troop mobilization. Adenovirus types 4 and 7 have been reported in most outbreaks in the USA, but types 14 and 21 have also been implicated. ARD is marked by malaise, fever, chills, and headache. Respiratory manifestations include nasopharyngitis, hoarseness, and dry cough. The disease may resemble streptococcal pharyngitis with exudate on the faucial pillars and posterior pharyngeal wall. Cervical adenopathy is present, but the nodes are not as tender as in streptococcal pharyngitis. A fine, erythematous macular rash may appear on the body, and viremia and viruria may be shown, but this viruria does not produce symptoms like those of the epidemic hemorrhagic cystitis that occurs as a primary disease with type 11. Physical signs are minimal except in about 10% of patients, who develop rales and x-ray evidence of pneumonia. Fever usually subsides within 2 to 4 days; convalescence, while uneventful, may require another 10 to 14 days. In immunocompromised persons, chronic viremia and virus shedding can occur.

Viral pneumonia of infants, due chiefly to type 7, is a rare but specific clinicopathologic entity. Small outbreaks have occurred in France, South Africa, the USA, China, and Japan, with fatalities resulting from extensive pneumonia. Onset is sudden, affecting babies from a few days or weeks old up to 2 to 3 yr, with high fever and rapid upper and lower respiratory tract involvement. The pneumonia is lobular but may be sufficiently extensive to suggest lobar pneumonia. In several fatal cases, patients developed a maculopapular rash and encephalitis, with focal necrosis apparent in the brain, skin, and lungs.

Acute pharyngoconjunctival fever (APC) produces the clinical triad of fever, pharyngitis, and conjunctivitis. Infection is sometimes waterborne. The incubation period is 5 to 8 days. Adenovirus types 3, 4, and 7 have been reported in nearly all outbreaks. In a typical outbreak, ≥ 50% of the patients have all 3 components, while others may have only 1 or 2. The conjunctivitis is initially unilateral and sometimes painful. Lower respiratory tract involvement may occur in addition to pharyngitis. The illness usually subsides within a week, but follicular conjunctivitis may persist for another week.

Conjunctivitis without constitutional symptoms is a common manifestation of infection with several different adenovirus serotypes. It occurs most often in young adults, chiefly parents of children with APC, and is self-limited and benign. Onset is sudden and usually unilateral. Symptoms and signs include a foreign-body sensation in the eye, lacrimation, and focal erythema of the palpebral and bulbar conjunctiva. The discharge is mucoid but not purulent. In about half the patients, the other eye is subsequently involved, usually less severely. Persistent follicular enlargement of submucous lymphoid tissue under the palpebral conjunctiva, even resembling early trachoma, may be seen about 2 to 4 days after onset. Preauricular and posterior cervical lymphadenopathy, more prominent on the same side as the more involved eye, is usual. A mild sore throat occasionally develops, often on the same side as the affected eye. The course is usually mild, though focal conjunctival hemorrhages and extensive periorbital edema occasionally occur.

Epidemic keratoconjunctivitis (EKC) is a specific, sometimes severe, epidemic disease caused by adenovirus, especially type 8. Observed for many years in Japan, it became epidemic in the USA during World War II, chiefly among shipyard workers on both coasts. It has occurred only sporadically in this country since then, but widespread epidemics have occurred in Europe and Asia. Onset is sudden, one eye showing redness and chemosis followed by peri-orbital swelling, preauricular lymphadenopathy, and superficial corneal opacities. Unlike herpetic keratitis, it does not result in corneal ulceration; however, local pain like that from foreign-body irritation is usual. The other eye may become involved within a week. Systemic symptoms and signs are mild or absent. The illness usually lasts 3 or 4 wk, though opacities may persist much longer and vision may be permanently impaired.

Mild, transient corneal involvement has been observed in eye infections (eg, APC) with other adenoviruses (types 3, 4, and 7), but the opacities are seldom noticeable except to an ophthalmologist.

Diagnosis

Clinical identification of adenoviral infection is only presumptive, except in typical APC, EKC, and ARD in military recruits; in these conditions, the clinical or epidemiologic characteristics, or both, are unique. During the acute stages of adenoviral illnesses, the virus can be isolated for 7 to 10 days from respiratory and ocular secretions and frequently from feces and urine. Several serologic procedures (CF, HI, and neutralization tests) can be performed on serum specimens from acute and convalescent stages. A four-fold rise in the serum antibody titer indicates recent adenoviral infection. The CF test is group-specific for any adenovirus serotype. HI and neutralization tests are type-specific. Commercial antigen is available for the CF test but not for the other 2. An enzyme-linked immunosorbent assay **(ELISA)** based on the group (hexon) antigen may also be useful in serologic testing.

Prognosis and Prophylaxis

Adenoviral infections are generally benign and of relatively short duration. Except for rare cases of fulminating primary pneumonia, predominantly in infants and military recruits, even severe adenoviral pneumonia is not fatal.

Live types 4 and 7 adenovirus vaccine, given orally in an enteric-coated capsule, has markedly reduced ARD in military populations. The vaccine virus can spread among family members with intimate contact, but this is of no apparent importance. The vaccine, however, is neither recommended nor available for civilian use. Vaccines for other serotypes have not been developed. Among civilians, adenoviruses causing outbreaks of conjunctivitis are spread by contact with contaminated objects (towels, instruments, etc), by secretions, or by finger transmission. Practicing proper sterilization techniques, changing gloves and washing hands before and after examining infected patients, and avoiding multiple patient exposures to ophthalmologic instruments are recommended to prevent transfer of virus.

Treatment

Treatment is symptomatic and supportive. Bed rest at home or hospitalization may be required during the acute febrile period. Aspirin is not recommended unless headache and malaise are distressing; for children, acetaminophen may be preferred because of concerns about developing Reye's syndrome; analgesics such as codeine are rarely necessary. Severe pneumonia in infants and EKC require early hospitalization and close supervision to prevent death in the former and permanently impaired vision in the latter. Topical corticosteroids relieve symptoms and shorten the course of EKC and adenoviral conjunctivitis. Such therapy is dangerous in ulcerative corneal conditions, however, and should always be supervised by an ophthalmologist.

RESPIRATORY SYNCYTIAL VIRUS (RSV)

RSV is one of the most important causes of lower respiratory illness (including bronchiolitis and pneumonia) in infants and young children; it can be fatal. Often, the sudden death of a baby with respiratory disease is believed to be due to RSV infection. In healthy adults and older children, RSV usually causes milder respiratory illness, but it is also an important cause of the influenza syndrome, bronchopneumonia, and exacerbations of chronic bronchitis. Elderly persons and those with underlying pulmonary diseases may be quite susceptible to infection with RSV.

Etiology and Epidemiology

RSV is an RNA virus, classified as a pneumovirus. Two subgroups (designated A and B) have been identified serologically. Biologically and behaviorally, RSV resembles influenza and parainfluenza viruses more than other taxonomically related virus groups, but serologically and in other ways (eg, by its failure to grow in eggs or produce hemagglutinin), it is distinct from them.

RSV is associated with a sharp outbreak of acute respiratory disease occurring annually in late autumn or in winter. Like influenza, it increases morbidity and mortality from bronchitis and pneumonia. The annual recurrence of RSV subgroups indicates that reinfection, with illness, occurs. Although about 70% of persons have serum antibodies against RSV by age 5, infections continue to occur in persons of all ages. The poor protective effect of serum antibody against infection is exemplified by the illness seen in infants < 6 mo old; though they have maternal antibody, they develop severe lower respiratory tract disease that causes an appreciable number of deaths.

Symptoms and Signs

The clinical manifestations of RSV infection are variable and generally differ with age, previous exposure to RSV, and underlying diseases (especially respiratory conditions). The clinical syndrome has few specific signs that identify RSV as the cause of the infection, but along with epidemiologic data, symptoms can heighten suspicion of RSV. Dyspnea, cough, and wheezing are the most prominent symptoms, usually appearing several days after upper respiratory signs, which may include fever in infants. Bronchopneumonia and/or bronchiolitis are often apparent on chest x-ray. The leukocyte count is expected to be normal, but elevations occur and granulocytes may be moderately increased. In adults and older children, RSV infections may be inapparent or manifested only as an afebrile URI (the common cold), but they also can mimic influenza and they account for 15% of hospital admissions for acute exacerbations of chronic bronchitis. Secondary bacterial pneumonia (most commonly pneumococcal) may signify a preceding RSV infection.

Diagnosis

RSV can be isolated from respiratory secretions in susceptible tissue cultures. Since the virus does not tolerate freezing and thawing well unless protected by special media, storing or shipping specimens may be difficult. RSV infection is usually confirmed serologically. A rise in serum antibody levels can be detected by CF with a standard antigen. However, serologic findings may be difficult to evaluate. Very young infants often have maternal antibody, children may show acquired antibody in serum from the early phase of RSV, young children may not show a rise in antibody levels, and adults may have mild disease with no increase in antibody titer. An enzyme-linked immunosorbent assay (ELISA) has a sensitivity and specificity of 98 and 96%, respectively, in a diagnostic laboratory. When applied in a clinic, the assay's sensitivity remains and the specificity is 85%. It is a convenient technique for detecting RSV antigens in secretions and for titration of antibody. Immunofluorescent detection of RSV antigen in infected cells from the respiratory tract has been 88% sensitive and 100% specific when the preparation contains an adequate number of cells.

Treatment

Mild and inapparent infections are probably quite frequent and resolve without special attention. Severe disease in infants and children requires hospitalization and close observation to ensure adequate respiration. Hypoxemia is a common pathophysiologic event in infants infected with RSV. Arterial blood O_2 measurements and/or oximetry give objective information about the severity of the infection and need for intensive care. In studies of infants with bronchiolitis or pneumonia caused by RSV, ribavirin (a newer antiviral drug) reduced virus shedding and accelerated recovery in those with severe disease. Ribavirin 10 mg/kg was administered as a small-particle aerosol over 12 h for 3 to 5 days. Practical problems in administration of the aerosol are common; skin reactions and other symptoms of exposure have occurred among health care workers. Pregnant women should avoid exposure to ribavirin. Adults with bronchopneumonia and acute bronchitis may also require respiratory support.

ENTEROVIRAL DISEASES

(See also TABLE 32–11)

A group of diseases caused by enteroviruses (polio-, coxsackie-, and echoviruses).

Etiology and Epidemiology

Because of similar biologic, chemical, and physical properties, the **enteroviruses** and the rhinoviruses are placed together taxonomically as subgroups of the Picornaviridae family (*pico*, small; *rna*, their characteristic nucleic acid component). For a discussion of the polioviruses, see POLIOMYELITIS, below.

The **coxsackieviruses** are an antigenically heterogeneous group divided into groups A (23 types) and B (6 types). They resemble the polioviruses in size, resistance to physical and chemical agents, prevalence during summer and fall, and chiefly person-to-person spread. They have been isolated from oral secretions, stool, blood, and CSF.

The **echoviruses** (enteric cytopathic human orphan), like the coxsackieviruses, are small, heterogeneous, most prevalent in summer and

fall, and widely distributed geographically; 31 serotypes are recognized. These viruses have been isolated from the pharynx, feces, blood, CSF, and CNS tissues.

More recently identified enteroviruses have growth and host characteristics that variably overlap with coxsackieviruses and echoviruses. These are simply classified as higher-numbered enteroviruses (types 68 to 72).

RECOGNIZED DISEASE ENTITIES

Herpangina

Numerous group A coxsackieviruses and, occasionally, other enteroviruses may cause herpangina. It tends to occur in epidemics, most commonly in infants and children, and is characterized by sudden onset of fever with sore throat, headache, anorexia, and frequently, pain in the neck, abdomen, and extremities. Vomiting and convulsions may occur in infants. Within 2 days after onset, a few (rarely > 12) small (1 to 2 mm in diameter), grayish, papulovesicular lesions with erythematous areolae appear, most frequently on the tonsillar pillars but also on the soft palate, tonsils, uvula, or tongue. During the next 24 h, the lesions become shallow ulcers, seldom > 5 mm in diameter, that heal in 1 to 5 days. Complications are unusual, and the patient is generally asymptomatic by the 7th day. Lasting immunity to the infecting strain follows infection, but repeated episodes caused by other group A viruses are possible. Coxsackievirus A10 has been shown to cause a similar disease, but oral and pharyngeal lesions are raised, whitish to yellowish nodules. This entity is called **lympho-nodular pharyngitis.**

Diagnosis is based on the symptoms and characteristic oral lesions. It is best confirmed by isolating the virus from the lesions or by demonstrating a rise in specific antibody titer. Differential diagnosis includes herpetic stomatitis (which occurs during any season and shows larger, more persistent ulcers) and recurrent aphthae and Bednar's aphthae (which rarely occur in the pharynx and generally are not associated with systemic symptoms).

Treatment is symptomatic.

Hand-Foot-and-Mouth Disease

This is usually associated with coxsackievirus A16 and occurs particularly among young children. The course is similar to that of herpangina, but a vesicular exanthem is distributed over the

TABLE 32–11. SYNDROMES CAUSED BY ENTEROVIRUSES

Syndrome	Serotypes Most Often Implicated	Comments
Herpangina	Coxsackievirus A2, 4–6, 8, 10; probably 3 and others	Most common in infants and children; characteristic palatal and pharyngeal lesions
Hand-foot-and-mouth disease	Coxsackievirus A16 Enterovirus 71	Most common in young children; vesicular exanthem usually brief and benign
Epidemic pleurodynia (Bornholm disease)	Coxsackievirus B1–6	Most common in children, but any age group may be affected
Aseptic meningitis	Coxsackievirus A2, 4, 7, 9, 23, and others; B1–6 Poliovirus 1–3 Echovirus 4, 6; others less commonly	Most common in infants and children; course usually benign
Paralysis	Poliovirus 1–3 Coxsackievirus A7 and others Echovirus 4, 6, and others Enterovirus 71	See POLIOMYELITIS, below
Myocarditis Pericarditis	Coxsackievirus B2–5 Coxsackievirus A23, B1–5 Echovirus 1, 6, 8, 16	May occur at any age; myocarditis neonatorum has high mortality
Exanthems: With fever alone	Coxsackievirus A23, B2, 3, 5; A4–6, 9, 16 also implicated Echovirus 4; 2, 6, 11, 14, 16, 18, 30 also implicated	Course usually benign
With aseptic meningitis	Coxsackievirus A16, 23; B4 Echovirus 4, 16	Course usually benign
Respiratory disease	Echovirus 4, 8, 20, and others Coxsackievirus A21, B1, 3, 4, 5 Poliovirus 1–3	Most common in infants and children; course usually mild
Gastroenteritis	Echovirus 6, 14, and 18 proved to be cause in newborns; many other enteroviruses suspected in immunocompromised patients	Probably most important in newborn or preterm nursery
Conjunctivitis	Enterovirus 70 Coxsackievirus A24 Echovirus 7	Outbreaks of hemorrhagic conjunctivitis most common with enterovirus 70

buccal mucosa and palate, with similar lesions appearing on the hands and feet and occasionally in the diaper area. **Treatment** is symptomatic.

Epidemic Pleurodynia (Bornholm Disease)

This disease may occur at any age, but it is most common in children. It may be caused by any of the 6 group B coxsackieviruses and is characterized by sudden onset of severe, frequently intermittent (often pleuritic) pain in the epigastrium or lower anterior chest, with fever and often headache, sore throat, and malaise. Local tenderness, hyperesthesia, muscle swell-

ing, and myalgias of the trunk and extremities may occur. The disease usually subsides in 2 to 4 days, but relapse may develop within a few days and symptoms may recur for several weeks. In some cases, symptoms continue for a few weeks. Complications include orchitis, fibrinous pleuritis, pericarditis, and rarely aseptic meningitis.

Diagnosis is obvious during an epidemic. However, in sporadic cases or in the early stages of an epidemic, the disease may be mistaken for poliomyelitis, myocardial infarction, spontaneous pneumothorax, acute appendicitis, pancreatitis, costochondritis, a perforated viscus, or an influenza-like respiratory infection. Laboratory diagnosis consists of isolating the virus from the throat or stool or demonstrating a rise in specific neutralizing antibody titers.

Prognosis is good in uncomplicated cases, although a few deaths have been reported. Repeated infections with other group B coxsackieviruses are possible.

Treatment is symptomatic.

Aseptic Meningitis

Aseptic meningitis in infants and young children is frequently caused by a group A or B coxsackievirus or an echovirus; viruses other than enteroviruses are often responsible in older children and adults (see ACUTE VIRAL ENCEPHALITIS AND ASEPTIC MENINGITIS and ARBOVIRUS ENCEPHALITIDES, below). Headache, pain and stiffness in the neck and back, and muscular aches may be abrupt in onset or preceded by prodromal fever, malaise, anorexia, and vomiting. Kernig's and Brudzinski's signs usually are positive. Symptoms generally subside by the end of a week, but fatigue and irritability may persist for months. CSF findings consist of a normal or slightly elevated protein level, a normal glucose level, and a cell count usually < 500/µL; neutrophils may predominate in the early stages, but lymphocytes are more common in 1 to 2 days. Encephalitic signs occasionally develop and may be severe.

Meningitis due to coxsackie- or echovirus is usually impossible to differentiate clinically from other viral meningitides during the acute stages. Occasionally a patient presents with CSF hypoglycorrhachia in addition to a neutrophil predominance, suggesting bacterial meningitis. If an associated petechial rash is also present, further confusion can result. **Diagnosis** is made by isolating the virus from the throat, stool specimens, or occasionally the CSF or by demonstrating a rise in neutralizing antibody titer.

Prognosis is generally good, but death may occur in the newborn. **Treatment** should follow that for nonparalytic poliomyelitis (see POLIOMYELITIS, below), since the 2 diseases are clinically indistinguishable in the acute stages.

Paralysis

Certain group A and B coxsackieviruses (especially A7), several echoviruses, and enterovirus type 71 may produce muscle weakness or paralysis that is clinically indistinguishable from paralytic poliomyelitis. The causative virus can be identified by laboratory techniques; **treatment** is the same as for paralytic poliomyelitis.

Myocarditis; Pericarditis

Myocarditis neonatorum, caused by group B coxsackieviruses and some echoviruses, occurs in newborns infected after birth (rarely in utero). Usually, several days of well-being are followed by sudden onset of fever, feeding difficulties, pharyngitis, tachycardia, cyanosis, and tachypnea; associated cardiac murmurs and hepatomegaly also frequently occur. The ECG may show signs of myocarditis. CNS, hepatic, pancreatic, or adrenal lesions may be present concomitantly. Recovery may occur within a few weeks, but death from circulatory collapse is not uncommon.

Myocarditis and pericarditis in older children or adults also may be due to a group B coxsackievirus, and in a few instances, to a group A coxsackievirus or an echovirus. Symptoms and signs are usually localized only to the myocardium or pericardium, and complete recovery is usual.

Diagnosis is made, as in other coxsackievirus infections, by virus isolation or antibody titer studies. **Treatment** is symptomatic, including strict bed rest and control of heart failure and arrhythmias. Corticosteroids have not been beneficial; their use is best reserved for severe cases of myocarditis with associated cardiac failure. Other treatments directed at specific T cell suppression are being evaluated.

Exanthems With or Without Aseptic Meningitis

Certain echo- and coxsackieviruses may cause a rash that is generally discrete, nonpruritic, nondesquamative, and usually confined to the face, neck, and chest. The rash is sometimes maculopapular or morbilliform, occasionally hemorrhagic, petechial, or vesicular. Fever is common. Aseptic meningitis may develop. The disease is usually epidemic, with exanthems predominating among infants and children, but sporadic cases occur. The course is usually benign.

Respiratory Disease

Enteroviruses have been implicated in some infants' and children's respiratory illnesses characterized by fever, coryza, and pharyngitis, sometimes with diarrhea and vomiting. Bronchitis and interstitial pneumonia have occasionally occurred in infants. **Treatment** is symptomatic.

Diarrhea; Gastroenteritis

Enteroviruses are occasionally isolated from the stools of newborn infants with acute diarrheal disease and from immunocompromised patients with protracted diarrhea, but their overall importance in the etiology of these illnesses is questionable. **Treatment** of enteric infections is symptomatic (see ACUTE INFECTIOUS GASTROENTERITIS under BACTERIAL INFECTIONS in this chapter, above).

Conjunctivitis

Acute hemorrhagic conjunctivitis has occurred rarely in epidemics in the USA, but importation from Africa, Asia, and Mexico, where outbreaks have occurred, is considered to be more likely in the future. The disease, associated with infection by enterovirus 70, is characterized by rapid onset of eyelid swelling, with congestion, pain, and increased lacrimation. Some patients also develop subconjunctival hemorrhages and epithelial keratitis. Systemic illness is unusual, although a few cases of transient lumbosacral radiculomyelopathy or poliomyelitis-like illness have been recorded. Recovery is usually complete within 1 to 2 wk of onset. Other enteroviruses associated with conjunctivitis include some strains of coxsackievirus A24 and echovirus 7; these are usually not associated with hemorrhagic manifestations.

Treatment is symptomatic.

POLIOMYELITIS
(Infantile Paralysis;
Acute Anterior Poliomyelitis)

An acute viral infection with a wide range of manifestations, including nonspecific minor illness, aseptic meningitis (nonparalytic poliomyelitis), and flaccid weakness of various muscle groups (paralytic poliomyelitis).

Etiology and Epidemiology

Poliovirus is an enterovirus belonging to the Picornaviridae, whose major properties include a single-stranded RNA genome, small size (22 to 30 nm), lack of an envelope, and insensitivity to ether and other lipid solvents. Of the 3 immunologically distinct poliovirus serotypes, type 1 is the most paralytogenic and the most common cause of epidemics.

Man is the only natural host for polioviruses. The infection occurs through direct contact and is highly contagious. Inapparent infections (the main source of spread) are common in unimmunized populations, but overt disease is rare; even in epidemics, the ratio of inapparent infections to clinical cases exceeds 100:1. The paralytic disease had been thought to be uncommon in developing (mainly tropical) countries, but recent surveys of lameness indicate an incidence as high as in the peak years in the USA before introduction of vaccines. In such areas, where sanitation and hygiene are poor, virus circulation is extensive and occurs year-round; infection and immunity are acquired in the first few years of life; there are no epidemics; and > 90% of paralytic cases are confined to children < 5 yr. In contrast, as sanitation and hygiene improved in economically developed countries, infection was delayed; many older children and young adults remained susceptible; and summer epidemics involving increasingly older age groups occurred. Extensive use of vaccines has almost eliminated the disease in developed countries. The International Task Force for Disease Eradication has deemed that worldwide eradication is technically possible by the year 2000.

Pathology and Pathogenesis

Virus enters the mouth and primary multiplication occurs in lymphoid tissues in the oropharynx and intestinal tract, mainly the ileum. Small amounts of virus reach the blood and are carried to other sites in the reticuloendothelial system, where extensive multiplication occurs. Secondary viremia is followed by invasion of the CNS. Under certain circumstances, the virus may also reach the CNS via autonomic nerve fiber endings in the alimentary tract. The agent is present in blood, throat, and feces during the incubation period, and after onset it persists in throat washings for 1 to 2 wk and in feces for 3 to 6 wk or longer. Viremia lasts several days but disappears by the time of onset, when antibodies have already developed.

The spinal cord and brain are the only sites of significant virus-induced pathology. The motor neurons of the anterior horn of the spinal cord, the medulla, and to a lesser degree certain other parts of the brain, including the cerebellum and the motor cortex, are involved. Damage to neurons by the virus, the primary event, elicits an intense inflammatory reaction and eventually neuronophagia. The site and severity of paralysis are determined by the distribution of the neuronal lesions. Factors predisposing to serious neurologic damage include increasing age, recent tonsillectomy, inoculations (most often DTP), pregnancy, and physical exertion concurrent with onset of the CNS phase.

Symptoms and Signs

Clinical forms vary, but the 2 basic patterns are the minor illness (abortive type) and the major illness (which may be paralytic or nonparalytic). The **minor illness**, accounting for 80 to 90% of clinical infections, occurs chiefly in young children, is mild, and does not involve the CNS. Symptoms are slight fever, malaise, headache, sore throat, and vomiting, which develop 3 to 5 days after exposure. Recovery occurs within 24 to 72 h.

Symptoms of the **major illness** may follow several days of well-being but more commonly appear without a previous minor illness, particularly in older children and adults. Incubation is usually 7 to 14 days; rarely, longer. Fever, severe headache, stiff neck and back, deep muscle pain, and sometimes hyperesthesias and paresthesias may be present. There may be no further progression from this picture of aseptic meningitis, or the disease may go on, with loss of selective tendon reflexes and asymmetric weakness or paralysis of muscle groups, depending on the location of lesions in the spinal cord or medulla. Dysphagia, nasal regurgitation, and nasal voice are early signs of bulbar involvement. Encephalitic signs occasionally predominate. The CSF glucose is normal, the protein is slightly elevated, and the cell count commonly ranges from 10 to 300 cells/μL (predominantly lymphocytes). The peripheral WBC counts may be normal or moderately increased.

Diagnosis and Differential Diagnosis

Asymmetric flaccid limb paralyses or bulbar palsies without sensory loss during an acute febrile illness in a child or young adult almost always indicate poliomyelitis, though rarely certain coxsackieviruses and echoviruses may produce the same clinical picture (see above in this chapter in the general discussion of enteroviral diseases). In the Guillain-Barré syndrome (see in Ch. 43), often confused with paralytic poliomyelitis, there is usually no fever, muscle weakness is symmetric, sensory findings coexist in 70% of cases, and CSF protein is usually elevated in the presence of a normal cell count. CNS involvement due to mumps or herpesviruses, tuberculous meningitis, or brain abscess should also be considered, and in certain geographic areas, meningoencephalitis due to arboviruses. Nonparalytic poliomyelitis cannot be distinguished clinically from aseptic meningitis due to other agents; virus isolation from throat and/or feces or demonstration of a rise in specific antibody is required to confirm the diagnosis.

Prognosis

In the abortive and nonparalytic forms, recovery is complete. In paralytic poliomyelitis, < 25% of patients suffer severe permanent disability, about 25% have mild disabilities, and > 50% recover with no residual paralyses. The greatest return of muscle function occurs in the first 6 mo, but improvement may continue for 2 yr. Mortality is 1 to 4% but may increase to 10% in adults or those with bulbar disease. Recently, a **postpoliomyelitis syndrome** has been described, characterized by muscle fatigue and decreased endurance, often accompanied by weakness, fasciculations, and atrophy in selective muscles. The syndrome occurs many years after an attack of paralytic poliomyelitis, affecting especially older and initially more severely involved patients. The cause is thought to be associated with aging changes and further loss of anterior horn cells in a population of neurons already depleted by earlier poliovirus infection.

Prophylaxis

Active immunization is recommended for all infants and children (see IMMUNIZATION PROCEDURES THROUGHOUT CHILDHOOD in Ch. 23). Two vaccines have been used: **Salk inactivated poliovirus vaccine (IPV)**, given in a series of injections with periodic booster doses, and **Sabin live attenuated oral poliovirus vaccine (OPV)**. An enhanced form of IPV, which evokes a more potent antibody response, has recently been approved. Where available, it is preferable to the standard IPV, but supplies may be somewhat limited. Both OPV and IPV induce circulating antibodies, but OPV also induces alimentary tract resistance associated with local secretory (IgA) antibody production that blocks virus implantation. Because of its immunologic superiority and logistic simplicity, trivalent OPV is recommended for routine childhood immunization in the USA. Very rarely, OPV has been associated with paralytic poliomyelitis. OPV is contraindicated in immunodeficient persons, who should receive IPV, and in families with an immunodeficient member because of the possibility of contact infection from recipients who excrete the virus. Because poliomyelitis incidence in the USA is extremely low, primary vaccination of adults (> 18 yr) is not recommended. Adults who have never been immunized and are traveling to endemic or epidemic areas should be given a course of IPV; if the time is too short to permit at least 2 doses of IPV, a single dose of trivalent OPV is indicated.

Treatment

Therapy is symptomatic. Patients with abortive or mild nonparalytic poliomyelitis need only bed rest for several days. Analgesics and antipyretics may be useful. During active myelitis, rest on a firm bed (with footboards, to help prevent footdrop) is indicated. Muscle spasm and pain may be relieved by several 20-min applications per day of hot, moist packs. Urinary retention, a frequent complication in patients with leg paralysis, may respond to a parasympathomimetic such as bethanechol 5 to 30 mg orally or 0.6 mg/kg/day s.c. in divided doses q 6 to 8 h. An intermittent catheterization program is often preferable, though, to decrease the possibility of developing UTI. If infection occurs, treatment with an appropriate antibiotic and a high fluid intake is indicated to prevent formation of urinary calcium phosphate stones. Physical therapy is the most important part of management of paralytic poliomyelitis during convalescence.

Respiratory failure may result from spinal cord involvement causing paralysis of the muscles of respiration or from damage by the virus to the respiratory centers in the medulla and paralysis of muscles innervated by the cranial nerves. Artificial respiration is the treatment for both types. In patients with pharyngeal muscle weakness, difficulty in swallowing, inability to cough, and pooling of bronchotracheal secretions, postural drainage and suction should be instituted. Intubation or tracheostomy is frequently required to keep the airway clear. Pulmonary atelectasis is common in respiratory failure, and bronchoscopy and aspiration are often necessary. Antimicrobial agents are not recommended unless bacterial infection occurs.

MUMPS
(Epidemic Parotitis)

An acute, contagious, generalized viral disease, usually causing painful enlargement of the salivary glands, most commonly the parotids.

Etiology and Incidence

The causative agent, a paramyxovirus, is spread by infected droplets or direct contact with materials contaminated by infected saliva. The virus probably enters through the mouth. It may be found in saliva for 1 to 6 days before the salivary glands swell and for the duration of glandular enlargement (usually 5 to 9 days). It has been isolated from patients' blood and urine and from the CSF in patients with CNS involvement.

Mumps is endemic in heavily populated areas but may occur in epidemics when many susceptible individuals are crowded together. It is less communicable than measles or chickenpox. Incidence peaks in late winter and early spring. Although the disease may occur at any age, most cases are in children aged 5 to 15 yr; the disease is unusual in children < 2 yr, and infants up to 1 yr ordinarily are immune. One attack usually confers permanent immunity, even though only one salivary gland has been enlarged. About 25 to 30% of cases are clinically inapparent.

Symptoms, Signs, and Course

After a 14- to 24-day incubation period, onset occurs with chilly sensations, headache, anorexia, malaise, and a low- to moderate-grade fever that may last 12 to 24 h before salivary gland involvement is noted. These prodromal symptoms may be absent in mild cases. Pain on chewing or swallowing, especially on swallowing acidic liquids such as vinegar or lemon juice, is the earliest symptom of parotitis. There is marked sensitivity to pressure over the parotid or other involved salivary glands. With development of parotitis, the temperature frequently rises to 39.5 or 40° C (103 or 104° F). Gland swelling reaches maximum about the 2nd day and is associated with tissue edema extending beyond the parotid in front of and below the ear.

Both parotid glands are involved in most cases. Occasionally, the submaxillary and sublingual glands also swell; more rarely, these are the only glands affected. Neck swelling beneath the jaw occurs in such cases; with submaxillary gland involvement, suprasternal edema may develop. The oral duct openings of the involved glands are "pouting" and slightly inflamed. The skin over the glands may become tense and shiny. Involved glands are acutely tender during the 24- to 72-h febrile period. The WBC count may be normal, though a slight leukopenia with a reduction in granulocytes is usual.

Prognosis is excellent in uncomplicated mumps, although rarely a relapse occurs after about 2 wk.

Complications

Particularly in postpubertal patients, the disease may involve organs other than the salivary glands. Symptoms may precede, accompany, or follow salivary gland involvement or may occur without primary sialadenitis.

Orchitis: About 20% of postpubertal male patients have testicular inflammation, usually unilateral. Some testicular atrophy may ensue, but sterility is a rare outcome and hormonal function is not lost. Gonadal involvement in females (oophoritis) is less commonly recognized, is far less painful, and has not been associated with subsequent infertility.

Meningoencephalitis: Headache, stiff neck, and CSF pleocytosis is common in mumps; CSF glucose levels are usually normal but occasionally low, between 20 and 40 mg/dL, mimicking bacterial meningitis. More severe encephalitic signs occur in about 5 to 10% of patients, with drowsiness or even coma or convulsions that may develop abruptly. About 30% of CNS mumps infections occur without associated parotitis. The prognosis is favorable in most cases with CNS involvement and considerably better than in measles encephalitis, although permanent sequelae, such as unilateral (rarely bilateral) nerve deafness or facial paralysis, may result. As in other viral diseases, a para- or postinfectious form of encephalitis may occur in mumps, but this is uncommon. Other unusual manifestations include postinfectious acute cerebellar ataxia, transverse myelitis, and polyneuritis.

Pancreatitis: Toward the end of the first week, a few patients may have sudden severe nausea and vomiting, with abdominal pain that is most severe in the epigastrium, suggesting pancreatitis. These symptoms disappear in about a week, and the patient completely recovers.

Miscellaneous: Prostatitis, nephritis, myocarditis, mastitis, polyarthritis, and lacrimal gland involvement are seen occasionally. Inflammation of the thyroid and thymus glands may cause edema and swelling over the sternum, but this is more common secondary to submaxillary gland involvement.

Diagnosis

Diagnosis of typical cases during an epidemic is easy, but sporadic cases are more difficult to detect. Mumps-induced swelling of the parotid or other salivary glands must be distinguished from (1) bacterial parotid involvement in streptococcal throat infections, diphtheria, or debilitation associated with poor oral hygiene, typhoid, or typhus fever; (2) Mikulicz's syndrome—a chronic, usually painless parotid and lacrimal gland swelling of unknown etiology that occurs with TB, sarcoidosis, SLE, leukemia, and lymphosarcoma; (3) malignant and benign salivary gland tumors; (4) drug-related parotid enlargement (eg, from iodides or guanethidine); and (5) obstruction produced by a calculus in Stensen's duct. Enlarged lymph nodes along the mandible may be mistaken for swollen salivary glands. Mumps meningoencephalitis, sometimes the only clinical manifestation, must be differentiated from other viral meningitides.

Paired serum specimens from acute and convalescent phases permit diagnosis by CF test, preferably with both soluble (S) and viral (V) antigens. S antibodies increase in the first week of infection and drop rapidly, often disappearing after 6 to 8 mo; V antibodies usually increase later than S antibodies but drop slowly to a plateau. A single serum specimen is occasionally diagnostic if both CF antigens are used. Other serologic tests are also available. An elevated serum amylase level may also suggest the diagnosis. If virologic diagnostic services are available, the virus can be readily isolated from the throat, CSF, and occasionally the urine.

Prophylaxis

The patient should remain in isolation until glandular swelling subsides. Susceptible contacts should be followed closely from the 14th to the 28th day after exposure. Mumps immune globulin and immune serum globulin are not helpful.

Live mumps virus vaccine is the agent of choice for active immunization (see IMMUNIZATION PROCEDURES THROUGHOUT CHILDHOOD in Ch. 23). This vaccine produces no significant local or systemic reaction and requires only one injection. It is not yet clear whether revaccination is required to maintain lifelong immunity. Postexposure vaccination does not protect against mumps from that exposure.

Treatment

Treatment is symptomatic. A soft diet reduces pain caused by chewing. Acidic substances (eg, citrus fruit juices) may also cause discomfort and should be avoided. Analgesics may be used for headache and general malaise.

Complications are also treated symptomatically. Patients with orchitis require bed rest. Supporting the scrotum in cotton on an adhesive-tape bridge between the thighs to minimize tension, or applying ice packs, often helps relieve pain.

If nausea and vomiting of pancreatitis are severe, oral feedings should be withheld and fluid balance restored by administering IV dextrose and saline solutions.

Corticosteroids are not usually necessary, although they may diminish pain and swelling in acute orchitis.

CROUP
(Acute Laryngotracheobronchitis)

An acute viral inflammation of the upper and lower respiratory tracts, characterized by inspiratory stridor, subglottic swelling, and respiratory distress that is most pronounced on inspiration.

Etiology, Epidemiology, and Pathophysiology

Croup is primarily a disease of children aged 6 mo to 3 yr, though it occasionally occurs earlier or later. The parainfluenza viruses, especially type 1, are the major pathogens. Less common causes are respiratory syncytial virus **(RSV)** and influenza A and B viruses, followed by adeno-, entero-, rhino-, and measles viruses and *Mycoplasma pneumoniae*. Croup caused by influenza may be particularly severe and may occur in a broader age range of children. Seasonal outbreaks are common; cases due to parainfluenza viruses tend to occur in the fall, and those due to RSV and influenza viruses are likely to occur in the winter and spring. Spread is usually by the airborne route or by contact with infected secretions.

The infection produces inflammation of the larynx, trachea, bronchi, bronchioles, and lung parenchyma. However, obstruction, caused by swelling and inflammatory exudate, is most pronounced in the subglottic region. Obstruction increases the work of breathing and, as the child tires, results in hypercapnia. Hypoxemia without hypercapnia commonly occurs as a result of accompanying parenchymal pulmonary infection. Atelectasis may occur concurrently if the bronchioles become obstructed.

Symptoms and Signs

Croup is usually preceded by a URI. A barking, often spasmodic, cough and hoarseness may mark the acute onset of inspiratory stridor, commonly at night. The child may awaken during the night with respiratory distress, tachypnea, and supraclavicular, suprasternal, substernal, and intercostal inspiratory retractions. In severe cases, cyanosis with increasingly shallow respirations may develop as the child tires. The obvious respiratory distress and the harsh inspiratory stridor are the most dramatic physical findings. Auscultation reveals prolonged in-spiration and stridor, often with some expiratory rhonchi and wheezes. Rales also may be present. Breath sounds may be diminished with atelectasis. Fever is present in about ¹/₂ the children. Leukocytosis with increased polymorphonuclear cells may be present initially, with a subsequent shift to leukopenia and lymphocytosis. With involvement of the lung parenchyma, arterial blood gas analysis reveals hypoxemia with or without hypercapnia. Hypoxemia is present in about 80% of patients who are hospitalized. Subepiglottic narrowing may be seen on anteroposterior neck x-ray. The child's condition may appear improved in the morning but may worsen again at night. The illness usually lasts 3 to 4 days. Recurrent episodes are often called **spasmodic croup.** Allergy or airway reactivity may play a role in spasmodic croup, but the clinical manifestations cannot be differentiated from those of viral croup, and spasmodic croup is also usually initiated by a viral infection.

Differential Diagnosis

Croup must be differentiated from **epiglottitis.** Distinguishing features are given under Acute Epiglottitis, above. **Bacterial tracheitis** is a separate and unusual entity that is most likely to be confused with epiglottitis because of its rapid onset and severe, progressive course. It is characterized by the acute onset of fever, dyspnea, and stridor in young and older children. Although it rarely follows viral croup, it should be differentiated from this disease by the greater degree of toxicity and respiratory distress, the left shift of the WBC count, the thick secretions, and the shaggy, exudative laryngeal membrane, which may be visualized on x-ray or directly. Specimens of the membrane or deep tracheal secretions obtained by suctioning are most likely to grow a pure culture of *Staphylococcus aureus* or Group A β-hemolytic streptococcus. *Streptococcus pneumoniae* and *Hemophilus influenzae* type b are less frequent causes. A **foreign body** may cause respiratory distress and a typical croupy cough, but fever and a preceding URI are absent. X-rays of the neck may show a foreign body, but indirect and direct laryngoscopy may be required to confirm the diagnosis. **Diphtheria** is excluded by a history of adequate immunization or confirmed by identification of the organism in special cultures of scrapings from the typical grayish diphtheritic pharyngeal or laryngeal membrane. Rarely, **retropharyngeal abscess** presents with stridor. Diagnosis may be made by direct visualization, lateral x-ray of the neck, or CT.

Treatment

Home therapy: The mildly ill child may be cared for at home with supportive measures. The child should be made comfortable and kept well hydrated. Rest is important, as fatigue and crying can aggravate the condition. Home humidification devices (eg, "cold-steam" vaporizers or humidifiers) may ameliorate upper airway drying, but the water droplets produced are too large to help mobilize secretions in the lower respiratory tract. Increasing or persistent respiratory distress, tachycardia, fatigue, cyanosis, or dehydration indicates need for hospitalization.

Hospital therapy: Since moderate hypoxemia may exist without cyanosis, arterial blood gas analysis is indicated initially in all hospitalized croup patients. If the Pa_{O_2} is initially < 60 mm Hg, humidified O_2 should be administered. A 30 to 40% inspired O_2 concentration is usually adequate. CO_2 retention ($Pa_{CO_2} > 45$ mm Hg) generally indicates fatigue and necessitates close surveillance of the patient. *The need for intubation should be anticipated, and equipment and personnel should be ready.* The need for airway intervention is indicated by (1) increasing CO_2 retention despite adequate oxygenation, nebulized mist therapy, and hydration; (2) hypoxemia that is unresponsive to O_2 administration; and (3) secretions that cannot be mobilized by coughing. Nasotracheal intubation, if performed early by skilled personnel, causes fewer complications than does tracheostomy.

The viscosity of tracheobronchial secretions may be reduced and their clearance enhanced by mist therapy. Standard jet-type nebulizers improve laryngeal humidification, but bronchiolar humidification requires use of an ultrasonic nebulizer fitted to a mask or an O_2 tent.

The viruses that most commonly cause croup do not usually predispose to secondary bacterial infection, and antibiotics are rarely indicated. Nebulized racemic epinephrine offers symptomatic improvement and relieves fatigue. However, it should be used only with the understanding that the effects are transient; that the course of the illness, the underlying viral infection, and the Pa_{O_2} are not altered by its use; and that tachycardia and other side effects may occur. The use of corticosteroids remains controversial, but many

physicians use them early in the course of severe, hospitalized cases of viral croup.

BRONCHIOLITIS

An acute viral infection of the lower respiratory tract affecting infants and young children and characterized by respiratory distress, expiratory obstruction, wheezing, and crackles.

Bronchiolitis often occurs in epidemics and mostly in children < 18 mo of age, with a peak incidence in infants < 6 mo—the ages of predilection for respiratory syncytial virus (**RSV**) and parainfluenza type 3 virus. The annual incidence in the first year of life is estimated to be 11 cases/100 children.

Etiology and Pathophysiology

The major pathogens of bronchiolitis are RSV and parainfluenza 3 virus; influenza A and B, parainfluenza 1 and 2, and adenoviruses are less frequent causes. Rhinoviruses, enteroviruses, measles virus, and *Mycoplasma pneumoniae* are uncommon etiologic agents.

The infecting virus spreads from the upper respiratory tract to the medium and small bronchi and bronchioles, causing epithelial necrosis. The developing edema and exudate result in partial obstruction, which is most pronounced on expiration and leads to air trapping within the alveoli. Complete obstruction and absorption of the trapped air may lead to multiple areas of atelectasis.

Symptoms and Signs

Typically, an affected infant has had a preceding URI, followed by rapid onset of respiratory distress with tachypnea, tachycardia, and a hacking cough. Increasing distress is evidenced by circumoral cyanosis; deepening retractions of the subcostal, intercostal, and suprasternal areas; and audible wheezing. The child often appears markedly lethargic, but fever is not always present. Dehydration may develop from vomiting and decreased oral intake. With fatigue, respirations may become more shallow and ineffective, leading to respiratory acidosis. The chest is hyperresonant on percussion, and auscultation reveals wheezing, prolonged expiration, and often, fine moist crackles. X-ray usually shows hyperinflated lungs, depressed diaphragm, and prominent hilar markings. Infiltrates may be present from atelectasis as well as RSV pneumonia, which is relatively common with RSV bronchiolitis.

Diagnosis

Initial laboratory findings are *not* diagnostic. About 2/3 of the children have WBC counts of 10,000 to 15,000. Most have 50 to 75% lymphocytes. In severe cases, serum BUN and electrolyte levels reveal the degree and type of dehydration; blood gas levels are likely to show hypoxemia. Specific etiologic diagnosis is made by viral isolation or rapid diagnostic techniques, such as immunofluorescence and enzyme-linked immunosorbent assay **(ELISA)**.

Asthma is the major consideration in the differential diagnosis and is the more likely diagnosis in a child > 18 mo of age, especially if previous episodes of wheezing and a family history of allergy have been documented. Gastric reflux with aspiration of gastric contents may also produce the clinical picture of bronchiolitis; multiple episodes in an infant may be a clue to this diagnosis. Foreign body aspiration occasionally causes wheezing and should be considered if the history or epidemiologic setting is suggestive and if the onset is sudden and not associated with prior upper respiratory tract signs (eg, nasal congestion).

Prognosis and Treatment

Most children can be treated at home and recover in 3 to 5 days without sequelae. The mortality rate is < 1% when medical care is adequate. Increasing respiratory distress, cyanosis, fatigue, and dehydration are indications for hospitalization. Children with underlying conditions such as cardiac disease, immunodeficiency, or bronchopulmonary dysplasia, which put them at high risk for severe or complicated disease, should be followed closely and considered candidates for hospitalization early in the course of illness.

Oxygenation: *Recognizing and treating hypoxemia is most important.* In the hospital, arterial blood gas determinations are performed, since the degree of hypoxemia cannot be accurately defined clinically. Adequate levels of oxygenation (Pa_{O_2} > 60 mm Hg) are usually attained with a 30 to 40% O_2 mixture delivered by tent or face mask. Endotracheal intubation is indicated if progressive CO_2 retention occurs, if the child cannot clear bronchial secretions, or if hypoxemia is unresponsive to O_2 administration. Following intubation, O_2 administration should be continued, secretions should be cleared (by postural drainage and tracheal suctioning), and the lower tracheobronchial tree should be humidified with ultrasonic nebulization.

Fluids: At home, hydration is maintained with frequent small feedings of clear liquids. In the hospital, fluids should be given IV initially, and the level of hydration should be monitored by urine output and specific gravity or serum electrolyte determinations.

Pharmacologic agents: Corticosteroids are valueless, and sedatives are contraindicated. Antibiotics should be withheld unless a secondary bacterial infection (a rare sequela) occurs. Bronchodilators are usually ineffective, and repeated administration may harm the young infant. An antiviral agent, ribavirin, is administered as a small-particle aerosol with equipment using a generator run by compressed air. Ribavirin, usually given for 12 to 18 h/day for 3 to 5 days, should be considered for hospitalized infants who are premature, have underlying conditions that place them at high risk for severe disease, or have moderate to severe disease. Since ribavirin aerosol may precipitate in ventilator tubing, precautions should be taken (eg, using filters and one-way valves). Infants receiving mechanical ventilation should be treated with ribavirin only in centers experienced in its use.

HUMAN IMMUNODEFICIENCY VIRUS (HIV) INFECTION IN CHILDREN
(See also Ch. 20)

Infection caused by a cytopathic human retrovirus, resulting in a continuously changing and progressive spectrum of immunologic deterioration and associated clinical conditions, of which the end stage is acquired immunodeficiency syndrome (AIDS). Infection rates have been epidemic since the virus was introduced in the USA.

AIDS was first described in adults in the USA in 1981, although cases had occurred since at least the mid-1970s. In retrospect, cases in children occurred almost as early as those in adults. In the USA, HIV infection and AIDS occur primarily in young adults; only 2% of all cases reported have been in children or adolescents.

Etiology and Epidemiology

The primary cellular receptor for HIV is the **CD4 molecule;** therefore, the cells most commonly infected are T4 lymphocytes and monocytes-macrophages. Once a cell has been infected with HIV, proviral genome is integrated into the host cell DNA, establishing a persistent chronic infection. The complex gene structure of HIV includes regulatory genes that control the timing and rate of viral replication, but the details of this regulatory mechanism within the infected cell are not yet fully understood.

Two major HIV types have been identified to date: HIV-1 and HIV-2. HIV-1 is the predominant cause of HIV infection worldwide, while infection caused by HIV-2 is restricted primarily to a few countries of West Africa and adjacent islands. Although selected regions of the envelope genes of HIV-1 mutate relatively rapidly, giving rise to numerous strains, virtually all HIV-1–strain antibodies react with commercially available diagnostic tests.

Humans are the only known reservoir of HIV, and the **virus is transmitted** by (1) sexual contact (male homosexual or heterosexual) with an infected person; (2) injection of infected blood, usually during IV injection of illicit drugs but occasionally through accidental needlestick injury (eg, to a health care worker) or through transfusion of contaminated blood or blood products (in the USA, current risk of new infections via this route is negligible); or (3) congenital or perinatal transmission from an infected pregnant woman to her fetus or, at delivery, to her infant. The disease in infants and young children is largely congenital or perinatal. However, under certain circumstances, an infant also may become infected through breast-feeding.

Transmission by other means (eg, through food or water, fomites, or casual contact in a household, workplace, or school setting) has not been documented. A few cases have been reported (in health care settings only) in which HIV appears to have been transmitted by contact with infected blood on the skin of hands or face; however, in most instances the skin was not intact (ie, abrasions or open sores were present). Transmission by bite has been of particular concern to many people because HIV has been isolated from saliva of some infected persons, but transmission by saliva has not been reported.

HIV infection in older children and adolescents, like that in adults, is often latent or low grade for months or years. Onset of chronic, clinically apparent disease typically occurs years after infection. About 1/2 of infected adults meet the surveillance criteria for a diagnosis of AIDS (see TABLE 20–1) 8 to 10 yr after infection.

Infants and children at highest risk for HIV infection and AIDS are those born to women who use drugs or are sexual partners of drug users or bisexual men. Boys with hemophilia who received clotting factor concentrates before the mid-1980s are also at high risk, and children who

received a blood transfusion before 1985 had a significant risk of having been infected. Since 1985 all donated blood has been screened for HIV antibody, and since the mid-1980s major improvements have been made in the safety of clotting factor concentrates, with the result that in the USA today new infection by these routes is extremely rare.

AIDS in the USA in children < 13 yr continues to increase rapidly; > 3000 cases cumulatively and 700 to 800 cases annually were reported as of early 1991. Congenital or perinatal transmission accounted for 85% of the cases diagnosed in 1990. Cases associated with infection by blood transfusion have declined (6% of cases in 1990, compared with 17% in the mid-1980s), while the proportion of cases in children with hemophilia appears to have achieved a plateau (4% of cases). In about 5% of cases, no source of infection currently can be identified.

Projections from serologic studies suggest that about 6000 HIV-infected women in the USA annually give birth, resulting in about 2000 infected infants. In 1990, the mean prevalence of HIV infection among women of childbearing age in the USA was about 0.15%, but in some areas, such as New York City and the inner cities of northern New Jersey, as many as 1 to 3% of pregnant women were infected. There is no area of the USA in which the risk of HIV infection for women is zero.

The sexes are equally affected by congenital or perinatal HIV infection, but racial and ethnic group distribution is highly disproportionate. Nearly 52% of affected children are black, 26% are Hispanic, and only 22% are white, reflecting the distribution and frequency of HIV infection in the mothers. The risk to the infant of congenital or perinatal infection from an infected mother ranges from 20 to 40% in most studies. Factors associated with transmission or protection of an infant are being studied.

Symptoms, Signs, and Clinical Course

Congenital or perinatal infection usually is not apparent immediately after birth; problems often are manifested during the 1st or 2nd yr of life, although they may not appear until years later. On the basis of prospective studies, it is estimated that about 1/2 of perinatally infected children are diagnosed with AIDS by their 3rd birthday.

HIV has a highly variable clinical course, characterized by a wide range of complications and conditions that progress as immune system function deteriorates. **Common early manifestations** include failure to thrive or wasting; fever; chronic or recurrent diarrhea without definable specific cause; generalized lymphadenopathy, hepatosplenomegaly, and parotitis; persistent or recurrent oral or perineal candidiasis; and a variety of recurrent infections, including sepsis, otitis media, pneumonia, and meningitis, usually of bacterial origin. The most common bacterial pathogens include *Streptococcus pneumoniae*, *Salmonella* spp, and *Hemophilus influenzae*. Various opportunistic viral, fungal, and parasitic infections also occur (see TABLE 20–1). Bleeding secondary to immune thrombocytopenia has been reported.

CNS involvement occurs in about 50 to 60% of HIV-infected children, resulting in developmental delay or loss of milestones, intellectual impairment, and acquired microcephaly. While the neurologic deficit in some children remains relatively static, progressive encephalopathy with loss of social and language skills as well as motor function may occur in as many as 20% of affected children. Focal neurologic abnormalities, including pyramidal tract signs, paresis, ataxia, and rigidity, also occur, and cerebral atrophy with ventricular enlargement and calcification of the basal ganglia can be demonstrated.

Cardiomyopathy, hepatitis, and nephropathy occur in some children. Malignancies associated with AIDS are uncommon in children, although non-Hodgkin's lymphoma and primary CNS lymphoma have been described, and Kaposi's sarcoma occurs extremely rarely.

Lymphocytic interstitial pneumonitis (also known as pulmonary lymphoid hyperplasia) of unknown origin occurs in ≥ 30% of infected children, usually during the first several years of life. Cough, digital clubbing, lymphadenopathy, hepatosplenomegaly, and markedly elevated serum immunoglobulin levels are frequent findings. The illness tends to progress less rapidly in these children than in those with significant infections, but superimposed bacterial or viral pneumonia may occur.

Pneumonia caused by *Pneumocystis carinii* is the most frequently described opportunistic infection in AIDS. In children with congenital or perinatal HIV infection, it commonly occurs in the first 15 mo of life, is diagnosed at some point in > ½ of the children, and is a major cause of mortality. Although it may present with an indolent course, it is more likely to be acute. Fever, tachypnea, cough, and abnormal auscultatory findings are typical. The disease often progresses rapidly, and ventilatory support may be necessary.

Disseminated mycobacterial infections also occur, most often caused by *Mycobacterium avium-intracellulare*. Pulmonary and nonpulmonary TB, increasingly common among adults with HIV infection in selected populations, also occurs in children. Disseminated cytomegalovirus infection, chronic or recurrent mucocutaneous herpes simplex, ulcerative varicella-zoster infection, cryptococcal meningitis, fatal measles, and an array of other opportunistic infections often occur as multiple simultaneous problems late in the course of AIDS.

In children who have later onset of disease, acute complicating infections may be interspersed with periods during which the child functions relatively normally. As the disease progresses, multiple organ system involvement and multiple infections or conditions may occur simultaneously.

Laboratory Findings and Diagnosis

In infants and younger children, **abnormalities of humoral immunity** precede those of cell-mediated immunity. Serum immunoglobulin levels, especially IgG, often are markedly elevated, and B cells may be increased in number, with spontaneous secretion of antibody. Despite this, poor primary and decreased secondary responses to antigens such as toxoid or polysaccharide vaccine can be documented, and the in vitro lymphocyte proliferative response to pokeweed mitogen is abnormal. Circulating immune complexes often are present. A late manifestation may be hypogammaglobulinemia.

Abnormalities of cell-mediated immunity, characteristic of HIV infection in adults, also occur in children. A typical finding is a decrease in ratio of T4 (helper/inducer) to T8 (suppressor/cytotoxic) lymphocytes, with a continuing decline in the number of T4 cells over time; the absolute number of T8 cells often is above normal. However, CD4+ counts and percentages are quite different in infants and young children from those found in adults (see TABLE 32–12); therefore, recommendations for initiation of prophylaxis of pneumonia caused by *P. carinii* must be based on age-related criteria (see FIG. 32–1). The in vitro lymphocyte response to mitogen stimulation with phytohemagglutinin and concanavalin A is poor. Paradoxically, in children the T4:T8 ratio may be normal or increased, and response to lymphocyte mitogen and antigen stimulation may be normal despite a clinically severe

TABLE 32–12. AGE-ADJUSTED CD4+ LYMPHOCYTE PARAMETERS
FOR NORMAL, HEALTHY CHILDREN AND ADULTS

Parameter	Age				
	1–6 mo	7–12 mo	13–24 mo	25–74 mo	Adult
Number tested	106	28	46	29	327
Absolute CD4+ count					
Median (cells/μL)	3211	3128	2601	1668	1027
5–95 percentile (cells/μL)	1153–5285	967–5289	739–4463	505–2831	237–1817
Percentage CD4+ cells					
Median (%)	51.6	47.9	45.8	42.1	50.9
5–95 percentile (%)	36.3–67.1	32.8–63.0	31.2–60.4	32.2–52.0	34.7–67.1
CD4:CD8 ratio					
Median	2.2	2.1	2.0	1.4	1.7
5–95 percentile	0.9–3.5	0.8–3.4	0.6–3.4	0.7–2.1	0.4–3.0

From "Guidelines for prophylaxis against *Pneumocystis carinii* pneumonia for children infected with human immunodeficiency virus." *Morbidity and Mortality Weekly Report* 40(RR-2):1–11, 1991.

bacterial or other opportunistic infection. Cutaneous anergy is typical.

Anemia, leukopenia, and thrombocytopenia are frequent findings, although lymphopenia may not occur in infants. Liver function abnormalities are also common.

A diagnosis of HIV infection or AIDS in infants and young children depends on establishing the presence of HIV infection, defining the immunologic status of the child, and diagnosing the pattern of clinical illnesses that occur secondary to the infection and loss of immune function. Commercially available diagnostic tests have facilitated the distinction of HIV-induced immune dysfunction from other primary immunodeficiency disorders.

Infants born to HIV-infected mothers will almost always be seropositive on HIV antibody tests because of the passive placental transfer of maternal IgG antibody, even though most of these infants will not be infected. Though maternal antibody is lost at a variable rate, it may be present in some infants for ≥ 15 mo. If these infants are asymptomatic, diagnosis of HIV infection is complex and may require confirmation by viral culture, HIV antigen assay, or laboratory evidence of immune impairment. To date, IgM antibody assays have not been helpful. New tests and procedures such as polymerase chain reaction for HIV-specific nucleic acids, serial antibody profiles to detect acquisition of specific antibody, and in situ hybridization with complementary DNA probes for HIV on cultured mononuclear cells from the infant are being studied.

Loss of HIV antibody in an asymptomatic infant with normal immune function is presumptive evidence that the infant is not infected, but it is not definitive; some infants with demonstrable infection do not have detectable antibody for various reasons. Infants with HIV antibody who have infections or other symptoms compatible with the case definition for AIDS, or who have cellular and humoral immunodeficiency plus clinical involvement, are presumed to be infected.

In an asymptomatic child 15 to 18 mo of age or older, HIV infection is diagnosed by a positive HIV antibody test or other positive tests of HIV in blood or tissue. In a child of any age, complicating infections or clinical conditions compatible with AIDS should suggest a diagnosis of HIV infection, regardless of known risk.

Serologic tests for HIV infection are highly sensitive and specific if performed by a reliable laboratory with proper precautions; confirmation of screening test results by an assay such as the Western blot is essential, and special problems that may impair test accuracy (eg, immunologic tolerance or hypogammaglobulinemia) should be kept in mind.

The Centers for Disease Control (CDC) classification system for HIV infection in children describes the various clinical findings and complications in a systematic form that aids diagnosis (see TABLE 32–13).

Prognosis and Treatment

Two survival patterns based on time and manner of clinical presentation have been de-

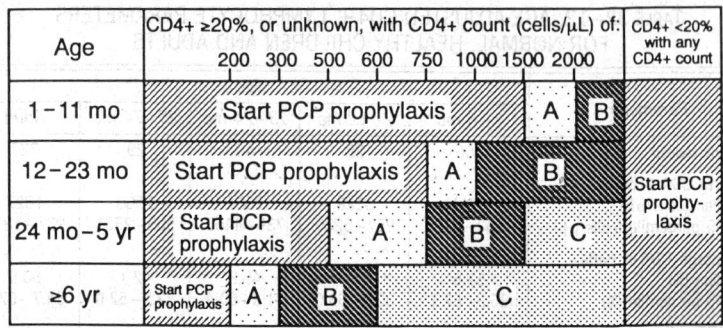

Age	CD4+ ≥20%, or unknown, with CD4+ count (cells/μL) of:									CD4+ <20% with any CD4+ count
	200	300	500	600	750	1000	1500	2000		
1–11 mo	Start PCP prophylaxis						A	B		
12–23 mo	Start PCP prophylaxis			A		B			Start PCP prophylaxis	
24 mo–5 yr	Start PCP prophylaxis		A		B		C			
≥6 yr	Start PCP prophylaxis	A	B		C					

FIG. 32–1. Recommendations for initiation of prophylaxis for *Pneumocystis carinii* pneumonia (PCP) for children ≥ 1 mo old who are HIV-infected, HIV-seropositive, or < 12 mo old and born to an HIV-infected mother. A CD4+ cell count and CD4+ percentage should be obtained for each child; results and child's age should be used as criteria for starting PCP prophylaxis. A = No prophylaxis is recommended at this time; recheck CD4+ count in 1 mo. B = No prophylaxis is recommended at this time; recheck CD4+ count at least every 3 to 4 mo. C = No prophylaxis is recommended at this time; recheck CD4+ count at least every 6 mo. (From "Guidelines for prophylaxis against *Pneumocystis carinii* pneumonia for children infected with human immunodeficiency virus." *Morbidity and Mortality Weekly Report* 40(RR-2):1–11, 1991.)

scribed: (1) Children whose major disease manifestations are opportunistic infections, especially *P. carinii* pneumonia, characteristically have an earlier onset of disease, often during the 1st yr, and a rapidly fatal course with a median survival of ¹/₂ yr after onset. (2) Children whose primary clinical presentation is lymphocytic interstitial pneumonitis frequently are > 1 yr of age at onset and diagnosis and have a more slowly progressive course with a median survival of > 18 mo after onset. Children with progressive encephalopathy also tend to have a poor prognosis.

Therapy for HIV infection and the complicating infections is evolving rapidly, and current recommendations should be sought. In general, the most successful approach has been to provide thorough medical and supportive care and adequate nutrition, with rapid diagnosis and aggressive treatment of infections as they occur. Successful treatment of the complex problems posed by AIDS often requires a multidisciplinary team approach, including home health care and social services involvement to keep the children at home as much as possible rather than in a hospital environment.

Zidovudine (ZDU, also called azidothymidine **[AZT]**) is available for treatment of HIV infection associated with AIDS in children. It is currently not used in children to treat asymptomatic or mildly symptomatic HIV infection associated with

significant immune impairment, as it may be in adults. Clinical trials are under way to determine the most effective timing, dose, and route of administration. In late 1991, a second drug, dideoxyinosine **(DDI)**, was approved for children and adults who cannot tolerate ZDU or whose T cell levels are falling dangerously low even though they are taking ZDU. Other antiretroviral agents also are being tested and some are available on a compassionate-use basis. Because all of these agents have a significant toxicity, close monitoring of the child is essential.

Periodic administration of IV immunoglobulin (IVIG) to HIV-infected children has been advocated by some, but a definitive assessment of its efficacy is not yet available. Prophylaxis against *P. carinii* pneumonia with trimethoprim-sulfamethoxazole **(TMP/SMX)** is recommended for infants at least 1 mo old and children with significantly impaired immune function (see FIG. 32–1). If TMP/SMX is not tolerated, alternative regimens using aerosolized pentamidine (for children ≥ 5 yr old) or dapsone (for those ≥ 1 mo) may be tried. If these agents are not tolerated, some clinicians recommend IV pentamidine.

The American Academy of Pediatrics and the Immunization Practices Advisory Committee of the CDC have published recommendations for **immunization against other** diseases for children with HIV infection; current recommendations should be consulted (see also IMMUNIZATION

TABLE 32-13. CDC CLASSIFICATION SYSTEM FOR HIV INFECTION IN CHILDREN

Class P-0: Indeterminate Infection
Infants < 15 mo born to infected mothers but without definitive evidence of HIV infection or AIDS

Class P-1: Asymptomatic Infection
Subclass A: Normal immune function
Subclass B: Abnormal immune function—hypergammaglobulinemia, T4 lymphopenia, decreased
  T4:T8 ratio, or absolute lymphopenia
Subclass C: Immune function not tested

Class P-2: Symptomatic Infection
Subclass A: Nonspecific findings (≥ 2 for ≥ 2 mo)—fever, failure to thrive, generalized lymphade-
  nopathy, hepatomegaly, splenomegaly, enlarged parotid glands, persistent or recurrent diarrhea
Subclass B: Progressive neurologic disease—loss of developmental milestones or intellectual ability,
  impaired brain growth, or progressive symmetrical motor deficits
Subclass C: Lymphoid interstitial pneumonitis
Subclass D: Secondary infectious diseases
  Category D-1: Opportunistic infections in the CDC case definition
    Bacterial: mycobacterial infection (noncutaneous, extrapulmonary, or disseminated); nocardiosis
    Fungal: candidiasis (esophageal, bronchial, or pulmonary), coccidioidomycosis, disseminated
      histoplasmosis, extrapulmonary cryptococcosis
    Parasitic: *Pneumocystis carinii* pneumonia, disseminated toxoplasmosis with onset ≥ 1 mo
      of age, chronic cryptosporidiosis or isosporiasis, extraintestinal strongyloidiasis
    Viral: cytomegalovirus disease (onset ≥ 1 mo of age), chronic mucocutaneous/disseminated
      herpes (onset ≥ 1 mo age), progressive multifocal leukoencephalopathy
  Category D-2: Unexplained, recurrent, serious bacterial infections (≥ 2 in a 2-yr period)—sepsis,
    meningitis, pneumonia, abscess of an internal organ, bone/joint infections
  Category D-3: Other infectious diseases—persistent oral candidiasis, recurrent herpes stomatitis
    (≥ 2 episodes in 1 yr), multidermatomal or disseminated herpes zoster, etc
Subclass E: Secondary cancers
  Category E-1: Cancers in the AIDS case definition—Kaposi's sarcoma, B-cell non-Hodgkin's
    lymphoma, or primary lymphoma of brain
  Category E-2: Other malignancies possibly associated with HIV
Subclass F: Other conditions possibly due to HIV infection—hepatitis, cardiopathy, nephropathy,
  hematologic disorders, dermatologic diseases, etc

CDC = Centers for Disease Control.

PROCEDURES THROUGHOUT CHILDHOOD in Ch. 23). Both symptomatic and asymptomatic children with HIV infection should receive diphtheria and tetanus toxoids and pertussis vaccine (DTP), measles-mumps-rubella vaccine, *inactivated* polio vaccine (IPV), and *Hemophilus* b conjugate vaccine (HbCV), following the routine immunization schedule. In general, live viral (eg, oral polio vaccine [OPV]) and bacterial (eg, bacille Calmette-Guérin [BCG]) vaccines should not be given to these children, but measles-mumps-rubella vaccine is recommended since measles can cause severe or fatal illness in HIV-infected children and no adverse effects from the vaccine have been reported. Pneumococcal vaccine, polyvalent, is suggested for children > 2 yr old, and annual influenza virus vaccine should be given to children ≥ 6 mo. Since children with symptomatic HIV infection often have a poor immunologic response to vaccines, they are candi-

dates for postexposure prophylaxis (eg, with immune globulin for measles exposure or with varicella-zoster immune globulin for varicella exposure).

Children with HIV infection need close medical supervision as their condition progresses, but they should be managed in the least restrictive environment possible.

Adolescent Cases

HIV infection and AIDS have been hidden problems in adolescents for 2 related reasons: The number of cases has been small (< 700 cumulatively through 1990, and < 200 annually reported), and the long latent period between infection and disease disguises and underestimates the number of individuals who have become infected during adolescence. In contrast, the number of AIDS cases reported in young adults (age 20 to 24 yr) is > 10 times higher than those reported in adolescents, but many, if not most, of these young adults probably were infected as adolescents.

The means of infection in adolescents is the same as in adults: sexual intercourse, both male homosexual (24% of recent cases) and heterosexual (20% of recent cases), and sharing of injection equipment during IV drug use (11% of recent cases). The proportion of cases in adolescent females is higher than in adult females (23%, compared with 10% in adults), and cases in nonwhite persons are disproportionately high (71% of affected adolescent females and 49% of affected adolescent males are black or Hispanic). In younger adolescents, previous treatment with clotting factor concentrates for hemophilia is a prominent cause of infection, accounting for 31% of cases.

Diagnosis, clinical features, and treatment of infection in adolescents are similar to those in adults (see Ch. 20). Prevention depends on education, behavior patterns, and peer support in adopting and maintaining a life-style that is low in risk for HIV infection.

Public Health Issues

No vaccine against HIV infection or AIDS is currently available, nor is one likely to be available for years. Prevention depends on knowing the routes of infection and taking appropriate steps to avoid exposure. Broad-based, effective education programs are essential, including comprehensive health education in schools and programs to reach adolescents no longer in school.

Public health prevention programs have focused on personal knowledge and behavior choices through self-identification of risk behaviors, counseling, antibody testing to determine infection status, and referral of sex and needle-sharing partners for counseling and antibody testing (see also Prevention in Ch. 20).

The most effective means of preventing congenital and perinatal HIV infection is to prevent infection in women of childbearing age; secondary prevention requires HIV-infected women to avoid pregnancy—a step that is difficult, given the restricted access to medical care and the personal, social, and economic circumstances of many of these women. Despite the risks, many infected women and couples in which one or both partners are infected decide for personal reasons to have a child.

Although the risk of acquiring HIV infection through breast-feeding is relatively low for infants under most circumstances, in the USA and other developed countries where alternative nutrition for infants is readily available and safe, infected mothers are routinely advised to avoid breast-feeding. In countries where alternative nutrition poses greater risks of malnutrition or infectious diarrhea for infants, the benefits of breast-feeding far outweigh any additional risk of HIV infection.

School and child-care centers: The American Academy of Pediatrics and the CDC have published guidelines for foster care, day care, and schooling of HIV-infected infants and children. In general, these children should be in the least restrictive environment possible, and attending school is encouraged. The child's physician should be involved in placement decisions to determine risk of exposure to serious infectious diseases.

Day-care placement for younger HIV-infected children is more difficult; each case should be decided on an individual basis by qualified persons, including the physician. Factors to be considered include the type of care the child will receive, potential exposure to infectious diseases, and potential risk of HIV transmission to others. Young children who have open skin lesions or potentially dangerous behaviors such as biting may not be suitable candidates for child-care centers in which other small children are present. Since HIV infection causes neurologic impairment and developmental delays, placement decisions should be based on developmental stage rather than chronologic age. Periodic reassessment of the child is important. Testing of all children for HIV antibody before admission to a day-care center or after an infected child is discovered is not justified.

Since a child may not be known to be infected with HIV (or other blood-borne infectious agents such as hepatitis B virus), all child-care centers should adopt reasonable policies and procedures for managing accidents such as a nosebleed and for cleaning and disinfecting surfaces contaminated with blood. A barrier should be used to prevent skin contact with blood; gloves may be useful but are unnecessary if paper towels or folded cloths are used. Contaminated surfaces should be cleaned and disinfected with a freshly prepared bleach solution (1:10 dilution). All center personnel should be aware of these procedures and have access to necessary supplies.

Social and Ethical Issues

The AIDS epidemic has raised numerous social and ethical issues regarding potentially serious implications and problems. Social ostracism and discrimination resulting in loss of job, housing, and medical insurance are unfortunate but frequent by-products. Consequently, issues such as confidentiality of medical information, informed consent, and full explanation of the implications of various decisions are extremely important.

HIV antibody testing should be presented as a useful diagnostic procedure for a person at risk but should be carried out only as a voluntary procedure, after informed consent is obtained, accompanied by counseling and education about the significance of the results, risk behaviors, and prevention.

In a school or child-care setting, only persons directly involved with the care of an HIV-infected child and who have a need to know should be informed of an infected child's status; they also should be instructed about the rights of the child and family to privacy and confidentiality.

AIDS can be viewed as a family disease, with many social implications attendant to the diagnosis. An infected adult can transmit the disease sexually to the spouse, and an infected woman can transmit the disease to her fetus or newborn. A diagnosis of congenital or perinatal HIV infection in a child is tantamount to a diagnosis in the mother. Many infected infants are abandoned as "boarder babies" in hospitals by parents unable or unwilling to care for them. Even infants born to infected parents, but who are not also infected, will need to be cared for when the parents become ill or die, resulting in additional children who need foster or adoptive homes.

Because of the large number of people already infected, the AIDS epidemic will continue for the foreseeable future. HIV infection can be prevented by people who know how the virus is transmitted, how it is not, and how to protect themselves. The general population as well as health care personnel need to become informed and involved if this epidemic is to be curtailed and those already affected given appropriate care.

CYTOMEGALOVIRUS (CMV) INFECTION

(Cytomegalic Inclusion Disease)
(See also CONGENITAL AND PERINATAL CYTOMEGALOVIRUS INFECTION under NEONATAL INFECTIONS in Ch. 27)

A virus infection occurring congenitally, postnatally, or at any age, and ranging in severity from a silent infection without consequences, through disease manifested by fever, hepatitis, pneumonitis, and (in neonates) severe brain damage, to stillbirth or perinatal death. The restrictive appellation "cytomegalic inclusion disease" refers to the intranuclear inclusions found in enlarged infected cells.

Etiology and Epidemiology

The human CMV (salivary gland virus) is a member of the herpes group of viruses, all of which have the propensity for remaining latent in man. Molecular analysis of the DNA of CMV isolates reveals minor strain-specific differences that are useful markers in epidemiologic investigation. CMV is highly host-specific and cannot be propagated in laboratory animals or in most nonhuman cell cultures.

CMV is ubiquitous. Infected persons may excrete virus in urine or saliva for months; virus may also be found in human cervical secretions, semen, feces, and milk; fresh blood or organs (eg, kidneys) from asymptomatic infected donors may produce disease in susceptible recipients. Infection may be acquired transplacentally, during birth, or by contact with infected secretions or excretions at any time thereafter. High infection rates may occur among children in closed populations, such as orphanages and infant daycare centers, and are the rule in male homosexuals with multiple sexual partners. Prevalence in the general population increases gradually with age; 60 to 90% of adults have had CMV infection.

Symptoms and Signs

Congenital infection: The extent of the pathologic process is highly variable. Infection may be manifested only by cytomegaloviruria in an otherwise apparently normal infant. At the other extreme, CMV infection may cause abortion, stillbirth, or postnatal death from hemorrhage, anemia, or extensive hepatic or CNS damage (see CONGENITAL AND PERINATAL CYTOMEGALOVIRUS INFECTION under NEONATAL INFECTIONS in Ch. 27).

Acquired infection: Infections acquired postnatally or later in life are often asymptomatic. An acute febrile illness, termed **cytomegalovirus mononucleosis** or **cytomegalovirus hepatitis,** may result from iatrogenic or spontaneous contact with CMV. **Postperfusion syndrome** develops 2 to 4 wk after transfusion with fresh blood containing CMV and is characterized by fever lasting 2 to 3 wk, hepatitis of variable degree with or without jaundice, a characteristic atypical lymphocytosis resembling that of infectious mononucleosis, and occasionally a rash. Patients receiving immunosuppressive therapy who have CMV infections, acquired or due to reactivation of a latent process, may have pulmonary, GI, CNS, or renal involvement. This important complication has a 50% attack rate and high associated mortality in patients undergoing transplantation. Disseminated CMV infection commonly causes retinitis, encephalitis, or ulcerative disease of the colon or esophagus in the terminal phase of AIDS.

Diagnosis

CMV may be isolated from urine, other body fluids, or tissues by inoculation of human fibroblastic cell cultures. However, CMV may be excreted for months or years after infection and cytomegaloviruria must be interpreted accordingly. The appearance of specific CF antibodies during illness provides supportive evidence. New, more rapid approaches based on demonstrating CMV in secretions or tissues by immunofluorescence with commercially available monoclonal antibodies, or by in situ hybridization, are promising.

Congenital infection must be differentiated from bacterial, viral (eg, rubella), and protozoan (eg, toxoplasmosis) infections. Diagnosis is best made by urine culture, preferably during the first 3 wk of life. Acquired infection must be differentiated from viral hepatitis and infectious mononucleosis. The absence of pharyngitis or lymphadenopathy and a negative heterophil antibody test are more typical of primary CMV mononucleosis than of illnesses caused by Epstein-Barr virus or *Toxoplasma gondii.*

Treatment

Ganciclovir, the first antiviral agent licensed in the USA for treatment of life- or sight-threatening infections due to CMV, has improved symptoms of CMV retinitis in patients with AIDS. However, its effects are limited to the duration of administration, and continued treatment is necessary to prevent relapses. In patients undergoing bone marrow transplantation, it has resulted in virologic improvement, although mortality rates have not been affected. For CMV retinitis, ganciclovir is given IV 5 mg/kg q 12 h for 14 to 21 days, followed by 5 mg/kg once daily or 6 mg/kg once daily for 5 days/wk. It does not affect latency or viral reactivation. Its use in severe symptomatic congenital infections has not been established. In patients who do not respond to ganciclovir, foscarnet should be considered.

RABIES
(Hydrophobia)

An acute infectious disease of mammals, especially carnivores, characterized by CNS irritation followed by paralysis and death.

Etiology and Epidemiology

The etiologic agent is a neurotropic virus often present in the saliva of rabid animals. The use of monoclonal antibodies has revealed that isolates of rabies virus collected from different animal species and from different parts of the world are distinct; such information is particularly valuable in epidemiology and vaccine production.

Rabid animals transmit the infection by biting animals or humans. Rabies is rarely acquired by exposure of a mucous membrane or fresh skin abrasion to infected saliva. Four cases of apparent respiratory infection have been reported: 2 following laboratory exposure and 2 from the atmosphere of a bat-infested cave. Worldwide, rabid dogs still present the highest risk to man. Rabies in dogs is prevalent in most countries of Latin America, Africa, and Asia. In the USA, where vaccination has largely eliminated canine rabies, bites of infected wild animals have caused most of the infrequent cases of human rabies that have occurred since 1960.

Infected dogs may have either **furious rabies,** characterized by agitation and viciousness, followed by paralysis and death; or **dumb rabies,** in which paralytic symptoms predominate. Rabid wild animals may show "furious" behavior, but less obvious changes (diurnal activity of normally nocturnal bats, skunks, and foxes; lack of normal fear of humans) are more likely.

Pathology

The virus has an affinity for nervous tissue. It travels from the site of entry via peripheral nerves to the spinal cord and the brain, where it multiplies; subsequently, it continues through efferent nerves to the salivary glands and into the saliva. Postmortem examination shows vessel engorgement and associated punctate hemorrhages in the meninges and brain; microscopic examination shows perivascular collections of lymphocytes but little destruction of nerve cells. The presence of intracytoplasmic inclusion bodies **(Negri bodies)**, usually in the cornu Ammonis, is pathognomonic of rabies, but these are not always found.

Symptoms and Signs

In man, the incubation period varies from 10 days to > 1 yr (average, 30 to 50 days). It is usually shortest in patients with extensive bites or bites about the head or trunk. The disease commonly begins with a short period of mental depression, restlessness, malaise, and fever. Restlessness increases to uncontrollable excitement, with excessive salivation and excruciatingly painful spasms of the laryngeal and pharyngeal muscles. The spasms, which result from reflex irritability of the deglutition and respiration centers, are easily precipitated—eg, by a slight breeze or an attempt to drink water. As a result, the patient cannot drink, though thirst is great (hence, "hydrophobia"). Death from asphyxia, exhaustion, or general paralysis previously occurred within 3 to 10 days, but with modern supportive care, the course may be altered.

Diagnosis

The fluorescent antibody test and virus isolation have replaced examination of the animal's brain for Negri bodies as the preferred method of diagnosis. An asymptomatic dog or cat that bites a human should, when practicable, be confined and observed by a veterinarian for 10 days. If the animal remains healthy, one can safely conclude that it was not infectious at the time of the bite. If the biting animal was apparently rabid or was a wild animal, it should be killed and its brain should immediately be submitted to a diagnostic laboratory, since a biting animal must be proved uninfected to avoid human treatment.

In patients, diagnosis is suggested by a history of a compatible animal bite (infrequently absent) and confirmed by viral testing once characteristic clinical symptoms appear. The diagnosis should be considered in patients with severe, progressive encephalitis or ascending paralysis with encephalitis. The latter presentation occurs in 20% of human rabies cases, appearing more often after exposure to rabid bats. Hysteria due to fright may follow a bite and give the impression of rabies, but the symptoms should subside promptly once the patient is assured that there is

no immediate danger and protection from rabies can be provided.

Control

Prevention and control require that dogs be restrained by their owners and stray dogs be impounded. Immunizing 70% or more of the canine population has effectively restricted transmission of the disease, even in areas where rabies is endemic among wildlife.

Controlling rabies in wildlife reservoirs is more difficult, especially when the wildlife host population is dense. Locally, rabies becomes self-limiting because it decimates susceptible hosts. Adequate systematic reductions of host species yield the same result and prevent spread; however, these expensive control efforts are best limited to locales where human contact with wildlife is high (eg, campgrounds).

Prophylaxis

Postexposure: Rabies rarely occurs in man if proper local and systemic prophylaxis is carried out immediately after exposure. **Local wound treatment** may be the most valuable preventive measure. The contaminated area should be cleansed immediately and thoroughly with a 20% solution of medicinal soft soap. Deep puncture wounds should be flushed with a catheter and soapy water. Cauterizing or suturing the wound is not advised.

Systemic postexposure prophylaxis (see TABLE 32–14) should be started immediately if (1) the animal is rabid or develops rabies during confinement or (2) a domestic animal that is not available for observation or examination was behaving in an atypical manner or its biting was unprovoked *and* rabies is present in the area. Among wild animals, skunks, raccoons, foxes, and bats are particularly suspect and, unless proved uninfected by examination, their bites generally necessitate rabies treatment. Rabbits and rodents (including squirrels, chipmunks, rats, and mice) are rarely infected, and their bites seldom justify rabies treatment. State or local health departments may be consulted on these decisions.

Administration of rabies immune globulin or antirabies serum for **passive immunization** followed by vaccine for **active immunization** gives the best specific postexposure prophylaxis. Both passive and active immunizing products should be used concurrently but never administered in the same anatomic site. The preferred products are rabies immune globulin **(RIG)** for passive im-

TABLE 32–14. RABIES POSTEXPOSURE PROPHYLAXIS GUIDE

Animal Type	Evaluation and Disposition of Animal	Postexposure Prophylaxis Recommendations*
Dogs and cats	Healthy and available for 10 days' observation	Do not begin prophylaxis unless animal develops symptoms of rabies[†]
	Rabid or suspected rabid	Vaccinate immediately
	Unknown (escaped)	Consult public health officials
Skunks, raccoons, bats, foxes, and most other carnivores; woodchucks	Regarded as rabid unless geographic area is known to be free of rabies or until animal proven negative by laboratory tests[‡]	Vaccinate immediately
Livestock, rodents, and lagmorphs (rabbits and hares)	Consider individually	Consult public health officials; bites of squirrels, hamsters, guinea pigs, gerbils, chipmunks, rats, mice, other rodents, rabbits, and hares almost never require antirabies treatment

* Clean bites with soap and water.

† During the 10-day holding period, begin treatment with rabies immune globulin (RIG) and human diploid cell vaccine (HDCV) or rabies vaccine, adsorbed (RVA) at first sign of rabies in a dog or cat that has bitten someone. The symptomatic animal should be killed immediately and tested.

‡ The animal should be killed and tested as soon as possible. Holding for observation is not recommended. Discontinue vaccine if immunofluorescence test results of the animal are negative.

Adapted from "Rabies Prevention—United States, 1991: Recommendations of the Immunization Practices Advisory Committee (ACIP)." *Morbidity and Mortality Weekly Report* 40(RR-3):1–19, 1991.

munization and human diploid cell rabies vaccine (HDCV) or rabies vaccine, adsorbed (RVA) for active immunization. HDCV produces a superior immune response and fewer adverse reactions than older vaccines. RVA has similar advantages and is given in generally the same manner and dosage as HDCV but *should not be given intradermally*. If RIG is unavailable, antirabies serum (ARS) of equine origin may be substituted; however, RIG is preferred because it has a lower risk of adverse reactions. For **passive immunization**, RIG is given only once—at the beginning of antirabies prophylaxis. The recommended dose is 20 IU/kg. If possible, up to $^1/_2$ of the total dose is infiltrated around the wound; the remainder is given IM. If ARS is used, 40 u./kg is given in the same manner.

Active immunization with HDCV or RVA should also begin immediately. The vaccine is given in a series of five 1-mL IM injections (the deltoid area is preferred) beginning on the day of exposure, followed by injections on days 3, 7, 14, and 28. Because antibody response has been uniformly satisfactory following this regimen, routine serologic testing is not recommended

unless the patient is thought to be immunosuppressed by disease or drugs. The World Health Organization also recommends that a 6th injection be given 90 days after the 1st injection. Local reactions at the injection site are usually minor, and systemic reactions are rarely associated with primary immunization. Prophylaxis should not be interrupted because of minor adverse reactions that can be managed with antihistamine, anti-inflammatory, and antipyretic agents; for serious systemic or neuroparalytic reactions, consideration should be given to evaluating the patient's risk of developing rabies before discontinuing vaccination. Testing the patient's serum for rabies antibody titer may provide essential information in such cases. Individual assistance in each situation may be sought from the state health department or the Centers for Disease Control, Atlanta, GA 30333.

Preexposure: Because of the relative safety of HDCV and RVA, prophylactic vaccination of persons with a high risk of exposure to rabid animals is justified. Such persons include those in frequent contact with potentially rabid animals (eg, veterinarians, animal handlers, spelunkers), laboratory workers handling tissues infected with rabies virus, and individuals who reside or stay for an extended period (> 30 days) in developing countries where rabies in dogs is prevalent. HDCV is given in the deltoid area in a series of three 0.1-mL intradermal injections, with the 2nd injection 7 days after the 1st, and the 3rd one 2 or 3 wk later. RVA is not given intradermally. Persons receiving RVA, or those who received chloroquine for malaria prophylaxis 30 days before or during the vaccination regimen, require 1-mL IM injections. Routine confirmation of antibody titer following these regimens is not required. However, any person with a continued high risk of exposure should have serum tested for antibody at 2-yr intervals and a booster dose of HDCV if the titer is inadequate. Hypersensitivity reactions, presumed to be type III, have occurred in about 5% of those given these booster doses. A previously immunized person (postexposure or preexposure regimen) bitten by a rabid animal should receive two 1-mL IM injections of vaccine, one dose immediately and another 3 days later. Passive immunization is not given. Preexposure immunization gives greater protection and reduces the postexposure regimen; it does *not* eliminate the need for prompt postexposure prophylaxis.

Treatment

If rabies develops, treatment is symptomatic. Vigorous supportive treatment is recommended, and expert consultation should be sought to assist in clinical management. Although death from rabies was once considered inevitable if symptoms developed, recovery has occurred following aggressive, vigorous, supportive treatment to control respiratory, circulatory, and CNS symptoms.

ACUTE VIRAL ENCEPHALITIS AND ASEPTIC MENINGITIS

Encephalitis: *An acute inflammatory disease of the brain due to direct viral invasion or to hypersensitivity initiated by a virus or other foreign protein.* **Encephalomyelitis:** *The same disorder affecting spinal cord structures as well as the brain.* **Aseptic meningitis:** *A febrile meningeal inflammation characterized by CSF mononuclear pleocytosis, normal glucose, mild elevations in protein, and an absence of bacteria on examination and culture.*

Etiology

Viral infection may cause encephalitis as a primary manifestation or as a secondary complication. Viruses causing **primary encephalitis** may be epidemic (arbo-, polio-, echo-, and coxsackieviruses) or sporadic (herpes simplex, varicella zoster, mumps). Mosquito-borne arboviral encephalitides (St. Louis, eastern and western equine, and California) infect man only during warm weather (see below).

Secondary encephalitis, usually a complication of viral infection, is considered to have an immunologic mechanism. Examples are the encephalitides following measles, chickenpox, rubella, smallpox vaccination, vaccinia, and many other less well defined viral infections. These **parainfectious** or **postinfectious encephalitides** (sometimes called **acute disseminated encephalomyelitis**) typically develop 5 to 10 days after onset of illness and are characterized (at autopsy) by perivascular demyelination; a virus has rarely been isolated from the brain. In mumps, both primary and postinfectious CNS involvement may occur.

Meningitis with CSF findings of pleocytosis, normal glucose, and no evidence of bacterial organisms (hence, "aseptic") may be caused by infections from viruses (see also ENTEROVIRAL DISEASES, above) and other organisms as well as noninfectious causes (see TABLE 32–15).

Very rarely, encephalitis or other encephalopathies occur as a late consequence of viral infections. The best known of these are **subacute sclerosing panencephalitis (SSPE,** see above), associated with the measles virus; **kuru,** a "slow virus" infection seen in New Guinea, and **Creutzfeldt-Jakob disease,** a rare dementia of middle age transmitted by a slow virus.

Pathology

Cerebral edema is present, and numerous petechial hemorrhages are scattered throughout the hemispheres, brainstem, cerebellum, and occasionally the spinal cord. Direct viral invasion of the brain is likely to be associated with neuron necrosis, and, frequently, with visible inclusion bodies. In para- and postinfectious encephalomyelitis, perivenous demyelinating lesions are characteristic.

Symptoms and Signs

CNS viral infections may take 3 forms: (1) **Asymptomatic:** Fever and malaise may be present without meningeal signs. However, the CSF may be abnormal, with lymphocytic pleocytosis,

TABLE 32-15. CAUSES OF ASEPTIC MENINGITIS (INCLUDING COMMON ENCEPHALITIDES)

Infectious causes

Viral: Mumps, echovirus, poliovirus, coxsackievirus, lymphocytic choriomeningitis, herpes simplex, varicella zoster, eastern and western equine encephalitis, St. Louis encephalitis, infectious hepatitis, infectious mononucleosis, HIV

Postinfectious: Measles, rubella, varicella, smallpox, vaccinia

Bacterial: TB, syphilis, partially treated bacterial meningitis

Miscellaneous infections: Leptospirosis, toxoplasmosis, torulosis, trichinosis, syphilis, coccidioidomycosis, mycoplasma, lymphogranuloma venereum, cat-scratch disease, brucellosis, rickettsia, cysticercosis, malaria, amebas, cerebral Whipple's disease

Noninfectious causes

Parameningeal disease: Brain tumor, stroke, multiple sclerosis, abscess, chronic sinusitis or otitis

Reaction to intrathecal injections: Chemotherapeutic agents, antibiotics, iophendylate and other dyes, air

Poison: Lead

Vaccine reactions: Many, especially rabies, pertussis, smallpox

Meningeal disease: Sarcoidosis, meningeal leukemia, meningeal carcinomatosis

Drugs: Trimethoprim/sulfamethoxazole, azathioprine, carbamazepine, NSAIDS (eg, ibuprofen, naproxen)

and (rarely) a virus may be isolated from the CSF. (2) **Meningitis:** Fever, headache, vomiting, malaise, and stiff neck and back may predominate. (3) **Encephalitis:** Meningitis may be associated with cerebral dysfunction (alteration in consciousness, personality change, seizures, paresis) and cranial nerve abnormalities. The distinction between aseptic meningitis and encephalitis is based on the extent and severity of cerebral dysfunction, independent of signs of meningeal inflammation.

Diagnosis

Viral CNS infections must be differentiated from other infectious and noninfectious causes (see TABLE 32-15); the major problem is to distinguish viral from acute or partially treated bacterial meningitis (see ACUTE BACTERIAL MENINGITIS under BACTERIAL INFECTIONS, above). Diagnosis usually is based on the CSF characteristics, including normal glucose and failure to grow bacteria on culture. Viruses occasionally are isolated directly from the CSF or from other tissues, but even ideally, viruses causing aseptic meningitis and encephalitis are identified in fewer than half the cases. Precise diagnosis usually requires the use of paired sera documenting a rise in specific antibodies. Culture of peripheral sites (eg, nasopharynx, stool) may be helpful, as is attention to epidemic agents in the community. Since many forms of encephalitis and aseptic meningitis have important public health implications, serum

should be drawn and preserved whenever the diagnosis of encephalitis or aseptic meningitis of uncertain etiology is first suspected. Information regarding more precise viral diagnosis can be obtained from local departments of health.

Although **herpes simplex encephalitis** is clinically similar to other viral encephalitides, repeated seizures occurring early in the course, and localizing signs indicating temporal or frontal lobe involvement, strongly suggest herpes simplex as the cause. The presence of RBCs in the CSF following an atraumatic spinal tap also suggests herpes simplex infection. The virus is rarely isolated from the CSF, and although paired sera may detect a rise in herpes simplex IgM during the first 10 to 12 days of illness, the serologic changes occur too late for any practical use in making therapeutic decisions. MRI, however, may detect temporal lobe inflammation before EEG, CT, or radionuclide brain scanning and can prompt antiviral therapy before neurologic deterioration occurs. MRI can also exclude brain abscess, subdural empyema, subdural hematoma, tumor, and sagittal sinus thrombosis, which can clinically mimic viral encephalitis. Brain biopsy can establish the diagnosis (by recovery of the virus or by its immunologic detection) but its morbidity must be justified on a case-by-case basis against the relatively low morbidity of acyclovir therapy (see below). Biopsy is usually indicated only in patients with an undiagnosed lesion on CT or MRI and a poor response to acyclovir.

Prognosis and Treatment

Even desperately ill patients may recover completely. The mortality rate varies with the etiology, and epidemics with the same virus vary in severity in different years. Permanent cerebral sequelae are more likely to occur in infants, but young children show improvement over a longer period than adults with similar infections.

Acyclovir 10 mg/kg IV q 8 h must be started promptly (before the patient lapses into coma) and continued for at least 10 days to derive a maximal therapeutic benefit. Acyclovir is relatively nontoxic, but can cause abnormal liver function, bone marrow suppression, and transient renal failure. To avoid nephrotoxicity, acyclovir should be given IV slowly over 1 h.

Supportive therapy is as for acute bacterial meningitis (see above). Fluid balance should be maintained but overhydration avoided.

ARBOVIRUS ENCEPHALITIDES

The arboviruses (**ar**thropod-**bo**rne viruses) number > 250; at least 80 immunologically distinct arboviruses cause disease in humans. Arboviruses are transmitted among vertebrates by biting insects, chiefly mosquitoes and ticks. Birds are often sources of infection for mosquitoes, which then transmit the infection to horses, other domestic animals, and humans. Man is a "dead-end" host (ie, incidental to the natural cycle and ineffective in virus perpetuation) for most of the agents but a definitive host (ie, part of the natural cycle and necessary for transmitting the infection) in urban yellow fever, phlebotomus fever, chikungunya, and dengue. The agents are widely distributed throughout the world, depending on the availability of lower vertebrate hosts and appropriate vectors.

In the USA, western equine encephalitis (WEE) occurs throughout the country in all age groups, but a disproportionate number of cases occur in children < 1 yr old. Eastern equine encephalitis (EEE) occurs in the eastern USA, mainly in young children and persons > 55 yr, and has a higher mortality rate than WEE. In children < 1 yr old, WEE and EEE tend to be severe, with permanent neurologic sequelae. Epidemics of both WEE and EEE are associated with epizootics in horses. Urban and rural outbreaks of St. Louis encephalitis have occurred throughout the USA; morbidity and mortality are greatest in older age groups. The California encephalitis virus group is distributed primarily in the North Central States and New York and affects mainly children in rural or suburban areas.

Symptoms, Signs, and Treatment

Arboviruses may cause CNS syndromes (including aseptic meningitis and encephalitis), minor nonspecific febrile illnesses, and most commonly, inapparent infection. Except in epidemics, the clinical findings in meningitis and encephalitis rarely permit specific identification. Headache, drowsiness, fever, vomiting, and stiff neck are the usual presenting symptoms. Tremors, mental confusion, convulsions, and coma may develop rapidly. Paralysis of the extremities occasionally occurs. Ribavirin IV (2-gm loading dose followed by 1 gm q 6 h for 4 days, then 0.5 gm q 8 h for 6 days) is effective in Lassa fever, Korean hemorrhagic fever, Rift Valley fever, and Crimean-Congo hemorrhagic fever. Treatment for most is supportive, as in other viral encephalitides (see above).

MISCELLANEOUS INFECTIONS

FEVER OF UNKNOWN ORIGIN (FUO) IN CHILDREN

A rectal temperature (or its equivalent) of 38.5° C (101.3° F) or higher measured on at least 4 occasions over a minimum period of 2 wk. This definition excludes most of the brief, self-limited, febrile illnesses that account for about 30% of pediatric outpatient visits in the USA. FUO in children is not as well delineated as that in adults because of a paucity of data, but certain differences are apparent.

Etiology

As with FUO in adults, the etiology of FUO in children depends partly on locale; the data presented here are derived from children living in the temperate zone of the USA.

Infection accounts for about 50% of FUO in children; in almost 50% of these cases, viruses are the presumptive cause. The type of infection varies with age: Upper respiratory tract and viral infections are most common in children < 2 yr, while endocarditis and infectious mononucleosis are more common in those > 6 yr. Of all children with an FUO due to infection, 65% are ≤ 6 yr old. Children tend to have more viral and common bacterial diseases, whereas TB, occult abscesses, and diseases from less common organisms are more likely to occur in adults.

Collagen-vascular diseases (CVD) account for about 20% of FUO in children. Again, age helps in differential diagnosis. Of the children with CVD who present with FUO, including almost all of those with inflammatory bowel disease (Crohn's disease of the small or large intestine, ulcerative colitis), 80% are > 6 yr. Juvenile RA is also a common cause of FUO in children with CVD.

Neoplasia causes 10% of FUO in children (leukemia being the most common disease) and affects children of all ages. In adults, neoplasia accounts for 20% of FUO, with solid tumors predominating (eg, lymphoma, disseminated carcinomatosis).

Miscellaneous causes (eg, milk allergy, Behçet's and diencephalic syndromes, thyroiditis) account for about 10% of FUO in children. The cause of FUO remains **unknown** in about 15% of children (7% of adults), despite exhaustive diagnostic investigation.

Symptoms, Signs, Diagnosis, and Prognosis

Nonspecific symptoms (eg, anorexia, weight loss, fatigue, chills, sweats) are common and have little differential diagnostic or prognostic value. In contrast, cutaneous symptoms and signs (eg, pruritus, rash, pigmentary changes) are more likely to signal a serious illness (malignancy or CVD) with a poor prognosis. Chest pain, dyspnea, significant heart murmur, arthropathy, and cyanosis are similarly associated with serious underlying diseases (eg, bacterial endocarditis, SLE). Localized findings are present in only 60% of patients with FUO but in nearly all patients with a fatal outcome.

Rare diseases are uncommon causes of FUO in children; in > 85% of cases, a cause can be pinpointed—usually a common childhood disease. Sophisticated, often invasive, and usually expensive diagnostic procedures requiring hospitalization are needed less often in evaluating children than adults with FUO.

Routine CBC, urinalysis, and chest x-ray are not often helpful in detecting a serious illness or identifying a specific cause of FUO. On the other hand, an elevated ESR and reversed albumin: globulin ratio are found in about 75% of patients with CVD or malignancy, while only 10% of patients with viral or benign illnesses have these abnormalities.

The physician's skills in obtaining a history, performing a physical examination, selecting laboratory screening tests, and synthesizing available clinical information are especially important in evaluating the child with FUO; the data obtained suggest further diagnostic evaluation. Bone marrow examination may be particularly helpful in diagnosing infection (by culture, particularly in *Salmonella* infections) or certain malignancies; it may reveal plasma cell predominance, suggesting CVD, or show an increase in the myeloid:erythroid ratio, suggesting infection. Tissue biopsies (eg, lymph node, skin lesions) are diagnostic in about 40% of children. Laparotomy and selective angiographic and radioisotopic techniques are needed less frequently for diagnosis in children than in adults (although they may be helpful in selected patients), primarily because of the different causes of FUO in children. Ultrasonography, CT, and gallium 67 scanning help to define lesions usually already suspected on clinical grounds and should be used selectively in this way rather than for screening patients in diagnostic evaluations of FUO.

At some time during their illness, 80% of children with FUO receive antibiotics and nearly 100% receive antipyretics. These therapies are not generally helpful in diagnosis, as they may mask the underlying process.

Prognosis is related to the underlying cause. The rate of expected complete recovery for children with FUO due to infection is 90%; due to CVD, 10%; due to undiagnosed causes, 33%. In malignancy, the outcome depends on the type and stage of the tumor when the diagnosis is made.

REYE'S SYNDROME

The syndrome of acute encephalopathy and fatty infiltration of the viscera that tends to follow some acute viral infections.

Reye's syndrome was first characterized as a distinct clinical and pathologic entity in 1963. The cause is unknown, but viral agents (eg, influenza A or B, varicella virus), exogenous toxins (eg, *Aspergillus flavus* aflatoxin), salicylates, and intrinsic metabolic defects have been implicated as associated or interrelated factors.

Epidemiology

The syndrome usually is seen in children under age 18 yr but has occasionally been reported in patients in their 6th or 7th decade. In the USA, most cases occur in late fall and winter. Both geographic and temporal clusters, as well as sporadic cases, have been described. Widespread outbreaks have occurred in association with influenza and varicella. Epstein-Barr, entero-, and myxoviruses have been associated with sporadic cases. In Thailand, the syndrome has been associated with aflatoxin ingestion. An increased incidence among siblings has been noted, but whether environmental factors (eg, common exposure to exogenous toxins or viruses) or genetic predispositions (eg, an inherited enzyme deficiency) account for the familial clustering is unknown. Salicylate use during an acute influenza illness can increase the risk for developing Reye's syndrome by as much as 35-fold. In fact, the use of salicylates in persons under 18 yr of age, except for a few specific diseases, is considered dangerous because of its predisposition to development of Reye's syndrome.

Pathology

With light microscopy, uniform intracytoplasmic panlobular microvesicular fatty infiltration of the liver is seen, which stains with oil-red-O (a Sudan dye) on frozen section. Fatty accumulation in the pancreas, heart, kidney, spleen, and lymph nodes, and pulmonary histiocytes have also been described. Fatty infiltration is thought to be neutral lipid (probably triglyceride), and hepatic inflammation is generally absent or slight. An occasional patient, especially one who has had significant hypotension, may show zonal hepatic necrosis, typically central in the hepatic lobule. On electron microscopy, sections of liver show mitochondrial injury that varies with the severity of the disease but includes glycogen depletion, smooth endoplasmic reticulum proliferation, peroxisome damage, and mitochondrial matrix swelling. Histologic abnormalities of the liver usually return to normal by 8 to 12 wk after onset of the disease.

CNS findings are generally nonspecific and include cerebral edema, gyral flattening, swollen white matter, and ventricular compression. On microscopy, perineuronal and perivascular clear spaces with swollen astrocytes are seen.

Symptoms and Signs

Severity of the disease varies greatly, but the syndrome is characterized by a biphasic illness: Initially a viral infection, usually a URI (occasionally exanthematous), is followed on about day 6 by the onset of *pernicious* nausea and vomiting and by a sudden change in mental status. When associated with varicella, the encephalopathy usually develops on the 4th to 5th day of the rash. The changes in mental status may vary from a mild amnesia and noticeable lethargy to intermittent episodes of disorientation and agitation that often progress rapidly to deepening stages of coma manifested by progressive unresponsiveness, decorticate and decerebrate posturing, seizures, flaccidity, fixed dilated pupils, and respiratory arrest. Focal neurologic findings are usually not present. Hepatomegaly occurs in about 40% of cases, but jaundice is rare.

Complications include electrolyte and fluid disturbances, diabetes insipidus, syndrome of inappropriate ADH secretion, hypotension, cardiac arrhythmias, bleeding diatheses (especially GI), pancreatitis, respiratory insufficiency, and aspiration pneumonia. In fatal cases, the mean time from hospitalization to death is 4 days.

Diagnosis and Laboratory Findings

Reye's syndrome should be suspected in any child exhibiting the acute onset of an encephalopathy (without known heavy metal or toxin exposure) *and pernicious vomiting associated with hepatic dysfunction.* Liver biopsy provides the definitive diagnosis and is especially useful in sporadic cases and young children. The diagnosis may also be made when the typical clinical findings and the history are associated with a constellation of laboratory findings: increased liver transaminases (AST [SGOT], ALT [SGPT] > 3 times normal), usually normal bilirubin, increased blood ammonia level, and prolonged prothrombin time. CSF examination usually shows increased pressure, < 8 to 10 WBC/μL, and normal protein values; the CSF glutamine level may be elevated. Hypoglycemia and hypoglycorrhachia are seen in 15% of cases, especially in children under age 4 yr.

Signs of widespread metabolic derangements also may be present, including elevated serum levels of the amino acids glutamine, alanine, lysine, and α-amino-N-butyrate and of the medium-chain free fatty acids; acid-base disturbances, usually hyperventilation with mixed respiratory alkalosis and metabolic acidosis; and other electrolyte abnormalities such as hyper- and hypo-osmolality, hypernatremia, hypokalemia, and hypophosphatemia.

Differential diagnosis includes other causes of coma and hepatic dysfunction, such as sepsis or hyperthermia (especially in infants); potentially treatable inborn abnormalities of urea synthesis or of fatty acid oxidation—eg, systemic carnitine deficiency or medium-chain acyl-CoA dehydrogenase **(MCAD)** deficiency, with episodic hypoglycemia and hyperammonemia; inborn errors of carbohydrate metabolism (also especially in infants); aminoacidurias (eg, lysinuric protein

TABLE 32–16. STAGING OF REYE'S SYNDROME

Signs	Stages				
	I	II	III	IV	V
Level of consciousness	Lethargy, follows verbal commands	Combative or stuporous	Coma	Coma	Coma
Posture	Normal	Normal	Decorticate	Decerebrate	Flaccid
Response to painful stimuli	Purposeful	Purposeful or nonpurposeful	Decorticate	Decerebrate	None
Pupillary reaction	Brisk	Sluggish	Sluggish	Sluggish	None
Doll's eyes (oculocephalic reflex)	Normal	Conjugate deviation	Conjugate deviation	Inconsistent or absent	None

From "NIH Consensus Development Conference, Diagnosis and Treatment of Reye's Syndrome." *Journal of the American Medical Association* 246:2441–2444, November 27, 1981.

intolerance); phosphorus or carbon tetrachloride intoxication; acute encephalopathy caused by salicylism or other drugs or poisons; viral encephalitis or meningoencephalitis; and acute hepatitis. Similar light microscopy findings on liver biopsy may be seen with idiopathic steatosis of pregnancy and tetracycline liver toxicity.

Prognosis

Outcome is related to the severity and rate of progression of coma, severity of the increased intracranial pressure, and degree of blood ammonia elevation. A recommended staging system for evaluating Reye's syndrome patients is shown in TABLE 32–16. Progression from stage I to higher stages can be anticipated when the initial blood ammonia level exceeds 100 μg/dL (60 μmol/L) and the prothrombin time is $\geq$ 3 sec longer than that of the control. Fatality rates average 21% but range from < 2% among patients in stage I to > 80% in patients in stage IV or V. Fortunately, most patients are diagnosed while in stage I, and early intervention is believed to ameliorate or prevent progression. Fatality rates are especially high in patients who have seizures, flaccidity, and respiratory arrest. Prognosis for survivors usually is good. Recurrences are uncommon. The incidence of neurologic sequelae (mental retardation, seizure disorders, cranial nerve palsies, motor dysfunction) is as high as 30% among those who developed convulsions or decerebrate posturing during hospitalization.

Treatment

Since the cause of the syndrome is uncertain and widespread metabolic derangements are

present, no universally accepted therapy exists. Early diagnosis and prompt institution of intensive supportive care are the mainstays of treatment. Meticulous and constant attention to the neurologic, electrolyte, metabolic, cardiovascular, respiratory, and fluid status is essential to cope with rapid changes. Treatment includes IV fluid and electrolyte solutions containing glucose, usually 5 to 10% but occasionally up to 50%; judicious use of cathartics and nonabsorbable antibiotics (eg, neomycin 100 mg/kg/day orally in divided doses q 6 h); and vitamin K_1 5 mg/day IV or IM. Increased intracranial pressure must be controlled with such agents as mannitol 0.5 to 1.0 gm/kg given IV over 45 min, dexamethasone 0.5 mg/kg/day IV, or glycerol 3 to 6 gm/kg/day by gastric tube; close monitoring of intracranial pressure may help to guide this therapy. Common procedures include monitoring arterial blood gas levels, blood pH, and BP by arterial catheters; inserting an endotracheal tube; and controlling ventilation. Other treatment modalities, eg, exchange transfusion, hemodialysis, and induction of deep coma with the use of barbiturates (to reduce intracranial pressure), have not been proved effective. Attempts to alleviate urea-cycle defects with agents such as L-carnitine are being evaluated.

SUBACUTE AND CHRONIC MENINGITIS

Meningeal inflammation (without antibiotic use) that lasts > 2 wk (subacute) or > 1 mo (chronic).

Etiology

Subacute and chronic meningitis may occur with fungal infections, TB, sarcoid, Lyme disease, AIDS, syphilis, and neoplasm (eg, leukemia, lymphomas, melanomas, carcinomas, and gliomas). Chronic meningitis must be distinguished from acute meningitis or encephalitis in which recovery is protracted and from recurrent meningitis (eg, craniopharyngioma leakage, posttraumatic).

The growing use of immunosuppressive therapy and the AIDS epidemic have increased the incidence of CNS fungal infections. *Cryptococcus* is the most common offender, complicating AIDS, Hodgkin's disease, lymphosarcoma, and chronic high-dose steroid therapy. *Coccidioides, Mucor, Candida, Actinomyces, Histoplasma*, and *Aspergillus* are encountered less often.

Neoplastic meningitis with diffuse leptomeningeal involvement is a continuing problem in acute lymphoblastic leukemia, especially in leukemic children being treated with antileukemic drugs, which do not cross the blood-brain barrier. Neoplastic meningitis also may occur with gliomas (particularly glioblastoma, ependymoma, or medulloblastoma) or with carcinoma metastatic to the brain. Rarely, the first sign of malignant disease may be a subacute meningeal inflammation.

Symptoms and Signs

Manifestations are similar to those in acute meningitis, but the illness evolves more slowly—over weeks rather than days. Fever may be minimal. In neoplastic meningitis, headache, dementia, backache, and cranial and peripheral nerve palsies are common. Chronic communicating hydrocephalus may be a complication. The course may be progressive and fatal within a few weeks or months.

Diagnosis

Because of the slow evolution of cerebral symptoms, the differential diagnosis includes structural lesions (eg, brain tumors, abscesses, and subdural effusions). Active TB elsewhere in the body or a known malignancy suggests the etiology, but the CSF must be examined to establish a diagnosis unless contraindicated by evidence of increased intracranial pressure from an expanding lesion. The CSF cell count is generally < 1000/μL with lymphocytes predominant; glucose frequently is low except in syphilis, and protein may be high. Besides lymphocytic pleocytosis, CSF findings in neoplastic meningitis include low glucose, slightly elevated protein, and (frequently) elevated pressure; at times tumor cells may be found. Microscopic examination or culture of the CSF is needed to identify malignant cells or a causative organism. Fungi often can be identified by examination of a centrifuged sediment, TB by acid-fast or immunofluorescence staining. In syphilis, CSF pressure, cell count, and protein resemble findings in other subacute meningitides, but the CSF glucose usually is normal; CSF and blood Venereal Disease Research Laboratory (VDRL) tests and STS are positive in most patients. Since most causative infections must be treated over a prolonged period with highly specific drugs, precise identification of the organism is essential before therapy is begun.

Treatment

Syphilitic meningitis: See Ch. 21. **Lyme disease:** See under BACTERIAL INFECTIONS, above. **Leukemic meningitis:** See THE ACUTE LEUKEMIAS in Ch. 35.

Sarcoid meningitis: Prednisone 80 mg/day orally is given for 3 wk, then decreased by 5 mg/day every 3 days.

Actinomyces **meningitis:** The drug of choice is penicillin G, 20 million u./day IM or IV (200,000 u./kg/day divided q 4 h for children), given for at least 6 wk. Treatment may be continued for an additional 2 to 3 mo with penicillin V, 100 mg/kg/day orally divided q 6 h.

Fungal meningitis: Amphotericin B is the drug of choice for all fungi and yeasts. Starting at a 1-mg test dose, amphotericin B is given by slow IV infusion in gradually increasing doses up to 1 mg/kg/day as tolerated. (CAUTION: *Daily dosage should not exceed 1 mg/kg for adults or children.*) A total of 2 to 6 gm usually is given, but the optimal total dose is uncertain. For children, amphotericin B 0.25 mg/kg IV; a test dose is given in a 6-h infusion of 0.1 mg/mL in 5% D/W. The daily dosage is increased by 0.25 mg/kg to the maximum of 1 mg/kg. Treatment duration need not be > 10 wk if the blood level of amphotericin B can be maintained at a concentration at least twice that needed to inhibit growth of the fungus in culture. Although hazardous, intrathecal or intraventricular (via Ommaya reservoir) amphotericin B sometimes is necessary to eradicate the infection. **Cryptococcal meningitis:** The treatment of choice is a combination of amphotericin B 0.3 mg/kg plus 5-flucytosine 150 mg/kg/day divided q 6 h for 6 wk.

Fluconazole, a new antifungal drug, is effective against cryptococcal meningitis. It is less toxic than amphotericin B or flucytosine, and oral doses produce peak plasma concentrations that are comparable to IV doses. Whether fluconazole is more effective than amphotericin B (with or without flucytosine) is under study. The dosage is 400 mg on the first day, followed by 200 to 400 mg once/day for 10 to 12 wk after the CSF becomes negative. A maintenance oral dosage of 200 mg/day can prevent relapses (eg, in AIDS patients). A small number of children (> 3 yr old) have been safely treated with 3 to 6 mg/kg/day, but efficacy has not been established.

SUBDURAL EMPYEMA

A collection of pus between the dura and the arachnoid membranes.

Etiology and Pathology

Most cases are complications of sinus infections (especially frontal and ethmoid) but others follow ear infections, cranial trauma or surgery, and bacteremia due to pulmonary infections. The pathogens are similar to those causing brain abscess. In children < 5 yr old, subdural empyema is usually due to bacterial meningitis (eg, *Hemophilus influenzae*, gram-negative bacilli in neonates).

Symptoms, Signs, and Diagnosis

Headache, lethargy, focal neurologic deficits, and seizures evolve over several days and, without treatment, progress rapidly to coma and death. As with brain abscess, LP provides little useful information and may precipitate transtentorial herniation. CT and MRI are diagnostic. A subdural tap may be diagnostic in infants. Careful anaerobic cultures of blood and surgical specimens improve diagnostic yield and antibiotic management.

Treatment

Measures to reduce intracranial pressure (see cerebral edema under Treatment of ACUTE BACTERIAL MENINGITIS, above) should be coupled with immediate surgical drainage of the empyema (and of the underlying sinus to prevent recurrence). Pending culture results, antibiotic coverage is the same as for brain abscess except in young children, who require antibiotic coverage for the accompanying meningitis (see TABLE 32–2).

KAWASAKI SYNDROME
(Mucocutaneous Lymph Node Syndrome [MLNS])

A syndrome occurring usually in infants and children < 5 yr of age, consisting of a characteristic exanthem, enanthem, fever, lymphadenopathy, and polyarteritis of variable severity.

Etiology, Epidemiology, and Pathology

The etiology is unknown. Since the syndrome was first described in Japan in the 1960s, thousands of cases have been reported worldwide in diverse racial and ethnic groups, although children of Japanese descent have a higher incidence. Most patients are 2 mo to 5 yr of age, but the syndrome has also been reported in individuals up to 34 yr. The male:female ratio is about 1.8:1. No clear-cut seasonal or geographic pattern has been observed. In Japan, it has been suggested that genetic factors affect susceptibility to the syndrome; the histocompatibility antigen HLA-Bw22 was found in these patients about twice as often as in the general population (25% vs. 12%), but no single HLA antigen is common to all cases. Several persons in the same household can be affected. The estimated risk for a secondary case among siblings is 2% (8 to 9% for those < 2 yr of age).

The pathology is nearly identical to infantile periarteritis nodosa, with vasculitis primarily affecting large and medium-sized arteries. There is a particular predilection for the coronary vessels. An immunologic basis for the pathologic findings is suspected.

Symptoms and Signs

The illness tends to progress through stages, beginning with fever, usually remittent and > 39° C (102.2° F), associated with irritability, often lethargy, and occasional intermittent, colicky abdominal pain. Usually within a day of fever onset, a polymorphous, erythematous macular rash appears, primarily over the trunk, especially in the perineal region. The rash varies morphologically and may be urticarial. This is followed within several days by mucous membrane changes, including injected pharynx; reddened, dry, fissured lips; bilateral conjunctival injection; and a red strawberry tongue.

The most characteristic changes occur in the distal parts of the extremities. During the first week of illness, pallor of the proximal portion of the fingernails or toenails (leukonychia partialis) may be apparent. Erythema or a purple-red discoloration and variable edema of the palms and soles usually appear on about the 3rd to 5th day of illness. While edema may be slight, it is often tense, hard, and nonpitting. Periungual, palmar, and plantar desquamation begins on about the 10th day after onset. The superficial layer of the skin sometimes comes off in large casts, revealing new, normal skin. Cervical lymphadenopathy ($\geq$ 1 node $\geq$ 1.5 cm in size) is often present throughout the course. The illness may last from 2 to 12 wk or longer, and relapses may occur.

The most feared additional manifestations include those related to the heart, which usually begin about the 10th day, as the rash, fever, and other early acute clinical features begin to subside; ie, in a subacute phase of the syndrome. Inflammation of the coronary arteries occurs in 5 to 20% of all cases, sometimes associated with acute myocarditis with heart failure, arrhythmias, pericarditis, cardiac tamponade, thrombosis, infarction, or development of coronary artery aneurysms.

Other findings indicate involvement of many systems. Arthritis or arthralgias (mainly involving large joints) occur in about 1/3 of patients. Other clinical features may include pneumonia, aseptic meningitis, diarrhea, and tympanitis. Less common manifestations are hepatitis, hydrops of the gallbladder, anterior uveitis, encephalopathy, pleural effusions, tonsillar exudate, and unusual exanthems—petechial or vesicular.

Laboratory Findings

Leukocytosis, frequently with a marked increase in immature (band) cells, is common in the acute phase of the illness. Other hematologic findings include a mild anemia, thrombocytosis ($\geq$ 500,000/μL) in the 2nd or 3rd wk of illness, and elevated ESR. Serum immunoglobulins are characteristically increased, particularly IgE. Serum complement and transaminase values are often mildly elevated.

Other laboratory abnormalities may be observed, depending on the organ systems involved; these include pyuria, proteinuria, CSF pleocytosis, and ECG changes (arrhythmias, decreased voltage, or left ventricular hypertrophy). *Echocardiography*, for detection of coronary artery aneurysms, should be performed in all patients in about the 5th wk. Coronary arteriography is useful in selected cases.

Cultures for bacteria and viruses, as well as serologic tests for evidence of infection, have been unrevealing. Some patients have shown positive antibody responses to *Proteus* Ox-19 or Ox-K antigens, but specific rickettsial serologic tests have been negative.

Diagnosis

This is based on the clinical findings and reasonable exclusion of other diseases. The diagnosis is accepted if fever of $\geq$ 5 days has occurred and 4 of the 5 following criteria are noted: (1) bilateral conjunctival injection; (2) changes in the lips, tongue, or oral mucosa (injection, drying, fissuring, strawberry tongue); (3) changes in the peripheral extremities (edema, erythema, desquamation); (4) polymorphous truncal exanthem; (5) cervical lymphadenopathy. Some children with atypical illnesses that do not meet these criteria have developed coronary artery aneurysms.

The **differential diagnosis** includes bacterial diseases (especially scarlet fever, staphylococcal exfoliative syndromes, and leptospirosis), viral exanthems (eg, measles), rickettsial disease (eg, Rocky Mountain spotted fever), toxoplasmosis, acrodynia, Stevens-Johnson syndrome, juvenile RA, and infantile periarteritis nodosa.

Prognosis

The overall case-fatality rate is estimated at 1 to 2% and is most commonly related to cardiac complications. Unfortunately, the fatalities are unpredictable; > 50% occur during the first month after onset, 75% within 2 mo, and 95% within 6 mo. Death, reported as long as 10 yr later, can be sudden and unexpected, occurring at any time. However, if no coronary artery disease can be demonstrated, the prognosis for complete recovery is excellent. Aneurysms tend to regress within 1 yr, although it is not known whether residual coronary lesions remain.

Treatment

There is no specific therapy. During the acute, febrile phase, aspirin 80 to 150 mg/kg in divided doses q 6 h is thought to reduce the risk of coronary artery involvement. Doses are adjusted to achieve serum levels of 20 to 25 mg/dL. Following the febrile phase, aspirin 5 to 10 mg/kg once daily has been recommended, primarily for its antithrombotic effect. The duration of aspirin therapy is guided by the clinical course and is usually continued for several months. ECGs should be checked frequently; some authorities recommend close follow-up with two-dimensional echocardiography and consideration of coronary angiography whenever a coronary aneurysm is suspected. If coronary aneurysms develop, anticoagulation therapy with warfarin and dipyridamole may decrease the risk for coronary artery thrombosis.

In Japan and the USA, multicenter controlled trials comparing treatment with aspirin alone and treatment with aspirin and a 4-day course of IV immune globulin (IVIG) 400 mg/kg/day demonstrated significantly fewer coronary artery lesions in the group that received IVIG. Equivalent results have been obtained with a single dose of 2 gm/kg of IVIG. Early suspicion, diagnosis, and treatment are critical in decreasing the risk of aneurysm.

Corticosteroids are not recommended as routine therapy, as they may increase the risk of coronary aneurysm development.

GIARDIASIS

An infection of the small intestine caused by Giardia lamblia, a flagellated protozoan. It is often asymptomatic, but clinical manifestations may range from flatulence to malabsorption.

Etiology and Epidemiology

The infection is found worldwide, especially in children and particularly where sanitation is poor; rates > 50% have been noted in day-care centers. Infection rates are also high among travelers, male homosexuals, and patients with gastrectomies, decreased gastric acidity, chronic pancreatitis, and immunodeficiencies. In the USA, giardiasis is one of the most common intestinal infections; about 7% of stools submitted for parasitologic examination contain *G. lamblia* cysts.

The *G. lamblia* trophozoite attaches itself to the duodenal and jejunal mucosa by a ventral sucker; it multiplies by binary fission. The organisms are passed in normal stool as cysts. In this resistant form, the disease is spread from host to host by fecal-oral routes, either directly (as between children or sexual partners) or indirectly (via food or water). Documented water-borne epidemics involve sources that range from remote mountain streams to chlorinated but poorly filtered community systems. Both humans and wild animals may serve as reservoirs.

Pathogenesis, Symptoms, and Signs

Symptoms are commonly mild, but intermittent nausea; eructation; flatulence; epigastric pain; abdominal cramps; bulky, malodorous stools; and diarrhea may occur. In severe cases, malabsorption can lead to significant weight loss. The severity of the malabsorption is related to the degree of infection, but the pathogenesis of these manifestations is unknown. Mechanical blockade of the microvilli, damage to their brush border, altered motility, and mucosal invasion resulting in T-cell–mediated mucosal damage have all been suggested as possible mechanisms.

Diagnosis

Finding the organism in the stool or duodenal secretions is diagnostic. In acute infections, the parasite can be readily found in the stool; in chronic cases, excretion is irregular, requiring repeated stool examination. Alternatively, duodenal contents—obtained with a nylon string (Enterotest®) or by endoscopic aspiration—can be examined for trophozoites.

Treatment

Of the drugs available in the USA for giardiasis, the most frequently recommended is quinacrine 100 mg tid for 5 days for adults; 2 mg/kg tid (maximum 300 mg/day) for 5 days for children. Although it is highly effective (70 to 95% cure rate), it may produce GI disturbances and, rarely, toxic psychosis. Metronidazole 250 mg tid for 5 days for adults (15 mg/kg/day in 3 divided doses for 5 days for children) is also effective and better tolerated, but it is not currently licensed for use in giardiasis. Furazolidone (100 mg qid for 7 to 10 days for adults, 6 mg/kg/day in 4 doses for 7 to 10 days for children) is less effective than either of these agents but is available as a suspension, making it useful in children. Tinidazole (unavailable in the USA) has been reported to effect a good cure rate in adults with one 2-gm dose given orally.

Household and sexual contacts should be examined and, if infected, treated. Pregnant women should be treated (with paromomycin) only if they show significant symptoms.

TOXOPLASMOSIS

A generalized or CNS disease caused by Toxoplasma gondii. Asymptomatic infections are common; serologic surveys show that 7 to 80% of various populations are infected. The infection occurs worldwide; those at risk for severe disease are the developing fetus and the immunocompromised.

Etiology and Pathogenesis

T. gondii is a small intracellular protozoan parasite that can infect any warm-blooded animal. It invades and multiplies asexually within the cytoplasm of nucleated host cells. With development of host immunity, multiplication slows and tissue cysts form. Sexual multiplication occurs in the intestinal cells of cats (and apparently only cats); oocysts form and are shed in the stool. Transmission may occur transplacentally, by ingestion of raw or undercooked meat containing tissue cysts, or by exposure to oocysts in soil contaminated with cat feces.

Symptoms and Signs

Neonatal congenital toxoplasmosis (see also CONGENITAL TOXOPLASMOSIS under NEONATAL INFECTIONS in Ch. 27) is acquired transplacentally, the mother presumably having acquired a primary infection during pregnancy. Abortion may ensue if infection occurs early in pregnancy. Infection later in pregnancy may result in miscarriage or stillbirth or in the birth of a living child with clinical disease. The disease may be severe, fulminating, and rapidly fatal, or it may be asymptomatic. Symptoms of subacute infection may begin shortly after birth but more often appear months or several years later. Common manifestations of congenital infection are chronic chorioretinitis, severe jaundice, hepatosplenomegaly, thrombocytopenic purpura, intracerebral calcification, convulsions, opisthotonos, psychomotor disturbances, and hydrocephalus or microcephaly. Blindness and severe mental retardation may result.

Acquired toxoplasmosis is seldom symptomatic and is usually recognized serologically. However, symptomatic infection may present in any of 4 ways:

1. The more common **mild lymphatic form** may resemble infectious mononucleosis. It is characterized by cervical and axillary lymphadenopathy, malaise, muscle pain, and irregular low fever, which can last for weeks or months but is almost always self-limited. Mild anemia, hypotension, leukopenia, lymphocytosis, and slightly altered liver function may be present. More commonly, it presents as asymptomatic cervical lymphadenopathy.

2. **Chronic toxoplasmosis** causes retinochoroiditis (posterior uveitis); other symptoms are often vague and indefinite, making diagnosis difficult.

3. An acute, **fulminating, disseminated infection**—often with a rash, high fever, chills, and prostration—occurs primarily in patients with compromised immunity. Some patients may develop meningoencephalitis, hepatitis, pneumonitis, or myocarditis.

4. **In patients with AIDS,** disseminated infection may occur, but toxoplasmosis (as a result of reactivation of latent infection) most often occurs as **encephalitis** and has become one of the most common causes of encephalitis in the USA. Manifestations may be focal (eg, hemiparesis, sensory loss, tremor) or generalized (eg, headache, confusion, coma).

Diagnosis

The diagnosis is usually established serologically. IgM antibodies, detected by the indirect fluorescent antibody **(IFA)** procedure (IgM-IFA), appear during the first 2 wk of illness, peak within 4 to 8 wk, and typically revert to normal within several months. IgG antibodies arise more slowly, peak in 1 or 2 mo, and may remain high and stable for months to years. They are measured with the IgG-IFA technique or with the Sabin-Feldman dye, indirect hemagglutination, or CF test. A positive IgM-IFA test or a four-fold rise in one of the IgG tests usually indicates acute disease, which should also be suspected if the IgG-IFA or dye test titers exceed 1:1000 in the presence of lymphadenopathy in a pregnant woman or encephalitis in an immunocompromised host.

In immunocompromised patients with CNS manifestations (predominantly **AIDS patients with encephalitis**), serum antibody tests are less useful. Since most of these patients have reactivation of latent infection, IgM antibodies are not present. IgG titers are usually low and may be unreliable in diagnosing acute infection. CT and MRI scans are the most useful tests. Typical findings on CT scan are multiple dense, rounded lesions, which form "ring-enhancing" lesions when contrast is used. MRI is more sensitive than CT scan. Although these lesions are not pathognomonic, when associated with CNS symptoms they provide sufficient evidence to warrant a trial of chemotherapy (see below).

The parasite has been isolated during the acute phase of the disease by inoculating mice or tissue cultures with biopsy material from lymph nodes, muscle, or other tissues. However, since this requires up to 6 wk for completion, it is not useful in initial patient management.

Prognosis

The prognosis is poor in congenital toxoplasmosis acquired during the first trimester. Often, affected children die in infancy or suffer chronic destructive CNS lesions. Infections acquired during the 3rd trimester are usually asymptomatic. The prognosis in acquired postnatal toxoplasmosis is good. The general mildness of postnatally acquired infection is indicated by the large number of persons with latent or cured toxoplasmosis and by the fact that the disease is rarely fatal in adults. Reactivation of toxoplasmosis in immunosuppressed patients is often fatal.

Treatment

Acute toxoplasmosis of newborns, pregnant women, and immunosuppressed patients should be treated with standard oral doses of trisulfapyrimidines or sulfadiazine (2 to 6 gm/day for adults, 100 to 200 mg/kg/day for children) plus pyrimethamine 25 to 50 mg/day for 3 to 4 wk for adults (for children, 2 mg/kg for 3 days, then 1 mg/kg/day to a maximum of 25 mg/day for 4 wk). Congenitally infected infants should be given pyrimethamine every 2 or 3 days and sulfonamide daily for up to a year. Relapses are so common in AIDS patients that treatment should continue indefinitely. The hematologic toxicity of pyrimethamine can be minimized by daily administration of folinic acid 10 mg (for children, 5 mg on alternate days). However, treatment in pregnancy is controversial. The risks to the fetus at its stage of development must be weighed against the potential benefits of the reduced risk of infection. Other patients with active disease do not require specific therapy unless a vital organ (eye, brain, heart) is involved or constitutional symptoms are severe and persistent. Corticosteroids given with specific therapy are often useful for controlling inflammation. Periodic blood counts are needed during therapy to monitor pyrimethamine hematotoxicity.

TOXOCARIASIS
(Visceral Larva Migrans)

A widely distributed clinical syndrome resulting from invasion of human viscera by nematode larvae (eg, Toxocara canis and T. cati, normally intestinal parasites of dogs and cats), with subsequent prolonged migration of the larvae through the body. It usually occurs as a relatively benign disease in children aged 2 to 4 but may afflict older persons as well.

Etiology and Pathogenesis

The fully embryonated parasitic egg develops in soil contaminated by feces of infected dogs and cats. Children's sandboxes, attractive defecating sites for cats, are a potential hazard. Eggs may be transferred either directly to the mouth as the child plays in or eats the contaminated soil (geophagia) or indirectly through contaminated

food or other objects. The incubation period varies from weeks to several months, depending on the intensity and number of exposures and on the patient's sensitivity.

The eggs hatch in the intestine after ingestion. Liberated larvae penetrate the intestinal wall and are widely disseminated by the systemic circulation. Almost any tissue may be involved, particularly the CNS, eye, liver, lung, and heart. The larvae may remain alive for many months, causing damage by migrating to and sensitizing tissue. They produce a focal granulomatous reaction, though the larvae themselves may be difficult to find in tissue sections. The parasites do not complete their development in the human body.

Symptoms, Signs, and Diagnosis

Patients present with fever, cough or wheezing, and hepatomegaly. Skin rash, splenomegaly, and recurrent pneumonia occur in some patients. Eye lesions that may be mistaken for retinoblastoma may be seen in older children and adults, usually without other manifestations.

Marked eosinophilia ($>$ 60%), hepatomegaly, pneumonitis, fever, and hyperglobulinemia suggest the diagnosis. Liver biopsy and finding of a larva or its fragments in the typical granulomatous lesion may be helpful. Reliable serologic tests have been developed.

Prognosis, Prophylaxis, and Treatment

The **prognosis** is good; the disease is self-limited (6 to 18 mo without reinfection). Infected pet dogs and cats, particularly those $<$ 6 mo old, should be dewormed regularly starting before 4 wk of age (under veterinary direction), and sandboxes should be covered when not in use.

No proven treatment is available. Mebendazole 200 to 400 mg orally for 5 days is probably the treatment of choice; diethylcarbamazine 2 mg/kg tid orally after meals for 2 to 4 wk may be helpful. Prednisone 20 to 40 mg/day orally, with reduced dosage after 3 to 5 days, helps to control symptoms.

PINWORM INFESTATION
(Enterobiasis; Oxyuriasis)

An intestinal infestation by Enterobius vermicularis *characterized by perianal itching.* The pinworm is the most common parasite infesting children in temperate climates. The prevalence of *Enterobius* in the general childhood population is at least 20%; for institutionalized children, it is as high as 90%.

Etiology

Infestation usually results from finger transfer of eggs from the perianal area to fomites (clothing, bedding, toys), from which the ova are picked up by the new host, transmitted to the mouth, and swallowed. Airborne eggs may be inhaled and then swallowed. Reinfestation (or autoinfestation) easily occurs through finger transfer of eggs from the perianal area to the mouth.

The parasites reach maturity in the lower GI tract within 2 to 6 wk. The female worm migrates to the perianal region (usually at night) to deposit her eggs within the skin folds. The sticky, gelatinous substance in which the ova are deposited and the movements of the female worm cause pruritus. The ova can survive for as long as 3 wk at normal room temperature. However, the larvae may hatch quickly and migrate back within the rectum and lower intestine (retroinfestation).

Symptoms and Signs

Most individuals who harbor pinworms have no symptoms or signs. Some will, however, experience perianal itching and develop excoriations in this area from persistent scratching. Vaginitis in young girls may be due to irritation from pinworms. Abdominal pain, insomnia, convulsions, and many other conditions have been attributed to pinworm infestation, but a causal relationship has not been demonstrated. Appendicitis due to obstruction of the appendiceal lumen by pinworms occurs rarely; the presence of the parasites may be only coincidental.

Diagnosis

Pinworm infestation can be diagnosed by finding the female worm, which is about 10 mm long (males average 3 mm), in the perianal region 1 or 2 h after the child has been put to bed for the night or by low-power microscopic identification of the ova. The 50×30-μg ova are oval-shaped with thin shells that contain the curled-up larvae. The ova are obtained in the early morning before the child arises by patting the perianal skin folds with a strip of transparent adhesive tape placed sticky side out over the end of a tongue depres-

sor. The tape is then put sticky side down on a glass slide. A drop of toluene between tape and slide dissolves the mucilage and eliminates the air bubbles in the tape that can hamper identification of the ova.

Prognosis and Treatment

Since the parasitic relationship is seldom harmful, prevalence is high, and reinfestation is probable, treatment is usually not indicated. However, most parents are upset by the concept of infestation and actively seek treatment, even when their children have had pinworms many times. A single dose of mebendazole 100 mg orally is effective in about 90% of cases. Pyrantel pamoate in 1 dose of 11 mg/kg (maximum 1 gm) given orally and repeated after 2 wk also eradicates pinworms in about 90% of cases. Retro- and reinfestation are likely, since ova may be deposited for as long as 1 wk following therapy, and the ova deposited in the environment before therapy can survive for 3 wk. Treatment of only one family member is useless, since multiple infestations within the household are the rule. Meticulous handwashing and housekeeping have little effect on the control or treatment of pinworm infestation.

Carbolated petrolatum or other antipruritic creams or ointments used topically in the perianal region 2 to 3 times daily may relieve the itching.

When infestation recurs, complete eradication of pinworms for a single family would be possible in most instances under the following extreme regimen: (1) all family members receive the therapeutic dose of pyrantel pamoate; (2) all members move out of their home for 3 wk, preferably taking a vacation, during which time they stay at a different place each night; and (3) pyrantel pamoate is given to all again at the end of 2 wk.

Since only 20% of the general childhood population harbor pinworms, and a large percentage of those who encounter this parasite never receive treatment, there must be unknown means by which an individual rids himself of *Enterobius* or the organism gives up its parasitic relationship with humans.

---

33. IMMUNODEFICIENCY DISEASES

A group of diverse conditions caused by one or more immune system defects, and characterized clinically by increased susceptibility to infections with consequent severe, acute, recurrent, and chronic disease.

An immunodeficiency disorder should be considered in anyone with infections that are unusually frequent, severe, and resistant; without a symptom-free interval; from an unusual organism; or with unexpected or severe complications.

TABLE 33-1. DISORDERS WITH INCREASED SUSCEPTIBILITY TO UNUSUAL INFECTIONS

Type of Disorder	Examples
Circulatory disorders	Sickle cell disease, diabetes, nephrosis, varicose veins, congenital cardiac defects
Obstructive disorders	Ureteral or urethral stenosis, bronchial asthma, bronchiectasis, allergic rhinitis, blocked eustachian tubes, cystic fibrosis
Integumentary defects	Eczema, burns, skull fractures, midline sinus tracts, ciliary abnormalities
Unusual microbiologic factors	Antibiotic overgrowth, chronic infections with resistant organism, continuous reinfection (contaminated water supply, infectious contact, contaminated inhalation therapy equipment)
Foreign bodies	Ventricular shunts, central venous catheter, artificial heart valves, urinary catheter, aspirated foreign bodies
Secondary immunodeficiencies	Malnutrition, prematurity, lymphoma, splenectomy, uremia, immunosuppressive therapy, protein-losing enteropathy, chronic viral diseases
Primary immunodeficiencies	X-linked agammaglobulinemia, DiGeorge syndrome, chronic granulomatous disease, C3 deficiency

Modified from Stiehm ER: *Immunologic Disorders in Infants and Children*, ed. 3. Philadelphia, WB Saunders Company, 1989, p 158.

Since immunodeficiency disorders are relatively uncommon, other conditions leading to recurrent infection should be considered first (see TABLE 33-1); if they can be excluded, a defect in host defense should be suspected.

PRIMARY AND SECONDARY IMMUNODEFICIENCIES

Immunodeficiencies may be either secondary or primary. **Secondary immunodeficiency:** *an impairment of the immune system resulting from an illness in a previously normal person.* The impairment may be reversible if the underlying condition or illness is rectified. Secondary immunodeficiencies are considerably more common than primary immunodeficiencies and occur in many hospitalized patients; indeed, nearly every prolonged serious illness interferes with the immune system to some degree. A classification of the secondary immunodeficiencies is shown in TABLE 33-2.

The primary immunodeficiencies (*defects of B, T, or phagocytic cells or complement*) are classified into 4 main groups, depending on which component of the immune system is deficient. Over 70 primary immunodeficiencies have been described, and considerable heterogeneity may exist within each disorder. A classification of the primary deficiencies is given in TABLE 33-3 (unusual variants are excluded).

T cell defects include several disorders with associated B cell (antibody [Ab]) defects, which is understandable since B and T cells originate from a common primitive stem cell and T cells influence B cell function. Phagocytic diseases include disorders in which the primary defect is one of cell movement (**chemotaxis**) and those in which the primary defect is one of microbicidal activity.

Incidence of the primary immunodeficiencies: B cell or Ab defects predominate; IgA deficiency (mostly asymptomatic) may occur in 1:400 individuals. Excluding asymptomatic IgA deficiency, B cell defects account for 50% of the primary immunodeficiencies; T cell deficiencies, about 30%; phagocytic deficiencies, 18%; and complement deficiencies, 2%. The overall incidence of *symptomatic* primary immunodeficiency is estimated to be 1:10,000; about 400/yr new cases occur in the USA. Since many primary immunodeficiencies are hereditary and congenital, they appear initially in infants and children; about 80% are < 20 yr old and, owing to X-linkage, 70% occur in males.

Etiology

Immunodeficiency has no common cause, although a single gene defect is often implicated: The defect can lead to absence of an enzyme (eg, adenosine deaminase deficiency), absence of a protein (eg, complement component deficiencies), or developmental arrest at a specific differ-

TABLE 33-2. THE SECONDARY IMMUNODEFICIENCIES

Premature and newborn infants	Physiologic immunodeficiency due to immaturity of immune system
Hereditary and metabolic diseases	Chromosome abnormalities (eg, Down syndrome) Uremia Diabetes mellitus Malnutrition Vitamin and mineral deficiencies Protein-losing enteropathies Nephrotic syndrome Myotonic dystrophy Sickle cell disease
Immunosuppressive agents	Radiation Immunosuppressive drugs Corticosteroids Anti-lymphocyte or anti-thymocyte globulin Anti-T-cell monoclonal antibodies
Infectious diseases	Congenital rubella Viral exanthems (eg, measles, varicella) Cytomegalovirus infection Infectious mononucleosis Acute bacterial disease Severe mycobacterial or fungal disease
Infiltrative and hematologic diseases	Histiocytosis Sarcoidosis Hodgkin's disease and lymphoma Leukemia Myeloma Agranulocytosis and aplastic anemia
Surgery and trauma	Burns Splenectomy Anesthesia
Miscellaneous	Lupus erythematosus Chronic active hepatitis Alcoholic cirrhosis Aging Anticonvulsant drugs Graft-vs.-host disease

ential stage (eg, pre−B-cell arrest in X-linked agammaglobulinemia). In certain illnesses, intrauterine events may be implicated (eg, maternal alcoholism in some cases of DiGeorge syndrome); in others, drug ingestion (eg, phenytoin in IgA deficiency). The exact biologic abnormality in most of the illnesses is unknown.

Symptoms and Signs

Most manifestations of immunodeficiency result from frequent infections, usually beginning with recurrent respiratory infections. (However, many immunologically normal infants have 6 to 8 respiratory infections per year, particularly when exposed to older siblings or other children.) Further, most immunodeficient patients eventually develop one or more severe bacterial infections that persist, recur, or lead to complications; eg,

sinusitis, chronic otitis, and bronchitis often follow repeated episodes of sore throat or URI. Bronchitis may progress to pneumonia, bronchiectasis, and respiratory failure, the most common cause of death. Infections with opportunistic organisms (eg, *Pneumocystis carinii* or cytomegalovirus [CMV]) may occur, particularly in patients with T cell deficiencies.

Infection of the skin and mucous membranes also is common. Resistant thrush may be the first sign of T cell immunodeficiency. Oral ulcers and periodontitis also are noted, particularly in granulocytic deficiencies. Conjunctivitis occurs in many Ab-deficient adults. Pyoderma, alopecia, eczema, and telangiectasia are common.

Common symptoms include diarrhea, malabsorption, and failure to thrive. The diarrhea usually is noninfectious but may be associated with

TABLE 33–3. CLASSIFICATION, INHERITANCE, AND ASSOCIATED FEATURES OF THE PRIMARY IMMUNODEFICIENCIES

Disorder	Associated Findings
B CELL (ANTIBODY) DEFICIENCIES	
X-linked agammaglobulinemia	
Ig deficiency with hyper-IgM (XL)	Neutropenia, lymphadenopathy
IgA deficiency	Autoimmunity; respiratory or food allergy; respiratory infection, often asymptomatic
IgG subclass deficiencies	IgA deficiency
Ab deficiency with normal or elevated Igs	
Immunodeficiency with thymoma	Aplastic anemia
Common variable immunodeficiency	Autoimmunity
Transient hypogammaglobulinemia of infancy	Prematurity
X-linked lymphoproliferative syndrome	Epstein-Barr virus infection
T CELL (CELLULAR) DEFICIENCIES	
Predominant T cell deficiency	
DiGeorge syndrome	Hypocalcemia, peculiar facies, aortic arch abnormalities, heart disease
Chronic mucocutaneous candidiasis	Endocrinopathies
Combined immunodeficiency with Igs (Nezelof syndrome)	
Nucleoside phosphorylase deficiency (AR)	Bronchiectasis
Combined T and B cell deficiencies	
Severe combined immunodeficiency (AR or XL)	
Combined Ig and adenosine deaminase deficiencies (AR)	Skeletal abnormalities
Reticular dysgenesis	Pancytopenia
Bare lymphocyte syndrome	Absence of HLA Ags
Ataxia telangiectasia (AR)	Dermatitis, neurologic deterioration
Wiskott-Aldrich syndrome (XL)	Eczema, thrombocytopenia
Short-limbed dwarfism	Cartilage-hair hypoplasia
PHAGOCYTIC DISORDERS	
Defects of cell movement	
Hyperimmunoglobulinemia-E syndrome	Eczema, dermatitis
Leukocyte adhesion deficiency	Prolonged attachment of umbilical cord, leukocytosis, periodontitis
Defects of microbicidal activity	
Chronic granulomatous disease (XL or AR)	Lymphadenopathy
G6PD deficiency (XL)	
Myeloperoxidase deficiency (AR)	
Chédiak-Higashi syndrome (AR)	Oculocutaneous albinism, giant granules of neutrophils
COMPLEMENT DISORDERS	
Defects of complement components	
C1q deficiency	Combined immunodeficiency, SLE-like syndrome
C1r ⎫	
C4 ⎪	SLE-like syndrome, glomerulonephritis
C2 ⎬	
C3	Pyogenic infections
C5 ⎫(ACD)	
C6 ⎪	
C7 ⎬	Neisserial infection
C8 ⎪	
C9 ⎭	
Defects of control proteins	
C1 inhibitor deficiency (AD)	Angioedema, SLE
Factor I (C3b inactivator) deficiency (ACD)	Pyogenic infections
Factor II deficiency (ACD)	Hemolytic-uremic syndrome, glomerulonephritis
Properdin deficiency (XL)	Neisserial infections

Ab = antibody; ACD = autosomal codominant; AD = autosomal dominant; Ag = antigen; AR = autosomal recessive; Ig = immunoglobulin; XL = X-linked.

Giardia lamblia, rotavirus, CMV, or *Cryptosporidium*. In some patients the diarrhea may be exudative with loss of serum proteins and lymphocytes.

Less common manifestations of immunodeficiency include hematologic abnormalities (autoimmune hemolytic anemia, leukopenia, thrombocytopenia), autoimmune phenomena (vasculitis, arthritis, endocrinopathies), and CNS problems (eg, chronic encephalitis, slow development, seizures).

Diagnosis

A **family history** should be obtained for early death, related disease, autoimmune illness, allergy, early malignancy, and consanguinity. If this history is positive, a pedigree chart will help identify a hereditary pattern. A **past history** of adverse reactions to immunizations or viral infections should be noted as well as prior surgery (eg, tonsillectomy, adenoidectomy), radiation therapy to the thymus or nasopharynx, and prior antibiotic and immune globulin therapies and their apparent clinical benefit.

The **type of infection** may give some clue as to the nature of the immunodeficiency. Infections with major gram-positive organisms (pneumococci, streptococci) are noted in Ab (B cell) immunodeficiencies. Severe infections from viral, fungal, and other opportunistic organisms are common in cellular (T cell) immunodeficiencies. Recurrent staphylococcal and gram-negative infections are common in phagocytic deficiencies. Recurrent *Neisseria* infection is characteristic of patients with several complement component deficiencies. Certain opportunistic infections (eg, from *P. carinii*, *Cryptosporidium*, or *Toxoplasma*) may occur in several types of immunodeficiency.

The **age of onset** also may help in diagnosis; infants < 6 mo old usually have a T cell defect. However, onset of illness around 6 mo of age, when transplacentally acquired maternal Ab has disappeared, suggests congenital Ab deficiency.

Physical examination: Patients with immunodeficiency often appear chronically ill, with pallor, malaise, malnutrition, and a distended abdomen. The skin may reveal macular rashes, vesicles, pyoderma, eczema, petechiae, alopecia, or telangiectasia. Conjunctivitis is common, particularly in adults. Cervical lymph nodes and adenoid and tonsillar tissue typically are absent in B or T cell immunodeficiency, despite a history of recurrent throat infections. This can be confirmed by a lateral pharyngeal x-ray, which may show absence of adenoidal tissue. Occasionally the lymph nodes are enlarged and suppurative. The tympanic membranes often are scarred and/or perforated. The nostrils may be excoriated and crusted, indicative of purulent nasal discharge. There may be a postnasal drip and a decreased gag reflex. Often there is a chronic cough. Rales are often present, especially in adults with lifelong immunodeficiency. The liver and spleen frequently are enlarged. Muscle mass is diminished and fat deposits of the buttocks are diminished. In infants there may be excoriation around the anus as a result of chronic diarrhea. Neurologic examination may reveal delayed developmental milestones or ataxia.

A **characteristic constellation of findings** permits a tentative clinical diagnosis in a number of immunodeficiency syndromes. These include **newborns with DiGeorge syndrome** who have infections, tetany, peculiar facies, and congenital heart disease; **boys with Wiskott-Aldrich syndrome** who have pyogenic infections, eczema, and bleeding manifestations; **children with ataxia-telangiectasia** who have recurrent sinopulmonary infections, ataxia, and telangiectasia; and **redheaded girls with the Job variant of the hyper-IgE syndrome** who have fair skin, eczema, and recurrent staphylococcal infections. These disorders are further discussed below.

Laboratory tests: In all cases of immunodeficiency, selected tests are needed to confirm or establish the diagnosis; advanced tests often are necessary to subclassify the disorder before rational therapy (see TABLE 33–4). In general, screening tests can be done in most offices and hospitals and advanced tests in most large hospitals, but specialized tests are available only in laboratories or hospitals with a sophisticated immunology laboratory.

When immunodeficiency is suspected, the screening tests recommended include a CBC with differential and platelet count; determination of IgG, IgM, and IgA levels; assessment of Ab function; and infection evaluation. The CBC will establish the presence of anemia, thrombocytopenia, neutropenia, or leukocytosis. The total lymphocyte count should be noted; lymphopenia (< 1500/μL) is suggestive of T cell immunodeficiency. The peripheral smear should be examined for the presence of Howell-Jolly bodies and other unusual RBC forms suggestive of asplenia or poor splenic function. The granulocytes may show morphologic abnormalities (eg, granules of the **Chédiak-Higashi syndrome**).

Although immunoglobulin (**Ig**) levels also are part of the initial screen, IgD and IgE levels are

TABLE 33–4. LABORATORY TESTS IN IMMUNODEFICIENCY

Screening Tests (Office)	Advanced Tests	Special Tests
B cell deficiency		
IgG, IgM, IgA levels	B cell enumeration	Lymph node biopsy
Isoagglutinin titers	IgD and IgE levels	IgG subclass levels
Preexisting Ab titers (tetanus,	Ab responses to vaccines	Ig survival
diphtheria, rubella, rubeola)	(eg, typhoid, pneumococcal,	Secretory Ig levels
Schick test	or *Hemophilus influenzae*	In vitro Ig synthesis study
	polysaccharide)	Ab response to special Ags:
	Lateral pharyngeal x-ray	φ phage Ag, KLH
	IgG subclass levels	
T cell deficiency		
Lymphocyte count and	T cell and T subset enumeration	HLA typing
morphology	(CD3, CD4, CD8)	Lymphokine assays (eg, IL-2,
Thymus size by x-ray	Lymphocyte proliferative	IFN)
Delayed skin tests:	responses to mitogens, Ags,	Enzyme assays (eg, ADA, NP)
Trichophyton, mumps,	allogeneic cells	Cytotoxic assays (eg, NK,
Candida, tetanus toxoid		ADCC, CTL)
		Thymic hormone assays
		Other T cell surface Ag
		analysis (eg, CD1, DR, CD25)
Phagocytic cell deficiency		
WBC count, morphology	Special morphology	WBC response to
NBT dye test	Rebuck skin window	epinephrine, steroids,
IgE level	Random mobility and	polysaccharides
	chemotactic assay	Chemoluminescence
	Quantitative intracellular killing	Enzyme assays—MPO, G6PD
	assay	Surface glycoprotein assays
		with monoclonal Abs
		(eg, CD 11 [CR 3])
Complement deficiency		
CH₅₀ activity	Classical and alternative	Serum opsonic or chemotactic
C3 level	complement activity assays	activity
C4 level	Component assays—immuno-	Complement breakdown
	chemical or functional	product analysis
	Inhibitor assays—immuno-	
	chemical or functional	

Ab = antibody; ADA = adenosine deaminase; ADCC = antibody-dependent cellular toxicity; Ag = antigen; C = complement; CD = clusters of differentiation; CTL = cytotoxic T lymphocyte; IFN = interferon; HLA = human leukocyte antigen; KLH = keyhole-limpet hemocyanin antigen; MPO = myeloperoxidase; NBT = nitroblue tetrazolium; NK = natural killer; NP = nucleoside phosphorylase.

Modified from Stiehm ER: *Immunologic Disorders in Infants and Children*, ed. 3. Philadelphia, WB Saunders Company, 1989.

not done initially. Ig must be interpreted with care because of marked alterations with age; all infants 2 to 6 mo old are hypogammaglobulin-emic by adult standards. Thus levels must be compared with normal levels from age-matched controls (see TABLE 33–5). In general, Ig levels within 2 standard deviations for age are considered normal. A total Ig level (IgG + IgM + IgA) > 600 mg/dL or an IgG level > 400 mg/dL with normal screening functional Ab tests excludes Ab deficiency. A total Ig level < 200 mg/dL usually indicates significant Ab deficiency. Intermediate levels (ie, IgG levels 200 to 400 mg/dL, and total

Igs 400 to 600 mg/dL) are nondiagnostic and must be correlated with functional Ab tests.

Screening Ab tests also are recommended for the initial screen. IgM function is estimated by isoagglutinin titers (anti-A and/or anti-B). All patients except young infants and individuals of blood type AB will have natural Abs at a titer of 1:8 (anti-A) or 1:4 (anti-B) or greater. Abs to these and certain bacterial polysaccharides are selectively deficient in certain immunodeficiencies (eg, Wiskott-Aldrich syndrome, IgG2 deficiency). In the immunized patient, Ab titers to poliovirus, rubella virus, tetanus, or diphtheria antigens

TABLE 33-5. LEVELS OF IMMUNOGLOBULINS IN SERA
OF NORMAL SUBJECTS BY AGE*

Age	IgG		IgM		IgA		Total Ig	
	mg/dL	% of Adult Level	mg/dL	% of Adult Level	mg/dL	% of Adult Level	mg/dL	% of Adult Level
Newborn	1031±200†	89±17	11±5	11±5	2±3	1±2	1044±201	67±13
1-3 mo	430±119	37±10	30±11	30±11	21±13	11±7	481±127	31±9
4-6 mo	427±186	37±16	43±17	43±17	28±18	14±9	498±204	32±13
7-12 mo	661±219	58±19	54±23	55±23	37±18	19±9	752±242	48±15
13-24 mo	762±209	66±18	58±23	59±23	50±24	25±12	870±258	56±16
25-36 mo	892±183	77±16	61±19	62±19	71±37	36±19	1024±205	65±14
3-5 yr	929±228	80±20	56±18	57±18	93±27	47±14	1078±245	69±17
6-8 yr	923±256	80±22	65±25	66±25	124±45	62±23	1112±293	71±20
9-11 yr	1124±235	97±20	79±33	80±33	131±60	66±30	1334±254	85±17
12-16 yr	946±124	82±11	59±20	60±20	148±63	74±32	1153±169	74±12
Adult	1158±305	100±26	99±27	100±27	200±61	100±31	1457±353	100±24

* The values were derived from measurements made in 296 normal children and 30 adults. Levels were determined by the radial diffusion technique, using specific rabbit antisera to human immunoglobulins.
† One standard deviation.
From Stiehm ER, Fudenberg HH: "Serum levels of immune globulins in health and disease: A survey." Pediatrics 37:715, 1966; reproduced by permission of Pediatrics.

(Ags) can be used to estimate IgG function. An adequate Ab response to one or more of these Ags is evidence against Ab deficiency. Finally, screening should include a search for chronic infection. The ESR often is elevated, usually in proportion to the degree of infection. Appropriate x-rays (chest, sinus, etc) and cultures should be done.

If all these screening tests are normal, immunodeficiency (particularly Ab deficiency) usually can be excluded. However, if chronic infection is documented, if the history is unusually suspicious, or if the screening tests are positive, advanced tests must be done.

Tests for B cell (Ab) deficiency: If Igs are very low (total < 200 mg/dL), a diagnosis of Ab deficiency is established, and other procedures are indicated only to define the exact illness and identify other immunologic defects. If Ig levels and preexisting Ab titers are low but not absent, the Ab responses to one or more standardized Ags should be assessed. Ab titers are obtained before and 3 to 4 wk after immunization with tetanus toxoid or typhoid vaccines (for protein Ag responsiveness) or after immunization with pneumococcal or unconjugated Hemophilus influenzae vaccine (for polysaccharide Ag responsiveness). An inadequate response (less than a four-fold rise in titer) is suggestive of Ab deficiency regardless of Ig levels.

If Igs are low, B cell enumeration is done by assessing the percentage of lymphocytes with surface membrane Igs by staining with fluoresceinated anti-Ig antisera or a B-cell specific monoclonal Ab (ie, anti-CD20). Normally, 4 to 10% of peripheral blood lymphocytes are surface membrane Ig-positive (B cells). Disorders associated with low or absent B cells are shown in TABLE 33-3.

Next, serum levels of IgG subclasses, IgD, and IgE are obtained. IgG1 subclass levels (like IgG levels) are strongly age dependent. In general, after the age of 2 yr, an IgG1 level < 280 mg/dL, an IgG2 level < 50 mg/dL, an IgG3 level < 30 mg/dL, or an undetectable IgG4 level must be present to diagnose an IgG subclass deficiency. IgD and IgE (both high and low levels) are common in incomplete Ab deficiency syndromes. IgE levels are high in chemotactic disorders, partial T cell immunodeficiencies, allergic disorders, and parasitism. Isolated absences of IgD and IgE are rare and not significant clinically.

Special tests for B cell deficiencies (see TABLE 33-4) are indicated in certain circumstances. A lymph node biopsy (sometimes preceded by immunization in the adjacent extremity) is indicated in the presence of lymphadenopathy or to exclude malignancy. IgG subclass determinations are indicated if IgG levels are normal or near normal but Ab function is deficient. Selective deficiencies of one of the 4 subclasses may be present. If there is a suspicion of rapid IgG catabolism or IgG loss through the skin or the GI tract, an IgG survival study may be indicated, using isotope-labeled IgG; or if the patient has low levels of IgG, a large dose of immunoglobulin is given IV (**IGIV**) and the IgG levels are measured daily to determine the half-life. If local infections are severe, Ig levels in secretions (eg, tears or saliva) can be done. In vitro IgG synthesis and the Ab response to special Ags (eg, ϕX phage Ag or keyhole-limpet hemocyanin [KLH]) are done to determine the exact location of the synthetic block.

Tests for T cell deficiency: The presence of profound and prolonged lymphopenia is suggestive of a T cell immunodeficiency; however, lymphopenia is not usually present. A chest x-ray is a useful screening test in an infant; an absent thymic shadow in the newborn period is suggestive of T cell deficiency, particularly if done before the onset of infection or other stress that may shrink the thymus.

Delayed hypersensitivity skin tests are valuable screening tests: Mumps Ag, *Candida* Ag (1:100), fluid tetanus toxoid (1:10), and *Trichophyton* Ag are used; nearly all adults and most immunized infants and children will react to one or more of these Ags with erythema and induration (> 5 mm) at 48 h. The presence of one or more positive delayed skin tests generally indicates an intact T cell system.

The most valuable advanced test in cellular immunodeficiency is T cell and T subset (helper/inducer and suppressor/cytotoxic) enumeration, usually done by flow cytometry using T-cell–specific monoclonal murine Abs. Total T cells are measured using a pan T cell Ab (eg, anti-CD3, anti-CD2), T helper/inducer cells are measured using an anti-CD4 Ab, and suppressor/cytotoxic cells are measured using an anti-CD8 Ab. (Such assays have in general replaced sheep-cell rosetting techniques to enumerate T cells.) A total T cell (CD3) count < 500 cells/μL is highly suggestive of a T cell immunodeficiency and a CD3 count < 200 cells/μL indicates a profound T cell immunodeficiency. The ratio of CD4/CD8 (helper/suppressor) cells should be > 1.0; reversal of this ratio also suggests T cell immunodeficiency (eg, in AIDS, a progressive decrease in the CD4/CD8 ratio indicates progressive immunologic impairment). Monoclonal Abs also are available to identify activated cells (DR-CD25), natural killer cells (CD16), and immature T cell (thymocyte) Ags (CD1).

Another useful advanced test measures the ability of the patient's lymphocytes to proliferate and enlarge (transform) when cultured in the presence of mitogens (eg, phytohemagglutinin, concanavalin A), irradiated allogeneic WBCs (in the mixed leukocyte reaction), or Ags to which the patient has been previously exposed. Under these stimuli, normal lymphocytes undergo rapid division; this can be assessed either morphologically or by uptake of radioactive thymidine into dividing cells. Proliferation usually is reported as an index—the ratio of counts/min (**CPM**) of stimulated cells to CPM of an equal number of unstimulated cells. Patients with T cell immunodeficiency have low or absent proliferative responses in proportion to the degree of immune impairment. The proliferative responses to mitogens (which activate all cells) are considerably higher (stimulation index, 50 to 100) than the response to Ags or allogeneic cells (stimulation index, 3 to 30).

Special procedures also assess lymphokine production after mitogen or Ag stimulation. Although > 30 lymphokines exist, the 2 usually assayed are interferon gamma (**IFN-γ**) and interleukin-2 (**IL-2**). Certain patients have adequate proliferative responses but deficient lymphokine production (eg, migration inhibition factor [**MIF**] deficiency in chronic mucocutaneous candidiasis). Another group of tests assesses cytotoxic function. Different types of cytotoxicity (natural killer, Ab-dependent, or cytotoxic T cell) are measured using different tumor-cell or viral-infected target cells. Cytotoxic defects are variably present in cellular immunodeficiency. In some forms of combined immunodeficiency, enzymes of the purine pathway (adenosine deaminase, nucleoside phosphorylase) are deficient and can be assayed with RBCs. Levels of various thymic hormones (thymosin, facteur thymique serique) can be assessed; these are low in certain cellular immunodeficiencies. HLA typing can be valuable for assessing the presence of 2 populations of cells (chimerism) and for excluding deficiencies of HLA Ags (**bare lymphocyte syndrome**).

Tests for phagocytic and complement deficiencies: An investigation is indicated when a patient with a convincing history of immunodeficiency has normal B and T cell immunity. A lack of pus formation at the site of inflammation and delayed umbilical cord detachment without leukopenia are clues suggestive of a **chemotactic defect.**

In addition to the blood count, initial screening should include an IgE level, which is elevated in many chemotactic disorders, and a nitroblue tetrazolium **(NBT)** dye reduction test for chronic granulomatous disease **(CGD)**, the most common phagocytic disorder. The NBT test is based on the increased metabolic activity of granulocytes during phagocytosis and killing with reduction of colorless NBT to blue formazan. This color change, absent in CGD, can be assessed visually, microscopically, or by spectrophotometry.

The first special test is staining of the granulocytes for myeloperoxidase, alkaline phosphatase, or esterase. Absence of staining for these enzymes should be followed by quantitative assays. Next, cell movement can be assessed by a Rebuck skin window in which the skin is superficially abraded with a scalpel and coverslips are placed over the site; these are removed and replaced at intervals, and stained for migrating cells. An initial influx of polymorphonuclear cells should occur within 2 h, and then be replaced by monocytes within 24 h. A chemotactic abnormality can be confirmed by an in vitro chemotactic assay in which migration of granulocytes or monocytes is measured, using either a special chemotactic chamber (Boyden) or an agarose plate; cell movement toward a chemoattractant (eg, opsonized zymosan) is assessed.

Next, phagocytosis is tested by measuring uptake of latex particles or bacteria by isolated granulocytes or monocytes. Microbial killing is then assessed by mixing the patient's granulocytes in fresh serum with a known number of live bacteria, followed by serial quantitative bacterial assays over a 2-h period.

Other specialized tests define phagocytic defects: assays of granulocyte mobilization after giving corticosteroids, epinephrine, or endotoxin; quantitative assays of granulocyte enzymes (myeloperoxidase, G6PD, etc); assays for granulocyte oxidant products (chemoluminescence, superoxide); and assays of specific granulocyte proteins (cytochrome b_{559}, CR3 [CD11] adhesive glycoproteins).

A **complement abnormality** is screened by measuring the total serum complement activity (CH_{50}) and serum C3 and C4 levels. Low levels of any of these should be followed by titration of the classical and alternative complement pathways and the measurement of individual complement components. These latter use monospecific antisera or sensitized RBCs and solutions that contain all components except for the one to be assessed.

Antisera also are available to measure complement control proteins; hereditary angioedema is associated with deficiency of C1 inhibitor, and C3 deficiency with C3 hypercatabolism is associated with deficiency of factor I (C3 inhibitor). Assays of serum opsonic activity, serum chemotactic activity, or serum bactericidal activity measure complement function.

Principles of Treatment

Prevention of primary immunodeficiency is limited to genetic counseling when identified genetic inheritance patterns are known. Prenatal diagnosis using cultured amniotic cells or fetal blood is feasible for a few of these disorders, including X-linked agammaglobulinemia, Wiskott-Aldrich syndrome, severe combined immunodeficiency, combined immunodeficiency with adenosine deaminase deficiency, and chronic granulomatous disease. Sex determination also can be used to exclude X-linked disorders. Heterozygote inheritance in several of these disorders can be detected.

General management: Patients with immunodeficiency require an extraordinary amount of care to maintain optimal health and nutrition, prevent emotional problems related to their illness, manage infections, and cope with costs. They should be protected from unnecessary exposure to infection, sleep in their own beds, and preferably have their own rooms. Killed vaccines should be given regularly if there is evidence of some Ab function. The teeth should be kept in good repair.

Antibiotics are lifesaving for treating infections; selection and dosage are identical to those used normally. However, because immunodeficient patients may succumb rapidly to infection, fevers or other manifestations of infection are assumed to be secondary to bacterial infection, and antibiotic treatment is begun immediately. Throat, blood, or other cultures are obtained before most therapy; these are especially important when the infection does not respond to the initial antibiotic chosen and when the infectious organism is unusual.

Continuous prophylactic antibiotics often are beneficial in immunodeficiencies, particularly when there is the risk of sudden overwhelming infection (eg, Wiskott-Aldrich syndrome, asplenic syndromes); when other forms of immune therapy are unavailable (eg, in phagocytic disorders) or insufficient (eg, recurrent infection in agammaglobulinemia despite immune globulin therapy); and when there is a high risk for a specific infection (eg, *P. carinii* in cellular immunodeficiency disorders).

Precautions: Patients with either B or T cell immunodeficiencies should not be given live vaccines (eg, poliovirus, measles, mumps, rubella, BCG) because of the risk of vaccine-induced illness, and family members should not receive live poliovirus vaccine.

Patients with cellular immunodeficiency should not receive fresh blood products that may contain intact lymphocytes, because of the risk of graft-vs.-host disease (GVHD); thus, whole blood or blood fractions (eg, RBCs, platelets, granulocytes, and plasma) should be irradiated (15 to 30 Gy [1500 to 3000 rads]) before giving. Immune globulin or plasma usually should be avoided in patients with selective IgA deficiency because anti-IgA Abs may develop or cause reactions. Patients with splenomegaly should avoid contact sports. Patients with thrombocytopenia should avoid IM injections (eg, immune globulin). Antibiotics should be given at the time of surgery or dental work.

Immune globulin (IG) is effective replacement therapy in most forms of Ab deficiency. It is a 16.5% solution of IgG with trace quantities of IgM and IgA for IM injection, or a 3 to 6% solution for IV infusion (IGIV). The usual loading dose is 200 mg/kg (1.4 mL/kg of the 16.5% preparation, 4 mL/kg of a 5% preparation) followed at monthly intervals by 100 mg/kg (0.7 mL/kg of the 16.5% solution, 2 mL/kg of the 5% solution). Lesser doses are therapeutically ineffective. The recommended dosage of IG increases the serum IgG level to only about 200 mg/dL; some patients need larger or more frequent doses. The largest IM dose at one site is 10 mL in adults, 5 mL in children; accordingly, multiple injections at various sites may be necessary. High doses of IGIV (400 to 800 mg/kg/mo) can be given and are beneficial to some Ab-deficient patients not responding well to conventional doses, particularly those with chronic lung disease. The aim with high-dose IGIV is to keep IgG trough levels in the normal range (ie, > 500 mg/dL).

Plasma has been used as an alternative to IG, but because of the risk of disease transmission, it is rarely indicated. Plasma contains many factors in addition to Igs and has been of particular value in patients with protein-losing enteropathy, complement deficiencies, and refractory diarrhea. IgA-deficient plasma has been successful in patients acutely sensitive to IgA in IG preparations.

Other therapy: Immunologic-enhancing agents, including drugs (levamisole, isoprinosine), biologics (transfer factor, ILs, IFNs), and hormones (thymic) have been of limited value in treating cellular or phagocytic immunodeficiencies. Fetal thymic transplants, thymic epithelial cell transplants, and fetal liver transplants occasionally succeed, particularly fetal thymic transplants in the DiGeorge syndrome. Enzyme replacement with bovine adenosine deaminase conjugated to polyethylene glycol (PEG-ADA) has benefited a few patients with adenosine deaminase deficiency.

Transplantation: Complete correction of immunodeficiency can often be achieved by bone marrow transplantation (BMT). In severe combined immunodeficiency and its variants, BMT from an HLA-identical, mixed leukocyte culture-matched sibling has resulted in restored immunity in > 100 cases. In patients with intact or partial cellular immunodeficiency (eg, Wiskott-Aldrich syndrome), prior immunosuppression must be given to ensure engraftment. When a matched sibling donor is unavailable, a haploidentical (half-matched) BMT from a parent should be used. Under these circumstances, mature T lymphocytes that will cause GVHD must be removed from the parenteral marrow before its administration. This can be achieved by removal with soybean lectin agglutination or with T cell monoclonal Abs. These specialized procedures are available in only a few centers.

SPECIFIC IMMUNODEFICIENCIES

Transient Hypogammaglobulinemia of Infancy

A self-limited Ab deficiency of both sexes, with onset at age 3 to 6 mo. It persists usually for 6 to 18 mo. Sometimes there is an associated increased frequency of infection. The disorder results from a delay in the onset of Ig synthesis despite normal numbers of B cells. T helper cells may be reduced. Premature infants are especially at risk because of lower levels of transplacental IgG at birth. The disorder is not familial. **Treatment:** Despite low IgG levels (total < 400 mg/dL), many of these children do not require immune globulin (IG), particularly if there is some evidence of Ab function, if the IgG levels are increasing, and if infections are absent or trivial. Patients needing IG should receive full therapeutic doses for 3 to 6 mo, with frequent recheck of the IgG levels. Antibiotics are indicated with each infectious episode. The outlook is excellent for complete recovery. Newborns < 32 wk of gestation and/or < 1500 gm at birth have such predictably low levels of IgG that IGIV has been used in treating suspected bacterial sepsis or in preventing bacterial infection in the first months of life (see IMMUNOLOGIC STATUS OF THE FETUS AND NEWBORN under MANAGEMENT OF THE NORMAL NEWBORN in Ch. 23).

X-Linked Agammaglobulinemia
(Bruton's Agammaglobulinemia; Congenital Agammaglobulinemia)

Panhypogammaglobulinemia of male infants characterized by levels of IgG < 100 mg/dL and other Igs low or absent, low or absent B cells, intact cellular immunity, and onset of infections sometime after age 6 mo when maternal Ab disappears. These infants have recurrent pyogenic infections of the lungs, sinuses, and bones with such organisms as pneumococcus, hemophilus, and streptococcus. They also are susceptible to vaccine-induced poliovirus infection and chronic echovirus encephalitis. Some infants have arthritis that disappears with Ig therapy. X-linked inheritance is proved in about 20% of cases. The genetic defect seems to be one of inability to form B cells from pre-B cells. **Treatment** is lifelong IG given IM or IV in the lowest dose that prevents recurrent infection. Prompt, adequate antibiotic administration with each infection is crucial; continuous antibiotics are sometimes indicated. Despite these measures, many patients still develop persistent sinusitis, bronchitis, and bronchiectasis. Susceptibility to malignancy is increased.

Common Variable Immunodeficiency (CVID)
(Acquired Agammaglobulinemia)

A heterogeneous disorder occurring equally in both sexes and characterized by the onset of recurrent bacterial infections in the 2nd or 3rd decade as a result of markedly decreased Ig and Ab levels. The presence of normal numbers of B cells distinguishes CVID from X-linked agammaglobulinemia. Cellular immunity usually is intact but may be impaired in some patients; and in others, T cell immunoregulatory abnormalities are described. Autoimmune abnormalities including Addison's disease, thyroiditis, and RA are common in these patients and their relatives. Diarrhea, malabsorption, and nodular lymphoid hyperplasia of the GI tract sometimes are present. Bronchiectasis often develops. Immunologic ab-

normalities vary in different patients; eg, excessive T suppressor activity, deficient T helper activity, intrinsic defects of B cell function, and auto-Abs to B or T cells. **Treatment:** As with X-linked agammaglobulinemia, lifelong IG is required, and antibiotics should be used with each infectious episode.

IgG Subclass Deficiency

An Ab deficiency associated with increased susceptibility to infection and absence or severe reduction of 1 or 2 IgG subclasses, but with normal or increased levels of other subclasses. Most patients have normal or near-normal total IgG and other Ab levels but decreased Ab responsiveness to certain Ags. Chronic respiratory infections, otitis media, chronic lung disease, and recurrent meningitis have been described. Since IgG1 constitutes 70% of the total IgG, an isolated IgG1 deficiency is associated with panhypogammaglobulinemia and is not considered a subclass deficiency. Selective or combined deficiency of IgG2 or IgG3 with or without IgG4 deficiency is the most common subclass deficiency. Patients with IgG2 deficiency (selective or combined with another subclass deficiency) often have impaired Ab responses to polysaccharide Ags, and/or an associated IgA deficiency (<15 mg/dL). Patients with documented IgG subclass deficiencies may benefit from IG (see treatment for X-linked agammaglobulinemia, above). Subclass deficiencies in young children may be transient in nature and disappear with age. A few patients have been described who have **impaired polysaccharide responsiveness** but have normal levels of IgG subclasses.

Selective IgA Deficiency

The absence or marked reduction (< 15 mg/dL) of serum IgA with normal levels of other Igs and intact cellular immunity. Selective IgA deficiency is the most common (and mildest) immunodeficiency, occurring as often as 1:400 subjects. Selective IgA deficiency usually is sporadic but occasionally familial. It may occur as a result of phenytoin treatment and in persons with chromosome 18 abnormalities. It also may occur in relatives of patients with common variable immunodeficiency (see above).

Most patients are asymptomatic, and their defect is noted fortuitously. Others have recurrent respiratory infections, chronic diarrhea, allergy, or autoimmune disease. Patients with IgA deficiency lack IgA in their secretions but may compensate by secreting other Igs. Patients with IgA deficiency may develop anti-IgA Abs as a result of exposure to IgA in plasma or IG; *these Abs can cause anaphylactic reactions when IG or blood is subsequently given.* Some patients with IgA deficiency have an associated IgG2 subclass immunodeficiency; many such patients have recurrent infections.

Treatment is unnecessary in most cases. A Medic-Alert bracelet is recommended to prevent inadvertent plasma or IG administration with sensitization or reaction. Continuous antibiotics are needed for those with persistent respiratory infections. IgA replacement therapy is unavailable. IG injections usually are *contraindicated,* although a few patients who have IgA deficiency with IgG subclass deficiency have been given IG successfully. A few IgA-deficient patients remit spontaneously.

DiGeorge Syndrome
(Thymic Hypoplasia; Third and Fourth Pharyngeal Pouch Syndrome)

A congenital immunodeficiency characterized clinically by hypocalcemic tetany, congenital heart disease, characteristic facies, and increased susceptibility to infection; pathologically by absence or hypoplasia of the thymus and parathyroid glands; and immunologically by partial or complete T cell immunodeficiency but normal or near normal B cell immunity. Affected infants have low-set ears, midline facial clefts, a small receding mandible, hypertelorism, and a shortened philtrum. The onset of tetany is within 24 to 48 h of life. Both sexes are equally affected, and genetic factors usually are not present (however, chromosome 22 abnormalities are reported in a few cases). Recurrent infections begin soon after birth. The etiology seems to be an interruption of normal development of pharyngeal pouch structures near the 8th wk of gestation by a number of factors (eg, maternal alcoholism). The degree of immunodeficiency varies considerably from patient to patient, and sometimes T cell function improves spontaneously. **Treatment:** Bone marrow transplantation has been successful. Some success has been achieved with fetal thymic transplants. The severity of the heart disease often determines the eventual prognosis. Partial deficiency is compatible with prolonged survival.

Chronic Mucocutaneous Candidiasis

A cellular immunodeficiency characterized by persistent Candida infection of the mucous membranes, scalp, skin, and nails, and often associated with an endocrinopathy, particularly hypothyroidism. Onset may be in infancy with the occurrence of persistent thrush or may be delayed until late adulthood. The disorder is somewhat more frequent in females. The disease varies considerably in severity from involvement of a single nail to generalized mucous membrane and skin and hair involvement, and disfiguring granular lesions of the face and scalp. Systemic candidiasis and increased susceptibility to other infections do not occur. Several clinical patterns exist, including an autosomal recessive illness associated with hypoparathyroidism and Addison's disease (*Candida*-endocrinopathy syndrome). The characteristic immunologic findings are cutaneous anergy to *Candida,* absent proliferative responses to *Candida* Ag (but normal proliferative responses to mitogens), and good Ab responses to *Candida* and other Ags. Associated findings in some cases include bronchiectasis, hepatitis, and biotin deficiency with carboxylase enzyme deficiency.

Treatment consists of local (nystatin, clotrimazole) or systemic (ketoconazole, fluconazole, amphotericin B) antifungal drugs. Affected nails may have to be removed surgically. Immunotherapy with transfer factor, thymic epithelium, thymic hormones, or immune lymphocytes is not of permanent benefit. Bone marrow transplantation has been successful in a single case.

Combined Immunodeficiency (CID)

A group of disorders characterized by congenital and often hereditary deficiency of both B and T cell systems, lymphoid aplasia, and thymic dysplasia; ie: **severe combined immunodeficiency (SCID); Swiss agammaglobulinemia; thymic dysplasia; CID with adenosine deaminase or nucleoside phosphorylase deficiency; and CID with Igs (Nezelof syndrome).** Most patients have an early onset (within 3 mo of age) of infection with thrush, pneumonia, and diarrhea, and if left untreated, a fatal progressive course before age 2. Most patients have profound deficiency of B cells and Igs. Characteristically there are lymphopenia, low or absent T cell numbers, poor proliferative response to mitogens, cutaneous anergy, an absent thymic shadow, and diminished lymphoid tissue. *P. carinii* and other opportunistic infections are common.

A number of variants of the disorder exist. In 50% of cases an X-linked or autosomal recessive **(AR)** inheritance can be established. About 1/2 of patients with an AR inheritance have **adenosine deaminase (ADA)** deficiency, a purine salvage pathway enzyme that converts adenosine and deoxyadenosine to inosine and deoxyinosine, respectively. ADA deficiency results in elevated quantities of deoxyadenosine triphosphate (**deoxyATP**), which inhibits DNA synthesis. These children may be normal at birth but develop progressive immunologic impairment as deoxyATP accumulates. In **CID with Igs**, there is a profound cellular immunodeficiency but normal, near normal, or elevated levels of Igs—but with poor Ab function. The course may be only slightly less severe than in SCID. **CID with reticuloendotheliosis** is a variant with skin lesions resembling Letterer-Siwe disease, lymphadenopathy, and hepatosplenomegaly. Some of these infants may have graft-vs-host disease from maternal lymphocytes or from previous blood transfusions. In the bare lymphocyte syndrome, infants lack HLA class I and/or class II Ags.

Treatment with IG and antibiotics (including *P. carinii* prophylaxis) is indicated but is not curative. The treatment of choice is bone marrow transplantation. Patients with ADA deficiency have been treated successfully with polyethylene glycol conjugated to bovine ADA (PEG-ADA).

Wiskott-Aldrich Syndrome (WAS)

An X-linked recessive disorder of male infants, characterized by eczema, thrombocytopenia, and recurrent infection. The first manifestations often are hemorrhagic (usually bloody diarrhea), followed by development of recurrent respiratory infections. Malignancy (especially lymphoma and acute lymphoblastic leukemia) is common in survivors > 10 yr old. The characteristic immunologic defects include poor Ab responses to polysaccharide Ags, cutaneous anergy, partial T cell immunodeficiency, elevated levels of IgE and IgA, low levels of IgM, and hypercatabolism of IgG but normal IgG levels. Because of the combined deficiency in both B and T cell function, infections occur with pyogenic bacteria, viruses, fungi, and *P. carinii*. Hematologically, these patients have small platelets and increased splenic destruction of platelets; accordingly, splenectomy may alleviate the thrombocytopenia. **Treatment** consists of splenectomy, continuous antibiotics, immune globulin given IV (not IM, because of risk of hemorrhage), and bone marrow transplantation.

Ataxia-Telangiectasia

An AR progressive multisystem disorder characterized by cerebellar ataxia, telangiectasia of the conjunctiva and skin, recurrent sinopulmonary infections, and variable immunologic disease.

Both neurologic symptoms and evidence of immunodeficiency are variable in onset. Ataxia usually develops at about the time when children begin to walk, but may be delayed until age 4 yr. Its progression leads to severe disability. Speech becomes slurred, choreoathetoid movements and ophthalmoplegia occur, and muscle weakness usually progresses to muscle atrophy. Progressive mental retardation may occur. Telangiectasias develop between 1 and 6 yr of age, most prominently on the bulbar conjunctiva, ears, antecubital and popliteal fossae, and sides of the nose. The recurrent sinopulmonary infections, which result from the immunologic deficits, lead to recurrent pneumonia, bronchiectasis, and chronic obstructive and restrictive lung disease.

Endocrine abnormalities may occur, including gonadal dysgenesis, testicular atrophy, and an unusual form of diabetes mellitus characterized by marked hyperglycemia, resistance to ketosis, and a marked plasma insulin response to glucose or tolbutamide.

The disorder is associated with a high degree of malignancy (especially leukemia, brain tumors, and gastric cancer) and increased frequency of chromosome breaks, probably indicative of a defect in DNA repair. Patients often lack IgA and IgE and have cutaneous anergy and a progressive cellular immune defect. Serum α_2-fetoprotein is generally elevated. **Treatment** of the immunodeficiency with antibiotics or IG is of some value, but there is no effective treatment for the CNS abnormalities. Thus, the course is one of progressive neurologic deterioration with choreoathetosis, muscle weakness, dementia, and death.

Hyper-IgE Syndrome (Job-Buckley Syndrome)

An immunodeficiency syndrome characterized by recurrent staphylococcal infections, particularly of the skin, and markedly elevated levels of IgE. Some patients have an autosomal dominant inheritance. The staphylococcal infection may involve the skin, lung, joints, and other sites. Some patients have coarse features; some are fair and redheaded. Osteopenia and recurrent fractures are common. Many have neutrophil chemotactic defects. All have exceptionally elevated IgE levels (> 1000 IU/mL). Allergic manifestations (eg, eczema, rhinitis, and asthma) sometimes are present. Other laboratory features include subtle defects of B and T cell immunity and tissue and blood eosinophilia. The basic defect may be an immunoregulatory T cell abnormality. **Treatment** consists of intermittent or continuous antibiotics. Trimethoprim/sulfamethoxazole is a particularly effective prophylactic.

Chronic Granulomatous Disease (CGD)

An inherited disorder of WBC bactericidal function characterized by widespread granulomatous lesions of the skin, lungs, and lymph nodes; hypergammaglobulinemia, anemia, leukocytosis; and defective killing of certain bacteria and fungi. Most patients are males with an X-linked recessive inheritance; a few patients of either sex have an autosomal recessive inheritance. The **clinical pattern** is one of recurrent infections with catalase-producing organisms, eg, *Staphylococcus aureus, Serratia, Escherichia coli,* and *Pseudomonas,* which do not usually cause granulomas, but because of the bactericidal killing defect, the organisms survive intracellularly.

The disease usually begins in early childhood, but may be delayed until the early teens in a few patients. Clinical characteristics are suppurative lymphadenitis, hepatosplenomegaly, pneumonia, and hematologic evidence of chronic infection. Persistent rhinitis, dermatitis, diarrhea, perianal abscesses, stomatitis, osteomyelitis, brain abscess, obstructive GI and GU tract lesions (from granuloma formation) and delayed growth also occur.

WBCs from patients with CGD do not produce hydrogen peroxide, superoxide, and other activated O_2 species, probably because of deficient nicotinamide adenine dinucleotide phosphate (NADPH) oxidase activity. In the X-linked form, a deficiency of cytochrome b_{559} occurs. The gene controlling this protein is near the gene for Duchenne muscular dystrophy on the short arm of the X chromosome. Laboratory diagnosis is made by deficient nitroblue tetrazolium (NBT) dye reduction of granulocytes, or an in vitro bactericidal defect. **Treatment** consists of intermittent or continuous antibiotic use. Bone marrow transplantation also has been successful. IFN-γ therapy is under study.

Leukocyte Adhesion Deficiency
(MAC 1/LFA-1/CR3 Deficiency)

Leukocyte adhesion deficiency is an AR disorder of WBC function characterized by recurrent or progressive necrotic soft tissue infection, periodontitis, poor wound healing, leukocytosis, and delayed ($>$ 3 wk) umbilical cord detachment. Severely affected infants have multiple infections with a rapid progressive downhill course. Moderately affected patients with a less severe course have also been noted; severity is correlated with the degree of deficiency of specific glycoproteins on the surface of WBCs that anchor cells to surfaces, promote bacterial adherence, and serve as a receptor for opsonic complement component C3bc (CR3). As a result, their granulocytes (and lymphocytes) do not chemotax well, kill other cells in cytotoxic reactions, or phagocytose bacteria well. Diagnosis is established by showing an absence or severe deficiency of these Ags on the surface of WBCs, using monoclonal Abs (eg, anti-CD11) and flow cytometry. **Treatment** consists of vigorous (often continuous) antibiotic therapy. Bone marrow transplantation has been curative in a few cases.

Splenic Deficiency Syndromes

Susceptibility to infection because of splenectomy, congenital splenic absence or functional asplenia due to thrombosis of splenic vessels (sickle cell disease) or infiltrative diseases (storage disorders). The spleen is a major phagocytic organ of the reticuloendothelial (mononuclearphagocyte) system with trapping of circulating organisms. The spleen also serves as a major site of Ab synthesis. Asplenic patients, particularly young infants, are susceptible to rapid overwhelming bacterial infection with *H. influenzae, E. coli,* pneumococci, and streptococci, and to a lesser extent, to other infections. These patients should have continuous prophylactic antibiotics for at least the first 2 to 3 yr of life, and thereafter be given antibiotics at the onset of each febrile episode and with surgery. They should also receive pneumococcal polysaccharide, meningococcal, and *Hemophilus* vaccines.

Protein-Losing Immunodeficiencies
(Nephrosis, Burns, Enteritis)

Loss of serum proteins leading to secondary Ab deficiency with striking degrees of hypogammaglobulinemia. This can be due to loss through the kidney (nephrotic syndrome), skin (severe burns or dermatitis), or GI tract (protein-losing enteropathy, intestinal lymphangiectasia). There is simultaneous loss of albumin and other serum proteins. In GI protein-loss disorders, there may also be lymphocyte loss, resulting in lymphopenia and cellular immunodeficiency. These patients are susceptible to major gram-positive infections, but since a compensatory increase of Ab production occurs, infections may be relatively uncommon despite striking hypogamma-globulinemia. Correction of the underlying disease will correct the immunodeficiency. When this is impossible, medium-chain triglycerides may be of partial benefit to decrease the loss of Igs and lymphocytes from the GI tract.

Immunodeficiency and Malnutrition
(See also Ch. 39)

Malnutrition with immunodeficiency and infection is the world's leading cause of infant and child death. Malnutrition may be due to a deficiency of all nutrients (marasmus) or primarily of protein (kwashiorkor), usually with superimposed vitamin and mineral deficiencies (eg, vitamin A, iron, zinc). When malnutrition is severe enough to reduce weight to < 80% of the expected mean, some impairment of immune function is noted; when growth retardation is < 70% of the expected mean, severe impairment of immune function usually is seen. Most such patients (except those with anorexia nervosa) are extraordinarily susceptible to respiratory infection, viral disease, and gastroenteritis. These infections increase metabolic requirements and decrease appetite, leading to a vicious circle of more malnutrition and immunodeficiency. Poverty with inadequate food intake causes most malnutrition; less often it is due to ignorance (eg, strict vegetarianism), chronic disease (eg, shortgut, colitis), or psychiatric disturbance (anorexia nervosa). The immunologic defect is primarily a T cell immunodeficiency with cutaneous anergy, low T cell numbers, poor proliferative responses to mitogens and Ags, and deficiency of lymphokines (interferon) and cytotoxic activity. Secretory Ab levels may be diminished but serum Igs usually are normal or elevated, particularly IgE. The degree of immune impairment depends on the degree and duration of malnutrition, and on underlying illness (eg, infection, other nutritional deficiencies). With infectional rehabilitation, the immunologic defect reverses rapidly.

34. DISORDERS DUE TO HYPERSENSITIVITY

INTRODUCTION

Hypersensitivity reactions: *Pathologic processes that result from specific interactions between antigens* (Ags—exogenous or endogenous) *and either humoral antibodies* (Abs) *or sensitized lymphocytes.* This definition excludes disorders in which demonstrated Abs have no known pathophysiologic significance (eg, the Ab to heart tissue that follows heart surgery or MI), even though their presence may have diagnostic value.

Any classification of hypersensitivity is bound to be oversimplified. Some are based on the time required for symptoms or skin test reactions to appear after exposure to Ag (eg, immediate and delayed hypersensitivity), on the type of Ag (eg, drug reactions), or on the nature of organ involvement. Moreover, these classifications do not take into account that > 1 type of immune response may be occurring or that > 1 type may be necessary to produce immunologic injury.

The Gell and Coombs classification of reactions, consisting of 4 types, has come into general use over the last 20 yr; despite limitations, it remains the most satisfactory classification.

Type I: *Reactions in which Ags (allergens) combine with specific IgE Abs that are bound to* membrane receptors on tissue mast cells and blood basophils. *The Ag-Ab reaction causes the release of potent vasoactive and inflammatory mediators. Some are preformed (histamine, chemotactic factors), while others (eg, the leukotrienes and platelet activating factor [PAF]) are newly generated from membrane lipids. The mediators produce vasodilation, increased capillary permeability, glandular hypersecretion, smooth muscle spasm, and tissue infiltration with eosinophils and other inflammatory cells.*

Type II: *Cytotoxic reactions resulting when Ab reacts with antigenic components of a cell or tissue elements or with Ag or hapten that has become intimately coupled to a cell or tissue. The Ag-Ab reaction may activate certain cytotoxic cells (killer lymphocytes or macrophages) to produce "Ab-dependent cell-mediated cytotoxicity" (ADCC). Furthermore, it usually involves complement activation and may cause opsonic adherence through coating of the cell with Ab; the reaction develops by activation of complement components through C3 (with consequent phagocytosis of the cell), or by activation of the full complement system with consequent cytolysis or tissue damage.*

Type III: *Immune complex* (IC) *reactions resulting from deposition of soluble circulating Ag-*

Ab ICs in vessels or tissue. The ICs activate complement and thus initiate a sequence of events that results in polymorphonuclear cell migration and release of lysosomal proteolytic enzymes and permeability factors in tissues, thereby producing an acute inflammation. The consequences of IC formation depend in part on the relative proportions of Ag and Ab in the IC. With an excess of Ab the ICs rapidly precipitate where the Ag is located (eg, within the joints in RA) or are phagocytosed by macrophages and thus do no harm. With a slight excess of Ag, the ICs tend to be more soluble and may cause systemic reactions by being deposited in various tissues.

Type IV: *Cellular, cell-mediated, delayed, or tuberculin-type hypersensitivity reactions caused by sensitized T cell lymphocytes after contact with specific Ag.* Circulating Abs are not involved nor are they necessary for tissue injury to develop. Transfer of delayed hypersensitivity from sensitized to nonsensitized persons can be shown with peripheral WBCs or with a dialyzable extract of these cells (transfer factor), but not with serum.

The sensitized T lymphocyte that has been triggered or activated by contact with specific Ag may cause immunologic injury by a direct toxic effect or through the release of soluble substances (lymphokines). In tissue culture, activated T lymphocytes have been shown to destroy "target" cells following sensitization by direct contact. The cytokines released from activated T lymphocytes include several factors affecting the activity of macrophages, neutrophils, and lymphoid killer cells.

Following the Gell and Coombs classification as much as possible, hypersensitivity disorders will be discussed below. Disorders clinically similar to type I disorders, but of different or unknown mechanisms, will be included with the corresponding type I diseases.

DISORDERS WITH TYPE I HYPERSENSITIVITY REACTIONS

These disorders include the **atopic diseases** (allergic rhinitis, conjunctivitis, and asthma, and some cases of urticaria and GI food reactions) and **systemic anaphylaxis**. Recently, a marked increase in type I reactions has been noted in relation to exposure to water-soluble proteins in latex products (eg, rubber gloves, dental dams, condoms, tubing for respiratory equipment, catheters, enema tips with inflatable latex cuffs). As a rule, patients with atopic diseases (including **atopic dermatitis**) have in common an inherited predisposition to develop IgE Ab-mediated hypersensitivity to inhaled and ingested substances (allergens) that are harmless to people who are not atopic. Features similar to atopy have been identified in several mammalian species. IgE Abs usually mediate hypersensitivity symptoms, but atopic dermatitis is an exception. Although IgE-mediated food allergy may contribute to symptoms of atopic dermatitis in infants and young children, the condition is largely independent of allergic factors in older children and adults, even though most patients continue to have specific allergy as detected by skin testing and measurement of serum IgE.

GENERAL PRINCIPLES OF MANAGEMENT OF IgE−MEDIATED DISORDERS

Diagnosis

History: Review of the symptoms, their relation to the environment and to seasonal and situational variations, their clinical course, and the family history of similar problems should yield sufficient information to classify the disease as atopic. The history is more valuable than tests in determining whether a patient is allergic, and it is inappropriate to subject the patient to extensive skin testing unless reasonable clinical evidence exists for atopy. Age of onset may be an important clue (eg, childhood asthma is more likely to be allergic than asthma beginning after age 30). Also indicative are seasonal symptoms (eg, correlating with specific pollen seasons), or those that appear after exposure to animals, hay, or dust, or that develop in specific environments (eg, at home, at work). For advising the patient, it is also helpful to investigate the effects of nonspecific contributory factors (eg, tobacco smoke and other pollutants, cold air, exercise, alcoholic beverages, certain drugs, and life stresses).

Nonspecific tests: Eosinophilia in the blood and secretions is often associated with atopic conditions, particularly asthma and atopic dermatitis. Total IgE levels may help to diagnose atopic dermatitis, since they are elevated and will rise during exacerbations and fall during remissions. IgE levels usually are elevated in atopic asthma, often are normal in allergic rhinitis, but are not diagnostically useful in these conditions. Occasionally, very high IgE levels may help confirm the diagnosis of either allergic pulmonary aspergillosis or Buckley's syndrome (*hyper-IgE immunodeficiency with recurrent staphylococcal infections*).

Specific tests are used to confirm sensitivity to a particular allergen or allergens. For this purpose, **skin tests** are the most convenient: They should be selective and based on clues provided by the history as much as possible. Test solutions are made from extracts of inhaled, ingested, or injected materials (eg, wind-borne tree, grass, and weed pollens; house dust mites; animal danders and sera; insect venoms; foods; and a few drugs). For the **prick (puncture) test**, a drop of a 1:10 or 1:20 (weight/volume) dilution of an allergenic extract is placed on the skin, and then the skin is pricked or punctured through the extract. A common way to do this is to "tent" up the skin with the tip of a stylet or #27 needle held at a 20° angle until the tip pops loose. The **intradermal test** is done by injecting just enough of a 1:500 or 1:1000 dilution of a sterile extract (using a 0.5- or 1-mL syringe and a #27 short-bevel needle) to produce a 1- or 2-mm bleb. Each set of skin tests should include the diluent alone as a negative control and histamine (10 mg/mL of the base for the prick test or 0.1 mg/mL for the intradermal test) as a positive control. A skin test is considered positive if it produces a wheal-and-erythema reaction in 15 min with a wheal diameter at least 5 mm larger than the control.

It is common practice to do prick skin testing first. This is usually sufficient for detecting sensitivity to most allergens. The more sensitive intradermal testing can then be used to test suspected inhaled allergens that have produced negative or equivocal prick tests. For foods, prick tests alone are diagnostic. Intradermal tests to food are likely to produce positive reactions of no clinical significance, as determined by double-blind oral symptom-provoking challenge tests.

A **radioallergosorbent test (RAST)** may be done when direct skin testing is impossible because of generalized dermatitis, extreme dermographia, or the patient's inability to cooperate or to stop using antihistamines. The RAST detects the presence of allergen-specific serum IgE. A known allergen, in the form of an insoluble polymer-allergen conjugate, is mixed with the serum to be tested. Any IgE in the serum that is specific for the allergen will attach to the conjugate. Adding ^{125}I-labeled anti-IgE Ab and measuring the amount of radioactivity taken up by the conjugate will determine the quantity of allergen-specific IgE in the patient's circulation.

WBC histamine release, another in vitro test, detects allergen-specific IgE on sensitized basophils by measuring allergen-induced histamine release from the patient's WBCs. This valuable research tool has given insight into the kinetics of histamine release; like RAST, it provides no diagnostic information not provided by the skin test.

Provocative challenge may be done when a positive skin test has raised a question about the role of the particular allergen in the production of symptoms. The allergen may be applied to the eyes, nose, or lungs. **Ophthalmic testing** offers no advantage over skin testing and is rarely used. **Nasal challenge**, done occasionally, is primarily a research tool, as is **bronchial challenge**. Some allergists use bronchial challenge (when the clinical significance of a positive skin test is unclear or when skin test reagents are unavailable) to show that symptoms are related to materials to which a patient is exposed (eg, in occupationally related asthma). **Oral provocative tests** may be used when regularly occurring symptoms are suspected of being food-related and skin tests are of doubtful clinical significance. Provocative challenge is the only way to test food additives for which there are no reliable skin or immunologic tests. Elimination diets and challenge testing will be discussed further in the food allergy section below.

Tests of unproven effectiveness: No evidence supports the use of cutaneous or sublingual provocation testing or leukocytotoxic testing in allergy diagnosis.

TREATMENT

Avoidance

The preferred treatment is to eliminate the allergen; this may require a change of diet, occupation, or residence; withdrawal of a drug; or removal of a household pet. Some locales, free of allergens (eg, ragweed) are havens for afflicted persons. When complete avoidance is impossible, as in the case of house dust, exposure may be reduced by removing dust-collecting furniture, carpets, and draperies; using plastic covers over the mattress and pillows; frequent wet-mopping and dusting; reducing the high humidity favorable to breeding of dust mites; and installing a high-efficiency air filter.

Desensitization
(Hyposensitization; Allergen Immunotherapy)

When an allergen cannot be avoided or controlled sufficiently to relieve symptoms of atopic disease, desensitization can be tried by injecting an extract of the allergen s.c. in gradually increasing doses. Several specific effects can be shown, although no test correlates absolutely with clinical improvement. The titer of blocking (neutralizing) Ab increases proportionately to the dose given. Sometimes, particularly when high doses of pollen extract can be tolerated, the serum IgE level falls significantly. Also, peripheral blood basophil histamine release is reduced from pretreatment levels on incubation with Ag (or an increased amount of Ag is required to release 50% of the basophil histamine), and the lymphocyte responsiveness to Ag may also be diminished.

Results are most satisfactory when injections are continued year-round. Depending on the degree of sensitivity, the first dose is 0.1 mL of a high dilution (1:1,000,000 or 1:100,000). For allergens standardized by the FDA, the starting dose is 0.1 to 1.0 allergy units (**AU**). The dose is increased weekly or biweekly by $\leq$ 75% until a maximum tolerated concentration is reached (eg, 0.3 mL of a 1:100 dilution). For standardized pollen extracts, the maintenance dose is 1000 to 1500 AU. Once reached, the maximum dose can be maintained at monthly intervals year-round; even in seasonal allergies, perennial treatment is superior to preseasonal or coseasonal methods.

The major allergens used for desensitization are those that usually cannot be effectively avoided: pollens, house dust mites, molds, and venom of stinging insects. Insect venoms are standardized by weight; a typical starting dose is 0.01 μg; the usual maintenance is 100 μg. Animal dander desensitization is ordinarily limited to those who cannot avoid exposure (eg, veterinarians, laboratory workers). There is no indication for food desensitization.

Adverse reactions to desensitization: Patients often are extremely sensitive, particularly to pollen allergens, and if an overdose is given can experience constitutional reactions varying from a mild cough or sneezing to generalized urticaria, severe asthma, and anaphylactic shock. **Prevention:** To prevent such reactions, one must increase the dose by small increments, repeat the same dose (or even decrease it) if the local reaction from the previous injection is large ($\geq$ 2.5 cm in diameter), and reduce the dose when a fresh extract is used. Reducing the dose of pollen extract during the pollen season is often wise also. *IM and IV injection must be avoided.*

Despite all precautions, reactions occur occasionally. *Since the severe, life-threatening ones develop within 20 min, patients must remain under observation for that time.* **Manifestations** of an impending reaction may be sneezing, coughing, and chest tightness, or a generalized flush, tingling sensations, and pruritus. A tourniquet should be applied above the injection site at once, and the site infiltrated with 0.2 mL of epinephrine 1:1000 (0.01 mg/kg in children); the tourniquet should be released in 15 min. If the reaction is mild or moderate, a double dose of an oral antihistamine can then be given (eg, diphenhydramine 100 mg or chlorpheniramine 8 mg), and 0.3 mL of epinephrine 1:1000 (0.01 mg/kg in children) can be given s.c. in the opposite arm. *For manifestations of shock, IV fluids should be started; epinephrine 1:100,000, 5 to 10 μg/min IV, should be given over about 10 min; and other measures should be instituted to treat anaphylaxis* (see below). Glucocorticoids will not help during the acute reaction, but may help to prevent the late 4- to 6-h asthmatic or urticarial reaction that may develop after the patient has recovered from the first reaction and gone home. Following any generalized reaction, the next dose of allergen should be reduced to $^1/_3$ or $^1/_4$ of the previous dose, and later increments kept as small as is practicable (usually 0.03 to 0.05 mL).

Antihistamines

Symptomatic relief with drugs should not be neglected while the patient is being evaluated and specific control or treatment is being developed. The proper use of antihistamines, sympathomimetics, cromolyn, and glucocorticoids is outlined for each disease category in the discussions that follow. In general, early use of glucocorticoids is appropriate for potentially disabling conditions that are self-limited and of relatively short duration (seasonal flares of asthma; serum sickness; infiltrative lung disease; severe contact dermatitis), and prudent glucocorticoid use may be necessary when other measures are insufficient to manage chronic conditions.

Histamine is widely distributed in mammalian tissue. In man the highest concentrations are in skin, lungs, and GI mucosa. Histamine is present mainly in the intracellular granules of mast cells, but there is also an important extra-mast-cell pool in the gastric mucosa, with smaller amounts in the brain, heart, and other organs. The release of histamine from the mast-cell storage granules can be triggered by physical tissue disruption, various chemicals (including tissue irritants, surface active agents, and polymers), and most prominently by Ag-Ab interactions.

The specific homeostatic function of histamine remains unclear. Its actions, which in man are exerted primarily on the cardiovascular system, extravascular smooth muscle, and exocrine glands, appear to be mediated by 2 distinct receptors termed H_1 and H_2. This discussion will be limited to the H_1 receptors and their antagonists.

Histamine H_1 receptor effects: In the **cardiovascular system,** histamine is a potent arteriolar dilator that can cause extensive peripheral pooling of blood and hypotension. It also increases capillary permeability by distortion of the endothelial lining of the postcapillary venules, with widening of the gap between endothelial cells and exposure of basement membrane surfaces. This accelerates loss of plasma and plasma proteins from the vascular space and, combined with arteriolar and capillary dilation, can produce circulatory shock. Histamine also dilates cerebral vessels, which may be a factor in histamine headache.

The **"triple response"** is mediated by local *intracutaneous* histamine release, causing (1) local erythema from vasodilation, (2) wheal due to local edema from increased capillary permeability, and (3) flare from a neuronal reflex mechanism producing a surrounding area of arteriolar vasodilation. **Other smooth muscle:** In man, histamine may cause severe bronchoconstriction in susceptible individuals. Histamine also stimulates GI motility. **Exocrine glands:** Histamine increases salivary and bronchial gland secretions. **Endocrine gland:** Stimulation of catecholamine release from adrenal chromaffin cells also appears to be H_1-receptor–mediated. **Sensory nerve endings:** Local instillation of histamine may produce intense itching.

Histamine H_1 receptor antagonists (H_1 blockers): The conventional antihistamines possess a substituted ethylamine side-chain (similar to that of histamine) linked to one or more cyclic groups. The similarity between the ethylamine moiety of histamine and the substituted ethylamine structure of the H_1 blockers suggests that this molecular configuration is important in receptor interactions. H_1 blockers appear to act by competitive inhibition; they do not significantly alter histamine production or metabolism.

The H_1 blockers, given orally or rectally, are usually well absorbed from the GI tract. Onset of action usually occurs within 15 to 30 min, with peak effects attained in 1 h; duration of action is usually 3 to 6 h, but some blockers act considerably longer.

Antihistaminic effects of H_1 blockers are noted only in the presence of increased histamine activity. They block the effects of histamine on GI tract smooth muscle, but in man the allergic reaction of the bronchial smooth muscle is not dependent primarily on histamine release and does not respond effectively to antihistamines alone. H_1 blockers effectively block histamine-induced increased capillary permeability and sensory nerve stimulation, thus inhibiting the wheal, flare, pruritus, sneezing, and mucous secretion responses. However, these agents are only partially effective in reversing histamine-induced vasodilation and hypotension.

Clinically useful effects other than histamine antagonism are discussed below.

Therapeutic indications: In addition to blocking the effects of histamine, many antihistamines have other therapeutic uses. Pharmacologic differences among them are most apparent in their sedative, antiemetic, and other CNS effects, and in their anticholinergic, antiserotonin, and local anesthetic properties.

Antihistamines are useful to treat the symptoms of allergies, including seasonal hay fever, allergic rhinitis, and conjunctivitis. They are mildly effective in vasomotor rhinitis. Acute and chronic urticaria and certain pruritic allergic dermatoses respond well. They are also useful to treat minor transfusion incompatibility reactions and systemic reactions to IV x-ray contrast media. They provide little benefit in treating the common cold, but because of their anticholinergic effects (see below) they may control rhinorrhea.

TABLE 34–1 summarizes the dosage, route, and frequency for giving some commonly available H_1 blockers. Doses may need to be given more often to children than to adults because of shorter antihistamine half-lives (except as noted in the table). These agents all block H_1 receptors; their pharmacologic differences are primarily in the type and intensity of their other effects.

Other clinically useful effects: Since CNS depression and drowsiness are prominent with many H_1 blockers, occasionally one takes advantage of these potentially adverse effects to use H_1 blockers as sedatives and hypnotics. However, the alkylamines and 2 new agents, astemizole and terfenadine, having relatively little sedative effect, are useful when sedation is undesirable. The ethanolamines are significant CNS depressants; although less potent and dependable than the barbiturates and other central de-

TABLE 34–1. DOSAGE, ADMINISTRATION, AND PREPARATIONS OF SOME HISTAMINE H$_1$ RECEPTOR ANTAGONISTS

Agent	Route	Usual Adult Dosage	Usual Pediatric Dosage	Available Preparations
Alkylamines				
Brompheniramine maleate	Oral IM or IV	4–8 mg q 4–6 h 5–20 mg q 6–12 h	0.1 mg/kg/dose	4-, 8-, and 12-mg tablets 2 mg/5 mL elixir 8- and 12-mg tablets (timed-release) 10 mg/mL injection
Chlorpheniramine maleate	Oral	2–4 mg q 4–6 h	0.1 mg/kg/dose	2-mg chewable tablets 4-, 8-, and 12-mg tablets 2 mg/5 mL syrup 8- and 12-mg tablets, capsules (timed-release)
Dexchlorpheniramine maleate	Oral	2 mg tid or qid	0.05 mg/kg/dose	2-mg tablets 2 mg/5 mL syrup 4- and 6-mg tablets (extended-release)
Triprolidine HCl	Oral	2.5 mg q 4–6 h	0.05 mg/kg/dose	2.5-mg tablets 1.25 mg/5 mL syrup
Ethanolamines				
Clemastine fumarate	Oral	1.34 mg bid to 2.58 mg tid	0.14 mg/kg/dose	1.34- and 2.68-mg tablets 0.67 mg/5 mL syrup
Diphenhydramine HCl	Oral IV, deep IM	25–50 mg tid or qid 10–50 mg q 3–4 h	5 mg/kg/day divided q 6 h	25- and 50-mg capsules 12.5 mg/mL syrup 12.5 mg/5 mL elixir 10- and 50-mg/mL injection
Diphenylpyraline HCl	Oral	5 mg q 12 h	NA	5-mg capsules (sustained action)
Ethylenediamines				
Tripelennamine citrate	Oral	25–50 mg q 4–6 h	(1 mL citrate = 5 mg HCl salt)	37.5 mg/5 mL elixir
Tripelennamine HCl	Oral	25–50 mg q 4–6 h	5 mg/kg/day	25- and 50-mg tablets 100-mg tablets (timed-release)

Piperazines			
Hydroxyzine HCl	Oral	25–100 mg tid or qid	10-, 25-, 50-, and 100-mg tablets
	IM	25–100 mg q 4–6 h	10 mg/5 mL syrup
			25- and 50-mg/mL injection
Phenothiazines			
Methdilazine HCl	Oral	8 mg q 6–12 h	> 3 yr, 4 mg q 6–12 h	8-mg tablets
			4-mg chewable tablets
			4 mg/5 mL syrup
Promethazine HCl	Oral	12.5–25 mg bid	0.1 mg/kg q 6 h	12.5-, 25-, and 50-mg tablets*
	Rectal	12.5–25 mg q 4 h prn or q 6 h		6.25 and 25 mg/5 mL syrup
	IV or IM	12.5–25 mg q 6 h		12.5-, 25-, and 50-mg suppositories
	IM only	50 mg for sedation		25 mg/mL injection
				50 mg/mL injection (IM only)
Trimeprazine tartrate	Oral	2.5 mg qid	6 mo–3 yr, 1.25 mg hs or tid	2.5-mg tablets
			> 3 yr, 2.5 mg hs or tid	2.5 mg/5 mL syrup*
				5-mg capsules (timed-release)
Piperidines			
Azatadine maleate	Oral	1–2 mg bid	> 12 yr only	1-mg tablets*
Cyproheptadine HCl	Oral	4 mg tid or qid (not > 0.5 mg/kg/day)	0.25–0.5 mg/kg/day	4-mg tablets*
				2 mg/5 mL syrup
Nonsedating			
Astemizole	Oral	10 mg once daily	> 12 yr only	10-mg tablets*
Terfenadine	Oral	60 mg bid	6–12 yr, 30 mg bid	60-mg tablets*
			> 12 yr, adult dosage	

NA = not applicable; hs = hour of sleep.
* Do not increase the frequency in children.

pressants, they are useful as sedatives and hypnotics but have marked anticholinergic properties, and thus may be poorly tolerated by the elderly. The ethylenediamines produce less CNS depression but more GI side effects than the ethanolamines.

The ethanolamine derivative diphenhydramine and its chlorotheophyllinate salt dimenhydrinate, the phenothiazine congener promethazine, and the piperazines (cyclizine and meclizine) are all used to prevent or treat motion sickness and relieve the nausea and vertigo associated with labyrinthitis. Cyclizine, hydroxyzine, and meclizine have been implicated as teratogens in animals, *and probably should not be given during pregnancy.*

The phenothiazine group of H_1 receptor antagonists, notably promethazine, are useful as sedatives and are effective in controlling the nausea associated with radiotherapy and certain anticancer drugs; for this latter use they are less effective than prochlorperazine and chlorpromazine.

Most H_1 blockers have some anticholinergic properties that may account centrally for modest antiparkinsonian activity and peripherally for symptomatic relief of rhinorrhea in URIs. Combined with drugs for local anesthesia, some H_1 blockers have been applied to the skin in the form of creams and lotions to reduce itching. However, *topical application of ethylenediamine antihistamines incurs considerable risk of drug sensitization,* and they are no longer approved for this purpose.

Undesirable side effects and toxicity of the H_1 blockers include anorexia, nausea, vomiting, constipation, diarrhea, epigastric distress, decreased alertness, impaired ability to concentrate, drowsiness, and muscular weakness. Blood dyscrasias (eg, leukopenia, agranulocytosis, thrombocytopenia, hemolytic anemia) occur rarely. The manifestations of overdosage are dominated by anticholinergic effects: dry mouth, palpitations, chest tightness, urinary retention, visual disturbances, convulsions, hallucinations, and later, respiratory depression, fever, hypotension, and mydriasis.

ATOPIC DISEASES

ALLERGIC RHINITIS

A symptom complex including hay fever and perennial allergic rhinitis, characterized by seasonal or perennial sneezing, rhinorrhea, nasal congestion, pruritus, and often conjunctivitis and pharyngitis.

Hay Fever

The acute seasonal form of allergic rhinitis **(pollinosis),** is generally induced by wind-borne pollens. The spring type is due to tree pollens (eg, oak, elm, maple, alder, birch, juniper, olive); the summer type, to grass pollens (eg, Bermuda, timothy, sweet vernal, orchard, Johnson) and to weed pollens (eg, Russian thistle, English plantain); the fall type, to weed pollens (eg, ragweed). Occasionally, seasonal rhinitis is caused primarily by airborne fungal spores. Important geographic regional differences occur.

Symptoms and signs: The nose, roof of the mouth, pharynx, and eyes begin to itch gradually or abruptly after onset of the pollen season. Lacrimation, sneezing, and clear, watery nasal discharge accompany or soon follow the pruritus. Frontal headaches, irritability, anorexia, depression, and insomnia may occur. The conjunctiva is injected, and the nasal mucous membranes are swollen and bluish-red. Coughing and asthmatic wheezing may develop as the season progresses. Many eosinophils are present in the nasal mucus during the season.

Diagnosis: The history indicates the nature of the allergic process and often the pollens responsible. Diagnosis is supported by the physical findings and eosinophils in the nasal secretions. Skin tests may be useful to confirm or identify the responsible pollens.

Treatment

Symptoms may be diminished by avoidance of the allergen (see above). **Oral antihistamines** relieve most patients; if the usual ones are too sedating, a nonsedating but more expensive one may be used (see Antihistamines, above). Topical treatment is another alternative (see below). Sympathomimetics are often given with antihistamines. Phenylpropanolamine, phenylephrine, or pseudoephedrine are available in many antihistamine-decongestant preparations. Because oral sympathomimetics can raise the BP, patients with a tendency to hypertension should not use them without periodic monitoring.

If antihistamines are unsatisfactory, then 4% **cromolyn sodium** may be given by nasal spray (delivered by a finger-activated pump). The usual dosage is one spray (5.2 mg) tid to qid. Because cromolyn acts by blocking the reaction of allergen with tissue mast cells, it is more effective to prevent rather than to relieve acute symptoms. Since cromolyn costs more and its effect is limited to the nose, it usually is not the first drug to try for hay fever.

When nasal symptoms are inadequately relieved by antihistamines, **intranasal glucocorticoid spray** usually is effective. Two sprays bid to qid are used initially. Beclomethasone dipropionate is available in 2 forms. One is freon-propelled; the other is finger-activated. Both deliver 0.042 mg (42 μg)/dose). Flunisolide 0.025% (0.025 mg/dose) is delivered by a finger-activated pump. When symptoms have been relieved, dosage is reduced to 1 dose bid for the rest of the season. Severe intractable extranasal symptoms may require a short course of **systemic corticosteroids** (prednisone 30 mg/day with gradual reduction in dosage over 1 wk to zero or to 10 mg on alternate days).

Desensitization treatment (see above) is advised if drug treatment is poorly tolerated, if systemic glucocorticoids are needed during the season, or if asthma develops. If the patient is allergic to pollens, therapy should begin soon after the pollen season has ended to prepare for the next season.

Perennial Rhinitis

In contrast to hay fever, **symptoms** of perennial rhinitis vary in severity (often unpredictably) throughout the year. Extranasal symptoms (eg, conjunctivitis) are uncommon, but chronic nasal obstruction is often prominent and may extend to eustachian tube obstruction. The resultant hearing difficulty is particularly common in children. The **diagnosis** of allergic rhinitis is supported by a positive history of atopic disease, the characteristic bluish-red mucosa, numerous eosinophils in the nasal secretions, and positive skin tests (particularly to house dust mites, feathers, animal danders, or fungi). Some patients have complicating sinus infections and nasal polyps.

Eosinophilic nonallergic rhinitis or **nonallergic rhinitis with eosinophilia:** Certain patients who have negative skin tests and numerous eosinophils in their nasal secretions suffer from chronic rhinitis, sinusitis, and polyps. These patients are not atopic, but often have sensitivity to aspirin and other NSAIDs; a subset suffers only from chronic rhinitis. Some patients with mild but annoying chronic continuous nasal obstruction or rhinorrhea have no demonstrable allergy and no polyps, infection, eosinophils, or

drug sensitivity; this condition is called **vasomotor rhinitis** (see Ch. 68).

Treatment

Management is similar to that for hay fever if specific allergens are identified, except that systemic glucocorticoids, even though effective, should be avoided because of the need for prolonged use. Surgery (antrotomy and irrigation of sinuses, polypectomy, submucous resection) may be necessary after allergic factors have been controlled or ruled out. The subset of patients with **eosinophilic nonallergic rhinitis** mentioned above usually respond best to a topical glucocorticoid. For patients with **vasomotor rhinitis**, the only treatment is reassurance, antihistamine and vasoconstrictor drugs, and advice to avoid topical decongestants, which produce after-congestion and, when used continuously for a week or more, may aggravate or perpetuate chronic rhinitis **(rhinitis medicamentosa)**. Some patients may benefit from frequent use of saline irrigation or nasal sprays.

ALLERGIC CONJUNCTIVITIS
(See also VERNAL KERATOCONJUNCTIVITIS in Ch. 79)

Atopic conjunctivitis of an acute or chronic catarrhal form is usually part of a larger allergic syndrome (eg, hay fever), but may occur alone through direct contact with airborne substances (eg, pollen, fungal spores, dusts, animal danders). **Symptoms and signs:** Prominent itching may be accompanied by excessive lacrimation. The conjunctiva is edematous and hyperemic. **Diagnosis:** The cause is often suggested by the history and may be confirmed by skin testing.

Treatment

An identified or suspected causative allergen should be avoided. Frequent use of a bland eyewash (eg, buffered 0.65% saline) may reduce the irritation. Contact lenses should not be worn. Oral antihistamines usually are helpful. Topical antihistamines are available (antazoline 0.5%, pheniramine 0.3, 0.5%, or pyrilamine 0.1%), but only combined with the vasoconstrictors naphazoline 0.025 to 0.05% or phenylephrine 0.125% as ophthalmic solutions. Topical antihistamine or the preservative in the preparation may be sensitizing, and most patients respond equally well or better to an oral antihistamine plus a topical vasoconstrictor alone than to the topical combination. Cromolyn sodium (4% ophthalmic solution) may be helpful, particularly to prevent the development of symptoms when allergen exposure is anticipated (see ALLERGIC RHINITIS, above). Indications for desensitization are similar to those for hay fever. A corticosteroid ophthalmic suspension (eg, medrysone 1% or fluorometholone 0.1% applied qid) may be used as a last resort in severe cases. *Intraocular pressure should be checked before and regularly during such treatment, which should be ended as soon as possible.*

OTHER ALLERGIC EYE DISEASES

The **lids** may be involved by angioedema or urticaria, contact dermatitis, or atopic dermatitis. Contact dermatitis of the eyelids, a cellular (delayed, type IV) hypersensitivity reaction, may be caused by various ophthalmic drugs or others conveyed by the fingers to the eyes (eg, antibiotics by drug handlers) or by face powder, nail polish, or hair dye. The **cornea** may become involved by extension of allergic conjunctivitis or by a variant of superficial punctate keratitis, leading rarely to scarring.

Pain, photophobia, lacrimation, and circumcorneal ciliary inflammation indicate probable **anterior uveitis.** The cause is usually unknown; it may rarely be due to a specific environmental allergen, and bacterial hypersensitivity of the cell-mediated (delayed) type may be suspected. **Sympathetic ophthalmia** is believed to be a hypersensitivity reaction to uveal pigment. **Endophthalmitis phacoanaphylactica** is *allergy to native lens protein.* This severe reaction occurs typically in the remaining lens after the other has been removed uneventfully, though it may follow trauma or inflammation involving the lens capsule. Prompt evaluation and treatment by an ophthalmologist is required in these serious conditions.

FOOD ALLERGY AND INTOLERANCE

Food allergy: *Reproducible symptoms occurring after ingestion of a specific food and for which an immunologic basis is proved or suspected.* **Food intolerance:** *Clinical GI reactions in which the mechanism is not immunologic or is unknown.*

Many common (probably psychophysiologic) adverse food reactions are attributed to food allergy when no convincing cause-and-effect evidence exists, at least of the type of allergy that can be evaluated by skin tests and is thus associated with specific IgE Abs to foods. Certain claims are controversial; eg, that intolerance (or

allergy) to food or food additives can be responsible for hyperactive children, the "tension-fatigue syndrome," and enuresis. Unsubstantiated claims blame food allergy for arthritis, obesity, suboptimal athletic performance, depression, etc.

Occasionally, cheilitis, aphthae, pylorospasm, spastic constipation, pruritus ani, and perianal eczema have been attributed to food allergy or intolerance, but the association is difficult to prove. Recently, food intolerance was found to be responsible for symptoms of some patients with the **irritable bowel syndrome,** confirmed by double-blind food challenge. Of additional interest was the increase in rectal prostaglandin levels when a reaction occurred. Preliminary information suggests that the same phenomenon may take place occasionally in patients with chronic ulcerative colitis. **Eosinophilic enteropathy,** which may be related to specific food allergy, is an unusual illness with pain, cramps, and diarrhea that is associated with blood eosinophilia, eosinophilic infiltrates in the gut, protein-losing enteropathy, and a history of atopic disease. Rarely, dysphagia occurs, indicating esophageal involvement.

Symptoms and Signs

True IgE-mediated food allergy usually develops in infancy, most likely in those with a strong family history of atopy. The first manifestation may be eczema (atopic dermatitis) alone or in association with GI symptoms. By the end of the first year, dermatitis usually is less of a problem as allergic respiratory symptoms begin to develop. Asthma and allergic rhinitis can be aggravated by allergy to foods that can be identified by skin testing. However, as the child grows, foods become less important, and he reacts increasingly to inhaled allergens. By the time the child with asthma and hay fever is 10 yr old, it is rare for a food to provoke respiratory symptoms, even though positive skin tests persist. If atopic dermatitis persists or appears in the older child or adult, its activity seems to be largely independent of IgE-mediated allergy, even though atopic patients with extensive dermatitis have much higher IgE levels in the serum than those who are free of dermatitis.

Some patients very sensitive to potent allergens (eg, allergens in nuts, legumes, seeds, and shellfish) may react violently to ingesting even a trace of such foods, with explosive urticaria and angioedema, and even anaphylaxis. Anaphylaxis may occur in patients with a lower level of sensi-

TABLE 34–2. ELIMINATION DIETS—ALLOWABLE FOODS

Foodstuff	Diet No. 1* (No beef, pork, fowl, milk, rye, corn)	Diet No. 2* (No beef, lamb, milk, rice)	Diet No. 3* (No lamb, fowl, rye, rice, corn, milk)
Cereal	Rice products	Corn products	
Vegetable	Lettuce, spinach, carrots, beets, artichokes	Corn, tomatoes, peas, asparagus, squash, string beans	Lima beans, beets, potatoes (white and sweet), string beans, tomatoes
Meat	Lamb	Chicken, bacon	Beef, bacon
Flour (bread or biscuits)	Rice	Corn, 100% rye (ordinary "rye" bread contains wheat)	Lima beans, soybeans, potatoes
Fruit	Lemons, pears, grapefruit	Peaches, apricots, prunes, pineapple	Grapefruit, lemons, peaches, apricots
Fat	Cottonseed oil, olive oil	Corn oil, cottonseed oil	Cottonseed oil, olive oil
Beverage	Tea, coffee (black), lemonade		Tea, coffee (black), lemonade, juice from approved fruit
Miscellaneous	Tapioca pudding, gelatin, cane sugar, maple sugar, salt, olives	Cane sugar, gelatin, corn syrup, salt	Tapioca pudding, gelatin, cane sugar, maple sugar, salt, olives

*Diet No. 4: Should symptoms persist when on the above 3 elimination diets, the daily diet may be restricted to an elemental diet, such as Vivonex®.

tivity only if they exercise after eating the offending food.

Milk intolerance is sometimes caused by an intestinal disaccharidase deficiency and is expressed by GI symptoms. In other patients, milk causes GI, and even respiratory, symptoms for no identifiable reason. **Food additives** can produce systemic symptoms (monosodium glutamate); asthma (metabisulfite, tartrazine—a yellow dye); and possibly urticaria (tartrazine). A few patients suffer from food-induced or aggravated migraine, confirmed by blinded oral challenge.

That digestion effectively prevents food allergy symptoms in most adults is shown by allergic patients who react on inhalation or contact but not on ingestion (eg, **bakers' asthma**—the affected workers wheeze on exposure to flour dust and have positive skin tests to wheat and/or other grains, yet have no problem eating grain products).

After dietary overindulgence, development of urticaria is a common experience. Since the responsible food can be eaten in moderation later on with no problem, the reaction can best be

classed as a toxic one, although the mechanism is unknown.

Diagnosis

Severe food allergy is usually obvious to the patient. When it is not, diagnosis may be difficult and the condition must be differentiated from functional GI problems.

In persons suspected of having reactions to foods hours after eating, the relationship of symptoms to foods is determined by an **elimination diet** and, if symptoms improve, by reexposure to the food to determine if it is capable of inducing symptoms. All positive challenges are best confirmed by introducing the food in a fashion not recognized by the patient or known by the person administering the challenge (double-blind). The basic diet is determined by eliminating foods suspected by the patient of causing symptoms or by placing the patient on a diet composed of relatively nonallergenic foods (see TABLE 34–2).

Commonly incriminated food allergens include milk, eggs, shellfish, nuts, wheat, peanuts, soybeans, and chocolate, and all products containing one or more of these ingredients. Most common allergens and all suspected foods must be eliminated from the starting diet. No foods or fluids may be consumed other than those specified in the starting diet. Eating in restaurants is not advisable, since the patient (and physician) must know the exact composition of all meals. Furthermore, one must always be certain that pure products are used; eg, ordinary rye bread contains some wheat flour.

If no improvement occurs after 1 wk on a given diet, another should be tried. If symptoms are relieved, one new food is added to the diet and eaten in more than the usual amount for > 24 h or until symptoms recur. Alternatively, small amounts of the food to be tested are eaten in the physician's presence, and the patient's reactions observed. Aggravation or recrudescence of symptoms following the addition of a new food is the best evidence of allergy to that item. Such evidence should be verified by noting the effect of removing that food from the diet for several days, then restoring it.

Treatment

Except for elimination of the offending foods, there is no specific treatment. Elimination diets can be used for both diagnosis and treatment. When only a few foods are involved, abstinence is preferred. Sensitivity to one or more foods may disappear spontaneously. Oral desensitization (by first eliminating the offending food for a time and then giving small, daily increased amounts) has not been proved effective nor has the use of sublingual drops of food extracts. Heating certain foods (eg, milk) may reduce their antigenicity by protein denaturation. Antihistamines are of little value except in acute general reactions with urticaria and angioedema. Oral cromolyn sodium has been used with apparent success in other countries, but the oral form is approved for use in the USA only for mastocytosis (see below). Prolonged glucocorticoid treatment is not indicated except in eosinophilic enteropathy.

For treatment of the severe, potentially fatal acute attack, see ANAPHYLAXIS, below.

ALLERGIC PULMONARY DISEASE

The lungs are involved in known or suspected allergic reactions in several ways, depending on the nature of the allergen and its route of entry. See also ASTHMA in Ch. 37.

ANAPHYLAXIS

Generalized anaphylaxis is an acute, often explosive, systemic reaction that occurs in a previously sensitized person who again receives the sensitizing Ag. This IgE-mediated reaction occurs when Ag (proteins, polysaccharides, and haptens coupled with a carrier protein) reaches the circulation. The most common causative Ags are foreign serum, parenteral enzymes, blood products, β-lactam antimicrobials and many other drugs, desensitizing injections, and insect stings. β-Adrenergic blockers, even as eyedrops, may aggravate anaphylactic reactions. Anaphylaxis can be aggravated or even induced de novo by exercise, and some patients suffer from recurrent symptoms for no identifiable reason. Histamine, leukotrienes, and other mediators are generated or released when the Ag reacts with IgE on basophils and mast cells. These mediators cause the smooth muscle contraction (responsible for wheezing and GI symptoms) and vascular dilation that characterize anaphylaxis. Vasodilation and escape of plasma into the tissues causes urticaria and angioedema and results in a decrease in effective plasma volume, which is the major cause of shock. Fluid escapes into the lung alveoli and may produce pulmonary edema. Obstructive angioedema of the upper airway may also occur. Arrhythmias and cardiogenic shock may develop if the reaction is prolonged.

Anaphylactoid reactions are clinically similar to anaphylaxis, but may occur after the *first* injection of certain drugs (polymyxin, pentamidine, opioids, contrast media), and have a dose-related, toxic-idiosyncratic mechanism rather than an immunologically mediated one. Aspirin and other NSAIDs can cause reactions in susceptible patients.

Symptoms and Signs

Typically, in 1 to 15 min, the patient feels uneasy, becomes agitated and flushed, and complains of palpitation, paresthesias, pruritus, throbbing in the ears, coughing, sneezing, urticaria-angioedema, and difficulty breathing owing to laryngeal edema or bronchospasm. Nausea, vomiting, abdominal pain, and diarrhea are less common. The manifestations of shock may develop within another 1 or 2 min, and the patient may become incontinent, convulse, become unresponsive, and die. Primary cardiovascular collapse can occur without respiratory symptoms.

Prophylaxis

Patients with the greatest risk of a drug anaphylaxis are those who have reacted previously to that drug, but anaphylactic death may occur without such a history. *Since the risk of a reaction to xenogenic antiserum is high, routine skin testing before giving the serum is mandatory,* and prophylactic measures may be needed. Routine skin testing before other drug treatment is neither practicable nor reliable, except for penicillin (tests are discussed under Mechanisms of Drug Hypersensitivity, below).

Long-term desensitization is effective and appropriate in preventing anaphylaxis from insect sting, but has rarely been tried in patients with a history of drug or serum anaphylaxis. Instead, if treatment with a drug or serum is essential, rapid desensitization must be carried out under carefully controlled conditions (see HYPERSENSITIVITY TO DRUGS, below).

A patient with a previous reaction to an x-ray contrast agent, even an anaphylactoid one, can be given an agent again with reasonable safety (if the study is essential) by pretreatment with prednisone 50 mg orally q 6 h for 3 doses, diphenhydramine 50 mg orally 1 h beforehand, and ephedrine (if no contraindication) 25 mg orally 1 h beforehand (adult dosage).

Treatment

Immediate treatment with epinephrine is imperative. It is a pharmacologic antagonist to the effects of the chemical mediators on smooth muscle, blood vessels, and other tissues.

For mild reactions (eg, generalized pruritus, urticaria, angioedema, mild wheezing, nausea, and vomiting) 0.3 to 0.5 mL of aqueous epinephrine 1:1000 should be given s.c. (0.01 mL/kg in children). If an Ag injected in an extremity has caused the anaphylaxis, a tourniquet should be applied above the injection site and $1/2$ of the above dose of epinephrine also injected into the site to reduce systemic absorption of the Ag. A second injection of epinephrine s.c. may be needed. After symptoms resolve, an oral antihistamine should be given for 24 h.

For more severe reactions, with massive angioedema but without evidence of cardiovascular involvement, patients should be given diphenhydramine 50 to 100 mg IV (for an adult) in addition to the above treatment, to forestall laryngeal edema and to block the effect of further histamine release. When the edema is responding, 0.3 mL of an aqueous suspension of long-acting epinephrine 1:200 s.c. (0.005 mL/kg in

children) can be given for its 6- to 8-h effect, an oral antihistamine should be given for the next 24 h, and possibly a glucocorticoid should be given to suppress the late phase of a dual reaction.

For asthmatic reactions that do not respond to epinephrine, IV fluids should be started and aminophylline 6 mg/kg IV should be given over 10 to 20 min, followed by 0.5 mg/kg/h, more or less, to maintain a theophylline blood level of 10 to 20 μg/mL. Endotracheal intubation or tracheostomy may be needed, with O_2 at 4 to 6 L/min.

The most severe reactions usually involve the cardiovascular system, causing severe hypotension and vasomotor collapse. IV fluids should be started and the patient should be recumbent with legs elevated. Epinephrine (1:100,000) should be given slowly IV (5 to 10 μg/min) with close observation for development of side effects, including headache, tremulousness, nausea, and arrhythmias. The underlying severe hypotension may be due to vasodilation, hypovolemia from loss of fluid, myocardial insufficiency (rarely), or a combination of these. Each has a specific treatment, and often the treatment of one exacerbates the others. The appropriate therapy may be clarified if central venous pressure (CVP) and left atrial pressure can be obtained. A low CVP and normal left atrial pressure indicate peripheral vasodilation and/or hypovolemia. Vasodilation should respond to the epinephrine (which will also retard the loss of intravascular fluid).

Hypovolemia is usually the major cause of the hypotension. The CVP and left atrial pressure are both low, and large volumes of saline must be given, with BP monitored until the CVP rises to normal. Colloid plasma expanders (eg, dextran) are rarely necessary. Only if fluid replacement does not restore normal BP should one initiate treatment *cautiously* with vasopressor drugs (eg, metaraminol).

In the rare instance of myocardial insufficiency, both CVP and left atrial pressure will be elevated. Isoproterenol 1 mg in 500 mL of 5% dextrose is infused at 0.5 to 1 mL/min. *The patient should be monitored carefully, for the isoproterenol may cause cardiac arrhythmias and hypotension due to peripheral vasodilation.*

Cardiac arrest may occur, requiring immediate resuscitation (see CARDIOPULMONARY RESUSCITATION in Ch. 30). Further therapy depends on ECG findings.

When all the above measures have been instituted, diphenhydramine (50 to 75 mg IV slowly over 3 min) and glucocorticoids may then be given for treatment of slow-onset urticaria, asthma, laryngeal edema, or hypotension. Methylprednisolone 40 mg IV (or equivalent) should be given and repeated if necessary 8 h later. Complications (eg, MI, cerebral edema) should be watched for and treated specifically. Patients with severe reactions should remain in a hospital under observation for 24 h after recovery to ensure adequate treatment in case of relapse.

Anyone who has had an anaphylactic reaction to a stinging insect should be provided with a kit containing a pre-filled syringe of epinephrine and an epinephrine nebulizer (the latter is for topical therapy of upper airways angioedema) to allow prompt self-treatment of any future reaction. Such a person should also be evaluated for venom immunotherapy (desensitization).

DISORDERS OF VASOACTIVE MEDIATORS

Disorders having manifestations of vasoactive mediators derived from mast cells and other sources (even though an IgE-mediated or other immunologic mechanism may not be involved).

Urticaria; Angioedema
(Hives; Giant Urticaria; Angioneurotic Edema)

Urticaria: *Local wheals and erythema in the dermis.* **Angioedema:** *An eruption similar to urticaria, but with larger edematous areas that involve both dermis and subcutaneous structures.*

Etiology

Acute urticaria and angioedema are essentially anaphylaxis limited to the skin and subcutaneous tissues and can be due to drug allergy, insect stings or bites, desensitization injections, or ingestion of certain foods (particularly eggs, shellfish, nuts, or fruits). Some reactions occur explosively following ingestion of minute amounts. Others (eg, reactions to strawberries) may occur only after overindulgence, and possibly result from direct (toxic) mediator liberation. Urticaria may accompany or even be the first symptom of several viral infections, including hepatitis, infectious mononucleosis, and rubella. Some acute reactions are unexplained, even when recurrent. If acute angioedema is recurrent, progressive, and never associated with urticaria, a hereditary enzyme deficiency should be suspected (see HEREDITARY ANGIOEDEMA, below).

Chronic urticaria and angioedema lasting > 3 wk are more difficult to explain, and only in exceptional cases can a specific cause be found. The reactions are rarely IgE-mediated. Occasionally, chronic ingestion of an unsuspected drug or chemical is responsible; eg, from penicillin in milk; from the use of nonprescription drugs; or from preservatives, dyes, or other food additives. Chronic underlying disease (SLE, polycythemia vera, lymphoma, or infection) should be ruled out. Though often suspected, controllable psychogenic factors are rarely identified. Urticaria caused by physical agents is discussed in PHYSICAL ALLERGY, below. A few patients with intractable urticaria are hyperthyroid. Occasionally, urticaria may be the first or only visible sign of cutaneous vasculitis.

Symptoms and Signs

In **urticaria**, pruritus (generally the first symptom) is followed shortly by the appearance of wheals that may remain small (1 to 5 mm) or may enlarge. The larger ones tend to clear in the center and may be noticed first as large rings (> 20 cm across) of erythema and edema. Ordinarily, crops of hives come and go; a lesion may remain in one site for several hours, then disappear, only to reappear elsewhere. If a lesion persists ≥ 24 h, one should think of the possibility of vasculitis. **Angioedema** is *a more diffuse swelling of loose subcutaneous tissue:* dorsum of hands or feet, eyelids, lips, genitalia, mucous membranes. Edema of the upper airways may produce respiratory distress, and the stridor may be mistaken for asthma.

Diagnosis

The cause of acute urticaria is usually obvious. Even when it is not, a diagnostic investigation is seldom required because of the self-limited, nonrecurrent nature of these reactions. In chronic urticaria, an underlying chronic disease should be ruled out by a careful history and physical examination and routine screening tests. Eosinophilia is uncommon in urticaria. Other tests (eg, stool examination for ova and parasites, serum complement, antinuclear Ab, and sinus or dental x-rays) are not usually worthwhile without additional clinical indications.

Treatment

Acute urticaria is a self-limited condition that generally subsides in 1 to 7 days; hence, treatment is chiefly palliative. If the cause is not obvious, all nonessential drugs should be stopped until the reaction has subsided. Symptoms usually can be relieved with an oral antihistamine (eg, diphenhydramine 50 to 100 mg q 4 h, hydroxyzine 25 to 100 mg bid, or cyproheptadine 4 to 8 mg q 4 h). A glucocorticoid (eg, prednisone 30 to 40 mg/day orally) may be necessary for the more severe reactions, particularly when associated with angioedema. Topical glucocorticoids are of no value. Epinephrine 1:1000, 0.3 mL s.c., should be the first treatment for **acute pharyngeal or laryngeal angioedema**. This may be supplemented with topical treatment; eg, nebulized epinephrine 1:100, and an IV antihistamine (eg, diphenhydramine 50 to 100 mg). This usually prevents airways obstruction, but one must be prepared to intubate or perform a tracheostomy and give O$_2$.

In **chronic urticaria**, spontaneous remissions occur within 2 yr in about $1/2$ of cases. Control of stress often helps reduce the frequency and severity of episodes. Certain drugs (eg, aspirin) may aggravate symptoms, as will alcoholic beverages, coffee, and tobacco smoking; if so, they should be avoided. When urticaria is produced by aspirin, sensitivity to related NSAIDs and to the food- and drug-coloring additive tartrazine should be investigated (see also PERENNIAL RHINITIS, above). Oral antihistamines with a tranquilizing effect are usually beneficial (eg, hydroxyzine 25 to 50 mg bid or cyproheptadine 4 to 8 mg q 4 to 8 h for adults; for children hydroxyzine 2 mg/kg/day divided q 6 h, and cyproheptadine 0.25 to 0.5 mg/kg/day divided q 6 to 8 h). Doxepin 25 to 50 mg bid may be the most effective agent for some adult patients. All reasonable measures should be used before resorting to glucocorticoids, which are frequently effective but, once started, may have to be continued indefinitely.

Hereditary Angioedema

A form of angioedema transmitted as an autosomal dominant trait and associated with a deficiency of serum inhibitor of the activated first component of complement. In 85% of cases, the deficiency is due to a lack of the C1 esterase inhibitor **(C1 INH)**; in 15%, to C1 INH malfunction. A positive family history is the rule, but there are exceptions. The edema is typically unifocal, indurated, painful rather than pruritic, and unaccompanied by urticaria. Attacks are often precipitated by trauma or viral illness, and are aggravated by emotional stress. The GI tract is often involved, with nausea, vomiting, colic, and even signs of intestinal obstruction. The condition may cause fatal upper airways obstruction. **Diagnosis** may be made by measuring C4, which is low even between attacks, or more specifically by showing C1 INH deficiency by immunoassay, and by a functional assay if the former is unexpectedly normal.

Treatment

The edema progresses until complement components have been consumed. Acute attacks that threaten to produce airways obstruction therefore should be treated promptly by establishing an airway. ε-Aminocaproic acid 8 gm q 4 h may succeed in ending the attack. The use of fresh frozen plasma is controversial. Epinephrine, an antihistamine, and a glucocorticoid should be given, but there is no proof that these drugs are effective.

For short-term prophylaxis of the previously untreated patient (as before a dental procedure, endoscopy, or surgery) 2 u. of fresh frozen plasma can be given. Although theoretically a complement substrate in the plasma might provoke an attack, this has not been observed in symptom-free patients. Recently, a partially purified C1 INH fraction of pooled plasma has been shown to be safe and effective for prophylaxis, but it is unavailable for general use. If time permits, it is preferable to treat the patient for 3 to 5 days with an androgen (see below).

For long-term prophylaxis, androgens are effective. One of the impeded androgens should be used. Treatment is begun with oral stanozolol 2 mg tid or danazol 200 mg tid. Stanozolol is less expensive. Once control is achieved, the dosage should be reduced as much as possible to reduce the cost and, in women, to minimize masculinizing side effects. These drugs not only are effective but also have been shown to raise the low C1 INH and C4 toward normal.

Mastocytosis

A condition of unknown etiology characterized by an excessive accumulation of mast cells in various body organs and tissues. Normally, tissue mast cells contribute to host defense by releasing potent preformed mediators (eg, histamine) from their granules and by generating newly formed mediators (eg, leukotrienes) from membrane lipids. Normal tissue mast cells also mediate the symptoms of common allergic reactions by means of IgE Abs attached to specific surface receptors.

Mastocytosis can occur in 3 forms: **mastocytoma** (*a benign cutaneous tumor*); **urticaria pigmentosa** (*multiple small cutaneous collections of mast cells that develop as salmon-colored or brown macules and papules, which ur-*

ticate when stroked and may become vesicular or even bullous); and **systemic mastocytosis** (*mast cell infiltrates in the skin, lymph nodes, liver, spleen, GI tract, and bones*).

Symptoms, Signs, and Diagnosis

Patients with **systemic mastocytosis** have arthralgias, bone pain, and anaphylactoid symptoms. Other symptoms are caused by stimulation of H_2 histamine receptors (increased gastric acid and mucus secretion). Thus, peptic ulcer disease and chronic diarrhea are common problems. The histamine content of tissue biopsies can be extremely high, commensurate with the elevated mast cell concentration. The urinary excretion of histamine and metabolites is high in systemic mastocytosis, and plasma histamine may be elevated. Increased plasma levels of heparin and prostaglandin D_2 (**PGD₂**) have also been reported.

Prognosis and Treatment

Cutaneous mastocytosis usually develops in childhood. The solitary mastocytoma should involute spontaneously; **urticaria pigmentosa** either clears completely or is substantially improved before adolescence. These conditions rarely, if ever, progress to systemic mastocytosis. Treatment of pruritus with an H_1 antihistamine (see URTICARIA, above) is usually all that is needed.

The symptoms of **systemic mastocytosis** should be treated with an H_1 and an H_2 antihistamine. Because prostaglandins, especially PGD₂, are thought to contribute to mast cell–related symptoms, aspirin therapy may be tried, but cautiously; while inhibiting prostaglandin synthesis, this and similar drugs may enhance leukotriene production. If GI symptoms are inadequately controlled, oral cromolyn sodium 200 mg qid (100 mg qid for children 2 to 12 yr old) should be given. There is no effective treatment available to reduce the number of tissue mast cells.

Physical Allergy

A condition in which allergic symptoms and signs are produced by exposure to physical stimuli, eg, cold, sunlight, heat, or mild trauma.

Etiology

The underlying mechanism is unknown in most cases. Photosensitivity (see Ch. 113 and CONTACT DERMATITIS in Ch. 90) may sometimes be induced by drugs or topical agents, including certain cosmetics. Cold and light sensitivity in some cases can be passively transferred with serum that contains a specific IgE Ab, suggesting an immunologic mechanism involving a physically altered skin protein as Ag. An alternative mechanism is suggested by the recent finding of IgG and IgM auto-Abs in some patients with cold urticaria. The serum of a few patients with cold-induced symptoms contains cryoglobulins or cryofibrinogen; these abnormal proteins may be associated with a serious underlying disorder (eg, malignancy, collagen-vascular disease, chronic infection). Cold may aggravate asthma or vasomotor rhinitis, but cold urticaria is independent of any other known allergic tendencies. Heat sensitivity usually produces cholinergic urticaria, which is also induced in the same patients by exercise, emotional stress, or any stimulus that causes sweating. **Dermographism** (*a wheal-and-flare reaction seen after scratching or firmly stroking the skin*) is usually idiopathic but occasionally is the first sign of an urticarial drug reaction. The sensitivity of about $1/2$ the idiopathic cases studied can be passively transferred by serum and appears to be IgE-mediated. Urticaria has also occurred following a persistent, vibratory stimulus (familial), after water exposure ("aquagenic"), and as an immediate or late (4 to 6 h, occasionally 24 h) reaction to pressure.

Symptoms and Signs

Pruritus and unsightly appearance are the most common complaints. Cold sensitivity is usually manifested by urticaria and angioedema, which develop most typically following exposure to cold and during or after swimming or bathing. Bronchospasm and even histamine-mediated shock may occur in extreme cases and result in drowning. Sunlight may produce urticaria or a more chronic polymorphous skin eruption. The possibility of protoporphyria should be considered (see in Ch. 40).

The skin lesions in cholinergic urticaria are small, highly pruritic, discrete wheals surrounded by a large zone of erythema. Cholinergic urticaria appears to be caused by an unusual sensitivity to acetylcholine. A skin test using methacholine 1:5000 may reproduce the lesions, but in only about $1/3$ of cases. The most reliable test is to provoke symptoms with exercise, using occlusive garments to promote sweating.

Prophylaxis and Treatment

The use of drugs or cosmetics should be reviewed with the patient, particularly if photosensitivity is suspected. Protection from the physical stimulus is necessary.

For relief of itching, an antihistamine with sedative effects should be given orally (diphenhydramine 50 mg qid; cyproheptadine 4 to 8 mg qid). Cyproheptadine has been noted to be the most effective in cold urticaria. Hydroxyzine 25 to 100 mg orally qid is the preferred drug for cholinergic urticaria; anticholinergic drugs are ineffective at tolerable doses. Prednisone 30 to 40 mg/day orally should be given in severe light eruptions other than urticaria to shorten the clinical course; the dosage is gradually reduced as the patient improves.

DISORDERS WITH TYPE II HYPERSENSITIVITY REACTIONS

Examples of cell injury in which antibody (Ab) reacts with antigenic components of a cell are Coombs-positive hemolytic anemias, Ab-induced thrombocytopenic purpura, leukopenia, pemphigus, pemphigoid, Goodpasture's syndrome, and pernicious anemia. These reactions occur in patients receiving incompatible transfusions, in hemolytic disease of the newborn, and in neonatal thrombocytopenia, and they also may play a part in multisystem hypersensitivity diseases (eg, SLE).

The mechanism of injury is best exemplified by the effect on RBCs. In hemolytic anemias the RBCs are destroyed either by intravascular hemolysis or by macrophage phagocytosis, predominantly within the spleen. In vitro studies have shown that in the presence of complement some complement-binding Abs (eg, the blood group Abs anti-A and anti-B) cause rapid hemolysis; others (eg, anti-LE) cause a slow cell lysis; still others do not damage cells directly but cause their adherence to and phagocytosis by phagocytes. By contrast, Rh Abs on RBCs do not activate complement, and they destroy cells predominantly by extravascular phagocytosis.

Examples in which the antigen (Ag) is a component of tissue include *early acute* (hyperacute) graft rejection of a transplanted kidney, which is due to the presence of Ab to vascular endothelium, and Goodpasture's syndrome, which is due to reaction of Ab with glomerular and alveolar basement membrane endothelium. In experimental Goodpasture's syndrome, complement is

an important mediator of injury, but the role of complement has not been clearly determined in early acute graft rejection.

Examples of reactions due to **haptenic coupling** with cells or tissue include many of the drug hypersensitivity reactions, (eg, penicillin-induced hemolytic anemia—see HYPERSENSITIVITY TO DRUGS, below).

Antireceptor hypersensitivity reactions *alter cellular function as a result of the binding of Ab to membrane receptors.* In a number of diseases (eg, myasthenia gravis, Graves' and Raynaud's diseases, type B insulin-resistant diabetes, and asthma), Abs to cell membrane receptors have been reported. In myasthenia gravis, the production of Abs by immunization to the acetylcholine receptor in a number of animals has resulted in the typical muscle fatigue and weakness noted in humans. In humans, this Ab also is shown in the serum and on muscle membranes. In addition, when serum or the IgG fraction from patients with myasthenia gravis is transfused into nonhuman primates, a self-limiting myasthenic syndrome is produced. This Ab prevents the binding of endogenously produced acetylcholine to its receptor, thereby preventing muscle activation. In some diabetics with extreme insulin resistance, Abs to insulin receptors have been shown, thus preventing the binding of insulin to its receptor. In patients with Graves' disease, an Ab to the thyroid-stimulating hormone (TSH) receptor has been identified that simulates the effect of TSH on its receptor, resulting in hyperthyroidism. Abs also have been shown to the β_2-adrenergic receptor in asthma and Raynaud's disease, but their role in these diseases is not determined.

Ab-mediated cytotoxicity *reactions occur when an Ab-coated cell is injured by K (killer) cells.* Techniques are available for determining B and T cell subsets of circulating lymphocytes. Another subset does not have B or T cell markers; these are called **null cells** and include **K** and **NK (natural killer)** cells. The K cells bind to cells coated with IgG by their Fc receptors and are capable of destroying the target cell. NK cells do not require Ab coating of the cell for recognition and are capable of lysing tumor cells, virus-infected cells, and fetal cells. These mechanisms have been shown in animal models and in vitro studies of hypersensitivity, but their role in human disease is not established.

Diagnostic Tests

Tests to support this mechanism of immunologic injury include (1) detecting the presence of Ab or complement on the cell or on tissue, or (2) detecting the presence, in serum, of Ab to a cell surface Ag, a tissue Ag, a receptor, or a foreign (exogenous) Ag. Although complement often is required for type II cell injury, and may be detected on the cell or in the tissue, total serum hemolytic complement activity is not depressed as it often is in immune complex (type III) hypersensitivity reactions.

The **direct antiglobulin (Coombs')** and **anti—non-γ-globulin tests** detect Ab and complement on RBCs, respectively. These tests use rabbit antisera, one to immunoglobulin (**Ig**) and the other to complement. When these reagents are mixed with RBCs coated with Ig or complement, agglutination occurs. Abs eluted from these cells have shown both a specificity for RBC blood group Ags and an ability to fix complement, thus showing that they are true auto-Abs and account for the complement present on the RBCs in the direct non-γ-globulin test.

The **indirect antiglobulin test** detects the presence of a circulating Ab to RBC Ags. The patient's serum is incubated with RBCs of the same blood group (to preclude false results due to incompatibility); the antiglobulin test is then done on these RBCs. Agglutination confirms the presence of circulating Ab to RBC Ags.

In penicillin-induced hemolytic anemia the patient has a positive direct Coombs' test while receiving penicillin but has a negative indirect antiglobulin test using RBCs of the same type as the patient. The patient's serum, however, will agglutinate the indirect-test RBCs if they are coated with penicillin.

Fluorescence microscopy is most commonly used to detect the presence of Ig or complement in tissue (by the direct technique) and also can be used to determine the specificity of a circulating Ab (by the indirect technique). In the **direct immunofluorescence technique**, animal Ab specific for human Ig or complement is labeled with a fluorescent dye (usually fluorescein) and then layered on tissue. When the tissue is examined under the fluorescence microscope, a typical fluorescent color (green for fluorescein) indicates the presence of human Ig or complement in the tissue. Direct immunofluorescence also can be used to detect the presence of other serum proteins, tissue components, or exogenous Ag as long as specific animal Abs to them can be produced. The technique itself does not indicate a cell-specific Ag unless the Ab can be eluted from the tissue and its specificity for tissue Ags determined.

In Goodpasture's syndrome the immunofluorescence pattern is seen as a linear fluorescence on kidney and lung basement membrane. When Ab is eluted from the kidney of a patient with Goodpasture's syndrome and layered on normal kidney or lung, it attaches to the basement membrane and gives the same linear fluorescence pattern when tested with fluorescein-labeled Ab to human γ globulin (**indirect immunofluorescence**).

In pemphigus the direct immunofluorescence technique reveals Ab to an Ag present in the intercellular cement of the prickle-cell layer; in pemphigoid, to an Ag in the basement membrane. In both diseases serum Ab is detectable by the indirect immunofluorescence technique. The indirect immunofluorescence technique is used to detect tissue-specific circulating Abs in many other disorders; eg, thyroiditis (antithyroid Abs) and SLE (antinuclear and anticytoplasmic Abs).

Antireceptor tests to detect Ab to the acetylcholine receptors are commercially available, but tests for the insulin and thyroid receptors are not. The clinical significance of the test for detection of Ab to the β_2-adrenergic receptor has not been determined. There are no clinical situations in which the **Ab-dependent cytotoxicity test** is necessary.

See also AUTOIMMUNE DISORDERS, below.

DISORDERS WITH TYPE III HYPERSENSITIVITY REACTIONS

Clinical conditions in which immune complexes (ICs) appear to play some role are serum sickness due to serum, drugs, or viral hepatitis antigen (**Ag**); SLE; RA; polyarteritis; cryoglobulinemia; hypersensitivity pneumonitis; bronchopulmonary aspergillosis; acute glomerulonephritis; chronic membranoproliferative glomerulonephritis; and associated renal disease. In bronchopulmonary aspergillosis, drug- or serum-induced serum sickness, and some forms of renal disease, an IgE-mediated reaction is thought to precede the type III reaction.

The standard laboratory examples of type III reactions are the local Arthus reaction and experimental serum sickness. In the **Arthus reaction** (typically a local skin reaction), animals are first hyperimmunized to induce large amounts of circulating IgG antibodies (Abs) and are then given a small amount of Ag intradermally. The Ag precipitates with the excess IgG and activates complement, so that a highly inflammatory, edematous, painful local lesion rapidly appears (by 4 to 6 h), which may progress to a sterile abscess containing many polymorphonuclear cells, and then to tissue necrosis. A necrotizing vasculitis with occluded arteriolar lumina can be seen microscopically. No lag period precedes the reaction because Ab is present already.

In **experimental serum sickness**, a large amount of Ag is injected into a nonimmunized animal. After a lag period, Ab is produced; when this reaches a critical level (10 to 14 days in man), Ag-Ab complexes form that are deposited in endothelial vessels, where they produce widespread vascular injury characterized by the presence of polymorphonuclear leukocytes. During the appearance of the vasculitis, a fall in serum complement can be detected, and Ag, Ab, and complement can be found in the areas of vasculitis. The Ag-Ab complexes are incapable of inducing injury by themselves, however, but require the presence of increased vascular permeability such as occurs in IgE-mediated (type I) reactions and when complement is activated to enhance vascular deposition of the IC.

Diagnostic Tests

Type III reactions can be suspected in human disease when a vasculitis occurs. In polyarteritis the presence of vasculitis is the only clinical evidence to support a role for ICs. Further support may be obtained by direct immunofluorescence tests (as described above), which may indicate the presence of Ag, immunoglobulin (Ig), and complement in the area of vasculitis.

In experimental studies, fluorescence microscopy shows a coarse granular deposit ("lumpy bumps") along the basement membrane when animal glomeruli are stained for the presence of Ig and complement. A similar distribution can be seen in type III human renal diseases. The electron microscope also can be used to detect electron-dense deposits (similar to those seen in experimental serum sickness), which are believed to be the Ag-Ab complexes. Rarely, the presence of both Ag and Ab can be detected by immunofluorescence in the inflamed tissue—this has been shown in the renal disease of SLE and the vasculitic lesions of hepatitis-Ag–associated serum sickness.

Further evidence to support a type III reaction is demonstration of circulating Ab to Ag such as horse serum, hepatitis Ag, DNA, altered IgG (RF), and some molds. In SLE, for example, a rise in Ab to native undenatured, double-stranded DNA and a fall in serum complement occur during exacerbations of renal disease. If the Ag is unknown, levels of total serum complement and of the early components (C1, C4, or C2) can be tested; a depressed level indicates classic complement activation and therefore that a type III reaction is occurring.

In allergic pulmonary aspergillosis an intradermal skin test with aspergillus Ag may produce an IgE wheal-and-flare reaction followed by an Arthus-like reaction.

Until recently, detection of ICs in serum was by cryoprecipitation (using the property of some complexes to precipitate in the cold). Sophisticated equipment also could detect soluble complexes by analytic ultracentrifugation and sucrose density gradient centrifugation. Several tests detecting circulating ICs now have been developed that depend on the ability of complexes to react with complement components (eg, **C1q-binding assays**) and the ability of complexes to inhibit the reaction between monoclonal RF and IgG. Assays such as the **Raji cell assay** are based on the interaction of ICs containing complement components with cellular receptors (eg, a C3 receptor on the Raji cell). Other assays are available, but the 3 mentioned are used most commonly. No single test detects all ICs, and their use in clinical medicine is limited to following the activity of certain diseases.

AUTOIMMUNE DISORDERS

Disorders in which the immune system produces auto-Abs to an endogenous Ag, with consequent injury to tissues.

Considered here are the pathogenetic immunologic mechanisms underlying autoimmune diseases (see also TABLE 34–3). Clinical aspects of the specific disorders are presented elsewhere in THE MANUAL.

Development of the Autoimmune Response

Although precise details of the autoimmune response are incompletely understood, the outcome of antigenic stimulation, whether Ab formation or activated T cells or tolerance, seems to depend on the same factors with auto-Ag as with exogenous Ag. Four possible mechanisms for de-

TABLE 34-3. PUTATIVE AUTOIMMUNE DISORDERS

	Disorder	Mechanism or Evidence
Highly probable	Hashimoto's thyroiditis	Cell-mediated and humoral thyroid cytotoxicity
	Systemic lupus erythematosus	Circulating and locally generated immune complexes
	Goodpasture's syndrome	Anti-basement membrane Ab
	Pemphigus	Epidermal acantholytic Ab
	Receptor autoimmunity	
	Graves' disease	TSH receptor Ab (stimulatory)
	Myasthenia gravis	Acetylcholine receptor Ab
	Insulin resistance	Insulin receptor Ab
	Autoimmune hemolytic anemia	Phagocytosis of Ab-sensitized RBCs
	Autoimmune thrombocytopenic purpura	Phagocytosis of Ab-sensitized platelets
Probable	Rheumatoid arthritis	Immune complexes in joints
	Scleroderma with anti-collagen Abs	Nucleolar and other nuclear Abs
	Mixed connective tissue disease	Ab to extractable nuclear Ag (ribonucleoprotein)
	Polymyositis	Nonhistone ANA
	Pernicious anemia	Antiparietal cell, microsomes, and intrinsic factor Abs
	Idiopathic Addison's disease	Humoral and (?) cell-mediated adrenal cytotoxicity
	Infertility (some cases)	Antispermatozoal Abs
	Glomerulonephritis	Glomerular basement membrane Ab, or immune complexes
	Bullous pemphigoid	IgG and complement in basement membrane
	Sjögren's syndrome	Multiple tissue Abs, a specific nonhistone ANA (SS-B)
	Diabetes mellitus (some)	Cell-mediated and humoral islet cell Abs
	Adrenergic drug resistance (some with asthma or cystic fibrosis)	β-Adrenergic receptor Ab
Possible	Chronic active hepatitis	Smooth muscle Ab
	Primary biliary cirrhosis	Mitochondrial Ab
	Other endocrine gland failure	Specific tissue Abs in some cases
	Vitiligo	Melanocyte Ab
	Vasculitis	Some cases: Ig and complement in vessel walls, low serum complement
	Post-MI, cardiotomy syndrome	Myocardial Ab
	Urticaria, atopic dermatitis, asthma (some cases)	IgG and IgM Abs to IgE
	Many other inflammatory, granulomatous, degenerative, and atrophic disorders	No reasonable alternative explanation

ANA = antinuclear antibody; Ab = antibody; Ag = antigen; Ig = immunoglobulin; TSH = thyroid-stimulating hormone.

veloping an immune response to auto-Ags are recognized:

1. **Hidden or sequestered Ags (eg, intracellular substances) may not be recognized as "self"**; if released into the circulation they may induce an immune response. This occurs in sympathetic ophthalmia with the traumatic release of an Ag normally sequestered within the eye. Auto-Ab alone may not produce disease because it

cannot combine with the sequestered Ag. For example, Abs to sperm and heart muscle Ags are blocked by the basement membrane of the seminiferous tubules and myocardial cell membrane, respectively. Immunologically active T cells may lack such restrictions and would produce injury more effectively.

2. **The "self" Ags may become immunogenic because of chemical, physical, or bio-

logic alteration. Certain chemicals couple with body proteins and render them immunogenic (as in contact dermatitis). Drugs can produce several autoimmune reactions (see HYPERSENSITIVITY TO DRUGS, below). Photosensitivity exemplifies physically induced autoallergy: ultraviolet light alters skin protein, to which the patient becomes allergic. Biologically altered Ags occur in New Zealand mice that develop autoallergic disease resembling SLE when persistently infected with an RNA virus known to combine with host tissues, altering them enough to induce Ab.

3. **Foreign Ag may induce an immune response that cross-reacts with normal "self"** Ag; eg, the cross-reaction that occurs between streptococcal M protein and human heart muscle; the encephalitis that can follow rabies vaccination in which an autoimmune cross-reaction probably is initiated by animal brain tissue in the vaccine.

4. **Auto-Ab production may result from a mutation in immunocompetent cells.** This may explain the monoclonal auto-Abs seen occasionally in patients with lymphoma.

Finally, autoimmune phenomena may be epiphenomena, and the primary pathogenesis the result of an immune response to an obscure Ag (eg, a virus).

Probably the autoimmune reaction is normally held in check by the action of a population of specific suppressor T cells. Any of the above processes could lead to or be associated with a suppressor T cell defect. Perhaps a perturbation in the regulation of Ab activity by anti-idiotype Abs (Abs to the Ag combining site of other Abs) may play a role.

The roles of other complex mechanisms demonstrable experimentally still need clarification. For example, nonantigenic adjuvants (eg, alum, bacterial endotoxin) enhance the antigenicity of other substances. Freund's complete adjuvant, an emulsion of Ag in mineral oil with heatkilled mycobacteria, is usually required to produce autoimmunity in experimental animals.

Genetic factors play a role: Relatives of patients with autoimmune disorders often show a high incidence of the same type of auto-Abs, and the incidence of autoimmune disease is higher in identical than in fraternal twins. Women are affected more often than men. The genetic contribution appears to be one of predisposition. In a predisposed population a number of environmental factors could provoke disease; eg, in SLE these might be latent virus infection, drugs, or tissue injury such as occurs with ultraviolet light

exposure. This situation would be analogous to the development of hemolytic anemia as a consequence of environmental factors in persons with G6PD deficiency, a predisposing genetically determined biochemical abnormality.

Pathogenesis

The pathogenetic mechanisms of autoimmune reactions are, in many cases, better understood than the way in which autoimmune Abs develop. In some autoimmune hemolytic anemias, the RBCs become coated with cytotoxic (type II) auto-Ab; the complement system responds to these Ab-coated cells just as it does to similarly coated foreign particles, and the interaction of complement with the Ab complexed to the cell-surface Ag leads to RBC phagocytosis or cytolysis.

Autoimmune renal injury can occur as the result of either an Ab-mediated (type II) or immune complex (type III) reaction. The Ab-mediated reaction occurs in Goodpasture's syndrome, in which lung and renal disease is associated with the presence of an anti-basement membrane Ab. The best known example of autoimmune injury associated with soluble Ag-Ab complexes (immune complexes) is the nephritis associated with SLE. Another example is a form of membranous glomerulonephritis that is associated with an immune complex containing renal tubular Ag. Although it is possible that poststreptococcal glomerulonephritis could be due in part to streptococcus-induced cross-reacting Abs, there is as yet no proof.

A variety of auto-Abs are produced in **SLE** and other systemic (as opposed to organ-specific) autoimmune diseases. Abs to formed elements in the blood account for autoimmune hemolytic anemia, thrombocytopenia, and possibly leukopenia; anticoagulant Abs may cause bleeding problems. Abs to nuclear material result in deposition of Ag-Ab complexes, not only in glomeruli but also in vascular tissues and in skin at the dermal-epidermal junction. Synovial deposition of aggregated IgG-rheumatoid factor (**RF**)-complement complexes occurs in **RA**. RF is usually an IgM (occasionally IgG or IgA) with specificity for a receptor on the constant region of the heavy chain of autologous IgG. The IgG-RF-complement aggregates can also be found within neutrophils, where they cause the release of lysosomal enzymes that contribute to the inflammatory joint reaction. Plasma cells are also present in large numbers within the joint, and may synthesize anti-IgG Abs. T cells and lymphokines are also found in rheumatoid joints and may contribute to the inflammatory process. The process that sets off the immunologic events is unknown; it could be a bacterial or viral infection. In SLE the low serum complement level reflects the widespread immunologic reactions taking place; in RA, by contrast, serum complement is normal but intrasynovial complement levels are low.

In **pernicious anemia**, auto-Abs capable of neutralizing intrinsic factor are found in the GI lumen. Auto-Abs against the microsomal fraction of gastric mucosal cells are even more common. It is postulated that a cell-mediated autoimmune attack against the parietal cells results in the atrophic gastritis that, in turn, reduces the production of intrinsic factor but still allows absorption of sufficient vitamin B_{12} to prevent the megaloblastic anemia. If auto-Abs to intrinsic factor should also develop in the GI lumen, however, B_{12} absorption would cease and pernicious anemia would develop.

Hashimoto's thyroiditis is associated with auto-Abs to thyroglobulin, the microsomes of thyroid epithelial cells, a thyroid cell-surface Ag, and a second colloid Ag. Tissue injury and eventual myxedema may be mediated both by the cytotoxicity of the microsomal Ab and by the activity of specifically committed T cells. Low-titered Abs are also found in patients with primary myxedema, suggesting that it is the end result of unrecognized autoimmune thyroiditis. An autoimmune reaction is also involved in thyrotoxicosis **(Graves' disease)**, and about 10% of patients eventually develop myxedema spontaneously; many more do so after ablative therapy. Other Abs unique to Graves' disease are called thyroid-stimulating Abs. They react with thyroid-stimulating hormone **(TSH)** receptors in the gland and have the same effect on thyroid cell function that TSH normally has.

DISORDERS WITH TYPE IV HYPERSENSITIVITY REACTIONS

Examples of clinical conditions in which type IV reactions are believed to be important are contact dermatitis, hypersensitivity pneumonitis, allograft rejection, granulomas due to intracellular organisms, some forms of drug sensitivity, thyroiditis, and encephalomyelitis after rabies vaccination. Evidence for the last 2 is based on experimental models, and in human disease on the appearance of lymphocytes in the inflammatory exudate of the thyroid and brain.

Diagnostic Tests

A type IV reaction can be suspected when an inflammatory reaction is characterized histologically by perivascular lymphocytes and macrophages. Delayed-hypersensitivity skin tests (see discussion of tests for T cell deficiency in Ch. 33) and patch tests are the most readily available methods of testing for delayed hypersensitivity.

Patch tests are used to identify allergens causing a contact dermatitis, but are not done until the contact dermatitis has cleared, in order to prevent its exacerbation. The suspected material (in appropriate concentration) is applied to the skin under a nonabsorbent adhesive patch and left for 48 h. If burning or itching develops earlier, the patch is removed. A positive test consists of erythema with some induration and, occasionally, vesicle formation. Because some reactions do not appear until after the patches are removed, the sites are reinspected at 72 and 96 h.

Blastogenesis of lymphocytes or thymidine incorporation after stimulation with specific Ag are in vitro tests that can be done in a patient with a negative skin test, when the Ag is known, to determine whether the defect is an inability of the skin to react to lymphokines or an inability of T cells to produce lymphokines. The best correlate with type IV delayed hypersensitivity as a measure of immune competence, however, is the blastogenesis of lymphocytes and the production of certain lymphokines in the mixed lymphocyte culture. (For a discussion of these tests, see Ch. 33.)

HYPERSENSITIVITY TO DRUGS

Drug eruptions are discussed in Ch. 97. Discussed here are other hypersensitivity reactions that can follow oral or parenteral drug administration. Contact dermatitis, which is a cellular (delayed, type IV) hypersensitivity reaction that follows topical use, is discussed in Ch. 90; and drug reactions that result from other than immunologic mechanisms are also discussed in Ch. 138.

Before attributing a given reaction to a drug, one should appreciate the fact that *placebos* also may cause unwanted effects. Nausea, tachycardia, excessive sweating, epigastric disturbance with diarrhea, dry mouth, headache, easy fatigue, somnolence, and even skin rashes have been reported by persons taking inert substances in double-blind studies. Nevertheless, true drug reactions constitute a major medical problem. The literature on specific drugs should be consulted for the most likely adverse reactions.

With a **drug overdosage**, toxic effects occur in direct relation to the total amount of drug in the body, and can occur in any patient if the dose is large enough. **Absolute overdosage** results from an error in the amount or frequency of individual doses. **Relative overdosage** may be seen in patients who, because of liver or kidney disease, do not metabolize or excrete the drug normally.

In **drug intolerance**, the adverse reaction develops on the first use of the drug. It may be the same toxic reaction ordinarily expected at higher doses or it may be an exaggeration of a common mild side effect (eg, antihistaminic sedation). **Idiosyncrasy** is *a condition in which the adverse reaction on first use of the drug is pharmacologically unexpected and unique.* Reactions due to genetically determined enzyme deficiencies are being identified in increasing numbers (eg, hemolytic anemia, which develops in patients with G6PD deficiency during treatment with any of several drugs; succinylcholine apnea; isoniazid peripheral neuropathy; see also ADVERSE DRUG REACTIONS in Ch. 138).

Most toxic and idiosyncratic reactions differ sufficiently from allergic reactions to cause no confusion. There are a few exceptions. Toxic or idiosyncratic reactions from drugs with a direct histamine-releasing action (eg, radiographic contrast media, opiates, pentamidine, polymyxin B) may present as urticaria or even as anaphylactoid reactions. Hemolytic anemia may be allergic (eg, penicillin, stibophen) or due to G6PD deficiency. Drug fever may be allergic, toxic (eg, amphetamine, tranylcypromine), or even pharmacologic (eg, etiocholanolone).

Characteristics of allergic reactions: (1) The reaction occurs only after the patient has been exposed to the drug (not necessarily for therapy) one or more times without incident. (2) Once hypersensitivity has developed, the reaction can be produced by doses far below therapeutic amounts, and usually below those levels that give idiosyncratic reactions. (3) Clinical features are restricted in their manifestations. Skin rashes (particularly urticaria), serum sickness, unexpected fever, anaphylaxis, and eosinophilic pulmonary infiltrates appearing during drug therapy are almost always due to hypersensitivity; some cases of anemia, thrombocytopenia, or agranulocytosis may be. Rarely, vasculitis devel-

ops after repeated exposure to a drug (eg, sulfonamides, iodides, penicillin), and interstitial nephritis (eg, methicillin) and liver damage (eg, halothane) have been reported in circumstances consistent with development of specific hypersensitivity.

The standard example of drug hypersensitivity is **serum sickness**, which is an allergic reaction usually appearing 7 to 12 days after administration of a foreign serum or certain drugs (eg, penicillin). Reactions from horse serum occur in at least 5% of persons given it for the first time. It is still used in managing diphtheria, botulism, and venomous snake and spider bites; and antilymphocyte or antithymocyte serum from horses and other species is used to suppress immune reactions to transplanted organs.

Injected serum is slowly excreted, so that it remains in the circulation long enough to stimulate production of specific IgG Abs that form soluble complexes with the Ag to cause an immune complex (type III) reaction; IgE Abs and consequently an IgE-mediated reaction also are produced. Little evidence exists for an IgG immune complex mechanism in serum-sickness–type reactions caused by low-mol-wt drugs.

Onset of symptoms is usually several days after injection of the serum or drug but may be much sooner than the usual 7 days if the patient has been exposed previously (**accelerated serum sickness**). Urticaria is the usual skin manifestation. Less often, the rash may be multiform or morbilliform; rarely, it is scarlatiniform or purpuric. Most patients have polyarthritis or periarticular edema. Temporomandibular arthritis may be severe, and has been confused with tetanus. When fever occurs, it is mild and lasts for only 1 or 2 days. Adenopathy develops in the region draining the injection site and may become generalized. Splenomegaly is sometimes present. Occasionally, abdominal pain and diarrhea may accompany other symptoms. Myocarditis is rare. Peripheral neuritis is the only complication that may cause irreversible injury. Surprisingly, glomerulonephritis, so prominent in experimental serum sickness in animals, is rarely a problem.

Mechanisms of Drug Hypersensitivity

Protein and large polypeptide drugs can stimulate specific Ab production by straightforward immunologic mechanisms. Perhaps the smallest molecule that is potentially antigenic is **glucagon**, with a mol wt of about 3500. Most drug molecules are much smaller and cannot act alone as Ags. However, as **haptens**, some bind covalently to proteins, and the resulting conjugates stimulate Ab production specific for the drug. The drug, or one of its metabolites, must be chemically reactive with protein, and must form a stable covalent bond. The usual serum-protein binding common to many drugs is much weaker and of insufficient strength for antigenicity.

The specific immunologic reaction has been determined only for benzylpenicillin. This drug does not bind firmly enough with tissue or serum proteins to form an antigenic complex, but its major degradation product, benzylpenicillenic acid, can combine with tissue proteins to form benzylpenicilloyl (**BPO**), the **major antigenic determinant** of penicillin. Several **minor antigenic determinants (MDM)** are formed in relatively small amounts, by mechanisms that are less well defined. IgE Abs to the BPO determinant cause the urticaria that follows penicillin administration, while IgE Abs to minor determinants are usually responsible for anaphylaxis as well as urticaria. In addition, IgG Abs have been shown to the major but not to the minor determinants. It is thought that these act as "blocking Abs" to BPO, modifying or even preventing a reaction to BPO, while the lack of blocking IgG Abs to the *minor* determinants seems to explain the ability of these determinants to induce anaphylaxis.

A BPO-polylysine conjugate (benzylpenicilloyl-polylysine) is commercially available for **skin testing**. The minor determinants have not been approved by the FDA as skin testing reagents for penicillin allergy. Fortunately, almost all MDM-sensitive patients will react with one of the reagents, penicillin G, which can be used for skin testing in a concentration of 1000 u./mL. Skin testing is first performed by the prick technique. If the patient gives a history of a severe explosive reaction, the reagents should be diluted 100-fold for initial testing. Negative prick tests may be followed by intradermal testing. If skin tests are positive, the patient risks an anaphylactic reaction if treated with penicillin. Negative skin tests minimize but do not exclude the risk of a serious reaction. Although there is no evidence in man that the penicillin skin test has ever induced de novo sensitivity, it is prudent in most instances to test the patient to rule out penicillin allergy only immediately before essential penicillin therapy is begun. Since they detect only IgE-mediated reactions, skin tests will not predict the occurrence of morbilliform eruptions or hemolytic anemia.

All semisynthetic penicillins (eg, amoxicillin, carbenicillin, ticarcillin) cross-react with penicillin, so that penicillin-sensitive patients often (though not always) react to them as well. Cross-reactions occur with cephalosporins to a lesser degree. Treatment with a cephalosporin should be started with great *caution* if the patient gives a history of a severe reaction (eg, anaphylaxis) to penicillin.

Hematologic Ab-mediated (cytotoxic, type II) drug reactions may develop by any of 3 mechanisms, examples of which follow: (1) In penicillin-induced anemia, the Ab reacts with the hapten, which is firmly bound to the RBC membrane, producing agglutination and increased destruction of RBCs. (2) In stibophen- and quinidine-induced thrombocytopenia, the drug forms a soluble complex with its specific Ab. The complex then reacts with nearby platelets (the "innocent bystander" target cells) and activates complement, which alone remains on the platelet membrane and induces cell lysis. (3) In other hemolytic anemias, the drug (eg, methyldopa) appears to alter the RBC surface chemically, thereby uncovering an Ag that induces and then reacts with an auto-Ab, usually of Rh specificity.

Diagnosis

Toxic-idiosyncratic and **anaphylactic reactions** are sufficiently unique in kind or in time that the offending drug is usually easily identified. **Serum-sickness—type reactions** are most often due to the penicillins, but occasionally sulfonamides, hydralazine, sulfonylureas, or thiazides are responsible. **Photosensitization** is characteristic of chlorpromazine, certain antiseptics in soaps, sulfonamides, psoralens, demeclocycline, and griseofulvin. All drugs except those deemed absolutely essential should be stopped. When **drug fever** is suspected, the most likely drug is stopped (eg, allopurinol, penicillin, isoniazid, sulfonamides, barbiturates, quinidine). Reduction in fever within 48 h implicates that drug. If fever is accompanied by granulocytopenia, drug toxicity is more likely than allergy and is a much more serious matter.

Allergic pulmonary reactions to drugs are usually infiltrative, with eosinophilia, and can be produced by gold salts, penicillin, and sulfonamides, among others. The most common cause of an acute infiltrative pulmonary reaction is nitrofurantoin. This is probably allergic but usually not eosinophilic.

Hepatic reactions may be primarily cholestatic (phenothiazines and erythromycin estolate are most frequently involved) or hepatocellular (allopurinol, hydantoins, gold salts, isoniazid, sulfonamides, valproic acid, and many others). The usual **allergic renal reaction** is interstitial nephritis, most commonly due to methicillin; other antimicrobials and cimetidine have also been implicated.

A syndrome similar to SLE can be produced by several drugs, most commonly hydralazine and procainamide. The syndrome is associated with a positive test for antinuclear Ab and is relatively benign, sparing the kidneys and CNS. Penicillamine can produce SLE and other autoimmune reactions, most notably myasthenia gravis.

Diagnosis of any drug hypersensitivity reaction can be confirmed by challenge, ie, by readministering the drug; but reproducing most allergic reactions to confirm the relationship may be risky, and is seldom warranted.

Laboratory tests for specific drug hypersensitivity (eg, RAST, histamine release, basophil or mast cell degranulation, lymphocyte transformation) are either unreliable or remain experimental. Tests for hematologic drug reactions are an exception (see Diagnostic Tests under DISORDERS WITH TYPE II HYPERSENSITIVITY REACTIONS). For treatment by desensitization, see below.

Skin tests for immediate-type (IgE-mediated) hypersensitivity help in diagnosis of reactions to penicillin (as noted above), enzymes, xenogenic serum, and some vaccines and polypeptide hormones, but for most drugs they are unreliable. For xenogenic serum, a patient who is not atopic and who has not received horse serum previously should first be given a **prick test** with a 1:10 dilution; if this is negative, 0.02 mL of a 1:10 dilution is injected intracutaneously. A wheal > 0.5 cm in diameter will develop within 15 min if the patient is sensitive. All patients who may have received serum previously (*whether or not they reacted*) and those with a suspected allergic history should be tested first with a 1:1000 dilution. Negative skin test results make anaphylaxis (IgE-mediated reaction) unlikely but do not predict the incidence of subsequent serum sickness.

It is usually necessary to stop treatment with the offending drug if the reaction appears to be allergic, in contrast to toxic reactions, where the dose often can be reduced and still be effective without causing a reaction. Most allergic reactions clear within a few days after a drug is stopped. Treatment usually can be limited to control of pain or itching. The arthralgias of serum sickness usually can be controlled with aspirin or another NSAID. Conditions such as drug fever, a nonpruritic skin rash, or mild organ system reactions require no treatment. However, if a patient is acutely ill, with signs of multiple system involvement, or with exfoliative dermatitis, intensive glucocorticoid treatment is required (eg, prednisone 40 to 80 mg/day orally). More information on treatment of specific clinical reactions is found in the pertinent chapters throughout THE MANUAL.

Sometimes a drug that may be lifesaving must be continued despite allergic manifestations; eg, treatment of bacterial endocarditis with penicillin may be continued despite the appearance of a morbilliform eruption, urticaria, or drug fever. Urticaria is treated in the usual manner, including a glucocorticoid if necessary.

Treatment by Desensitization

Rapid desensitization to a drug may be necessary if sensitivity has been established by history and positive challenge or (for penicillin, insulin, antisera) a positive skin test, and if treatment is essential and no alternative exists. As examples, desensitization to penicillin will be described here, and foreign serum desensitization is described below. **Penicillin desensitization** is most likely to be needed to prepare an allergic person for treatment of bacterial endocarditis. This should be done if possible with the collaboration of an expert consultant. If only the intradermal skin test is positive, then the first dose should be given IV: 100 u. (or µg)/mL in a 50-mL bag. It is run in very slowly at first. If no symptoms appear, the flow rate can be increased gradually until the bag is empty after 20 to 30 min. This is then repeated with concentrations of 1,000 and 10,000 u./mL, followed by the full therapeutic dose. If any allergic symptoms develop, the flow rate should be slowed, and the patient given appropriate drug treatment (see ANAPHYLAXIS, above). IV desensitization is safer than s.c. or IM desensitization because both amount and rate of drug administration are under control. **Oral desensitization** also is safe and effective. The first dose is 100 u. (or µg); the following doses are doubled q 15 min, and symptoms are relieved with suitable anti-anaphylactic drugs if they occur. Whichever route is used, the starting dose should be a thousandfold lower if the prick test for penicillin is positive, but this practically never happens.

Desensitization to foreign serum: If the skin test is positive, risk of anaphylaxis is high. If serum treatment is essential, then desensitization is necessary first. Skin tests, using weaker concentrations prepared by serial dilution, are done to determine the proper starting dose for desensitization, which is at the concentration that gave a weak or negative reaction. One-tenth mL of this is injected s.c. or slowly IV; although not the standard method, the IV approach, as with penicillin desensitization, gives the physician control over both concentration and rate of delivery. If no reaction occurs in 15 min, the dose is doubled q 15 min until 1 mL of undiluted serum is given. This dose is repeated IM, and if no reaction occurs in another 15 min, the full dose can be given. If a patient does react, it may still be possible to proceed cautiously by cutting back the dose, treating with an antihistamine and glucocorticoid given as for acute urticaria, and then increasing with smaller increments.

Whenever desensitization is to be carried out, O_2, epinephrine, and resuscitation equipment must be at hand to initiate prompt treatment of anaphylaxis.

35. HEMATOLOGIC DISORDERS

ANEMIAS

Decreases in numbers of RBCs or Hb content because of blood loss, impaired production, increased RBC destruction, or a combination of these alterations.

ANEMIAS DUE TO ALTERATIONS OF RED CELL MEMBRANE

Analysis of the RBC membrane cytoskeleton shows that most inherited or acquired structural alterations result from changes in membrane proteins. Studies of these cytoskeletal proteins (α- and β-spectrin, protein 4.1, F-actin, ankysin) have shown quantitative and functional abnormalities in these hemolytic anemias. Often a familial pattern has been seen in the congenital cases. The mechanism whereby these structural protein alterations result in hemolysis is unknown.

CONGENITAL RED CELL MEMBRANE DISORDERS

(See also CONGENITAL ERYTHROPOIETIC PORPHYRIA under ANOMALIES IN PIGMENT METABOLISM in Ch. 40)

Hereditary elliptocytosis (ovalocytosis): *A rare autosomal dominant disorder in which RBCs are oval or elliptical; hemolysis is usually absent or slight, with little or no anemia; and splenomegaly is often present.* The RBC abnormality appears to be due to altered membrane proteins. Splenectomy relieves hemolysis, but is required only in patients with anemia or a clinical complex as seen in hereditary spherocytosis. The clinical features are similar to those seen in the more common hereditary spherocytoses.

Hereditary spherocytosis (chronic familial icterus; congenital hemolytic jaundice; chronic acholuric jaundice; familial spherocytosis; spherocytic anemia): *A chronic disease, inherited as a dominant trait, characterized by hemolysis of spheroidal RBCs, anemia, jaundice, and splenomegaly.* Although usually one or more family members have had jaundice, anemia, or splenomegaly, one or more generations may be skipped because of variations in the degree of gene penetrance.

Etiology and Pathogenesis

In hereditary spherocytosis, the cell membrane surface area is decreased out of proportion to the intracellular content. Several different RBC membrane protein abnormalities result in spherocyte change. The decreased surface area of the cell impairs the flexibility needed to traverse the spleen's microcirculation, and RBCs are trapped there and destroyed.

Symptoms and Signs

Symptoms and signs are usually mild. Moderate jaundice and symptoms of anemia are present in severe cases. Aplastic crises due to intercurrent infection may exacerbate the anemia. Splenomegaly is almost invariable, but rarely causes abdominal discomfort. Hepatomegaly may be present, and cholelithiasis is common. Congenital skeletal abnormalities (eg, tower-shaped skull and polydactylism) are seen occasionally.

Laboratory Findings

Anemia varies greatly in degree. The RBC count, usually between 3 and 4 million/μL, may fall during an aplastic crisis to < 1 million and the Hb level drops proportionately. Since RBCs are spheroidal and the MCV is normal, the mean corpuscular diameter is somewhat below normal, and RBCs resemble microspherocytes. Reticulocytosis of 15 to 30% and leukocytosis are common.

The osmotic fragility of RBCs is characteristically increased, but in mild cases it may be normal unless sterile defibrinated blood is first incubated at 37° C (98.6° F) for 24 h. Direct antiglobulin (Coombs') test is negative. Glucose can correct an increased autohemolysis.

Prognosis and Treatment

Splenectomy, the only treatment, is indicated in patients under age 45—especially when anemia exists, episodes of jaundice or biliary colic occur, or the patient has had episodes of erythroblastopenia (aplastic crisis). At surgery a gallbladder with stones or evidence of disease should be removed. After splenectomy, symptoms usually abate, the RBC count rises, and the reticulocyte count returns to normal; since spherocytosis persists, the osmotic fragility of the blood is still increased, but the patient is improved because the removal filter (spleen) for these abnormal cells is absent.

ACQUIRED RED CELL MEMBRANE DISORDERS

Stomatocytosis: *Condition of RBCs in which a mouth- or slit-like pattern replaces the normal central zone of pallor.* These cells are associated with both congenital and acquired hemolytic anemia.

The rare congenital form is best characterized and can be used to describe some aspects of this anemia in the acquired form; it has autosomal inheritance. The RBC membrane is considered very "leaky" with hyperpermeability to monovalent cations; movement of divalent cations and anions is normal. Circulating RBCs (20 to 30%) are stomatocytic; osmotic fragility is increased, as is autohemolysis with inconstant correction with glucose. Splenectomy results in amelioration of the anemia in some.

Acquired stomatocytosis with hemolytic anemia occurs primarily with recent excessive alcoholism. Stomatocytes in the peripheral blood and the accelerated RBC destruction disappear within 2 wk of alcohol withdrawal.

Anemia due to hypophosphatemia: RBC pliability depends upon intracellular ATP, Ca, and

Mg levels. Since ATP in RBCs is related to the serum P concentration, hypophosphatemia (serum levels < 0.5 mg/dL) results in erythrocyte ATP depletion; the complex metabolic sequelae of hypophosphatemia also include 2,3-DPG depletion, a shift to the left in the O_2 dissociation curve, decreased glucose utilization, and lactate production. The resultant rigid, nonyielding RBCs are susceptible to injury in the capillary circulatory bed, leading to a hemolytic anemia with membrane injury and microspherocytosis.

Severe hypophosphatemia may occur in alcoholic withdrawal states, diabetes mellitus, the recovery (diuretic) phase after severe burns, hyperalimentation, severe respiratory alkalosis, or in uremic patients on dialysis being treated with antacids. Since these changes are prevented or reversed if cellular ATP is maintained with phosphate supplements, therapy should be directed toward protection against hypophosphatemia in the potential clinical setting and phosphate administration when depletion is recognized.

ANEMIAS DUE TO DISORDERS OF RED CELL METABOLISM
(Hereditary Enzyme Deficiencies)

The prime energy source for RBCs is glucose. After it enters the RBC, glucose is converted to lactate either by anaerobic glycolysis (the Embden-Meyerhof pathway) or via the hexose monophosphate shunt. Hemolytic anemias may result from hereditary deficiencies in the enzyme systems involved in these metabolic pathways.

EMBDEN-MEYERHOF PATHWAY DEFECTS

Embden-Meyerhof pathway defects are relatively rare and share the following characteristics: the trait is autosomal recessive, and hemolytic anemia occurs only in homozygotes; spherocytes are absent, but small numbers of crenated spheres may be present; and hemolysis and anemia persist after splenectomy, though there may be some improvement. The most common form is that of pyruvate kinase deficiency due to a deficient or defective enzyme. Deficiencies in virtually every enzyme reaction are associated with a congenital hemolytic anemia. The exact mechanism of RBC destruction is unknown. In general, assays of ATP and diphosphoglycerate help identify the presence of a metabolic defect and assist in localizing the sites in the pathway for further biochemical characterization.

HEXOSE MONOPHOSPHATE SHUNT DEFECTS

The only important defect in this pathway is caused by glucose-6-phosphate dehydrogenase (G6PD) deficiency. In some cases this is an abnormal enzyme, a form of genetic polymorphism. Clinically, the most common form is that of drug sensitivity.

G6PD deficiency—drug-sensitive variety: This X-linked disorder (see also under PHARMACO-GENETICS in Ch. 137) is fully expressed in males and homozygous females and variably expressed in heterozygous females. It occurs in about 10% of American black males and fewer black females, and in low frequency among people from the Mediterranean basin (eg, Italians, Greeks, Arabs, and Sephardic Jews).

In affected blacks and most affected whites, hemolysis occurs in older RBCs after exposure to drugs or other substances that produce peroxide and cause oxidation of Hb and RBC membranes. These include primaquine, salicylates, sulfonamides, nitrofurans, phenacetin, naphthalene, some vitamin K derivatives, and in some whites, fava beans. In current clinical practice, fever, acute viral and bacterial infections, and diabetic acidosis are the most common precipitating events. Anemia, jaundice, and reticulocytosis develop. Heinz bodies may be seen early during the hemolytic episode, but since they are removed by the spleen, they do not persist in a patient with an intact spleen. Often the best diagnostic clue is the presence in the peripheral blood of RBCs that appear to have had one or more bites (1 μm in size) taken from the cell periphery (**bite cells**), possibly as a result of Heinz body removal by the spleen. Since older cells are selectively destroyed, in most episodes hemolysis is self-limited, affecting < 25% of the RBC mass in blacks; in whites the deficiency is more severe, and profound hemolysis may lead to hemoglobinuria and acute renal failure. Whether the patient will develop a compensated hemolytic state or lethal hemolysis if the offending drug is continued depends on the degree of G6PD deficiency in the patient and the oxidant potential of the drug. Chronic congenital hemolysis (without drug use) occurs in some whites.

Many screening tests are available. Following hemolysis, false-negative results may occur owing to the lack of older, more deficient RBCs and the presence of reticulocytes rich in G6PD. Specific enzyme assays are the best diagnostic tests.

Affected patients should be advised to eliminate drugs or substances that initiate this deficiency.

ANEMIAS DUE TO DEFECTIVE HEMOGLOBIN SYNTHESIS
(Hemoglobinopathies)
(Hemoglobinopathies in pregnancy are discussed in Ch. 17)

Genetic abnormalities of the Hb molecule shown by changes in chemical characteristics, electrophoretic mobility, or other physical properties.

The normal adult Hb molecule (Hb A) consists of 2 pairs of polypeptide chains designated α and β. Fetal Hb (Hb F, in which γ chains replace β chains) is present at birth, but gradually decreases in the first months of life until it makes up < 2% of total Hb in adults. In certain disorders of Hb synthesis and in aplastic and myeloproliferative states, Hb F may be increased. Normal blood also contains ≤ 2.5% of Hb A2 (composed of α and δ chains).

The types of chains and the chemical structure of individual polypeptides in the chains are controlled genetically. Defects may result in Hb molecules with abnormal physical or chemical properties; some result in anemias that are severe in homozygotes but mild in heterozygous carriers. Some persons may be heterozygous for 2 such abnormalities and show an anemia with characteristics of both traits.

Abnormal Hbs, distinguished by electrophoretic mobility, are designated by letters; the first was sickle cell Hb, named Hb S. Since then designations follow the alphabet in order of discovery; thus, C, D, E, G, H, etc. Structurally different Hbs with the same electrophoretic mobility are named also by the city where they were discovered (eg, Hb C$_{Harlem}$, Hb S$_{Memphis}$). In the USA, important hemoglobinopathies are those due to Hb S, Hb C, and the thalassemias; recent immigration of Southeast Asians has led to the common recognition of Hb E in clinical practice. By laboratory tradition the electrophoretic Hb of greatest concentration is named first (ie, AS in sickle cell trait, SA in sickle cell β-thalassemia, etc).

SICKLE CELL DISEASES
(Hemoglobin S Disease; Drepanocytic Anemia; Meniscocytosis)

A chronic hemolytic anemia occurring almost exclusively in blacks and characterized by sickle-

shaped RBCs due to homozygous inheritance of Hb S.

Etiology, Incidence, and Pathogenesis

Homozygotes have sickle cell anemia (about 0.3% of blacks in the USA); heterozygotes (8 to 13% of blacks) are not anemic, but the sickling trait (sicklemia) can be demonstrated in vitro.

In Hb S, valine is substituted for glutamic acid in the sixth amino acid of the β-chain. This decreases its electrical charge, and it moves more slowly toward the anode than Hb A on electrophoresis. Deoxy-Hb S is much less soluble than deoxy-Hb A; it forms a semisolid gel of rodlike tactoids that cause RBCs to sickle at sites of low P_{O_2}. Distorted, inflexible RBCs plug small arterioles and capillaries, which leads to occlusion and infarction. Because sickled RBCs are too fragile to withstand the mechanical trauma of circulation, hemolysis occurs after they enter the circulation.

Symptoms and Signs

In homozygotes, clinical manifestations are due to both anemia and vaso-occlusive events resulting in tissue ischemia and infarction. Anemia is usually severe but highly variable from patient to patient; most have mild jaundice with bilirubin levels of 2 to 4 mg/dL. Anemia may be exacerbated in children by acute sequestration of sickled cells in the spleen. More common is the **aplastic crisis** in both children and adults occurring when marrow RBC production slows during acute infections (especially viral). The vaso-occlusive lesion, which appears due to an abnormal RBC membrane, results in cellular adherence to endothelium and subsequent obstruction. Long bone pain (eg, pretibial) is a common clinical complaint; in children severe pain in the hands and feet (eg, **"hand-foot" syndrome)** is both common and typical. Episodes of arthralgia with fever may occur, and avascular necrosis of the femoral head is common. Chronic punched-out ulcers about the ankles are a recurrent problem. Episodes of severe abdominal pain with vomiting may simulate severe abdominal disorders; such **painful crises** are usually associated with back and joint pain. Hemiplegia, cranial nerve palsies, and other neurologic disturbances may result from occlusion of major intracranial vessels. Infections, particularly pneumococcal, are common, especially in early childhood and are associated with a high mortality rate. Progressive decreases in lung and kidney function may be seen in older patients. Priapism is a seri-

ous complication most commonly seen in the young adult.

Patients may be poorly developed and often have a relatively short trunk with long extremities and a tower-shaped skull. Chronic marrow hyperactivity causes typical bone changes that can be seen on x-ray: widening of the diploic spaces of the skull and the "sun-ray" appearance of the diploic trabeculations are characteristic. The long bones often show cortical thickening, irregular densities, and evidence of new bone formation within the medullary canal. Hepatosplenomegaly is common in children, but because of repeated infarctions and subsequent fibrosis, the spleen in adults is rarely palpable. The heart is usually enlarged, with a prominent pulmonary conus. Heart murmurs may simulate rheumatic or congenital heart disease. Cholelithiasis is common.

In the heterozygous state, affected individuals are normal and do not experience hemolysis, painful crises, or thrombotic complications. There may be an increased incidence of rhabdomyolysis and sudden death in patients with AS trait involved in sustained, exhausting exercise. Hyposthenuria is common. Unilateral hematuria (by unknown mechanisms and usually from the left kidney) occurs but is self-limited. Recognition of the heterozygous sickle cell state should provide understanding of the unilateral bleeding and thus avoid needless nephrectomy. Typical renal papillary necrosis also occurs with increased frequency in sickle cell disease.

Laboratory Findings and Diagnosis

RBCs are normocytic with the count usually between 2 and 3 million/μL and Hb reduced proportionately. Dry stained smears may show only a few sickled cells. The pathognomonic finding is sickling (crescent-shaped RBCs, often with elongated or pointed ends) in an unstained drop of blood that has been prevented from drying or has been treated with a reducing agent (eg, sodium metabisulfite). It may also be produced by reduced O_2 tension. Sealing a drop of blood under a coverslip with petroleum jelly provides such an environment, which may be viewed microscopically. A rapid tube test that depends upon the differential solubility of Hb S is widely used for screening.

Normoblasts are frequently seen in the peripheral blood, and a reticulocytosis of 10 to 40% or more is common. Leukocytosis may rise to 35,000/μL with a shift to the left during either crisis or bacterial infection. Platelets are usually increased. Bone marrow is hyperplastic, with normoblasts predominating; it may become aplastic during sickling crises or severe infections. Serum bilirubin is usually elevated, and fecal and urinary urobilinogen values are high. The ESR is low.

Diagnosis of the homozygous state is made by demonstrating only Hb S with a variable amount of Hb F by electrophoresis. The heterozygote is recognized by the presence of both Hb A and S (with more A than S) on electrophoresis. Hb S must be distinguished from other Hbs that migrate similarly by electrophoresis. This is accomplished by the sickling phenomenon that is negative with other Hbs of similar electrophoretic mobility. This difference is important for genetic counseling. Currently, prenatal screening with recombinant DNA technology is done; the availability of the polymerase chain reaction has remarkably improved sensitivity of prenatal diagnosis.

Prognosis and Treatment

The life span of homozygous patients has steadily increased to > 40 yr. Common causes of death are intercurrent infections, multiple pulmonary emboli, occlusion of a vessel supplying a vital area, and renal failure.

Therapy is symptomatic, since no effective in vivo anti-sickling agent exists. Splenectomy and hematinics are valueless. Transfusions should be given only for anemia that is more severe than usual (eg, during aplastic crises accompanying severe infections); there is little reason to use them in treating painful crises. In general, crises should be managed with vigorous oral or IV hydration and analgesics, including narcotics for pain. Accepted indications for transfusions include cardiopulmonary symptoms (particularly when Hb is < 5 gm/dL) or signs (eg, high output cardiac failure or hypoxemia with $P_{O_2} < 65$ mm Hg) or when other life-threatening events exist and improved O_2 delivery would be of benefit (eg, sepsis, severe infection, cerebrovascular accident, organ failure). Transfusions and RBC exchanges are recommended before general anesthesia and surgery. Reduction in surgical morbidity has been seen when Hb A content is maintained at $> 50\%$ by this approach. Finally, chronic transfusion therapy appears to limit recurrences of cerebrovascular bleeding and is recommended in those < 18 yr old who have had a stroke; therapy is given for at least 3 yr. It is also recommended in patients with recalcitrant leg ulcers, and probably during pregnancy. Since the goals of such programs should be to achieve sickle cell concentrations $< 30\%$ with a Hct not $> 46\%$, partial exchange transfusions are usually the best procedure. A partial exchange or hypertransfusion may break a cycle of closely spaced painful crises. Neither urea nor cyanate therapy has been proved efficacious.

Prophylactic antibiotics, pneumococcal vaccine, early identification and treatment of serious bacterial infection, and general prophylaxis have reduced mortality, particularly during childhood. A recent study showed a marked reduction in the occurrence of pneumococcal septicemia in infants given prophylactic penicillin starting by age 4 mo, suggesting that this should become standard procedure.

Recent trials of hydroxyurea therapy appear to provide an increment in Hb content and a decrease in incidence of pain crisis.

HEMOGLOBIN C DISEASE

The degree of anemia is variable, but can be moderately severe. From 2 to 3% of American blacks show the trait. Heterozygotes are usually not anemic. Symptoms in homozygotes are due to the anemia. The spleen is usually enlarged, and arthralgia is common. There may be abdominal pain but the abdominal crises of sickle cell anemia do not occur. The patient may be mildly jaundiced. Episodes of splenic sequestration with left upper quadrant pain and abrupt decreases in RBC values may occur; if they are severe, splenectomy may be required.

In the homozygote, anemia is normocytic, with 30 to 100% target cells, associated spherocytes, and rarely, crystal-containing RBCs seen in the smear. Reticulocytes are increased slightly, and nucleated RBCs may be present. The RBCs do not sickle. Electrophoresis shows that all the Hb is type C. Serum bilirubin is slightly elevated, and urobilinogen is increased in the stools and urine. There is no specific treatment. Anemia is usually not severe enough to require blood transfusion. In the heterozygote, the only finding is many normochromic cells with central targets.

HEMOGLOBIN S-C DISEASE

Since 10% of blacks carry the Hb S trait, the incidence of the heterozygous S-C combination is much greater than that of the homozygous Hb C disease. Many cases of anemia in patients with sicklemia may represent undetected examples of the S-C combination. The anemia in Hb S-C disease is like that of Hb C disease but milder; some patients even have normal Hb levels. Most symptoms are those of sickle cell anemia, but they are usually less frequent and less severe. However, gross hematuria, retinal hemorrhages, and aseptic necrosis of the femoral head are common. Stained blood smears show target cells and a rare sickle cell. All cells sickle in a sickling preparation.

HEMOGLOBIN E DISEASE

Hb E ($\alpha_2\beta_2^{26glu\rightarrow lys}$) is the 3rd most prevalent Hb worldwide (after A and S), primarily in Southeast Asian (> 15%) and black populations, but rarely in Chinese.

In the heterozygote (Hb AE) no peripheral blood abnormalities are found. Hb electrophoresis reveals about 30% E (found near the origin where A₂, C, and O_Arab occur) and 70% A. On agar gel electrophoresis at acid pH, E comigrates with A, thereby separating it from C and O_Arab. The relative percentage of E decreases in association with α-thalassemia or in the presence of Fe deficiency. Homozygous E is associated with a mild hypochromic-microcytic anemia with prominent targeting. Double heterozygotes for E and β-thalassemia have a hemolytic disease more severe than S-thalassemia.

THALASSEMIAS
(Mediterranean Anemia; Hereditary Leptocytosis; Thalassemia Major and Minor)

A group of chronic, inherited, microcytic anemias characterized by defective Hb synthesis and ineffective erythropoiesis; they are particularly common in persons of Mediterranean, African, and Southeast Asian ancestry. They are one of the most common inherited disorders in man. Prenatal diagnosis by the recombinant DNA approaches of gene mapping has become standard.

Etiology and Pathogenesis

Thalassemia results from unbalanced Hb synthesis due to defective production rates of one or more of the normal globin polypeptide chains (α, β, γ, δ).

β-Thalassemia results from decreased synthesis of β-polypeptide chains. The disease is autosomal dominant: Heterozygotes are carriers and have asymptomatic mild-to-moderate microcytic anemia (thalassemia minor); the typical symptoms occur in homozygotes (thalassemia major). α-Thalassemia, which results from decreased α-chain synthesis, has a more complex inheritance pattern, since genetic control of α-chain synthesis involves 2 pairs of structural genes. Heterozygotes for a single gene defect ("α-thalassemia-2 [silent]") are usually free of

clinical abnormalities. Heterozygotes for a double gene defect or homozygotes for a single gene defect ("α-thalassemia-1 [trait]") tend to manifest a clinical picture similar to heterozygotes for β-thalassemia. Inheritance of both a single gene defect and a double gene defect results in a more severe impairment of α-chain synthesis. The deficiency of α-chains results in the formation of tetramers of excess β-chains (Hb H) or, in infancy, γ-chains (Bart's Hb). Homozygosity for the double-gene defect is *lethal*, since Hb lacking α-chains does not transport O₂. In African-Americans, the gene frequency for α-thalassemia is about 25% and the phenotypic (clinical) expression is seen in 10%.

Symptoms and Signs

Clinical features of all thalassemias are similar but vary in degree. Symptoms of severe anemia occur in β-thalassemia major (Cooley's anemia). Clinical features result from anemia, markedly expanded marrow space, and transfusional and absorptive Fe overload. Patients are jaundiced, and leg ulcers and cholelithiasis occur (as in sickle cell anemia). Splenomegaly is common, and the spleen may be huge. If splenic sequestration develops, the survival time of transfused, normal RBCs is shortened. Bone marrow hyperactivity causes thickening of the cranial bones and malar eminences, producing "hemolytic facies." Long-bone involvement makes pathologic fractures common. Growth rates are impaired, and puberty may be significantly delayed or absent. Fe deposits in heart muscle may cause dysfunction and ultimately heart failure. Hepatic siderosis occurs typically, leading to functional impairment and cirrhosis. Patients with Hb H disease often have symptomatic hemolytic anemia and splenomegaly.

Laboratory Findings
(See TABLE 35–1)

In thalassemia major, anemia is severe, often with Hb ≤ 6 gm/dL. The RBC count is elevated. *The blood smear is virtually diagnostic,* with large numbers of nucleated erythroblasts, target cells, small pale RBCs, and punctate and diffuse basophilia.

Serum bilirubin is increased and the serum-Fe and -ferritin levels are well above normal. The bone marrow reveals florid erythroid hyperplasia. In thalassemia minor (β or α) the usual finding is mild-to-moderate microcytic anemia. Serum-Fe and -ferritin determinations will help rule out Fe deficiency.

TABLE 35–1. CHARACTERISTICS OF THE THALASSEMIAS

Category	Anemia	MCV	% Hb A$_2$	% Hb F
β-Thalassemia				
Heterozygous	Mild	↓	↑	Variable
Homozygous	Severe	↓	Variable	↑ up to 90%
β-δ–Thalassemia				
Heterozygous	Mild		N or ↓	> 5%
Homozygous	Moderate–severe	↓	Absent	100%
α-Thalassemia				
Single gene defect	None	N– ↓	N	N
Double gene defect	Mild	↓ ↓	N– ↓	< 5%
Triple gene defect	Moderate	↓ ↓	N– ↓ (Hb H or Bart's present)	Variable

↓ = decreased; ↑ = increased; N = normal; MCV = mean corpuscular volume.

Diagnosis

Quantitative Hb studies are used for routine clinical diagnosis, and the abnormality depends on the type of thalassemia. In homozygous β-thalassemia, Hb F is usually increased, sometimes to as much as 90%; Hb A$_2$ is also usually elevated to > 3%. Elevation of Hb A$_2$ is the diagnostic test for heterozygous β-thalassemia. The percentages of Hb A$_2$ and F are generally normal in the α-thalassemia syndromes and the diagnosis often is one of exclusion of other causes of microcytic anemia. Hb H disease can be diagnosed by demonstrating the fast-migrating Hb H or Bart's fractions on Hb electrophoresis. The specific molecular defect can now also be characterized, but to date such effort does not alter the clinical approach. Recombinant DNA technology (particularly using the polymerase chain reaction) has been quite important in prenatal diagnosis and genetic counseling.

In β-thalassemia homozygotes, skeletal x-rays show findings characteristic of chronic marrow hyperactivity. The cortices of the skull and the long bones are thinned, and the marrow space is widened. The diploic spaces in the skull may be accentuated, with the trabeculae giving a sun-ray appearance. In the long bones, areas of osteoporosis may occur. The vertebral bodies and the skull may have a granular or "ground glass" appearance. The phalanges may lose their normal shape and appear rectangular or even biconvex.

Prognosis

The outlook varies. Some patients with β-thalassemia major live to puberty or beyond. Life

expectancy is normal for persons with thalassemia minor.

Treatment

Children with thalassemia major should receive as few transfusions as possible, since Fe overload can ultimately result. However, suppression of abnormal hematopoiesis by chronic RBC hypertransfusion may be valuable in severely affected patients; to prevent or delay hemochromatosis, excess (transfusional) Fe must then be removed (eg, by use of chronic Fe-chelation therapy). Transfusing relatively younger fractions of RBCs appears to provide a further advantage at decreasing the rate of Fe overload. Splenectomy may help patients with splenomegaly when superimposed hemolysis of RBCs may occur in the spleen; the benefit is primarily a decrease in transfusion requirements. Thalassemia minor requires no treatment.

HEMOGLOBIN S–β-THALASSEMIA DISEASE

Because of the increased frequency of both Hb S and β-thalassemia genes in similar population groups, inheritance of both defects is relatively common. Clinically, the disorder produces symptoms of moderate anemia and many signs of sickle cell anemia, which are usually less frequent and less severe. Laboratory findings are mild-to-moderate microcytic anemia, some sickled RBCs on stained blood smears, and reticulocytosis. The Hb A$_2$ is > 3%. Hb S predominates on electrophoresis and Hb A is decreased or absent. Hb F increase is variable. Treatment is the same as for sickle cell anemia, although most patients will generally have a milder clinical course.

VASCULAR DISORDERS

Vascular disorders may cause petechiae, purpura, and bruising, but seldom lead to serious blood loss. Tests of hemostasis are usually normal. The diagnosis is made from other clinical findings.

HEREDITARY HEMORRHAGIC TELANGIECTASIA
(Rendu-Osler-Weber Disease)

A hereditary disease of vascular malformation transmitted as an autosomal dominant trait affecting both men and women. Diagnosis is made on physical examination by the discovery of characteristic small, red-to-violet telangiectatic lesions on the face, lips, oral and nasal mucosa, and the tips of the fingers and toes. Similar lesions may be present throughout the mucosa of the GI tract and result in major episodes of GI bleeding. Patients also experience repeated, profuse nosebleeds. Some patients may have associated pulmonary arteriovenous fistulas. Laboratory studies are usually normal except for evidence of an iron-deficiency anemia in most patients.

Treatment is nonspecific. Accessible lesions may be treated with pressure, styptics, and topical hemostatics. Blood transfusions may be needed for acute hemorrhage. Most patients require continuous iron therapy to replace iron lost in repeated mucosal bleeding.

EHLERS–DANLOS SYNDROME AND OTHER HEREDITARY CONNECTIVE TISSUE DISORDERS

Bleeding may result from deficiencies of vascular and perivascular collagen in Ehlers-Danlos syndrome and other rare hereditary connective tissue disorders, eg, pseudoxanthoma elasticum, osteogenesis imperfecta, and Marfan's syndrome (see in INHERITED DISORDERS OF CONNECTIVE TISSUE in Ch. 42).

ALLERGIC PURPURA
(Henoch-Schönlein or Anaphylactoid Purpura)

An acute or chronic vasculitis affecting primarily small vessels of the skin, joints, GI tract, and kidney. The disease affects primarily young children, but older children and adults with allergic purpura are also seen. An acute respiratory infection precedes the purpura in a high proportion of affected young children. Less commonly, a drug appears to be the inciting agent, and a drug history should always be obtained.

Pathology and Pathogenesis
The serum often contains immune complexes with an IgA component. Biopsy of an acute skin lesion reveals an aseptic vasculitis with fibrinoid necrosis of vessel walls and perivascular cuffing of vessels with polymorphonuclear leukocytes. Granular deposits of Ig reactive for IgA and of complement components may be seen on immunofluorescent study. Therefore, deposition of IgA-containing immune complexes with consequent activation of complement is thought to represent the pathogenetic mechanism for the vasculitis. The typical renal lesion is a focal, segmental proliferative glomerulonephritis.

Symptoms, Signs, and Clinical Course
The disease begins abruptly with the sudden appearance of a purpuric skin rash involving primarily the extensor surfaces of the feet and legs, a strip across the buttocks, and the extensor surfaces of the arms. Lesions may start as small areas of urticaria that progress to become indurated, palpable, purpuric spots. Crops of new lesions may appear over days to several weeks. Most patients also have fever and polyarthralgia with associated periarticular tenderness and swelling affecting the ankles, knees, hips, wrists, and elbows. Many patients also develop edema of the hands and feet. GI findings are common and include colicky abdominal pain, abdominal tenderness, and melena or stool tests positive for occult blood. From 25 to 50% of patients develop hematuria and proteinuria. The disease usually remits after about 4 wk but often recurs one or more times after a disease-free interval of several weeks. In most patients the disorder then subsides without serious residual consequences; however, in some patients the renal lesion progresses to chronic renal failure.

Diagnosis, Prognosis, and Treatment
The diagnosis is based largely on recognition of the clinical findings. Prognosis: Renal biopsy may help define the prognosis of the renal lesion. The finding of diffuse glomerular involvement or of crescentic changes in most glomeruli predicts progressive renal failure.

Treatment, except for the elimination of a possible offending drug, is primarily symptomatic. Corticosteroids (eg, prednisone 2 mg/kg up to a total of 50 mg/day) may help to control edema, joint pain, and abdominal pain, but have no effect upon the course of acute renal involvement. Immunosuppressive therapy (with azathioprine or cyclophosphamide) has been used with questionable benefit in patients who develop chronic renal disease.

PLATELET DISORDERS

IMMUNOLOGIC IDIOPATHIC THROMBOCYTOPENIC PURPURA (ITP)

In children, usually a self-limited disorder that follows a viral infection; in most adults, a chronic disorder with no apparent predisposing cause. In childhood ITP, viral antigen (**Ag**) is thought to trigger synthesis of antibody (**Ab**) that may react with viral Ag that has come down onto the platelet surface or that may come down onto the platelet as viral Ag-Ab immune complexes. In contrast, adult ITP usually results from development of an Ab directed against a structural platelet Ag (an auto-Ab). In both forms, physical examination is negative except for petechiae, purpura, and mucosal bleeding, which may be minimal or extensive. Peripheral blood is normal except for reduced platelet numbers with a relative increase in large forms. Bone marrow examination usually reveals increased numbers of megakaryocytes in an otherwise normal marrow.

Treatment in the adult is usually begun with large doses of an oral corticosteroid (eg, prednisone 40 mg bid). In the patient who responds, the platelet count will rise to normal within 2 to at most 6 wk. The corticosteroid dosage is then gradually tapered. Unfortunately, most patients either fail to respond adequately initially or relapse as the adrenal steroid is tapered. Splenectomy can achieve a remission in 50 to 60% of those who fail to respond to adrenal steroid therapy or who relapse after a steroid response. Use of a synthetic androgen, danazol, or immunosuppressive therapy with azathioprine, vincristine, cyclophosphamide, or cyclosporine has been variably effective in patients refractory to steroids and splenectomy.

In the patient with ITP and life-threatening bleeding, an attempt should be made to suppress mononuclear phagocytic clearance of Ab-coated platelets rapidly by giving high-dose immune globulin IV (**IGIV**). The IGIV is given in a dosage of 1 gm/kg on 2 successive days. In most patients this will cause the platelet count to rise rapidly but for only a short period, eg, 2 to 4 wk.

Unfortunately, high-dose IGIV is very expensive. It was recently reported (but unconfirmed) that high-dose methylprednisolone 1 gm/day IV for 3 days, a less costly treatment, is as effective as IGIV in inducing a rapid rise in the platelet count. As already discussed, the patient with ITP and life-threatening bleeding should also be given platelet concentrates.

HEMOLYTIC-UREMIC SYNDROME (HUS)

A disorder characterized by the sudden onset of thrombocytopenia and hemolysis with fragmented RBCs and acute anuric renal failure.

HUS occurs primarily in infants and small children and pregnant or postpartum women, and occasionally in older children and nonpregnant adults. Its pathogenesis is debated. In some patients, a gram-negative infection (eg, an episode of diarrheal illness due to *Escherichia coli* 0157:H7) appears to be an initiating event, and then the syndrome may represent a clinical equivalent of the **generalized Shwartzman reaction**; ie, endotoxemia may trigger an episode of DIC that results in fibrin deposition within the glomerular capillary bed and the onset of acute renal failure. A syndrome resembling HUS may also occur in patients treated with cytotoxic agents, particularly those given mitomycin or cyclosporine. Its pathogenesis is unclear, but presumably involves drug-induced renovascular endothelial cell injury.

Pathogenesis: Although HUS resembles TTP, it differs in that the kidney is primarily affected with the resultant sudden onset of anuria. A characteristic focal renal lesion is found: Its major feature is fibrin thrombi in glomerular arterioles and capillaries. This may lead to fibrinoid necrosis of afferent glomerular arterioles and to areas of frank cortical necrosis. Marked fibrosis of glomerular arterioles may be noted in older lesions. Fibrin thrombi in vessels of other organs are rare. Since the initiating episode of DIC is transient, blood coagulation tests indicative of continuing intravascular coagulation are not found when the usual patient is first seen. This concept of the pathogenesis of HUS does not preclude a role for local factors (eg, glomerular endothelial cell damage as a consequence of fibrin deposition) in the progression of HUS. Fibrin thrombi in small vessels in organs other than the kidneys are rare in HUS.

Prognosis: With conservative management including dialysis, most infants and children with

HUS will recover. (Since some features of HUS resemble TTP, plasmapheresis and plasma exchange have been tried without clear evidence of its efficacy.) The prognosis for recovery in adults is less certain. Postpartum women often do not recover renal function. Most patients with HUS induced by mitomycin die of complications of HUS within a few months.

HEREDITARY DISORDERS OF PLATELET FUNCTION

When a patient's childhood history reveals easy bruising, and bleeding after tooth extractions, tonsillectomy, or other surgical procedures, the finding of a normal platelet count but a prolonged bleeding time suggests a hereditary disorder affecting platelet function. The cause will be either (1) von Willebrand's disease (VWD), *the most common hereditary hemorrhagic disease*, see below, or (2) a hereditary intrinsic platelet disorder, which is much less common. Special studies (eg, measurement of VW antigen (Ag), platelet aggregation studies) are needed to establish the diagnosis. It is important to do so because treatment differs. Bleeding in VWD is managed with infusions of desmopressin, an analog of vasopressin that stimulates release into the plasma of VW factor stored within the Weibel-Palade bodies of endothelial cells, and with cryoprecipitate, a plasma concentrate rich in VW factor. Serious bleeding in a patient with an intrinsic platelet disorder may require transfusion of platelet concentrates. Whatever the cause of platelet dysfunction, drugs that may further impair platelet function should be avoided—particularly aspirin and other NSAIDs used in arthritis. Acetaminophen may be used for analgesia, as it does not inhibit platelet function.

VON WILLEBRAND'S DISEASE (VWD)

An autosomal dominant bleeding disorder resulting from a quantitative (type I) or qualitative (type II variants) abnormality of VW factor (VWF), a plasma protein secreted by endothelial cells that circulates in plasma in multimers of up to 20,000,000 daltons. VWF has 2 known hemostatic functions: (1) The very large multimers are required for platelets to adhere normally to subendothelium at sites of vessel wall injury (see Physiology of Hemostasis, above). (2) Multimers of all sizes form complexes in plasma with factor VIII; formation of such complexes is required to maintain normal plasma factor VIII levels. (Note, therefore, that 2 hereditary disorders may cause

factor VIII deficiency: hemophilia A, described below, in which the factor VIII molecule is not synthesized in normal amounts or is synthesized abnormally, and VWD, in which the VWF molecule is not synthesized in normal amounts or is synthesized abnormally.)

Symptoms and Signs

A typical person with VWD may be of either sex with a positive maternal or paternal history. Bleeding manifestations will be mild to moderate and include easy bruising, bleeding from small skin cuts that may stop and start again over hours, increased menstrual bleeding (in some women), and abnormal bleeding after surgical procedures (eg, tooth extraction and tonsillectomy). Screening coagulation tests will reveal a long bleeding time and sometimes a slightly prolonged PTT reflecting a moderately reduced plasma factor VIII level.

Vasoactive stimuli induced by stress or exercise may temporarily elevate plasma VWF through release of endothelial stores. Hormonal changes associated with stress or pregnancy and an acute phase response to inflammation or infection stimulate increased synthesis of VWF, which will also elevate VWF in plasma. Thus, in persons with mild VWD, plasma level variation may cause screening tests to be normal on some occasions and abnormal on others, making diagnosis difficult; in this circumstance an aspirin-sensitized bleeding time may bring out the abnormality.

Diagnosis

A definitive diagnosis requires measuring (1) total plasma VWF Ag as the height of the "rocket" obtained on electrophoresis of plasma through agarose containing an antibody to VWF; (2) the ability of the plasma to support agglutination of normal platelets by ristocetin (ristocetin cofactor activity), a phenomenon that depends on presence of the intermediate-sized multimers of VWF; and (3) the plasma factor VIII level. In patients with the common type I form of VWD, results will be *concordant;* ie, VWF Ag, ristocetin cofactor activity, and factor VIII coagulant activity will all be depressed to the same extent. The degree of depression will vary in different patients from about 15 to 60% of normal and determines the severity of a patient's abnormal bleeding. (It has recently been noted that a significant number of presumably normal blood donors of blood group O have VWF Ag levels in the 40 to 60% range. This observation requires further study to determine whether such persons should be viewed as having a mild form of VWD.)

Patients with type II variants of VWD synthesize abnormal VWF molecules with a resultant selective deficiency of the very large multimers of VWF. A type II variant is suspected when tests for VWF Ag do not fit with results of a screening test of agglutination of the patient's plasma with different concentrations of ristocetin. Diagnosis may be confirmed by an abnormal precipitin arc on crossed immunoelectrophoresis due to a selective deficiency of the large multimers or by a reduced concentration of large multimers on agarose gel electrophoresis.

Treatment

Replacement of VWF by infusing cryoprecipitate (see under THE HEMOPHILIAS, below) controls or prevents bleeding in either the type I variant or the type II variants of VWD. Dosage is selected empirically (eg, 1 bag/10 kg q 8 to 12 h for several days to prevent excessive bleeding after major surgery). A "pasteurized" intermediate-purity factor VIII concentrate called Humate-P® contains the large multimers of VWF and has not been found to transmit HIV infection or hepatitis. Therefore, it provides a safe alternative to cryoprecipitate. Other intermediate-purity factor VIII concentrates are a less reliable source of VWF when Humate-P® is unavailable. (High-purity factor VIII concentrates prepared by immunoaffinity chromatography contain no VWF and are not used for replacement therapy.)

Desmopressin has an important place in the treatment of type I VWD but is of no value for most patients with type II variants (and may even have paradoxical deleterious effects in the patient with a type IIb variant). When given in a dose of 0.3 μg/kg in 50 mL 0.9% sodium chloride solution IV over 15 to 30 min, desmopressin may cause plasma levels of VWF and factor VIII to rise sufficiently for the patient with mild type I VWD to undergo tooth extraction or minor surgery without the need for replacement therapy. Levels of VWF and factor VIII will revert to baseline according to an intravascular half-life of about 8 to 10 h. ε-Aminocaproic acid (EACA) 75 mg/kg orally qid, or tranexamic acid 25 mg/kg tid, should also be given to suppress fibrinolysis. About 48 h must elapse for new endothelial stores of VWF to accumulate and so permit a second injection of desmopressin to be as effective as an initial dose. In some instances combining the use of desmopressin and cryoprecipitate may substantially reduce the amount of the latter needed to control or prevent bleeding.

AUTOSOMAL RECESSIVE VON WILLEBRAND'S DISEASE

A rare, autosomal recessive form of VWD (type III variant) in which the homozygote (or double heterozygote) has a severe bleeding diathesis and barely measurable (< 1% of normal) plasma levels of VW factor (VWF) and factor VIII. The parents usually have no history of excessive bleeding and at most only a minimal abnormality of VWF on testing. Patients with the type III variant often develop antibodies to VWF after replacement therapy, which complicates management.

HEREDITARY PLATELET DISORDERS

The most common of the hereditary platelet disorders are a group of mild bleeding disorders that may be considered *disorders of amplification of platelet activation.* They may result from a decreased content of ADP in the platelet dense granules (storage pool deficiency), from an inability to generate thromboxane A_2 from arachidonic acid released from the membrane phospholipids of stimulated platelets, or from an inability of platelets to respond normally to thromboxane A_2. They present with a common pattern of platelet aggregation test results: (1) impaired-to-absent aggregation following exposure to collagen, epinephrine, and a low concentration of ADP; and (2) normal aggregation following exposure to a high concentration of ADP. Aspirin and other NSAIDs may produce the same pattern of platelet aggregation test results in normal individuals. Since aspirin's effect can persist several days, one must be sure that a patient has not taken aspirin for several days before being tested to avoid confusion with a hereditary platelet defect.

Thrombasthenia and the Bernard-Soulier syndrome are other rare but important hereditary platelet defects that affect platelet surface membrane glycoproteins. Persons with **thrombasthenia** may experience severe mucosal bleeding (eg, nosebleeds that stop only after nasal packing and transfusions of platelet concentrates). Their platelets, lacking 2 surface membrane glycoproteins (GP IIb and GP IIIa), fail to bind fibrinogen during platelet activation and thus fail to aggregate. Typical laboratory findings are (1) failure of platelets to aggregate with any physiologic aggregating agent including a high concentration of exogenous ADP, (2) absence of clot retraction, and (3) single platelets without small platelet aggregates on a peripheral blood smear of capillary blood obtained from a finger stick.

Bernard-Soulier syndrome: *A rare disorder in which unusually large platelets are found that do not agglutinate with ristocetin but aggregate normally with the physiologic aggregating agents ADP, collagen, and epinephrine.* A surface membrane glycoprotein (**GP Ib**) that contains a receptor for VWF is missing from the platelet surface membrane in this disorder. Therefore, the platelets do not adhere normally to subendothelium despite normal VWF levels in plasma. Large platelets associated with functional abnormalities also may be found in the **May-Hegglin anomaly,** a thrombocytopenic disorder with abnormal WBCs, and in the **Chédiak-Higashi** syndrome.

HEREDITARY COAGULATION DISORDERS

THE HEMOPHILIAS

Most common of bleeding disorders due to hereditary clotting factor deficiencies. Hemophilia A (*factor VIII deficiency*), which affects about 80% of hemophiliacs, and hemophilia B (*factor IX deficiency*) have identical clinical manifestations, screening test abnormalities, and sex-linked genetic transmission. Specific factor assays are required to distinguish the two.

Genetic Manifestations
(See also Ch. 48)

Hemophilia may result from many different mutations of the genes for factors VIII (hemophilia A) and IX (hemophilia B): point mutations involving a single nucleotide, deletions of parts of the gene, and mutations affecting gene regulation. Because both factor VIII and factor IX genes are located on the X chromosome, hemophilia affects males almost exclusively. All daughters of hemophiliacs will be obligatory carriers, but all sons will be normal. Each son of a carrier will have a 50% chance of being either normal or a hemophiliac and each daughter will have a 50% chance of being either normal or a carrier. By measuring factor VIII level and comparing it with the level of von Willebrand factor (**VWF**) antigen (**Ag**), it is often (not always) possible to determine whether a female in a pedigree at risk for being a carrier is a true carrier of hemophilia A. Similarly, measuring the factor IX level will often identify the carrier of hemophilia B. Rarely, random inactivation of 1 of the 2 X chromosomes in early embryonic life will result in a carrier's having a low enough factor VIII or IX level to experience abnormal bleeding.

Analysis of the DNA in the factor VIII gene amplified from lymphocytes by the polymerase chain reaction is available at a few specialized centers. With increased accuracy, this allows identification of the hemophilia A carrier, either directly by recognition of the specific genomic defect when the gene defect in the pedigree is known, or indirectly through study of restriction fragment length polymorphisms (RFLP) linked to the factor VIII gene. These techniques have also been applied to the diagnosis of hemophilia A in the 8- to 11-wk fetus from a biopsy of chorionic villi.

Symptoms and Signs

Different abnormal allelic hemophilic genes support different levels of factor VIII or IX activity. The patient with a factor VIII or IX level < 1% of normal will have severe bleeding episodes throughout his lifetime. The first episode will usually occur before age 18 mo. Minor trauma can result in extensive tissue hemorrhages and hemarthroses, which, if improperly managed, can result in crippling musculoskeletal deformities. Bleeding into the base of the tongue with airway compression may be life-threatening and requires prompt, vigorous replacement therapy. Even a trivial blow to the head requires prophylactic replacement therapy to prevent intracranial bleeding.

Patients with factor VIII or IX levels in the 5% of normal range have mild hemophilia. They rarely have "spontaneous" hemorrhages; however, they will bleed seriously (even fatally) after surgery if not managed correctly. Occasional patients have even milder hemophilia with a factor VIII or IX level in the 10 to 25% of normal range. Such patients may also bleed excessively after surgery or dental extraction.

Laboratory Findings

Typical screening test findings in hemophilia are a prolonged partial thromboplastin time (**PTT**), a normal bleeding time, and a normal prothrombin time (**PT**). Specific assays of factors VIII and IX will determine the type and severity of the hemophilia. Since factor VIII levels may also be reduced in VWD (see above), VWF Ag should also be measured in patients with newly discovered hemophilia A, particularly the patient with mild hemophilia A in whom a family history of sex-linked transmission cannot be obtained.

After transfusion therapy about 15% of patients with hemophilia A develop factor VIII antibodies (Abs) that act as anticoagulants inhibiting the coagulant activity of further factor VIII given to the patient. Patients should be screened for factor VIII anticoagulant activity (eg, by measuring the degree of shortening of the PTT immediately after mixing the patient's plasma with equal parts of normal plasma and after incubation for 1 h at room temperature), especially before an elective procedure that requires replacement therapy.

Treatment

A list of treatment centers and other information about hemophilia care can be obtained from the National Hemophilia Foundation, 110 Greene Street, New York, NY 10012.

Patients with hemophilia should avoid using aspirin; acetaminophen is recommended for analgesia. In some patients disabling pain from musculoskeletal complications may require judicious use of the NSAID ibuprofen, which has a lesser, more transient effect than aspirin on platelet function. Prophylactic dental care on a regular basis is essential to prevent tooth extractions and other dental surgery. All drugs should be given either orally or IV; IM injections can cause large hematomas. Newly diagnosed hemophiliacs should be vaccinated against hepatitis B.

As described above for VWD, use of desmopressin may temporarily raise factor VIII levels in the patient with mild hemophilia A (basal factor VIII levels of 5 to 10%), and such patients should be tested for the response of their factor VIII plasma level to desmopressin. Its use in a responsive patient after minor trauma or before elective dental surgery may obviate or reduce the need for replacement therapy. Desmopressin is uniformly ineffective in severe hemophilia A.

Preparations used for replacement therapy: Fresh frozen plasma contains both factors VIII and IX. However, unless plasma exchange is done, sufficient whole plasma cannot be given to patients with severe hemophilia to raise factor VIII or IX concentrations to levels that effectively prevent or control bleeding episodes. **Plasma concentrates** are available: For hemophilia A, treatment is cryoprecipitate and lyophilized factor VIII concentrate; for hemophilia B, a single concentrate, prothrombin complex concentrate, which contains not just factor IX but all of the vitamin K–dependent clotting factors, is currently available, but a pure factor IX concentrate is expected to become available.

Cryoprecipitate is prepared from single donors by a freeze-thaw technique that removes the thawed plasma before the last ice crystals (which contain factor VIII, VWF, and fibrinogen) are dissolved. Bags of cryoprecipitate are stored frozen and their contents dissolved in 10 mL of 0.9% sodium chloride solution before use. Factor VIII activity is expressed in units, with 1 u. being defined as the amount of factor VIII in 1 mL of normal plasma. The concentration in individual bags varies, but to calculate the number of bags needed for replacement therapy, one may assume that a bag contains 80 u. of factor VIII. Cryoprecipitate is often the replacement therapy of choice in infants and small children.

Lyophilized factor VIII concentrate, prepared from plasma pools of several thousand donors, is of 2 types: intermediate preparations and high-purity preparations prepared by affinity chromatography using monoclonal Abs. The preparations are heat-treated in solution or treated with solvent detergent to inactivate viruses. Concentrates so treated do not transmit HIV (and may not transmit hepatitis, although prospective studies involving larger numbers of patients are needed to verify this). Units of factor VIII are given on the label of the bottle. The lyophilized material is reconstituted in sterile diluent according to the manufacturer's instructions and given IV usually over 5 to 10 min. Lyophilized factor VIII concentrates are particularly useful for home care; patients can give themselves concentrate at the first indication of bleeding. Recombinant factor VIII is being evaluated in patients and presumably will become available for general use. If its price makes widespread use feasible, it could replace plasma factor VIII in the management of hemophilia A.

Calculation of dosage for replacement therapy in hemophilia A: The factor VIII level should be raised transiently to about 0.3 u. (30%) to protect against bleeding after dental extraction or to abort a beginning joint hemorrhage; to 0.5 u. (50%) if major joint or IM bleeding is already evident; and to 1.0 u. (100%) in life-threatening bleeding or before major surgery. Repeat infusions at 50% of the initial calculated dose should be given q 8 to 12 h to keep trough levels above 0.5 u. (50%) for several days in a life-threatening bleeding episode and for 10 days after major surgery.

Dosage is calculated by multiplying the patient's weight in kg by 44 (or lb by 20) and by the desired plasma level in units. Thus, to raise the factor VIII level of a man who weighs 68 kg (150 lb) from essential zero to 1 u./mL, the dosage needed would be 68 × 44 × 1 (150 × 20 × 1) or 3000 u. of factor VIII, whereas to raise the level to 0.33 u./mL would require 150 × 20 × 0.33 or 1000 u. of factor VIII.

Calculation of dosage for replacement therapy in hemophilia B: When dosage of factor IX for replacement therapy is calculated as described above and given as prothrombin complex concentrate, the plasma factor IX level rises to only ½ of that expected from the number of factor IX units listed on the bottle. This may reflect binding of infused factor IX to vascular endothelium. Because prothrombin complex concentrate may contain variable amounts of activated clotting factors, patients receiving repeated doses of factor IX concentrate are, paradoxically, at increased risk for thrombosis. For this reason, factor IX levels are often not raised to 100% before major surgery, but are allowed to fluctuate between about 60 and 30% of normal. Heparin 5 to 10 u. is usually added to each mL of reconstituted prothrombin complex concentrate. Moreover, if a patient must receive replacement therapy for a number of days after a surgical procedure, the amount of concentrate used is reduced by giving the patient fresh frozen plasma as a supplemental source of factor IX.

An antifibrinolytic **(AF)**—ε-aminocaproic acid 2.5 to 4 gm qid for 1 wk or tranexamic acid 1.0 to 1.5 gm tid or qid for 1 wk—should be given to prevent late bleeding after dental extraction or other causes of oropharyngeal mucosal trauma (eg, tongue laceration). *However, because prothrombin complex concentrate may contain activated clotting factors, an AF should not be given immediately after prothrombin complex but only after 10 h has elapsed.* An AF may also be useful in selected patients with other types of bleeding but should not be given to patients with hematuria because of the possibility of formation of clots resistant to lysis within the GU system.

Treatment of bleeding in hemophiliacs who develop a factor VIII inhibitor is difficult and should be undertaken in consultation with someone experienced in such care. In patients with a low initial Ab titer, a large dose of factor VIII, calculated to overcome the inhibitor and temporarily raise plasma factor VIII concentration, may be given. If this does not control the bleeding, further factor VIII infusion will usually be useless because of the rapid rise in Ab titer that the initial infusion induces in most patients. The factor VIII Abs responsible for inhibitor activity are heterogeneous and in some patients do not inhibit or

only minimally inhibit porcine factor VIII. A high-purity porcine factor VIII preparation has proved useful in controlling bleeding in such patients. Prothrombin complex concentrate, which contains variable amounts of an activity bypassing the role of factor VIII in coagulation, has also been used to manage serious bleeding in patients with a high-titer inhibitor, but again runs the risk of inducing hypercoagulability and a paradoxical thrombotic event. The factor VIII inhibitor bypassing material in prothrombin complex concentrate may be factor VIIa. Recombinant factor VIIa in repeated high doses (eg, 50 to 75 u./kg) has recently been reported to control bleeding in a limited number of patients with a factor VIII inhibitor without inducing a hypercoagulable state; if these observations are substantiated in a larger number of patients, then recombinant factor VIIa will become the treatment of choice.

HIV infection in hemophiliacs: Most hemophiliacs treated with plasma concentrates in the early 1980s are infected with HIV. Their care should include instruction on safe sexual practice to minimize the possibility of HIV transmission to a sexual partner. An occasional patient has become thrombocytopenic secondary to HIV infection, which increases the difficulty of managing bleeding episodes. Many patients with positive HIV serology and reduced T4 lymphocyte counts take zidovudine in the hope of delaying disease progression. Unfortunately, an increasing number of seropositive hemophiliacs, particularly those who are older, have developed AIDS (see Ch. 20).

UNCOMMON HEREDITARY HEMORRHAGIC DISORDERS

Other hereditary coagulation disorders are summarized in TABLE 35-2; most are rare, autosomal recessive states producing disease only in the homozygote. Included is an important disorder resulting from a deficiency of a plasma protease inhibitor, α_2-antiplasmin, the major physiologic inhibitor of plasmin. A homozygote for **hereditary α_2-antiplasmin deficiency** will bleed as severely as a hemophiliac after trauma or surgery. The only screening test that will be abnormal is lysis of the plasma clot on incubation overnight in saline. A euglobulin lysis time will be normal. A specific α_2-antiplasmin assay will reveal values in the 1 to 3% of normal range. Prophylaxis with ε-aminocaproic acid or tranexamic acid will correct the bleeding tendency. A hetero-

TABLE 35–2. HEREDITARY DISORDERS OF BLOOD COAGULATION FACTORS

Deficiency	Screening Test Results	Comments
Factor XII **HMWK** **PK**	PTT long PT normal	Test tube abnormality without clinical bleeding. Must be distinguished by specific assays from factor XI deficiency in which postoperative bleeding may occur
Factor XI	PTT long PT normal	AR. Increased frequency in Ashkenazic Jews. No excess bleeding after trauma. May have negative bleeding history after earlier surgery, yet still bleed excessively after next surgery. Diagnosis by specific assay. Therapy for bleeding: Keep factor XI level > 30% with fresh frozen plasma 5–20 mL/kg/day
Factor VIII **Factor IX**	PTT long PT normal	Factor VIII deficiency = hemophilia A; factor IX deficiency = hemophilia B. Sex-linked transmission. Severe bleeding. For therapy, see text
Factor VII	PTT normal PT long	AR, rare. Severe deficiency (< 2%) associated with serious bleeding including CNS bleeding. Levels > 5% associated with mild or no bleeding. Therapy: plasma 3–5 mL/kg. Check availability of recombinant factor VIIa, which will become the therapy of choice
Factor V, X, or prothrombin	PTT long PT long	AR, rare. Bleeding may be mild or severe. Heavy menstrual flow in women. Distinguish by specific assays. Therapy for factor V deficiency: fresh plasma, platelet concentrates (supply platelet factor V). Therapy for factor X or prothrombin deficiency: fresh plasma or prothrombin complex concentrate for life-threatening bleeding
Fibrinogen	In afibrinogenemia (fibrinogen < 10 mg/dL) no clotting in PTT, PT because machine endpoint not triggered. In hypofibrinogenemia (fibrinogen 70–100 mg/dL) PT often ≅ 2 sec prolonged, PTT normal, thrombin time long	Severe bleeding in afibrinogenemia (homozygous state), minimal early bleeding after surgery in hypofibrinogenemia (heterozygous state). Therapy: cryoprecipitate (4 gm fibrinogen as 16 bags of cryoprecipitate)
Dysfibrinogenemia	Thrombin time long PTT often prolonged PT slightly prolonged	Manifestations vary: there may be excessive bleeding, tendency to thrombosis, wound dehiscence. Fibrinogen low by clotting assay but normal by immunologic assay
Factor XIII	PTT normal PT normal Thrombin time normal Clot dissolves in 5M urea	AR, rare. There may be severe bleeding with hemarthrosis, delayed postsurgical bleeding, poor wound healing. Spontaneous abortions in women. Therapy: plasma (1 u. is effective because of long half-life of factor XIII)
Protein C **Protein S**	PTT normal PT normal Thrombin time normal	Heterozygote state (≅ 50%) associated with increased tendency to venous thrombosis. Homozygous protein C deficiency causes neonatal purpura fulminans. Diagnosis: usually by immunoassay of plasma antigen level. Activity assays are becoming available

AR = autosomal recessive; HMWK = high molecular weight kininogen; PK = prekallikrein; PTT = partial thromboplastin time; PT = prothrombin time.

TABLE 35–3. CLINICAL IMPORTANCE OF CHARACTERISTIC
CHROMOSOMAL CHANGES IN ACUTE LEUKEMIA

Karyotype Feature	Clinical Implication
Acute myeloid leukemia	
t(15;18)	M 3
t(8;21)	M 2, better prognosis
inv 16 (p13q22)	M 4 with eosinophilia
−7	Poor prognosis
−5	Poor prognosis
Acute lymphoblastic leukemia	
t(1;19)	Pre-B
t(8;14)	L 3, poor prognosis
t(9;22)	Poor prognosis

zygote with an α_2-antiplasmin level in the 30 to 40% of normal range can also experience excessive surgical bleeding, if an untoward event (eg, a hypotensive episode) triggers an unusual degree of fibrinolytic activity.

THE LEUKEMIAS

Malignant neoplasms of the blood-forming tissues.

Etiology and Pathogenesis

Although viruses cause several forms of leukemia in animals, the cause in humans is undefined; only 2 viral associations are identified: The Epstein-Barr virus, a DNA virus, is associated with Burkitt's lymphoma (see below), and the human T-cell lymphotropic virus, called human acute leukemia/lymphoma virus (HTLV-1), an RNA retrovirus, has been linked to some T cell leukemias and lymphomas. Exposure to ionizing radiation and certain chemicals (eg, benzene and some antineoplastics) is associated with an increased risk of leukemia. Some genetic defects (eg, Down syndrome) and some familial disorders (eg, Fanconi's anemia) predispose to leukemia.

Whatever the etiologic agent, transformation to malignancy appears to occur in a single cell through 2 or more steps with subsequent proliferation and clonal expansion. In some leukemias, specific chromosomal translocations (t) have been identified with consistent leukemia cell morphology and special clinical features (see TABLE 35–3). Usually, transformation occurs at the pluripotential stem cell level, but sometimes it may involve a committed stem cell with capacity for more limited differentiation. The clone tends to be genetically unstable with features of heterogeneity and phenotypic evolution. In general, leukemic cell populations divide with longer cell cycles and smaller growth fractions than normal bone marrow cells. Clonal growth advantage occurs because of the accumulation of leukemic cells defective in differentiation and maturation. Clinical and laboratory features of leukemia are caused by suppression of normal blood cell formation and organ infiltration. Inhibitory factors produced by leukemic cells or replacement of marrow space may suppress normal hematopoiesis, with ensuing anemia, thrombocytopenia, and granulocytopenia. Organ infiltration results in enlargement of the liver, spleen, and lymph nodes, with occasional kidney and gonadal involvement. Meningeal infiltration results in clinical features associated with increasing intracranial pressure.

Classification

The original basis for designating leukemias as acute or chronic was life expectancy; these terms now refer to cellular maturity. Thus, acute leukemias are predominantly undifferentiated cell populations and chronic leukemias more mature cell forms.

Acute leukemias are divided into **lymphoblastic (ALL)** and myeloid **(AML)** types. They may be further subdivided by morphologic and cytochemical appearance according to the French-American-British **(FAB)** classification or according to type and degree of differentiation (see TABLE 35–4). The currently available panel of specific B- and T-cell and myeloid-antigen monoclonal antibodies are most helpful for classification, especially with the availability of flow cytometry for analysis. In some patients, progressive bone marrow failure is associated with a smaller proportion of blast cells insufficient for a definite diagnosis of AML. These patients are classified as having myelodysplastic syndromes or refractory anemias

TABLE 35-4. CLASSIFICATION OF ACUTE LEUKEMIAS

Cell Lineage	Description
Acute lymphoblastic leukemia (ALL)	
Functional classification	
B cell	Immunoglobulin gene rearrangements
Undifferentiated	CALLA-negative
Common	CALLA-positive
Pre-B	CALLA-positive cytoplasmic immunoglobulin (CIg)
B	Surface immunoglobulin (SIg), FAB L 3 morphology
T cell	Antigen–receptor-gene rearrangements
Pre-T	T-antigen–positive; sheep-erythrocyte–receptor-negative
T	T-antigen–and sheep-erythrocyte–receptor-positive
FAB classification	
L 1	Lymphoblasts with uniform, round nuclei and scant cytoplasm
L 2	More variability of lymphoblasts; nuclei may be irregular with more cytoplasm than L 1
L 3	Lymphoblasts have finer nuclear chromatin and blue-to-deep-blue cytoplasm with cytoplasmic vacuolization
Acute myeloid leukemia (AML)	
FAB classification	
M 1	Undifferentiated myeloblastic; no cytoplasmic granulation
M 2	Differentiated myeloblastic; a few to many cells may have sparse granulation
M 3	Promyelocytic; granulation typical of promyelocytic morphology
M 4	Myelomonoblastic; mixed myeloblastic and monocytoid morphology
M 5	Monoblastic; pure monoblastic morphology
M 6	Erythroleukemic; predominantly immature erythroblastic morphology, sometimes megaloblastic appearance
M 7	Megakaryoblastic; cells have shaggy borders that may show some budding

CALLA = common acute lymphoblastic leukemia antigen; FAB = French-American-British.

with excess blasts. In time, a frankly leukemic picture may develop.

Chronic leukemias are described as being lymphocytic (CLL) or myelocytic (CML). CLL is characterized by the appearance of mature lymphocytes in blood, bone marrow, and lymphoid organs. Most CLL patients have clonal expansion of lymphocytes with B cell characteristics; occasionally CLL of the T cell type is found. In CML the characteristic feature is the predominance of granulocytic cells of all stages of differentiation in blood, bone marrow, liver, spleen, and other organs. While the granulocytic series predominates in the expression of this leukemia, RBCs, platelets, monocytes, and even some lymphocytes can be demonstrated to be produced by the same stem cell clone. Orderly differentiation of the granulocytic series is a feature of the early

phase of CML with acceleration of the disease process and eventual blast transformation as the result of clonal evolution.

The diagnosis and appropriate classification of leukemia are usually simple. General features of the 4 common forms are shown in TABLE 35–5. (For details regarding clinical and laboratory features, see specific leukemias, below.)

Treatment Principles

The very nature of hematopoietic cancer necessitates using systemic chemotherapy as the primary treatment modality. Drugs selected according to sensitivities of specific leukemias are usually given in combination. Radiation may be used as an adjunct to treat local accumulations of leukemic cells. Surgery is rarely indicated as a primary treatment modality but may be used in

TABLE 35-5. FINDINGS AT DIAGNOSIS
IN THE 4 MOST COMMON TYPES OF LEUKEMIA

	Acute Lymphoblastic	Acute Myeloid	Chronic Myelocytic	Chronic Lymphocytic
Peak age incidence	Childhood	Any age	Young adulthood	Middle and old age
WBC concentration	H in 50% N or L in 50%	H in 60% N or L in 40%	H in 100%	H in 98% N or L in 2%
Differential WBC count	Many lympho-blasts	Many myelo-blasts	Entire myeloid series	Small lymphocytes
Anemia	In > 90%, severe	In > 90%, severe	In 80%, but mild	In about 50%, mild
Platelets	L in > 80%	L in > 90%	H in 60%; L in 10%	L in 20–30%
Lymphadenopathy	Commonly seen	Occasionally seen	Infrequently seen	Commonly seen
Splenomegaly	60%	50%	Usual and severe	Usual and moderate
Other features	50% CNS occurrence after 1 yr	Rare CNS occurrence; Auer rods may be seen in myeloblasts	Leukocyte alkaline phosphatase low; Philadelphia chromosome positive in 85%	Occasional hemolytic anemia and hypogamma-globulinemia

L = low; N = normal; H = high.

managing some complications. Bone marrow transplantation **(BMT)** from an HLA-matched sibling is sometimes indicated. Autologous BMT (with "purging" of residual leukemic cells) is moving from a research mode to clinical core in selected circumstances. For details, see under specific headings, below.

The goals for treating patients with acute leukemias are to eradicate leukemic cell populations and to restore normal hematopoiesis. For patients with chronic leukemias, the intensity of therapy needed to eradicate the leukemic cells carries a great risk with no evident survival benefits; thus, the goals are to limit the leukemic clone size and to maintain the patient in an asymptomatic state as long as possible. Recent experience with BMT in CML is beginning to change this concept and approach. In addition, general supportive therapy is needed as described below under treatment of the acute leukemias.

THE ACUTE LEUKEMIAS
(Acute Lymphoblastic Leukemia [ALL]; Acute Myeloid Leukemia [AML])

Usually rapidly progressing forms of leukemia characterized by replacement of normal bone marrow by blast cells of a clone arising from malignant transformation of a hematopoietic stem cell. Classification as to cell type—ALL as op-posed to AML—is critical in treatment planning and prognosis. Other names are sometimes used for ALL (eg, acute lymphocytic leukemia) and AML (eg, acute myelocytic, myelogenous, myeloblastic, myelomonoblastic).

Incidence

ALL predominates as the most common malignancy in children, with a peak incidence from ages 3 to 5 yr. It also occurs in adolescents and less commonly in adults.

AML occurs at all ages and is the more common acute leukemia in adults; this form rarely may be associated with irradiation as a causative agent, and it occurs as a second malignancy following cancer chemotherapy.

Pathology

Leukemic cells accumulate in the bone marrow, replace normal hematopoietic cells, and spread to the liver, spleen, lymph nodes, CNS, kidneys, and gonads. Since the cells are blood-borne, they can accumulate in and affect any organ or site. The accumulation can often be identified with specific acute types (eg, T cell ALL often involves the CNS; acute monoblastic leukemia, the gums; acute myeloid leukemia, lo-calized collections in skin or around the head and neck [**chloromas**]). Leukemic infiltration appears as sheets of undifferentiated round cells with usually minimal disruption of organ function except for the CNS and bone marrow. Meningeal infiltration results in increasing intracranial pressure, and replacement of normal hematopoiesis in the bone marrow causes anemia, thrombocytopenia, and granulocytopenia.

Symptoms and Signs

The presenting findings usually represent the consequences of failure of normal hematopoiesis: bleeding, pallor, and fever. Bleeding is usually manifested by petechiae and easy bruisability with mucous membrane hemorrhage (eg, epistaxis). Hematuria and GI bleeding are uncommon. Initial CNS involvement may be associated with headaches, vomiting, and irritability. Sometimes bone and joint pain may be the dominant complaint. Granulocytopenia may be associated with an obvious bacterial infection; more commonly, if fever is present, its cause cannot be found. Sometimes an insidious onset is associated with progressive weakness, lethargy, and pallor.

Diagnosis

Diagnosis is established by laboratory findings. Some degree of anemia and thrombocytopenia is almost always found. The total WBC count may be decreased, normal, or increased. Leukemic blast cells are inevitably found in the blood smear unless the WBC count is markedly decreased. Although the diagnosis can usually be made from the smear, a bone marrow examination should always confirm it. Sometimes a bone marrow aspiration yields such a hypocellular specimen that a needle biopsy is required; its examination should include both touch preparations for cytology and sections for cellularity. Aplastic anemia should be considered in the differential diagnosis of severe pancytopenia, but bone marrow biopsy should be definitive, and an experienced observer will not confuse the atypical lymphocytes of infectious mononucleosis with leukemic cells. It is important to distinguish the blasts of ALL from AML. In addition to smears with the usual stains, para-aminosalicylic acid (PAS), myeloperoxidase, Sudan Black B, and specific and nonspecific esterase histochemical stains are frequently helpful.

Prognosis

Before treatment was available, the average person survived about 4 mo after diagnosis.

Now, cure is the realizable goal for both ALL and AML.

Several features help to predict the prognosis of patients with ALL. Favorable factors include an age of 3 to 7 yr, total WBC counts < 25,000/μL, FAB L 1 morphology, a leukemic cell karyotype with > 50 chromosomes and no CNS disease at diagnosis. Unfavorable factors include total WBC counts > 25,000/μL, a leukemic cell karyotype with chromosomes that are normal in number but abnormal in morphology (pseudodiploid), age of > 20 yr, and leukemic blast cells with cytoplasmic immunoglobulin.

Regardless of risk factors, the likelihood of initial remission is ≥ 90% in ALL patients. Fifty percent of children should have continuous disease-free survival for 5 yr. Depending on the presence of risk factors mentioned above, expectations may be better or worse. Most regimens select patients with poor risk factors for more intense therapy with the understanding that the increased risk from treatment is outweighed by the greater risk of treatment failure.

For patients with AML, reported remission induction rates range from 50 to 85%. Failure to achieve remission can be related to drug resistance or death from infection or bleeding during the period of hypoplasia. The FAB classification has not proved useful to predict risk of failure. The most important prognostic feature is age; patients > 50 yr are less likely to achieve remission.

Long-term disease-free survival currently is reported to occur in 20 to 40% of patients. Bone marrow transplantation (BMT) is reported to result in 40 to 50% long-term disease-free survival. Patients who develop AML following chemotherapy and irradiation have the poorest prognosis. It is clear that some patients with AML can achieve long-term disease-free survival and probably cure, which should be the therapeutic goal for every patient.

Treatment

The first goal is to achieve complete remission, which is associated with resolution of abnormal clinical features, return to normal blood counts, and hematopoiesis in the bone marrow with < 5% blast cells. Biologically, remission is associated with disappearance of the leukemic clone and restoration of normal polyclonal hematopoietic proliferation. It is possible here to give only a general outline for achieving and maintaining remission. Concepts of both specific and supportive therapy are constantly being revised and improved. Treatment programs and clinical situations are complex and, for optimal outcome, require an experienced team. The responsible physician should be knowledgeable and aware of current treatment opportunities. Whenever possible, patients should be treated at specialized medical centers, particularly during critical phases.

To characterize leukemic cells, one must take full advantage of available laboratory studies, including cytogenetics and immunophenotyping. In addition to the histochemical studies mentioned above that help delineate ALL and AML, the subclassification of ALL according to cell type and the observations of the leukemic karyotype can further identify the patient's risk status. In general, high-risk patients are assigned to more intensive regimens.

Although basic principles in treating ALL and AML are similar, details of the regimens and drugs differ. Because patients with AML usually undergo an initial phase of marrow hypoplasia that is more intense and more extended before recovery of normal hematopoiesis, they need greater supportive therapy.

Supportive care requires blood bank, pharmacy, laboratory, and nursing services. Bleeding, usually the consequence of thrombocytopenia, generally responds to platelet administration. In acute promyelocytic leukemia, disseminated intravascular coagulation (DIC) may occur as leukemic cell lysis releases procoagulant; in some centers, heparinization is routine during initial therapy. Fever in the neutropenic patient has been mentioned; after appropriate studies and cultures are obtained, combination antibiotic therapy should be given promptly. Anemia is treated with packed RBC transfusions unless caused by massive bleeding, in which case whole blood may be indicated to restore blood volume. Neutropenic patients with gram-negative sepsis may be helped with granulocyte transfusions. Prophylactic granulocyte transfusions are of no benefit. For the leukemic who is also at risk from opportunistic infections associated with drug-induced immunosuppression, trimethoprim/sulfamethoxazole (TMP/SMX) 5/25 mg/kg/day for 1 mo should be given to prevent Pneumocystis carinii pneumonia.

Infections are serious in the neutropenic, immunosuppressed patient. The febrile, neutropenic patient should have appropriate studies and cultures according to clinical findings. Because of the likelihood of a bacterial sepsis even without clinical evidence of infection, patients with neutrophil counts < 500/μL should be started on combination antibiotic treatment (which usually should include a semisynthetic penicillin and an aminoglycoside) after cultures are obtained. Fungal infections may be difficult to diagnose, and in some situations empiric treatment with fungicidal agents is indicated. In the patient with pneumonitis, the diagnosis of P. carinii should be suspected and confirmed, then treated with TMP/SMX 20/100 mg/kg/day in oral doses divided qid, or parenterally, if needed. Too little experience with newer antiviral agents is available to know their specific roles.

In patients undergoing rapid lysis of leukemic cells associated with initial therapy, metabolic abnormalities may occur, including hyperuricemia, hyperphosphatemia, and hyperkalemia. If rapid cell lysis is anticipated, careful attention to hydration, urine alkalinization, and electrolyte balance must be maintained to avoid the complication of uric acid nephropathy. Hyperuricemia can be minimized by giving allopurinol (a xanthine oxidase inhibitor) before starting chemotherapy to reduce the conversion of xanthine to uric acid.

ALL: Several regimens emphasize early introduction of an intensive multiple drug regimen. Remission can be induced with daily oral prednisone and weekly IV vincristine with the addition of a third agent, either an anthracycline or asparaginase. Other drugs and combinations that may be introduced early in treatment are cytarabine and etoposide, cyclophosphamide and doxorubicin, and asparaginase. In some regimens, IV methotrexate is given in an intermediate dose with leucovorin rescue. The combinations and their dosages are modified according to the presence of factors that predict a high risk of treatment failure. An important site of leukemic infiltration is the meninges (see SUBACUTE AND CHRONIC MENINGITIS in Ch. 32); treatment may include intrathecal methotrexate plus cranial irradiation or intermediate dose IV methotrexate. CNS prophylaxis is usually given after completion of remission induction.

Most regimens include maintenance therapy for continued suppression of leukemic cells and reduction of their numbers to a point consistent with cure. Treatment usually lasts from 2½ to 3 yr. Some regimens that are more intensive in earlier phases may use shorter total therapy durations. For the patient who has been in continuous complete remission for 2½ yr, the risk for relapse after cessation of therapy is about 20%, usually within 1 yr. Thus, when therapy can be stopped, most patients are cured.

Relapse occurs most often in the bone marrow but may also happen in the CNS or testes. Bone marrow relapse is an ominous event. Although remissions can be reinduced in 80 to 90% of patients, subsequent remissions tend to be brief, and patients usually have already been exposed to the most effective drugs. If an HLA-matched sibling is available, BMT is advocated for patients in second remission. A small proportion of patients who have bone marrow relapses, however, can achieve long disease-free second remissions and may even be cured. CNS disease may be the first evidence of relapse, even in those who have had effective CNS prophylaxis. Treatment includes intrathecal injection of methotrexate (with or without cytarabine) 1 or 2 times/wk until all signs disappear. Most regimens include systemic chemotherapy in the form of a reinduction regimen because of likelihood of systemic spread of blast cells. The role of continued intrathecal drug or CNS irradiation is not clear. Testicular relapse may be evident clinically with painless firm swelling of the testis, or it may be identified on routine biopsy. Clinical evidence of unilateral testicular involvement should always be an indication to biopsy the apparently uninvolved testis. Treatment is by irradiation and administration of systemic reinduction therapy as noted above for isolated CNS relapse.

AML: The initial approach to therapy, the prompt induction of a remission, is identical to that for ALL. The major difference in treatment is that ALL responds to a wider variety of drugs, some of which are not particularly myelsuppressive. In AML, treatment usually results in significant myelosuppression; thus, patients often get clinically worse before they improve. The period of myelosuppression before marrow recovery requires meticulous anticipatory and supportive care. The basic induction regimen includes cytarabine given by continuous IV infusion or s.c. q 12 h for 5 to 7 days. Daunorubicin is given IV for 3 days during this time. Some regimens include 6-thioguanine or vincristine and prednisone, but their contribution is unclear. After remission is achieved, many regimens contain a phase of intensification with these or other agents. CNS prophylaxis is usually not given because it has no demonstrated contribution to remission duration or survival. With better systemic disease control, CNS leukemia might become a more frequent complication. There is no demonstrated role for

maintenance therapy in AML. Extramedullary sites are infrequently involved in isolated relapse. BMT early after a remission has been achieved would be recommended for younger patients with HLA-matched siblings. As mentioned above, AML of the acute promyelocytic type should be carefully observed for DIC. Most centers would recommend prophylactic heparinization before beginning therapy.

MALIGNANT LYMPHOMAS: NON–HODGKIN'S LYMPHOMA (NHL)

A heterogeneous group of diseases consisting of neoplastic proliferation of lymphoid cells that usually disseminate throughout the body. The old terms lymphosarcoma and reticulum cell sarcoma have been replaced by nomenclature that reflects the cell of origin and biology of the disease (see below). Their courses vary from rapidly fatal to indolent and initially well tolerated. A leukemia-like picture may develop in up to 50% of children and about 20% of adults with some types of NHL.

Incidence and Etiology

NHL occurs more often than Hodgkin's disease. Annually in the USA, 8,000 to 10,000 new cases are diagnosed in all age groups, the incidence increasing with age. Its cause is unknown, although, as with the leukemias, substantial experimental evidence suggests a virus. Close association of a human **type C retrovirus** with some adult leukemias and lymphomas composed of peripheral T cells has been shown recently. The virus, called **HTLV-I** (human T-cell leukemia-lymphoma virus), has been isolated and appears to be endemic to southern Japan, the Caribbean, South America, and the southeastern USA. The acute illness is characterized by a fulminating clinical course with skin infiltrates, lymphadenopathy, hepatosplenomegaly, and leukemia. The leukemic cells are mainly immature lymphoid cells, many with convoluted nuclei. Hypercalcemia often develops, related to humoral factors rather than direct bone invasion. An increased incidence of lymphomas, particularly immunoblastic and undifferentiated or Burkitt types, has been seen in AIDS patients. Primary CNS involvement and disseminated disease have been reported. In about 30% of cases, the lymphomas are usually preceded by generalized lymphadenopathy, suggesting that polyclo-

TABLE 35-6. CHROMOSOME ABNORMALITIES IN LYMPHOMA

Histologic Type	Immunophenotype	Cytogenetics
Nodular (follicular)	B cell	t(14;18)
Diffuse	B cell	Abnormal 17
High grade	B cell (rare T cell)	Trisomy 3
Burkitt's	B cell	t(8;14)

A shorter survival has been noted with presence of abnormalities of chromosome 5 or involvement of breakpoint 14 q11-12, +5, +6, +18, or with 6 q11-16 breakpoints (also increased incidence of B symptoms) and 3 q21-25; 13 q21-14 breakpoint (also seen with bulky disease).

nal stimulation of B cells results in the emergence of immortalized but not fully transformed B cell clones. C-myc gene rearrangements are characteristic of AIDS-associated lymphomas. Response to modern therapy is possible, but toxicity is common and opportunistic infections continue to occur, resulting in short survival.

Recent advances in molecular biology have allowed for detailed analysis of the DNA sequences that are located at certain translocations. Recurring cytogenetic abnormalities generally correlate with clinical morphologic and immunophenotypic features (see TABLE 35-6).

Pathology

Recent histopathologic classification systems, although complex, offer reasonable means of distinguishing clinical subgroups with different prognoses and providing guidelines for management. In general, longer survival is related to a follicular or nodular nodal architecture and smaller lymphoid cell size; larger cell types or undifferentiated cells are usually diffuse and have a poorer prognosis, although modern intensive chemotherapy has reversed this.

The Rappaport classification for the histopathology of NHL is based on the degree of differentiation of the tumor and on whether the growth pattern is diffuse or nodular. Large immature cells are designated as histiocytes and smaller ones as lymphocytes or undifferentiated cells. NHL is classified as (1) malignant lymphoma, undifferentiated Burkitt's type, or non-Burkitt's (pleomorphic) type; (2) malignant lymphoma, histiocytic; (3) malignant lymphoma, mixed lymphocytic-histiocytic; (4) malignant lymphoma, lymphocytic (well differentiated or poorly differentiated); or (5) malignant lymphoma, lymphoblastic. All classes are further divided into nodular or diffuse except for (1) and (5), which occur only in a diffuse pattern. Nodular involvement is characterized by fibrous strands that separate the lymphoma infiltrate into nodules.

The Lukes and Collins classification, based upon the cell of origin, divides NHL into T cell (thymus-derived) types that include immunoblastic sarcoma and convoluted cell lymphoma, similar to lymphoblastic lymphoma (about 15% of all cases), or B cell (bone-marrow–derived) types that include well-differentiated lymphocytic, plasmacytic, follicular center cell (small and large cleaved and noncleaved cell type) lymphomas, and a B cell immunoblastic sarcoma (about 75% of cases). A third category includes rare cases of "true" histiocytic (or monocytic) origin (5%), while a fourth category includes unclassifiable cases (5%).

The International Panel Working Formulation (of the National Cancer Institute) separates NHL into categories, each incorporating the above classifications and having therapeutic implications, as follows (NOTE: *The prognostic designations are based on untreated disease and may not accurately reflect outcomes in patients undergoing modern therapy,* as discussed under Treatment, below):

I. **Low-grade or favorable-prognosis lymphomas** (38%): diffuse, well-differentiated; nodular, poorly differentiated lymphocytic; and nodular-mixed types.

II. **Intermediate-grade or -prognosis lymphomas** (40%): nodular histiocytic; diffuse, poorly differentiated, lymphocytic; and diffuse-mixed types.

III. **High-grade or unfavorable-prognosis lymphomas** (20%): diffuse histiocytic lymphoma (diffuse large cell, cleaved, noncleaved, and immunoblastic types); diffuse undifferentiated (Burkitt's and non-Burkitt's type); and lymphoblastic T cell lymphoma.

IV. **Miscellaneous lymphomas** (2%): composite lymphomas, mycosis fungoides, true histiocytic, other, and unclassifiable types.

Modern immunophenotyping, using fresh tumor tissue, reveals that 80 to 85% of NHLs arise from B lymphocytes, 15% from T lymphocytes, and < 5% from true histiocytes (monocyte-macrophages) or undefined null cells. Furthermore, immunologic studies have shown that lymphomas arise from different stages of normal lymphoid activation and differentiation. However, except in certain T cell lymphomas, immunologic classification has not played a major role in treatment strategy.

For a correlation of type of lymphoma, cell of origin, and cytogenetic findings, see TABLE 35–6.

Symptoms and Signs

While a variety of clinical manifestations exist, many patients present with asymptomatic adenopathy involving cervical or inguinal regions, or both. Enlarged lymph nodes are rubbery and discrete and later become matted. Local disease is apparent in some patients, but most have multiple areas of involvement. Waldeyer's ring (especially the tonsils) is an occasional site of disease. Mediastinal and retroperitoneal lymphadenopathy may cause pressure symptoms on various organs. Extranodal sites may dominate the clinical picture (eg, gastric involvement can simulate GI carcinoma, and intestinal lymphoma may cause a malabsorption syndrome). The skin and bones are initially involved in 15% of patients with large cell (histiocytic) lymphoma and 7% of patients with lymphocytic lymphoma. Histiocytic lymphoma rarely remains localized to bone; the marrow is invaded in about 50% of cases. When extensive abdominal or thoracic disease is present, about 33% of patients develop chylous ascites or pleural effusion, respectively, owing to lymphatic obstruction. Weight loss, fever, night sweats, and asthenia indicate disseminated disease.

Anemia is present initially in about 33% of patients and eventually develops in most. It may be due to bleeding from GI involvement or low platelet levels, hemolysis due to hypersplenism or Coombs-positive hemolytic anemia, bone marrow infiltration by lymphoma, or marrow suppression by drugs or irradiation. A leukemic phase develops in 20 to 40% of lymphocytic lymphomas and 10% of histiocytic lymphomas. Hypogammaglobulinemia due to progressive decrease in immunoglobulin production occurs in 15% of patients and may predispose to serious bacterial infection.

Recently 1 subset of high-grade lymphoma (termed Ki-1 positive large cell lymphoma) affecting both children and adults has been codified by the Ki-1 (CD30) antigen (Ag) on the malignant cells. The Ki-1 Ag is expressed on Reed-Sternberg cells and on activated B and T cells. The lymphoma is heterogeneous, with immunophenotypic studies showing 75% of cases of T cell origin, 15% of B cell origin, and 10% unclassified. Patients have rapidly progressive skin lesions, adenopathy, and visceral lesions. It may be mistaken for Hodgkin's disease or metastatic carcinoma.

In children, NHL may be of the undifferentiated, diffuse histiocytic, or lymphoblastic type. These childhood lymphomas present special problems (eg, GI involvement) and require different management approaches from those seen in adults. The lymphoblastic type represents a variation of acute lymphoblastic leukemia (T cell type), since both have a predilection for marrow, peripheral blood, skin, and CNS involvement; and patients often present with mediastinal adenopathy (Sternberg sarcoma) and superior vena cava syndrome. Nodular lymphomas are rarely seen in children.

Diagnosis

NHL must be differentiated from Hodgkin's disease, acute and chronic leukemia, metastatic carcinoma, infectious mononucleosis, TB (especially primary TB with hilar adenopathy), and other causes of lymphadenopathy, including pseudolymphoma due to phenytoin. Diagnosis can be made only by histologic study of excised tissue. Destruction of normal lymph node architecture and invasion of the capsule and adjacent fat by characteristic neoplastic cells are the usual histologic criteria. Immunologic surface marker studies to determine cell of origin will identify specific subtypes and help to define prognosis, and may be of value in management decisions (see below). Demonstration of the presence of the leukocyte common antigen (LCA) CD45 by immunoperoxidase rules out metastatic carcinoma, which is often in the differential diagnosis of "undifferentiated" malignancies. The test for LCA can be done on fixed tissues, while most surface marker studies require fresh tissue.

Staging

Localized NHL does occur, but the disease is disseminated in about 90% of nodular lymphomas and 70% of diffuse lymphomas when first recognized. Clinical staging procedures similar to those for Hodgkin's disease (see above) are indicated, except that laparotomy and splenectomy are rarely required. CT scans of the abdomen and pelvis have largely replaced lymphangiograms. The final staging is more often based upon clinical findings than is the case in Hodgkin's disease, in which pathologic stage is critical for management decisions.

Initially, constitutional symptoms tend to be less common in NHL than in Hodgkin's disease and do not usually alter prognosis. Organ infiltration is more widespread, and the bone marrow and peripheral blood may be involved. Bone marrow biopsy to determine marrow involvement should be done in all patients.

Treatment and Prognosis

The histopathology, the stage of disease, and (in some reports) the results of surface marker studies significantly influence the prognosis and response to treatment. Patients with T cell lymphomas generally have a worse prognosis than those with B cell types, although results of recent intensive treatment programs lessen these differences. Other factors that adversely affect prognosis are poor performance status, age > 70, elevated LDH level, bulky tumor masses > 10 cm in diameter, and > 2 extranodal sites of disease.

Treatment of early disease (stages I and II): With low- and intermediate-grade lymphomas ("favorable-prognosis" types), patients rarely present with localized disease, but when they do, regional radiotherapy offers long-term control and sometimes cure. They have median survivals of > 5 to 7½ yr; unfortunately, most eventually die from the disease. Patients with "intermediate-prognosis" lymphomas have median survivals of 2 to 5 yr. Patients with "unfavorable-prognosis" or high-grade lymphomas untreated die in 6 to 12 mo. With intensive multiagent chemotherapy (and regional radiation) treatment, the cure rate is > 50%.

Treatment of advanced disease (stages III and IV): Treatment varies considerably in patients with low-grade or "favorable-prognosis" lymphomas. A watch-and-wait approach, treatment with a single alkylating agent, or 2- and 3-drug programs may be used. Interferon and other biologic response modifiers may be of benefit in some cases. While survival may be prolonged, cure rates are generally < 20 to 25% and relapse eventually occurs; ie, paradoxically, long-term prognosis is unfavorable.

In patients with intermediate-grade lymphomas, combinations of cyclophosphamide, vincristine, and prednisone, with or without adriamycin (COP, CVP, CHOP, C-MOPP) result in complete regression of disease in 50 to 70% of patients. Only 20 to 30% are cured, and continuous late relapse usually occurs.

Patients with lymphomas of "unfavorable-prognosis" histology (diffuse "histiocytic" or large cell types) usually have rapid tumor growth (high grade); however, intensive programs of combination chemotherapy have dramatically reversed the designation of "unfavorable" to "favorable." Use of 4-, 5-, and 6-drug programs with acronyms (eg, BACOP, CHOP-Bleo, m-BACOD, COMLA, ProMACE-MOPP, ProMACE-CytaBOM, COP-BLAM, MACOP-B) that use the above drugs plus others (bleomycin, methotrexate with leucovorin rescue, cytarabine, procarbazine) have resulted in complete remission rates of 50 to 75% with about 40 to 60% of patients being cured. Newer, effective drugs include cisplatinum, epipodophyllotoxin (VP-16), and large doses of cytarabine.

With highly specific monoclonal antibodies directed at lymphoma cells, and improved techniques in bone marrow preservation, new intensive programs are under investigation in selected patients who relapse from standard regimens. Thus, autologous marrow (from the patient) or allogeneic marrow (from an HLA-matched sibling or donor) can be purged of tumor cells and preserved for reinfusion (rescue) after high-dose chemotherapy and total-body radiotherapy (designed to eradicate recurrent lymphoma). The best results are achieved in patients < 55 yr old who have a minimal tumor burden at the time of BMT (about 30 to 60% of patients may be cured, but death from toxicity occurs in 10 to 30% of patients). The need for bone marrow purging is under investigation.

Patients with T cell lymphoblastic lymphoma are managed in similar fashion to those with acute childhood T cell leukemia, with intensive drug regimens including prophylactic treatment of the CNS. Results are encouraging, with an estimated 50% cure rate.

BURKITT'S LYMPHOMA

A highly undifferentiated B cell lymphoma that tends to involve sites other than the lymph nodes and reticuloendothelial system.

Etiology

Burkitt's lymphoma, unlike other lymphomas, has a specific geographic distribution. Rare in the USA, it is most common in Central Africa, where its distribution appears to be determined by climatic factors, suggesting an unidentified insect vector and an infectious agent. Strong evidence points to the herpes-like Epstein-Barr virus (see also INFECTIOUS MONONUCLEOSIS in Ch. 47).

Symptoms and Signs

Burkitt's lymphoma occurs in all age groups but is unusual in adults. It is more common in children and young adults, particularly in males. Most patients present with large abdominal masses due to involvement of the bowel or retroperitoneum. Other presenting features include adenopathy or painful jaw masses (especially in African patients), or anemia due to bone marrow involvement. Unless therapy is carried out, the disease is rapidly progressive.

Diagnosis

Lymph node or other tissue biopsy reveals diffuse replacement by characteristic small-to-intermediate–sized noncleaved cells that have a high nuclear:cytoplasmic ratio and mitotic count. Nuclei are immature and contain prominent nucleoli, while the cytoplasm is basophilic with several conspicuous vacuoles. Under low-power magnification a "starry-sky" pattern is evident in virtu-

ally all cases due to the presence of background reactive phagocytic histiocytes. Immunologic studies show the presence of B cell surface markers (usually IgM, either κ or λ light chain), while cytogenetic studies reveal t(8;14) or, less commonly, t(8;2), and t(8;22).

Staging and Treatment

Stages A and B indicate single or multiple extra-abdominal sites. Stage C is defined by intra-abdominal disease including kidneys or gonads. Stage D disease is similar to C but with involvement of extra-abdominal sites including bone marrow or CNS. Prognosis is improved when bulky abdominal tumor can be resected.

Intermittent intensive chemotherapy (high doses of cyclophosphamide combined with methotrexate, vincristine, and often adriamycin or cytarabine) produces long-term disease-free survival in 70 to 80% of patients with stage A or B disease, and in 30 to 40% of patients with stages C and D disease. Treatments under investigation include high-dose drugs with bone marrow transplantation.

36. NEOPLASMS

Childhood neoplasms are also discussed in Ch. 35.

WILMS' TUMOR
(Nephroblastoma)

An embryonal adenomyosarcoma of the kidneys with heterogeneous carcinomatous elements; the tumor occurs fetally and may not manifest itself clinically for years. A genetic defect has been associated in some cases (see under GENETICS OF MALIGNANT DISEASE in Ch. 48).

Symptoms, Signs, and Diagnosis

The diagnosis usually is made in children < 5 yr of age, but the tumor occasionally can be detected in older children and rarely in adults. The most frequent presenting finding is a palpable abdominal mass; other findings include abdominal pain, hematuria, fever, anorexia, nausea, and vomiting. Hematuria (15 to 20% of cases) indicates invasion of the collecting system. Hypertension may occur secondary to ischemia from renal pedicle or parenchymal compression.

The intrarenal tumor usually distorts the functioning parenchyma. Abdominal ultrasonography

defines the cystic or solid nature of the mass and whether the renal vein or vena cava is involved, and excretory urography usually is diagnostic. Renal arteriography, vena cavography, or retrograde pyelography seldom is required. CT scan of the abdomen is helpful in determining the extent of the tumor but may be difficult to perform in small children. Chest x-rays (and possibly CT scans) are indicated, since metastatic pulmonary involvement may be present at the time of initial diagnosis. Bilateral synchronous Wilms' tumors occur in about 4% of cases. Congenital anomalies (eg, aniridia and hemihypertrophy) are associated with an increased incidence of Wilms' tumor.

Prognosis and Treatment

Prognosis depends on the histologic appearance of the tumor, the stage at the time of diagnosis, and the age of the patient (younger is better).

Prompt surgical exploration of potentially resectable lesions is indicated, with examination of the contralateral kidney. Chemotherapy with actinomycin D and vincristine, with or without radiation therapy, is used, depending on the stage of the disease. The National Wilms' Tumor Study

NEUROBLASTOMA

A common solid tumor of childhood, arising mainly in the adrenal gland but also from any portion of the extra-adrenal sympathetic chain, including in the retroperitoneum or chest. It can occur very rarely as a primary CNS tumor. A familial incidence of neuroblastoma is observed (see under GENETICS OF MALIGNANT DISEASE in Ch. 48). Many neuroblastomas are functional, producing elevated levels of serum or urinary catecholamines. **Ganglioneuroma** is a benign neoplasm that occasionally represents maturation of neuroblastoma; ganglioneuroma usually occurs in adults.

Symptoms, Signs, and Diagnosis

About 75% of these tumors are diagnosed in children < 5 yr of age. About 50% begin in the abdomen; 15 to 20%, in the thorax. Presenting symptoms and signs depend on the site of origin and disease stage. A palpable abdominal mass or evidence of a metastatic lesion to liver, lung, or bone, especially to the skull in the orbital region, may be the initial presentation. If bones are involved, bone pain may be present. Bone marrow involvement may cause pallor (anemia), petechiae (thrombocytopenia), and leukopenia. Other metastatic sites are uncommon and include the skin and brain. Hemorrhage and necrosis into the tumor occur, and abdominal tumors may cross the midline. **Differential diagnosis** includes Wilms' tumor, renal masses, rhabdomyosarcoma, hepatomas, leukemia, and tumors of GI and genital origins. **Diagnostic tests** include ultrasonography, bone marrow examination, IVU, and bone and CT scans. Urinary vanillylmandelic acid **(VMA)** is elevated in ≥ 65% of patients; elevated VMA together with elevated homovanillic acid identifies > 90% of patients. Twenty-four-hour urine collections are used.

Prognosis and Treatment

Surgical excision of localized primary lesions provides the best chance for cure. For more advanced disease, a staging procedure is necessary. However, most patients (especially if > 1 yr old) present with metastases to the liver, lung, or bone. Chemotherapeutic agents (eg, vincristine, cyclophosphamide, doxorubicin, and cisplatin) are used, as well as radiation therapy for ad-

vanced disease. Spontaneous regression of neuroblastomas has been reported with hemorrhage and necrosis. The younger the child at the time of diagnosis (< 2 yr), the better the prognosis for cure, partly because younger children tend to have less disseminated disease.

RETINOBLASTOMA

A malignant tumor that arises from the immature retina. It occurs in 1/15,000 to 1/30,000 live births and represents about 2% of childhood malignancies. The disease may be inherited or result from a new germinal mutation. About 10% of patients have a family history of retinoblastoma and another 20 to 30% have bilateral disease; all of these (ie, 30 to 40% of the patients) may pass the trait to their children in an autosomal dominant fashion. These patients appear to have a constitutive genetic abnormality, which in at least 25% appears to be a deletion involving chromosome 13q14 (smaller, undetectable abnormalities may be present in all of these patients). A mutation in the other chromosome 13 ("second hit") is thought to result in the tumor. Most of the remaining 60% of patients, with unilateral disease and no family history of retinoblastoma, have nonheritable disease. However, about 5% of these patients may also carry the "retinoblastoma gene," with the risk of passing the trait to their children (see also under GENETICS OF MALIGNANT DISEASE in Ch. 48).

Diagnosis is usually made before age 2 yr when a white reflex from the pupil (cat's-eye pupil) or strabismus is investigated. Both fundi must be carefully examined by indirect ophthalmoscopy with the pupils widely dilated and the child under anesthesia. The tumors appear as single or multiple gray-white elevations in the retina; tumor seeds may be visible in the vitreous. In almost all tumors, calcification can be detected by CT scan.

Treatment: If diagnosed when the tumor is intraocular, > 90% can be cured. Unilateral retinoblastoma is managed by enucleation with removal of as much of the optic nerve as possible. For those patients with bilateral disease, preservation of vision usually can be achieved with bilateral coagulation or unilateral enucleation and photocoagulation, cryotherapy, or radiation of the other eye. Systemic chemotherapy may be helpful, particularly when the disease has disseminated beyond the globe. Ophthalmologic reexamination of both eyes and retreatment, if necessary, are required at 2- to 4-mo intervals. Studies of spinal fluid and bone marrow for malignant cells are conducted concomitantly. Patients with the hereditary form of retinoblastoma have an increased incidence of second malignancies, about 50% of which arise within the irradiated area. By 30 yr from the time of diagnosis, 70% have developed a second tumor.

Screening: Family members of patients with retinoblastoma should be informed about the genetic implications and risks. Penetrance of the retinoblastoma gene is not necessarily complete (80 to 100%, with some carriers having an undiagnosed retinocytoma). Immediate family members of any child with retinoblastoma should have at least one ophthalmologic examination to exclude retinoblastoma (young children) or retinocytoma (older individuals). Recombinant DNA probes may be useful to detect asymptomatic carriers.

INTRACRANIAL NEOPLASMS
(Brain Tumors)

An expanding intracranial lesion may be a granuloma, parasitic cyst, hemorrhage (intracerebral, extradural, or subdural), aneurysm, abscess, or neoplasm (metastatic or primary). Neoplasms are common and are frequently misdiagnosed.

Primary intracranial neoplasms are divided into 6 classes: tumors of (1) the skull (osteoma, hemangioma, granuloma, xanthoma, osteitis deformans); (2) the meninges (meningioma, sarcoma, gliomatosis); (3) the cranial nerves (glioma of the optic nerve, schwannoma [neurilemoma] of the 8th and 5th cranial nerves); (4) the neuroglia (gliomas) and ependyma (ependymomas); (5) the pituitary or pineal body (pituitary adenoma, pinealoma); and (6) congenital origin (craniopharyngioma, chordoma, germinoma, teratoma, dermoid cyst, angioma, hemangioblastoma).

Metastases may involve the skull or any intracranial structure.

Pathology and Incidence

Generally, CNS changes result from invasion and destruction by the tumor and from its secondary effects (increased intracranial pressure, cerebral edema, and compression of brain tissue, cranial nerves, and cerebral vessels). Rarely, remote neurologic effects occur as "paraneoplastic syndromes."

Brain tumors are found in about 2% of routine autopsies. They may occur at any age but are most common in early adult or middle life. Common primary childhood tumors are cerebellar astrocytomas and medulloblastomas, ependymomas, gliomas of the brainstem and optic nerve, germinomas (pinealomas), and congenital tumors. The most common metastatic invaders in childhood are neuroblastoma (usually epidural) and leukemia (meningeal). Primary adult tumors include meningiomas, schwannomas, gliomas of the cerebral hemispheres (particularly the malignant glioblastoma multiforme, anaplastic astrocytoma, and the more benign astrocytoma and oligodendroglioma). Metastatic tumors in adults arise most commonly from bronchogenic carcinoma, adenocarcinoma of the breast, and malignant melanoma.

The relative frequency of various types of intracranial tumors is gliomas 45%, pituitary adenomas 15%, meningiomas 15%, schwannomas 7%, congenital tumors 3%, metastatic and other types 15%. Overall incidence in males and females is about equal, but cerebellar medulloblastoma and glioblastoma multiforme are more common in males; meningioma and schwannoma, in females. The incidence of primary lymphomas of the nervous system is increasing in both AIDS and non-AIDS patients.

How lethal a brain tumor is depends on its size, location, rate of growth, and histologic grade of malignancy. Benign intracranial tumors grow slowly, with few mitoses, no necrosis, and no vascular proliferation. They may achieve considerable size before producing symptoms, in part because there is often no associated cerebral edema. Malignant tumors are characterized by more rapid growth, invasiveness, frequent mitotic figures, necrosis, vascular proliferation, and endothelial hyperplasia. However, "benign" brain tumors that cannot be entirely excised because of size or location are usually lethal. "Malignant" brain tumors rarely metastasize out of the CNS and cause death by inexorable local growth. Thus, the distinction between "benign" and "malignant" is less important for intracranial neoplasms than for systemic cancer.

The techniques of molecular biology permit tumors to be studied at the genotypic level. Data from studies of low-grade astrocytomas concerning chromosomes support the histopathologic finding of its relative homogeneity compared to the glioblastoma multiforme. Most astrocytoma cells contain near-diploid chromosome numbers (42 to 50 chromosomes/metaphase). In comparison to these findings, cytogenetic analysis of most high-grade tumors shows extensive heterogeneity with numerous subpopulations and isolated cell types. There are both a greater range of chromosome ploidy (35 to 200 chromosomes/metaphase) and more chromosome rearrangement than in low-grade tumors. In addition, some laboratories also report the frequent occurrence of **double minutes** (DMs, *doublet fragments of DNA*) thought to be associated with gene amplification.

The oncogene c-*erb*-B is often amplified in gliomas, and the product of this gene, epidermal growth factor receptor **(EGFR)**, may be overproduced. The actual role of EGFR amplification is unknown. Platelet-derived growth factor **(PDGF)** has been shown to be produced by some malignant gliomas. The specific role of PDGF in glial tumor growth is under active investigation.

Symptoms and Signs

General manifestations result from increased intracranial pressure. This may be due to the space-occupying tumor mass itself or to associated cerebral edema, obstructed flow of CSF (occurring early in 3rd ventricle or posterior fossa tumors), obstructed dural venous sinuses (especially by bony or extradural metastatic tumors), or obstructed CSF absorption mechanisms (as in leukemic or carcinomatous involvement of the meninges). Headache and vomiting result, as may mental symptoms. Papilledema develops in about 25% of patients with brain tumor and may not be an early sign; its absence does not rule out a tumor or elevated intracranial pressure. In young children, elevated intracranial pressure may enlarge the head. Intracranial pressure is usually normal in patients with small tumors of the cerebral hemispheres, pituitary adenomas, or brainstem tumors that do not obstruct the aqueduct of Sylvius. Changes in temperature, pulse or respiratory rate, or BP are unusual except terminally.

Convulsive seizures, either focal or generalized, occur with cerebral hemisphere tumors and may precede other symptoms by months or years. They are more frequent with meningiomas and slowly growing astrocytomas than with malignant gliomas. Focal seizures help to locate the tumor.

Mental symptoms (eg, drowsiness, lethargy, obtuseness, personality changes, disordered conduct, impaired mental faculties, psychotic episodes) may appear at any time. They are the initial symptoms in 25% of malignant brain tumors.

Special (focal) manifestations are due to localized destruction or compression of nerve tissue or to altered endocrine function, and depend on the tumor's location.

Tumors of the cerebral hemispheres: Frontal lobe tumors (commonly meningiomas or gliomas) involving the frontal convexity are characterized by progressive hemiplegia, focal or generalized seizures, and mental changes. Expressive aphasia may accompany a tumor of the dominant hemisphere. A tumor at the base of the frontal lobes (particularly meningioma of the olfactory groove) produces ipsilateral anosmia. A tumor on the medial surface of a frontal lobe may cause precipitate urination. Mental changes (especially inattention and loss of motivation) and ataxic gait are common when the tumor spreads across the corpus callosum to both frontal lobes. Meningioma of the tuberculum sellae may compress the optic chiasm, producing a visual field defect similar to that of a pituitary adenoma (see discussion of tumors of the pituitary and suprasellar region, below). Meningioma of the inner third of the sphenoid ridge may cause exophthalmos and unilateral amblyopia. Meningioma of the outer part of the sphenoid ridge may invade the temporal lobe (see discussion of temporal lobe tumors, below).

Parietal lobe tumors may produce either generalized convulsions or sensory focal seizures. Cutaneous tactile, pain, and temperature senses are unimpaired, but stereognosis and the cortical sensory modalities (position sense, 2-point discrimination) are impaired contralaterally. Contralateral homonymous hemianopia, apraxia, and anosognosia (nonrecognition of bodily defects) may also be present. Denial of illness is characteristic, especially if obtundation is present. Speech disturbances, agraphia, and finger agnosia may occur when the tumor involves the dominant hemisphere.

Temporal lobe tumors, particularly in the nondominant hemisphere, are often relatively "silent" except when they cause convulsive seizures. A tumor deep in the temporal lobe may cause contralateral hemianopia, psychomotor seizures, or convulsive seizures preceded by an olfactory aura or visual hallucinations of complex formed images. Tumors involving the surface of the dominant temporal lobe produce mixed expressive and receptive aphasia or dysphasia, chiefly anomia.

Occipital lobe tumors usually cause a contralateral quadrant defect in the visual field or a hemianopia with sparing of the macula. Associated convulsions may be preceded by an aura of flashing lights, but not formed images.

Subcortical tumors commonly involve the internal capsule and produce contralateral hemiplegia. They may invade any lobe of the hemisphere, producing corresponding symptoms. Thalamic invasion produces contralateral cutaneous sensory impairment. Invasion of the basal ganglia usually does not produce parkinsonian symptoms, but athetosis, bizarre tremors, or dystonic postures occasionally result. Hypothalamic tumors may produce eating disorders or precocious puberty in children.

Cranial extradural or subdural metastatic tumors, by compressing or invading the underlying cortex, may produce the same localizing signs that a primary cortical tumor would cause.

Herniation syndromes may develop as lesions enlarge and brain tissue is pushed through the fixed intracranial openings (eg, the medial surface of a hemisphere may be forced beneath the falx cerebri). **Transtentorial herniation** occurs when brain tissue is displaced through the tentorial notch. In **central herniation,** there is symmetric bilateral tissue displacement, while **temporal lobe herniation** is an asymmetric displacement of a cone of temporal lobe tissue through the tentorial notch. Both types of herniation compress vital brainstem structures. Central herniation leads to coma, midposition fixed pupils, altered respiration, loss of oculocephalic and oculovestibular reflexes (failure of the eyes to move in response to head rotation or to caloric stimulation, respectively), and bilateral motor paralysis (decerebrate rigidity or flaccidity). Temporal lobe herniation may produce an early 3rd nerve palsy (unilateral dilated fixed pupil and extraocular paralysis) in addition to the central signs. Less commonly, a cerebellar cone may be forced through the foramen magnum, producing abrupt respiratory and cardiac arrest.

False localizing signs may accompany prolonged elevated intracranial pressure. They include uni- or bilateral lateral rectus palsy from 6th nerve compression, hemiplegia on the same side as the tumor from compression of the opposite cerebral peduncle against the tentorium, and visual field defect on the same side as the tumor from compromise of the opposite posterior cerebral artery.

Tumors of the pituitary and suprasellar region: Pituitary adenomas may present as intrasellar secretory or nonsecretory masses, or masses with extrasellar extension. Secretory adenomas produce hormones that cause specific endocrinopathies. Traditionally, adenomas with particular histologic staining characteristics have been associated with specific endocrinopathies; eg, **acidophilic adenoma** overproduces growth hormone, leading to gigantism before puberty and acromegaly after puberty; **basophilic adenoma** overproduces ACTH, leading to Cushing's syndrome. **Chromophobe adenomas** are known to be responsible for most endocrinopathies caused by pituitary tumors. The most common endocrine hypersecretion is prolactin, producing amenorrhea and galactorrhea in women and, less frequently, impotence and gynecomastia in men. Many secretory tumors are microadenomas, found only after an endocrinopathy is discovered.

Enlarging pituitary adenomas cause headache. As the tumor grows out of the sella, it compresses the optic chiasm, nerves or tracts, and the hypothalamus. The common visual field defect is bitemporal hemianopia, but unilateral optic atrophy, contralateral hemianopia, or any combination of the 3 may occur. Hypothalamic compression usually causes diabetes insipidus from injury to the supraoptic-pituitary tract. The tumor may destroy functioning glandular tissue and cause pituitary deficiency. MRI and CT scans have advanced the radiologic diagnosis of pituitary adenoma. MRI best delineates microadenomas. The CT scan is most helpful when the tumor extends above the sella, but high-resolution CT scanning can also be used to diagnose microadenomas. If the tumor is large, skull x-rays may show a balloon-shaped sella.

Other tumors in the region of the sella turcica (eg, meningiomas, craniopharyngiomas, metastases, dermoid cysts) or aneurysms may compress the optic chiasm, invade the sella, and produce symptoms similar to those of chromophobe adenoma.

Pineal tumors (usually germinomas) occur at any age but are most common in childhood. Precocious puberty may result, especially in boys. The tumor compresses the aqueduct of Sylvius, causing hydrocephalus, papilledema, and other signs of increased intracranial pressure. The pretectum rostral to the superior colliculi is also compressed, resulting in paralysis of upward gaze, ptosis, and loss of pupillary light and accommodation reflexes.

Tumors of the brainstem: Gliomas of the brainstem are usually astrocytomas. Common symptoms, resulting from destruction of nuclear masses, are unilateral or bilateral paralysis of the 5th, 6th, 7th, and 10th cranial nerves, and paralysis of lateral gaze. Damage to the motor or sensory pathways causes hemiplegia, hemianesthesia, or cerebellar disturbances (ataxia, nystagmus, intention tremor). Increased intracranial pressure appears late in brainstem tumors.

Posterior fossa tumors: Tumors of the 4th ventricle and cerebellum (usually medulloblastomas, gliomas, ependymomas, or metastases) interfere with CSF circulation, and symptoms of increased intracranial pressure appear early. Ataxic gait, intention tremor, and other signs of cerebellar dysfunction follow.

Cerebellopontine angle tumors, particularly neurilemomas (acoustic neurinomas, schwannomas), are characterized by tinnitus, unilateral hearing impairment, and sometimes vertigo. Pressure on the adjacent cranial nerves, brainstem, and cerebellum produces loss of corneal reflex, facial palsy and anesthesia, palatal weakness, signs of cerebellar dysfunction, and, rarely, contralateral hemiplegia or hemianesthesia. Loss of vestibular response to caloric stimulation, enlargement of the porus acusticus as shown by x-ray, and high CSF protein content suggest an acoustic neurilemoma (see also ACOUSTIC NEURINOMA in Ch. 67).

Meningiomas: *Benign tumors that appear to arise from arachnoidal cells and therefore can occur wherever there is dura.* The most common locations are over the convexities near the venous sinuses, along the base of the skull, and in the posterior fossa. Rarely, meningiomas may arise within the ventricles, presumably from cells migrating in along with the choroid plexus. Meningiomas < 2 cm in diameter are among the most common tumors found at biopsy. While a variety of pathologic types have been described, they are not usually associated with different clinical courses. Meningiomas occur more commonly in women and are the only intracranial neoplasms to do so. They tend to occur between ages 40 and 60 yr, but can present in childhood. Meningiomas may be multiple and may be become malignant, especially the hemangiopericytoma variant.

Meningiomas are one of the few tumors that present characteristic changes in plain skull x-rays. The CT scan is the most specific diagnostic tool, but most meningiomas can be visualized on MRI. Convexity meningiomas often give rise to focal seizures and ultimately to signs of mass effect in the hemispheres. Radiographically they may produce skull atrophy, dilated blood vessels, and occasionally hyperostosis. Parasagittal or falx meningiomas may produce a progressive spastic weakness or numbness, usually beginning in the leg opposite the lesion, but occasionally extending to both legs. The resulting paraparesis may be confusing and lead the physician incorrectly to believe that the patient has a spinal cord lesion. Differing from supratentorial tumors in their presentation, tumors along the base of the skull primarily produce visual disturbances and exophthalmos, while tumors in the posterior fossa usually produce hydrocephalus. Olfactory groove meningiomas impair the sense of smell and may produce papilledema and visual loss. Tuberculum sellae meningiomas produce visual loss and are characterized by bony changes. Sphenoid wing meningiomas may arise in the medial, middle, or lateral aspect of the sphenoid wing. If medial, they tend to grow into the cavernous sinus; if in the middle portion, they may grow anteriorly into the orbit, and in the lateral portion, may grow into the temporal bone, producing either a globular mass or a meningioma *en plaque* (ie, spread into the dura, with dural thickening and invasion of adjacent bone). Posterior fossa meningiomas may occur as a tentorial tumor that grows above and below the tentorium and principally produces hydrocephalus. Clivus and apical petrous bone meningiomas produce gait instability and limb ataxia as well as abnormalities of cranial nerves 5, 7, and 8. Meningiomas around the foramen magnum produce suboccipital pain on the ipsilateral side along with a characteristic weakness that begins in the ipsilateral arm, progresses to the ipsilateral leg, and then to the opposite leg and arm. A Lhermitte's sign, similar to that which occurs in multiple sclerosis, may be seen. Cranial nerve involvement may produce dysphagia, difficulty speaking, nystagmus, diplopia, and sensory changes in the face.

Diagnosis

A brain tumor should be considered and neurologic consultation requested for patients with slowly progressive signs of focal cerebral dysfunction, focal or generalized convulsions, headaches of recent onset, or other evidence of increased intracranial pressure (eg, vomiting, papilledema).

Studies should include a complete neurologic examination, testing of visual fields and acuity, audiometry, a CT scan, and chest x-rays (for a source of metastases). MRI may detect low-grade astrocytomas before they are visible on CT scans. Cerebral angiography may be necessary preoperatively, but less often for diagnosis.

CSF examination is unnecessary if the diagnosis is obvious but may be useful if the diagnosis or nature of the lesion is unclear after preliminary studies; it is essential to diagnose chronic or subacute neoplastic meningitis or benign intracranial hypertension (**pseudotumor cerebri**). Lumbar puncture (**LP**) is *contraindicated* in the presence of papilledema if an expanding lesion is suspected, since the sudden pressure change can precipitate a herniation syndrome. Since tumors in the pineal region are often germinomas, CSF assay for β-human chorionic gonadotropin or α-fetoprotein may provide histologic characterization.

Treatment

Treatment of brain tumor is often multimodal, depending on the pathology and location. Surgical excision should be used to effect a diagnosis, remove tumor, and improve symptoms. It may be curative in benign tumors. Radiation therapy is required for residual tumors and for most infiltrating neuroectodermal tumors. Chemotherapy appears to benefit some patients with infiltrating gliomas.

The treatment of meningiomas is surgical removal if at all possible. When tumors are small or when they occur in the elderly, surgery may be deferred because of the risk to life. Generally, tumors of medium-to-large size can be removed safely and completely, but very large tumors may encroach on vascular elements, especially the surrounding veins, making them especially difficult to remove. There may be value in irradiation for residual or recurrent meningioma. Schwannomas should be removed surgically.

The management of malignant gliomas should be based on the rationale of cytoreduction through multimodality therapy including surgery, irradiation, and chemotherapy. Surgical resection of as much tumor as is neurologically safe should be the initial step. After surgery, patients should receive radiation therapy to a full tumor dose of 60 Gy (6000 rads). Chemotherapy with a nitrosourea (eg, carmustine, 200 mg/m^2 IV q 6 to 8 wk; lomustine, 130 mg/m^2 orally q 6 to 8 wk) should be given. Referral of such patients to centers specializing in investigative programs

(eg, radioactive seed implants, new chemotherapy) may be offered. The prognosis for such patients is guarded. In national studies the median survival after surgery, irradiation, and chemotherapy is about 1 yr and 25% of patients survive 2 yr. Favorable prognostic variables include age (< 45 yr), pathology of anaplastic astrocytoma rather than glioblastoma multiforme, and better clinical status and little or no residual tumor after initial resection.

Low-grade gliomas (astrocytoma, oligodendroglioma) should be resected if possible, or undergo needle biopsy if resection is too dangerous, and then receive radiotherapy. There is some debate about timing of the radiation. MRI permits early diagnosis, when radiation might offer better treatment, but might also expose the brain to damage (from irradiation) earlier than necessary. The overall prognosis is considerably better than with malignant gliomas. Patients might be expected to live 3 to 5 yr before the tumor recurs.

For **medulloblastoma**, radiation therapy consists of whole-head irradiation to about 35 Gy, a posterior fossa boost of 15 Gy, and spinal cord irradiation, also of about 35 Gy. In recent years, chemotherapy has been added both as adjunctive therapy and for recurrent disease. Whereas several agents have been reported to be effective in treating recurrent medulloblastoma, an adjunctive chemotherapy regimen has yet to be shown consistently effective, although high-risk patients may benefit. Drugs that have been reported as useful include the nitrosoureas, procarbazine, vincristine alone and in combination, intrathecal methotrexate and polychemotherapy (MOPP). Prognostically, at least 50% of these patients will survive 5 yr, and perhaps 40% for 10 yr.

The common **intracranial ependymoma** arises in the 4th ventricle, usually in children, and obstructs CSF flow, producing headache, vomiting, and ultimately cranial nerve palsies and ataxia. While most of these tumors are benign, malignant degeneration does occur and the tumor may seed along CSF pathways in a manner similar to medulloblastoma. Ependymomas are usually approached surgically with the same goals as for medulloblastoma, ie, to remove as much tumor as is neurosurgically safe and to open the CSF pathways. The incidence of seeding varies with different reports, and thus treatment protocols have differed among treatment centers. One recommendation is to use whole-brain irradiation for all patients with supratentorial low-grade ependymomas, whole brain plus cervical cord extensions for low-grade infratentorial ependymomas without evidence of CSF seeding, and craniospinal irradiation for all high-grade ependymomas or low-grade tumors with evidence of seeding. Prognostically, one study reports a 10-yr survival of 69% for patients with intracranial ependymomas (75% for low-grade, 67% for high-grade), although these figures are more optimistic than others.

Metastatic tumors may be irradiated with good short-term results. Patients with solitary metastases may achieve longer survival and more rapid return to neurologic normality if the tumors are resected before irradiation.

If neurologic or neurosurgical consultation is not readily available, temporary measures may be necessary to relieve increased intracranial pressure and prevent herniation. Mannitol 25 to 100 gm infused IV is given to relieve pressure immediately, and should be accompanied by a corticosteroid (eg, dexamethasone 16 mg/day orally or parenterally, or prednisone 60 to 80 mg/day orally, in divided doses) to maintain the reduced pressure. LP is *contraindicated* to reduce intracranial pressure accompanying brain neoplasms.

37. PULMONARY DISORDERS

CYSTIC FIBROSIS (CF)

(Mucoviscidosis; Fibrocystic Disease of the Pancreas; Pancreatic Cystic Fibrosis)

An inherited disease of the exocrine glands, primarily affecting the GI and respiratory systems, and usually characterized by the triad of chronic obstructive pulmonary disease, exocrine pancreatic insufficiency, and abnormally high sweat electrolytes.

Etiology and Incidence

CF, the most common lethal genetic disease in the white population, occurs in the USA in about 1/2400 white and 1/17,000 black live births; it is rare in Orientals. In the USA, 25% of patients are adults. CF is carried as an autosomal recessive trait by about 5% of the white population. The gene responsible for CF has been localized to 250,000 base pairs of genomic DNA on chromosome 7q (the long arm). It encodes a membrane-associated protein called the cystic fibrosis transmembrane conductance regulator (**CFTR**). The most common gene mutation is found in about 70% of patients with CF; a large number of less common mutations account for the remaining 30%. Although the function of CFTR remains unknown, it appears to be closely involved with chloride transport across epithelial membranes. Heterozygotes may show subtle abnormalities of epithelial transport but are clinically unaffected.

Pathology and Pathophysiology

Nearly all exocrine glands are affected in varying distribution and degree of severity. Involved glands fall into 3 types: (1) those that become obstructed by viscid or solid eosinophilic material in the lumen (pancreas, intestinal glands, intrahepatic bile ducts, gallbladder, submaxillary glands); (2) those that produce an excess of histologically normal secretions (tracheobronchial and Brunner's glands); and (3) those that are normal histologically but secrete excessive Na and Cl (sweat, parotid, and small salivary glands). Duodenal secretions are viscid and contain an abnormal mucopolysaccharide. Aspermia and infertility are seen in 98% of adult men secondary to maldevelopment of the vas deferens. In women fertility is decreased secondary to viscid cervical secretions, but many women with CF have carried pregnancies to term. However, maternal complications and fetal wastage show an increased incidence.

Evidence suggests that the lungs are normal at birth. The pulmonary lesion is probably initiated by diffuse obstruction in the small airways by abnormally thick mucus secretions. Secondary to obstruction, there is bronchiolitis and mucopurulent plugging of the airways. Bronchial changes are more common than parenchymal changes. Emphysema is not prominent. Early in the course, *Staphylococcus aureus* is the pathogen most often isolated from respiratory tract secretions, but as the disease progresses, *Pseudomonas aeruginosa* is most frequently isolated. A mucoid variant of *Pseudomonas* is uniquely associated with CF. Colonization with *P. cepacia* is often associated with rapid pulmonary deterioration. As the pulmonary process progresses, bronchial walls thicken, the airways remain filled with purulent, viscid secretions, areas of atelectasis develop, and hilar lymph nodes enlarge. Chronic hypoxemia results in muscular hypertrophy of the pulmonary arteries, pulmonary hypertension, and right ventricular hypertrophy. Some of the pulmonary damage may be caused by immune-mediated inflammation secondary to the release of proteases by neutrophils in the airways. Death usually results from a combination of respiratory failure and cor pulmonale.

Symptoms and Signs

Meconium ileus due to obstruction of the ileum by viscid meconium is the earliest sign (see under GASTROINTESTINAL DEFECTS in Ch. 28), which is present at birth in 7 to 10% of affected infants. It is often associated with volvulus, perforation, or atresia and, with rare exceptions, is always followed by the other signs of CF. In the newborn period, CF may also be associated with delayed passage of meconium and with the **meconium plug syndrome**, a transient form of distal intestinal obstruction secondary to 1 or more plugs of inspissated meconium in the anus or colon.

In infants without meconium ileus, onset is frequently heralded by a delay in regaining birthweight and inadequate weight gain at 4 to 6 wk of age. Pancreatic insufficiency is clinically apparent in 85 to 90% of patients. It is usually present early in life but may be progressive. Manifestations include the passage of frequent, bulky, foul-smelling, oily stools; abdominal protuberance; and poor growth pattern with decreased subcutaneous tissue and muscle mass, despite a normal or voracious appetite. Rectal prolapse occurs in 20% of untreated infants and toddlers. Clinical signs may be related to deficiency of the fat-soluble vitamins; CF should be considered in every infant with hypoprothrombinemia. Infants with CF who have been on soy protein formula or breast milk may develop hypoproteinemia with edema and anemia secondary to protein malabsorption. Excessive sweating (as in hot weather or with fever) may lead to episodes of hypotonic dehydration and circulatory failure. In arid climates infants may present with chronic metabolic alkalosis. Findings of salt crystal formation on the skin and a salty taste on the skin are highly suggestive of CF.

Fifty percent of all patients present with **pulmonary manifestations** usually consisting of chronic cough and wheezing associated with recurrent or chronic pulmonary infections. Cough is the most troublesome complaint, often accompanied by gagging, vomiting, and disturbed sleep. With disease progression, there are intercostal retractions, use of accessory muscles of respiration, a barrel-chest deformity, digital clubbing, and cyanosis. Upper respiratory tract involvement includes nasal polyposis and opacification of the paranasal sinuses. Teenagers may have retarded growth, delayed onset of puberty, and a declining tolerance for exercise. Pulmonary complications in adolescents and adults include pneumothorax, hemoptysis, and right heart failure secondary to pulmonary hypertension. Insulin-requiring diabetes develops in 2 to 3% of patients, and multinodular biliary cirrhosis with varices and portal hypertension develops in 4 to 5% of adolescents and adults. Chronic and/or recurrent abdominal pain may be related to intussusception, peptic ulcer disease, periappendiceal abscess, pancreatitis, gastroesophageal reflux, esophagitis, gallbladder disease, or episodes of partial intestinal obstruction secondary to abnormally viscid fecal contents.

Laboratory Findings

Since meconium in most neonates with CF contains large amounts of serum proteins (especially albumin), meconium examination has been used as the basis of a newborn screening test. However, since such testing does not detect the 10 to 15% of patients with normal or near-normal pancreatic enzymes, it is not recommended for mass screening. Pancreatic insufficiency is present in about 85% of patients with CF. The duodenal fluid is abnormally viscid and shows absence or diminution of enzyme activity and decreased HCO_3^- concentration; stool trypsin and chymotrypsin are absent or diminished. Tests of fat absorption, including 72-h fecal fat excretion, provide an indirect assessment of pancreatic exocrine function. Patients with normal exocrine pancreatic function fail to produce HCO_3^- following IV secretin stimulation. About 40% of patients show a diabetic oral glucose tolerance curve secondary to a reduced and delayed insulin response, but < 3% develop diabetes mellitus. Fasting blood levels of carotenoids, vitamins A and E, essential fatty acids, and cholesterol are reduced in patients with steatorrhea. Total serum protein is initially normal, but with advanced disease, the α_1-, α_2-, and γ-globulin fractions are elevated and albumin is decreased.

The serum concentration of immunoreactive trypsin is elevated in newborns with CF. A radioimmunoassay has been developed for use with dried blood spots routinely collected for newborn metabolic screening and is now being used in newborn screening programs. However, the diagnosis of CF should never be based solely on this test.

Chest x-ray findings may be helpful in suggesting the diagnosis of CF. Hyperinflation and bronchial wall thickening are the earliest findings. Subsequent changes include areas of infiltrate, atelectasis, and hilar adenopathy. With advanced disease, segmental or lobar atelectasis, cyst formation, bronchiectasis, and pulmonary artery and right ventricular enlargement are seen. Branching, finger-like opacifications that represent mucoid impaction of dilated bronchi are characteristic. Pulmonary function tests reveal hypoxemia and reduction in forced vital capacity (FVC), forced expiratory volume in 1 sec (FEV₁), and FEV₁/FVC ratio, and an increase in residual volume and the ratio of residual volume to total lung capacity. Fifty percent of patients have evidence of airways hyperreactivity.

Diagnosis

In families with a previously affected child, mutation analysis can be used for prenatal diagnosis and carrier testing. Analysis for the common Δ F508 mutation can also be used for carrier detection and prenatal diagnosis in the general population, but it is not recommended for population-based screening. The diagnosis of CF is usually confirmed in infancy or early childhood, but 10% of patients escape detection until adolescence or early adulthood.

The diagnosis of CF is suggested by the clinical and laboratory features described above and then confirmed by demonstrating an elevation of Na and/or Cl concentrations in sweat. The only reliable test is the **quantitative pilocarpine iontophoresis sweat test**: Localized sweating is stimulated pharmacologically, the amount of sweat collected is measured, and the electrolyte concentration is determined. In patients with a suggestive clinical picture or a positive family history, a Na or Cl concentration > 60 mEq/L confirms the diagnosis. It is estimated that $< 1/1000$ patients with CF will have a sweat chloride < 50 mEq/L. False-negative results are rare but may occur in the presence of edema and hypoproteinemia or with inadequate quantities of sweat. False-positive results are usually related to technical errors or use of inappropriate equipment. Transient elevation of sweat electrolyte concentrations can occur in association with environmental deprivation and in patients with anorexia nervosa. Although results of the sweat test are valid after the first 24 h of life, it may be difficult to obtain an adequate sweat sample (> 50 mg) before 3 to 4 wk of age. Concentrations of electrolytes in sweat normally increase slightly

with age; nevertheless, the sweat test is valid in adults.

A small subset of patients, labeled as **CF variants,** have chronic *Pseudomonas* bronchitis, normal pancreatic function, and intermediate sweat Cl concentrations in the range of 40 to 60 mEq/L.

Patients with CF have increased nasal transepithelial potential differences owing to increased Na reabsorption across epithelium, which is relatively impermeable to Cl. This may be a diagnostic adjunct to the sweat test immediately after birth and in patients with borderline sweat electrolyte values.

Prognosis

The course of CF, largely determined by the degree of pulmonary involvement, varies greatly from patient to patient. However, deterioration is inevitable, leading to debilitation and eventual death. The prognosis has steadily improved over the past 4 decades, mainly owing to institution of aggressive treatment before the onset of irreversible pulmonary changes. Median survival is to 28 yr of age. Long-term survival is somewhat better in males, blacks, patients without pancreatic insufficiency, and those who present with isolated GI symptoms. Early colonization with *Pseudomonas* and airways hyperreactivity are associated with a somewhat worse prognosis. Over the course of the illness, care givers, including physicians, nurses, physical therapists, counselors, and social workers, have the opportunity to form the kind of supportive environment for these patients and their families that will make their condition more tolerable. With this support, most patients can make an age-appropriate adjustment at both home and school. Despite myriad problems, the occupational and marital successes of these patients are impressive. Most patients work or attend school until shortly before death.

Genetic counseling can be useful for at-risk families to explain the inheritance pattern, risk figures, and to outline the possibilities for prenatal diagnosis and carrier detection.

Treatment

A comprehensive and intensive therapy program is essential, directed by an experienced, available physician with the services of personnel in nursing, nutrition, physical and respiratory therapies, and counseling. The goals of therapy include maintenance of adequate nutritional status, prevention or aggressive therapy of pulmonary complications, encouragement of physical activity, and provision of adequate psychosocial support.

Obstruction in uncomplicated meconium ileus can sometimes be relieved with enemas containing a hyperosmolar radiopaque contrast material, with surgical intervention if needed. After the newborn period, episodes of partial intestinal obstruction (**"meconium ileus equivalent"**) can be treated with enemas containing a hyperosmolar radiopaque contrast material or acetylcysteine, or by oral administration of a balanced intestinal lavage solution. Dioctyl sodium sulfosuccinate, lactulose, or acetylcysteine given orally may be helpful in preventing such episodes. When **pancreatic insufficiency** is present, pancreatic enzyme replacement in the form of powder, tablets, or capsules should be given with each meal; the dosage varies with the size of the meal, potency of the preparation, and stool pattern. The most effective enzyme preparations consist of pancrelipase in pH-sensitive, enteric-coated microspheres.

Diet therapy includes (1) sufficient calories and protein to promote normal growth—exceeding usual Recommended Dietary Allowance requirements (of the Food and Nutrition Board of the National Research Council) by 50%, (2) a normal-to-high total fat intake to increase the caloric density of the diet, (3) multivitamins in double the recommended daily allowance, (4) supplemental vitamin E in water-miscible form, and (5) salt supplementation during periods of thermal stress and increased sweating. Infants being given broad-spectrum antibiotics and patients with liver disease and hemoptysis should be given vitamin K supplements. Formulas containing protein hydrolysates and medium-chain triglycerides may be used instead of modified whole milk for infants with severe pancreatic insufficiency. Glucose polymers and medium-chain triglyceride supplements can be used to increase caloric intake. In patients who fail to maintain adequate nutritional status, **enteral supplementation** via a nasogastric tube, gastrostomy, or jejunostomy may restore normal growth and stabilize pulmonary function.

Prophylaxis against respiratory infections consists of maintenance of pertussis and measles immunity, and annual influenza vaccination. In unvaccinated patients, amantadine can be used for prophylaxis against influenza A. There has been no demonstrated increase in susceptibility to or morbidity from pneumococcal infections, and routine use of pneumococcal vaccine is *not* advocated.

Aerosol therapy with the antiviral agent ribavirin should be used in infants with respiratory syncytial viral infections.

Treatment of pulmonary manifestations includes prevention of airway obstruction and control of infection. Chest physical therapy consisting of postural drainage, percussion, vibration, and assisted coughing is recommended at the first indication of pulmonary involvement. If there is evidence of reversible airway obstruction, bronchodilators may be given orally and/or by aerosol. O_2 therapy is indicated in patients with severe pulmonary insufficiency and hypoxemia. In general, assisted ventilation is not indicated for CF patients with chronic respiratory failure. Its occasional use should be restricted to the patient with good baseline status in whom acute respiratory failure develops, or in association with pulmonary surgery.

Pneumothorax can be treated by closed chest tube thoracostomy in combination with the intrapleural instillation of a sclerosing agent to create adhesions between the visceral and parietal pleural surfaces; eg, quinacrine 2% (100 mg in 50 mL isotonic saline) instilled daily for 3 days. Open thoracotomy with resection of pleural blebs and sponge abrasion of the pleural surfaces is also effective in creating pleural adhesions.

Aerosolized mucolytics and oral expectorants are widely used, but few data support their efficacy. Home mist tents are no longer recommended, as studies of aerosol deposition, pulmonary function, chest x-ray changes, and sputum viscosity fail to show any benefit. Tracheobronchial lavage provides temporary improvement in some patients, but results are not superior to those obtained with intensive chest physical therapy and IV antibiotics. The use of IPPB devices is not recommended because of the possibility of causing a pneumothorax.

Oral glucocorticoids are indicated in infants with a prolonged bronchiolitic syndrome and in those patients with refractory bronchospasm, allergic bronchopulmonary aspergillosis, and inflammatory complications (eg, arthritis and vasculitis). Long-term use of alternate-day glucocorticoid therapy is under investigation, but it is not yet recommended for routine use. Patients receiving glucocorticoids need to be closely monitored for evidence of carbohydrate abnormalities and linear growth retardation.

Antibiotics: In symptomatic outpatients, bacterial pathogens in the respiratory tract should be treated with drugs determined appropriate by culture and sensitivity testing. Penicillinase-resistant penicillins (eg, cloxacillin or dicloxacillin) or a cephalosporin (eg, cephalexin) is the agent of choice for staphylococci. Erythromycin, ampicillin, tetracycline, trimethoprim/sulfamethoxazole, or occasionally chloramphenicol may be used individually or in combination for protracted ambulatory therapy of pulmonary infection due to a variety of organisms. In adult patients colonized with sensitive strains, the fluoroquinolone antibiotic ciprofloxacin is an effective oral anti-_Pseudomonas_ agent. For severe pulmonary exacerbations, especially in patients colonized with _Pseudomonas_, treatment with parenteral antibiotic therapy is advised. This usually requires hospital admission, but in older patients may be carried out safely at home. Combinations of an aminoglycoside with an anti-_Pseudomonas_ penicillin are frequently used by the IV route. Some of the newer cephalosporins with anti-_Pseudomonas_ activity may be useful. Serum aminoglycoside concentrations should be monitored and dosage adjusted to achieve a peak level of 8 to 10 μg/mL and a trough value of < 2 μg/mL. Patients with CF may require high doses of aminoglycosides to achieve acceptable serum concentrations. They also show enhanced renal clearance of some penicillins and may require large doses to achieve adequate serum levels. The goal of treating pulmonary infections should be to improve the clinical picture sufficiently so that continuous use of antibiotics is unnecessary. However, in some ambulatory patients with frequent pulmonary exacerbations, long-term use of antibiotics may be indicated. In selected patients chronic anti-_Pseudomonas_ therapy delivered by aerosol may be effective.

Massive or recurrent hemoptyses are treated by embolization of the involved bronchial arteries. Patients with symptomatic **right heart failure** should be treated with diuretics, salt restriction, and O_2.

Surgery may be indicated for the following: localized bronchiectasis or atelectasis that cannot be effectively treated medically; nasal polyps; chronic sinusitis; bleeding from esophageal varices secondary to portal hypertension; gallbladder disease; and intestinal obstruction due to a volvulus or an intussusception that cannot be medically reduced. Liver transplants have been performed successfully in patients with end-stage liver disease. In patients with advanced cardiopulmonary disease, heart-lung and double-lung transplants have been carried out successfully.

ASTHMA

(See also discussion of asthma in pregnancy in Ch. 17)

A lung disease characterized by (1) airways obstruction that is reversible (but not completely in some patients), either spontaneously or with treatment, (2) airways inflammation, and (3) increased airways responsiveness to a variety of stimuli.

Epidemiology

About 10 million asthmatics live in the USA. From 1980 to 1987 prevalence rates of asthma increased 29%, and from 1970 to 1987 hospital discharge rates for asthma nearly tripled. Blacks were more than twice as likely as whites to need hospitalization. Increasing mortality from asthma is worldwide; from 1980 to 1987 in the USA the death rate increased by 31%.

Pathophysiology

The airways obstruction in asthma is due to a combination of factors that include (1) spasm of airways smooth muscle; (2) edema of airways mucosa; (3) increased mucus secretion; (4) cellular, especially eosinophilic, infiltration of the airways walls; and (5) injury and desquamation of the airways epithelium.

Formerly, attention was focused on bronchospasm due to smooth muscle contraction as the major contributor to the airways obstruction. More recently, it is appreciated that asthma, particularly in its chronic form, is truly an inflammatory disease of the airways. Bronchoalveolar lavage (**BAL**) and biopsy studies, even of patients with mild asthma, show the presence of an inflammatory response involving infiltration with eosinophils and lymphocytes in particular, and epithelial cell desquamation. Typically, all asthmatics with active disease have hyperresponsive or hyperreactive airways, manifest as exaggerated bronchoconstrictor response to many different stimuli. The degree of hyperresponsiveness is closely linked to the extent of inflammation. Both are highly correlated with the severity of the disease and the need for drugs. Research on the pathophysiology of asthma over the past decade has focused on the inflammatory cells and their mediators, neurogenic mechanisms, and vascular abnormalities involved.

The mast cell seems important in the acute bronchoconstrictive response to inhaled allergens and perhaps to exercise, but less important in the pathogenesis of chronic inflammation than other cells, especially the eosinophil, which contains proteins capable of damaging airways epithelium. The number of eosinophils in both peripheral blood and BAL fluid correlates closely with the degree of bronchial hyperresponsiveness. Macrophages, lymphocytes, and their secretory products may help perpetuate airways inflammation. The role of neutrophils is unknown.

Many inflammatory mediators identified in the airways secretions of patients with asthma contribute to bronchoconstriction, mucus secretion, and microvascular leakage. The latter, a constant component of inflammatory reactions, leads to submucosal edema, increases airways resistance, and contributes to bronchial hyperresponsiveness. Inflammatory mediators are either released or formed as a consequence of allergic reactions in the lung; they include histamine, products of arachidonic acid metabolism (leukotrienes and prostaglandins, both of which can cause transient increase in airways hyperresponsiveness) and, perhaps most important, platelet activating factor (PAF). Upon inhalation, PAF, a lipid-derived substance, can cause a prolonged state of bronchial hyperresponsiveness (up to 4 wk) in nonasthmatics.

Earliest speculations about neurogenic influences on the pathogenesis of asthma led to the cholinergic theory. While cholinergic reflex bronchoconstriction probably occurs in the acute bronchoconstrictive response to inhalation of irritant substances, recent interest in neurogenic mechanisms has focused on neuropeptides released from sensory nerves by an axon reflex pathway. These peptides, which include substance P, neurokinin A, and calcitonin-related peptide, have (respectively) vascular permeability and mucus secretagogue activity, bronchoconstrictor activity, and a bronchial vascular dilation effect.

Inflammatory cells, mediators released by these cells or synthesized by other cells, and biologically active molecules released from sensory nerves act on the pulmonary airways and their microvasculature, and contribute to the special kind of airways inflammation that is characteristic of asthma.

Symptoms and Signs

The pathophysiologic changes described above lead to airways obstruction of varying degree and ventilation that is typically nonuniform.

Continued blood flow to some areas of hypoventilation leads to ventilation/perfusion imbalance, resulting in arterial hypoxemia, which is almost always present in attacks severe enough to require medical attention. Hyperventilation typically occurs early in an attack and results in a decrease in Pa_{CO_2}. As the attack progresses, the patient's capacity to compensate by hyperventilation of unobstructed areas of the lung is further impaired by more extensive airways narrowing and muscular fatigue due to the substantial work of breathing. Arterial hypoxemia worsens and Pa_{CO_2} begins to rise, leading to respiratory acidosis. At this point the patient is said to be in respiratory failure, stage IV of an acute attack (see TABLE 37-1). Early in the acute attack there may be only a modest decrease in the forced expiratory flow between 25 and 75% of the vital capacity ($FEF_{25-75\%}$). As the attack progresses, the forced vital capacity (FVC) and the forced expiratory volume during the first second (FEV_1) progressively decrease; associated air trapping and increased residual volume result in hyperinflation of the lungs. Abnormalities in flow rates have been shown to persist *many weeks* after an acute attack.

The symptoms of each asthmatic differ greatly in frequency and degree. Some asthmatics are symptom-free, with an occasional episode that is mild and brief. Others have mild coughing and wheezing much of the time, punctuated by severe exacerbations of symptoms following exposure to known allergens, viral infections, exercise, or nonspecific irritants. Psychologic factors, particularly those associated with crying, screaming, or hard laughing, may precipitate symptoms.

Especially in children, an itch over the anterior neck or upper chest may be an early prodromal symptom, and dry cough, particularly at night and with exercise, may be the sole presenting symptom. However, an attack usually begins acutely with paroxysms of wheezing, coughing, and shortness of breath, or insidiously with slowly increasing manifestations of respiratory distress. In either case, the asthmatic usually first notices dyspnea, tachypnea, cough, and tightness or pressure in the chest, and may even notice audible wheezes. The episode may subside quickly or persist for hours to days. Pulmonary function abnormalities (see under Laboratory Findings, below) may persist weeks after an acute attack, even without symptoms.

The cough during an acute attack sounds "tight" and is generally nonproductive of mucus.

TABLE 37-1. STAGING OF THE SEVERITY OF AN ACUTE ASTHMA ATTACK

Stage	Symptoms and Signs	FEV₁ or FVC	pH	Paco₂	Pao₂ (Room air)
I (mild)	Mild dyspnea, diffuse wheezes, adequate air exchange	50–80% of N	N or slightly ↑	N or ↓	Occasionally N or most often ↓
II (moderate)	Respiratory distress at rest, hyperpnea, use of accessory muscles, marked wheezes, air exchange N or ↓	50% N	N or ↑	Generally ↓	↑
III (severe)	Marked respiratory distress, cyanosis, use of accessory muscles, marked wheezes or absent breath sounds; check for pulsus paradoxus 20–30 mm Hg	25% N	Most often ↓	N or ↑	↓ ↓
IV (respiratory failure)	Severe respiratory distress, lethargy, confusion, prominent pulsus paradoxus 30–50 mm Hg, use of accessory muscles	10% N	↓ ↓	↑ ↑	↓ ↓ ↓

N = normal; ↓ = diminished; ↑ = increased.

Except in young children, who rarely expectorate, tenacious mucoid sputum is produced as the attack subsides.

On physical examination during an acute attack, the patient shows varying degrees of respiratory distress, depending on the severity and duration of the episode. Tachypnea, tachycardia, and audible wheezes are often present. Because of sweating and increased insensible water loss from the lungs secondary to tachypnea, variable degrees of dehydration may occur during prolonged episodes. The patient prefers to sit upright or even leans forward, uses accessory muscles of respiration, is anxious, and may appear to struggle for air. Chest examination shows a prolonged expiratory phase with relatively high-pitched wheezes throughout inspiration and most of expiration. The chest may appear quite hyperinflated owing to air trapping. Although coarse rhonchi may accompany the wheezes, fine crackles are not heard unless pneumonia, atelectasis, or cardiac decompensation is also present.

In more severe episodes, the patient may be unable to speak more than a few words without stopping for breath. Fatigue and severe distress

are evident in rapid, shallow, ineffectual respiratory movements. Cyanosis becomes evident as the attack worsens. Confusion and lethargy may indicate the onset of progressive respiratory failure with CO₂ narcosis. In such patients, *less wheezing* may be heard on auscultation, because extensive mucous plugging and patient fatigue result in marked reduction of air flow and gas exchange. In an asthmatic with a quiet-sounding chest, an inexperienced examiner may mistakenly attribute the anxiety and respiratory distress to emotional factors or may underestimate the severity of obstruction. *Such a patient may actually have a more severe problem than one with audible wheezes. Extensive small airways obstruction may be present with few auscultatory findings.*

Thus, the presence, absence, or prominence of wheezes does not correlate precisely with the severity of the attack. The most reliable signs include the degree of dyspnea at rest, cyanosis, difficulty in speaking, pulsus paradoxus of > 20 to 30 mm Hg, and the use of accessory muscles of respiration. The severity of an attack can be most precisely assessed by arterial blood gas (ABG) levels.

Between acute attacks, breath sounds may be normal during quiet respiration. However, fine wheezes may be audible during forced expiration or after the patient exercises. Low-to-moderate grade wheezing may be heard at any time in some patients, even when they claim to be completely asymptomatic. With long-standing severe asthma, especially if dating from childhood, there may be evidence of secondary effects of chronic hyperinflation on the chest wall (eg, "squared off" thorax, anterior bowing of the sternum, depressed diaphragm).

Complications During an Acute Attack of Asthma

Pneumothorax may present as a sudden worsening of respiratory distress, accompanied by sharp chest pains and, on physical examination, a shift of the mediastinum. X-ray examination confirms the diagnosis. **Mediastinal and subcutaneous emphysema** due to alveolar rupture and dissection of air along vessels is occasionally observed. **Atelectasis,** usually involving the right middle lobe or even an entire lung, is more common. Unless a substantial amount of tissue collapses, the atelectasis is usually diagnosed only as a result of x-ray examination. **Bronchiectasis** is rare. While evidence of acute **cor pulmonale** can occasionally be noted on an ECG, chronic cor pulmonale secondary to asthma is rare. Contrary to popular opinion, uncomplicated asthma rarely leads to chronic obstructive emphysema, especially in a nonsmoker.

Laboratory Findings

Eosinophilia (> 250 to 400 cells/μL) is common regardless of whether allergic factors can be shown to have an etiologic role. In many asthmatics, the degree of eosinophilia may correlate with the asthma's severity. The extent that corticosteroids can suppress eosinophilia (as measured by total eosinophil counts) has been used as an index of the adequacy of corticosteroid dosage.

Determination of **ABGs and pH** is essential to the adequate evaluation of a patient with asthma of sufficient severity to warrant hospitalization. (See TABLE 37–1.)

Sputum in a patient with uncomplicated asthma is highly distinctive. Grossly, it is tenacious, rubbery, and whitish; in the presence of infection, especially in adults, it may be yellowish. Many eosinophils, often arranged in sheets, are found microscopically; large numbers of histiocytes and polymorphonuclear leukocytes are also present. Eosinophilic granules from disrupted cells may be seen throughout the sputum smear. Elongated dipyramidal crystals (**Charcot-Leyden**) originating from eosinophils are commonly found. When bacterial respiratory infection is present, and particularly when there is a bronchitic element, polymorphonuclear leukocytes and bacteria predominate. In uncomplicated asthma, sputum cultures rarely show pathogenic bacteria.

Chest x-ray findings vary from normal to hyperinflation. Lung markings are commonly increased, particularly in chronic disease. Atelectasis, most often involving the right middle lobe, is common in children and may be recurrent. Small areas of segmental atelectasis, often observed during acute exacerbations, may be misinterpreted as pneumonitis, but their rapid clearing suggests atelectasis. An esophagogram should be considered part of the evaluation of an infant or young child with suspected asthma to rule out congenital anomalies, which might cause manifestations of airways obstruction by compression of the trachea or bronchi. Inspiratory and expiratory chest x-rays help to diagnose foreign-body aspiration as a cause of wheezing in children. The expiratory film will show impaired exit of air from the affected lung; this film is especially important in cases of a nonopaque foreign body (see foreign-body obstruction, below).

Pulmonary function tests are valuable in differential diagnosis, and in known asthmatics to assess the degree of airways obstruction and disturbance in gas exchange, to measure the airways' response to inhaled allergens and chemicals (bronchial provocation testing), to quantify the response to drugs, and for long-term follow-up. Pulmonary function testing is most valuable when done before and after giving an aerosolized bronchodilator to determine the degree of reversibility of the airways obstruction.

Static lung volumes and capacities reveal various combinations of abnormalities, although these may not be detected when mild disease is in remission. Of the tests most often used clinically, total lung capacity (**TLC**), functional residual capacity (**FRC**), and residual volume (**RV**) are usually increased. Vital capacity (**VC**) may be normal or decreased.

Dynamic lung volumes and capacities, an index of airways obstruction, are reduced in asthmatics and return toward normal after inhalation of an aerosolized bronchodilator. In mild, asymptomatic asthmatics, these tests may be normal. Since expiratory flow (EF) is determined by the diameter of the airways and also by the elastic recoil forces of the lung, flow at high lung volumes will exceed flow at low lung volumes. Tests that measure flow at relatively large lung volumes ($FEV_{0.5}$ and peak expiratory flow [PEF]) are, to a considerable degree, effort-dependent and are less satisfactory than tests that measure flow over a larger range of lung volume. These include FEV_1 and the mean $FEF_{25-75\%}$, which is particularly valuable, since it is considered to reflect small airways obstruction. EF measurements at large lung volumes are insensitive to changes in peripheral airways resistance and reflect abnormalities principally in central airways. The EF-volume curve, in which expired lung volume is plotted against flow rate, is probably of greatest value; this curve gives a graphic picture of flow at large and small lung volumes and presumably, therefore, reveals abnormalities in both central and peripheral airways. In the past, probably too much was made of these distinctions. The FEV_1 provides most of the information needed to manage an asthmatic. Before spirometry, patients should withhold inhaled adrenergic bronchodilators for at least 4 h, and theophylline products (particularly sustained-release preparations) for at least 12 h.

Distribution of ventilation in asthmatics is often abnormal; ie, various lung units fill and empty asynchronously. This maldistribution is quantified by the single-breath N_2 test and the 7-min N_2 washout test. Measurements of lung elasticity (lung compliance), by use of an esophageal balloon to estimate pleural pressure, have shown a loss of elastic recoil (particularly during acute asthma attacks), which is often reversible upon remission of asthma. Diffusing capacity for CO (DL_{CO}) is generally normal in asthma; it is low in emphysema (in which there is loss of a functioning alveolar capillary bed with increased lung volume).

Other laboratory tests: Assessment of etiologic factors is more difficult. Nonspecific irritant factors, particularly cigarette smoke, and evidence of infection (usually viral) should be evaluated. Exacerbations related to environmental allergen exposures, history of rhinitis, or family history of atopic disorders suggests the likelihood of extrinsic allergic factors. Confirmation is best accomplished by an allergy evaluation that includes **allergy skin testing** with extracts to detect IgE antibody (**Ab**) to common inhalants (pollens, molds, epidermals [epidermal scales of furred animals like dogs and cats; in the case of

cats, the antigen is in the saliva, which represents a serious problem because cats groom themselves regularly], house dust mite) suggested by the patient's history. Bronchodilators containing adrenergic agents should be discontinued for 12 h and antihistamines for 48 h (even longer with some of the newer long-lasting agents), but a corticosteroid may be continued (eg, prednisone up to 40 to 60 mg/day) without interfering with the immediate skin test response. Negative skin test responses to a suitable battery of appropriate allergens strongly rule against an allergic component. Positive skin tests indicate the presence of IgE Ab to the test allergen and represent only the *potential* for allergic reactivity to the allergens in question. Their clinical significance is determined when results are correlated with the pattern of symptoms and related to environmental exposures.

Specific IgE Ab to inhalants may also be detected by in vitro methods (eg, **radioallergosorbent test [RAST]**—see in Ch. 34) or similar tests on the patient's serum, but in vitro tests are expensive, subject to laboratory error, and offer little advantage over properly done and interpreted skin tests. Measurement of total serum IgE or specific IgE Abs to a small panel of common allergens by one of several in vitro methods may be useful in establishing the atopic constitution of the patient. **Inhalational bronchial challenge testing** has been used (1) with allergens to establish the clinical significance of positive skin tests, (2) with methacholine or histamine to assess the degree of airways hyperactivity in known asthmatics, or (3) to aid in diagnosis when the symptoms are atypical, ie, patients with persistent cough but no wheeze as in cough-variant asthma. **Exercise testing** using a treadmill or bicycle ergometer has been used, particularly in children, to confirm equivocal diagnoses of asthma. Over 90% of children with asthma will develop a postexercise fall in pulmonary function after 7 min of appropriate treadmill or bicycle ergometer exercise.

Diagnosis and Staging

Asthma should be considered in anyone who wheezes; it is the likeliest diagnosis when typical paroxysmal wheezing starts in childhood or early adulthood and is interspersed with asymptomatic intervals. A family history of allergy or asthma can be elicited in most asthmatics. Difficulties occur in diagnosis when asthma presents initially in adults, especially those over age 50, or when atypical symptoms (eg, cough without audible wheezing), physical findings, or chest x-rays are noted. A number of other disorders may produce wheezing.

Children with congenital malformations of the vascular system (vascular rings and slings) and of the GI and respiratory tracts (tracheoesophageal fistula) may present with wheezing. The presence of other congenital malformations, special attention to infants whose symptoms begin before age 1 yr, x-ray studies, and a high index of suspicion will lead to a correct diagnosis.

Foreign-body obstruction must be considered, particularly in children with unilateral wheezing or sudden onset of wheezing without a history of respiratory symptoms. Opaque foreign bodies are readily visible on x-ray. With nonopaque foreign bodies, the diagnosis can be established by a history of sudden onset of cough and wheezing in a previously well child, combined with asymmetric diaphragmatic movement or mediastinal shifts on inspiratory and expiratory chest x-rays.

Viral URI involving the epiglottis, glottis, and subglottis generally causes signs and symptoms of croup (inspiratory stridor, high-pitched cough, and hoarseness) that are distinct from the lower airways signs and symptoms of asthma (see CROUP under VIRAL INFECTIONS in Ch. 32). *When epiglottitis is suspected, direct examination of the epiglottis should be done with great care and with the capability for immediate intubation if acute airways obstruction should develop during examination.* Primary bacterial infection of the lower airways, without an underlying predisposing disease, is rare in infants and children. On the other hand, viruses, particularly respiratory syncytial virus, can cause **bronchiolitis** with a clinical picture virtually identical to asthma during infancy. Bronchiolitis, particularly that due to respiratory syncytial virus, may be a forerunner of subsequent asthma. If tested, about 50% of infants with bronchiolitis will show pulmonary function abnormalities and abnormal bronchial responses to provocation with histamine and methacholine. However, it is rare for an infant or young child to have > 1 or 2 episodes of infectious bronchiolitis, and a history of recurrent episodes of obstructive airways symptoms should strongly suggest the diagnosis of asthma. Since chronic bronchitis as a primary diagnosis is rare in children, underlying disorders (eg, cystic fibrosis, immunodeficiency disease, and ciliary dyskinesia syndrome) should always be considered. These may be ruled out by a careful history, sweat test, in vivo and in vitro evaluation of immunologic

competence, and biopsy of respiratory mucosa with electron microscope study of cilia. Most children with a diagnosis of chronic bronchitis based on chronic cough will be shown to have asthma.

In **adults**, manifestations of airways obstruction due to upper airways disorders may be clarified by a flow-volume curve. Upper airways obstruction due to vocal cord dysfunction may be diagnosed by flexible bronchoscopy during an attack. Chronic obstructive pulmonary disease and heart failure are the main considerations in the differential diagnosis of wheezing, although multiple small pulmonary emboli frequently present with wheezing. Patients with hypersensitivity pneumonitis have a superficial clinical resemblance to asthmatics, but generally have more constitutional symptoms after exposure to the offending substance and typically do not wheeze, except in allergic bronchopulmonary aspergillosis. Patients with bronchial obstructions secondary to malignancy, aortic aneurysm, endobronchial TB, or sarcoidosis may occasionally present with wheezing.

Patients with allergic bronchopulmonary aspergillosis may present with typical asthmatic symptoms. The diagnosis of aspergillosis is confirmed by the findings of high peripheral blood eosinophilia, immediate skin test reactivity to *Aspergillus* antigen, precipitating Abs against *Aspergillus* antigen, increased serum IgE concentrations (which appear to fluctuate with the activity of the disease), pulmonary infiltrates (transient or fixed), and a peculiar central type of bronchiectasis.

Other rare disorders that may simulate asthma include carcinoid syndrome, Churg-Strauss allergic angiitis and granulomatosis, and eosinophilic pneumonias (including tropical eosinophilia and other parasitic infestations that involve the lung during some phase of the disease). In all, the history is usually sufficiently atypical of asthma to suggest that another disorder is causing the airways obstruction.

Physical examination should search for heart failure and signs of chronic hypoxemia (clubbing of the fingers). Nasal polyposis should suggest aspirin intolerance. Unilateral wheezing should provoke a search for obstruction by a foreign body, vascular malformation, aneurysm, or tumor. In tracheal obstruction, an inspiratory wheeze (stridor) is present over the upper airway.

Staging of the severity of the asthma attack is critical after the diagnosis is established. This is accomplished by a combination of evaluation of respiratory distress, monitoring of ABGs, and spirometry. TABLE 37–1 illustrates one staging method.

Prophylaxis

The role of **environmental factors** (generally animal danders, house dust mite, airborne molds, and pollens) should be rigorously investigated. If suspected, allergy skin tests should confirm the history. Allergens that can be controlled by avoidance (animal danders, house dust mite) should be eliminated (mattress and box springs should be placed in an impermeable zippered casing and the carpet should be removed, particularly in a warm, moist climate that favors the propagation of house dust mites. Other allergens (dust mite, mold, and pollens) may be selected for a trial of allergy immunotherapy (formerly termed hyposensitization). Improvement should be noted within 12 to 24 mo after beginning treatment. If no significant improvement is noted within this time, immunotherapy should be stopped. When improvement occurs, the optimum duration of therapy is unknown, but at least 3 yr is recommended.

Nonspecific exacerbating factors (eg, cigarette smoke especially, odors, irritant fumes, and changes in temperature, atmospheric pressure, and humidity) should also be investigated and controlled if possible. Aspirin should be avoided, particularly by patients with nasal polyposis, because of a significant incidence of aspirin-induced asthma. A few aspirin-intolerant asthmatics also react adversely to indomethacin and other NSAIDs, and rarely to tartrazine (FD and C yellow No. 5). Sensitivity to sulfites (used widely as food preservatives) is suggested by attacks that follow eating from a salad bar or drinking red wine or beer.

Treatment

Treatment may be conveniently considered as management of the acute attack and day-to-day therapy. Drug therapy enables most patients to lead relatively normal lives with few adverse drug effects. The detailed approach described below is one of a number that may be tried, but several general principles are important regardless of the particular drug or drugs used. (1) Staging of the severity of the attack (see above) is paramount, especially if it has been prolonged (> 12 h) or if the patient is unfamiliar to the examiner. (2) Bronchodilators should be used in orderly progression, with the patient under close observation during initial therapy. Treatment to alleviate acute respiratory distress without maintenance follow-up treatment often results in a return of acute symptoms within 24 h. (3) Although most asthmatics may benefit from inhalation of nebulized bronchodilators, some cannot inhale aerosol effectively and require parenteral drugs.

Drug therapy: Five groups are useful.

1. **β-Adrenergic agents** cause bronchial smooth muscle relaxation and modulate inhibition of mediator release, at least in part by stimulating the adenylate cyclase-cAMP system. They also protect against challenge with various bronchoconstrictor substances and may inhibit microvascular leakage into the airway. These drugs include epinephrine, isoproterenol, and some more selective β_2-adrenergics (relatively more bronchodilatory β_2 effect and less cardiostimulatory β_1 effect). The latter commonly used β_2-adrenergics include metaproterenol, terbutaline, isoetharine, albuterol, bitolterol, and pirbuterol. In general, epinephrine s.c. and one of the inhaled β_2-agents are most useful in treating the acute attack. After inhalation, the β_2-agents have rapid onset of action (within minutes) but are active for only 4 to 6 h at most. β_2-Agonists are the drugs of choice to relieve acute exacerbations of asthma and prevent bronchoconstriction following exercise or other stimuli. Adverse effects are dose-related; they are more common after oral than aerosol administration because of the manyfold higher dose required for oral drugs. Sustained-release (**SR**) oral formulations help prevent nocturnal asthma.

2. **Theophylline (a methylxanthine)** relaxes bronchial smooth muscle. Its mechanism of action is unclear but theophylline appears to inhibit intracellular release of Ca, decreases microvascular leakage into the airways mucosa, inhibits the late response to allergens, and may inhibit mast cell release of chemical mediators. It does not inhibit mediator release from eosinophils and neither prevents bronchial hyperresponsiveness following allergen challenge nor decreases bronchial hyperresponsiveness in asthma after long-term use. Theophylline is a valuable adjunct to adrenergic drugs for management of acute episodes, especially in patients who do not respond to optimal aerosol bronchodilator therapy. SR theophylline is very useful for management of nocturnal asthma.

3. **Corticosteroids** inhibit attraction of polymorphonuclear leukocytes to the site of an allergic reaction, stimulate synthesis of β_2-receptors, and block leukotriene synthesis. Very impor-

tantly, corticosteroids, particularly when given by aerosol, block the late response (but not the early response) to inhaled allergens and subsequent bronchial hyperresponsiveness. With long-term therapy, bronchial hyperresponsiveness also gradually decreases. While systemic corticosteroids are exceptionally effective, they are reserved for more difficult episodes because of their potential for adverse effects. Short-term use in high dosage (eg, for 5 to 7 days to abort an attack) is unassociated with significant problems. The new surface-active inhaled steroids are useful for maintenance therapy, but not for managing acute episodes, although this is under active investigation.

4. **Cromolyn sodium** (disodium cromoglycate—DSCG), used prophylactically, appears to inhibit mediator release and reduce airways hyperreactivity. DSCG is primarily useful in children and some adults *for maintenance therapy only and has no place in treatment of the acute attack.* Cost and problems with patient compliance appear to have limited its use in the USA. It is the safest of all drugs used to treat asthma.

5. **Anticholinergic agents** (eg, atropine and its derivative ipratropium bromide) block cholinergic pathways that cause airways obstruction. They may provide added bronchodilator effect in patients who have already received inhaled β_2-agents for acute asthma. The role of anticholinergics in day-to-day treatment has not been defined. Measurement of FEV_1 and PEF, especially after therapy, is a very useful predictor of need for hospitalization. For example, improvement in FEV_1 of $< 40\%$ of predicted indicates, along with other factors, the need to hospitalize the patient.

Treatment of the Acute Attack

Drug therapy: Patients with acute asthma presenting in stage I or II (see TABLE 37–1) may be treated effectively with an aerosolized bronchodilator (eg, albuterol 0.5%) using compressed air for nebulization. In adults with acute asthma, albuterol from a metered-dose inhaler with a spacer (InspirEase®) has been shown in some studies (but not all) to be as effective as a compressor-generated aerosol. Alternatively, epinephrine 1:1000 in a dose of 0.01 mL/kg s.c. up to a maximum of 0.2 mL in children and 0.3 mL in adults, repeated once or twice in 20 to 30 min, if indicated, may be given. Terbutaline, an alternative to epinephrine in the same dosage, may be preferred in adults because of somewhat less cardiovascular effect. If there is no response af-

ter 3 adrenergic aerosol treatments and/or epinephrine injections, theophylline (as aminophylline) should be given IV. Although a number of studies indicate that in an emergency room setting IV aminophylline given to patients who receive optimal β_2-agonist therapy (treatments q 20 min for 3 times) adds nothing but adverse effects, many experienced clinicians believe that aminophylline is still indicated. If the patient does not have an optimal response to inhaled β_2-agonists and needs to be hospitalized, the use of IV aminophylline would be recommended by most experienced clinicians, although this too has become controversial.

Different schedules for giving aminophylline are used because each patient varies in susceptibility to its beneficial or adverse effects. Serum levels of 10 to 20 μg/mL of theophylline are most effective. Most regimens start with an IV loading dose of aminophylline 6 mg/kg (at a concentration of 25 mg/mL, diluted 1:1 with IV fluids) for children or adults given over about 20 min; then a continuous infusion is begun (0.45 mg/kg/h in adults and 0.8 to 1.0 mg/kg/h in children < 12 yr of age). Serum levels should be monitored at 1, 12, and 24 h after starting the infusion. If continuous infusion is unfeasible, then aminophylline 4 to 6 mg/kg IV over 20 min q 6 h is an acceptable alternative. ABGs should be obtained, especially if there is no sign of a prompt response (within about 30 min), if the patient is in severe distress or worsening, or if there is uncertainty about the stage of illness.

For any patient presenting in stage III, an ABG determination should be obtained immediately and IV aminophylline started. For a patient in severe distress, continuous infusion doses may be raised to the limit of 1 mg/kg/h in young or middle-aged adults and 1.25 mg/kg/h in children. To prevent toxicity, monitoring of serum theophylline levels is essential. Greater caution is necessary and lower dosages (by $^1/_3$ to $^1/_2$) should be used in a patient with heart failure, liver disease, or one who is elderly. Patients who take drugs known to reduce serum theophylline clearance (eg, cimetidine, erythromycin, ciprofloxacin) should have the dosage reduced by 25 to 50% and serum concentrations should be monitored carefully. O_2 at an inspired flow (F_{IO_2}) appropriate to correct hypoxemia should be given.

While corticosteroids may be advantageous in stage II of an attack, when patients present in stage III and show no improvement or worsen despite one dose of aminophylline, IV corticosteroids are mandatory. Criteria for hospitalization vary, but definite indications are (1) failure to improve, (2) relapse after repeated adrenergic therapy and aminophylline, and (3) significant decrease in Pa_{O_2} ($<$ 50 mm Hg) or increase in Pa_{CO_2} ($>$ 50 mm Hg), indicating progression to respiratory failure. Far too many patients with severe asthma attacks are sent home from hospital emergency rooms.

Any patient presenting in or reaching stage IV should immediately be given methylprednisolone 1 to 2 mg/kg IV q 4 to 6 h or hydrocortisone sodium succinate 4 mg/kg IV q 2 to 4 h. IV corticosteroids in these doses (or double the maintenance dose, whichever is greater) are also indicated immediately for any acute attack if the patient had taken maintenance corticosteroids any time within the previous 6 to 12 wk.

Patients in stage IV who show no favorable response to aggressive bronchodilator and antiinflammatory therapy and who evidence fatigue and progressive deterioration in ABGs and pH should be considered candidates for endotracheal intubation and respiratory assistance. Such patients should be hospitalized in an intensive care unit (ICU).

Children in stage III or IV may be given isoproterenol 0.08 to 2.7 μg/kg/min by continuous IV infusion with a suitable infusion pump. This procedure requires ECG and ABG monitoring in an ICU and supervision by clinicians experienced in monitoring asthmatic children. Terbutaline in an initial dose of 0.5 mg given over 20 min by constant infusion has also been used in this setting. If improvement occurs without adverse effects (eg, drop in diastolic BP, arrhythmia) the same dose or one that is even higher may be given if the patient again becomes dyspneic. IV albuterol, used effectively in England and Canada, is unavailable in the USA. Because of the increased potential for arrhythmias in adults, IV isoproterenol should probably not be used.

IV aminophylline and corticosteroids should be continued until the patient's condition has stabilized and there is no danger of progression to respiratory failure. Continuous nebulization of albuterol 0.5% solution in a concentration of 0.833 mg/mL in saline is used successfully in pediatric ICUs for children with severe status asthmaticus. O_2, rather than room air, should be used as the aerosolizing gas. Sedatives and cough suppressants are **contraindicated**.

Anxiety may be extreme, because of hypoxia and the feeling of asphyxiation. Treatment of the underlying respiratory problems, including judicious use of O_2 therapy (see below), is the preferred approach, especially when conducted by calm, attentive, supportive medical personnel.

Fluid and electrolyte balance requires attention, especially when the episode lasts $>$ 12 h, because these patients may be dehydrated. Therapy replaces previous and current fluid losses, not with an arbitrary amount/24 h, but by constant infusion of amounts sufficient to result in a urine output adequate for the patient's age and size. Overhydration may cause pulmonary edema. Humidification of inhaled air or O_2 reduces excess loss from the respiratory tract.

With progressive severity and duration of the episode, respiratory acidosis may supervene; the arterial pH may drop alarmingly to ranges of pH 7 to 7.1. Most adults are intubated at this stage and started on assisted ventilation, because *the acidosis mainly reflects a respiratory mechanical problem that must be relieved.* Use of alkaline solutions (eg, sodium bicarbonate) in the IV fluid should be limited to maintain the pH between 7.2 and 7.3, since there is some evidence that adrenergic agent resistance is reversed by normalizing the pH. While there are theoretic objections to adding bicarbonate to a closed system, sodium bicarbonate has been safely and successfully used in children and adults with status asthmaticus. It should be used only with careful ABG and pH monitoring.

Supplemental K may need to be added to the infusion, since K shifts occur with changes in arterial and tissue pH and fluid turnover in a dehydrated patient. In addition, high doses of hydrocortisone (more so than methylprednisolone) given during therapy promote urinary K loss.

O_2 therapy is always indicated, since severe asthmatics are invariably hypoxemic. The F_{IO_2} is guided by ABG levels; Pa_{O_2} should be maintained at $>$ 60 mm Hg—in the 70 to 90 mm Hg range, if possible. O_2 may be given effectively with nasal prongs or, if tolerated, a Venturi mask. In the occasional patient who will not tolerate a mask, use of nasal prongs with low F_{IO_2} (2 to 4 L/min) may achieve the same result. Since O_2 may dry the mucosa, it should always be humidified.

Respiratory tract infections that exacerbate asthma are predominantly viral; bacterial infections rarely play a significant role, especially in children. However, if the patient expectorates yellowish, green, or brown sputum, and Wright's stain of the sputum shows a predominance of polymorphonuclear WBCs, antibacterial therapy is given empirically. This is especially appropriate in adults with a known tendency to have chronic or recurrent bronchitis. The antibiotic should be chosen according to bacteriologic findings, but ampicillin is usually most useful. If the patient is allergic to β-lactam antibiotics, erythromycin or tetracycline (the latter should not be given to young children) or trimethoprim/sulfamethoxazole as well may be given. Gram stain of the sputum, noting intracellular bacteria, and chest x-rays are useful guides to therapy.

Although not all physicians agree, many believe that **chest x-ray** is indicated in most hospitalized asthmatics. Spontaneous pneumothorax and subcutaneous and mediastinal emphysema are complications of acute asthma, particularly in children. A large pneumothorax requires immediate treatment. Mediastinal and subcutaneous emphysema rarely cause difficulty, even when large. Rarely, **compression of the glottis** may occur with extreme extravasation of air into the soft tissues of the neck.

Maintenance Therapy for Asthma

Appropriate drug use keeps most asthmatics out of the emergency room and hospital. Drug selection is based upon the severity of illness. When symptomatic, patients with mild intermittent asthma may be successfully managed with β2-agonists given from a metered-dose inhaler **(MDI)**. If symptoms become persistent, adrenergic aerosols may be required on a regular basis in a dose of 2 inhalations tid to qid. A recent well-designed study in New Zealand suggests that regular use of inhaled β2-agonists may increase the morbidity of asthma. If these results are confirmed, the use of inhaled β2-agonists like albuterol may be relegated to acute or prn use. Patients must be carefully instructed in the proper use of the MDI. For those unable to use the MDI properly, prescription of one of several types of spacers or holding chambers (InspirEase® or Aerochamber®) will be very helpful. If despite correct use of the MDI tid to qid, the patient's symptoms remain unacceptable (poor exercise tolerance, significant nocturnal symptoms), another drug should be added: cromolyn or inhaled corticosteroids. Cromolyn, marketed as a powder in capsules for inhalation, as an MDI, or in solution, is particularly useful in children when given tid to qid. In infants and preschool children subject to asthma precipitated by viral respiratory infection, prophylaxis with cromolyn solution (2 mL) with or without albuterol (0.25 to 0.5 mL) as a compressor-generated aerosol reduces the frequency of exacerbations. While cromolyn blocks exercise-induced asthma, it is less effec-

tive in this regard than a β2-agonist. During an exacerbation, it is unnecessary to discontinue use of the solution or metered-dose aerosol as is recommended with the powder, which may act as an irritant. Instead, many physicians will prescribe theophylline to supplement the regular therapy of β2-agonist inhalation.

Oral theophylline formulations are available as tablets, capsules, or liquids. Anhydrous preparations are preferred to theophylline combinations. Sustained-release **(SR)** formulations maintain the serum theophylline level in the therapeutic range when given tid, bid, or even once/day in particularly slow theophylline metabolizers. Since children, in particular, metabolize theophylline rapidly, serum level peaks (which may cause toxic symptoms) and troughs (which may be therapeutically ineffective) often occur with the conventional rapidly absorbed formulations. SR formulations overcome this problem and are convenient for adults and older children. Because capsules may be opened and the pellet contents mixed with moist food, they are useful in young children. Neither tablets nor pellets should be chewed. As with IV use, toxic symptoms may be noted at serum concentrations > 20 μg/mL. Nausea, vomiting, and CNS stimulation should be watched for, serum theophylline measured, and the dosage or interval modified accordingly. Inhaled corticosteroids have become increasingly popular in recent years as very effective maintenance therapy for both children and adults with asthma. The drugs are extraordinarily safe and effective for patients with significant degrees of asthma that cannot be managed with bronchodilators alone.

The importance of education for patients cannot be overemphasized: The more they know about asthma, including precipitating factors, what drug to use when, and the importance of early intervention with corticosteroids when asthma worsens, the better they will do. Asthma education programs that incorporate the use of peak flow meters for measurement of PEF bid or tid at home are particularly valuable. Use of a peak flow meter is useful to follow the day-to-day fluctuation in disease activity and as a guide for patients in terms of when to increase drugs or consult with the physician.

Surgical procedures should be done when the patient's pulmonary state is optimum. Corticosteroids may be required; short-term use is safer than a compromised respiratory status. Procedures involving nasal and tracheal manipulation are particularly troublesome, and polypectomies in aspirin-sensitive asthmatics may require a week's pretreatment with prednisone 50 to 60 mg/day orally.

ACUTE BRONCHITIS

Acute inflammation of the tracheobronchial tree, generally self-limited and with eventual complete healing and return of function. Though commonly mild, bronchitis may be serious in debilitated patients and those with chronic lung or heart disease. Pneumonia is a critical complication.

Etiology

Acute infectious bronchitis, most prevalent in winter, is often part of an acute URI. It may develop after a common cold or other viral infection of the nasopharynx, throat, or tracheobronchial tree, often with secondary bacterial infection. *Mycoplasma pneumoniae* and *Chlamydia* (Taiwan acute respiratory agent) also cause acute, infectious bronchitis, often in young adults. Exposure to air pollutants and possibly chilling, fatigue, and malnutrition are predisposing or contributory factors. Recurrent attacks often complicate chronic bronchopulmonary diseases, which impair bronchial clearance mechanisms. Repeated infections may be associated with chronic sinusitis, bronchiectasis, bronchopulmonary allergy, or, in children, hypertrophied tonsils and adenoids.

Acute irritative bronchitis may be caused by various mineral and vegetable dusts; fumes from strong acids, ammonia, certain volatile organic solvents, chlorine, hydrogen sulfide, sulfur dioxide, or bromine; the environmental irritants ozone and nitrogen dioxide; or tobacco or other smoke.

Cough-variant asthma, asthma in which the degree of bronchoconstriction is not sufficient to produce overt wheezing, may be caused by allergen inhalation in an atopic individual, or chronic exposure to an airways irritant when airways hyperreactivity is relatively mild. (For inhalational challenge testing, see ASTHMA, above.) Its management is similar to that of ordinary asthma.

Pathology and Pathophysiology

Hyperemia of the mucous membranes is the earliest change, followed by desquamation, edema, leukocytic infiltration of the submucosa, and production of sticky or mucopurulent exudate. The protective functions of bronchial cilia, phagocytes, and lymphatics are disturbed, and bacteria may invade the normally sterile bronchi with consequent accumulation of cellular debris and mucopurulent exudate. Cough, though distressing, is essential to eliminate bronchial secretions. Airways obstruction may result from edema of the bronchial walls, retained secretions, and, in some cases, spasm of bronchial muscles.

Symptoms and Signs

Acute infectious bronchitis is often preceded by symptoms of a URI: coryza, malaise, chilliness, slight fever, back and muscle pain, and sore throat. Onset of cough usually signals onset of bronchitis. The cough is initially dry and nonproductive, but small amounts of viscid sputum are raised after a few hours or days; it may later become more abundant and mucoid or mucopurulent. Frankly purulent sputum suggests superimposed bacterial infection. In a severe uncomplicated case, fever to 38.3 or 38.8 C° (101 or 102° F) may be present for up to 3 to 5 days, following which acute symptoms subside (though cough may continue for several weeks). Persistent fever suggests complicating pneumonia. Dyspnea may be noted secondary to the airways obstruction.

Pulmonary signs are few in uncomplicated acute bronchitis. Scattered high- or low-pitched rhonchi may be heard, as well as occasional crackling or moist rales at the bases. Wheezing, especially after cough, is commonly noted. Persistent localized signs suggest development of bronchopneumonia.

Serious complications are usually seen only in patients with an underlying chronic respiratory disorder. In such patients, acute bronchitis may lead to severe blood gas abnormalities (acute respiratory failure).

Diagnosis

Diagnosis is usually based on the symptoms and signs, but a chest x-ray to rule out other diseases or complications is indicated if symptoms are serious or prolonged. Arterial blood gases should be monitored when serious underlying chronic respiratory disease is present. In persons who do not respond to antibiotic therapy, or in special circumstances (eg, immunosuppression), Gram stain and sputum culture should be done to determine the causative organism.

Treatment

General: Rest is indicated until fever subsides. Oral fluids (up to 3 or 4 L/day) are urged during the febrile course. An antipyretic analgesic (eg, for adults aspirin 600 mg or acetaminophen 500 mg q 4 to 6 h; for children acetaminophen 10 to 15 mg/kg q 4 to 6 h) relieves malaise and reduces fever.

Antibiotics are indicated when there is concomitant chronic obstructive pulmonary disease, when purulent sputum is present, or when high fever persists and the patient is more than mildly ill. For adults oral tetracycline or ampicillin 250 mg q 6 is a reasonable first choice for most cases. Tetracycline should be withheld in children < 8 yr old; instead give amoxicillin 40 mg/kg/day in divided doses tid. When symptoms persist or recur, or in unusually severe disease, smear and sputum culture are indicated. The antibiotic is then chosen according to the predominant organism and its sensitivity. If *M. pneumoniae* is thought to be the causative agent, erythromycin 250 to 500 mg orally qid can be given. Trimethoprim/sulfamethoxazole (160/800 mg orally bid) may be used as an alternative to tetracycline.

BRONCHIECTASIS

Irreversible, focal bronchial dilation, usually accompanied by infection. Most often acquired, it is associated with diverse conditions, including some that are congenital and/or hereditary.

Etiology and Pathogenesis

Congenital bronchiectasis: *A rare condition in which the lung periphery fails to develop, resulting in cystic dilation of developed bronchi.* **Acquired bronchiectasis** results from (1) direct bronchial wall destruction after infection, inhalation of noxious chemicals, immunologic reactions, or vascular abnormalities that interfere with bronchial nutrition or (2) mechanical alterations secondary to atelectasis or loss of parenchymal volume leading to bronchial dilation and secondary infection. Bacterial endotoxins, proteases (eg, neutrophil elastase), release of superoxide radicals, and antigen-antibody complexes may facilitate bronchial wall damage.

Conditions commonly leading to bronchiectasis are severe pneumonia (especially one complicating measles, pertussis, or certain adenovirus infections in children); necrotizing infections at any age due to *Klebsiella*, staphylococci,

influenza virus, fungi, mycobacteria, and perhaps mycoplasma; and bronchial obstruction from any cause (eg, foreign body, enlarged lymph nodes, mucus impaction, or lung cancer). Miscellaneous chronic fibrosing lung diseases (eg, those following aspiration pneumonia, inhalation of injurious gases or irritant or immunologically active particles [eg, silica, talc, or bakelite]) also predispose to bronchiectasis. Immunologic deficiencies and various congenital and/or hereditary abnormalities that increase host susceptibility to infection or impair respiratory defenses and clearance of bronchial secretions are also important. Although incidence and mortality have decreased with widespread use of antibiotics and immunizations in children, bronchiectasis as a manifestation of cystic fibrosis **(CF)** is still common (see above). With situs inversus and sinusitis, bronchiectasis is also a feature of **Kartagener's syndrome,** a subgroup of the **primary ciliary dyskinesia (PCD) syndrome,** in which various structural or functional abnormalities in the cilial organelles result in defective mucociliary clearance that leads to suppurative bronchial infections and bronchiectasis, as well as chronic rhinitis, otitis, male sterility, corneal abnormalities, headaches, and poor sense of smell. Bronchiectasis has also been reported in patients with **Young's syndrome,** which is characterized by obstructive azoospermia, chronic sinopulmonary infections, normal spermatogenesis, dilated epididymal head filled with spermatozoa, and amorphous material without spermatozoa in the region of the corpus. Absent are the ciliary ultrastructural or functional abnormalities seen in the PCD syndrome and the electrolyte abnormalities characteristic of CF. An unusual pattern of bronchiectasis occurs in allergic bronchopulmonary mycosis: Dilation occurs in the proximal segmental or subsegmental bronchi (rather than in the peripheral bronchi as in idiopathic bronchiectasis). The bronchial wall damage is thought to be due to an immunologic response to a fungus in the bronchial lumen, most commonly *Aspergillus fumigatus.*

Pathology

Bronchiectasis may be uni- or bilateral; it is most common in the lower lobes, though the right middle lobe and lingular portion of the left upper lobe may often be involved. It may be described as cylindrical, varicose, or saccular, depending on the pathologic and radiographic appearance. In cylindrical bronchiectasis, the bronchi, instead of tapering normally, end squarely because of mucus plugging or fibrous obliteration. In saccular and varicose bronchiectasis, the distal bronchi are obliterated and the bronchi have a ballooned appearance. However, these distinctions are of little clinical value. In all types of bronchiectasis, the manifestations and course are similar.

Bronchial walls show extensive inflammatory destruction, chronic inflammation, increased mucus, and loss of cilia. Where adjacent interstitial and alveolar areas are destroyed, tissue reorganization and fibrosis result in loss of volume. Bronchiectasis is associated with chronic bronchitis and/or emphysema. Extensive anastomoses between the bronchial and pulmonary arteries may be seen with markedly enlarged bronchial arteries. Anastomoses between bronchial and pulmonary veins also enlarge. The resultant increased flow, right-to-left shunts, and hypoxemia lead late in the disease to pulmonary hypertension and cor pulmonale.

Symptoms and Signs

Bronchiectasis can develop at any age; it begins most often in early childhood, but symptoms may not be apparent until much later. Their severity and characteristics vary widely from patient to patient, and from time to time in an individual, depending largely on the extent of the disease and the extent and presence of complicating chronic infection. Although a patient may be completely asymptomatic, chronic cough and sputum production are the most characteristic and common symptoms. They often begin insidiously, usually after a respiratory infection, and tend to worsen gradually over a period of years. Severe pneumonia with incomplete clearing of symptoms and residual persistent cough and sputum production is a common mode of onset. As the condition progresses, the cough tends to become more productive; it occurs with typical regularity in the morning on arising, late in the afternoon, and on retiring, but many patients are relatively free of cough during intervening hours. The sputum usually is similar to that of bronchitis and is not characteristic. Less commonly, in long-standing cases, sputum may be abundant and on standing may separate into 3 layers: frothy at the top, greenish and turbid in the middle, and thick with pus at the bottom. Hemoptysis is common and may be the first and only complaint. Recurrent pneumonia is also common; its investigation may lead to the diagnosis of bronchiectasis. Wheezing, shortness of breath and other manifestations of respiratory insufficiency and right heart failure from cor pulmonale may occur in advanced cases with associated chronic bronchitis and emphysema.

Physical findings are nonspecific, but persistent crackles over any part of the lungs suggest bronchiectasis. Clubbing of the fingers sometimes occurs with extensive disease and persistent chronic infection. Pulmonary functional and hemodynamic changes depend largely on the extent of accompanying pathologic changes (eg, diffuse chronic bronchitis, pulmonary emphysema, or pulmonary fibrosis). They may include reduction in lung volumes and airflow rates, ventilation/perfusion defects, hypoxemia, and in severe cases, pulmonary hypertension and cor pulmonale.

Diagnosis

Bronchiectasis must be suspected in anyone with the above symptoms and signs. Standard chest x-rays may show increased bronchovascular markings from peribronchial fibrosis and intrabronchial secretions, crowding from intervening atelectatic lung, "tram tracking," areas of honeycombing, or cystic areas with or without fluid levels, but often they are normal. Experienced interpretation of thin-section CT (eg, 1.5-mm cuts) of the chest may make bronchography unnecessary, but the latter should be considered to confirm the diagnosis and extent, particularly in puzzling cases or when surgery is contemplated. It should be done when the patient's state is stable and after vigorous bronchial hygiene. Excessive secretions or blood in the bronchial tree, or acute bronchopneumonia can lead to misinterpretation. The reversible dilation that occurs when there is air space consolidation (eg, in pneumonia) should not be confused with true bronchiectasis. Bronchography should not be done in an iodine-sensitive patient or one with significant functional lung impairment. Chronic bronchitis and mycobacterial and fungal infections should be ruled out. When disease is unilateral or of recent onset, fiberoptic bronchoscopy is indicated to rule out tumor, foreign body, or other localized endobronchial abnormality. Fiberoptic bronchoscopy can also be combined with bronchography; dye is injected through a catheter that has been passed through the bronchoscope into the area of interest in the lung *or* a catheter is passed over a guide wire that had been first inserted and positioned through a bronchoscope.

A search for associated conditions should be made, particularly CF (which is increasingly seen in adults), immune deficiencies, and predisposing congenital abnormalities.

CF should be suspected if the abnormalities on x-ray are predominantly apical or upper lobe. Although a feature in children, pancreatic insufficiency is not common in adults, in whom the pulmonary manifestations predominate. A sweat chloride test (quantitative pilocarpine iontophoresis) showing chloride > 60 mEq/L in children or > 80 mEq/L in adults is diagnostic. Values between 45 and 60 mEq/L in children and 50 to 80 mEq/L in adults justify retesting. Measurement of nasal transepithelial electrical potential difference (PD) may also help to distinguish CF from other conditions having similar symptoms. The negative PD is 2 to 3 times greater in CF (eg, 45 mv) than in normals, patients with Young's syndrome, or bronchiectasis (17 to 20 mv).

Young's syndrome, more common than CF or PCD syndromes, should be suspected in men with chronic recurrent sinopulmonary symptoms and infertility. Normal spermatozoa, testicular function tests, and sweat chloride distinguish this from CF or PCD syndromes.

PCD may be present in 11% of children with chronic respiratory disease. Diagnosis is confirmed by ultrastructural and functional (motility, beat frequency) examination of nasal or other respiratory cilia obtained by biopsy or brushing, and by nasal ciliary clearance time, measured by instilling saccharin above the inferior turbinate of the nose and noting the time it takes for the subject to first taste it (normal is 12 to 15 min). Ultrastructural examination of a number of biopsy (tissue) sections to exclude nonspecific ciliary defects, which can be present in $\leq 10\%$ of cilia in patients with acquired pulmonary disease and normals, recognition that infection can cause transient dyskinesia, and realization that overlap between patients' and controls' ciliary characteristics has been observed are important considerations when interpreting abnormalities.

Immunoglobulin (Ig) deficiencies may be identified by serum Ig measurements (see Ch. 33). α_1-Antitrypsin deficiency may be suspected when α_1-globulin is low and confirmed by phenotyping by crossed immunoelectrophoresis. Congenital abnormalities of tracheal or bronchial cartilage and connective tissue are usually detected on x-ray. In tracheobronchomegaly, the tracheal width is about twice normal. In the rare Williams-Campbell syndrome, total or partial absence of cartilage beyond the main segmental bronchi produces wheezing and dyspnea early in infancy, and bronchography shows inspiratory ballooning and collapse on expiration of the affected bronchi.

The yellow nail syndrome, believed to be due to a congenital hypoplasia of the lymphatic system, is recognized by the thickened, curved, yellowish-to-greenish nails and primary lymphedema; some patients manifest exudative pleural effusion and bronchiectasis.

Allergic bronchopulmonary aspergillosis may be suspected when there is a wheal and flare reaction to fungal antigens, serum IgE is high, serum precipitins for Aspergillus fumigatus or some other fungus are elevated, and the clinical picture suggests it. Blood and sputum eosinophilia are often present.

Prophylaxis

Awareness and early identification of conditions frequently associated with bronchiectasis may permit earlier therapy to prevent its development and severity. When there is a family history of CF, prenatal diagnosis by immunoreactive trypsinogen assay or DNA analysis may be useful. Childhood immunization against pertussis and measles, widespread use of antibiotics, improved living conditions, and nutrition have helped to reduce the prevalence, morbidity, and mortality of bronchiectasis. Influenza vaccine yearly and pneumococcal vaccine one time in those at particular risk and likely to respond may be helpful. Early treatment of respiratory syncytial virus (RSV) with ribavirin aerosol, and of mycoplasmal infections with erythromycin for 7 to 10 days (adults: 250 to 500 mg orally qid; children: erythromycin base 40 mg/kg q 6 h, erythromycin estolate 30 to 40 mg/kg q 8 to 12 h, or erythromycin succinate 40 mg/kg q 6 h) may lessen their damaging potential. Immunoglobulin replacement in deficiency states; early detection and bronchoscopic, surgical, or other appropriate measures to remove foreign bodies and eliminate localized bronchial obstructions; and treatment of recurrent sinusitis and of gastroesophageal reflux may prevent repeated chest infections that lead to bronchiectasis. Inhalation of noxious gases and particulates, including cigarette smoke, should be avoided totally or minimized by use of effective environmental controls or personal protective devices.

Treatment

Treatment is directed to control of acute and chronic infection, secretions, airways obstruction, and complications (eg, hemoptysis, hypoxemia, respiratory failure, and cor pulmonale).

To control infection, therapy includes antibiotics, bronchodilators, and physical therapy to promote bronchial drainage. Flora in the sputum usually are mixed gram-positive and gram-negative microorganisms, and anaerobes commonly inhabit bronchiectatic cysts. A broad-spectrum antibiotic (eg, ampicillin 250 to 500 mg orally q 6 h [50 to 100 mg/kg/day in divided doses q 6 to 8 h in children with a maximum dose of 2 to 3 gm in large children] or tetracycline 250 to 500 mg orally q 6 h) is often used until the sputum is nonpurulent and less voluminous, about 1 to 2 wk. Trimethoprim/sulfamethoxazole (TMP/SMX) 320/1600 mg orally q 12 h for 14 days has also been successful to reduce volume and eliminate pathogens; for children, TMP/SMX (6 to 12/30 to 60 mg/kg/day) is given in divided doses q 12 h, depending on the size of the child and severity of the infection. Antibiotics should be repeated at the first sign of returning infection (change in volume or increase in purulence of the sputum). If infection recurs often, prolonged chemoprophylaxis with ampicillin or tetracycline may be tried but is generally disappointing. In severe cases, high-dose amoxicillin (3 gm orally bid) is reported to achieve higher serum and sputum concentrations than equal doses of ampicillin. For bronchopneumonia or serious respiratory infection, parenteral antibiotics guided by Gram stain, cultures, and sensitivity studies are indicated.

Treatment of CF is discussed above.

Patients with bronchiectasis should avoid cigarette smoke and other irritants, and refrain from using sedatives or antitussives. Postural drainage, clapping, and vibration done regularly may be helpful; in some cases, sputum clearance is facilitated. Diffuse chronic bronchitis, often accompanying bronchiectasis, should be treated accordingly. β_2-Agonists, theophylline, and occasionally corticosteroids may decrease airflow obstruction. If asthma or allergic bronchopulmonary aspergillosis is also present, corticosteroids may be beneficial.

Chronic hypoxemia should be treated with O_2, particularly if the Pa_{O_2} in a stable patient is < 55 mm Hg on room air or if there is evidence of pulmonary hypertension or secondary polycythemia. Respiratory failure and cor pulmonale should also be treated as in other patients with chronic airways obstructive disease. Intubation and mechanical ventilation should, if possible, be avoided, as the ability to cough is lost and the risk of inadequate evacuation of secretions by suctioning alone and promotion of further infection is enhanced.

Surgical resection is rarely necessary but should be considered when response to conservative management is unacceptable, as demonstrated by recurrent pneumonia, disabling bronchial infections, or frequent hemoptysis, and the disease is sufficiently localized and stable. For massive pulmonary hemorrhage, emergency resection or embolization of the bleeding vessel (usually bronchial artery) has been lifesaving.

ATELECTASIS

A shrunken, airless state of the lung that may be acute or chronic, complete or partial; the affected area is often composed of a complex mixture of airlessness, infection, bronchiectasis, destruction, and fibrosis.

Etiology

In adults the chief cause of **acute or chronic atelectasis** is intraluminal bronchial obstruction that is often due to plugs of tenacious bronchial exudate, endobronchial tumors, granulomas, or foreign bodies. Atelectasis may also be due to bronchial distortions or kinkings; external compression of a bronchus by enlarged lymph nodes, tumor, or an aneurysm; and external pulmonary compression by pleural fluid or gas (eg, due to pleural effusion, pneumothorax). Surfactant, a complex mixture of phospholipids and lipoproteins, covers the surface of the alveoli, reduces surface tension, and contributes to alveolar stability. Interference with surfactant production or its effectiveness also promotes atelectasis in O_2 toxicity, pulmonary edema, the adult and neonatal respiratory distress syndromes (see under RESPIRATORY DISORDERS in Ch. 27), pulmonary embolism, and probably during general anesthesia and mechanical ventilation.

Acute massive lung collapse is usually a postoperative complication, most often after upper abdominal procedures and heart operations with heart-lung bypass (endothelial cell damage by hypothermia and the intravascular cardioplegic solution have been postulated to contribute to atelectasis). Large doses of opiates or sedatives, high O_2 concentrations during anesthesia, tight dressings, abdominal distention, and immobility of the body also favor atelectasis because of limited thoracic movement, elevated diaphragm, accumulated viscid bronchial secretions, and suppressed cough reflex. Other conditions also can produce shallow breathing that interferes with cough and effective clearance of secretions: CNS depressive disorders, thoracic cage abnormalities, pain and muscle spasm, and neuromuscular diseases. Blood hyperosmolality observed in diabetics with ketoacidosis and occult mucus plugging may be another factor, presumably increasing the retention of viscous secretions.

In the **middle lobe syndrome,** *a form of chronic atelectasis,* the middle lobe collapses, usually from bronchial compression by surrounding lymph nodes. Acute pneumonia, usually with delayed, incomplete resolution, may develop. Infection with partial bronchial obstruction may lead to chronic atelectasis and ultimately to chronic pneumonitis because of poor drainage. However, the syndrome has been reported without abnormal bronchoscopic findings; the length and narrow caliber of the right middle lobe bronchus, and ineffective collateral ventilation may explain the atelectasis.

Pathology and Pathophysiology

Following a bronchial obstruction, circulating blood absorbs peripheral alveolar gas, and consequent lung retraction produces airlessness within a few hours; lung shrinkage or collapse may be complete without infection. In early stages, blood perfuses the airless lung, with consequent arterial hypoxemia. Capillary and tissue hypoxia may result in transudation of fluid and pulmonary edema; alveolar spaces fill with secretions and cells, preventing complete collapse of the atelectatic lung. Although distention of uninvolved surrounding lung may partially compensate for the volume loss, in cases of extensive collapse, the diaphragm may become elevated and the chest wall may flatten. Volume loss from atelectasis of an entire lung may cause the heart and mediastinum to shift to the affected side.

Hyperventilation and dyspnea are common. A decrease in Pa_{O_2} is usual and, if the atelectatic area is large, may be considerable; Pa_{O_2} often improves during and after the first 24 h, presumably as blood flow decreases to the atelectatic area. Pa_{CO_2} is usually normal or low owing to increased ventilation of the remaining normal lung parenchyma.

If the obstruction is relieved, air enters, any complicating infection subsides, and (depending on the magnitude of the infection) the lung eventually returns to normal. If the obstruction remains and infection is present, lack of air and circulation initiates changes leading to fibrosis and bronchiectasis. Even without obstruction, changes in alveolar surface tension, reduction in alveolar size, and changes in airway-to-pleural pressure relationships can lead to inadequate regional ventilation and small areas of **patchy atelectasis** or **diffuse microatelectasis.** Mild to severe disturbances in gas exchange may result. **Acceleration atelectasis,** occurring in military pilots, results from absorption of trapped alveolar gas when high accelerative forces close dependent airways and keep them closed.

Symptoms and Signs

Symptoms and signs depend upon the speed of the bronchial occlusion, the extent of lung affected, and the presence of infection. **Rapid occlusion with massive collapse,** particularly with infection, causes pain on the affected side, sudden onset of dyspnea and cyanosis, a drop in BP, tachycardia, elevated temperature, and sometimes shock. Chest examination reveals dullness to flatness over the involved area and diminished or absent breath sounds. Chest excursion in the area is reduced or absent and the trachea and heart are deviated toward the affected side. **Slowly developing atelectasis** may be asymptomatic or cause minor pulmonary symptoms. The **middle lobe syndrome** is also often asymptomatic, though a severe, hacking, nonproductive cough may result from irritation in the right lower and middle lobe bronchi. Chest examination discloses the same findings as in rapid occlusion.

Chest x-rays may show an airless lung area whose size and location depend on the bronchus involved. If only a segment is affected, the shadow will be triangular, with its apex toward the hilum. When small areas are involved, surrounding tissue distention causes them to appear curiously discoid, particularly in subsegmental lower lobe atelectasis. If the atelectasis is lobar, the entire lobe is airless. The trachea, heart, and mediastinum may be deviated toward the affected area, the diaphragm on that side may be elevated, and rib spaces are narrowed. **Diffuse microatelectasis,** an early manifestation of O_2 toxicity and the acute respiratory distress syndrome, is usually not visible initially but is recognized or suspected by its effects: arterial hypoxemia, decreased lung compliance, and reduced lung volume.

Diagnosis

Diagnosis is usually made from clinical findings plus x-ray evidence of diminished lung size (indicated by retracted ribs, elevated diaphragm, and deviated mediastinum) and of a solid, airless opacity. A cause for obstruction should always be sought regardless of the patient's age. With the fiberoptic bronchoscope it is possible to see segmental and subsegmental divisions. CT can help to clarify the mechanism of collapse; an experienced interpreter can distinguish atelectasis secondary to endobronchial obstruction from compression atelectasis due to fluid or air, and scars resulting from chronic inflammation. Massive effusion may also cause dyspnea, cyanosis, weakness, flatness to percussion over the involved area, and absent breath sounds, but shift of the heart and mediastinum away from the involved area and absence of chest wall flattening distinguish it from massive atelectasis.

Spontaneous pneumothorax produces similar symptoms, but the percussion note is tympanitic, the heart and mediastinum are pushed to the opposite side, and x-rays showing air in the pleural space are diagnostic.

An unusual form of peripheral lobar collapse, **rounded atelectasis** or "folded lung," is often mistaken for tumor. Most commonly a complication of asbestos-induced pleural disease, it has a characteristic appearance on x-ray that distinguishes it from tumor. The lung density is round and immediately subpleural, with an acute angle between it and the pleura, and it frequently has a "comet tail" extending toward the hilum, thought to represent compressed vessels and bronchi that enter the atelectatic area. CT scan may improve reliability of diagnosis and in some cases obviate the need for diagnostic thoracotomy. Needle biopsy often has not been helpful, but can be attempted before resorting to thoracotomy when the distinction between rounded atelectasis and a subpleural tumor is less certain.

Prophylaxis

Acute massive atelectasis may be avoidable. Since preexisting chronic bronchitis and heavy smoking increase the risk of postoperative atelectasis, preoperative cessation of smoking and measures to improve bronchial toilet should be encouraged. Long-acting anesthetics should be avoided and narcotics should be used sparingly after surgery, since they depress the cough reflex. When anesthesia is ended, the lungs should be left filled with some air, not 100% O_2. The patient must be turned hourly and should be encouraged to cough and breathe deeply; early ambulation is important. A combined approach is most effective: encouragement of coughing and deep breathing, use of nebulized bronchodilators and aerosols of water or saline to liquefy and facilitate removal of secretions, and tracheal suc-

tioning as necessary. The relative merits of IPPB, incentive spirometry (in which a simple device is used to encourage voluntary maximum sustained [3 to 5 sec] inspiratory maneuvers), and the components of physical therapy (percussion, vibration, postural drainage, and deep breathing) are disputed. If it is to be effective, each modality must be used appropriately with adjunctive measures. Chest percussion in the postoperative patient may actually enhance the risk of atelectasis if it increases pain and muscular splinting.

Patients with a tendency to hypoventilate or to have prolonged shallow breathing because of thoracic cage abnormality, neuromuscular weakness or paralysis, or CNS disorders, or who are on prolonged mechanical ventilation are at special risk for atelectasis and should be monitored for early signs: tachypnea, hypoxemia, decreasing lung volume (eg, reduced vital capacity), and x-ray signs.

Treatment

Acute atelectasis (including postoperative acute massive lung collapse) requires removal of the underlying cause. When a mechanical obstruction is suspected, but relief is not obtained by coughing or suctioning and a 24-h trial of vigorous respiratory and physical therapeutic measures, or when the patient is unable to cooperate with such measures, fiberoptic bronchoscopy should be done. Once bronchial obstruction is established, therapy is directed at the obstruction and the infection usually present. Often mucus plugs or inspissated secretions can be removed through the bronchoscope and the involved lung will reinflate, but vigorous chest physical therapy and other measures noted above should be continued. If foreign body aspiration is suspected, bronchoscopy should be done promptly; removal of the foreign body may require use of a rigid bronchoscope.

Patients with atelectasis should (1) lie with the involved side uppermost to promote drainage, (2) have appropriate physical therapy, and (3) be encouraged to cough. Subsequently they should be encouraged to move from side to side and breathe deeply. Frequent (q 1 to 2 h) supervised use of IPPB or an incentive spirometer may help to ensure deep breaths. If the atelectasis occurred outside the hospital (eg, foreign body aspiration), a broad-spectrum antibiotic (eg, ampicillin 500 mg orally or 1 gm parenterally q 6 h or 50 to 100 mg/kg/day in divided doses q 6 to 8 h in children) should be given at the outset, if there are clinical and laboratory findings of infection or the clinical circumstances suggest a strong likelihood of infection. If the patient is seriously ill in hospital, antimicrobial therapy should be based on the known local pathogens and drug susceptibility profiles of that hospital. The regimen might include a penicillin (eg, ampicillin) or clindamycin 1200 to 2700 mg/day IV (for infants > 1 mo and children, 25 to 40 mg/kg/day IM or IV tid or qid) and an aminoglycoside (eg, amikacin 15 to 30 mg/kg/day IM or IV in 3 equal doses or gentamicin 3 to 7.5 mg/kg/day IM or IV in 3 equal doses) or a 2nd- or 3rd-generation cephalosporin (eg, cefuroxime 0.75 to 1.5 gm q 8 h IV [for infants > 1 mo and children, 75 to 150 mg/kg/day IM or IV in divided doses q 6 to 8 h] or cefamandole 0.5 to 1 gm q 4 to 6 h IV). Dosage in the elderly may need adjustment, and caution should be used in patients with a history of GI disease or severe renal or hepatic impairment. If a specific pathogen is subsequently isolated from sputum or bronchial secretions, the antibiotic should be modified accordingly.

Patients with recurrent atelectasis (eg, neuromuscular disease) may benefit from a trial of nasal continuous positive airway pressure (CPAP) at 5 to 15 cm H_2O.

Chronic atelectasis: The longer the lung remains unexpanded, the more likely it is to develop destructive, fibrotic, and bronchiectatic changes. Since secondary atelectasis usually becomes infected regardless of the cause, a broad-spectrum antibiotic (eg, ampicillin or tetracycline or others based on Gram stain and culture results) should be given when sputum volume and purulence increase. Surgical resection of the atelectatic segment or lobe should be considered, particularly when the patient has had recurrent disabling respiratory infections or recurrent hemoptysis from the affected area. When a tumor causes the obstruction, its cell type and extent, the overall condition of the patient, and his pulmonary function will determine whether the obstruction can best be relieved by surgery, radiation, or chemotherapy. In selected cases, laser therapy has effectively reduced obstruction from an endobronchial lesion.

HISTIOCYTOSIS X
(Letterer-Siwe Disease; Hand-Schüller-Christian Disease; Eosinophilic Granuloma)

A group of disorders characterized by proliferation of histiocytes. Granulomatous lesions may occur in many organs, especially the lungs and bones. The etiology is unknown. Pathologically, changes begin with progressive proliferation of

histiocytes and infiltration with eosinophilic granulocytes. A fibrotic phase with little cellular infiltration finally supervenes. The lungs show varying degrees of granulomatosis, fibrosis, and honeycombing. Histiocytosis X bodies, seen on electron microscopy, are characteristic of this disorder and may be recognized within histiocytes or alveolar macrophages on examination of alveolar lavage fluid.

Letterer-Siwe disease occurs before age 3 yr and, *without therapy, is usually fatal.* Skin, lymph nodes, bone, liver, and spleen are frequently involved. Pneumothorax is a common complication. Without therapy, the disease is always fatal. **Hand-Schüller-Christian syndrome** most often begins in early childhood but can appear even in late middle age. The lungs and bones are most frequently involved, though other organs may be affected. A triad of bone defects, exophthalmos, and diabetes insipidus occurs rarely. **Eosinophilic granuloma** occurs most commonly between ages 20 and 40 and characteristically involves bone, though about 20% of patients have lung infiltration and the lungs sometimes may be involved exclusively. Patients with Hand-Schüller-Christian syndrome or eosinophilic granuloma may recover spontaneously. Death usually results from respiratory or cardiac failure. **Treatment** of the lung involvement in the 3 disorders is with corticosteroids. Therapy for bone lesions is discussed in Ch. 42.

IDIOPATHIC PULMONARY HEMOSIDEROSIS

A rare disease of unknown etiology characterized by episodes of hemoptysis, hemorrhage into the lung, pulmonary infiltration, and secondary iron-deficiency anemia. It must be distinguished from Goodpasture's syndrome and from lung hemorrhage in SLE or rarely Wegener's granulomatosis. It is most common in young children but can occur in adults. Diffuse infiltration with hemosiderin-containing macrophages is characteristic, though hemosiderin deposition is found in many other disorders. Pulmonary hemorrhages, which determine the clinical course, vary from mild to severe but are most often mild and continuous. Blood in the interstitial spaces leads to pulmonary fibrosis. Patients may live for several years, developing pulmonary fibrosis and insufficiency along with chronic secondary anemia. **Treatment** is symptomatic and supportive. Death often occurs as a result of massive pulmonary hemorrhage.

38. GASTROINTESTINAL DISORDERS

RECURRENT ABDOMINAL PAIN (RAP)

Three or more episodes of abdominal pain over at least 3 mo. The persistence, recurrence, and chronicity of RAP distinguish it from the presentation of children with an acute abdomen. Incidence in the general population is slightly > 10%; the ratio of girls to boys is 4:3. RAP is rare in children < 4 to 5 yr old and most common between ages 8 and 10 yr, with a second peak noted among girls in early adolescence.

There are 3 distinct types of RAP depending upon whether it arises secondary to organic disease, a dysfunctional state, or stress that results in psychogenic pain.

RAP OF ORGANIC ORIGIN

An organic cause for symptoms is found in only 5 to 10% of children with RAP, although there is a wide variety of possible causes. TABLE 38–1 lists the most commonly occurring organic causes to be considered. Of these conditions, inflammatory bowel disease, chronic appendicitis, peptic ulcer disease, *Helicobacter pylori* infection, parasitism (especially in endemic areas), urinary tract disease, and sickle cell disease are found most frequently. In adolescent girls, pelvic inflammatory disease and ovarian cyst should be considered.

Symptoms, Signs, and Diagnosis

Pain from organic disease has distinctive characteristics. It is commonly described as constant or cyclical (associated with certain activities or related to diet); is well localized, especially to areas other than the periumbilical region; and may penetrate to the back. It frequently may wake the child from sleep. Associated findings that vary according to the underlying disease include recurrent or persistent fever; jaundice; changes in bowel consistency, color, or elimination pattern; blood in the stools; vomiting; hematemesis; abdominal distention; joint symptoms; change in appetite; and weight loss.

Two entities deserve particular attention because their presentation can be confusing: (1) **Peptic ulcer disease** is often missed because the typical relationship of food intake to pain sensation and the usual epigastric location of the pain, as seen in adults, are seen infrequently in

children (see CHILDHOOD PEPTIC ULCER, below). (2) **UTI**, in which the pain may be described by the child as abdominal or pelvic in origin with no referral to the flank or the urethra, will be missed unless tested for specifically.

Treatment

When an underlying organic disorder is suspected, appropriate testing (see TABLE 38–1) should be done immediately and specific therapy instituted accordingly.

RAP ARISING FROM A DYSFUNCTIONAL STATE

Pain arising from a nondiseased organ as a result of interaction between constitutional and environmental factors. The exact incidence in RAP of this relatively new classification is unknown; it probably occurs as often as organic disease. It is important because it contains a number of entities, each with a clear-cut pathophysiologic basis for the pain that usually responds well to specific therapy, eg, diet change or drugs.

Etiology

Why some persons with dysfunctional states develop abdominal pain and others do not is unknown. Perhaps anxiety alters autonomic and intestinal function, which then becomes expressed as pain in persons with a constitutionally defined temperament prone to experience pain when stressed.

Diagnosis

Differential diagnosis of RAP arising from a dysfunctional state includes conditions secondary to inappropriate diet, ineffective toilet training, or improperly sized toilet facilities that lead to constipation or fecal retention and incontinence; dysmenorrhea; mittelschmerz (see Ch. 5); and lactose intolerance secondary to the normal physiologic decline in lactase activity seen in many population groups > 4 to 5 yr old. Because pain may not occur for up to 2 h after ingestion of milk or a milk product, this cause may not be suspected initially.

A careful history defining associated symptoms or precipitating factors (eg, a 24-h diet recall to investigate food allergy or dietary indiscretion; menstrual history; etc) is the most important diagnostic tool. Once the underlying dys-

TABLE 38-1. ORGANIC CAUSES OF RECURRENT ABDOMINAL PAIN

Cause	Diagnostic Approach
GU disorders	
Congenital abnormalities	IVU and/or ultrasound
UTI	Urine culture
Pelvic inflammatory disease	Pelvic examination
Ovarian cyst, endometriosis	Gynecologic consultation
GI disorders	
Hiatus hernia	Barium swallow, fluoroscopy
Hepatitis	Liver function tests
Cholecystitis	Cholangiogram, ultrasound
Pancreatitis	Serum amylase level
Peptic ulcer disease	Upper GI series, endoscopy, silver stain for *Helicobacter pylori*, stool for occult blood
Parasitic infestation (eg, giardiasis)	Stool examination for ova, parasites
Meckel's diverticulum	Technetium scan
Granulomatous enterocolitis	ESR, barium enema
Intestinal TB	Tuberculin test
Ulcerative colitis	Sigmoidoscopy, rectal biopsy
Postoperative adhesive bands	Upper GI series
Pancreatic pseudocyst	Ultrasound
Chronic appendicitis	Abdominal x-ray, ultrasound
Systemic disorders	
Lead intoxication	Blood lead, free erythrocyte protoporphyrin levels
Henoch-Schönlein purpura	History, urinalysis
Sickle cell disease	Sickle preparation, Hb electrophoresis
Food allergy	Elimination diet
Abdominal epilepsy	EEG
Porphyria	Urine uroporphyrin level
Familial Mediterranean anemia, familial angioneurotic edema, migraine equivalent	Family history

Adapted from Barbero GJ: "Recurrent abdominal pain." *Pediatrics in Review* 4:30, 1982; reproduced by permission of *Pediatrics*.

functional state has been identified, therapy should be directed toward habit or diet change, or analgesics and patient/family education.

RAP OF PSYCHOGENIC ORIGIN

In 80 to 90% of cases, RAP is psychogenic. Its pathophysiology is unknown, but it appears to be linked to stress and anxiety or depression.

Symptoms and Signs

Pain may occur daily or several times a week or month. Occasionally, the child is symptom-free for weeks or months. Rarely sharp, the pain is generally vague and ill-defined but sometimes is reported as crampy or colicky. Awakening during the night with pain is unusual, although some patients awaken early because of discomfort.

Pain is most often periumbilical, and it has been suggested that the farther the pain is from the umbilicus, the greater the likelihood of an organic disorder. However, this tendency is not diagnostic, and psychogenic pain can mimic *any* symptom complex. Thus, frequency, nature, and localization of pain are not reliable discriminators between the different types of RAP. Any change in the location or pattern of pain deserves immediate evaluation, because an acute organic condition can intervene.

Diagnosis and Differential Diagnosis

Distinguishing children with underlying organic conditions from those with dysfunctional or psychogenic abdominal pain can be difficult. Psychogenic pain, not a diagnosis of exclusion, must be documented by historic, personality, and family characteristics, findings on physical examination, and laboratory results consistent with the diagnosis.

The history: A most significant finding with psychogenic abdominal pain is that symptoms progress little or not at all; the child will become no worse. It is important to begin with the first attack of pain, documenting its frequency, nature, and location; relationship to meals, defecation, and voiding; and results of any treatment including position change, home remedies, and OTC and prescription drugs. Important characteristics that suggest, but are not pathognomonic of, psychogenic pain include *lack* of consistent bowel symptoms, fever, weight loss, or growth failure. Associated symptoms are common and can include headache, dizziness (not vertigo), facial pallor, and diaphoresis. Fatigue, anorexia, nausea, vomiting, diarrhea, constipation, and limb pain occur occasionally but are less common in psychogenic pain than with RAP of organic or dysfunctional cause.

Psychosocial characteristics include evidence of immaturity, unusual dependence on parents, anxiety or depression, apprehension, tension, and perfectionism. Often parents see the child as special, either because of the position in the family (only child, youngest sibling, or only male or female child in a large sibship) or because of an early problem (colic or eating difficulty) or a minor unrelated medical condition. Parents are often described as anxious, overprotective, authoritarian, and preoccupied with the child. Data should be obtained regarding the occurrence of any possible precipitating factor such as illness, family discord, separation and loss, or school-related stress; evidence of primary gain (what the child avoided because of pain) or secondary gain (what psychosocial benefits may be derived from being sick); and the child's personality.

It is helpful to meet with both parents (and any stepparents) during the initial data-gathering stage. Differences in perception about what precipitates the pain and how the pain is used provide insight into family dynamics; such insight can be useful in developing an approach to pain management that is consistent, yet comfortable for each parent. Inclusion of each parent also underlines the importance of the role each plays in the child's life in precipitating, perpetuating, and eventually overcoming the pain.

Records obtained directly from the school provide information about the impact of the pain on daily functioning in the classroom. Early involvement of school personnel, particularly the school nurse (who may suspect psychogenic pain but is unable to act without direction from a physician), is a key element in fostering a comprehensive treatment plan.

The family history frequently is positive for chronic somatic complaints or pain, peptic ulcer disease, headaches, "nerves," or depression; questions should be included about similar or related illnesses in other members, especially the parents at a similar age.

What constitutes a **stressful situation** is relative; these patients appear to be stressed easily. The physician can usually detect specific precipitating events at home (recent illness, financial problems, separation or loss) or at school (concern about performance or interpersonal relationships with teachers or peers). The illness itself may cause stressful problems (eg, significant school absenteeism, isolation from peers), or it may compound preexisting problems (eg, increased sibling rivalry).

Physical examination: Most children are seen initially when symptom-free. Therefore, before making a final diagnosis, an evaluation should be done during a pain episode to observe for bowel distention and to be reassured that no signs of an organic disorder are overlooked. Except for evidence of periumbilical discomfort on palpation of the abdomen, findings on examination are typically negative. Once the physician is certain of the findings, frequently repeated examinations are to be avoided lest they focus on or magnify the physical complaints or instill or perpetuate the idea that the physician lacks confidence in the diagnosis.

Laboratory studies should be ordered promptly to allay patient and parent anxiety. However, initial investigation should be limited to a search for the most likely organic or dysfunctional causes of RAP. Appropriate tests to consider include Hb, Hct, blood smear, WBC count, and ESR; urinalysis and urine culture; examinations of the stool for ova, parasites, *H. pylori*, blood, pH, and reducing substances; a tuberculin test; liver function studies; serum amylase levels; and a plain x-ray of the abdomen. A test for sickle cell disease is appropriate in selected at-risk patients. Specific, well-documented food intolerances such as that for lactose should be evaluated appropriately (eg, by a trial of a lactose-free diet). Further evaluation, including contrast studies of the GI or urinary tract, EEG, or endoscopy, should be reserved for patients with specific indications.

Treatment

Management begins with the initial evaluation, when the tone of the relationship between physician and family is established. Parents and child should be interviewed separately, and then together; all should be asked what they think (or fear) might be causing the problem. Parental reaction to the pain and perceptions of their child's reactions to pain should be elicited.

In younger children, the complete physical examination generally should be performed with the parents present, to impress upon them its care and thoroughness. In preadolescent and older children, the parent of the same sex may be asked to stay for the examination if comfortable for the patient. Regardless, findings should be shared in detail with the patient and both parents. The list of laboratory studies to be obtained and the reason why each has been selected also should be shared with the family.

During the initial visit, it is premature to suggest specific treatment, even if the physician is fairly certain that the primary problem is psychogenic. Most parents are concerned about an organic cause; this concern must be addressed adequately or they are unlikely to react favorably or consistently to a behavioral management plan. Rather, between the initial evaluation and the follow-up visit, it helps if the child and family keep a record of any pain: its nature, intensity, and duration; precipitating factors; diet; defecation pattern; and any remedies applied and the results obtained. Use of a diary often reveals inappropriate behavior patterns and exaggerated responses to pain, facilitating cooperation in a behaviorally oriented management strategy.

A follow-up appointment should be scheduled as soon as possible after test results are available, so that findings can be reported and put into perspective, and a management plan outlined. Each parent's and child's specific concerns should be addressed and appropriate reassurance provided that the child is not in physical danger. The physician must redefine the problem by reviewing the data that established the diagnosis, explaining clearly the nature of the problem, and clarifying how the pain is generated and how the child perceives it.

In describing how the symptoms appear to be related to stress and tension, the difficulty should not be ascribed to an "emotional problem," which families erroneously interpret as meaning that the child is imagining pain or is "crazy"—fears and defensiveness about this issue may lead to resistance to further advice or therapy. Instead, by using the analogy of a stress- or tension-related headache (experienced by most people at one time or another), the explanation is more likely to be understood and accepted.

A useful way to interpret the child's RAP is that he or she has a constitutional tendency to feel pain at times of stress. Almost invariably, another family member will be identified as having a similar problem. Even if the pain is manifested through another body organ (headaches, back pain), this model can be used to show a familial pattern and thus help to remove guilt. It is important to remember that some families have difficulty talking about feelings (especially negative emotions such as anger or sadness) and, instead, are more comfortable focusing on somatic complaints. In such families, the patient has a problem that he or she is unable to complain about; developing an illness allows the child to express discomfort with the situation indirectly. Although parents in such families frequently are reluctant to admit that they themselves cannot express negative feelings, they often are able to accept this personality characteristic in their child. Such insight can free them from unnecessary concern about an organic etiology for the symptom and facilitate their willingness to withdraw the secondary gain that the child derives from being sick. Failure to withdraw the secondary gain acts as a disincentive to recovery.

The primary goal of treatment is to avoid perpetuating the negative psychosocial aspects of chronic pain (eg, prolonged absences from school or withdrawal from peer activities) and to promote age-appropriate activities and increase independence and self-reliance. Such strategies foster the attitude that the child can either control or learn to live with the symptoms while participating fully in everyday activities. It is important to point out that as the parents change their attitude and stop treating the child as special or ill, *the symptoms may become worse for a period of time before they abate.*

The next step is to engage the family's cooperation in removing as many sources of excessive stress and tension as possible and helping the child to cope with unavoidable stress in a more effective way. Involvement of school personnel is especially critical for children whose RAP interferes with school attendance or functioning. The goal of the school-based portion of the intervention plan is to promote attendance despite pain. The school nurse can assist by providing a place for the child to rest or lie down for short intervals during the school day, with the expectation that the child will return to class after 15 to 30 min. The nurse can also be authorized to dispense a mild analgesic (eg, acetaminophen) as necessary. In some instances, the nurse can allow the child to call a parent who will then provide encouragement to stay in school. Typically, a child will request time in the nurse's office one or more times daily during the first week or two of the treatment phase. This behavior diminishes over time.

Periodic follow-up visits for support should be scheduled (weekly, monthly, or bimonthly, depending upon the family's needs) until the problem has resolved *and* for some months after. Psychiatric referral may be required (up to 50% of families in some reports) when the symptom persists despite supportive counseling, especially when there is evidence of depression in the child or chronic marital conflict or serious psychologic difficulties in the parents.

Drugs are not recommended; none has proved effective, and they may reinforce hypochondriasis or lead to dependency.

Hospitalization is usually reserved for patients whose families have difficulty accepting a nonorganic diagnosis or in whom further studies (including psychologic evaluation and family interaction observation) are necessary. The hospitalization should be brief and goal-directed, to avoid reinforcing symptoms or unduly magnifying any aspect of the problem.

Prognosis

Long-term prognosis is guarded, and no single treatment regimen is universally successful. Some children later develop a variety of other somatic complaints or emotional difficulties.

CHILDHOOD PEPTIC ULCER

Peptic ulcer is not commonly diagnosed in infants and children, possibly because a satisfactory history cannot be obtained in this age group. In the neonatal period, perforation and hemorrhage may be the first recognized manifestation. Hemorrhage may also be the first recognized sign in later infancy and early childhood, although repeated vomiting or evidence of abdominal pain may be a clue. A family history is present in 50 to 60% of children with duodenal ulcer. School-aged children may be better able to localize and describe the pain and relate it to time of

day and eating. Relationship of the pain to eating and its occurrence at night suggest an ulcer, although this typical pattern may not be present in children.

To establish the **diagnosis**, a barium x-ray study should be done first. If it is negative and ulcer is still suspected, 2 options are open. The first and the best for definitive diagnosis is fiberoptic endoscopy, which, in children < 8 yr old, requires general or narcoleptic anesthesia. The second option, if endoscopy is not feasible and after excluding other possible causes of ulcerlike pain (see RECURRENT ABDOMINAL PAIN, above), is to treat the child for a presumptive diagnosis of ulcer with antacids or histamine H_2 antagonists as below.

Treatment follows the principles of adult care. Basal and stimulated gastric secretion per kilogram and per unit time in children are not different from adults, and pharmacokinetics and pharmacodynamics of ranitidine and cimetidine in children are also not different from those in adults. Thus the regimens for oral (or where needed, IV) dosage should follow those recommended for adults. As a general principle, adult dosage of H_2 receptor antagonists should be used for children with duodenal or gastric ulcer who weigh $\geq$ 40 kg. Below that weight, the dosage of ranitidine given orally is 4 mg/kg/day and cimetidine 20 mg/kg in 2 divided doses q 12 h. Efficacy for healing of peptic ulcer with once-a-day full dosage instead of half dosage q 12 h has not been established. For esophageal reflux disease, the dosage should be divided at least q 12 h and preferably q 8 h. It is prudent to limit therapy to 6 to 8 wk. Recurrences and complications may occur as in adults (but obstruction is rare).

MECKEL'S DIVERTICULUM

A congenital sacculation of the distal ileum, found in about 2% of adult surgical patients, usually located within 91.5 to 183 cm (3 to 6 ft) of the ileocecal valve, and varying in length from 2.5 to 15.2 cm (1 to 6 in.).

Pathophysiology

In early fetal life the vitelline duct runs from the terminal ileum to the umbilicus and yolk sac; this duct is normally obliterated by the 7th wk. Failure to atrophy leads to several abnormalities: a fibrous band running from the diverticulum to the umbilicus; an umbilical cyst; an ileoumbilical fistula; a Meckel's diverticulum (the most common) is formed when all of the duct except the portion to the ileum is obliterated. Arising from the antimesenteric margin of the intestine, this true congenital diverticulum contains all coats of the normal bowel. At least 25% of diverticula removed by surgery contain heterotopic tissue of the stomach (which contains parietal cells that secrete hydrochloric acid), pancreas, or intestine.

Symptoms, Signs, and Diagnosis

Diagnosis is difficult and usually is based on the symptoms and signs, which are more common in infants and children. In children repeated episodes of severe, bright-red bleeding occur because of formation of a peptic ulcer in the adjacent ileum. Bleeding tends to be acute and profuse but usually is not severe enough to produce shock. In adolescents and adults, intestinal obstruction, manifested by cramps and vomiting, is most common; it occurs from adhesions, intussusception, angulation from retained foreign bodies, volvulus, tumors, or incarceration in a hernia (Littre's). Acute diverticulitis may occur at any age. It is diagnosed by localized abdominal pain and tenderness below or to the left of the umbilicus; it is acute, often accompanied by vomiting, and is similar to appendicitis except for location of the pain.

Occasionally a diverticulum can be seen on a small bowel barium x-ray. Presence of acid-secreting cells permits the use of technetium pertechnetate scanning; this method is effective in about 50% of cases with rectal bleeding.

Treatment

A bleeding diverticulum with an indurated area in the adjacent ileum requires a resection of this section of the bowel as well as the diverticulum. In symptomatic patients without ileal induration, only the diverticulum is excised. Small, asymptomatic diverticula encountered incidentally at laparotomy need not be removed. *Whenever a normal appendix is found during an exploration for appendicitis, a search should be made for a Meckel's diverticulum.* Intestinal obstruction is a dangerous complication since torsion and gangrene can lead to a fatal outcome if early operation is not done.

APPENDICITIS

Acute inflammation of the vermiform appendix.

Etiology and Incidence

Although acute appendicitis is by far the most common disease of this organ, other pathology may be caused by swallowed foreign bodies, pinworms, fecaliths, carcinoid tumors, cancer, villous adenomas, and diverticula; it may also be involved in idiopathic ulcerative colitis or the ileocolitis of Crohn's disease.

Except for hernia, acute appendicitis is the most common cause for an attack of acute abdominal pain and for abdominal operations in the USA. Because symptoms and signs vary widely, and because the hazards of delay before operation are so high, it is accepted that nearly 15% of operations with this diagnosis lead to other findings at laparotomy or even to finding no pathology at all.

Symptoms and Signs

Typical symptoms and signs of acute appendicitis appear in $< 1/2$ of patients; they consist of sudden onset of epigastric or periumbilical pain followed by brief nausea and vomiting and, after a few hours, shifting of pain to the right lower quadrant. Direct tenderness in the right lower quadrant, rebound tenderness felt in the right lower quadrant, localized pain on cough, low-grade fever (rectal temperature 37.7 to 38.3° C [100 to 101° F]) and leukocytosis (12,000 to 15,000/μL) characterize the syndrome.

Classic right lower quadrant tenderness is located at **McBurney's point** (*junction of the middle and outer thirds of the line joining the umbilicus to the anterior superior spine*). **Rovsing's sign** (*pain felt in the right lower quadrant resulting from palpation in the left lower quadrant*) suggests the possibility of appendicitis. The presence of the **psoas sign** (*an increase in pain from passive extension of the right hip joint that stretches the iliopsoas muscle*) or **adductor pain** (*that produced by passive internal rotation of the flexed thigh*) may suggest both the anatomic location of the appendix and progression of the inflammatory process.

Many variations occur. Pain, particularly in infants and children, may not be localized. Tenderness may be diffuse or noted only on rectal or pelvic examination; in rare instances tenderness can be absent so that abdominal pain, persistent fever, and leukocytosis are the only signs. Bowel movements are usually decreased in frequency or absent; if diarrhea is a sign, a retrocecal appendix should be suspected. A few RBCs may be present in the urine. Atypical symptoms are also common in the elderly and in pregnant women;

in particular, pain is less severe, and local tenderness less acute.

Diagnosis

Usually diagnosis must be based on clinical examination, and operation must follow rapidly to avoid perforation and peritonitis. In early appendicitis, essentially no diagnostic aid is furnished by x-ray or by ultrasound **(US)** or CT scan; barium enemas can be dangerous. In late stages of the disease, US and CT scans can be very helpful in the diagnosis of abscesses, particularly in pelvic and subphrenic areas. Laparoscopy can be of aid in some cases, particularly in women with pelvic inflammatory disease **(PID)**.

Alternative diagnoses must be rapidly considered—immediate operation is necessary for perforated peptic ulcer, acute gangrenous cholecystitis, and acute intestinal obstruction; at laparotomy, if a normal appendix is found in a woman, careful inspection of the pelvic organs for an ovarian cyst, salpingitis, or ectopic pregnancy should be done first. In both men and women, the distal small bowel is examined for a distance of about 2 m (6 ft) to rule out a Meckel's diverticulum or ileitis (Crohn's disease or *Yersinia* enteritis). Mesenteric adenitis (hyperplastic lymph nodes) may be found in the mesentery of the terminal ileum. Operation should be avoided for renal colic, ruptured ovarian follicle (unless there is serious bleeding), early PID in women, or acute gastroenteritis.

Prognosis

With early operation, the mortality is low, the patient is usually discharged within a few days, and convalescence is normally rapid and complete. With complications (rupture and either formation of an abscess or peritonitis that can be local or general), the prognosis is more serious; although antibiotics have lowered mortality to nearly zero in many institutions, repeated operations and long convalescence often follow.

Treatment

Since perforation may occur in < 24 h after the onset of symptoms, laparotomy is the only safe procedure when appendicitis is a reasonable diagnosis. The treatment of acute appendicitis is appendectomy; the surgeon nearly always can remove the appendix, even in the presence of perforation or some other pathology. Occasionally it is difficult to locate; then it usually lies behind the cecum or the ileum and mesentery of the right colon. The operation should be preceded by antibiotics given IM or IV; they are repeated during the operative procedure and continued for 48 h. Third-generation cephalosporins are preferred.

Alternative procedures may be required. When a large inflammatory mass is found involving the appendix, terminal ileum, and cecum, a resection of the entire mass and ileocolostomy is preferable. In some late cases a pericolic abscess already has formed; it can be drained either by percutaneous catheter guided by US or by open operation with appendectomy to follow at a later date. Unless the procedure is prevented by extensive inflammation about the appendix, a Meckel's diverticulum should be removed concomitantly with the appendectomy. A contraindication to appendectomy is inflammatory bowel disease involving the cecum. However, if terminal ileitis is found and the cecum is normal, the appendix usually is removed.

Suspected acute appendicitis should not be treated by antibiotics alone unless an operation is impossible.

Perforated appendix is the most common cause of peritonitis in children and young adults, but it occurs at any age. In children, because of a poorly developed omentum, peritonitis is likely to be generalized; in adults, local peritonitis and abscess formation are more common. Tenderness in either the right lower quadrant or over the entire abdomen will indicate the extent of inflammation. In children a high fever should be reduced if possible before operation. Antibiotic options include cefoxitin 80 to 160 mg/kg/day in divided dosage qid, or amikacin 15 mg/kg/day in divided dosage tid plus clindamycin 20 to 40 mg/kg/day in divided dosage qid or tid in adults with corresponding dosage in children. A nasogastric tube is inserted and urine output assured by adequate IV fluids and electrolytes. In late cases several hours may be required to improve the patient's condition. If an abscess or an inflammatory mass has formed, operation may be limited to drainage of the abscess; whenever possible, the appendix should be removed as well.

CELIAC DISEASE
(Nontropical Sprue; Gluten Enteropathy; Celiac Sprue)

A chronic intestinal malabsorption disorder caused by intolerance to gluten, characterized by a flat jejunal mucosa with clinical and/or histologic improvement following withdrawal of dietary gluten.

Etiology and Prevalence

This hereditary disorder is caused by sensitivity to the gliadin fraction of gluten, a cereal protein found in wheat and rye and to a lesser degree in barley and oats. Gliadin, acting as antigen, combines with antibodies to form an immune complex in the intestinal mucosa that promotes the aggregation of K (killer) lymphocytes. In some way these lymphocytes cause mucosal damage with loss of villi and proliferation of crypt cells. The prevalence of celiac disease varies from about 1:300 in southwest Ireland to 1:5000 or more in North America. There is no single genetic marker.

Symptoms and Signs

Celiac disease may be symptomatic or asymptomatic and present at any age, often without diarrhea or steatorrhea. Primary symptoms and signs may be short stature, infertility, anemia, recurrent aphthous stomatitis, or dermatitis herpetiformis.

Family studies show that typical mucosal abnormalities appear in apparently healthy siblings of affected patients. The disease may present for the first time in infancy or adulthood, but it should not be assumed that an adult presentation is the first manifestation. Although the patient may have no knowledge of childhood disease, his mother may recall abdominal symptoms. If the adult patient is significantly smaller than his siblings and has evidence of mild bowing deformities of the long bones, the likelihood of latent or undiagnosed childhood disease is increased.

In **infancy,** symptoms are absent until the child eats food containing gluten. The child fails to thrive, begins to pass pale, malodorous, bulky stools, and suffers painful abdominal bloating. Iron deficiency anemia develops and, if hypoproteinemia is severe enough, edema appears. Celiac disease is strongly suspected in a pale, querulous child, with wasted buttocks and a pot belly, who has an adequate diet (thus ruling out protein-calorie malnutrition or kwashiorkor).

In **adults,** celiac disease is usually diagnosed when malabsorption is found in conjunction with a flat jejunal biopsy not due to some recognizable cause (eg, tropical sprue, neomycin intake) and gluten is shown to be of etiologic significance. Family incidence is a valuable clue. It may present, apparently for the first time, at any age. The disease may be unmasked after partial gastrectomy and drainage. The average age of presentation in women is 10 to 15 yr earlier than in men, because amenorrhea or anemia in pregnancy may heighten clinical suspicion.

There is no single typical presentation. Many symptoms (eg, anemia, weight loss, bone pain, paresthesia, edema, and skin disorders) are secondary to deficiency states. If overt alimentary symptoms (eg, diarrhea, abdominal discomfort, and distention) also occur, the real diagnosis is unlikely to be missed. Without these direct clues, malabsorption may not be suspected.

Laboratory Findings

There tends to be iron-deficiency anemia in children and folate deficiency anemia in adults. Depending on severity and duration, there can be any combination of low albumin, Ca, K, and Na, and elevated alkaline phosphatase and prothrombin time. The 5 gm D-xylose test (see discussion of absorption tests, above) will usually be abnormal, and most patients will have steatorrhea that can range from mild to massive (7 to 50 gm [20 to 150 mEq] fatty acid/day).

In the immune protein system, levels of C3 and C4 are low in the untreated patient and rise with gluten withdrawal. The serum IgA level is usually normal or increased in untreated patients, and in $^1/_3$ to $^1/_2$, the IgM level is reduced. Serum antigliadin antibody titers have been proposed as a screening test for celiac disease.

Diagnosis

Diagnosis is suspected on the basis of the symptoms and signs, enhanced by the laboratory and x-ray studies, and confirmed by biopsy showing a flat mucosa and clinical and histologic improvement on a gluten-free diet. Jejunal biopsy can be performed even in small infants, but to obviate the risk of bowel perforation, only an experienced investigator should do the test. If a biopsy cannot be done, the diagnosis may have to depend on the clinical and laboratory response (including xylose absorption) to a gluten-free diet.

Prognosis and Natural History

While gluten withdrawal has transformed the prognosis for children and substantially improved it for adults, there is still some mortality from the disease, mainly among adults whose condition is severe from the beginning. An important cause of death is the development of lymphoreticular disease (especially intestinal lymphoma). It is not known whether this risk is diminished by scrupulous adherence to a gluten-free diet. Some patients can tolerate the reintroduction of gluten into the diet. It is not certain whether this means that some mild cases can achieve complete remission (unlikely) or whether the gluten toxicity is a nonspecific effect on a mucosa previously damaged by an acute bacterial or viral enteritis. In any case, apparent clinical remission is often associated with histologic relapse that is detected only if review biopsies are performed.

Treatment

Dietary gluten must be excluded: Ingesting even small amounts may prevent remission or induce relapse. Gluten is so widely used (eg, in commercial soups, sauces, ice creams, hot dogs) that patients need detailed lists of foodstuffs to avoid and expert advice from a dietitian familiar with the problems of celiac disease.

Supplementary vitamins, minerals, and hematinics may be given, depending on the degree of deficiency. In mild cases no supplementation may be necessary. In severe cases comprehensive replacement may be required. For adults this includes ferrous sulfate 300 mg/day, folic acid 5 to 10 mg/day, calcium gluconate 5 to 10 gm/day, and any standard multivitamin preparation, all orally. Only if the prothrombin time is abnormal should vitamin K 10 mg IM be given. Proportional doses are given to children. Sometimes children (but rarely adults) who are seriously ill on first diagnosis may require a period of IV feeding. This should be carried out in accordance with the general principles of total parenteral nutrition.

A few patients respond poorly or not at all to gluten withdrawal, either because the diagnosis is incorrect or because the disease has entered a refractory phase. In the latter case, a response may be induced by a period of treatment with oral corticosteroids (eg, prednisone 10 to 20 mg bid).

ALPHA$_1$–ANTITRYPSIN (AAT) DEFICIENCY

AAT, a glycoprotein produced by the liver, makes up 80 to 90% of the α_1-globulin in serum and provides most of the serum's ability to inhibit trypsin. AAT is present in saliva, duodenal

fluid, pulmonary secretions, tears, nasal secretions, and CSF. Numerous phenotypes vary in physical structure and (possibly) functions. Each person has 2 alleles labeled alphabetically according to electrophoretic separation on starch gel: Fast-moving proteins are labeled with beginning letters of the alphabet, the slowest with Z. In this protease inhibitor system (**Pi**), PiM is the predominant normal type with serum AAT values from 200 to 400 mg/dL. Genetic deficiency associated with liver disease is linked to PiZZ, a homozygous phenotype with circulating levels 10 to 15% of normal. There is also a marked tendency to adult panacinar emphysema.

Pathogenesis

The AAT deficiency results from amino acid substitution in the nucleic acid chain, leading to secondary changes in the carbohydrate side chains. Defective glucosylation impedes the release of the AAT from the hepatocytes, which are retained as amorphous periodic acid-Schiff (**PAS**)–positive globules. The pathogenesis of liver injury is unknown but probably relates to the uninhibited action of proteases, perhaps from Kupffer cells, leading to cell destruction. Why only 15 to 30% of infants with phenotype ZZ develop cholestasis and only a few have cirrhosis in childhood or adulthood is unknown.

Symptoms, Signs, and Diagnosis

Prenatal diagnosis can now detect PiZZ, using amniotic cells.

A low serum globulin and particularly a reduced AAT level (to 10% of normal) are characteristic of AAT deficiency. Confirmatory diagnosis is revealed by finding eosinophilic globules on hematoxylin and eosin stains of liver biopsy specimens. These globules are PAS-positive. In neonates with cholestasis, there may be hepatocellular damage without marked inflammatory cell infiltrate, portal fibrosis with duct proliferation, or ductal hypoplasia. Cirrhosis is a late finding.

Prognosis and Therapy

Of children with PiZZ AAT deficiency, up to 25% develop cirrhosis and portal hypertension and die of complications before age 12 yr; another 25% will die of the same process by age 20 yr, while 25% more will have liver fibrosis and minimal hepatic dysfunction and can live into adulthood. The remaining 25% show no evidence of progressive disease; their late adult life is not clear. These figures may overestimate the true frequency of liver disease. Neonatal hepatitis is the earliest presentation, and many will progress to cirrhosis by the second decade. The long-term consequences of those with PiZZ without neonatal hepatitis is unclear.

Adult AAT deficiency is associated with chronic pulmonary emphysema (in 60%) and cirrhosis of the liver (in 12%). Conversely, $2/3$ of patients with liver disease have lung disease. In adults, the most common manifestation of AAT deficiency is a symptomatic cirrhosis that may progress from a micro- to a macronodular state and eventually be complicated by the development of hepatocellular carcinoma. Liver disease presenting for the first time in adulthood is usually associated with a previous history of neonatal jaundice.

Therapy: Standard therapy should be directed at the lung disease, including education not to smoke, relief of any reversible component of airways obstruction, elimination and prevention of bronchopulmonary infection, and general health measures. Liver transplantation is the only successful therapeutic management for severe hepatic injury. The recipient phenotype changes to that of the donor. AAT-like products are not yet in clinical trials.

INTESTINAL LYMPHANGIECTASIA
(Idiopathic Hypoproteinemia)

A syndrome affecting children and young adults, characterized by telangiectasia of the intramucosal lymphatics of the small intestine. A congenital malformation of the lymphatics is most likely when onset occurs at birth. In acquired cases the defect may be secondary (eg, to retroperitoneal fibrosis, pancreatitis, constrictive pericarditis).

Symptoms, Signs, and Diagnosis

Early manifestations include massive, often asymmetric, edema and mild intermittent diarrhea with nausea, vomiting, and abdominal pain. Chylous effusions and ascites may be present. Lymphocytopenia occurs, and marked reductions of serum albumin, IgA, and IgG. Cholesterol may be low. A few patients have mild to moderate steatorrhea, but D-xylose absorption is normal. Intestinal protein loss can be demonstrated using chromium 51-labeled albumin. Jejunal biopsy shows the characteristic dilation and telangiectasia of the lymphatic vessels that distinguish

this condition from other protein-losing disorders (eg, Crohn's and Whipple's diseases).

Treatment

Some patients improve on a low-fat diet (< 30 gm/day), supplements of medium-chain triglycerides, and occasionally by resection, if the lesion is localized.

DYSPHAGIA LUSORIA

Dysphagia due to compression of the esophagus by a congenital vascular abnormality (usually an aberrant right subclavian artery arising from the left side of the aortic arch). The dysphagia may occur in childhood or may develop later due to arteriosclerotic changes in the aberrant vessel. Esophageal x-ray studies show the extrinsic compression above the aortic arch, at the third thoracic vertebra. Arteriography is necessary for absolute diagnosis. Surgical correction is only rarely indicated.

FOREIGN BODIES

From time to time foreign bodies are swallowed by children and deranged or inebriated adults. Denture wearers especially are prone to swallow chicken or fish bones. Probably most intragastric foreign bodies could be ignored, but the temptation to retrieve an object from the esophagus, stomach, or duodenum will prove irresistible to most endoscopists. There can be little quarrel with the attempt to remove an object from as far down as the duodenum, if only to forestall further x-ray surveillance. Sharp objects should be retrieved, if possible, but small round ones (eg, coins) can probably be watched without undue apprehension.

Foreign objects that have passed into the small intestine usually traverse the GI tract without problem, even if they take weeks or months to do so. They tend to be held up just before the ileocecal valve or at any site of narrowing, as in Crohn's disease. Smugglers, who sometimes swallow drug-filled balloons to escape detection, have developed intestinal obstruction as the balloons come up against a stricture. Sometimes objects like toothpicks remain within the GI tract for many years, only to turn up in a granuloma or abscess, particularly at a clinicopathologic conference.

39. NUTRITIONAL DISORDERS

NUTRITIONAL STATUS OF CHILDREN

Although frank deficiency states are rare in children of advanced Western societies, marginal undernutrition is common in families living in poverty or consuming restricted diets for alleged health reasons. Growth is primarily affected, usually resulting in a greater decline in weight gain than in height gain. Deviations can be detected by measurements at regular intervals and the use of standard growth charts. Single observations are insignificant, as individual children vary in their growth potential. Additionally, blood levels of vitamins A and C, thiamine, riboflavin, iron, and transferrin saturation are low in a significant proportion of these children. Zinc deficiency may be responsible for retarded growth and loss of taste.

Children suspected of being nutritionally impaired should have a careful dietary history taken, including any suspected food intolerance (see FOOD ALLERGY AND INTOLERANCE in Ch. 34). A general physical examination should be made, and systemic disease that causes undernutrition and impaired growth should be excluded. Specific vitamin or trace element measurements are necessary only if the history or physical examination is indicative. In the absence of any evident cause for poor growth, reassurance is given, growth is observed at regular intervals, and dietary intake is monitored. (See TABLES 39–1 and 39–2 for recommended daily allowances.)

ESSENTIAL FATTY ACIDS (EFA)

Unsaturated fatty acids that cannot be synthesized in the body and therefore must be provided by the diet. EFAs are essential for many physiologic processes, including growth, the integrity of cell membranes, and the synthesis of prostaglandins (see Ch. 142). The 3 most important EFAs are linoleic, linolenic, and arachidonic acids.

In infants, EFA deficiency has been observed after prolonged administration of fat-free diets or total parenteral nutrition and may result in a scaly dermatitis, thrombocytopenia, failure to thrive, poor wound healing, and increased sus-

ceptibility to infection. Low plasma levels of linoleic and arachidonic acids are diagnostic of early EFA deficiency.

For the maintenance of proper health, 2 to 3% of the total calories in the diet should be in the form of EFAs. Common vegetable oils (eg, corn, cottonseed, and soybean) are excellent sources of linoleic and linolenic acids. Arachidonic acid can be synthesized in the body from linoleic acid. In deficiency states, up to 10 gm/day of EFA may be required.

INFANTILE SCURVY

Scurvy: *An acute or chronic disease characterized by hemorrhagic manifestations and abnormal osteoid and dentin formation and caused by a deficiency of ascorbic acid.* Primary deficiency in infants is due to lack of supplementary vitamin C.

Symptoms and Signs

Infantile scurvy usually occurs between the 6th and 12th mo of life. Early symptoms include irritability, anorexia, and failure to gain weight. The infant screams when moved and may keep his legs motionless because of pain from subperiosteal hemorrhage. Advanced cases show angular enlargements of the costochondral junctions (scorbutic rosary), swelling over the ends of the long bones (especially at the lower end of the femur), and a tendency to hemorrhage, as shown by swollen hemorrhagic gums surrounding erupting teeth. Skin hemorrhages at this age are rare, and gingivitis does not develop until teeth have erupted. Fever, anemia, and increased pulse and respiration rates are common. The anemia is usually normocytic and normochromic; however, macrocytosis and a megaloblastic bone marrow may be seen, due either to a combined deficiency of vitamin C and folic acid or to oxidation of tetrahydrofolates to 10-formylfolic acid in the absence of vitamin C.

X-ray findings are characteristic. The ends of the long bones show a transverse thickening and increased density—the **white line**. Immediately shaftward of the white line is a localized area of rarefaction, first evident at the lateral margins and appearing in the x-ray as a small fracture. The trabecular markings of the shaft become indistinct, giving it a ground-glass appearance. Af-

TABLE 39–1. RECOMMENDED DIETARY
FOOD AND NUTRITION BOARD, NATIONAL ACADEMY

Category	Age (yr) or Condition	Weight[†] (kg)	(lb)	Height[†] (cm)	(in)	Protein (gm)	Fat-Soluble Vitamins			
							Vitamin A (μg RE)[‡]	Vitamin D (μg)[§]	Vitamin E (mg α-TE)**	Vitamin K (μg)
Infants	0.0–0.5	6	13	60	24	13	375	7.5	3	5
	0.5–1.0	9	20	71	28	14	375	10	4	10
Children	1–3	13	29	90	35	16	400	10	6	15
	4–6	20	44	112	44	24	500	10	7	20
	7–10	28	62	132	52	28	700	10	7	30
Males	11–14	45	99	157	62	45	1000	10	10	45
	15–18	66	145	176	69	59	1000	10	10	65
	19–24	72	160	177	70	58	1000	10	10	70
	25–50	79	174	176	70	63	1000	5	10	80
	51+	77	170	173	68	63	1000	5	10	80
Females	11–14	46	101	157	62	46	800	10	8	45
	15–18	55	120	163	64	44	800	10	8	55
	19–24	58	128	164	65	46	800	10	8	60
	25–50	63	138	163	64	50	800	5	8	65
	51+	65	143	160	63	50	800	5	8	65
Pregnant						60	800	10	10	65
Lactating	1st 6 mo					65	1300	10	12	65
	2nd 6 mo					62	1200	10	11	65

* The allowances, expressed as average daily intakes over time, are intended to provide for individual variations among most normal persons as they live in the USA under usual environmental stresses. Diets should be based on a variety of common foods to provide other nutrients for which human requirements have been less well defined.

† Weights and heights of Reference Adults are actual medians for the US population of the designated age, as reported by NHANES II (National Health and Nutrition Examination Survey [1976–1980], National Center for Health Statistics). The median weights and heights of those 19 yr were taken from Hamill et al (Am J Clin Nutr, 1979). The use of these figures does not imply that the height-to-weight ratios are ideal.

ter 7 to 10 days of therapy (see below), some calcification results; x-ray shows a club-like swelling extending from the white line to the middle of the shaft (never into the joint). The blood is resorbed, and the bone resumes its normal shape as treatment proceeds.

Differential Diagnosis

Infantile scurvy must be differentiated from rickets, poliomyelitis, osteomyelitis, rheumatic fever, and hemorrhagic disorders (eg, blood diseases, severe anemias, allergic purpuras). Rickets often occurs before the 5th mo, scurvy almost never before the 6th. The diseases rarely occur simultaneously. Hemorrhagic manifestations are absent in rickets. The costochondral junctions are enlarged in either condition; in scurvy the swellings are angular, while in rickets they tend to be rounded. Poliomyelitis is often considered because the infant does not move his legs and cries when moved; in scurvy, the ab-

sence of neurologic changes, the presence of bleeding, and bone changes permit differentiation. Joint involvement may suggest rheumatic fever, but this disease is uncommon before age 2. The bone swellings in scurvy never extend into the joint. Other bleeding disorders can usually be excluded by their characteristic tests. In doubtful cases, a therapeutic trial of ascorbic acid 300 to 500 mg orally will stop the pain of infantile scurvy within 24 to 48 h and will decrease gingival swelling and bleeding within 72 h.

Prophylaxis

In industrialized countries proprietary infant formulas are fortified with vitamin C, and liquid multivitamin preparations are readily available. Alternatively, unboiled orange juice, beginning with 1 tsp daily in the 2nd to 4th wk of life, with progressive increases until at 5 mo the intake is 2 to 3 oz, may be given. Tomato juice at 3 times these doses may be used.

ALLOWANCES,* REVISED 1989
OF SCIENCES—NATIONAL RESEARCH COUNCIL

Water-Soluble Vitamins							Minerals						
Vita-min C (mg)	Thia-mine (mg)	Ribo-flavin (mg)	Niacin (mg NE)††	Vita-min B$_6$ (mg)	Fo-late (µg)	Vita-min B$_{12}$ (µg)	Cal-cium (mg)	Phos-phorus (mg)	Mag-nesium (mg)	Iron (mg)	Zinc (mg)	Iodine (µg)	Sele-nium (µg)
30	0.3	0.4	5	0.3	25	0.3	400	300	40	6	5	40	10
35	0.4	0.5	6	0.6	35	0.5	600	500	60	10	5	50	15
40	0.7	0.8	9	1.0	50	0.7	800	800	80	10	10	70	20
45	0.9	1.1	12	1.1	75	1.0	800	800	120	10	10	90	20
45	1.0	1.2	13	1.4	100	1.4	800	800	170	10	10	120	30
50	1.3	1.5	17	1.7	150	2.0	1200	1200	270	12	15	150	40
60	1.5	1.8	20	2.0	200	2.0	1200	1200	400	12	15	150	50
60	1.5	1.7	19	2.0	200	2.0	1200	1200	350	10	15	150	70
60	1.5	1.7	19	2.0	200	2.0	800	800	350	10	15	150	70
60	1.2	1.4	15	2.0	200	2.0	800	800	350	10	15	150	70
50	1.1	1.3	15	1.4	150	2.0	1200	1200	280	15	12	150	45
60	1.1	1.3	15	1.5	180	2.0	1200	1200	300	15	12	150	50
60	1.1	1.3	15	1.6	180	2.0	1200	1200	280	15	12	150	55
60	1.1	1.3	15	1.6	180	2.0	800	800	280	15	12	150	55
60	1.0	1.2	13	1.6	180	2.0	800	800	280	10	12	150	55
70	1.5	1.6	17	2.2	400	2.2	1200	1200	320	30	15	175	65
95	1.6	1.8	20	2.1	280	2.6	1200	1200	355	15	19	200	75
90	1.6	1.7	20	2.1	260	2.6	1200	1200	340	15	16	200	75

‡ Retinol equivalents. 1 retinol equivalent = 1 µg retinol or 6 µg β-carotene. See text for calculation of vitamin A activity of diets as retinol equivalents.

§ As cholecalciferol. 10 µg cholecalciferol = 400 IU of vitamin D.

** α-Tocopherol equivalents. 1 mg d-α tocopherol = 1 α-TE. See text for variation in allowances and calculation of vitamin E activity of the diet as α-tocopherol equivalents.

†† Niacin equivalents. 1 niacin equivalent = 1 mg niacin or 60 mg dietary tryptophan.

From *Recommended Dietary Allowances*, © 1989 by the National Academy of Sciences, National Academy Press, Washington, DC.

Treatment

Ascorbic acid 50 mg qid should be given orally for 1 wk in infantile scurvy, then 50 mg tid for 1 mo, with prophylactic doses thereafter. In vomiting or diarrhea, one half the recommended oral dose may be given IM or IV as sodium ascorbate.

PROTEIN–ENERGY MALNUTRITION (PEM)
(Protein-Calorie Malnutrition)

Classification and Etiology

PEM is classified according to *degree* of severity as 1st (mild), 2nd (moderate), or 3rd (severe). Mild PEM is characterized by growth failure in the child or wasting in the adult; moderate PEM by superimposed biochemical changes (see Laboratory Findings, below); and severe PEM by the development of additional clinical signs.

Meeting energy requirements is basic to survival, and the way in which this is accomplished from protein or nonprotein sources determines the *type* of severe PEM produced. A diet with excessive nonprotein calories from starch or sugar, but deficient in total protein and essential amino acids, results eventually in **kwashiorkor.** Severe inadequacy of energy and nutrients causes total inanition, which in the young child is called **marasmus,** but does not differ in essence from semistarvation in the adult. Intermediate forms are termed **marasmic-kwashiorkor.**

Epidemiology

Marasmus is the predominant form of PEM throughout most developing countries. It is associated with the early abandonment or failure of breast-feeding and with consequent infections, most notably those causing infantile gastroenteritis. These infections result from lack of hygiene and proper knowledge of infant rearing that are

TABLE 39–2. ESTIMATED SAFE AND ADEQUATE DAILY DIETARY INTAKES OF SELECTED VITAMINS AND MINERALS*

	Vitamins		Trace Elements†				
Age (yr)	Biotin (μg)	Pantothenic Acid (mg)	Copper (mg)	Manganese (mg)	Fluoride (mg)	Chromium (μg)	Molybdenum (μg)
Infants							
0–0.5	10	2	0.4–0.6	0.3–0.6	0.1–0.5	10–40	15–30
0.5–1	15	3	0.6–0.7	0.6–1.0	0.2–1.0	20–60	20–40
Children and adolescents							
1–3	20	3	0.7–1.0	1.0–1.5	0.5–1.5	20–80	25–50
4–6	25	3–4	1.0–1.5	1.5–2.0	1.0–2.5	30–120	30–75
7–10	30	4–5	1.0–2.0	2.0–3.0	1.5–2.5	50–200	50–150
11+	30–100	4–7	1.5–2.5	2.0–5.0	1.5–2.5	50–200	75–250
Adults	30–100	4–7	1.5–3.0	2.0–5.0	1.5–4.0	50–200	75–250

* Because there is less information on which to base allowances, these figures are not given in TABLE 39–1 but are provided here in the form of ranges of recommended intakes.

† Since the toxic levels for many trace elements may be only several times usual intakes, the upper levels for the trace elements given in this table should not be habitually exceeded.

From *Recommended Dietary Allowances*. © 1989 by the National Academy of Sciences, National Academy Press, Washington, DC.

prevalent, especially in the rapidly growing slums of developing countries.

Kwashiorkor is less common and is usually manifest as the intermediate marasmic-kwashiorkor state. It tends to be confined to those parts of the world (rural Africa, the Caribbean and Pacific islands) where staple and weaning foods such as yam, cassava, sweet potato, or green banana are protein deficient and excessively starchy.

Pathophysiology

In marasmus, energy intake is insufficient to match requirements and the body draws on its own stores. Liver glycogen is exhausted within a few hours, and skeletal muscle protein is then used by gluconeogenesis to maintain adequate plasma glucose. At the same time, triglycerides in fat depots give rise to free fatty acids that contribute to the energy needs of most tissues except the nervous system. In prolonged starvation, fatty acids are incompletely oxidized to ketone bodies that can be used by the brain and other organs as an alternative energy source. Thus in the severe energy deficiency of marasmus, adaptation is facilitated by high cortisol and growth hormone levels and depression of insulin and thyroid hormone secretion.

In kwashiorkor, increased carbohydrate intake with decreased protein intake leads to decreased visceral protein synthesis. The resulting hypoalbuminemia causes dependent edema; and the impaired β-lipoprotein synthesis produces fatty liver. Insulin is stimulated and epinephrine and cortisol reduced. Fat mobilization and release of amino acids from muscle are reduced. As in marasmus there is poor insulin response to a glucose load, possibly due to chromium deficiency.

Total body protein synthesis is about 300 gm/day in the average adult male. The daily obligatory loss is only about 30 to 90 gm, as 80 to 90% is reused. The daily allowance of protein recommended for an adult is about 0.8 gm/kg body wt (see Table 39–1). Of this dietary protein, about 20% of the constituent amino acids should be essential amino acids (see Table 39–3), since these cannot be synthesized in adequate amounts by the body and must be present in the diet. The degree to which the essential amino acid pattern of the dietary protein approximates that of the body's requirement determines **protein quality**.

In protein deficiency, adaptive enzyme changes occur in the liver, amino acid synthetases increase, and urea formation diminishes, thus conserving nitrogen and reducing its loss in the urine. Homeostatic mechanisms initially operate to maintain the level of plasma albumin and other transport proteins. The rates of synthesis and catabolism soon decrease. Albumin shifts from the extravascular to the intravascular compartment and eventually plasma levels fall, leading to reduced oncotic pressure and edema. Growth, immune response, repair, and production of enzymes and hormones are all impaired in severe protein deficiency.

Symptoms and Signs

Mild and moderate PEM may be classified by calculating weight as a percentage of expected weight/length (normal, 90 to 110%; mild PEM, 85 to 90%; moderate, 75 to 85%; severe, < 75%) using international standards.

Marasmic infants show hunger, gross weight loss, growth retardation, and wasting of subcutaneous fat and muscle. Kwashiorkor is characterized by generalized edema, "flaky paint" dermatosis, thinning and decoloration of the hair, enlarged fatty liver, and petulant apathy in addition to retarded growth. In developing countries, severely malnourished children may also be HIV positive.

Laboratory Findings

Mild or moderately severe cases of PEM may show slight depression of plasma albumin and a lowering of the urinary excretion of urea, due to decreased protein intake, and of hydroxyproline, reflecting impaired growth. Increased urinary 3-methylhistidine reflects muscle breakdown. In both marasmus and kwashiorkor, the percentage of body water, extracellular water, and plasma volume is increased. Electrolyte depletion (especially K and Mg), anemia (usually Fe deficiency), low levels of some enzymes and circulating lipids, falling blood urea, and metabolic acidosis are also present. Diarrhea is sometimes related to intestinal disaccharidase deficiency, especially lactase. Kwashiorkor is characterized by low plasma levels of albumin (10 to 25 gm/L), transferrin, essential amino acids (especially the branched-chain), β-lipoprotein, glucose, and an "overflow" aminoaciduria. Plasma cortisol and growth hormone levels are high, but insulin secretion is depressed.

Diagnosis

Differential diagnosis includes secondary growth failure due to malabsorption, congenital defects, or deprivation. Skin changes in kwashi-

TABLE 39-3. ESSENTIAL AMINO ACID (EAA) REQUIREMENTS
IN MG/KG BODY WEIGHT

Requirement	Infant (Holt)	Child, 10-12 yr (Nakagawa)	Adult Male		Adult Female (Hegsted)
			(Rose)	(Inoue)	
Histidine	(25)	—	—	—	—
Isoleucine	111	28	10	11	10
Leucine	153	49	11	14	13
Lysine	96	59	9	12	10
Methionine and cystine	50	27	14	11	13
Phenylalanine and tyrosine	90	27	14	14	13
Threonine	66	34	6	6	7
Tryptophan	19	4	3	3	3
Valine	95	33	14	14	11
Total EAA (excluding histidine)	680	261	81	85	80

Adapted from Munro HN: "Amino acid requirements and metabolism and their relevance to parenteral nutrition," in *Parenteral Nutrition*, edited by AW Wilkinson. Edinburgh, Churchill Livingstone, 1972; used with permission.

orkor differ from those of pellagra where they occur on parts exposed to light and are symmetrical. Edema in nephritis, nephrosis, and cardiac failure is accompanied by features of these diseases. Hepatomegaly from disorders of glycogen metabolism and cystic fibrosis must be differentiated.

Treatment

Fluid and electrolyte balance should be restored and maintained. All but the most severely ill respond to a diet based on milk; dilute milk feedings can usually be introduced after 24 h.

Low-lactose formulas have been helpful in some cases in controlling excessive diarrhea caused by lack of disaccharidases. Lactic acid—fortified milk (0.125 mL/oz of milk) is preferred by some. Sufficient milk should be given to infants and small children to supply 2 gm, increasing slowly to 5 gm of protein/kg/day. At this stage, more calories in the form of sugar and cereal or locally acceptable oil, eg, arachis, may be added to the milk diet to provide 150 to 250 kcal/kg/day. Increased dietary allowances soon become possible, and the diet is supplemented with high-energy foods such as candies, cake, puddings, meats, eggs, and fruit juices. Prepared nutritional supplements are available commercially. Bulky or low-caloric vegetables or fruits should be avoided and those containing 10 to 20% carbohydrate used. Supplementary vitamins may be advisable. Small, frequent feedings around the clock are tolerated best in the early stages of recovery. Antibiotics may be indicated.

Unless urgent, treatment of malaria or other parasitic infections should be postponed until the patient is clinically improved. Anemia is usually mild and responds to oral protein, iron, and folic acid supplements. If severe (Hb < 6 gm/dL), transfusion is indicated with packed RBCs (15 to 20 mL/kg) given slowly to avoid circulation overload as evidenced by rise in venous pressure, tachycardia, hypotension, tachypnea, pulmonary edema, and cyanosis.

Prognosis

Mortality varies between 15 and 40%. Death in the first days of treatment is usually due to electrolyte imbalance, infection, hypothermia, or heart failure. Stupor, jaundice, petechiae, low serum Na, and low serum vitamin A are ominous signs. Recovery is more rapid in kwashiorkor than in marasmus; disappearance of apathy, edema, and anorexia is a favorable sign.

Long-term effects of malnutrition in childhood are not fully understood. In the adequately treated case the liver probably recovers fully without subsequent cirrhosis, but some GI malabsorption and pancreatic deficiency may remain. Persistent chromosomal breaks observed in malnourished children have not been shown to be due to the malnutrition per se. Humoral immunity is usually unimpaired. Cell-mediated immunocompetence is markedly compromised in the acute phase but is restored with recovery. Behavioral development may be markedly retarded in the severely malnourished child. The degree of mental impairment is related to the duration of malnutrition and age of onset. The infant with marasmus is affected more severely than the older child with kwashi-orkor. Prospective studies suggest that a relatively mild degree of mental retardation persists into school age.

40. ENDOCRINE AND METABOLIC DISORDERS

CONGENITAL GOITERS

An enlarged thyroid gland present at birth, with or without hypothyroidism. There are 4 types of congenital goiter. **Type 1** involves a defect in iodide transport, probably secondary to an alteration in synthesis of cell surface proteins necessary for transport. **Type 2** is associated with several defects in iodination mechanisms within the thyroid. One involves the absence of the enzyme peroxidase, necessary for the organification of iodine, which can result in goitrous cretinism. Another defect, which is inherited as an autosomal recessive trait, appears to involve hydrogen peroxide generation and is associated with deaf-mutism, a complex known as **Pendred's syndrome**. These patients are usually euthyroid; therefore, the deafness is not secondary to hypothyroidism. A third defect, associated with abnormal peroxidase, allows sufficient compensation for maintenance of a euthyroid state. **Type 3** congenital goiters are found in patients with dehalogenase defects. Although the precise biochemical abnormality is unclear, patients have complete or partial deiodination defects of monoiodotyrosine and diiodotyrosine within thyroglobulin. **Type 4** congenital goiters are associated with defects in the synthesis of thyroglobulin. **Athyreotic cretinism** is found in children born without a thyroid gland.

HYPOTHYROIDISM

A deficiency of thyroid activity. Hypothyroidism in the young produces symptoms and signs that differ from adult hypothyroidism. **Neonatal hypothyroidism (cretinism)** is characterized by respiratory distress, cyanosis, jaundice, poor feeding, hoarse cry, umbilical hernia, and retardation of bone growth. Diagnosis requires a high index of suspicion and is greatly aided by routine determination of serum thyroxine (T_4) and thyroid-stimulating hormone (TSH) in umbilical cord blood, or filter paper blood spots taken at 2 to 5 days of age. Prompt treatment with exogenous thyroid (no later than the first 7 to 10 days

of the postnatal period) prevents or markedly reduces deficiencies in mental development. Appropriate doses of thyroid hormone in the first year of life range from 25 to 90 μg L-thyroxine sodium orally/day (infants aged 0 to 3 mo, 10 μg/kg/day; infants 3 to 6 mo, 7 to 10 μg/kg/day; infants 6 to 12 mo, 6 to 8 μg/kg/day). Treatment is monitored by measuring serum T_4 and TSH and changes in the symptoms and signs associated with hypothyroidism, such as macroglossia and slow growth rate, which may take many months to normalize. Caution must be taken not to overtreat and produce hyperthyroidism. **Childhood (juvenile) hypothyroidism** is characterized by growth retardation, delayed dentition, and mental deficiency. Treatment is with L-thyroxine sodium orally—average doses for 1- to 5-yr-olds are 4 to 6 μg/kg/day; for 6- to 12-yr-olds, 3 to 5 μg/kg/day. Symptoms and signs of **adolescent hypothyroidism** are similar to those of adults; additionally there may be short stature and precocious puberty with an enlarged sella turcica.

HYPERTHYROIDISM

Neonatal Graves' disease is a potentially life-threatening occurrence in infants born of mothers who have or have had Graves' disease. The mothers often are under treatment for Graves' disease during the pregnancy and almost invariably have high blood titers of thyroid-stimulating antibodies (**TSAb**), which presumably cross the placenta and stimulate the infant's thyroid gland. Clinical manifestations of neonatal Graves' disease may occur as early as several days after birth and differ in several respects from those observed in juvenile or adult hyperthyroidism. Feeding problems, vomiting, and diarrhea can result in significant electrolyte imbalance; the thyroid goiter may cause respiratory difficulty, and tachycardia may result in heart failure. Ophthalmopathy is rare.

Affected infants generally recover within 3 or 4 mo, although occasionally the course is prolonged—6 mo to 1 yr or more. Disease duration appears to be a function of the concentration of TSAb in the infant's blood following birth and the rate that TSAb is metabolized; but with TSAb half-life of about 2 wk, disease persisting > 3 or 4 mo after birth is difficult to explain on the basis of passive transfer of TSAb. Therefore, infants with neonatal Graves' disease are probably a heterogeneous group with different pathogenetic mechanisms for hyperthyroidism.

Persistent elevations of thyroid hormone may result in premature fusion of cranial sutures, impaired intellect, hyperactivity later in childhood, and growth retardation. The mortality may be as high as 15 to 20%. Intrauterine Graves' disease also may result in death of the fetus in utero, stillbirth, or premature birth. Thus, the possibility of neonatal Graves' disease must be considered in advance in any pregnant woman with active Graves' disease or a history of Graves' disease, and titers of TSAb should be determined during pregnancy.

Treatment: During the hyperthyroid phase, the cornerstone of therapy is oral propylthiouracil 5 mg/kg/day in 3 divided doses. Strong iodine solution (Lugol's) may be given in a dose of 6 to 12 mg/day (1 drop q 8 h). Infants with severe cardiovascular manifestations may require digitalis and/or a β-adrenergic blocking drug such as propranolol 2 mg/kg/day in 3 divided doses. Severe cases, with high titers of TSAb, may require exchange transfusion.

PITUITARY DWARFISM

Abnormally slow growth and short stature with normal proportions due to hypofunction of the anterior pituitary. Height is less than the 3rd percentile, growth velocity is ≤ 4 cm/yr, and bone age is ≥ 2 yr behind chronologic age.

Etiology

The potential etiology of pituitary dwarfism is varied, as detailed in TABLE 40–1; in most children with short stature, it is currently not possible to identify a specific pituitary disorder. Although endocrine disorders constitute a minority of all causes of growth retardation, it is important to try to identify them because they are treatable.

Children with hypopituitarism most commonly have either a pituitary tumor (generally a craniopharyngioma) or no demonstrable etiology (idiopathic hypopituitarism). In some patients, the combination of lytic lesions of

bone in the skull and diabetes insipidus will suggest Hand-Schüller-Christian disease (see HISTIOCYTOSIS X in Ch. 37). Isolated growth hormone (GH) deficiency may occur in association with midline defects, such as cleft palate, absence of the septum pellucidum, optic nerve hypoplasia, and nystagmus. GH deficiency, either alone or in association with other abnormalities, is hereditary in 10% of cases. (See also FAILURE TO THRIVE in Ch. 29.)

Symptoms and Signs

Growth retardation with normal proportions is the hallmark of hypopituitarism in childhood. Children with hypopituitarism will also fail to begin pubertal development. Those with isolated GH deficiency have normal body proportions, undergo normal (although sometimes delayed) pubertal development, and have normal reproductive potential.

Determination of bone age from hand x-rays is important in evaluating growth problems, as is the careful recording of height and weight over time on any of several available growth charts (see GROWTH AND DEVELOPMENT FROM BIRTH THROUGH CHILDHOOD in Ch. 23). In pituitary dwarfism, epiphyseal maturation is usually retarded to the same extent as height. Evaluation of the sella turcica with CT or MRI is indicated to rule out calcification and neoplasms. In addition, the sella is abnormally small in 10 to 20% of children with pituitary GH deficiency.

Diagnosis

The great majority of children below the 3rd percentile for stature have normal levels of GH and insulin-like growth factor I (IGF-I, also termed somatomedin-C). Both the bone and height ages are generally somewhat retarded. A family history of short stature or delayed puberty is common. Such children are generally diagnosed as having either hereditary (familial) short stature or constitutional (physiologic) delayed puberty. As diagnostic tests improve, some of these children may prove to have somatomedin receptor and postreceptor defects. The short stature of certain racial groups, as exemplified by the African pygmy, is due in part to a failure of IGF-I to increase at puberty.

Levels of IGF-I are a useful indirect measure of GH secretion. Normal IGF-I levels in children > 6 yr of age can exclude severe GH deficiency. In younger children, the difference between normal and low IGF-I levels may be too small to permit reliable screening. Reported mean (± SE) levels

TABLE 40-1. MAJOR ENDOCRINE CAUSES OF SHORT STATURE

Decreased GH secretion
  Hypothalamic causes
    Decreased secretion of GRH
    Organic lesions
  Pituitary causes
    Decreased secretion of GH alone or with other pituitary hormones
    Organic lesions
  Functional GH deficiency (emotional deprivation)

Defective GH action
  Defective GH receptors (Laron dwarfism)
  Secretion of abnormal forms of GH
  Nutritional impairment of GH-induced somatomedin formation (kwashiorkor)

Impaired skeletal response to somatomedin (or GH)
  Constitutional short stature
  Gonadal dysgenesis (Turner's syndrome)
  Primary cartilaginous or bone disease
  Chronic renal disease
  Chronic inflammatory disease
  Corticosteroid excess
    Pituitary and adrenal disorders
    Treatment with pharmacologic doses of corticosteroids

Hypothyroidism (primary or secondary)

Precocious puberty
  Organic
    Central (CNS) ("true precocious puberty" with early epiphyseal closure)
    Pseudoprecocious puberty
  Idiopathic ("true precocious puberty")

Diabetes mellitus

Adrenocortical insufficiency

GH = growth hormone; GRH = growth hormone–releasing hormone.

of IGF-I established by one reference laboratory (Nichol's Institute) are: age 2 to 6, 0.64 ± 0.55 U/mL; age 6 to 10, 1.21 ± 0.75 U/mL; and age 10 to 17, 1.72 ± 1.01 U/mL. However, since IGF-I levels are low in conditions other than GH deficiency (eg, protein malnutrition), the diagnosis should be confirmed with provocative tests of GH secretion.

Basal GH values are highly variable. A value of > 6 ng/mL generally excludes GH deficiency, but normal values must be determined for each center. Not enough is known about endogenous GH secretion to rely on GH determinations alone for diagnosis, so provocative GH-stimulating tests are commonly used. Reduced GH responses to provocative stimuli (using arginine, insulin, levodopa, clonidine, exercise, or sleep) indicate GH deficiency. If diminished GH release is confirmed, then the secretion of other pituitary hormones must also be evaluated. Prolactin levels may be increased in children with craniopharyngiomas.

Children with normal levels of GH and very low levels of IGF-I have also been described. Since such children do show increases in IGF-I and growth velocity when given exogenous GH, it is suspected that they secrete biologically inactive GH.

Dwarfism secondary to environmental factors: Extreme emotional deprivation may also retard growth, apparently by hypothalamic inhibition of growth hormone–releasing hormone (GRH) release. Characteristically the family environment is poor and disordered. The child may be neglected, isolated, and abused. Resumption of normal growth occurs rapidly after removing the child from the oppressive environment (see also FAILURE TO THRIVE in Ch. 29, and Ch. 31).

Patients with **Laron dwarfism** have severe proportionate growth retardation, elevated GH levels, and low IGF-I levels. After administration of exogenous GH, IGF-I levels and growth velocity do not increase, implying a defect in the GH receptor.

In **hypothyroidism**, growth retardation is not proportionate; the extremities are particularly short in comparison to the rest of the body.

In **Turner's syndrome**, the short stature is often confused with pituitary dwarfism. Turner's syndrome may be strongly suspected in short girls with primary amenorrhea, webbed neck, a low nuchal hairline, short fourth metacarpal or metatarsal bones, a shield-like chest with widely spaced nipples, and cardiac abnormalities, especially coarctation of the aorta. Rarely, girls with short stature and gonadal dysgenesis have none of the stigmas usually associated with Turner's syndrome. Patients with these disorders have abnormalities involving the X chromosome as discussed in Gonadal Dysgenesis under Syndromes Associated with Sex Chromosome Aberrations in Ch. 48. Thus, chromosomal evaluation should be a part of the assessment of short girls who have no obvious cause of growth retardation.

The possibility of an occult **chronic inflammatory disease** also should be considered. Children with juvenile RA, rheumatic fever, and inflammatory bowel disease often present with growth failure. A thorough evaluation will usually suggest the cause. **Corticosteroids** should be used to treat affected children when indicated, bearing in mind that excess glucocorticoids from any source also inhibit skeletal growth.

A number of **congenital and hereditary diseases of the skeleton** must be considered, but disproportionate growth is generally easily recognized (see Musculoskeletal Defects in Ch. 28, and Ch. 42).

Many **renal diseases**, including chronic renal insufficiency, renal tubular acidosis, and Bartter's syndrome, are also associated with growth retardation. Since clinical signs may be absent in many such patients, all individuals in whom growth failure is unexplained should undergo tests to screen for renal disease.

Children with severe congenital **heart disease** and mentally retarded children with **CNS disease** may also suffer from retarded growth.

Treatment

Replacement therapy with exogenous human GH is indicated for all children with short stature who have documented GH deficiency. Semi-purified GH, prepared from human pituitary glands, has been banned because its use has transmitted fatal Creutzfeldt-Jacob disease. Purification procedures did not include steps known to exclude and inactivate agents causing the subacute spongiform viral encephalopathies. (The potential for transmission of infectious diseases with other purified hormones derived from human sources must always be remembered.)

Two synthetic human GH products of recombinant DNA origin—somatrem and somatropin—are available to replace the natural product. Results with synthetic GH appear to be identical to those obtained with highly purified monomeric pituitary human GH. Dosing is usually 3 times/wk, but optimal regimens have yet to be determined. Some reports have used s.c. dosing daily, and total weekly dosage varies. Larger doses may lead to more rapid growth. It has been suggested that the growth response is directly proportional to the logarithm of the dose between 30 and 100 mIU/kg. Increases in height of 10 to 15 cm frequently occur in the first year of treatment, but the growth rate may slow thereafter. Tripling the dose from 0.1 IU/kg to 0.3 IU/kg 3 times/wk is often effective in restoring the growth rate.

With the availability of synthetic GH, the question arises whether short children with normal GH levels and normal provocative tests of GH secretion, who may also have low IGF-I levels for their age, should be treated. The question is complicated, because current testing cannot detect all levels and forms of GH *functional* deficiencies; many short, slow-growing children respond well to synthetic GH administration; and there is abundant evidence that height discrimination occurs in the USA (ie, to be short is to be stigmatized). It has been suggested that such children be given a short-term trial of synthetic GH to determine therapeutic response. Increases in growth rate of at least 2 cm/yr greater than the pretreatment rate are considered a satisfactory response and a possible indication for long-term GH supplementation. However, the use of exogenous GH to treat individuals who do not have documented GH deficiency is controversial, and most authorities recommend against such use. The cost is high ($\approx$ $20,000/year), the optimal dose has not been determined, and there is little or no information on long-term results and any adverse effects. Such data should be accumulated in controlled trials. The use of GH in children with short stature from other causes has not been established, but GH-treated girls with Turner's syndrome grow faster and several have exceeded their previously predicted adult height.

Replacement of cortisol and thyroid hormone should be provided whenever indicated. Overtreatment of thyroid and adrenal deficiencies must be avoided or will impair the response to

GH. Replacement with gonadal steroids is not indicated until normal puberty occurs, treatment with exogenous GH is completed, or pubertal development needs to be induced because of hypogonadism. These steroids in high doses initiate epiphyseal closure, thereby *limiting* ultimate height.

CONGENITAL ADRENAL HYPERPLASIA

(See also discussion under Amenorrhea in Ch. 6)

The term congenital adrenal hyperplasia covers a group of disorders caused by defects in hydroxylation of cortisol precursors (see TABLE 40-2). The resulting low levels of cortisol induce increased secretion of corticotropin (ACTH), causing adrenal hyperplasia. In the most common forms, 21-hydroxylase and 11-hydroxylase defects, the net effect is an increased secretion from the adrenal gland of cortisol precursors and androgens. Hypersecretion of adrenal androgens during intrauterine life causes masculinization of the female external genitalia (pseudohermaphroditism)—see INTERSEX STATES in Ch. 28. Differentiation of ovaries, tubes, and uterus remains normal. If hypersecretion occurs before 12 wk gestation, there may be a persistent genitourinary sinus, a single opening for vagina and urethra, and even labioscrotal fusion. After 12 wk, only clitoral hypertrophy is produced. (Synthetic progestational agents or androgens taken during the first trimester of pregnancy may also cause masculinization of the external genitalia.) The phallus is enlarged in boys (macrogenitosomia), but the testes and prostate remain small at puberty because of suppression of luteinizing or interstitial-cell–stimulating hormone (LH or ICSH) and follicle-stimulating hormone (FSH) by excessive androgens. These children grow at an accelerated rate when young, but show advanced skeletal maturation. Because of premature closing of the epiphyses, their ultimate height is below average. If the defect in cortisol production is sufficiently severe, and especially if aldosterone production is also blocked, the neonate may develop life-threatening adrenal failure immediately after birth, which requires immediate treatment with cortisol and mineralocorticoid as well as appropriate fluid and electrolyte therapy. In patients with 11-hydroxylase block, an excess of the mineralocorticoid deoxycorticosterone is produced, which causes hypertension but protects against early adrenal failure.

Other defects, especially of 17-hydroxylase, cause phenotypic feminization of genetically male infants, in association with other characteristics of excessive mineralocorticoid activity.

Elevated urinary 17-ketosteroids (17-KS), especially dehydroepiandrosterone (DHEA) and its sulfate (DHEAS) as well as androsterone, with normal or decreased 17-hydroxycorticosteroids (17-OHCS), such as free cortisol, suggest the diagnosis of 11-hydroxylase or 21-hydroxylase defect. Amniotic fluid obtained between 14 and 20 wk gestation shows increased 17-OH progesterone and Δ^4-androstenedione levels in fetuses with the 21-hydroxylase defect. This should be confirmed by finding HLA type Bw47; HLA Bw51, Bw53, Bw60, and Dr7 are less positive supportive evidence. High 11-deoxycortisol is found in the 11-hydroxylase defect. After birth, raised serum 17-OH progesterone is found in patients with the 21-hydroxylase defect. The presence of excessive urinary pregnanetriol excretion gives strong support to the diagnosis of 21-hydroxylase defect, whereas in 11-hydroxylase block, excessive amounts of tetrahydro-S and tetrahydro deoxycorticosterone are excreted and serum deoxycorticosterone and deoxycortisol levels are elevated. Plasma testosterone levels are elevated in both defects. Plasma renin activity is elevated in patients with a mineralocorticoid defect (eg, 21-hydroxylase).

The female genotype in pseudohermaphrodite girls can be confirmed by leukocyte karyotyping. In boys with macrogenitosomia, true precocious puberty (see under DEVELOPMENTAL CONDITIONS in Ch. 47) must be ruled out. All of the defects are transmitted as autosomal recessive characteristics. The 21-hydroxylase defect is linked to HLA genes on chromosome 6; the others are not known to be HLA-linked. The gene for 11-hydroxylase is located on chromosome 8.

Treatment

Therapy with hydrocortisone arrests the disorder. Administration of hydrocortisone 0.3 mg/kg/day or 10 to 20 mg/m^2/day in divided doses s.c. in infants for 3 days reduces 17-KS (DHEA and DHEAS) by > 50%. In patients old enough to take tablets, hydrocortisone may be given orally, starting at 25 mg bid or 20 to 25 mg/m^2/day.

TABLE 40–2. TYPES OF METABOLIC BLOCKS
IN CONGENITAL ADRENAL HYPERPLASIA

Missing Enzyme	Deficiency	Excess	Phenotype
Desmolase	All steroid hormones	Lipid in adrenal	Adrenal insufficiency
3β-OL Dehydrogenase	Corticoids Aldosterone	Dehydroepiandrosterone Pregnenolone 17-Hydroxypregnenolone	Sodium loss, adrenal insufficiency Male: hypospadias Female: mild virilism
17-Hydroxylase	Androgens Estrogens Cortisol Aldosterone	Corticosterone 11-Deoxycorticosterone	Immature female; ambiguous genitalia in males Hypertension Low potassium Alkalosis
21-Hydroxylase	Aldosterone Corticoids	Androgens	Masculinization Sometimes sodium loss, adrenal insufficiency
11-Hydroxylase	Corticoids Aldosterone	Androgens 11-Deoxycorticosterone	Masculinization Hypertension
18-Hydroxylase	Aldosterone	Corticosterone	Sodium loss

Modified from *Metabolic Control and Disease* (formerly *Duncan's Diseases of Metabolism*), ed. 8, edited by PK Bondy and LE Rosenberg. Philadelphia, WB Saunders Company, 1980; used with permission.

Prednisolone 5 mg bid can be substituted. Patients with sodium-losing syndromes may require desoxycorticosterone or fludrocortisone as in adrenocortical insufficiency. Dosage should be titrated to maintain normal plasma 17-OH progesterone levels (< 50 ng/dL in childhood) or excretion levels of DHEAS (< 10 μg/24 h for each year of age until puberty). For simplicity, some prefer to follow total 17-KS (< 0.5 mg/24 h for each year of age until puberty). Serum electrolyte levels and BP should be followed closely, especially if the patient has a sodium-losing form of the disease (eg, 21-hydroxylase defect). Adequate treatment will reduce the plasma renin value to low-normal levels, a useful way to monitor mineralocorticoid replacement. The rate of growth should be monitored at least twice/yr, and bone age should be checked every few years. Ordinarily, these will be within normal limits if steroid suppression has been maintained. Surgical reconstruction of the external genitalia is often necessary in girls. Hydrocortisone therapy permits feminization of girls; menstruation occurs, and some treated patients have had normal pregnancies. Hydrocortisone suppresses androgen secretion in boys and permits secretion of LH and FSH at puberty so that testicular development and spermatogenesis may take place.

THE TESTES

MALE HYPOGONADISM

Decreased functional activity of the testes (either endocrinologic, gametogenic, or both), which results in retardation of growth and sexual development and/or reproductive insufficiency.

The testes have 2 functional components: interstitial (Leydig) cells that synthesize and secrete testosterone, and seminiferous tubules in which sperm production takes place. This discussion deals with problems that lead to androgen deficiency. For syndromes of androgen resistance, see INTERSEX STATES in Ch. 28; for congenital disorders of the testes and scrotum, see under RENAL AND GENITOURINARY DEFECTS also in Ch. 28.

Testicular Development and Function

During the 7th wk of male fetal development, the gonad differentiates into a testis, presumably under the influence of the H-Y antigen, a protein product of the Y chromosome that binds to receptors present on gonadal cells. Leydig cells appear during the 8th wk of intrauterine life. These cells actively secrete testosterone, initially under the influence of **human chorionic gonadotropin (HCG)** and later through stimulation by fetal pituitary **luteinizing hormone (LH)**. Testosterone stimulates development of the wolffian duct structures that include the epididymis, vas deferens, seminal vesicles, and ejaculatory ducts. Testosterone is taken up by the external genital tissue primordia and converted by the enzyme 5α-reductase to **dihydrotestosterone**, which brings about fusion of labioscrotal folds, resulting in the formation of the scrotum and penile urethra. This process takes place by the 12th wk of gestation. Sertoli cells in the fetal testes secrete **müllerian duct inhibitory factor**, a protein that brings about regression of the müllerian duct structures, thus preventing the development of the fallopian tubes, uterus, and upper third of the vagina in a normal male.

During the first several months following birth, serum concentrations of LH, **follicle-stimulating hormone (FSH)**, and testosterone are generally elevated above prenatal and early childhood levels. After about 6 mo, concentrations of the gonadotropins and testosterone remain low until puberty. About 99% of American males enter puberty between the ages of 9 and 14 yr. As gonadotropins rise, testicular enlargement ensues, primarily owing to rapid growth of the seminiferous tubules, which comprise > 80% of testicular volume. The earliest sign of puberty is enlargement of the testicles to > 2.5 cm in longest diameter (volume > 5 mL). Secondary sexual development, which includes deepening of the voice, growth of pubic and facial hair, male muscle development, growth of the scrotum, and linear growth spurt, normally takes place during the next 2 to 4½ yr and reflects increasing secretion of testosterone by the Leydig cells.

Postpubertally, testicular function is maintained through a complex interplay between the hypothalamus, pituitary, and testes. The hypothalamus secretes **gonadotropin-releasing hormone (GnRH)** in a pulsatile fashion every 90 to 120 min. GnRH in turn stimulates the gonadotropins in the anterior pituitary to secrete LH and FSH. LH circulates in the blood and binds with membrane receptors on the Leydig cells and, through an adenosine 3':5'-cyclic phosphate (**cAMP**)—mediated mechanism, promotes the conversion of cholesterol to pregnenolone, the first step in gonadal steroid biosynthesis. The end result is increased secretion of testosterone, which feeds back in a negative fashion, either directly or through conversion to estradiol, on the

pituitary and hypothalamus. FSH binds to membrane receptors on Sertoli cells and stimulates the secretion of androgen-binding protein and inhibin. **Androgen-binding protein** captures testosterone secreted by adjacent Leydig cells and allows the developing sperm cells to be bathed in a high concentration of testosterone required for normal maturation. **Inhibin**, a protein related to transforming growth factor-beta, enters the blood and inhibits the pituitary release of FSH. Thus, damage to the Leydig compartment results in low testosterone and a compensatory increase in LH, while damage to the seminiferous tubules may result in oligo- or azoospermia, deficient inhibin production, and elevation of serum FSH concentrations. Disorders of the hypothalamus or pituitary may be associated with low gonadotropins, low testosterone, and deficient sperm production (see below).

Symptoms and Signs

The age of onset of androgen deficiency dictates the clinical presentation. Early (< 12 wk) prenatal androgen deficiency or defects in androgen action result in inadequate differentiation of the external genitalia along male lines, leading to ambiguous genitalia ranging from mild hypospadias to fully developed female external genitalia (male pseudohermaphroditism). Androgen deficiency occurring at later stages of gestation may result in microphallus and inadequate descent of the testes.

Postnatal but prepubertal androgen deficiency results in inadequate secondary sexual development, including retention of a high-pitched voice; poor muscle development; inadequate growth of the phallus, testes, or scrotum; sparsity of axillary or pubic hair and failure to develop body hair; and the attainment of eunuchoidal proportions (span greater than height by 2 in., pubic to floor length greater than crown to pubic length by ≥ 2 in.), due to failure of the epiphyses to fuse with continued growth of the long bones under the influence of growth hormone.

Postpubertal testosterone deficiency has varied manifestations depending on the degree and length of deficiency. Decreased libido, potency, and overall strength are common. Testicular atrophy, fine wrinkling of the skin around the eyes and lips, and sparse body hair may be found with long-standing hypogonadism. Osteopenia may also be present. If hypogonadism is due to primary testicular failure, gynecomastia may occur.

Laboratory Assessment of Testicular Function

1. Semen analysis: A sample collected by masturbation following 2 days of abstinence from ejaculation provides an excellent index of seminiferous tubular function. A normal semen has a volume of 1 to 6 mL, $> 20 \times 10^6$ sperm/mL, of which 60% are of normal morphology and are motile.

2. Serum testosterone concentrations: Serum testosterone levels fluctuate throughout the day and, therefore, 3 blood samples at 20-min intervals should be obtained with equal aliquots of the sera combined for testosterone measurement. About 98% of testosterone is bound to serum proteins, leaving 2% capable of entering target tissues. Alterations in binding protein levels will alter total testosterone, and therefore in individuals with borderline-low testosterone concentrations, free testosterone measurements may be useful. Normal adult male values for total testosterone are generally > 300 ng/dL and for free testosterone > 50 pg/mL.

3. Serum gonadotropins: Serum concentrations of LH and FSH should be measured in pooled serum samples as described above. Although the normal range of both LH and FSH is generally 2 to 15 mIU/mL, some normal individuals will have undetectable gonadotropins at times. In the presence of a low testosterone, elevated gonadotropins indicate primary testicular disease, while low or normal gonadotropins suggest a pituitary hypothalamic disorder.

4. Chorionic gonadotropin stimulation test: Because HCG closely resembles LH, it binds to Leydig cell receptors and stimulates the secretion of testosterone. Following an injection of 500 IU/1.7 m^2 in adults or 100 IU/kg in children, testosterone levels should at least double after 72 to 96 h (1 IU = 1 USP u.).

5. Clomiphene citrate stimulation test: Clomiphene citrate is a weak estrogen that inhibits the binding of estradiol at various estrogen receptor sites. Since estradiol is an important inhibitor of serum gonadotropin secretion, occupancy of the estradiol receptors by a weak estrogen should result in decreased inhibition of gonadotropin secretion by estrogens. Normal individuals have a 50 to 250% increase in LH, a 30 to 200% increase in FSH, and a 30 to 220% increase in testosterone after 10 days of clomiphene citrate 100 mg orally bid. Patients with pituitary or hypothalamic problems may not have a rise in LH and FSH or testosterone.

6. Gonadotropin-releasing hormone test: The administration of 100 μg of GnRH by rapid IV injection directly stimulates the pituitary gonadotropes to secrete LH and FSH. A normal response is a two- to five-fold increase in LH over baseline concentration and a two-fold increase of FSH between 15 and 60 min after the injection. Patients with pituitary disease generally do not show a rise in gonadotropins, while patients with hypothalamic disease may have a normal or insufficient rise, the latter owing to gonadotroph atrophy from insufficient endogenous stimulation by GnRH. In patients with hypothalamic disease, the repeated pulsatile administration of GnRH may restore gonadotroph function to normal.

7. Testicular biopsy: This is rarely needed to establish the diagnosis of hypogonadism. It is generally restricted to men who have azoospermia with normal-sized testes in order to distinguish between ductal obstruction and failure at spermatogenesis.

Classification of Hypogonadism

Hypogonadism can be classified into 3 categories: hypothalamic-pituitary disorders (secondary hypogonadism), gonadal abnormalities (primary hypogonadism), and defects in androgen action. The latter group of disorders is discussed under INTERSEX STATES in Ch. 28.

HYPOTHALAMIC-PITUITARY DISORDERS

Panhypopituitarism may occur on a congenital basis due either to structural abnormalities in the pituitary or to hypothalamic-releasing hormone deficiencies. Acquired causes of panhypopituitarism include pituitary tumors, vascular disorders, infiltrative diseases such as sarcoidosis or histiocytosis involving the hypothalamus or pituitary, infectious destruction of the pituitary, trauma, hypothalamic neoplasms, and metastatic disease. Such patients present with multiple hormone deficiencies. If the patient is prepubertal, growth delay as well as secondary hypothyroidism and secondary hypoadrenalism may be found along with persistent sexual infantilism. Postpubertally, symptoms and signs of hypothyroidism and hypoadrenalism are mixed with impotence, decreased libido, and testicular atrophy.

LH and FSH deficiency (hypogonadotropic hypogonadism) may be associated with a normal sense of smell or with hyposmia or anosmia **(Kallmann's syndrome).** Although this syndrome is familial, multiple inheritance patterns have been described, including X-linked inheritance as well as autosomal dominant and autosomal recessive patterns. Other manifestations of the syndrome include short fourth metacarpals, syndactyly, and midline skeletal defects. The primary defect in these patients is an absence of the formation or release of GnRH by the hypothalamus. Pulsatile administration of GnRH mimicking the normal pulsatile patterns of every 90 to 120 min leads to increases in LH and FSH and virilization in the affected male.

Constitutional delay in adolescence: A complete absence of pubertal development in a boy of age 14 is considered to be delayed pubescence. In many instances there is a family history of delay in sexual development in a parent or sibling. The majority of boys obtain some degree of sexual maturation by age 18 or when the skeletal age reaches 12 yr. In addition to deficient sexual maturation, such boys usually exhibit short stature because of the absence of gonadal steroid-induced epiphyseal growth and closure. There are no reliable means other than watchful waiting to differentiate delayed puberty from Kallmann's syndrome.

Isolated LH deficiency (fertile eunuch syndrome): Some patients have a monotropic loss of LH secretion while FSH secretion remains normal. At puberty these boys have growth of the testes, since the vast majority of testicular volume is made up of seminiferous tubules responsive to FSH. Spermatogenesis may occur as tubular development proceeds. However, the absence of LH results in Leydig cell atrophy and prepubertal testosterone levels. Therefore, these boys do not develop normal secondary sexual characteristics and continue to grow, attaining eunuchoidal proportions since they do not have androgen-induced closure of their epiphyses.

Other syndromes: Several complex hypothalamic syndromes have been associated with secondary hypogonadism. These include the Prader-Willi and Laurence-Moon-Biedl syndromes. Acute illnesses as well as chronic systemic disorders may be associated with hypogonadotropic hypogonadism, which improves following recovery from the underlying disorder.

PRIMARY HYPOGONADISM

Klinefelter's syndrome (see also under SYN-DROMES ASSOCIATED WITH SEX CHROMOSOME ABERRATIONS in Ch. 48): The most frequent cause of primary hypogonadism is XXY seminiferous tubule dysgenesis, in which an extra X chromosome is acquired through maternal (and to a lesser extent paternal) meiotic nondisjunction. Most pa-

tients escape detection until puberty, when there is a variable degree of sexual maturation, with the spectrum going from virtually no sexual development to development that overlaps with normal males. The testes are small (< 2 cm), firm, and fibrotic. Gynecomastia is present in the majority of individuals, and these patients have abnormal skeletal proportions with a greater pubic to floor height than crown to pubic bone height. These patients may also demonstrate dyssocial behavior, chronic pulmonary disease, varicose veins, glucose intolerance, primary hypothyroidism, and breast cancer. Gonadotropins are elevated, testosterone levels are in the low-normal to low range, and a female type of buccal smear and an XXY karyotype is present.

Bilateral anorchia (vanishing testes syndrome): About 1:20,000 males have testes that presumably were present and then were resorbed prior to birth or postnatally. Since these individuals have normal external genitalia, normal wolffian duct structures, and absence of müllerian duct structures, testicular tissue must have been present during the first 12 wk of gestation in order to secrete sufficient testosterone to bring about male sexual differentiation as well as müllerian duct inhibitory substance to cause regression of the müllerian duct structures. These patients present a clinical picture similar to that of bilateral cryptorchidism (see below) but, unlike patients with cryptorchidism, fail to have a rise in testosterone following HCG injections.

Leydig cell aplasia: Congenital absence of Leydig cells is a cause of male pseudohermaphroditism associated with ambiguous genitalia. Although there is some wolffian duct development, there is insufficient testosterone production to provide for normal external genitalia differentiation. Müllerian duct structures are absent because of normal Sertoli cell production of the inhibitory factor. Elevated serum gonadotropins and low testosterone concentration are found, and there is no testosterone increase following HCG administration.

Cryptorchidism (see also UNDESCENDED TESTES under RENAL AND GENITOURINARY DEFECTS in Ch. 28): At birth about 3% of male infants have cryptorchidism, most of whom have resolution by 1 yr of age. Long-standing bilateral cryptorchidism is associated with oligospermia and infertility, possibly owing to the increased testicular temperature found when the testicles are in an intra-abdominal or inguinal position. Early correction of the disorder is indicated to try to prevent this complication, as well as testicular torsion, and to reduce the risk of testicular neoplasms.

Noonan's syndrome (male Turner's syndrome) is a complex disorder that may occur sporadically or as an autosomal dominant familial problem. It is associated with a number of somatic abnormalities, including hyperelasticity of the skin, webbing of the neck, hypertelorism, ptosis, low-set ears, short stature, shortened fourth metacarpals, high-arched palate, and cardiovascular abnormalities including pulmonary stenosis, supravalvular pulmonary artery stenosis, atrial septal defect, and coarctation of the aorta. Testes are often small and are associated with low testosterone and high gonadotropin levels.

Myotonic dystrophy: About 80% of males with myotonic dystrophy have primary testicular failure, with testicular biopsies that show derangements of spermatogenesis, hyalinization, and fibrosis. In addition to the muscle weakness and atrophy, frontal balding, mental retardation, cataracts, diabetes mellitus, primary hypothyroidism, and cranial hyperostosis may be found. As with other causes of primary hypogonadism, gonadotropins are elevated with testosterone levels being low or low-normal.

Adult seminiferous tubular failure: Oligospermia or azoospermia associated with infertility may be found in men who have idiopathic seminiferous tubular failure or who have developed such failure following testicular infections (eg, mumps or gonorrhea), cryptorchidism, uremia, antineoplastic agents, alcoholism, irradiation, vascular damage, or trauma. In addition to an abnormal semen analysis, serum FSH levels may be elevated, although with mild oligospermia the levels may be normal. Serum testosterone and LH concentrations are usually in the normal range, although there may be an excessive rise in LH following GnRH stimulation, suggesting mild androgen deficiency.

Enzymatic defects: Multiple defects in the enzymatic pathways leading to testosterone production have been described. These congenital problems are associated with marked ambiguity of the genitalia and are a cause of male pseudohermaphroditism.

Treatment

Patients with hypogonadotropic hypogonadism should receive therapy directed toward the underlying pituitary-hypothalamic disorder, if any is found. Boys with delayed onset of puberty, who have marked psychosocial adjustment problems

because of their inadequate sexual development, may be given a 3-mo course of testosterone enanthate or testosterone cypionate 100 mg IM once a month. This will bring about some degree of virilization and height increase without significantly compromising final adult height.

Androgen deficiency per se in adults should be treated with a long-acting testosterone preparation such as testosterone enanthate or testosterone cypionate. Either may be given in doses of 200 mg IM q 2 wk to achieve optimal adult therapeutic levels. Major side effects include fluid retention, acne, and occasionally transient gynecomastia. Oral androgen preparations should not be used, since they are less effective and carry a risk of hepatocellular dysfunction or tumor formation. Men with hypogonadotropic hypogonadism who want to develop spermatogenesis may be given menopausal gonadotropins that contain 75 IU each of FSH and LH at a dose of 1 to 2 vials IM 3 times/wk along with 2000 IU of HCG IM 3 times/wk. This therapy must be given for at least 3 mo to achieve an effect on spermatogenesis. Alternatively, pulsatile administration of GnRH through a portable infusion pump may be tried if sufficient gonadotroph reserve is present.

Patients with primary hypogonadism should be given testosterone replacement therapy unless there is a major contraindication. Therapy with testosterone cypionate or enanthate 200 mg IM q 2 wk is adequate replacement therapy and should reduce the likelihood of osteopenia, vasomotor instability, decreased libido, and impotence developing. There are no uniformly good medical therapies for the treatment of idiopathic oligospermia. However, if the sperm concentration is sufficient, sperm obtained from ejaculated specimens that are washed and capacitated may be tried for in vitro fertilization of harvested eggs. (See also Ch. 3.)

POLYGLANDULAR DEFICIENCY SYNDROMES
(Autoimmune Polyglandular Syndromes; Polyendocrine Deficiency Syndromes)

Concurrent subnormal function of several endocrine glands.

Etiology and Pathogenesis

Endocrine deficiency can be caused by infection, infarction, or tumor destroying all or a large part of the gland. However, the activity of an en-

TABLE 40-3. CHARACTERISTICS OF TYPE I AND TYPE II
POLYGLANDULAR DEFICIENCY SYNDROMES

Characteristic	Type I	Type II
Age at onset	Childhood (peak 12 yr)	Adult (peak 30 yr)
HLA types	A28, A3	Primarily B8, DW3, DR3, DR4; others in specific diseases
Female/male	1.4/1.0	1.8/1.0
Clinical manifestations (% involved)		
Addison's disease	67%	100%
Thyroid disease*	10–11%	69%
Pernicious anemia	13–15%	< 1%
Diabetes mellitus (insulin-dependent)	2–4%	52%
Gonadal failure	45%	3.5%
Hypoparathyroidism	82%	Not seen
Vitiligo	4%	5–50%
Chronic mucocutaneous candidiasis	73–78%	Not seen
Chronic active hepatitis	11–13%	Not seen
Alopecia	26–32%	Not seen
Malabsorption	22–24%	Not seen
Celiac disease and myasthenia gravis	Not seen	Incidence uncertain

* Usually chronic lymphocytic thyroiditis, but includes also Graves' disease.
Adapted from Trence DL, Morley JE, Handwerger BS: "Polyglandular autoimmune syndromes." *American Journal of Medicine* 77(1):107–116, 1984; and from Leshin M: "Polyglandular autoimmune syndromes." *American Journal of Medical Sciences* 290(2):77–88, 1985; used with permission.

docrine organ is most often depressed as a result of an autoimmune reaction that produces inflammation, lymphocyte infiltration, and partial or complete destruction of the gland. Autoimmune disease affecting one organ is frequently followed by impairment of other glands, resulting in multiple endocrine failure. Two major patterns of failure have been described (see TABLE 40-3).

In type I, onset usually occurs in childhood, and hypoparathyroidism is the most frequent manifestation, followed by adrenal cortical failure. Chronic mucocutaneous candidiasis is also commonly present, and diabetes mellitus seldom occurs. This pattern is associated with HLA types A3 and A28. The pattern of inheritance is not clear, but some kinships appear to have an autosomal recessive pattern.

In type II, glandular failure generally occurs in adults, with peak incidence at age 30. It always involves the adrenal cortex and frequently also the thyroid gland (Schmidt's syndrome) and the pancreatic islets, producing insulin-dependent diabetes mellitus (IDDM). Antibodies against the target organs are frequently present, but their role in producing glandular damage is unclear. Some patients have thyroid-stimulating antibodies and initially present with the clinical picture of hyperthyroidism. The glandular destruction seen in these patients is chiefly a result of cell-mediated autoimmunity, probably because of depressed suppressor T-cell function. In addition, reduced cell-mediated immunity is frequently present, manifested by poor response on skin testing to standard antigens such as *Candida*, *Trichophyton*, and tuberculin. Depressed reactivity is also found in about 30% of first-degree relatives with normal endocrine function. There is a characteristic HLA pattern, and it has been suggested that the specific HLA types in type II are associated with susceptibility to certain viruses that induce the destructive reaction.

An additional group, type III, occurs in adults and does not involve the adrenal cortex, but includes at least 2 of the following: thyroid deficiency, IDDM, pernicious anemia, vitiligo, and alopecia. Since the diagnosis of the type III pattern depends on the absence of adrenocortical insufficiency, it may merely be a wastebasket of combined disease that is converted to type II if adrenal failure develops.

Symptoms, Signs, and Diagnosis

The clinical appearance of patients with polyglandular deficiency syndromes is the sum of the picture of each of the individual deficiencies.

There is no specific sequence for appearance of individual glandular damage. Measurement of the levels of circulating antibody against the endocrine organs or their components does not appear to be useful, since such antibodies may persist for years without development of clinical endocrine failure. However, the presence of antibodies is clearly helpful in differentiating autoimmune from tuberculous hypoadrenalism and determining the cause of hypothyroidism. The presence of multiple endocrine deficiencies may raise a question of hypothalamic-pituitary failure. In almost all instances, elevated plasma levels of pituitary tropic hormones will demonstrate the peripheral nature of the defect; but rare instances of hypothalamic-pituitary insufficiency have also been reported as a part of the type II syndrome.

Treatment

Treatment of the various glandular deficiencies is the same as for sporadic examples of the individual diseases discussed elsewhere in THE MANUAL, but the interaction of multiple deficiencies (eg, adrenal cortical insufficiency combined with diabetes mellitus) may complicate clinical management. Patients manifesting hypofunction of one organ should be observed during follow-up over a period of years for development of additional defects. Gonadal failure does not respond, and chronic mucocutaneous candidiasis is usually resistant to treatment.

DIABETES MELLITUS (DM)
(See also DIABETES MELLITUS in Ch. 17)

A syndrome characterized by hyperglycemia resulting from impaired insulin secretion and/or effectiveness, associated with risks for diabetic ketoacidosis (DKA) or nonketotic hyperglycemic-hyperosmolar coma (NKHHC) and a group of late complications including retinopathy, nephropathy, atherosclerotic coronary and peripheral arterial disease, and peripheral and autonomic neuropathies. DM has diverse genetic, environmental, and pathogenic origins.

Classification and Pathogenesis

Current classifications are based on clinical criteria, eg, the presence or absence of a propensity to DKA, as well as on ancillary criteria used to segregate specific pathogenic forms of DM (see TABLE 40-4).

Insulin-dependent diabetes mellitus (IDDM, type I DM) accounts for 10 to 15% of all cases of DM and is clinically characterized by hyperglycemia and a propensity to DKA. Its control requires chronic insulin treatment. Although it may occur at any age, it most commonly develops in childhood or adolescence and is the predominant type of DM diagnosed before age 30. The term IDDM (or type I DM) is also used more restrictively to refer to the subset of patients with DKA-prone DM diagnosed prior to age 30, in which specific HLA phenotypes are associated with detectable serum islet cell cytoplasmic antibodies (ICA) and/or islet cell surface antibodies (ICSA) in about 80% of cases at diagnosis. In these patients, IDDM results from a genetically conditioned, immune-mediated, selective destruction of > 90% of their insulin-secreting β cells. If these patients die shortly after the onset of IDDM, their pancreatic islets exhibit **insulitis**, which is characterized by an infiltration of T lymphocytes accompanied by macrophages and B lymphocytes and by the loss of most of the β cells, without involvement of the glucagon-secreting α cells. Cell-mediated immune mechanisms are believed to play the major role in the β-cell destruction.

The ICA and ICSA present at diagnosis usually become undetectable after 1 to 2 yr; they may be primarily a response to β-cell destruction, but some are cytotoxic for β cells and may contribute to their loss. Cytotoxicity is particularly associated with islet cell autoantibodies that selectively bind to β cells (many ICA are not β cell specific). Glutamic acid decarboxylase (GAD) was recently found to be the autoantigen for one of the β cell–specific autoantibodies present at diagnosis in ~80% of IDDM patients. (GAD, the enzyme that synthesizes the neurotransmitter γ-aminobutyric acid, is found in high levels only in pancreatic islet β cells and in the brain.) The clinical onset of IDDM is characteristically abrupt, but it may occur in some patients years after the insidious onset of the underlying autoimmune process. (Detectable ICA and subclinical alterations in glucose tolerance have been found in some siblings and parents of IDDM patients, years before these first-degree relatives developed IDDM.)

In white populations there is a strong association between IDDM diagnosed before age 30 and specific HLA-D phenotypes (HLA-DR3, HLA-DR4, and HLA-DR3/HLA-DR4), and one or more genes that convey susceptibility to IDDM are believed to be located near or in the HLA-D locus on chro-

TABLE 40–4. GENERAL CHARACTERISTICS OF THE MAJOR CLINICAL
TYPES OF DIABETES MELLITUS (DM)

Characteristic	Insulin-Dependent DM (IDDM, Type I DM)	Non–insulin-Dependent DM (NIDDM, Type II DM)
Age at onset	Most commonly < 30 yr	Most commonly > 30 yr
Associated obesity	No	Very common
Propensity to ketoacidosis requiring insulin treatment for its control	Yes	No
Endogenous insulin secretion	Extremely low to undetectable plasma insulin and C-peptide levels	Significant but variable levels of insulin secretion that are low relative to plasma glucose levels and accompanied by insulin resistance
Twin concurrence	< 50%	> 90%
Associated with specific HLA-D antigens	Yes	No
Islet cell antibodies at diagnosis	Yes	No
Islet pathology	Insulitis, selective loss of most β cells	Smaller, normal-appearing islets; amyloid (amylin) deposition common
Associated risks for retinopathy, nephropathy, neuropathy, and atherosclerotic coronary and peripheral vascular disease in most Western populations	Yes	Yes
Hyperglycemia responds to sulfonylureas	No	Yes, initially in many patients

mosome 6. Specific HLA-DQ alleles appear to be more intimately related to risks for or protection from IDDM than HLA-D antigens, and current evidence suggests that genetic susceptibility to IDDM is probably polygenic. Only 10 to 12% of newly diagnosed children with IDDM have a first-degree relative with IDDM. The concordance rate for IDDM in monozygotic twins is ≤ 50%, and in genetically susceptible individuals some environmental factor, probably a virus (congenital rubella, mumps, and coxsackie B viruses have been postulated), appears to incite the development of autoimmune β-cell destruction and IDDM.

Non–insulin-dependent diabetes mellitus (NIDDM, type II DM) is characterized clinically by hyperglycemia that is not associated with a propensity to DKA, but some patients intermittently or persistently require insulin to control or prevent symptomatic degrees of hyperglycemia, which might lead to NKHHC. NIDDM is usually the type diagnosed in patients > 30 yr of age, but it also occurs in children and adolescents. It

is commonly associated with obesity. The concordance rate for NIDDM in monozygotic twins is > 90%, and genetic factors appear to be the major determinants of its development. No association between NIDDM and specific HLA phenotypes or ICA has been demonstrated (an exception is a subset of nonobese adults with detectable ICA who carry one of the HLA phenotypes and who may eventually develop IDDM). The pancreatic islets in NIDDM retain β cells in ratios to α cells that are not consistently altered, and normal β-cell mass appears to be preserved in most patients. Pancreatic islet amyloid, resulting from a deposition of amylin, is found in a high percentage of NIDDM patients at autopsy, but its relationship to the pathogenesis of NIDDM is unknown.

NIDDM is a heterogeneous group of disorders in which hyperglycemia results from both an impaired insulin secretory response to glucose and decreased insulin effectiveness (**insulin resistance**). Most patients retain a significant, but variable, insulin secretory capacity but exhibit a decreased insulin secretory response to glucose, which is most pronounced in patients with both fasting and postprandial hyperglycemia. Recent studies using an assay that is highly specific for insulin have demonstrated that there is a considerable overlap in fasting plasma insulin levels in NIDDM patients and age- and weight-matched controls, but that both obese and nonobese NIDDM patients have a delayed and *decreased* rise in plasma insulin following glucose ingestion despite their higher plasma glucose levels. The degree of abnormality in the peripheral plasma insulin response to glucose ingestion in both obese and nonobese NIDDM patients correlates with the degree of fasting hyperglycemia.

Persistent hyperglycemia has a "toxic" effect on β cells, which may augment the primary abnormality in insulin secretion and explain why many NIDDM patients show some improvement in the insulin secretory response to ingested glucose after a period of vigorous insulin control of the hyperglycemia or aggressive diet therapy. Some primary β-cell abnormality may be necessary for the development of NIDDM, but an acquired (eg, obesity related) or genetically determined insulin resistance appears to be required. NIDDM patients exhibit decreased insulin effectiveness in restraining hepatic glucose output and in stimulating glucose uptake by skeletal muscle, which are important in normal plasma glucose regulation. Obesity and inadequate insulin secretion can cause similar manifestations of insulin resistance, and the existence of a primary genetically determined insulin resistance in most NIDDM patients is controversial. The insulin resistance does not appear to result from genetic alterations in insulin receptor numbers or function, but a role for genetically determined postreceptor defects is possible. In obese NIDDM patients, improvement in the insulin secretory response to glucose is frequently observed after a period of weight reduction associated with decreased hyperglycemia or after rigorous insulin treatment.

Insulinopathies: Rare cases of DM, with the clinical characteristics of NIDDM, result from the heterozygous inheritance of a defective gene, leading to secretion of insulin that does not bind normally to the insulin receptor. These patients have greatly elevated plasma immunoreactive insulin (**IRI**) levels associated with normal plasma glucose responses to exogenous insulin.

Maturity-onset diabetes of young people (MODY) is NIDDM with an autosomal dominant inheritance found in successive generations of some families, frequently in asymptomatic, nonobese, young adolescents.

Diabetes attributed to pancreatic disease: Chronic pancreatitis, particularly in alcoholics, is frequently associated with diabetes. In Asia, Africa, and the Caribbean, malnutrition-related DM is commonly observed in young, severely emaciated patients with severe protein deficiency and pancreatic disease, who are not DKA-prone but who may require insulin treatment.

Diabetes associated with other endocrine diseases: DM can be a secondary manifestation of Cushing's syndrome, acromegaly, pheochromocytoma, glucagonoma, primary aldosteronism, or somatostatinoma, resulting from the influence of the primary endocrine abnormality on insulin effectiveness and/or secretion. Patients with certain autoimmune endocrine diseases, eg, Graves' disease, Hashimoto's thyroiditis, and idiopathic Addison's disease, have an increased prevalence of IDDM (see POLYGLANDULAR DEFICIENCY SYNDROMES, above).

Insulin-resistant DM associated with acanthosis nigricans (type A and type B insulin resistance syndromes): Two rare syndromes result from marked insulin resistance at the insulin receptor level associated with acanthosis nigricans. Type A results from genetic alterations in the insulin receptor. Type B results from circulating antibodies to the insulin receptor and may be associated with other evidence of autoimmune disease.

Lipoatrophic diabetes, a rare syndrome in which insulin-resistant DM is associated with an extensive symmetrical or virtually complete disappearance of subcutaneous adipose tissue, has been linked to genetic alterations in the insulin receptor.

Diabetes induced by β-cell toxins: Vacor™, a rodenticide commonly used in suicide attempts in Korea, is cytotoxic for human islets and commonly causes IDDM in survivors. The use of streptozocin in treating pancreatic islet carcinomas rarely causes diabetes, although this β-cell toxin can induce experimental diabetes in rats.

Symptoms and Signs

DM has diverse initial presentations. IDDM patients usually present with symptomatic hyperglycemia or DKA. NIDDM may initially present with symptomatic hyperglycemia or NKHHC, but is frequently diagnosed in asymptomatic patients during a routine medical study or when patients present with clinical manifestations of a late complication.

Symptomatic hyperglycemia: Polyuria, polydipsia, and weight loss, despite a normal or sometimes increased dietary intake, occur when elevated plasma glucose levels cause marked glucosuria and an osmotic diuresis, resulting in dehydration. Polyuria is the initial manifestation. In IDDM there also is usually a rise in plasma ketones, frequently followed by DKA, sometimes within hours. In NIDDM symptomatic hyperglycemia may persist for days or weeks before medical attention is sought; in women it is frequently associated with itching due to vaginal candidiasis.

Acute complications: see below under Diagnosis and Treatment of Diabetic Ketoacidosis (DKA); and Diagnosis and Treatment of Nonketotic Hyperglycemic-Hyperosmolar Coma (NKHHC).

Late complications: The risks of a late clinical complication vary markedly in individuals but generally increase with increasing duration of DM. Hyperglycemia causes the initial metabolic alterations and early functional alterations in the kidney, peripheral nerves, and retina in diabetics; but evidence suggests that once these structural alterations reach a given stage, factors other than hyperglycemia determine the subsequent course. The symptoms and signs of late complications of DM mimic those of pathologically similar or indistinguishable disease in the same organ or system in nondiabetics. These manifestations may be present at diagnosis in those with NIDDM, but not in those with IDDM.

Atherosclerotic coronary artery disease (manifested by angina and/or myocardial infarction) and peripheral atherosclerotic vascular disease (manifested by intermittent claudication and gangrene) are more common in diabetics than in nondiabetics and occur at an earlier age.

Diabetic retinopathy (see also DIABETIC RETINOPATHY in Ch. 83): Background retinopathy (the initial retinal changes seen on ophthalmoscopic examination or in retinal photographs) does not significantly alter vision, but it can lead to processes that cause blindness (eg, macular edema or proliferative retinopathy with retinal detachment or hemorrhage). *Patients with background retinopathy require regularly scheduled examinations by an ophthalmologist, since specific retinal findings are indications for prompt retinal laser photocoagulation therapy to prevent or control macular edema or proliferative retinopathy.* Evidence of retinopathy, rarely present at diagnosis in IDDM, is present in up to 20% of NIDDM patients at diagnosis. About 85% of all diabetics eventually develop some degree of retinopathy.

Diabetic nephropathy is usually asymptomatic until end-stage renal disease develops, but it can cause the nephrotic syndrome prior to the development of uremia. Nephropathy develops in 30 to 50% of IDDM patients and in a smaller percentage of NIDDM patients. In patients with IDDM, persistent clinically detectable albuminuria ($\geq$ 300 mg/L) unexplained by other urinary tract disease can predict a progressive decrease in GFR and the development of end-stage renal disease within 3 to 20 yr (median, 10 yr). Albuminuria is absent during the first 5 yr of IDDM; its incidence increases and peaks during the 2nd decade and then declines. In NIDDM albuminuria is occasionally present at diagnosis. Albuminuria is almost 2.5 times higher in IDDM patients with diastolic BP $>$ 90 mm Hg than in those in whom it is $<$ 70 mm Hg. Whether the higher BPs result from more advanced renal disease or whether clinical nephropathy develops primarily in patients with a predisposition to essential hypertension is controversial, but hypertension accelerates the progression to end-stage renal disease.

Diabetic neuropathy: The most common form is a distal, symmetric, predominantly sensory **polyneuropathy** that causes sensory deficits with a stocking-glove distribution, which begin and are usually most marked in the feet and legs. Diabetic polyneuropathy is frequently asymptomatic but may be associated with numbness, tingling, and paresthesias in the extremities, and less often with debilitating, severe, deep-seated pain and hyperesthesias. Ankle jerks are usually decreased or absent. Symptoms and signs of polyneuropathy can be present at diagnosis in patients with NIDDM but are not usually found in those with recently diagnosed IDDM. Other causes of polyneuropathy must be excluded. Acute, painful **mononeuropathies** affecting the 3rd, 4th, or 6th cranial nerve, which may spontaneously improve over a period of weeks to months, occur more frequently in older diabetics and are attributed to nerve infarctions. **Autonomic neuropathy** occurs primarily in diabetics with polyneuropathy and can cause postural hypotension, disordered sweating, impotence and retrograde ejaculation in men, impaired bladder functions, delayed gastric emptying, esophageal dysfunction, constipation or diarrhea, and nocturnal diarrhea. Alterations in the cardiac rate response to the Valsalva maneuver or on standing and in heart rate variation during deep breathing are evidence of autonomic neuropathy in diabetics.

Foot ulcers are an important cause of morbidity in DM. The major predisposing cause is diabetic polyneuropathy—the sensory denervation impairs the perception of trauma from common causes (ill-fitting shoes, pebbles, etc), and alterations in proprioception lead to an abnormal pattern of weightbearing and in some instances to the development of typical Charcot's joints.

Infections commonly result from manipulation of an ingrown toenail, plantar corn, or callus. A mycotic infection may be the initial process, leading to wet interdigital lesions, cracks, fissures, and ulcerations that favor secondary bacterial invasion. Patients with infected foot ulcers frequently feel no pain because of neuropathy and have no systemic symptoms until late in a neglected course. The infection may extend into the deeper soft tissues and result in osteomyelitis of foot bones. Cultures of samples from superficial and deep tissues usually demonstrate mixed bacterial flora, including aerobic gram-positive cocci and gram-negative enteric bacteria and anaerobic organisms, particularly *Bacteroides* sp and various anaerobic gram-positive cocci; differences in the specific components of the flora at the 2 sites are common. Deep ulcers and particularly those associated with any detectable cellulitis require immediate hospitalization, since there are risks of developing systemic toxicity and permanent disability, and early surgical debridement is an essential part of appropriate management.

Diagnosis

The principal aim of diagnosis is to identify patients at risk for symptomatic hyperglycemia, for DKA or NKHHC, and for late clinical complications, ruling out those who have fluctuations only in the upper range of their plasma glucose levels, which may not convey the risks associated with DM. Symptomatic hyperglycemia, DKA, or NKHHC unequivocally establishes a diagnosis of DM. In asymptomatic patients, DM is established when the diagnostic criteria for fasting hyperglycemia recommended by the National Diabetes Data Group (NDDG) are met: a plasma (or serum) glucose level of $\geq$ 140 mg/dL after an overnight fast on 2 occasions in an adult or child (the glucose concentration in venous samples of whole blood is about 15% lower than that in plasma). If these criteria are met, an **oral glucose tolerance test (OGTT—see below) is unnecessary.**

The major indication for an OGTT is to exclude or diagnose NIDDM in those suspected of having diabetes although fasting or symptomatic hyperglycemia is absent; eg, in patients with a clinical condition that might be related to undiagnosed DM (eg, polyneuropathy, retinopathy). However, an OGTT diagnosis of DM does not necessarily predict the subsequent development of fasting or symptomatic hyperglycemia. Various conditions (other than DM) and drugs can cause abnormalities in the OGTT. The NDDG criteria (see below and in TABLE 40–5) for an OGTT diagnosis of DM apply only to healthy patients who do not have infections, acute cardiovascular or cerebrovascular disease, endocrine disease that impairs glucose tolerance, or hepatic, renal, or CNS disease. These criteria also do not apply to patients treated with drugs that can impair glucose tolerance (eg, thiazides, phenytoin, glucocorticoids, indomethacin, nicotinic acid, oral contraceptives containing synthetic estrogens) or to patients who develop nausea, sweating, faintness, or pallor during the test. (The effects of **pregnancy** on the OGTT and the diagnosis of gestational diabetes are discussed under DIABETES MELLITUS in Ch. 17.)

No special dietary preparation is required for an OGTT unless the patient has been ingesting < 150 gm/day of carbohydrate. The test should be done in the morning after a 10- to 14-h fast, without prior coffee or smoking, with the patient seated upright. A chilled solution containing 75 gm of glucose is used in adults; the test dose in children is 1.75 gm/kg ideal body wt up to a maximum of 75 gm. Commercial solutions, flavored for palatability, may be used. Blood samples are obtained fasting and at 30-min intervals over 2 h from the initial swallow of the glucose solution. A diagnosis of DM in a nonpregnant adult is justified if the plasma glucose level at both 2 h and one other time between 0 and 2 h is $\geq$ 200 mg/dL. The criteria for the OGTT diagnosis in asymptomatic *children* are stricter (because of the greater risk of overdiagnosing DM) and also require a fasting plasma glucose $\geq$ 140 mg/dL. A final diagnosis of DM based solely on an OGTT requires a repeated positive test.

As indicated in TABLE 40–5, the NDDG also recommends criteria for the diagnosis of impaired glucose tolerance (IGT) in individuals who do not meet the OGTT diagnostic criteria for DM, but whose plasma glucose values are higher than normal. Patients with IGT may be at increased

TABLE 40-5. DIAGNOSTIC CRITERIA OF THE NATIONAL
DIABETES DATA GROUP

	Criteria for Diagnosis of Diabetes Mellitus and Impaired Glucose Tolerance (All plasma glucose values in mg/dL)						Criteria for Diagnosis of Gestational Diabetes (100 gm OGTT)
	Normal		Diabetes Mellitus		Impaired Glucose Tolerance		Venous Plasma Glucose
	Adult	Child	Adult	Child	Adult	Child	Fasting ≥ 105 mg/dL
FPG	< 115	< 130	≥ 140	≥ 140	115–139	130–139	1 h ≥ 190 mg/dL
OGTT	< 140	< 140	≥ 200	≥ 200	140–199	140–199	2 h ≥ 165 mg/dL
							3 h ≥ 145 mg/dL

FPG = fasting plasma glucose; OGTT = oral glucose tolerance test (at least 2 values).
From Harris M, et al for the National Diabetes Data Group: "Classification and diagnosis of diabetes mellitus and other categories of glucose intolerance." *Diabetes* 28:1049, 1979. Copyright 1979 by American Diabetes Association, Inc.; reprinted with permission.

risk of developing fasting or symptomatic hyperglycemia, but in many patients the IGT does not progress or reverts to normal.

Treatment

General considerations: There is good evidence that hyperglycemia conveys risks for all of the common late complications of DM, which are the major causes of excess morbidity and mortality in diabetics. However, there is no generally applicable and consistently effective means of maintaining persistently *normal* plasma glucose fluctuations in diabetics, and efforts to do so entail significant risks of causing frequent or severe hypoglycemic episodes, particularly in IDDM patients. Treatment regimens differ in the priorities assigned to keeping the risks for hypoglycemia *minimal* and to keeping the diurnal plasma glucose fluctuations in a normal to near-normal range. Regimens are effective in preventing symptomatic hyperglycemia and DKA or NKHHC under most circumstances, but their ability to reduce the risks for the common late complications of DM is unknown.

The recommended target maximum acceptable plasma glucose levels vary, but postprandial plasma glucose levels > 200 mg/dL should be avoided whenever possible with minimal risk of hypoglycemia. This stems from the observation in the Pima Indian population, 40% of whom have NIDDM, that diabetic complications are rare in individuals whose 2-h plasma glucose level during an OGTT is < 200 mg/dL. Many authorities add the recommendation that fasting levels be kept ≤ 130 mg/dL. These goals are possible in most NIDDM patients and some IDDM patients, but they must be individualized and should be

modified when circumstances make any risk of hypoglycemia unacceptable (eg, in patients with a short life expectancy, those with cerebrovascular or cardiac disease) or increase the risks of being hypoglycemic (eg, in patients who are unreliable or who have autonomic neuropathy).

Patient education is essential to ensure the effectiveness of the prescribed therapy, to recognize indications for seeking immediate medical attention, and to carry out appropriate foot care. On each physician visit, the patient should be assessed for symptoms or signs of complications, including a check of the feet and the pulses and sensation in the feet and legs, and a urine test for albumin. The BUN or serum creatinine levels should be assessed regularly (at least yearly), and an ECG and complete ophthalmologic evaluation should be performed at least yearly (see DIABETIC RETINOPATHY in Ch. 83). Coexistent hypertension or hypercholesterolemia increases the risks for specific late complications and requires special attention and appropriate treatment (see ANOMALIES IN LIPID METABOLISM, below). Psychologic problems are frequently seen in children and adolescents with IDDM and their families as a result of the associated stresses, and professional assistance is often helpful.

Because there is an increased risk of acute renal failure in diabetics, x-ray studies that require IV injection of contrast dyes should be performed only when absolutely necessary and only when the patient is well hydrated.

Although β-adrenergic blockers (eg, propranolol) can be used safely in most diabetics, they can mask the β-adrenergic symptoms of insulin-induced hypoglycemia and delay an appropriate patient response. In some insulin-treated patients, they can contribute to severe hypoglycemia by impairing the normal counterregulatory response.

In treating IDDM, chronic insulin therapy is always required, but the degree of hyperglycemia aimed for varies, as described below under Insulin Treatment Regimens. **Patients with NIDDM exhibit varying propensities to symptomatic hyperglycemia.** Many obese patients with NIDDM are seldom symptomatic, including some who intermittently or fairly persistently maintain plasma glucose levels around 300 mg/dL. For such patients, weight reduction alone is preferred, because it avoids the risks associated with insulin or an oral hypoglycemic agent. If improvement in hyperglycemia is not achieved by diet, some authorities institute insulin therapy; others prefer an initial trial with an oral hypoglycemic agent. Other NIDDM patients, usually obese, become symptomatic in association with infections, trauma, exposure to drugs that impair glucose tolerance, following binge eating and rapid weight gain, or for reasons that are not apparent. Insulin treatment is the most rapid and predictably effective means of correcting the hyperglycemia and avoiding the risk of NKHHC in such patients. Many physicians prefer to continue insulin treatment after recovery from such acute episodes, but this is a matter of clinical preference, for it is frequently possible to resume maintenance of the desired degree of hyperglycemia restriction with diet alone or with an added oral hypoglycemic agent. Finally, some (usually nonobese) NIDDM patients cannot be adequately controlled without insulin. Many physicians underestimate the risks associated with symptomatic hyperglycemia in NIDDM, because its progression to NKHHC is less predictable and usually less rapid than the progression of symptomatic hyperglycemia to DKA in IDDM, but NKHHC has a mortality rate of > 50%.

Plasma Glucose Monitoring

All patients should be instructed in self–glucose-monitoring, and insulin-treated patients should be taught to adjust their insulin dosages accordingly. A variety of commercial reagent strips are available for determining the glucose concentrations in a drop of fingertip blood; the results are determined by comparing the strip with a color chart provided by the manufacturer or by using a reflectance meter that provides a numeric read-out (glucose concentration in fingertip blood is equivalent to that in venous plasma). A spring-powered lancet is recommended to obtain the fingertip blood sample. The patient's testing technique should be evaluated at regular intervals. The frequency of testing is determined individually. IDDM patients usually monitor their plasma glucose fasting, 1 h after each meal, and at bedtime daily or at least twice weekly. In patients with NIDDM, similar monitoring weekly is desirable.

Most physicians periodically determine **glycosylated hemoglobin (Hb A$_{1c}$)** to estimate plasma glucose control during the preceding 3 mo. Hb A$_{1c}$ is the stable product of nonenzymatic glycosylation of the β-chain of Hb by plasma glucose, which is formed at rates that increase with increasing plasma glucose levels. Thus, the test is an index of long-term blood glucose control. *The results must be evaluated in terms of normal values for the testing laboratory. Some laboratories use methods that are not specific for Hb A$_{1c}$, and information on this point should be requested.* In most laboratories, the normal Hb A$_{1c}$ value is about 6%, and in poorly controlled diabetics the values range from 9 to 12%.

Patients with IDDM should be instructed in **testing for urine ketones** with commercially available reagent strips and advised to test for urine ketones whenever they first develop symptoms of a cold, flu, or other intercurrent illness; nausea, vomiting, or abdominal pain; polyuria; or if they find an unexpectedly high plasma glucose level on self–glucose-monitoring. Tests for ketones in all urine samples are recommended in IDDM patients who exhibit persistent, rapid, and marked fluctuations in their degree of hyperglycemia.

Insulin Preparations

Preparations of purified porcine insulin, purified bovine insulin, semisynthetic human insulin, and biosynthetic human insulin (all 99% pure, < 10 parts per million [ppm] proinsulin) are now available; they have equivalent biologic activities. Detectable insulin antibody levels, usually very low, develop in most insulin-treated patients, including those receiving human insulin preparations. Human or purified porcine insulin is often preferred in initiating insulin treatment, because these are less antigenic than purified bovine insulin. Patients who develop insulin allergy, fat atrophy, or immunologic insulin resistance (see Complications of Insulin Treatment, below) after treatment with bovine or porcine insulin are usually switched to human insulin. Insulin requirements may change when the species of insulin is switched, and a 20% decrease in dosage

TABLE 40–6. TIME COURSE OF ACTION OF INSULIN PREPARATIONS*

Insulin Preparation	Onset of Action†	Peak Action (h)	Duration of Action (h)
Rapid-acting regular	15–30 min	2–4	6–8
Rapid-acting Semilente® (prompt insulin zinc suspension)	1½–2 h	4–9	10–16
Intermediate-acting (NPH and Lente®)	1–3 h	6–12	18–26
Long-acting (Ultralente® and PZI)	4–8 h	14–24	28–36

* Extreme variability between different persons accounts for the broad ranges indicated.
† Subcutaneous injection.
NPH = neutral protamine Hagedorn; PZI = protamine zinc insulin.

at the time of the switch is recommended to reduce the risk of hypoglycemia; but patients switched from intermediate-acting purified porcine insulin to an intermediate-acting human insulin preparation may require a subsequent increase in dosage.

Insulin is routinely provided in preparations containing 100 u./mL (U-100 insulin) and is injected s.c. with disposable insulin syringes calibrated for use with U-100 insulin, which are commercially available with maximal capacities of 100 u. (1 mL), 50 u. (0.5 mL), and 30 u. (0.3 mL). The smaller syringes are generally preferred by patients who routinely inject doses of ≤ 50 u., because they are more easily read and facilitate the accurate measurement of smaller insulin doses. A multiple-dose insulin injection device (NovolinPen®), commonly referred to as an insulin pen, is designed to use a cartridge containing several days' dosage of a semisynthetic human insulin preparation. Some diabetics who take multiple daily insulin injections (see below) prefer its convenience in transporting their insulin supplies. Insulin should be refrigerated *but never frozen;* however, most insulin preparations are stable at room temperature for months, which facilitates their use at work and when traveling.

Insulin preparations are classified as **short-acting** (rapid-acting), **intermediate-acting**, or **long-acting.** The usual onset of action, time of peak action, and duration of action of the most commonly used preparations are listed in TABLE 40–6; *these data should be used only as rough guidelines,* because there is considerable variation in individual patients and with different doses of the same preparation in the same patient. All insulin preparations are designed for s.c. injection. **Regular insulin (insulin injection),** *a rapid-acting preparation of zinc insulin crystals in a neutral, nonbuffered, suspending*

solution, is the only insulin preparation that can be given IV. **Semilente® insulin,** another rapid-acting insulin preparation, contains zinc insulin microcrystals in an acetate buffer. The critical determinant of the onset and duration of action of an insulin preparation is the rate of insulin absorption from the injection site. The 2 common long-acting preparations use different means to slow absorption. **Protamine zinc insulin (PZI)** is a long-acting preparation containing insulin that is negatively charged, combined with an excess of positively charged fish sperm protamine. **Ultralente®,** a long-acting preparation, contains large zinc insulin crystals in an acetate buffer. **Neutral protamine Hagedorn (NPH)** is intermediate acting; it contains a stoichiometric mixture of regular and PZI insulin. **Lente®** is an intermediate-acting preparation that contains 30% Semilente® insulin and 70% Ultralente® insulin in an acetate buffer.

Mixtures of insulin preparations with different onsets and durations of action are frequently given in a single injection, by drawing measured doses of 2 preparations into the same syringe immediately before use. The manufacturers recommend that Semilente® be mixed only with Lente® or Ultralente® to maintain the same buffer solution. However, individually measured doses of regular insulin and NPH or Lente® insulin are commonly drawn up into the same syringe to provide a combination of rapid- and intermediate-acting insulin in a single injection. A preparation that contains a mixture of 70% NPH and 30% regular human semisynthetic insulin (Novolin 70/30®) is also available, but its fixed ratio of intermediate- to rapid-acting insulin restricts its use. *PZI must always be injected separately,* because it contains an excess of protamine. The cartridges for use with the insulin pen contain semisynthetic human insulin in the form of NPH insulin, regular insulin, or a mixture of 30% regular and 70% NPH.

Insulin Treatment Regimens

Conventional insulin treatment (CIT) refers to the common practice of treating with 1 or 2 injections/day of intermediate-acting insulin, with or without smaller added doses of rapid-acting insulin in the same syringe. When determining the goal of hyperglycemia restriction, CIT gives priority to minimizing the number of daily injections and the risk of hypoglycemia. Most patients with NIDDM who are not acutely ill can be safely started on insulin on an outpatient basis with adequate patient education and close physician follow-up. Patients with IDDM usually start treatment in the hospital. They require close monitoring during efforts to develop an appropriate insulin treatment regimen, and the patients or their care givers require detailed education in their responsibilities and proficiency in them before home management is safe. The assistance of a visiting nurse is frequently required during the initial period of home management.

NIDDM patients are usually started on a single daily s.c. injection of intermediate-acting insulin 30 to 60 min before breakfast. An initial total daily dose of 0.2 to 0.5 u./kg is usually safe in both children and adults. The higher dosage is usually given to obese NIDDM patients because of the degree of insulin resistance they commonly exhibit. In adults, treatment is commonly started with a single s.c. injection of 10 to 25 u. and adjusted after several days on the basis of plasma glucose levels found under fasting and 1- to 2-h postprandial conditions. Increases in the dosages of intermediate-acting insulin are usually restricted to 5 to 10 u. The plasma glucose evaluations and insulin adjustments are repeated after several days. A small quantity of rapid-acting insulin (usually not more than 5 u. initially and increased subsequently by 2 to 5 u. if necessary) added to the morning injection may be required to restrict hyperglycemia after breakfast. Many physicians prefer to avoid a 2-dose regimen in patients with NIDDM until some arbitrary maximum morning dose of intermediate-acting insulin (eg, 50 u.) has proved inadequate to maintain the desired range of diurnal plasma glucose levels.

Most NIDDM patients are treated with one-injection regimens. However, when excessive levels of fasting hyperglycemia persist at total daily intermediate-acting insulin dosages in the range of 35 to 50 u., giving ⅔ of the dose before breakfast and ⅓ in a second injection 30 to 60 min before the evening meal may significantly improve the quality of plasma glucose control. However, giving an evening dose of intermediate-acting insulin increases the risk of causing hypoglycemia during the night. Therefore, patients on a 2-injection regimen should routinely take a bedtime snack. If adjustments in the evening dose of intermediate-acting insulin maintain the fasting glucose levels in the desired range but plasma glucose levels tend to increase excessively after the evening meal, small doses of rapid-acting insulin are added to the evening injection.

CIT treatment of IDDM refers to the common practice of treating IDDM patients with 2 daily injections of mixtures of intermediate- and rapid-acting insulin. The specific doses of each type of insulin are initially selected from trials conducted when the patient is hospitalized. The starting insulin doses vary with the circumstances under which the patient presents, and *the starting insulin doses cited below do not apply in patients who present in DKA.*

Starting insulin doses are individualized, and examples of doses in different situations are described below. After the initial dose is selected, adjustments in the amounts, types, and timing are made based on closely monitored plasma glucose determinations. **Plasma glucose is determined** before meals, at bedtime, and between 2 to 4 AM, and the insulin dose is adjusted daily to maintain preprandial plasma glucose between 80 and 150 mg/dL. Increments in insulin dose are generally restricted to 10% at a time, and the effects are assessed over about 3 days before any further increment is made. More rapid adjustments of regular insulin are indicated if hypoglycemia threatens. The fact that the severity of IDDM is subject to change at the outset must be kept in mind.

Children who present at an early stage of IDDM with moderate hyperglycemia but without ketonuria or acidosis are the main exception to the generalization that all IDDM patients require > 1 insulin injection/day from the outset of treatment. Some pediatricians prefer to start with a single daily s.c. injection of 0.3 to 0.5 u./kg of intermediate-acting insulin alone, because in many such children this is adequate to maintain near-normal diurnal plasma glucose levels, at least for a time. Otherwise, plasma glucose is monitored and dosage adjustments are made as described above.

In children who present with both hyperglycemia and ketonuria but who are not acidotic or dehydrated, treatment is started by giving 0.5 to 0.7 u./kg of intermediate-acting insulin and then supplemented by s.c. injections of 0.1 u./kg of regular insulin at 4- to 6-h intervals. Plasma glucose monitoring, the goal of treatment, and dosage adjustments are as described above. When the patient has been metabolically stable for a few days, treatment is switched to 2 daily injections of mixed intermediate- and rapid-acting insulin given before breakfast and supper. The previous total daily insulin dose is split, $2/3$ is given before breakfast and $1/3$ before supper, and about $1/3$ of each dose is given as rapid-acting insulin. The insulin doses are then adjusted with the aim of maintaining preprandial plasma glucose levels between 80 and 150 mg/dL; some pediatricians make efforts to maintain preprandial plasma glucose levels between 80 and 120 mg/dL, but in either case the avoidance of hypoglycemia is a priority. (This is obviously not the case if the patient develops an intercurrent infection and a sudden marked increase in hyperglycemia associated with ketonuria.)

Adults with previously undiagnosed IDDM most commonly present in incipient or overt DKA; following recovery from the acute episode and maintenance on injections of regular insulin at 4- to 6-h intervals for 24 to 48 h (see treatment of DKA, below), they are, if metabolically stable, switched to 2 daily injections of mixtures of intermediate- and rapid-acting insulin as described above. The general principles involved in adjusting the morning and evening doses are similar to those outlined for 2-injection CIT of NIDDM. However, the critical difference is that *in patients with IDDM, small changes in insulin dosage can have profound effects on plasma glucose, and there is a much smaller margin for error in adjusting insulin doses without causing inadequate hyperglycemia restriction or hypoglycemia.*

The **dawn phenomenon** refers to the normal tendency of the plasma glucose to rise in the early morning hours before breakfast, which is frequently exaggerated in patients with IDDM and in some patients with NIDDM. In patients with NIDDM receiving CIT, a persistent tendency toward high fasting glucose levels is usually treated by adding an evening dose of intermediate-acting insulin or by increasing the evening dose. However, in some patients with IDDM, increases in the evening insulin dose may induce nocturnal hypoglycemia, followed by a marked increase in fasting plasma glucose (rebound hyperglycemia) that may be associated with an increase in plasma ketones; this is termed the **Somogyi phenomenon.** The frequency with which this phenomenon actually occurs is disputed, but it appears to be increased in patients with IDDM receiving multiple-dose insulin regimens (see below). Particularly in patients with IDDM, a trial of reducing the evening insulin dose should be instituted.

Aggressive or intensive hyperglycemia control refers to *treatment regimens in which the specific aim is to persistently maintain normal to near-normal diurnal plasma glucose fluctuations,* in hopes of preventing late complications. **Multiple subcutaneous insulin injections (MSI)** are designed to maintain normal or near-normal plasma glucose levels throughout the day in patients with IDDM, and a variety of MSI regimens are used. Such treatment carries increased risks for frequent and severe episodes of hypoglycemia. It should be tried only in selected patients who are highly motivated, well educated in DM, informed of the risks and uncertain benefits, competent in self–glucose-monitoring, and under the supervision of a physician experienced in its use. Close patient supervision, intensive patient education, and assured patient access to medical care on a 24-h basis are essential. In one MSI regimen, about 25% of the total daily dose is given as intermediate-acting insulin at bedtime, with additional doses of rapid-acting insulin before each meal (a 4-dose regimen). The patient adjusts daily dosage on the basis of self–glucose-monitoring before each meal and at bedtime; the plasma glucose level between 2 and 4 AM is assessed at least once/wk. In a 3-dose regimen, intermediate- or long-acting insulin is given before the evening meal (supplemented with rapid-acting insulin), and rapid-acting insulin is given before breakfast and lunch. The insulin doses are adjusted daily on the basis of multiple self–glucose determinations, as previously described for the 4-dose regimen.

Continuous subcutaneous insulin infusion (CSII): This mode of intensive insulin treatment in patients with IDDM involves a small battery-powered infusion pump worn by the patient, which provides a continuous s.c. infusion of rapid-acting insulin through a small needle inserted in the abdominal wall. The pump is programmed to infuse a selected basal rate of insulin, supplemented by increased rates before each meal. Multiple self–glucose determinations are made daily to adjust the dosage. The quality of plasma glucose control obtainable with CSII is superior to that obtainable with CIT, but MSI often provides comparable control in experienced hands. CSII increases the risk of hypoglycemia, particularly during sleep, and frequent undetected pump malfunctions may lead to the development of DKA. CSII, like MSI, should be used only by highly trained physicians and only in carefully selected patients.

Insulin treatment of brittle diabetes: Brittle diabetics are *a subgroup of IDDM patients who exhibit frequent, rapid swings in glucose requirements without apparent cause and have a pattern of plasma glucose control that fluctuates erratically between marked hyperglycemia and frequent episodes of symptomatic hypoglycemia.* Many of these patients improve when switched to a modified MSI regimen that provides most of the daily insulin as rapid-acting insulin in daily adjusted dosages before each meal, with some intermediate-acting insulin before the evening meal or at bedtime. The aim is not to maintain the diurnal plasma glucose fluctuations in a near-normal range, but to stabilize the fluctuations in a range that prevents symptomatic hyper- and hypoglycemia.

Brittle diabetes is most common in patients with no residual insulin secretory capacity, in whom insulin therapy is a crude and grossly inadequate substitute for a normal insulin secretory mechanism. The metabolic processes through which insulin affects the plasma levels of glucose, albumin-bound free fatty acids, and ketones are normally regulated by shifts in the balance between the effects of insulin and the opposing effects of glucagon (in liver) and the adrenergic autonomic nervous system. These **counterregulatory mechanisms** are independently regulated and normally increased during fasting, exercise, and other conditions that require protection against hypoglycemia (exercise increases skeletal muscle glucose uptake in a way that does not require insulin). Insulin doses must be adequate to deal with a sudden increase in counterregulatory mechanisms and to prevent rapidly developing symptomatic hyperglycemia and hyperketonemia, but this frequently produces transient plasma insulin excess. Counterregulatory responses to hypoglycemia become impaired in some chronic IDDM patients, limiting the patient's capacity to adapt to transient plasma insulin excesses.

Complications of Insulin Treatment

An insulin reaction (hypoglycemia) is an inherent risk that may occur because of an error in insulin dosage, a missed meal, unplanned exercise (patients are usually instructed to reduce their insulin dose or to increase their carbohydrate intake before planned exercise), or without apparent cause. (The symptoms and signs are discussed under HYPOGLYCEMIA, below.) Patients are taught to recognize symptoms of hypoglycemia, which usually respond rapidly to the ingestion of carbohydrate-containing fluids or foods. All diabetics should carry candy or lumps of sugar. An identification card, bracelet, or necklace indicating that the patient is an insulin-treated diabetic aids recognition of hypoglycemia in emergencies.

Local allergic reactions (at the site of insulin injections) are less common with purified porcine and human insulins. There is often immediate pain and burning, followed after several hours by local erythema, pruritus, and induration, the latter sometimes persisting for days. Most reactions spontaneously disappear after weeks of continued insulin injection and require no specific treatment, although antihistamines are sometimes used.

Generalized insulin allergy (usually to the insulin molecule) is rare but can occur when treatment is discontinued and restarted after a lapse of months or years. Such reactions may occur with any type of insulin, including human biosynthetic insulin. Symptoms usually develop shortly after an injection and may include urticaria, angioedema, pruritus, bronchospasm, and, in some instances, circulatory collapse. Treatment with antihistamines may suffice, but epinephrine and IV glucocorticoids are frequently required. *Insulin treatment should be stopped immediately.* If continued insulin treatment is required after the condition stabilizes, skin testing with a panel of purified insulin preparations (while hospitalized) and desensitization by a physician experienced in the management of this problem should be performed.

Immunologic insulin resistance: Most patients treated with insulin for 6 mo have antibodies to insulin. The relative antigenicity of purified insulin preparations is bovine > porcine > human (biosynthetic or semisynthetic), but genetic factors also affect individual response. Circulating insulin-binding antibodies can modify the pharmacokinetics of free insulin absorbed from a s.c. or IV injection, but in most patients

TABLE 40-7. CHARACTERISTICS OF SULFONYLUREA AGENTS

Generic Name	Daily Dosage Range (mg)	Duration of Action (h)	Tablet Size (mg)	Doses/day
Tolbutamide	500-3000	6-12	250, 500	2-3
Chlorpropamide	100-750	60	100, 250	1
Acetohexamide	250-1500	12-18	250, 500	1-2
Tolazamide	100-1000	12-24	100, 250, 500	1-2
Glyburide	2.5-20	Up to 24	1.25, 2.5, 5	1-2
Glipizide	5-40	Up to 24	5, 10	1-2

Modified from Melander A: "The clinical pharmacology of glipizide." *American Journal of Medicine* 75 (Suppl 5B):41-45, 1983; and from Skillman TG, Feldman JM: "The pharmacology of sulfonylureas." *American Journal of Medicine* 70:363, 1981; used with permission.

they have no adverse effect on treatment. When resistance occurs, requirements are usually < 500 u./day, but some patients require > 1000 u./day. Increases in insulin to ≥ 200 u./day associated with marked increases in the plasma insulin-binding capacity indicate a diagnosis of immunologic insulin resistance. If the patient has been treated with bovine or mixed bovine-porcine preparations, switching to purified porcine or human insulin may lower the requirement. A concentrated preparation (U-500) of purified porcine, regular insulin is available. Remission may be spontaneous or may be induced in some NIDDM patients who can stop insulin treatment for 1 to 3 mo. Prednisone may decrease insulin requirements within 2 wk; treatment is usually initiated with about 30 mg bid and is tapered as the requirements decrease.

Local fat atrophy or hypertrophy at sites of s.c. insulin injection is relatively rare and usually improves by switching to human insulin and injecting it directly into the affected area. No specific treatment of local fat hypertrophy is required, but injection sites should be rotated in all patients because repeated insulin injections at the same site can induce local fat hypertrophy.

Oral Hypoglycemic Agents

Oral hypoglycemic agents are not used to treat IDDM because they cannot prevent symptomatic hyperglycemia or DKA in such patients. There are 2 classes of oral hypoglycemic agents—sulfonylureas and biguanides (eg, phenformin). **Biguanides** are not currently approved for treatment of NIDDM in the USA (phenformin was linked to an increased frequency of lactic acidosis). The **sulfonylureas** lower plasma glucose primarily by stimulating insulin secretion and also by enhancing insulin ef-

fects in some target tissues and inhibiting hepatic glucose synthesis. Sulfonylureas differ in potency and duration of action (see TABLE 40-7); they bind to plasma proteins by ionic and nonionic interactions. Tolbutamide, chlorpropamide, acetohexamide, and tolazamide bind ionically, and their durations of action can be altered by the administration of drugs that can displace them (phenylbutazone, salicylates, sulfonamides). All of the sulfonylureas are metabolized in the liver, but only tolbutamide and tolazamide are inactivated exclusively by the liver. About 30% of chlorpropamide is normally disposed of by urinary excretion, and the principal hepatic metabolite of acetohexamide is highly active and excreted in urine; both drugs carry an increased risk of hypoglycemia in patients with impaired renal function.

Authorities differ in the extent to which they recommend sulfonylureas. Some prefer to use insulin whenever any treatment for hyperglycemia in addition to weight reduction is indicated in an NIDDM patient. They note that the sulfonylureas do not provide a rapid and consistently effective means of treating or preventing *symptomatic* hyperglycemia in NIDDM patients, and, in *asymptomatic* obese NIDDM patients, they are not consistently effective either in decreasing the hyperglycemia or in maintaining the commonly recommended target levels of plasma glucose. Other authorities place a priority on avoiding insulin treatment in NIDDM, whenever possible. This stems from the view that most NIDDM patients are already hyperinsulinemic and that hyperinsulinemia is a cause of atherosclerotic complications, but the grounds for this view have been challenged. Other reasons for using sulfonylureas are the preference for oral over injection treatment and that they cause hypoglycemia less frequently than does insulin, although sulfonylureas can cause severe and prolonged hypoglycemia (see complications of sulfonylurea treatment, below). Most authorities agree that a trial of sulfonylurea treatment is acceptable in asymptomatic obese NIDDM patients whose hyperglycemia does not respond adequately to efforts at weight reduction. However, the sulfonylureas are generally most effective in NIDDM patients in whom weight reduction alone causes some improvement in the hyperglycemia, and, in all sulfonylurea-treated patients, continued efforts should be made to reduce obesity and maintain a normal weight. If the sulfonylurea treatment has no effect on the hyperglycemia or if it fails to maintain the recommended target plasma glucose levels, it should be stopped and insulin treatment started.

For the initial choice of a sulfonylurea, many authorities prefer the shorter-acting agents, and most do not recommend using a combination of different sulfonylureas. **Allergic reactions and other side effects** (eg, cholestatic jaundice) are relatively uncommon. Chlorpropamide and acetohexamide should not be used in patients with impaired renal function, and chlorpropamide should not be used in elderly patients because it can cause the syndrome of inappropriate antidiuretic hormone secretion **(SIADH)**, hyponatremia, and a deterioration in mental status (which in an elderly patient might not be recognized as a drug-induced effect).

Treatment is started with a low dose, which is adjusted after several days until a satisfactory response is obtained or the maximum recommended dosage is reached. About 10 to 20% of patients fail to respond to a trial of treatment (primary failures), and patients who fail to respond to one sulfonylurea often fail to respond to others. In patients who initially respond, secondary failures occur in 5 to 10% of patients/yr.

Complications of sulfonylurea treatment: Hypoglycemia is the most important complication; estimates of its incidence vary markedly, the highest being 19/1000 patients/yr in one prospective study. Hypoglycemia can occur in patients treated with any of the sulfonylureas but is most frequent with long-acting sulfonylureas (glyburide, chlorpropamide). Increased age; renal, hepatic, and cardiovascular disease; and decreased food intake are predisposing factors. *Sulfonylurea-induced hypoglycemia can be severe and may last or recur for days after treatment is stopped,* even when it occurs in tolbutamide-treated patients, whose usual duration of

action is 6 to 12 h. A mortality rate of 4.3% in patients hospitalized with sulfonylurea-induced hypoglycemia has recently been reported. *Therefore, all sulfonylurea-treated patients who develop hypoglycemia should be hospitalized, for even if they respond rapidly to initial treatment for hypoglycemia, they must be closely monitored for 2 to 3 days.*

Diet Management

In **insulin-treated diabetics,** diet management aims to restrict variations in the timing, size, or composition of meals, which could make the prescribed insulin regimen inappropriate and result in hypoglycemia or marked postprandial hyperglycemia. To buffer the effects of evening and morning injections of intermediate-acting insulin when they most commonly cause hypoglycemia, bedtime and/or late afternoon snacks are usually incorporated into the diet. All insulin-treated patients require detailed diet management. Diet management includes prescribing total daily caloric intake; proportions of carbohydrate, fat, and protein in the diet; and distribution of the calories into the individual meals and snacks. The continuing aid of a professional dietitian and tailoring the diet plan and patient education to individual needs are most effective.

Total calories are determined on the basis of the patient's ideal weight and estimates (available in most diet manuals) on the number of calories/kg/day required to maintain, increase, or decrease weight in patients of a given age, sex, and level of physical activity. Most physicians provide for 1.0 to 1.5 gm/kg of protein, assuming that protein provides 4 kcal/gm, and the remainder of the daily caloric intake is distributed into carbohydrate (4 kcal/gm) and fat (9 kcal/gm). About 40 to 60% of the total calories should consist of carbohydrate and $\leq$ 30% of fat, although some diets have carbohydrate contents $\geq$ 60%. Carbohydrate is usually provided in the form of complex carbohydrates, but prohibiting sucrose in moderation is not justified. Moderate amounts of sucrose in a mixed meal do not usually cause exaggerated postprandial hyperglycemia. A restricted intake of eggs and dairy fat, as well as red and organ meat, in adults to limit the intake of cholesterol and saturated fat is also prudent (see ANOMALIES IN LIPID METABOLISM, below). Diets with high fiber contents (10 to 15 gm/day) derived from bran, beans, and other legumes are recommended by some physicians, but they commonly cause flatulence and abdominal discomfort and do not consistently improve glycemic control. Publications are available from the American Diabetes Association and other sources for diet planning and patient education. Exchange lists providing information on the carbohydrate, protein, fat, and calorie contents of individual servings are used to translate the dietary prescription into a diet plan, *which should contain foods that the patient likes to eat, provided there is no specific reason to exclude a particular food.* Foods with similar exchange values (ie, similar calories and contents of carbohydrate, protein, and fat) do not necessarily have equivalent effects on postprandial hyperglycemia in any individual diabetic. However, exchange lists are helpful in reducing the variation in the size and composition of the patient's usual breakfasts, lunches, suppers, and snacks.

In **obese NIDDM patients**, the aims of diet management are weight reduction and improved control of hyperglycemia. The diet should meet the patient's minimum daily protein requirement (0.9 gm/kg) and be designed to induce a gradual and sustained weight loss ($\sim$ 2 lb/wk) until ideal body weight is approached and maintained. Total calories are based on the patient's age, sex, weight, usual daily activity, and ideal body weight, using *A Guide for Professionals* published by the American Diabetes and Dietetic Associations or similar publications. A decrease in fat intake is an inherent part of most weight reduction diets; other general nutritional recommendations for obese nondiabetics should be followed. Efforts to change the eating habits of obese NIDDM patients and to curb intake of sucrose-containing soft drinks, cakes, and other desserts are important. However, the actual degree of caloric restriction that can be attempted with a reasonable hope of long-term compliance varies markedly in individual patients, and the assistance of a dietitian is helpful in developing a diet that the patient will follow. *An increase in physical activity in sedentary obese NIDDM patients* is a valuable adjunct, and over a period of time may decrease their degree of insulin resistance.

Management of Diabetics During Surgery

Surgical procedures (including the prior emotional stress, the effects of general anesthesia, and the trauma of the procedure) can markedly increase plasma glucose in diabetics and induce DKA in IDDM patients. In patients who normally take 1 or 2 daily injections of insulin, a common technique is to give 1/3 to 1/2 the usual morning dose in the morning before surgery and to start an IV infusion of 5% glucose in either 0.9% so-

dium chloride solution or water at a rate of 1 L (50 gm of glucose) over 6 to 8 h. After surgery, the plasma glucose level and the plasma reaction for ketones are checked. Unless a change in dosage is indicated, the preoperative dose of insulin is repeated when the patient has recovered from the anesthesia and the glucose infusion is continued. Plasma glucose and ketones are monitored at 2- to 4-h intervals, and regular insulin is given q 4 to 6 h (no less frequently in patients with IDDM) as needed to maintain the plasma glucose level between 100 and 250 mg/dL. This is continued until the patient can be switched to oral feedings and a 1- or 2-dose insulin schedule.

Some authorities prefer to give no s.c. insulin on the day of surgery and to add 6 to 10 u. of regular insulin to 1 L of 5% glucose in 0.9% sodium chloride solution or water infused initially at 150 mL/h on the morning of surgery following a plasma glucose determination. This is continued through the surgical procedure and recovery, with adjustments in the insulin dose based on plasma glucose determinations obtained in the recovery room and at 2- to 4-h intervals thereafter. The aim is to maintain plasma glucose in the range of 100 to 250 mg/dL. In diabetics who have maintained satisfactory plasma glucose control by diet alone or in combination with a sulfonylurea prior to surgery, insulin is not required, but plasma glucose levels should be determined pre- and postoperatively and q 6 h while they are dependent on IV fluids. Complacency is not warranted just because patients have been identified as having "mild diabetes."

Diagnosis and Treatment of Diabetic Ketoacidosis (DKA)

DKA results from grossly deficient insulin modulation of glucose and lipid metabolism. In IDDM patients, it is commonly precipitated by a lapse in insulin treatment or by an acute infection, trauma, or infarction that makes their usual insulin treatment inadequate. In DKA, the effects of marked hyperglycemia (osmotic diuresis, excessive urinary losses of water, Na, K, and volume contraction) are augmented by those resulting from increases in hepatic ketone body synthesis and release in amounts grossly exceeding peripheral tissue requirements for energy. The major ketone bodies, acetoacetic acid and β-hydroxybutyric acid, are strong organic acids; the hyperketonemia induces a metabolic acidosis and respiratory compensation, and the marked increases in urinary excretion of acetoacetic acid and β-hydroxybutyric acid obligate additional losses of Na and K. Acetone derived from the spontaneous decarboxylation of acetoacetic acid accumulates in plasma and is slowly disposed of by respiration; it is a CNS anesthetic, but the cause of coma in DKA is unknown.

The abnormal ketogenesis in DKA results from the loss of insulin's normal modulating effect on **free fatty acid (FFA)** released from adipose tissue and on hepatic FFA oxidation and ketogenesis. Plasma FFA levels and FFA uptake by liver are greatly increased. In liver, insulin normally regulates FFA oxidation and ketogenesis by indirectly inhibiting the transport of coenzyme A derivatives of long-chain FFA across the inner mitochondrial membrane into the mitochondrial matrix. Long-chain fatty acid-CoA that enters the matrix is rapidly oxidized, and an increase in hepatic fatty acid oxidation beyond a given rate automatically induces an increase in acetoacetic acid synthesis and release; a large and variable part of the acetoacetic acid (determined by the mitochondrial ratio of reduced to oxidized nicotinamide adenine dinucleotide [NADH/NAD]) is reduced to β-hydroxybutyric acid before it is released in plasma. Glucagon stimulates hepatic long-chain fatty acid-CoA transport and oxidation and ketogenesis in mitochondria, and in DKA the normal opposing effect of insulin is lost. The plasma ratio of β-hydroxybutyric acid:acetoacetic acid is normally 3:1 and is usually increased in DKA, sometimes reaching 8:1. *Commercially available reagent strips and tablets react with acetoacetic acid (and weakly with acetone) but do not react with β-hydroxybutyric acid.*

The initial symptoms are polyuria, nausea, vomiting, and, particularly in children, abdominal pain. Lethargy or somnolence is a common later development and, in untreated patients, progression to coma over varying periods is predictable. A small percentage of patients present in coma. In patients with no previous history of IDDM, DKA may not be considered initially, since the patient may not volunteer or emphasize a history of polyuria. DKA may be mistaken for an acute surgical abdomen in children, because it can cause severe abdominal pain and leukocytosis. In uncomplicated DKA the temperature is usually normal or low. Signs of dehydration are usually present, and some patients are hypotensive on admission. Kussmaul's respiration may be present, and acetone may be detected on the breath.

Diagnosis of DKA requires the demonstration of hyperglycemia, hyperketonemia, and a metabolic acidosis. However, a presumptive bedside diagnosis is justified if the urine is strongly positive for both glucose and ketones when tested by reagent strips or tablets, or if hyperglycemia detected by a reagent strip is associated with a strongly positive reaction for ketones in a 1:1 plasma dilution. The initial plasma glucose level is usually 400 to 800 mg/dL, but can be lower. Plasma pH and bicarbonate are decreased, and the calculated anion gap is increased. Although reported series of DKA are usually limited to patients with initial plasma bicarbonate levels < 10 mM, higher levels may be present, particularly in compliant IDDM patients who recognize the significance of their symptoms, take additional insulin, and rapidly seek medical attention. The initial serum Na level is usually slightly decreased, while initial serum K is usually elevated or high-normal. K values ≤ 4.5 mEq/L should be considered evidence of marked K depletion that will require rapid attention. The initial BUN is frequently increased to the degree expected with prerenal azotemia. The serum amylase is typically elevated, but pancreatitis in association with DKA is rare.

A thorough search for a treatable infection must be made. In unconscious patients, other causes of coma should be excluded. Coma associated with DKA can be distinguished from hypoglycemic coma within 2 min using a reagent strip determination of blood glucose. If an IV infusion of 5% glucose in 0.9% sodium chloride solution is started with the same needle used to draw the blood specimen, hypoglycemia can usually be excluded before 50% glucose is injected, thus preventing its administration in cases of DKA.

In **treatment** the major considerations are (1) rapid fluid volume expansion to stabilize the circulation and maintain adequate urine production, (2) IV administration of regular insulin in doses adequate to correct the hyperglycemia and hyperketonemia, (3) prevention of hypokalemia during treatment, and (4) identification and treatment of any associated bacterial infection. Rapid correction of the pH by bicarbonate administration is not required in most patients (those with a plasma pH > 7), and such treatment carries significant risks of inducing alkalosis and hypokalemia. *Close physician supervision is required, since frequent clinical and laboratory assessments of the course of DKA and appropriate adjustments in treatment are necessary.* The mortality rate is about 10%; hypotension or coma on admission adversely affects the prognosis. The major causes of death are circulatory collapse, hypokalemia, and infection.

No evidence shows that any aspect of DKA treatment significantly alters the risk for **acute cerebral edema,** a rare and frequently fatal complication that occurs primarily in children and less often in adolescents and young adults. Some physicians believe that rapid reduction of plasma glucose (> 50 mg/dL/h) should be avoided to minimize rapid osmotic changes. Some patients have premonitory symptoms (eg, sudden headache, rapid decreases in level of consciousness), but in others acute respiratory arrest is the initial manifestation. Hyperventilation, steroids, and mannitol have been used but are usually ineffective after the onset of respiratory arrest; however, isolated instances of recovery, often with persistent neurologic deficits, have been reported.

IV fluid therapy: In adults, a rapid infusion of 0.9% sodium chloride (eg, 1 L over 30 min) is given and then reduced to about 1 L/h if the BP is stable and urine flow is adequate. Usually, the fluid deficits are 3 to 5 L, and the water deficits exceed the electrolyte deficits. Initially, 0.9% sodium chloride is used to obtain rapid expansion of the intravascular compartment (usually 1 or 2 L); later, when the BP is stable and adequate urine flow is restored, 0.45% sodium chloride with K added as a phosphate salt is commonly used to provide free water and initiate K replacement. After the initial infusion, IV fluid therapy must be adjusted individually on the basis of urine output, clinical assessments of hydration and circulation, and frequent determinations of plasma electrolytes. A well-maintained flow sheet is essential. There is a propensity to hypokalemia during the treatment of DKA; the deficits of K are usually 3 to 5 mmol/L. In most patients the initial serum K is high-normal or elevated, and the initiation of K replacement (20 to 40 mmol/h) usually can be deferred for 2 h, using hourly serum measurements as a guide. However, in patients whose initial K is ≤ 4.5 mEq/L despite the existing metabolic acidosis, K replacement should be started earlier, usually as soon as urine production is adequate, and the serum K must be closely monitored. The use of bicarbonate is not recommended unless the plasma pH is ≤ 7.0, and should be restricted to efforts to raise the pH to between 7.1 and 7.2. Usually, the effects of adding 44 mEq of sodium bicarbonate to 1 L of infusion fluid should be evaluated before any additional bicarbonate is given.

Insulin treatment: DKA can be treated with low-dose insulin regimens; eg, initial IV administration of 10 to 20 u. of regular insulin followed by continuous IV infusion of 10 u./h in 0.9% sodium chloride solution. Such treatment is adequate **in most adults,** but others require significantly higher doses. For this reason, some authorities prefer to give 50 u. of regular insulin IV initially, followed by doses of 20 to 25 u./h. **In most children,** a priming IV injection of regular insulin (0.1 to 0.25 u./kg) is given, followed by a continuous IV infusion of regular insulin in 0.9% sodium chloride at a rate of 0.1 u./kg/h controlled by an infusion pump; in some children 0.2 to 0.3 u./kg/h is required. The plasma glucose should be monitored hourly to assess the efficacy of the insulin regimens and make appropriate adjustments to induce a progressive decline in plasma glucose, which is usually associated with a parallel decline in plasma FFA, followed by a progressive gradual decline in total plasma ketones. Because the reagent strips and tablets used to assess plasma and urine ketones react primarily with acetoacetic acid, they cannot reliably assess the adequacy of insulin in decreasing total plasma ketones during the first several hours; the ratio of plasma β-hydroxybutyric acid:acetoacetic acid usually falls during treatment, and the plasma levels of acetoacetic acid may remain unchanged or may increase despite a significant fall in plasma β-hydroxybutyric acid.

If insulin is given in sufficient doses to lower plasma glucose, it will correct the hyperketonemia within several hours. Plasma pH and bicarbonate usually improve significantly within 6 to 8 h, but the restitution of a normal plasma bicarbonate level may take 24 h. When plasma glucose falls to 250 to 300 mg/dL, 5% glucose is added to the IV fluids to reduce the risk of hypoglycemia. At that point, the insulin dosage can be reduced, but the continuous IV infusion of regular insulin should be maintained until the plasma and urine are persistently negative for ketones. The patient may then be switched to s.c. regular insulin q 4 to 6 h. Any lapse in insulin therapy during the first 24 h after recovery from DKA may result in a rapid resurgence of the hyperketonemia. Oral fluids can be given when tolerated.

Alcoholic Ketoacidosis

Some chronic alcoholics are predisposed to repeated episodes of *severe vomiting and abdominal pain, ketoacidosis that is accompanied* by mild hyperglycemia (the plasma glucose is commonly < 150 mg/dL and rarely > 300 mg/dL), and the absence of an elevated blood alcohol level. The characteristic history is of a binge that ended in vomiting and caused the cessation of alcohol or food intake for ≥ 24 h. During this period of starvation, the vomiting is repeated and severe and abdominal pain develops, leading the patient to seek medical attention. When this syndrome occurs in a patient known to have previous episodes of alcoholic ketoacidosis or when the history is characteristic and the degree of hyperglycemia clearly makes DKA improbable (eg, plasma glucose < 150 mg/dL), it is treated by an IV infusion of 5% glucose in 0.9% sodium chloride, with added thiamine and other water-soluble vitamins and with K replacement as required. The ketoacidosis and GI complaints usually respond rapidly. (The use of insulin in patients in whom there is any question of atypical DKA is appropriate.) Evidence of pancreatitis is found in > 50% of patients, and many exhibit impaired glucose tolerance or mild NIDDM after recovery from the acute episode. This syndrome is ascribed to the combined effects of alcohol withdrawal and starvation on endogenous insulin secretion and on stimuli for increased FFA release and ketogenesis in patients who probably have an underlying impairment in insulin secretion.

Diagnosis and Treatment of Nonketotic Hyperglycemic-Hyperosmolar Coma (NKHHC)

NKHHC is a syndrome characterized by impaired consciousness, sometimes accompanied by seizures, extreme dehydration, and extreme hyperglycemia that is not accompanied by ketoacidosis. It is a complication of NIDDM and has a mortality rate > 50%. NKHHC is most commonly a complication of previously undiagnosed or medically neglected NIDDM; it usually develops after a period of symptomatic hyperglycemia in which fluid intake is inadequate to prevent extreme dehydration from the hyperglycemia-induced osmotic diuresis. The precipitating factor may be a coexisting acute infection or some other circumstances (eg, elderly patient living alone). In some series, an infection, particularly pneumonia or gram-negative sepsis, is the most common initiating event; but NKHHC can also result from giving drugs that impair glucose tolerance or increase fluid loss (eg, glucocorticoids, phenytoin, immunosuppressive drugs, diuretics) to patients with undiagnosed or neglected NIDDM. NKHHC can also be induced by perito-

neal or hemodialysis, by tube feeding, and by giving large IV glucose loads.

The consistent and diagnostic features of NKHHC are CNS alterations, extreme hyperglycemia, dehydration and hyperosmolarity, mild metabolic acidosis without marked hyperketonemia, and prerenal azotemia (or preexisting chronic renal failure). The state of consciousness on presentation varies from mental cloudiness to coma. Seizures are not uncommon (in contrast to DKA) and may be either focal or generalized. Transient hemiplegia may also occur. The plasma glucose is usually in the range of 1000 mg/dL (much higher than in most cases of DKA). The calculated serum osmolality on admission averaged 384 mOsm/kg in one large series, while the normal value is about 290 mOsm/kg. The initial plasma bicarbonate averaged 17 and 22 mmol/L in 2 large series, and the plasma generally does not give a strongly positive reaction for ketones. Both the serum Na and K are usually in a normal range, but markedly increased levels of BUN and serum creatinine are characteristically present on admission.

In autopsied cases a frequent finding is widespread in situ thrombosis, and in some cases bleeding ascribed to disseminated intravascular coagulation or gangrenous-appearing digits has been observed.

Treatment of NKHHC: The average fluid deficit is 10 L, and acute circulatory collapse is a common terminal event in NKHHC. The immediate aims of treatment are to rapidly expand the contracted intravascular volume in order to stabilize the BP, improve the circulation, and improve the rate of urine production. Treatment is started by infusing 2 to 3 L of 0.9% sodium chloride over 1 to 2 h; if this suffices to stabilize the BP and circulation and restore good urine flow, the IV fluid can be changed to 0.45% sodium chloride to provide some free water. The rate of the 0.45% sodium chloride infusion must be adjusted in accordance with frequent assessments of BP, cardiovascular status, and the balance between fluid input and output. The aim of this phase of IV fluid therapy is not to attempt to rapidly correct the total fluid deficit or the hyperosmolarity, but rather to maintain stable circulation and renal function and to progressively replenish water and sodium at rates that do not threaten or cause acute fluid overload. Serum K should be closely monitored throughout treatment, since K replacement is required and hypokalemia may develop. K replacement is usually started by adding 20 mmol/L of K as a phosphate salt to the initial L of the IV-infused 0.45% sodium chloride, provided that urine flow is good and that the resulting initial rate of K infusion does not exceed 20 to 40 mmol/h.

Insulin treatment in NKHHC is started by giving IV regular insulin; the recommended doses vary. Many authorities routinely use the same insulin treatment regimens as for treating DKA (see insulin treatment for DKA, above). Other authorities recommend smaller doses of insulin (eg, 10 to 30 u. of IV regular insulin q 2 to 3 h or a continuous IV infusion of 5 to 10 u./h of regular insulin without a priming IV bolus). This is because they believe patients with NKHHC are often very sensitive to insulin, and larger doses might cause precipitous decreases in plasma glucose and its contribution to plasma osmolality, which could reduce intravascular fluid and predispose to cerebral edema. This view is not universally accepted, and many obese NIDDM patients with NKHHC require larger insulin doses to induce a progressive decrease in their marked hyperglycemia. When the plasma glucose reaches the range of 250 mg/dL, 5% glucose should be added to the IV fluids to avoid the risk of hypoglycemia. Following recovery from the acute episode, patients are usually switched to adjusted doses of s.c. regular insulin at 4- to 6-h intervals. When they are able to eat, this is changed to a 1- or 2-injection CIT regimen (see above).

HYPOGLYCEMIA

A syndrome characterized by symptoms of sympathetic nervous system stimulation or of CNS dysfunction that are provoked by an abnormally low plasma glucose level, which has many potential causes (see TABLE 40–8).

Pathophysiology

The brain depends on plasma glucose as its major metabolic fuel under most conditions, because the blood-brain barrier protects it from exposure to plasma albumin-bound free fatty acids (FFA) and because the rate of ketone body transport into the brain is too inadequate to contribute significantly to its energy requirements, unless the normal fasting plasma ketone body levels are markedly increased (eg, by prolonged fasting). Plasma glucose is normally regulated to maintain a level that ensures glucose transport into brain at adequate rates. Brain glucose utilization is not regulated by insulin. CNS centers

monitor plasma glucose levels and react to a potential deficiency by rapidly increasing adrenergic nervous system activity, which includes epinephrine release from the adrenal medulla, and also by increasing growth hormone and cortisol secretion. Hypoglycemia increases glucagon secretion and decreases insulin secretion; these effects are amplified by the increased sympathetic activity. These neural and hormonal responses to hypoglycemia increase hepatic glucose output and decrease glucose utilization by nonneural tissues (in part by providing increased levels of alternative substrates, eg, FFA and ketones). Adrenergic stimulation and glucagon play critical roles in the acute response to hypoglycemia, while growth hormone and cortisol secretion are delayed and less critical; but chronic deficiencies of these hormones can impair the normal **counterregulatory response** to hypoglycemia. If the potential for a profound CNS glucose deficiency develops, higher brain center activity decreases to reduce brain energy requirements. If the hypoglycemia in unconscious patients is not rapidly treated, seizures and true brain energy deficiency may develop, leading to irreversible neurologic deficits or death.

Disorders that cause abnormal restrictions on hepatic glucose output and/or abnormal increases in glucose uptake by nonneural tissues are responsible for the hypoglycemic syndromes. Hepatic glucose release is the major source of plasma glucose in the postabsorptive period. During a short-term fast (up to about 12 h), glycogenolysis is the major source of the glucose released from liver; thereafter, hepatic glucose release depends on gluconeogenesis. Drugs (eg, alcohol) and genetic enzymatic deficiencies that selectively inhibit gluconeogenesis cause hypoglycemia only under fasting conditions.

Classification of Hypoglycemic Syndromes

Hypoglycemic syndromes are divided into **drug-induced** (the most common cause) and nondrug-related. The latter are divided on the basis of clinical characteristics into **fasting hypoglycemia,** characterized by CNS manifestations, usually during fasting or exercising, and **reactive hypoglycemia,** characterized by adrenergic symptoms that occur only when provoked by a meal. Reactive hypoglycemia is usually associated with less marked and briefer decreases in plasma glucose than fasting hypoglycemia. Some disorders that cause symptomatic hypoglycemia characteristically present in childhood

TABLE 40–8. MAJOR CAUSES OF CLINICAL HYPOGLYCEMIA

Drugs (the most common cause)
  Insulin, alcohol, and sulfonylureas > 50% of all hospitalized cases. Occasional causes: salicylates, propranolol, pentamidine, disopyramide, hypoglycine A (unripened akee fruit), quinine in falciparum malaria

Nondrug-induced
  Fasting hypoglycemia
    Characteristically present in infancy or childhood
      Nesidioblastosis
      Ketotic hypoglycemia
      Inherited hepatic enzyme deficiencies that restrict hepatic glucose release:
        glucose-6-phosphatase; phosphorylase; pyruvate carboxylase; phosphoenolpyruvate carboxykinase; fructose-1, 6-diphosphatase; glycogen synthetase
      Inherited defects in fatty acid oxidation including systemic carnitine deficiency
      Inherited defects in ketogenesis
    Characteristically or more commonly present in adults
      Islet cell adenoma or carcinoma
      Hypoglycemia associated with large mesenchymal tumors
      Autoimmune hypoglycemia in nondiabetics
      Insulin-receptor antibody hypoglycemia
      Severe liver disease
      Severe renal disease
    Less age-restricted causes
      Cachexia
      Endotoxic shock
      Hypopituitarism with deficiency of both growth hormone and cortisol
  Reactive hypoglycemia
    Characteristically present in infancy or childhood
      Hereditary fructose intolerance
      Galactosemia
      Leucine sensitivity
    Characteristically present in adults
      Alimentary hypoglycemia
      Idiopathic alimentary hypoglycemia
      Early noninsulin-dependent diabetes mellitus (?)

or infancy, whereas others more commonly present in adult life.

Drug-induced hypoglycemia: Insulin, alcohol, and sulfonylureas account for 50% of hospitalized cases (see above under Complications of Insulin Treatment and under Oral Hypoglycemic Agents). **Alcoholic hypoglycemia** is characterized by impaired consciousness, stupor, or coma that is attributable primarily to hypoglycemia in a patient with a significantly elevated blood alcohol level. It is frequently associated with elevated plasma lactate and ketone levels and a metabolic acidosis. The syndrome occurs in individuals who ingest alcohol after fasting sufficiently long enough to make their hepatic glucose output dependent on gluconeogenesis. *It can be induced by blood alcohol levels well below the common legal driving limit of 100 mg/dL.* Alcoholic hypoglycemia requires prompt treatment. (NOTE: Po-

licemen and emergency room workers may fail to recognize that stuporous individuals with alcohol on their breath can be hypoglycemic rather than just inebriated.)

Hepatic alcohol oxidation increases the cytosolic ratio of reduced to oxidized nicotinamide adenine dinucleotide (NADH/NAD) and inhibits hepatic glucose release by inhibiting the use of the major plasma gluconeogenic substrates (lactate, alanine) for glucose synthesis, resulting in a fall in plasma glucose that stimulates increases in plasma FFA and ketones. Prompt improvement in the level of consciousness and subsequent resolution of the metabolic acidosis usually occur after a rapid IV infusion of 50 mL of 50% glucose followed by IV 5% glucose in 0.9% sodium chloride (thiamine is usually added).

Other drugs that less commonly cause hypoglycemia include salicylates (most often in children), propranolol, pentamidine, disopyramide, and hypoglycine A found in unripened akee fruit (Jamaican vomiting sickness). Quinine is considered a possible cause in patients with falciparum malaria.

Fasting hypoglycemia:

Causes usually diagnosed in infancy or childhood include **inherited liver enzyme deficiencies that restrict hepatic glucose release** (deficiencies of glucose-6-phosphatase, fructose-1,6-diphosphatase, phosphorylase, pyruvate carboxylase, phosphoenolpyruvate carboxykinase, or glycogen synthetase). **Inherited defects in fatty acid oxidation**, including that resulting from systemic carnitine deficiency, and **inherited defects in ketogenesis** (3-hydroxy-3-methylglutaryl-CoA lyase deficiency) cause fasting hypoglycemia by restricting the extent to which nonneural tissues can derive their energy requirements from plasma FFA and ketones during fasting or exercise. This results in an abnormally high rate of glucose uptake by nonneural tissues under these conditions. **Ketotic hypoglycemia in infants and children** is characterized by recurrent episodes of fasting hypoglycemia with elevated plasma levels of FFA and ketones, usually normal lactate levels, and low plasma alanine levels (alanine is a major substrate for gluconeogenesis). In normal infants and young children, the duration of a fast required to cause an abnormally low plasma glucose level is very much shorter than in adults; in patients with ketotic hypoglycemia this period is further reduced and is ascribed to a quantitative defect in the capacity to mobilize substrate for hepatic gluconeogenesis. **Nesidioblastosis** is characterized by a diffuse budding of insulin-secreting cells from pancreatic duct epithelium and pancreatic microadenomas of such cells; it is a rare cause of fasting hypoglycemia in infants and an extremely rare cause in adults.

Causes usually diagnosed in adults: Islet cell adenoma or carcinoma (insulinoma) is an uncommon but important cause of fasting hypoglycemia because it is usually curable. It may occur as an isolated abnormality or as a component of the type I multiple endocrine neoplasia **(MEN)** syndrome. Carcinomas account for only 10% of insulin-secreting islet cell tumors. Hypoglycemia in patients with islet cell adenomas results from impaired modulation of insulin secretion during fasting and exercise and is not usually associated with greatly elevated plasma insulin levels. In **large noninsulin-secreting tumors**, most commonly malignant mesenchymal tumors in the retroperitoneum or chest, fasting hypogly-

cemia may be the initial manifestation and most prominent symptom over a prolonged course. The hypoglycemia is corrected when the tumor is completely or partially removed, and usually recurs when the tumor regrows to a large size. Some patients have elevated plasma levels of an insulin-like growth factor, but the cause of the hypoglycemia is unknown. **Extensive liver disease** resulting from cardiac cirrhosis, fulminating viral hepatitis and acute hepatic necrosis, or hepatoma can cause fasting hypoglycemia. (Forms of cirrhosis other than cardiac rarely cause hypoglycemia.) **Autoimmune hypoglycemia** (a rare form) occurs in nondiabetics with spontaneously developed insulin antibodies and a large pool of circulating insulin-antibody complexes when episodic increases in insulin dissociation occur. Patients with insulin-resistant diabetes due to insulin-receptor antibodies and acanthosis nigricans sometimes develop **insulin-receptor antibodies that mimic insulin effects** and cause fasting hypoglycemia.

Reactive hypoglycemia: Hereditary fructose intolerance, galactosemia, and **leucine sensitivity of childhood,** usually diagnosed in infancy or childhood, are disorders in which the ingestion of a specific normal food component provokes clinical manifestations that include symptomatic hypoglycemia. In hereditary fructose intolerance and galactosemia, an inherited deficiency of a hepatic enzyme causes acute inhibition of hepatic glucose output when fructose or galactose is ingested. Leucine provokes an exaggerated insulin secretory response to a meal and reactive hypoglycemia in patients with leucine sensitivity of childhood.

Alimentary hypoglycemia is characterized by adrenergic symptoms provoked by normal meals, which are associated with an abnormally low plasma glucose level and are specifically corrected by carbohydrate ingestion. It occurs in patients who have had prior upper GI surgery (gastrectomy, gastrojejunostomy, vagotomy, pyloroplasty) that allows rapid glucose entry and absorption in the intestine, provoking excessive insulin response to a meal. Very rare cases of **idiopathic alimentary hypoglycemia** occur in patients who have not had GI surgery. **Reactive hypoglycemia associated with early NIDDM** is characterized by adrenergic symptoms occurring 4 to 5 h after eating that are associated with an abnormally low plasma glucose level after an initial period of postprandial hyperglycemia. This is ascribed to a delayed and exaggerated rise in plasma insulin. Isolated cases have been reported, but these were based on inferences drawn from observations made during a 5-h oral glucose tolerance test (OGTT). Some practitioners question its existence.

Other causes of hypoglycemia: Fasting hypoglycemia occasionally develops in patients with chronic renal failure; a specific cause is not usually identifiable. The development of renal disease in insulin-treated diabetics can cause hypoglycemia by decreasing renal insulin degradation and decreasing insulin requirements. Cachexia and endotoxin shock can cause fasting hypoglycemia at any age. Hypopituitarism with a deficiency of both growth hormone and cortisol can cause fasting hypoglycemia. Addison's disease (primary adrenocortical deficiency) rarely causes hypoglycemia in nondiabetics, but it occurs with increased frequency in IDDM patients, in whom its development frequently causes hypoglycemia and decreases in insulin requirements.

Symptoms and Signs

Two distinct patterns are distinguished: (1) sweating, nervousness, tremulousness, faintness, palpitations, and sometimes hunger are termed **adrenergic symptoms** and are attributed to increased sympathetic activity and epinephrine release (they can occur in adrenalectomized patients); and (2) confusion, inappropriate behavior (which can be mistaken for inebriation), visual disturbances, stupor, coma, and seizures are **CNS manifestations.** Hypoglycemic coma is commonly associated with an abnormally low body temperature. Adrenergic symptoms are usually associated with acute, less marked decreases in plasma glucose than those that cause CNS manifestations, but the plasma levels at which symptoms of either type develop vary markedly in individual patients.

Diagnosis

The approach to diagnosis depends on whether the patient presents with unexplained CNS manifestations or unexplained adrenergic symptoms. In either case, diagnosis requires evidence that the symptoms occur in association with an abnormally low plasma glucose level and are corrected by raising the plasma glucose. Symptom-producing plasma glucose levels vary in individuals and in different physiologic states. Abnormally low plasma glucose is usually defined as < 50 mg/dL in men or < 45 mg/dL in women (below the lower limits seen in normal men and women after a 72-h fast) and < 40 mg/

dL in infants and children. (See also HYPOGLYCEMIA under METABOLIC PROBLEMS IN THE NEWBORN in Ch. 27.) The majority of cases of hypoglycemia occur in patients treated with insulin or a sulfonylurea or who have recently ingested alcohol, and the diagnosis in such patients is rarely a problem.

A reagent strip blood glucose test should be performed on any patient with unexplained impairment of consciousness (or seizures), using drops of the blood sample obtained when a needle is inserted to start an IV fluid infusion. If an abnormally low blood glucose level is found, glucose is rapidly infused (see Treatment, below); prompt improvement in the CNS manifestations with a rise in blood glucose (which occurs in most patients) confirms the diagnosis of fasting or drug-induced hypoglycemia. A portion of the initial blood sample should be saved as frozen plasma to determine the initial plasma insulin, proinsulin, and C-peptide levels or to perform a drug scan when necessary. Blood lactate and pH should be determined and the plasma checked for ketones with a reagent strip. The initial assessment frequently suggests a probable cause; eg, alcohol on the breath, a history of drug use that can cause hypoglycemia, evidence of extensive liver or renal disease, the finding of a large retroperitoneal or chest tumor, or a history of an inherited cause of fasting hypoglycemia.

Patients with insulin-secreting pancreatic tumors **(insulinomas, islet cell carcinomas)** usually have increased proinsulin and C-peptide levels that parallel the insulin levels. In patients taking a **sulfonylurea,** an increased C-peptide level would be expected, but a significant blood level of the drug should be detectable. Patients with **hypoglycemia induced by exogenous insulin injections** (commonly health care workers or family members of a diabetic) have normal proinsulin levels and suppressed C-peptide levels. In the rare cases of **autoimmune hypoglycemia,** the plasma-free insulin during a hypoglycemic episode is usually markedly elevated, plasma C-peptide suppressed, and plasma insulin antibodies readily detectable. Distinguishing autoimmune hypoglycemia from surreptitious insulin administration requires special studies.

Patients with an insulinoma differ from those with other causes of fasting hypoglycemia in that they frequently are asymptomatic when they finally seek medical attention because of isolated episodes of sudden confusion or unconsciousness that have occurred over a period of years and have become more frequent. The episodes characteristically occur in a postabsorptive period or after an overnight fast and are sometimes precipitated by exercise (eg, rapid walking before eating breakfast); they may resolve spontaneously, but a history of rapid improvement when the patient was given fluid or food containing carbohydrate can frequently be elicited and is a critical diagnostic point.

An initial plasma insulin level > 6 $\mu U/mL$ and certainly > 10 $\mu U/mL$ associated with hypoglycemia is inappropriately high and strongly suggests an insulin-secreting tumor if surreptitious use of insulin or a sulfonylurea can be excluded. Plasma insulin levels usually fall to background levels when plasma glucose falls to abnormally low levels, and insulin levels in a normal range are inappropriately high. Conditions that predispose to fasting hypoglycemia, other than an insulin-secreting tumor, can usually be excluded by an outpatient study.

If other causes of episodic CNS symptoms are not apparent, the patient is hospitalized and subjected to a fast to reproduce the symptoms, while plasma glucose, insulin, proinsulin, and C-peptide levels are monitored. Within 48 h, 79% of patients with an insulinoma develop symptoms, and 98% develop them within 72 h. The fast is terminated at 72 h or when symptoms develop. If the fast reproduces the patient's symptoms, which respond rapidly to glucose administration, and if the symptoms are associated with an abnormally low plasma glucose level and an inappropriately high plasma insulin level, a presumptive diagnosis of an insulin-secreting tumor is warranted. Other diagnostic procedures (eg, IV tolbutamide infusion) should be used only in referral centers with experience in their use and interpretation; they are rarely required. Insulinomas are usually too small to be detected by standard x-rays or CT scans, but some insulin-secreting islet cell carcinomas are detectable. Because pancreatic exploration involves significant risks for inducing pancreatitis and other complications, and because identification of a small insulin-secreting tumor at surgery requires experience in this area, patients with a presumptive diagnosis should be sent to a referral center for evaluation by experienced physicians prior to surgery.

Alimentary (reactive) hypoglycemia should be considered only in patients with prior upper GI surgery who have postprandial adrenergic symptoms that are selectively corrected by carbohydrate ingestion. The relationship between the symptoms and the plasma glucose level is assessed by home blood glucose monitoring (eg, 1 and 2 h postprandially and whenever symptoms occur for at least 1 wk) to confirm the presumptive diagnosis.

Idiopathic (reactive) hypoglycemia is extremely rare; a diagnosis should be considered only when the patient is emotionally stable and the history clearly indicates that recurrent adrenergic symptoms are selectively provoked by meals and are rapidly corrected only by carbohydrate ingestion. The diagnosis requires the demonstration by home blood glucose monitoring that when eating normal meals and carrying out normal activities there is a consistent relationship between the spontaneous occurrence of symptoms and an abnormally low postprandial glucose level. *Erroneous diagnoses of "reactive (alimentary) hypoglycemia" in patients without prior upper GI surgery are common.* Postprandial adrenergic symptoms that are not selectively corrected by ingesting carbohydrate are common, frequently occurring during emotional stress, and can become the focus of an anxiety state. The history usually distinguishes these patients, but many are needlessly subjected to a 5-h OGTT and misdiagnosed as having reactive hypoglycemia because of one of the variations in OGTT that occur in many asymptomatic, normal patients. *The OGTT is not a valid means of diagnosing alimentary hypoglycemia.*

Treatment

Acute adrenergic symptoms are usually relieved by the immediate ingestion of glucose or sucrose. Patients treated with insulin or a sulfonylurea are advised to drink a glass of fruit juice or water with 3 tbsp of table sugar added, and to teach their family members to give such treatment if they suddenly exhibit confusion or inappropriate behavior. Insulin-treated children are advised to carry sugar lumps, candy, or glucose tablets at all times. Each glucose tablet contains 5 gm of glucose, and patients should take or be given 10 to 20 gm of glucose if they have an insulin reaction. Most insulin reactions can be handled by continued oral ingestion of glucose or sucrose over several hours. However, in patients treated with a sulfonylurea, hypoglycemia may recur over several days, and even if their symptoms respond to glucose or sucrose ingestion, patients should be instructed to seek immediate medical attention since hospitalization is indicated.

The families of insulin-treated children, as well as diabetics who are unusually susceptible to frequent insulin reactions (eg, the elderly and those attempting stringent insulin control of their blood glucose by MSI or CSI regimens), are commonly given glucagon to keep at home.

Adults with CNS manifestations of hypoglycemia who do not respond adequately to oral sugar or glucagon injection are initially treated with an IV injection of 50 or 100 mL of 50% glucose, followed by a continuous infusion of 10% glucose (20 or 30% glucose may be needed). Blood glucose levels are monitored within a few minutes after the start of the 10% glucose infusion and frequently thereafter with reagent strips, and the rate of infusion is adjusted to maintain a normal plasma glucose level. In children with CNS manifestations, treatment is started by infusing 10% glucose at a rate of 3 to 5 mg/kg/min, and the rate is adjusted to rapidly restore and maintain a normal plasma glucose level. *In general, pediatricians do not recommend the use of an IV bolus of 50% glucose or the use of IV fluids containing > 10% glucose in infants and children because they can have pronounced osmotic effects, and in some patients may induce marked hyperglycemia and a marked stimulation of insulin secretion.* (See HYPOGLYCEMIA under METABOLIC PROBLEMS IN THE NEWBORN in Ch. 27 for treatment of hypoglycemia in newborns and infants.) In adults and children, oral feeding is instituted when feasible, but the IV glucose infusion should be continued at decreasing rates and changed to 5% glucose until it clearly can be stopped safely.

Hypoglycemia associated with a large non-insulin-secreting mesenchymal tumor frequently responds to surgical excision of most of the tumor burden, and the patient can remain free of symptomatic hypoglycemia for relatively long periods (years in some instances) on frequent carbohydrate-containing meals, including meals at bedtime and during the night. Surgery is recommended when the patient's general health and life expectancy make this appropriate. Where surgical removal of most of the tumor is unfeasible or when the tumor regrows to a large size with recurrence of fasting hypoglycemia, a gastrostomy for continuous feeding of the sometimes enormous amounts of carbohydrate required throughout the day and night is frequently helpful in controlling the hypoglycemia.

When hypoglycemia is caused by an insulin-secreting islet cell tumor, surgery in a referral center is recommended. Most often, a single insulinoma is found, and its enucleation is curative; but the tumor (or all of the tumors in the 14% of cases with multiple insulinomas) may not be located, resulting in a second operation or a blind partial pancreatectomy. Medical treatment is sometimes required to prepare the patient for surgery or to control hypoglycemia if the insulinoma(s) is not located and removed at surgery. Two drugs that inhibit insulin secretion are available, diazoxide and octreotide (a long-acting octapeptic analog of somatostatin); both drugs have other effects, and consultation with a physician experienced in their use is recommended. Patients with insulin-secreting islet cell carcinomas generally have a poor prognosis; to control their hypoglycemia, diazoxide or octreotide, along with frequent carbohydrate-containing meals and IV glucose infusions, is used.

Hypoglycemia provoked by the ingestion of fructose, galactose, or leucine is treated by removing or limiting the offending substance. Alimentary hypoglycemia that occurs after GI surgery or that is idiopathic is managed with frequent small feedings of a high-protein, low-carbohydrate diet.

GENETIC ABNORMALITIES OF CARBOHYDRATE METABOLISM

GALACTOSEMIA

Inborn errors of galactose metabolism characterized by elevated levels of galactose in the blood, which arise from the inability to convert galactose to glucose. The enzymes involved in this conversion are shown in FIG. 40–1. Clinical manifestations depend on the site of the defect.

Galactokinase deficiency is a rare disorder, associated with early development of cataracts unless diagnosed soon after birth and treated by permanent exclusion of galactose from the diet. The consequent accumulation of galactose and its reduction to galactitol cause osmotic damage to the lens fibers. The diagnosis is made by finding galactose in the blood or urine of infants after the first few milk feeds that contain lactose, a sugar hydrolyzed in the gut to galactose and glucose. Liver damage or neurologic disturbances do not occur in this disorder because galactose-containing cerebrosides can be synthesized from glucose.

Classic galactosemia is inherited as an autosomal recessive trait caused by the absence of the enzyme galactose-1-phosphate uridyl transferase. It occurs in about 1/80,000 births, giving a gene frequency of 1/150 of the population.

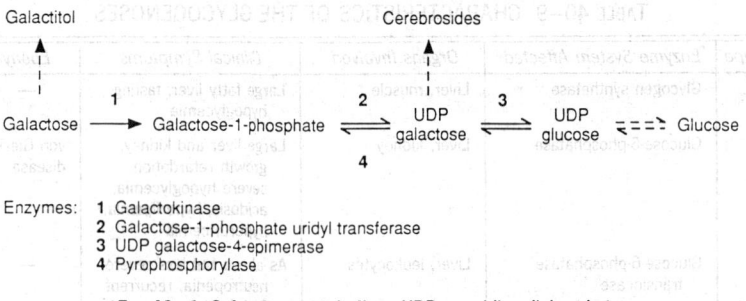

FIG. 40–1. Galactose metabolism. UDP = uridine diphosphate.

At birth, the newborn appears normal, but within a few days or weeks of being fed with milk, the infant becomes anorexic, vomits, becomes jaundiced, and stops growing normally. The liver enlarges, protein and amino acids appear in excess in the urine, and later edema and ascites develop. If treatment is delayed, the child remains physically stunted and mentally retarded; many also have cataracts. The severe abnormalities are due to the intracellular accumulation of galactose-1-phosphate, which interferes with many normal metabolic processes. The **diagnosis** may be suspected from the presence of non-glucose-reducing substances (galactose and galactose-1-phosphate) in the urine and confirmed by the absence of the transferase enzyme in cells and tissues, such as erythrocytes and liver. If galactosemia is suspected before birth (eg, because of family history), the diagnosis can be made at the time of birth by analyzing erythrocytes from a few drops of cord blood for decreased concentrations of galactose-1-phosphate uridyl transferase and increased concentrations of galactose-1-phosphate. Justification for diagnosis early in prenatal life remains a matter of debate. If a galactosemic mother has high blood galactose levels, the fetus may develop cataracts in utero; but unless it too has the enzyme defect, its brain development will not be impaired because the mother's galactose-1-phosphate does not cross the placenta.

Treatment

Milk and milk-containing foods must be eliminated from the diet, preferably during pregnancy in women known to be carriers of the trait. Synthetic galactose and lactose-free milk substitutes are available. Dietary restriction of galactose must be lifelong. Early treatment results in normal physical growth and development; but al-

though their IQ is within the normal range, children with galactosemia tend to remain underachievers. This may be caused by the synthesis of galactose-1-phosphate from uridine diphosphate (UDP) galactose by the action of pyrophosphorylase, which may accumulate to excess.

GALACTOSE EPIMERASE DEFICIENCY

A rare inherited metabolic disorder that may be restricted to erythrocytes without significant clinical abnormalities, or may exist in a generalized form, clinically indistinguishable from classic galactosemia.

A deficiency of UDP galactose 4-epimerase activity results in accumulation of galactose-1-phosphate in the affected cells through its conversion from UDP galactose by pyrophosphorylase (see FIG. 40–1).

GLYCOGEN STORAGE DISEASES
(Glycogenoses)

A group of hereditary disorders caused by lack of one or more of the many enzymes involved in glycogen synthesis or breakdown, and characterized by the deposition of abnormal amounts or types of glycogen in the tissues (see TABLE 40–9 for classification and characteristics). Symptoms and signs arise either through accumulation of glycogen or other intermediate metabolites or through lack of an end product of glycogen breakdown, particularly glucose. Glycogen and some of the intermediate metabolites deposited in tissues can be detected noninvasively by MRI. The incidence of all forms of glycogen storage diseases is 1/40,000, but this may be a considerable underestimate because some forms of glycogenosis cause only minimal disturbances and may therefore remain undiagnosed. Varia-

TABLE 40–9. CHARACTERISTICS OF THE GLYCOGENOSES

Type	Enzyme System Affected	Organs Involved	Clinical Symptoms	Eponym
0	Glycogen synthetase	Liver, muscle	Large fatty liver, fasting hypoglycemia	—
Ia	Glucose-6-phosphatase	Liver, kidney	Large liver and kidney, growth retardation, severe hypoglycemia, acidosis, hyperlipemia, hyperuricemia	von Gierke's disease
Ib	Glucose-6-phosphatase translocase	Liver, leukocytes	As above but less severe; neutropenia, recurrent GI infections	—
II	Lysosomal glucosidase (various types)	All organs	Large liver and heart, no abnormal blood chemistry	Pompe's disease
III	Debrancher enzyme system	Liver, muscle, heart, leukocytes	Enlarged liver, fasting hypoglycemia, variable muscle involvement	Forbes' disease
IV	Brancher enzyme system	Liver, muscle, and most tissues	Progressive cirrhosis in juvenile type, myopathy and heart failure in late-onset type	Andersen's disease
V	Muscle phosphorylase	Skeletal muscle	Cramps on exercise with no rise in blood lactate	McArdle's disease
VI	Liver phosphorylase	Liver	Enlarged liver, fasting hypoglycemia but often no symptoms at all	Hers' disease
VII	Phosphofructokinase	Skeletal muscle, erythrocytes	Cramps on exercise but no rise in blood lactate, hemolysis	Tarui's disease

VIII, IX, X, XI: Rare disorders involving various components of the liver phosphorylase activating–deactivating cascade

tions in severity and age of onset of clinical manifestations are due to involvement of different isoenzymes or other components of the affected enzyme systems. Inheritance is autosomal recessive, except in type IX, which is X-linked. Types 0, I, IV, and VI mainly affect the liver. Types II and III involve most tissues. Types V and VII are restricted to skeletal muscle (see Glycogen Storage Diseases of Muscle under MUSCULAR DYSTROPHIES AND OTHER MYOPATHIES in Ch. 43); type II also affects the myocardium.

Diagnosis is made by demonstrating absence of the specific enzyme in a biopsy of the affected tissue. **Treatment** in types 0, I, and III is directed toward preventing hypoglycemia and lactic acidosis by frequent small carbohydrate feedings: Uncooked cornstarch, 2 gm/kg/meal given q 4 or 6 h day and night, has proved particularly helpful in

maintaining a steady blood glucose level. With it, catch-up growth and reduction of lactic acidemia, hyperuricemia, and hyperlipidemia can be achieved. Alternatively, continuous overnight feeding of a high dextrin preparation (eg, Vivonex®) through a nasogastric tube may be attempted, but this method carries with it the risk of accidental aspiration of the feed. Allopurinol may be required to prevent gout and renal urate stones. Limiting anaerobic (ischemic) exercise reduces the muscle symptoms of types V and VII. No effective treatment is known for the other types.

HEREDITARY FRUCTOSE INTOLERANCE

A metabolic inability to utilize fructose caused by absence of the enzyme phosphofructoaldolase and inherited as an autosomal recessive trait. The incidence of this disorder is 1/20,000 in Switzerland, where it was first described. Fructose-1-phosphate accumulates in the body, inhibiting glycogenolysis and gluconeogenesis. Ingestion of more than very small amounts of fructose or sucrose (which on hydrolysis yields glucose and fructose) induces hypoglycemia, with sweating, tremor, confusion, nausea, vomiting, abdominal pain, and possibly convulsions and coma. With prolonged ingestion of fructose, proximal renal tubular acidosis may occur with urinary loss of phosphate and glucose; cirrhosis of the liver and mental deterioration may also develop. Patients protect themselves by developing a strong dislike for sugar-containing sweets and fruit; as a result their teeth are usually completely free of caries.

Diagnosis is suggested by the onset of symptoms in infancy and finding fructose in the urine. It is confirmed by demonstrating the absence of the enzyme in a liver biopsy or by demonstrating a fall in blood glucose 5 to 40 min after giving fructose 250 mg/kg IV, followed by the administration of IV glucose as soon as the fall in blood glucose has been documented. It has recently become possible to make the diagnosis and identify heterozygous carriers of the mutated gene coding for the enzyme by direct analysis of genomic DNA from a few cells obtained from mouth washes.

Treatment is to exclude fructose (found chiefly in sweet fruits), sucrose, and sorbitol from the diet. Attacks of fructose-induced hypoglycemia are treated with glucose.

FRUCTOSURIA

A harmless excretion of fructose in the urine, caused by an autosomal recessive lack of the enzyme fructokinase. The incidence in the general population is about 1/130,000. This benign asymptomatic defect prevents normal utilization of ingested fructose, resulting in abnormal levels in the blood and urine. Fructosuria may lead to an incorrect diagnosis of diabetes mellitus (fructose will reduce copper sulfate but will not react with glucose oxidase). No treatment is required.

FRUCTOSE-1,6-DIPHOSPHATASE DEFICIENCY

A rare metabolic disorder caused by a deficiency of fructose-1,6-diphosphatase, a key enzyme of gluconeogenesis. This results in hypoglycemia and acidosis owing to the accumulation of gluconeogenic precursors—certain amino acids,

lactic acid, and ketoacids. The symptoms can be relieved by giving glucose orally, or IV if hypoglycemia is severe.

PENTOSURIA

A harmless autosomal recessive metabolic derangement characterized by the excretion of L-xylulose in the urine due to absence of the enzyme L-xylulose dehydrogenase. It occurs almost exclusively in Jews, with an incidence of 1/2500 in American Jews. As with fructosuria, its only importance is the danger that the presence of xylulose in the urine may lead to an erroneous diagnosis of diabetes mellitus. Treatment is not required.

INHERITED ABNORMALITIES OF PYRUVATE METABOLISM

Pyruvate appears in the metabolic pathway of carbohydrates, fats, and amino acids. Inborn errors of pyruvate metabolism can therefore cause a wide variety of disturbances.

Deficiency of the pyruvate dehydrogenase complex: Deficiency of one of the proteins in this multienzyme complex results in inadequate production of acetyl-CoA and subsequently of acetylcholine, which is essential in the normal development of the nervous system. Clinical manifestations are predominantly ataxia and psychomotor retardation. This deficiency may be one of the causes of Reye's syndrome. There is no known treatment for this disorder.

Pyruvate carboxylase deficiency: The absence of this enzyme results in inadequate production of oxaloacetate; gluconeogenesis is therefore reduced and causes fasting hypoglycemia, lactic acidosis, and ketoacidosis. Amino acid synthesis is also impaired and results in reduced formation of amino acid neurotransmitters with a variety of neurologic symptoms. Hypoglycemia and acidemia may be relieved by frequent feeding with carbohydrate-containing foods, but there are no reports of specific replacement with neurotransmitters (eg, dopamine, tyrosine) for treatment of the neurologic symptoms.

Mitochondrial abnormalities: Pyruvate is a major substrate for mitochondrial energy metabolism. Patients with defects in the oxidative phosphorylation pathway or the respiratory chain present with clinically and biochemically heterogeneous features. They may present at any time in early infancy to late adulthood with myopathies, mental retardation or seizures, lactic acidosis, and cardiac, respiratory, hepatic, or renal failure. Exacerbations, brought on by exercise, infections, or alcohol, result in severe lactic acidosis, requiring treatment with IV sodium bicarbonate.

Maternal transmission of the defect is 10 times more common than paternal transmission because many of the enzymes involved in mitochondrial metabolism are encoded by mitochondrial DNA, which is exclusively inherited through the maternal line.

ANOMALIES IN AMINO ACID METABOLISM

Anomalies of amino acid metabolism may be categorized as those of transport and those of catabolism. Both are determined genetically. Although the latter are usually considered the only true metabolic anomalies, defects in amino acid transport in the renal tubule (see ANOMALIES IN KIDNEY TRANSPORT in Ch. 28) or GI mucosa are also metabolic because they too are caused by enzyme defects. *Elevated plasma levels of various metabolites occur in the catabolic group but are absent in the transport group.* Newly discovered entities and recognition of variations in many of the original or classic types are leading to the definition of increasing numbers of catabolic disorders.

The salient features of catabolic amino acid diseases are listed in TABLE 40–10. Phenylketonuria as a prototype is discussed in greater detail below.

PHENYLKETONURIA (PKU)
(Phenylalaninemia; Phenylpyruvic Oligophrenia)

An inborn error of metabolism, characterized by a virtual absence of phenylalanine hydroxylase activity and an elevation of plasma phenylalanine, which frequently results in mental retardation.

Etiology and Incidence

Excess phenylalanine, an essential amino acid, is normally eliminated from the body by hydroxylation to tyrosine. The enzyme phenylalanine hydroxylase is essential for this reaction. If it is inactive, phenylalanine accumulates in the blood and is mainly excreted in excess in the urine; some is transaminated to phenylpyruvic acid, which may be further metabolized to phenylacetic, phenyllactic, and o-hydroxyphenylacetic

acids; all are excreted in the urine. The exact cause of the mental retardation is not known, but it is a consequence of the biochemical defect. This enzyme defect, transmitted as an autosomal recessive trait, is found in most population groups but is rare in Ashkenazi Jews and in blacks. Incidence in the USA of the typical variety is about 1/16,000 live births.

Clinical Features

Clinical symptoms of PKU are usually absent in the newborn period, hence *laboratory screening tests are mandatory for its detection.* Rarely an infant may be lethargic or may feed poorly. The majority of untreated patients manifest some degree of mental retardation, usually severe, which is the most important symptom. They tend to have lighter colored skin, hair, and eyes than unaffected family members. Some infants may have a rash similar to infantile eczema.

Many neurologic symptoms and signs, especially affecting reflexes, occur. Both petit and grand mal seizures are common in older children, and the incidence of abnormal EEGs is 75 to 90%. Children manifest extreme hyperactivity and psychoses and often exhibit an unpleasant "mousy" body odor caused by phenylacetic acid in the urine and sweat.

Diagnosis

Early diagnosis depends on detecting a high plasma phenylalanine level and a normal or low plasma tyrosine level. The exact plasma level that serves as a cut-off point between classic PKU and its variants cannot be fixed, although 20 mg/dL (1.2 mM/L) has been proposed. Better methods of differentiation are required. Prenatal diagnosis is now possible in the majority of PKU families; DNA isolated from cultured amniotic cells or chorionic villus samples is analyzed by restriction fragment length polymorphism, and the profiles are compared with those of the parents and the proband.

After consuming a moderate amount of milk (the source of phenylalanine) for at least 48 h, the newborn should be screened for PKU. The **Guthrie inhibition assay test** is usually used. A strain of phenylalanine-dependent *Bacillus subtilis* is cultured in a medium, on which is placed a filter paper disk impregnated with several drops of capillary blood and other disks containing varying amounts of phenylalanine (controls). The zone of growth around the disk containing the blood sample is proportional to the phenylalanine content. After 4 to 6 wk of age, abnormal levels of phenylalanine metabolites may appear in the urine, including phenylpyruvic acid, phenyllactic acid, phenylacetic acid, and *o*-hydroxyphenylacetic acid. **Another screening test** involves the addition of a few drops of 10% ferric chloride solution to a urine sample or wet diaper (a paper test strip is commercially available). A deep bluish-green color indicates the presence of phenylpyruvic acid in the urine. Urine testing is done *after* the neonatal period and should be repeated at regular intervals for 1 yr if the infant has a family history of PKU. The results of all screening must be confirmed by more exact tests using fluorometric methods or ion exchange column chromatography.

Variants

Screening has detected a number of infants with abnormally high phenylalanine levels. In many, the finding is secondary to neonatal (developmental) tyrosinemia, which can be distinguished by abnormal plasma tyrosine levels. The remaining cases can be divided into classic PKU and mild and severe forms of **hyperphenylalaninemia**. Mild forms usually exhibit plasma levels of < 8 to 10 mg/dL while on a normal diet; the severe forms are associated with greater elevations. The distinction between severe hyperphenylalaninemia and classic PKU cannot be made by plasma phenylalanine measurements alone. Exact differentiation requires assay of liver phenylalanine hydroxylase activity, which is virtually absent in classic PKU and present in amounts varying from 5 to 15% of normal in the hyperphenylalaninemias. The liver is normally the only place where measurable quantities of phenylalanine hydroxylase may be found.

No sequelae to the mild variants are expected. The consequences of the more severe forms are not known, and these patients should be treated the same as those with classic PKU until more information is available.

Elevated plasma phenylalanine levels may also occur as a result of **tetrahydrobiopterin deficiency**. Dietary therapy can correct the abnormal plasma phenylalanine level, but severe neurologic deterioration continues. This occurs because tetrahydrobiopterin is a cofactor in the synthesis of dopamine and serotonin; deficiency of these neurotransmitters may account for the neurologic symptoms. Tetrahydrobiopterin deficiency may occur either as a result of a defect in the synthesis of biopterin or as a deficiency of dihydropteridine reductase, which reduces

biopterin to its active form, tetrahydrobiopterin. Substitution therapy with levodopa, carbidopa, 5-OH tryptophan, and tetrahydrobiopterin, in addition to dietary treatment, may have a beneficial effect on these variants if started early in life.

Maternal phenylketonuria, if left untreated, has a profound effect on the fetus. The majority of such pregnancies result in an infant with mental and physical retardation, and there is a high incidence of microcephaly and congenital heart disease. Control of the maternal blood phenylalanine level before pregnancy may prevent these sequelae, but experience is too limited to be certain of the complete efficacy of early treatment.

Treatment

Treatment consists of limiting the phenylalanine intake of the child so that essential amino acid requirements are met but not exceeded, allowing normal growth and development but preventing accumulation of phenylalanine and its abnormal end products in the body. Monitoring of the child's plasma phenylalanine levels is required. Since all natural protein contains about 4% phenylalanine, it is impossible to satisfy the protein requirement without exceeding the phenylalanine requirement. Hence, casein hydrolysates (treated to remove the phenylalanine) or mixtures of amino acids should constitute the protein moiety of the diet. Lofenalac®, a widely used product in the USA, is a complete food, except for its phenylalanine content, and is used in place of milk in the diet. Low-protein natural foods, such as fruits, vegetables, certain cereals, etc, are allowed. The phenylalanine requirement is supplied by measured quantities of natural protein and the residual phenylalanine content of Lofenalac® (80 mg/100 gm of dry powder). Requirements in terms of body wt decrease with age, varying from 60 to 90 mg/kg/day during the first months of life to 20 to 30 mg/kg/day by the end of the first year. Dietary products completely free of phenylalanine are now available. They facilitate control of the blood phenylalanine level and allow a little more leeway in the use of natural foods. Phenyl-free (Mead Johnson) is a complete food except for phenylalanine; PKU-1, PKU-2 (Milupa), and Maxamaid (Scientific Hospital Supplies) do not contain fat and hence provide fewer calories than the other preparations.

Treatment must be initiated during the first days of life to prevent mental retardation. Early and well-maintained treatment makes normal

TABLE 40–10. ANOMALIES IN AMINO ACID METABOLISM

Disease	Amino Acid Affected	Enzyme Defect	Prenatal Diagnosis*	Clinical Features	Treatment
Phenylketonuria	Phenylalanine	Phenylalanine hydroxylase	RFLP analysis	Neurologic symptoms, mental retardation	Controlled phenylalanine intake
Tyrosinosis	Tyrosine	Tyrosine α-ketoglutarate aminotransferase (?)		One reported case, probably benign	
Tyrosinemia	Tyrosine	Tyrosine aminotransferase		Mental retardation, keratitis, dermatitis	Controlled phenylalanine and tyrosine intake
Tyrosinemia	Tyrosine and methionine	Fumarylacetoacetate hydrolase	Enzyme assay, succinyl acetone accumulation	Fanconi's syndrome, hepatic cirrhosis, fulminating hepatic failure	Controlled phenylalanine, tyrosine, and methionine intake; liver transplant
Albinism	Tyrosine	Tyrosinase		Absent pigment in skin, hair, eyes	Protection of skin and eyes from actinic radiation
Alkaptonuria	Tyrosine	Homogentisate oxidase		Arthritis, dark urine	
Histidinemia Classic	Histidine	L-Histidine ammonia lyase (liver and skin)	Enzyme assay	Retardation, neurologic manifestations; frequently benign	Low-protein diet, controlled histidine intake
Variant	Histidine	L-Histidine ammonia lyase (liver only)		As above	As above
Maple syrup urine disease (branched-chain ketoaciduria) Classic	Leucine Isoleucine Valine Alloisoleucine	Branched-chain keto acid decarboxylase	Enzyme assay	Reflex changes, hypertonicity, odor of urine and perspiration, convulsions, coma, death	Controlled intake of branched-chain amino acids, peritoneal and/or hemodialysis for acute episodes
Intermittent	Same	Same, but some activity		Symptoms only with stress (fever, infection)	Same for acute episodes, none necessary between episodes
Intermediate	Same	Degree of activity between classic and intermittent		Retardation, neurologic symptoms; full-blown picture develops with stress	Protein intake limited to requirement or controlled intake of branched-chain amino acids
Thiamine-responsive	Same	Cofactor stabilizes the enzyme		Similar to mild picture of intermediate	Thiamine—large doses; dietary restriction also necessary
Valinemia	Valine	Valine aminotransferase		Retardation	Controlled valine intake

	Amino acid	Enzyme defect	Prenatal diagnosis	Clinical symptoms	Treatment
Homocystinemia	Methionine	Cystathionine synthetase 1. Pyridoxine-responsive 2. Non–pyridoxine-responsive		Skeletal abnormalities, ectopia lentis, retardation, thromboembolic disease	1. Massive doses of pyridoxine 2. Controlled intake of methionine and cystine supplementation, also folic acid supplementation
Cystinosis	Cystine	Defective lysosomal membrane protein	Cystine accumulation by ^{35}S pulse labeling	Cystine accumulation throughout RE system, WBC, cornea; Fanconi's syndrome; renal failure	Symptomatic for Fanconi's syndrome; renal transplant for failure Cysteamine
Cystathioninemia	Methionine	Cystathionase		Retardation (?), large number of persons have no clinical symptoms—benign trait	Large doses of pyridoxine
Glycinemia (nonketotic)	Glycine	Glycine cleavage enzyme system	Enzyme assay in chorionic villus (not amniocyte)	Convulsions, retardation	Low-protein diet, strychnine (?), sodium benzoate
β-Alaninemia	β-Alanine	β-Alanine-α-ketoglutarate aminotransferase		Seizures, somnolence, death	Pyridoxine (?)
Prolinemia, type I	Proline	Proline oxidase		Hereditary nephritis, nerve deafness (?)	May be benign trait
Prolinemia, type II	Proline	Δ^1Pyrroline-5-carboxylate dehydrogenase		Convulsions, mental retardation	Low-protein diet, low proline and glutamic acid
Hydroxyprolinemia	Hydroxyproline	Hydroxyproline oxidase		Mental retardation, CNS symptoms	Low-protein diet (?), benign (?)
Lysinemia	Lysine	Lysine ketoglutarate reductase		Muscle weakness, retardation, benign in some instances	Controlled lysine intake (?)
Lysine intolerance	Lysine Arginine	L-Lysine:NAD oxidoreductase (deaminating)		Vomiting, coma	Low-protein diet, controlled lysine intake
Saccharopinuria	Lysine	Aminoadipic semialdehyde–glutamate reductase		Retardation	Controlled lysine intake
Pipecolicacidemia	Lysine	Pipecolate oxidase	Very long chain fatty acid level, plasmalogen synthesis (Zellweger's)	Usually a manifestation of cerebrohepatorenal (Zellweger) syndrome	Reduced intake of very long chain fatty acids
N-Acetylglutamate synthetase deficiency	Ammonia	N-Acetylglutamate synthetase		Lethargy, coma, vomiting	Low-protein diet, arginine, sodium benzoate, sodium phenylacetate

(Continued)

TABLE 40–10. ANOMALIES IN AMINO ACID METABOLISM *(Cont'd)*

Disease	Amino Acid Affected	Enzyme Defect	Prenatal Diagnosis*	Clinical Features	Treatment
Carbamoyl phosphate synthetase deficiency	Ammonia	Carbamoyl phosphate synthetase	RFLP analysis	Vomiting, lethargy, acidosis, coma, death	Low-protein diet; essential amino acid mixture, ketoacid analogs of amino acids; arginine; sodium benzoate; sodium phenylacetate
Ornithine-transcarbamylase deficiency	Ammonia	Ornithine transcarbamoylase	RFLP analysis	Recurrent vomiting, irritability, lethargy, coma, seizures, X-linked, lethal in the male	Low-protein diet; essential amino acid mixture, ketoacid analogs of amino acids; arginine; sodium benzoate; sodium phenylacetate
Citrullinemia	Citrulline	Argininosuccinic acid synthetase	Enzyme assay, RFLP analysis	Vomiting, coma, convulsions	Low-protein diet; essential amino acid mixture, ketoacid analogs of amino acids; arginine; sodium benzoate; sodium phenylacetate
Argininosuccinicacidemia	Argininosuccinic acid	Argininosuccinase	Enzyme assay	Seizures, retardation, coma, vomiting, hepatomegaly, trichorrhexis nodosa	Low-protein diet; essential amino acid mixture, ketoacid analogs of amino acids; arginine; sodium benzoate; sodium phenylacetate
Argininemia	Arginine	Arginase	Enzyme assay, RFLP analysis	Retardation, seizures, spasticity	Essential amino acid mixture
Ornithinemia	Ornithine	Ornithine keto-acid transaminase	Enzyme assay	Gyrate atrophy of choroid and retina	Low-protein diet, low arginine; proline supplement
Syndrome of hyperornithinemia, hyperammonemia, and homocitrullinemia	Ornithine Ammonia Homocitrulline	Transport defect into mitochondria (?)		Seizures, retardation	Low-protein diet
Sarcosinemia	Sarcosine	Sarcosine dehydrogenase		Mental retardation (?), no symptoms	May be benign trait, no treatment indicated
Glutamicacidemia	Glutamic acid	?		Mental and physical retardation, seizures, trichorrhexis nodosa	?

Pyroglutamic acidemia	Pyroglutamic acid	5-Oxoproline glutathione synthetase	Enzyme assay	Acidosis, increased hemolysis, episodic vomiting, retardation	?
Isovaleric acidemia	Leucine	Isovaleryl-CoA dehydrogenase	Enzyme assay	Vomiting, lethargy, acidosis, retardation, sweaty feet odor, neonatal death	Controlled leucine intake; glycine
β-Hydroxyisovaleric aciduria	Leucine	β-Methylcrotonyl-CoA carboxylase	Enzyme assay, elevated BOH, isovaleric acid	Retardation, muscle atrophy, unpleasant urine odor	Controlled leucine intake
HMG-CoA lyase deficiency	Leucine	3-Hydroxy-3-methylglutaryl CoA lyase	Enzyme assay; elevated 3-hydroxy-3-methyl-glutaric, 3-methyl-glutaric, and 3-hydroxyisovaleric acids in maternal urine	Acidosis, hypoglycemia, hypotonia, lethargy	Low-protein diet, controlled leucine intake, control of hypoglycemia
α-Methylacetoacetate accumulation	Isoleucine	Acetyl-CoA thiolase	Enzyme assay	Episodes of acidosis, coma; retardation	Low-protein diet, controlled isoleucine intake
Propionicacidemia (form of ketotic glycinemia)	Threonine, Isoleucine, Methionine, Valine	Propionyl-CoA carboxylase 1. Apoenzyme deficiency 2. Coenzyme deficiency	Enzyme assay	Acidosis, lethargy, coma, mental and physical retardation	Low-protein diet, controlled intake of threonine, valine, isoleucine, methionine, and carnitine
Multiple carboxylase deficiency	Leucine, Isoleucine, Valine, Threonine	1. Holocarboxylase synthetase 2. Biotinidase	Enzyme assay	Acidosis, skin rash, alopecia, hypotonia, defective T- and B-cell immunity, hearing loss	Biotin 5–10 mg/day
Methylmalonic acidemia (form of ketotic glycinemia)	Isoleucine, Valine, Threonine, Methionine	Methylmalonyl-CoA mutase 1. Apoenzyme deficiency 2. Vitamin B₁₂ cofactor deficiency Methylmalonyl-CoA racemase (?)	Enzyme assay	Acidosis, lethargy, coma, mental and physical retardation	1. Low-protein diet, controlled intake of isoleucine, valine, threonine, methionine, and carnitine 2. Massive doses of vitamin B_{12} .... Same as (1) above
Methylmalonic acidemia – homocystinuria	Isoleucine, Valine, Threonine, Methionine	Methylmalonyl-CoA mutase and homocysteine: methyl tetrahydrofolate methyl transferase	Enzyme assay	Retardation, failure to thrive, seizures, megaloblastic anemia	Hydroxocobalamin

NAD = nicotinamide-adenine dinucleotide; RE = reticuloendothelial; RFLP = restriction fragment length polymorphism.
* Advances are occurring so rapidly that molecular biologic techniques may soon be available for the diagnosis of many more disorders.

development possible and prevents CNS involvement. Treatment started after 2 to 3 yr of age may be effective only in controlling the extreme hyperactivity and intractable seizures. The length of time that treatment should be continued is still not completely resolved. Although it was formerly considered safe to discontinue treatment when brain myelinization is virtually complete, reports of a drop in IQ and the development of learning and behavior problems have led to a reconsideration of this recommendation. An increasing number of physicians now believe that therapy should be continued for life and are trying to continue therapy indefinitely.

ANOMALIES IN PIGMENT METABOLISM

THE PORPHYRIAS

A group of disorders of heme biosynthesis in which the activities of the enzymes of the heme biosynthetic pathway are partially or almost completely deficient. Abnormally elevated levels of porphyrins or their precursors (eg, δ-aminolevulinic acid [ALA] and porphobilinogen [PBG]) are produced, accumulate in tissues, or are excreted in urine and stool.

Heme Biosynthetic Pathway

Outline of the pathway: The steps involved in the heme biosynthetic pathway are illustrated in FIG. 40–2. In animal cells, the first step and the last 3 steps take place in mitochondria; the intermediate steps occur in the cytosol. For example, heme is made in erythroblasts or reticulocytes that still contain mitochondria, while circulating erythrocytes lack the ability to form heme.

1. Formation of δ-aminolevulinic acid (ALA): ALA synthase, the first enzyme of the heme biosynthetic pathway, catalyzes the condensation of glycine and succinyl coenzyme A (CoA) to form ALA. The enzyme is localized in the inner membrane of mitochondria and requires pyridoxal 5'-phosphate as a cofactor. Separate genes encode erythroid and nonerythroid ALA synthases.

2. Formation of porphobilinogen (PBG) from ALA: Two molecules of ALA are converted by a cytosolic enzyme, **ALA dehydratase**, to a monopyrrole, PBG, with the removal of 2 molecules of water. Lead inhibits ALA dehydratase activity by displacing zinc (the metal essential for enzyme activity) from the enzyme. The most potent inhibitor of the enzyme is succinylacetone, a structural analog of ALA, which is found in urine and blood of patients with hereditary tyrosinemia.

3. Formation of hydroxymethylbilane (HMB) from PBG: PBG deaminase catalyzes the condensation of 4 molecules of PBG to yield a linear tetrapyrrole, HMB. In the absence of the subsequent enzyme, uroporphyrinogen (Uro') III cosynthase (CoS), the bilane is spontaneously cyclized into the first tetrapyrrole, Uro' I. In the presence of the CoS enzyme, Uro' III, which has a reversed D-ring pyrrole, is formed. There are 2 isozymes of PBG deaminase; one is present exclusively in erythroid cells, whereas the other is in nonerythroid cells. The 2 isoforms of PBG deaminase are encoded by distinct messenger RNAs (mRNAs) that are transcribed from a single gene by alternate transcription and splicing.

4. Formation of Uro' III from HMB: Uro'CoS catalyzes the formation of Uro' III from HMB. This involves an intramolecular rearrangement that affects only ring D of the porphyrin macrocycle.

5. Formation of coproporphyrinogen (Copro') from Uro': A cytosolic enzyme, **Uro' decarboxylase**, catalyzes the sequential removal of the 4 carboxylic groups of the carboxymethyl side chains in Uro' to yield Copro'.

6. Formation of protoporphyrinogen (Proto') from Copro': Copro' oxidase in mammalian cells is a mitochondrial enzyme that catalyzes the removal of the carboxyl group and 2 hydrogens from the propionic groups of pyrrole rings A and B of Copro' to form vinyl groups at these positions.

7. Formation of protoporphyrin from Proto': The oxidation of Proto' to protoporphyrin is mediated by **Proto' oxidase**, which catalyzes the removal of 6 hydrogen atoms from the porphyrinogen nucleus.

8. Formation of heme from protoporphyrin: The final step of heme biosynthesis is the insertion of iron into protoporphyrin. This reaction is catalyzed by a mitochondrial enzyme, **ferrochelatase**.

Control of Heme Synthesis

Regulation of hepatic ALA synthase: Biosynthesis of heme in the liver is controlled largely by the rate of formation of ALA synthase. The enzyme activity in normal liver cells is very low, while its level increases dramatically when the liver needs to make more heme in response to various chemical treatments. The synthesis of the enzyme is also regulated in a feedback fash-

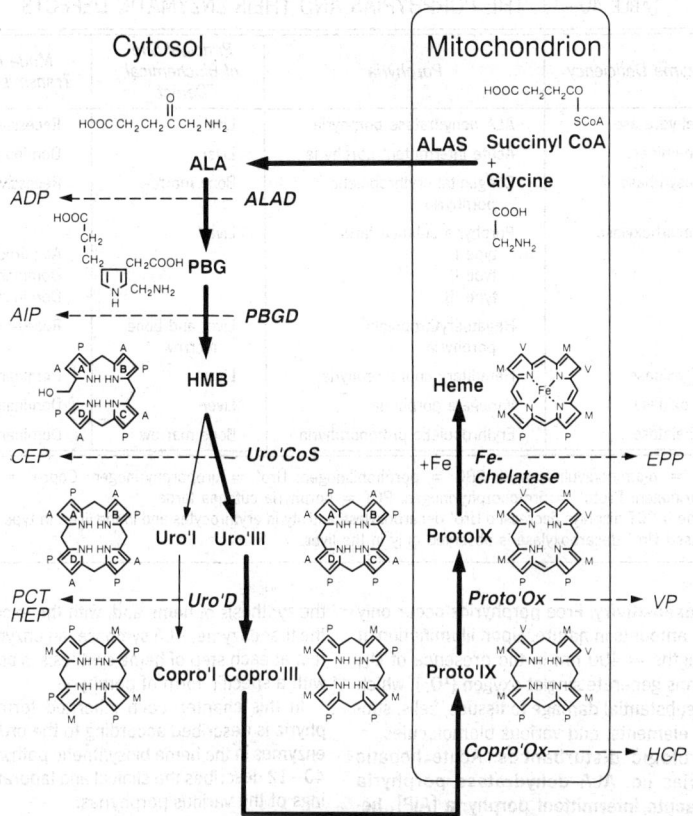

FIG. 40–2. **Enzymes and intermediates in the heme biosynthetic pathway.** Pyrrole ring designation is shown in the structures of hydroxymethylbilane, uroporphyrinogen I and III. In uroporphyrinogen III, β-substituent groups in ring D have undergone "flipping," ie, the ring is reversed. ADP = δ-aminolevulinic acid dehydratase porphyria; AIP = acute intermittent porphyria; ALA = δ-aminolevulinic acid; ALAD = δ-aminolevulinic acid dehydratase; ALAS = δ-aminolevulinic acid synthase; CEP = congenital erythropoietic porphyria; Copro' = coproporphyrinogen; Copro'Ox = Copro' oxidase; EPP = erythropoietic protoporphyria; HCP = hereditary coproporphyria; HEP = hepatoerythropoietic porphyria; HMB = hydroxymethylbilane; PBG = porphobilinogen; PBGD = porphobilinogen deaminase; PCT = porphyria cutanea tarda; Proto' = protoporphyrinogen; Proto'Ox = Proto' oxidase; Uro' = uroporphyrinogen; Uro'CoS = Uro'III cosynthase; VP = variegate porphyria. A: −CH₂COOH; M: −CH₃; P: −CH₂CH₂COOH; V: −CH=CH₂.

ion by heme. At higher heme concentrations than those that repress the synthesis of ALA synthase, heme induces microsomal heme oxygenase, resulting in an enhancement of its own catabolism. Thus, the hepatic heme concentration is maintained by a balance between the synthesis of ALA synthase and heme oxygenase, both under the regulatory influence of heme. In contrast, ALA synthase in erythroid cells is re-

fractory to or little influenced by heme treatment. Regulation of heme synthesis in erythroid cells appears to be different from that in the liver.

Pathophysiology of Porphyrins and Porphyrin Precursors

Two cardinal symptoms of porphyrias are photosensitivity and neurologic disturbances.

TABLE 40–11. THE PORPHYRIAS AND THEIR ENZYMATIC DEFECTS

Enzyme Deficiency	Porphyria	Principal Site of Biochemical Defect	Mode of Transmission
ALA dehydratase	ALA dehydratase porphyria	Liver	Recessive
PBG deaminase	Acute intermittent porphyria	Liver	Dominant
Uro' cosynthase	Congenital erythropoietic porphyria	Bone marrow	Recessive
Uro' decarboxylase	Porphyria cutanea tarda	Liver*	
	type I		Acquired
	type II		Dominant
	type III		Dominant
	Hepatoerythropoietic porphyria	Liver and bone marrow	Recessive
Copro' oxidase	Hereditary coproporphyria	Liver	Dominant
Proto' oxidase	Variegate porphyria	Liver	Dominant
Ferrochelatase	Erythropoietic protoporphyria	Bone marrow	Dominant

ALA = δ-aminolevulinic acid; PBG = porphobilinogen; Uro' = uroporphyrinogen; Copro' = copro-porphyrinogen; Proto' = protoporphyrinogen; PCT = porphyria cutanea tarda.
* Type II PCT displays decreased Uro' decarboxylase activity in erythrocytes and in the liver; in type III PCT, decreased Uro' decarboxylase is observed only in the liver.

Photosensitivity: Free porphyrins occur only in small amounts in nature. Upon illumination at wavelengths ≃ 400 nm in the presence of O_2, porphyrins generate singlet oxygen ($^1O_2$), which causes substantial damage to tissues, cells, subcellular elements, and various biomolecules.

Neurologic disturbances: Acute hepatic porphyrias (ie, **ALA dehydratase porphyria [ADP]**, **acute intermittent porphyria [AIP]**, **hereditary coproporphyria [HCP]**, and **variegate porphyria [VP]**) are characterized by neurologic disturbances. Most commonly observed symptoms are abdominal pain, disordered intestinal motility (eg, diarrhea and constipation), dysesthesia, muscular paralysis, and respiratory failure, which can often be fatal. Several mechanisms for the neurologic disturbances have been postulated; eg, the involvement of excessive ALA and PBG, deficient heme synthesis, or increased tryptophan in the CNS due to decreased hepatic tryptophan pyrrolase activity. However, the exact cause and nature of the neurologic disturbances remain unclear.

Classification of Porphyrias

Porphyrias are classified as either hepatic or erythropoietic depending on the principal site of expression of the specific enzymatic defect (see TABLE 40–11). There are 8 enzymes involved in

the synthesis of heme and, with the exception of the first enzyme, ALA synthase, an enzymatic defect at each step of heme synthesis is associated with a specific form of porphyria.

In this chapter, each inherited form of porphyria is described according to the order of the enzymes in the heme biosynthetic pathway. TABLE 40–12 describes the clinical and laboratory findings of the various porphyrias.

ALA DEHYDRATASE PORPHYRIA (ADP)

An autosomal recessive disorder resulting from a homozygous ALA dehydratase deficiency. This is the rarest form of the porphyrias; only 4 cases have been reported to date. The clinical findings are similar to those seen in acute intermittent porphyria (see below) and are exacerbated following stress, alcohol use, or decreased food intake. An infant with ADP was reported who had symptoms of acute hepatic porphyria from birth, which included general muscle hypotonia and respiratory insufficiency.

Laboratory Findings

Urinary ALA excretion is markedly elevated, whereas urinary PBG excretion is little affected. Urinary and erythrocyte porphyrins are also markedly elevated (one hundredfold); no satisfactory explanation has yet been advanced to ac-

TABLE 40–12. CLINICAL AND LABORATORY FINDINGS OF THE PORPHYRIAS

Porphyria	Clinical Symptoms	Laboratory Findings*			
		Red Cells	Plasma	Urine	Stool
AIP	Neurologic Nausea, vomiting, abdominal pain, diarrhea, constipation, ileus, dysuria, muscle hypotonia, respiratory insufficiency, sensory neuropathy, seizures	—	—	ALA, PBG	—
ADP	Neurologic (same as AIP)	Zn-PP	—	ALA	
CEP	Photosensitivity Bullae, crusts, scar formation, sclerodermoid, hyper- and hypopigmentation, hypertrichosis, erythrodontia, hemolytic anemia, splenomegaly	Uro I, Copro I	Uro I, Copro I	Uro I, Copro I	—
PCT	Photosensitivity Skin fragility, bullae, crusts, sclerodermoid, hyper- and hypopigmentation, hypertrichosis	—	Uro, 7-carboxyl	Uro, 7-carboxyl	Uro, 7-carboxyl, Isocopro
HEP	Photosensitivity (same as CEP)	Zn-PP	Uro, 7-carboxyl	Uro, 7-carboxyl	Uro, 7-carboxyl, Isocopro
HCP	Neurologic and photosensitivity (same as AIP and PCT)	—	Copro	ALA, PBG, Copro	Copro
VP	Neurologic and photosensitivity (same as AIP and PCT)	—	Proto	ALA, PBG	Proto
EPP	Photosensitivity Burning sensation, edema, erythema, itching, scarring, vesicles	Proto	Proto	—	Proto

ADP = δ-aminolevulinic acid dehydratase porphyria; AIP = acute intermittent porphyria; ALA = δ-aminolevulinic acid; CEP = congenital erythropoietic porphyria; Copro = coproporphyrin; EPP = erythropoietic porphyria; HCP = hereditary coproporphyria; HEP = hepatoerythropoietic porphyria; PCT = porphyria cutanea tarda; PBG = porphobilinogen; Proto = protoporphyrin; Uro = uroporphyrin; VP = variegate porphyria; Zn-PP = Zn-protoporphyrin.
* Laboratory findings show increased levels, which are abnormal. It is difficult to provide approximate values, since normal values vary depending upon laboratory.

count for this observation. Fecal porphyrin excretion is normal or marginally elevated. Patients with ADP display little activity of ALA dehydratase in erythrocytes or in nonerythroid cells (≤ 2% of normal), while their parents show about 50% decreases in enzyme activity.

Diagnosis and Treatment

Definitive diagnosis is dependent upon the demonstration of impaired ALA dehydratase activity and deficiency of enzyme protein in erythrocytes. Supporting evidence for the diagnosis includes massive elevations in urinary ALA, substantial elevations of porphyrins in urine and erythrocytes, and perhaps modest elevations in fecal porphyrins. Clinical symptoms of ADP occur only in homozygous patients, while heterozygous patients (ie, parents and certain siblings of the probands) remain clinically unaffected. Treatment of ADP is the same as for AIP (see below).

ACUTE INTERMITTENT PORPHYRIA (AIP)
(Swedish Porphyria; Pyrroloporphyria)

An autosomal dominant disorder resulting from a deficiency in PBG deaminase activity. The deficient enzyme activity ($\approx$ 50% of normal) is found in all tissues, including erythrocytes, in the majority of patients (> 85%). This is consistent with the heterozygous state of affected individuals. However, a subset of patients (< 15%) show deficient enzyme activity only in nonerythroid cells. The majority ($\approx$ 90%) of individuals with this genetic enzyme deficiency remain biochemically and clinically normal. Clinical expression of the disease is usually linked to environmental or acquired factors; eg, nutritional status, drugs, steroids, and other chemicals of endogenous or exogenous origin. The cardinal pathobiology of the disease is a neurologic dysfunction that may affect the peripheral, autonomic, or central nervous system; the resulting neuropathic symptoms may be highly diverse.

Incidence

AIP is probably the most common of the genetic porphyrias. The highest incidence occurs in Lapland, Scandinavia, and the United Kingdom, although it has been reported in other population groups. The incidence of the defective gene in the USA has been estimated at between 5 and 10/100,000. The incidence of AIP in psychiatric populations is somewhat higher than in the normal population. The disorder is expressed clinically after puberty and more commonly in women than in men.

Symptoms and Signs

Abdominal pain is almost always present and is often the initial symptom of an acute attack. It may be generalized or localized, and in severe cases can be confused with an "acute surgical abdomen." Other GI features may include nausea, vomiting, constipation or diarrhea, abdominal distention, and ileus. Urinary retention, incontinence, dysuria, and frequency may be observed. Tachycardia and hypertension, and less frequently fever, sweating, restlessness, and tremor are also observed. In up to 40% of patients, hypertension may become sustained between acute attacks.

Neuropathy is a common feature of AIP. Muscle weakness often begins proximally in the legs but may involve the arms or the distal extremities; involvement may be symmetric, asymmetric, or focal, and may occasionally be associated with a decrease or loss of tendon reflexes. Motor neuropathy may also involve the cranial nerves (most commonly the 7th and 10th) or lead to bulbar paralysis, respiratory deficiency, and death. Sensory patchy neuropathy also occurs when motor neuropathy is severe. Acute attacks of AIP may be accompanied by seizures, especially in patients with hyponatremia due to vomiting, inappropriate fluid therapy, or the syndrome of inappropriate antidiuretic hormone release. The course of an acute attack of AIP is highly variable both in individuals and between patients, with attacks lasting from a few days to several months.

Precipitating factors: Asymptomatic heterozygotes ($\approx$ 90% of subjects with documented PBG deaminase deficiency) may display neither abnormalities in concentrations of heme pathway intermediates nor clinical symptoms. Individuals with both latent or previously clinically expressed AIP may be precipitated into an acute attack by endogenous or exogenous environmental factors. Most, if not all, precipitating factors in AIP can be related to an associated increase in the activity of ALA synthase in liver. The clinical disease is more common in women, especially perimenstrually; a subset of female patients experiences regular cyclical premenstrual exacerbations of their disease. Reduced calorie intake often leads to exacerbations of AIP. Many chemicals that exacerbate porphyria are thought to have the potential to induce cytochrome P-450, and the resultant enhanced demand for de novo heme synthesis is presumed to lead to induction of hepatic ALA synthase activity. These chemicals include sex steroids, barbiturates, and other foreign chemicals. Stress is also considered to exacerbate AIP. Similarly, intercurrent illnesses, infections, alcoholic excess, and surgery may all contribute to the genesis of an acute attack of this disorder. Glucose administration is effective in attenuating ALA synthase induction in rat liver as well as in decreasing urinary ALA and PBG excretion in patients. The mechanism of the glucose effect remains unclear.

Laboratory Findings

Patients with clinically expressed AIP, as well as a few individuals with latent AIP, excrete variably increased amounts of ALA and PBG in the urine between attacks. In the majority of cases, the onset of an acute attack is accompanied by further marked to massive increases in excretion of these precursors. Acute attacks may also be associated with elevations in the serum concentrations of ALA, PBG, and porphyrins, which are normally undetectable. In severe cases, the urine develops a port-wine color due to a high content of porphobilin, an auto-oxidized product of PBG. Urine may also contain elevated levels of porphyrins that are formed by nonenzymatic cyclization of PBG. Stool porphyrins are usually normal or only slightly elevated. The Watson-Schwartz test is widely used as a screening test for urinary PBG. However, it is neither as sensitive nor as specific as the quantitative column method of Mauzerall and Granick, which should be used to verify positive results from screening tests. There are no abnormalities in Hb or bilirubin production in AIP.

Diagnosis

Diagnosis can be made by the demonstration of decreased PBG deaminase activity in erythrocytes in the majority of patients ($> 85\%$); the distinction between carrier or latent status and clinically expressed AIP depends upon the demonstration of elevated urinary excretion of PBG and ALA and upon the natural history of the individual patient. Elevated levels of both ALA and PBG may also be seen in hereditary coproporphyria (HCP) and variegate porphyria (VP); measurement of urinary and stool porphyrins will usually differentiate these conditions from AIP. The subset of AIP patients expressing the PBG deaminase gene defect only in nonerythroid tissues ($< 15\%$ of all AIP) is due to a single-base substitution at the first position of the intron, which results in abnormal splicing leading to an aborted gene product in nonerythroid cells. This mutation, however, does not affect the transcription of the erythroid PBG deaminase mRNA, since the transcription of the erythroid mRNA starts downstream from the mutated site. Diagnosis of the latter group of patients requires the demonstration of either PBG deaminase deficiency in nonerythroid cells or DNA hybridization using allele-specific oligonucleotides.

Treatment

The treatment of AIP as well as ADP, HCP, and VP is essentially identical. Treatment between attacks comprises adequate nutritional intake, avoidance of drugs known to exacerbate porphyria, and prompt treatment of other intercurrent diseases or infections. Unresponsive severe cases should be treated with IV dextrose to provide a minimum of 300 gm of carbohydrate/day. IV hematin 4 mg/kg q 12 to 24 h is also effective in reducing ALA and PBG excretion as well as in curtailing acute attacks. It has also been used prophylactically (200 mg/wk) to abol-

ish cyclical perimenstrual porphyria attacks. Nasal or s.c. administration of long-acting agonistic analogs of luteinizing hormone releasing hormone has been shown to inhibit ovulation and greatly reduce the incidence of perimenstrual attacks of AIP in some women with cyclic exacerbations of the disease. Synthetic heme analogs, eg, Sn-mesoporphyrin, have also been shown to diminish the output of ALA, PBG, and porphyrins in AIP and VP patients.

CONGENITAL ERYTHROPOIETIC PORPHYRIA (CEP)

(Günther's Disease; Erythropoietic Porphyria; Congenital Porphyria; Congenital Hematoporphyria; Erythropoietic Uroporphyria)

An inherited autosomal recessive disorder wherein the primary abnormality is a decreased activity of Uro'CoS, which results in accumulation and hyperexcretion of type I porphyrins. Clinically, this enzymatic defect is already expressed in utero as brownish amniotic fluid due to excessive amounts of porphyrins and, after birth, in cutaneous photosensitivity, hemolysis, and a decreased life expectancy. The primary site of expression is the bone marrow wherein fluorescence secondary to porphyrin accumulation is variably distributed but invariably present. Most marrow normoblasts display fluorescence, principally localized in the nuclei of the cells. Massive elevations of systemic porphyrins in CEP are derived from porphyrin-laden erythrocytes, which accounts for the multiple pathologies of the integument.

Incidence: Less than 200 cases have been reported, and some of these may really have been porphyria cutanea tarda or hepatoerythropoietic porphyria. There is no clear racial or sexual predominance.

Symptoms and Signs

The first clue suggesting the diagnosis of CEP may be pink to dark-brown staining of diapers in infants due to large amounts of porphyrins in urine. Early onset of cutaneous photosensitivity is characteristic and is exacerbated by exposure to sunlight. Subepidermal bullous lesions progress to crusted erosions that heal with scarring and either hyperpigmentation or, less commonly, hypopigmentation. Hypertrichosis and alopecia are frequent, and erythrodontia (with red fluorescence under UV light) is virtually pathognomonic of CEP. Patients may display symptoms and signs of hemolytic anemia with splenomegaly and porphyrin-rich gallstones. Bone marrow shows erythroid hyperplasia, which may result in pathologic fractures or vertebral compression-collapse and shortness of stature. Although the onset of symptoms of CEP is most often observed in early infancy, a few patients may first present as adults.

Laboratory Findings

Urinary porphyrins are always elevated (twenty to sixtyfold) above normal levels. Uroporphyrin and coproporphyrin are mostly type I isomers (see TABLE 40–12). Occasionally anemia may be severe and require transfusion.

Diagnosis

Pink urine and/or the onset of severe cutaneous photosensitivity in infancy (or rarely in adults) suggests the diagnosis of CEP. Demonstration of elevated urinary, fecal, and erythrocyte porphyrins, with elevated type I isomers of uro- and coproporphyrin, establishes the diagnosis of CEP. Demonstration of a deficiency of Uro'CoS activity constitutes the definitive diagnosis.

Treatment

The avoidance of sunlight, trauma to the skin, and infections is the most important preventive measure in CEP. Topical sunscreens may be of some help, as may oral treatment with β-carotene. Transfusions with packed erythrocytes transiently decrease hemolysis and its attendant drive to increased erythropoiesis, and also decrease porphyrin excretion. Splenectomy has been used fairly frequently and has produced short-term reductions in hemolysis, porphyrin excretion, and skin manifestations, but not all cases respond. Hematin infusions have been given to a woman with CEP and were reported to reduce porphyrin output with about the same efficacy as packed erythrocyte transfusions but over a shorter duration.

PORPHYRIA CUTANEA TARDA (PCT)

(Symptomatic Porphyria; Porphyria Cutanea Symptomatica; Idiosyncratic Porphyria)

A heterogeneous group of porphyrias that may be inherited (familial, or type II and III) or, more commonly, acquired (sporadic, or type I). Both forms of the disease are heterozygous and display reductions in the activity of Uro' decarboxylase. In type II the enzyme is deficient in all tissues, whereas in type I the defect is confined to the liver. Type I typically presents in adults, either spontaneously or more commonly in conjunction with precipitating environmental factors such as alcohol, estrogen or drug use, or in association with other disorders. Recently another form, type III, has been reported in which normal erythrocyte Uro' decarboxylase activity and concentrations were found in more than one member in a single family, but with decreased hepatic Uro' decarboxylase activity (see TABLE 40–11). The hallmark of all types of PCT is cutaneous photosensitivity due to increased production of uroporphyrin and 7-carboxylic porphyrin.

Epidemiology

PCT is probably the most common of all the porphyrias, genetic and acquired combined, but its exact incidence is not clear. The disease is recognized worldwide and there is no racial predilection except among the Bantus in South Africa, probably secondary to their high incidence of hemosiderosis. Type I PCT is generally more common than type II in Europe, South Africa, and South America, although the trend may be less obvious in North America. Previously, PCT was held to be more common in men than women, perhaps secondary to higher alcohol intake, but the incidence in women has increased lately to the level seen in men, perhaps due to increased use of oral contraceptives, postmenopausal estrogens, and alcohol.

Symptoms and Signs

Cutaneous lesions in the light-exposed areas, including skin fragility, vesicle and bullae formation, atrophic changes, and scar formation, are often followed by hyper- and hypopigmentation, hypertrichosis, and pseudosclerodermoid changes. Phototoxic porphyrins in the skin may be largely derived from the liver and, to some extent, formed locally in the skin. Activation of the complement system after irradiation has been demonstrated in PCT patients both in vivo and in vitro in sera and is presumed to result from the generation of reactive O_2 species, most likely $^1O_2$. Bullous fluid is known to contain prostaglandin E_2, and photoactivation of uroporphyrin damages lysosomes; inflammation and autolysis may be attributable in part to these factors. Liver from patients with PCT almost invariably displays siderosis with fatty changes, necrosis, chronic inflammatory changes, and granuloma formation. Iron, estrogens, alcohol, and chlorinated hydrocarbons, which are all potential hepatotoxins, may also aggravate PCT. The incidence of hepatitis B infection may also be higher than normal in PCT patients. Any or all of these factors or porphyrins themselves may predispose the liver of PCT patients to neoplastic changes, and the incidence of hepatocellular carcinoma in PCT is known to be greater than in the general population. Rarely, primary hepatomas may secrete porphyrins and simulate PCT. Several patients with AIDS were first recognized as having PCT, preceding the terminal phase of the syndrome.

Laboratory Findings

Increased concentrations of uroporphyrin (mainly isomer I) and 7-carboxylic porphyrins (mainly isomer III) are found in the urine of patients with PCT, with lesser increases of coproporphyrin and 5- and 6-carboxylic porphyrins. Small quantities of isocoproporphyrin may be detected in serum or in urine, but in feces this is often the dominant porphyrin excreted and represents the most important diagnostic criterion for PCT (see TABLE 40–12). Concentrations of coproporphyrin, 7-carboxylic porphyrin, uroporphyrin, and fecal X-porphyrins (ether–acetic acid insoluble, extracted with urea-triton), a heterogeneous group of porphyrin-peptide conjugates, may all be increased in PCT. Total daily fecal porphyrin excretion exceeds total urinary porphyrin excretion. Skin porphyrins are increased, especially in areas that are protected from photoactivation. Serum iron and ferritin concentrations are frequently elevated.

Diagnosis

The clinical picture in PCT is fairly specific but can be confused with other porphyric (eg, VP) and nonporphyric (eg, SLE) diseases. Urinary fluorescence under UV light and quantitation of porphyrins and separation and identification of porphyrins by chromatography will assist the diagnosis. Plasma porphyrins are elevated in PCT in other photosensitizing porphyrias. Fecal porphyrins are often elevated; isocoproporphyrin (or an isocoproporphyrin:coproporphyrin ratio ≥ 0.1) is virtually diagnostic of PCT. In type II PCT patients, the catalytic activity and the concentration of immunoreactive Uro' decarboxylase are both about 50% of normal, and the enzyme deficiency segregates as an autosomal dominant trait in patients' families. In contrast, patients with type I PCT show normal erythrocyte Uro' decarboxylase activity and concentrations, and no familial occurrence of the disorder. However, patients with type III PCT show familial

occurrence also with normal erythrocyte Uro' decarboxylase activity.

Treatment

In type I PCT, the identification and avoidance of precipitating factors is the first line of treatment. The clinical response to cessation of alcohol ingestion is highly variable; nonetheless, abstinence should be recommended. Phlebotomy is usually effective in reducing urinary porphyrin concentrations and in inducing clinical remissions. There is strong evidence that the beneficial effects of phlebotomy result from a diminution in the stores of body iron. If phlebotomy is ineffective or contraindicated owing to the presence of other diseases such as anemia, low-dose chloroquine therapy may be effective. Efficacy of chloroquine therapy and phlebotomy is probably similar, and a combined approach may diminish the incidence of side effects. The mechanism of action of chloroquine therapy is thought to be related to its ability to chelate porphyrins in a water-soluble and hence more easily excretable form.

HEPATOERYTHROPOIETIC PORPHYRIA (HEP)

A rare form of porphyria probably resulting from a homozygous defect in Uro' decarboxylase activity, which is clinically indistinguishable from CEP and characterized by the childhood onset of severe photosensitivity and skin fragility. Less than 20 cases have been reported worldwide.

Symptoms and Signs

These are very similar to those seen in CEP. Pink urine, severe photosensitivity leading to scarring and mutilation of sun-exposed areas of skin, sclerodermoid changes, hypertrichosis, erythrodontia, anemia (often hemolytic), and hepatosplenomegaly characterize HEP. Onset is usually in early infancy or childhood, but adult onset has also been described. In contrast to type I PCT patients, serum iron concentrations have usually been normal, and phlebotomy has no beneficial effects in HEP patients. The incidence of bone marrow and liver fluorescence, anemia, and evidence of abnormal liver function and histology are highly variable. Skin biopsies show subepidermal bullae and other findings similar to the lesions of PCT.

Laboratory Findings

Elevations in urinary porphyrins, predominantly uroporphyrin of isomer type I, with lesser quantities of mainly type III 7-carboxylic porphyrins, are commonly found. Isocoproporphyrin concentrations equal to or greater than coproporphyrin are also found in urine and feces. Elevated erythrocyte Zn-protoporphyrin is commonly observed (see TABLE 40–12). Anemia and biochemical evidence of impaired hepatic function are highly variable. Cloning and sequencing of a cDNA of the mutated gene in a patient with HEP revealed the enzymatic defect to be due to a mutation of a Gly (GGG) to Glu (GAG) in the amino acid sequence at position 281. This point mutation results in an unstable protein.

Diagnosis

The diagnosis must be suspected in patients with severe photosensitivity and especially considered in the differential diagnosis of CEP. Diagnostic criteria include elevated levels of fecal or urinary isocoproporphyrin and erythrocyte Zn-protoporphyrin. Included in the differential diagnosis is erythropoietic protoporphyria (EPP), in which erythrocyte protoporphyrin is also elevated but, in contrast to HEP, urinary porphyrins are normal. EPP is also clinically milder than HEP. Measurement of erythrocyte or fibroblast Uro' decarboxylase activities typically shows reductions to 2 to 10% of normal control values with intermediate reductions of Uro' decarboxylase activities in family members.

Treatment

Avoidance of the sun and the use of topical sunscreens are essentially all that can be offered these patients. Response to phlebotomy has not been seen, although this is perhaps not surprising, as serum iron levels, in contrast to those in type I patients, are invariably normal.

HEREDITARY COPROPORPHYRIA (HCP)

A disease caused by a heterozygous deficiency of Copro' oxidase activity that is inherited in an autosomal dominant manner. Clinically, the disease is similar to ADP or AIP, although it is often milder; additionally, HCP may be associated with photosensitivity. Expression of the disease is variable and influenced by the same precipitating factors responsible for the exacerbation of AIP. Very rarely, homozygous deficiency of this enzyme may occur and is associated with a more severe form of the disease.

Incidence: Clinically expressed HCP is much less common than is clinically expressed AIP but,

as with the latter disease, latent HCP or HCP gene carriers are being recognized with greater frequency since the advent of improved laboratory techniques for their detection.

Symptoms and Signs

Neurovisceral symptomatology is predominant and is essentially indistinguishable from that of ADP or AIP. Abdominal pain, vomiting, constipation, neuropathies, and psychiatric manifestations are common. Cutaneous photosensitivity occurs in about 30% of cases. Attacks can be precipitated by pregnancy, the menstrual cycle, and oral contraceptives, but the most common precipitating factor is drug administration, most notably of phenobarbital.

Laboratory Findings

The biochemical hallmark of HCP is hyperexcretion of coproporphyrin (predominantly type III) into the urine and feces (see TABLE 40–12). Hyperexcretion of ALA, PBG, and uroporphyrin into the urine may accompany exacerbations of the disease, but in contrast to AIP, these findings generally normalize between attacks. Copro' oxidase activity, which can be measured in fibroblasts or in lymphocytes, is typically reduced by about 50% in heterozygotes and by about 90 to 98% in homozygotes. The latter also show elevations in urinary ALA, PBG, and uroporphyrin. Additionally, patients with harderoporphyria, a variant of HCP, have elevated erythrocyte protoporphyrin and higher total fecal porphyrins, of which about 60% is harderoporphyrin, ie, a tricarboxylate porphyrin.

Diagnosis and Treatment

The diagnosis of HCP should be suspected in patients who have the symptoms, signs, and clinical course characteristic of the acute hepatic porphyrias (ADP, AIP, HCP, and VP) but in whom PBG deaminase activity is normal. Urinary excretion of heme precursors is similar in HCP and VP, but the predominant or exclusive presence of fecal coproporphyrin is more suggestive of HCP than VP, in which fecal coproporphyrin and protoporphyrin concentrations are usually approximately equal. Fecal or urinary predominance of harderoporphyrin, with greatly reduced Copro' oxidase activity, indicates harderoporphyria.

Treatment of acute attacks is the same as for AIP (see above).

VARIEGATE PORPHYRIA (VP)
(Porphyria Variegata; Protocoproporphyria; South African Genetic Porphyria; Royal Malady)

VP is caused by a heterozygous deficiency in Proto' oxidase activity and is inherited in an autosomal dominant manner. Patients with this disorder may show neurovisceral symptoms, photosensitivity, or both. Very rare forms of VP are seen with homozygous deficiencies in Proto' oxidase activity.

Epidemiology: The incidence of VP of 3/1000 in South Africa is substantially higher than elsewhere. In 1980, it was estimated that there were 10,000 affected individuals in South Africa, and there is good evidence to suggest that they all are descendants of a single union between 2 Dutch settlers in 1680. However, the disease is recognized worldwide and, with the exception of South Africa, there is probably no racial or geographic predilection. The incidence in Finland is reported at 1.3/100,000. Outside of South Africa, VP is probably less common than AIP.

Pathogenesis of the clinical findings: Proto' oxidase activity is decreased in patients with VP. Homozygous VP has been documented by virtual absence of Proto' oxidase activity in 3 patients and suspected in another. Symptoms were severe photosensitivity, growth and mental retardation, and marked neurologic abnormalities in 2 cases; onset was in childhood in all cases.

Symptoms and Signs

The neurovisceral symptomatology is indistinguishable from that observed in ADP, AIP, and HCP, which has been described above. Photosensitivity is more common and the resulting lesions tend to be more chronic in VP than in HCP. Cutaneous manifestations include vesicles, bullae, hyperpigmentation, milia, hypertrichosis, and increased skin fragility. Lesions are clinically and histologically indistinguishable from PCT and, in the absence of neurovisceral symptoms, the diagnosis of VP is easily overlooked. Skin manifestations are seen less frequently in cold climates than in hot climates. The same spectrum of factors that leads to activation of ADP, AIP, and HCP may also exacerbate VP. Thus, barbiturates, lead from "moonshine" whiskey, oral contraceptives, pregnancy, and decreased carbohydrate intake have been reported to induce or exacerbate VP.

Laboratory Findings

The biochemical hallmark of VP is elevated fecal porphyrin excretion, usually, but not invari-

ably, with protoporphyrin exceeding coproporphyrin (mostly isomer III). While fecal porphyrin excretion may be normal, the concentration in bile may be more distinctively elevated. Fecal meso- and deuteroporphyrins may also be elevated. Fecal X-porphyrins are elevated in VP more than in any other type of porphyria. Urinary coproporphyrin (type III), ALA, and PBG are often normal between attacks but may become markedly elevated during acute attacks. Plasma invariably shows a fluorescence emission maximum that probably represents a protoporphyrin-peptide conjugate characteristic of this disorder.

Diagnosis

VP should be considered in the differential diagnosis of acute porphyria, especially if PBG deaminase activity is normal. Characteristic plasma porphyrin fluorescence, having a fluorescence emission maximum different from PCT, is seen in VP. The differentiation of VP from HCP is usually possible following fecal or bile porphyrin analysis and in patients with only cutaneous manifestations. The demonstration of urinary 8- and 7-carboxylic porphyrins and isocoproporphyrin in PCT is usually sufficient for differentiation from VP. Proto' oxidase deficiency can be demonstrated in fibroblasts or lymphocytes.

Treatment

Identification and avoidance of precipitating factors are essential. Photosensitivity can be minimized by protective clothing. The treatment of neurovisceral symptoms is identical to that described for AIP.

ERYTHROPOIETIC PROTOPORPHYRIA (EPP)
(Protoporphyria; Erythrohepatic Protoporphyria)

EPP is associated with decreased activity of ferrochelatase and is inherited in an autosomal dominant fashion. Biochemically, this defect results in massive accumulations of protoporphyrin in erythrocytes, plasma, and feces. Clinically, the disease is characterized by the childhood onset of cutaneous photosensitivity in light-exposed areas, but skin lesions are milder and less disfiguring than those seen in CEP, PCT, HEP, and VP.

Prevalence: EPP is the most common form of erythropoietic porphyria. Three hundred case reports were published as of 1976. There is no racial or sexual predilection, and onset is typically in childhood.

Pathogenesis of the clinical findings: The peak light absorption range for porphyrins corresponds well to the wavelength of light (about 400 nm) known to trigger photosensitivity reactions in the skin of EPP patients. Light-excited porphyrins generate free radicals and $^1O_2$. Such radicals, notably $^1O_2$, may lead to peroxidation of lipids, and cross-linking of membrane proteins which, in erythrocytes, may result in reduced deformability and hence hemolysis. Interestingly, protoporphyrin, but not Zn-protoporphyrin, is released from erythrocytes following irradiation, which may explain why, unlike EPP, lead intoxication and iron deficiency are not associated with photosensitivity. Forearm irradiation in EPP patients leads to complement activation and polymorphonuclear chemotaxis. Similar results have been obtained in vitro, and these events may also contribute to the pathogenesis of skin lesions in EPP.

Symptoms and Signs

Symptoms are usually worse during spring and summer and occur in light-exposed areas, especially on the face and hands. Within 1 h of exposure to the sun, stinging or painful burning sensations in the skin occur and are followed several hours later by erythema and edema. Petechiae or, more rarely, purpura, vesicles, and crusting may develop and persist for several days after sun exposure. Some patients experience burning sensations in the absence of such objective signs of cutaneous phototoxicity. Artificial lights may also cause photosensitivity, especially operating theater lights. Intense and repeated exposure to the sun may result in oncolysis, leathery hyperkeratotic skin over the dorsae of the hands, and mild scarring. Gallstones, sometimes presenting at an unusually early age, are fairly common. Hepatic disease, although unusual, may be severe and associated with significant morbidity. Anemia is uncommon. There are no known precipitating factors and no neurovisceral manifestations.

Laboratory Findings

The biochemical hallmark of EPP is excessive concentrations of protoporphyrin in erythrocytes, plasma, bile, and feces but not in urine, owing to its poor water solubility. The bone marrow and the newly released reticulocyte/erythrocyte appear to be the major source of elevated protoporphyrin concentrations, although the liver may contribute in certain cases. Mild anemia with hypochromia and microcytosis may oc-

casionally be seen. Mild hypertriglyceridemia also occurs with increased frequency in patients with EPP.

Diagnosis

Photosensitivity and the demonstration of elevated concentrations of free protoporphyrin in erythrocytes, plasma, and stools with normal urinary porphyrins establish the diagnosis. Fluorescent reticulocytes on examination of peripheral blood smear may also suggest the diagnosis.

Treatment

Avoidance of the sun and use of topical sunscreen agents may be helpful. Oral administration of β-carotene 120 to 180 mg/day may afford systemic photoprotection resulting in improved, though highly variable, tolerance to the sun. The recommended serum β-carotene level is 600 to 800 μg/dL; beneficial effects are typically seen 1 to 3 mo after the onset of therapy. The mechanism probably involves quenching of activated O_2 radicals.

ANOMALIES IN LIPID METABOLISM

Abnormal levels of blood or tissue lipids resulting from metabolic disorders that may be inborn or due to endocrinopathy, specific organ failure, or external causes.

TYPE I HYPERLIPOPROTEINEMIA (HLP)
(Exogenous Hypertriglyceridemia; Familial Fat-Induced Lipemia; Hyperchylomicronemia)

A relatively rare congenital deficiency of either lipoprotein lipase activity or the lipase-activating protein apolipoprotein C-II. In either case the ability to remove or "clear" chylomicrons from the blood is impaired.

Symptoms, Signs, and Diagnosis

This disease is manifested in children or young adults by pancreatitis-like abdominal pains; pinkish-yellow papular cutaneous deposits of fat (eruptive xanthomas), especially over pressure points and extensor surfaces; lipemia retinalis and hepatosplenomegaly. Symptoms and signs are exacerbated by increased dietary fat that accumulates in the circulation as chylomicrons.

Diagnosis: Spectacular plasma Tg levels cause marked lactescence. Chylomicrons, which refract light and produce lactescence, accumulate as a floating cream layer on standing overnight in the refrigerator. This cream layer overlying an otherwise clear plasma is often diagnostic, as is the failure of the lipoprotein lipase activity to increase after injection of IV heparin (postheparin lipolytic activity).

Prognosis

Pancreatitis is the principal sequela. Abdominal pain that recurs during periods of fat indulgence may be marked by severe and sometimes fatal hemorrhagic pancreatitis. Avoidance of dietary fat prevents serious sequelae and allows for an otherwise normal life. There is no evidence that type I HLP predisposes to atherosclerosis.

Treatment

The goal is to reduce circulating chylomicrons to avoid episodes of acute pancreatitis. Since hypertriglyceridemia is promoted by ingesting fat, whether saturated, unsaturated, or polyunsaturated, a diet markedly restricted in *all* common sources of fat is effective. Calories can be supplemented and palatability enhanced by using 20 to 40 gm of medium chain (C_{12} or less) Tgs a day. These fatty acids are not transported via chylomicron formation, but are bound to albumin and pass directly through the portal system to the liver.

TYPE II HYPERLIPOPROTEINEMIA (HLP)

(Familial Hypercholesterolemia; Hyperbetalipoproteinemia; Familial Hypercholesterolemic Xanthomatosis)

A genetic disorder of lipid metabolism characterized by elevated serum TC in association with xanthelasma, tendon and tuberous xanthomas, arcus juvenilis, accelerated atherosclerosis, and early death from myocardial infarction (MI). This disorder occurs most often in a familial pattern of a dominant gene with complete penetrance and is much more severe in homozygotes than in heterozygotes. It appears to be caused by absent or defective LDL cell receptors, resulting in delayed LDL clearance, increased levels of plasma LDL, and accumulation of LDL cholesterol over joints, pressure points, and in blood vessels.

Symptoms, Signs, and Diagnosis

The patient may be asymptomatic, or any of the aforementioned manifestations may be present. Xanthomas are usually in the Achilles, patellar, and digital extensor tendons. A family history of premature CAD (before age 55) may be present.

The plasma TC elevation in the presumed heterozygote may be as much as 2 to 3 times normal, all secondary to increased LDL. The plasma is usually translucent, since LDL does not refract light, regardless of its concentration, and Tg levels are normal or slightly increased. In the rare presumed homozygote with this disorder, TC levels of 500 to 1200 mg/dL occur and are usually associated with xanthomas before age 10 yr. A normal free cholesterol:cholesterol ester ratio and phospholipid level differentiate this disorder from the marked hypercholesterolemia (with clear plasma) seen in obstructive liver disease.

Prognosis

The incidence of xanthomas and other external stigmas will increase with each decade in the presumed heterozygote with this disorder. Sometimes, especially in females, an Achilles tendinitis will recur. Atherosclerosis, especially of the coronary vessels, is markedly accelerated, particularly in males. Of type II men, 1 in 6 will have a heart attack by age 40, and 2 in 3 by age 60. Homozygotes may develop and succumb to CAD and its sequelae before age 20.

Treatment

With lowered cholesterol, unsightly xanthomas will cease growing and regress or disappear. However, the major reason for therapy is to decelerate premature development of atherosclerosis and lessen the likelihood of CAD and MI. **For mild or moderate elevations of LDL cholesterol**, an altered diet is usually sufficient and represents step 1 in treatment. Dietary changes usually should be tried for at least 6 mo before determining that a drug is also needed. **For severe hypercholesterolemia** (eg, TC > 240 mg/dL, LDL > 160 mg/dL) **or familial disease**, it is appropriate to add a drug sooner.

The basic premise of today's dietary programs is that ingestion of saturated fats and cholesterol suppresses hepatic LDL receptor activity and thus retards the clearance of LDL from plasma, which leads to its accumulation. Saturated fats in the diet may be reduced in 4 ways: (1) Replace saturated fats with monounsaturated fats. This will lower LDL levels without altering HDL levels. (2) Replace saturated fats with polyunsaturated fats. While apparently having some independent effect on further lowering LDL levels, this also can reduce HDL levels disproportionately when consumed in excess. (3) Replace saturated fats with carbohydrates, which will in some instances raise Tg concentrations to high levels and will often lower HDL levels. (4) Recommend a weight reduction regimen for overweight patients. Obesity and the intake of excess calories lower HDL levels and can also elevate LDL levels by increasing the rate of secretion of VLDL, the precursor of LDL. Individual cultural preferences often determine the choice of the options.

Diet: The most effective diet to lower serum LDL and TC has been strict avoidance of foods containing cholesterol and saturated fatty acids. In the **stage 1 diet,** the total amount of fat for the average adult should be limited to $\leq 30\%$ of the 24-h calorie intake. Cholesterol intake should be reduced to 300 mg/day and saturated fat to 10% of calories. Meat (especially organ meats and obvious fat), egg yolks, whole milk, cream, butter, cheeses, lard, and other saturated cooking fats are eliminated and replaced with foods low in saturated fat and cholesterol (eg, fish, vegetables, poultry) and supplemented when necessary with mono- or polyunsaturated oils, margarines, and mayonnaise. Most vegetable oils (eg, corn oil, safflower oil) are poor in saturated fat and relatively rich in polyunsaturated fat, but some (eg, coconut and palm oils) are relatively rich in saturated fat.

A more rigorous diet is advised for patients whose LDL levels remain elevated after following the stage 1 diet. The **stage 2 diet** further reduces cholesterol intake to 200 mg/day and saturated fats to 7% of calories. To assist the patient's understanding and compliance, consultation with a registered dietitian is helpful.

Drugs lower elevated lipid levels by several known mechanisms (see TABLE 40–13): (1) Bile acid sequestrants (cholestyramine and colestipol) and 3-hydroxy-3-methylglutaryl coenzyme A (**HMG-CoA**) reductase inhibitors (lovastatin, pravastatin, simvastatin, and fluvastatin) stimulate the clearance of LDL via receptor-mediated mechanisms. (2) Nicotinic acid (niacin) reduces the rate of synthesis of VLDL, the precursor of LDL. (3) Fibric acid derivatives (gemfibrozil and clofibrate in the USA and fenofibrate and bezafibrate in Europe) accelerate the clearance of VLDL. (4) Probucol, a bis-phenol, stimulates the clearance of LDL via nonreceptor mechanisms. In published clinical trials, bile acid sequestrants, nicotinic acid, and gemfibrozil have been shown to prevent CAD, and nicotinic acid has been shown to reduce overall mortality.

Cholestyramine and colestipol effectively lower serum TC, especially when coupled with diet. A dosage of 12 to 32 gm orally in 2 to 4 divided daily doses will lower LDL levels by 25 to 50%. Side effects (eg, constipation and unpalatability) may limit general patient acceptance. Cholesterol reduction with cholestyramine reduces the number of events from CAD (eg, development of a positive exercise test, anginal episodes, sudden cardiac death). **Niacin** (nicotinic acid) may also be useful in type II HLP, but the high dosage required (3 to 9 gm/day orally in divided doses with meals) coupled with its side effects (gastric irritability, hyperuricemia, hyperglycemia, flushing, and pruritus) often restricts its use. Niacin is most effective when combined with cholestyramine in the type II homozygote or severe heterozygote. **Lovastatin** (an HMG-CoA reductase inhibitor) 20 to 80 mg orally in 1 to 2 daily doses can remarkably lower LDL level in type II heterozygotes. Its effectiveness can be further enhanced when combined with cholestyramine and/or niacin. Overt side effects with lovastatin are uncommon. They can include hepatitis and myositis. *The risk of myositis and rhabdomyolysis that can result in renal failure increases when lovastatin is combined with gemfibrozil, clofibrate, or niacin.* Therefore, such combinations should be used only in special situations that warrant the risks, and then only with careful supervision, monitoring, and immunosuppressives (eg, cyclosporine). **Probucol** 500 mg orally bid may lower LDL levels 10 to 15% when added to diet, but it often has the additional undesirable side effect of lowering HDL levels. Thyroid analogs like D-thyroxine effectively lower LDL levels but are contraindicated in patients with suspected or proven heart disease. **Clofibrate** has little effect on plasma TC or LDL levels in this disorder, may produce gallstones and other metabolic problems, and usually is not indicated. Other agents are generally less effective than strict dietary management.

Familial combined hypercholesterolemia is an apparently less common genetic cause of hypercholesterolemia that is sometimes confused with familial hypercholesterolemia. It is transmitted in a dominant manner but is often not chemically manifest until after adolescence. It appears to be due to excessive hepatic production of apolipoprotein B. Since apolipoprotein B is the major protein of VLDL and LDL, this disorder can lead to excess LDL, VLDL, or both, dependent upon clearance. One often finds different lipoprotein patterns in different affected

TABLE 40–13. LIPID–LOWERING DRUGS

Drug	Dosage	Side Effects	Indications	Primary Effect	Effect on Lipoprotein Metabolism
Bile acid sequestrants (cholestyramine and colestipol)	Cholestyramine 12–32 gm/day Colestipol 12–32 gm/day	Constipation, abdominal pain, nausea, bloating, drug interactions	High LDL	Bind bile acids in intestine, interrupting enterohepatic circulation of bile acids	Enhance LDL clearance via increased apolipoprotein B, E receptor activity
3-Hydroxy-3-methylglutaryl coenzyme A reductase inhibitors (lovastatin, simvastatin, pravastatin, and fluvastatin)	Lovastatin 20–80 mg/day	Hepatitis, myositis, rhabdomyolysis, increase of hepatic enzymes	High LDL	Competitively inhibit the early stage of cholesterol biosynthesis	Enhances LDL clearance via increased apolipoprotein B, E receptor activity
Nicotinic acid	1–3 mg tid	Hepatitis, gout, hyperglycemia, ulcerogenesis, acanthosis nigricans, ichthyosis	High LDL, high VLDL, and low HDL	Possibly inhibits lipolysis in adipocytes and possibly inhibits hepatic triglyceride production	Decreases synthesis of VLDL and clearance of HDL
Fibric acid derivatives (clofibrate, gemfibrozil, and fenofibrate)	Gemfibrozil 600 mg bid Clofibrate 1 gm bid	Cholelithiasis, hepatitis, high LDL, decreased libido, myositis, ventricular arrhythmia, increased appetite, abdominal pain, nausea	Low HDL, high VLDL, and high LDL	Possibly increase activity of lipoprotein lipase	Enhance nonsplanchnic catabolism of VLDL and possibly increase synthesis of HDL
Probucol	500 mg bid	Prolonged QT, low HDL, diarrhea, bloating, nausea, abdominal pain	Homozygous familial hypercholesterolemia	Unknown	Enhances LDL clearance not via apolipoprotein B, E receptor pathway and decreases synthesis of HDL

LDL = low-density lipoproteins; HDL = high-density lipoproteins; VLDL = very low-density lipoproteins.
Modified from Blum CB, Levy RI: "Current therapy for hypercholesterolemia." *Journal of the American Medical Association* 261(24):3582–3587, 1989; copyright 1989, American Medical Association; used with permission.

members of the same family. Xanthomas are very uncommon in familial combined hypercholesterolemia, but there is a marked predilection to premature CAD. Dependent on the lipoprotein excess present, the disorder responds well to weight reduction, restriction of saturated fat and cholesterol, and followed when necessary by niacin 3 gm/day, lovastatin 20 to 40 mg/day, or a combination of cholestyramine with niacin or gemfibrozil.

Polygenic hypercholesterolemia is probably a heterogeneous group of disorders and accounts for the largest number of patients with genetic elevation of LDL. Some of these patients possess an abnormal LDL that binds poorly to receptors, resulting in retarded clearance of LDL from plasma. However, most patients with polygenic hypercholesterolemia exhibit impaired clearance of LDL for other reasons. Some are sensitive to dietary restriction of saturated fat and cholesterol. When this fails, therapy with lovastatin, cholestyramine, or niacin will usually totally reduce the elevated LDL to normal levels.

LIPIDOSES

GAUCHER'S DISEASE
(Glucosylcerebroside Lipidosis)

A familial autosomal recessive disorder of lipid metabolism resulting in an accumulation of abnormal glucocerebrosides in reticuloendothelial cells, and manifested clinically by hepatosplenomegaly, skin pigmentation, skeletal lesions, and pingueculae. Although uncommon, it is the lipidosis most frequently seen by physicians.

Etiology and Pathology

The underlying defect appears to be a lack of glucocerebrosidase activity, which normally hydrolyzes glucocerebroside to glucose and ceramide. The onset usually occurs in childhood, but may be in infancy or adult life. The typical pathologic finding is widespread reticulum cell hyperplasia. The cells are filled with glucocerebroside and a fibrillar cytoplasm, vary in shape, and have one or several small eccentrically placed nuclei. They are found in the liver, spleen, lymph nodes, and bone marrow.

Symptoms, Signs, Diagnosis, and Prognosis

There are 3 major clinical forms due to differential cellular enzyme deficiency: type I, the **adult chronic nonneuronopathic form**, which is the most common, manifested primarily by hypersplenism, splenomegaly, and bone lesions;

type II, the acute **infantile neuronopathic form,** associated with splenomegaly and severe neurologic abnormalities; and type III, the **juvenile form,** which may occur anytime in childhood and combines the features of the adult chronic form with slowly progressive but usually milder neurologic dysfunction. Infants usually die within a year. Patients who survive to adolescence may live for many years.

Splenomegaly is the outstanding sign. Hepatomegaly and occasionally lymphadenopathy occur. Bone involvement may result in pain, and swelling of adjacent joints sometimes appears. Pingueculae and brown pigmentation of the skin may be present. Onset is more acute in infants (cerebral form); nuchal rigidity and opisthotonos may be noted. Splenic and marrow involvement frequently leads to pancytopenia. Epistaxis or other hemorrhages due to thrombocytopenia may occur. X-rays show flaring of the ends of the long bones and thinning of the cortex.

Diagnosis is based on finding typical cells in bone marrow, splenic aspiration, or liver biopsy specimens and may be confirmed by demonstrating the lack of glucocerebrosidase activity in cell culture. Dependable prenatal detection of affected cases uses amniocytes or chorionic villi.

Treatment

Enzyme replacement by purified placental glucocerebrosidase (alglucerase), modified for efficient delivery to the lysosomes of macrophages and given IV, has produced objective clinical improvement in patients with type I disease. Although it is currently administered by IV infusion over a 1- to 2-h period, usually once q 2 wk (dosage is individualized, with an initial dosage up to 60 U/kg per infusion), definitive dosing schedules are still being developed.

Splenectomy may be indicated in cases with anemia, leukopenia, or thrombocytopenia, or when the size of the spleen causes discomfort. Blood transfusions may be given for the anemia.

NIEMANN-PICK DISEASE
(Sphingomyelin Lipidosis)

A familial disorder of lipid metabolism in which sphingomyelin (ceramide phosphorylcholine) accumulates in the reticuloendothelial cells. There are at least 5 forms of this lipidosis characterized by different levels of sphingomyelinase. The enzyme is absent in the severe juvenile form. Demyelination and neurologic symptoms may be seen. The infantile and juvenile forms are inherited as recessive traits, appearing most often in

Jewish families. Patients may show xanthomas, pigmentation, hepatosplenomegaly, lymphadenopathy, and mental retardation. Pancytopenia is common. Diagnosis may be made by tissue biopsy and confirmed by enzyme assay. Prenatal diagnosis of some forms is done by sampling amniocytes or chorionic villi. Absence of the sphingomyelin-cleaving enzyme can be shown in both biopsy specimens and tissue culture. Plasma lipids usually are normal. Treatment is supportive and nonspecific.

FABRY'S DISEASE
(Angiokeratoma Corporis Diffusum Universale; α-Galactosidase Deficiency)

A rare, familial, X-linked disorder of lipid metabolism in which glycolipid (galactosylgalactosylglucosyl ceramide) accumulates in many tissues. The metabolic abnormality is due to lack of the lysosomal enzyme α-galactosidase A needed for normal catabolism of trihexosylceramide. Clinical recognition in males results from typical skin lesions (angiokeratomas) over the lower trunk. Patients may have corneal opacities, febrile episodes, and burning pain in the extremities. Death results from renal failure or from cardiac or cerebral complications of hypertension or other vascular disease. Prenatal diagnosis is possible by the assay of a galactosidase activity in amniocytes or chorionic villi. Heterozygous females may have an attenuated form most likely with corneal opacities. Replacement of the deficient enzyme by transfusion is being explored. Treatment is supportive, especially during periods of pain and fever.

WOLMAN'S DISEASE
(Acid Cholesteryl Ester Hydrolase Deficiency)

An autosomal recessive disease characterized by hepatosplenomegaly, steatorrhea, and adrenal calcification manifested in the first weeks of life. Large amounts of neutral lipids, particularly cholesteryl esters and glycerides, accumulate in the body tissues. Deficiency of an acid lipase has been described. There is no specific therapy, and death usually occurs by age 6 mo.

CHOLESTERYL ESTER STORAGE DISEASE

An extremely rare autosomal recessive disease characterized by hepatomegaly and accumulation of cholesteryl esters and Tgs mainly in lysosomes in the liver, spleen, lymph nodes, and other tissues. Hyperbetalipoproteinemia is common, and premature atherosclerosis may be se-

vere. A deficiency in cholesteryl ester hydrolase has been described. Patients may be asymptomatic. Diagnosis is made by liver biopsy. There is no proven treatment. Recently, the suppression of cholesterol synthesis induced by HMG-CoA reductase inhibition has been shown to reduce at least the plasma levels of LDL.

CEREBROTENDINOUS XANTHOMATOSIS
(van Bogaert's Disease)

A rare recessive disorder characterized by progressive ataxia, dementia, cataracts, and tendon xanthomas. Cholestanol (dihydrocholesterol), which is usually barely detectable in the body, is found in increased concentrations in the nervous system, lungs, blood, and xanthomas. The underlying defect involves deficiency of a hepatic enzyme that catalyzes the 24S hydroxylation of an intermediate sterol in the bile acid synthetic pathway. Though plasma TC levels are usually low or normal, premature atherosclerosis also occurs. Disability is progressive, but often not manifested until after age 30 yr. Treatment with chenodiol (chenodeoxycholic acid) 0.5 to 1.5 gm/day orally, which inhibits normal bile acid synthesis, reduces plasma TC and may prevent further disease progression.

β-SITOSTEROLEMIA AND XANTHOMATOSIS

A rare recessive familial disease characterized by the accumulation of plant sterols in the blood and tissues and by the occurrence of tendon and tuberous xanthomas, premature atherosclerosis, and abnormal RBCs. Increased intestinal absorption of dietary β-sitosterol has been shown. Treatment consists of reducing intake of foods rich in plant sterols (eg, vegetable oils) and giving cholestyramine resin to promote sterol excretion.

REFSUM'S SYNDROME
(Phytanic Acid Storage Disease)

A rare recessive familial disorder of phytanic acid metabolism characterized clinically by peripheral neuropathy, cerebellar ataxia, retinitis pigmentosa, and bone and skin changes. The disorder is due to a deficiency of phytanic acid hydroxylase, an enzyme that metabolizes phytanic acid, and is associated with marked accumulation of phytanic acid in the plasma and tissues (see also TABLE 43–4). A diet deficient in phytanic acid ("chlorophyll free") is beneficial. Serial plasmapheresis may help reduce phytanic acid levels.

OTHER LIPIDOSES

Several rare inheritable lipidoses have been shown with sophisticated techniques of tissue culture and enzyme analysis. The more common ones are described. Diagnosis of these disorders may be made *prenatally* from sampling of amniotic fluid or chorionic villi (see also GENETIC COUNSELING IN HEREDITARY DISORDERS and GENETIC COUNSELING IN CHROMOSOME ANOMALIES in Ch. 48). No specific therapy is known.

Tay-Sachs disease (GM₂ gangliosidosis) is characterized by very early onset, progressive retardation in development, paralysis, dementia, blindness, cherry red retinal spots, and death by age 3 or 4 yr. This recessive disorder is most common in families of Eastern European Jewish origin; it is caused by deficiency of the enzyme hexosaminidase A, resulting in accumulation of gangliosides (complex sphingolipids) in the brain.

Generalized (GM₁) gangliosidosis is an infantile disorder often fatal by age 2 yr in which the ganglioside GM₁ accumulates in the nervous system.

In sulfatide lipidosis (metachromatic leukodystrophy) there is a deficiency of the enzyme cerebroside sulfatase, causing metachromatic lipids to accumulate in the white matter of the CNS, peripheral nerves, kidney, spleen, and other visceral organs. It is characterized by progressive paralysis and dementia usually beginning before age 2 yr and fatal by age 10.

Galactosylceramide lipidosis, also known as Krabbe's disease or globoid leukodystrophy, is a fatal infantile disorder characterized by progressive retardation, paralysis, blindness, deafness, and pseudobulbar palsy. This familial condition is secondary to a deficiency of galactocerebroside β-galactosidase.

41. RENAL DISORDERS

GLOMERULAR DISEASES

A group of diverse conditions including, but not limited to, glomerulonephritis (GN), in which the disease process appears mainly to affect the glomerulus. Structural, functional, and clinical similarities exist within the group because of the limited number of ways that renal tissue can respond to injury and give rise to symptoms and signs. Clear-cut differentiation may be impossible. Although pathologic differences may provide an understanding of the glomerular disease, correlations between morphologic changes and clinical features are not completely reliable with regard to prognosis and response to treatment.

Glomerular damage produces changes in glomerular capillary permeability, resulting in various degrees of proteinuria, hematuria, leukocyturia, and urinary casts. Microthrombosis, commonly accompanied by epithelial "crescents" (formed within Bowman's space from epithelial cell hyperplasia, probably mediated by growth factors from stimulated macrophages), may occur and, if damage is severe, hemodynamic changes produce oliguria. Commonly, tubular function is deranged by inflammatory changes in the interstitium. Measurable changes consist of reduction in urinary concentrating capacity and acid excretion and varying disturbances in nephron solute exchange. Because there is some inherent capacity for glomerular hypertrophy, such defects in tubular function usually occur before the GFR is much reduced. As glomerular derangement progresses, however, the total filtration surface is significantly reduced, the GFR falls, and azotemia occurs.

These varied glomerulopathies, which may be either primary or secondary to systemic disease, can be grouped into 5 major syndromes based on their clinical presentation: (1) acute nephritic syndrome—acute onset and early resolution; (2) rapidly progressive nephritic syndrome—acute onset and rapid progression; (3) nephrotic syndrome; (4) primary renal hematuric/proteinuric syndrome—persistent, asymptomatic, minimal urinary abnormalities; and (5) chronic nephritic/proteinuric syndrome.

ACUTE NEPHRITIC SYNDROME
(Acute Glomerulonephritis [AGN]; Postinfectious Glomerulonephritis [PIGN])

A disease characterized pathologically by diffuse inflammatory changes in the glomeruli and clinically by the abrupt onset of hematuria with RBC casts, mild proteinuria, and, in many cases, hypertension, edema, and azotemia.

Etiology and Pathogenesis

The prototypic glomerular disease of acute onset is poststreptococcal glomerulonephritis

TABLE 41-1. DISEASES ASSOCIATED WITH ACUTE NEPHRITIC SYNDROME

Primary glomerular diseases
Membranoproliferative GN
Mesangiocapillary GN
Intramembranous dense deposit disease
Mesangial proliferative GN
IgA nephropathy
Pauci-immune rapidly progressive GN (RPGN)
Renal-limited ANCA-associated crescentic GN

Secondary (multisystem disease–associated) glomerular diseases
Postinfectious GN
Acute bacterial infections
Group A β-hemolytic streptococcal infection
Staphylococcal infections
Pneumococcal pneumonia
Acute viral infections
HBV, EBV, HZV
Coxsackievirus
Parasitic infections
Toxoplasmosis
Falciparum malaria
Collagen-vascular diseases
Polyarteritis nodosa
Systemic lupus erythematosus
Wegener's granulomatosis
Necrotizing vasculitis
Hematologic dyscrasias
Henoch-Schönlein purpura
Hemolytic-uremic syndrome
Thrombotic thrombocytopenic purpura
Mixed IgG-IgM cryoglobulinemia
Serum sickness
Glomerular basement membrane diseases
Alport's syndrome
Goodpasture's syndrome

GN = glomerulonephritis; ANCA = antineutrophil cytoplasmic autoantibodies; HBV = hepatitis B virus; EBV = Epstein-Barr virus; HZV = herpes zoster virus.

(PSGN). In this immune complex (IC) disease, Group A β-hemolytic streptococcal antigens (nephritis strains 1, 4, 12, 29) provoke an antibody response, and the resulting antigen-antibody complexes, whether circulating or formed in situ, are deposited in the glomerular capillary walls. These complexes activate a cascade of events. PSGN may occur during epidemics of streptococcal infection or sporadically. The streptococcal infection is most often in the upper respiratory tract; however, infections at other sites (skin, middle ear) may precede nephritis, particularly in the first decade of life. Cultures of urine and renal tissue grow no streptococci. Antibiotics do not halt progression of the nephritis, unlike their effect in rheumatic fever.

Clinically, **PIGN due to other infections** is indistinguishable from PSGN. Other infections

thought to induce immunologic injury include the glomerulopathy associated with bacterial endocarditis, infected prosthetic material, pneumonia, visceral abscesses, varicella, infectious hepatitis (HBsAg-positive), syphilis, and malaria (see TABLE 41-1). The last 3 infections may cause a sclerosing lesion and severe proteinuria (**nephrotic syndrome**—see below) rather than acute glomerular disease, possibly because of chronic but low-level antigenemia.

Pathology

The lesion is confined mainly to the glomeruli, which become enlarged and hypercellular, initially with numerous neutrophils and/or eosinophils and later with relatively large numbers of mononuclear cells. Epithelial cell hyperplasia is a common early, transient feature after onset of the clinical syndrome, and cellular crescents may be found in a few glomeruli. Endothelial cells increase in number and, due to swelling, the usual fenestration of their cytoplasm may not be apparent. The mesangial regions often are greatly expanded by edema and contain neutrophils, dead cells, cellular debris, and deposits of electron-dense material (ICs from the circulation or formed in situ).

The most notable feature of the glomerular basement membrane (GBM) is the large number of deposits in its epithelial side, chiefly near or in mesangial regions (see FIG. 41–1). Experimental evidence indicates that these are probably formed in situ. The epithelial cells swell over the deposits so that the foot processes appear fused or effaced. Fluorescence microscopy shows diffuse granular deposits of IgG and C3 distributed irregularly along the GBM and in the mesangium.

Symptoms, Signs, and Diagnosis

PSGN is most common in children > 3 yr and in young adults, but 5% of cases occur after age 50. There is a latent period of 1 to 6 wk (average, 2 wk) between the infection and the onset of nephritis. The presenting complaints are edema, oliguria, dark urine (blood content), and, if fluid retention is severe enough, hypervolemia. Headaches and visual disturbances may occur secondary to hypertension. A history of a sore throat, impetigo, or, better yet, a culture-proven streptococcal infection 1 to 6 wk before onset of these symptoms, and elevated serum titer of antistreptococcal antibodies, are clues to the diagnosis. The course is not stereotyped. About 50% of patients are symptom-free. In many cases, the first indicator is the incidental discovery of gross or microscopic hematuria. Transient renal insufficiency is common; in the majority of patients, the symptoms and signs gradually abate. In severe cases, complications include hypertension, with or without heart failure, and hypertensive encephalopathy. The nephrotic syndrome develops in about 30% of patients. In an unfortunate few, onset of the disease is with anuria, severe hypervolemia, and hyperkalemia; death may occur unless the patient is dialyzed.

Other forms of PIGN usually are easier to diagnose than PSGN, having a much shorter lag period or being present when the infection is apparent. However, the nephritis of SBE can pose a diagnostic enigma: a wide spectrum of renal involvement is possible; the systemic manifestations often mimic other diseases (eg, SLE or polyarteritis nodosa); and blood cultures may be sterile.

Laboratory Findings

The urine may be scanty and appears brown, smoky, or frankly bloody. From 0.5 to 2 gm of protein/m^2/day may be excreted, or a random urinary protein:creatinine ratio < 2 may be found. The urinary sediment contains RBCs, WBCs, and renal tubular cells; casts containing RBCs and Hb are characteristic, and WBC casts and granular casts (protein droplets) are common. The RBC cast is pathognomonic of any form of glomerulitis but, in association with the clinical picture just described, is strongly indicative of glomerular disease of acute onset.

The antibody titer against the causal infectious agent usually rises within 1 to 2 wk. In particular, the increase in antibodies to streptococcal antigenic products can be measured: antistreptolysin-O (ASO), antistreptokinase (ASKase), antihyaluronidase (AHase), and antideoxyribonuclease B (ADNase B). ASO is the best indicator of upper respiratory infections; AHase and ADNase B, of pyoderma. Serum complement levels (C3, C4, CH50) usually are diminished during the active phase of the disease (see TABLE 41–2). Complement levels return to normal within 6 to 8 wk in 80% of PSGN, but virtually never in membranoproliferative GN. Cryoglobulinemia usually persists for several months, whereas circulating ICs are detectable for only a few weeks. Ultrasound studies may help to distinguish acute disease (usually normal or slightly enlarged kidneys) from an exacerbation of chronic disease (small kidneys). Renal function (GFR) can be estimated from the serum creatinine concentration or urinary creatinine clearance. Although the GFR usually returns to normal over 1 to 3 mo, proteinuria may persist for 6 to 12 mo and microscopic hematuria for several years. Transient changes in urinary sediment may recur with minor respiratory infections.

Course and Prognosis

IC glomerular disease of acute onset such as PSGN usually carries a good prognosis if the initial renal damage is not severe and the source of antigenemia can be reduced or removed. However, in some cases (1% in children, 10% in adults), the acute nephritic syndrome evolves into rapidly progressive glomerulonephritis (RPGN). In patients with remittent disease, renal cellular proliferation disappears within weeks, but the severity of the inflammatory response

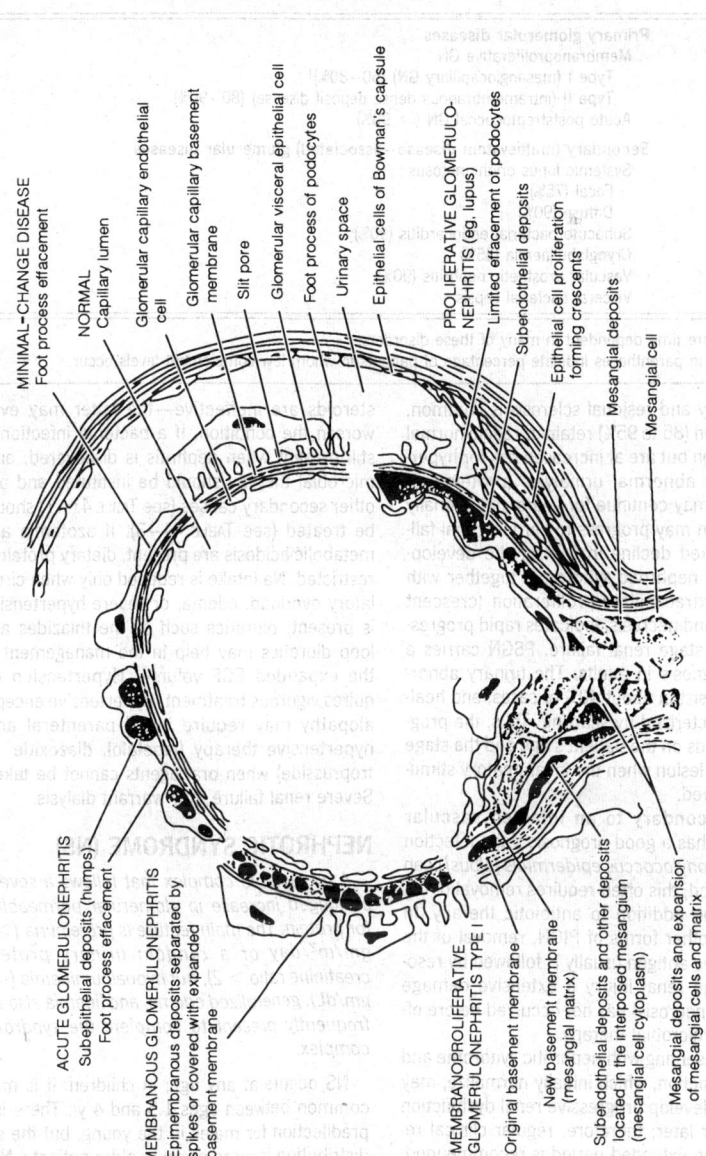

Fig. 41–1. Schematic representation of electron microscopic features in immunologic glomerular diseases.

TABLE 41–2. LOW SERUM COMPLEMENT LEVELS IN DISEASES
ASSOCIATED WITH ACUTE NEPHRITIC SYNDROME*

Primary glomerular diseases
Membranoproliferative GN
Type I (mesangiocapillary GN) (50–80%)†
Type II (intramembranous dense deposit disease) (80–90%)
Acute poststreptococcal GN (> 90%)
Secondary (multisystem disease–associated) glomerular diseases
Systemic lupus erythematosus
Focal (75%)
Diffuse (90%)
Subacute bacterial endocarditis (90%)
Cryoglobulinemia (85%)
Vascular prosthetic nephritis (90%)
Visceral bacterial sepsis

* C levels are time dependent in many of these disorders.
† Numbers in parentheses indicate percentage of patients in whom low complement levels occur.

varies widely and residual sclerosis is common. Most children (85 to 95%) retain or regain normal renal function but are at increased risk for hypertension. An abnormal urinalysis (proteinuria, hematuria) may continue for years; occasionally the condition may progress to chronic renal failure. A marked decline in GFR or the development of the nephrotic syndrome, together with extensive extracapillary proliferation (crescent formation) and necrosis, indicates rapid progression to end-stage renal failure. PSGN carries a poorer prognosis in adults. The urinary abnormalities persist in about 40% of cases, and healing is characterized by scarring. Thus, the prognosis depends on the patient's age and the stage of the renal lesion when the inflammatory stimulus is removed.

PIGN secondary to an infected vascular prosthesis has a good prognosis if the infection (usually *Staphylococcus epidermidis [albus]*) can be eradicated; this often requires removal of the prosthesis in addition to antibiotic therapy. In SBE, as in other forms of PIGN, removal of the source of the antigen usually is followed by resolution of the renal injury if extensive damage (crescents, necrosis) has not occurred before effective antimicrobial therapy.

PIGN presenting with nephrotic syndrome and renal dysfunction, which initially normalize, may ultimately develop progressive renal dysfunction 10 to 20 yr later; therefore, regular clinical review over an extended period is recommended.

Treatment

No specific treatment is available in most cases. Immunosuppressive agents and cortico-steroids are ineffective—the latter may even worsen the condition. If a bacterial infection is still present when nephritis is discovered, antimicrobial therapy should be instituted and any other secondary causes (see TABLE 41–1) should be treated (see TABLE 41–3). If azotemia and metabolic acidosis are present, dietary protein is restricted. Na intake is reduced only when circulatory overload, edema, or severe hypertension is present; diuretics such as the thiazides and loop diuretics may help in the management of the expanded ECF volume. Hypertension requires vigorous treatment. Hypertensive encephalopathy may require initial parenteral antihypertensive therapy (labetalol, diazoxide, nitroprusside) when oral agents cannot be taken. Severe renal failure may warrant dialysis.

NEPHROTIC SYNDROME (NS)

A predictable complex that follows a severe, prolonged increase in glomerular permeability for protein. The main feature is proteinuria (> 2 gm/m^2/day or a random urinary protein:creatinine ratio > 2), but hypoalbuminemia (< 3 gm/dL), generalized edema, and lipemia also are frequently present to complete the syndrome complex.

NS occurs at any age; in children, it is most common between ages 1.5 and 4 yr. There is a predilection for males in the young, but the sex distribution is more equal in older patients. New cases of NS are more common in children than in adults. The literature contains conflicting reports of the percentages of **minimal-change disease** (**MCD**—formerly termed lipoid nephrosis or "nil

TABLE 41-3. THERAPY FOR THE GLOMERULOPATHIES

Disease	Treatment
Postinfectious GN (PIGN)	Antimicrobial agents specific for infection
Rapidly progressive GN (RPGN)	
ANCA-associated GN	High-dose IV methylprednisolone; if fulminant disease, same as anti-GBM therapy
Immune complex–mediated GN	High-dose IV methylprednisolone
Anti-glomerular basement membrane (anti-GBM)–mediated GN	Plasmapheresis + maintenance prednisone + cyclophosphamide or chlorambucil
IgA nephropathy	Resistant to known therapeutic agents; trial of antibiotics/dietary changes
Minimal-change disease (MCD)	Initial: prednisone; maintenance: alternate-day prednisone Corticosteroid-resistant or frequent relapses: prednisone on alternate days + daily cyclophosphamide; or cyclosporine
Focal glomerulosclerosis (FGS)	Usually corticosteroid-resistant; trial of prednisone ± cyclophosphamide; or cyclosporine
Membranous GN (MGN)	Prednisone alternating monthly with chlorambucil
Membranoproliferative GN (MPGN)	No specific treatment; trial of high-dose alternate-day corticosteroids; or cyclosporine
Mesangial proliferative GN	Mainly corticosteroid-resistant; trial of high-dose alternate-day prednisone
Goodpasture's syndrome	Plasmapheresis + maintenance prednisone + cyclophosphamide or chlorambucil
Systemic lupus erythematosus	Low-dose corticosteroids + monthly cyclophosphamide; plasmapheresis in resistant cases
Wegener's granulomatosis	Cyclophosphamide ± prednisone
Thrombotic thrombocytopenic purpura/hemolytic-uremic syndrome	Plasmapheresis + antiplatelet inhibitors (dipyridamole and aspirin)
Henoch-Schönlein purpura	No specific therapy; trial of plasmapheresis
Renal allograft rejection	
Acute	High-dose corticosteroids; muromonab-CD3; ALG; ATG; irradiation
Chronic	Prednisone; cyclosporine; azathioprine; cyclophosphamide

ALG = antilymphocyte globulin; ANCA = antineutrophil cytoplasmic autoantibodies; ATG = antithymocyte globulin; GN = glomerulonephritis.

disease") in various age groups. The variations depend on selection of patients and referral patterns, local incidence of **focal glomerulosclerosis (FGS)**, and geographic prevalence of predisposing diseases (eg, schistosomiasis in Egypt, malaria in Nigeria).

Etiology and Classification

NS may be due to primary glomerular disease (eg, MCD, immune complex nephritides, focal segmental and mesangial diseases). It also is associated with a vast array of systemic diseases—metabolic (diabetes mellitus), neoplastic (carci-nomas, lymphomas, leukemias), collagen-vascular (SLE)—as well as infections (HIV) and drugs.

Familial nephrotic syndromes occur. Congenital NS (Finnish type) is hereditary (autosomal recessive), rapidly progressive, and usually requires dialysis within 1 yr. A simplified classification of diseases associated with NS is in TABLE 41–4; the disorders touch almost every branch of medicine.

Pathology

Proteinuria is thought to occur through functional derangement of 2 mechanisms: the **size-selective barrier** leaks large protein molecules,

TABLE 41-4. DISEASES ASSOCIATED WITH THE NEPHROTIC SYNDROME

		Approximate Incidence	
		Children	Adults
Primary renal disease		90%	75%
Minimal-change disease (MCD)		65	15
Focal glomerulosclerosis (FGS)		10	15
Membranous glomerulonephritis (MGN)		5	30
Membranoproliferative glomerulonephritis (MPGN)		10	7
Others: mesangial proliferative glomerulonephritis, IgA nephropathy, rapidly progressive glomerulonephritis (RPGN)		10	3
Secondary disease		10%	25%
Metabolic	Diabetes mellitus, amyloidosis		
Immunogenic	Systemic lupus erythematosus, Henoch-Schönlein purpura, polyarteritis nodosa, Sjögren's syndrome, sarcoidosis, serum sickness, erythema multiforme		
Neoplastic	Leukemias, lymphomas, Hodgkin's lymphoma, multiple myeloma, carcinoma (bronchus, breast, colon, stomach, kidney), melanoma		
Nephrotoxic/drugs	Gold, penicillamine, NSAIDs, lithium, street heroin		
Allergenic	Insect stings, snake venoms, antitoxins, poison ivy, poison oak		
Infective	Bacterial—postinfective glomerulonephritis, vascular prosthetic nephritis, infective endocarditis, leprosy, syphilis		
	Viral—hepatitis B, Epstein-Barr, herpes zoster, HIV		
	Protozoa—malaria		
	Helminthic—schistosomiasis, filariasis		
Congenital nephrotic syndrome	Finnish type		
Heredofamilial	Alport's syndrome, Fabry's disease		
Miscellaneous	Toxemia of pregnancy, malignant hypertension		

and the **charge-selective barrier** fails to retain lower molecular weight proteins.

MCD is thought to be caused by an imbalance in T-lymphocyte subpopulations. Morphologic change is apparent only on electron microscopy, which shows edema with diffuse swelling (effacement) of foot processes of the epithelial podocytes, proportionate to proteinuria (see FIG. 41–1). Vacuoles, lysozymes, and increased numbers of organelles may be detected; mesangial hypercellularity occurs in about 5%.

In **FGS**, segmental hyalinization and IgM and C3 occur in a nodular and coarse granular pattern with diffuse loss of the foot processes. FGS begins in the juxtamedullary glomeruli and thus is easily missed on biopsy sampling. **Global sclerosis** may occur, leading to atrophic glomeruli.

In **membranous glomerulonephritis (MGN)**, ICs are seen as dense deposits by electron microscopy (see FIG. 41–1). Subepithelial dense deposits occur with early disease, with spikes of lamina densa between the deposits. Later, the deposits appear within the basement membrane,

and marked thickening of the glomerular basement membrane **(GBM)** occurs. There is a diffuse and granular pattern of IgG along the GBM, but no cellular proliferation, exudation, or necrosis. SLE glomerulonephritis is characterized by subendothelial, intramembranous, or subepithelial deposits. Wherever immune complexes **(ICs)** are deposited, immunofluorescence staining is positive for complement **(C)** and for IgG, IgA, and IgM in varying proportions. A C receptor has been identified on the epithelial podocyte.

Based on differences in the glomerular ultrastructure, 3 forms of idiopathic **membranoproliferative glomerulonephritis (MPGN)** are recognized. In **type I MPGN** (mesangiocapillary GN), glomerular deposits, predominantly C3 and IgG, are subendothelial, and the GBM is intact (see FIG. 41–1). In **type II MPGN** (intramembranous dense deposit disease), deposits of C3 are present in a discontinuous linear pattern on either side of the capillary wall, in the tubular basement membrane, and in Bowman's capsule. **Type III MPGN** (probably a variant of type I) is characterized by both subendothelial and sub-epithelial deposits; basement membrane–like material formed on the surface of these deposits eventually produces a GBM that has a fenestrated and duplicated appearance. The glomerular sclerosis that leads to renal failure in all 3 types appears to be caused by chronic deposition of ICs in the glomeruli.

In **mesangial proliferative GN**, mesangial cells and matrix are increased and contain IgM or IgA and C3 deposits.

Proliferation may be focal or diffuse in the NS associated with acute PIGN, RPGN, Henoch-Schönlein purpura, Goodpasture's syndrome, and other glomerulonephritides. Most of the other etiologies of NS have distinctive lesions; eg, with diabetic nephropathy, there is diffuse or nodular intercapillary glomerulosclerosis; amyloidosis has a fibrillar infiltrate that is diagnostic on electron microscopy and on polarizing microscopy with Congo red.

HIV-associated nephropathy is another form of FGS. Rare in whites, it is mostly a disease of blacks in whom heroin use and HIV infection coexist. In these instances, HIV nephropathy may occur with symptoms of AIDS or AIDS-related complex (**ARC**). At presentation, mild azotemia and severe proteinuria are often found; the kidneys are enlarged and highly echogenic on ultrasonography. Light microscopy shows capillary collapse and dilated tubules, but interstitial fibrosis and tubular atrophy are absent. Tubular reticular inclusions, similar to those in SLE, are found within endothelial cells in this variant of FGS. There is rapid progression to end-stage renal disease within 3 to 4 mo, with normotension and enlarged kidneys invariably persisting as an unusual differentiating feature.

Symptoms and Signs

An early sign of NS, noted by patients, is frothy urine. At presentation, proteinuria is usually > 2 gm/m^2/day, or a random urine protein:creatinine ratio is > 2. Symptoms and signs include anorexia, malaise, puffy eyelids, retinal sheen, abdominal pain, wasting of muscles, and edema. Anasarca with ascites and pleural effusions is not uncommon.

Focal edema may be the reason for seeking help for such varied complaints as difficulty breathing (pleural effusion or laryngeal edema), substernal chest pain (pericardial effusion), scrotal swelling, swollen knees (hydroarthrosis), swollen abdomen (ascites), and (in children) abdominal pain from edema of the mesentery. Most of-

ten the edema is mobile—detected in the eyelids in the morning and in the ankles after ambulation. Fluid accumulates primarily by Starling forces (dependent on the relationship between hydraulic and oncotic pressure in capillaries and interstitium) and by systemic factors that increase fractional reabsorption of Na, such as the renin-angiotensin-aldosterone mechanism. Parallel white lines in fingernail beds are a clinical finding of uncertain etiology.

Orthostatic hypotension and even shock may develop in children. Adults may be hypo-, normo-, or hypertensive depending on the degree of stimulation of their angiotensin II production. It is important to be alert for muscle wasting, which may be masked by edema. Oliguria and even acute renal failure may develop because of hypovolemia and diminished perfusion; occasionally, oliguric acute renal failure occurs.

Complications

A wide variety of clinical syndromes may develop in prolonged NS: nutritional deficiencies, including protein malnutrition resembling kwashiorkor; brittle hair and nails; alopecia; stunted growth; demineralization of bone; glucosuria; hyperaminoaciduria of various types; potassium-depletion syndromes; myopathy; decreased total Ca; tetany; and hypometabolism. Spontaneous peritonitis may occur, and opportunistic infections are prevalent. The high incidence of infection is thought to be due to the loss of immunoglobulins (**Ig**). Coagulation disorders, together with decreased fibrinolytic activity and episodic hypovolemia, are a serious thrombotic risk (notably, renal-vein thrombosis). Hypertension with cardiac and cerebral complications is most likely in diabetics and patients who have collagen-vascular diseases.

Laboratory Findings

The initial urinalysis shows marked proteinuria, with an excretion of 2 gm/m^2/day or, more simply, a random urinary protein:creatinine ratio > 2. The urine sediment usually contains hyaline, granular, fatty, waxy, and epithelial-cell casts. Microscopic hematuria and RBC casts also may be present depending on the etiology of the glomerular disease. Leukocytes are prominent in exudative diseases and SLE. Amyloid fibrils may be seen on electron microscopy.

Hypoalbuminemia is detected by chemical measurement or quantitative electrophoresis. Albumin often is < 2.5 gm/dL, and in children it is sometimes < 1 gm/dL; values as low as 0.2 gm/

dL have been recorded. Certain carrier proteins are lost in the urine in nephrosis. Usually low are α and γ globulins, adrenocortical and thyroid hormones, as well as ceruloplasmin, transferrin, ASO protein, other Igs, and complement. By contrast, in SLE the IgG level usually is elevated; in FGS the IgG levels frequently are depressed; and in MGN the C3 level is normal. Serum urea nitrogen or creatinine concentrations vary according to the degree of renal impairment.

Urine Na concentration often is < 1 mmol/L in the accumulation phase of nephrotic edema. **Urine K** usually is high; the K:Na ratio > 1. **Aldosterone** secretion is elevated during this stage but may be normal at other times despite the continued presence of edema. Nephrotic patients excrete a salt load poorly, indicating a defect in the renal handling of Na.

Lipemia may be detectable visually as lactescent sera. Such patients have lipoprotein-lipase deficiency (transiently correctable by heparin) or a problem in converting high- to low-density lipoprotein. In the laboratory, lipemia is documented by increased total cholesterol, triglycerides, free and esterified cholesterol, and phosphatides. Unesterified fatty acids are normal. Greatly increased lipid levels (up to or even exceeding 10 times normal) are associated with severe hypoalbuminemia.

Lipiduria is determined by Sudan staining of casts containing lipid granules, identifying macrophages and renal tubular cells containing fatty droplets (oval fat bodies), and finding anisotropic crystals (doubly refractile fat bodies) with polarized light microscopy.

Microcytic anemia may be present because of the urinary loss of transferrin. **Coagulation disorders** are common, perhaps because of the loss of factors IX, XII, and thrombolytic factors (urokinase and antithrombin III) in the urine and increased serum levels of factor VIII, fibrinogen, and platelets.

Diagnosis

Diagnosis of NS is based on the clinical features and laboratory findings but definitely by renal histology. **Severe proteinuria** (> 2 gm/m^2/day; urinary protein:creatinine ratio > 2) is the cardinal finding and is essential to the diagnosis. The selection of a single value for the separation of nephrotic- and nonnephrotic-range proteinuria is arbitrary. However, it is useful because diseases that principally affect the extraglomerular vasculature and/or tubulointerstitial areas do not commonly evoke proteinuria of

this magnitude. Patients with primary NS have heavy proteinuria and its biochemical consequences as the main clinical problem; renal failure rarely is a presenting finding. However, renal insufficiency may occur in primary NS after a lengthy illness. Thus, heavy proteinuria in the nephritic patient often indicates that the disease is far advanced and is, therefore, an ominous sign. By contrast, patients with NS in association with a secondary cause of NS frequently have renal insufficiency at the time of onset or acquire it soon thereafter.

MCD occurs most commonly in children and is characterized by NS without hematuria, hypertension, or azotemia. By contrast, **MPGN**, also mainly a disease of children, presents with NS in 60 to 80%, with macroscopic hematuria in 50%, and with azotemia and hypertension in a smaller percentage. However, MPGN can be asymptomatic, with only hematuria and proteinuria. **FGS** commonly presents with hematuria, hypertension, and renal dysfunction in association with NS. In **MGN**, NS of insidious onset occurs, often with microscopic hematuria and sometimes associated with other conditions (eg, chronic IC disease, chronic infection, drug-induced states, neoplasm, and collagen-vascular disease). With **mesangial proliferative GN**, NS occurs in $> 75\%$ of cases, microscopic hematuria in 20%, and hypertension in 35%.

Secondary causes of NS, including drugs (see TABLE 41-4), should be sought. Urinary and serum protein electrophoresis and immunoelectrophoresis differentiate glomerular from tubular proteinuria and detect light chains (Bence Jones protein) or a monoclonal gammopathy. Screening for common underlying systemic diseases, such as diabetes mellitus, amyloidosis, multiple myeloma, and SLE, should be performed. If the histology confirms MGN, and particularly if the patient has lost weight or is elderly, a search for malignancy should be undertaken. HB$_s$Ag is present in 22% of primary glomerulopathies associated with MGN, MPGN, and IgA nephropathy.

Prognosis

Prognosis varies with specific etiology. Complete remissions may occur if NS is secondary to treatable disorders (eg, infection, malignancy, drug-induced states), which occur in about 50% of cases in childhood but at a lower rate in adulthood. The prognosis generally is favorable in the corticosteroid-responsive disorders and in patients who are immunosuppressed and frequently relapse (see Treatment, below). Certain of these diseases, such as MGN, remit spontaneously even after 5 yr.

MCD has the best prognosis, with 90% of children and nearly as many adults responding to therapy. Relapses are common, but progression to renal failure is rare. It has been suggested that after a year of remission a recurrence is unlikely during pregnancy.

MGN, a disease mainly of adults, runs an indolent course, progressing to renal failure in 50% of patients over 15 yr; 50% will be in remission or have persistent proteinuria or NS with adequate renal function. The majority of children will have complete spontaneous remission of proteinuria within 5 yr of diagnosis.

FGS and MPGN respond poorly to therapy, and the prognosis is guarded. Over 50% of patients with FGS have renal failure within 10 yr; in 20% the course is more malignant, with endstage renal disease occurring within 2 yr; and the disease is more rapidly progressive in adults than in children. Similarly, 50% of patients with MPGN progress to renal failure within 10 yr, with remission in only a few ($< 5\%$). Those with mesangial proliferative GN are virtually always nonresponsive to corticosteroids. In SLE, amyloidosis, and diabetic nephropathy, treatment is chiefly palliative, although newer treatment protocols are improving the prognosis for SLE. In diabetic NS, end-stage renal disease usually develops within 3 to 5 yr.

In all cases of NS, the prognosis may be altered drastically by infection, hypertension, significant azotemia, hematuria, or thromboses in cerebral, pulmonary, peripheral, or renal veins.

There is a high recurrence rate of NS in transplanted kidneys in patients who have FGS, SLE, IgA nephropathy, and especially type II MPGN, but less so in type I MPGN patients. Recurrence in transplants also occurs in some cases of MGN and mesangial proliferative GN.

Treatment

Treatment of NS is directed at the underlying pathogenetic process and is dependent on the renal pathology determined from biopsy tissue (see TABLE 41-3).

In MCD, spontaneous remissions do occur, but several drug regimens have proved effective, and children especially experience a predictable, rapid recovery. Response to treatment is indicated by cessation of proteinuria and a diuresis if edema is present. Ninety percent of children respond to initial therapy (prednisone 60 mg/m^2 or 2 mg/kg/day orally for 4 wk), but 75% of these relapse. Adults are less responsive to corticosteroid therapy (prednisone 1.0 to 1.5 mg/kg/day orally for not more than 4 to 6 wk), and responders relapse at about the same rate as children. Adults are more prone to iatrogenic complications, particularly with increasing age and hypertension. For all patients who respond, after continuing medication for another 2 wk, a change is made to a maintenance regimen: prednisone 2 to 3 mg/kg on alternate days (to minimize toxicity) for 4 wk, tapering off during the next 4 mo. All patients should be carefully observed for signs of relapse.

For both corticosteroid nonresponders and frequent relapsers, prolonged remission may be obtainable with the combination of prednisone on alternate days with a cytotoxic agent (usually cyclophosphamide 2 to 3 mg/kg/day for 8 wk, or chlorambucil 0.2 mg/kg/day for 12 wk). An alternative approach is oral cyclosporine, 5 mg/kg/day in 2 divided doses, adjusted to obtain a whole blood trough concentration between 150 and 300 μg/L using monoclonal antibody radioimmunoassay. Some initial responders may relapse when dosage is reduced.

Cytotoxic agents pose the hazards of gonadal suppression (most serious in prepubertal adolescence) and, if cyclophosphamide is used, hemorrhagic cystitis. Dosage should be monitored by frequent blood counts, and cystitis should be excluded by urinalysis. In MCD, the risks of therapy should be weighed against the advantages of reducing proteinuria, possibly without influencing the outcome of other manifestations of NS.

For FGS, treatment usually is ineffective, although in some patients the disorder remits spontaneously or responds to a course of corticosteroids. If it improves only slightly or relapses with this therapy, the addition of cyclophosphamide may induce remission. Proteinuria may be improved in the short term with an 8-wk course of cyclophosphamide and prednisone. Therefore, a 4-wk course of corticosteroid therapy probably is acceptable to delineate the few responders. The usefulness of anticoagulants and antithrombotics has not been established. An improvement in GFR and a reduction in proteinuria may occur with cyclosporine, given as described above for MCD. An investigational drug, FK 506, has, when tried in a small number of patients, reduced proteinuria.

In MGN, patients benefit significantly from a 6-mo course of methylprednisolone alternating with chlorambucil each month, starting before the onset of renal insufficiency. Methylprednisolone 1 gm IV is given for 3 days, followed by oral methylprednisolone 0.4 mg/kg/day for 27 days. Chlorambucil is given orally at a dosage of 0.2 mg/kg/day. In adults with type I MPGN, a randomized prospective trial of the platelet inhibitors dipyridamole 225 mg/day and aspirin 975 mg/day stabilized renal function. In children with MPGN, alternate-day prednisone 2.5 mg/kg (maximum, 80 mg) as a single dose appears to prolong renal survival. Recently cyclosporine has been shown to be beneficial. In **mesangial proliferative GN,** spontaneous remissions are frequent, but the condition is corticosteroid-resistant (5 to 20% response).

In the **secondary causes of NS** (eg, Hodgkin's lymphoma and other neoplasms), remission of the renal manifestations can occur with specific therapy. Treatment of infectious antigens may cure NS (eg, staphylococcal and *Streptococcus viridans* endocarditis, vascular prosthetic nephritis, malaria, syphilis, and schistosomiasis). Heroin addicts with NS due to FGS can experience complete remission of the NS if they cease taking heroin early in the disease. Relentless progression to end-stage renal disease generally occurs in HIV-associated FGS. Colchicine produces favorable results in some cases of amyloid NS associated with familial Mediterranean fever. Careful desensitization may reverse NS associated with nephroallergens such as poison oak or ivy and insect antigens. Removal of nephrotoxins such as gold, penicillamine, and NSAIDs may be followed by remission.

Congenital nephrosis is rarely compatible with life beyond 1 yr, but a few patients have been supported nutritionally to the stage of renal failure and then managed with dialysis or transplantation.

Supportive therapy requires nutritional guidance to provide a diet that is normal in protein and K (1 mmol/kg/day) and low in saturated fat and Na (< 100 mmol/day). Excessive protein intake aggravates proteinuria. Angiotensin converting enzyme **(ACE)** inhibitors usually reduce the degree of proteinuria and lipemia. (CAUTION: *ACE inhibitors may exacerbate hyperkalemia in patients with moderate to severe renal dysfunction.*) Graded exercise should be instituted.

If **hyponatremia** is present, fluid intake is restricted. If a brisk diuresis occurs and edema remits, Na may need to be liberalized. If ascites is present, frequent small meals may be helpful. To **control symptomatic edema,** judicious use of thiazide or loop diuretics is recommended (CAUTION: *Diuretics, by reducing plasma volume further, may compromise renal function and predispose to thrombosis.*) If **hypovolemia** is severe and life-threatening, an infusion of plasma or albumin may be justified. **Hypertension** should be treated, usually with diuretics; occasionally other agents may be necessary. **Infections** (especially bacteriuria, endocarditis, and peritonitis) are life-threatening; they should be sought and treated promptly. **Thrombosis** is frequent and should be sought (particularly deep-vein thrombosis and pulmonary emboli); anticoagulants may be helpful.

With alteration in serum protein levels, binding of many drugs may be changed, altering the degree of therapeutic efficacy. Sunlight, routine immunization, nephroallergens, insect bites, and potentially nephrotoxic drugs may have to be avoided in hypersensitive persons.

Children and their families should be counseled to avoid the **deprived sibling syndrome,** which may occur when a nephrotic child dominates parental energies, and to deal with other psychologic aspects, such as cosmetic effects of the disease and corticosteroid therapy. Management of a child with chronic disability is discussed in Ch. 24.

IDIOPATHIC PRIMARY RENAL HEMATURIC/PROTEINURIC SYNDROME
(IgA Nephropathy [Berger's Disease])

A group of disorders featuring recurrent episodes of macroscopic hematuria, mild proteinuria, glomerular changes, with or without progression to renal failure.

These conditions have in common various degrees of hematuria with or without nonnephrotic-range proteinuria; the hematuria may be microscopic or macroscopic, persistent or recurrent. Isolated proteinuria has been described. Initially, parameters of renal function are normal, but eventually symptomatic renal disease may intervene. Causes of primary hematuria/proteinuria include mesangial proliferative glomerulonephritis **(GN)** and membranoproliferative GN (see TABLE 41–5). Mesangial proliferative GN is associated with a pattern of glomerular injury characterized by differing degrees of mesangial hypercellularity or mesangial matrix expansion; commonly, mesangial deposits of immune complexes **(ICs)** are detected. Although fitting this

TABLE 41-5. DISEASES ASSOCIATED WITH RENAL
HEMATURIC/PROTEINURIC SYNDROMES

Primary glomerular diseases
Mesangial proliferative glomerulonephritis
  IgA mesangial deposits (IgA nephropathy)
  IgM mesangial deposits (IgM nephropathy)
  IgG mesangial deposits (IgG nephropathy)
  C3 mesangial deposits
  Without mesangial deposits
Membranoproliferative glomerulonephritis

Secondary (multisystem disease–associated) glomerular diseases
Heredofamilial disorders
  Alport's syndrome
  Fabry's disease
  Thin basement membrane disease
  Sickle cell disease
Immunologic disorders
  Henoch-Schönlein purpura
  Systemic lupus erythematosus
  Systemic vasculitis
  Wegener's granulomatosis
  Complement deficiency syndromes
Infective disorders
  Bacterial endocarditis
  Resolving postinfectious glomerulonephritis

morphologic description, the discussion excludes many well-characterized heredofamilial, immunologic, and infectious disorders (see TABLE 41-5).

IgA nephropathy **(Berger's disease)**, the most important of the primary renal group, occurs at all ages but is most common in children and young adults. It affects 6 times as many males as females and is rare in blacks. Its prevalence compared with all primary glomerular diseases is 5% in the USA, 10 to 20% in southern Europe and Australia, and 30 to 40% in Asia.

Pathology

About 50% of patients with recurrent renal hematuria demonstrate prominent mesangial IgA deposits, and about half of these patients have increased serum IgA. **IgA nephropathy** can be differentiated from other causes of primary renal hematuria by immunofluorescence study of renal biopsy tissue. Distinguishing features are granular deposition of IgA and C3 in the expanded mesangium, with foci of segmental proliferative or necrotizing lesions. IgA nephropathy is associated with major histocompatibility HLA and certain other genetic markers; HLA-DR4 is detectable in about 50% of patients. Alterations in subsets of T cells have been reported. Available evidence suggests that IgA nephropathy occurs from either increased production or reduced clearance of polymeric IgA–antigen complexes that are ultimately demonstrated within the mesangium and activate the classical complement pathway. Polymeric IgA is supposedly derived from IgA-rich mucosal surfaces. Mesangial IgA deposits may occur in other diseases, such as Henoch-Schönlein purpura and chronic alcoholic hepatic cirrhosis (see TABLE 41-6).

Symptoms, Signs, and Diagnosis

There appear to be at least 2 forms of presentation: either **recurring macroscopic hematuria** (90% of involved children) or **asymptomatic microscopic hematuria** with mild proteinuria. Although many patients are not truly asymptomatic when the urinary abnormality is first detected, few if any symptoms are readily referrable to the kidney. In a few patients, acute or chronic renal failure, severe hypertension, or nephrotic syndrome **(NS)** may be the presenting feature. The syndrome usually begins 1 or 2 days after a febrile mucosal (upper respiratory, sinus, enteral) illness, thus mimicking postinfectious glomerulonephritis, except that the onset of the hematuria is coincident with the febrile illness. Mild proteinuria (< 1 gm/day) is typical, but NS can develop in $\le 20\%$ of patients who have IgA nephropathy. Microscopic hematuria is always present, but RBC casts are infrequent, at least

TABLE 41-6. DISEASES ASSOCIATED WITH MESANGIAL IgA DEPOSITS

Primary glomerular diseases
    Mesangial proliferative glomerulonephritis
    IgA nephropathy (Berger's disease)

Secondary (multisystem disease–associated) glomerular diseases
    Hepatic disorders
        Chronic alcoholic liver disease
        Portosystemic shunts
    Gastrointestinal disorders
        Celiac disease
        Crohn's disease
        Adenocarcinomas
        Mucin-secreting carcinoma
        Pancreatic carcinoma
    Respiratory disorders
        Chronic obstructive bronchiolitis
        Idiopathic interstitial pneumonia
        Pulmonary hemosiderosis
        Adenocarcinoma of lung, pharynx
    Dermatologic disorders
        Dermatitis herpetiformis
    Arthropathic disorders
        Ankylosing spondylitis
        Reiter's syndrome
        Psoriasis
        Relapsing polychondritis
        Sjögren's syndrome
    Vasculitic disorders
        Henoch-Schönlein purpura
        Buerger's disease
        Familial immunothrombocytopenia
    Neoplastic disorders
        IgA monoclonal gammopathy
        Mycosis fungoides
        Sézary syndrome
    Infective disorders
        Leprosy
        Toxoplasmosis
        Schistosomiasis
        Recurrent mastitis
    Ophthalmic disorders
        Episcleritis
        Anterior uveitis

initially. Loin pain may accompany the hematuria. Hypertension is unusual at the time of diagnosis. The serum creatinine and complement (C) levels are usually normal, but the IgA level is commonly increased.

Prognosis and Treatment

IgA nephropathy usually progresses, albeit slowly, with renal insufficiency and hypertension developing within 10 yr in 15 to 20% of patients. Older age at onset of disease, persistent heavy proteinuria, absence of recurrent macroscopic hematuria, reduced GFR, diffuse proliferative GN, and focal glomerulosclerosis with tubular at-rophy are unfavorable prognostic findings. When diagnosed in children, prognosis is usually benign. Should hematuria persist, however, then hypertension, proteinuria, and renal insufficiency invariably develop.

Therapeutic interventions have proved disappointing. Short- or long-term antibiotic therapy or dietary manipulations to reduce antigen loads may be of value in a few patients. Plasmapheresis has been tried in those with rapidly progressive disease. Renal transplantation has been successful, although immunologic evidence of IgA nephropathy recurrence is not unusual. Long-term nephrologic follow-up is essential.

NEPHROGENIC DIABETES INSIPIDUS (NDI)

A disease in which renal function is normal except for an inability to concentrate the urine owing to lack of response of the renal tubules to ADH.

NDI occurs as an X-linked, probably recessive, disease. Affected males are completely unresponsive to **antidiuretic hormone (ADH, vasopressin)**. Heterozygous females show normal or slightly impaired responsiveness to ADH.

Normally the kidney alters the concentration of urine to maintain the osmolality of plasma and the volume of ECF. In the presence of ADH and a medullary osmotic gradient (established by the countercurrent mechanism), water resorption by the collecting duct is increased and a concentrated urine is excreted. Without ADH, a large amount of dilute urine is excreted.

In NDI, the formation and secretion of ADH by the posterior pituitary are normal, but the nephron is unresponsive to the hormone. The consequences are polydipsia, polyuria, and hypotonic urine, the same features as are seen in pituitary DI, from which the disease must be distinguished. Usually the disease appears soon after birth. Since the infant cannot communicate its thirst, severe water depletion may result, with hypernatremia, fever, vomiting, and convulsions. *Brain damage with permanent mental retardation may occur if the cause of the symptoms is not recognized.* Urine osmolality is usually 50 to 100 mOsm/kg but may rise to 280 mOsm/kg during a solute diuresis. Other evidence of abnormal tubular function is lacking, and the GFR is normal. Physical growth is often retarded because of frequent episodes of dehydration.

An **NDI syndrome** may be seen in disorders preferentially affecting the medulla or distal nephrons, resulting in impaired ability to concentrate the urine and apparent insensitivity to ADH: medullary and polycystic disease; sickle cell nephropathy; release of obstructing periureteral fibrosis; medullary pyelonephritis; hypokalemic, hypercalcemic, and hypomagnesemic nephropathies; the nephrotic syndrome; amyloidosis; Sjögren's syndrome; and myeloma. Certain nephrotoxins, especially aminoglycosides, lithium, and demeclocycline, also are causes.

The diagnosis of NDI is made with a **water deprivation test**. The test examines the maximum urine-concentrating ability and the response to exogenous ADH. With water deprivation, the maximal osmolality of urine in NDI patients is abnormally low ($<$ 800 mOsm/kg), and there is only a small increase in urine osmolality (of $<$ 50 mOsm/kg) following administration of exogenous ADH (vasopressin).

Treatment of NDI consists of ensuring that the patient has an adequate free water intake. As long as the patient can increase his water intake in response to thirst, serious sequelae seldom occur, but polyuria and polydipsia may be nuisances. Na restriction, thiazide diuretics, and indomethacin or tolmetin may be helpful.

BARTTER'S SYNDROME

A combination of fluid, electrolyte, and hormonal abnormalities characterized by renal K, Na, and Cl wasting; hypokalemia; hyperaldosteronism; hyperreninemia; and normal BP. The syndrome usually appears in childhood, either as a sporadic or a familial, usually autosomal recessive, disorder.

Etiology, Pathophysiology, and Symptoms and Signs

Bartter's syndrome results from a complex disturbance of renal electrolyte handling. The underlying renal tubular disorder (or disorders) has not been defined. The proximal tubule, the ascending thick limb of the loop of Henle, and the distal nephron have all been suggested as possible sites of transport defects, which might be etiologic. K, Na, and Cl wasting occurs, each contributing to the stimulation of renin release, which is accompanied by hyperplasia of cells of the juxtaglomerular apparatus. Elevated levels of aldosterone are present. K depletion is not eliminated by correction of the hyperaldosteronism. Na wasting results in a chronically low plasma volume, which is reflected by a normal BP despite high levels of renin and angiotensin and by an impaired pressor response to angiotensin infusion. Metabolic alkalosis often develops. Platelet aggregation is inhibited. Hyperuricemia and hypomagnesemia may occur.

Excretion of prostaglandins and kallikrein in the urine is increased. Inhibition of prostaglandin synthesis results in correction of most of the abnormalities, but K depletion is only partially eliminated.

Affected children have poor growth rates and appear malnourished. Muscle weakness, polydipsia, polyuria, and mental retardation may be present.

Diagnosis and Treatment

Bartter's syndrome is distinguished from other diseases associated with hyperaldosteronism by the absence of hypertension (as in primary hyperaldosteronism) and edema (as in secondary aldosteronism). When the features of the dis-

ease are first seen in adults, vomiting or surreptitious diuretic abuse must be explicitly eliminated as causes.

Potassium supplementation plus spironolactone, triamterene, amiloride, propranolol, or indomethacin will correct most features, but no drug completely eliminates K wasting. Indomethacin 1 to 2 mg/kg/day usually maintains the plasma K level close to the lower limit of normal.

42. MUSCULOSKELETAL AND CONNECTIVE TISSUE DISORDERS

RHEUMATIC FEVER (RF)

A nonsuppurative acute inflammatory complication of Group A streptococcal infections, characterized mainly by arthritis, chorea, or carditis appearing alone or in combination, with residual heart disease as a possible sequela of the carditis. Subcutaneous tissues (nodules) and the skin (erythema marginatum) also can be involved.

Etiology and Incidence

Group A streptococcus is the etiologic precursor, but the role of the host's constitutional and environmental susceptibility has not yet been clarified. Low income, malnutrition, and overcrowding seem to predispose to the infections and subsequent rheumatic episodes. The attack rates of RF range from 0.1% in untreated people with mild or asymptomatic streptococcal infections to as high as 3% in those with febrile exudative pharyngitis. It occurs most often during school age, with first attacks rare before age 4 and uncommon after 18. Familial susceptibility is of significant but not paramount importance. For unknown reasons, RF is relatively rare in the USA, even when streptococcal pharyngitis is not treated, but has increased in frequency since 1985 and is less associated with poverty and crowding.

Exact incidence rates of acute RF are difficult to determine because the physician does not see many episodes, particularly those with only mild asymptomatic carditis. Though incidence rates have declined in recent years in most developed countries, RF flourishes in developing countries. The contribution of antibiotics is difficult to separate from a reduction due to the use of more specific diagnostic criteria. The prevalence of rheumatic heart disease is also difficult to determine because clinical diagnostic criteria are not stan-

dardized, and autopsy is not done routinely. Recent reports indicate a resurgence of RF in the USA. An outbreak was detected in 1985 in Salt Lake City and nearby mountainous states; smaller clusters were detected in Ohio and Pennsylvania. Surprisingly, cases tended to occur in white middle class children living in suburban or rural areas. A mucoid M type 18 Group A streptococcus seemed prevalent in these cases; this type had been associated previously with RF but had been uncommon in the USA for several decades. An outbreak was also reported from a military camp in 1989; 3 of 10 adult men with the disease developed carditis.

Pathology

The histopathology of acute RF is difficult to assess because few patients die during the acute attack. Aschoff lesions are often, but not consistently, found in the myocardium and other parts of the heart of the patient with carditis. Biopsy of subcutaneous nodules shows certain features resembling Aschoff lesions, but no characteristics distinguish the nodules from those of RA. Biopsy of inflamed synovial membrane shows nonspecific edema and hyperemia; erythema marginatum has no specific histopathologic lesions. Only hyperemia has been found in the brains of patients who died either during an acute episode of chorea or years later.

The most characteristic and potentially dangerous anatomic lesion of rheumatic inflammation is the gross effect on cardiac valves. The mitral valve is involved most commonly; the aortic valve, often; the tricuspid valve, infrequently; and the pulmonic valve, rarely. An acute interstitial valvulitis may cause edema, thickening, fusion, and retraction or other destruction of leaflets and cusps, leading to stenotic or regurgitant functional changes. Similar involvement can shorten, thicken, or fuse chordae tendineae, adding to the regurgitation of damaged valves or producing regurgitation of a valve that is itself unaffected. Dilation of valve rings may be a 3rd mechanism causing regurgitation. Regurgitation and stenosis are the usual effects on the leaflets of mitral and tricuspid valves; the aortic valve generally becomes regurgitant initially and stenotic only later.

Fibrinous nonspecific pericarditis, sometimes with effusion, is seen only in the presence of endocardial inflammation and almost always subsides without permanent damage.

Symptoms and Signs

Because the 5 major manifestations of RF (carditis, migratory polyarthritis, chorea, erythema marginatum, and subcutaneous nodules) can appear alone or in combination, RF has many clinical patterns. Cutaneous and subcutaneous features are uncommon and almost never occur alone, usually developing in a patient who already has arthritis, chorea, or carditis. Fever is a prominent symptom, but is not specific.

1. Arthritis is the most common clinical manifestation. Joints become painful and tender and may also be red, hot, and swollen, sometimes with effusion. Involved joints usually are the ankles, knees, elbows, or wrists. The shoulders, hips, and small joints of hands and feet also may be involved, but almost never alone. If vertebral joints are affected, other disease should be suspected. Rheumatic arthropathy can be mono- or polyarticular, and the typical pattern of migratory polyarthritis is now seen mainly when bed rest and anti-inflammatory therapy have not been started promptly. Tenosynovitis may develop at the site of muscle insertions.

2. Chorea can occur alone or with other rheumatic manifestations (see SYDENHAM'S CHOREA in Ch. 43).

3. Carditis has its own spectrum of manifestations, with the appearance, alone or in various combinations, of pericardial rub, murmurs, cardiac enlargement, or heart failure. In first attacks of RF, carditis is present in about 50% of patients with arthritis. In the absence of arthritis (or chorea), a patient with carditis will seek medical attention only if sufficiently febrile, if pericarditis is present and painful, or if cardiac decompensation produces respiratory, peripheral, or abdominal manifestations. In the absence of these provocations, the cardiac damage may not be discovered until much later, when the patient is found to have "rheumatic heart disease without a his-

tory of RF." In about 50% of adults, the carditis develops in this insidious manner.

Since murmurs are the most frequent manifestation of carditis, careful auscultatory techniques and rigorous interpretative criteria are required to avoid errors. The soft diastolic blow of aortic regurgitation (heard best along the lower left sternal border) and the presystolic murmur of mitral stenosis (heard focally above or medial to the apex) may be undetected when present.

Cardiac decompensation in acutely ill children may be undiagnosed because its manifestations may be different from those expected in adults. Children's symptoms may be dyspnea without rales, nausea and vomiting (due to gastric hyperemia), a right upper quadrant or epigastric ache (due to distention of the hepatic capsule), and a hacking nonproductive cough (due to pulmonary congestion).

4. Subcutaneous nodules, which occur most frequently on the extensor surfaces of large joints, usually coexist with evidence of carditis. Ordinarily, the nodules are painless, transitory, and responsive to whatever agent is used for the associated joint or heart inflammation.

5. Erythema marginatum, a serpiginous, flat, painless rash, is transient, sometimes lasting < 1 day. Its appearance is often delayed after the inciting streptococcal infection; if it appears as (or even after) other aspects of rheumatic inflammation subside, it should not be mistaken for a new attack.

Other manifestations: Abdominal pain and **anorexia** can occur in RF either via the hepatic mechanism described under cardiac decompensation, above, or via a concomitant mesenteric adenitis. Because of the elevated WBC count and abdominal guarding, the situation may resemble acute appendicitis, particularly when other rheumatic manifestations are absent. A prompt response to diuretic or anti-inflammatory agents may confirm the diagnosis.

The arthralgias ("growing pains") often attributed to RF are due to nonspecific myalgia or tenodynia in the para-articular zone and can be distinguished from rheumatic arthropathy by the absence of tenderness during passive movement of the allegedly involved joint. Isometric contraction of the neighboring muscles or tendons often reproduces the pain.

The lethargy, malaise, or fatigue often ascribed to RF can be caused by heart failure. Rheumatic pneumonia or pleurisy is no longer regarded as specific to RF. The manifestations may be caused by other diseases (eg, RA or SLE) or by conventional types of pulmonary infection or infarction associated with decompensated rheumatic heart disease.

Laboratory Findings

The clinical pathology of RF is manifested in systemic and local indexes of acute inflammation. Systemically, the ESR is elevated, often to levels > 120 mm/h (Westergren) and > 50 (uncorrected Wintrobe test). The WBC count reaches values of 12,000 to 20,000/μL and may go higher with corticosteroid therapy. Serum C-reactive protein is abnormally high; since it rises and falls faster than the ESR, a negative test is useful to confirm the absence of inflammation in a patient whose ESR remains elevated for some time after an acute rheumatic episode has subsided clinically.

Local indexes of inflammation are found in synovial fluid, although aspiration is seldom necessary for diagnosis or therapy. The fluid is usually clear and sterile, with normal mucin concentration, an elevated WBC count, and a ropy acetic acid precipitate.

Prolongation of the PR interval is the most common ECG abnormality. This finding has *not* correlated well with prognosis or with other evidence of carditis, and it is now regarded as due to a nonspecific abnormality, unrelated to cardiac inflammation, that chemically causes delayed atrioventricular electrical conductivity in about 30% of patients with poststreptococcal complications. Other ECG abnormalities may be due to pericarditis, enlargement of ventricles or atria, or cardiac arrhythmias.

Diagnosis

No single test or other evidence is pathognomonic of RF. Diagnosis usually is based on the modified Jones criteria, which require at least 1, and preferably 2, of the 5 major manifestations cited earlier, together with evidence not only of recent Group A streptococcal infection (scarlet fever, positive throat culture, or elevated antistreptolysin O or other streptococcal antibody titers), but also of such "minor" manifestations of acute inflammation as fever and an elevated ESR or WBC count.

Gout, sickle cell anemia, leukemia, SLE, embolic bacterial endocarditis, serum sickness, drug reactions, traumatic arthritis, or gonococcal arthritis usually can be distinguished by history or specific laboratory tests. The main diagnostic source of confusion is juvenile RA (see below), which sometimes begins with a relatively

abrupt onset, occasionally with rheumatoid cardiac involvement, and often without positive serologic tests for rheumatoid factor. The absence of an antecedent streptococcal infection and the long clinical course of an arthropathic episode usually distinguishes rheumatoid from rheumatic arthritis.

Congenital heart disease with murmurs, cardiomegaly, or heart failure in children and adolescents is distinguished by characteristic murmurs and by cyanosis, when present; echocardiography, cardiac catheterization, or angiography can be used to verify difficult diagnoses. Subendocardial fibroelastosis has been increasingly recognized as an uncommon mimic of rheumatic cardiac abnormalities; it can be suspected when there is no convincing evidence of rheumatic or congenital lesions.

Clinical Course and Prognosis

Except for carditis, all manifestations of RF subside without residual effects. Joint pain and fever usually subside within 2 wk, often more rapidly, and seldom last > 1 mo; the ESR usually returns to normal within 3 mo in the absence of carditis. Patients with carditis generally have overt acoustic evidence of it when first encountered; if no worsening occurs during the next 2 to 3 wk, new manifestations of carditis seldom occur thereafter. Since murmurs often do not disappear and new cardiac phenomena are uncommon, inflammatory rather than cardiac manifestations are the best indexes of therapeutic response. The evidence of acute inflammation, including ESR, usually subsides within 5 mo in uncomplicated carditis.

About 5% of rheumatic patients have prolonged attacks (8 mo or longer) with clinical and laboratory manifestations of inflammation appearing in spontaneously recurrent episodes unrelated to intervening streptococcal infection or to cessation of anti-inflammatory therapy. Such recurrent attacks are more likely to be associated with carditis.

RF does not seem to produce chronic "smoldering" cardiac inflammation. Scars left by acute valvular damage may contract and change, and secondary hemodynamic difficulties may develop in the myocardium without the persistence of acute inflammation.

The long-term outcome depends on the severity of the initial carditis. Patients without carditis seldom develop valvular damage, are less likely to have rheumatic recurrences, and are unlikely to develop carditis during recurrences.

Those with severe carditis during the acute episode are usually left with residual heart disease that is often worsened by the rheumatic recurrences to which they are particularly susceptible. Murmurs eventually disappear in about ½ of the patients whose acute episodes were manifested by mild carditis without major cardiac enlargement or decompensation. Susceptibility to recurrences in this group is intermediate, between the low risk of the "no carditis" and the high risk of the "severe carditis" patients, but the recurrences may create permanent or further cardiac damage.

Treatment

In patients with **arthritis only**, therapy is directed toward relief of pain. In mild cases, codeine, other analgesics, or relatively small doses of aspirin are adequate. In more severe situations, complete **salicylization** is necessary. Aspirin is given in an escalating pattern, resembling that of digitalization, until clinical effectiveness has been attained or toxicity supervenes. Measurements of blood or urinary levels of salicylate are necessary only to help deal with signs of toxicity. The starting dosage of aspirin for children and adolescents is 60 mg/kg (about 30 mg/lb), divided into 4 daily doses. If not effective overnight, the dosage is increased to 90 mg/kg the next day, 120 mg/kg on the following day, and 180 mg/kg on the day after. High doses can be divided into 5 or 6 doses/day. Aspirin should be abandoned in favor of a corticosteroid if a therapeutic effect has not been produced after the 4th day.

Enteric-coated, buffered, or complex salicylate molecules appear to have no advantages over ordinary aspirin. Local gastric reactions can be avoided (or treated, when they occur) by giving milk or antacids ½ h after ingestion of the aspirin. Systemic toxicity of salicylate is manifested by tinnitus, headache, or tachypnea and may not appear until after a week or more of fixed dosage. Toxicity is managed by reducing the dosage if the drug appears therapeutically effective, or by abandoning the drug.

Carditis: The goal is to suppress inflammation while avoiding a posttherapeutic rebound. **Salicylate** is the first choice, because an 8-wk course is seldom followed by a rebound, and adverse effects are less serious than those of high-dosage corticosteroid therapy. However, with severe carditis, particularly when heart failure is present, salicylates may be ineffective. A **corticosteroid program** then should be started promptly. One useful regimen consists of prednisone 40 to 80 mg/day (0.5 to 2 mg/kg/day) given q 6 or 12 h, depending on the size of the patient. If inflammation is not suppressed after 2 days at this dosage, a total daily amount of 120 to 160 mg may be needed. The fully suppressive dose should be maintained until the ESR has remained normal for ≥ 1 wk; the dose is then halved for the next week. To prevent poststeroid rebounds, an overlap of full-scale salicylate therapy is begun simultaneously, maintained throughout the tapering of the corticosteroid, which may proceed at the rate of 5 mg every 2 days, and continued until 2 wk after the corticosteroid has been stopped.

Cardiac arrhythmias or decompensation should be treated with appropriate agents. A posttherapeutic rebound manifested only by fever or joint pain often subsides spontaneously, but heart failure in a rebound, if uncontrollable by cardiotonic agents, requires resumption of anti-inflammatory therapy. In patients with prolonged, spontaneously recurrent attacks with carditis, treatment with immunosuppressive agents may be effective.

Other therapeutic procedures: The acutely ill patient's choice of **physical activities** is usually as wise as arbitrary medical decisions. Patients generally limit themselves appropriately if symptomatic with arthritis, chorea, or heart failure. In the absence of carditis, no restrictions are needed after the acute episode subsides. Advice about physical restrictions is most difficult for asymptomatic patients with carditis; strict bed rest has no proved value, and its enforcement may create undesirable psychologic reactions. **Physical restrictions** seem advisable only in patients with symptomatic heart failure to reduce or remove the symptoms.

Though poststreptococcal inflammation is well developed by the time a rheumatic patient is detected, an eradicating course of **antibiotics** is useful to remove any lingering organisms. Appropriate regimens are described under STREPTOCOCCAL INFECTIONS in Ch. 32.

Antistreptococcal prophylaxis should be maintained continuously after an attack of acute RF (or chorea) to prevent recurrent attacks. The most effective method is benzathine penicillin G in a monthly IM injection of 1.2 million u., but the injections are painful and require monthly medical attention. Sulfadiazine, in a single oral dose of 1 gm/day (500 mg/day in patients < 27 kg [60 lb]), is as effective as other oral regimens. The daily prophylactic dose of oral penicillin G is 400,000 u. or of penicillin V is 250 mg.

TABLE 42–1. PROPHYLAXIS FOR BACTERIAL ENDOCARDITIS IN CHILDREN AT RISK*

Indication	Drug	Dosage
Dental, oral, and upper respiratory tract procedures†		
Standard regimen	Amoxicillin	50 mg/kg (max. 3 gm‡) orally 1 h before procedure; then ½ the dose 6 h after initial dose. (Alternative initial dose: < 15 kg, 750 mg; 15–30 kg, 1.5 gm; > 30 kg, 3 gm)
For patients allergic to amoxicillin or penicillin	Erythromycin ethylsuccinate *or*	20 mg/kg (max. 800 mg) orally 2 h before procedure; then ½ the dose 6 h after initial dose
	Erythromycin stearate *or*	20 mg/kg (max. 1 gm) orally 2 h before procedure; then ½ the dose 6 h after initial dose
	Clindamycin	10 mg/kg (max. 300 mg) orally 1 h before procedure; then ½ the dose 6 h after initial dose
For patients initially unable to take drugs orally	Ampicillin§	50 mg/kg (max. 2 gm) IV or IM 30 min before procedure; then ½ the dose (or amoxicillin 25 mg/kg orally) 6 h after initial dose
For patients initially unable to take drugs orally who are allergic to ampicillin, amoxicillin, or penicillin	Clindamycin	10 mg/kg (max. 300 mg) IV 30 min before procedure; then ½ the dose (IV or orally) 6 h after initial dose
For high-risk patients who are not candidates for the standard regimen	Ampicillin, gentamicin, and amoxicillin	Ampicillin 50 mg/kg (max. 2 gm) plus gentamicin 2 gm/kg** (max. 80 mg) IV or IM 30 min before procedure; then amoxicillin 25 mg/kg orally 6 h after initial dose. Alternatively, the parenteral regimen may be repeated 8 h after initial dose
For high-risk patients who are allergic to ampicillin, amoxicillin, or penicillin	Vancomycin	20 mg/kg (max. 1 gm) IV over 1 h, starting 1 h before procedure; no repeat dose necessary
GU and GI procedures		
Standard regimen	Ampicillin, gentamicin, and amoxicillin	Ampicillin 50 mg/kg (max. 2 gm) plus gentamicin 2 mg/kg** (max. 80 mg) IV or IM 30 min before procedure; then amoxicillin 25 mg/kg orally 6 h after initial dose. Alternatively, the parenteral regimen may be repeated once, 8 h after initial dose
For patients allergic to ampicillin, amoxicillin, or penicillin	Vancomycin and gentamicin	Vancomycin 20 mg/kg (max. 1 gm) IV over 1 h plus gentamicin 2 mg/kg** (max. 80 mg) IV or IM 1 h before procedure; may be repeated once, 8 h after initial dose

(Continued)

TABLE 42–1. PROPHYLAXIS FOR BACTERIAL ENDOCARDITIS
IN CHILDREN AT RISK* (Cont'd)

Indication	Drug	Dosage
GU and GI procedures (Cont'd) Alternative regimen for patients at low risk	Amoxicillin	50 mg/kg (max. 3 gm) orally 1 h before procedure; then $1/2$ the dose 6 h after initial dose

* Recommendations of the American Heart Association, 1990.

† Includes those with prosthetic heart valves and other high-risk patients.

‡ Maximum doses in parentheses throughout table are equivalent to adult doses; *total pediatric dose should
not exceed total adult dose.*

§ Ampicillin is recommended because parenteral amoxicillin is not available in the USA.

** The adult dose for gentamicin is 1.5 mg/kg (max. 80 mg).

NOTE: Antibiotic regimens used to prevent the recurrence of rheumatic fever are *inadequate* for the prevention of bacterial endocarditis. Moreover, they may encourage the growth of resistant organisms in the oral cavity. Patients on such therapy with a penicillin should be prescribed erythromycin or another of the alternative regimens shown above (*not* amoxicillin or another of the penicillins) for endocarditis prophylaxis.

Adapted from Dajani AS, Bisno AL, Chung KJ, et al: "Prevention of bacterial endocarditis: Recommendations by the American Heart Association." *Journal of the American Medical Association* 264(22):2919–2922, 1990. Copyright 1990, American Medical Association.

The optimum duration of antistreptococcal prophylaxis is uncertain. Some authorities believe it should be maintained for life in every patient who has had RF or chorea, or as long as they have close contact with children, who have higher rates of carriage of Group A streptococci. Others recommend prophylaxis only for the first few years after an acute attack in all patients under age 18, and for life only in patients with severe cardiac damage.

In patients with mild cardiac damage (ie, murmurs but no cardiomegaly or decompensation, prophylaxis can be maintained or discontinued in favor of early treatment of future streptococcal infections. In patients with known or suspected rheumatic valvular disease, prophylaxis against bacterial endocarditis should be instituted for dental or oral surgical procedures like to cause gingival bleeding, for surgery on the upper respiratory tract, and for surgery or instrumentation of the GU and lower GI tras (see TABLE 42–1).

JUVENILE RHEUMATOID ARTHRITIS (JRA)

Arthritis beginning before 16 yr of age. JRA similar in many respects to adult rheumatoid arthritis (RA), but it can be divided into 3 subs (systemic, pauciarticular, polyarticular), in presenting with different clinical featur/e disease tends to affect both large and small

joints, which may result in interference with growth and development. Micrognathia (receded chin) due to impaired mandible growth may be seen.

About 20% of children have a **systemic onset** (often called **Still's disease**). High fever, rash, splenomegaly, generalized adenopathy, serositis, and a striking neutrophilic leukocytosis frequently are present. At times these systemic features precede appearance of the arthritis. Rheumatoid factor **(RF)** usually is absent. **Pauciarticular onset** affects about 40% of children. Girls, especially, with this type of onset often have antinuclear antibodies and a high incidence of chronic iridocyclitis. Iridocyclitis often is asymptomatic and is detected only with periodic slit-lamp examinations. A subgroup of boys with pauciarticular onset includes many who have HLA-B27 antigen; most of them subsequently develop classic clinical features of one of the seronegative spondyloarthropathies. The remaining 40% of children with JRA have a **polyarticular onset** that often is similar to adult RA. RF usually is negative, but some patients, mostly adolescent girls, have a positive RF. In this latter group, prognosis is less favorable. Outlook in general is better than in adults. In fact, complete remissions occur in up to 75% of patients.

Treatment

Therapy is somewhat similar to that for adults. Aspirin is well tolerated and effective, provided large and anti-inflammatory doses (80 to 130 mg/kg/day) are prescribed; serum salicylate levels should be checked for therapeutic levels (20 to 30 mg/dL) with the higher doses. Elevated AST (SGOT) levels may occur, but they return to normal once aspirin is stopped. In children under age 15, only aspirin, naproxen, and tolmetin are approved for use in the USA, but if these drugs prove to be toxic or ineffective, other NSAIDs may be tried. Reye's syndrome is an occasional complication of aspirin use in children. Systemic corticosteroids usually can be avoided except for treatment of severe systemic disease. Growth retardation is the major hazard of using prolonged corticosteroids in children. Intra-articular corticosteroids can be given, the dosage being adjusted to the smaller size of affected joints. IM gold salts are administered to children who do not respond to aspirin or other NSAIDs. Dosage is built up gradually with precautions, as in adults, being adjusted in younger children to the body weight: 1 mg/kg weekly initially, then slowly weaned to 1 mg/kg/mo if it is effective. Although penicillamine and hydroxychloroquine are not approved for use in children, they may be effective in patients in whom gold salts are ineffective or not tolerated.

Active exercises, splints, and other supportive measures help to prevent flexion contractures. Adaptive devices can help children live as normal lives as possible. Ophthalmologic examinations should be given semiannually to detect asymptomatic iridocyclitis (anterior uveitis—see Ch. 82), thereby facilitating early treatment with ophthalmic corticosteroid drops (and mydriatics).

POLYMYOSITIS/ DERMATOMYOSITIS

A systemic connective tissue disease characterized by inflammatory and degenerative changes in the muscles (polymyositis) and frequently also in the skin (dermatomyositis), leading to symmetric weakness and some degree of muscle atrophy, principally of the limb girdles. Certain clinical findings are shared with progressive systemic sclerosis (PSS) or, less frequently, SLE or vasculitis.

Classification of the types of myositis includes primary idiopathic polymyositis; childhood dermatomyositis or polymyositis; primary idiopathic dermatomyositis in adults; inclusion body myositis (IBM); dermatomyositis or polymyositis associated with malignant neoplasms; polymyositis or dermatomyositis associated with various connective tissue disease overlap syndromes, including mixed connective tissue disease and sclerodermatomyositis.

Etiology and Incidence

The etiology is unknown. The disease may be caused by an autoimmune reaction; deposits of IgM, IgG, and the 3rd component of complement have been found in the blood vessel walls of skeletal muscle (with particularly high frequency in childhood dermatomyositis). A cell-mediated immune reaction to muscle plays a role. Viruses may participate: Picornavirus-like structures have been found in muscle cells, and tubular inclusions resembling paramyxovirus nucleocapsid have been identified by electron microscopy in myocytes and endothelial cells of vessels in the skin and muscle. The association of malignancy with dermatomyositis suggests that a neoplasm may incite myositis as the result of an autoimmune reaction directed against a common antigen in muscle and tumor.

The disease is not rare; it is less common than SLE or PSS, but more frequent than polyarteritis nodosa. The female:male ratio is 2:1. The disease may appear at any age but occurs most commonly from age 40 to 50 or, in children, from age 5 to 15.

Pathology

Microscopic examination of the skin may show epidermal atrophy, basal cell liquefaction and degeneration, vascular dilation, and lymphocytic infiltration of the dermis. Structural changes in affected muscle vary greatly. The most frequent abnormalities consist of necrosis; phagocytosis; regenerative activity reflected by basophilia, large vesicular nuclei, and prominent nucleoli; atrophy and degeneration of muscle fibers, especially a perifascicular distribution in patients with dermatomyositis; internal migration of nuclei; vacuolation; fiber-size variation; and a lymphocytic infiltrate, often most prominent in a perivascular location. There is an increase in endomysial and later perimysial connective tissue. Recently identified as a subset of the inflammatory myopathies, inclusion body myositis (IBM) on muscle biopsy shows less fiber necrosis and perivilar inflammation but more frequently show pertrophied fibers containing vacuoles rimmed with basophilic granules. In childhood, there may be widespread ulceration and infarction in the GI tract related to necrotizing arteritis. Intimal proliferation and thrombosis of small arteries also follow.

Symptoms and Signs

Onset may be acute or insidious. Symptoms in children and adults are similar, the only distinction being that childhood onset is more likely to be very acute, and adult onset more insidious. An acute infection may precede or incite the initial symptoms, which consist of proximal muscle weakness (in patients with IBM, distal weakness is equal to or greater than proximal weakness), muscle tenderness and pain, rash, polyarthralgias, Raynaud's phenomenon, dysphagia, and constitutional complaints, most notably fever, fatigue, and weight loss.

The **muscle weakness** may appear suddenly and progress over weeks to months. Patients may have difficulty raising the arms above the shoulders, climbing steps, or arising from a sitting position, and be unable to raise the head from the pillow. Patients may become wheelchair- or bedridden because of weakness of pelvic and shoulder girdle muscle groups. The flexors of the neck may be severely affected. Weakness of the laryngeal musculature is responsible for dysphonia. Involvement of the striated muscle of the pharynx and upper portion of the esophagus leads to dysphagia and regurgitation. A diminution in peristaltic activity and dilation of the lower esophagus and small intestine may be indistinguishable from that found in PSS. (The diagnosis in patients with such GI changes, who are described as having minimal or mild scleroderma, may in fact be PSS with CREST syndrome.) The muscles of the hands, feet, and face escape involvement. Contractures of limbs may develop late in the chronic stage.

The **cutaneous eruption** tends to be dusky and erythematous and to have an SLE-like butterfly distribution on the face. Periorbital edema with a heliotrope hue is pathognomonic. The skin rash may be slightly elevated and smooth or scaly, and may appear on the forehead, V of the neck and shoulders, chest and back, forearms and lower legs, elbows and knees, medial malleoli, and dorsum of the proximal interphalangeal and metacarpophalangeal joints. The base and sides of the fingernails may be hyperemic. The skin lesions frequently fade completely but may be followed by brownish pigmentation, atrophy, scarring, or vitiligo. Muscular pain, tenderness, and induration tend to be associated with the rash. The skin changes suggest scleroderma in a few patients. Subcutaneous calcification may occur, particularly in childhood: This is similar in distribution to that encountered in PSS but tends to be more extensive (**calcinosis universalis**),

particularly in untreated or undertreated disease.

Polyarthralgia, accompanied at times by swelling, joint effusions, and other evidence of nondeforming arthritis, occurs in about ⅓ of patients. These rheumatic complaints tend to be mild and respond well to corticosteroids. **Raynaud's phenomenon** occurs with particularly high frequency in those patients in whom polymyositis coexists with other connective tissue disorders.

Visceral involvement (with the exception of the pharynx and esophagus) is relatively uncommon in polymyositis compared to the high frequency of internal changes in other connective tissue diseases, such as SLE and PSS, but occasionally precedes weakness with presenting symptoms. **Interstitial pneumonitis** (manifested by dyspnea and cough) occurs and may dominate the clinical picture. **Cardiac involvement**, detected chiefly in the ECG (arrhythmias, conduction disturbances, abnormal systolic time intervals), has been reported with increasing frequency. Acute **renal failure** as a consequence of severe rhabdomyolysis with myoglobinuria (crush syndrome) has been reported. **Sjögren's syndrome** occurs in some patients. **Abdominal symptoms**, more common in children, may be associated with hematemesis or melena from GI ulcerations that may progress to perforation and require surgical intervention.

An associated **malignancy** occurs in about 15% of men (and a smaller proportion of women) over age 50. There is no characteristic type or site.

Laboratory Findings

Laboratory studies are helpful but nonspecific. The ESR frequently is elevated. Antinuclear antibodies and/or LE cells are found in a few patients, most often those with another connective tissue disease. About ⅔ of patients have antibodies to a thymic nuclear antigen designated PM-1 or whole thymus and thymic nuclear extracts (Jo-1). The relationship between these autoantibodies and disease pathogenesis remains unclear. Serum muscle enzymes, especially the transaminases, creatine kinase (**CK**), and aldolase, are usually elevated; the most sensitive and useful is CK. Periodic enzyme determinations are helpful in monitoring treatment: Elevated levels decrease with effective therapy. However, these enzymes may be normal despite active disease in patients with chronic myositis and widespread muscle atrophy.

Diagnosis

Five major criteria are useful in diagnosis: proximal muscle weakness; a characteristic skin rash; elevated muscle enzymes in the serum; muscle biopsy changes (often the definitive test); and a characteristic triad of electromyographic abnormalities: (1) spontaneous fibrillations and positive sharp potentials, with increased insertional irritability; (2) polyphasic short potentials during voluntary contraction; and (3) bizarre, repetitive, high-frequency discharges during mechanical stimulation. Preferred sites for biopsy are muscles that show electrical abnormalities, usually the deltoid and quadriceps femoris, but on the opposite extremities to avoid sites previously explored.

A malignancy should be considered in any adult with dermatomyositis, following up on clues in the basic assessment, but not pursuing extensive, invasive blind studies.

Prognosis

Relatively satisfactory and long remissions, even apparent recovery, have been reported, especially in children. Death in adults follows severe and progressive muscle weakness, dysphagia, malnutrition, aspiration pneumonia, or respiratory failure with superimposed pulmonary infection. Polymyositis tends to be more severe and resistant to treatment in those individuals with cardiac or pulmonary involvement. Death in children usually is a result of vasculitis of the bowel. The prognosis for patients with malignancy-associated myositis generally is determined by the malignancy prognosis.

Treatment

The patient's activities should be curtailed until the inflammation subsides. Corticosteroids are the drugs of choice initially. For acute disease, prednisone is given 40 to 60 mg or more/day, together with antacids and potassium supplements. Serial measurements of muscle enzyme activity in serum (especially CK) provide the best guide of therapy effectiveness, falling toward or reaching normal values in most patients in 4 to 6 wk. This is followed by an improvement in muscle strength. Once the enzyme levels have returned to normal, the dose of prednisone is reduced slowly; if muscle enzymes rise, the dose is increased. In adults, maintenance therapy with prednisone (10 to 15 mg/day) usually is necessary indefinitely. Children require high initial doses of prednisone (30 to 60 mg/m²/day). Occasional patients treated chronically with high

doses of corticosteroids become increasingly weak because of a superimposed **corticosteroid myopathy;** the corticosteroids must then be discontinued and another agent (eg, an immunosuppressant) substituted. In childhood, it may be possible to discontinue prednisone after a year or more, with apparent remission. The myositis associated with nonresectable tumors, metastatic disease, or IBM usually is more refractory to corticosteroids.

Immunosuppressive agents, including methotrexate, cyclophosphamide, chlorambucil, and azathioprine have been beneficial in patients who fail to respond to corticosteroids alone. Some patients have received methotrexate for ≥ 5 yr for the control of this disease. Effectiveness of IV immunoglobulins is being evaluated; preliminary data are encouraging. Malignancy-associated myositis often remits if the tumor is removed.

INFECTIOUS ARTHRITIS

Arthritis resulting from infection of the synovial tissues with pyogenic bacteria or other infectious agents.

Etiology and Pathogenesis

Any pathogenic microbe may infect a joint. **Bacteria** are most often the etiologic agents, typically producing an acute arthritis. In young children, the predominating pathogens are staphylococci, *Hemophilus influenzae*, and gram-negative bacilli. Older children and adults are most commonly infected with gonococci, staphylococci, streptococci, or pneumococci. Acute arthritis at any age may be associated with **viral infections** (eg, rubella, mumps, human parvovirus, human immunodeficiency virus (HIV), or hepatitis B). Chronic arthritis may be caused by *Mycobacterium tuberculosis* and other **mycobacteria or fungi** such as *Sporothrix schenckii, Coccidioides immitis, Blastomyces dermatitidis,* and *Candida albicans.*

Microbes usually reach the joint hematogenously; however, direct inoculation of bacteria or fungi into the joint may occur during surgery or drug injection, or secondary to trauma. Patients with RA and chronically inflamed joints are particularly susceptible to bacterial arthritis.

Symptoms and Signs

An infant with septic arthritis is irritable and has a fever. Examination usually reveals failure to move a limb spontaneously, tenderness, or pain

TABLE 42-2. INITIAL ANTIMICROBIAL PROGRAMS RECOMMENDED
FOR ACUTE BACTERIAL ARTHRITIS

Gram Stain	Antimicrobial
Gram-positive cocci	Nafcillin 30 mg/kg q 4 h IV
Gram-negative cocci	Penicillin G 50,000 u./kg q 4 h IV
Gram-negative bacilli	Gentamicin 1.5 mg/kg q 8 h IM
	plus
	Piperacillin 50 mg/kg q 4 h IV
No organism present	
Gonococcal infection suspected	Penicillin, as above
Other bacterial possibilities	Nafcillin and gentamicin, as above

with passive motion of the involved joint. Older children and adults with nongonococcal bacterial arthritis complain of acute joint pain (most often the knee, followed by the shoulder, wrist, hip, phalanges, and elbow) and stiffness. On examination, the joint is warm, tender, and swollen, with evidence of effusion. Other signs of infection (eg, fever, chills, or leukocytosis) usually are present. However, patients receiving anti-inflammatory drugs may show little systemic or local response. A history of recent urethritis, salpingitis, or hemorrhagic vesicular skin lesions suggests gonococcal arthritis (see under GONORRHEA in Ch. 21). Mycobacterial and fungal arthritides are typically chronic and monarticular.

Diagnosis

The diagnosis requires a high index of suspicion, particularly in patients with underlying chronic joint disease. *Even the remote possibility that a joint might be septic demands aspiration of synovial fluid from the involved joint and a search for the infecting organism by Gram stain and culture.* Since acute bacterial arthritis is often a manifestation of bacteremia, cultures should be taken from all likely sources of infection, such as blood, sputum, spinal fluid, and abscesses. For patients with nongonococcal bacterial arthritis, the synovial fluid culture is almost always positive unless antibiotics have recently been taken. For patients with gonococcal arthritis, the organism often is not recovered early in the synovial fluid; blood cultures are positive in only about 20% of cases. For those patients in whom an infecting agent is not recovered early, diagnosis of infectious arthritis may be supported by the following joint fluid characteristics: WBC count > 10,000/μL; > 90% polymorphonuclear leukocytes; synovial fluid:blood glucose ratio < 0.5; poor mucin clot; and absence of uric acid or calcium pyrophosphate dihydrate crys-

tals. Bacteria that may cause acute arthritis, but that are difficult to isolate on culture, include the spirochetes causing syphilis and Lyme arthritis.

Mycobacterial and fungal agents should be considered in any case of chronic monarticular arthritis. These agents are difficult to isolate from synovial fluids, and successful diagnosis often depends on their demonstration by microscopic examination and culture of synovial biopsy tissue. When usual culture methods are unsuccessful, the recovery of viruses, mycoplasma, or chlamydia should also be considered.

Treatment

Acute bacterial arthritis is a medical emergency; the joint may be destroyed if not promptly treated. Successful therapy depends on **early and appropriate antibiotic use,** which may have to be started before isolating the infecting organism and evaluating its antimicrobial sensitivity pattern. Early antibiotic choice depends on an estimate of the likely infecting organism—eg, penicillin for a sexually active healthy young person; broad-spectrum antibiotics for an elderly, immunocompromised person. The appropriate antimicrobial (see TABLE 42-2) should be given parenterally, since absorption of oral antimicrobials may be inadequate. When antimicrobial sensitivities are available, therapy may be changed to the least toxic and least expensive antimicrobial agent. Intra-articular antimicrobials may cause synovitis and are rarely indicated.

Treatment should be continued for ≥ 2 wk after all symptoms and signs of inflammation have disappeared. **The joint should be aspirated and cultured daily or more often** to confirm sterilization of the joint fluid and to remove accumulated pus. If a clinical response and sterilization of the joint fluid are not apparent after 48 h of therapy, the choice and dosage of antimicrobials should be adjusted until bactericidal activity of the joint fluid against the infecting organism can be demonstrated at a dilution of 1:8 or greater. **Surgical drainage** is indicated when needle aspiration of the joint is difficult, as in hip infections, or if the infection is not controlled after 48 h. **Splinting** is useful for pain relief during the acute stage. Physical therapy is indicated during convalescence to ensure optimal return of function.

Antimicrobial therapy for mycobacterial or fungal arthritis is the same as for other serious infections with these agents. Viral arthritis is usually self-limited and responds to symptomatic therapy.

OSTEOMYELITIS

An infection of bone, usually caused by bacteria (occasionally mycobacteria), but sometimes by fungi.

Pathogenesis

Hematogenous osteomyelitis may arise from a clinically evident infection or from an unknown source via bacteremia. This osteomyelitis usually develops in bones with a good blood supply and a rich marrow. In children, the most common sites are the long bones, particularly near the epiphyseal plate at the end of the shaft. Because fat replaces the marrow in these sites during adolescence and the vasculature substantially diminishes, hematogenous osteomyelitis of the long bones in adults is rare. Instead, vertebrae are the most common location. Especially predisposed to hematogenous osteomyelitis are hemodialysis patients and drug abusers, in whom the osteomyelitis occasionally occurs in other sites, such as the pubic bone or the clavicle.

Infection spread to bone from adjacent soft tissue suppuration: Typically, the infection has persisted for several days to weeks in an area damaged by trauma, radiation therapy, malignancy, or other causes. In patients with diabetic or atherosclerotic arterial insufficiency of the lower extremities, organisms usually reach the bone by entering the soft tissues through a cutaneous foot ulcer. Osteomyelitis of the skull typically arises from sinus or dental infections.

Organisms enter the bone directly with open fractures, surgical reduction of closed fractures, penetrating trauma, or operative procedures for nontraumatic bone and joint disorders. Most infections of orthopedic prostheses occur from bacterial contamination during surgery.

Because of the rigidity of bone, inflammation in the medullary cavity causes increased intracavitary pressure, leading to diminished vascular flow, ischemia, vascular thrombosis, and bone necrosis. *Fragments of devitalized bone* are called **sequestra.** The infection may extend through the cortex to cause subperiosteal suppuration and may perforate the periosteum to form soft tissue abscesses or draining sinuses through the skin. With persistent infection in the long bones, the periosteum may form new bone (**involucrum**) around the inflammation.

Symptoms, Signs, and Radiographic Findings

In children, acute hematogenous osteomyelitis appears as pain in the affected bone and fever that sometimes precedes the pain by several days. There may be a history of preceding trauma in the area. Tenderness and soft tissue swelling over the bone may develop, accompanied by pain on motion. Elevated WBC count and ESR are usual. Except in infants, radionuclide scanning with technetium phosphate is nearly always positive, even early in the disease, while x-ray changes of bone destruction usually take ≥ 3 wk to appear.

Vertebral osteomyelitis usually has an insidious onset and a gradually progressive course of persistent back pain unrelieved by rest, heat, or analgesics, and worsened by movement. Fever typically is minimal or absent. Tenderness to palpation and percussion over the affected bone, paravertebral muscle spasm, and guarding and splinting on motion are the usual physical signs. The WBC count typically is normal, but the ESR nearly always is elevated (distinguishing vertebral osteomyelitis from many other causes of back pain). Radionuclide scans with technetium phosphate are positive early in the disease, but tumors, fractures, and other conditions also may give positive results. The major x-ray changes, appearing several weeks after the infection begins, include erosion of the subchondral bony plate, narrowed intervertebral disk space, and bony destruction with loss of vertebral height. CT may be helpful in (1) demonstrating bone destruction when the plain films are equivocal; (2) more accurately delineating the extent of bony involvement; and (3) disclosing complications of the infection, eg, paravertebral abscess. MRI in acute osteomyelitis will reliably demonstrate a focal abnormal signal intensity in the bone marrow but does not accurately distinguish between infection and trauma.

Posttraumatic osteomyelitis and osteomyelitis from a contiguous source cause, in varying combinations, local pain, draining sinuses, and soft tissue inflammation or abscesses overlying the affected bone. Fever commonly is absent, and the WBC count and ESR usually are normal. In patients with infected orthopedic prostheses, persistent pain and loosening of the appliance typically are present. X-ray changes in these forms of osteomyelitis include bony destruction with formation of radiolucent areas, radiopaque sequestra, and involucra. An infected prosthesis may show radiographic evidence of loosening. Injection of contrast material into a sinus may delineate the location and extent of the infection. CT may do so more accurately and identify certain complications such as sequestra. In suspected osteomyelitis from a contiguous source, MRI may help distinguish soft tissue infection alone from osteomyelitis by demonstrating whether or not there is abnormal signal intensity in the bone. Radionuclide imaging with technetium phosphate commonly is unhelpful, since it accumulates in many noninfectious circumstances, such as fracture sites, uninfected nonunions of fractures, periosteal new bone, overlying cellulitis, and aseptic loosening of prostheses.

With unsuccessful treatment of acute osteomyelitis, **chronic osteomyelitis** may develop, usually causing episodic bone pain, intermittent or persistent drainage from sinus tracts, or overlying soft tissue infections. Acute exacerbations of pain and the development of subcutaneous abscesses may occur when closure of the sinuses obstructs the drainage. Sometimes the osteomyelitis is quiescent for months to years.

Diagnosis and Treatment

Diagnosis requires isolation of the responsible organisms, which permits specific antibiotic treatment. In **acute hematogenous osteomyelitis in children,** blood cultures often are positive. Other sources include pus from soft tissue abscesses, synovial fluid aspirated from an affected adjacent joint, or material from needle aspiration or bone biopsy. If these tests are unrevealing or not indicated, the child should receive antibiotics, such as oxacillin or nafcillin, effective against *Staphylococcus aureus,* the usual pathogen. Parenteral therapy is advisable initially, but most of the 4- to 6-wk course can

be with oral agents if the clinical response is rapid. Surgery usually is unnecessary with prompt antibiotic administration; the main indication is drainage of subperiosteal or subcutaneous abscesses.

In **vertebral osteomyelitis,** blood cultures occasionally are positive, but diagnosis usually requires needle aspiration of the appropriate intervertebral disk space (if it appears infected), percutaneous needle biopsy of the infected bone, or open biopsy at surgery. Although *S. aureus* is the most common isolate, enteric gram-negative rods also are frequent. Moreover, fungal and tuberculous vertebral osteomyelitis may be indistinguishable from a pyogenic cause except by culture results. The treatment of vertebral osteomyelitis is bed rest and 6 to 8 wk of an appropriate antimicrobial agent. Surgery is reserved for drainage of paravertebral or epidural abscesses or stabilization of an unstable cervical spine.

In patients with **chronic osteomyelitis, posttraumatic osteomyelitis,** or **osteomyelitis from a contiguous site of infection,** the diagnosis depends on both aerobic and anaerobic cultures of bone, tissue, or pus from a deep abscess. These infections commonly are polymicrobial. Material obtained from draining sinuses is unreliable, because the tract may harbor skin organisms not present in the deep sites. The main treatment for these forms of bone infection is a combination of surgery and antimicrobials. Antibiotics alone rarely are curative. Surgical goals include removal of all devitalized tissue and elimination of dead space, achieved by (1) open packing, allowing granulation tissue to fill the defect; (2) packing the cavity with cancellous bone grafts; (3) transfer of a pedicle of skeletal muscle into the cavity; (4) skin grafting directly onto the granulating bone surface; and (5) transfers of vascularized bone segments from the fibula or iliac crest. The patient usually receives a minimum of 3 wk of antimicrobial therapy following surgery.

Infection of a prosthesis generally requires its removal, thorough debridement, and appropriate antibiotic administration. With indolent infections, a new appliance may be implanted at the same operation. With active infection, a period of intense antibiotic treatment precedes replacement of the prosthesis. Alternatively, the patient may require arthrodesis or, in certain cases, amputation.

Cutaneous ulcers and osteomyelitis due to vascular insufficiency or diabetes often yield predominantly staphylococci on culture; however, with extensive **soft tissue suppuration** and involvement of multiple bones of the **feet**, the process is commonly polymicrobial, with both anaerobic and aerobic bacteria, including aerobic gram-negative bacilli. Initial antimicrobial therapy for such severe infections should include agents such as cefoxitin, cefotetan, or a combination of an aminoglycoside and clindamycin. Cure of these infections often requires amputation of the involved bones. The radiographic diagnosis of osteomyelitis in diabetics may be difficult, however, because overlying soft tissue infection or unrecognized trauma associated with a severe sensory neuropathy can cause osteopenia of the bones of the feet, even without bone infection; only bone biopsy and culture will distinguish among these. When osteomyelitis is absent, these radiographic abnormalities will often stabilize or improve with appropriate treatment of the soft tissue infection or with use of protective footwear when the changes are neuropathic.

COMMON FOOT AND LEG PROBLEMS IN CHILDREN AND ADOLESCENTS

As children develop, the musculoskeletal system changes dramatically, with varying angulations, rotations, and longitudinal growth. Many lower extremity problems relate to these variations and either improve or worsen as growth occurs. For example, in infancy, external rotation of the hip (femoral retroversion), medial rotation of the tibia (tibial torsion), and metatarsus adductus are common. With time and conservative treatment, improvement generally occurs.

Evaluation for foot and leg problems in children requires cooperation and sequential individual analysis of each part of the extremity. Asymmetric findings or progressive deformity is *not* typical of normal variation, and a neurologic cause should be sought (myelodysplasia, cerebral palsy, etc). The range of mobility at each joint should be tested, and angulation or rotation of femur, knees, and feet checked with the patient standing, sitting, and lying prone. **To assess tibial torsion**, seat the patient with knees flexed 90° and the legs hanging free. Next align the longitudinal tibial axis and tibial tubercle with the 2nd metacarpal. Now imagine a line between the 2 malleoli. The angle at which these 2 lines intersect, as seen looking along the tibia, will approximate the degree of internal or external tibial torsion. Gait also should be evaluated.

Hips and femurs: Internal torsion of the femur is common in children, and femoral anteversion decreases from 40° to 15° between birth and teen age. Marked **femoral anteversion** results in "kissing knees," toeing-in, and clumsiness. Sitting in the "W" position or sleeping prone with the legs extended or flexed (knee-chest) and internally rotated may contribute to the problem and should be avoided. If marked findings persist after age 8 yr, orthopedic referral is needed. **External femoral torsion** is commonly seen before children walk and apparently is due to an abduction/external rotation soft-tissue contracture following in utero positioning. Sleeping prone with the legs externally rotated can prolong the condition. Internally rotating the lower extremities with diaper changes may be helpful, but most cases begin to correct spontaneously when the child walks. A careful check for hip dislocation is indicated (see MUSCULOSKELETAL DEFECTS in Ch. 28).

Hip pain and limp are characteristic of a slipped femoral capital epiphysis in adolescents, or avascular necrosis of the femoral head (Legg-Calvé-Perthes disease, discussed below under THE OSTEOCHONDROSES) in younger children. The pain sometimes is referred to the knee or anterior thigh. Early diagnosis of a **slipped epiphysis** dramatically improves the outcome. Slippage generally is slow and occurs most commonly in obese teenage boys. It is bilateral in 20% of patients. The cause is unknown, but hormonal factors are suspected. X-rays confirm the diagnosis and exclude acetabular dysplasia or arthritic changes. Treatment is surgical.

Knee or femoral-tibial angular deformities are of 2 major types: (1) bowlegs (genu varus) and (2) knock-knees (genu valgus). Both variations can result in adult osteoarthritis of the knee if untreated. **Bowlegs** are common in toddlers and usually correct spontaneously by age 18 mo. If bowlegs persist or increase in severity, then **Blount's disease** (tibial osteochondrosis) should be suspected. Early diagnosis of Blount's disease is difficult, since x-rays may be normal. Rickets should be ruled out. Treatment using the Danish night splint can be effective if started early; surgery is often needed. **Knock-knees** are less common, and even severe degrees usually correct spontaneously by age 9 yr. Skeletal dysplasia or hypophosphatasia should be excluded. Treatment involves surgical stapling of the medial distal femoral epiphysis if marked deformity persists after age 10 yr.

Knee pain with swelling over the tibial tubercle in adolescence usually is due to **Osgood-Schlatter disease** (see below under THE OSTEOCHONDROSES). Adolescents also are prone to develop **chondromalacia patellae** (*softening of the patellar articular cartilage*). Angular or rotational changes in the leg apparently produce this by unbalancing elements of the quadriceps with patellar misalignment during movement. Knee pain occurs when climbing, especially up or down stairs. Treatment consists of isometric quadriceps strengthening, aspirin, and avoiding pain-producing activities.

Tibial twisting or torsion occurs with growth, going from 0° of lateral external rotation at birth to 20° by adult life. External tibial torsion rarely is a problem. Internal or medial tibial torsion is common at birth but improves with growth. It is associated with toeing-in and bowlegs. Rickets or a neuromuscular problem should be excluded. Occasionally, passive exercises (external rotation of the foot) or corrective shoes (wedges on inner heel and outer sole, Thomas or torque heel) may be useful. Torsion persisting after age 7 yr requires orthopedic care.

Forefoot abnormalities occur in 1 of every 100 births. Fortunately most are functional, such as metatarsus adductus, rather than structural, such as partial clubfoot (talipes varus) or metatarsus varus. In **metatarsus adductus**, the forefoot can be passively abducted and everted beyond the neutral position and lacks inversion, and when the sole is stimulated lateral movement of the forefoot is seen. Resolution without treatment usually occurs in the first year of life. **Metatarsus varus** may require treatment with corrective casting by an orthopedist. **Pronation, flatfoot,** and **pes planovalgus** are recognized by a flattened medial longitudinal arch with outward rolling of the foot. There is eversion of the hindfoot and eversion and abduction of the forefoot. Most children have some pronation when they begin to walk because of ligament laxity and a wide-based gait, but the pronation corrects without treatment by age 2½ yr. Infants often appear falsely flatfooted because of a fat pad below the medial longitudinal arch. The arch usually is restored when standing on tiptoe if the deformity is functional. If there are pains or cramps in the feet, then treatment with corrective shoes is indicated (arch support or shoes with a long medial counter and a Thomas heel).

INHERITED DISORDERS OF CONNECTIVE TISSUE

EHLERS–DANLOS SYNDROME (EDS)

(See also under VASCULAR DISORDERS in Ch. 35)

An inherited connective tissue disorder characterized by articular hypermobility, dermal hyperelasticity, and widespread tissue fragility. Though usually inherited as an autosomal dominant condition, EDS is heterogeneous based on different gene mutations affecting the structure or assembly of different collagens, and 9 varieties have been described including uncommon X-linked and recessive forms (see TABLE 42–3). In the common dominant forms, no specific biochemical or histologic changes have been demonstrated, though cross-linking of the collagen fibrils is thought to be defective.

Symptoms, Signs, and Diagnosis

Clinical findings vary widely, depending on the specific gene mutation and resultant phenotype. This discussion covers the range of possibilities that occur in varying degrees in individual patients.

The skin can be stretched several centimeters but returns to its normal position on release. Wide papyraceous scars are often present over bony prominences, particularly the elbows, knees, and shins. The extent of joint hypermobility varies but may be marked. Affected individuals have become the "elastic ladies" or "India rubber men" of circus side shows. A bleeding tendency may be present but is troublesome in only a minority of patients (see under VASCULAR DISORDERS in Ch. 35). Fleshy outgrowths (molluscoid pseudotumors) frequently form on top of scars or at pressure points. Subcutaneous calcified spherules may be palpated or demonstrated radiologically.

Minor trauma may cause wide gaping wounds but little bleeding; wound closure may be difficult, since sutures tend to tear out of the fragile tissue. Surgical complications arise because of deep tissue fragility. Synovial effusions, sprains, and dislocations occur frequently. Spinal kyphoscoliosis is present in 25% of patients, thoracic deformity in 20%, talipes equinovarus in 5%, and congenital dislocation of the hip in 1%. Pes planus is present in 90% of adult patients. GI hernias and diverticula are common. Spontaneous hemorrhage and perforation of portions of the GI

TABLE 42–3. NOMENCLATURE OF INHERITED DISORDERS OF CONNECTIVE TISSUE, SHOWING MODE OF INHERITANCE, CLINICAL FEATURES, AND BASIC DEFECT

Type	General Designation	Subcategories	Inheritance	Clinical Features
EDS I	Gravis type		AD	Cardinal clinical features in severe degree
EDS II	Mitis type		AD	Cardinal clinical features in mild degree
EDS III	Hypermobile type		AD	Marked articular hypermobility; moderate dermal hyperextensibility; minimal scarring
EDS IV	Vascular type		Heterogeneous	Variable stigmas; severe bruising and/or scarring; thin skin with prominent venous plexus; vascular rupture; characteristic facies
		IV-A: acrogenic type	AD	
		IV-B: acrogenic type	AR	
		IV-C: ecchymotic type	AD	
		IV-D: others	AD/AR	
		(All forms have defective type III collagen except IV-D,AR)		
EDS V	X-linked type		XL	Cardinal clinical features in moderate degree
EDS VI	Ocular-scoliotic type		AR	Cardinal clinical features in severe degree; ocular involvement (microcornea, scleral perforation, retinal detachment); scoliosis
		VI-A: decreased lysyl hydroxylase activity		
		VI-B: normal lysyl hydroxylase activity		
EDS VII	Arthrochalasis multiplex congenita		Heterogeneous	Cardinal clinical features with marked articular hypermobility; short stature and micrognathia
		VII-A: structural defect of pro alpha 1(1) collagen	AD	
		VII-B: structural defect of pro alpha 2(1) collagen	AD	
		VII-C: procollagen N-proteinase deficiency?	AR	
EDS VIII	Periodontosis type		AD	Cardinal clinical features in moderate degree; aggressive periodontitis, gingival recession, early tooth loss
EDS IX	Vacant (formerly occipital horn syndrome, or X-linked cutis laxa, now recategorized)		—	

(Continued)

TABLE 42–3. NOMENCLATURE OF INHERITED DISORDERS
OF CONNECTIVE TISSUE, SHOWING MODE OF INHERITANCE,
CLINICAL FEATURES, AND BASIC DEFECT *(Cont'd)*

Type	General Designation	Subcategories	Inheritance	Clinical Features
EDS X	Fibronectin abnormality		AR	Cardinal clinical features but skin texture normal; petechiae; platelet aggregation defect corrected by fibronectin
EDS XI	Vacant (formerly familial joint instability, now recategorized)		—	

EDS = Ehlers-Danlos syndrome; AD = autosomal dominant; AR = autosomal recessive; XL = X-linked.
Adapted from Beighton P, de Paepe A, Danks D: "International nosology of heritable disorders of connective tissue, Berlin, 1986." *American Journal of Medical Genetics* 29:581–594, 1988. Copyright © 1988; reprinted by permission of John Wiley & Sons, Inc.

tract occur rarely, as do dissecting aneurysm of the aorta and spontaneous rupture of large arteries. Medullary sponge kidney has been reported in a very small proportion of EDS patients. Tissue extensibility in an affected mother may cause premature birth; fetal membrane fragility and consequent early rupture may occur if the fetus is affected. Maternal tissue fragility may complicate episiotomy or cesarean section. Ante-, peri-, and postnatal bleeding may occur. Epicanthus is common in children; myopia in adults. Scleral fragility and perforation of the globe of the eye have been described in the ocular-scoliotic form of EDS.

Prognosis and Treatment

Although numerous and varied complications may occur, the life span usually is normal. The prevalence of lethal complications may be very high in a minority of kindreds.

There is no specific treatment. Trauma should be minimized. Protective clothing and padding may be helpful. If an operation is performed, hemostasis must be meticulous. Wounds should be carefully sutured and tissue tension avoided. Obstetric supervision during pregnancy and delivery is mandatory. Genetic counseling should be provided.

MARFAN'S SYNDROME

An inherited disorder of connective tissue transmitted as an autosomal dominant trait, resulting in ocular, skeletal, and cardiovascular abnormalities. The marfanoid hypermobility syndrome and congenital contractual arachnodactyly are uncommon variants. An abnormality of the aortic media is the principal structural defect in the great vessels, the histologic changes re-

sembling those of Erdheim cystic medial necrosis. Despite extensive research, the basic biomolecular defect remains unknown. Preliminary evidence suggests an abnormality of a connective tissue protein known as microfibrillin.

Symptoms and Signs

Severity varies greatly. Patients are taller than average for age and family, with arm span exceeding height. The digits are disproportionately long and thin (arachnodactyly). Deformity of the sternum—outward displacement (pectus carinatum) or inward displacement (pectus excavatum)—is frequent. Hyperextensibility of joints, backward curvature of the legs at the knees (genu recurvatum), flat feet, and kyphoscoliosis occur often. Hernias are common. Subcutaneous fat usually is sparse. The palate is often high-arched.

Ocular findings include subluxation or dislocation of the lens (ectopia lentis) and iridodonesis (tremulousness of the iris). The margin of the dislocated lens often can be seen through the undilated pupil. High-grade myopia may be present, and spontaneous detachment of the retina sometimes occurs.

Cardiovascular changes are associated with weakness of the aortic media in areas subject to the greatest hemodynamic stress. The ascending aorta undergoes progressive dilation or acute dissection beginning in the coronary sinuses as early as the 1st or as late as the 5th decade of life. Aortic regurgitation may precede x-ray evidence of aortic dilation. Bacterial endocarditis may develop. Mitral valve prolapse or regurgitation due to redundant cusps and chordae tendinae may occur, producing systolic clicks and a late systolic murmur. Cystic disease of the lungs and recurrent spontaneous pneumothorax have occurred.

Diagnosis

This is made by recognition of the cardiovascular, ocular, and skeletal manifestations, especially with a positive family history. Diagnosis can be difficult because many patients have few major features, specific histologic or biochemical changes are lacking, and there are no objective tests for diagnostic confirmation. There are numerous "partial" cases of Marfan's syndrome, in whom the precise diagnosis remains uncertain. Homocystinuria may be confused with Marfan's syndrome because of similar clinical features, but it can be differentiated by demonstrating homocystine in the urine.

Appropriate genetic counseling is indicated. At present, antenatal diagnosis is not feasible.

Prognosis and Treatment

In general, the liability to complications relates to the severity of the abnormalities.

For girls who are very tall, induction of precocious puberty by age 10 with estrogens and progesterone may reduce ultimate height. Reserpine or propranolol reduces the abruptness of ventricular ejection and has been prescribed in an attempt to prevent aortic dilation and dissection. The results have been promising, but there is no general agreement on this form of therapy. The ascending aorta has been replaced successfully in some patients.

PSEUDOXANTHOMA ELASTICUM (PXE)
(Grönblad-Strandberg Syndrome)

A generalized connective tissue disorder characterized by premature dermal infiltration and laxity in the flexural creases of skin, angioid streaks in the ocular fundi, and hemorrhagic arterial degeneration. PXE is heterogeneous, with 5 distinct types. The most common forms are inherited as autosomal recessive.

Histologic change begins in the elastin fibers (basophilia, calcification, and fragmentation) of the skin, the media of intermediate- and small-sized arteries, and occasionally the endo- and pericardium. Similar changes with subsequent cracking of Bruch's membrane cause retinal angioid streaks.

Symptoms, Signs, and Diagnosis

The skin of the neck, axillae, and inguinal and periumbilical areas is thickened, grooved, inelas-

tic, lax, and redundant, with yellowish pebbly nodules in the later stages. The skin changes resemble those in actinic (senile) elastosis, but only exposed areas are involved in the latter. Brownish or gray angioid streaks, wider than retinal veins but similarly coursing over the fundus, are characteristically present in the retina. Retinal hemorrhage and severe vision loss may occur. Weak or absent pulses, intermittent claudication, and easy fatigability occur in the extremities. Arterial calcification may be radiographically apparent at an early age. Angina pectoris and hypertension are common. Uterine, GU tract, nasal, and subarachnoid hemorrhage may occur.

Prognosis and Treatment

The clinical course varies with the severity and location of vascular involvement. Blindness due to retinal involvement is frequent in adults with PXE type 5 (the Afrikaner form). Deaths from the disease or its complications have been reported in patients aged 30 to 70. Treatment is conservative and symptomatic.

CUTIS LAXA

A rare disorder characterized by lax skin hanging in loose folds. A comparatively benign form of cutis laxa is inherited as an autosomal dominant condition; a potentially lethal form with cardiorespiratory complications, as an autosomal recessive condition. A relatively benign variety of cutis laxa with developmental retardation and joint laxity has recently been delineated as autosomal recessive. Acquired cutis laxa occurs rarely.

In all forms of cutis laxa, histologic examination of the skin shows fragmented elastin. The underlying defect is unknown.

Symptoms and Signs

Inherited forms: Dermal laxity may be present at birth or may develop later, occurring wherever the skin is normally loose and hanging but most obviously on the face. Affected children have a mournful or "Churchillian" facies because of the lax skin folds. A "hooked nose" is characteristic. Hernias and diverticula of the GI tract are common. Progressive pulmonary emphysema may precipitate cor pulmonale in severely affected patients.

Acquired cutis laxa is clinically distinct from the genetic forms (late onset, different distribution and appearance of skin abnormality, no "hooked nose"). It may develop insidiously during adulthood and sometimes leads to death from aortic rupture and pulmonary complications. It also may develop following a severe illness involving fever, polyserositis, and erythema multiforme, usually in children or adolescents.

Differential Diagnosis

The dermal fragility and articular hypermobility of **Ehlers-Danlos syndrome** are absent in typical cutis laxa. Localized areas of loose skin are sometimes found in other disorders; eg, **Turner's syndrome** (see also Ch. 48), in which the affected newborn female's folds of lax skin at the base of the neck tighten and resemble webbing as the child grows older; and **neurofibromatosis** (see also in Ch. 43), in which pendular plexiform neuromas occasionally develop that are unilateral and have a configuration and texture distinguishing them from cutis laxa.

Treatment

There is no specific therapy. Plastic surgery considerably improves appearance in inherited cutis laxa; healing usually is uncomplicated, but dermal laxity may recur. Plastic surgery is less successful in acquired cutis laxa. Cardiorespiratory complications should be treated appropriately.

THE MUCOPOLYSACCHARIDOSES (MPS)

Genetic conditions characterized by increased urinary mucopolysaccharide excretion and variable systemic manifestations, including a typical facies, skeletal dysplasia, mental deficiency, corneal opacity, and hepatosplenomegaly. Each MPS has distinct clinical features, a specific genetic biochemical defect, and a predictable prognosis (see TABLE 42–4). The disorders are designated MPS I through MPS VII (with specific eponyms) by identifying the excess urinary mucopolysaccharide. The primary enzyme defect has been identified in some instances.

Symptoms, Signs, and Diagnosis

The clinical features of MPS are not usually apparent at birth. During infancy and childhood, short stature, bony dysplasia, hirsutism, and abnormal development become apparent; diagnosis is further suspected in the presence of the characteristic coarse facies, with thick lips, an open mouth, and a flattened nasal bridge. Family history can be helpful. With the exception of MPS II, which is X-linked, all forms of MPS are inherited as autosomal recessive.

The MPS group of conditions can be diagnosed antenatally by estimation of enzymatic activity in cultured amniotic fluid cells or chorionic villus biopsy specimens. Postnatal urine screening tests must be interpreted cautiously, since false-negative and false-positive results are common. Even in severely affected individuals, tests may be negative in early infancy. The diagnosis is confirmed by estimation of specific enzymatic activity in leukocytes, cultured fibroblasts, or, in some conditions, serum. Radiologic skeletal changes are typical of dysostosis multiplex; they vary in severity with the form of MPS and may be sufficiently specific to allow a precise diagnosis. However, these radiologic features vary considerably throughout childhood and must be interpreted cautiously.

Prognosis and Treatment

For prognosis, see TABLE 42–4.

At present, no worthwhile therapy is available. Attempts at replacement of the deficient enzyme by plasma infusion or skin grafting have had only limited and temporary success. Bone marrow transplantation has produced a biochemical remission in some instances, but impairment of intellectual function has persisted. A high rate of morbidity and mortality accompanies bone marrow transplantation, and its value in these disorders is questionable.

THE OSTEOCHONDRODYSPLASIAS

A group of inherited disorders in which growth abnormalities of bone or cartilage lead to skeletal maldevelopment; dwarfism is a feature of many of them. **Achondroplasia** is the most common and best known, but many other distinct forms of short-limbed dwarfism have been described. These differ widely in genetic background, course, and prognosis, and diagnostic precision is essential. Genetic counseling can be effective, since the pattern of inheritance in most of the osteochondrodysplasias is known. Antenatal diagnosis is possible in some cases by fetoscopy or ultrasonography (including conditions in which fetal limb shortening is severe). New radiographic and molecular techniques have future promise; type II collagen has been shown to be implicated in a few rare entities, but the basic defect is still unknown in the majority of these conditions. Features of the most important disorders in this group are summarized in TABLE 42–5.

Management: Surgical intervention (eg, prosthetic joint replacement of the hip) has proved to

TABLE 42-4. GENETIC MUCOPOLYSACCHARIDOSES (MPS)

	Designation	Clinical Features	Excessive Urinary Mucopolysaccharide	Enzyme Deficiency
MPS I H	Hurler's syndrome*	Early clouding of cornea; grave manifestations; death usual before age 10	Dermatan sulfate Heparan sulfate	α-L-Iduronidase (formerly called Hurler corrective factor)
MPS I S	Scheie's syndrome	Stiff joints; cloudy cornea; aortic regurgitation; normal intelligence; ?normal lifespan	Dermatan sulfate Heparan sulfate	α-L-Iduronidase
MPS I H/S	Hurler-Scheie compound	Phenotype intermediate between Hurler and Scheie	Dermatan sulfate Heparan sulfate	α-L-Iduronidase
MPS II	Hunter's syndrome (severe and mild forms)	No clouding of cornea; milder course than in MPS I H, but death usual before age 15 In the mild form, survival to age 30 to 50; fair intelligence	Dermatan sulfate Heparan sulfate	Iduronosulfate sulfatase
MPS III	Sanfilippo's syndrome (several forms)	Identical phenotype: mild somatic and severe CNS effects	Heparan sulfate	Heparan sulfate sulfatase N-Acetyl-α-D-glucosaminidase in some forms
MPS IV	Morquio's syndrome	Severe bone changes of distinctive type; cloudy cornea; aortic regurgitation	Keratan sulfate	N-Acetylhexosaminidase-6-SO4 sulfatase
MPS IV A	Morquio's syndrome, type A (severe, intermediate, and mild forms)	Severe bone changes of distinctive type; cloudy cornea; aortic regurgitation	Keratan sulfate	N-Acetylhexosaminidase-6-SO4 sulfatase
MPS IV B	Morquio's syndrome, type B	Moderate bone changes causing dwarfism and spinal malalignment; few visceral ramifications		β-Galactosidase
MPS V	Vacant			
MPS VI	Maroteaux-Lamy syndrome (severe and mild forms)	Severe osseous and corneal change; normal intellect	Dermatan sulfate	Arylsulfatase B
MPS VII	β-Glucuronidase deficiency (more than 1 allelic form?)	Hepatosplenomegaly; dysostosis multiplex; WBC inclusions; mental retardation	Dermatan sulfate	β-Glucuronidase

* Other rare metabolic disorders such as the mucolipidoses bear a clinical resemblance to Hurler's syndrome, but they may be differentiated biochemically.
Modified from *Heritable Disorders of Connective Tissue*, ed. 4, by VA McKusick. St. Louis, CV Mosby Co, 1972; used with permission.

TABLE 42–5. FORMS OF DISPROPORTIONATE DWARFISM

Disorder	Additional Clinical Manifestations	Usual Mode of Inheritance	Reported Cases
Achondroplasia	Bulky forehead, saddle nose, lumbar lordosis, bow legs	AD	Common
Hypochondroplasia	Resembles achondroplasia in mild degree; heterogeneous ?	AD	100
Pseudoachondroplasia	Normal facies; dwarfism and kyphoscoliosis vary in degree; heterogeneous	AD/AR	200
Diastrophic dysplasia	Severe dwarfing with rigid hitchhiker thumb and fixed talipes equinovarus	AR	200
Multiple epiphyseal dysplasia	Mild dwarfism; spine and face normal; digits sometimes stubby; often presents with hip dysplasia; very heterogeneous	AD	Common
Spondyloepiphyseal dysplasia	Kyphoscoliosis is a major feature; myopia and a "flat" facies are sometimes present; heterogeneous	AD/AR/XL	100
Metaphyseal chondrodysplasia	Many different eponymous types (eg, Jansen, Schmid, McKusick); associated features in some include malabsorption, neutropenia, and thymolymphopenia	AR/AD	200
Mesomelic dysplasia	Shortening of the forearms and shanks predominates; face and spine are normal; several eponymous forms (eg, Nievergelt, Langer)	AD/AR	50
Chondrodysplasia punctata	All forms have pug nose, ichthyotic skin lesions, and radiographic epiphyseal stippling		
1. Rhizomelic form	Marked proximal limb shortening; lethal in infancy	AR	30
2. Conradi-Hünermann form	Mild asymmetric limb shortening; benign	AD/XL dominant	100
Chondroectodermal dysplasia (Ellis-van Creveld syndrome)	Distal limb shortening; postaxial polydactyly; structural cardiac defects	AR	100

AD = autosomal dominant; AR = autosomal recessive; XL = X-linked.

be of value in certain disorders. Hypoplasia of the odontoid process is an inconsistent feature of many of these conditions, which predisposes to subluxation of the 1st and 2nd cervical vertebrae and compression of the spinal cord. For this reason, the status of the odontoid should be evaluated preoperatively by x-ray studies, and, if abnormal, the patient's head should be carefully supported when hyperextended for endotracheal intubation during anesthesia.

Organizations such as the Little People of America provide social contact for affected individuals and act as a pressure group on their be-

half. Similar societies are active in Australia and Great Britain.

LETHAL SHORT–LIMBED DWARFISM

Osteochondrodystrophies that present as lethal (or potentially lethal) short-limbed dwarfism in the newborn. Characteristic x-ray changes are diagnostic, and a whole-baby x-ray study should be obtained in every newborn short-limbed dwarf. This is important even if the infant is stillborn, as diagnostic precision is essential for ge-

TABLE 42–6. FORMS OF LETHAL SHORT–LIMBED DWARFISM*

Disorder	Additional Features	Mode of Inheritance	Reported Cases
Achondrogenesis	Gross limb shortening; hydropic head and trunk; heterogeneous	AR	50
Thanatophoric dysplasia	On AP x-rays, vertebrae are H-shaped and femora have a "telephone receiver" configuration	Polygenic	Common
Asphyxiating thoracic dysplasia (Jeune's syndrome)	Constriction of upper thorax; polydactyly sometimes present; prognosis variable	AR	50
Short rib–polydactyly syndromes	Thoracic constriction; polydactyly; invariably lethal; heterogeneous	AR	50
Campomelic dysplasia	Marked bowing of lower limbs; heterogeneous	AR	30
Osteogenesis imperfecta congenita	Limb deformity due to multiple fractures (see also MUSCULOSKELETAL DEFECTS in Ch. 28)	AR/AD	
Hypophosphatasia lethalis	Multiple fractures	AR	50
Fibrochondrogenesis	Short limbs; "dumbell-shaped" tubular bones; platyspondylia with vertebral clefting	AR	10
Hypochondrogenesis	Delayed vertebral and pelvic ossification	AR	20
Atelosteogenesis	Short limbs; club feet; cleft palate	?	10
Dyssegmental dysplasia	Short limbs; articular rigidity; gross vertebral malsegmentation	AR	20
Boomerang dysplasia	Short limbs; bowing of long bones	?	3
De la Chapelle dysplasia	Severe micromelia; limb bowing; cleft palate	AR	5
Schneckenbecken's dysplasia	"Snail-shaped" pelvis	AR	10

AP = anteroposterior; AD = autosomal dominant; AR = autosomal recessive.
* For chondrodysplasia punctata (severe rhizomelic form), see TABLE 42–5.

netic prognostication. These conditions are summarized in TABLE 42–6.

Specific histologic abnormalities have been recognized in some osteochondrodysplasias, and further subdivision and delineation are anticipated on the basis of these findings.

THE OSTEOPETROSES
(Albers-Schönberg Disease; Marble Bones)

Increased bone density and abnormalities of skeletal modeling characterize these genetic disorders. Formerly loosely grouped under the above nonspecific terms, the disorders can now be categorized by predominance of bone sclerosis or defective skeletal modeling: **osteoscleroses, craniotubular dysplasias,** and **craniotubular hyperostoses.** Since some disorders are comparatively benign and others progressive and fatal, diagnostic accuracy is crucial; there is no specific therapy for most of them. Surgical decompression may be required to relieve elevated intracranial pressure or for trapped facial or auditory nerves. Malocclusion of the teeth may require specialized orthodontic measures. Facial distortion due to bone overgrowth is sometimes severe and may cause psychologic problems.

The most important of the disorders are summarized below.

Osteoscleroses

Increased skeletal density with little disturbance of modeling.

Osteopetrosis with delayed manifestations (in childhood, adolescence, or young adulthood): **Albers-Schönberg disease** strictly pertains to the *autosomal dominant (AD) delayed, tarda, or benign form of osteopetrosis*, which is relatively common with wide geographic and ethnic distribution. Affected persons may be totally asymptomatic, the diagnosis often reached by chance when x-ray studies are taken for some unrelated purpose. The facies, physique, mentality, and life span are normal, and general health is unimpaired. Occasionally the presenting feature is facial palsy or deafness resulting from cranial nerve compression by bone overgrowth. A mild anemia is an infrequent complication.

The skeleton usually is radiologically normal at birth, bone sclerosis becoming increasingly apparent as childhood progresses. Bony involvement is widespread but patchy, and the extremities are sometimes spared. The calvaria is dense, and the sinuses may be obliterated. In the spine, sclerosis of the vertebral endplates gives rise to the characteristic "rugger jersey" or "rugby shirt" (horizontal banding) appearance.

Osteopetrosis with precocious manifestations (*the autosomal recessive [AR] precocious, malignant, or congenita form of osteopetrosis presenting in infancy*) is an uncommon, potentially lethal disorder clinically and genetically distinct from the benign AD type. Bone overgrowth is associated with marrow dysfunction, and presenting symptoms include failure to thrive, spontaneous bruising, abnormal bleeding, and anemia. Hepatosplenomegaly develops, and palsies of the optic, oculomotor, and facial nerves occur in later stages. Death from anemia, overwhelming infection, or hemorrhage usually occurs in the first year of life.

Generalized bone density is the predominant radiologic feature. Penetrated films of long bones reveal transverse bands in the metaphyseal regions and longitudinal striations in the shafts. As the condition progresses, the ends of the long bones, particularly the proximal humerus and distal femur, develop a flask-shaped configuration. Endobones form in the vertebrae, pelvis, and tubular bones; the skull becomes thickened; and the spine shows the "rugger jersey" appearance.

Bone marrow transplantation has produced excellent initial results in a few infants, but the long-term outcome is unknown.

Osteopetrosis, immediate type: This AR condition is compatible with survival into adulthood. Entrapment of facial and auditory nerves, bone fragility, and a propensity to osteomyelitis of the jaws are the most important features.

Osteopetrosis with renal tubular acidosis: Affected children show weakness, stunted stature, and failure to thrive. The skeleton is radiologically dense, renal tubular acidosis is present, and red cell carbonic anhydrase activity is defective.

Pyknodysostosis (AR inheritance): Short stature becomes evident in early childhood; adult height does not exceed 150 cm (5 ft). Other manifestations (enlarged skull, short and broad hands and feet, dystrophic nails, and blue sclerae) usually are recognized in infancy. Affected individuals resemble each other closely, having small faces, receding chins, and carious, misplaced teeth. The cranium bulges, and the anterior fontanelle remains patent. The terminal phalanges are short and the fingernails dysplastic. Pathologic fractures are an important complication.

On x-ray, bone sclerosis appears during childhood, but neither bone striations nor endobones are seen. The calvaria is not particularly dense, but fontanelles are patent and multiple wormian bones are present. Facial bones and paranasal sinuses are hypoplastic, and the mandibular angle is obtuse. Clavicles may be gracile, with underdevelopment of their lateral portions; the distal phalanges are rudimentary.

Craniotubular Dysplasias

Abnormal skeletal modeling, with minor bone sclerosis.

Metaphyseal dysplasia (Pyle's disease) is a rare AR disorder often confused semantically with craniometaphyseal dysplasia (see below). Persons with metaphyseal dysplasia are clinically normal, apart from valgus knee deformities, although scoliosis and bone fragility are occasional complications. Diagnosis usually is reached by chance following x-ray studies for an unrelated purpose.

In contrast to the mild clinical signs, x-ray changes are striking. The long bones are undermodeled and bony cortices generally thin. Tubular bones of the legs have gross "Erlenmeyer flask" flaring, particularly in the distal portions of the femora. The skull is virtually spared, apart from a supraorbital prominence; the mandibular angle is obtuse; and the bones of the pelvis and thoracic cage are expanded.

Craniometaphyseal dysplasia (AD inheritance) is relatively common compared with the other conditions in this group. Paranasal bossing develops during infancy, and progressive expansion and thickening of the skull and mandible distort the jaw and face. Bone encroachment leads to entrapment and dysfunction of the cranial nerves, particularly the 7th and 8th. Malocclusion of the jaws may be troublesome, while partial obliteration of the sinuses predisposes to recurrent nasorespiratory infection. Height and general health are normal, but progressive elevation of intracranial pressure is an infrequent and serious complication.

X-ray changes are age-related and usually evident by age 5. The main feature in the skull is sclerosis, which is maximal in the base although the cranium is always involved to some degree. Long bones have widened metaphyses with a club-shaped configuration, particularly at the lower end of the femur. However, these changes are much less severe than in Pyle's disease. The spine and pelvis are uninvolved.

Frontometaphyseal dysplasia: Distinct AD and X-linked forms may exist. The disorder becomes evident in early childhood. The supraorbital ridge is prominent, resembling a knight's visor. The mandible is hypoplastic, with anterior constriction. Dental anomalies are common, and deafness develops in adulthood because of sclerotic narrowing of the internal acoustic foramina and the middle ear. Long bones of the legs are moderately bowed. Progressive contractures in the digits may simulate RA. General health is good and height is normal.

On x-ray, bone overgrowth of the frontal region is obvious; patchy sclerosis is present in the cranial vault. The vertebral bodies are dysplastic but not sclerotic. The iliac crests are abruptly flared and the pelvic inlet distorted. Femoral capital epiphyses are flattened, with expansion of the femoral heads and coxa valga deformity. Finger bones are undermodeled, with erosions and loss of joint space.

Craniotubular Hyperostoses

Overgrowth of bone, causing both alteration of contour and increase in skeletal density.

Endosteal hyperostosis (van Buchem's disease): The classic form is inherited as AR. A mild AD variety has also been reported. Overgrowth and distortion of the mandible and brow become evident in mid childhood. Subsequently, entrapment of the cranial nerves leads to facial palsy and deafness. The life span is not compromised, stature is normal, and the bones are not fragile. Major x-ray features are widening and sclerosis of the calvaria, cranial base, and mandible. Endosteal thickening is present in the diaphyses of the tubular bones.

Sclerosteosis (AR inheritance) is most prevalent in the Afrikaner population of South Africa. Overgrowth and sclerosis of the skeleton, particularly the skull, develop in early childhood. Height and weight are often excessive, and deafness and facial palsy due to cranial nerve entrapment may be a presenting feature. Distortion of the facies, apparent by age 10, eventually becomes severe. In adults, elevation of intracranial pressure may cause headache, and several sudden deaths have occurred from impaction of the brainstem in the foramen magnum. Cutaneous or bony syndactyly of the 2nd and 3rd fingers distinguishes sclerosteosis from the other disorders in this group.

Predominant x-ray features are gross widening and sclerosis of the calvaria and mandible. The vertebral bodies are spared, although their pedicles are dense. Pelvic bones are sclerotic but with normal contours. Cortices of the long bones are sclerosed and hyperostotic and their shafts undermodeled.

Diaphyseal dysplasia (Camurati-Engelmann disease) is a comparatively well-known AD disorder that presents in mid childhood with muscular pain, weakness, and wasting, typically in the legs. These symptoms usually resolve by age 30. Cranial nerve compression and raised intracranial pressure are occasional complications. The manifestations are variable; some patients are severely handicapped, whereas others are virtually asymptomatic.

The predominant x-ray feature is marked thickening of the periosteal and medullary surfaces of the long bones' diaphyseal cortices. The medullary canals and external bone contours are irregular. The extremities and the axial skeleton usually are spared. Infrequently, the skull is involved, with calvarial widening and basal sclerosis. As with the clinical features, the x-ray changes are quite variable. Corticosteroid therapy may be effective in relieving bone pain and improving muscle power.

THE OSTEOCHONDROSES

A group of disorders affecting the epiphyses during childhood characterized by noninflammatory, noninfectious derangements of the normal process of bony growth occurring at various ossification centers at the time of their greatest developmental activity. Etiology is unknown. The osteochondroses do not have a simple genetic basis. They differ in their anatomic distribution, course, and prognosis; their importance lies in their orthopedic implications. Rare osteochondroses include Freiberg's disease (head of 2nd metatarsal), Panner's disease (capitulum), Sever's disease (calcaneus), and Johansson-Larsen syndrome (patella).

Legg-Calvé-Perthes Disease

Idiopathic aseptic necrosis of the femoral capital epiphysis. The disease is by far the most common of the osteochondroses, has a maximum incidence between the ages of 5 and 10 yr, with a predilection for males, and is usually unilateral.

Symptoms, signs, and diagnosis: Major symptoms are pain in the hip joint and disturbance of gait, usually of gradual onset and slow progression. Joint movements are limited, and the thigh muscles may become wasted. X-rays initially reveal flattening and, later, fragmentation of the femoral head, which contains areas of lucency and sclerosis.

Differential diagnosis: The inherited skeletal disorders, notably multiple epiphyseal dysplasia, frequently are misdiagnosed as Legg-Calvé-Perthes disease. In any atypical bilateral or familial case, a skeletal survey to exclude conditions of this type is *mandatory*, as the prognosis and optimal form of management differ in these various disorders. Hypothyroidism, sickle cell anemia, and trauma also must be excluded.

Prognosis: The untreated case usually follows a prolonged but self-limited course (2 to 3 yr). When the condition eventually becomes quiescent, residual distortion of the femoral head and acetabulum predisposes to secondary degenerative osteoarthritis. For the treated case, these sequelae are less severe.

Treatment is orthopedic and includes prolonged bed rest, mobile traction, slings, and containment of the femoral head by abduction plaster casts and splints. Some authorities advocate subtrochanteric osteotomy with internal fixation and early ambulation.

Osgood-Schlatter Disease

Osteochondritis of the tibial tubercle is usually unilateral, occurs between ages 10 and 15 yr, and is more common in boys. The etiology is thought to be trauma from excessive traction by the patella tendon on its immature epiphyseal insertion.

Symptoms, signs, and diagnosis: Major features are pain, swelling, and tenderness over the tibial tubercle at the patellar tendon insertion. There is no systemic disturbance. Lateral radiographs of the knee show fragmentation of the tibial tubercle.

Treatment: Resolution is usually spontaneous after a course of weeks or months. Relief of pain and avoidance of sport and excessive exercise, especially deep knee bending, are the only necessary measures. Immobilization in plaster, intralesional injection of hydrocortisone, surgical removal of loose bodies, drilling, and grafting are procedures required infrequently.

Scheuermann's Disease

A relatively common condition in which backache and kyphosis are associated with localized changes in the vertebral bodies. It presents in adolescence (boys are more frequently affected) and probably is heterogeneous (ie, not a single entity but a group of conditions sharing similar features), but the etiology and pathogenesis are a matter of debate. Osteochondritis of the upper and lower cartilaginous vertebral endplates has been incriminated, but trauma sometimes is a causative factor. Some affected persons have a marfanoid habitus (disproportionality between trunk and limb length); some show a familial tendency.

Symptoms, signs, and diagnosis: A "round-shouldered" posture and persistent low-grade backache are the usual presenting features. Mild cases often are recognized during routine screening of schoolchildren for spinal deformity. The major clinical finding is an increase of the normal thoracic kyphosis, which may be diffuse or localized. The course is long (very variable—often several years) but mild; trivial spinal malalignment often persists when the disorder has become quiescent.

Lateral x-rays of the spine show anterior wedging of the vertebral bodies, usually in the lower thoracic and upper lumbar region. The endplates become irregular and sclerotic in later stages. Spinal malalignment is predominantly kyphotic, but an element of scoliosis sometimes is present. The x-ray changes often are inconsistent, possibly reflecting underlying heterogeneity. In atypical cases, a generalized skeletal dysplasia and spinal tuberculosis must be excluded.

Treatment: Mild nonprogressive cases can be treated by reduction of weight-bearing stress and by avoidance of strenuous activity. Occasionally, when the kyphosis is more severe, a spinal brace or rest and recumbency on a rigid bed are indicated. Surgical stabilization and correction of malalignment are infrequently required for progressive cases.

Köhler's Disease

A rare form of osteochondritis of the navicular bone of the tarsus. The disease affects children between ages 3 and 5 yr and has an increased incidence in boys.

Symptoms, signs, and diagnosis: The foot becomes swollen and painful, with tenderness maximal over the medial longitudinal arch. Weight-bearing and walking increase the discomfort, and the gait is disturbed. The condition has a chronic course but rarely persists for > 2 yr.

On x-ray, the navicular bone initially is flattened and sclerotic and later becomes fragmented, prior to reossification. The condition is unilateral, and comparative x-rays of the unaffected side are valuable for assessment of progression.

Treatment is symptomatic, requiring rest, pain relief, and avoidance of excessive weight-bearing. In the acute case, a few weeks in a below-knee walking plaster cast, well molded under the longitudinal arch, may be helpful in early stages.

PRIMARY MALIGNANT TUMORS OF BONE

Osteogenic sarcoma (osteosarcoma), except for myeloma, is the most common primary bone tumor and is highly malignant, with a tendency to metastasize to the lungs. Osteosarcoma is most common in persons aged 10 to 20, though it can occur at any age. About half the lesions are located in the region of the knee but can be found in any bone. Pain and a mass are the usual symptoms. X-ray findings vary greatly, with no characteristic appearance, and the tumor may be predominantly sclerotic or lytic. Accurate diagnosis rests on pathologic examination of representative biopsy tissue.

Once a definite diagnosis has been established, oncology consultation should be obtained to consider either preoperative **(neoadjuvant)** chemotherapy or postoperative **(adjuvant)** chemotherapy. If neoadjuvant treatment is instituted, the course of the disease can be followed by x-ray, pain level (it usually abates), and level of serum alkaline phosphatase (it usually goes down). After several courses of chemotherapy,

surgery can proceed. Many lesions are amenable to limb salvage procedures; ie, using newer surgical techniques the tumor may be resected and the limb reconstructed, instead of requiring amputation as in the past. Neoadjuvant treatment also allows study of the resected tumor to determine the extent of necrosis caused by chemotherapy; lesions that show nearly complete necrosis have the best outlook. Some oncologists prefer adjuvant chemotherapy. With either form of treatment, 75% of patients survive for ≥ 5 yr. Numerous clinical studies are under way to improve survival even further.

Fibrosarcomas have the same characteristics as osteogenic sarcomas, above, and pose the same problems.

Malignant fibrous histiocytoma behaves clinically in a manner similar to osteosarcoma and fibrosarcoma. Treatment is the same as for osteosarcoma.

Chondrosarcomas, malignant tumors of cartilage, are clinically, therapeutically, and prognostically *unlike* osteogenic sarcomas. They develop in > 10% of patients with multiple benign osteochondromas. However, 90% of chondrosarcomas are primary, arising de novo. **Diagnosis** can be made only by biopsy. Many chondrosarcomas can be graded histologically from 1 to 4. Grade 1 lesions are slow-growing with a good prognosis for cure; grade 4 lesions grow more rapidly and are much more likely to metastasize. Regardless of grade, the outstanding feature is their ability to "seed" or implant in surrounding soft tissues.

Treatment is total surgical resection. Neither radiation nor chemotherapy is effective in either primary or adjunctive treatment. Because of the potential to seed, the biopsy wound should be closed and ablative surgery carried out meticulously. Care must be taken to avoid entry into the tumor and spillage of tumor cells into the soft tissues of the wound, since recurrence is inevitable if this happens. With no spillage of tumor contents, the cure rate is ≥ 50%, depending on the grade of the tumor. When surgical ablation with maintenance of function is impossible, amputation is obligatory.

Mesenchymal chondrosarcoma is a rare but histologically distinct type of chondrosarcoma with a great potential for metastasizing; the cure rate is low.

Ewing's tumor (Ewing's sarcoma) is a radiosensitive round-cell bone tumor. Males are affected more frequently than females. Ewing's tumor appears at a younger age than any other primary malignant bone tumor, with a peak incidence between 10 and 20 yr. Most of the tumors develop in the extremities, but any bone may be involved. Microscopically, the lesion consists of solidly packed, small round cells. Pain and swelling are the most common symptoms. Ewing's tumor tends to be extensive, sometimes involving the entire shaft of a long bone. Generally, more of the bone is pathologically involved than is apparent from the x-rays (CT scans and MRI are often helpful in further defining disease extent). Lytic destruction is the most common finding, but there may be multiple layers of subperiosteal reactive new bone formation, giving the "onion-skin" appearance once considered a classic diagnostic sign. **Diagnosis** depends on biopsy, since many other malignant bone tumors produce an identical appearance. **Treatment** includes various combinations of surgery, multimodal chemotherapy, and radiation therapy. At the present time, > 60% of patients with primary localized Ewing's sarcoma of bone may be cured by this multimodal approach.

Malignant lymphoma of bone is a small round-cell tumor that affects adults, usually in their 40s and 50s. It may arise in any bone. While the lesion may be referred to as **reticulum cell sarcoma,** a mixture of reticulum cells, lymphoblasts, and lymphocytes is common in these neoplasms. When malignant lymphoma involves bone, one of 3 clinical conditions may be found: (1) The lymphoma may be primary in bone, without evidence of disease elsewhere. (2) In addition to the bone lesion, similar disease may be found in other osseous or soft tissue sites. (3) A patient with known soft tissue lymphomatous disease may subsequently have metastatic spread into any bone.

Pain and swelling are the usual symptoms. On x-ray, bone destruction is predominant. Depending on the stage, the involved bone may be mottled or patchy, or, in more advanced disease, the entire outline of the affected bone may be lost. Pathologic fracture is common.

When malignant lymphoma is primary in bone and no disease is present elsewhere, the 5-yr survival rate is $\geq$ 50%. The tumors are radiosensitive. Combination radiation and chemotherapy is as effective in achieving cure as amputation or other extensive ablative surgery. Amputation is indicated only when function is lost because of pathologic fracture or extensive soft tissue involvement.

Multiple myeloma is a tumor of hematopoietic derivation and is the most common bone neoplasm. The neoplastic process is regularly multicentric and often involves the bone marrow so diffusely that bone marrow aspiration usually is diagnostic.

Malignant giant cell tumor is rare; even its existence is controversial. The lesion usually is located at the extreme end of a long bone. The classic features of malignant destruction (predominantly lytic destruction; cortical destruction; soft tissue extension; pathologic fracture) are seen on x-ray. To be sure of diagnosis, zones of typical benign giant cell tumor must be demonstrated in a malignant neoplasm or in previous tissue obtained from the neoplasm. A sarcoma that develops in a previously benign giant cell tumor is characteristically radioresistant. The same principles of treatment apply as in osteogenic sarcoma, above, but the cure rate is low.

Many other types of primary malignant bone tumors exist, most of them so rare as to be medical curiosities. **Chordoma** develops from the remnants of the primitive notochord. It has a predilection for the ends of the spinal column and usually is located in the sacrum or near the base of the skull. Pain is a virtually constant feature of a chordoma located in the sacrococcygeal region. When located in the base of the occipital region, the symptoms may be referred to any of the cranial nerves, but symptoms resulting from involvement of the nerves to the eye are most common. The duration of symptoms varies from months to several years before diagnosis. A chordoma is seen on x-ray as an expansile, destructive bone lesion that may be associated with a soft tissue mass. Hematogenous metastasis is unusual. Local recurrence is often more troublesome than metastatic spread. Chordomas located in the spheno-occipital region usually are inaccessible to surgery but may respond to radiation therapy. In the sacrococcygeal region they may be cured by radical en bloc excision.

CONDITIONS THAT COMMONLY SIMULATE PRIMARY TUMORS OF BONE

Many non-neoplastic conditions of bone may simulate bone tumors, either clinically or radiologically. **Heterotopic ossification (myositis ossificans)** or **exuberant callus** after fracture may be mistakenly interpreted as a malignant neoplasm; histopathologic tissue examination differentiates the conditions.

Simple **unicameral bone cysts** occur in the long bones in children. Most come to the clinician's attention when pathologic fracture occurs. Small ones heal and may obliterate themselves in the process of fracture healing. Larger ones may require evacuation and bone grafting.

Fibrous dysplasia is a cystic bone lesion probably resulting from an anomaly in bone development. The lesion may appear in one or several bones during childhood. When several bones are involved and cutaneous pigmentation and endocrine abnormalities are present, the condition is called **Albright's syndrome.** On x-ray, the lesions appear cystic and may be extensive and deforming. The lesions commonly stop growing at puberty. Spontaneous malignant degeneration is rare. Treatment should be conservative, though deformity in the long bones may require surgical correction.

Aneurysmal bone cyst is a cystic lesion of unknown cause that usually appears before age 20. The cyst may occur in the metaphyseal region of the long bones, but almost any bone may be affected. Pain and swelling occur. The lesion may be present for a few weeks to a few years before diagnosis. It tends to increase slowly in size until therapy is begun. The appearance on x-ray often is characteristic: The rarefied area usually is well

circumscribed, eccentric, and associated with soft tissue extension produced by periosteal bulging. Periosteal new bone formation tends to delimit the periphery of the tumor. Surgical removal of the entire lesion is the most successful treatment, but complete regression after incomplete removal sometimes occurs. Radiation is the treatment of choice *only* in surgically inaccessible vertebral lesions that are compressing the spinal cord, since postirradiation sarcomas occasionally occur.

Histiocytosis X (Letterer-Siwe disease, Hand-Schüller-Christian disease, eosinophilic granuloma) is also discussed in Ch. 37. Solitary or multiple reticuloendothelial osseous lesions occur and are usually well defined on x-ray. When the lesion is solitary with periosteal new bone formation, the x-ray may suggest a malignant bone tumor; diagnosis depends on biopsy. When only one or a few osseous lesions are present, local radiation therapy can produce cure, but the prognosis is ominous in patients < 3 yr old or at any age with more than 8 bones involved, and particularly in those with hemorrhagic manifestations and enlarged spleens. More extensive involvement, particularly skull lesions, may occur, and extreme widespread involvement may produce fulminating, rapidly fatal disease, with death usually the result of respiratory or cardiac failure.

43. NEUROLOGIC DISORDERS

SEIZURE DISORDERS

(Epilepsy)

(See also SEIZURE DISORDERS
IN THE NEWBORN in Ch. 27)

Epilepsy: *A recurrent paroxysmal disorder of cerebral function characterized by sudden, brief attacks of altered consciousness, motor activity, sensory phenomena, or inappropriate behavior caused by abnormal excessive discharge of cerebral neurons.* **Convulsive seizures,** the most common form of attacks, begin with loss of consciousness and motor control, and tonic or clonic jerking of all extremities, but any recurrent seizure pattern may be termed epilepsy.

Etiology

Epilepsy is classed etiologically as symptomatic or idiopathic: **Symptomatic** implies that a

probable cause has been identified that at times permits a specific course of therapy to eliminate that cause; **idiopathic** means that no obvious cause can be found, which is the case in about 75% of young adults and a smaller percentage of children under age 3. Epilepsy due to a microscopic scar in the brain resulting from birth trauma or other injury may be misclassified during life as idiopathic but show evidence of a causative lesion at autopsy or surgery for epilepsy. In such patients, positron emission tomography **(PET)** or single proton emission computerized tomography **(SPECT)** may show local areas of brain dysfunction when CT and MRI are normal. Unexplained, predominantly inherited neuronal abnormalities probably underlie most idiopathic cases.

Idiopathic epilepsy generally begins between ages 2 and 14. Seizures before age 2 are usually related to developmental defects, birth injuries, or a metabolic disease affecting the brain; those beginning after age 25 are usually secondary to cerebral trauma, tumors, or other organic brain disease. Focal brain diseases can cause seizures at any age.

Seizures may be associated with a variety of cerebral or systemic disorders, as a result of a focal or generalized disturbance of cortical function. These include **hyperpyrexia** (acute infection, heat stroke), **CNS infections** (meningitis, AIDS, encephalitis, brain abscess, neurosyphilis, rabies, tetanus, falciparum malaria, toxoplasmosis, cysticercosis of the brain), **metabolic disturbances** (hypoglycemia, hypoparathyroidism, phenylketonuria), **convulsive or toxic agents** (camphor, chloraquine, pentylenetetrazol, strychnine, picrotoxin, lead, alcohol, cocaine), **cerebral hypoxia** (Adams-Stokes syndrome, carotid sinus hypersensitivity, anesthesia, CO poisoning, breath-holding), **expanding brain lesions** (neoplasm, intracranial hemorrhage, subdural hematoma in infancy), **brain defects** (congenital, developmental), **cerebral edema** (hypertensive encephalopathy, eclampsia), **cerebral trauma** (skull fracture, birth injury), **anaphylaxis** (foreign serum or drug allergy), and **cerebral infarct or hemorrhage**. Convulsions may also occur as a withdrawal symptom after chronic use of alcohol, hypnotics, or tranquilizers. **Hysterical patients** occasionally simulate convulsive attacks.

The seizures are transient in many of these conditions and do not recur once the illness ends. However, convulsions may recur at intervals for years or indefinitely if there is a permanent lesion or scar in the CNS, in which case a diagnosis of epilepsy is made.

Pathogenesis

Convulsive seizures result from a generalized disturbance in cerebral function. In some instances, a small focus of dysfunctional tissue in the cerebrum discharges abnormally in response to endogenous or exogenous stimuli, and spread of the discharge to other portions of the cerebrum results in convulsive phenomena and loss of consciousness. In primary generalized epilepsy, the seizures are generalized from the outset, beginning as a diffuse abnormal discharge affecting all cerebral cortical areas simultaneously.

Given a sufficient stimulus (eg, convulsant drugs, hypoxia, hypoglycemia), even the normal brain can discharge in a diffusely synchronous fashion and produce a seizure. In susceptible persons, seizures may occasionally be precipitated by exogenous factors (sound, light, cutaneous stimulation).

Classification and Incidence

Epileptic seizures can be classified according to several different criteria. TABLE 43–1 gives a current internationally agreed-upon classification. **Partial seizures** begin focally with a specific sensory, motor, or psychic aberration that reflects the affected part of the cerebral hemisphere where the seizure originates. TABLE 43–2 gives some of the characteristic manifestations and their sites of origin. **Auras** (*focal manifestations that immediately precede complex or generalized seizures*) reflect where the seizure begins. Sometimes a focal lesion of one part of a hemisphere activates the entire cerebrum bilaterally so rapidly that it produces a generalized grand mal seizure before any focal sign appears. **Generalized seizures** usually affect both consciousness and motor function from the outset. The seizure itself frequently has a genetic or metabolic cause.

Seizures affect about 2% of the population; chronically recurring seizures (epilepsy) are perhaps ¼ that frequent. Most patients have only 1 type of seizure; about 30% have 2 or more types. About 90% experience grand mal seizures, either alone (60%) or with other seizures (30%). Absence (petit mal) attacks occur in about 25% (4% alone, 21% with others). Psychomotor attacks occur in 18% (6% alone, 12% with others).

Symptoms and Signs

Simple partial (focal, local) seizures begin with specific motor, sensory, or psychomotor focal phenomena without loss of consciousness. Isolated epileptic auras are simple partial seizures with a single sensory symptom (often olfactory) preceding a complex or generalized seizure. Common manifestations are given in TABLE 43–2. In **jacksonian seizures** (*focal motor symptoms begin in one hand or foot and then "march" up the extremity, or spread similarly from a corner of the mouth*), the dysfunction may remain localized or may spread to other parts of the brain, with consequent loss of consciousness and generalized convulsive movements.

Complex partial (psychomotor) seizures are characterized by a variety of patterns of onset (see TABLE 43–1). In most instances, the patient has a 1- to 2-min loss of contact with the surroundings. The patient at first may stagger,

TABLE 43-1. INTERNATIONAL CLASSIFICATION OF EPILEPTIC SEIZURES

I. Partial (focal, local) seizures
   A. Simple partial seizures (consciousness not impaired)
      1. With motor signs (includes jacksonian seizures)
      2. With somatosensory or special-sensory symptoms (hallucinosis)
      3. With autonomic symptoms or signs
      4. With psychic symptoms (includes dysphasic, dysmnesic, cognitive, and affective symptoms)
   B. Complex partial seizures
      1. Any simple partial seizure onset followed by impairment of consciousness
      2. Impairment of consciousness only
II. Generalized seizures
   A. Absence seizures
      1. With impairment of consciousness only
      2. With clonic components
      3. With atonic components
      4. With tonic components
      5. With automatisms
      6. With autonomic components
   B. Myoclonic seizures
   C. Clonic seizures
   D. Tonic seizures
   E. Tonic-clonic seizures
   F. Atonic seizures
III. Unclassified seizures due to incomplete data

Modified from Bancaud J, Henriksen O, Rubio-Donnadieu F, et al: "Proposal for revised clinical and electroencephalographic classification of epileptic seizures." *Epilepsia* 22:489–501, 1981; used by permission of Raven Press.

perform automatic purposeless movements, and utter unintelligible sounds. He does not understand what is said and may resist aid. Mental confusion continues for another 1 or 2 min after the attack is apparently over. **Psychomotor attacks** may develop at any age and are usually associated with structural pathology (eg, mesial temporal sclerosis, low-grade astrocytomas). **Status psychomotor epilepsy** may occur, in which affected subjects act in a slow, bewildered, and sometimes confused state for hours or, rarely, days.

Complex partial seizures of temporal lobe origin are *not* characterized by unprovoked aggressive behavior. If restrained, however, such a patient occasionally may lash out at the person restricting his movement, as may a patient in a postictal confused state after a generalized seizure. No satisfactory evidence suggests that premeditated or unprovoked aggression can ever be attributed to attacks of temporal lobe epilepsy.

Patients with temporal lobe epilepsy experience a higher incidence of interictal psychiatric disorders than does the normal population. Selection factors in evaluation make exact figures difficult to be sure of, but some studies show as many as 33% of patients with temporal lobe epilepsy having substantial psychologic difficulties, with up to 10% showing symptoms of schizophreniform or depressive psychoses.

Generalized seizures can be minor or major in their motor manifestations. Generalized seizures may be primarily generalized (bilateral cerebral cortical involvement at onset), or secondarily generalized (local cortical onset with subsequent bilateral spread). **Absence (petit mal) attacks** are *brief, primarily generalized seizures manifested by a 10- to 30-sec loss of consciousness, with eye or muscle flutterings at a rate of 3/sec, and with or without loss of muscle tone.* The patient suddenly stops any activity in which he is engaged and resumes it after the attack. Petit mal seizures are genetically determined and occur predominantly in children: they never begin after age 20. The attacks are likely to occur several or many times a day, often when the patient is sitting quietly. They are infrequent during exercise. Between seizures, patients are normal.

Infantile spasms (salaam seizures) are *primarily generalized seizures characterized by sudden flexion of the arms, forward flexion of the trunk, and extension of the legs.* The attacks last only a few seconds but may be repeated many

TABLE 43-2. FOCAL MANIFESTATIONS OF PARTIAL SEIZURES
AND SITES OF THE ASSOCIATED CEREBRAL DYSFUNCTION

Focal Manifestation	Site of Dysfunction
Localized twitching of muscles (jacksonian seizure)	Frontal lobe (motor cortex)
Localized numbness or tingling	Parietal lobe (sensory cortex)
Chewing movements or smacking of lips	Anterior temporal lobe
Olfactory hallucinations	Anteromedial temporal lobe
Visual hallucinations (formed images)	Temporal lobe
Visual hallucinations (flashes of light)	Occipital lobe
Complex automatic behaviorisms	Temporal lobe

times a day. They are restricted to the first 3 yr of life, often to be replaced by other forms of attacks. Brain damage is usually evident.

Tonic-clonic (grand mal) seizures *occasionally begin with a partial "aura" of epigastric discomfort, followed by an outcry; the seizure continues with loss of consciousness; falling; and tonic, then clonic, contractions of the muscles of the extremities, trunk, and head.* Urinary and fecal incontinence may occur. The attack usually lasts 2 to 5 min. It may be preceded by a prodromal mood change, and may be followed by a postictal state, with deep sleep, headache, muscle soreness or, at times, focal motor or sensory phenomena. The attacks may appear at any age.

Akinetic seizures are *brief, primarily generalized seizures seen in children and characterized by complete loss of muscle tone and consciousness.* The child falls or pitches to the ground, so that attacks carry the risk of serious trauma, particularly head injury.

Febrile seizures occur primarily in children from 3 mo to 5 yr old, in association with fever without evidence of intracranial infection or other defined cause. Up to 4% of all children are affected, and there is a genetic predisposition. "Benign" or "simple" febrile convulsions are brief, solitary, and generalized; "complicated" febrile seizures are either focal, last > 15 min, or recur 2 or more times in < 24 h. The occurrence of febrile seizures overall is associated with a slightly increased incidence of subsequent afebrile recurrent seizures (2% develop epilepsy); the incidence of later epilepsy and the risk for recurrent febrile seizures are much greater among children with complicated febrile seizures, pre-existing abnormal neurologic examination, onset before age 1 yr, or family history of epilepsy.

In status epilepticus, *motor, sensory, or psychic seizures follow one another with no intervening periods of consciousness.* Grand mal status epilepticus may persist for hours or days and may be fatal. It may occur spontaneously or result from too rapid withdrawal of anticonvulsants. Partial continuous epilepsy is a form of rare focal (usually hand or face) motor seizures in which the attacks recur at intervals of a few seconds or minutes, lasting from days to weeks at a time.

Diagnosis

Idiopathic epilepsy must be distinguished from symptomatic epilepsy. The type of seizure seen in the newborn is not helpful in distinguishing between structural and metabolic causes. In older children and adults, focal seizures or focal postictal symptoms generally imply a focal structural lesion in the brain, while generalized seizures are more likely to have a metabolic cause.

The history should include an eyewitness account of a typical attack and information on the frequency of seizures and the longest and shortest intervals between attacks. A history of prior trauma (eg, cranial injury producing unconsciousness, birth trauma), infection (eg, meningitis, encephalitis, pertussis), or toxic episodes (eg, excessive alcohol or drug consumption and its relation to seizures) must be sought and evaluated. A family history of convulsions or neurologic disorders is significant.

Fever and stiff neck accompanying convulsions of recent onset should suggest meningitis or subarachnoid hemorrhage. Focal cerebral symptoms and signs in association with seizures suggest brain tumor, cerebrovascular disease, or residual traumatic abnormalities. Grand mal seizures, particularly in an adult, always require a diagnostic search for an unsuspected focal lesion.

Appropriate studies include serum glucose and Ca, and EEG. If these are focally abnormal, and in all cases of adult-onset seizures, CT or MRI is indicated.

The interictal EEG in primarily generalized grand mal attacks is characterized most often by relatively symmetric bursts of sharp and slow (4- to 7-sec) activity. Unilateral or focal discharges occur in secondarily generalized seizures. In petit mal, spikes and slow waves appear at the rate of 3/sec. Interictal temporal lobe foci (spikes or slow waves) are frequent with psychomotor epilepsy. The presence of a focal EEG abnormality may aid in the differential diagnosis of brain disease, as may the presence of a characteristic bilateral abnormality. Since an EEG taken during a seizure-free interval is normal in about 15% of patients, one normal EEG does not exclude epilepsy. In rare cases even repeated EEGs may be normal and the diagnosis of epilepsy as opposed to a behavioral disorder may have to be made on clinical grounds.

Prognosis

Drug therapy can completely control grand mal seizures in 50% of cases and greatly reduce the frequency of seizures in another 35%, can control petit mal seizures in 40% and reduce the frequency in 35%, and can control psychomotor attacks in 35% and reduce the frequency in 50%. Among patients with well-controlled seizures, about 50% can eventually discontinue drugs without seizure relapse.

Most patients with epilepsy are normal between attacks, although overuse of anticonvulsants can dull alertness. Progressive mental deterioration is usually related to an accompanying neurologic disease that itself caused the seizures; only rarely do seizures per se impair mental abilities. The outlook is better when no brain lesion is demonstrable. About 70% of noninstitutionalized patients with epilepsy are mentally normal, 20% show a slight reduction in intellect, and 10% have a moderate to pronounced impairment.

Management and Treatment

1. General principles: In idiopathic epilepsy, treatment is primarily control of seizures. In symptomatic epilepsy, the associated disease must be treated as well; continued anticonvulsant treatment is usually needed after surgical removal of cerebral lesions.

A normal life should be encouraged. Moderate exercise is recommended; such sports as swimming and horseback riding are permitted with proper safeguards. Movies, dancing, and other social activities should be encouraged. Most state licensing agencies permit driving after seizures have stopped for 1 yr. Alcoholic beverages are **contraindicated.**

Family members must be taught a commonsense attitude toward the patient. Instead of overprotection and oversolicitude, sympathetic support should be directed against feelings of inferiority, self-consciousness, and other emotional handicaps, and emphasis placed on preventing invalidism. Vocational rehabilitation may help. Institutional care is advisable only for severely retarded patients or for those whose attacks are frequent, violent, and uncontrolled by drugs.

2. Management of a convulsion, whatever its etiology, is limited to preventing injury. Attempts to protect the tongue should not be undertaken: Teeth may be damaged. A finger should not be inserted to straighten the tongue; this is dangerous and unnecessary. Clothing about the neck should be loosened, and a pillow placed under the head. The patient should be rolled onto his side to prevent aspiration. A responsible fellow worker may be trained to give emergency aid if the patient agrees.

3. Elimination of causative or precipitating factors: The first rule in treating seizure disorders is to seek and treat progressive organic lesions of the brain (eg, tumors and abscesses). After surgical removal of organic lesions, continued medical treatment usually is necessary. Physical disorders (eg, infections, endocrine abnormalities) should be corrected.

4. Drug therapy: No single drug controls all types of seizures, and different drugs are required for different patients. Rarely do patients require several drugs. For the newly diagnosed patient with a seizure disorder, the single first drug of choice for the particular type of epilepsy is selected, starting with relatively low dosage, increasing over a week or so to the standard therapeutic dosage. After about a week at such dosage, **blood levels** are obtained to determine the patient's pharmacokinetic response and, if appropriate, whether the effective therapeutic level has been reached. If seizures continue, the daily dosage is increased by small increments as dosage rises above the usual. If toxic blood levels or symptoms occur before seizures are controlled, a second anticonvulsant is added slowly, again guarding against toxicity, since interaction between agents can interfere with their rate of metabolic degradation. The initial failed antiepileptic drug then is withdrawn gradually. Once seizures are brought under control, the drug should be continued *without interruption* at least 1 seizure-free year. At that time, discontinuation of drug should be considered, since about 50% of such patients will remain seizure free without drugs. Patients whose attacks initially were difficult to control, those who failed a therapy-free trial, and those with important social reasons for avoiding seizures should be treated indefinitely.

The most effective **anticonvulsants** for chronic use in children and adults are given in TABLE 43–3. Estimates of drug concentrations in blood are useful (1) to indicate the particular response to specific drugs (patients can vary widely); (2) if abnormally high, to warn against toxicity in susceptible patients; and (3) if abnormally low, to reflect the patient's noncompliance in taking the drug. Despite these potential advantages, management must give first attention to the patient's epilepsy. Once the drug response is known, blood levels become substantially less useful to follow than the clinical course. Some patients have clinical toxicity at low levels; others tolerate high levels without toxic symptoms.

For generalized motor (grand mal) or **partial motor (focal) seizures,** phenytoin, carbamazepine, or valproate isthe drug of choice. For adults, phenytoin 300 mg/day orally can be given in divided doses or at bedtime. If seizures continue, dosages can be increased cautiously to 500 mg/day with blood level monitoring. At higher dosage, divided daily doses may reduce toxic symptoms. Carbamazepine 200 mg qid to 400 mg tid can be given but should be started slowly. Effective valproate dosages typically are 250 to 500 mg tid to qid. Phenobarbital 100 mg/day at bedtime or primidone up to 1500 mg/day can be added *slowly* to minimize drowsiness.

For partial complex (psychomotor) seizures, treatment begins with carbamazepine, phenytoin, primidone, or valproate; carbamazepine is the drug of choice. Primidone is particularly effective, but is not the first choice because it may cause drowsiness.

For absence (petit mal) seizures, ethosuximide orally is preferred. Valproate and clonazepam orally also are effective, but the latter shows a high incidence of tolerance. Acetazolamide 250 mg tid is reserved for otherwise refractory cases. A ketogenic diet may be helpful but is difficult to maintain.

Akinetic seizures, myoclonic seizures, and infantile spasms are difficult to treat. Valproate is preferred, followed (if unsuccessful) by clonazepam. Ethosuximide sometimes is effective, as is acetazolamide (in dosages as for petit mal). Phenytoin has only limited effectiveness. For infantile spasms, corticosteroids given for a total of 8 to 10 wk are often effective. Prednisone 2 mg/kg/day orally is given for 4 wk, then reduced to about half this amount for maintenance; ACTH 20 to 60 u./day IM may also be used. The optimal corticosteroid treatment regimen remains controversial. Carbamazepine may worsen patients with primary generalized epilepsy and multiple seizure types.

For seizures during pregnancy medical treatment results in the **fetal antiepileptic drug syndrome** in 2% of children of epileptic mothers (cleft lip, cleft palate, cardiac defects, microcephaly, growth retardation, developmental delay, abnormal facies, digital hypoplasia). Uncontrolled generalized seizures during pregnancy lead to an even higher incidence of congenital defects, but should be treated. Women in the child-bearing age group should be made aware of these data before they become pregnant. Trimethadione and valproic acid are specifically teratogenic and should be *avoided* during pregnancy.

For status epilepticus, diazepam 10 to 20 mg (for adults) is given IV; alternatively, diazepam 10 mg IV q 15 min for up to 1 h may be given. In children, diazepam up to 0.3 mg/kg IV is given. To prevent recurrence, in adults 500 mg to 1 gm of phenytoin may be given IV at a rate of 50 mg/min for the first 500 mg and 100 mg/30 min thereafter. Children are given phenytoin 20 mg/kg IV in 2 doses divided 30 min apart. Giving the full amount in one successively administered "loading" dose as noted produces better results than divided doses. Lorazepam 0.1 mg/kg IV q 8 h is an alternative to diazepam and phenytoin for the acute treatment of status epilepticus; this must be followed by addition of one of the antiepileptic drugs for chronic use described above. Anesthetic doses of pentobarbital (IV or rectally) may be necessary in some refractory cases; in such instances, intubation and O_2 therapy are desirable to prevent hypoxemia.

Acute convulsive seizures from febrile illnesses, ingestion of alcohol or other toxins, or acute metabolic disturbance require emergency

TABLE 43-3. DRUGS USED IN EPILEPSY

Drug	Indications	Daily Dosage		Blood Levels			Toxicity
		Child	Adult	Therapeutic	Toxic		
Phenytoin	Generalized motor, partial motor, partial complex seizures	5–10 mg/kg p.o. divided bid or qid	300–500 mg	10–20 µg/mL	> 25 µg/mL		Nystagmus, ataxia, dysarthria, lethargy, megaloblastic anemia, gingival hyperplasia Idiosyncratic: rash, exfoliative dermatitis, grand mal convulsions (rare)
Phenobarbital	Generalized motor, partial motor seizures	3–5 yr: 4–6 mg/kg divided bid; follow levels	5 yr to adult: 150–300 mg	10–30 µg/mL	> 35 µg/mL		Sedation, nystagmus, ataxia, learning difficulties Idiosyncratic: anemia, rash, hyperkinesis
Primidone	Partial complex, generalized motor seizures	10–20 mg/kg divided bid to qid Increase slowly	750–1500 mg Increase slowly	5–12 µg/mL	> 15 µg/mL		See phenobarbital
Carbamazepine	Partial complex, partial motor, generalized motor seizures	< 6 yr: Initially 7–8 mg/kg for 3 days, then increase to 12 mg/kg divided bid 6–12 yr: 20–30 mg/kg divided bid Increase slowly	800–1200 mg Increase slowly	4–12 µg/mL	> 14 µg/mL		Nystagmus, diplopia, dysarthria, lethargy, nausea Idiosyncratic: granulocytopenia, thrombocytopenia, liver toxicity

				Therapeutic level	Toxic level	Side effects
Ethosuximide	Petit mal seizures	20 mg/kg divided bid	500 mg qid (maximum: 1500 mg except with strict monitoring)	40–100 µg/mL	> 100 µg/mL	Nausea, lethargy, dizziness, headache Idiosyncratic: leuko- or pancytopenia, dermatitis, SLE
Clonazepam	Petit mal, atypical petit mal, and akinetic seizures; infantile spasms	Initial: 0.005–0.01 mg/kg Maintenance: 0.03–0.06 mg/kg	Initial: 0.5 mg tid Maintenance: up to 5–7 mg tid (maximum: 20 mg/day)	20–80 ng/mL (preliminary)		Drowsiness, ataxia, behavioral abnormalities Serious reaction rare, but partial or complete tolerance to beneficial effects usual in 1–6 mo
Valproate	Petit mal, myoclonic, generalized motor, akinetic, partial motor, and complex seizures; infantile spasms	15–30 mg/kg	15–30 mg/kg (Total given in doses divided tid. Start slowly, especially if other drugs are being taken.)	50–100 µg/mL (before AM dose)	> 130 µg/mL	Nausea and vomiting, transient drowsiness, transient neutropenia, hyperammonemic encephalopathy

therapy, especially for the causative condition as well as for the convulsion. Status epilepticus should be treated at once. If there has been only one seizure, phenytoin or phenobarbital should be given in full dosage (see TABLE 43–3) for 7 to 10 days. However, anticonvulsants are of little value to prevent alcoholic withdrawal seizures.

Benign febrile convulsions do not require treatment, owing to the favorable prognosis compared with potential toxic antiepileptic drug effects for the young child. For patients with complicated febrile seizure or other risk factors for recurrence listed above, recurrence rates for seizures associated with high fever can be reduced by continuous prophylactic treatment with phenobarbital 5 to 10 mg/kg/day. However, there is no evidence that treatment of complicated febrile seizures in this way prevents the subsequent development of recurrent nonfebrile seizures (epilepsy).

Undesirable side effects of drug therapy: At therapeutic blood levels, phenobarbital and primidone often cause incapacitating drowsiness and may produce paradoxical hyperactivity in children. Phenytoin may result in gingival hyperplasia, osteopenia, hirsutism, adenopathy, and megaloblastic anemia. When treatment is first initiated, carbamazepine often produces diplopia, dizziness, and GI upset; this drug commonly lowers the WBC count to 3000 to 4000/μL. Aplastic anemia may occur rarely as an idiosyncratic reaction to carbamazine and phenytoin. Valproate may cause GI intolerance, and it can induce hyperammonemic encephalopathy as an idiosyncratic reaction. Rarely, this drug has caused fatal hepatic necrosis in young children with neurologic impairment who are being treated with multiple antiepileptic drugs. All antiepileptic drugs may cause an allergic scarlatiniform or morbilliform rash. At high blood levels, phenytoin produces drowsiness, irritability, nausea, vomiting, unsteady gait, and confusion.

Patients receiving carbamazepine should have a CBC once/month for the first year of therapy. If the WBC or RBC counts decrease significantly, the drug should be **discontinued immediately.** Patients receiving valproate should have liver function tests checked monthly for 1 yr; if significant elevation in transaminases or ammonia occurs (> 2 times normal), the drug should be discontinued. Modest elevations in ammonia levels up to 1.5 times the upper limit of normal can be tolerated safely.

When an overdose reaction occurs, one reduces the amount of drug until the intoxication subsides. When more serious acute poisoning occurs, the patient is given ipecac syrup or, if obtunded, is lavaged. After emesis or lavage, activated charcoal is administered, followed by a saline cathartic, eg, magnesium citrate. The suspect drug should be discontinued and a new anticonvulsant substituted at the same time.

Surgical therapy: About 10 to 20% of patients have seizures that are refractory to medical management. If a local area of abnormal brain function is responsible for the seizures, most of these patients are markedly improved by surgical resection of the epileptic focus, and some are completely cured. Since extensive monitoring and skilled medical-surgical teamwork are required, these patients are best managed in specialized centers.

SYDENHAM'S CHOREA
(Chorea Minor; Rheumatic Chorea; St. Vitus' Dance)

A CNS disease, often of insidious onset but of finite duration, characterized by involuntary, purposeless, nonrepetitive movements, and subsiding without neurologic residua.

Etiology

Sydenham's chorea is generally regarded as an inflammatory complication of Group A β-hemolytic streptococcal infections. The illness is probably immune-mediated: Streptococcal antigens resemble neuronal tissue antigens, and cross-reactive antibodies bind to nerve tissue, which is damaged by lymphocytes. After the infection, the time interval before onset of chorea (sometimes up to 6 mo) is longer than that of other rheumatic manifestations, and the chorea may begin as (or after) other clinical and laboratory features have returned to normal. If it is a sole clinical feature of poststreptococcal inflammation, Sydenham's chorea may thus appear to be an isolated, unrelated event.

The disease is more common in girls than boys; in childhood; and (for temperate climates) in the summer and early fall, after the spring and early summer peak incidence of rheumatic fever. Chorea occurs in up to 10% of rheumatic attacks.

Symptoms and Signs

The patient develops rapid, purposeless, nonrepetitive, involuntary movements that disappear with sleep and may involve all muscles except the eyes. Voluntary movements are abrupt, with impaired coordination. Facial grimacing is common. The patient may appear clumsy in mild cases and may have slight difficulties in dressing and feeding. In extreme cases, the patient may need vigorous sedation and protection to avoid self-injury from flailing arms or legs. The neurologic examination shows no defect in muscle strength or sensory perception except for an occasionally pendulous knee jerk.

The course of chorea is variable and difficult to measure because of its insidious onset and gradual cessation. A month or more may elapse before the movements become intense enough to make the patient or his parents seek medical attention. The episode may end within another 3 mo but, occasionally, may last 6 to 8 mo.

Diagnosis

The athetoid movements of chorea are pathognomonic. They resemble those of cerebral palsy, from which they can be distinguished by the history of recent onset. Other conditions that must be differentiated are habit spasms, which are repetitive, and the movements of hyperkinetic children, which are purposeful. Huntington's chorea is usually associated with a family history and appears in adulthood. The Parkinson-like side effects of tranquilizers, given to control the apparently hyperactive child, may confuse the diagnosis of chorea until the drugs are discontinued and the unaltered choreic movements can be noted.

Aside from occasional lingering evidence of previous streptococcal infection, chorea has no characteristic laboratory features. The CSF is usually unremarkable, and the EEG shows no more than nonspecific dysrhythmias.

Treatment

No drug is consistently effective. Sedation with a barbiturate may be attempted when the movements are severe, in dosage adequate to make the patient barely drowsy. A tranquilizer (eg, diazepam 5 mg 4 to 6 times/day) may be effective if barbiturates fail. If both of these agents fail, a salicylate or a corticosteroid may be given in the dosage described for rheumatic fever (see in Ch. 42).

Chorea is best regarded and treated as a transitory, reversible form of cerebral palsy. It is important to reassure patients and those who deal with them—family, friends, nurses, teachers, classmates—that the ailment is self-limited, that it will ultimately subside without residual damage, and that the temporary impairment of mo-

tor functions will not affect intellectual capacity. Patients should miss school only if movements are uncontrollably severe and should return to school as soon as they can manage the necessary locomotion and residual dysfunction is minimal. Many of the so-called psychologic effects ascribed to chorea in the past were due not to the disease itself, but to the associated scholastic deprivation and to the patients' anxiety and dismay at the bizarre movements and at the reactions they invoke in people who do not understand.

Severe cardiac involvement is seldom present in patients with active chorea but, if present, can be managed as described for rheumatic fever (see in Ch. 42). After completion of an attack, antistreptococcal prophylaxis against recurrences of chorea (or rheumatic fever) should be maintained as described for rheumatic fever.

TOURETTE SYNDROME (TS)
(Gilles de la Tourette's Syndrome)

An autosomal dominant multiple tic disorder with variable penetrance that begins in childhood, often with simple tics, and progresses to multiple, complex movements including respiratory and vocal tics. The syndrome is more prevalent in males (3:1). Vocal tics may begin as grunting or barking noises and evolve into compulsive utterances. **Coprolalia** (*involuntary, scatologic utterances*) occurs in 50% of patients. Severe tics and coprolalia may be physically and socially disabling.

Diagnosis and Treatment

Tics tend to be more complex than myoclonus, but less flowing than choreic movements (from which they must be differentiated), and the patient may voluntarily suppress them for seconds or minutes.

Simple tics may respond to benzodiazepine anxiolytics. For TS, haloperidol 0.5 to 40 mg/day is the drug of choice. Side effects of dysphoria, parkinsonism, and akathisia may be limiting. Whenever treatment with neuroleptic drugs is initiated in a chronic neurologic disorder, the potential for development of a tardive dyskinesia syndrome must be recognized. The risk for development of drug-induced involuntary movements in TS patients may not differ from that in the psychiatric population. Thus, caution should be used when instituting such therapy, and patients should be informed of potential adverse outcomes. In situations where the tics are mild or not disabling, consideration may be given to the use of anxiolytic agents, which may reduce tic frequency. Clonidine 0.1 to 0.6 mg/day or pimozide 1 to 20 mg/day may be as effective as haloperidol in some patients. Clonidine lacks the potential for causing tardive dyskinesias with long-term use; its limiting side effect is hypotension. Intermediate-acting benzodiazepines (eg, lorazepam 0.5 to 2.5 mg tid or qid) may be useful as adjuvant treatment.

CEREBRAL PALSY (CP) SYNDROMES

A broad term used to describe a number of motor disorders resulting from prenatal developmental abnormalities or perinatal or postnatal CNS damage occurring before age 5 yr and characterized by impaired voluntary movement. The term is not a diagnosis, but provides a useful therapeutic classification for children with nonprogressive spasticity, ataxia, or involuntary movements who will require complex training and therapy to attain their optimum potential.

Etiology and Incidence

Between 0.1 and 0.2% of children have CP syndromes; up to 1% of premature babies or those small for gestational age are afflicted. The cause often is hard to establish, but in utero disorders, neonatal jaundice, birth trauma, and neonatal asphyxia play important roles. Recent studies indicate that asphyxia and birth injury account for ≤ 15% of cases of CP. Spastic paraplegia is especially common after premature birth, spastic quadriparesis after perinatal asphyxia, and athetoid and dystonic forms after perinatal asphyxia or kernicterus. CNS trauma or severe systemic disease during early childhood (eg, meningitis, sepsis, dehydration) may also cause a CP syndrome.

Symptoms and Signs

A number of the syndromes described are grouped into 4 main categories: spastic, athetoid, ataxic, and mixed forms.

Spastic syndromes represent about 70% of cases. The spasticity is due to upper motor neuron involvement and may mildly or severely affect motor function. **Hemiplegia** connotes involvement of both limbs on one side; the arm usually is affected more severely. **Paraplegia** connotes involvement of both legs, with relative or complete sparing of the arms. **Quadriplegia** or **tetraplegia** connotes involvement of all limbs to a similar degree. **Diplegia** refers to a form intermediate between para- and quadriplegia, with predominant involvement of the legs.

Affected limbs usually are underdeveloped and show increased deep tendon reflexes and muscular hypertonicity, weakness, and a tendency to contractures. A "scissors gait" and toewalking are characteristic. In mildly affected children, impairment may be seen only during certain activities (eg, running). With quadriplegia, an associated corticobulbar impairment of oral, lingual, and palatal movement, with consequent dysarthria, is common.

Athetoid or **dyskinetic syndromes** occur in about 20% of patients and result from basal ganglia involvement. The resultant slow, writhing, involuntary movements may affect the extremities (athetoid), or the proximal parts of the limbs and the trunk (dystonic); abrupt, jerky, distal movements (choreiform) also may occur. The movements increase with emotional tension and disappear during sleep. Dysarthria is present and often severe.

Ataxic syndromes are uncommon (about 10%) and result from involvement of the cerebellum or its pathways. Weakness, incoordination, and intention tremor produce unsteadiness, a wide-based gait, and difficulty with rapid or fine movements.

Mixed forms are common: most often, spasticity and athetosis; less often, ataxia and athetosis.

Associated disorders: Convulsive seizures occur in about 25% of patients, most often in those with spasticity. Strabismus and other visual defects may be seen. Children with athetosis due to kernicterus commonly display nerve deafness and paralysis of upward gaze. Children with spastic hemiplegia or paraplegia frequently have normal intelligence and a good prognosis for social independence; spastic quadriplegia and mixed forms often are associated with disabling mental retardation. Short attention span and hyperactivity are commonly seen in children with CP.

Diagnosis

It is rarely possible to establish the presence of CP during early infancy. Nevertheless, early diagnosis and therapy are highly desirable, and children known to be at high risk (those with evidence of birth trauma, asphyxia, jaundice, or meningitis, or with a neonatal history of seizures, hypertonia, hypotonia, or reflex suppression) should have close follow-up surveillance.

Specific forms of CP often cannot be characterized until age 2 yr. Before the specific motor syndrome develops, the child will show lagging motor development and often persistent infantile reflex patterns, hyperreflexia, and altered muscle tone. It is important to distinguish the specific CP syndromes from progressive hereditary neurologic disorders or those requiring surgical or other specific forms of neurologic treatment. The relatively uncommon ataxic forms are particularly hard to distinguish, and many ataxic children ultimately are found to have progressive cerebellar degenerative disease.

Laboratory tests are useful to exclude certain progressive biochemical disorders that involve the motor system (eg, Tay-Sachs disease, metachromatic leukodystrophy, and the mucopolysaccharidoses). Other progressive disorders (eg, infantile neuroaxonal dystrophy) cannot be excluded by laboratory tests and must be diagnosed by clinical or pathologic criteria. Children with pronounced mental retardation and symmetric motor abnormalities should be evaluated for amino acid and other metabolic abnormalities.

Athetosis, self-mutilation, and hyperuricemia in boys identify the Lesch-Nyhan syndrome. Cutaneous or ocular abnormalities may indicate tuberous sclerosis, neurofibromatosis, ataxia-telangiectasia, von Hippel-Lindau disease, or Sturge-Weber syndrome; these disorders are occasionally progressive. Infantile spinal muscular atrophy, spinocerebellar degenerations, and the muscular dystrophies generally lack signs of cerebral disease. Adrenoleukodystrophy has an onset later in childhood.

Brain imaging studies (MRI, CT) are useful when there is uncertainty regarding diagnosis or cause of a CP syndrome.

Treatment

CP is a lifelong condition. The treatment goal is for patients to develop maximal independence within the limits of their motor and associated handicaps; with proper management, many patients, especially those with spastic paraplegia or hemiplegia, can lead near-normal lives. Seizures require the use of anticonvulsants for control (see SEIZURE DISORDERS, above). Physical therapy, occupational therapy, bracing, orthopedic surgery, and speech training may all be required. Attendance in a regular school class is desirable when intellectual and physical handicaps are not severe.

Complete social independence is not a realistic goal for many who will require varying degrees of lifelong supervision and assistance. For these children, special schooling is highly desirable. Even the severely affected can profit from training in activities of daily living (eg, washing, dressing, and feeding) that increase independence and self-esteem and greatly reduce the burden for families or chronic-care facilities.

As with all chronically handicapped children, the parents need continuing assistance and guidance in understanding the child's status and future potential, and in relieving their own feelings (see MANAGEMENT OF CHRONIC DISABILITY in Ch. 24). These children will reach their maximal potential only with the support of stable, sensible parental care and the assistance of public and private agencies (eg, community health agencies, vocational rehabilitation organizations, and lay health organizations such as the United Cerebral Palsy Association).

CEREBELLAR AND SPINOCEREBELLAR DISORDERS

Disorders of the cerebellum and its inflow or outflow pathways produce deficits in the rate, range, and force of movement. Anatomically, the cerebellum has 3 subdivisions. The oldest phylogenetically, the **archi-** or **vestibulocerebellum**, comprises the flocculonodular lobe, is concerned with the maintenance of equilibrium and eye-head-neck movements, and is closely interconnected with the vestibular nuclei. The midline **vermis (paleocerebellum)** helps coordinate movement of the trunk and legs. Vermis lesions result in abnormalities of stance and gait. The lateral hemispheres, which make up the **neocerebellum**, exert control over both ballistic and finely coordinated limb movements, predominantly of the upper extremities.

The signs of cerebellar disease are **ataxia** (*reeling, wide-based gait*); **dysmetria** (*inability to control range of movement*); **dysdiadochokinesia** (*inability to perform rapid alternating movements*); **hypotonia** (*decreased muscle tone*); **decomposition of movement** (*inability to sequence properly fine, coordinated acts*); **tremor**, which may occur with intention or with sustention; **dysarthria** with slurring, inappropriate phrasing, and lack of modulation of speech volume (scanning speech); and nystagmus, with the fast component maximal toward the side of the cerebellar lesion.

STRUCTURAL LESIONS OF THE CEREBELLUM

Vascular lesions (infarcts) and tumor deposits producing manifestations appropriate to their locus within the cerebellum. As infarcts, hemorrhages, or tumors enlarge, they may acutely cause hydrocephalus or increased intracranial pressure with papilledema because of obstruction of CSF outflow pathways. The midline cerebellum is the most common site of primary brain tumors (medulloblastoma, cystic astrocytoma) in childhood. Demyelinating plaques of multiple sclerosis may arise anywhere in the cerebellar white matter and can give rise to a variety of cerebellar deficits. The Arnold-Chiari malformation and platybasia/basilar impression also cause cerebellar manifestations.

Alcoholism with nutritional deprivation can cause degeneration of the vermis and anterior cerebellum with profound gait ataxia. Other acquired cerebellar syndromes include those caused by hypothyroidism, various toxins (CO, heavy metals, phenytoin), hyperpyrexia, and repeated head trauma. Rarely, reversible pancerebellar dysfunction may follow viral infections in children. A rare, profound cerebellar degeneration may accompany certain malignancies in adults.

SPINOCEREBELLAR DEGENERATIONS
(Hereditary Ataxias)

A group of degenerative disorders characterized by progressive ataxia due to degeneration of the cerebellum, brainstem, spinal cord, and peripheral nerves, and occasionally the basal ganglia. Many of these syndromes are hereditary; others occur sporadically. The spinocerebellar degenerations can be thought of in 3 broad groups: the predominantly spinal ataxias, the cerebellar ataxias, and multiple systems degenerations (see Table 43–4). Patterns of clinical involvement usually breed true, but great variability may be found among affected members of ataxic kindreds. There is no treatment.

Friedreich's ataxia is the prototypal spinal ataxia. Inheritance is autosomal recessive. The gene responsible is located on chromosome 9. Gait unsteadiness begins between the ages of 5 and 15 and is followed by upper extremity ataxia and dysarthria. Tremor, if any, is a minor feature.

Patients are areflexic and there is loss of large-fiber sensory modalities (vibration and position sense). Pes cavus and scoliosis are common, as is progressive cardiomyopathy. Although Bassen-Kornzweig syndrome (abetalipoproteinemia, vitamin E deficiency) and Refsum's disease (phytanic acid storage disease) share some clinical features with Friedreich's ataxia, the metabolic basis of the latter remains unknown.

Cerebellar cortical degenerations generally begin between ages 30 and 50. Clinically, only signs of cerebellar dysfunction can be detected, and pathologic changes are restricted to the cerebellum and occasionally the inferior olives. Both sporadic and dominantly inherited cases have been reported.

In the multiple systems degenerations (olivopontocerebellar atrophies), ataxia occurs in young to middle adult life in varying combinations with spasticity and extrapyramidal, sensory, lower motor neuron, and autonomic dysfunction. Optic atrophy, retinitis pigmentosa, ophthalmoplegia, and dementia occur in some kindreds. These syndromes include Menzel's dominant disorder (with cranial nerve findings and spasticity); the Dejerine-Thomas sporadic or recessive syndrome in which parkinsonism is prominent; and Azorean motor systems degeneration (Machado-Joseph disease).

Miscellaneous disorders: Ataxia also may occur in systemic disorders of unknown pathogenesis. Ataxia-telangiectasia is discussed in Ch. 33. In the mitochrondial multisystem disorders, ataxia is seen in varying combinations with ophthalmoplegia, heart block, and myopathy. Muscle biopsy reveals characteristic "ragged red fibers." Decreased activity of several respiratory chain enzymes and mitochondrial DNA deletions have been described in some patients with these disorders.

INHERITED SPINAL MUSCULAR ATROPHIES (SMA)
(Werdnig-Hoffmann Disease; Wohlfart-Kugelberg-Welander Disease)

Disorders beginning in infancy or childhood, characterized by skeletal muscle wasting due to progressive degeneration of anterior horn cells in the spinal cord and motor nuclei in the brainstem. Most cases are inherited, and 3 main variants are recognized.

TABLE 43–4. MAJOR CLINICAL FEATURES OF SOME SPINOCEREBELLAR DISORDERS

Syndrome	Weakness & Atrophy	Extrapyramidal	Cranial Nerve	Sensory Loss	Areflexia	Peripheral Neuropathy	Optic Atrophy	Retinitis Pigmentosa	Skeletal Changes	Onset	Heredity	Miscellaneous
Spinal ataxia												
Friedreich's ataxia	+	–	–	+	+	+	±	–	+	J	R	Cardiomyopathy, pes cavus
Cerebellar cortical degenerations												
Holmes	–	–	–	–	–	–	±	–	–	A	D	Hypogonadism
Marie (LCCA)	–	–	–	–	–	–	–	–	–	A	R/S	
Multiple systems degenerations												
Menzel	–	±	±	–	–	–	±	–	–	A	D	
Dejerine-Thomas	–	±	–	–	–	±	–	–	–	A	R/S	
Shy-Drager	±	±	±	–	–	–	–	–	–	A	S	Autonomic insufficiency
Machado-Joseph	+	±	±	–	–	–	–	–	–	A	D	
Systemic disorders												
Refsum's disease	+	–	–	+	+	+	±	+	–	J	R	Ichthyosis, decreased phytanic acid
Abetalipoproteinemia	+	+	+	+	+	+	±	+	+	J	R	Steatorrhea
Ataxia-telangiectasia	+	±	–	–	+	–	–	–	–	J	R	Telangiectasias, decreased IgA, infections
Mitochondrial multi-system disorder	+	–	±	–	–	–	–	±	–	J/A	S	Ophthalmoplegia, heart block, "ragged red fibers"

R = recessive; D = dominant; S = sporadic; J = juvenile; A = adult; LCCA = late cortical cerebellar atrophy; + = always present; – = absent; ± = variable.

Symptoms and Signs

Acute SMA (Werdnig-Hoffmann disease) is an autosomal recessive disorder, symptomatic by 2 to 4 mo of age. Most infants are hypotonic at birth. All affected infants have delayed motor milestones by 6 mo.

In **intermediate SMA**, infants and children are symptomatic by age 2, and most at about 6 to 12 mo; < 25% learn to sit, and none walk or crawl. Regardless of the age of onset, children are hypotonic with flaccid muscle weakness, absent deep tendon reflexes, and fasciculations that may be hard to see in young children. Dysphagia may be present. The disease often is fatal in early life, frequently from respiratory complications. However, spontaneous arrest can leave the child with a chronic, nonprogressive weakness.

Chronic SMA (Wohlfart-Kugelberg-Welander disease) begins between 2 and 17 yr of age with similar pathologic findings and mode of inheritance, but a slower evolution and longer life expectancy. Weakness and wasting are most evident in the legs, with onset in the quadriceps and hip flexors. Later, the arms are affected. Weakness often progresses from proximal to distal parts. Some familial cases may be secondary to specific enzyme defects (eg, hexosaminidase deficiency).

Diagnosis and Treatment

Diagnosis usually is confirmed by demonstration of denervation without peripheral nerve involvement, chiefly by electromyography (abnormal) and nerve conduction velocity studies (normal). Muscle biopsy is used occasionally. Serum enzymes (CK, aldolase) may be mildly increased. Amniocentesis is *not* diagnostic.

There is no specific treatment. By preventing scoliosis and contractures, physical therapy, bracing, and special appliances can benefit patients with static or slowly progressive disease.

GUILLAIN–BARRÉ SYNDROME (GBS)

(Acute Polyneuropathy; Acute Polyradiculitis; Infectious or Acute Idiopathic Polyneuropathy; Landry's Ascending Paralysis; Acute Segmentally Demyelinating Polyradiculoneuropathy)

An acute, usually rapidly progressive form of inflammatory polyneuropathy characterized by muscular weakness and mild distal sensory loss that about ²/₃ of the time begins 5 days to 3 wk after a banal infectious disorder, surgery, or an

immunization. GBS is the most frequently acquired demyelinating neuropathy. The **cause** is unknown, although an autoimmune basis is probable. Histologically, focal areas of segmental demyelination with perivascular and endoneurial infiltration of lymphocytes and monocytes are scattered along the peripheral nerves, roots, and cranial nerves. In severe lesions, axonal degeneration accompanies the segmental demyelination.

Symptoms and Signs

Relatively symmetric weakness accompanied by paresthesias usually begins in the legs and progresses to the arms. Weakness always is more prominent than sensory symptoms or signs, and may be most prominent proximally. Deep tendon reflexes are lost. Sphincters usually are spared. More than 50% of severely involved patients have weakness of facial and oropharyngeal muscles, and 5 to 10% require intubation for respiratory failure. Autonomic dysfunction, including BP fluctuations, inappropriate ADH secretion, cardiac arrhythmias, and pupillary changes occur in more severely involved patients. The respiratory paralysis and the autonomic defects may be life-threatening. Despite advances in respiratory care, up to 5% of patients die; 90% of patients reach their maximal degree of weakness in 3 wk, most in the first 2 wk.

In an unusual variant of acute idiopathic polyneuropathy, patients may develop only ophthalmoparesis, ataxia, and areflexia. It is important in such cases to rule out myasthenia gravis, acute thiamine deficiency, and, rarely, botulism.

Diagnosis

Diagnosis of acute GBS is based on the clinical syndrome. Laboratory studies include increased protein without increased cells in the CSF. Electrophysiologic abnormalities support the diagnosis, but the latter are hardly necessary in typical cases. Two-thirds of patients will have slow nerve conduction velocities and evidence of segmental demyelination at the time of onset. F-wave latencies, evidence of proximal demyelination, tend to be prolonged. Antecedent mononucleosis, or cytomegalovirus infections, mumps, or rubella can be excluded by appropriate serologic tests but do not change the prognosis.

Differential diagnosis includes toxins that act at the neuromuscular junction (eg, organic phosphates, and botulism—see under BACTERIAL INFECTIONS in Ch. 32). Acute poliomyelitis occurs in epidemics and produces fever, malaise, and pleocytosis in the CSF. Serologic studies are available. Tick infestation of the scalp causes an acute ascending motor neuropathy, mainly in children. Deep tendon reflexes are lost; sensation is normal. Removal of the tick results in resolution of all symptoms.

Prognosis and Treatment

Severe acute polyneuropathy is a medical emergency, requiring constant monitoring and vigorous support of vital functions. The airway must be kept clear, and vital capacity should be measured frequently, so that respiration can be assisted if necessary. Fluid intake should be sufficient to maintain a urine volume of at least 1 to 1.5 L/day; serum electrolytes should be monitored to prevent water intoxication. The extremities should be protected from trauma and from pressure of bedclothes. Heat helps relieve pain and permits early physical therapy. Immobilization may cause ankylosis and is to be avoided: Passive full-range joint movement should be started immediately and active exercises begun when acute symptoms subside. Heparin 5000 u. s.c. bid may be beneficial while the patient is bedridden.

Corticosteroids worsen the outcome in GBS and should *not* be used. **Plasmapheresis** has been shown to be beneficial when carried out early in the disease and is the treatment of choice in patients acutely ill with GBS. It is a relatively safe procedure that shortens the disease course, lowers mortality, lessens the incidence of permanent paralysis, and abbreviates hospitalization.

Considerable improvement over a period of months is usual; about 30% of adults have residual weakness at 3 yr and the percentage is higher in children. Residual defects may require retraining, orthopedic appliances, or operation. About 10% of patients relapse after initial improvement and enter a chronic state **(chronic relapsing polyneuropathy)**. Pathology and laboratory data are similar to acute cases, but the weakness may be more asymmetric and progress more slowly. Nerves eventually become palpable from repeated episodes of segmental demyelination and remyelination. Corticosteroids improve weakness in the chronic state, and prolonged therapy may be necessary. Immunosuppressive agents (azathioprine) and plasmapheresis benefit some patients.

HEREDITARY NEUROPATHIES

Hereditary neuropathies are classified as either hereditary sensory-motor neuropathies **(HSMN)** or hereditary sensory neuropathies **(HSN)**. (The hereditary motor neuropathies are discussed under motor neuron diseases. Neurofibromatosis, a distinct hereditary neuropathy with prominent skin involvement, and Charcot-Marie-Tooth disease, the most common HSMN, previously known as peroneal muscular atrophy, are described separately, below.) Other less common HSMN begin from birth, and patients are more disabled. HSN are rare. Loss of distal pain and temperature modalities are more prominent than vibratory and position loss. The main problem in these patients is pedal mutilation due to insensitivity to pain with frequent infections and osteomyelitis. Good foot care is mandatory.

PERONEAL MUSCULAR ATROPHY; HYPERTROPHIC INTERSTITIAL NEUROPATHY
(Charcot-Marie-Tooth Disease; Dejerine-Sottas Disease)

Peroneal muscular atrophy (Charcot-Marie-Tooth [CMT] disease) is a relatively common hereditary (usually autosomal dominant) disorder of the peripheral nervous system characterized by weakness and atrophy, primarily in peroneal and distal leg muscles. Other degenerative diseases (eg, Friedreich's ataxia) may be present in these patients or in the same family pedigrees.

Symptoms and Signs

Type 1 patients present in middle childhood with foot drop and slowly progressive distal muscle atrophy producing "stork leg deformity." Intrinsic muscle wasting in the hand begins later. A stocking-glove decrease in vibration, pain, and temperature is present. Deep tendon reflexes are absent. Foot deformities, ie, high pedal arches or hammer toes, may be the only signs in less affected family members who carry the trait. Type 1 patients have slow nerve conduction velocities with prolonged distal latencies. Pathologic specimens show segmental demyelination and remyelination. Enlarged peripheral nerves may be palpated. The disease progresses slowly and is compatible with a normal life span. Patients with **type 2 CMT** disease usually develop weakness later in life, and the process is slower in evolution. They have relatively normal nerve conduction velocities but low amplitude evoked potentials, and biopsies reveal wallerian degeneration.

Hypertrophic interstitial neuropathy (Dejerine-Sottas disease), a rare autosomal recessive disorder of the peripheral nerves, presents in

TABLE 43–5. DIAGNOSTIC CRITERIA FOR THE NEUROFIBROMATOSES

Neurofibromatosis 1 may be diagnosed when 2 or more of the following are present:

    6 or more café au lait macules whose greatest diameter is > 5 mm in prepubertal patients and
        > 15 mm in postpubertal patients
    2 or more neurofibromas of any type, or one plexiform neurofibroma
    Freckling in the axillary or inguinal region
    Optic glioma
    2 or more Lisch nodules (iris hamartomas)
    A distinctive osseous lesion (eg, sphenoid dysplasia or thinning of long-bone cortex), with or without
        pseudarthrosis
    A parent, sibling, or child with neurofibromatosis 1 according to the above criteria

Neurofibromatosis 2 may be diagnosed when 1 of the following is present:

    Bilateral 8th-nerve masses seen with appropriate imaging techniques (CT or MRI)
    A parent, sibling, or child with neurofibromatosis 2 and either unilateral 8th-nerve mass or any 2 of
        the following: neurofibroma, meningioma, glioma, schwannoma, or juvenile posterior subcapsular
        lenticular opacity

From Martuza RL, Eldredge R: "Neurofibromatosis 2." *The New England Journal of Medicine* 318:684–688, 1988; reprinted by permission of *The New England Journal of Medicine.*

childhood with progressive weakness and sensory loss with absent deep tendon reflexes. It initially resembles CMT disease, but motor weakness progresses at a faster rate. This is also a demyelinating-remyelinating disorder with enlarged peripheral nerves and "onion bulbs" on biopsy.

Diagnosis and Treatment

The characteristic distribution of motor weakness, foot deformities, family history, and electrophysiologic abnormalities confirm the diagnosis. No specific treatment is available. Vocational counseling to anticipate disease progression may be useful in young patients. Bracing helps correct foot drop; orthopedic surgery to stabilize the foot may be of value.

NEUROFIBROMATOSIS

A pair of autosomal dominant disorders designated type 1 (sometimes called von Recklinghausen's disease) and carried on chromosome 17, and type 2 characterized by bilateral acoustic neuromas (see TABLE 43–5).

Symptoms, Signs, and Diagnosis

One third of patients with neurofibromatosis type 1 are asymptomatic and discovered on routine examination. In 1/3 of patients cosmetic problems are the initial complaints. Characteristic skin lesions, apparent at birth or in infancy in > 90% of patients, are medium-brown (café au lait) macules distributed most commonly over the trunk, pelvis, and flexor creases of elbows

and knees. The presence of 6 or more of these freckle-like lesions with one > 1.5 cm is diagnostic of neurofibromatosis. Multiple cutaneous tumors, flesh-colored and of variable size and shape, appear in late childhood. There may be only a few or thousands of these lesions. Subcutaneous nodules or amorphous overgrowth of subcutaneous tissues **(plexiform neuromas)** and underlying bone may produce grotesque deformities (which are rare). Skeletal anomalies include absence of the greater wing of the sphenoid bone (posterior orbital wall) with consequent pulsating exophthalmos, fibrous dysplasia, subperiosteal bone cysts, vertebral scalloping, scoliosis, and pseudarthrosis.

The remaining 1/3 of patients present with neurologic problems. **Neurofibromas** (tumors of Schwann cells and nerve fibroblasts), which rarely appear before puberty, can be felt along the course of subcutaneous peripheral nerves. These tumors may involve spinal nerve roots, characteristically growing through an intervertebral foramen to produce intraspinal and extraspinal masses ("dumbbell" tumor). The intraspinal component may cause spinal cord compression. Plexiform neuromas may involve peripheral nerves producing deficits distal to the lesion. Tumors of cranial nerves may produce progressive blindness (optic glioma) or dizziness, ataxia, and deafness (acoustic neuroma). A study of neurofibromatosis showed a 40 (male) to 87 (female) times increase in risk for neural tumors vs. the general population. The type 1 neurofibromatosis tumors, ranging in number from one or two to hundreds, occur in 5 to 10%. Recurrence is common and, in most cases, the disease is progressive.

The rarer type 2 neurofibromatosis is characterized by bilateral acoustic neuromas, which become symptomatic when the patient is about 20 yr old. Family members may show gliomas or meningiomas and some have juvenile cataracts.

Treatment

Tumors are treated by surgical removal or radiation when severely symptomatic, but usually surgery requires sacrificing the function of the involved nerve. The underlying cellular disorder is unknown and no general treatment is available. Genetic counseling is advisable.

MUSCULAR DYSTROPHIES AND OTHER MYOPATHIES

(Malignant hyperthermia is discussed under PHARMACOGENETICS in Ch. 137)

Duchenne Dystrophy (DD)

An X-linked recessive disorder typically presenting in boys aged 3 to 7 yr as proximal muscle weakness causing waddling gait, toe-walking, lordosis, frequent falls, and difficulty in standing up and climbing stairs. DD is caused by a mutation at the Xp21 locus, which results in the absence of the gene product dystrophin. This protein is normally localized to the sarcolemma of muscle cells.

The pelvic girdle is affected first, then the shoulder girdle. Serum enzymes, notably CK, are markedly elevated (up to 50 to 100 times normal) even early in the disease or during the first year of life, before symptoms develop. Progression is steady and most patients are confined to a wheelchair by age 10 or 12. Cardiac involvement is common; 90% of patients show ECG abnormalities. A firm pseudohypertrophy of the calves is due to fatty and fibrous infiltration of the muscle. The average IQ in DD is 1 standard deviation below the mean. Flexion contractures and scoliosis ultimately occur, and most patients die by age 20 yr.

Becker muscular dystrophy (BMD) is a clinical variant. It is also an X-linked disorder with the same genomic mutation at Xp21, but the BMD patients have dystrophin of abnormal molecular weight. Clinically this illness is less severe. Very few patients are in wheelchairs by age 16 yr and > 90% are alive at age 20 yr.

Patients with a still milder clinical course of X-linked muscular dystrophy have reduced amounts of a normal-sized dystrophin protein.

Diagnosis depends on characteristic clinical findings, age of onset, and family history, supported by electromyography, muscle biopsy findings, and dystrophin immunoblotting. Nerve conduction velocities are normal; electromyography reveals rapidly recruited myopathic motor units without spontaneous activity. Muscle biopsy shows necrosis and variation in muscle fiber size. Later, fibrous tissue and fat replace muscle tissue. Dystrophin is absent in DD.

Carrier detection and prenatal diagnosis are possible for many families using a combination of conventional studies (pedigree analysis, CK determinations, fetal sex determination) and the powerful techniques of recombinant DNA analysis and dystrophin immunoblotting. Referral to major medical centers specialized in these areas is recommended.

Treatment: There is no specific therapy. Exercise should be encouraged as long as possible, and corrective surgery considered in slowly progressive forms. Passive exercises may extend the period of ambulation in severely affected patients. The added burden of obesity should be avoided; caloric requirements are likely to be less than normal. Isolated reports suggest that prednisone improves functional capabilities. Random controlled trials are under way.

Genetic counseling is indicated (see GENETIC COUNSELING IN HEREDITARY DISORDERS in Ch. 48).

Other Muscular Dystrophies

A group of inherited, progressive muscle disorders of unknown cause. The different types are distinguished primarily on clinical grounds.

Facioscapulohumeral (Landouzy-Dejerine) muscular dystrophy is *an autosomal dominant form characterized by weakness of the facial muscles and shoulder girdles,* usually beginning at age 7 to 20 yr. Difficulty with whistling, eye closure, and elevation of the arms are early symptoms. Anterior tibial and peroneal weakness develops in some kindreds, and although foot drop develops, ambulation is rarely lost. Life expectancy is normal.

Limb-girdle muscular dystrophy describes patients with *weakness of pelvic* (Leyden-Möbius [pelvifemoral] type) *and shoulder* (Erb [scapulohumeral] type) *girdles.* This is a mixed population, involving myopathic and neurogenic pedigrees, usually presenting in adults.

Mitochondrial myopathies are inherited through maternal, nonmendelian inheritance. Some mitochondrial myopathies cause only progressive external ophthalmoplegia (ocular myopathy); others also cause patients to develop limb weakness and multisystem disorders, predominantly involving brain and muscle.

Diagnosis is made either by finding biochemical abnormalities of mitochondria or "ragged red fibers" in muscle biopsy specimens stained with modified Gomori's trichrome stain. This appearance is due to excessive accumulation of mitochondria. Mitochondrial DNA deletions have been described recently in some of these patients.

Congenital myopathies have been named by their characteristic findings on muscle biopsy (**central core disease, centronuclear myopathy, nemaline myopathy**). These children present with *delayed walking and mild proximal muscle weakness that is not progressive.* The biochemical defect is unknown.

Myotonic Myopathies

A group of conditions characterized by abnormally slow relaxation after voluntary muscle contraction, due to a muscle membrane abnormality.

Myotonic dystrophy (Steinert's disease) is *an autosomal dominant disorder that combines dystrophic muscular weakness with myotonia.* The gene for this disorder has been localized to 19q. It occurs at any age and is variable in severity. Myotonia is prominent in the hand muscles, and ptosis is common even in mildly affected individuals. Severe cases show marked peripheral muscular weakness associated with a high incidence of cataracts, testicular atrophy, premature balding, cardiac muscle conduction defects, hatchet facies, and endocrine abnormalities, ie, diabetes mellitus. Mental retardation occurs frequently. Death occurs in the early 50s in severely affected families.

Myotonia congenita (Thomsen's disease) is *a rare, autosomal dominant myotonia that begins usually in infancy. The myotonia produces symptoms most troublesome in the hands, legs, and eyelids. Weakness is usually minimal.* Muscles may become hypertrophied, but muscle stiffness is the most important problem.

Diagnosis usually is established by the characteristic physical appearance, by inability to relax the handgrip rapidly after opening and closing the hand, and by sustained muscle contraction after direct muscle percussion. The myotonic phenomena causes a typical dive-bomber sound in electromyography studies. Family pedigrees are important.

Treatment: In myotonia congenita, oral therapy with phenytoin 5 mg/kg/day; quinine sulfate 300 to 600 mg bid or tid; or procainamide, beginning with small amounts and increasing to 4 to 6 gm/day, may diminish the muscle stiffness and cramping. However, in myotonic dystrophy quinine or procainamide may increase cardiac conduction defects. Recently a Ca-channel blocker, nifedipine, was reported to treat myotonia unresponsive to other drugs. The weakness of myotonic dystrophy does not respond to therapy, but active and passive exercises, as in other dystrophies, may be helpful.

Glycogen Storage Diseases of Muscle
(See also GENETIC ABNORMALITIES OF CARBOHYDRATE METABOLISM in Ch. 40)

Rare autosomal recessive diseases, characterized by abnormal accumulation of glycogen in skeletal muscle due to a specific biochemical defect in carbohydrate metabolism.

These diseases can be clinically mild or severe. The more severe **Pompe's disease** (absence of α-1,4-glucosidase or acid maltase) is evident in the first year of life and fatal by age 2. Glycogen accumulates in liver, muscle, nerve, and heart tissue. In a less severe form, adult patients may present with proximal limb weakness and respiratory involvement causing hypoventilation. Myotonic discharges are seen on electromyogram but myotonia does not occur clinically.

Four other enzyme deficiencies (see TABLE 40-9) are relatively mild in their clinical impact. After exercise, painful cramps develop, followed by myoglobinuria. The diagnosis is supported by an ischemic exercise test and confirmed by demonstrating a specific enzyme abnormality. Diuresis is important during episodes of myoglobinuria to prevent renal failure. Most patients learn to limit their activities and to drink fluids after exercise.

Familial Periodic Paralysis

A rare group of autosomal dominant disorders of unknown cause characterized by episodes of flaccid paralysis with loss of deep tendon reflexes and failure of the muscle to respond to electrical stimulation. There is no alteration in consciousness. **Hypokalemic** and **hyperkalemic** forms have been described. (**Normokalemic** is probably the same as the hyperkalemic form.)

Symptoms and signs: In the **hypokalemic** variety, attacks usually begin before age 16 yr. The day after vigorous exercise, the patient often awakens with weakness, which may be mild and limited to certain muscle groups or involve all 4 limbs. Oropharyngeal and respiratory muscles are spared. Serum and urine K are decreased. Weakness lasts 24 to 48 h. In the **hyperkalemic** form, the attacks often begin at an earlier age and usually are shorter, more frequent, and less severe. They often are accompanied by myotonia. (Myotonic lid lag may be the only symptom in asymptomatic family members.)

Diagnosis: The best clue is a history of the typical attack. During an episode, documentation of serum K level is important. Attacks can be provoked by glucose and insulin (hypokalemic form) or potassium chloride (hyperkalemic form), but this should be done only by experienced physicians in medical centers, since respiratory paralysis or cardiac conduction abnormalities may occur. The differential diagnosis includes persistent hypokalemia from any cause and hyperthyroidism, especially in Oriental males.

Treatment: Acetazolamide 250 to 2000 mg/day orally may prevent both hyper- and hypokalemic attacks, perhaps by inducing a mild metabolic acidosis. Potassium chloride 2 to 10 gm orally in an unsweetened 10 to 25% aqueous solution should be given during hypokalemic attacks.

44. NOSE AND THROAT DISORDERS
(See also §5)

FOREIGN BODIES

Common in young children, foreign bodies in the nose cause a foul-smelling, bloody, unilateral discharge. Mineral salts are deposited on a long-retained foreign body, producing a rhinolith. **Treatment:** Removal usually requires general anesthesia in a child. Vasoconstriction with a topically applied sympathomimetic amine (eg, 10 drops of phenylephrine 0.25%) may facilitate removal. A blunt hook is placed behind the foreign body and then drawn forward. Attempts to grasp smooth, firm foreign bodies with forceps tend to push them farther posteriorly. Rhinoliths are difficult to remove because their shape tends to conform to the contour of the nasal passage.

JUVENILE ANGIOFIBROMA

A benign tumor arising from the connective tissue in the nasopharyngeal vault and occurring almost exclusively in males at puberty. The angiofibroma is red and firm; it is composed of fibrous tissue and numerous thin-walled vessels without contractile elements. Epistaxis is the major symptom. The angiofibroma may obstruct the nasal cavity, encroach upon the paranasal sinuses, and invade the orbit and the cranial cavity. The pterygomaxillary fissure is frequently widened by extension of the tumor into the infratemporal fossa. The widening of the fissure may be determined radiographically; the extent of the tumor may be determined with CT or MRI. The source of the blood supply and the presence of intracranial extension are determined with bilateral selective internal and external carotid angiography.

Although angiofibromas usually involute with maturity, **treatment** is often necessary. Angiographic embolization followed by excision is the more definitive method of treatment, but radiation therapy is the treatment of choice for patients with intracranial or orbital extension. Estrogen therapy with diethylstilbestrol 5 mg orally tid for 6 wk prior to excision reduces the size and vascularity of the tumor.

JUVENILE PAPILLOMAS

Benign tumors of the larynx may grow so exuberantly at multiple sites that tracheotomy is required to maintain an adequate airway. Papillomas are of viral origin, and they may appear as early as 1 yr of age and occur in epidemics. They cause hoarseness (that may progress to aphonia) and upper respiratory obstruction characterized by inspiratory stridor and intercostal, supraclavicular, suprasternal, and subxiphoid retractions. The diagnosis is made at direct laryngoscopy and confirmed by histopathologic examination. **Treatment** is by periodic excision or laser vaporization. Recurrence is common, and regression usually occurs spontaneously at puberty.

45. OPHTHALMOLOGIC DISORDERS

(Disorders of the eye are also discussed in §6, and under CONGENITAL EYE DEFECTS in Ch. 28.)

STRABISMUS
(Squint; Cross-Eyes; Heterotropia)

Deviation of one eye from parallelism with the other. **Paralytic (nonconcomitant) strabismus,** resulting from paralysis of one or more ocular muscles, may be caused by a specific oculomotor nerve lesion. It is characterized by limitation of eye motion and increasing diplopia in the fields of action of the paralyzed muscles. Diplopia is not present if the paralysis is congenital, since vision in the deviated eye is suppressed. **Nonparalytic (concomitant) strabismus** usually results from unequal ocular muscle tone caused by a supranuclear abnormality within the CNS. A concomitant strabismus may be convergent **(esotropia),** divergent **(exotropia),** or vertical **(hyper- or hypotropia).** The deviation from parallelism does not vary with ocular movements and the function of individual muscles is usually intact, unless secondary contraction occurs. **Latent strabismus (phoria)** is concomitant and may occur as **esophoria, exophoria,** or **hypo- or hyperphoria.** In phorias, the muscle imbalance is overcome by the neurologic (central) tendency to fuse the images from each eye. Phorias, unless large, rarely cause symptoms and are apparent only when fusion is suppressed artificially.

Examination for strabismus can be initiated by having the patient fix on a pencil or flashlight held in front of the examiner. By alternately covering and uncovering one eye, the examiner can detect a shift in the eye's position when it is uncovered and proceeds to fix on the object. In the presence of exotropia, the eye that was covered turns *in* to achieve fixation; in esotropia, it turns *out* to fixate. The amount of tropia can be estimated by using prisms oriented in such a way that the deviating eye need not move to fixate. The power of the prism (in diopters) used to prevent deviation also quantitates the tropia.

Amblyopia (reduced visual acuity due to an abnormal visual experience early in life) usually results from cortical suppression of the image in the deviating eye to avoid confusion and diplopia. Disuse of an eye, as in cases of severe refractive error or impaired vision due to disease, may also result in strabismus.

Treatment

Since strabismus may be the result of serious ocular or neurologic disease, complete evaluation of the eyes (corneas, lenses, retinas, and optic nerves) and neurologic status of the patient, regardless of age, is mandatory. Ocular deviation, if constant, should be investigated shortly after birth; if intermittent, by age 6 mo. It should never be merely observed on the assumption that it will be outgrown, since serious disease may be overlooked. Early treatment of amblyopia by patching the normal eye may result in improved vision, leading to a better prognosis for development of binocular vision and more stability if surgery is performed. If muscle imbalance alone is responsible, strabismus should be treated early with corrective glasses or contact lenses, miotics (eg, echothiophate iodide 0.03% bid), orthoptic training (eg, eye exercises), botulinum toxin, or surgical restoration of the muscle balance. Permanent loss of vision can occur if strabismus and its attendant amblyopia are not treated before age 4 to 6 yr, with intermittent follow-up examinations at least until age 10 yr.

46. PSYCHIATRIC CONDITIONS IN CHILDHOOD AND ADOLESCENCE

CHILDHOOD PSYCHOSIS

Psychoses are manifested by pathology in all areas of mental function: behavior, cognition, and affect. They are relatively rare (4 to 10 cases/10,000 children), but they pose significant problems for medical care. They can be differentiated into 3 major categories, each differing in age of onset, course, and prognosis: (1) infantile autism and childhood-onset pervasive developmental disorder, (2) disintegrative psychosis, and (3) childhood schizophrenia.

INFANTILE AUTISM
(Kanner's Syndrome)

A syndrome of early childhood characterized by (1) abnormal social relationships; (2) language disorder with impaired understanding, echolalia, and pronominal reversal (particularly using "you" instead of "I" or "me" when referring to one's self); (3) rituals and compulsive phenomena (an insistence on the preservation of sameness); and (4) uneven intellectual development, in most cases.

The ratio of male:female cases ranges from 2:1 to 4:1. An epidemiologic study of all cases in England in which autism was known to have occurred in at least one of a pair of twins revealed that the concordance rate in monozygotic twins was significantly greater than that in dizygotic pairs; this points to an important role for genetic factors. When the syndrome was originally identified, its differentiation from mental deficiency and from manifest brain injury was emphasized; however, it is now defined by its behavioral manifestations. The level of intellectual function and the presence or absence of neurologic damage are recorded separately using a multiaxial diagnostic system.

Symptoms, Signs, and Diagnosis

Infantile autism usually is manifest in the first year of life; its onset is not later than age 30 mo. The syndrome is characterized by extreme aloneness (lack of attachment, failure to cuddle, avoidance of eye gaze); insistence on sameness (resistance to change, rituals, morbid attachment to familiar objects, repetitive acts); speech and language disorder (which varies from total muteness through delayed onset of speech to markedly idiosyncratic use of language); and uneven intellectual performance. Autistic children are difficult to test; they usually do better on performance than on verbal items in standard IQ tests and may show instances of age-appropriate performance despite retardation in most areas. Nonetheless, in the hands of an experienced examiner, an IQ test provides a useful predictor of outcome. Those children with IQ < 50 have an almost uniformly poor prognosis; about half of those who test higher can do moderately well. The disorder tends to maintain a consistent symptomatic picture throughout development, with some individuals acquiring symptoms of schizophrenia (delusions and hallucinations) in adolescence or young adulthood.

Neurologic examination commonly yields nonfocal findings, although about 20 to 40% of the children (particularly those with IQ < 50) develop seizures before adolescence. EEG examination usually is uninformative. CT scans have isolated a subgroup of autistic children with enlarged ventricles. Use of MRI recently identified a subgroup of autistic adults with hypoplasia of the cerebellar vermis. Individual cases of autism have been associated with the congenital rubella syndrome, cytomegalic inclusion disease, phenylketonuria, and the fragile X syndrome.

Treatment

For the most severely impaired children, systematic application of behavior therapy, a technique that can be taught to parents, helps to manage the child in the home and at school. These benefits are considerable for autistic children who try the patience of the most loving parents and the most devoted teachers. Butyrophenones provide limited benefit, mainly in controlling the most severe forms of aggressive and self-destructive behavior; they do not resolve the psychosis. The use of fenfluramine, a serotonergic antagonist, to control unmanageable behavior remains controversial. Electric shock, tried in the past, was of no help. Speech therapy should begin early. For mute children, the value of learning sign language is not yet established.

Children in the near-normal or higher IQ range often benefit from psychotherapy and special education.

CHILDHOOD—ONSET PERVASIVE DEVELOPMENTAL DISORDER

A syndrome similar to infantile autism but with a later age of onset (30 mo to 12 yr). It is characterized by abnormal social relations (eg, aloofness, inappropriate affect, and a lack of skill in making friendships) and by bizarre mannerisms, which commonly include oddities of motor movement, strange gestures, and unusual speech patterns. The disorder is not fully expressed until after age 30 mo, although some features may appear earlier. As with autism, delusions and hallucinations are characteristically absent.

Except for a later age of onset, the syndrome appears to be a variant of autism. The disorder often coexists and tends to become blurred with symptoms of Tourette's disorder, obsessive-compulsive disorder, and hyperactivity. Treatment and prognosis are similar to those described for autism, above.

DISINTEGRATIVE PSYCHOSIS

A heterogeneous collection of syndromes with onset after age 3 yr and a history of prior normal development. The typical history is that of a child with normal development to age 3 or 4 (including the acquisition of speech, toilet training, and adequate social behavior). Following a period of vague illness and mood change in which the child is irritable and complaining, he undergoes marked regression with loss of the developmental landmark achievements previously acquired. The child deteriorates to a grossly defective level. Disintegrative psychosis includes some cases that later may be identifiable as specific neurodegenerative syndromes (eg, slow virus diseases, juvenile cerebromacular degeneration) as well as those in which no cause can be identified. The course is inexorably grave, and the child will require lifelong care as a severe mental defective; longevity may not be impaired in the cases where etiology is unclear. At present, there are no specific treatments for any of the disorders within this category.

CHILDHOOD SCHIZOPHRENIA
(See also Ch. 58)

Psychotic states with onset after age 7 yr and with behavioral similarities to adult schizophrenia. Evidence concerning cause suggests that environmental stress precipitates manifest illness in individuals with a genetic predisposition. Although biochemical hypotheses implicating abnormalities of dopamine metabolism have been tested, results have been inconclusive.

The prevalence of this disorder increases with age. Whereas infantile autism and childhood-onset pervasive developmental disorder are distinctly different from the adult schizophrenias, childhood schizophrenia forms a continuum with the adolescent and adult forms of the disorder. It is characterized by withdrawal of interest, flat affect, thought disorder (blocking and perseveration), ideas of reference, hallucinations and delusions, and complaints of thought control. Di-agnosis is based on descriptive clinical phenomena.

Treatment
Combined psychotropic and psychotherapeutic treatment is required. Phenothiazines (eg, thiothixene 0.10 to 0.40 mg/kg/day) and butyrophenones (eg, haloperidol 0.15 to 0.30 mg/kg/day) may be effective in controlling acute psychotic symptoms, but relapse is common.

(Because children are susceptible to extra-pyramidal side effects with those drugs, they must be used with caution.) Hospitalization is useful in the management of acute exacerbations; some children require continuing inpatient psychiatric care.

AFFECTIVE DISORDERS (DEPRESSION AND MANIA)
(See also Ch. 57)

Severe affective (mood) disorders, comparable to those seen in adults, are relatively rare among children. However, in recent years, attention has been drawn to the recognition of depression in school-aged children. When symptoms are severe, association with a family history of depressive disorder is likely. Studies of adults support the belief that there is a major genetic component in affective disease, with a higher incidence in the pedigree than in the general population.

Symptoms, Signs, and Diagnosis
The symptoms of **depression** include a sad and unhappy appearance, apathy and withdrawal, reduced capacity for pleasure, feeling rejected and unloved, difficulty in sleeping, somatic complaints (headaches, abdominal pain, insomnia), episodes of clowning or foolish behavior, and persistent self-blame. Chronic depressive reactions are associated with anorexia, weight loss, despondency, and suicidal ideation. Some contend that depression may be "masked" by overactivity and aggressive, antisocial behavior.

Bipolar affective disorder (manic-depressive psychosis) is exceedingly rare before puberty and unknown in early childhood. Some children do manifest marked mood swings (cyclothymic temperament), but these do not reach psychotic proportions, except when they are the result of exposure to toxins and drugs.

Treatment
Evaluation of the family and social setting is required to identify stresses that may have precipitated these disorders. Appropriate measures directed at the family and school must accompany direct treatment of the child, focusing on enhancing his self-esteem. Brief hospitalization may be necessary in acute crises. Although controlled studies remain to be done, most clinicians believe that tricyclic antidepressants (eg, imipramine 1 to 2.5 mg/kg/day) are useful adjuncts to

treatment. Given individual variation in pharmacokinetics of tricyclic antidepressants, monitoring plasma concentration is useful in determining optimal dosage levels. A plasma level of 125 to 250 ng/mL is considered the range of therapeutic effectiveness, although an upper level in children has not been firmly established. Prior to starting therapy with a tricyclic antidepressant, an ECG should be obtained. Throughout treatment, PR and QRS characteristics should be monitored.

Whether lithium is useful in preventing recurrence has yet to be established; its use in children remains experimental because there are no data on possible toxic effects on the developing organism, particularly on the kidney, thyroid, and brain.

GENDER IDENTITY DISORDER OF CHILDHOOD

The essential features of this disorder are a persistent feeling of discomfort and inappropriateness in a prepubertal child about his or her anatomic sex and a desire to be, or a conviction that he or she is, of the opposite sex. Apparently rare, the disorder must be differentiated from the much more frequent rejection of stereotypical sex-role behavior (eg, tomboyishness in girls or sissyish behavior in boys). Children with a gender identity disorder have a profound disturbance of the normal sense of maleness or femaleness, and will strongly and persistently state a desire to be of the other sex, or will insist that they are. (Individuals who develop **transsexualism** [see in Ch. 54] often have evidenced gender identity problems as children.)

Girls regularly have male peer groups and are avidly interested in sports and rough-and-tumble play; they are not interested in playing with female-type dolls or in playing house. They insist on wearing stereotypical masculine clothing. Boys invariably are preoccupied with female stereotypical activities, such as dressing in girls' or women's clothes, or have a compelling desire to participate in girls' games. They choose toys and games that are most usually favored by girls and frequently demonstrate gestures and actions usually regarded as feminine. They encounter considerable male peer-group teasing and rejection.

Of the boys who cross-dress, 75% begin prior to their 4th birthday. Doll-playing begins during the same period. Social ostracism and conflict become significant at about age 7 or 8; about $1/3$ become homosexuals. The age of onset in females is also early, but a majority give up this pattern in late childhood or adolescence. A minority of the girls remain identified as males, and some of these develop a homosexual arousal pattern. A smaller number from each sex may later develop transsexualism. The condition may be reversible with long-term psychotherapy and family therapy; the data are not yet conclusive.

Intersexuality

Confusion over gender identity may arise if the child is born with ambiguous genitalia. These children are sometimes called **hermaphrodites**, although most are **pseudohermaphrodites**. Male pseudohermaphrodites have testicular tissue; females have ovarian tissue. In true hermaphrodites, both testicular and ovarian tissues coexist.

The sex of rearing should be determined by the probable course of development at adolescence. If corrective surgery is recommended, it should be carried out very early, whenever possible prior to 18 mo of age. Intersex states are discussed in more detail in Chs. 28 and 48.

ADOLESCENT PSYCHIATRIC CONDITIONS

Adolescents have no more psychiatric illness than any other age group. The mistaken assumption that psychopathology is typical in adolescence leads to both over- and underdiagnosis (if all teenagers are "disturbed," disturbance is normal). Follow-up studies suggest that adolescents seen in clinics and emergency departments for behavioral problems are different from the great majority of their peers and are likely to remain so without adequate intervention.

Some problems typical of adolescence are discussed here, but detailed information on psychiatric conditions occurring in all groups can be found in §4. Suicide in adolescents is discussed separately, below.

Adjustment Disorder

An acute response to environmental stress by an adolescent with a basically good adaptive capacity; symptoms abate as stress diminishes. This diagnosis often is misapplied to chronic difficulties of adjustment and to more serious psychopathology because of reluctance to give an unfavorable label and prognosis to adolescents.

However, it is appropriate when there is little evidence of an underlying disorder and when the environmental stress is impressive.

Occasionally, a generally stable adolescent who experiences an unusually distressing event may suffer **posttraumatic stress disorder** (see also in Ch. 56), with recurrent recollections of the event, marked efforts to avoid recalling it, and a persistent state of anxiety and arousal, with extreme and even bizarre symptoms and behavior. Crisis intervention is necessary. While prompt displays of empathy, support, and guidance may lead to rapid remission, individual, family, and group therapy over an extended period are sometimes required.

Conferences with parents or family group therapy may help, but with some older adolescents or in instances of insoluble family pathology, the teenager should be treated alone. Referral to a social agency, with arrangements for reporting to the physician, may be used. Psychiatric referral may be necessary.

Substance Use Disorders
(See also Ch. 53)

Patterns of adolescent substance abuse change. Daily use of marijuana and experimentation with a variety of compounds have diminished since the late 1970s, while alcohol use may be slightly less, and cocaine, crack, and other stimulants are used more frequently. Reported rates are unreliable and probably underestimated. Although substances in favor change, the susceptible adolescent is the same: less able in school, more invested in recreation, more likely to have a job and money. There is commonly a progression of use from alcohol through marijuana to other compounds, a rise in alcohol use in mid-to-late adolescence, and a relatively stable pattern of use thereafter. Most persons begin serious abuse before age 20 yr, but adolescent preventive programs have not been as effective as hoped. However, the gradual diminution in male adolescent tobacco use suggests that behavioral change can be induced. At the individual level, substance abuse may be self-medication for depression or dysphoria; therapeutic intervention—group or individual therapy and/or antidepressant medication—may then be helpful. Detailed information on alcohol and substance abuse should be sought in confidence during the course of a routine examination, particularly when academic and behavioral problems are reported in previously well-adjusted youngsters or in families with a history of substance abuse.

Conduct Disorder

This disorder is more frequent and more difficult to treat than adjustment disorder. Persons with **solitary aggressive** conduct disorder show selfishness, a failure of normal bonds with others, and a lack of appropriate guilt. Those with **group conduct disorder** demonstrate peer loyalty, often at the expense of outsiders. **Undifferentiated conduct disorder** is a mixture of the 2 types, while **oppositional defiant disorder** demonstrates negative, angry, defiant behavior without actual violation of the rights of others; it often evolves into conduct disorder. Adolescents with conduct disorders tend to have higher-than-expected incidences of medical pathology and psychotic illness at follow-up. Treating medical, neurologic, and psychiatric conditions may improve the patient's self-esteem and control. Moralizing or dire admonitions are ineffective and should be avoided. Often, only separation from a damaging environment and external discipline offer hope of success.

Attention Deficit Disorder
(See under LEARNING DISORDERS in Ch. 29)

Somatoform Disorders

These disorders are also discussed in Ch. 56 and under PSYCHOSOMATIC MEDICINE in Ch. 51. However, they deserve mention here because they often begin at early adolescence, often occur together, are underdiagnosed, and may be inadvertently reinforced by vigorous medical intervention. **Conversion disorder** occurs when unacceptable psychic conflict is expressed as a somatic symptom, often as a neurologic disease. Incidence in children is equal in both sexes but is more common in girls by midadolescence. Subsequent development of **somatoform pain disorder** is common. The diagnosis in somatization disorder requires a multitude of symptoms in patients—nearly all female—who make illness a way of life. These conditions occur more frequently if parents and other family members are symptomatic, providing models for a youth's symptomatology. Each disorder may afford both "primary gain" (by keeping the basic conflict unconscious) and "secondary gain" (by avoiding an undesired situation or by affording extra attention). Although once synonymous with hysteria, both conditions actually occur in a wide range of psychopathology: depression, particularly, but schizophrenia, retardation, and many personality disorders as well.

When these disorders are suspected, the physician should avoid extensive laboratory evaluations, which suggest diagnostic uncertainty and may be seen by the patient as confirmation of a physical problem, and decisive medical or surgical intervention, which may entrench symptomatology. A psychiatric referral often will be unacceptable, since it threatens the patient's symptomatic solution. However, relatively short visits, with reassurance and inquiries into nonmedical areas, may gradually wean the patient away from the condition. Reassurance and support of family members help to minimize somatic symptoms as the "ticket" for continued medical attention.

SUICIDE IN CHILDREN AND ADOLESCENTS
(See also Ch. 60)

Suicide has increased in childhood, at least in boys, and has particularly increased in adolescents (2nd only to accidents as the leading cause of adolescent death). In the 15- to 24-yr age group, male suicide has increased 50% since 1970; female suicide, only slightly. For all adolescents 15 to 24 yr, the 1989 suicide rates were 13.8/100,000 (the male:female ratio was 4:1). Suicide rates for all children between ages 5 and 14 were 0.5/100,000 in 1989. These preliminary rates represent minimum incidence figures because official designation of a death as suicide requires proof of intention. Thus, many deaths attributed to accidents (eg, motor vehicle and firearms) are suicides.

Identifying the suicidal patient: Suicidal incidents often are preceded by medical visits, when recent changes in behavior may be revealed (eg, despondent mood, low self-esteem, sleep and appetite disturbances, inability to concentrate, truancy from school, somatic complaints, and suicidal preoccupation). Statements such as "I wish I had never been born" or "I'd like to go to sleep and never wake up" should be taken seriously as possible indications of suicidal intent. Directly questioning pediatric patients about suicide diminishes the risk. **Predisposing factors** include a history of suicide in family members or close friends, recent deaths in the family, substance abuse, and conduct disorders (see above under ADOLESCENT PSYCHIATRIC CONDITIONS) because of the associated potential for suicidal action. **Precipitating factors** often involve losses: eg, of self-esteem, as in family arguments, a humiliating disciplinary episode, pregnancy, or

school failure; of a boyfriend or girlfriend; of familiar surroundings (school, neighborhood, friends) due to a geographic move. Other factors may be a lack of structure and boundaries, leading to an overwhelming feeling of lack of direction, or the intense pressure to succeed in certain families, and the belief by the child or adolescent that he is falling short of expectations. A frequent motive for a suicide attempt is the effort to manipulate or punish others with the fantasy "You'll be sorry after I'm dead." Publicity around dramatic suicides often is followed by similar episodes. A rise in suicides among self-identified populations (eg, a single high school, a college dormitory) also indicates the importance of suggestion. Early community intervention with a stated intention of supporting youths who have suicidal thoughts can be helpful.

Responding to suicidal behavior: *A suicidal threat or attempt represents an important communication about the intensity of experienced despair.*

When somatic complaints bring a child or adolescent to the physician's office, early recognition of the risk factors mentioned above may help prevent a suicide attempt. In responding to these early cues, or when confronted with threatened or attempted suicide or severe risk-taking behavior, vigorous intervention is appropriate and patients should be directly questioned about their unhappy or self-destructive feelings. The physician should not provide reassurance without fully understanding the circumstances, since this can undermine his credibility and/or lower the youngster's self-esteem even further.

Every suicide attempt is a medical emergency. Once the immediate threat to life has been removed, a decision must be made on the need for hospitalization. This depends on the balance between the degree of risk and the family's capacity to provide support. Lethality of suicidal intent can be assessed by the degree of forethought evidenced (eg, writing a suicide note), the method used (firearms are usually more lethal than pills), the degree of self-injury sustained, and the circumstances or immediate precipitating factors surrounding the attempt. A negative or unsupportive parental response is ominous. If the family response shows love and concern, a positive outcome is more likely. If necessary, hospitalization (even on an open ward, with special duty nursing) is the surest form of protection and usually is indicated if severe depression and/or psychosis is suspected. Psychiatric referral is most successful if continuity with the primary caretaker is assured. Essential to the follow-up treatment process is the rebuilding of morale and the restoration of emotional equilibrium within the family.

47. PHYSICAL CONDITIONS IN ADOLESCENCE

The most common health problems of adolescents relate to growth and development, appearance, increased socialization, and certain metabolic and infectious disorders. Periodic medical evaluations are important to document and evaluate growth and development and maintain a favorable doctor-patient relationship. For immunization procedures in adolescents, see Ch. 23.

Accidents (many due to motor vehicle mishaps) are the leading cause of death during adolescence. Nonfatal accidents, eg, burns and multiple fractures, are responsible for many teenage hospitalizations. A detailed, comprehensive history should be obtained, because premorbid behavioral problems are common in adolescents who experience serious injuries. A significant history of behavioral problems, eg, running away, depression, or truancy, requires further psychologic evaluation (see ADOLESCENT PSYCHIATRIC CONDITIONS in Ch. 46).

DEVELOPMENTAL CONDITIONS
(See also Osgood-Schlatter disease under THE OSTEOCHONDROSES in Ch. 42)

NORMAL GROWTH AND DEVELOPMENT

Adolescent physical growth includes both somatic and sexual maturation. The age of onset and rapidity of development vary with each individual and are influenced by genetic and environmental factors. Maturity begins at an earlier age today than a century ago, probably because of improvements in nutrition, general health, and living conditions. For example, the age at menarche in the USA decreased 3 to 4 mo/decade during that time, although it has now leveled off.

Somatic growth of both males and females includes attainment of adult height and weight, musculoskeletal growth, and increased size of all organs, except the lymphatics, which decrease in size, and the brain, the weight of which plateaus during adolescence. The growth spurt in boys occurs between ages 13 and 15½ yr; a gain of 4 in.

can be expected in the year of peak velocity. For girls, the growth spurt begins at about age 11 yr, may reach 3½ in. in the year of peak velocity, and is almost completed by 13½ yr. In general, boys are heavier and taller than girls when growth is complete because they have a longer growth period. At age 18, growth is 99% complete for girls; about 2 cm of growth remain for boys, slightly less for girls. One adolescent may develop early, another late, but both may reach the same height. Factors that control bone age progression also exert a considerable influence over menarche and, to a lesser extent, over pubic hair development.

Once **sexual changes** begin, they proceed in an established sequence in both boys and girls. **In the male,** sexual changes begin with growth of the scrotum and testes and lengthening of the penis, followed by the appearance of pubic hair and growth of the seminal vesicles and prostate. The height spurt usually begins a year after the testes start growing. Axillary and facial hair appear about 2 yr after pubic hair. The median age for first ejaculation (between 12½ and 14 yr in the USA) is affected by psychologic, cultural, and biologic factors. First ejaculation takes place about 1 yr after the accelerated penis growth. Mature spermatozoa appear between ages 14 and 16 yr, but maximum fertility is not reached until the late teens or early 20s. Uni- or bilateral gynecomastia is common in young teenage boys and usually resolves within 1 yr.

In the female, sexual changes chronologically are bony pelvis growth; breast development; uterine, vaginal, labial, and clitoral growth; secondary sexual hair appearance; and menarche. Menarche occurs about 2 to 2½ yr after onset of breast development and when growth in height slows after reaching its peak. The stages of breast growth and pubic hair development can be detailed using Tanner's criteria (see FIGS. 6−1 and 6−2). If the order of sexual changes is disturbed, growth is abnormal and the physician should suspect pathologic reasons.

See below for discussions of delayed sexual maturation and precocious puberty.

IDIOPATHIC SCOLIOSIS

A structural lateral curvature of the spine.

Sixty to 80% of cases occur in girls. Scoliosis may first be suspected when one shoulder seems higher than the other or when clothes do not hang straight. An initial complaint may be fatigue in the lumbar region after prolonged sitting or standing. This may be followed by muscular backaches in areas of strain, such as the lumbosacral angle. Pain, a late manifestation, may become more persistent as irritation of the ligaments increases. Of the 4% of children age 10 to 14 yr with detectable scoliosis, $1/2$ will necessitate treatment or continuing medical observation; $1/2$ can be screened in school for progression.

The teenager should bend forward for examination, because the spinal curve is more pronounced in that position. Most curves are convex to the right in the thoracic area and to the left in the lumbar area, so that the right shoulder is higher than the left. One hip may be more prominent than the other. X-ray examination should include anteroposterior and lateral views of the spine with the patient standing.

The prognosis depends on the site and severity of the curve and the age of onset of symptoms. The type of curve is related to the complications. The greater the curve, the greater the likelihood of progression after skeletal maturity. Prompt referral to an orthopedist is indicated, so that the means of preventing further deformity (a cast or Milwaukee brace) or correcting the deformity (surgery or electrospinal stimulation) can be instituted. Scoliosis and its treatment threaten the teenager's self-image. Wearing a brace or a cast can cause concern about being different from peers, and hospitalization and surgery challenge the youngster's independence, but the alternative is a significant deformity. Counseling and support are the major components of the family physician's care of teenagers with scoliosis.

SLIPPED CAPITAL FEMORAL EPIPHYSIS

Etiology is not known but may be related to the effects of growth hormone and estrogen on the thickness of the epiphyseal plate. The disorder is often seen in overweight teenagers, usually boys. Onset is usually insidious, and symptoms are associated with the stage of slippage. Initially there may be hip stiffness that improves with rest. This is followed by a limp and then by hip pain that radiates down the anteromedial thigh to the knee. Examination of the hip in the early stages may reveal no pain or limitation of movement. In more advanced stages, there may be pain on motion of the affected hip, with limited flexion, abduction, and medial rotation; knee pain, without specific knee findings; and a limp. The affected leg is externally rotated. If the blood supply to the area is compromised, avascular necrosis and collapse of the epiphysis may occur.

Early diagnosis is vital, as treatment becomes more difficult in the more advanced stages. Anteroposterior and "frog-leg" lateral x-rays of both hips should be obtained. X-rays of the affected hip show widening of the epiphyseal line or displacement posteriorly and inferiorly of the femoral head. Orthopedic referral is important to confirm the diagnosis and evaluate the need for corrective surgery. Surgical treatment requires immobility, which limits the adolescent's independence.

DELAYED SEXUAL MATURATION
(See also PITUITARY DWARFISM in Ch. 40)

Delayed sexual maturation is present in boys if there is no testicular enlargement by age $13^{1}/_{2}$ or if there are > 5 yr between the initial and complete growth of the genitalia. For girls, no breast development by age 13 or a period of > 5 yr between the beginning of breast growth and menarche indicates delayed maturation, as does short stature in both boys and girls.

The major causes of delayed puberty are (1) **constitutional delay**, occurring in the teenager whose family has a history of late growth (the youngster's prepubertal growth rate is normal and his skeletal growth and adolescent growth spurt are delayed; he experiences late, but normal, sexual maturation); (2) **genetic disorders**, including Turner's syndrome (gonadal dysgenesis) in the female and Klinefelter's syndrome (primary testicular dysfunction) in the male; (3) **CNS conditions**, such as a destructive tumor of the pituitary, which results in decreased gonadotropin secretion; and (4) **chronic illnesses**, eg, diabetes mellitus, chronic renal disease, and cystic fibrosis.

PRECOCIOUS PUBERTY

The onset of sexual maturation before age 8 in a girl and age 10 in a boy.

True precocious puberty is activation of the hypothalamic-pituitary axis with consequent enlargement and maturation of the gonads and the development of secondary sexual characteristics, adult serum gonadal steroid levels, and spermatogenesis or oogenesis. In **pseudoprecocious puberty**, by contrast, secondary sexual characteristics develop because of high circulating levels of androgens or estrogens, usually secreted from a gonadal or adrenal tumor, but the gonads remain immature and spermatogenesis or oogenesis does not occur. Other causes of pseudoprecocious puberty in boys are human chorionic gonadotropin (**HCG**)–secreting tumors, such as hepatoblastomas and rare pineal tumors. In girls, causes of persistent or recurrent pseudoprecocious puberty include follicular cysts of the ovary; granulosa and/or thecal cell tumors; and, rarely, feminizing adrenal tumors.

The incidence of true precocious puberty is 2 to 5 times greater in females. About 80% of cases in girls $\geq$ age 6 have no identifiable abnormality, but CNS lesions such as hamartomas are frequently found in girls $<$ 4 yr. In contrast, 60% of male cases have identifiable underlying disease. Organic causes in either sex include lesions of the hypothalamus (hamartomas, rarely craniopharyngiomas), intracranial tumors (pinealomas), neurofibromatosis, and a few rare diseases.

In a recently recognized syndrome, a small group of boys has been identified with apparently autonomous, **gonadotropin-independent, Leydig-cell function (familial male precocious puberty)**. In this syndrome, both gametogenesis and steroidogenesis are stimulated in the absence of any increase in gonadotropin secretion.

Precocious puberty associated with polyostotic fibrous dysplasia and café au lait pigmentation is the classic triad seen in a child presenting with **McCune-Albright syndrome (MAS)**. Generally the hypothalamic-pituitary axis is prepubertal, with ovarian cysts accounting for the sexual maturation.

Precocious pubarche refers to *the appearance of pubic hair alone prior to age 8 in a girl and age 10 in a boy*; **precocious adrenarche** refers to *the appearance of axillary and pubic hair alone prior to age 8 in a girl and age 10 in a boy*; and **precocious thelarche** refers to *the onset of breast development prior to age 8 in a girl*. These conditions may herald the onset of precocious puberty, but precocious pubarche, adrenarche, and thelarche may occur independently of any further development. When these conditions do occur and there is no pubertal progress, they are generally benign. Variant forms of congenital adrenal hyperplasia (**CAH**) should be excluded

with the development of hair. Occasionally a girl may present with sporadic vaginal bleeding associated with an ovarian cyst, but minimal or no breast development or pubic hair. Bone age is either normal or slightly advanced. Further progression into puberty does not always occur, even with intermittent episodes of vaginal bleeding. Careful follow-up of affected children with any of these conditions is warranted, especially to assess progression of pubertal development.

Symptoms, Signs, and Diagnosis

In both true and pseudoprecocious puberty, boys exhibit facial, axillary, and pubic hair; penile growth; and increased masculinity. Girls develop breasts and pubic and axillary hair. Girls begin to menstruate more commonly with true precocious puberty, but vaginal bleeding may also occur with pseudoprecocious puberty (such as MAS). Body odor and acne as well as adolescent-type behavior may be present in both sexes. Linear growth is initially rapid in both sexes, but the adult height is shortened by premature closure of the epiphyses. Testicular or ovarian enlargement, which occurs in true precocious puberty, is usually absent in pseudoprecocious puberty; but ovarian cysts may occur in some cases of MAS or in association with sporadic vaginal bleeding.

Laboratory evaluation should include β-HCG, serum estradiol, testosterone, dehydroepiandrosterone sulfate, 17-hydroxyprogesterone, luteinizing hormone (**LH**), follicle-stimulating hormone (**FSH**), and prolactin levels. Diagnostic imaging studies should include an x-ray of the left hand and wrist for bone age, as well as pelvic and adrenal ultrasonography. MRI or CT scanning of the brain is indicated in all cases of precocity. Gonadotropin-independent precocious puberty can be documented by establishing prepubertal gonadotropin responses to exogenous gonadotropin-releasing hormone (**GnRH**, also known as luteinizing hormone–releasing hormone [**LHRH**]) in boys or girls with no neoplasm or other obvious cause for early development. A pubertal response to the GnRH stimulation test is useful to avoid exploratory laparotomy in girls with large ovarian cysts.

Treatment

For true precocious puberty: A GnRH agonist (an analog of GnRH)—such as D-Trp^6-Pro^9-NEt-GnRH (deslorelin) or D-His^6-Pro^9-NEt-GnRH (histrelin acetate) at a dose of 8 to 10 μg/kg/day s.c.; or D-Ser(tBU)^6-NEt-GnRH (1-9) ethylamide 400 to 1200 μg/day intranasally in 2 to 4 divided doses; or nafarelin acetate 800 to 1600 μg/day intranasally in single or divided dose q 12 h; or triptorelin (D-Trp[6] GnRH) 60 μg/kg/mo IM microcapsule or leuprolide acetate 30 μg/kg/day s.c. (maximum 50 μg/kg/day) or 7.5 to 11.25 mg IM depot q 3 to 4 wk—can be given until the time of normal puberty and will suppress pituitary gonadotropin (LH and FSH) secretion after transient stimulation of LH and FSH, thereby halting precocious puberty. Treatment has been successful in all cases of true precocious puberty in boys and girls.

For gonadotropin-independent precocious puberty, androgen antagonists (eg, spironolactone 1.5 mg/kg/day in 3 divided oral doses or cyproterone acetate 75 to 100 mg/m² in 3 divided oral doses) ameliorate the effects of the excess androgen. The antifungal agent ketoconazole 30 μg/kg/day orally in 2 to 3 divided doses will reduce testosterone in boys with gonadotropin-independent Leydig cell function. Testolactone, an inhibitor of aromatase, 20 to 40 μg/kg/day orally in 4 divided doses, will reduce serum estradiol and effectively treat girls with MAS. Finally, in advanced cases of pseudopuberty associated with these latter conditions or CAH, activation of the hypothalamicpituitary axis may occur, necessitating the use of a GnRH analog in conjunction with the therapeutic regimen.

Excision of hormone-producing tumors, especially granulosa cell tumors in girls, which is the most common ovarian neoplasm, is curative. However, prolonged follow-up is necessary in case of recurrence in the contralateral ovary. Excision is also an option for the various neoplasms causing pseudopuberty in males. However, these tumors are generally aggressively malignant and associated with high mortality rates.

ANABOLIC STEROID ABUSE

Anabolic steroids (AS) are synthetic derivatives of testosterone. Controversy centers on their ability to improve athletic performance and on the resultant ethical and safety issues. The problem is serious in many power-related sports, despite a ban on AS use by amateur and professional sports organizations worldwide supported by all major medical and sports associations.

This discussion will address the problem as it affects adolescents and young adults. The reported incidence in the USA ranges from 6 to 11% of high-school–aged males and includes an unexpected number of nonathletes. In a national survey, the second most common reason given for AS use was to improve appearance (27%), and 35% of users were not participating in school-sponsored athletics.

The typical profile of an AS user is a male (95%) athlete (65%), most probably a football player, heavyweight wrestler, or weight lifter. He is more likely to attend a metropolitan school of > 700 students and to be a minority student. He is less likely to have a parent who finished high school. He is more likely to have received his steroids from a black-market source (60%).

Primary care physicians are generally more familiar with patients and their families than are other physicians, allowing them to be more aware of changes in the patient, to have a greater rapport with the family, and to enable more timely diagnosis and treatment.

Symptoms and Signs

The most characteristic sign of AS abuse is a dramatic and rapid change in body bulk. If the patient is involved in a weight-training regimen and eats a high-calorie, high-protein diet while taking AS, an increase in muscle bulk and strength is usually produced. Increases in energy level and libido (in men) are established but are more difficult to identify by family or physician.

Psychologic effects are often noticed by the family; eg, wide and erratic mood swings, irrational behavior, and increased aggressiveness (commonly termed "steroid rage").

Increased acne is a common complaint and is one of the few side effects for which an adolescent may seek medical attention. Another possible skin sign is jaundice, indicating liver dysfunction.

Other potential side effects include musculotendinous injuries, accelerated closure of the bony epiphyses in prepubertal and pubertal patients, gynecomastia, azoospermia, liver dysfunction or tumors (benign and malignant), and increased cardiovascular risk through hypertension, increased LDL, and decreased HDL cholesterol.

Adverse effects in females include some potentially irreversible virilizing ones; eg, alopecia, enlarged clitoris, hirsutism, and hoarse voice. Others are decreased breast size, some atrophy of the vaginal mucosa, changes in menstrual cycles (menstruation may stop) and in libido (may increase or less commonly decrease), increased aggressiveness and appetite, and acne.

Diagnosis

Detection of abuse can be accomplished up to 6 mo (even longer for some types of AS) after drug use has ended by testing for AS metabolites in urine. An AS urine drug screen will detect abuse in most patients.

Prevention

Preventive measures should start by the beginning of middle school, as the largest group to report first use was < 15 yr of age. Specific measures include peer counseling groups, counseling by primary care physicians (eg, during sports physicals), and school presentations by physicians, exercise physiologists, coaches, and athletes. School principals, team coaches (especially football, wrestling, basketball, track and field), and school health care officials should be targeted for education as well as adolescents and their parents.

Treatment

Because many patients are abusers of other drugs, in-patient rehabilitation should be strongly considered. Treatment should be individualized to the type and severity of physical and psychologic effects (see also Ch. 53).

TEENAGE PREGNANCY AND CONTRACEPTION

In 1987, 472,623 infants were born to teenagers in the USA (an estimated 12% of all births). Of these, 64% were born out of wedlock. About 10,311 babies were born to mothers under age 15. About 400,000 therapeutic abortions are performed on teenagers annually. The divorce rate for teenage marriages is 50% within 2 yr, 80% by 5 yr. Many teenage mothers have histories of school failure and psychologic problems and are likely to have repeated pregnancies.

Prenatal management should include rigorous medical and psychosocial care, while planning with the adolescent about her future. Pregnant teenagers, particularly the very young, may have a higher incidence of anemia and toxemia than do women in their 20s; but, if they receive prepartum care, they should not experience greater obstetric morbidity than adult women of similar background. Infants of young mothers (especially those < 15 yr) have an increased incidence of prematurity and low birth weight.

Teenagers are in a developmental transition, and pregnancy or marriage usually adds emotional stress. Pregnant girls and their partners tend to drop out of school or vocational training, thus increasing their economic problems, loss of self-esteem, and strain on interpersonal relationships. Easy access to abortion does not remove the psychologic problems of the unwanted pregnancy for the girl or the boy. Emotional crises may occur when pregnancy is diagnosed, when the decision to have an abortion is made, during the postabortal period, the date when the baby would have been born, and on anniversaries of that date. Follow-up care is imperative and should include family counseling, psychosocial planning, and contraceptive education for both the boy and the girl.

Despite sexual activity, many adolescents are ignorant of the risk of fertility and of how they may become pregnant. Nonpregnant, sexually active older adolescents who seek information should be counseled and given contraceptives, if indicated (see Ch. 4). Areas of concern include irregularity of pill taking; the wish to think of intercourse as unplanned and spontaneous, which complicates the use of contraceptives; the tendency for "accidents" to occur; concerns about the pill, often because of misinformation; and limited options for birth control methods, since the diaphragm, in particular, requires preplanning and must be in place prior to intercourse. New methods, such as subdermal implants (polysiloxane capsules containing levonorgestrel) which act continuously over 5 yr, ensure compliance and may be more successful than other methods. Despite many difficulties, even young teenagers can effectively manage contraceptive techniques with adequate professional guidance.

EATING DISORDERS

ANOREXIA NERVOSA

A disorder characterized by a disturbed sense of body image, marked weight loss, morbid fear of obesity, and amenorrhea in women. Only about 5% of cases are male. Onset is usually in adolescence, occasionally prepubertal, and less commonly in adulthood. A high percentage of patients are of middle and upper socioeconomic status. The incidence appears to be increasing in Western society.

Anorexia nervosa may be mild and transient, but it can also be severe and of long duration. Long-term follow-up studies have reported mortality rates of 10 to 20%. However, since most mild cases are probably undiagnosed, the true prevalence of the disorder and its mortality rates are not really known.

The etiology is unknown, but anorexia nervosa is rare where there is a genuine shortage of food. Social factors appear to play an important role. Emphasis on the desirability of being thin pervades our society, and obesity is associated with a wide variety of undesirable traits. Recent surveys reveal that 80 to 90% of prepubertal children are aware of these attitudes, and > 50% of these girls attempt diets and other measures to control their weight. Since only a small percentage develops anorexia nervosa, other factors must be important. Some are probably predisposed because of as-yet-undefined psychologic, genetic, and metabolic vulnerability.

Symptoms and Signs

Even before the onset of illness, many patients are described as being meticulous, compulsive, and intelligent, with very high standards for achievement and success. The first specific indications of the impending disorder are a concern about body weight (even if the patient is lean, which most of them are) and the start of restricting food intake. Preoccupation and anxiety about weight increase even as emaciation develops, and denial of the illness is a prominent feature. Patients do not complain of anorexia or weight loss, usually resist treatment, and are brought to the physician's attention by their families, by intercurrent illness, or by complaints about other symptoms (eg, bloating, abdominal distress, constipation).

Anorexia is a misnomer, as appetite remains unless the patient becomes cachectic. Patients are preoccupied with food: They study diets and calories; hoard, conceal, and waste food; collect recipes; and prepare elaborate meals for others. Binge eating (**bulimia**—see below) followed by induced vomiting and the use of laxatives and diuretics (**binge-purge behavior**) occurs in 50% of anorectics. **Amenorrhea** is universal in female anorectics and often appears before appreciable weight loss. In men and women, there is usually a loss of interest in sex. Other common findings include bradycardia, low BP, hypothermia, the development of lanugo hair or frank hirsutism, and edema. Remarkably, even patients who appear cachectic tend to remain very active (including pursuing vigorous exercise programs) and free of symptoms of nutritional deficiencies or unusual susceptibility to infections. Depression is common, and patients tend to be very manipulative.

They often lie about food intake and conceal behavior such as induced vomiting.

Many endocrine changes have been reported, including pre- or early pubertal patterns of luteinizing hormone secretion, low levels of thyroxine and triiodothyronine, and increased cortisol secretion. Dysfunction may be found in virtually every major organ system in the severely malnourished patient, but the most dangerous are cardiac and fluid and electrolyte disorders. There is decreased cardiac muscle mass, chamber size, and output. Dehydration, metabolic acidosis, and low serum K may be present; all are aggravated when the patient induces vomiting and uses laxatives and/or diuretics. Sudden death is not rare, most likely due to ventricular tachyarrhythmias. Some patients have been found to have prolonged QT intervals (corrected for heart rate), which, in addition to the risks imposed by hypokalemia, may predispose to such arrhythmias.

Diagnosis

Anorexia nervosa usually is apparent from the constellation of symptoms described above, particularly the association of loss of $\geq$ 15% of body weight in a young person who fears obesity, becomes amenorrheic, denies illness, and otherwise appears well. The key to diagnosis is eliciting the central fear of obesity, which is not diminished by weight loss. In severe cases, marked depression or symptoms suggesting another disorder such as schizophrenia may require differentiation or may be additional diagnostic criteria.

Treatment

Treatment can be divided into 2 distinct phases—short-term intervention to restore body weight and save life, and long-term therapy to ameliorate long-standing personality and family problems.

When weight loss has been severe or rapid, or when weight has fallen below some arbitrary level (eg, 80% of ideal), prompt restoration of weight becomes the overriding consideration, and hospitalization is imperative. When in doubt, hospitalize. Simply removing the patient from her home sometimes reverses a downhill course, but more energetic psychiatric treatment is often required. Tube feeding or parenteral alimentation is rarely necessary. Patients who are depressed may benefit from antidepressant medication.

Once the patient's nutritional and water and electrolyte status has stabilized, there begins a difficult treatment, complicated by the patient's abhorrence of weight gain, denial of illness, and manipulative behavior. The physician should attempt to provide a calm, concerned, stable relationship, while encouraging a reasonable caloric intake. Combined management by a family doctor and psychiatrist is often useful, and consultation with or referral to a specialist in eating disorders is wise. Individual psychotherapy—behavioral, cognitive, or psychodynamic—is helpful, as is family therapy for younger patients.

BULIMIA NERVOSA

Bulimia nervosa has been designated a discrete diagnostic entity in *Diagnostic and Statistical Manual of Mental Disorders*, Third Edition—Revised (**DSM-III-R**) published by the American Psychiatric Association (1987). The disorder is characterized by *recurrent episodes of binge eating during which the patient experiences a loss of control over eating and engages in either self-induced vomiting, use of laxatives and/or diuretics, or rigorous dieting or fasting to overcome the effects of the binges.* Patients show a persistent overconcern with body shape and weight.

Bulimia nervosa, like anorexia nervosa, afflicts primarily females of upper and middle socioeconomic status. Although there has been considerable notice of bulimia in the popular press and even talk of an "epidemic," much of the attention has focused on relatively benign instances of binging. Careful epidemiologic studies have shown a prevalence of < 2% of true bulimia nervosa among college women, the group believed to be at highest risk.

Symptoms and Signs

Binge eating can cause acute gastric dilatation and even rupture. Induced vomiting is associated with erosion of dental enamel, parotid gland enlargement, esophagitis, and esophageal rupture. Aspiration pneumonia occurs when induced vomiting is associated with reduced consciousness (during drug or alcohol use). Hypokalemia can result from vomiting and purging, and death has been reported from abuse of ipecac taken to induce vomiting.

People with bulimia tend to be more aware of and remorseful or guilty about their behavior than those with anorexia and are more likely to admit their concerns when questioned by a sympathetic physician. They appear to be less introverted than patients with anorexia nervosa and more prone to impulsive behavior, drug and alcohol abuse, and overt depression.

Bulimia may be suspected in patients expressing marked concern about weight gain and manifesting wide fluctuations in weight, especially if there is evidence of excessive use of laxatives or unexplained hypokalemia. Suspicion is also aroused by swollen parotid glands, scars on the knuckles of the hand (from induced vomiting), and dental erosion. However, the diagnosis depends on the patient's description of binge-purge behavior.

A frequency of 2 binge-eating episodes/wk for at least 3 mo is required for the diagnosis according to DSM-III-R. Typically, a binge involves rapid consumption of food (especially of high caloric value). Binges may consist of thousands of kcal, but at least half of them are relatively small—fewer than 1000 kcal. Binges tend to be episodic, are often triggered by psychosocial stress, and may occur as often as several times a day; they are carried out in secret. Although bulimic patients express concern about becoming obese and some are obese, they usually tend to fluctuate around a normal body weight. Except for those with concomitant anorexia nervosa, they tend not to become emaciated.

Treatment

The 2 approaches to treatment are cognitive-behavioral and pharmacologic. Cognitive-behavioral therapy, usually administered by psychologists, is effective and is currently the focus of intensive research. Antidepressant medication is often effective in controlling bulimia, even in the absence of overt depression, but its withdrawal is all too often followed by relapse. The often intractable nature of the disorder and the rather specialized treatment that is required make it desirable to refer the patient to a specialist in eating disorders should the condition persist.

OBESITY

Arbitrarily, body weight 20% over standard height-weight tables. Severe obesity: > 100% overweight.

Obesity in adolescence, as at any age, is difficult and discouraging to treat and is one of the most common presenting complaints in adolescent clinics. Primary endocrine or metabolic disorders are uncommon, but some secondary medical problems seen in overweight adults may be evident (eg, hypertension, knee and back problems). Frequently, a mildly obese adolescent rapidly gains weight during the teenage years and becomes significantly obese. Untreated, obesity continuing throughout adulthood is likely. The obese adolescent usually has a poor self-image and becomes more sedentary and socially isolated. Parents often are overprotective and may subtly encourage overeating.

Treatment approaches are numerous, but long-term success rates are low. School is an appropriate place for specialized education in nutrition and physical activity. There are few programs designed for overweight adolescents. Currently available drugs should be avoided because they are not helpful in the long run. Surgical approaches such as operations to reduce stomach size may be used in severe obesity. Behavior modification is best because it encourages the factors essential to long-term success: reduction and control of caloric intake with well-balanced choices of ordinary foods, permanent changes in eating habits, and increased physical activity (walking, biking, swimming, and dancing are excellent).

INFECTIOUS MONONUCLEOSIS

*An acute disease due to the **Epstein-Barr virus (EBV)**, characterized by fever, pharyngitis, and lymphadenopathy; it is usually associated with heterophil antibodies and an atypical lymphocytosis.*

Etiology

EBV is a ubiquitous herpesvirus with a host range limited primarily to B lymphocytes and nasopharyngeal cells of humans and certain non-human primates. After initial replication in the nasopharynx, the virus infects B lymphocytes, which are induced to secrete immunoglobulin. Among the specificities of these immunoglobulins are antigens present on sheep and beef erythrocytes. Antibodies to these antigens, termed **heterophil antibodies,** are useful diagnostically (see Laboratory Findings and Diagnosis, below).

The EBV-transformed B lymphocytes are the target of a multifaceted immune response. The **humoral immune response** may be used to document primary infection; the **cellular immune response,** consisting partly of induction of activated T lymphocytes of the CD8 surface phenotype, accounts mainly for the atypical lymphocytosis associated with primary EBV infection. Thus, the cell-mediated immune response plays a major role in preventing ongoing proliferation of EBV-transformed B lymphocytes during primary infection and in reversing EBV-induced polyclonal B cell activation.

Epidemiology

Primary EBV infection may occur during childhood, adolescence, or adulthood; about 50% of children have had such infection before the age of 5 yr. In most of these children, the infection is subclinical. In adolescents or adults, it may be subclinical or it may be recognized as a clinical syndrome (infectious mononucleosis), depending somewhat on the clinical setting. In prospective studies of university students, primary EBV infection was recognized as infectious mononucleosis in 30 to 70% of cases of seroconversion, but in similar studies among Peace Corps volunteers and military recruits, the infection was not clinically apparent in up to 90% of cases. Most individuals have acquired the virus by early adulthood, but even when primary EBV infection is delayed until late adulthood, it may be associated with typical symptoms of infectious mononucleosis.

After primary infection, EBV remains within the host for life and is intermittently shed from the oropharynx. The virus is detectable in oropharyngeal secretions of 15 to 25% of healthy EBV-seropositive adults on any given day. Oropharyngeal shedding is increased in frequency and titer in immunocompromised patients (eg, organ allograft recipients and persons with HIV infection). Reactivation of EBV, unlike that of herpes simplex or varicella zoster virus, is generally subclinical.

EBV is relatively labile, has not been recovered from environmental sources, and is not very contagious. Only about 5% of patients can give a history of recent contact with someone who has infectious mononucleosis. The incubation period is believed to be 30 to 50 days in most cases. Transmission may occur by transfusion of blood products but is much more frequently accomplished by oropharyngeal contact (kissing) between an uninfected and a healthy EBV-seropositive individual who is asymptomatically shedding the virus from the oropharynx. Early childhood transmission occurs more frequently among members of lower socioeconomic groups or under conditions of crowding.

EBV has also been associated with African Burkitt's lymphoma, certain B cell neoplasms in immunocompromised patients (especially those with organ allografts, HIV infection, or ataxia-telangiectasia), and nasopharyngeal carcinoma. These associations are based on serologic evidence of increased EBV activity and on the demonstration of EBV nuclear antigens **(EBNA)** and DNA in tumor biopsies. It has been postulated that EBV plays a role in certain B cell lymphomas by transforming and polyclonally stimulating B cells, making them more susceptible to subsequent chromosomal translocation and evolution of oligoclonal or monoclonal lymphoproliferation. Although EBNA have been demonstrated within nasopharyngeal cells and EBV receptors have been detected on nasopharyngeal epithelial cells, the precise role of EBV in the pathogenesis of nasopharyngeal carcinoma is not yet understood.

Over the past several years, a number of investigators have identified patients with an illness characterized by fatigue, mild cognitive dysfunction, and in some cases low-grade fever and lymphadenopathy. This illness, termed **chronic fatigue syndrome,** is observed primarily among adults between the ages of 20 and 40. In most clinical studies, females outnumber males by at least 2:1. Although some have speculated that EBV plays a role in the pathogenesis of chronic fatigue syndrome, little objective evidence supports this hypothesis. Thus, EBV-specific serologic studies are not indicated in evaluation of symptoms restricted to fatigue. Occasional case reports have supported an association between **chronic EBV infection** and a syndrome of fever, interstitial pneumonitis, pancytopenia, and uveitis. These patients with chronic EBV infection should be clearly distinguished from those with chronic fatigue syndrome who have no objective symptoms or signs.

Symptoms and Signs

Infectious mononucleosis typically consists of a tetrad of **fatigue, fever, pharyngitis,** and **lymphadenopathy;** however, patients may have all or only some of these features. Usually, a patient presents with malaise lasting several days to a week, followed by fever, pharyngitis, and adenopathy. The pharyngitis may be severe, painful, and exudative and may resemble streptococcal pharyngitis. The lymphadenopathy may involve any group of nodes but is usually symmetric; anterior and posterior cervical adenopathy is often prominent. Enlargement of a solitary node or group of nodes may be the sole clinical manifestation; in such cases, heterophil antibody studies may obviate the need for a lymph node biopsy or help in interpretation of rather worrisome histopathologic findings. Fever usually peaks in the afternoon or early evening,

with a temperature around 39.5° C (103° F), though it may reach 40.5° C (105° F). Fatigue is usually maximal in the first 2 to 3 wk. When fever and fatigue predominate (the so-called **typhoidal form** of the illness), onset and resolution may be much slower.

Splenomegaly, observed in about 50% of cases, is maximal during the 2nd and 3rd wk and is usually confined to a splenic tip palpable just below the left costal margin. Mild **hepatomegaly** and hepatic percussion tenderness may also be observed. Less frequent findings include maculopapular eruptions, jaundice, periorbital edema, and palatal enanthema.

Complications

Though most cases resolve uneventfully, complications may be dramatic and could overshadow other clinical manifestations.

CNS complications include encephalitis, seizures, Guillain-Barré syndrome, peripheral neuropathy, aseptic meningitis, myelitis, cranial nerve palsies, and psychosis. EBV-associated encephalitis may present with cerebellar manifestations, or it may be global and rapidly progressive, mimicking herpes simplex encephalitis. Unlike the latter, however, EBV-associated encephalitis is usually self-limited and fully reversible.

Hematologic complications include splenic rupture, granulocytopenia, thrombocytopenia, and hemolytic anemia. Splenic rupture results from splenic enlargement and capsular swelling, which is maximal 10 to 21 days after presentation. Though most patients note abdominal pain, splenic rupture is occasionally painless, and patients may present with hypotension. A history of trauma is present only about half of the time. Mild granulocytopenia or thrombocytopenia is observed transiently in about 50% of patients; severe cases, associated with bacterial infection or bleeding, are observed less frequently. Hemolytic anemia is usually due to antibodies of anti-i specificity. Hematologic manifestations are usually self-limited and do not require specific therapeutic intervention.

Pulmonary complications involve airway obstruction or interstitial pulmonary infiltration. Airway obstruction due to pharyngeal or paratracheal lymphadenopathy is an indication for hospitalization and possible surgical intervention, if corticosteroids fail to control the process. Interstitial pulmonary infiltrates are reported more frequently in pediatric cases, are usually found on radiography, and remain clinically silent.

Hepatic complications are signaled by abnormalities in liver function tests. Elevated hepatocellular enzyme levels (about 2 to 3 times normal, returning to baseline over 3 to 4 wk) are seen in about 95% of cases. If jaundice or more severe enzyme elevations are encountered, a search for other causes of hepatitis should be undertaken.

Overwhelming infection with EBV occurs sporadically, but a family history may also be encountered. In particular, an X-linked condition, termed **X-linked lymphoproliferative syndrome** or **Duncan's syndrome**, has been delineated in several kindreds. In these kindreds, primary EBV infection may be associated with uncontrolled lymphoproliferation, with aplastic anemia, or with hypogammaglobulinemia.

Laboratory Findings and Diagnosis

Although the clinical syndrome of infectious mononucleosis and its epidemiologic setting may be so stereotypical that the diagnosis seems certain, there is sufficient overlap with other illnesses to recommend laboratory testing.

Hematologic findings: In most patients, a mild leukocytosis is observed, usually accompanied by a more pronounced relative and absolute lymphocytosis, resulting from reactive lymphocytes that are morphologically atypical to varying degrees. Atypical lymphocytes may be absent or may account for up to 80% of the differential count. Individual lymphocytes may have such extremely bizarre morphologic characteristics that a hematologic malignancy may be suspected. However, the heterogeneity of such atypical lymphocytes distinguishes EBV infection from leukemia, which has more homogeneous morphologically atypical lymphocytes.

Serologic findings: Heterophil antibodies are directed at antigens present on erythrocytes obtained from sheep, horses, or cattle. These antibodies may be detected in only 50% of patients < 5 yr but are observed in 90% of adolescents and adults with primary EBV infection. The standard tube heterophil titer, in which serum is preabsorbed by guinea pig kidney (Forssman) antigens, is less sensitive, more labor-intensive, and of little additional diagnostic value compared with the wide variety of card-agglutination (Monospot) tests commercially available. The titer and prevalence of heterophil antibodies rise during the 2nd and 3rd wk of illness. Thus, if the diagnosis of infectious mononucleosis is strongly suspected on clinical grounds but the heterophil antibody test is negative, repeating the test after

7 to 10 days of symptoms is quite reasonable. Heterophil antibodies may persist for 6 to 12 mo after recovery from the illness.

Antibodies to EBV antigens are usually demonstrable when patients develop symptoms and present with primary EBV infection; they may also be used diagnostically. If a typical clinical syndrome is accompanied by detectable heterophil antibodies, EBV-specific serologic studies are not indicated. However, in children ≤ 4 yr, in whom heterophil antibodies may never turn positive, antibodies to the EBV viral capsid antigen **(VCA)** are helpful diagnostic aids. Appropriate use of EBV-specific antibodies requires a knowledge of when they appear in relation to primary EBV infection. EBV-VCA antibodies usually emerge during the incubation period. IgG antibodies to VCA persist for life in titers sufficiently high that detection of these antibodies is generally not helpful in determining whether a patient has primary EBV infection or another illness and a former EBV infection. However, IgM antibodies to VCA are present in all patients with primary EBV infection and disappear 2 to 3 mo after recovery; thus, demonstration of these antibodies is diagnostic of primary EBV infection. Since some commercial laboratories lack the capabilities to perform assays for IgM antibodies to VCA, consulting a reference laboratory may be useful if the diagnosis is in doubt. Antibodies to early antigens of 2 specificities (diffuse and restricted) are termed **anti-EAD** and **anti-EAR antibodies,** respectively. Anti-EAD antibodies are encountered in about 70% of adolescents and adults with infectious mononucleosis and are associated with more severe clinical manifestations and with nasopharyngeal carcinoma. Anti-EAR antibodies are less common and are associated with African Burkitt's lymphoma. **Antibodies to EBNA** generally appear later in primary EBV infection than do anti-VCA antibodies and thus occasionally may be more readily detectable than IgM antibodies to VCA.

Differential Diagnosis

The clinical syndrome of infectious mononucleosis may be induced by bacterial or other viral pathogens. The pharyngitis, lymphadenopathy, and fever may be clinically indistinguishable from that caused by Group A β-hemolytic streptococci; however, detection of this organism in the oropharynx does not rule out a diagnosis of infectious mononucleosis. The most common cause of heterophil-negative mononucleosis is cytomegalovirus **(CMV)**. Though CMV mononucleosis is less likely to be associated with severe pharyngitis, it may be associated with atypical lymphocytosis as well as hepatosplenomegaly and hepatitis. Diagnosis of primary CMV infection depends on demonstration of IgM anti-CMV antibodies and/or isolation of the agent from peripheral blood (see CYTOMEGALOVIRUS INFECTION under VIRAL INFECTIONS in Ch. 32). Heterophil-negative mononucleosis may also be associated with *Toxoplasma gondii,* hepatitis B, or rubella infection, and atypical lymphocytes may be associated with adverse drug reactions. A mononucleosis-like illness has also been observed in association with primary HIV infection. In most of these cases, other clinical features of the syndrome are helpful in establishing the correct diagnosis.

Prognosis

Infectious mononucleosis is usually self-limited. The duration of the illness is variable; the acute phase lasts about 2 wk. Patients are generally able to resume usual activities after this but may find that full resolution of the fatigue takes several more weeks. Prospective studies among military and university populations have established that 20% of patients can return to school or work within 1 wk and 50% within 2 wk. Occasionally fatigue, which is usually intermittent and of moderate intensity, lasts for months; such chronicity of symptoms occurs in only 1 to 2% of cases.

Death occurs in < 1% of cases and is most often associated with complications of primary EBV infection (eg, encephalitis, splenic rupture, airway obstruction).

Treatment

Treatment is largely supportive. Unless complications ensue, additional laboratory studies are generally not needed because recovery is not correlated with the persistence or titer of heterophil antibodies, the presence of atypical lymphocytes in the peripheral blood, or hepatocellular enzyme elevations. Patients should be encouraged to rest during the acute phase of the illness but should be quickly mobilized as the fever, pharyngitis, and malaise abate. Because of the risk of splenic rupture, heavy lifting and contact sports should be avoided for 2 mo after presentation, even if there is no splenomegaly.

Acetaminophen is preferable to aspirin as an analgesic and antipyretic because of the rare association of EBV with Reye's syndrome. **Corticosteroids** have been shown to hasten defervescence and relieve pharyngitis, but they should be used only to treat specific complications such as impending airway obstruction. Their efficacy in treating thrombocytopenia and hemolytic anemia is less well established. Oral or IV **acyclovir** decreases oropharyngeal shedding of EBV, but there is no convincing evidence to warrant its use in uncomplicated cases. Its usefulness in patients with overwhelming infection or transplant-associated B cell lymphoproliferative syndromes has not yet been established.

48. GENERAL PRINCIPLES OF MEDICAL GENETICS

The development of an individual depends on the interacting influences of genetic factors and environment. An individual's genetic composition, or **genome,** is established at conception; thereafter, a complex interaction of genes and environment (both internal and external) shapes his development. Though the genes remain largely unaltered, environmental experiences are constantly changing and may even alter the genome through **mutation,** or inheritable alteration of a gene.

Some genetic component probably exists in almost all diseases, but the extent of this component varies. For example, bacterial diseases are considered purely environmental, yet the human male is slightly more susceptible to most of them than the female. There is little doubt that genetic factors play a role, though the precise role is not known. Conversely, diseases such as Down syndrome and phenylketonuria are due to specific genetic defects, and the environment plays a relatively small role. Between the extremes is a host of conditions wherein genetic and environmental factors interact (eg, to produce birth defects or metabolic disorders).

Genes (molecules of DNA) are the basic units of heredity. The capacity of DNA to replicate itself constitutes the basis of hereditary transmission. DNA also provides the **genetic code,** which determines the development and metabolism of cells by controlling RNA synthesis. The sequential order of the components that make up RNA determines the amino acid composition of proteins, which in turn determines the functions of proteins and thereby of cells.

The many thousands of genes are carried by

the **chromosomes** (rod-like structures in the cell nuclei). In man, each somatic or non-germ cell normally has 46 chromosomes, arranged in 23 pairs. One pair, the **sex chromosomes**, determines the sex of the individual. The female has two X chromosomes in every somatic cell nucleus; the male has one X and one Y. The male sex chromosomes are **heterologous**, since the 2 members of the pair are not identical: The X chromosome is larger and carries genes responsible for many hereditary traits as well as for sex determination; the Y chromosome is small, is shaped differently, and carries primarily genes concerned only with male sex determination. The remaining 22 pairs of chromosomes, the **autosomes**, are **homologous**, since both members of a pair are usually identical in size, shape, and genetic loci.

The genes are arranged linearly along the chromosomes, each gene having its specific **locus**. The number and arrangement of loci on homologous chromosomes are identical, and genes that occupy homologous loci are called **alleles**. Each person has 2 alleles for each kind of gene, one on each chromosome of a pair, with the exception of most genes on the X and Y chromosomes in males. A person possessing a pair of identical alleles for a particular gene is a **homozygote**; one with a dissimilar pair of alleles is a **heterozygote**. If a gene exerts its effect when present on only 1 chromosome, the gene is **dominant**. A **recessive** gene is expressed only when present in both members of a chromosome pair (or in the single X of a normal male or a 45,X female). The gene, or its corresponding trait, is **X-linked** if it is located on the X chromosome; otherwise it is **autosomal.**

Three types of genetically determined disorders are (1) **mendelian** or **single-gene mutations**, which are inherited in recognizable patterns; (2) **polygenic** or **multifactorial conditions**, in which genetic mutations involving more than one gene and nongenetic factors interact in ways that are not always clearly recognizable; and (3) **chromosomal aberrations** or **abnormalities**, which include both structural defects and deviations from the normal number.

INHERITED DISORDERS

CONSTRUCTION OF THE PEDIGREE

In man, the chief method of genetic study is to observe family trees or **pedigrees**, which show the distribution of genetic traits in kindreds. A careful family history must be taken and a pedigree constructed in order to determine the inheritance pattern. Some familial disorders with identical **phenotypes**, or observable features, are inherited in different patterns. For example, cleft palate may be due to an autosomal dominant, an autosomal recessive, or an X-linked recessive gene, or it may be a multifactorial condition (ie, familial but with no precisely predictable inheritance pattern).

FIG. 48–1 shows the symbols used to construct a pedigree chart. As illustrated in the various pedigrees (FIGS. 48–2 to 48–5), the generations are numbered with Roman numerals, with the earliest at the top and the most recent at the bottom. Within each generation, individuals are numbered from left to right with Arabic numerals. Thus, each individual in the pedigree can be specifically identified by 2 numbers (eg, II, 4). A spouse who is included in the pedigree chart is also assigned an identifying number (eg, II, 6 in FIG. 48–2). Siblings are usually ranged by age, with the oldest on the left.

The study of a trait or a disease in a particular family begins with an affected person (the **proband, propositus**, or **index case**). When taking a family history, the pedigree must be drawn as the various relatives are being described. The inquiry begins with the siblings of the proband and proceeds to the parents; then to relatives of the parents, including brothers and sisters and their children; then to the grandparents; and so on. The number of relatives included in the pedigree is determined by the inheritance pattern of the condition and by the extent of the informant's memory or knowledge.

SINGLE–GENE HUMAN DEFECTS

Genetic disorders determined by a single gene are easiest to analyze and thus are the ones most fully studied. Single-gene defects may be autosomal or X-linked, dominant or recessive.

AUTOSOMAL DOMINANT INHERITANCE

A typical pedigree is shown in FIG. 48–2. In general, the following rules apply: (1) Every affected person has at least one affected parent. (2) An affected person marrying a normal individual has, on the average, an equal number of affected and normal children. (3) Normal children of an affected parent have normal children and grandchildren. (4) Males and females are equally likely to be affected. (5) The trait can ap-

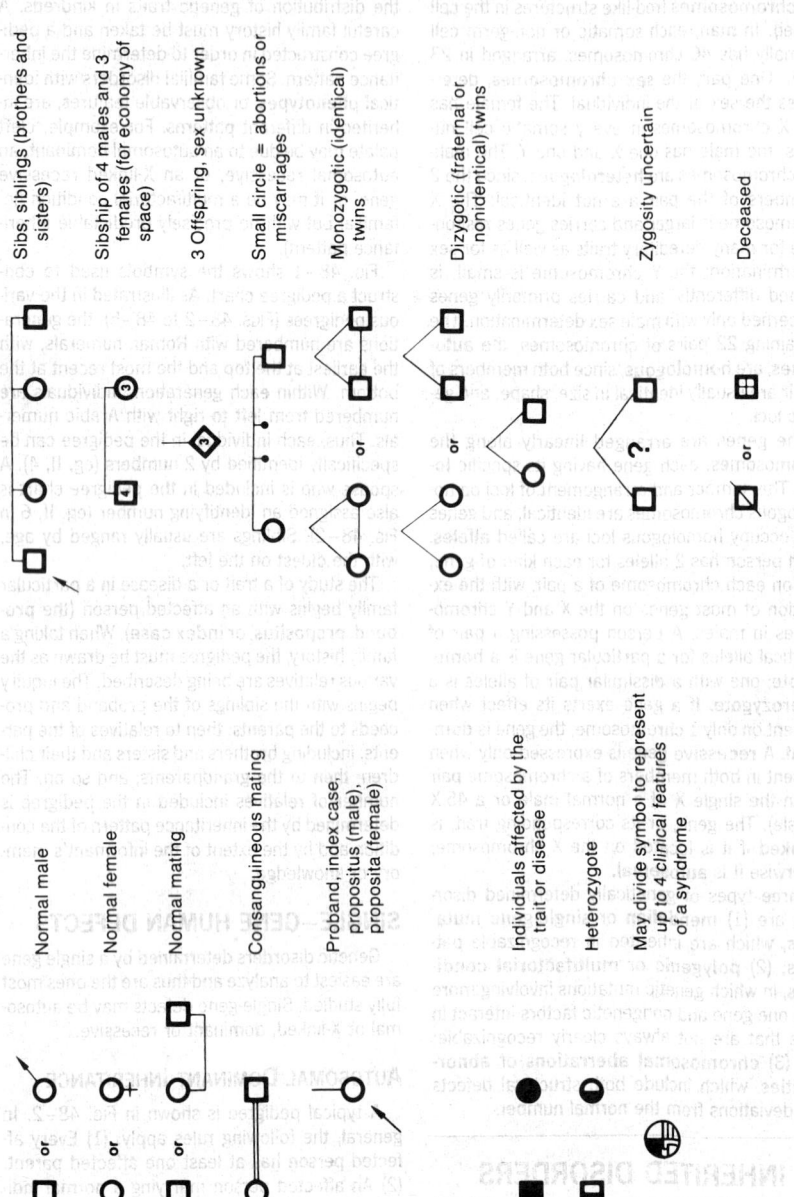

Fig. 48—1. Symbols used in constructing a pedigree chart.

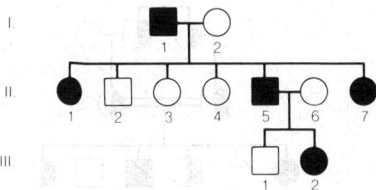

FIG. 48–2. Autosomal dominant inheritance.

pear in every generation. (6) Heterozygotes are affected.

Variations in the above rules are as follows:

1. Expressivity and penetrance: The effects of a single gene may be influenced both by the individual's environment and by the thousands of other genes that may alter the phenotypic expression (or expressivity) of the gene in question. Thus, even within a single family, affected individuals may manifest widely variable phenotypes. In **Waardenburg syndrome,** a condition characterized by white forelock, deafness, hypertelorism, and heterochromia of the iris, < 20% of cases have significant hearing loss. Some, with none of the features except white forelock, have had children with serious congenital deafness. Rarely, the expressivity of a dominant gene is so modified that no clinical abnormality can be detected, yet the individual can pass the gene to offspring, who may develop the full clinical picture. In this case, expressivity of the individual's gene is nil, and in the pedigree the gene will appear to skip a generation. This rare phenomenon is known as **lack of penetrance.** On the other hand, some cases of apparent lack of penetrance are due to the examiner's failure to recognize or to become familiar with the minor manifestations of the dominant condition. Cases with minimal expressivity are sometimes referred to as a **forme fruste** of the disease.

2. Pleiotropy (literally, "many forms"): A single-gene defect may produce multiple anomalies. For example, in **osteogenesis imperfecta** (an abnormality of connective tissue), various structures are affected (see under MUSCULOSKELETAL DEFECTS in Ch. 28), including fragile bones because they cannot be normally calcified and hypermobile joints that tend to dislocate. Minor manifestations of other pleiotropic genes may easily be missed.

3. Mutations arise spontaneously from time to time. An autosomal dominant pedigree begins with a fresh mutation, and fresh mutations are

surprisingly common in autosomal dominant disorders. For example, in a population of unrelated achondroplastic dwarfs, about 80% would have no family history and would thus presumably represent fresh mutations. Almost all would be able to transmit the freshly mutated genes to offspring. In general, the unaffected parents are not at increased risk of having additional affected offspring. However, in a few families, nondwarf parents have had 2 or even 3 typical achondroplastic dwarfs. The explanation is a germline mutation—an event that can occur early in the embryonic life of one parent when only a handful of germ cell precursors is present. The cell possessing the new mutation could then contribute a large number of cells to the developing gonad. In such cases it is impossible to predict the risk for subsequent pregnancies. Fortunately this is a fairly rare occurrence, but the existence of germline mutations has been confirmed through molecular studies of the actual gene mutation in parents and offspring.

4. Phenocopies: Very rarely, an individual appears with a syndrome indistinguishable from that caused by a fresh mutation, but does not transmit the condition to his offspring and apparently does not have the mutant gene—ie, the syndrome appears to be due to nongenetic phenomena or at least to a different genotype. A phenocopy is indistinguishable from an individual with an abnormal dominant gene who, by chance, fails to pass the gene to his offspring.

5. Sex-limited inheritance: A trait that appears in only one sex is **sex-limited.** Males are almost always the sex affected, usually because of X-linked inheritance (see below). However, sex hormones and other physiologic differences between males and females may greatly alter the expressivity of an allele. For example, premature baldness is almost certainly inherited as an autosomal dominant trait; but, presumably as a result of female sex hormones, the condition is rarely expressed in the female and then usually only af-

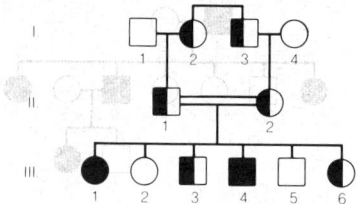

FIG. 48–3. Autosomal recessive inheritance.

ter menopause. Thus, sex-limitation, or perhaps more correctly, sex-influenced inheritance, is a special case of limited expressivity and penetrance.

6. Homozygous dominant genotype: This can occur in the offspring of 2 individuals who are heterozygous (or homozygous) for the same dominant gene (eg, the offspring of 2 achondroplastic dwarfs). In theory, the homozygote for the dominant gene is phenotypically indistinguishable from the heterozygote. However, in the few known marriages between persons with the same autosomal dominant abnormality, some offspring have had much more severe anomalies than either parent, suggesting that a pair of dominant alleles may have a worse effect than one. Also, in some of these matings, an increased number of spontaneous abortions and stillborn infants with multiple malformations has occurred, suggesting that the presence of 2 dominant alleles may at times be lethal. In contrast, the availability of gene markers for Huntington's disease has shown that there are no phenotypic differences between heterozygotes and homozygotes for this dominant condition. A homozygote would have 100% of offspring affected.

AUTOSOMAL RECESSIVE INHERITANCE

A typical pedigree is shown in FIG. 48–3. In general, the following rules apply: (1) If an affected person is born to normal parents, both parents are heterozygotes, and, on the average, $1/4$ of their offspring will be affected, $1/2$ will be heterozygotes, and $1/4$ will be normal. (2) If affected siblings come from a consanguineous marriage, there is strong evidence of recessive inheritance. (3) If an affected person and a genotypically normal person marry, all of their children will be phenotypically normal heterozygotes. (4) If an affected person and a heterozygote marry, on the average $1/2$ of their children will be affected and $1/2$ will be heterozygotes. (5) If 2 affected people marry, all of their children

will be affected. (6) Males and females are equally likely to be affected. (7) Heterozygotes are phenotypically normal but are carriers of the trait. Where a defect of a specific protein (eg, an enzyme) is recognized as the cause of the disease, the carrier usually has a reduced amount of that protein.

Most diseases due to homozygosity for autosomal recessive mutant genes are rare (eg, most inborn errors of metabolism). Affected individuals are homozygous, and each parent is a heterozygote or carrier.

Consanguinity becomes an important factor in autosomal recessive diseases since related individuals are much more likely to share the same mutant allele. A detailed family history taken from both parents may disclose an unknown or forgotten consanguinity.

X-LINKED RECESSIVE INHERITANCE

A typical pedigree is shown in FIG. 48–4. In general, the following rules apply: (1) Nearly all affected persons are males. (2) The trait is always transmitted through the heterozygous mother, who is phenotypically normal. (3) An affected male never transmits the trait to his sons. (4) All daughters of an affected male will be carriers. (5) The carrier female transmits the trait to $1/2$ of her sons. None of her daughters will show the trait, but $1/2$ will be carriers.

More than 300 traits, most of which are diseases (eg, inborn errors of metabolism), are a result of mutant genes on the X chromosome. Since the human male has only one X chromosome, the term **hemizygous** is applied. In males, all genes on the X chromosome, whether recessive or dominant, are expressed; this explains the predominance of males in X-linked recessive conditions. An affected female (with rare exceptions) must be homozygous for the mutant allele; ie, it must be present in both X chromosomes. This can happen only if her father is affected and her mother is either heterozygous or else homo-

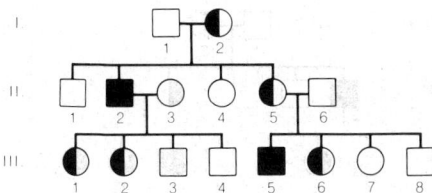

FIG. 48–4. X-linked recessive inheritance.

zygous for the mutant allele. Since most X-linked mutants are rare, affected females are very rare (the incidence in females is the square of that in males). In addition, on the average, $1/2$ of the maternal uncles of the proband will be affected, and since $1/2$ of the maternal aunts will be carriers, some of the proband's male maternal first cousins will also be affected.

On occasion, females known to be heterozygous for X-linked mutations show varying degrees of expression, but rarely as severely as the affected (hemizygous) male (see The Lyon Hypothesis under SYNDROMES ASSOCIATED WITH SEX CHROMOSOME ABERRATIONS, below). In addition, a structural chromosomal rearrangement (eg, an X-autosome translocation) can result in an affected female even though she is a heterozygote.

X-LINKED DOMINANT INHERITANCE

A typical pedigree is shown in FIG. 48–5. In general, the following rules apply: (1) Affected males transmit the trait to all of their daughters but none of their sons. (2) Affected heterozygous females transmit the condition to $1/2$ of their children regardless of sex. (3) Affected homozygous females transmit the trait to all of their children.

X-linked dominant mutants are very rare, with females usually more mildly affected than males. For example, in nephrogenic diabetes insipidus, females show mild degrees of polydipsia and polyuria. In incontinentia pigmenti, the X-linked gene appears to be lethal in males and causes a peculiar swirling pattern of melanin pigmentation and other anomalies in affected females.

Since it is difficult to distinguish X-linked dominant from autosomal dominant inheritance, large pedigrees are required with particular attention given to the offspring of affected males, since male-to-male transmission rules out X-linkage. However, the new gene technology (see ADVANCES IN MOLECULAR GENETICS, below) is providing the means to solve this problem. For example, Alport's syndrome (*hereditary nephritis with deafness*) was believed to be an autosomal dominant trait. One of the problems is that affected males become sicker from the kidney disease earlier and more severely than affected females, and very few males have reproduced. Recently, an X-linked probe clearly showed that the gene is on the X chromosome. Similarly, gene probes can now distinguish between the X-linked and the autosomal dominant forms of Charcot-Marie-Tooth disease (peroneal muscular atrophy). Genetic counseling is more accurate and more helpful as a result of these advances.

CODOMINANT INHERITANCE

Only a *trait* or *disease* can be dominant or recessive, not the *gene* itself, since most often both alleles at a genetic locus produce some product. Codominance can only be observed if the phenotypes are qualitatively different, as with the blood group antigens (AB, MN), the WBC antigens, and serum proteins differing in electrophoretic mobility (albumin, haptoglobin, etc). Confusion occurs where heterozygotes are clinically normal and the condition is usually considered recessive, as in sickle cell disease. However, if the basis for the phenotype is taken to be the sickle cell preparation, which is positive in heterozygotes as well as homozygotes, the disorder could be considered dominant. Or, the condition can be thought of as codominant if one looks at the Hb electrophoresis, since the ratio of sickle Hb to normal Hb in the heterozygote is roughly 40:60.

MULTIFACTORIAL INHERITANCE

Close relatives tend to resemble each other with respect to a number of quantitative or measurable characteristics (eg, height, weight, size and shape of nose and other facial features, BP, and "intelligence"). Many of these traits have a distribution that fits the familiar bell-shaped curve known as the normal curve, a phenomenon that is compatible with determination of the trait by a number of genes. Each gene adds to or subtracts from the trait, and each acts in an addi-

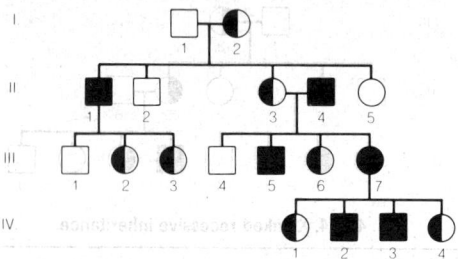

FIG. 48–5. X-linked dominant inheritance.

tive manner independently of the others with no dominance. There are few individuals at the extremes of the distribution and many in the middle, since an individual is unlikely to inherit a large number of factors all acting in the same direction. In addition, a number of environmental factors, each adding to or subtracting from the final result, will also produce a normal distribution. Most of the time, the variation in the population results from a number of genes and environmental factors acting together to determine the final result. This is termed **multifactorial inheritance.**

A large number of relatively common congenital anomalies and diseases that are clearly familial do not fit the expectations for mendelian inheritance. More likely these conditions result from multifactorial inheritance of a continuously distributed variable, with a threshold separating the affected individual from the normal. Thus, the affected patient has a liability or predisposition to the condition representing the sum of genetic and environmental influences.

This concept explains the relatively high risk of the trait in first-degree relatives (siblings and children), who share 50% of their genes, and the much lower risk to the more distant relatives, who are likely to inherit only a few of the high-liability genes.

The **neural tube defects** (anencephaly, encephalocele, myelomeningocele), often referred to collectively as **spina bifida**, are a common example. In the North American white population they occur with a combined incidence of about 1.5/1000 live births. The parents of an affected infant, now identified as carrying a relatively large number of high-liability genes, have about a 1/30 chance of producing a 2nd affected offspring (this 3% risk has been calculated mathematically and confirmed by empiric data from population studies). Similarly, the patient with a neural tube defect, if able to have children, has a 3 to 4% chance of having an affected child. In the relatively rare instance where a couple has had 2 affected children, the risk for a 3rd rises further (7 to 8%). For the neural tube defects, environmental factors unquestionably play a role. For example, the incidence approaches 1/100 in areas in the western part of the United Kingdom, and clusters of cases have appeared in some neighborhoods. When people from these high-risk areas emigrate to North America, their risk falls but remains higher than that of the American population. A recent multicenter international study indicated that daily oral supplementation with folic acid before conception and during early pregnancy substantially reduces the recurrence of neural tube defects. Whether folic acid deficiency is the sole environmental factor or one of several factors remains to be determined.

Other examples of multifactorial inheritance, with similar risks for siblings and offspring of affected individuals, are congenital anomalies of the heart (see in Ch. 28), idiopathic epilepsy (petit or grand mal), congenital megacolon (Hirschsprung's disease), most cases of cleft lip with or without cleft palate, and many forms of cancer (see below). Congenital pyloric stenosis provides an interesting variation on the multifactorial theme. There is a striking male:female ratio of 5:1, suggesting that the threshold for girls is higher. Thus, the female apparently requires more potent liability genes in order to develop the condition, and should have more affected sibs and a greater risk of producing affected offspring than a male with pyloric stenosis. Family studies confirm this.

Currently, attention is being focused on a group of common disorders with multifactorial cause (eg, arteriosclerotic heart disease, diabetes mellitus, cancer, and arthritis). Genetically determined predisposing factors, including positive family history and biochemical and molecular parameters, are being used to identify individuals at increased risk who would be most likely to benefit from preventive measures (eg, drugs, special diets, changes in life-style, and changes in occupation; see PREVENTION OF GENETIC DISORDERS, below).

GENETIC HETEROGENEITY

The tremendous capacity of the human organism to vary both phenotypically and genotypically should be emphasized. Heterogeneity occurs in almost all inborn errors of metabolism, resulting from different alleles or mutations at different loci; eg, > 12 mutations are now known to produce the phenotype of Hurler's syndrome (see TABLE 42–4). Over 60 specific causes of congenital deafness have been identified; some are genetic, others result from rubella virus and other environmental agents. There is growing concern about the teratogenic effects of drugs taken during pregnancy. Women who consume large quantities of alcohol during pregnancy have a high risk of producing infants with severe intrauterine growth and mental retardation, as well as congenital malformations (the fetal alcohol syndrome—see under METABOLIC PROBLEMS IN THE NEWBORN in Ch. 27).

Thus, phenotypically similar conditions may be due to different mutations, nongenetic factors, or combinations of both. In order to establish the cause of the patient's problem and determine the risk for future offspring as accurately as possible, the physician must take a thorough family history, including an inquiry into possible environmental teratogens, keeping heterogeneity in mind.

MITOCHONDRIAL DNA ABNORMALITIES

Mitochondria are *intracellular organelles that generate energy via a series of respiratory chain complexes.* They contain a unique circular chromosome that codes for 13 proteins, a variety of RNAs, and several regulating enzymes. However, > 90% of the mitochondrial proteins are coded by nuclear genes.

Although the first human mitochondrial disease was identified > 30 yr ago, it was not until 1988 that the first association between mitochondrial DNA abnormalities (large deletions) and human disease, chronic progressive external ophthalmoplegia **(CPEO)** and its variant, the multisystem **Kearns-Sayre syndrome** (*CPEO, heart block, retinitis pigmentosa, and CNS degeneration*) was made. Similar deletions are found in **Pearson syndrome** (*sideroblastic anemia, pancreatic insufficiency, and progressive liver disease that begins in the first few months of life and is frequently lethal in infancy*). Several other clinical syndromes have been recently identified as probably related to mitochondrial failure, including **Leber's hereditary optic neuropathy** (*a variable but often devastating bilateral visual loss that often occurs in the teenage years and is due to a point mutation in mitochondrial DNA*).

Maternal inheritance characterizes abnormalities of mitochondrial DNA since mitochondria are passed on via the ova. Thus, all offspring of an affected female should be affected and none of the offspring of an affected male. Variability in the clinical manifestations is the rule and may be due to variable mixtures of mutant and normal mitochondrial genomes within cells and tissues.

Mitochondrial pathology extends into more common disorders (eg, large mitochondrial deletions in the cells of the basal ganglia of patients with Parkinson's disease). Perhaps of greater interest is the demonstration of decreasing respiratory chain efficiency and progressive accumulation of mitochondrial DNA deletions with age, leading to the possibility of a role for mitochondria in the natural aging process.

GENETICS OF MALIGNANT DISEASE

(Neurofibromatosis [von Recklinghausen's disease] is discussed in Ch. 43)

Little is known of the genetics of most types of cancer, but the pieces of the puzzle are slowly falling into place. The new techniques of molecular genetics have confirmed the existence of **oncogenes**—literally, tumor genes—which at least in some instances are normal genes that were responsible for control of embryonic or fetal development and are present in everyone. Normally they are inactivated and remain so. It is now clear, however, that the human genome is not as stable as once was thought, and when some of these "regulatory" genes are relocated or rearranged as a result of a chromosomal translocation, inversion, or even simple breaking, they may act to initiate a malignancy. The rearrangements may be induced by a variety of environmental agents or by genetically determined events that are poorly understood.

In some families there seem to be many instances of various and apparently unrelated malignancies, while few cases of cancer appear in other families from similar environments. Most malignancies seem to occur in genetically predisposed individuals who are at some time exposed to environmental carcinogens (many of them as yet unknown). However, some malignancies clearly show mendelian or multifactorial inheritance.

Familial polyposis of the colon: This well-known autosomal dominant condition is a good example of the potential for prevention using the new molecular genetic technology. At the moment, individuals at risk must undergo regular rectosigmoidoscopy, colonoscopy, and barium enemas in order to detect the premalignant polyps as early as possible. Removal of the affected part of the bowel will prevent malignancy. In the near future, gene probes will be able to detect the relatives who have actually inherited the gene, and the bowel investigations will not be required for those who did not.

Even more important has been the association between mutations at or near the gene locus that causes familial polyps and some forms of carcinoma of the colon unassociated with polyps. This raises the possibility of the use of probes to identify individuals in the general population who, because of their inheriting a certain predisposing gene or genes, are at increased risk of developing colonic carcinoma, a disease with an incidence of about 5%.

Retinoblastoma, a relatively common tumor, accounts for 2% of childhood malignancies. Its multiple occurrence in about 40% of families indicates that some cases are due to an autosomal dominant gene, especially when the tumor is bilateral. Recent studies have demonstrated a deletion of a segment of chromosome 13q in some retinoblastoma patients, and the gene has been mapped to the 13q14 band and cloned (see discussion of nomenclature under CHROMOSOME ABERRATIONS, below). Gene probes have already been found for identification of potentially affected newborns, but until they are widely available, careful and repeated eye examinations of subsequent offspring are mandatory. With early diagnosis and treatment, survival and preservation of sight (even in the affected eye) can be anticipated. The closely related and more common childhood malignancy, **neuroblastoma,** is beginning to show a similar but less frequent familial incidence as more patients survive and have children. Urinary catecholamine levels should be determined in siblings and offspring at ages 6 and

12 mo. Similarly, a small fraction of **Wilms' tumors** is due to an inherited mutation, and the aniridia–Wilms' tumor syndrome invariably occurs in individuals with a specific chromosomal deletion (11p13).

Xeroderma pigmentosum is a rare, disfiguring syndrome inherited as an autosomal recessive trait. Areas of depigmentation, hyperpigmentation, telangiectasia, and epidermal scarring occur, and epidermal carcinomas frequently develop (particularly on exposure to sunlight).

Immunologic deficiency diseases (the inherited agamma- and dysgammaglobulinemias) carry an increased risk of malignancies of the lymphoid system, particularly lymphomas and leukemias.

In patients with Down syndrome (see below), **leukemia** develops about 15 times more often than in the normal population. Similarly, a group of **"chromosome instability"** syndromes (eg, Fanconi's anemia, Bloom's syndrome, ataxia telangiectasia) exists that are characterized by increased chromosome breakage and a high risk of leukemia or lymphoma; each is inherited as an autosomal recessive trait.

Carcinoma of the breast occurs significantly more often in daughters of similarly affected women than in the general population. Presumably, this is an example of multifactorial inheritance. Females at risk should be apprised of this, and regular self-examination of the breasts and mammography should be emphasized.

Carcinoma of the lung: First-degree relatives of individuals with lung cancer appear to be significantly more at risk, especially if they smoke cigarettes.

POPULATION GENETICS

Knowing the incidence of various mutations in different populations is important. For example, when a case of phenylketonuria (PKU) occurs, family members who are carriers of the abnormal gene will want to know their risk of marrying another carrier. This risk depends on the frequency with which that particular gene occurs in the population. Furthermore, many genes that cause serious human disease occur with a different frequency in different racial and ethnic groups. For instance, Tay-Sachs disease is nearly 100 times more frequent among Ashkenazi Jews than among non-Jews, and the incidence of heterozygotes in Ashkenazis is 1/30 (see DIAGNOSTIC

AND SCREENING PROCEDURES under PREVENTION OF GENETIC DISORDERS, below).

In the study of human genetics, representative samples of populations are surveyed to calculate gene frequencies. With autosomal dominant genes, the frequency in a given population can be calculated merely by identifying cases of the disease. The gene frequency for X-linked recessive genes can be calculated by determining the frequency of affected males in a male population. In autosomal recessive conditions, usually only the homozygote or affected individual can be detected with certainty; the asymptomatic carrier is seldom positively identifiable. However, the frequency of the carrier for autosomal recessive conditions can be determined from the frequency of the homozygote by using the following mathematical procedure. For any 2 alleles, A and a, there are 3 possible genotypes: AA, Aa, and aa. If the proportion of "A" genes in the population is represented as p and the proportion of "a" genes as q, then p plus q must equal 100%. Since gene frequencies are expressed as a fraction of unity, the equation is written $p + q = 1$. With random mating, the various combinations of gametes can be represented as a simple binomial expansion, and the frequencies of the various offspring will be in the proportion p^2 (AA), $2 pq$ (Aa), and q^2 (aa). This distribution of genotypes remains essentially the same from generation to generation (the **Hardy-Weinberg law**).

The analysis is more than an exercise in algebra because, by knowing the ratio of the various genotypes (p^2, $2 pq$, q^2), their frequency can be determined if the frequency of the affected homozygote is known. For example, cystic fibrosis (aa) has a frequency, among whites, of about 1/2500 live births. Thus:

$$q^2 = 1/2500$$
$$\text{therefore } q = 1/50$$
$$\text{but} \quad p = 1 - q$$
$$\text{therefore } p = 1 - 1/50$$
$$= 49/50$$
$$\simeq 1$$

$$
\begin{aligned}
\text{The frequency} & \\
\text{of carriers (Aa)} &= 2\,pq \\
&= 2 \times 1 \times 1/50 \\
&= 1/25
\end{aligned}
$$

This simple example shows that *carriers of a recessive condition are much more common than affected individuals.* Since most recessively in-

herited diseases are rare, p can be considered as 1, and the carrier frequency can be quickly estimated by calculating q and multiplying by 2.

When **cystic fibrosis** has occurred in one or more siblings in a family, each normal sibling has a 2:3 chance of being a heterozygote. These normal siblings should know their risk of having affected children. If a normal sibling marries an unrelated individual, that individual has a 1:25 chance of being a carrier. If 2 heterozygous individuals marry, their chance of having an affected child is 1:4. Therefore, the risk of having an affected child is 2:3 × 1:25 × 1:4, or about 1:150. Since the gene for cystic fibrosis has been cloned, these risks can now be modified by appropriate family studies (see under DIAGNOSTIC AND SCREENING PROCEDURES, below).

Consanguinity is a common indication for genetic counseling; autosomal recessive conditions are the major concern. Every human being is heterozygous for 6 to 8 alleles that would, in the homozygous state, lead to one of the several hundred known recessive diseases. Among incestuous unions where 50% of the genome is shared (eg, parent-child or brother-sister), abnormal offspring are common. Yet for the more often encountered first-cousin unions, in which 1:8 genes are shared, the risk of genetically determined disease is 3 to 5%, as compared to a risk of about 2% for nonconsanguineous parents. Some studies suggest an increased incidence of spontaneous abortions, stillbirths, prematurity, cerebral palsy, multifactorial conditions (eg, congenital dislocation of the hip), and infertility for first-cousin marriages, but the increases have been small and usually not statistically significant. For couples less closely related than first cousins, data are sparse, and the risks seem little if any increased over those for the nonconsanguineous population. Thus, there is little reason to discourage first-cousin marriages and no reason to discourage unions between less closely related couples, unless dealing with highly inbred groups (eg, the Amish or Mennonites) where heterozygosity for deleterious genes is often greatly increased.

GENETIC COUNSELING IN HEREDITARY DISORDERS

Physicians must recognize the hereditary nature of many human illnesses, and must impart this information to the patient or the family. Genetic counseling should be no different from counseling by a physician for any other illness. The facts should be clearly presented to all concerned family members so that they can make a rational decision about further pregnancies. Patients often misunderstand and misinterpret genetic information during the counseling session. Follow-up visits and written communications are usually very helpful. In addition, there is a remarkably large number of parent and family support groups related to specific genetic diseases (eg, the National Neurofibromatosis Foundation and the Williams Syndrome Association). Most publish informative brochures and newsletters, and many hold regular meetings with chapters in numerous locales.

Genetic counseling centers have been established at all medical schools in the USA and Canada, and private genetics programs are also appearing. Patients and families can be referred for diagnosis, counseling, and management, and the staff will provide physicians with up-to-date information should the referring physician wish to undertake the counseling himself. A working relationship with a genetics center has become essential for the practicing physician, in large part because of the rapidly developing applications of molecular genetics to patient care, particularly in early diagnosis, carrier detection, and prevention (see PREVENTION OF GENETIC DISORDERS, below).

SINGLE-GENE DEFECTS

More than 4000 conditions have been identified as single-gene defects for which the risk of producing affected offspring can be predicted mathematically.

Autosomal Dominant Conditions

The statistical risk of recurrence is 50%, regardless of the outcome of previous pregnancies; usually there is no sex predilection. If the family history is negative and the case is presumed to be a fresh mutation, the risk to siblings is nearly zero, but the affected individual risks transmitting the dominant mutant to $1/2$ of his offspring. (This is not true of phenocopies.)

Huntington's disease (HD) exemplifies a major problem posed by some autosomal dominant diseases. Though the abnormal gene is present at conception, its manifestations are usually delayed until the mid 30s or later. By this time, the unsuspecting victim may already have produced offspring, $1/2$ of whom have inherited the HD gene and will eventually develop the disease. Most physicians feel, therefore, that all individuals at risk—all children and all siblings of an affected individual—should consider not having children. These are individual decisions, how-

ever, and the physician must not allow personal biases to interfere. Recent developments in molecular genetics have provided new options for HD families (see PREVENTION OF GENETIC DISORDERS, below).

Autosomal Recessive Conditions

The risk to siblings of an affected individual is 25% and, again, families must realize that the same risk applies to each pregnancy. The analogy with drawing cards from a deck is useful: the chance of drawing a heart, club, spade, or diamond is 1:4, but it is not uncommon to draw 2 or even 3 cards of the same suit in a row.

Since consanguinity increases the risk, a family pedigree should be constructed before counseling, and the patient should be advised of the hazard of marrying a close relative. Heterozygote detection (see below) is also an important factor in autosomal recessive conditions.

X-Linked Recessive Conditions

A heterozygous female has a 25% chance of having an affected child, since the chance of having a male child is 50%, and 50% of male offspring are affected. Since heterozygous females have normal girls, prenatal detection of fetal sex by amniocentesis is a possible means of prevention. However, the rapidly increasing availability of X-linked gene probes has made detection of the affected male fetus a reality for several diseases (see PREVENTION OF GENETIC DISORDERS, below).

X-Linked Dominant Conditions

Of the children of affected females, $1/2$ will be affected regardless of sex; ie, the risk for offspring of affected females is the same as for autosomal dominant traits. *All* of the daughters and none of the sons of an affected male will be affected.

MULTIFACTORIAL CONDITIONS

Many congenital anomalies and syndromes are of multifactorial origin. The low recurrence risk is discussed above, and the possibility of prevention through prenatal diagnosis and selective abortion must be presented to couples at risk (see PREVENTION OF GENETIC DISORDERS, below, and Ch. 13).

HETEROZYGOTE DETECTION

This is a neglected, but extremely important, aspect of genetic counseling, especially in X-linked recessive conditions. In such families, female siblings of affected boys, as well as maternal aunts, run a high risk of being heterozygotes, and thus may themselves have affected children. It is the physician's responsibility to point this out to families and to keep up with the molecular genetic approaches to carrier detection.

Heterozygotes for X-Linked Conditions

Muscular dystrophy (Duchenne or pseudohypertrophic type; see also in Ch. 43): In affected males, the diagnosis is made from the clinical picture, muscle biopsy, and high serum concentrations of enzymes released from damaged muscle. The most useful is the serum creatine kinase (**CK**). In heterozygotes, CK levels lie between those of affected males and those of normal individuals. Unfortunately, CK values in normal and heterozygous females overlap considerably, so that only about 70% of heterozygous females can be positively identified. Today, however, Duchenne and the less severe Becker type muscular dystrophy are among the diseases for which DNA probes are available. They now provide the long-awaited means for accurate carrier detection and prenatal diagnosis of affected male fetuses (see PREVENTION OF GENETIC DISORDERS, below).

Hemophilia: Affected males have very low levels of serum antihemophilic globulin (**AHG**). Heterozygous females have, on the average, 50% of normal amounts of AHG, and tests combining AHG activity with immunologic quantitation of AHG protein appear to detect > 90% of heterozygotes. New methods of therapy using self-administered AHG concentrates, and in the very near future, pure AHG produced by recombinant DNA technology, are changing the prognosis in hemophilia. Prenatal detection of the hemophilias using gene probes is now available, and prevention by selective abortion of males is a clinical reality. Ethical issues must be discussed with each family.

Hunter's syndrome (X-linked mucopolysaccharidosis): The affected hemizygous male and heterozygous female can both be detected biochemically with close to 100% accuracy, and the affected male is detectable prenatally through enzyme assay or by X-linked gene probes in cultured amniotic fluid cells and chorionic villi (see Amniocentesis under DIAGNOSTIC AND SCREENING PROCEDURES, below).

Lesch-Nyhan syndrome (hereditary hyperuricemia): Usually, affected males are severely mentally and physically retarded, have marked hyperuricemia, and exhibit a peculiar propensity to self-mutilation by chewing their lips and fingertips, which leads to tissue loss and scarring. The basic enzymatic defect is known, and cases and carriers are detectable with almost 100% accuracy through biochemical studies on cultured cells. Affected males can be detected prenatally, as with Hunter's syndrome.

Autosomal Recessive Conditions

Heterozygote detection in autosomal recessive conditions is less vital than in X-linked conditions. Most autosomal recessive mutant genes that cause disease are rare, and thus, even though 2:3 of the phenotypically normal siblings of an affected person are heterozygotes, the chance of marrying a carrier of the same mutant is remote, and the chance of having affected offspring is even more remote. However, a consanguineous marriage greatly increases the risk of affected offspring. The actual risk for these situations can be calculated by using the formula given in POPULATION GENETICS, above. Heterozygote detection is important when the gene frequency is high, as occurs among certain ethnic and racial groups (see Screening Programs, below).

CHROMOSOME ABERRATIONS

Today it is relatively simple to culture cells and obtain chromosome preparations from many human cells and tissues, including circulating blood lymphocytes. Physicians in any location can mail a few milliliters of heparinized venous blood to a cytogenetics laboratory. Specimens should not be refrigerated, but must be packaged in a well-insulated container to avoid freezing or breakage. In the laboratory, the RBCs are sedimented out and the leukocytes are incubated in culture medium for 2 to 3 days. A bean extract, phytohemagglutinin, both accelerates the precipitation of RBCs and stimulates the division of lymphocytes. Then colchicine, a drug that arrests mitosis during metaphase, is added to the culture. Thus a large number of cells accumulate in metaphase, the time during the cell cycle when chromosomes are best visualized. Each chromosome has replicated (made a copy of itself) and appears as 2 chromatids attached at the centromere or central constriction. A variety of chromosome staining techniques is available, and after the treated cells are spread onto micro-

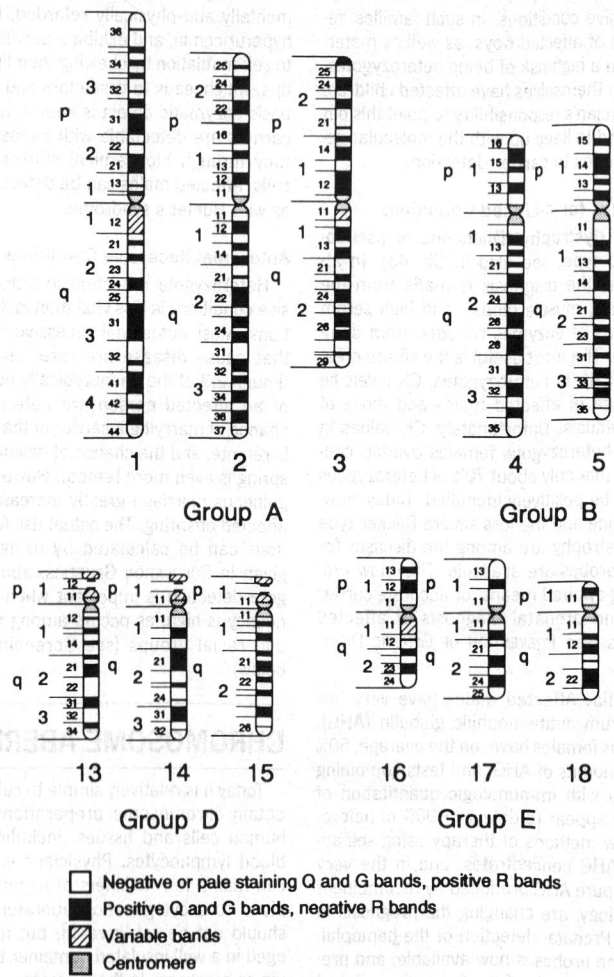

Group A

Group B

Group D

Group E

☐ Negative or pale staining Q and G bands, positive R bands

■ Positive Q and G bands, negative R bands

▨ Variable bands

▧ Centromere

FIG. 48–6. A diagrammatic representation of chromosome bands as observed with the Q-, G-, and R-staining methods; centromere representative of Q-staining method only. Each chromosome appears as a single strand joined at the centromere or central construction. The 23 pairs of chromosomes are sorted by size, position of centromere, and specific banding pattern; and the autosomes are numbered

scope slides, the chromosomes from single cells are photographed. Individual chromosomes can be cut out of the print and pasted onto a piece of paper. This chromosome picture is called a **karyotype**. Chromosomes can be stained using the Giemsa or G banding technique. The banding pattern produced by this procedure and a related technique using quinacrine mustard as the

stain (the Q banding technique, yielding fluorescent bands) permits identification of each chromosome in the human complement. Additional staining procedures and new techniques for extending chromosome length have greatly increased the precision of cytogenetic diagnosis (see FIG. 48–6 for a diagrammatic illustration of the standard chromosome bands).

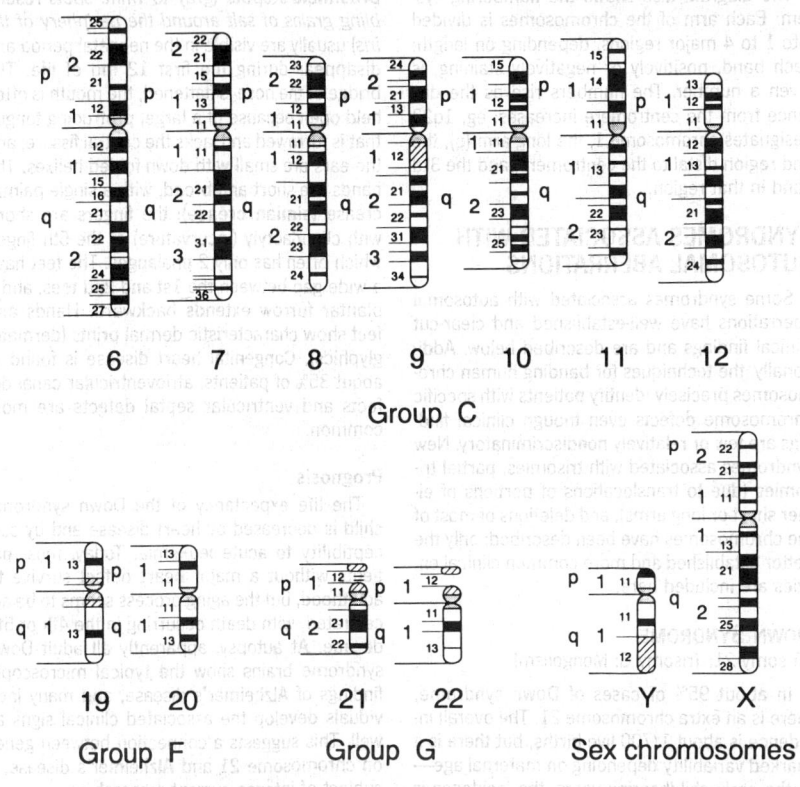

6   7   8   9   10   11   12

Group C

19   20   21   22   Y   X

Group F   Group G   Sex chromosomes

from 1 to 22. The chromosomes retain the classic X and Y designations. The older groupings of the chromosomes by letter, which was done before banding techniques were introduced, are also shown. (Adapted from McKusick VA: *Mendelian Inheritance in Man*, ed. 8, Appendix B—The Human Gene Map, pp xlii–xliii. Baltimore, The Johns Hopkins University Press, 1988; used with permission.)

The nomenclature for describing the human karyotype requires a brief explanation. The normal male and female are designated as 46,XY and 46,XX, respectively. In Down syndrome, when there is an extra chromosome 21 (trisomy 21), the notation for a female is 47,XX,21+ and for a male 47,XY,21+. When a chromosome has a structural abnormality, it is necessary to spec-

ify whether the long or short arm is affected; the letter p represents the short arm, q represents the long arm, and t represents a translocation. Thus, for a deletion of the short arm of chromosome 5 (as in the cat-cry syndrome) the female karyotype is 46,XX, 5p–. The typical 14/21 "balanced translocation carrier" parent (mother, in this example) of a translocation Down syndrome patient is written 45,XX, t(14q;21q): The translocation chromosome is formed from 14q and 21q; the short arms are lost.

The diagram also shows the numbering system: Each arm of the chromosomes is divided into 1 to 4 major regions, depending on length; each band, positively or negatively staining, is given a number. The numbers rise as the distance from the centromere increases; eg, 1q23 designates chromosome 1, the long arm (q), the 2nd region distal to the centromere, and the 3rd band in that region.

SYNDROMES ASSOCIATED WITH AUTOSOMAL ABERRATIONS

Some syndromes associated with autosomal aberrations have well-established and clear-cut clinical findings and are described below. Additionally, the techniques for banding human chromosomes precisely identify patients with specific chromosome defects even though clinical findings are few or relatively nondiscriminatory. New syndromes associated with trisomies, partial trisomies (due to translocations of portions of either short or long arms), and deletions of most of the chromosomes have been described; only the better established and more common clinical entities are included here.

DOWN SYNDROME
(Trisomy 21; Trisomy G; Mongolism)

In about 95% of cases of Down syndrome, there is an extra chromosome 21. The overall incidence is about 1/700 live births, but there is a marked variability depending on maternal age—in the early childbearing years, the incidence is about 1/2000 live births; for mothers over age 40, it rises to about 1/40 live births (see also TABLE 13-1). Just over 20% of infants with Down syndrome are born to mothers > 35 yr, yet these older mothers have only 7 to 8% of the children. However, the number of women having babies after age 35 has been rising quite rapidly in the last few years. The extra chromosome 21 comes from the father in 1/4 to 1/3 of the cases.

Symptoms and Signs

Infants tend to be placid, rarely cry, and demonstrate muscular hypotonicity. Nuchal lymphedema, similar to that seen in Turner's syndrome, also occurs in Down syndrome and is being detected with increasing frequency prenatally by fetal ultrasonography. Physical and mental development are retarded; the mean IQ is about 50.

Microcephaly, brachycephaly, and a flattened occiput are characteristic. The eyes are slanted, and epicanthal folds usually are present. **Brushfield's spots** (gray to white spots resembling grains of salt around the periphery of the iris) usually are visible in the neonatal period and disappear during the first 12 mo of life. The bridge of the nose is flattened, the mouth is often held open because of a large, protruding tongue that is furrowed and lacks the central fissure, and the ears are small with down-folded helixes. The hands are short and broad, with a single palmar crease (**simian crease**); the fingers are short, with clinodactyly (incurvature) of the 5th finger, which often has only 2 phalanges. The feet have a wide gap between the 1st and 2nd toes, and a plantar furrow extends backward. Hands and feet show characteristic dermal prints (dermatoglyphics). Congenital heart disease is found in about 35% of patients; atrioventricular canal defects and ventricular septal defects are most common.

Prognosis

The life expectancy of the Down syndrome child is decreased by heart disease and by susceptibility to acute leukemia. Today, most patients without a major heart defect survive to adulthood, but the aging process seems to be accelerated, with death occurring in the 4th or 5th decade. At autopsy, apparently all adult Down syndrome brains show the typical microscopic findings of Alzheimer's disease, and many individuals develop the associated clinical signs as well. This suggests a connection between genes on chromosome 21 and Alzheimer's disease, a subject of intense current research.

Chromosomal Variants

1. **Translocation (t):** Some individuals with Down syndrome have 46 chromosomes. However, these children actually have the genetic material of 47 chromosomes—the additional chromosome 21 has been translocated. Most commonly, the additional chromosome 21 is transferred and attached to a chromosome 14—t(14;21). In about half the cases, both parents will have normal karyotypes, indicating a de novo translocation in the child. Among the remaining couples, one parent (almost always the mother), although phenotypically normal, has only 45 chromosomes, one of which is the t(14;21). Theoretically, the chance is 1:3 that a mother with a t(14;21) will have a Down syndrome child, but for unknown reasons the actual

risk is lower (about 1:10); if the father carries this translocation, the chance is only 1:20, and the reason for this is not known.

The next most common translocation is t(21;22). In this case, the chance that the carrier will have a Down syndrome child is also about 1:10, and the risk for carrier fathers is small. In extremely rare instances, a parent may have a t(21;21). In this case, 100% of surviving offspring will have Down syndrome.

2. Mosaics: Presumably as a result of nondisjunction in the fertilized zygote, some cases of Down syndrome have 2 cell lines, one normal and one with 47 chromosomes. The relative proportion of each cell line is highly variable, both from individual to individual and within different tissues and organs in the same individual. The prognosis, as far as intelligence is concerned, becomes difficult and presumably depends on the proportion of trisomy 21 cells in the brain. A few mosaic Down syndrome patients have been found with barely recognizable clinical signs and normal intelligence, and thus the incidence of this variant is unknown. Curiously, in some cases both the physical stigmas and the intellectual deficit lessen as the affected child ages. The risk of having trisomy 21 offspring when either parent is a mosaic is increased by an incalculable factor depending on the degree of mosaicism in the gonads.

TRISOMY 18
(Edwards' Syndrome)

An additional chromosome 18 occurs in 1/3000 live births with a small but significant maternal age effect. There is a peculiar sex ratio—3 females:1 male.

The newborn infant is premature or small for gestational age, with marked hypoplasia of skeletal muscle and subcutaneous fat and hypotonia. The cry is weak, and response to sound is decreased. There is often a history of feeble fetal activity, polyhydramnios, a small placenta, and a single umbilical artery.

The occiput is prominent, and there is a narrow bifrontal diameter with hypoplasia of the orbital ridges, short palpebral fissures, small mouth, and micrognathia, all of which give the face a pinched appearance. Microcephaly, epicanthal folds, low-set malformed ears, and cleft lip and/or palate are common. The peculiar clenched fist with the index finger overlapping the 3rd and 4th fingers is almost pathognomonic. Absence of the distal crease on the 5th finger is

common, as is a low-arch dermal ridge pattern on the fingertips. The nails are hypoplastic, and the big toe is shortened and frequently dorsiflexed. Hypoplastic or absent thumbs, clubfeet, rocker-bottom feet, and syndactyly are also seen.

Ventricular septal defect, patent ductus arteriosus, atrial septal defect, anomalous pulmonary and/or aortic valves, and congenital anomalies of lung, diaphragm, kidneys, and ureters are frequent. Hernias and/or diastasis recti, cryptorchidism in the male, and redundant skin folds (particularly over the posterior aspect of the neck) also are common.

Survival for more than a few months is rare, and mental retardation is severe in those who do survive.

TRISOMY 13
(Patau's Syndrome)

This syndrome, caused by trisomy of chromosome 13, occurs in about 1/5000 births and is characterized by midline anomalies. Infants tend to be small at birth. Apneic spells in early infancy are frequent, and mental retardation is severe. Many appear to be deaf. Moderate microcephaly with sloping forehead, wide sagittal sutures, and widely patent fontanelles are present. Gross anatomic defects of the brain, especially **holoprosencephaly** (*failure of the forebrain to divide properly*), are common. Myelomeningocele is found in almost 50% of cases. Microphthalmia, colobomas (fissures) of the iris, and retinal dysplasia occur frequently. The supraorbital ridges are shallow and the palpebral fissures usually are slanted. Cleft lip, cleft palate, or both are present in most cases. The ears are abnormally shaped and usually low-set.

Simian crease, polydactyly, and hyperconvex narrow fingernails are common. The fingers tend to be flexed, but not in the characteristic manner seen in trisomy 18. The feet show posterior prominence of the heel, and there may be a rocker-bottom foot. About 80% of cases show the congenital cardiovascular anomalies described under TRISOMY 18, above. Dextrocardia is common as well.

Capillary hemangiomas, especially on the forehead in the midline, are common. Other midline defects include dermal sinuses of the scalp and loose folds of skin over the posterior aspect of the neck. The genitalia are frequently abnormal in both sexes; cryptorchidism and abnormal scrotum occur in the male, and bicornuate uterus is found in the female. Hematologically, there is an increased frequency of nuclear projections in polymorphonuclear leukocytes and a persistence of fetal Hb. Most patients (70%) are so severely affected that they die before age 6 mo; < 20% survive beyond age 1 yr.

PARTIAL TRISOMY 22
(The Cat-Eye Syndrome)

The association between coloboma of the iris (cat eye) or anal atresia, or both, with an extra small chromosome 22 (22q+) has been confirmed. In addition, anomalies such as severe psychomotor retardation, hypertelorism, eyes with an antimongoloid slant, abnormal ears with preauricular tags or fistulas, and congenital heart disease occur. Full trisomy 22 has been reported in a few patients with a similar phenotype, but frequently microcephaly, micrognathia, and hypotonia occur as well.

DELETION SYNDROMES

The rare cat-cry syndrome (cri-du-chat syndrome, 5p− syndrome) is characterized by a high-pitched, mewing cry, closely resembling the cry of a kitten, which is heard in the immediate newborn period, lasts several weeks, and then disappears. Affected infants often show low birth weight, microcephaly, facial asymmetry and/or a peculiar round or moon face with wide-set eyes, antimongoloid or downward-sloping palpebral fissures with or without epicanthal folds, strabismus, and a broad-based nose. The ears are low-set and abnormally shaped and frequently have narrow external canals and preauricular tags. A short neck and varying degrees of syndactyly are present; heart defects are frequent and the infants are hypotonic. Mental and physical development are markedly retarded. A significant number survive to adulthood, when facial asymmetry and malocclusion often lead to a grotesque appearance.

The 4p− deletion syndrome is extremely rare and the syndrome shares many of the features of the cat-cry syndrome but lacks the cat-like cry. Mental retardation is profound. In addition, there are midline scalp defects, ptosis and colobomas, beaked nose, cleft palate, delayed bone age, and, in males, hypospadias and undescended testes. A high mortality rate occurs during infancy; the relatively few survivors develop susceptibility to infections and epilepsy. Rare individuals, alive in their 20s, are all severely handicapped.

Contiguous gene syndromes: *Microdeletions of contiguous genes on a chromosome,* detectable as a result of techniques to extend chromosomes, cause syndromes such as Prader-Willi, Miller-Dieker, DiGeorge. Almost all cases are sporadic. Often the microdeletion cannot be shown cytogenetically, but its presence may be confirmed by DNA probes specific to the deleted area.

SYNDROMES ASSOCIATED WITH SEX CHROMOSOME ABERRATIONS
The Lyon Hypothesis (X-Inactivation Theory)

Sex determination in humans is controlled by a unique pair of chromosomes, the X and the Y. The female has two X chromosomes, and the male has one X plus one Y. The Y chromosome is among the smallest of the 46 chromosomes, and geneticists have been able to detect only a few non−sex-related genes in it. On the other hand, the X is one of the largest chromosomes in group C and contains hundreds of genes, most of which have nothing to do with sex.

This situation would seem to create a genetic "dosage" problem, since the normal female has 2 loci for every X-linked gene as compared to the male's single locus. However, according to the **Lyon hypothesis,** *one of the two X chromosomes in each somatic cell of the female is genetically inactivated* early in the life of the embryo. It is evident that the **Barr body,** or **sex chromatin mass,** seen within the nuclei of female somatic cells represents all (or at least most) of the 2nd X chromosome. In fact, no matter how many X chromosomes are present in the genome, all but one seem to be inactivated. Thus, the number of sex chromatin masses is one less than the total number of X chromosomes.

X-inactivation has interesting implications in clinical medicine. For example, X chromosome anomalies are relatively benign, compared with analogous autosomal anomalies. Females with three X chromosomes are often normal physically and mentally, and are apparently fertile. In contrast, all of the known autosomal trisomies (eg, Down syndrome and trisomies 18 and 13) have devastating effects. The relatively benign nature of additional X chromosomes presumably results from inactivation of most of the extra chromosomal material. Similarly, the total absence of an autosome is lethal, whereas the total absence of one X chromosome, though it leads to a specific syndrome (Turner's syndrome), is relatively benign.

The symptomatic heterozygote for an X-linked recessive disorder may also be explained on the basis of this theory. Females who are heterozygous for hemophilia or muscular dystrophy occasionally show bleeding tendencies or muscle weakness, respectively. The Lyon hypothesis also suggests that X-inactivation is a random event and, therefore, in each individual, 50% maternal and 50% paternal X-inactivation should occur. However, a random process follows the normal distribution curve, and most of the maternal Xs may be inactivated in specific tissues of some females, and the paternal Xs in other females. If, by chance, nearly all cells had the normal allele inactivated in a given tissue of a heterozygote, the disease in that individual and in the hemizygous affected male might be similar.

GONADAL DYSGENESIS
(Turner's Syndrome;
Bonnevie-Ullrich Syndrome)

This syndrome is due, in general, to the complete or partial absence of one of the two X chromosomes in the female. Its incidence is about 1/3000 live female births. Many affected newborns present with marked dorsal lymphedema of the hands and feet, and with lymphedema or loose folds of skin over the posterior aspect of the neck. This appearance is almost pathognomonic, but nuchal edema is occasionally seen in Down syndrome.

The full picture in the older child or adult consists of short stature, webbing of the neck, low hairline on the back of the neck, ptosis, a wide chest with broad-spaced nipples, multiple pigmented nevi, short 4th metacarpals and metatarsals, hypoplasia of the nails, coarctation of the aorta, amenorrhea, failure of breast development, and juvenile external genitalia. The ovaries are replaced by bilateral streaks of fibrous stroma that are usually devoid of developing ova.

Renal anomalies and hemangiomas are frequent. Occasionally, telangiectasia occurs in the GI tract, with resultant intestinal bleeding. Mental deficiency is rare, but many patients suffer from spatial disorientation and thus score poorly in performance tests and in mathematics, even though they score average or above in verbal IQ.

Variants: (1) Mosaics: A number of patients with Turner's syndrome are mosaics (eg, 45,X/46,XX or 45,X/47,XXX). The phenotype varies from that of a typical Turner's syndrome to normal, and many are fertile. (2) Ring chromosomes: Occasionally, affected individuals have one normal X and one abnormal X that forms a ring chromosome. For that to happen, there must be a piece lost from both the short and the long arm of the abnormal X. (3) Long arm isochromosomes: Some patients have one normal X and one long arm isochromosome formed by the loss of short arms and development of a chromosome consisting of just the long arms. These individuals tend to have the complete syndrome, so that deletion of the short arm of the X chromosome appears to be the most important factor in the syndrome. (4) Turner phenotype with normal sex chromosomes (Noonan's syndrome): In several families, both females and males have many characteristics of Turner's syndrome, though their chromosomes are 46,XX or 46,XY. This is apparently due to homozygosity for an autosomal recessive mutant in some cases, and to autosomal dominant inheritance in others. However, most cases are sporadic, presumably with multifactorial etiology. There are phenotypic differences, primarily a more normal stature, normal sexual development and fertility, pectus excavatum, and more frequent involvement of the right side of the heart (pulmonic stenosis) rather than coarctation of the aorta. Mental retardation occurs frequently but usually is not severe.

A cytogenetic analysis must be obtained on all patients with gonadal dysgenesis in order to rule out mosaicism with a Y-bearing cell line; eg, 46,XY/45,X. These patients are usually phenotypic females who have variable features of Turner's syndrome, although some are intersex. They are at high risk of developing gonadal malignancy, especially gonadoblastoma, and should have the gonads removed prophylactically during early childhood.

THE TRIPLE X SYNDROME (47,XXX)

These individuals have 3 X chromosomes and 2 Barr bodies or sex chromatin masses. This condition, found initially in hospitals for the mentally retarded, has also been discovered in about 1/1000 apparently normal females during routine surveys of newborn populations. Though sterility sometimes occurs, several normal XXX females have had offspring who have been both chromosomally and phenotypically normal. Follow-up studies of the unselected infants ascertained in newborn surveys have revealed mildly impaired intellect with IQ scores averaging just below 90 and associated school problems in all subjects when compared with siblings. Some have moderate-to-severe deficits in language areas, reflecting their difficulties with visual-motor and sensory perceptual integration.

RARE ANOMALIES OF THE X CHROMOSOME

Although rare, 48,XXXX or 49,XXXXX females have been found. There is no consistent phenotype, though the risk of mental retardation and congenital abnormalities increases markedly with an increase in number of X chromosomes, especially when there are > 3. The genetic imbalance early in embryonic life before X-inactivation may cause anomalous development.

KLINEFELTER'S SYNDROME (47,XXY)

This relatively common chromosome anomaly occurs in about 1/700 live male births. In the past, 47,XXY individuals were thought to be mentally retarded, and surveys of mental institutions have disclosed an incidence of about 1/50 mentally retarded male patients. The typical affected individual is tall and eunuchoid, with small, firm testes and gynecomastia. Puberty usually occurs at the normal time, but often facial hair growth is light; a small proportion may require testosterone supplements. Clinical variation is great, and it is now known that most 47,XXY males are normal in appearance and intellect and are found in the course of an infertility work-up (probably all are sterile) or in cytogenetic surveys of normal populations. Boys from the latter group have been followed developmentally. There has been no mental retardation but many have specific deficits in verbal IQ and reading. They are inefficient in their use of language and slow in auditory processing; speech and language therapy have been beneficial and they eventually do well in school. There is no increased incidence of homosexuality. Testicular development varies from hyalinized nonfunctional tubules to some production of spermatozoa, and urinary excretion of follicle-stimulating hormone (FSH) is frequently increased.

Variants: Some patients with Klinefelter's syndrome have 3, 4, and even 5 X chromosomes along with the Y. In general, as the number of X's increases, the severity of mental retardation and of malformations also increases. Again, genetic imbalance before X-inactivation may be significant. A few individuals appear to be 46,XX; these cases probably result from a translocation of a minute, and therefore microscopically undetectable, fragment of a Y chromosome to one of the X's or to another chromosome. Gene probes for the Y chromosome now confirm the presence of Y chromosomal DNA in virtually all cases. There are also rare mosaic individuals with Klinefelter's syndrome.

THE 47,XYY SYNDROME

This chromosome anomaly was first described in 1961 in a 6-ft white male with no particular problems. A number of males with this syndrome, particularly those who are aggressive or violent, are found in institutions for criminals with subnormal IQ, and it has been suggested that extra Y chromosomal material predisposes males to criminal aggressive tendencies. More recent data show that nearly all of these men came from very poor socioeconomic situations. Furthermore, 47,XYY individuals are also found in normal populations with about the same high frequency as 47,XXY, and the role of the extra Y chromosome in criminal tendencies is questionable. Early test results on the boys identified by newborn screening show increased language dysfunction similar to that of the 47,XXY males.

X-LINKED MENTAL RETARDATION
(Fragile X Syndrome)
(See also MENTAL RETARDATION in Ch. 29)

Among persons institutionalized because of mental retardation, a 30 to 50% excess of males is well documented. Family studies often reveal affected male sibs and maternal uncles, leaving no doubt that a group of X-linked mutant genes causes mental retardation without major congenital anomalies. This at least in part accounts for the excess of retarded males. Some of these males have an X chromosome with a constriction near the end of the long arm, resulting in what looks like a small knob separated from the main portion of the chromosome by a thin stalk. The stalk, often broken in preparing the karyotype, is referred to as a fragile site, and its presence can be detected by using special cell culture techniques. The clinical features include large testes, especially after puberty, large protuberant ears, and prominent chin and forehead. When affected males have this fragile X chromosome, often, but not always, the fragile X can be shown in the carrier female. Some carriers are also mentally retarded, and, curiously, some of the males are mentally normal. Thus, although the fragile X can be reliably detected in cultured chorionic villi or amniotic fluid cells, prenatal diagnosis is problematic for both sexes. Accurate pre- and postnatal detection will be provided when the fragile X gene is cloned and characterized. The fragile X syndrome is of major importance because, next to Down syndrome, it is the most common cause of mental retardation that can be specifically diagnosed.

INTERSEX STATES
(See also in Ch. 28)

Genetic disorders may be responsible for intersex states in a variety of ways. A useful diagnostic approach in cases of ambiguous genitalia is based on the results of chromosome analysis, and many patients can be placed into 1 of 3 categories:

1. **Chromosome abnormalities.** Sex chromosome abnormalities include a variety of mosaics with or without a Y chromosome, the gonadal dysgenesis syndromes (may be 46,XX or 46,XY) and true hermaphroditism (often 46,XX in lymphocytes but mosaic in the ovotestis). Ambiguous genitalia may also occur in trisomies 13 and 18 and in other autosomal chromosome disorders.

2. **Masculinization of 46,XX females (female pseudohermaphrodites).** A common cause is congenital virilizing adrenal hyperplasia **(adrenogenital syndrome),** a group of disorders due to enzyme deficiencies in the adrenal cortical biosynthetic pathways, each of which is inherited as an autosomal recessive trait. Exogenous androgen from maternal ingestion or maternal tumors may also masculinize a fetus.

3. **Undermasculinization of 46,XY males (male pseudohermaphrodites).** Some of the enzyme deficiencies in congenital adrenal hyperplasia lead to production of abnormal androgens that fail to fully masculinize the male fetus. In addition, there is a group of **"androgen resistance syndromes"** due to deficiencies of cell membrane androgen receptors (total resistance causes the **testicular feminization syndrome),** most of which are X-linked.

It is important to note that most cases of ambiguous genitalia occur as components of multiple malformation syndromes or as developmental defects, often associated with anomalies of the genitourinary tract and/or lower intestinal tract. If the adrenogenital syndrome is suspected, the infant must be carefully monitored for sodium depletion or hypertension while awaiting results of assays for urinary steroid metabolites.

INDICATIONS FOR CHROMOSOME ANALYSIS

1. **Congenital malformations.** Infants with multiple congenital anomalies of unknown cause often have chromosome anomalies (see above). Single malformations, even when severe (eg, congenital heart defects, neural tube defects), are rarely associated with chromosome aberrations, but minor defects that are easily overlooked must be carefully sought. Frequently the radiologist will find unsuspected skeletal anomalies, and therefore x-rays are part of the work-up of any patient who may have a syndrome. Similarly, patients with **nonspecific mental retardation,** infants who **fail to thrive,** and **small-for-gestational age** newborns provide a low yield of abnormal karyotypes but may still constitute indications for analysis; the discovery of the chromosome anomaly may prompt a more detailed search for malformations, some of which may be correctable (eg, early diagnosis of a urinary tract obstruction or abnormal vertebrae could greatly benefit the patient).

2. **Fetal anomalies detected by ultrasonography.** Chromosome abnormalities are found most commonly in fetuses with nuchal hygromas, limb defects, omphaloceles, duodenal stenosis, hydrocephalus/holoprosencephaly, and facial anomalies (eg, clefts). If 2 malformations of any type or 1 malformation in association with intrauterine growth retardation or variation in amniotic fluid volume is found, the risk of a chromosome anomaly rises severalfold. Fetal blood sampling has become a major component of a modern prenatal diagnostic unit (see Percutaneous Umbilical Blood Sampling, below).

3. **Ambiguous external genitalia** (see INTERSEX STATES, above, and in Ch. 28). Because of the wide variety of chromosomal variation that may lead to ambiguity, the buccal smear is no longer acceptable for even a presumptive diagnosis of either sex. In the rare event where the biologic sex must be obtained quickly (eg, to avoid serious psychologic problems for parents), a bone marrow aspirate may be used for immediate preparation of karyotypes.

4. **Habitual abortion.** Although a major chromosome anomaly is found in only 3 to 5% of couples who have had 3 or more spontaneous abortions, karyotyping both parents is part of the work-up.

5. **Infertility.** After anatomic defects are excluded as the cause, the couple should be karyo-

typed. Again, the buccal smear is inadequate. Both 47,XXY males and females with a variety of X chromosome anomalies may appear perfectly normal, but they may be sterile.

6. Sperm or ova donors. Individuals participating in donor programs should be karyotyped to rule out a translocation or other heritable chromosome anomaly.

7. X-linked mental retardation. Special chromosome studies for the fragile X are indicated.

8. Cancer cytogenetics. Data from chromosome analyses are being used in the diagnosis and management of an increasing number of malignancies, especially leukemias and lymphomas.

GENETIC COUNSELING IN CHROMOSOME ANOMALIES

Fortunately, most syndromes associated with chromosome anomalies occur only once in a family, and an optimistic prognosis for future offspring can usually be given after appropriate studies are completed. Parental karyotypes are essential for all patients with a translocation or deletion syndrome to be sure that the rearrangement was not inherited. When either parent is found to be a balanced carrier of any chromosome rearrangement, the siblings of both the patient and the affected parent are at risk and additional chromosome studies are indicated. The availability of prenatal diagnosis and prevention through selective abortion must be presented to those at risk (see below).

Patients with **Down syndrome** due to trisomy 21 present unique problems. Surprisingly, most familial cases are trisomy 21 rather than translocations, and only a few result from parental mosaicism (mosaicism may lead to multiple cases but only within one sibship). Thus, regardless of maternal age, the parents of any child with Down syndrome are at an increased risk (close to 1%) of having another affected child and should be made aware of the availability of prenatal diagnosis. The siblings of these parents, however, are not at increased risk as long as there are no other close relatives with trisomy 21.

PREVENTION OF GENETIC DISORDERS

The goal of the medical geneticist is to identify individuals who, because of their particular hereditary background, conditioned by their lifetime of special experiences, are unsuited for the environment in which they find themselves. In most instances, neither genes nor environment alone causes disease, and when individuals at high risk are identified, methods are becoming increasingly available to mitigate the effects of both the genome and the uniquely offensive components of the environment. For conditions not yet treatable or detectable prenatally, prevention by contraception may be necessary, with adoption or artificial insemination as options (the latter is becoming more acceptable and should be discussed when appropriate).

ADVANCES IN MOLECULAR GENETICS

The speed with which the new DNA technology is being moved from the laboratory bench to the care of patients is without precedent in the history of medicine. A few of the main acts in this rapidly developing drama are highlighted below.

The isolation of human genes: Techniques for purification of DNA and RNA, separation of the 2 polynucleotide strands of the double helix, and understanding the triplet code for translating the sequence of bases in the genetic material to the corresponding sequence of amino acids in polypeptide chains were crucial. For example, the gene for human insulin was synthesized by first purifying the 2 polypeptide chains of the hormone itself. The sequence of amino acids yielded the sequence of bases that coded them, and the appropriate bases were chemically linked together in the correct order in vitro. The genes for the α- and β-hemoglobin polypeptide chains were synthesized from purified messenger RNA (**mRNA**). The specific RNA was relatively easy to purify from human erythroid precursor cells because about half of their total mRNA is for Hb production. Transcription from an RNA template to DNA occurs, thanks to the enzyme reverse transcriptase. Several additional methods for purifying and analyzing human genes have been developed, and it turns out that a gene is not simply a segment of DNA coding for the amino acid sequence of a polypeptide chain. Instead, it consists of coding sequences called **exons** that are interspersed by noncoding intervening sequences known as **introns**. The introns are transcribed initially but are spliced out of the messenger RNA before it leaves the cell nucleus. The function of the introns is unknown, but many of the mutations that cause β-thalassemia, for example, lie within them. In addition, there are flanking sequences on both sides of structural genes that regulate their activity and provide start and stop signals for their transcription.

Restriction endonucleases are bacterial enzymes that break the genetic material into thousands of pieces; each specific endonuclease breaks the DNA or RNA only when there is a very specific sequence of bases. For example, one endonuclease might recognize the sequence G-C-C-T-A-A and break the chain between the T and the A (the 4 bases that make up the DNA are Cytosine, Guanine, Thymidine, and Adenine). This sequence will occur by chance over and over again in the human genome and thus produce the many fragments of varying lengths, as shown in Fig. 48–7.

Cloning the genes is the vital step whereby a piece, eg, of human DNA, be it a purified gene or not, is inserted into a cloning vehicle, often a bacterial **plasmid** (*a circular bit of DNA present naturally in bacteria*), and then the bacterium is cultured. Each newly produced plasmid contains the human DNA, and literally billions of copies of the human gene or DNA segment can be produced in this bacterial factory. The circular plasmids can be opened for insertion of foreign DNA using restriction endonucleases. The combination of bacterial plasmid and a human DNA segment is one example of recombinant DNA.

The gene probe: Any segment of DNA or RNA will bind to its complementary sequence. That is how the **double helix** is formed from a single strand in the first place—G always binds to C, and A to T. Thus, if one takes the many copies of one of the cloned genes described above and adds a radioactive label to each copy, one has a labeled probe. The probe will seek out its complementary segment of DNA, which can then be found by autoradiography. A probe added to a chromosome spread can actually locate a gene in a specific chromosome or use it to identify a piece of DNA in a Southern blot, as illustrated in Fig. 48–7.

The Southern blot, a procedure named after the investigator who devised it, is the cornerstone of the applications of recombinant DNA to prevention of genetically determined disease. The technique is outlined in Fig. 48–7. Briefly, DNA is extracted from cells of the patient and fragmented by one of the restriction endonucleases. The fragments are electrophoresed, which separates them primarily by size, the smaller ones moving more rapidly through the pores of the gel. The fragments are then blotted onto nitrocellulose filter paper and overlaid with a labeled probe. The probe will bind only to its complementary sequence and thus identify the gene of interest as a band or bands on the paper.

Restriction fragment length polymorphisms (RFLPs): The various available restriction endonucleases have revealed a remarkable amount of variability in the human genome. If just 1 base substitution occurs in the sequence recognized by the endonuclease, the DNA will not break at that site and, instead of 2 small fragments, there will be 1 big one. The different-sized fragments will move to different places in the Southern blot procedure and the probe will identify the different-sized fragments, as shown in Fig. 48–8. Since these variants are so common, they have provided us with an almost unending series of markers known as RFLPs. If the base substitution occurs within the gene in question, and coincidentally at the site of the mutation that causes the disease, as is the case for sickle cell anemia, the marker will identify an individual's genotype without family studies. If the variant flanks the gene in question but is very close to it, as in Huntington's disease **(HD)**, family studies are required to determine which sized fragment is associated with the HD gene in a given family.

Gene amplification: The polymerase chain reaction (PCR) for DNA amplification is a remarkable innovation whereby a specific segment of DNA, including a specific gene, can be amplified in vitro > 200,000-fold in a matter of hours. The DNA in a single cell is sufficient, and the amounts produced are large enough so that DNA stains can be used in place of radioactive probes after electrophoresis. With this technique, molecular diagnosis should soon become available in clinical diagnostic laboratories.

Medical applications: The techniques above have already led to extraordinary advances in mapping the human genome, and it is just a matter of time for the development of probes for most of the human diseases resulting from single gene mutations even though the nature of the genetic defect is unknown. This will permit precise identification of genotype, including heterozygotes and homozygotes, and provide the means for diagnosis before birth and before the development of detectable clinical signs in such conditions as HD. Genes whose function is unknown (eg, the HD gene) will soon be isolated and sequenced and their products deduced, which

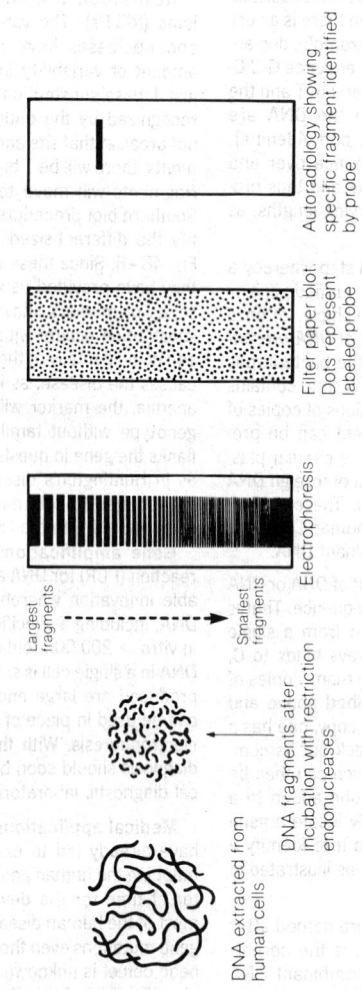

Autoradiology showing specific fragment identified by probe

Filter paper blot. Dots represent labeled probe

Electrophoresis

Largest fragments

Smallest fragments

DNA fragments after incubation with restriction endonucleases

DNA extracted from human cells

Fig. 48–7. The Southern blot technique.

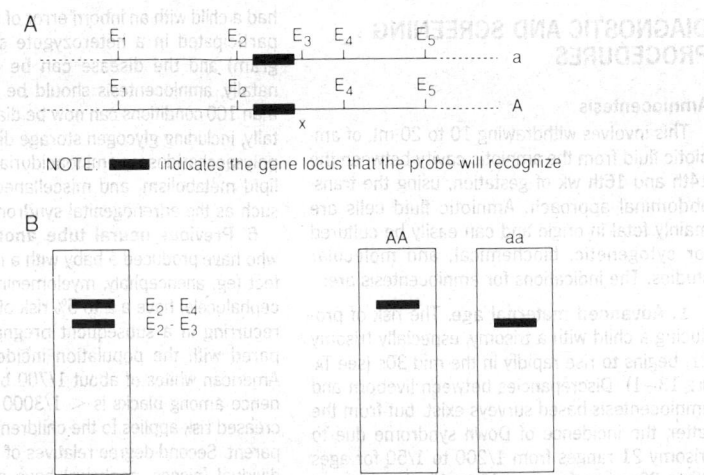

NOTE: ▬▬ indicates the gene locus that the probe will recognize

FIG. 48–8. Detection of restriction fragment length polymorphism (RFLP).

A. Depicted are small sections of 2 homologous chromosomes, **a** and **A**. E_1, E_2...E_5 are the breakpoints caused by a restriction endonuclease, E.

In chromosome A, a base substitution is present at the site marked x; thus, the site is not recognized by E. No break occurs and a large fragment results. The probe will bind to both the E_2-E_3 fragment of chromosome **a** and the E_2-E_4 fragment of chromosome A, the latter being the larger. After Southern blotting and autoradiography, the probe will identify both fragments (see *B*).

B. Some people will be homozygous AA and others aa. AA individuals will have only the large E_2-E_4 fragment; aa individuals, the E_2-E_3.

could lead to understanding of the basic defect and eventually to treatment approaches. This process is known as "reverse genetics" and it has recently led to the discovery of "dystrophin," a product of the X-linked gene that specifies this muscle protein, abnormalities of which cause Duchenne or Becker muscular dystrophy. Already available are probes for the genes causing the hemophilias, Duchenne muscular dystrophy, myotonic dystrophy, neurofibromatosis, adult-onset polycystic disease of the kidneys, the hemoglobinopathies, phenylketonuria, α_1-antitrypsin deficiency, cystic fibrosis, HD, and dozens of others. These probes provide the means for both presymptomatic and prenatal diagnosis: The ethical issues warrant serious consideration in every situation.

Additional applications include the use of recombinant DNA techniques in the production of scarce human replacement products, including growth hormone and pure factor VIII, both of which are currently commercially available. The practicality of actual gene replacement therapy, the ultimate genetic engineering, remains a distant possibility because of the many

hurdles yet to jump. We know very little about the nature or even the location of the crucial regulatory genes; we have no idea as to how to direct genes to specific sites in the genome, and in the wrong locale they could have serious deleterious effects.

Among the most exciting discoveries have been the markers for several genetically influenced, probably multifactorial, conditions that both are common and represent serious medical problems. These include the specific HLA associations with specific forms of arthritis and diabetes, the development of probes specific for mutations involved in control of serum and intracellular lipid levels, and probes for mutations associated with common malignancies (eg, carcinoma of the colon; see GENETICS OF MALIGNANT DISEASE, above). Early identification of these high-risk subgroups may permit interventions to delay or even prevent the effects of the disease.

Molecular genetics service laboratories are being developed in association with genetics centers to provide up-to-date information as well as diagnostic services for practicing physicians.

DIAGNOSTIC AND SCREENING PROCEDURES

Amniocentesis

This involves withdrawing 10 to 20 mL of amniotic fluid from the amniotic cavity between the 14th and 16th wk of gestation, using the transabdominal approach. Amniotic fluid cells are mainly fetal in origin and can easily be cultured for cytogenetic, biochemical, and molecular studies. The indications for amniocentesis are:

1. **Advanced maternal age.** The risk of producing a child with a trisomy, especially trisomy 21, begins to rise rapidly in the mid 30s (see TABLE 13–1). Discrepancies between liveborn and amniocentesis-based surveys exist, but from the latter, the incidence of Down syndrome due to trisomy 21 ranges from 1/200 to 1/50 for ages 35 to 39, while for ages 40 to 45, the risks are between 2 and 6/100. Most physicians believe that women who will be > 35 at the time of delivery should be told of the risk and offered amniocentesis. There is a minor paternal age effect but it is of little practical importance (eg, the husband of a 34-yr-old woman would have to be 70 to increase her risk to that of a 35-yr-old woman).

2. **Previous trisomic offspring.** When a couple has produced a still- or liveborn child with any trisomy, the risk in a subsequent pregnancy is increased.

3. **Translocation carriers.** When one parent carries a chromosome translocation, 5 to 100% of the offspring may be aborted or liveborn with multiple malformations, depending on which parent and which chromosomes are involved. In general, in nonhomologous translocations the risk is greater when the mother is the carrier.

4. **Sex determination.** The karyotype constructed from cultured fetal cells permits determination of fetal sex before birth. When the mother has been identified as a carrier of an X-linked mutant and a specific test for the affected fetus is unavailable, fetal sex determination may be carried out with the option to abort males, although half of them will be normal. The availability of specific X chromosome DNA probes now permits identification of the affected male for many X-linked diseases (see above). Prenatal sex determination should not be offered to couples who wish to have a child of a specific sex for nongenetic reasons.

5. **Metabolic diseases.** If both parents have been identified as carriers of the same abnormal autosomal recessive gene (ie, they have already had a child with an inborn error of metabolism or participated in a heterozygote screening program) and the disease can be detected prenatally, amniocentesis should be offered. More than 100 conditions can now be diagnosed prenatally, including glycogen storage diseases, mucopolysaccharidoses, aminoacidurias, diseases of lipid metabolism, and miscellaneous conditions such as the adrenogenital syndrome.

6. **Previous neural tube anomaly.** Couples who have produced a baby with a neural tube defect (eg, anencephaly, myelomeningocele, or encephalocele) have a 2 to 5% risk of such a defect recurring in a subsequent pregnancy, as compared with the population incidence in North American whites of about 1/700 births. The incidence among blacks is < 1/3000. The same increased risk applies to the children of an affected parent. Second-degree relatives of an affected individual (nieces, nephews) have about a 1/100 risk; for first cousins, the risk is about 1/200. There is little if any increased risk for other family members. α-Fetoprotein is elevated in about 99% of the amniotic fluids of fetuses with open neural tube defects, and this test is used to screen pregnancies at high risk. Today most geneticists suggest amniocentesis and high resolution ultrasonography (US) for 1st-degree relatives, and maternal serum α-fetoprotein with US for 2nd- and 3rd-degree relatives. Other conditions (eg, presence of fetal blood, threatened abortion, twins, omphalocele, exstrophy of the bladder, fetal death, Turner's syndrome, congenital nephrosis, duodenal atresia) also result in elevated α-fetoprotein, necessitating confirmation of diagnosis by US and assay of amniotic fluid for acetylcholinesterase activity of neurologic origin. Neither spina bifida occulta nor isolated congenital hydrocephalus is considered to be a neural tube defect.

7. **Other congenital defects.** The techniques for prenatal diagnosis of kidney anomalies such as renal agenesis (Potter's syndrome) and polycystic disease, lethal forms of short-limbed dwarfism (thanatophoric dwarf, achondrogenesis), anomalies of the gut (diaphragmatic hernia, obstruction), and micro- and hydrocephalus are being provided by improved resolving power of ultrasonography.

8. **Maternal insulin-dependent diabetes.** There is up to a ten-fold increase in the risk of a neural tube defect, which brings the incidence to between 1 and 2%. In addition, the risk of other congenital anomalies, particularly those involving the sacrum and lower limbs, is increased. However, it is now clear that careful control of blood

glucose, particularly before conception through embryogenesis, will significantly lower the risk of fetal malformations. Detailed US examinations of the fetus at 16 and 18 wk along with maternal serum α-fetoprotein should be offered.

Complications of amniocentesis at 16 wk are uncommon. Fetal loss due to the procedure occurs in about 1/200 amniocenteses, but other serious injury to the fetus has not been reported. Infection is rare. Although amniotic fluid leak, hemorrhage (fetal or maternal), or both occur in 1 to 2% of cases, they usually cease after a short period of bed rest. Cell culture failures and incorrect cytogenetic diagnosis are very rare in experienced laboratories.

Chorionic Villus Sampling (CVS)

A sample of chorionic villi can be obtained by inserting a flexible catheter through the vagina and cervix, and advancing it to the site of fetal implantation under direct US guidance or by transabdominal needle (also with US guidance). About 10 to 30 mg of villi are then aspirated into a syringe; any contaminating maternal tissue is removed under a dissecting microscope. Karyotypes are obtained after short-term (3 to 5 days) and long-term (10 days to 2 wk) culture. The latter is now believed to reflect more accurately the karyotype of the fetus. Most, if not all, of the enzymes present in cultured amniotic fluid cells are also measurable in extracts of chorionic villi or cultured villus cells, and DNA can be extracted from these fetal cells for molecular genetic studies.

Important advantages of CVS are these: It is done at 8 to 10 wk of gestation, which is 2 mo earlier than amniocentesis, and results are available more quickly. Thus, if a couple elects termination of pregnancy because of an abnormal result, a 1st-trimester abortion is easier and safer than one at 20 wk.

A problem with CVS is the risk; data currently indicate a miscarriage rate of between 1 and 2% as a direct result of the procedure. There is no evidence that CVS causes harm to the fetus that goes on to term after CVS. However, 1 to 2% of patients who have CVS go on to require amniocentesis because of uninterpretable cytogenetic findings (eg, mosaicism). The patient must be made aware of this possibility before having the procedure.

Percutaneous Umbilical Blood Sampling (PUBS)

A sample of fetal blood can be obtained by a needle inserted through the maternal abdomen into a placental blood vessel at the site of attachment of the umbilical cord. Previously requiring fetoscopy, it is now done under US guidance from as early as 12 wk gestational age until term. PUBS is useful for obtaining a rapid karyotype (2 to 3 days) after US detection of congenital anomalies or for WBC, serum, or Hb disorders not yet detectable by enzyme assay or molecular techniques. The risk of fetal loss is 1 to 5%.

Screening Programs

Newborn: Screening of newborn infants for phenylketonuria to detect the condition before significant CNS damage occurs is almost worldwide. When the diagnosis is confirmed, dietary treatment is started, so that mental retardation is prevented. Screening tests using dried blood spots on filter paper have been automated and expanded to permit early detection of other inborn errors of metabolism amenable to treatment (eg, galactosemia, maple syrup urine disease, and some forms of homocystinuria). The same patient specimens have been adapted to detect congenital hypothyroidism, a relatively common cause of mental retardation (1/3000 births) for which early institution of therapy is crucial. Screening programs are under way throughout North America.

Screening for heterozygotes: Tay-Sachs disease, the model for this approach to prevention of genetic disease, is inherited as an autosomal recessive condition and occurs with highest frequency among the Ashkenazi (Eastern European) Jews and a French Canadian isolate in the province of Quebec. The disease can be diagnosed with precision, both pre- and postnatally, and the carrier or heterozygote can also be accurately detected. Screening programs in several urban centers determined the carrier frequency to be between 1/20 and 1/30 Ashkenazi Jews. Many couples at risk have been identified, several affected fetuses have been detected prenatally by amniocentesis and have been aborted. Since only a fraction of the Jewish community has been screened, the physician should apprise every Ashkenazi Jewish couple of the risk of Tay-Sachs disease, preferably before any pregnancy occurs. The couple should then have the opportunity to be tested if they wish. Information for both doctor and patient is available from the Tay-Sachs Foundation. This approach has resulted in the near disappearance of Tay-Sachs disease in the Jewish population.

Sickle cell disease, thalassemia, and other hemoglobinopathies are now preventable. The populations at risk have been identified (Southern Italians, Greeks, and other Mediterranean peoples for β-thalassemia; orientals for α-thalassemia variants; and blacks for sickle cell disease and thalassemias), and carrier detection is readily available, accurate, and relatively inexpensive. Molecular techniques using restriction endonucleases, Southern blots, and/or polymerase chain reaction can identify affected fetuses through studies of DNA from amniotic fluid cells and chorionic villi (see above); fetal blood specimens obtained by PUBS are only rarely necessary for prenatal diagnosis of most hemoglobinopathies. Today physicians have both an ethical and a legal responsibility to inquire about the racial/ethnic origins of patients and to inform them about their risks and what they can do about it.

Cystic fibrosis (CF), with an incidence of about 1/2500 and a carrier frequency of about 1/25 in the white population, is a disease in which prenatal homozygosity and 70 to 85% of carriers can be detected. The gene has been isolated and a mutation consisting of a deletion of 3 base pairs has been found to account for 70% of the mutant genes that cause CF. Intrafamilial screening for carrier status among close relatives of an individual with CF is established, and general population screening is proposed.

Screening for neural tube defects: Since 9 of 10 infants with such defects are born to couples with no prior history of an affected baby, amniocentesis for high-risk couples can have little effect on the incidence. However, in > 80% of cases, α-fetoprotein is significantly elevated in maternal serum at 16 to 18 wk gestation. Several pilot research projects in Canada, the USA, and the United Kingdom have shown that maternal serum α-fetoprotein screening for all pregnant women who wish to participate is feasible, sufficiently accurate, cost effective, and acceptable to a large proportion of the population. Today serum screening is available throughout most of North America and the UK. However, the physician must exercise great care in the choice of laboratory or center that he uses. Interpretation of serum and amniotic fluid α-fetoprotein levels requires experience and the collaboration of a skilled ultrasonographer, both for the confirmation of gestational age and for the detailed sonography required when the serum α-fetoproteins are consistently elevated. It should be noted that an unexplained high α-fetoprotein identifies a pregnancy at increased risk of intrauterine growth retardation, fetal loss, prematurity, and other congenital anomalies.

Screening for Down syndrome: Recently obtained data indicate that in most pregnancies in which the fetus has Down syndrome, the maternal serum α-fetoprotein at 16 to 18 wk gestation is below the median. Cutoff points, below which amniocentesis for fetal karyotyping is indicated, have been determined for various maternal ages. This test, along with other serum assays (eg, chorionic gonadotropin and estriol) may permit detection of up to 70% of fetuses with Down syndrome and other serious trisomies in women < 35. It could also be used to reduce the number of amniocenteses for women > 35.

Ethics of Genetic Screening in the Workplace

This new concept is causing considerable conflict between labor and management. The issue is the employee or potential employee who, because of some genetically determined trait, is less suited to some specific job than an individual who does not have that trait. Many feel that such screening interferes with the individual's freedom of choice, could be considered an unfair labor practice, and would insist that the workplace be made safe for everyone, regardless of his or her genetic makeup.

On the other hand, this genetic approach may be reasonable for individuals making career or life-style decisions. First, however, unequivocal associations must be established between "deleterious genes" and specific environmental factors, and then interventions proved to be effective must be developed.

TERATOLOGY

Exposures to potentially teratogenic drugs (see also DRUGS IN PREGNANCY in Ch. 14), various forms of radiation, and industrial pollutants have become a major problem for physicians managing pregnancies. Up-to-date information pertaining to humans is difficult to find and interpret, and much of the available data have not been critically appraised. However, most genetics centers in North America have access to well-designed, computerized teratogen information services that provide the latest information on both animal and human studies. Physicians would be well advised to find out about the availability of such a service in their areas and to use it whenever the questions arise.

§4. PSYCHIATRIC DISORDERS

49. INTRODUCTION

Psychiatry, a branch of medicine, is responsible for the study, diagnosis, treatment, and prevention of human behavior disorders. Abnormal behavior may be determined or modified by genetic, physicochemical, psychologic, and social factors.

The psychiatrist must master the knowledge and skills not only of objective observation but also of subjective, participant, and self observation. His background in natural science has fostered objective observation, but as he learns other types he finds this differentiation of his role function is necessary for understanding the relationship to his patient and for growth in his capacity for human intimacy. Only then can the general notion of personality and its underlying principles be learned: the genetic and ontogenic factors in growth, development, and decline; recognition of unconscious and preconscious factors as determinants of behavior; the idea that the personality is integral and indivisible; and recognition that man is a social animal and that the emerging stages of the life cycle reflect coordination between the evolving individual and his social environment.

Recent Historic Developments

The introduction of rauwolfia and the phenothiazines in the early 1950s contributed to the effective treatment and symptomatic management of many severely psychotic patients, reduced the duration of hospital stays, and increased the percentage of patients discharged from hospitals after acute episodes, making deinstitutionalization (see below) possible.

Concern increased that psychotic patients (including those chronically disabled) be cared for properly in the hospital or community, and that they be viewed as family and community members. Awareness has grown regarding the reciprocal relations between patient and family that may enhance health or provoke illness. The patient's family has become more involved in therapy, and the family physician's important role in rehabilitation has been recognized. In hospitals, new psychosocial methods have led to the minimal use of seclusion and restraint and to earlier discharge. Attempts to break down administrative and other barriers between hospital and community have increased, as have attempts to reform the internal social organization within the hospital.

Other developments include large-group techniques, such as the therapeutic community; upgrading of the education of nonprofessionals; and movement toward greater precision in diagnosis (see Classification and Diagnosis of Mental Disease, below), better understanding of genetic factors in psychopathology, and more appropriate use of psychoactive drugs—antipsychotic, antidepressant, antianxiety, and antimanic. Pharmacologic investigation of these agents has led to biochemical studies of the neurotransmitters and their possible role in the cause or course of mental illness.

Recently, several noninvasive brain imaging techniques have become available. These include computed tomography, magnetic resonance imaging, measurement of regional cerebral blood flow and single photon emission computed tomography to assess functional activity, and positron emission tomography. These techniques are being used to map brain structure and function in normal humans and are enlarging our knowledge of the pathophysiology of mental illnesses.

Deinstitutionalization has increased, reinforced by more stringent legal mechanisms required to institutionalize a person against his wishes or, in hospitalized patients, to administer therapy. These measures protect against abuse of civil rights, but they also make it more difficult to provide treatment to patients who may be very irrational. Psychiatrists must understand and cope with the complexity of these issues, the sometimes competing demands for protection of individual rights vs. optimal therapy, and the need to assist society in developing better means of resolving these issues.

Psychotherapy is *the treatment of disorders of the mind or personality by psychologic or psychophysiologic methods.* The principal thrust of the modern theory of psychologic motivation emerged from Freud's study of neurotic patients, which drew attention to the conflict of competing needs and drives for expression or compromise. Formerly the province of psychiatrists and psychoanalysts, psychotherapy is now also practiced by nonpsychiatrists; eg, clinical psychologists, social workers, nurses, clergymen, and many paraprofessionals. Former patients may also act as psychotherapists; their credentials are that they have experienced distress similar to that experienced by those for whom they care—particularly, drug abusers, alcoholics, delinquents, and criminals. There are > 130 different psychotherapeutic modes, classified into 4 major schools: analytically oriented, behavioral, humanistic, and transpersonal. Others, such as many group and community-oriented therapies, may be classified as pantheoretical; some, such as primal therapy, defy classification.

Partly as a result of the broad range of those conducting psychotherapy, a new role has emerged, ie, as an aid in coping with the travails of ordinary life rather than only with deep, crippling psychologic disorders. People are being helped who do not fit into the traditional diagnostic categories of psychosis and neurosis; ie, normal persons seeking therapy for life problems (eg, employment problems, bereavement, or family illness). Methods of short-term therapy involve a therapist who is more active than was the case in traditional psychoanalysis. Jerome Frank proposed the following 6 features as common to all psychotherapies: (1) an intense, emotionally charged, confiding relationship with a helping person, often with the participation of a group; (2) a rationale or myth that includes an explanation of the cause of the patient's distress and a method for relieving it; (3) provision of new information concerning the nature and source of the patient's problems and possible alternatives for dealing with them; (4) strengthening the patient's expectations of help through the personal qualities of the therapist, enhanced by his status in society and the setting in which he works; (5) provision of success experiences that further heighten the patient's hopes and also enhance his sense of mastery, interpersonal competence, or capability; and (6) facilitation of emotional arousal, which seems to be a prerequisite to attitudinal and behavioral changes.

Hypnosis in medicine has had a resurgence of interest. In selected patients, it is valuable in managing pain, as an alternative or adjunctive method of anesthesia, and in treating psychosomatic disorders. Hypnotic approaches range from direct symptom modification to investigations of psychodynamic issues.

The cult movement must interest psychiatrists, who need to understand how cult members are recruited, what happens to them when they are in cults (ie, methods of indoctrination), and how to understand and treat the problems of former members and their families. Clinical studies have identified specific cult-related emotional problems with which ex-members must cope during their reentry into society.

Self-help/mutual-aid groups have been with us for over 50 yr, although in a broader sense they are quite ancient—mutual aid has been practiced since families first existed. Each of us requires a social network to satisfy our needs to be cared for, accepted, and emotionally supported, particularly in times of stress.

In this century social changes have diminished this traditional support, and today the help not always provided by natural or professional support systems is supplemented or complemented by mutual-aid groups, eg, self-care groups for those suffering from physical or mental illnesses, reform groups for addictive behaviors, and advocacy groups for certain minorities (handicapped persons, the elderly, homosexuals, etc). Although professionals have launched many groups, most are not dependent on (but can and do work well with) professionals or professional agencies. Psychiatrists can help group leaders to avoid the risks of unrealistic goals or excessive hope and also to learn more about the essential psychologic mechanisms of inspiration and hope inherent in the self-help movement. Psychiatrists have a serious responsibility in advising and supporting the families of the mentally ill.

In spite of these real advances, understanding of the basic causes of mental illness has yet to be achieved and requires continued and vigorous research in all fields relevant to the determinants of abnormal human behavior.

Classification and Diagnosis of Mental Disease

In all medical disciplines, classification of disease is a dynamic process, ever changing to incorporate new knowledge. Access to the brain and techniques for measuring and evaluating its functions, particularly mental activities, are still limited because our understanding of the etiology and pathogenesis of mental disorders is scant. Nevertheless, attempts to categorize mental illness for the past half century have included theoretical concepts of causality, mixed with descriptive criteria. As a result, terminology and definitions of terms have varied widely among different psychiatrists and in different places. Since diagnosis implies prognosis and determines choices of therapy, and since standardization of diagnostic categories is essential to research design, the need for revision of psychiatric nomenclature and classification has been great.

TABLE 49–1. DSM-III-R DIAGNOSES WITH DIFFERENT ICD-9-CM CODES

DSM-III-R	Diagnoses	ICD-9-CM
294.80	Organic mental disorder NOS	294.9
305.30	Hallucinogen hallucinosis	292.12
307.40	Parasomnia NOS	307.47
312.39	Impulse control disorder NOS	312.30
780.50	Hypersomnia related to known organic factor	780.54
780.50	Insomnia related to known organic factor	780.52
780.54	Primary hypersomnia	307.44
v40.00	Borderline intellectual functioning	v62.89

DSM-III-R = *Diagnostic and Statistical Manual of Mental Disorders* of the American Psychiatric Association (3rd Edition, Revised); ICD-9-CM = *International Classification of Diseases*, 9th Revision, Clinical Modification; NOS = not otherwise specified.

Adapted from *Psychiatric News* 24(9):24, 1989; used with permission of the American Psychiatric Association.

The American Psychiatric Association introduced a new *Diagnostic and Statistical Manual of Mental Disorders* (**DSM-I**) in 1952. The Third Edition (**DSM-III**) was published in 1980 and revised as **DSM-III-R** in 1987. This classification attempts to rely entirely on descriptions of symptoms and signs; ie, what the patient says and does as indicators of how he thinks and feels. Specific diagnostic criteria (based on current clinical impressions and not yet fully validated) are suggested for the various disorders. DSM-III also inaugurated a 5-axis evaluation system for coding information. The first 3 axes constitute the diagnostic assessment. Axis I codes the clinical syndromes and some additional codes; Axis II, personality disorders and specific developmental disorders; Axis III, potentially relevant physical disorders and conditions. Axis IV codes the severity of psychosocial stressors; Axis V, the highest level of functioning during the past year.

Often patients have multiple problems. A multiaxial system helps ensure that some of these are not overlooked and that the presenting problem does not shut out awareness of other important issues; eg, the presence of schizophrenia or depression should not preclude awareness of important personality and physical illnesses.

In this edition of THE MERCK MANUAL, most of the contributions use DSM-III (1980) and DSM-III-R (1987) terminology.

In the USA, physicians must include diagnosis codes on Medicare Part B claim forms to be paid for their services. The Health Care Financing Administration (**HCFA**) has specified that for consistency all physicians must use the numeric codes of the *International Classification of Diseases, 9th Revision, Clinical Modification* (**ICD-9-CM**), published by the World Health Organization (**WHO**). Psychiatrists will be able to use the codes in DSM-III-R with slight modifications. They will merely have to drop the 4th and 5th digit zeros from some 60 codes in DSM-III-R and substitute new codes for 8 diagnostic categories. TABLE 49–1 lists those DSM-III-R diagnoses with different ICD-9-CM codes.

50. THE PSYCHIATRIC INTERVIEW

Although detail and emphasis in psychiatric and medical interviews differ, the purposes and techniques are similar: to establish a therapeutic physician-patient relationship, upon which accurate data collection and effective treatment depend. The initial interview is therefore a particularly significant encounter.

Approach to the Patient

Sources of clinical data include the patient's verbal content (what he says), manner of speaking (how he says it), and nonverbal communication (body language) and associated somatic clues, as well as the interviewer's own emotional responses. Often overlooked but important are dress, posture, gait, facial expression, complexion, weight, and movement. These different sources of data are evaluated simultaneously in the psychiatric interview, a difficult but rewarding process that improves with the physician's increasing experience and sophistication. A mental posture of free-floating attention to the entire gestalt of the patient-interviewer interactions is the most effective way to obtain information from all levels. That is, while listening carefully to the patient, the interviewer is equally observant of the patient's facial expressions, gestures, postural changes, as well as his own emotional reactions toward the patient. Data at one level will often augment, modify, or even contradict data at another level; eg, the patient who shifts position or fidgets with his watch while verbally denying concern about the subject being discussed. Blushing, blanching, perspiring, increase in respiratory rate, and increase in tics or mannerisms all indicate emotional arousal. Often a subtle cue—a shift of gaze or slight change of expression—suggests covert emotions, fantasies, or impulses. Body language may communicate more eloquently than words the pain of a deep depression, the terror of acute anxiety, or the eroticism of seductive behavior.

The patient's behavior is determined by the reality of the present situation, his past experiences, his personality, and his outlook on life. Commonly, he will have mixed feelings; while he usually acknowledges his need for help and is relieved to share his concern with a potentially helpful professional, he may also fear rejection, criticism, or humiliation. Thus, his perceptions of and reactions to the interviewer contain both rational and irrational elements, and his behavior may appear inconsistent, puzzling, or inappropriate. With psychotic illness or severe organic brain syndrome, these aberrations of perception and behavior may be extreme.

A **spouse, relative, or friend** often accompanies a patient, who usually is seen first. Sometimes, however (eg, when there is an organic problem or language difficulty, or when the patient is an elderly person or a child), seeing the relative first or even both the patient and relative together may be preferable; but permission should be obtained from the patient, if appropriate. The opportunity to interview someone who knows the patient can add valuable perspective, but the confidentiality of each source must be respected.

The physician's attitude, while attentive, friendly, and encouraging, should retain an appropriate objectivity in relation to the patient and his problems. Total emotional neutrality is neither possible nor desirable, but the physician should be especially aware of feelings of irritability, impatience, or special attraction toward the patient. Other emotions that may be experienced by the physician are anxiety, sadness, sympathy, indifference, or resentment. Recognizing these emotions, learning what in the patient's behavior elicited them, and preventing them from disrupting the interview are essential.

The temptation to outdo the patient by recounting personal experiences, moralizing about the patient's behavior, giving gratuitous advice, or providing dogmatic opinions should be resisted. Questions generally should be turned back to the patient ("Well, what do you think yourself?"), although at times it is beneficial to answer a question directly and then promptly return the interview focus to the patient.

Interview Setting, Direction, and Length

The tone for the entire interview is established within the first few minutes. While not always available, a quiet, comfortable, and private **setting** lends dignity to the encounter and encourages free discussion. Regardless of the setting, the interviewer should communicate professionalism, concern, and willingness to take the necessary time. The physician greets the patient by name, performs introductions, indicates the purpose of the interview, and inquires regarding the patient's comfort at the moment.

Direction of the interview is established next. Needless controversy has existed concerning interviewing technique, with the two extremes represented by an entirely physician-directed interview and a totally open-ended interview directed entirely by the patient. The important points are that doctor and patient are constantly cueing each other (verbally and nonverbally) and every interview is "directed"; the style of direction by the physician may vary, and he should be aware of what is going on. No technique is uniformly successful under all circumstances, since the time available, the specific purpose of the interview, and the patient's clinical state will require appropriate modifications. Open-ended questions that permit the patient to respond in his own words have the virtue of eliciting unexpected information and often the most reliable data. Specific questions, as in a system review, provide important data that might not otherwise be obtained; eg, about sexual behavior, alcohol and drug abuse, suicidal ideas and plans, and hallucinations. The approach described below under Obtaining the History usually is applicable and productive.

The interview length must be flexible. With some patients 15 min may be ample, as in cases of severe delirium, psychosis, or dementia. Conversely, an hour may be insufficient in a complex case where the patient is articulate and cooperative. In crisis situations with an acutely agitated patient, or when the patient is otherwise incapable of supplying a complete history, the interview goals must be realistically limited. Time constraints include the patient's tolerance for fatigue and anxiety and the physician's own time limits. However, too brief an interview may prevent establishment of the bond necessary for the patient to communicate openly. The initial psychiatric interview usually requires at least 30 min; more often, 45 or 60 min. When there are time constraints, the patient should be assured of further opportunity to complete the assessment.

Termination of the interview usually is straightforward, although a loquacious or demanding patient may require firm interruption. The patient's questions should be encouraged and answered truthfully. Overly optimistic reassurance or unjustified guarantees of treatment efficacy should be avoided; the attempt to provide comfort and hope must be tempered with realism.

Obtaining the History

Inquiry should begin by asking the patient to identify the problem (in broad outline) for which he is seeking help. Questions such as "What has been the problem that brought you here?" or "Please tell me what has led you to come to see me today" are useful. Comments such as "Um-humm" or "Tell me more about that" at this stage encourage the patient to talk freely, as does repeating with a questioning inflection a key word or phrase spoken by the patient. As the patient talks, clarification is sought of key words such as depression, panic, nervousness, and anxiety, since these terms mean different things to different people. However, premature efforts to determine the exact details and their chronologic order at the very beginning of the interview may inhibit and distract the patient and reduce the information available to the interviewer. In this early phase of the interview, the major focus is to learn what is significant to the patient himself, how he narrates his story, what emotions are manifest, and what nonverbal cues he communicates, as well as areas of vagueness, inconsistency, or confusion. Exceptions to this approach occur in some psychotic and organic states, where it is obvious immediately that the patient needs structure and direction in order to furnish useful information.

Once the patient has related his difficulties in his own words, a more structured approach is used to **follow up leads** in the original narrative and to **open up new areas** for discussion. Again, questions should be initially open-ended in order to encourage elaboration by the patient. For each problem area, one must clarify the time and mode of onset and get a detailed description of the symptoms or situations, chronology of events, aggravating and alleviating factors, and associated elements or manifestations. Progressively more directed, specific questions are required to obtain all pertinent information, including queries about some symptoms merely to establish that the patient does not have them, eg, hallucinations or suicidal thoughts.

Personal and family histories are obtained next, to provide a background against which the illness can be viewed and to find clues to the genesis of the illness and to possible therapeutic approaches. **Work history, social relationships, other interests,** and future goals complete this section of the interview. The interviewer should observe evidence of emotional arousal or conflict in the patient during this review and encourage further elaboration in sensitive areas.

Recording the History

In contrast to the flexibility used in obtaining a history, a particular format should be followed to record it. The schema shown in TABLE 50-1 is commonly used; but the developmental approach is also acceptable, starting at birth or with the family history so that the illness is described in the perspective of the patient's life story.

Mental Status Examination

The distinction between history and examination is even more blurred in psychiatry than in general medicine. Most (and frequently all) of the mental status examination is carried out while the history is being obtained. It is unnecessary to demand from an intelligent, coherent young adult the names of the last six heads of state, a recitation of long sequences of numbers, or the interpretation of proverbs and fables. However, when a formal mental status test is *required* to document the patient's mental state, the interviewer tactfully requests cooperation. The results may be recorded as shown in TABLE 50-2.

Formulation

Essential to the psychiatric evaluation is *a concise statement of the interviewer's understanding of and plans for the case:* the formulation. It begins with a summary of the relevant data from the history and mental status examination organized

TABLE 50–1. FORMAT FOR RECORDING THE PSYCHIATRIC HISTORY

Category	Pertinent Details
Identifying characteristics	Name, age, sex, race, marital status, occupation, source of referral
Presenting problems	A brief verbatim statement

History of present illness	Chronologic account of the current symptoms and behavioral changes, together with coincident life events and their relationships
	
	    Events are dated as accurately as possible
	    Symptoms are recorded in the patient's own words, with qualifying details
	
	Previous treatments and responses to them are noted, and the present degree of disability is estimated

Personal history	Birth and infancy
	    Nature of delivery; temperament and habits; ages at passing milestones (walking, talking, toilet training)
	Childhood
	    Emotional adjustment, neurotic symptoms, physical illnesses, relationships with peers and siblings
	Education
	    Duration and details of schooling; achievements, attitudes, and adjustments
	Work record
	    List of jobs, reasons for changing, achievements, adjustments
	Legal
	    Criminal record, current legal status
	Religious
	    Affiliation, attendance, and activity
	Sexual maturation
	    Date of menarche or puberty
	    Growth of sexual interest and practice
	    Courtship, marriage, and children
	    Emotional and sexual compatibility with mate

Previous medical history	Physical and psychiatric illnesses
Personality and social patterns prior to illness	Social relationships within the home, at work, and in the community Individual and social activities and interests Predominant moods Character traits, strengths and weaknesses, coping style, methods of handling challenge and stress, temperament Religious and moral standards Ambitions and aspirations Habits, including drinking, drug use, smoking
Family history	Details of each parent and sibling regarding age, health, occupation, personality, relationship with the patient Familial diseases, including psychiatric illness For a deceased relative, the date and cause of death are recorded

TABLE 50–2. RECORDING OF MENTAL STATUS

Category	Pertinent Details
Appearance and behavior	Dress, posture, facial expression, motor activity such as agitation, impulsivity, mannerisms, retardation, relationship to the interviewer
Stream of talk (thought processes)	Poverty or rigidity of thought Pace and progression of speech Whether speech is logical and to the point or confusing and irrelevant Presence of thought disorder, flight of ideas, obsessional qualification, distractibility The stream of talk is recorded verbatim if relevant
Thought content	Special preoccupations, obsessional ideas, misinterpretations, ideas of reference or influence, delusions, derogatory or grandiose ideas
Perceptual abnormalities	Auditory, visual, or tactile hallucinations Depersonalization Derealization
Affect	Happiness, elation, sadness, depression, irritability, anger, suspicion, perplexity, fear, anxiety Blunting or incongruity of affect Lability or reactivity of mood Appropriateness to context
Cognitive functions	Sensorium (level of consciousness) Memory and orientation: immediate recall; memory for recent and remote events; digit span; orientation in time, place, person Concentration: serial sevens, months of the year in reverse order General information: the Presidents, capitals, distances, etc Intelligence: compatibility of school and work records with current performance, interpretation of proverbs, general vocabulary, calculations Insight and judgment, especially with regard to present illness and future plans Psychometric testing may be necessary

as an explanatory hypothesis of the patient's condition. Included is an assessment of the patient's personality strengths and vulnerabilities, as well as identification of those factors contributing to the origin and evolution of the illness. A differential diagnosis, necessary further investigations, an outline of an initial treatment plan, and a statement of prognosis complete the formulation.

51. PSYCHIATRY IN MEDICINE

PSYCHIATRIC CONSIDERATIONS IN THE MEDICAL INTERVIEW

Whether a physician is involved in primary care or in subspecialist consultative care, an organ- and disease-specific approach to diagnosis and care often goes awry when the *person* with the organs and disease is ignored. Relating a patient's complaints and disabilities to his personal-

ity and social circumstances helps to form a sound clinical judgment about the nature and causes of the disorder.

To form a picture of the individual patient's personality, the physician has only to listen attentively and show interest in the patient as a person (see also Ch. 50). A rigid interview conducted hastily and in an emotionally indifferent way with close-ended, branching system review queries will more likely prevent the patient from revealing relevant information than help him divulge it. Tracing the history of the presenting illness with open-ended questions that permit the patient to tell his story in his own words takes no longer, but it is important to note comments that describe associated social circumstances and emotional reactions, as well as attitudes toward physicians and medicines.

Attention then should turn to the patient's social background, previous medical and psychiatric history, and adjustment at different stages of his life. Parental characteristics and the family atmosphere during his childhood are important because personality features that influence the way a person handles illness and adversity are partly determined early in life. The way the patient has handled different family and social roles provides important clues. His behavior in schooling, manner of handling puberty and adolescence, stability and effectiveness at work, sexual adaptation, pattern of social life, and quality and stability of marriage provide information valuable in appraising his personality. Use or abuse of alcohol and tobacco, behavior while driving, and any tendencies to antisocial conduct should be tactfully inquired after. The patient's responses to the usual vicissitudes of life—failures, setbacks, losses, previous illnesses—are important; he may have endured stresses and misfortunes with courage and resilience, or his history may suggest a poor capacity for tolerating frustration.

The **personality profile** that emerges from these inquiries may reveal traits such as self-centeredness, immaturity, excessive dependency, anxiety, tendencies to deny illness, histrionic behavior—or conscientiousness, modesty, and adaptability. In particular, the history may reveal **patterns of repetitive behavior** that the patient exhibits under stressful conditions; ie, whether distress is expressed in somatic symptoms (eg, headache, abdominal pain), in psychologic symptoms (eg, phobic behavior, depression), or in social behavior (eg, withdrawal or rebelliousness). **Attitudes** should be noted; eg, toward the taking of medicines in general or specific types of drugs (steroids, sedatives), toward physicians or hospitals, etc. With this information the physician can better interpret the patient's complaints, anticipate his reactions to his illness, and plan appropriate therapy.

Observation during the interview also provides valuable data. A patient may be depressed and pessimistic, or cheerful, facile, and prone to deny illness; he may be friendly and warm, or reserved, cold, and suspicious. Nonverbal communication may reveal attitudes and affects denied by the patient's words. For example, a patient who "chokes up" or becomes tearful when discussing a parent's death is revealing that it was a significant loss; the possibility that unresolved grief is still a problem should occur to the physician. A tear in the eye, overt weeping, or other such manifestations of emotion should be considered as **physical signs** and should be recorded as such in the patient's chart.

Similarly, when a patient denies being angry, anxious, or depressed while his posture, gestures, and facial expression reveal these emotions, further inquiry may reveal stresses and emotionally depressing circumstances possibly related to the evolution of the present illness. However, the physician should be cautious and remember the possibility of error in such inquiries. Discriminating and experienced judgment is needed to assess whether psychologic conflicts are highly significant, of limited importance, or perhaps merely coincidental to the patient's physical illness.

Referral for a psychiatric opinion: About 10% of patients admitted to a hospital are referred for a psychiatric consultation. Many of these patients have attempted suicide, and a substantial proportion have other conspicuous psychologic disturbances that require appraisal and treatment. Particularly important are delirium, dementia, and functional psychiatric syndromes due to organic or metabolic brain disorders. In or out of the hospital, awareness of each patient's personality and its relation to his somatic complaints will aid in managing physically ill patients and increase the physician's awareness of psychiatrically ill or disturbed persons. Many of these patients suffer from complex, difficult, or refractory problems that will require referral to a psychiatrist.

An infrequently used, but very helpful, procedure is for the primary care physician to discuss the situation with a psychiatric colleague *before* making a referral. Advice obtained in such an exchange may obviate the need for referral or help to make the referral in the most appropriate manner. When referral is planned, it should be discussed openly and sensitively with the patient.

PSYCHOSOMATIC MEDICINE
(Biopsychosocial Medicine)

Psychologic factors may contribute directly or indirectly to the etiology of some physical disorders; in others, psychiatric symptoms may be a direct expression of a lesion involving neural or endocrine organs. Psychologic symptoms also may occur as a reaction to a physical illness. The use of the term "psychosomatic" to encompass these possibilities is a diffuse concept, but it draws attention to the ubiquity of emotional disturbances and psychologic interrelationships with somatic disease and disability.

In more limited use, "psychosomatic" refers to conditions in which psychologic factors have etiologic importance. Even in these disorders, however, the etiology is always complex and multifactorial, and psychologic factors are *not* the only contributors to the illness. It is useful to consider a *necessary* **biologic** component (eg, the genetic tendency to non−insulin-dependent diabetes mellitus) that, when combined with **psychologic** reactions (eg, depression) and **social** stress (eg, loss of a loved person), results in a set of conditions *sufficient* to produce the illness; hence, the term **biopsychosocial.** The stressful environmental events and psychologic reactions may be viewed as triggers or precipitants of illness. These reactions are *nonspecific* and have been noted in association with a wide variety of diseases, such as diabetes mellitus, SLE, leukemia, and multiple sclerosis. Furthermore, the importance of psychologic factors is relative and varies widely in different patients with the same disorder (eg, asthma, in which genetic factors, allergy, and infection, as well as the patient's emotions, interact to varying degrees).

The fact that psychologic stress can precipitate or alter the course of even major organic diseases has long been apparent but very difficult for physicians to accept and comprehend. Emotions obviously can affect the autonomic nervous system and, secondarily, cardiac rate, sweating, or bowel peristalsis. But can a reaction affecting the mind (brain) alter immune responses mediated by lymphocytes and lymphokines? And if so, what are the mechanisms? The answer to the first question is becoming clear. **Psychoimmunology** is now an established area of scientific research, and both animal and human studies have demonstrated the interrelationship. For example, the immune response of mice has been clearly reduced in response to conditioned stimuli; and in humans the ability to reduce the delayed hypersensitivity skin response and even in vitro stimulation of lymphocytes to varicella zoster has been demonstrated. However, the pathways and mechanisms by which the brain and immune system interact remain to be elucidated.

Indirect effects of psychologic factors may influence the course of a variety of illnesses. Commonly a patient's need to deny illness (or, more subtly, to deny the seriousness of an illness) may lead to noncompliance with medical regimens or refusal to accept therapeutic recommendations. In diabetes, for example, a patient may become depressed over his endless dependence on insulin injections and careful dietary management and may neglect his therapy. The result is an apparent or pseudo-brittle diabetes, which cannot be properly managed unless the patient's conflicts about independence are dealt with. Other common examples are patients with hypertension or epilepsy who fail to take medication, and patients who reject diagnostic procedures or operations.

Increasingly, physicians are dealing with disorders that result in chronic disability or that are likely to recur; eg, myocardial infarction, hypertension, cerebrovascular disease, diabetes mellitus, malignancy, RA, and chronic respiratory illness. Psychologic and social stress are entwined with these disorders; however, cause and effect are difficult associations to disentangle. Psychosocial pressures may alter the clinical course of these disorders, commonly interacting with the individual's hereditary predisposition, personality features, and the autonomic and endocrine effects that arise in response to individual vicissitudes.

Somatic Symptoms Reflecting Psychic States

Psychosocial stress producing conflict and requiring an adaptive response may appear *disguised in somatic form* with what appear to be symptoms of organic disease. The emotional disturbance is often overlooked or even denied by the patient and sometimes by the doctor. The cause and mechanism of symptom formation may be fairly obvious; eg, anxiety and adrenergic-mediated phenomena such as tachycardia and sweating. However, the mechanisms responsible for psychogenic symptoms are often unclear, although they are generally ascribed to tension, acting directly (eg, increased muscle tension) or through a conversion process.

Conversion is *the unconscious process of transforming psychic conflict and anxiety into a somatic symptom.* The term was traditionally linked to hysterical (histrionic) behavior (see HYSTERICAL NEUROSIS in Ch. 56), but in primary care medicine it should be considered separately, as it occurs in both sexes and in patients of any personality type. This type of symptom formation is seen virtually every day in a busy primary care practice but unfortunately is poorly understood and seldom recognized. As a result, patients may be subjected to multiple, tedious, expensive, and sometimes dangerous investigations in search of an elusive organic illness.

Virtually any symptom that can be imagined may become a conversion symptom, and the history usually reveals how the patient "selected" his particular symptom. Commonly, the patient will have **previously experienced the symptom on an organic basis**; eg, a painful fracture, angina pectoris, or a ruptured lumbar disk. At a time of psychosocial stress, the symptom reappears (or pe[sists following adequate treatment) as a psychogenic symptom. Alternatively, the patient may "borrow" the symptom from another person; eg, the medical student who imagines his lymph nodes are swollen while caring for a patient with lymphoma, or the person who presents with chest pain after an associate or relative has a myocardial infarction. In each case, the patient has **identified with someone else who had the symptom**. Finally, the symptom may have been unconsciously selected by the patient because of its **value as a metaphor** for his psychosocial condition; eg, the patient with chest pain following rejection by a lover ("broken heart"), or the patient with back pain who feels that his burdens are too difficult to carry. Pain of one sort or another is the most common conversion symptom; eg, atypical facial pain, vague headaches, poorly localized abdominal discomfort and colic, backache or neck pain, limb pain that sometimes simulates intermittent claudication, dysuria, dyspareunia, or dysmenorrhea.

An interesting variation of this mechanism has commonly been reported under the rubric of **mass hysteria** or **epidemic hysteria**, in which a group of people suddenly become concerned about, for example, food poisoning or a toxic substance in the air and develop symptoms in imitation of those who imagined the problem first. Reports have been most common about preadolescent and adolescent children who become ill at school, but similar phenomena occur in other settings. Such episodes may be dramatic and troublesome to distinguish early on, but they usually become obvious and have a benign outcome.

Anxiety and **depression** are commonly seen affects elicited by psychic stress and may be expressed as symptoms in any body system. No diagnostic difficulties are encountered if several body systems are involved and the patient also describes his personal anguish and apprehension. But if the patient expresses symptoms through a single system and fails to emphasize emotional discomfort, diagnostic problems are created. Such cases are often described as **masked depression**, although in some instances **masked anxiety** would be a more appropriate term. Dysphoria and depressive symptoms such as insomnia, self-disparagement, psychomotor retardation, and a pessimistic outlook are common; but the patient may deny actual depression of mood. Alternatively, the patient may acknowledge the presence of depression or anxiety but may insist that it is secondary to some elusive physical condition.

Psychologic Reactions to Physical Illness

Patients will respond differently to being ill, and it is wise to keep in mind the psychologic effects of chronic illnesses, the effect of the patient's knowledge about or lack of understanding of the diagnosis, and the patient's response to the physician's attitudes and communications. Responses to the side effects of drugs are also highly variable.

Many patients with recurrent or chronic physical disorders experience depression that aggravates the disability and sets up a vicious circle. The gradual decline in well-being due to the physical disorder in Parkinson's disease, cardiac failure, or RA creates a depressive reaction that in turn lessens the sense of well-being still further. Antidepressant treatment in these cases often promotes improvement.

Patients with major losses of function or of body parts (eg, as a result of stroke, amputation, spinal cord injury) are particularly difficult to evaluate. A subtle distinction needs to be made between a reactive clinical depression that requires traditional psychiatric treatment and dysphoric emotional reactions that may be extreme but are appropriate to devastating physical illness. The latter are mood disorders or a constellation of grief, demoralization, withdrawal, and regression. They tend not to respond favorably to psychotherapy or antidepressant drugs, but to fluctuate with the patient's clinical state and improve over time if rehabilitation is successful or if the patient adapts to his changed status. In rehabilitation hospitals, it is not unusual for staff to diagnose depression when that is not the problem or to miss the diagnosis when it is present. Differential diagnosis is very difficult in this situation, and it is most helpful to have a consulting physician who is trained in psychiatry and experienced in dealing with patients with somatic disorders.

MUNCHAUSEN SYNDROME
(Pathologic Malingering; Chronic
Factitious Illness; Hospital Hobos)

Repeated fabrication of illness, usually acute, dramatic, and convincing, by a person who wanders from hospital to hospital for treatment. Many medical disorders may be closely mimicked; eg, individual patients have produced the clinical picture of myocardial infarction, hematemesis or hemoptysis, acute abdominal conditions, or a fever of unknown origin—all mimicked with uncanny skill. A patient's abdominal wall may be a criss-cross of scars, and a digit or a limb may have been amputated. Fevers are often due to self-inflicted abscesses, and the culture, usually *Escherichia coli,* clearly indicates the source of the infecting organism.

In a bizarre variant of the syndrome, *a child may be used as a surrogate patient.* (This has been referred to as "Munchausen by proxy.") The parent falsifies history and may injure the child with drugs, add blood or bacterial contaminants to urine specimens, etc—all in order to simulate disease.

Patients with Munchausen syndrome initially and sometimes interminably become the responsibility of medical or surgical clinics. Nevertheless, the disorder is primarily a psychiatric problem, is more complex than simple dishonest simulation of symptoms, and is associated with severe emotional difficulties. The patient's personality may show prominent histrionic features, but these individuals are usually quite intelligent and resourceful. They not only know how to mimic disease, they are sophisticated with regard to medical practices. Their deceits and simulations are conscious, but the motivations for their forgery of illness and quest for attention are largely unconscious.

Commonly, there is an early history of emotional and physical abuse. Patients appear to have problems with their identity, intense feelings, inadequate impulse control, a deficient sense of reality, brief psychotic episodes, and unstable interpersonal relationships. The need to be taken care of is at odds with the inability to trust authority figures, who are manipulated and

continually provoked or tested. Feelings of guilt and the associated need for punishment and expiation are obvious.

Factitious illnesses of various sorts bear a modicum of similarity to Munchausen syndrome. Patients may consciously produce the manifestations of a disease, eg, by traumatizing their skin or by exposing themselves to an allergen to which they know they are sensitive. They then present themselves for medical care, but they sabotage therapy with self-induced or self-perpetuated disease. These patients, however, are quite different from those with Munchausen: They tend to simulate only one disease; this is done only at a time of major psychosocial stress; they do not tend to wander from one hospital or physician to another. Most important, they usually can be treated successfully.

Treatment

In Munchausen patients with psychopathology of psychotic proportions encompassed within a characterologic disorder, successful treatment is rare. Acceding to the patients' manipulations will relieve their tension, but their provocations escalate, ultimately surpassing what physicians are willing or able to do. Refusal to meet treatment demands or confrontation results in angry reactions, and the patient generally moves on to another hospital. Psychiatric treatment is usually refused or circumvented, but consultation and follow-up care may be accepted, at least to help resolve a crisis. However, management is generally limited to early recognition of the disorder and avoidance of risky procedures as well as excessive or unwarranted medication.

Patients with factitious illness should be confronted with the diagnosis in a manner that avoids suggesting guilt or reproach. The status of legitimate illness must be preserved, while the physician indicates that he and the patient can cooperatively resolve the underlying problem. Often this will involve another member of the family, but it is best then to discuss the problem as an illness, not as a deception; ie, the family is not told the precise mechanism of the disease.

52. PERSONALITY DISORDERS

Disordered patterns of behavior characterized by relatively fixed, inflexible, and stylized reactions to stress, representing the individual's way

of dealing with other people and external events regardless of existing realities. **Personality traits** also are patterns of perceiving and relating to the environment and oneself; but the **disorders** are rigid and maladaptive, and damage social, interpersonal, and work relationships. The characteristic patterns of maladjustment are evident from childhood and through much of the life span.

Without environmental frustration, individuals with personality disorders tend to show little anxiety or mental or emotional symptoms, and they feel that their behavior patterns are "normal" and "right." Rarely seeking help because of their own anxiety and discomfort, they more often are referred by their families or by social agencies because of the difficulties their maladaptive behavior causes others. When they seek help, usually after environmental frustrations, these patients view their difficulties as *outside* of themselves, unlike neurotic persons, whose defense mechanisms trouble the user but not the observer.

Personality disorders are medically and psychiatrically important for three reasons: (1) Externalization of internal conflicts often leads to clashes with others in ways that bring the patient under medical observation. The result often is a maladaptive physician-patient relationship, with the patient refusing to take appropriate responsibility and the physician blaming, distrusting, and ultimately rejecting the patient. (2) Individuals with severe personality disorders are at high risk of becoming addicted to alcohol or drugs, of behaving in a self-destructive manner, of pursuing sexually deviant lives with which they cannot cope, and of clashing with society and its mores. (3) These persons are susceptible to breakdown on exposure to stress. The type of personality disorder may or may not determine the kind of psychiatric illness that complicates it; eg, a person with a hysterical personality may respond to excess emotional stress by hysterical conversion or dissociative symptoms, or a suicidal depression.

Diagnosis

Diagnosis is based on the presence of the typical rigid behavior patterns as well as the patient's lack of insight and resistance to change—his apparent inability to learn from experience. Certain **mental coping mechanisms** (see below) are used unconsciously at times by most people. The maladaptive behavior patterns seen in personality disorders tend to be exaggerations of these mechanisms, which may result in the diagnosis of a personality disorder when used chronically and maladaptively. Although these mechanisms cannot be breached by reason or interpretation,

they respond to supportive but forceful confrontation in prolonged psychotherapy or peer encounters, and to improved interpersonal relationships.

Dissociation (neurotic denial) effects temporary but drastic modification of one's personality or sense of personal identity. These modifications can include fugues, hysterical conversion reactions, short-term denial of responsibility for one's acts or feelings, trance states, chance-taking, and pharmacologic intoxication to numb unhappiness. **Projection** is the act of attributing one's own *un*acknowledged feelings to others; it leads to prejudice, rejection of intimacy through paranoid suspicion, overvigilance to external danger, and injustice-collecting. **Schizoid fantasy** is a tendency to use imaginary relationships and private belief systems for the purpose of conflict resolution and relief from loneliness. It is associated with eccentricity and global avoidance of interpersonal intimacy. In contrast to the psychotic person, the user of schizoid fantasy who has a personality disorder does not fully believe in or insists on acting out his or her fantasies. Unlike dissociation, the use of fantasy remakes the outer, not the inner, world. **Hypochondriasis** (see also Ch. 56) transforms reproaches toward others (which may have arisen from bereavement, loneliness, or anger) into unremitting somatic complaints, as an expression of the entrenched belief that some organic disease is present. In contrast to neurotic conversion reaction, in which distress is muted and the doctor is fascinated, in hypochondriasis the patient's distress is exaggerated, he is resistant to logical reassurance and treatment, and the physician feels helpless and resentful. **Turning against the self** allows aggression toward others to be expressed toward the self; such expression may be expressed indirectly and ineffectively through passivity. It includes failures and illnesses that affect others more than oneself, and silly, provocative clowning. The mechanism underlies most sadomasochistic relationships. **Acting out** is the direct behavioral expression of an unconscious wish or impulse in order to avoid being conscious of the affect—painful or pleasurable—that accompanies it. The object of the wish or impulse is often a complete stranger. Acting out includes many delinquent, impulsive, and deviant acts that seem motiveless because the actor is unaware of his or her own feelings. **Splitting** allows the user to divide people regarded ambivalently in his past life and/or current medical setting into all-good, idealized saviors and all-bad, devalued malefactors. Splitting avoids the discomfort of loving and being angry at the same person. Either the loved or the hated facet is inappropriately transposed to another person.

Classification

The following classification largely reflects the nomenclature suggested in the American Psychiatric Association's *Diagnostic and Statistical Manual of Mental Disorders,* Third Edition – Revised **(DSM-III-R).**

Paranoid personalities are characterized by projection of their own conflicts and hostilities onto others (see also Ch. 59). These persons are markedly sensitive in interpersonal relationships and tend to find hostile and malevolent intentions behind trivial, innocent, or even kindly acts by others. Often their suspicious attitudes lead to aggressive feelings or behavior or bring about rejection by others, which seems to justify their original feelings; however, they are unable to see their own roles in this cycle. Their behavior may be designed to prove their adequacy, while their sense of superiority becomes exaggerated and is accompanied by belittlement of others. In many spheres these persons may be highly efficient and conscientious, although envious and inflexible. They may be litigious, especially when they feel a sense of righteous indignation.

Paranoid tendencies are especially likely to develop among those who feel particularly inferior because of a defect or handicap that makes them noticeably different from their peers. Likewise, sensory impairment, particularly chronic deafness, has a similar effect because it reduces the capacity for reality testing and thus leads to the misinterpretation of being talked about or laughed at.

Schizoid personalities are introverted, withdrawn, solitary, emotionally cold, and distant. They are most often absorbed with their own thoughts and feelings and are fearful of closeness and intimacy with others. They are reticent, given to daydreaming, and prefer theoretic speculation to practical action. This personality pattern is found in about 40% of schizophrenic patients before they become ill. However, many schizoid people do not develop schizophrenia or other mental disorders. Fantasy (see above) is a common coping mechanism. Schizophrenia is discussed in Ch. 58.

Schizotypal personalities display oddities of thinking, perception, communication, and behavior that suggest schizophrenia but are never severe enough to meet the criteria for that disorder (see Ch. 58). These oddities in cognition may be expressed as magical thinking, ideas of reference, and paranoid ideation and, by definition, are more marked than those found in schizoid (see above) and avoidant (see below) personalities.

Histrionic (hysterical) personalities are conspicuously egocentric. Since winning the esteem and admiration of others is important to them, they show attention-seeking and theatrical behavior. Their emotional immaturity is expressed with an exaggerated, childish, emotional response to any wounding of their vanity. Inconsistencies in behavior arise because the histrionic personality can adopt whatever pattern of conduct will place him or her in a favorable light or boost self-esteem. In our culture this form of personality disorder is noted more often in women but also is seen in men.

A histrionic individual's lively manner lends itself to easily established superficial relationships, but these persons are rarely deeply involved emotionally. They may combine provocativeness or sexualization of nonsexual relationships with sexual dysfunction or fears. Their relationships are affected by a seemingly insatiable need for affection, and behind their sexually seductive behavior lies a childlike wish for nonsexual affection and protection; ie, they tend to be dependent. Promiscuous entanglements with many partners are possible because of the histrionic person's lack of real involvement with any of them. The crises that arise from these relationships are managed with manipulative behavior that may include suicidal threats and shrewd exploitation of emotional susceptibilities in other people. Insight fails to develop in histrionic persons because they can easily repress or forget unpleasant experiences; responsibility for misfortunes and failures usually is ascribed to others. Dissociation (see above and in Ch. 56) is a commonly used coping mechanism.

Narcissistic personalities have an exaggerated sense of self-importance and are absorbed by fantasies of unlimited success. Paradoxically, such persons are also often preoccupied with envy. They exhibitionistically seek constant attention. Extreme swings between overidealization and devaluation characterize the relationships of these persons, who also display marked entitlement, interpersonal exploitiveness, and oversensitivity to failure or to criticism. The primary care physician often is frustrated by their incessant and frequently urgent demands relating to what he views as minor problems. As in the case of the hypochondriacal patient, the complaints and entitlement of the narcissistic patient may be caused by genuine but assiduously concealed emotional pain and unhappiness. Like the dependent personality (see below), the narcissistic personality is seen so commonly in the other personality disorders that treating it as an independent disorder may prove ineffective.

Some patients with narcissistic personalities also are characterized by a tendency to complain of multiple somatic symptoms. These patients have been referred to under a variety of terms including **histrionic (hysterical) personality disorder, primitive hysteric, or somatization disorder (Briquet's syndrome).** This last disorder is discussed in Ch. 56.

Antisocial personalities (previously used designations: **psychopathic, sociopathic**) characteristically act out their conflicts and flout normal rules of social order. These persons are impulsive, irresponsible, amoral, and unable to forego immediate gratification. They cannot form sustained affectionate relationships with others, but their charm and plausibility may be highly developed and skillfully used for their own ends. They tolerate frustration poorly, and opposition is likely to elicit hostility, aggression, or serious violence. Their antisocial behavior shows little foresight and is not associated with remorse or guilt, since these people seem to have a keen capacity for rationalizing and for blaming their irresponsible behavior on others. Frustration and punishment rarely modify their behavior or improve their judgment and foresight. Owing to impulsivity, a person with an antisocial personality may attempt suicide if his aggressions become turned inward instead of being directed against others. Dishonesty manifested by lies, frequent geographic moves, and use of false identification are common.

This personality type often is associated with a history of alcoholism, drug addiction, sexual deviation, promiscuity, occupational failure, or imprisonment. In our culture men are more often labeled as antisocial and women as histrionic personalities, but the two patterns have much in common. In families of patients with both patterns, there may be antisocial and histrionic male and female relatives, and in both patterns there is frequently a history of parental strife and severe emotional deprivation in the formative years. Their life expectancy is diminished, but among those surviving there is some tendency to stabilization after age 40. The effects of either severe cerebral injury or undiagnosed alcoholism may closely simulate the picture of an antisocial personality. Unless repetitive antisocial behavior is observed before age 15 and the person is currently at least 18 yr old, the diagnosis of antisocial personality must be doubted.

Borderline personalities are unstable in several areas, including self-image, mood, behavior, and interpersonal relationships. Characteristics include frequent mood shifts, impulsivity, inappropriate and frequently uncontrolled intense anger, and uncertainty concerning identity. These persons are extremists for whom the world is either black or white, hated or loved—never neutral. They are oversensitive to perceived abandonment. To some extent, the borderline personality has features of all the personality disorders listed above and at times their reality testing is so poor that they resemble psychotic patients. For example, brief but frank delusions and hallucinatory experiences are common. Unlike the schizoid personality, however, interpersonal relationships are far more dramatic and intense; unlike the antisocial personality, there is more disturbance of formal thought processes, and aggression is more often turned against the self; and unlike the histrionic personality, there is greater expression of overt anger and greater confusion over sexual identity. Borderline personalities are commonly seen in primary care medical practices, where they tend to appear frequently with vague somatic complaints, often do not comply with therapeutic recommendations, and tend to be very frustrating to their physicians. Splitting, hypochondriasis, and projection are common coping mechanisms (see above).

Avoidant personalities usually are hypersensitive to rejection and fear starting relationships unless assured of uncritical acceptance; there is, however, a strong desire for affection and acceptance. Unlike schizoid personalities, these individuals are openly distressed by their lack of ability to relate comfortably with others. Unlike borderline personalities, they do not respond to rejection with temper tantrums; instead, they appear shy and timid.

Dependent personalities surrender responsibility for major areas of their lives to others and permit the needs of those on whom they are dependent to supersede their own needs. They lack self-confidence and initiative, and they feel intense discomfort when alone for more than brief periods. The features of this syndrome are commonly seen in other personality disorders and are frequently obscured by the more obvious aspects of them. For example, histrionic behavior patterns are quite striking and may mask severe underlying dependency.

Compulsive personalities (obsessive-compulsive) are conscientious and have high levels of aspiration, but they also tend to be perfectionistic and often are unable to gain adequate satisfaction from their achievements. They are reliable, dependable, orderly, and methodical, but their inflexibility often makes them incapable of adapting to changed circumstances. They are cautious and weigh all aspects of a problem; consequently, making decisions may be difficult for them. They bear responsibilities seriously but may suffer much anxiety over them. They pay attention to every detail and are therefore in danger of becoming entangled with means and forgetting the main purposes of their tasks. Compulsiveness is in tune with Western cultural standards, and when the disorder is not too marked, these people often are capable of high levels of achievement, especially in the sciences and other academic fields where order is desirable. On the other hand, they often feel a sense of isolation and have difficulties with interpersonal relationships in which their feelings are not under strict control, events are less predictable, and they must rely on others.

Passive-aggressive personalities are characterized by helplessness, clinging dependency, and procrastination. The apparent passivity is designed to gain attention and affection, to avoid responsibility, or to control or punish others covertly. Passive-aggressive behavior is characterized by obstinacy, inefficiency, and sullenness, often disguised under a superficial compliance. Frequently, individuals with this disorder agree to perform a task and then proceed to subtly undermine its completion with complaints and passive obstructionism. They also may be provocative and argumentative, especially with those in authority. Such behavior usually serves to deny or conceal both hostility and dependency needs. The behavior is maladaptive in that, ironically, it drives others away and prevents the individual from receiving even a normal amount of support. In most cases sadomasochism is seen as a variant of passive-aggressive behavior, but some clinicians believe that masochism and sadism should be classified as separate personality disorders. Hypochondriasis and turning against the self (see above) are common coping mechanisms.

Cyclothymic personalities (see also Ch. 57) fluctuate in their moods between states of high-spirited buoyancy and states of gloom and pessimism, each sustained for weeks or longer. Characteristically, the rhythmic mood changes are regular and predictable and occur either without apparent external cause or in response to trivial events. In one common variant of this disorder, the mood is predominantly marked by elation, energy, an infectious gaiety, and optimism; the depressive phases are relatively short-lived and unnoticed. In other individuals the depressive phase is the predominant one. It is uncertain whether the cyclothymic personality disorder lies on a continuum with manic-depressive illness or is a different entity. Many gifted and creative individuals have personalities conforming to a cyclothymic pattern.

Treatment

While the specific problems encountered with individual personality disorders and the techniques of treatment may differ, several general concepts can be considered. Motivation for therapy often comes from someone other than the person involved, and the patient often feels that the reasons for therapy are foreign to him or that he is being victimized. The physician's job is to contain the patient's externalization through setting limits, confrontation, and avoiding his own tendency to become over involved—first to rescue and then to condemn. The temptation of both physician and patient to hope that drugs will relieve the patient's distress must be recognized and rejected. Over the long term, the anxiety and depression of personality disorders are rarely abolished by pharmacotherapy, while drug abuse and suicide attempts are common complications of prescribing drugs to these patients. The two exceptions to this generalization are that antidepressants may be helpful if there is an associated depression, and serotonin reuptake blocking agents (eg, clomipramine, fluoxetine) may help compulsive disorders.

Patients need to be confronted with the way their behavior affects other people. Frequently, limits on behavior need to be set and reality issues dealt with. In many cases the family should be involved, since group pressure seems to be effective. Group and family treatment, group living situations, therapeutic social clubs, self-help groups, milieu hospital therapy—all can be valuable in treatment. The patient's self-esteem can be supported while his maladaptive modes of behavior are confronted. It is also important that those who undertake treatment be aware of the difficulties and avoid the disappointment, annoyance, and moral judgments that tend to creep in.

The middle years tend to bring maturation for those with personality disorders, and this process can sometimes be given a helping hand.

53. DRUG DEPENDENCE
(Substance Use Disorders; Drug Addiction; Drug Abuse; Drug Habituation)

A single definition for drug dependence is neither desirable nor possible. The term **drug dependence of a specific type** emphasizes that different drugs have different effects, including the type and hazard of the dependence they produce. **Addiction** refers to a style of living characterized by compulsive use and overwhelming involvement with a drug; it may occur in the absence of physical dependence. Addiction also implies the risk of harm and the need to stop drug use, whether the addict understands and agrees or not.

Drug abuse is definable only in terms of societal disapproval and involves different types of behavior: (1) experimental and recreational use of drugs, which usually carries the hazard of illegal behavior; (2) unwarranted use of psychoactive drugs to relieve problems or symptoms; (3) use of drugs at first for the above reasons but development later of dependence and continuation at least partially to prevent the discomfort of withdrawal.

Recreational drug use has increasingly become a part of our culture, although in general not sanctioned by society and often illegal. Users who apparently do not suffer harm tend toward episodic use involving relatively small doses, precluding clinical toxicity and the development of tolerance and physical dependence. The drugs used are often "natural"; ie, close to plant origin and containing a mixture of compounds, and are not isolated psychoactive chemicals (eg, crude opium, alcoholic beverages, marijuana products, coffee and other caffeine-containing beverages, hallucinogenic mushrooms, and coca leaf). The drugs are most often taken orally or are inhaled. The use of active potent compounds administered by injection is seldom easily controllable. Recreational use is also often accompanied by ritualization with a set of observed rules and is seldom practiced alone. Most drugs used in this fashion are psychostimulants or hallucinogens designed to obtain the "high" rather than to relieve psychic distress; depressant agents are seldom used in this controlled manner.

Two general aspects are common to most types of drug dependence: (1) **Psychologic dependence** (addiction) involves *feelings of satisfaction and a desire to repeat the administration of the drug to produce pleasure or avoid discomfort.* This mental state is a powerful factor involved in chronic use of psychotropic drugs, and with some drugs psychologic dependence may be the only factor involved in intense craving and compulsive use. (2) **Physical dependence** is defined as *a state of adaptation to a drug, accompanied by development of tolerance and manifested by a withdrawal or abstinence syndrome.* **Tolerance** is defined as *the need to increase the dose progressively in order to produce the effect originally achieved by smaller amounts.* Physical dependence and tolerance do not accompany all forms of drug dependence. A **withdrawal syndrome** is characterized by *untoward physiologic changes that occur when the drug is discontinued or when its effect is counteracted by a specific antagonist.*

Drugs that produce dependence act on the CNS and have one or more of the following effects: reduced anxiety and tension; elation, euphoria, or other mood changes pleasurable to the user; feelings of increased mental and physical ability; altered sensory perception; and changes in behavior. These drugs may be divided into (1) those causing chiefly psychic dependence and (2) those causing both psychic and physical dependence. Important drugs in the first category are cocaine, marijuana, amphetamines, bromides, and the hallucinogens, such as lysergic acid diethylamide (LSD), methylene dioxyamphetamine (MDA), and mescaline. A major stereotyped abstinence syndrome does not follow withdrawal of these drugs, but some cause tolerance, and in some cases reactions following withdrawal resemble an abstinence syndrome (eg, depression and lethargy following withdrawal of cocaine or amphetamine; characteristic changes in the EEG with amphetamine). TABLE 53–1 lists some commonly used psychoactive drugs and their potential for various types of dependence.

In the USA, the Comprehensive Drug Abuse Prevention and Control Act of 1970 and subsequent changes require the drug industry to main-

TABLE 53–1. COMMONLY USED SUBSTANCES WITH POTENTIAL FOR DEPENDENCE

Drug	Physical Dependence	Psychologic Dependence	Tolerance
CNS depressants			
Opioids	+ + + +	+ + + +	+ + + +
Synthetic narcotics	+ + + +	+ + + +	+ + + +
Barbiturates	+ + +	+ + +	+ +
Glutethimide	+ + +	+ + +	+ +
Methyprylon	+ + +	+ + +	+ +
Ethchlorvynol	+ + +	+ + +	+ +
Methaqualone	+ + +	+ + +	+ +
Alcohol	+ + +	+ + +	+ +
Anxiolytics			
Diazepam, chlordiazepoxide (long-acting)	+	+ + +	+
Alprazolam, oxazepam, temazepam (short-acting)	+ +	+ + +	+
Stimulants			
Amphetamine	?	+ + +	+ + + +
Methamphetamine	?	+ + +	+ + + +
Cocaine	0	+ + +	+ +
Hallucinogens			
LSD	0	+ +	+ +
Mescaline, peyote	0	+ +	+
Marijuana			
(low-dose Δ-9 THC)	0	+ +	0
(high-dose Δ-9 THC)	0	+ +	?

LSD = lysergic acid diethylamide; THC = tetrahydrocannabinol; 0 = no effect; + = slight, to + + + + = marked, effect.

tain physical security and strict record-keeping over certain types of drugs, and divide controlled substances into 5 schedules (or classes) on the basis of their potential for abuse, accepted medical use, and accepted safety under medical supervision. Substances included in Schedule I are those with a high potential for abuse, no accepted medical use, and a lack of accepted safety. Those in Schedules II through V decrease in potential for abuse. Placing a drug into one of these schedules determines the nature of control that must be exercised. Prescriptions for drugs in all these schedules must bear the physician's Federal Drug Enforcement Administration (DEA) license number.

Etiology

The development of drug dependence is complex and unclear. At least 3 components require consideration: the addictive drugs, predisposing conditions (including a genetic predisposition), and the personality of the user. The psychology of the individual and drug availability determine the choice of addicting drug and the pattern and frequency of use.

Drug dependence is partly related to cultural patterns and socioeconomic classes; the progression from experimentation to occasional use and the development of tolerance and physical dependence are poorly understood processes. Factors leading to increased use and habituation or addiction appear to include peer or group pressure and emotional distress that is symptomatically relieved by specific drug effects. Factors involved in the mechanisms leading to drug abuse include sadness, low self-esteem, social alienation, and environmental stress, particularly if accompanied by feelings of impotence to effect change or to accomplish goals. The medical profession may rarely contribute to harmful psychoactive drug use inadvertently through overzealous drug application to the problems of living and through failure to prevent the diversion of drugs by ruse. Advertising in mass media may contribute to social expectations that drugs can safely relieve distress or gratify needs.

Pharmacologic factors: Persons who become addicted or dependent have no proven biochemical, drug dispositional, or physiologic responsiveness differences from those who do not, although many efforts have been made to find such differences. However, the data that indicate a *diminished* physical response to alcohol in genetic relatives of those identified as alcoholic cannot be ignored. After 2 to 3 days of treatment with full doses of a narcotic analgesic, some physical dependence may exist. Such patients have a mild withdrawal syndrome, scarcely noted or described as a case of influenza; they do not become addicted. Even patients with chronic pain problems requiring long-term administration usually are not addicts, although they may experience some problems with tolerance and physical dependence. Some substances have a high potential for physiologic dependence and are more prone to abuse even when used in a social or recreational setting. Pharmacologic effects are important, but not exclusive, factors in the development of drug dependence.

Personality factors: The "addictive personality" has been described variously by behavioral scientists, but there is little scientific evidence that characteristic personality factors exist. Some have concluded that addicts are basically escapists, persons who cannot face confronting realities and who "run away." Others have described addicts as schizoid individuals who are fearful, withdrawn, and depressed, and who have a history of frequent suicide attempts and numerous self-inflicted injuries. Addicts have also been described as basically dependent and grasping in their relations, frequently exhibiting overt and unconscious rage and immature sexuality. These descriptions may have a genesis in the describer's attitudes. Clinicians, patients, and the culture are prone to highlight drug abuse in the matrix of a dysfunctional life or life episode and choose to place blame on the drug or drug use.

Abuse of prescription drugs and avoidance of illegal drugs may occur in persons with an advanced education and professional status. Before developing the drug dependence, they did not demonstrate the pleasure-oriented, irresponsible behavior usually prejudicially attributed to addicts. Sometimes the patient justifies the use of medication because of a crisis, job pressure, or family catastrophe that produces temporary anxiety or depression. Most of these patients abuse alcohol or another drug at the same time and may have repeated hospital admissions for overdose, adverse reactions, or withdrawal problems.

DEPENDENCE ON ALCOHOL

The development of characteristic deviant behaviors associated with prolonged consumption of excessive amounts of alcohol. **Alcoholism** is considered a chronic illness of undetermined etiology with an insidious onset, showing recognizable symptoms and signs proportionate to its severity.

The discussion of alcoholism needs 2 separate foci. Consumption of large amounts of ethyl alcohol is usually accompanied by significant clinical toxicity and tissue damage, the hazards of physical dependence, and a dangerous abstinence syndrome. Additionally, the term alcoholism is applied to the social impairment occurring in the lives of addicted individuals and their families. Usually, the 2 foci are recognized simultaneously, but occasionally one predominates to the apparent exclusion of the other.

An **alcoholic** is identified by severe dependence or addiction and a cumulative pattern of behaviors associated with drinking. (1) Frequent intoxication is obvious and destructive; it interferes with the individual's ability to socialize and to work. Drunkenness may lead to (2) marriage failure and eventually, after work absenteeism becomes intolerable, to (3) being fired. Alcoholics may (4) seek medical treatment for their drinking. They may (5) suffer physical injury, (6) be apprehended for driving while intoxicated, or (7) be arrested by the police for drunkenness. Eventually, they may (8) be hospitalized for delirium tremens or cirrhosis of the liver. Women alcoholics have been, in general, more likely to drink alone and are less likely to experience some of the social stigmas.

The frequency and severity of these 8 symptoms and the age at which they occur are accepted as defining the alcoholic. The earlier in life these behaviors are evident, the more crippling is the disorder.

Incidence of diagnosed alcoholism among women, children, adolescents, and college students is increasing. The male:female ratio is now about 4:1. It is generally assumed that 75% of American adults drink alcoholic beverages, and 1 in 10 will experience some problem with alcoholism.

Etiology

The cause of alcoholism is unknown. Psychologic hypotheses have noted the frequent incidence of certain personality traits, including schizoid qualities (isolation, loneliness, shyness); depression; dependency; hostile and self-destructive impulsivity; and sexual immaturity. Families of alcoholics tend to have a higher incidence of alcoholism, and many clinicians now believe that alcoholism usually occurs in the context of a necessary genetic or biochemical predisposition. However, genetic or biochemical defects leading to alcoholism have not been clearly demonstrated, although a higher incidence of alcoholism has been consistently reported in biologic children of alcoholics, as compared to adoptive children. Some recent data suggest that persons who become alcoholics are less easily intoxicated, ie, have a higher threshold to CNS effects. Societal factors affect patterns of drinking and consequent behavior, the attitudes transmitted through the culture or child rearing. Alcoholics frequently have histories of broken homes and disturbed relationships with parents. Some authorities separate alcohol abuse, which may occur in any heavy drinker, from the chronic syndrome, which occurs only in the genetically predisposed.

Physiology and Pathology

Alcohol is absorbed into the blood, principally from the small intestine. It accumulates in the blood because absorption is more rapid than oxidation and elimination. Depression of the CNS is a principal effect of alcohol: A **blood alcohol level** of 50 mg/dL produces sedation or tranquility; 50 to 150 mg/dL, lack of coordination; 150 to 200 mg/dL, intoxication (delirium); and 300 to 400 mg/dL, unconsciousness. Blood levels > 400 mg/dL may be fatal. The legal driving level is 100 mg/dL or less in most states, and intoxication is often defined as present at this level. From 5 to 10% of ingested alcohol is excreted unchanged in urine, sweat, and expired air; the remainder is oxidized to CO_2 and water at a rate of 5 to 10 mL/h (of absolute alcohol), each mL furnishing about 7 kcal. Blood alcohol is not always actually measured; it is estimated from the amount present in expired air.

The most common forms of specific organ damage seen in alcoholics are cirrhosis of the liver, peripheral neuropathy, brain damage, and cardiomyopathy, often accompanied by arrhythmias. Gastritis is common and pancreatitis may also develop. Alcohol seems to have a direct

hepatotoxic effect, although inadequate nutrition secondary to heavy alcohol intake may aggravate this effect. Irreversible impairment of liver function occurs in some alcoholics; this may prevent adequate glycogen storage and promote a tendency to hypoglycemia from inability to mobilize glucose. Symptomatic hypoglycemia may result from the absence of adequate food intake. Both the direct action of alcohol and the accompanying nutritional deficiencies (particularly of thiamine) are considered responsible for the frequent peripheral nerve degeneration and brain changes. Alcoholic cardiomyopathy may develop after about 10 yr of heavy alcohol abuse and is attributed to a direct toxic effect of alcohol on the heart muscle, independent of nutritional deficiencies. It is manifested clinically as cardiomegaly and congestive heart failure and pathologically usually as diffuse myocardial fibrosis and hypertrophy with glycoprotein infiltration. In addition, thiamine deficiency associated with alcohol abuse can produce a cardiomyopathy ("beri-beri heart disease") in which high output failure is prominent, and cardiac conductive disturbances can occur related to electrolyte imbalance. The presence of ECG abnormalities and the occurrence of sudden death in youthful alcoholics raise the possibility that alcohol in excess may have a significant arrhythmic effect. Gastritis in alcoholics may be related to the effect of alcohol on gastric secretions, which are increased in volume and acidity while the pepsin content remains low.

Tolerance, Physical Dependence, and Abstinence Syndromes

Individuals who drink large amounts of alcohol repetitively become somewhat **tolerant** to its effects, a phenomenon also noted with other CNS depressants (opioids, barbiturates, meprobamate, etc); later doses do not have the same intoxicating effect as earlier ones. This tolerance is not based primarily on changes in drug disposition or metabolism but is caused by adaptational changes of CNS cells (cellular or pharmacodynamic tolerance). Those persons tolerant to alcohol may have incredibly high blood alcohol concentrations; a few have survived concentrations of > 700 mg/dL. Even so, the tolerance is incomplete, and individuals can always manifest some degree of intoxication and impairment with a high enough dose. In fact, in tolerant animals, the *lethal* dose increases minimally. The **physical dependence** accompanying tolerance is profound, and withdrawal produces a series of adverse effects that may lead to death. Individuals tolerant to alcohol are cross-tolerant to many other CNS depressants (barbiturates, nonbarbiturate hypnotics, and benzodiazepines).

Alcohol withdrawal syndrome: A continuum of symptoms and signs accompanies alcohol withdrawal, usually beginning 12 to 48 h after cessation of intake. The mild withdrawal syndrome includes tremor, weakness, sweating, hyperreflexia, and GI symptoms. Some patients may suffer generalized grand mal seizures, usually not more than 2 in short succession ("**alcoholic epilepsy**" or "**rum fits**").

Alcoholic hallucinosis follows prolonged excessive use of alcohol. The symptoms are auditory illusions and hallucinations, frequently accusatory and threatening; the patient usually is apprehensive and may be terrified. The condition resembles schizophrenia, but there is generally no thought disorder and the history is not typical of schizophrenia. The symptoms do not resemble the delirious state of an acute organic brain syndrome as much as do delirium tremens or the other pathologic reactions associated with withdrawal. Consciousness remains clear, and the signs of autonomic lability seen in delirium tremens usually are absent. When the syndrome occurs, it generally precedes delirium tremens, and frightening dreams may occur in this stage. The hallucinosis usually is transient and responds to treatment with moderately large doses of phenothiazines. Chlorpromazine or thioridazine 100 to 300 mg qid is recommended. Recovery usually occurs in 1 to 3 wk; recurrence is likely if the patient resumes drinking.

Delirium tremens (the severe withdrawal syndrome) begins with anxiety attacks, increasing confusion, poor sleep (accompanied by frightening dreams), marked sweating, and a profound depression. Autonomic lability, evidenced by diaphoresis and increased pulse rate and temperature, accompanies the delirium and parallels its progress. Mild delirium is usually accompanied by marked diaphoresis, a pulse rate of 100 to 120/min, and a temperature of 37.2 to 37.8° C (99 to 100° F). Marked delirium, with gross disorientation and cognitive disruption, is associated with significant restlessness, a pulse > 120/min, and temperature over 37.8° C (100° F).

Initially, fleeting hallucinations and nocturnal illusions that arouse fear and restlessness may occur. Typical of these delirious, confused, and disoriented states is a return to a habitual activity—eg, the patient frequently imagines that he

is back at work and attempts to perform some related activity. Visual hallucinations are frequent and often incite terror. The patient is suggestible to all sensory stimuli and particularly to objects seen in dim light. Vestibular disturbances may cause him to believe that the floor is moving, the walls are falling, or the room is rotating. As the delirium progresses, a persistent coarse tremor of the hand at rest develops, sometimes extending to the head and trunk. Marked ataxia is present; care must be taken to prevent self-injury. Symptoms vary among patients but are usually the same with each recurrence for a particular patient.

Temperature may be elevated during the withdrawal of any agent that has caused physical dependence, but elevated temperature in alcohol withdrawal is a poor prognostic sign. Although death may occur in delirium tremens, the course usually is self-limited, terminating in a long sleep. The acute period persists from 2 to 10 days but can be more prolonged in severe withdrawal syndromes. Delirium tremens should begin to clear within 12 to 24 h, and if improvement is not marked within this interval, other conditions such as subdural hematoma, a systemic disorder, or other disturbances of mentation should be suspected.

Patients with **cirrhosis and impending hepatic coma** become dull, lethargic, and stuporous and develop a "flapping" tremor of the extended arms (**asterixis**). The apprehension, panic, and restlessness seen in delirium tremens are absent. These patients are extremely ill and require immediate medical intervention.

Korsakoff's syndrome is characterized by *a gross disturbance in recent memory, often compensated for by confabulation.* The syndrome usually is associated with excessive alcohol intake, chronic malnourishment, and a diet deficient in the B vitamins, particularly thiamine, but may occur with other organic brain diseases. Korsakoff's syndrome may begin insidiously or may suddenly follow bouts of delirium tremens. The prognosis is poor because the patient usually does not alter his previous pattern of excessive alcohol intake. The outcome is graver if **Wernicke's disease or encephalopathy** (ocular palsy, impaired mentation, ataxia, and polyneuropathy) also develops.

Pathologic intoxication is a rare syndrome characterized by repetitive and automatic movements and the occurrences of extreme excitement with aggressive, uncontrolled irrational behavior after ingesting a relatively small amount of alcohol. The episode may last for minutes or hours and is followed by a prolonged sleep with amnesia for the event upon awakening.

Treatment

Medical evaluation is needed initially to detect any intercurrent illness that might complicate withdrawal and to rule out any CNS symptoms from injury that might mimic or be masked by the withdrawal syndrome. It is especially important to differentiate delirium tremens from the mental changes found in acute hepatic insufficiency because of the difference in management.

Delirious patients are extremely suggestible and respond well to reassurance. They generally should not be restrained. Fluid balance must be maintained and large doses of vitamin C and B-complex vitamins, particularly thiamine, must be given promptly. A dehydrated alcoholic patient should be given 1000 mL of 5% dextrose in 0.9% sodium chloride followed by 1000 mL of 10% dextrose in distilled water.

Some drugs frequently used to treat alcohol withdrawal are similar to alcohol in pharmacologic effects. In fact, the most useful agents are apparently those to which alcohol induces cross-tolerance. All patients entering withdrawal are candidates for CNS-depressant drugs, but not all need them. Nondrug "detoxification" can be used in many patients if proper attention is paid to psychologic support, reassurance, and a non-threatening approach and environment. Unfortunately, most of these are not readily available in a general hospital or emergency room venue.

Rapidly acting barbiturates (pentobarbital and secobarbital) are seldom used today, but phenobarbital is quite useful. However, benzodiazepines have become the mainstay of therapy. **Chlordiazepoxide** is recommended in most situations in initial 50- to 100-mg oral doses that may need repetition q 3 h. **Diazepam** is a useful alternative, given 5 mg IV or orally hourly until sedation occurs. (NOTE: Alcoholics may achieve intoxication and even physical dependence and withdrawal with diazepam or chlordiazepoxide.) Isolated seizures need no specific therapy, and repeated seizures will respond to 1- to 3-mg doses of IV diazepam. **Phenothiazines** are not recommended because they may not control severe delirium tremens and they lower the seizure threshold. The routine administration of **phenytoin** is not necessary. Outpatient therapy with phenytoin is almost always a waste of time and drug, because these seizures occur only under the stress of alcohol withdrawal, and withdrawing (or heavily drinking) patients do not take their antiseizure medication.

The first treatment phase consists of complete withdrawal of alcohol. The delirious state that may accompany withdrawal and its management has been described above. After correction of any nutritional deficiencies associated with excessive alcohol intake, the patient's behavior must be changed to eliminate drunkenness. Maintaining sobriety once it has been established is difficult because the patient has fixed patterns of nonsobriety. The patient should be warned that after a few weeks, when he has recovered from his last bout, he is likely to find some excuse to take a drink. He should also be told that he may be able to drink in a controlled manner for a few days or, rarely, even for a few weeks, but with depressing regularity he will repeat the pattern and again drink without control.

Various types of psychotherapy have been recommended for alcoholism, but a general belief is that group processes are superior to one-on-one processes. Newer behavioral techniques may hold promise.

Alcoholics Anonymous (AA): No other approach has benefited so many alcoholics as effectively as the help they have offered themselves through AA. The patient must find an AA group in which he is comfortable, preferably one in which he has common interests with the other members in addition to his alcohol problem; eg, in some metropolitan areas there are AA groups of physicians and dentists. These groups provide the patient with nondrinking friends who are always available as well as an area in which to socialize—away from the tavern. The patient also hears others, more expert than he, confess before the group every rationalization the patient has ever thought up privately to justify his own drinking. Finally, the help he gives to other alcoholics may afford him the self-esteem and confidence formerly found only in alcohol.

Disulfiram therapy: Disulfiram interferes with the metabolism of acetaldehyde (an intermediary product in the oxidation of alcohol) so that acetaldehyde accumulates, producing toxic symptoms and great discomfort. Drinking alcohol within 12 h after taking disulfiram produces facial flushing in 5 to 15 min, then intense vasodilation of the face and neck with suffusion of the conjunctivae, throbbing headache, tachycardia, hyperpnea, and sweating. Nausea and vomiting follow in 30 to 60 min and may be so intense as to lead to hypotension, dizziness, and sometimes fainting and collapse. The reaction lasts 1 to 3 h. Discomfort is so intense that few patients will risk taking alcohol as long as they are taking disulfiram. The patient should also avoid medications that contain alcohol (eg, tinctures, elixirs, some OTC liquid cough/cold preparations, which contain as much as 40% ethanol).

Disulfiram may be given on an outpatient basis after the patient has been free of alcohol for 4 or 5 days. The initial dose is 0.5 gm orally once/day for 1 to 3 wk. The maintenance dose is adjusted individually; 0.25 to 0.5 gm once/day is usually adequate, but some patients may require more. Both patient and relatives should be warned that the effects of disulfiram may persist for 3 to 7 days following the last dose. The patient must want to be helped, must cooperate, and should be seen periodically by the physician to encourage his continuing to take disulfiram as part of an abstinence program.

Few studies convincingly indicate a general usefulness of the drug, and many patients are noncompliant. However, when patients succeed they are often users of disulfiram, and the lack of proof should not interfere with its availability to patients and therapists. Disulfiram therapy is contraindicated in pregnancy and in decompensated cardiac patients.

DEPENDENCE OF THE OPIOID TYPE

A strong psychic dependence manifested as an overpowering compulsion to continue taking opioids, the development of tolerance so that the dosage must be continually increased in order to obtain the initial effect, and physical dependence that increases in intensity with increased dosage and duration of use. The physical dependence necessitates continued administration of the same opioid or a related drug to prevent withdrawal. Withdrawal of the drug or administration of an antagonist precipitates a characteristic and self-limited abstinence syndrome.

Tolerance and physical dependence on the opioids (natural or synthetic) develop rapidly; therapeutic doses taken regularly over a 2- to 3-day period can lead to some tolerance and dependence, and the user may show symptoms of withdrawal when the drug is discontinued. Opioid drugs induce cross-tolerance. Abusers may substitute one for another. With increased use of methadone in detoxification and maintenance

programs, illicitly obtained methadone has become an abused drug. People who have developed tolerance may show few signs of drug use and function normally in their usual activities. Tolerance to the various effects of these drugs frequently develops unevenly; eg, a meperidine user may tolerate large doses but show many of the stimulant and atropine-like side effects. Heroin users may become largely tolerant to the euphoric and lethal effects but will still have constricted pupils and constipation.

Symptoms and Signs

Acute intoxication with opioids is characterized by euphoria, flushing, itching of the skin, miosis, drowsiness, decreased respiratory rate and depth, hypotension, bradycardia, and decreased body temperature.

The withdrawal syndrome from an opioid generally includes symptoms and signs opposite to the drug's pharmacologic effects (eg, CNS hyperactivity). The severity of the withdrawal syndrome increases with the size of the opioid dose and the duration of dependence. Symptoms begin to appear as early as 4 to 6 h after withdrawal and reach a peak within 36 to 72 h for heroin. The initial anxiety and craving for the drug are followed by other symptoms increasing in severity and intensity. A reliable early sign of abstinence is an increased resting respiratory rate, > 16/min, usually accompanied by yawning, perspiration, lacrimation, and rhinorrhea. Other symptoms include mydriasis, piloerection ("gooseflesh"), tremors, muscle twitching, hot and cold flashes, aching muscles, and anorexia. The withdrawal syndrome in persons who have been taking methadone develops more slowly and is overtly less severe than heroin withdrawal, although users may perceive it as worse.

Complications

Many but not all complications of heroin addiction are related to unsanitary administration of the drug. The more frequent complications include pulmonary problems, hepatitis, arthritic conditions, immunologic alterations, and neurologic disorders. The effect of heroin addiction on pregnancy (see below) merits special mention.

Pulmonary problems: Pulmonary conditions found in narcotic addicts include aspiration pneumonitis, pneumonia, lung abscess, septic pulmonary emboli, atelectasis, and pulmonary fibrosis from talc granulomatosis. Chronic heroin addiction results in a decreased vital capacity and a mildly to moderately decreased pulmonary diffusion capacity. These effects are distinct from the unusual pulmonary edema that may be associated with overdose. In addition, many addicts smoke one or more packages of cigarettes/day. As a result, the addict is particularly susceptible to a variety of pulmonary infections.

Liver disturbance: Heroin addicts have a higher incidence of viral hepatitis, both type A and type B. The combination of viral hepatitis and the frequently high alcohol intake may account for a high incidence of liver dysfunction.

Musculoskeletal conditions: The most common problem is osteomyelitis (particularly lumbar vertebral), probably due to hematogenous spread of organisms from unsterile injections. Infectious spondylitis and sacroiliitis have been reported. **Myositis ossificans ("drug abuser's elbow")** is extraosseous metaplasia of muscle damaged by inept needle manipulation; injury to the brachialis muscle is followed by replacement of the muscle bundle by a calcific mass.

Immunologic abnormalities: Hypergammaglobulinemia, involving both IgG and IgM, may be detected in up to 90% of addicts. The reason for the immunologic changes is unknown, but they may reflect repeated antigenic stimulation, either from infections or from the daily parenteral injection of foreign substances. Most importantly, heroin addicts and other injectors of IV drugs are at extremely high risk for HIV infection and AIDS. In communities where sharing of needles and syringes is common, the spread of AIDS has become devastating (see Ch. 20).

Neurologic disorders that occur in heroin addicts are usually noninfectious complications of coma and cerebral anoxia. They may suffer from toxic amblyopia (apparently due to quinine contamination of heroin), transverse myelitis, and a variety of mono- and polyneuropathies, as well as Guillain-Barré syndrome. Cerebral complications include those secondary to bacterial endocarditis (bacterial meningitis, mycotic aneurysm, brain abscess, and subdural and epidural abscesses), acute cerebral falciparum malaria, and the cerebral complications of viral hepatitis and tetanus. Some neurologic complications are thought to be due to allergic responses to the heroin-adulterant mixture.

Other complications include superficial cutaneous abscesses, cellulitis, lymphangitis, lymphadenitis, and phlebitis from contaminated needles. Many heroin addicts begin with subcutaneous injections ("skin popping"). They may re-

turn to this mode when extensive scarring makes their veins no longer accessible. As addicts become more desperate, cutaneous ulcers in unlikely sites may be found. Contaminated needles and inoculum may also lead to bacterial endocarditis, hepatitis, and HIV infection.

Pregnancy and opioid addiction: Problems of the heroin-addicted mother are transferred to the fetus; because heroin and methadone freely cross the placental barrier, the fetus readily becomes drug-dependent. The mother infected with HIV or hepatitis B virus may transmit the virus to her neonate. Pregnant addicts seen early enough should be encouraged to enter a methadone maintenance program. Obviously, such plans should include the obstetrician and pediatrician who will treat the dependent infant. Pregnant women withdrawn from heroin or methadone late in the 3rd trimester risk the precipitation of labor. Pregnant women seen at or near term may best be stabilized on methadone. Abstinence would be better for the fetus, but experience indicates that withdrawn mothers often revert to heroin and withdraw from prenatal care. The methadone-maintained mother may nurse her newborn without apparent clinical problems in the child, and the minimal concentrations in breast milk have been confirmed. The infants of opioid-dependent mothers may present with tremors, a high-pitched cry, jitters, convulsions, and tachypnea. For a discussion of problems of the neonate, including **drug withdrawal** and **fetal alcohol syndromes,** see METABOLIC PROBLEMS IN THE NEWBORN in Ch. 27 and DRUGS IN LACTATING MOTHERS under FEEDING in Ch. 23. See also DRUGS IN PREGNANCY in Ch. 14.

Treatment

The clinical management of opioid addicts is extremely difficult. Physicians treating addicts must be fully aware of federal, state, and local regulations. Few physicians have had formal training or experience in dealing with opioid addicts and their companions and families, as well as the attitudes of society (including law enforcement officers, other physicians, and allied health personnel) toward the treatment of such individuals. The physician should be aware of locally available resources and usually should refer opioid addicts to specialized treatment centers rather than attempt to care for them in an office. If there are no specialized centers, the physician can closely supervise the patient, with frequent contacts and close work with the patient's family and friends.

In order to legally use an opioid drug in treating an addict, the existence of a physiologic opioid dependence must be established. This is a difficult diagnosis, since many individuals who seek treatment have minimal physical dependence; the high incidence of psychologic heroin dependence has occurred because at times only low-grade heroin has been available and most addicts may not maintain a high enough level of heroin use to produce physiologic dependence. The following are helpful in assessing physiologic dependence: (1) a history of 3 or more narcotic injections/day, (2) the presence of fresh needle marks, (3) observation of withdrawal symptoms and signs, and (4) the presence of morphine in a properly obtained urine specimen. Morphine (and its glucuronoside metabolite) is the most abundant urinary opioid in heroin users.

Management of acute intoxication (overdose): Naloxone (0.4 to 0.8 mg) given IV is the drug of choice because it possesses no respiratory depressant properties (see also under Narcotics in TABLE 145−4). If the patient's unconsciousness is due to an opioid, dramatic recovery occurs immediately after the administration of this antagonist. Since some patients become agitated, delirious, and combative as they recover from their comatose state, secure physical restraints may be required and should be applied before the antagonist is given. All patients treated for overdose should be hospitalized and observed for at least 24 h, since the action of the opioid antagonist is relatively short and respiratory depression may recur within several hours (especially with methadone). Pulmonary edema that may be severe enough to cause death from hypoxia is usually not responsive to naloxone and has an unclear relationship to overdosage.

The opioid withdrawal syndrome is self-limited and, although severely discomforting, is not life-threatening. A patient admitted for withdrawal should be told that he will experience some unpleasant symptoms and should be reassured that they will not be allowed to progress to an odious level but that the medication he receives will be based on some objective physical signs of withdrawal. The patient's drug-seeking behavior usually begins with the first symptoms of withdrawal, and hospital personnel must always be alert to the possibility that he will try to obtain illicit supplies of drugs. Visitors may have to be restricted. Many patients with withdrawal symptoms have other medical problems that must be diagnosed and treated. Opioid users

may have **mixed addictions**, and although providing appropriate withdrawal measures for each drug is theoretically feasible, for practical purposes this is not required.

Currently, **methadone substitution** is the preferred method of opioid withdrawal. Methadone is given orally in the smallest amount that will prevent severe signs of withdrawal but not necessarily all signs. Close observation of the patient is important because his subjective symptoms are unreliable. Many of the symptoms of withdrawal can be mimicked by anxiety states. Generally, 20 mg/day of methadone will block the symptoms of severe withdrawal. Higher doses should be given only on direct observations of the physical signs of withdrawal, since addicts are unreliable in reporting the size of their habits. Doses of 25 to 45 mg can produce unconsciousness if the person has not developed tolerance for heroin or methadone. Once a suppressing dose has been established, it should be reduced progressively *by not more than 20% each day.* Patients commonly become emotionally upset and frequently request additional medication. Chloral hydrate 500 to 1000 mg may be given orally for several nights to improve sleep. The acute manifestations of withdrawal usually subside within 7 to 10 days, but patients often complain of weakness, insomnia, and a severe pervasive anxiety for several months. Minor metabolic and physiologic effects of withdrawal may persist for up to 6 mo. It is appropriate to treat heroin withdrawal with oral methadone, but the usual low-grade level of dependence can be treated with propoxyphene napsylate or even benzodiazepines, which are not cross-tolerant to opioids.

The central α-adrenergic drug **clonidine** can halt essentially all signs of opioid withdrawal. This probably relates to diminution of central adrenergic outflow secondary to stimulation of central receptors (the same mechanism by which clonidine lowers BP). This theory supports the importance of central adrenergic discharge in the evolution of the opioid withdrawal syndrome. However, clonidine is not a benign drug. Besides causing hypotension and drowsiness, its withdrawal may precipitate restlessness, insomnia, irritability, tachycardia, and headache. Its overall contribution to therapy is minor. Withdrawal is not a difficult problem for patient or clinician; abstinence, which clonidine does not aid, is.

Withdrawal from methadone: The abstinence syndrome induced by methadone is like that of heroin, but onset is more gradual and delayed, beginning 36 to 72 h after discontinuing the drug. Deep muscle aches ("bone pains") are frequent complaints. Because the abstinence syndrome begins gradually, methadone addicts may be initially observed on admission. A urine sample should be obtained to document the methadone habit, and methadone provided as symptoms develop. Methadone withdrawal for individuals coming from methadone maintenance programs may be particularly difficult because the addict's dose of methadone may be as high as 100 mg/day. In general, ambulatory detoxification should be started by reducing the dose to ≤ 60 mg/day over several weeks before attempting complete detoxification. Clonidine may be particularly useful in aiding withdrawal from methadone.

Treatment of chronic opioid dependence: No consensus exists regarding long-term treatment of opioid-dependent users. Thousands of American opioid addicts are in methadone maintenance programs. It was hoped that large enough doses of oral methadone in treating addicts (chiefly heroin) would enable them to move to socially productive lives because their supply problems would be met. Additionally, the methadone would block any effects of injected heroin and alleviate user's "drug hunger." For some, the plan has worked. For others, methadone just adds another drug problem to their alcohol use, intermittent heroin use, and desperate lives. Additionally, the widespread availability of methadone has established its role as an important drug of abuse in the culture.

Experiments with L-acetyl α-methadol (LAAM), a longer-acting synthetic opioid, give hope of help to some addicts and of removing the problem of expensive daily client visits or take-home medication, which ensures some diversion. The culture's loss of faith in methadone maintenance or at least the lessening commitment of public money has diminished the number of treatment facilities and the amount of research given to LAAM.

Naltrexone, an orally bioavailable opioid antagonist, has been released for general use. It has little agonist effect, and many opioid addicts will not voluntarily consume it. Motivated patients may do well. There are reports of its usefulness in health professionals addicted to opioids. The usual dose is 50 mg/day or 350 mg/wk in 2 or 3 divided doses.

Reports suggest that the agonist-antagonist **buprenorphine** may deserve a trial in maintenance of opioid addicts. It will block receptors

and interfere with heroin use, and it may provide a slight opioid effect to motivate continued use.

The therapeutic community concept emerged nearly 25 yr ago in response to the heroin problem. Daytop Village and Phoenix House pioneered this nondrug treatment in residential centers, and the movement has grown. It was hoped that the communal, relatively long-term (usually 15-mo) residential setting would, by training, education, and redirection, help users achieve new lives. Like methadone maintenance, this mode has helped, indeed transformed, some. How well it works, how widely it may be applied, and how much funding society will give remain unanswered.

The AIDS epidemic has motivated some to believe that exchange of used needles and syringes for clean ones should be part of caring for addicts. Both adverse public opinion and paraphernalia laws have prevented the widespread acceptance of this idea.

DEPENDENCE ON ANXIOLYTIC AND HYPNOTIC DRUGS
(See also Ch. 62)

Psychic dependence that may lead to periodic, as often as continuous, abuse; and a physical dependence that can be detected only after consumption of amounts considerably above the usual therapeutic levels. (Barbiturates and ethanol are strikingly similar in their syndromes of dependence, withdrawal, and chronic intoxication.) When intake is reduced below a critical level, a self-limited abstinence syndrome ensues. Symptoms of withdrawal from barbiturates and other sedative-hypnotics can be suppressed completely with a barbiturate. **Tolerance** develops irregularly and incompletely so that considerable behavioral disturbances and psychotoxicity persist, depending on the drug's pharmacodynamic effects. Some mutual but incomplete cross-tolerance exists between alcohol and the barbiturates as well as the nonbarbiturate sedative-hypnotics, including benzodiazepines.

Symptoms and Signs

Drug effects: In general, those persons dependent on sedatives and hypnotics, including barbiturates and benzodiazepines, prefer the rapid-onset drugs (eg, secobarbital and pentobarbital). The signs of progressive sedative intoxication are depression of superficial skin reflexes, fine lateral-gaze nystagmus, slightly decreased alertness with coarser or rapid nystagmus, ataxia and slurred speech, and a positive Romberg's sign. With progression there is nystagmus on forward gaze, somnolence, marked ataxia with falling, confusion, deep sleep, small pupils, respiratory depression, and ultimately death. Patients on large doses of depressants frequently have difficulty thinking and show slowness of speech and comprehension with some dysarthria, poor memory, faulty judgment, narrowed attention span, and emotional lability. In general, the combination of slow thinking, slurred speech, and bruises on the extremities from falling may suggest dependence on depressants.

Withdrawal effects: In susceptible patients, psychologic dependence on the drug may develop rapidly; and, after only a few weeks, attempts to discontinue it exacerbate any initial insomnia and result in restlessness, disturbing dreams, frequent awakening, and feelings of tension in the early morning. The extent of physical dependence is related to dose and the length of time that the drug has been taken; eg, pentobarbital 200 mg/day may be ingested for many months without significant tolerance developing; 300 mg/day may induce an abstinence syndrome on terminating medication if ingested for more than 3 mo; and 500 to 600 mg/day may provoke an abstinence syndrome after 1 mo.

An abrupt withdrawal syndrome from large doses of barbiturates or anxiolytics produces a severe, frightening, and potentially life-threatening illness essentially similar to delirium tremens. Withdrawal carries a significant mortality rate and should always be undertaken in the hospital. Once the withdrawal syndrome has begun, reversing it is difficult, but with a careful schedule the symptoms can be minimized. The reestablishment of CNS stability requires about 30 days. Occasionally, even after properly managed withdrawal over 1 to 2 wk, a seizure may occur in the following 2 wk. Within the first 12 to 20 h after the withdrawal of a short-acting barbiturate, the patient becomes increasingly restless, tremulous, and weak. By the 2nd day, the tremulousness becomes more prominent, the deep tendon reflexes may be increased, and the patient becomes weaker. During the 2nd and 3rd days, convulsions occur in 75% of all patients taking 800 mg/day or more. The convulsions may progress to status epilepticus and death. From the 2nd to the 5th day, the untreated abstinence syndrome includes delirium, insomnia, confusion, and frightening visual and auditory hallucinations. Hyperpyrexia and dehydration often occur.

A withdrawal syndrome similar to the barbiturate syndrome, although seldom as severe, may occur with benzodiazepines. (See also Ch. 62.) Many clinicians believe that misuse of benzodiazepines may focus on those that have a rapid absorption and quick decline in serum (eg, alprazolam and lorazepam). Many patients so described have been heavy users of alcohol. The syndrome with these agents may be very long in developing because of continued presence of the drugs in the body. A withdrawal syndrome of varying severity may occur in individuals taking normal doses.

Treatment

The procedure for treating dependence on depressants, particularly barbiturates, is to reintoxicate the patient and then withdraw the drug on a strict schedule, being alert for signs of marked withdrawal. Before beginning withdrawal, one can evaluate sedative tolerance with a test dose of pentobarbital 200 mg orally given to the nonintoxicated, fasting patient; 1 to 2 h later this test dose produces drowsiness or sleep with response to arousal in individuals with no tolerance to pentobarbital. Patients with intermediate levels of tolerance may show some impairment, whereas patients tolerant to 900 mg or more show no signs of intoxication. If the 200-mg dose has no effect, the tolerance level can be determined by repeating the test q 3 to 4 h with a larger dose. Severe anxiety or agitation may increase the patient's tolerance. Once the 24-h dose to which the patient is tolerant has been ascertained, that dose of pentobarbital is usually given qid for 2 or 3 days to stabilize the patient and is then decreased by 10%/day.

Alternatively, phenobarbital can be used: it does not produce the "high" of the more rapidly acting drugs, its action is prolonged so that it provides smoother sedation, and it is the anticonvulsant of choice. Rapid-onset barbiturates or other sedative-hypnotics or minor anxiolytics can be replaced by a dose of phenobarbital equivalent to ⅓ the average daily dose of the drug on which the patient has become dependent (see TABLE 53–2). Phenobarbital is given orally qid, and the initial phenobarbital dose is reduced by 30 mg/day until the patient is drug-free; eg, if the patient has been taking secobarbital 1000 mg/day, the stabilizing dose of phenobarbital is 300 mg/day or 75 mg q 6 h. Since the initial daily dose must be estimated from the patient's his-

TABLE 53-2. DOSES OF SOME COMMON SEDATIVES AND ANXIOLYTICS
THAT HAVE PRODUCED PHYSICAL DEPENDENCE

Drug	Doses Producing Dependence (mg/day)	Time Necessary to Produce Dependence (days)	Dosage Equivalent to 30 mg Phenobarbital (mg)
Secobarbital	500–600	30	100
Pentobarbital ("yellow jackets")	500–600	30	100
Amobarbital ("blues")	500–600	30	100
Amobarbital-secobarbital combination ("rainbows")	500–600	30	100
Glutethimide	1250–1500	60	500
Methyprylon	1200–1500	60	300
Ethchlorvynol	1500–2000	60	500
Meprobamate	2000–2400	60	400
Chlordiazepoxide	200–300	60	25
Diazepam	60–100*	40	10
Methaqualone	1800–2400	30	300
Chloral hydrate	2000–2500	30	500

* See also discussion of withdrawal effects, above.

tory, there is obviously a large margin of error, and the patient must be observed closely for the first 72 h. If he remains agitated or anxious, the dosage should be increased; if he is drowsy, dysarthric, or has nystagmus, the dosage should be decreased. While patients are being detoxified, other sedatives and psychotropic medications should be avoided. However, if the patient is also taking antidepressant medications, especially the tricyclics, the antidepressant should not be abruptly discontinued but should be reduced over 3 to 4 days. Methaqualone, a pervasively misused drug, has been moved to Federal Schedule I and is no longer legally available in the USA. Fake methaqualone (usually imitating Quaalude®) contains OTC antihistamines or, rarely, large doses of diazepam.

DEPENDENCE OF THE CANNABIS (MARIJUANA) TYPE

*Chronic or periodic administration of cannabis or cannabis substances producing some psychic dependence because of the desired subjective effects, but no physical dependence; there is no abstinence syndrome when the drug is discontinued. Cannabis can be used on an episodic but continuous basis without evidence of social or psychic dysfunction. In many users the term de-*pendence, with its obvious connotations, probably is misapplied.

Use of the drug is widespread. However, the surveys that continually showed an increased prevalence and increasing daily use by high school students in recent years shown a diminution of use. In the USA it is commonly used in the form of cigarettes made from the dried plant, *Cannabis sativa,* or as hashish, the pressed resin of the plant. Synthetic Δ-9 tetrahydrocannabinol (THC), an active constituent of marijuana, is available for research and limited clinical use (eg, to treat nausea and vomiting associated with cancer chemotherapy); despite claims of dealers and users, THC does not appear on the street.

In recent years, critics of marijuana use have become prominent and have enlisted much scientific data in support. A movement opposed to decriminalization and the easy acceptance of the drug in American society has emerged. Most of the claims regarding severe biologic impact are still uncertain; although many dangers of marijuana are frequently cited, there is still little evidence of biologic damage, even among relatively heavy users. This is true even in the areas intensively investigated, such as immunologic and reproductive function. However, high-dose users of marijuana may develop pulmonary damage in the absence of tobacco-cigarette use. Pregnant users may deliver children of lower birth weight than nonsmokers.

Symptoms and Signs

Cannabis produces a dreamy state of consciousness in which ideas seem disconnected, uncontrollable, and freely flowing. Time, color, and spatial perceptions may be distorted and enhanced. In general, there is a feeling of well-being, exaltation, excitement, and inner joyousness that has been termed a "high." Many of the psychologic effects seem to be related to the setting in which the drug is taken. An occasional panic reaction has occurred, particularly in naive users, but these have become unusual as the culture has gained increasing familiarity with the drug. Communicative and motor abilities are decreased during the use of these drugs. Difficulty in depth perception and altered sense of timing, both of which are particularly hazardous during automobile driving, have been demonstrated. There are now several published reports of the exacerbation of schizophrenic symptoms by marijuana, even in patients being treated with antipsychotic medication (eg, chlorpromazine).

The persistence of Δ-9 THC and its metabolites will cause **urine tests** for the reactive cannabinoids to remain positive for days, weeks, or rarely months in regular users. Because urine testing is now so commonly applied in work and other settings, detection of previously secret, illegal behavior may provoke important deleterious social consequences. The testing that identifies an inactive carboxylic acid metabolite only identifies use. It has no correlation with dysfunction, and the smoker may be free of effect by the time his urine is positive. The ability of testing to identify extremely small amounts also means that a positive test is of little value in identifying pattern of use (high dose vs. low dose).

DEPENDENCE OF THE COCAINE TYPE

Psychic dependence, sometimes leading to profound psychic addiction, produced by high doses of this stimulant drug that cause euphoric excitement and, occasionally, hallucinatory experiences, properties highly esteemed by drug users. Tolerance does occur, but physical dependence has not been conclusively demonstrated and there is no abstinence syndrome when the drug is withdrawn. The tendency to continue taking the drug is strong.

Probably a majority of users are episodic recreational users who voluntarily curtail their use, or find that the drug's high cost mandates episodic

use. However, cocaine use and the development of addictive behavior in some users has continued to increase in North America in recent years.

The smoking of "free-base" cocaine (one version is now widely labeled as "**crack**") has become popular. This necessitates the conversion of the hydrochloride salt to the more volatile form. A flame is held to the converted material and the smoke inhaled. The speed of onset is shortened and the intensity of the high is magnified. This phenomenon has changed the way we view this drug. Currently urban use and the criminal market for volatile cocaine have become the most feared problems of drug abuse.

Procaine when snorted produces local sensations not unlike cocaine and may even produce some "high." Powdered procaine is widely used to cut cocaine and is occasionally mixed with mannitol or lactose and sold as cocaine. It is widely sold by mail-order suppliers and is sometimes called "synthetic cocaine."

Symptoms and Signs

Effects differ strikingly with different modes of use. When injected IV or inhaled, cocaine produces a condition of hyperstimulation, alertness, euphoria, and feelings of great power. The excitation and "high" are similar to that produced by injection of large doses of amphetamine. Because cocaine is a very short-acting drug, heavy users may resort to injecting it IV q 10 or 15 min. With this repetition, toxic effects such as tachycardia, hypertension, mydriasis, muscle-twitching, formication ("cocaine bugs"), miniaturized visual hallucinations, sleeplessness, and extreme nervousness appear. Hallucinations and paranoid delusions may develop, as well as violent behavior; the individual may be dangerous at this time. The action of the drug, however, is sufficiently brief to prevent sustained aggressive activity. The pupils are maximally dilated, and elevations of heart rate, BP, and respiration result from the drug's sympathomimetic effect. An **overdose** of cocaine produces tremors, convulsions with a temporal lobe seizure pattern, and delirium. Deaths are becoming increasingly common, due to arrhythmias and cardiovascular collapse or respiratory failure. Since the removal of cocaine from plasma requires intact serum esterase, there is speculation that patients with extreme clinical toxicity may, on a genetic basis, have diminished (atypical) serum cholinesterase.

Severe toxic effects occur in the compulsive heavy user, who often also has a history of heroin use. Volatile cocaine may stand in relationship to sniffed cocaine as IV heroin does to swallowed or smoked opium. Smoking delivers the drug rapidly to the brain and provokes a seductive and evanescent high. Repeated high-dose use has led to serious toxic consequences, both cardiovascular and behavioral.

Treatment

Many nonspecific therapies, including support and self-help groups, have emerged, and cocaine "hotlines" have generated much publicity. Extremely expensive in-patient therapy is available to those whose wealth enabled them to purchase enormous amounts of cocaine initially.

Treatment of acute cocaine intoxication is generally unnecessary because of the extremely short action of the drug. If an overdose requires intervention, IV barbiturates or diazepam may be used; but close observation and supportive care as needed is the current management approach. Anticonvulsants do not effectively prevent convulsions in cocaine overdose. Although rare, hyperthermia or significantly elevated BP must be treated. Discontinuing the chronic and sustained use of cocaine requires considerable assistance, and the depression that may occur requires close supervision and treatment.

For a discussion of the treatment of **infants born to cocaine-addicted mothers**, see COCAINE ABUSE AND WITHDRAWAL under METABOLIC PROBLEMS IN THE NEWBORNin Ch. 27.

DEPENDENCE OF THE AMPHETAMINE TYPE

Some psychic dependence produced by these widely used stimulants and anorexiants that cause elevated mood, increased wakefulness, alertness, concentration, and physical performance, and induce a feeling of well-being. Illicit synthesis of methamphetamine and its use in a variety of formats continue and have increased. This is the chief source of abused amphetamine in North America.

Symptoms and Signs

The **withdrawal** syndrome, if one exists, is not severe. Withdrawal is followed by a state of mental and physical depression and fatigue. Qualitatively, the psychologic effects are similar to those produced by cocaine; the psychologic dependence is variable. Amphetamine induces **tolerance**, but it develops slowly; a progressive increase in dosage can occur and permits the eventual ingestion or

injection of amounts several hundredfold greater than the original therapeutic dose. The tolerance to various effects develops unequally, so that nervousness and sleeplessness persist and psychotoxic effects, such as hallucinations and delusions, may occur. However, even massive doses are rarely fatal. Chronic drug users have reportedly injected as much as 15,000 mg of amphetamine in 24 h without observable acute illness. For neophytes, however, rapid injection of 120 mg *may be fatal,* although some individuals have survived 400 to 500 mg.

Abusers of amphetamine are prone to accidents because of the excitation and grandiosity produced and the accompanying excessive fatigue of sleeplessness. IV administration may lead to serious antisocial behavior and can precipitate a schizophrenic episode. **Adverse reactions** to continued high doses of methamphetamine include (1) anxiety reactions during which the person is fearful and tremulous and concerned about his physical well-being; (2) an amphetamine psychosis in which the person misinterprets others' actions, hallucinates, and becomes unrealistically suspicious; (3) an exhaustion syndrome, involving an intense feeling of fatigue and need for sleep, that comes after the stimulation phase; and (4) a prolonged depression during which suicide is a possibility.

A **paranoid psychosis** almost inevitably results from long-term use of high IV doses but also can result from large oral doses. This psychosis may rarely be precipitated either by a single large dose or by chronic moderate doses. Typical features of the amphetamine psychosis include delusions of persecution, ideas of reference, and feelings of omnipotence. Those who use high IV doses usually accept that sooner or later they will experience paranoia and are often able to cope with it. Nevertheless, when drug use becomes very intense, or toward the end of a long run, even well-practiced intellectual awareness may fail, and the user may respond to a delusional system. Recovery from even prolonged amphetamine psychosis is usual. The slow but complete recovery of users who have become thoroughly disorganized and paranoid is a striking phenomenon. The more florid symptoms fade within a few days or weeks, although some confusion and memory loss and some delusional ideas commonly persist for months.

Treatment

There are no specific symptoms associated with withdrawal, but EEG changes are seen that may fulfill physiologic criteria for dependence. Abrupt discontinuance of amphetamine is not without complications; withdrawal can uncover an underlying depression, or it may precipitate a depressive reaction, often with a suicidal potential. In many persons whose amphetamine intake masks chronic fatigue, withdrawal is followed by 2 or 3 days of intense tiredness or sleepiness. Patients recovering from an amphetamine psychosis may demonstrate severe anxiety and extreme restlessness. Therefore, withdrawal generally should be undertaken in a drug-free environment where hospital and nursing facilities are available.

The acute agitated psychotic state with paranoid delusions and auditory and visual hallucinations responds remarkably to phenothiazines; chlorpromazine 25 to 50 mg IM rapidly reverses the toxic psychotic conditions but may produce severe postural hypotension. Haloperidol 2.5 to 5 mg IM has been used effectively because it rarely produces hypotension, but it greatly increases the risk of an alarming acute extrapyramidal motor reaction. Usually, reassurance and a quiet, nonthreatening environment will permit the patient to recover. Acidification of the urine with ammonium chloride 500 mg orally q 4 h aids amphetamine excretion.

DEPENDENCE OF THE HALLUCINOGEN TYPE

Hallucinogens include lysergic acid diethylamide **(LSD)**, psilocybin, mescaline, peyote, 2,5-dimethoxy-4-methylamphetamine (DOM, "STP"), 3,4-methylenedioxymethamphetamine **(MDMA)**, and other substituted amphetamines. Generally, other than LSD, the listed hallucinogen exotica are not available on the street, despite the beliefs of dealers and users, although in recent years a number of samples of a street product called "ecstasy" have contained relatively pure MDMA.

Symptoms and Signs

These substances induce a state of excitation of the CNS and central autonomic hyperactivity, manifested as changes in mood (usually euphoric, sometimes depressive) and perception. True hallucinations apparently rarely occur. Psychic dependence on hallucinogens varies greatly but usually is not intense. No evidence of physical dependence can be detected when the drugs are abruptly withdrawn. A high degree of **tolerance** to LSD develops and disappears rap-

idly. Individuals tolerant to any of these drugs are cross-tolerant to the others. Chief dangers to the individual are the psychologic effects and impairment of judgment, which can lead to dangerous decision-making or accidents.

Responses to the hallucinogens depend on several factors, including the individual's expectations, the setting, and his ability to cope with the perceptual distortions. Untoward reactions to LSD apparently have become rare. **Adverse reactions** to hallucinogens appear as anxiety attacks, extreme apprehensiveness, or panic states. Most often, these reactions quickly subside with appropriate management in a secure setting. However, some individuals (especially after using LSD) remain disturbed and may even show a **persistent psychotic state**. It is unclear whether the drug use has precipitated or uncovered a preexisting psychotic potential or whether this can occur in previously stable individuals.

Some persons, especially among those who are chronic or repeated users of hallucinogenic drugs and particularly with the use of LSD, may experience drug effects after they have discontinued use of the drug. Referred to as **"flashbacks,"** these episodes most commonly consist of visual illusions but can include distortions of virtually any sensation (including perceptions of time, space, or self-image) or hallucinations. Such episodes can be precipitated by use of marijuana, alcohol, or barbiturates, by stress or fatigue, or they may occur without apparent reason. The mechanisms that produce flashbacks are not known, but they tend to subside over a period of 6 to 12 mo.

Treatment

Reassurance that the bizarre thoughts, visions, and sounds are due to the drug and not to a "nervous breakdown" usually suffices in acute adverse reactions to hallucinogens. **Phenothiazines must be used with extreme caution** because of the danger of hypotension, particularly if phencyclidine (see below) has been ingested. Short-acting barbiturates or minor anxiolytics such as chlordiazepoxide or diazepam may help reduce overwhelming anxiety.

For heavy users of hallucinogens, withdrawal of the drug is the simplest part of treatment; some may need psychiatric treatment for associated problems. Frequent contact and establishing a helpful relationship with a physician can be beneficial. Maintaining the patient's social functioning (eg, school or work performance) may be more realistic than aiming for complete abstinence.

Persistent psychotic states or other psychologic disorders require appropriate psychiatric care. Flashbacks may be transient and not unduly distressing to the patient, requiring no special treatment. However, they may be associated with anxiety and depression and may require therapy similar to that for the acute adverse reactions.

DEPENDENCE ON PHENCYCLIDINE (PCP)

PCP has emerged and declined as a frequently used drug of abuse. It is not easily classified and should be considered separately from the hallucinogenic drugs. It has a bewildering number of effects on the CNS, and its neuropharmacology is only poorly understood.

PCP was tested as an anesthetic agent in humans in the late 1950s because of an ability to isolate humans from noxious sensory input (dissociative anesthesia). It was withdrawn because individuals often experienced severe anxiety, delusional states, or frank psychosis postoperatively. Clinical testing stopped in 1962, and PCP appeared as a street drug in 1967. Initially sold deceptively as "THC," in recent years it has established its own market. Although once available as a veterinary anesthetic, essentially all street material results from illegal synthesis, not difficult to perform. Occasionally injected or ingested, it is most frequently sprinkled on smoking material (parsley, mint leaves, tobacco, marijuana), combusted, and inhaled. In recent years, much random violence and crime has been attributed to users of this drug, although as with past drug horror stories, this is not often well documented. Since the frequent reports of problems with PCP in 1978, the number of reports has declined significantly. Its current use and the attention directed to that use have declined.

Symptoms and signs: A giddy euphoria usually occurs with lower doses, often followed by bursts of anxiety or mood lability. Effects of higher doses include a withdrawn catatonic state, ataxia, dysarthria, muscular hypertonicity, and myoclonic jerks. Excessive salivation can distinguish PCP use from use of high-dose CNS stimulants, which produce xerostomia. Rotatory nystagmus is often present and helps in making the diagnosis. Cardiovascular status is usually unaffected. At very high doses, coma, convulsions, severe hypertension, and death may occur, although fatalities are unusual. Prolonged psychotic states have apparently followed use of this drug.

In treatment, diazepam often is helpful, and it is mandatory when seizure activity is present. Some clinicians believe that haloperidol is useful. Hypotension may occur when chlorpromazine is used. Diazoxide may be used when severe hypertension is present. PCP is highly lipid-soluble and may have a prolonged biologic persistence. It or its metabolites may remain in the CNS for lengthy periods. The alkaline character of the drug leads to surprisingly high secretion into the stomach, and prolonged gastric lavage has recovered large amounts of PCP. Lavage must be accompanied by acidification with ammonium chloride (or other agents) because this maneuver results in dramatic ionic trapping in the stomach and urine. Anecdotally, street users may resort to cranberry juice to hasten urinary excretion.

DEPENDENCE ON VOLATILE SOLVENTS

A state of intoxication achieved by use of industrial solvents and aerosol sprays continues to be an endemic problem among juveniles. These volatile solvents (eg, aliphatic and aromatic hydrocarbons, chlorinated hydrocarbons, ketones, acetates) along with ether, chloroform, and alcohol produce temporary stimulation before depression of the CNS occurs. Partial tolerance to the fumes develops with daily use, as does psychologic dependence, but an abstinence syndrome does not occur.

Acute **symptoms** of dizziness, drowsiness, slurred speech, and unsteady gait are seen early. Impulsiveness, excitement, and irritability may occur. As the CNS becomes more deeply affected, illusions, hallucinations, and delusions develop. The user experiences a euphoric dreamy "high," culminating in a short period of "sleep." Delirium with confusion, psychomotor clumsiness, emotional lability, and impairment of thinking are seen. The intoxicated state may last from minutes to an hour or more.

Complications may result from the effect of the solvent or from other toxic ingredients such as lead in gasoline. Carbon tetrachloride may cause a syndrome of hepatic and renal failure. Injuries to brain, liver, kidney, and bone marrow occur and may be the effects of heavy exposure or hypersensitivity. Death most often occurs from respiratory arrest, cardiac arrhythmias, or asphyxia due to occlusion of the airway.

Treatment of solvent-dependent children is difficult, and relapse is frequent. Intensive attempts to improve the patient's self-esteem and status in family, school, and society may be helpful. See also TABLE 145-4.

DEPENDENCE ON VOLATILE NITRITES

Inhalation of amyl nitrite ("poppers") to alter consciousness and enhance sexual pleasure has emerged in recent years. This use has been particularly prominent in urban male homosexual society. When amyl nitrite was returned to the prescription drug category, entrepreneurs began to market other nitrites (butyl, isobutyl) under a variety of trade names; eg, "Locker Room," "Rush," and others. At this time there is little evidence that the products have significant hazard, although they produce a predictable nitrite vasodilating effect with brief hypotension, dizziness, and flushing, followed by reflex tachycardia. See also TABLE 145-4.

54. PSYCHOSEXUAL ISSUES

Accepted norms of sexual behavior and attitudes vary greatly within and among different cultures. **Masturbation,** once widely regarded as a perversion and a cause of mental disease, is now recognized as a normal sexual activity throughout life and is considered a symptom only when it suggests an inhibition of partner-oriented behavior. Its cumulative incidence is about 97% in males and 80% in females. While masturbation per se is harmless, guilt created by disapproving and punitive attitudes may cause considerable distress and damage the capacity for sexual performance. Guilt and shame may also be induced by the discomfort of "forbidden" (eg, sadomasochistic or fetishistic) fantasies. Certain autoerotic practices, eg, partial asphyxiation, are dangerous and result in hundreds of fatalities.

About 8 to 10% of the population are preferentially **homosexual** for their entire lives. Some countries have passed laws permitting homosexual relationships between consenting adults. Since 1973, the American Psychiatric Association has not considered homosexuality a disease. **Frequent sexual activity with many partners,** often one-time-only encounters, indicates diminished capacity for pair-bonding. The fear of AIDS has caused a decrease in casual sex. **Extramarital sexuality** is discouraged by most cultures, but **premarital coitus** is accepted as normal by most. In the USA most people have intercourse prior to marriage, in keeping with a recent shift in developed countries toward more freedom of sexual expression. **Dysfunctions of desire, arousal, and orgasm** in the male and female are discussed in Ch. 55. **Illegitimacy** (unwed teenage pregnancies are discussed in Ch. 47) arouses disapproval and causes social disadvantage in many countries, while in others a high proportion of children are born out of wedlock and are well tolerated. Illegitimate children reared by a single parent or by surrogates, who may not form a close emotional bond with the child in the formative years, may be less likely to mature normally and may be more susceptible to developing emotional disorders or frank mental illness. Data show a slight risk of increased mental illness in selected groups of children; eg, young children (not illegitimate) raised by a single, divorced parent. The prognosis is better when the single parent has a support system.

Individuals whose sexual practices include small amounts of **fetishism** and **sadomasochism** generally have normal love relationships. Such tendencies may excite anxiety and distress but call for reassurance rather than therapy. However, if sexual drives are absorbed almost entirely in submission to flagellation, are vented mostly on articles of clothing, or are expressed to a great extent in **exhibitionism** or **voyeurism,** the individual's capacity for establishing love relationships is stunted, and other aspects of his personal and emotional adjustment suffer.

Physicians, provided they can become well informed themselves, can offer sensitive, disciplined advice on sexual matters and should not miss opportunities for helpful intervention, keeping in mind the influence of cultural diversity. The strength of the sexual drive, the needs of individuals, and the frequency of sexual contact are subject to great variation.

Etiology and Incidence

Etiology is complex and highly variable among individuals. Inherited or subtle constitutional factors probably play a part. The important role of fetal androgens in preparing the brain for later sexual activity suggests that interference with this process may render a person vulnerable to damaging environmental influences during childhood psychosexual development. Parental attitude toward sexual behavior is important. A forbidding, puritanical rejection of physical sexuality, including touching, engenders guilt and shame and inhibits the capacity for enjoying sex and developing healthy adult relationships.

In forming a secure **gender identity** (*sense of maleness or femaleness*) and **gender role** (*the public expression of gender identity*—see below), the character of the parents' emotional bond and the relationship that each of them has with the child are important. The parent of the same sex must be a person with whom the child can identify. The opposite-sex parent must engender enough love and trust so that the child later feels comfortable with members of the opposite sex. Relations with parents may be damaged by excessive emotional distance, by punitive behaviors, or by seductiveness and exploitation. Children exposed to hostility, rejection, and cruelty are liable to sexual maladjustment. The child needs to feel accepted and lovable. Establishing the individual's confidence that he is capable and worthy of being loved for himself is one of the goals of therapy.

These potentially damaging parent-child relationships can contribute to disorders of gender identity such as transsexualism, to one of the paraphilias, possibly to homosexuality (all discussed below), or to dysfunctions in sexual performance (see Ch. 55). For gender identity disorders in children, see Ch. 46. **Dissociation of sexual behavior** also may occur, in which emotional bonds can be formed with others from the individual's own social class or intellectual circle, but physical sexual relationships are possible only with those considered as inferiors, such as prostitutes, with whom the individual has no affinity and no emotional ties. In this type of maladjustment the sexual act with one's spouse is associated with guilt and anxiety, and sexual release is found in relationships or practices in which tender, caring feelings are not aroused.

Paraphilias are far more common among males than females, and this unequal distribution has been found in most cultures studied. Since reproductive competence in the female is of decisive importance for the species, and less so in the male, biologic reasons for the unequal distribution may exist. Developmentally, males must transfer their infantile identification with their mothers to their fathers during the preschool or oedipal period, from about the age of 3 to about 6, whereas females need not pass through this process of changing identification. The need to "disidentify" during a critical period of psychosexual development creates greater vulnerabilities for the male, hence the enormous preponderance of males affected by the paraphilias.

The pattern of erotic arousal is fairly well developed before puberty; therefore, if something goes awry, the causes for gender or paraphilic disorders should be sought in the prepubertal years. Three general factors present are (1) anxiety interferes with normal psychosexual development; (2) a displacement to another pattern of arousal allows the person to avoid the standard pattern of erotic arousal while retaining the capacity for sexual pleasure; and (3) the pattern of sexual arousal often has both symbolic and conditioning facets (eg, the fetish chosen symbolizes the object of arousal but may have developed by an accidental association of the fetish with sexual curiosity, desire, and excitement). Whether *all* transsexual or paraphilic development is created by these psychodynamic processes is still controversial. In many instances, perhaps in most, genetic endowment and fetal brain development produce the potential for responses to faulty environmental influences, especially family dynamics.

GENDER IDENTITY DISORDERS

The American Psychiatric Association's *Diagnostic and Statistical Manual of Mental Disorders,* Third Edition—Revised (**DSM-III-R**), states that the "essential feature of the disorder . . . is an incongruence between assigned sex (ie, the sex that is recorded on the birth certificate) and gender identity. Gender identity is a sense of knowing to which sex one belongs, that is, the awareness that 'I am a male,' or 'I am a female.' Gender identity is the private experience of gender role, and gender role is the public expression of gender identity. Gender role can be defined as everything that one says and does to indicate to others or to oneself the degree to which one is male or female."

When sex labeling and rearing are confusing, children will become uncertain about their gender identity. However, even the presence of ambiguous genitalia usually will not affect the child's gender identity if sex labeling and rearing are unambiguous. Transsexuals (see below) usually have had gender identity problems as children (see GENDER IDENTITY DISORDER OF CHILDHOOD in Ch. 46).

Transsexualism

A transsexual believes that he is the victim of a biologic accident, cruelly imprisoned within a body incompatible with his real sexual identity. The majority of transsexuals are males who consider themselves to have feminine gender identity and regard their genitalia and masculine features with repugnance. Their primary objective in seeking psychiatric help is not to obtain psychologic treatment but to secure surgery that will give them as close an approximation as possible to a female body. The diagnosis is made only if the disturbance has been continuous (not limited to periods of stress) for at least 2 yr. Rarely is it associated with genital ambiguity or genetic abnormality. Differential diagnosis must separate transsexuals from transvestites, cross-dressing homosexuals, and schizophrenics.

In true **male transsexuals** the condition begins in early childhood with indulgence in girls' games, fantasies of being female, avoidance of rough and tumble play and of competitive games, repugnance at the physical changes that attend puberty, and thereafter a quest for a feminine gender identity. Many transsexuals acquire skills enabling them to adopt a feminine gender identity. Some patients are satisfied with achieving a more feminine appearance, together with employment and an identity card allowing them to work and live in society as women. Others are not content with changing their social identity but can be helped to achieve a more stable adjustment with small doses of feminizing hormones. Many transsexuals request feminizing operations in spite of the sacrifices entailed. The decision for surgery often raises grave social and ethical problems. Since a few follow-up studies have provided evidence that some genuine transsexuals achieve more happy and productive lives with the aid of surgery, it is justified only in highly motivated true transsexuals with stable social and work records. After surgery, the patients need assistance with movement, gesture, and voice production. A few homosexual men, schizophrenics, or those with serious personality problems request reallocation surgery. The results in these patients are unsatisfactory from both a medical and social viewpoint.

Female transsexuals increasingly appear in medical and psychiatric practice. The patient asks for mastectomy, hysterectomy, and oophorectomy and also wants androgenic hormones to alter her voice and promote a more masculine appearance. She may ask for an artificial phallus to be fashioned by plastic surgery. Patients with stable and effective personalities whose social adaptation in most spheres of their lives has been successful may sometimes be helped to achieve greater satisfaction through surgical help. These patients must be carefully selected, because anatomic results of heroic surgery are often less satisfactory than in the male-to-female procedure.

PARAPHILIAS

Gross impairment in the capacity for affectionate sexual activity between adult human partners (see also under Etiology and Incidence, above). Many of the paraphilias are rare, and all occur mostly in males. Long-term psychotherapy usually is necessary but is not always successful. It is less useful when coercive, eg, by court order. **Group therapy** for some sex offenders is helpful, as is **anti-androgen treatment** for pedophiliacs, rapists, and lust murderers. The diagnosis of a paraphilia can be made in the absence of paraphilic *behavior,* according to DSM-III-R, if the patient is markedly distressed by "recurrent intense sexual urges and sexually arousing fantasies of at least 6 mo duration" involving the particular sexual deviation, eg, fetishism, pedophilia.

Fetishism

The use of physical objects as the preferred method of producing sexual excitement, usually beginning in adolescence. (The diagnosis of transvestism rather than fetishism should be made when a male is sexually stimulated and gratified by wearing, rather than simply fondling, some feminine garment, usually underclothing.) The fetish may replace sexual activity with a partner or may be integrated into sexual behavior with a partner. When the latter occurs, the fetish is usually required for erotic arousal. Commonly used fetishes are female undergarments, shoes, and boots—less commonly, parts of the human body such as hair or nails. Minor fetishistic behavior incorporated into heterosexual behavior is not aberrant. More intense fetishistic arousal patterns may generate serious problems in a relationship. When the fetish becomes the sole object of sexual desire, normal sexual relations are avoided.

Transvestism

Dressing by heterosexual males in female clothes, generally beginning in childhood or early adolescence. Transvestites usually achieve a certain amount of sexual excitement, and public display may give them much satisfaction. Despite their deviation, many transvestites have reasonably happy marriages. When their wives are cooperative, men have intercourse in feminine attire. When their wives are not cooperative, anxiety, depression, guilt, and shame associated with the desire to cross-dress are common. Few transvestites seek treatment unless there is marital conflict.

Pedophilia

(See also Ch. 31)

A preference for repetitive sexual activity with prepubertal children. Arbitrarily, the age difference between the adult with this disorder and the child victim is set at 5 yr or more. The age of the child is generally ≤ 13 yr. The age of the person with this diagnosis is arbitrarily set at ≥ 16 yr. For late adolescents, no precise age difference is specified; reliance is on clinical judgment. When the child is postpubertal, the disorder frequently is labeled as child molestation rather than pedophilia, but the distinction often is arbitrary. Pedophiliacs prefer opposite-sex children to same-sex children 2:1. Heterosexually oriented males tend to prefer girls aged 8 to 10 yr; in most cases, the adult is known to the child. Looking or touching seems to be more prevalent than genital contact. With homosexually oriented males, the preferred partner's age is 10 to 13 yr, and acquaintanceship is more casual than in the heterosexually oriented group. Bisexual adult pedophiles usually choose children under the age of 8 yr.

Sexual offenses against children constitute a significant proportion of reported criminal sexual acts. The recidivism rate for homosexual pedophilia is second only to exhibitionism, and ranges from 13 to 28% of those apprehended—roughly twice the rate of heterosexual pedophilia.

Exhibitionism

Repetitive acts of genital exposure to an unsuspecting stranger for the purpose of producing sexual excitement. Peak age at onset is in the mid 20s; rarely the first act occurs at either end of a spectrum that ranges from preadolescence to middle age. Further sexual contact is almost never sought. About 30% of apprehended male sex offenders are exhibitionists. These persons have the highest recidivism rate of all sex offenders; about 20% get rearrested. The victim almost always is a female adult or child. Most exhibitionists are married, but the marriage often is troubled by poor sexual adjustment, including frequent psychosexual dysfunction. A very few cases of exhibitionism in females have been reported—many females have exhibitionistic tendencies (usually not to strangers) sanctioned by society. Folklore has it that "women exhibit everything but the genitals; men, nothing but" (Romano).

Voyeurism

Sexual arousal by looking at unsuspecting females who are naked, disrobing, or engaging in sexual activity. Age at onset usually is early adulthood. Adolescent voyeurism generally is reported leniently; few teenagers are arrested. The essential feature is a repetitive seeking-out of these situations. Orgasm usually produced by masturbation may occur during the voyeuristic activity. The voyeur does not initiate further sexual contact. The disorder has to be differentiated from normal sexual curiosity occurring between people who know each other.

Sexual Masochism

Intentional participation in an activity in which the individual is physically harmed or the individual's life is threatened in order to produce sexual excitement; often the preferred or exclusive mode of producing sexual excitement is to be humiliated, bound, beaten, or otherwise made to suffer. Age at onset commonly is early adulthood. Fantasies are fairly frequent, whereas masochistic behavior is relatively uncommon. A potentially dangerous form entails various types of physical self-constraint and partial asphyxiation ("hypoxyphilia") by hanging or other means of O_2 deprivation, which can lead to accidental death. A few cases have been reported in women, but the vast majority with this disorder are men.

Sexual Sadism

The inflicting of physical or psychologic suffering on the sexual partner as a method of stimulating sexual excitement and orgasm. Age at onset commonly is early adulthood, although sadistic fantasies often occur during childhood. Generally there are insistent and persistent fantasies in which sexual excitement is produced as a result of suffering inflicted on the partner. The diagnosis is warranted whether the partner is consenting or not. Sadism is different from minor manifestations of aggression in normal sexual activity. At the extreme end of the spectrum of intensity for sexual sadism are individuals who brutally rape or torture victims. Even more extreme are lust murderers, in whom sexual excitement is produced by the death of the victim.

According to DSM-III-R, "In most cases of rape, however, the rapist is not motivated by the prospect of inflicting suffering." Fewer than 10% receive the diagnosis of sexual sadism, although in many, sexual excitement is increased "by coercing or forcing a nonconsenting person to engage in intercourse." Rape is a complex amalgam of sex and power-control over the victim in which the victim's suffering usually does not increase the rapist's sexual excitement.

HOMOSEXUALITY

Homosexuality is no longer regarded as a mental disorder by the American Psychiatric Association. Society is slowly accepting homosexuality as a sexual variant, but great hostility and prejudice (homophobia) are still widely prevalent.

A transient stage of homosexual conduct in puberty and adolescence is common ($^1/_3$ of male adolescents), but almost all persons who experience this, even those who engage in some form of physical contact, later become exclusively heterosexual in their preferences. Approximately 8 to 10% of males are exclusively homosexual during their entire lives. A majority report some heterosexual contact that was soon abandoned after initial experiences. Two-thirds of male homosexuals and a similar percentage of female homosexuals (lesbians) are capable of heterosexual performance and even pleasure, although they are preferentially homosexual. About 20% of homosexual men and 33% of homosexual women marry, but their heterosexual marriages tend to be unstable.

Seventy percent of male homosexuals reported having had sex with a married man, and 20% said they had had sex with 6 or more married men. In addition, 45% of lesbian women said they had sex with men since 1980, during the age of AIDS. If the spread of AIDS is to be diminished, specific unprotected sexual behavior should be the focus of behavioral research and educational intervention rather than a high-risk group label. Sexual behavior passes across identification boundaries.

Preferential or exclusive homosexuality should be distinguished from situational (facultative) homosexuality, frequently exhibited by males and females confined for long periods with members of their own sex, as on board ship or in prison. Usual sexual behavior is resumed on release from such environments.

Sexual acts between homosexuals consist of expressions of tenderness, fondling, caressing, and kissing that usually culminate in orgasm—achieved through mutual masturbation, fellatio, anal intercourse in the male, or cunnilingus in the female. It is uncommon for one partner to adopt an exclusively active or passive role, and most homosexuals participate in the relationship in a variety of ways.

About 25% of male homosexuals are capable of long-lasting partnerships. Casual, shallow contacts with strangers are more frequent; 28% of male homosexuals reported having had more than 1000 partners, although such behavior has substantially decreased because of AIDS. Contact with many partners has made sexually transmitted diseases (STDs) more frequent, but new cases of STDs, including AIDS and syphilis, are decreasing in the homosexual population. AIDS (see Ch. 20) is found predominantly among male homosexuals, although the incidence of both AIDS and syphilis is increasing rapidly among IV drug abusers and their heterosexual partners. Only 5% of homosexuals posture effeminately; most are repelled by such behavior. Most homosexuals are emotionally stable, conducting normal lives and considering themselves happy. Some indication exists that, unless they have formed "close-coupled" relationships, homosexuals suffer increasing isolation and rejection as they advance to middle or late life and are rejected by the homosexual culture, which seems to highly value youth and physical attractiveness.

Most female homosexuals are capable of close-coupled relationships and engage in casual sexual contacts far less frequently than their male counterparts. Psychiatric illnesses are also less common among lesbians than among male homosexuals. This may be intrinsic or due to more favorable societal reactions, or both.

The causes of homosexuality are not known. Constitutional factors involving hormonal programming of the brain during fetal life may be a significant factor. Some support for this hypothesis is to be found in the higher-than-expected prevalence of homosexual fantasies and behavior in women whose mothers received diethylstilbestrol (DES) during pregnancy.

Unless a homosexual requests help to change sexual orientation, treatment is not indicated. Some homosexuals seek treatment to alleviate distress due to problems with relationships, including sex (sexual dysfunctions are similar to those found in heterosexuals) or employment, and develop a motivation for change, but most have no wish to do so. Help in overcoming crises or mitigating emotional distress and simple psychotherapy to assist individuals in achieving realistic, satisfying adjustment to their social predicament are all that is needed in most cases. For those homo-

sexuals who are strongly motivated to change (and fundamental change is rarely possible even if motivation is high), the best therapy draws on both behavioral techniques and psychotherapy, including group therapy. The possibility for change is better with a history of heterosexual behavior and fantasies. In most instances, it is more helpful to assist the homosexual person to overcome the internal homophobia that has brought him or her into treatment. The greater the degree of commitment to a homosexual identity, the greater the person's psychological well-being.

55. DISORDERS OF SEXUAL FUNCTION

INTRODUCTION

The psychosexual disorders described in Ch. 54 include gender identity, the paraphilias, and homosexuality, although the latter is no longer considered a disorder. Sexual dysfunction, the most common of the psychosexual disorders encountered by the practicing physician, is discussed here.

Proper sexual functioning in men and women depends on an anticipatory mental "set" (the sexual motive state) or state of *desire,* effective vasocongestive *arousal* (erection in the male, swelling and lubrication in the female), and *orgasm.* The sensation of orgasm in the male includes emission followed by ejaculation. Emission produces a sensation of ejaculatory inevitability and is mediated by contractions of the prostate, seminal vesicles, and urethra. Orgasm in the female is accompanied by contractions, not always subjectively experienced as such, of the muscles that line the wall of the outer third of the vagina. In both sexes, generalized muscular tension, perineal contractions, and involuntary pelvic thrusting (at a periodicity of 0.8 sec) usually occur. Orgasm is followed by *resolution,* a sense of general relaxation, well-being, and muscular relaxation. During this phase men are physiologically refractory to further erection and orgasm for a variable period of time. In contrast, women may be able to respond to additional stimulation almost immediately.

The sexual response cycle is mediated by a delicate (or balanced) interplay between the sympathetic and parasympathetic nervous systems. Vasocongestion is largely mediated by parasympathetic (cholinergic) outflow, whereas orgasm is predominantly sympathetic (adrener-

gic). Ejaculation is almost entirely sympathetic, whereas emission involves a much more finely balanced combination of sympathetic and parasympathetic stimulation. All these reflex responses are easily inhibited by cortical influences or by impaired hormonal, neural, or vascular mechanisms; α- and β-adrenergic blocking agents may desynchronize emission, ejaculation, and the perineal muscle contractions occurring during orgasm.

The American Psychiatric Association's *Diagnostic and Statistical Manual of Mental Disorders,* Third Edition – Revised **(DSM-III-R)** states that **inhibitions in the response cycle** may occur at one or more of the sexual response phases, although inhibition in the resolution phase rarely is clinically significant. Generally, both the *subjective* dimensions of desire, arousal, and pleasure and the *objective* performance, vasocongestion, and orgasm are disturbed, although either component occasionally may occur alone.

All of the dysfunctions may be **primary** (lifelong, with effective performance never having been experienced in any situation, and generally due to intrapsychic conflicts) or **secondary** (acquired after a period of normal function); generalized or limited to certain situations or with certain partners; and total or partial (degree or frequency of disturbance). Most patients complain of anxiety, guilt, shame, and frustration, and many develop somatic symptoms. Although dysfunction usually occurs during sexual activity with a partner, it is useful to inquire about function during masturbation.

Etiologic factors for both primary and secondary dysfunction can be similar. Poor communication is always present. **Psychologic factors**

include *anger* directed toward the partner; *fear* of the partner's genitals, or of intimacy, losing control, dependency, or pregnancy; *guilt* following a pleasurable experience; *depression;* and *anxiety* created by marital discord, stressful life situations, aging, ignorance of behavioral norms (eg, frequency and duration of intercourse, oral-genital sex, or sexual practices), or sexual myths (eg, the assumed deleterious effects of masturbation, hysterectomy, or menopause). The so-called **immediate causes** of anxiety are the fear of failure, demand for performance, spectatoring (observing one's physical responses), an excessive wish to please the partner, and avoidance of sex and of talking about sexual concerns. These exacerbating factors additionally impair performance and satisfaction, and the further avoidance of sexual activity with impaired communication creates a vicious circle.

Other related inhibitory factors include ignorance (often the consequence of inhibited learning, itself based on anxiety, shame, or guilt) of the sex organs and their function; traumatic events in childhood or adolescence (eg, incest or rape); feelings of inadequacy; religious training; excessive modesty; and puritanical aversion to intercourse.

Interpersonal and situational causes include marital discord and boredom in the relationship and may be related to place, time, or a particular partner.

Physical factors are discussed under the individual disorders below. Even when these factors are identified, secondary psychogenic elements are almost always present and complicating.

HYPOACTIVE SEXUAL DESIRE DISORDER (HSD)

This disorder is defined by DSM-III-R as *persistently or recurrently deficient or absent sexual fantasies and desire for sexual activity in a woman or a man.*

Etiology

Sexual desire is a psychosomatic process based on brain activity (the "generator" or "motor" running in a rheostatic cyclic fashion) and cognitive scripting that includes sexual aspiration and motivation. Desynchronization of these components results in HSD. Acquired HSD is commonly caused by boredom in the relationship, depression (which leads more often to decreased interest in sex than it does to impotence

in the male or inhibited excitement in the female), psychoactive drugs, antihypertensive medication, and hormonal deficiencies. HSD also can be secondary to impaired sexual function. Lifelong generalized low levels of sexual desire are related to traumatic events in childhood or adolescence, the suppression of sexual fantasies, or, occasionally, insufficient levels of androgens. Generally, testosterone levels < 300 ng/dL in the male and < 10 ng/dL in the female are considered potential causes.

Symptoms and Signs

The patient complains of a lack of interest in sex, even in ordinarily erotic situations. The disorder usually is associated with infrequent sexual activity, often causing serious marital conflict. Some patients, however, have sexual encounters fairly often to please their partners and may not show any difficulty with performance but continue to have sexual apathy. When boredom is the cause, frequency of sex with the usual partner decreases, but sexual desire may be normal or even intense with others (real or fantasized). A generalized anhedonia (see below) may be present.

Treatment

Treatment is directed toward removing or alleviating the underlying cause; eg, marital conflict, depression, other sexual dysfunction, changing medications, and, in the occasional case of androgen insufficiency, administration of IM testosterone (see Treatment under SEXUAL AROUSAL DISORDER, below).

SEXUAL AVERSION DISORDER

DSM-III-R defines this disorder as *persistent or recurrent extreme aversion to and avoidance of all or almost all genital sexual contact with a sexual partner.* It occurs only occasionally in males, much more often in females.

Etiology and Diagnosis

If lifelong or primary, the aversion to sexual contact, especially to intercourse, may be the consequence of sexual trauma, such as incest, sexual abuse, or rape. In the absence of sexual trauma, one usually finds a very repressive atmosphere in the family, sometimes enhanced by orthodox and rigid religious training. A third possibility is that initial attempts at intercourse resulted in moderate to severe dyspareunia. Even after that has disappeared, painful memories may persist. If the problem is secondary, ie, after a period of normal functioning, the cause is either partner-related (interpersonal), trauma, or dyspareunia. If the aversion produces a phobic response, even panic, in addition to the causes listed above, less conscious and unrealistic fears of domination or of bodily damage may be present. A special situation occurs in which people attempt or are expected to have sexual relations not appropriate to their sexual orientation.

Treatment

Treatment is aimed at removing the underlying cause. The choice of behavioral or psychodynamic psychotherapy depends on the diagnosis. Marital therapy is indicated if the cause is interpersonal. The treatment of panic states can be enhanced by the use of antidepressants, either tricyclics or monoamine oxidase (MAO) inhibitors.

SEXUAL DYSFUNCTION IN THE MALE

SEXUAL AROUSAL DISORDER
(Erectile Dysfunction; Impotence)

Inability to attain or sustain an erection satisfactory for normal coitus. The dysfunction may be primary, which is rare and, if not organic, generally indicates severe psychopathology; or secondary, in which erectile dysfunction prohibits completion of successful sexual intercourse in about $\geq$ 25% of opportunities.

Etiology

Primary erectile dysfunction is almost always due to intrapsychic factors. In rare cases, biogenic factors, usually associated with low testosterone levels and reflecting disorders of the hypothalamic-pituitary-gonadal axis, provide the major etiology. Occasionally, vascular abnormalities are found. Intrapsychic factors include an abnormal fear of the vagina, sexual guilt, fear of intimacy, or depression. Of the **secondary** cases, about 50% are caused by psychic factors. A transient episode of erectile dysfunction for any reason may be followed by secondary psychologic factors labeled "immediate" causes (see above).

Erectile dysfunction may be situational, involving place, time, a particular partner, some perceived competitive defeat, or damage to self-esteem.

Physical factors include systemic diseases (eg, diabetes mellitus [the most common], syphilis, alcoholism, drug dependency, hypopituitarism, and hypothyroidism); local disorders (eg, congenital abnormalities and inflammatory diseases of the genitalia); vascular disturbances such as aortic aneurysm and atherosclerosis (eg, Leriche's syndrome); neurogenic disorders (eg, multiple sclerosis, spinal cord lesions, pituitary microadenoma with hyperprolactinemia, and cardiovascular accident); drugs such as hypertensives, sedatives, tranquilizers, and amphetamines; and surgical procedures such as sympathectomy. Prostatectomy and castration produce varying effects. Impotence is usually not induced by transurethral prostatectomy, whereas it almost always occurs after perineal prostatectomy. However, retrograde ejaculation is produced in the vast majority of men, irrespective of the type of prostatectomy.

Impotence is not inevitable with aging, even into the 70s or 80s. While the amount and force of the ejaculate and thus sexual tension and the need to ejaculate are decreased, the capacity for erection often is retained.

Diagnosis

Psychic factors are implicated if the patient has situational impotence, has morning erections, or can achieve a firm erection with masturbation. Because a combination of physical and psychic factors is possible, it must be determined whether the psychic factors are primary or secondary. Inability to have an erection under any circumstances requires a search for organic causes. A general medical evaluation includes history of drugs and alcohol, examination of the genitalia, neurologic evaluation, and search for signs of vascular or endocrine dysfunction; laboratory procedures include a glucose tolerance test and testosterone (total and "free"), luteinizing hormone (**LH**), follicle-stimulating hormone (**FSH**), and prolactin (**PRL**) levels (best taken at 9 AM to avoid diurnal variations).

Particularly important in evaluating cases in which the etiology is uncertain is the examination for nocturnal penile tumescence (**NPT**). Episodes of NPT accompany rapid-eye-movement (**REM**) sleep. Absence of erections during sleep strongly suggests, but does not prove, an organic basis. The patient can be monitored for nighttime erections in a special sleep laboratory. The number of erections, the duration of each erection, and the amount of penile vasocongestion during the course of a night's sleep can be evaluated to devise a quantitative estimate of erectile capacity. It is important to correct for artifacts by correlating erections with REM sleep and, usually, by direct observation.

Treatment

Psychic erectile dysfunction may respond to brief counseling to alleviate secondary factors. Every effort should be made to include the patient's partner. Reassurance following a careful physical examination and any necessary laboratory studies is a key first step. Education to dispel myths and misinformation and to help establish a nondemanding and mutually pleasurable situation may be sufficient. A specific technique is the 3-stage sensate focus method of Masters and Johnson, involving stepwise nongenital pleasuring, genital pleasuring, and nondemanding coitus. If about 6 counseling sessions do not bring results, referral to a sex therapist should be considered.

If physical abnormalities are found, therapy is directed toward alleviating the underlying disorder. If androgen levels are low (< 300 ng/dL), treatment with testosterone 200 mg IM every 2 wk for 3 to 4 mo should be tried. (First, however, PRL, FSH, and LH levels should be ascertained, since hyperprolactinemia can be successfully treated with bromocriptine.) Subcutaneous testosterone pellets are favored by some. There is often a short-lived positive placebo response to the administration of oral testosterone. Testosterone seems to increase sexual desire, especially spontaneous fantasies.

Men who do not respond to psychotherapy or in whom NPT testing demonstrates organic dysfunction can be administered a penile injection of a combination of papaverine and phentolamine, or of prostaglandin E_1. If the vascular supply to the penis is reasonably intact, and if the veins are not "leaking," the injection results in a firm erection that often lasts 1 h or longer. (This method can be also used to diagnose vascular disturbances of the penis.) If this is successful, the patient can be taught to inject himself. It is painless if done properly and does not affect ejaculation. Possible side effects are priapism (usually dose-related), penile plaques, or Peyronie's disease.

If the impotence does not respond to any of these treatments, or is not likely to, a penile prosthesis can be implanted and is usually successful.

ORGASM DISORDERS
(Premature Ejaculation)

Persistent or recurrent ejaculation before, upon, or shortly after penetration. Because specific criteria vary, it may also be defined as *ejaculation occurring before the individual wishes.* Since normal biologic response is to ejaculate within 2 min after vaginal penetration and since few women are able to reach orgasm within 2 min, most men must learn how to retard emission and ejaculation.

Etiology and Diagnosis

In the adolescent, premature ejaculation is common. It may be aggravated by a feeling of sinfulness about sex or by a fear of discovery, of impregnating the girl, or of getting a sexually transmitted disease, as well as by anxiety over performance. In the adult, similar concerns may persist, as well as interpersonal factors. Occult somatic factors are rare, although prostatitis or diseases affecting the neural pathways may be involved.

Treatment

Sometimes an explanation of the mechanism of premature ejaculation, reassurance, and simple advice are curative. Increasing the number of opportunities for ejaculation may decrease sexual tension. The "stop-and-start" technique involves stimulation of the penis either manually or during intercourse until the patient begins to recognize that he will soon ejaculate unless stimulation ceases. He signals his partner to cease stimulation, which is resumed after about 20 or 30 seconds. The partners rehearse this technique at first with manual stimulation, and later during coitus, stopping 3 times; with the 4th stimulation, they permit ejaculation to occur. With repetition, the patient learns ejaculatory control (for 5 or 10 min or even longer) in over 95% of the cases. Occasionally premature ejaculation masks deep-seated intrapsychic or interpersonal conflict, and the patient may have to be referred for individual psychotherapy or marital therapy.

INHIBITED ORGASM
(Retarded Ejaculation)

A relatively rare phenomenon in which intravaginal ejaculation does not occur or, more rarely, there is inability to masturbate to ejaculation. The etiology usually is psychologic, but diabetes mellitus, thioridazine and mesoridazine (piperidyl variants of the phenothiazines), or some antihypertensive drugs may impair ejaculation. Retarded ejaculation must be distinguished from the retrograde ejaculation that almost inevitably follows prostatectomy. Some drugs (amoxapine, desipramine, imipramine, and protriptyline) or neurologic disorders (eg, multiple sclerosis) can produce retrograde ejaculation or, rarely, erection or emission without ejaculation.

Treatment: The partner stimulates the patient to ejaculation outside the vagina, then at the lips of the vagina, and finally inside the vagina. Psychotherapy is indicated if this behavioral technique fails.

SEXUAL ANHEDONIA

Rarely, a patient experiences *erection and ejaculation with no pleasure during orgasm.* The cause is psychogenic penile anesthesia in either a hysterical or obsessive person. Psychiatric consultation is indicated unless there is evidence of spinal cord damage or peripheral neuropathy. Loss of tactile sensation over the penis is unlikely to be neurogenic unless there are also anesthetic areas around the anus or scrotum.

SEXUAL DYSFUNCTION IN THE FEMALE

SEXUAL AROUSAL DISORDER

Persistent or recurrent failure to attain or maintain the lubrication-swelling response of sexual excitement until completion of sexual activity. This inhibition occurs despite adequate sexual stimulation in focus, intensity, and duration. The disorder may be primary or, more frequently, secondary and restricted to the partner.

Etiology

Psychic, acquired factors cause most cases; eg, marital discord (about 80% of cases), depression, and stressful life situations (see also INTRODUCTION, above). Ignorance of genital anatomy and function is common, particularly of clitoral function and of effective arousal patterns and techniques. Association of sex with sinfulness, and sexual pleasure with guilt, may be lifelong. Fear of intimacy may also play a part.

The physical causes include localized diseases (eg, endometriosis, cystitis, vaginitis); systemic diseases (eg, hypothyroidism, diabetes mellitus—though its impact is greater on men); peripheral or CNS disorders (eg, multiple sclerosis); muscular disorders (eg, muscular dystrophy); drugs (eg, oral contraceptives, antihypertensives, tranquilizers have variable effects); and ablative surgery (eg, hysterectomy, mastectomy, which may have a negative impact on the woman's sexual self-image).

Aging: Although women can be orgasmic throughout their lives, sexual activity often decreases after age 60 because of the relative lack of partners, as well as untreated physiologic changes (eg, atrophy of the vaginal mucosa).

Diagnosis and Treatment

The history and physical examination help to establish (1) whether the origin of the condition is predominantly psychic, physical, or both; and (2) the degree of dysfunction. The physician should comfortably discuss sexual matters and elicit precise data, usually by asking questions that gradually move from the more general areas of concern to those of greater sensitivity. Organic factors are investigated by the physical examination and appropriate laboratory studies.

The patient's complaints are usually directed to the lack of orgasm, although it is not uncommon to hear women say, "I don't get turned on." The discussion of treatment appears in INHIBITED ORGASM, below, because inhibited sexual excitement almost invariably leads to inhibition of orgasm, and the treatment of both disorders is similar.

INHIBITED ORGASM

The essential feature of this disorder as indicated by DSM-III-R is *persistent or recurrent delay or absence of orgasm following the normal sexual excitement phase during sexual activity that is assessed as adequate in focus, intensity, and duration.* Frequently the patient has both an inhibition of sexual excitement and of orgasm. The disorder may be primary, secondary, or situational. About 10% of women do not attain orgasm through any source of stimulation or in any situation. Most women can attain orgasm with clitoral stimulation, but probably > 50% of women are unable to regularly attain orgasm *during coitus.* When a woman responds to noncoital clitoral stimulation but cannot attain coital orgasm, a thorough sexual evaluation and even a trial of treatment is required to judge whether it represents a normal variation of response or if psychopathology is present.

The **etiology** is similar to that of inhibited sexual excitement. However, if lovemaking is consistently terminated before the aroused woman reaches climax (eg, due to inadequate foreplay, ignorance of clitoral/vaginal anatomy and function, or premature ejaculation), the frustration created may result in resentment or aversion, and dysfunction. Also, women who have no difficulty developing adequate vasocongestion may be fearful of "letting go," especially during intercourse. This may be due to guilt following a pleasurable experience or to the fear of abandoning oneself to a pleasurable situation requiring dependency on the partner. It may also represent a fear of losing control.

Treatment

Organic disorders should be treated. When psychic factors predominate (see in INTRODUCTION, above), counseling to remove the secondary causes is helpful; usually both partners should attend these sessions.

The Masters and Johnson 3-stage sensate focus exercises that involve the couple in stepwise nongenital pleasuring, genital pleasuring, and nondemanding coitus are generally beneficial to women with all levels of sexual inhibition. Women accustomed to clitoral but not coital orgasms are less responsive to this treatment format. Individual psychotherapy or group therapy sometimes is useful.

A woman's knowledge of the function of her sexual organs and of her responses is essential. This includes understanding the best methods of stimulating the clitoris and the enhanced vaginal sensations possible by strengthening voluntary control of the **pubococcygeus muscle (PCG)**. The PCG, which also controls urine flow, contains the nerve endings that provide pleasurable sensations in the outer third of the vagina. **Kegel's exercises** develop control of the PCG, which is contracted 10 to 15 times tid. In 2 to 3 mo perivaginal muscle tone improves, as does the woman's sense of control.

Women classified as having lifelong inhibition of orgasm (with or without inhibitions of sexual desire or excitement) should be referred to a psychiatrist. In any case, the nonspecialist should limit himself to about 6 counseling sessions, referring complex situations to a sex therapist or a psychiatrist.

DYSPAREUNIA

Painful or difficult coitus.

Etiology

Primary dyspareunia appears during initial attempts at sexual intercourse and is usually introital. The cause may be psychogenic or due to local trauma such as hymenal tears, laceration of the fourchette, or bruising of the urethral meatus. Subsequent to the injury, painful superficial ulcerations may develop. Forceful pressure against a sensitive urethra during coitus may be a factor. Other causes include inadequate lubrication, usually secondary to improper or insufficient loveplay; improper intromission; introital lesions due to inflammatory conditions such as skenitis; infections (eg, abscesses of Bartholin's glands or ducts); inflammation of labial sweat glands; irritation due to the use of improperly fitted or inadequately lubricated prophylactics; allergic reactions to contents of contraceptive foams, jellies, etc; and abnormalities of the female genital tract (eg, congenital septum or a rigid hymen).

Secondary dyspareunia is unrelated to first coitus and often develops years later. Causes include menopausal involution with dryness and thinning of the mucosa, tight perineorrhaphies following an episiotomy or plastic repairs of the vagina, marked retroflection of the uterus with ovaries prolapsed into the cul-de-sac, endometriosis, vaginitis, suburethral diverticulum, and pelvic inflammatory disease. Radiation therapy for treatment of malignancy or sterilization may precipitate an acute onset. For psychogenic causes and related factors, see INTRODUCTION, above.

Diagnosis

Pain during or following coitus is the chief complaint. The location and nature of the pain may be helpful to the diagnosis; eg, pain on deep thrusting indicates lesions of the uterus and/or broad ligament. A general and sexual history and a physical and pelvic examination usually uncover the etiology. Local introital lesions and uterine displacements or other pelvic pathology can be detected by examination, for which anesthesia is sometimes required (see VAGINISMUS, below). Inadequate stimulation or psychic inhibition of arousal may result in inadequate vaginal lubrication and cause coital pain.

Prophylaxis

Premarital examination of both partners; a frank explanation of the reproductive organs, their functions, and physiologic and psychologic factors involved in sexual intercourse; and guidance in sexual techniques may prevent problems. Existing lesions or defects should be corrected, if possible. For example, the stretching of a rigid hymen is an office procedure. An anesthetic ointment (eg, 1% lidocaine) should be used before each treatment.

Treatment

Therapy of uncomplicated injuries is simple. Temporary avoidance of intercourse is important. A soothing ointment (eg, 1% dibucaine or 1% lidocaine) may be applied externally; sitz baths can also provide relief of vulval distress. Pain and spasm can usually be prevented by liberal use of a lubricant just before coitus; sometimes a more posterior intromission that avoids pressure on a sensitive urethra may help. For treatment of more severe vaginismus, see below. A local estrogenic preparation is helpful in postmenopausal vaginitis, although to avoid risk of endometrial or breast cancer, oral estrogen in low doses for 20 days followed by a progestin for 8 to 10 days is preferred.

Cysts or abscesses should be excised; inflamed labia must be kept clean and dry; leukorrhea is treated in the usual manner (see VULVOVAGINITIS in Ch. 5). If the vulva is swollen and painful, a wet dressing of dilute aluminum acetate solution may be applied locally. At times, codeine 30 to 60 mg orally q 4 h and sedation (eg, phenobarbital 15 or 30 mg orally tid) may be indicated. Uterine retroflexion and prolapsed ovaries often can be corrected by a pessary. If trauma to sacrouterine ligaments is caused by an ill-fitting diaphragm, adjustment or elimination of the diaphragm is indicated.

Educational discussions may be needed for both partners (see Prophylaxis, above). However, cases of long-standing dyspareunia or in which the underlying psychic factors cannot be uncovered should be referred to a psychiatrist.

VAGINISMUS

Spasm of the vagina, a conditioned involuntary contraction of the lower vaginal muscles resulting from a woman's unconscious desire to prevent penetration. Since intromission is often impossible, vaginismus is frequently seen in cases of unconsummated marriage. Some women with vaginismus enjoy clitoral orgasms.

Etiology

Vaginismus is often due to dyspareunia, the causes of which are listed above. Other causes are fear of pregnancy, of being controlled by the man, of losing control, or of being hurt during

coitus (a misconception of intercourse as a necessarily violent process). If these intrapsychic factors are present, the vaginismus is usually primary (lifelong). Even after the cause of dyspareunia has been removed, the memory of painful coitus can cause vaginismus.

Diagnosis

Observation of an involuntary vaginal spasm during pelvic examination and, sometimes, of an avoidance reaction by the patient as the examiner approaches confirms the diagnosis. The physical or psychogenic causes are established by history and physical examination. Anesthesia, local or general, may be required to overcome the spasm induced by even the gentlest vaginal inspection. The local injection of 1% xylocaine at the hymenal ring or a pudendal block may help some patients.

Treatment

Any painful physical disorders should be corrected (see DYSPAREUNIA, above). If vaginismus persists, techniques to eliminate the vaginal muscle spasm, such as the **graduated dilation technique,** have been successful. With the patient in the lithotomy position, well-lubricated rubber or glass dilators in graduated sizes starting with a wire-thin one are introduced into the vagina and allowed to remain in place for 10 min. A variation preferred by some is to use Young's rectal dilators because they are shorter than the vaginal ones and will cause less discomfort. A good practice, with usually less resistance on the patient's part, is to have the patient herself place the dilators in the vagina. It is helpful if the patient employs Kegel's exercises while the dilator is in place. By contracting the perivaginal muscles as long as possible and then relaxing them, while paying attention to the sensation when letting go, the patient develops a sense of mastery over her vaginal muscles. It is also useful to have the patient place one hand on her inner thigh and ask her to contract and relax those muscles. That generally relaxes both thighs and, in the process, the perivaginal muscles. The procedure should be carried out by the physician at least 3 times/wk, and self-insertion with her fingers should be practiced by the patient at home bid.

Intercourse is attempted after the patient has tolerated insertion of the larger dilators without discomfort (with the rectal dilators, usually No. 5). This procedure must be accompanied by educational counseling (see Prophylaxis under DYSPAREUNIA, above). It is often helpful, prior to instituting the technique of graduated dilation, to perform a sexologic examination. In the presence of the patient's partner, the physician points out the anatomic parts, letting the patient examine herself with the aid of a hand mirror. This often allays anxiety in both partners and encourages communication about sexual matters.

ATYPICAL SEXUAL DISORDERS

Coital pain in the male is now a specific DSM-III-R sexual dysfunction, but sexual anhedonia

(see above) is not. It could be classified here. Other examples are the female analog of premature ejaculation and genital pain during masturbation.

Other sexual disorders include persistent and marked distress about one's sexual orientation; distress over nonparaphiliac sexual addiction, eg, distress over or frequent compulsion to visit prostitutes, massage parlors or peep shows, or a compulsion to engage in casual sex with a succession of people ("sex objects"); and distress over feelings of inadequacy over the size or shape of penis, breasts, or other aspects of masculinity or femininity.

56. THE NEUROSES

Functional mental disorders in which specific, usually ego-dystonic, symptoms occur; ie, anxieties, phobias, obsessions, compulsions, hysterical conversion and dissociative phenomena, and certain symptoms relating to posttraumatic stress; reality testing is generally intact.

The neuroses comprise one of the 3 major categories of nonorganic psychiatric disorders, which also include the psychoses and personality (or character) disorders. Neurotic illness is not usually characterized by the major alterations in mental function and severe disturbances in cognitive and perceptual processes (eg, delusions, hallucinations) seen in the **psychoses;** also, the capacity to distinguish between fantasy and reality (reality testing) remains generally intact in neurotic illness, in contrast to its partial or complete absence in the psychoses. The significant aberrations in behavior patterns and personal relationships seen in the **personality disorders** also may occur in neurotic individuals (see Ch. 52).

Classification

In 1980, the American Psychiatric Association published the 3rd edition of its *Diagnostic and Statistical Manual of Mental Disorders (DSM-III)*, which revised the diagnostic classification of many of the mental illnesses. DSM-III omitted the diagnostic class of Neuroses, placing anxiety neurosis, phobic neurosis, and obsessive-compulsive neurosis under the general heading of Anxiety Disorders (see TABLE 56–1); and splitting hysterical neurosis between the DSM-III categories of Somatoform Disorder (which includes conversion hysteria, hypochondriasis, and somatization disorder) and Dissociative Disorder,

which comprises dissociative hysteria (including psychogenic amnesia or fugue, and multiple personality) and depersonalization neurosis. The recently published **DSM-III-R** (1987), a revision of DSM-III, generally follows the same classificatory scheme, differing from DSM-III in only minor details. The classification used here (which gives equal weight to the various neuroses) generally follows that set forth in the *International Classification of Diseases*, 9th Edition, Clinical Modification **(ICD-9-CM)**.

ANXIETY NEUROSIS
(Generalized Anxiety Disorder;
Anxiety Reaction)

A neurotic disorder characterized by chronic, unrealistic anxiety often punctuated by acute attacks of anxiety or panic. It afflicts 5% of the population, is characteristically a disorder of young adults, and affects women twice as often as men.

Etiology

Both psychologic and physiologic factors cause anxiety neurosis, and evidence of a genetic influence exists.

Psychologic factors: Emotional stress often precipitates anxiety (eg, threatened or actual changes in personal relationships). The precipitant is less obvious when inner emotional drives (sexual, aggressive, or dependency needs) cause conflict, because psychologic defenses keep them from the individual's conscious awareness. The drives are aroused by environmental events to which the person is especially sensitized, and anxi-

TABLE 56-1. ANXIETY DISORDERS

Disorder	Subcategories

Phobic disorders (phobic neuroses)	Agoraphobia
	  With panic attacks
	  Without panic attacks
	Social phobia
	Simple phobia

Anxiety states (anxiety neuroses)	Panic disorder Generalized anxiety disorder Obsessive-compulsive disorder (obsessive-compulsive neurosis)
Posttraumatic stress disorder	Acute Chronic or delayed
Atypical anxiety disorder	

ety represents the individual's fear of losing control of these drives and of his resulting actions.

Physiologically, the symptoms of anxiety (see below) are the direct manifestation of peripheral autonomic nervous system discharge often set in motion by the arousal of frightening fantasies, impulses, and emotions. In the CNS, noradrenergic neurotransmitters play a prominent role in the production of anxiety, and recent studies point to the locus ceruleus, with its widespread connecting neural pathways to the rest of the brain, as an important mediating center.

Symptoms and Signs

Anxiety is a symptom in all psychiatric disorders, but it occurs alone or as the primary symptom in anxiety neurosis. **Acute anxiety attacks (panic disorder)** form the cardinal feature of anxiety neurosis and are among the most painful life experiences. They may occur repetitively over a period of time and are self-limited, generally lasting a few minutes to an hour or 2. The patient experiences a subjective sense of terror that arises for no evident reason and a haunting dread of some nameless, imminent catastrophe, temporarily preventing rational thinking. Of the somatic symptoms integral to anxiety, the most common are cardiorespiratory, with tachycardia, palpitations, occasional premature beats, and precordial pain usually described as sharp or sticking in quality. Trembling, visible as a fine tremor of the outstretched hands, sweating, complaints of "butterflies in the stomach," and generalized motor weakness and dizziness are common; nausea and occasionally diarrhea occur. The patient may notice a feeling of unreality and loss of contact with people and objects in his environment. A sense of air hunger leading to hyperventilation often is experienced. This can re-

sult in a secondary respiratory alkalosis, varying degrees of muscular stiffness in the extremities, and a feeling of pins and needles or numbness around the mouth and in the fingers and toes—**hyperventilation syndrome.** These secondary symptoms compound the patient's anxiety and add to his frequent conviction that he is about to lose consciousness or die.

Chronic anxiety (generalized anxiety disorder): Symptoms are similar to those of acute anxiety attacks but are less intense and of longer duration, lasting days, weeks, or months. The patient is aware of a generalized tension and apprehension, a tendency to startle easily, an uneasiness and nervousness at work or with people, a vague, nagging uncertainty about the future that may be accompanied by chronic fatigue, headaches, insomnia, and a variety of subacute autonomic symptoms. Although the syndrome is not completely disabling, the patient is chronically uncomfortable in his daily activities and personal relationships and often finds his capacity for effective work compromised by chronic fatigue and difficulties in concentration.

Diagnosis

Because of the cardiac manifestations, anxiety attacks may be mistaken for myocardial infarction. Similarly, the autonomic symptoms secondary to a pheochromocytoma and the hyperarousal resulting from Graves' disease may imitate the clinical picture of anxiety neurosis. Appropriate physical and laboratory examinations usually establish the proper diagnosis.

Course and Prognosis

Mild anxiety tends to be chronic, punctuated by acute anxiety attacks of varying frequency and intensity. Roughly ⅓ of patients recover, with men having a better prognosis than women. Anxiety symptoms often become less severe and troublesome with middle age.

Treatment

Psychologic measures: Insight psychotherapy (in patients properly selected by the criterion of psychologic-mindedness), aimed at uncovering the unconscious conflicts, may bring about psychologic changes that lead to increased self-knowledge and tolerance of internal drives. **Supportive psychotherapy** may reduce symptoms through reassurance and the relationship with an understanding, sympathetic physician. **Relaxation techniques** permit some voluntary control over autonomic functions that diminish hyperactivity. **Meditation** is a specific and often effective form of relaxation. In persons with a capacity for entering hypnotic trance, **hypnosis** can potentiate the effects of the relaxation techniques.

Pharmacologic measures (see also Ch. 62): Medications that lower responsiveness to stress are helpful. As a rule, the symptoms of generalized chronic anxiety are responsive to benzodiazepines, whereas panic attacks respond to the tricyclic antidepressants and monoamine oxidase **(MAO)** inhibitors. As an exception to this differential response, the benzodiazepines alprazolam and clonazepam are effective in controlling panic attacks. However, the withdrawal of the latter 2 medications after long-term use can be difficult in many patients, dictating caution in their clinical use.

Medications (eg, benzodiazepines) generally should be used along with, not as a substitute for, appropriate psychotherapy, and care must be taken to avoid high dosage and prolonged use that may result in physiologic dependence.

PHOBIC NEUROSIS
(Phobic Disorders; Phobic Reactions)

A neurotic disorder characterized by the presence of irrational or exaggerated fear of objects, situations, or bodily functions not inherently dangerous or the appropriate source of the anxiety. Anxiety, both acute and chronic, is a prominent feature, but unlike the free-floating anxiety of anxiety neurosis, it is bound to and associated with exposure to specific environmental stimuli. Phobic disorders affect less than 1% of the population, account for about 5% of neuroses found in

patients > 18 yr, and occur more frequently in women.

Etiology

In many respects etiology is similar to that of neurotic anxiety in general; ie, phobias appear to be associated with an increased family history of anxiety disorders, and the anxiety itself is often a fearful reaction to the threatened emergence of forbidden, unconscious drives, a reaction that is expressed in excessive activity of the autonomic nervous system. However, further psychologic mechanisms **(projection, displacement)** focus the anxiety on specific external objects or situations, which then come to represent the underlying, original source of the anxiety. The shifting and binding of the anxiety to the external secondary symbol enable the individual to use the further defensive maneuver of **avoidance** of the object in order to control arousal of the painful anxiety. Choice of the phobic symbol is often determined by a chance exposure to the object at a time when the anxiety over a threatening inner impulse first appeared. In other words, the phobic object becomes a conditioned stimulus, and the phobic neurosis is, in effect, a learned response.

Symptoms and Signs

The very thought of the phobic object is sufficient to induce anxiety, and as the patient comes closer in reality to the phobic stimulus, the anxiety mounts to an intensity reaching panic. As a result, the patient protects himself from experiencing the anxiety by avoiding the phobic stimulus, which often leads to a disabling constriction in his daily life and capacity for normal functioning. In some phobic individuals, **counterphobic behavior** develops (*the active seeking out of exposure to phobic, often dangerous situations;* eg, the individual with a fear of heights who becomes an alpine rock climber).

Agoraphobia (*a fear of open, public places or of crowds*) is the most common (60%) of the phobic disorders. The individual's activities are severely restricted; in the extreme he cannot leave the security of his home. Agoraphobia often begins with the sudden onset of a panic attack in some public place; subsequently, anticipatory anxiety that the attack will recur causes the individual to avoid the site of the initial attack and to restrict himself to his home and its immediate environs in order to prevent a reemergence of the painful affect. Frequently, the agoraphobic patient can face the phobic situation without undue discomfort if in the company of someone with whom he has a close relationship—the so-called **obligatory companion**.

Phobias of objects (simple phobias) are *irrational fears of objects or situations other than those felt in agoraphobia or social phobias.* Simple phobias are commonly seen as transitory phenomena during early childhood (eg, fear of the darkness or of animals). Adults also may develop specific, localized neurotic fears (eg, dogs; insects; closed spaces—**claustrophobia**; or heights—**acrophobia**). If the objects or situations are uncommon or easily avoided, no serious disability results. However, great inconvenience may occur; eg, in a businessman with a phobia of flying whose work requires frequent air travel.

Phobias of function (social phobias), in which *anxiety is aroused by the presence of others and by the irrational fear of embarrassing or humiliating oneself in public,* are less common than the other types. The most frequent manifestations that cause the victim to shun social situations are a fear of blushing **(erythrophobia)** and a fear of eating in public.

Diagnosis

The sudden outbreak of severe phobias may herald the onset of a schizophrenic psychosis or occasionally may be seen in patients with a chronic schizophrenic disorder. The course of the latter illness and the presence of thought disorder and other psychotic features (hallucinations, delusions) suggest a psychosis (see Ch. 58). Phobic patients sometimes become depressed because of their failure to overcome their phobic avoidance, but this is secondary to the neurosis itself and disappears when it is resolved.

Course and Prognosis

Phobic disorders usually begin in early adulthood and have chronic courses of exacerbations and remissions. Agoraphobia is not only severely disabling but is the least likely of the phobic disorders to manifest significant remissions. Spontaneous remission of phobic neurosis is less likely in patients steadily symptomatic for over a year.

Treatment

Psychotherapy: Insight psychotherapy may be effective. However, despite significant changes in the patient's psychologic functioning and structure, the phobic symptoms may persist and require more active techniques focused specifically on bringing about their removal; eg, **behavior therapy**. These techniques decondition (desensitize) the patient to the phobic stimulus by requiring him to confront the stimulus while using relaxation techniques (including hypnosis) to combat the anxiety aroused by the stimulus (reciprocal inhibition). **Flooding** is an extreme behavioral desensitization based on the experimental observation that the fear aroused in animals confronted by a frightening conditioned stimulus tends to dissipate if the animal is not allowed to escape. Clinical flooding techniques require patients to imagine or actually confront the anxiety-provoking situation and to continue their exposure until the resulting intense anxiety abates. Because flooding is a highly painful procedure and, in clinical trials, generally produces no better therapeutic results than less intense forms of desensitization, it is not commonly used by behavior therapists.

Pharmacotherapy (see also Ch. 62): Minor tranquilizers (benzodiazepines, buspirone) are helpful in reducing the intensity of the anticipatory anxiety, enabling the patient to better face the phobic stimulus and work toward complete desensitization. Panic attacks may be effectively controlled by tricyclic antidepressants, MAO inhibitors, and the benzodiazepines alprazolam and clonazepam.

OBSESSIVE–COMPULSIVE NEUROSIS

(Obsessive-Compulsive Disorder; Obsessional Neurosis)

A disorder characterized by the presence of recurrent ideas and fantasies (obsessions) and repetitive impulses or actions (compulsions) that the patient recognizes as morbid and toward which he feels a strong inner resistance.

Anxiety is a central feature in the obsessive-compulsive neurosis, but in contrast to the phobias (where the patient is anxious in the face of external dangers of which he perceives himself to be the passive victim), the anxiety arises in response to internally derived thoughts and urges that the patient fears he may actively carry out despite his wishes not to. Recent epidemiologic studies suggest that the disorder is far more common than had previously been thought, reaching a lifetime prevalence rate of 1 to 2%.

Etiology

There is some evidence of a higher incidence in the families of obsessive-compulsive patients than in control populations.

Psychodynamic theory: The obsession is the ideational component of an underlying, forbidden impulse, most commonly aggressive in quality, that emerges into consciousness. Through the defense mechanism of **isolation**, the affective component of the drive is separated from the ideational content, so that the individual experiences only an insistent thought, unaccompanied by any awareness of a wish to realize the idea or that it stems from a hidden impulse. Despite the defense of isolation, the idea is too close to the forbidden drive. Therefore, the idea becomes the source of anxiety and motivates the further defensive maneuver of **undoing**, in the form of a secondary magical compulsive act.

Learning theory: An originally neutral thought becomes capable of arousing anxiety through its association with an unconditioned anxiety-provoking stimulus. When a subsequent action reduces that anxiety, the act becomes fixed as a compulsive ritual and a stable, but nonadaptive, learned psychologic structure is created.

Biologic factors: Recent research suggests that disturbances in the function of the basal ganglia, especially in their serotonin receptors, may be an important element in the appearance of obsessive-compulsive symptoms.

Symptoms and Signs

Obsessions: Ideas, words, and images, usually disconnected and unrelated to what the individual is doing, force themselves on his attention with a power and insistence that he cannot resist. They are often colored by an aggressive, sexual, or scatologic quality that the individual perceives as totally alien to himself as a person. The patient frequently is convinced that he has done something harmful or antisocial and feels considerable concern and anxiety. Despite this, he recognizes that the ideas are untrue and nonsensical, but at the same time spends considerable energy trying to resist them and banish them from his consciousness. His efforts may be momentarily successful; but inevitably the ideas return moments later, and the struggle is renewed.

Compulsions and compulsive acts: A compulsion has the same autonomous characteristics as an obsession, but rather than being merely an idea or image, it is an overwhelming urge to do something aggressive, disgraceful, or obscene. As with the obsessions, the patient experiences anxiety, recognizes the absurdity of the impulse, and resists putting it into action. Not infrequently, however, he does act on the compulsive urge and indulges in a repetitive behavioral pattern in the form of compulsive acts or rituals. These are often secondary to a primary obsessional idea and serve the function of combating or neutralizing its harmful qualities. A young man, for example, had the insistent thought every time he turned off an electric light: "My father will die" (obsession). To quell the anxiety associated with that thought, he would feel compelled to touch the light switch again and say to himself, "I take back that thought" (compulsion). The quality of **magical thinking** characterizes both obsessions and compulsions. Neither has anything to do with the real, physical world of cause and effect—a fact of which the patient is aware.

Diagnosis

The often bizarre quality of obsessive-compulsive ideas and rituals may at times resemble the similar bizarreness of schizophrenic thinking, but in the obsessional patient reality testing is intact.

Course and Prognosis

Onset of symptoms may occur in childhood, and in $1/3$ to $1/2$ of adult cases the disorder begins before the age of 15. It tends to run a chronic, remitting course, with symptomatic periods generally lasting < 1 yr before a remission brings relief. With treatment, about 25% of patients improve markedly; the rest are partially improved or unchanged. Prognosis is better for those patients who begin treatment early.

Treatment

Properly selected patients may respond to **insight psychotherapy** with disappearance of symptoms, but in many patients the symptoms are stubbornly resistant. **Supportive therapy,** with an emphasis on reassurance and encouragement to activity, may provide sufficient relief to enable patients to perform daily activities fairly comfortably. **Behavioral techniques,** especially those aimed at **flooding** (see under PHOBIC NEUROSIS, above) the patient with anxiety by forcibly preventing him from carrying out compulsive rituals, have been reported to be successful but are still experimental.

Pharmacotherapy (see also Ch. 62): The literature contains reports of relief from obsessions and compulsive rituals following the administration of tricyclic antidepressants and MAO inhibitors. Although the final appraisal of the general usefulness of these drugs must await controlled clinical studies, the initial findings are sufficiently promising to warrant a trial of such medication in obsessive-compulsive patients who are unresponsive to other forms of treatment. When depression is significantly present, its successful treatment with antidepressant medication may also be accompanied by the disappearance of the obsessive-compulsive symptoms. More recently, antidepressant drugs that block serotonin re-uptake by synapses have been reported to be especially effective in relieving obsessive-compulsive symptoms, even in the absence of overt depression. These drugs include clomipramine (the most extensively studied in this disorder), fluoxetine, and fluvoxamine.

POSTTRAUMATIC STRESS DISORDER

A neurotic disorder produced by exposure to an overwhelming environmental stress and characterized by recurrent episodes of reexperiencing the traumatic event, numbing of emotional responsiveness, and a dysphoric general hyperarousal. The pathogenic effects of exposure to emotionally traumatic stress have long been recognized, but the severity and prevalence of such reactions in some Vietnam war veterans have forced these reactions into prominence and have led to this DSM-III-R diagnostic category. The occurrence of the disorder is not accurately known, although figures as high as 80% have been reported in the survivors of some major civilian disasters.

Etiology

The etiologic sine qua non of the disorder is exposure to an overwhelming environmental stress. Since not every individual responds to such stress with a posttraumatic stress syndrome, a variety of factors in clinical combination are required to produce the pathologic state. These include (1) the suddenness and unexpectedness of the stress, as in major fires, explosions, and airplane crashes, or in natural disasters like floods, earthquakes, and tornadoes; (2) the bloody brutality and horror of events associated with active armed combat or terrorist attacks; (3) the more prolonged and chronic stress of exposure to inhumane treatment such as occurs in POW and concentration camps, with the frequently associated torture and atrocities; (4) the

psychologic and constitutional strengths and weaknesses of the victim; (5) concurrent bodily injury (especially of the head) suffered by the victim; and (6) the nature and availability of social supports.

Symptoms and Signs

A central feature is the reexperiencing of the trauma. This may occur in the form of intrusive, uncontrollable waking recollections or nightmares that reproduce the stressful events, or of dissociated states of consciousness in which the patient appears vividly to relive the traumatic experience as if it were actually taking place. These more discrete episodes occur against a background of chronic anxiety, hyperalertness, and insomnia, often accompanied by difficulty in concentrating or impairment of memory. Some individuals develop phobic reactions to situations that recall memories of the events, and forced exposure to such situations may cause an exacerbation of acute symptoms and precipitate a dissociative, fugue-like reproduction of the experience itself. Not infrequently patients are emotionally labile, irritable, restless, and tremulous, and on occasion may manifest explosive outbursts of violent behavior. Many patients resort to alcohol or other drug abuse in an apparent attempt to diminish their painful inner state of hyperarousal. Most patients, furthermore, complain of a numbing of their responsiveness to people, objects, and events in the world around them. They lose interest in their usual pursuits, feel emotionally dead and unreal, and experience detachment and estrangement from others.

Diagnosis

Posttraumatic stress disorder is to be differentiated from depressive, anxiety, and phobic disorders. Although the posttraumatic syndrome may include anxious, depressive, and phobic symptoms, these do not dominate the clinical picture and are clearly secondary to the trauma. A careful neurologic examination should be part of the evaluation of every patient with suspected posttraumatic stress disorder in order to rule out the presence of brain lesions underlying the changes in memory and the difficulty in concentration.

Course and Prognosis

Many patients experience the outbreak of symptoms a few days to a few weeks after the trauma, but onset also may be delayed for many months. The rapidly appearing acute form is often self-limited, the symptoms disappearing spontaneously within 6 mo. In others the disorder runs a chronic course, lasting months or years and frequently causing significant disability. In patients with a delayed onset or chronic symptoms the prognosis is generally poor, and recovery may be compromised by the secondary gain associated with receiving compensation for their trauma.

Treatment

Treatment is aimed largely at relieving the prominent hyperarousal and anxiety symptoms. Behavioral desensitization and relaxation techniques are particularly helpful, and where dissociative mechanisms underlie symptom formation, psychotherapy aimed at producing catharsis, abreaction, and insight may be useful. Antianxiety and antidepressant medications may be used adjunctively when necessary, but it should be remembered that this group of patients is particularly prone to develop drug dependency, so that prolonged pharmacotherapy generally is contraindicated.

HYSTERICAL NEUROSIS
(Conversion Reaction; Conversion Disorder; Dissociative Reaction; Dissociative Disorder)

A neurotic disorder characterized by a wide variety of somatic and mental symptoms resulting from dissociation, typically beginning during adolescence or early adulthood and occurring more commonly in women than men. Since the concept of hysteria as a disease is over 2000 yr old, its limits as a disorder have become blurred by a variety of definitions. Discussion is restricted to those phenomena classified as **conversion and dissociative disorders of consciousness,** which have a common basis in the mental phenomenon of dissociation.

Etiology

The concept of **dissociation,** *a process whereby specific internal mental contents (memories, ideas, feelings, perceptions) are lost to conscious awareness and become unavailable to voluntary recall,* is central to an understanding of the genesis of hysterical symptoms. Though unconscious, these mental contents can be recovered under special circumstances (eg, in dreams or a hypnotic trance). Furthermore, they are able to affect the individual's awareness and behavior

in a variety of ways. For example, the dissociation and loss from consciousness of memories of motor patterns lead to paralysis; the emergence of a fragment of a dissociated visual memory may produce an ego-alien visual hallucination; the emergence of a complex of mental associations forming a dissociated personality may effect a complete change in the individual's behavior. All phenomena of conversion and dissociative hysteria may be viewed as the effects of either the dissociation itself or the eruption into consciousness of portions of the dissociated mental contents of varying degrees of complexity. Proneness to dissociation may in part be genetic.

Two special aspects of dissociation should be noted: (1) It is closely correlated with hypnotizability, and individuals prone to spontaneous dissociation usually rate high on hypnotizability scales. (2) It may serve as a psychologic defense; ie, it provides a mechanism for banishing unpleasant, painful, and anxiety-provoking mental contents from consciousness. Recent clinical studies point to the particularly frequent presence of memories of major aggressive and sexual child abuse in patients with multiple personality disorders.

Symptoms and Signs

Conversion symptoms: Almost any organ disease symptom can be simulated on an hysterical basis; eg, symptoms mimicking the illness of a deceased relative. A variety of **sensorimotor symptoms** have been considered to be specific to and characteristic of hysterical neurosis. (Conversion symptoms are also commonly seen in nonpsychiatric practice in patients who do *not* have classic hysterical neurosis; see under PSYCHOSOMATIC MEDICINE in Ch. 51.) Weakness and paralysis of muscular groups are common; spasms and abnormal movements, less frequent. The motor disturbances are usually accompanied by altered sensibility, especially those involving touch, pain, temperature, and position sense. Especially characteristic are the "glove and stocking" distribution of the motor and sensory disturbances when these affect the limbs; ie, the distribution is determined by the body-image concept of a functional arm and leg rather than the dermatome innervation of the area affected. Another common distribution is complete hemianesthesia, which extends exactly to the midline of the body fore and aft. Less frequently, special senses and functions may be affected, such as in hysterical blindness, deafness, and aphonia;

both visual and auditory hallucinations may occur.

Dissociative phenomena: A variety of altered states of consciousness may result from the dissociative process. In **somnambulism**, the patient appears to be out of contact with his environment, is seemingly unresponsive to external stimuli, and in many cases appears to be living out a vivid, hallucinated drama, often the memory of some past emotionally traumatic event. In **amnesia**, the most common form of dissociative hysteria, the patient typically has a complete loss of memory for all past events covering a period of several hours to several weeks. **Anterograde amnesia** may occur, wherein the amnesia covers the memory of events as they are experienced, the patient forgetting continuously from moment to moment what he has just been thinking, feeling, and doing.

Far less common but more dramatic and eye-catching are the conditions of fugue states and multiple personalities. Central to both is a loss of personal identity. Typically, in a **fugue state** the individual suddenly loses all recollection of his past life and any awareness of who he is. He disappears from his usual haunts, leaving family and job, and traveling far from home, begins new work with a new identity, quite unaware of any change in his existence or life. Suddenly after a matter of days to weeks, he "comes to." Totally amnesic for the period of the fugue, he recaptures his former identity and, greatly distressed, wonders how he came to be in such strange surroundings. In the **multiple personality** a similar sudden change of identity occurs without, however, any wandering from home and with a frequent, unpredictable alternation between personalities. Two or more of such personalities may exist. The primary personality, often afflicted with disabling neurotic symptoms, has no awareness of the other secondary personalities. The latter, on the contrary, are fully aware of the thoughts and activities of the primary personality; ie, the amnesia is unidirectional.

Diagnosis

The sensorimotor symptoms of hysteria are distinguished from neurologic disease by the absence of pathologic neurologic signs, by recognition of precipitating psychosocial stress and conflict, and by the specific characteristics of the distribution of hysterical motor and sensory disturbances. Dissociative disorders of consciousness are differentiated from those caused by gross brain disease by the absence of positive

indications of the latter (eg, EEG changes, abnormal CT scan, pathognomonic changes in tests of cognitive functions). When the hysterical symptoms imitate those of medical diseases, the diagnosis is often more difficult. It is best established by the absence of findings pointing to disorders in organ functions and by the positive stigmas of hysteria, such as high hypnotizability, a previous history of clear-cut conversion or dissociative symptoms, and evidence that the symptoms represent a symbolic expression and resolution of psychologic conflicts.

Course and Prognosis

The paucity of studies on the natural history of hysteria precludes definite statements about its course and prognosis. Clinical experience suggests that it is a chronic illness. While patients may recover from specific symptoms, these are frequently replaced by others, especially during periods of emotional tension and stress, as a result of the propensity for dissociation.

Treatment

Psychoanalytic treatment, once thought to be specific for hysterical symptoms, is effective in a small number of hysterical patients who are capable of using the insights gained by psychoanalytic exploration. For others, family therapy, environmental manipulation (eg, job changes, homemaking assistance), reassurance, and a supportive physician relationship may be helpful. Hypnosis can remove specific symptoms, but a substitute symptom often arises. However, in patients with amnesia, hypnosis can be an effective tool to bring repressed ideas and feelings into consciousness, enabling the patient to face and resolve them more directly as the first step in the therapeutic process. Similarly, hypnosis can be helpful in raising the amnesia associated with fugue states and in eradicating the amnesic barriers between the various personalities of multiple personality disorders. Continued psychotherapeutic work is necessary to help the patient come to a more healthy and adaptive resolution of his problem.

SOMATIZATION DISORDER
(Briquet's Syndrome)

A neurotic illness characterized by the presence of multiple somatic symptoms, including those seen in classic conversion hysteria. Patients usually consult a physician other than a psychiatrist. Previously considered a form of hysteria and viewed by many as an hysterical personality disorder (see discussion of narcissistic personalities in Ch. 52), somatization disorder has been allocated a diagnosis of its own as a neurosis in DSM-III-R on the basis of phenomenologic clinical research. The disorder begins in adolescence or early adulthood, occurs predominantly in women (1 to 2% of the female population), and tends to be associated with sociopathy and alcoholism in male relatives.

Etiology

Etiology is not known, although the disorder often runs in families, and it is clear that the narcissistic personality structure of these patients (ie, their marked dependency needs and exaggerated rage when frustrated) is involved in their somatic complaints. The symptoms are a somatized message expressing a desperate plea for help and attention, and their intensity and persistence reflect the extreme degree of the wish to be cared for in every aspect of the patient's life.

Symptoms and Signs

Central to the disorder is the presence of multiple, vague somatic complaints that may be referable to any part of the body but most commonly take the form of headaches, nausea and vomiting, abdominal pain, bowel difficulties, dysmenorrhea, fatigue, syncope, dyspareunia, and sexual frigidity. Anxiety and depression are common accompaniments. The somatization appears to be part of a personality disorder, which has other characteristics. In their relationships with the physician and others, patients are seen to be dramatic and emotional in presenting their complaints, and they may be openly seductive and exhibitionistic. As the relationship develops, a marked, insatiable dependency emerges. Patients increasingly demand help and emotional support, may exhibit outbursts of rage when they feel that their needs are not gratified, and often attempt to manipulate others by threatening or attempting suicide. Often dissatisfied with their care, they go from physician to physician.

Diagnosis

Differentiation from hypochondriacal neurosis is discussed under that subchapter, below. Somatization disorder is distinguished from anxiety neurosis, hysterical neurosis, and depression by the predominance, multiplicity, and persistence of somatic complaints; the absence of the biologic signs and symptoms characterizing endogenous depression; and the gestural, manipulative nature of the suicidal behavior. The most difficult challenge lies in assessing the presence or absence of physical disease. Because such patients may develop concurrent physical illnesses, appropriate physical and laboratory examinations should be carried out during the initial clinical evaluation or whenever a significant shift occurs in the symptomatic picture.

Course and Prognosis

The disorder tends to run a fluctuating but chronic course. Complete relief of symptoms is rare, and unnecessary examinations and medical and surgical procedures may add to the patient's complaints or dysfunction. In some patients, depression becomes more prominent after many years, the frequent references and gestures relating to suicide become more ominous, and suicide may be carried out.

Treatment

Treatment usually is extraordinarily difficult, requiring tact and patience. The physician must walk a narrow clinical line between avoiding unnecessary diagnostic procedures and being alert to the possibility of developing physical disease. Medications do not help significantly, and attempts to provide insight with specific psychotherapeutic techniques usually fail. The patient needs a calm, firm, supporting relationship with a physician who provides reassurance and sets effective, appropriate limits to the patient's histrionically exaggerated behavior and demands.

HYPOCHONDRIACAL NEUROSIS
(Hypochondriasis; Atypical Somatoform Disorder)

A disorder characterized by a preoccupation with bodily functions and a morbid fear that one is suffering from serious disease. The peak incidence of onset is in the 30s in men, the 40s in women.

Etiology

Etiology is unknown, but some clinical evidence suggests that hypochondriasis, like somatization disorder, is related to a narcissistic character organization marked by excessive concern with self and with the gratification of dependency needs.

Symptoms and Signs

The hypochondriacal patient complains of symptoms in a wide variety of body parts, most commonly the abdominal viscera, chest, head, and neck. The specific symptom may be based on a heightened awareness of bodily sensation (heartbeat, peristaltic action) or minor disorders of function such as mild, localized pain or discomfort. The complaints often are described in minute, specific detail with respect to location, quality, and duration, but they follow no pattern recognizable as organic dysfunction and are usually not associated with abnormal physical findings. Although the symptoms described by the patient may be odd or bizarre, in *hypochondriasis*, as contrasted with hypochondriacal symptoms seen in psychotic disorders, they are not delusional in quality, and the patient exhibits no other signs of psychosis.

Diagnosis

Although hypochondriasis shares with somatization disorder a central complaint of somatic symptoms, the disorders differ in that hypochon-

driacal neurosis begins at a later age and the somatic complaints of the hypochondriac are richly detailed and sharply localized. Hypochondriacal symptoms are frequently associated with endogenous depressions, are then usually delusional in quality, and disappear when the affective disorder is relieved.

Course, Prognosis, and Treatment

The course is chronic—fluctuating in some, steady in others. Only a very small proportion of patients (perhaps 5%) recover permanently. The presence of hypochondriacal complaints in association with depression presages a poor prognosis for recovery from the basic affective illness.

Hypochondriasis is notoriously resistant to all forms of treatment, and all such measures are only palliative. Patients may gain some relief from a sympathetic, supportive relationship with a physician, and it is often helpful to work with the patient's family, giving them an awareness of the nature and course of the disorder so that they can provide a supportive home environment.

57. MOOD DISORDERS
(Affective Disorders)

Psychopathologic conditions in which a pervasive disturbance of mood constitutes the core manifestation. The term **affective disorder**, which in its broader usage also subsumes anxiety and related neuroses, is being replaced by the internationally preferred and more delimited concept of **mood disorder**. These conditions, especially the depressive forms, are heterogeneous and common in both psychiatry and general medicine.

Terminology and Classification

Moods are sustained emotions; **affects**, more short-lived expressions. Depression and elation tend to dominate the clinical picture in mood disorders; anxiety and anger are less constant manifestations.

Sadness and **joy** are part of the fabric of everyday life and should be differentiated from morbid depression and mania. Sadness, or normal depression, is a universal human response to defeat, disappointment, or other adverse situations; the response may be adaptive by permitting withdrawal to conserve inner resources. Transient depressive periods also occur as reactions to certain holidays or significant anniversa-

ries, as well as during the premenstrual phase and the first week postpartum. Such **holiday blues, anniversary reactions, premenstrual blues,** and **maternity blues** are not in themselves psychopathologic, but those predisposed to mood disorder may break down during such times.

Grief (normal bereavement), the prototype of **reactive depression,** also manifests with anxiety symptoms such as initial insomnia, restlessness, and autonomic nervous system hyperactivity. These reactions occur in response to significant separations and losses; eg, death, marital separation, romantic disappointment, leaving familiar environments, forced emigration, or civilian catastrophes. Like other adversities, bereavement and loss do not generally cause clinical depression, except in those persons predisposed to mood disorder.

Elation is popularly linked to success and achievement. However, paradoxical depressions also may follow such positive events, possibly because of the associated increased responsibilities that often have to be faced alone. Elation is sometimes conceptualized psychodynamically as a defense against depression or as a denial of the pain of loss; eg, the rare form of bereavement reaction in which elated hyperactivity may completely replace the expected grief. The concept of "flight into health" is invoked to explain the brief lucid and energetic periods encountered in dying patients or in those who need to take superhuman action in the face of unusual life duress. Again, in predisposed individuals, such reactions might be the prelude to clinical mania.

Morbid or clinical depression and mania are diagnosed when sadness or elation is overly intense and continues beyond the expected impact of a stressful life event; indeed, the morbid mood often arises without apparent or significant life stress. Furthermore, in different subtypes of mood disorder, symptoms and signs cluster into discrete syndromes that typically recur on an episodic basis or pursue a course of low-grade intermittent chronicity. Impaired functioning, arising from either the sustained severity of episodes or the continued chronicity of illness, is another characteristic that sets mood disorders apart from normal emotional reactions.

It is clinically useful to distinguish between **bipolar** (having depressive and elated or excited periods) and **unipolar** (depressions only) mood disorders. Unipolar depressive episodes tend to last 6 to 9 mo, though chronicity of ≥ 2 yr occurs in 15 to 20%. Bipolar disorder has younger age of onset, shorter duration of episodes (3 to 6 mo), and shorter **cycles** (*time from onset of one episode to that of the next*)—hence higher episode frequency and higher rates of disruption in developmental and social functioning. These prognostic features are particularly accentuated in **rapid-cycling** forms of bipolar disorder (*increased frequency of mood cycles of shorter duration, usually defined as ≤ 4 episodes/yr*).

Bipolar mood disorder *commonly begins with depression and is characterized by at least one elated period sometime during the course of the illness.* In **bipolar I disorder,** full-blown manic and major depressive episodes alternate. In **bipolar II disorder,** depressive episodes alternate with hypomanias (ie, mild, nonpsychotic periods of excitement) of relatively short duration. Although insomnia and poor appetite do occur during the depressive phase of bipolar illness, such atypical depressive signs as hypersomnia and overeating are more characteristic and may recur on a seasonal basis (eg, in the autumn or winter). As for hypomanic periods, they could be adaptive for some individuals, being associated with "supernormal" social functioning and, ordi-

narily, not leading to clinical referral; thus, the "high" periods of bipolar II disorder could be quite subtle, requiring expert evaluation for proper clinical diagnosis. Such expert evaluation is even more imperative in **cyclothymic disorder,** in which both elevated and depressive periods occur on a lower plane of severity, last typically a few days, and pursue an intermittently irregular course. Although cyclothymia is commonly the precursor of bipolar I and II disorders, in many individuals it pursues a lifelong course without superimposed major episodes.

Unipolar mood disorder (major depressive disorder) occurs as *syndromal depression, typically with several episodes over a lifetime.* The term **melancholia** is reserved for *the most full-blown expression of major depressive disorder with such manifestations as marked psychomotor slowing or agitation, weight loss, pathologic guilt, middle or early morning insomnia, diurnal variation in mood and activity with a nadir in the morning, and loss of the capacity to experience pleasure.* Other depressives may manifest the **reverse vegetative or atypical features** characterized by anxious-phobic symptoms, evening worsening, initial insomnia, hypersomnia that often extends into daytime hours, and hyperphagia. Unipolar illness is characteristically episodic with relatively asymptomatic phases between episodes; however, residual chronicity occurs in 15 to 20% of cases, most commonly in those with single-episode depression beginning after age 50 yr. In another pattern of chronicity, **dysthymic disorder,** depressive symptoms typically begin insidiously in childhood or adolescence and pursue an intermittent or low-grade course over many years or decades; superimposed major depressive episodes commonly complicate this disorder, usually with return to the low-grade depressive baseline upon recovery. This pattern is termed **double depression.**

The distinctions described above are not hard and fast because 1 of 5 patients with depressive illness, including those with dysthymia, eventually develops hypomania or mania. Almost all switches from unipolar to bipolar occur within a decade from the onset of clinically identifiable depressive manifestations. Predictors of bipolarity include early onset (ie, < 25 yr of age), intermittent or high episode-frequency illness, hypomania upon antidepressant administration, bipolar family history, and 3-generation consecutive affective pedigree. Recurrent unipolar depressions with bipolar family history (a condition known as **bipolar III**) are, in all likelihood, pseudounipolar (ie, genotypically bipolar), but they appear phenotypically unipolar because they have not yet expressed unequivocal periods of excitement. Subtle hypomanic tendencies can be seen in such a depressive individual's personality, which is driven, ambitious, and achievement-oriented.

Epidemiology

Although about 25% of all individuals experience some form of affective disturbance, the lifetime risk for clinically identifiable mood disorder is 8 to 9%. One third develop a chronic course and, of the remaining 5 to 6%, at least $2/3$ experience recurrent episodes. This means that for most sufferers, the illness will recur or pursue a protracted course. The rates are higher in women in a 2:1 ratio for the predominantly depressive forms of illness, and nearly even in bipolar disorder. Bipolar conditions, for which 1% of the population is at risk, usually begin in the teens, 20s, and 30s; unipolar conditions begin, on average, a decade later than their bipolar counterparts. Recent epidemiologic findings in the USA suggest a **cohort effect,** whereby those born in the latter part of this century have higher rates of depression and suicide, often associated with higher rates of substance abuse. Although some of this increase is probably due to easier ascertainment of depression in younger individuals, the comorbid substance abuse and poorly understood environmental factors may have contributed to the younger age shift.

Depression is among the most prevalent psychiatric conditions, varying from about 25% in public mental institutions to nearly 50% in outpatient and private psychiatric practice, and it may account for as much as 10% of all patients seen in nonpsychiatric medical settings.

Culture, social class, and race have not been shown to make significant differential contributions to the incidence of mood disorders. However, sociocultural factors seem to modify the clinical manifestations; eg, somatic complaints, worry, tension, and irritability are more common in the lower socioeconomic classes; guilty ruminations and self-reproach are more characteristic of depressions in Anglo-Saxon cultures; and in some Mediterranean and African countries, as well as in American blacks, mania tends to manifest itself more floridly.

Etiology and Pathogenesis

The syndromes of depression and mania, like many medical conditions (eg, congestive heart failure), represent the final common pathway of various processes.

Secondary affective states are chronologically superimposed on preexisting nonaffective disorders and are often understandable developments from them—somatically (see TABLE 57–1), psychologically, or via both mechanisms. Some, such as myxedema depression, are generally ascribed to physiochemical factors and thus are considered symptomatic depressions. Others, such as the chronic depressive states that accompany seriously debilitating cardiopulmonary diseases, are usually explained as depressive reactions to the limitations imposed by the underlying condition. More commonly both causes are operative; eg, in the depression of patients with AIDS, which could stem from cerebral factors as well as from the profound sense of demoralization imposed by a malignant mental disorder at the prime of life; or in the depressive psychosis of Cushing's disease, in which the changes in body image in a female afflicted with acne, hirsutism, obesity, striae, etc, are as relevant as the endocrine impact on the brain. Interestingly, excessive endogenous production of corticosteroids is often associated with depression, while exogenous administration of corticosteroids is more likely to lead to euphoria; corticosteroids are actually given to very sick individuals in whom some degree of "flight into health" is desirable.

Psychiatric conditions at high risk for depression include anxiety disorders, somatization hysteria, antisocial personality, alcoholism and other substance use disorders, schizophrenic disorders, and the early phase of cortical dementias. Bipolar disorder is rarely a complication of another psychiatric condition; if alcohol and substance abuse chronologically precede a bipolar disorder, they are most likely prodromal manifestations of mood swings that the patient has attempted to self-treat with available substances.

In mood states associated with nonaffective disorders, depression and mania are more likely to be partial syndromal expressions with frequent admixtures of anxiety, paranoia, delirium, or dementia. When a full-blown affective syndrome develops in the setting of a medical condition, etiologic factors important in the primary mood disorders are probably operative. For instance, the so-called reserpine depression is usually a pseudodepression that is partly attributable to the sedative side effects of the drug and is typically reversible upon discontinuation. Reserpine depressions refractory to such discon-

TABLE 57-1. COMMON CAUSES OF SYMPTOMATIC DEPRESSIONS AND ELATIONS

Type of Cause	Depressions	Elations
Pharmacologic	Steroidal contraceptives Reserpine; α-methyldopa; β blockers Anticholinesterase insecticides Amphetamine withdrawal Cimetidine; indomethacin Phenothiazine neuroleptics Thallium; mercury Cycloserine Vincristine; vinblastine	Corticosteroids Levodopa; bromocriptine Cocaine Amphetamines; methylphenidate Most heterocyclic antidepressants Monoamine oxidase inhibitors
Infectious	General paresis (tertiary syphilis) Influenza; viral pneumonia Viral hepatitis; infectious mononucleosis AIDS Tuberculosis	General paresis (tertiary syphilis) Influenza St. Louis encephalitis
Endocrinologic	Hypo- and hyperthyroidism Hyperparathyroidism Cushing's disease Addison's disease Hypopituitarism	Hyperthyroidism
Collagen-vascular	Systemic lupus erythematosis Rheumatoid arthritis	Systemic lupus erythematosis Rheumatic chorea
Neurologic	Multiple sclerosis Parkinson's disease Head trauma Complex partial seizures (temporal lobe) Cerebral tumors Stroke Sleep apnea	Multiple sclerosis Huntington's chorea Head trauma Complex partial seizures (temporal lobe) Diencephalic tumors Stroke
Nutritional	Pellagra Pernicious anemia	
Neoplastic	Cancer of the head of the pancreas Disseminated carcinomatosis	

tinuation are less frequent and are observed predominantly in predisposed individuals with family or personal history of mood disorder. This example highlights the arbitrary nature of the primary-secondary distinction and suggests a continuum of pathogenesis for all mood disorders. Although the removal of reversible medical or pharmacologic contributions does not always lead to the cure of the morbid mood state precipitated by them, their identification facilitates the planning of a joint medical-psychiatric approach to the patient.

Primary mood disorders arise in the absence of factors leading to secondary affective states. Thus, specific medical-pharmacologic factors are, by definition, absent. Exact patho-genetic mechanisms are unclear, but an interaction between several contributory causes is most likely.

Heredity is the most important predisposing factor, although sporadic (nonfamilial) forms are not uncommon, particularly in single-episode and less recurrent depressions where the evidence for genetic contributions is still controversial. There is greater convergence of evidence—based on adoption and twin data—for genetic factors in recurrent unipolar and bipolar disorders. The precise mode of inheritance is still uncertain, but single dominant genes (either X-linked or autosomal) have long been hypothesized and recently buttressed by molecular genetic approaches; alternatively, unipolar and bipolar disorders may lie on a hypothesized polygenic continuum of severity. The putative metabolic end results reflect some form of dysregulation in limbic-diencephalic neurotransmission, possibly at the level of receptors, but no direct evidence exists for specific neurotransmitter abnormalities in mood disorders. However, indirect neurophysiologic, pharmacologic, and endocrinologic evidence implicates midbrain abnormalities; eg, blunted growth hormone response to the α_2-agonist clonidine, shortened rapid eye movement **(REM)** latency and related circadian sleep disturbances, arecoline REM-induction, augmented melatonin suppression by light, blunted ACTH response to corticotropin-releasing hormone **(CRH)**, hypercortisolemia with disrupted diurnal rhythm and resistance to the dexamethasone suppression test **(DST)**, and blunted thyroid-stimulating hormone **(TSH)** response to synthetic thyrotropin (protirelin **[TRH]**). Cumulatively, these findings support the notion of dysregulation in cholinergic and catecholaminergic neurotransmission. Indirect evidence also is emerging for serotonergic dysregulation as measured by blunted growth hormone **(GH)** response to fenfluramine and by decreased serotonin uptake by platelets and decreased 5-hydroxyindoleacetic acid **(5-HIAA)** in the CSF of patients—whether clinically depressed or not—who engage in violent suicidal acts (see suicide under Complications, below).

Childhood loss of a parent does not place individuals at higher risk for a mood disorder, but such persons tend to have their depression at an earlier age, pursue an intermittently chronic course, exhibit greater personality disorder, and attempt suicide more often.

Stressors that provoke affective episodes can be psychologic or biologic. Thus, life events (especially separations) commonly precede depressive and manic episodes; however, such events may represent the prodromal manifestations of a mood disorder rather than its cause (eg, affectively ill persons often alienate their loved ones). The switch from depression to mania is often heralded by curtailed sleep over 1 to 3 days and can be experimentally induced by sleep or REM deprivation. Clinically, such switches are also commonly seen following therapy with antidepressants. Other biologic stressors possibly relevant to the onset of mania include stimulant abuse, sedative-hypnotic withdrawal, transmeridian travel beyond 2-h zones, and seasonal photoperiodic shifts.

Although any **personality type** can develop clinical depression, the personality attributes observed in the affectively ill more commonly represent temperamental inclinations toward dysthymia and cyclothymia. Thus, unipolar forms are more likely to arise from a background of introversion and anxious-neurotic tendencies. Such individuals are insecure, guilt- and anxiety-prone, and often lack the requisite social skills to adjust to significant departures from the routine imposed by life pressures, including the stress of being depressed; this means that such persons experience greater difficulty in recovering from a depressive episode. The personality structure in bipolar patients tends to be less "neurotic" but is subject to greater fluctuation in energy and mood, extroversion and achievement orientation; they more often use activity to combat depression, which may account for the shorter duration of bipolar depressions.

The higher vulnerability of women to depression is customarily traced to their presumed greater affiliative nature, passive-dependence, and helplessness in controlling their destiny in male-oriented societies. However, biologic vulnerabilities are at least as relevant: women have two X chromosomes (important in bipolar illness, if dominant X-linkage is involved); compared to men, have higher levels of monoamine oxidase (the enzyme that degrades the neurotransmitters considered important for mood) and whose gene has been recently located on the X chromosome; have more precarious thyroid function; may use depressant oral contraceptives; and undergo premenstrual and postpartum endocrine changes. Whatever the ultimate mechanisms for the differential gender rates of depression, recent data suggest that temperamental factors might mediate between gender and depression. Thus, clinically depressed women are more likely to conform to the introverted personality style observed among unipolars, whereas depressed men are significantly more likely to exhibit the extroverted tendencies observed among bipolars. This would in turn suggest that, once depressed, women would have greater difficulty recovering from their episodes.

Symptoms, Signs, and Diagnosis

Diagnosis is based on clinical grounds, symptomatic picture, course, family history, and sometimes on unequivocal response to somatic interventions. These approaches have been more recently buttressed by laboratory findings believed to tap limbic-diencephalic dysfunction, especially the TRH stimulation test, the dexamethasone suppression test (DST), and sleep EEG (REM latency).

The **TRH stimulation test** with either 500 μg or 200 μg, as some endocrinologists prefer, protirelin (synthetic TRH) given IV over 15 to 30 sec is a standard endocrine challenge test. A blunted TSH response (an increase of TSH < 5 μU/mL), which implicates hypothalamic disturbance, must be distinguished from an exaggerated TSH response (an increase of TSH > 20 μU/mL), indicating early failure at the level of the thyroid gland. Although the diagnostic usefulness of TSH blunting for primary mood disorder is still uncertain, an exaggerated TSH response might prove useful in identifying a biologic correlate of therapeutic nonresponse in certain mood disorder subtypes, eg, rapid-cycling bipolars. The interpretation of test findings is unreliable in the presence of other endocrine diseases, hepatic or renal failure, severe weight loss, cocaine abuse, alcohol intoxication or withdrawal, and use of estrogens, steroids, phenytoin, carbamazepine, and lithium.

The **DST protocol** in psychiatry is performed somewhat differently than in endocrinology. Dexamethasone 1 mg is given orally at 11 PM and serum cortisol is measured the next day at 4 PM and 11 PM; 50% of melancholics fail to suppress cortisol, giving rise to levels > 5 μg/dL (with competitive-protein binding) or > 4 mg/dL (with radioimmunoassay). False-positive results are obtained in pregnancy, high-dose estrogen use, Cushing's disease, severe weight loss, uncontrolled diabetes mellitus, during alcohol withdrawal, and with phenytoin, barbiturate, carbamazepine, and excessive caffeine intake. Finally, DST findings are less reliable in the outpatient setting; their specificity is higher in inpatient settings, with greater baseline prevalence of the melancholic subtype of major depression.

REM latency, *the time elapsed between onset of sleep and the first REM noted on sleep EEG,* has a mean duration of 90 min in normal persons (range 70 to 110 min, varying inversely with age). In a drug-free patient, when narcolepsy is excluded, shortening of this latency to less than the lower limit of the range for a given age group on consecutive nights is suggestive of primary mood disorder, especially in the presence of other sleep EEG findings such as concentration of REM in the first part of the night, increased REM density, curtailed delta sleep, and middle and terminal awakening.

Although there is no consensus on the sensitivities and specificities of these 3 tests, their judicious use can enhance conventional clinical wisdom in selected diagnostic, prognostic, and therapeutic decisions. The tests are not useful for screening and routine use, nor can they substitute for clinical examination and judgment. Because a negative test finding (eg, with the DST) does not exclude depressive illness, a positive result is potentially more significant clinically. For instance, DST nonsuppression can add weight to suggestive clinical findings for a mood disorder diagnosis and be used by the physician to convince a reluctant patient to accept somatic interventions. Furthermore, in a patient with known mood disorder, the failure of DST to normalize, despite apparent symptomatic improvement, strongly favors the need for continued biologic treatment of the depression.

Clinical depression: In the **depressive syndrome** (see TABLE 57–2), the mood typically is depressed, irritable, or anxious, or a combination thereof. However, in **masked depressions,** consciously experienced depression may be paradoxically absent. Instead, the patient complains of being somatically ill and may even wear a defensive mask of apparent cheerfulness (**smiling depression**). Other patients complain of various aches and pains, fears of calamity, and fears of becoming insane. Finally, in some the morbid mood is of such depth that tears dry up; the patient complains of an inability to experience usual emotions—including grief, joy, and pleasure—and a feeling that the world has become colorless, lifeless, and dead. In this type of depression, a return of the ability to cry usually is a sign of improvement.

The morbid mood in depressive illness is accompanied by related psychologic manifestations such as preoccupation with guilt, self-denigrating ideas, decreased ability to concentrate, indecisiveness, diminished interest in usual activities, social withdrawal, helplessness and hopelessness, and recurrent thoughts of death and suicide.

Marked psychomotor and vegetative signs occur in full-blown depressive conditions in both uni- and bipolar illness. Psychomotor retardation or slowing of thinking, speech, and general activity may progress to **depressive stupor,** in which all voluntary activities cease. More commonly, melancholia manifests with psychomotor agitation (eg, restlessness, wringing of the hands, and pressure of speech). Although special subgroups of depressives, especially those belonging to atypical, dysthymic, and bipolar categories, are often hypersomnolent, most melancholic patients complain of insomnia, with difficulty falling asleep, multiple arousals, or early morning awak-

TABLE 57–2. CLINICAL MANIFESTATIONS OF DEPRESSIVE AND MANIC STATES

	Depressive Syndrome	Manic Syndrome
Mood	Depressed, irritable, or anxious (the patient may, however, smile or deny subjective mood change and instead complain of pain or other somatic distress)	Elated, irritable, or hostile Momentary tearfulness (as part of mixed state)
	Crying spells (the patient may, however, complain of inability to cry or to experience emotions)	
Associated psychologic manifestations	Lack of self-confidence; low self-esteem; self-reproach	Inflated self-esteem; boasting; grandiosity
	Poor concentration; indecisiveness	Racing thoughts; clang associations (new thoughts triggered by word sounds rather than meaning); distractibility
	Reduction in gratification; loss of interest in usual activities; loss of attachments; social withdrawal	
	Negative expectations; hopelessness; helplessness; increased dependency	Heightened interest in new activities; increased involvement with people (who are often alienated because of the patient's intrusive and meddlesome behavior); buying sprees; sexual indiscretions; foolish business investments
	Recurrent thoughts of death and suicide	
Somatic manifestations	Psychomotor retardation; fatigue	Psychomotor accleration; eutonia (increased sense of physical fitness)
	Agitation	
	Anorexia and weight loss or weight gain	Possible weight loss from increased activity and inattention to proper dietary habits
	Insomnia or hypersomnia	
	Menstrual irregularities; amenorrhea	
	Anhedonia; loss of sexual desire	Decreased need for sleep
		Increased sexual desire
Psychotic symptoms	Delusions of worthlessness and sinfulness	Grandiose delusions of exceptional talent
	Delusions of reference and persecution	Delusions of assistance; delusions of reference and persecution
	Delusions of ill health (nihilistic, somatic, or hypochondriacal)	Delusions of exceptional physical fitness
	Delusions of poverty	
	Depressive hallucinations in the auditory, visual, and (rarely) olfactory spheres	Delusions of wealth, aristocratic ancestry, or other grandiose identity
		Fleeting auditory or visual hallucinations

ening. There is often loss of sexual desire, with orgasmic difficulties; amenorrhea can also occur. Anorexia and weight loss may lead to emaciation and secondary disturbances in electrolyte balance; overeating and weight gain are less common and more characteristic of milder atypical depressions.

Psychotic manifestations are present in 15% of depressions, most commonly in melancholia. Patients have delusions of having committed unpardonable sins or crimes; hallucinatory voices accuse them of various misdeeds or condemn them to death. The uncommon hallucinations of vision take the form of coffins or deceased relatives. Feelings of insecurity and worthlessness may lead some patients to believe that they are being observed, watched, and persecuted. Others think they harbor incurable and "shameful" illnesses, like cancer and sexually transmitted disease, and that they are contaminating other people. Rarely a patient may kill family members to "save" them from future misfortune and then commit suicide.

Diagnosis of a **melancholic episode** is usually not difficult; problems arise when the clinical picture is low-grade or chronic. Thus, patients with **incomplete recovery** from major unipolar illness may not manifest classic depressive symptoms but rather insomnia, hypochondriacal concerns, irritable morosity, and secondary interpersonal trouble in conjugal life. **Dysthymia**, like its nosologic precursor "neurotic depression," is characterized by milder subsyndromal and nonpsychotic depressive manifestations with less prominent somatic signs but marked disturbances in the personality domain. These patients are gloomy, pessimistic, humorless or incapable of fun; passive and lethargic; introverted; skeptical, hypercritical, or complaining; self-critical, self-reproaching, and self-derogatory; and preoccupied with inadequacy, failure, and negative events, sometimes to the point of morbid enjoyment of one's failures.

Clinical bipolar features: In the full-blown **manic psychosis,** the mood typically is one of elation, but irritability and frank hostility with cantankerousness are not uncommon. The morbid mood colors patients' entire experience and behavior to such an extent that they believe they are in their best mental state. Their lack of insight and inordinate capacity for activity lead to a dangerously explosive psychotic state, in which the individual is impatient, intrusive, and meddlesome and responds with aggressive irritability when crossed. Interpersonal friction results and may lead to secondary paranoid delusional interpretations of being persecuted. Acceleration of mental activity is experienced as racing thoughts by the patient and is observed as flight of ideas by the physician and, in the extreme, is difficult to distinguish from the loose associations of the schizophrenic patient. Attention is quite distractible, with the patient constantly shifting from one theme or endeavor to another. Thoughts and activities are expansive and may progress into frank delusional grandiosity; ie, false convictions of personal wealth, power, inventiveness, and genius, or temporary assumption of a grandiose identity. Patients may believe

they are being assisted or persecuted by external agents. Auditory and visual hallucinations are sometimes present, occur at the height of mania, and are usually understandably linked with the morbid mood. The need for sleep is decreased. Manic persons are inexhaustibly, excessively, and impulsively involved in various activities without recognizing the inherent social dangers. In the extreme, psychomotor activity is so frenzied that any understandable link between mood and behavior is lost (a kind of senseless agitation known as **delirious mania**). This counterpart of depressive stupor, which is rare today, constitutes a medical emergency, as patients may die from sheer physical exhaustion.

Mixed states are *labile mixtures between depressive and manic manifestations or rapid alternation from one to the other* and commonly occur in manic-depressives at one time or another. The most typical examples include momentary switches into tearfulness and suicidal ideation, seen at the height of mania, or racing thoughts in the context of a depressive state. In 10 to 30% of bipolars, the entire attack—or a succession of attacks—takes the form of mixed episodes, with dysphorically excited mood, severe insomnia, psychomotor restlessness, racing thoughts, suicidal ideation, grandiosity, persecutory delusions, auditory hallucinations, confusion, etc. Women are more vulnerable to mixed states. Furthermore, alcohol and sedative-hypnotic abuse often contribute to full-fledged mixed states. Antidepressant drugs, especially of the tricyclic type, also at times contribute to dysphoric-irritable mixed states, which may be protracted for many months beyond natural bipolar episodes.

An **alternation of major episodes of mania and depression in a cyclical pattern** is one of the most distinctive clinical pictures in medicine. Diagnostic difficulties arise when elated periods are of milder or hypomanic intensity. In diagnosing **bipolar II disorder,** emphasis should be placed on abrupt termination of episodes with brightening of mood, decreased need for sleep, and psychomotor acceleration beyond the patient's usual mode; often the switch into hypomania is induced by antidepressants.

In **cyclothymia,** the clinical manifestations are similar to those described for manic-depressive illness, but they are considerably attenuated. Most typically, there are brief cycles (usually lasting days) of alternating retarded depression with increased amounts of sleep and elevated periods

TABLE 57–3. VALIDATING CRITERIA IN THE DIFFERENTIATION
OF AFFECTIVE AND SCHIZOPHRENIC PSYCHOSES

Validating Criteria	Affective Psychosis	Schizophrenic Psychosis
Age	Any	Rarely begins after 40 yr
Premorbid traits	Anxiety-prone, dysthymic, cyclothymic, or hyperthymic	Schizoid or schizotypal
Onset	Usually abrupt	Usually insidious
Affect	Usually "infectious"	Rigid, blunted, or inappropriate
Thought processes	Usually intelligible: slowed down or accelerated	Typically difficult to follow (loose associations)
Delusions and hallucinations	Usually mood-congruent, but incidental Schneiderian symptoms can also occur	Typically idiosyncratic, bizarre, and involving multiple areas of the patient's life; commonly Schneiderian in form
Family history	Mood disorder; alcoholism	Schizophrenia
Course	Usually remitting or periodic; personality generally preserved	Usually unremitting; social functioning often deteriorated
Biologic tests	Shortened REM latency; abnormal DST; blunted TSH response to TRH	Normal results with these tests (except in some schizophreniform psychoses)

DST = dexamethasone suppression test; REM = rapid eye movement (sleep); TRH = thyrotropin-releasing hormone; TSH = thyroid-stimulating hormone.

Updated from Akiskal HS, Puzantian VR: "Psychotic forms of depression and mania." *Psychiatric Clinics of North America* 2(3):419–439, 1979; used with permission.

or labile irritability with shortened sleep. In another form, low-grade depressive features predominate; the bipolar tendency is shown primarily by the ease with which elation or irritability is elicited by the administration of antidepressants. In a form rarely seen clinically and termed **hyperthymic temperament** or **chronic hypomanic personality**, elevated periods predominate, with habitual reduction of sleep to < 6 h. The hyperthymic individual is characterized by the following lifelong traits: cheerful, overoptimistic, or exuberant, though irritability is not uncommon; overconfident, self-assured, boastful, bombastic, or grandiose; energetic, vigorous, full of plans, improvident, or rushing off with restless impulse; overtalkative; warm, people-seeking, or extroverted; overinvolved or meddlesome; and uninhibited or stimulus-seeking. Although both cyclothymia and hyperthymia might contribute to success in business, leadership, achievement, and artistic creativity in some individuals, it is important to recognize these temperamental dysregulations because their affective nature is often masked by serious interpersonal and social problems, such as uneven work and school records, dilettantism, geographic instability, episodic promiscuity, repeated roman-

tic breakups or marital failure, and an episodic pattern of alcohol and drug abuse. In about ⅓ of cyclothymics, these features represent the prelude to full-blown affective episodes.

Differential Diagnosis

The most common diagnostic errors equate affective psychosis with **schizophrenia** or **schizoaffective disorder** (see also Ch. 58). Differential diagnosis between affective and schizophrenic psychoses (see TABLE 57–3) is important clinically because of the relative specificity of lithium for treating recurrent mood disorders (and the potential for neurotoxicity in schizophrenia), and because affectively ill individuals should be protected from the unnecessary risk of tardive dyskinesia. No pathognomonic differentiating elements exist, and diagnosis must be based on the overall clinical picture, family history, course, and associated features. Not only mood-congruent psychotic features occur in mood disorders; mood-incongruent delusions or hallucinations are sometimes secondarily superimposed on the basic mood disorder because of the concomitant presence of alcoholic hallucinosis, sedative-hypnotic withdrawal, psychedelic-induced psychosis, or other systemic or brain

TABLE 57–4. CLINICAL FEATURES DIFFERENTIATING DEPRESSIVE "PSEUDODEMENTIA" FROM PRIMARY (DEGENERATIVE) DEMENTIA

Clinical Features	"Pseudodementia"	Primary Dementia
Onset	Acute	Insidious
Past affective episodes	Common	Uncharacteristic
Self-reproach	Common	Uncharacteristic
Diurnality	Worse in morning	Worse at night
Memory deficit	Recent = remote	Recent > remote
Other cognitive deficits	Circumscribed	Global
Responses to cognitive testing	"Don't know"	Near miss
Reaction to mistakes	Tend to give up	Catastrophic
Practice effects	Can be coached	Consistently poor
Response to sleep deprivation	Improvement	Worsening (?)

Modified from Akiskal HS: "Mood disturbances," in *Medical Basis of Psychiatry*, edited by G Winokur and P Clayton. Philadelphia, WB Saunders Company, 1986, pp 384–399; used with permission.

disease producing psychotic symptoms. In a remitting illness with affective and schizophrenic admixtures, a schizoaffective diagnosis should not be made unless such complicating factors are excluded. When in doubt, because of the better prognosis of mood disorders, **therapeutic trial** with a thymoleptic drug (an antidepressant or lithium carbonate) or electroconvulsive therapy **(ECT)** is indicated. TSH response to TRH is almost never blunted in nuclear schizophrenic conditions; such TSH blunting or DST nonsuppression, even in the presence of schizophreniform features, tends to predict good response to thymoleptic drugs.

Therapeutic trial with thymoleptics or ECT also is justified in the elderly to clarify the differential diagnosis between **early dementia** (which often presents with affective change) and **pseudodemented depression**. In the latter, psychomotor retardation, decreased concentration, and memory impairment contribute to the appearance of dementiform features. Because of the better prognosis of depressive illness, it should be preferentially diagnosed, especially when more classic affective episodes have occurred or when family history is suggestive. These and other clinical differentiating features are summarized in TABLE 57–4. Traditional laboratory tests (eg, blood chemistry, CT scan, EEG) are more informative in differential diagnosis than neuroendocrine and sleep EEG findings.

The dual and related concepts of **masked depression** and **affective equivalents** are often invoked to explain certain disorders with promi-

nent somatic symptoms or behavioral disturbance with minimal or absent mood change. These include antisocial acting out (especially in children and adolescents), substance use disorders, chronic pain, hypochondriasis, anxiety states, and psychophysiologic disorders. In the absence of clear-cut symptoms, the diagnosis of a mood disorder is not appropriate unless past affective episodes have occurred, the condition is periodic, and the family history is positive for mood disorder. DST and sleep EEG latency findings may serve as corollary data in this type of differential diagnosis. Therapeutic trial with an antidepressant drug also may be helpful in differential diagnosis if unequivocal response occurs.

The basic manifestations of **childhood depressive illness** (see also Ch. 46) are not radically different from those of adults. They are simply manifested in areas of typical concern to children and parents, such as school work and play. However, extremes of irritability and even frank aggressive behavior, rather than depressed mood per se, are quite common in childhood depressions, suggesting a higher incidence of mixed-manic features coexisting with depression. When such features coexist with more typical adult symptoms and signs of depression, the diagnosis of mood disorder should be made in preference to adjustment reactions or neurotic and behavior disorders; the latter often are given exaggerated prominence in child psychiatry. Conversely, when other affective symptoms are lacking, hyperactivity and behavioral disturbances alone should not be considered affective equivalents unless validating criteria as outlined above are present. Mood disorders, including bipolar psychoses, do occur in mentally retarded children and adults, in whom somatic symptoms and behavioral disturbances are especially likely to mask the basic mood disorder. A history of episodic occurrence of such disturbances and family history for bipolar illness may aid differential diagnosis in such cases. **Depressive manifestations in adolescents**, especially with stuporous or psychotic presentations, often herald the onset of bipolar illness. **Mania in adolescence**, which often takes the form of mixed attacks, is commonly confused with schizophrenia, but a cyclical pattern of retarded depression and an accelerated psychosis with good premorbid and intermorbid functioning strongly favor diagnosis of a mood disorder. The diagnostic status of laboratory tests is generally uncertain in juvenile mood disorders.

Unipolar depression is less often a cause of **alcoholism** and drug abuse than has been thought; indeed, alcohol is more likely to be abused by the manic patient (see also Ch. 53). While an attempt to treat the sleep disorder may be the motive in the abuse of alcohol in both depressed and manic patients, the latter sometimes seek drugs (eg, cocaine) to enhance excitement, with catastrophic effects on the course of their illness. Affective symptoms, especially depression, of a transient or intermittent nature (due to toxic effects, drug withdrawal, or social complications) which often accompany **substance use disorders** should not be confused with primary mood disorders that most typically have a sustained duration of several months. Differentiation from intermittently chronic mood disorders such as cyclothymia and dysthymia is more problematic. Although primary alcoholism, other substance use disorders, and antisocial personality are the most likely diagnoses in individuals with flagrant alcohol and drug histories, polysubstance abuse (including cocaine) in many teenagers and young adults, especially those with bipolar family history, may represent self-treatment for subsyndromal or cyclothymic mood swings. Finally, episodic substance abuse (especially that of alcohol—**dipsomania**) or onset after age 30 favors the diagnosis of primary mood disorder with secondary substance abuse. When in doubt, a therapeutic trial with thymoleptic agents is indicated, because neuroendocrine and sleep EEG testing is notoriously unreliable in the differential diagnosis of mood and substance use disorders. Unfortunately, some experts

frown upon the therapeutic use of any pharmacologic agents in substance-abusing patients; this total chemical abstinence tends to complicate the rational use of modern psychopharmacologic treatments for the difficult group of patients whose addictive illness represents self-medication.

Differentiation of mood disorders from severe personality disorders (eg, **borderline personality**) is more difficult, especially when the mood disorder is one with a chronic or intermittent course; eg, dysthymia, cyclothymia, and bipolar II disorder. Longitudinal course with affective manifestations, especially when biphasic, and family history for mood disorder support an affective diagnosis. DST nonsuppression, TSH blunting in response to TRH, and sleep EEG findings in many individuals diagnosed as borderline have been reported indistinguishable from those with primary mood disorders. In view of the greater gravity of missing an affective diagnosis in young patients with a tempestuous impulsive course that could culminate in suicide, therapeutic trials are recommended, in the controlled setting of a hospital, with such agents as lithium, monoamine oxidase inhibitors, and carbamazepine as an aid in differential diagnosis (see below).

Neurotic symptoms such as worrying, panic attacks, and obsessions are common in primary depressive disorders; they disappear when the depressive episode remits. In primary neurotic syndromes, conversely, there are usually irregular exacerbations and remissions of the anxiety symptoms beginning in early adulthood; remission of depressive symptoms does not typically result in a cure from the neurotic manifestations. However, neurotic conditions making their first appearance after age 40 are most likely to be secondary to a primary mood disorder. Differentiating neurotic and mood disorders is more problematic when mild symptoms common to both groups of illnesses coexist. Such conditions, variously referred to as **mixed anxiety-depression** or **anxious depression**, usually pursue chronically intermittent courses. Current evidence, based in part on sleep EEG findings and follow-up, suggests that patients with these mixed syndromes are more like anxiety neurotics than primary depressives.

Treatment of Unipolar and Bipolar Disorders

The clinical pharmacology of thymoleptic agents: Psychopharmaceuticals effective in the treatment of mood disorders can be grouped

TABLE 57-5. CLASSIFICATION OF SELECTED EFFECTS AND DOSAGE RANGE
OF THE HETEROCYCLIC ANTIDEPRESSANTS (HCAs)

HCA	Sedation	Anticholinergic	α_1 Adrenolytic	Usual Dosage Range (mg/day)
III° amine tricyclic antidepressants with II° amine metabolites				
Amitriptyline	+ + +	+ + +	+ + +	50–300
Nortriptyline*	+ +	+ +	+	25–125
Imipramine	+ +	+ +	+ + +	50–300
Desipramine*	+	+	+	50–300
Other tricyclic antidepressants				
Doxepin	+ + +	+ +	+ + +	50–300
Trimipramine	+ + +	+ +	+ + +	50–300
Clomipramine	+ +	+ + +	+ + +	50–225
Protriptyline	±	+ + +	+	10–60
Other cyclic antidepressants				
Amoxapine	+ +	+	+ +	150–400
Maprotiline	+ +	+	+	50–225
Trazodone	+ + +	0	+ +	50–400
Fluoxetine	±	0	0	10–60
Bupropion	0	±	0	75–450

* Arrows indicate biotransformed secondary amine tricyclic; such transformation is usually complete with imipramine and variable with amitriptyline.

into 3 classes: the heterocyclic antidepressants (HCAs), monoamine oxidase inhibitors (MAOIs), and lithium salts.

HCAs comprise the largest class of antidepressants (see TABLE 57-5), which include the classic tricyclic antidepressants (TCAs), the tertiary amines amitriptyline and imipramine, and their secondary amine metabolites nortriptyline and desipramine; other TCAs with modified ring structure or side-chains; and the newer cyclic antidepressants. Unlike amphetamine-type drugs, HCAs have no immediate euphoriant effects and hence no effect on normal sadness—probably why they pose no risk of abuse potential. Acutely, these agents increase the availability of the biogenic amines norepinephrine and/or serotonin (5-HT) by blocking re-uptake in the synaptic cleft. Upon chronic administration, they down-regulate β_1 adrenoreceptors on the postsynaptic membrane. Long hypothesized to be crucial for their antidepressant action, these acute and chronic effects are not shared by some of the newer antidepressants, eg, bupropion. Recent shift of thinking to serotonergic mechanisms of antidepressant action has not led to any definitive results on specific receptor changes, except

for the finding that an intact serotonergic system is necessary for the optimal functioning of the noradrenergic system and the antidepressants that act on the latter system. Other actions common to most, though not all, HCAs include anesthesia, increased cerebral capillary permeability, and suppression of REM sleep. The latter has also been hypothesized to be relevant to antidepressant action, because total sleep or REM deprivation by forceful waking has been shown to have transient antidepressant action.

Indications for HCAs: These drugs appear to be equally effective in about 70% of clinically depressed patients. The rate of response climbs to 90% in those with melancholic symptoms and signs. Other predictors of antidepressant response include previous response, family history of response, and, experimentally, euphoric response to a 20- to 30-mg single oral dose of dextroamphetamine, and REM suppression with 2 nights of HCA use. Most HCAs tend to precipitate hypomania in bipolar depressives and, even when combined with lithium, should not be used chronically in such patients.

Given the multiple pharmacologic properties of the HCAs, they have found clinical usefulness, though not necessarily supported in controlled studies, for a variety of conditions, including (1) treatment of school phobia and panic attacks (most studies have been with imipramine); (2) childhood enuresis (imipramine); (3) palliation of peptic ulcer in depressed patients (doxepin and trimipramine possess strong anticholinergic and histamine H_2 blocking properties); (4) symptomatic treatment of dermatologic allergies with pruritus (doxepin, trimipramine, amitriptyline, and maprotiline have strong histamine H_1 blocking properties); (5) idiopathic hypersomnia and sleep apnea (protriptyline given in the AM is not only useful for symptomatic alleviation of the hypersomnia, but might reduce the ventricular tachyarrhythmias associated with apnea); (6) bulimia (fluoxetine and desipramine); (7) cocaine dependence (desipramine); (8) narcolepsy manifesting predominantly with cataplexy (imipramine); (9) palliation or prevention of pain syndromes and migraine (trazodone and amitriptyline block serotonin S_2 receptors); (10) attention deficit disorder (imipramine); and (11) obsessive-compulsive disorder (clomipramine and fluoxetine, both of which enhance serotonergic mechanisms).

Side effects: In general, the secondary amine TCAs and the newer cyclic antidepressants have fewer side effects. However, this does not pertain to all side effects; eg, lowering of the seizure threshold, which is common to all the HCAs, is particularly accentuated with maprotiline and bupropion. The more common HCA side effects derive from their muscarinic-blocking and α_1-adrenolytic actions (see TABLE 57-5). Thus, even small doses could cause troublesome side effects such as tachycardia, postural hypotension, and quinidine-like cardiotoxicity. The newer agents fluoxetine, bupropion, and, to some extent, maprotiline are essentially safe from this perspective. Though postural hypotension represents a distinct risk for those with osteoporosis, cerebral arteriosclerosis, or ischemic heart disease, in a mildly hypertensive depressive individual free of such diseases, TCAs with high α_1 adrenolytic activity can control both the depression and the BP. Except for trazodone, fluoxetine, and bupropion, which possess no measurable anticholinergic activity, HCAs are commonly associated with blurred vision, xerostomia, tachycardia, constipation, and urinary hesitancy. Sedation (see TABLE 57-5), depending on its desirability from the point of view of sleep induction and maintenance, may or may not be considered a side effect and derives largely from serotonin S_2 and histamine H_1 blockade. Sedation

and weight gain are common side effects with most HCAs, being least problematic with fluoxetine, bupropion, desipramine, and protriptyline. Unlike neuroleptics, HCAs produce no appreciable blockade of dopamine D_2 receptors, except for amoxapine (derived from the neuroleptic loxapine), which has an increased risk of undesirable extrapyramidal effects.

Seizures and behavioral symptoms due to toxicity (excitement, confusion, hallucinations, or oversedation) are especially likely to occur in elderly patients with organic brain disease, dictating even lower initial and maintenance doses of HCAs. These considerations are pertinent to fluoxetine (which is prone to produce psychomotor excitement) and bupropion (particularly prone to lower the seizure threshold). These 2 new cyclic antidepressants, however, offer greater freedom and safety from the standpoint of the more troublesome anticholinergic, cardiotoxic, and hypotensive side effects that make other HCAs unsuitable for many patients with medical disorders, especially the elderly.

MAOIs inhibit the oxidative deamination of the 3 classes of biogenic amines—noradrenergic, dopaminergic, and 5-HT—as well as other phenylethamines. Those marketed as antidepressants in the USA (eg, phenelzine, isocarboxazid, and tranylcypromine) are irreversible and nonselective (inhibit both MAO-A and MAO-B) and can cause hypertensive crises if tyramine- or dopamine-containing food or sympathomimetic agents are ingested concurrently (most common with tranylcypromine). More selective and reversible MAOIs (eg, moclobemide, an inhibitor of MAO-A), which are not yet available for clinical use in the USA, may offer relative freedom from such interaction.

Indications for MAOIs: The efficacy of phenelzine is clearly established for panic disorder. Recent data that have reaffirmed its efficacy in selected affective subtypes with anxious or atypical features (especially in females) have rekindled motivation to prescribe it. However, even "typical" melancholias sometimes respond to phenelzine. Furthermore, tranylcypromine is useful for hypersomnic-retarded bipolar patients experiencing a relapse under lithium prophylaxis. Like the HCAs, MAOIs can precipitate hypomanic switches, usually in those with bipolar potential. Although the switchover is more frequent with MAOIs, recent data suggest that the excitement tends to be euphoric rather than aggressive and hence more easily manageable clinically. Despite such clinical activity in bipolar depressives, MAOIs have little or no effect on normal mood, and despite some direct amphetamine-like action possessed by tranylcypromine, MAOIs generally are safe from an abuse standpoint.

Side effects: MAOIs are underused in the USA because of clinicians' fears of paradoxical hypertension that might result from dietary or drug interactions. This is popularly known as the "cheese reaction" due to the high tyramine content of overripe and mature cheese. Actually, postural hypotension—and consequent lightheadedness—is more of a problem with these agents. (Indeed, pargyline, a MAO-B inhibitor, is marketed as an antihypertensive in the USA.) As with TCAs, a mildly hypertensive depressed patient who is a candidate for an MAOI can thereby benefit from the dual action of the MAOI on both the depression and BP. This could prove particularly useful in depressed bipolar patients taking lithium, in whom a diuretic is generally contraindicated. Other common side effects of MAOIs include erectile difficulties (least common with tranylcypromine), anxiety, nausea, dizziness, insomnia, edema, and weight gain. Potential for cardiotoxicity and anticholinergic side effects is minimal. Hepatotoxicity (the reason why the first MAOI, iproniazid, was withdrawn) is fortunately quite rare with the MAOIs in current use (least likely with tranylcypromine).

To avert paradoxical hypertensive crises with MAOIs, the patient should be instructed to avoid sympathomimetic drugs (including phenylpropanolamine and dextromethorphan found in many OTC nasal decongestants and cough suppressants), reserpine, and meperidine, as well as tyramine or L-dopa—containing beers, wine (including sherry) or liqueurs, and overripe aged foods with such content (eg, bananas, fava or broad beans, yeast extracts, canned figs, raisins, yogurt, cheese, sour cream, soy sauce, pickled herring, caviar, liver, and extensively tenderized meats). Inadvertent ingestion of such drugs or foods may lead to sudden rise in BP (hypertensive crisis) manifested by severe throbbing headache. It is best to supply patients with 25-mg tablets of the adrenolytic drug chlorpromazine and instruct them to take 1 or 2 tablets orally upon the earliest signs of such a reaction on their way to the nearest emergency room. Sublingual nifedipine 10 to 20 mg is another alternative; the capsule should be bitten and the liquid contents retained in the mouth. These precautions often bring down the BP by the time the patient arrives at the emergency room. Another precaution is to avoid combining an MAOI with an HCA, and ordinarily at least 1 wk should elapse between the use of the 2 classes of drugs (see below). Patients receiving MAOIs, and who also may need antiasthmatic, antiallergic, local anesthetic, and general anesthetic medication, should be treated with the joint expertise of a psychiatrist and an internist, dentist, or anesthesiologist with the requisite experience in neuropsychopharmacology.

Lithium is a naturally occurring alkali metal. By the early 1970s, its efficacy had been demonstrated and methods of safe administration established. Its precise mechanism of stabilizing the unpredictable, often explosive, mood swings and behavior of bipolar patients is unknown. It may be any or all of the following: reduction of neuronal Ca mobilization via activation of membrane phosphoinositide signaling system; hyperpolarization of the neuronal membrane; increased presynaptic deamination of norepinephrine and decreased norepinephrine release; blocking β-adrenoreceptor-stimulated adenyl cyclase; decreased dopaminergic turnover; increased tryptophan uptake and consequent stabilization of 5-HT synaptic dynamics; inhibition of the synthesis of prostaglandin E_1; and slowing of biologic rhythms.

Indications for lithium: Although lithium attenuates bipolar mood swings, it has no effect on normal mood. It also appears to have an antiaggressive action, but it is unclear whether this occurs in patients without a bipolar disorder. By its direct action, lithium produces no sedation nor, ordinarily, cognitive impairment; should the latter occur, it is often due to lithium-induced hypothyroidism. Lithium does not produce dependence.

Sixty to 70% of bipolar patients respond to lithium. Predictors of good response include a classic manic picture as part of primary mood disorder, episode frequency $< 2/yr$, and past and family history of lithium response. Promising therapeutic uses of lithium include cluster and migraine headaches, periodic alcoholism, polysubstance abuse, and episodic aggression—some of which might represent bipolar variants—and, experimentally, neutropenia (lithium regularly induces a modest leukocytosis).

Pharmacokinetics: Lithium, usually given as the carbonate, is rapidly and completely absorbed via the GI tract and peaks in the serum in $1^1/_2$ h. It is not biotransformed; 95% is excreted via the kidney, a process enhanced by a Na+ load. Thus, any condition that leads to Na loss—via disease or treatment with diuretics—poses a risk for toxicity. The elimination half-life is 24 h, which tends to increase with age and with the decreased GFR that accompanies kidney disease, dictating extreme caution and use of lower doses in patients at risk. Lithium carbonate is given orally as 300-mg tablets or capsules, up to 1200 to 1800 mg/day in acute cases, and 600 to 1500 mg/day during maintenance. Steady state is reached in 4 to 6 days—hence the latency in acute antimanic action. During a manic episode, the patient retains lithium and excretes Na; oral dosage and the blood level need to be higher during acute treatment compared with maintenance prophylaxis. Lithium **side effects and toxicity** are discussed below, under Bipolar illness.

Unipolar illness.

1. **Medical or neurologic causes should be excluded**, especially after age 40.

2. **Hospitalization:** Persistent suicidal ideation (particularly when family support is lacking), stupor, agitated-deluded depression, and physical debilitation or concurrent severe cardiovascular disease require hospitalization and, often, electroconvulsive therapy **(ECT)**; the response to 4 to 8 treatments in such cases usually is dramatic and may be lifesaving. For less ill patients, the physician can begin a 3- to 6-wk course with maximal doses of sedating HCAs, which, if necessary, can be buttressed with a neuroleptic (eg, thiothixene up to 30 mg/day orally or IM given in 2 to 3 divided doses). To avert the risk of tardive dyskinesia, the neuroleptic should be given in the lowest effective dose and discontinued as soon as possible. Continuation therapy with an HCA for 6 to 12 mo (and up to 2 yr in patients > 50 yr) usually prevents relapse in ECT- or drug-treated patients.

3. **General principles of clinical management:** Presently, most depressives are treated as outpatients. It is imperative to gently, but directly, inquire about suicidal ideation, plans, or activity (see Ch. 60). Pharmacotherapy is the treatment of choice for depressions of melancholic depth; nonmelancholic depressions are treated with either drugs or psychotherapy or, preferably, both. Initially, the patient is seen on a weekly or biweekly basis to provide support and education about the nature of the illness and to monitor progress. Because many are embarrassed and demoralized by the implications of having a mental disorder, especially one that seriously diminishes the capacity for work, it is extremely important to tell the patient, his family, and his employer (when appropriate and after obtaining informed consent from the patient) that depression is a self-limiting medical illness

with a generally good prognosis. An explanation also may be given in terms of our current understanding of the biologic aspects of depression. Because some patients are concerned about "taking drugs," it is important to reassure them that thymoleptic agents are not habit-forming. To reduce demoralization and ensure compliance, patients should also be told that the path to recovery often fluctuates.

4. **Guidelines for drug therapy:** The history of response to a specific MAOI or HCA guides drug choice. Prominence of phobic anxiety and reverse vegetative signs suggest using phenelzine or another MAOI. Otherwise, because of ease of administration, it is best to begin with an HCA. Although different HCAs are equally effective in the average case of depression, many experienced practitioners often begin the treatment with TCAs because of greater accumulated clinical wisdom about their usefulness and side effects. Thus, it is convenient to treat the agitated insomniac patient with a sedating TCA, eg, amitriptyline or trimipramine; the retarded insomniac patient with an even less sedating HCA, eg, imipramine or nortriptyline; and the hypersomnic retarded patient with an even less sedating TCA, eg, desipramine. For patients with cardiac disease, or those who cannot tolerate anticholinergic side effects because of severe constipation, or in whom such effects could lead to clinical catastrophes (eg, angle-closure glaucoma, neurogenic bladder, prostatic hypertrophy), several of the new cyclic antidepressants such as trazodone, fluoxetine, and bupropion offer almost complete freedom from cardiotoxic and anticholinergic side effects and are less likely to aggravate impotence (though it should be borne in mind that trazodone has been associated with priapism). These newer agents are also preferred in geriatric depressives who are vulnerable to confusion due to anticholinergic side effects. However, anticholinergic effects can be useful in depressed patients with parkinsonism, (though amoxapine should be avoided because of its dopamine-blocking action) and in those with chronic diarrhea or peptic ulcer. Amitriptyline and other sedating HCAs help the depressed patient with concurrent pain and insomnia while decreasing the need for analgesic and spasmolytic medication.

It is generally best to begin with the lowest unit dose marketed and to increase gradually over a period of 2 to 3 wk. Ordinarily, an average of $1/3$ to $1/2$ of the maximum listed in the dosage range in TABLE 57–5 will suffice, but some may need even higher doses for remission. It is likely that the relatively high doses recommended by research clinicians, especially in the USA, are based on experiences with relatively refractory patients.

Giving the entire dose at bedtime usually renders hypnotics unnecessary, minimizes side effects during daytime, and improves compliance; however, some elderly patients may better tolerate daily divided doses. Furthermore, some HCAs such as protriptyline and fluoxetine are activating for many depressives and should be given in the morning. Because of their relatively long half-lives, these 2 drugs are often prescribed (especially during maintenance) in the lowest dosage strength or even on an every-other-day basis. Therapeutic response to HCAs is seen in about 2 to 3 wk (it can be as early as 4 days or as late as 5 to 6 wk). Within 1 to 2 mo following response, a downward adjustment of dosage is customarily attempted, to be maintained at about 2/3 of the effective therapeutic dose for the natural duration of an episode. Abrupt withdrawal of TCAs should be *avoided* to prevent cholinergic rebound; eg, nightmares, nausea, colic.

The indications and dosage range of the HCAs for preadolescent depressions are not established; in a clinically depressed child, conservative doses and increments are best, as is true with the elderly (about 1/2 the adult dose or less). For reasons that are not entirely clear, adolescent depressives do not seem to respond as well to TCAs. Although experience with the new cyclic antidepressants is too recent to permit a definitive statement, clinical trial with fluoxetine is worthwhile.

Side effects of the HCAs are discussed above. TABLE 57–6 summarizes potentially serious interactions of the HCAs with various medical conditions and drugs. During the first 10 to 15 days, when the patient is largely reaping side effects and little therapeutic benefit, he should be informed that these effects are to be expected, are the prelude to therapeutic response, and will abate with time. The most serious (but fortunately rare) undesirable effects are precipitation of angle-closure glaucoma, urinary retention, and cardiac arrhythmias.

5. Resistant and refractory depressions: Where anxiety is prominent, response to TCAs is often suboptimal, and a benzodiazepine tranquilizer (eg, diazepam 2 to 5 mg orally bid or tid or lorazepam 1 to 2 mg orally bid or tid) can be added to the HCA regimen for 2 to 3 wk. It has been suggested that alprazolam, a more recent benzodiazepine with a tricyclic ring structure, in doses of 0.5 to 2 mg orally bid may be effective as monotherapy in controlling both anxiety and depression. As noted earlier, the MAOI phenelzine (up to 75 mg/day) is another alternative, particularly useful when anxious-phobic symptomatology coexists with reverse vegetative signs. Patients with pronounced obsessional features would benefit from clomipramine or fluoxetine.

Plasma level–therapeutic response relationships, which are most reliable for imipramine, desipramine, and nortriptyline, can be useful in determining causes of inadequate clinical response on standard oral doses in selected instances. Other uses of plasma level determination include pronounced side effects on small doses or when anticipated side effects might be dangerous because of heart disease or old age. HCA dosage should be titrated accordingly, thereby rendering a hitherto pharmacotherapy-resistant patient to a responder. Fluoxetine tends to raise the blood levels of other HCAs, which should be kept in mind when exchanging this drug with other HCAs. However, as fluoxetine may be associated with insomnia, small doses of trazodone 50 to 100 mg orally can be given at bedtime. Fluoxetine alone or in such combination often works in depressives resistant to classic antidepressants.

Patients not responding to the above measures are best treated in a specialized mood disorders unit or in consultation with a psychiatrist experienced in this area. ECT or a potent MAOI such as tranylcypromine 10 to 30 mg orally bid may be given for those who are poor risks with HCAs, cannot tolerate them, or fail to improve on full courses of 2 different HCAs for 4 to 6 wk each (after dosage adjustment suggested by plasma drug levels). Although liothyronine 25 to 50 μg/day has been advocated as a method to boost TCA responses in women with borderline thyroid indexes (eg, high baseline TSH, augmented TSH response to TRH), it is doubtful whether the method works in strictly unipolar patients. A lithium-HCA combination may be beneficial in patients in whom an eventual bipolar course is suspected because of family history or a cyclothymic temperament. Although some advocate TCA-MAOI combination in smaller doses (eg, amitriptyline 75 to 100 mg orally at bedtime with phenelzine 30 to 45 mg in the morning), there are lingering doubts about the safety and efficacy of this procedure, and therefore it is best reserved to physicians with expertise in this area.

TABLE 57–6. CLINICALLY SIGNIFICANT INTERACTIONS BETWEEN HCAs AND SELECTED SOMATIC OR PSYCHIATRIC CONDITIONS AND DRUGS

Condition/Drugs	Interaction	Clinical Recommendation
Cardiac disease	Conduction defect, arrhythmias, or heart failure	Coordinate treatment with cardiologist; maprotiline can be used in conduction defect, nortriptyline in ischemic heart disease and failure; fluoxetine and bupropion are generally safest; consider ECT
Hypotension	Potentiation	Consider bupropion or fluoxetine
Guanethidine	Decreased uptake by sympathetic neuron, thereby diminishing its hypotensive action	Trimipramine, trazodone, and fluoxetine have minimal effect on guanethidine pump
Clonidine or α-methyldopa	Inhibition of α_2-adrenergic receptors leads to abolition of antihypertensive action	Consider fluoxetine
Prazocin	Blockade of α_2-adrenergic receptors potentiates antihypertensive action	Consider fluoxetine, bupropion, desipramine, or protriptyline
Angle-closure glaucoma	Ocular hypertension	Coordinate with ophthalmologist; consider trazodone, fluoxetine, or bupropion
Prostatic hypertrophy	Urinary retention	Give urecholine; consider trazodone, fluoxetine, or bupropion
Esophageal hiatus hernia	Increased reflux	Reduce dose; consider trazodone, fluoxetine, or bupropion
Debilitated physical state	Sluggish reflexes predispose to postural hypotension	Fluoxetine; consider ECT
Pregnancy, 1st trimester	Teratogenic	Treat depression with psychotherapy; reserve ECT for severe cases
Parkinsonism	Anticholinergic effects potentiate antiparkinsonian drugs	Avoid amoxapine; use lowest doses of the least anticholinergic HCAs; consider ECT
Seizure disorder	Precipitation of seizure	Lower dose of HCA; avoid maprotiline, clomipramine, and bupropion; MAOIs best; consider use of antiepileptic medication
Chronic schizophrenia	Exacerbation of hyperactive aggressive psychotic state	Discontinue HCA; consider amoxapine; raise neuroleptic dose
Neuroleptics	Increased blood levels of both drugs	Avoid combination unless absolutely necessary
Bipolar depression	Precipitation of hypomania or mania	Discontinue HCA; consider lithium carbonate and/or bupropion
Ethanol	Potentiation of CNS depression	Do not prescribe HCAs to alcoholics unless depressive syndrome is sustained; consider fluoxetine
Advanced liver disease	Decreased degradation, increased blood level	Begin with very small doses; monitor plasma level of HCA
Heavy smoking, phenobarbital, and carbamazepine	Increased degradation, decreased blood level	Monitor plasma level; use higher HCA dose as needed
Cimetidine	Decreased degradation, increased blood level	Monitor plasma level; use lower HCA dose
Thyroid hormone	Potentiation of central effects; cardiotoxicity	Discontinue thyroid drug; reduce dosage of HCA

*ECT = electroconvulsive therapy; HCA = heterocyclic antidepressant; MAOI = monoamine oxidase inhibitor.

Updated from Akiskal HS: "Clinical overview of depressive disorders and their pharmacological management," in *Neuropharmacology of Central and Behavioral Disorders*, edited by G Palmer. New York, Academic Press, 1981; used with permission.

6. Brief individual psychotherapy (with interpersonal focus) or **cognitive-behavioral therapy** (either individual or group format) is best introduced when antidepressants have controlled melancholic signs. By providing support, guidance, removal of cognitive distortions that prevent adaptive action, and encouragement to gradually resume one's responsibilities, these therapies often improve coping and enhance the gains made through pharmacotherapy. **Couples' therapy** may further help diminish conjugal conflicts. Elaborate long-term psychotherapy is unnecessary except in the presence of significant personality disturbance.

Psychologic support is particularly important in refractory cases and should involve the patient as well as significant others whose lives are often seriously stressed.

7. Recurrent depressions occurring infrequently can be treated as outlined above for a single episode. Those with frequent relapses are often treated with maintenance HCAs, the dosage periodically adjusted with respect to mood level and side effects; however, recent research suggests that relapses are best prevented by maintaining the full therapeutic dosage used during the acute phase. Family history for bipolar illness is often positive in depression with high episode frequency, and patients must be observed for hypomania. As expected, maintenance with lithium carbonate alone (see below) is probably equally effective in such cases and may be the preferred prophylaxis to avoid rapid-cycling. Relapses are not uncommon with maintenance chemotherapy; supportive psychotherapy may therefore assist in boosting morale, improving coping skills, and identifying early manifestations of relapse.

Bipolar illness.

Many bipolar patients with recurrent depressions experience pleasant elevation of mood, usually at the tail end of a depression, but do not report it unless specifically questioned. In the absence of documented history for hypomanic or manic episodes, the **depressive phase** of bipolar illness may not be easily distinguishable from unipolar depression cross-sectionally. TCAs may sometimes overcorrect the mood in a hypomanic direction, giving a clue to the bipolar nature of the illness; such pharmacologic hypomania also is seen with MAOIs and probably all centrally acting sympathomimetic drugs, as well as with ECT. Lithium has a modest acute antidepressant effect in the depressive phase of bipolar illness and

can be given alone or in conjunction with an HCA or MAOI.

Manic psychosis often presents as a social emergency and is preferably managed on an inpatient basis, and **hypomania,** if it comes to clinical attention at all, on an outpatient basis. After preliminary laboratory tests (CBC, urinalysis, T_4, TSH, serum electrolytes, creatinine, and BUN), lithium carbonate is started 300 mg orally bid or tid and increased over a 7- to 10-day period until a serum level of 0.8 to 1.2 mEq/L is reached. Acutely manic patients have high tolerance for lithium and preferentially retain it during the first 10 days while excreting Na; regular diet is recommended. Teenagers, who enjoy excellent glomerular function, need higher doses of lithium to achieve the same level of equilibrium in the serum, while the reverse is true for elderly patients. Because lithium's onset of action has a 4- to 10-day latency period, it is sometimes initially necessary to coadminister haloperidol 5 to 10 mg orally as needed (up to 60 mg/day) or another suitable neuroleptic until the manic stage is under control. In extremely hyperactive psychotic patients with precarious food and fluid intake, it is preferable to give neuroleptics IM and supportive care for a week before initiating lithium. Lorazepam 1 to 2 mg tid IM or orally in the early days of acute management can boost the effects of the neuroleptic and reduce the dosage of the latter. **Mixed states** of manic-depressive illness can be similarly managed, though ECT would be preferable in severe cases. Carbamazepine up to 1200 mg/day orally is another alternative for such patients, especially in the presence of mood-incongruent psychotic features. Recent clinical experience also supports the usefulness of valproate up to 2000 mg/day orally in such cases.

Maintenance phase: Therapy for an isolated manic episode should continue for at least 6 mo, but most manias occur as part of recurrent bipolar illness. Maintenance lithium should be initiated after 2 classic bipolar episodes occur < 3 yr apart, or following a single manic episode or psychotic mixed state in an adolescent or young adult with bipolar family history. This less conservative approach is recommended for juveniles because prevention of disruptive psychotic episodes is important for achieving scholastic and vocational goals. The need for lithium maintenance can be reassessed after graduation from high school or college.

Serum lithium should be maintained between 0.3 and 0.8 mEq/L and is usually achieved with two to five 300-mg capsules/day. Doses of HCA (in the lower range as given in TABLE 57-5) can be added cautiously when needed, preferably for a few weeks at a time (see below), especially during the first 2 yr of maintenance therapy, to control moderate to severe depressive swings; and chlorpromazine or thioridazine 50 to 300 mg/day orally, again for a few days to a few weeks at a time, when disruptive psychomotor acceleration or mixed states supervene.

Rapid-cycling forms: There is growing concern that HCAs given to some bipolar patients, even when protected by lithium carbonate, may induce rapid-cycling. Low doses of MAOIs (eg, tranylcypromine 10 to 20 mg/day orally), though not entirely benign from a cycling standpoint, might be preferable in such patients. Other alternatives, possibly free of cycling effects (in combination with lithium), include trimipramine, trazodone, and, especially, bupropion, though more systematic data are needed in this regard. In the approach to bipolar depressives, it is best to continue lithium, to avoid TCAs for mild relapses, to limit MAOIs to the lowest possible dose for a few weeks in moderate relapses, and to treat severe cases with ECT. Because borderline hypothyroidism—disclosed with an exaggerated TSH response to TRH—also predisposes to rapid-cycling, hormone augmentation of lithium therapy (eg, with L-thyroxine [T4], 100 to 200 μg/day orally) is often beneficial in many rapid-cycling bipolar patients. The anticonvulsants carbamazepine and valproate can also be useful in many rapid-cycling patients; some psychiatrists have successfully combined one of these anticonvulsants with lithium, endeavoring to keep both drugs at 1/2 to 2/3 the usual dosage (see below).

Precautions in pregnancy: In women who wish to have a baby, it is best to wait for at least 2 yr of episode-free prophylaxis before prescribing a lithium holiday, which should come *before* giving up contraceptive measures. This is to avoid the risk of cardiovascular (Ebstein's) anomalies in the 1st trimester. For a serious relapse in the 1st trimester, ECT would be a safer alternative to antidepressant medication, which, if absolutely necessary, can be used at other times during pregnancy, but should be stopped 1 to 2 wk before delivery and resumed a few days postpartum. Such mothers should not nurse, as these drugs pass through the milk.

Side effects: The most common **acute benign side effects of lithium** consist of tremor, fasciculation, nausea, diarrhea, polyuria, polydipsia, and weight gain (partly attributed to high-calorie beverages). These effects usually are transient and often respond to a slight decrease in dosage (and use of diet soft drinks). They are minimized when the dosage is divided throughout the day (eg, tid) or when slow-release forms are used; this is convenient during the first 6 to 12 mo of stabilization. However, once the dosage is established for a given patient, it may be prudent in those at risk for kidney disease to give the entire dose following the evening meal—which may improve compliance despite possible peaking of side effects at night; the troughs in the blood level with single daily dose are believed to protect the kidneys. Empirically, some clinicians advocate short courses of a β blocker such as atenolol 25 mg orally daily or bid for incapacitating tremor.

Toxic effects are manifested initially by gross tremor, increased deep tendon reflexes, persistent headache, vomiting, and mental confusion and may progress to stupor, seizures, and cardiac arrhythmias. Apart from overdose, lithium toxicity is more likely in elderly patients and those with renal disease with decreased creatinine clearance and with Na loss that may result from fever, vomiting, diarrhea, or diuretics; nonsteroidal analgesics other than aspirin may also contribute to hyperlithemia. None of these represent absolute contraindications to lithium but may dictate assessment of baseline renal function (eg, creatinine clearance), lower doses, dietary Na supplementation, frequent serum lithium determinations, follow-up of renal function with 24-h urine volume, urine concentration, and creatinine clearance tests. It is likewise desirable to obtain TSH response to TRH challenge and other thyroid indexes when thyroid disease is suspected. Otherwise, in healthy patients with relatively stable mood, quarterly serum checks and weight recording—together with biannual determination of creatinine and TSH—usually are sufficient.

The more common **chronic side effects** of lithium include mild leukocytosis (of no functional significance), exacerbation of acne and psoriasis (which may require dermatologic management), hypothyroidism (successfully managed with thyroid supplementation), and nephrogenic diabetes insipidus (which may respond to reduction of dosage or temporary interruption of lithium therapy). Individuals with a history of parenchymal kidney disease may be at some risk for structural damage to the distal tubule. Therefore, serum lithium levels generally should be maintained at the lowest level compatible with freedom from incapacitating mood swings. As noted, giving the entire therapeutic dose at bedtime may further protect against kidney complications. For lithium overdose, see under Complications, below.

Alternatives to lithium: In the noncompliant, cantankerous manic patient, a **depot phenothiazine** such as fluphenazine decanoate 12.5 to 25 mg IM q 3 to 4 wk is customarily given (see TABLE 63–6). Because of the risks for tardive dyskinesia, lithium should be resumed as soon as feasible. In bipolar patients with mood-incongruent psychotic features beyond the usual boundaries of "pure" mood disorder, intermittent courses of depot uroleptics often prove to be necessary as well. Recent clinical experience suggests that the antiepileptic **carbamazepine** in doses of 400 to 1250 mg/day orally may be the drug of choice in such patients. As noted above, carbamazepine is also increasingly used in other refractory bipolar cases with rapid-cycling, mixed manic, or dysphonic features, especially those in whom sleep-deprived EEG or nasopharyngeal leads reveal abnormal temporal spiking. *Because of the risk of agranulocytosis, clinical vigilance and periodic CBCs are prudent. Valproate,* also an antiepileptic, in dosages of 250 to 1500 mg/day, is being explored clinically in such refractory bipolar patients and offers the advantage of hematologic safety; hepatic function should be monitored carefully though it is rarely a problem in adults. **Phototherapy** is a new approach to seasonal bipolars from the ranks of bipolar II (autumn-winter depression and spring-summer hypomania). All of these novel approaches to refractory cases are best reserved to physicians with special experience and expertise.

Psychotherapy: Enlisting the support of a family member is crucial for the success of lithium prophylaxis. Patients and their significant others are often placed in "lithium groups" devoted to psychoeducational sessions on the nature of bipolar illness, its social sequelae, lithium therapy, and its problems. Bipolar patients may complain of being overcontrolled and of being less alert and creative; therefore, considerable psychotherapeutic skills are needed to ensure compliance to maintenance doses of lithium. Actual decrease in creativity is relatively uncommon, because lithium generally offers the opportunity for more even performance, and patients are able to put order in their lives, such as in interpersonal, scholastic, professional, and artistic pursuits. Individual psychotherapy with a practical focus may further help patients to cope better with their living problems and adjust to their new self-identities. Interventions with the patient's spouse or family to abate interpersonal crises secondary to mercurial moods are also helpful. It is important to teach patients to avoid stimulant drugs and alcohol, to minimize sleep deprivation, and to recognize early signs of relapse. For those patients with financial extravagance, finances should be turned over to a trusted family member. Those with a tendency to sexual excesses should be made aware of conjugal consequences and the spectre of AIDS.

Treatment of Cyclothymic and Dysthymic Disorders

Cyclothymics should be taught how to live with the extremes of their temperamental inclinations, though this is not easy because of their stormy interpersonal relations. The decision to give a lithium trial depends on the functional impairment produced by the unpredictable mood swings, but this should be balanced against any social or creative benefits the patient might be getting from hypomanic swings and the potential adverse effects of lithium treatment. Antidepressants are best avoided in view of the cyclothymic's elevated risk for rapid-cycling.

For **dysthymia**, especially with a bipolar family history, a vigorous trial of a noradrenergic HCA such as desipramine (if necessary, augmented by adding lithium carbonate) may help. Sedating HCAs given at bedtime can benefit selected patients with anxious-insomniac features, though it is generally best to avoid minor tranquilizers in dysthymics. Vocational counseling is also important, because some dysthymics, by the nature of their work-oriented temperaments, are suited for certain types of vocations that involve much dedication to painstaking detail; such measures would obviously fail in more lethargic patients. Recent clinical experience supports the usefulness of fluoxetine in selected, especially lethargic-hypersomnic, dysthymics. A trial with tranylcypromine is also worthwhile for such patients. Although traditionally the domain of psychodynamically oriented psychotherapy, dysthymics are also being increasingly treated by behavioral and cognitive approaches.

Complications

Social consequences. Mood disorders, especially when recurrent or chronic, may poison family life and rob children of optimal parenting. Frequent episodes of bipolar illness, not well controlled often because of inadequate treatment or noncompliance with maintenance chemotherapy, result in uneven productivity, dilettantism, bankruptcy, ruined careers, and repeated marital breakdown. Early recognition and comprehensive approaches to the treatment of recurrent mood disorders minimize such complications.

Secondary alcoholism and sedative-hypnotic abuse, the latter often iatrogenically facilitated, as well as stimulant or cocaine abuse as self-treatment are common risks in inadequately treated or unrecognized recurrent mood disorders. Detection of mood disorders, especially in the children of bipolar adults, and knowledge of their pharmacologic management are important for primary care physicians. Finally, it is important to note that minor tranquilizers and sedative-hypnotics by themselves are of little therapeutic value in mood disorders.

Modest increase in mortality from cardiovascular causes occurs in bipolar illness, is not accounted for by cardiotoxicity from lithium and TCAs, and tends to involve nonaffective first-degree biologic relatives as well. The reasons for this are obscure.

Suicide, the most serious risk, causes 15% of deaths in untreated mood disorders and tends to occur within 4 to 5 yr from the first clinical episode. The recovery phase from depression (when psychomotor activity is returning to normal but the mood is still dark) is a major risk period, as are the premenstrual period and personally significant anniversaries. (See also Ch. 60).

Recent USA data indicate some decline of suicide in middle-aged men and increases in adolescent, young adult, and elderly men over age 30. Findings from mood and lithium clinics suggest that changes may be occurring in the epidemiology of suicide, in that lithium and ECT-treated patients are underrepresented in suicide statistics. This may be due to personalized follow-up strategies by such clinics or, more hypothetically, the lithium correction of the serotonergic deficit. Recent research has provided us with the provoca-

tive possibility of biochemical prediction of suicide; these experimental data suggest that those who have the lowest levels ($<$ 15 mg/mL) of CSF 5-hydroxyindoleacetic acid (5-HIAA), the major metabolite of serotonin, are at the highest risk for suicide. Other biologic risk factors include family history of suicide, even when the proband was raised away from the biologic relative. Family history in an individual who has made suicidal communication, along with traditional clinical risk factors and sociodemographic indicators (eg, substance-abusing men at any age, especially when unemployed and lacking social support) dictate greater clinical vigilance and specific preventive measures (eg, hospitalization, specific pharmacotherapy). (See also Ch. 60.)

Barbiturates are much less commonly used today, and all emergency physicians and those in primary care must be familiar with TCA and lithium overdose (see also TABLE 145-4), the most likely medications to be ingested by suicidal patients; alcohol often is a complicating factor. TCA overdose presents as a hyperactive coma with atropinism, and the usual causes of death are cardiac arrhythmias and status epilepticus. Because of protein-binding, forced diuresis and hemodialysis are useless and treatment effort centers on measures to stabilize cardiac and cerebral function. Similar effort also is vital with lithium overdose, but forced diuresis with sodium chloride or mannitol and alkalinization of urine and hemodialysis could prove lifesaving. Newer cyclic antidepressants such as fluoxetine and bupropion appear safe in suicidal overdoses. The prevention of suicidal behavior is theoretically possible by early diagnosis and rigorous clinical management of mood disorders, because unrecognized or inadequately treated depression contributes to at least 70% of all completed suicides. This question, though untested in a prospective design, is such a major public health concern that all physicians—especially those in primary care—should participate in the early detection and appropriate treatment of depressive disorders.

58. SCHIZOPHRENIC DISORDERS
(See also Ch. 46)

The schizophrenic disorders, as defined by the American Psychiatric Association's Diagnostic and Statistical Manual of Mental Disorders, Third Edition (DSM-III, 1980) and its revision, DSM-III-R (1987), are mental disorders with a tendency toward chronicity, which impair functioning and are characterized by psychotic symptoms involving disturbances of thought, perception, feeling, and behavior. Six specific criteria for the diagnosis include (1) certain psychotic symptoms, delusions, hallucinations, formal thought disorder; (2) deterioration from a previous level of functioning; (3) continuous signs of the illness for at least 6 mo; (4) a tendency toward onset before age 45; (5) symptoms not due to mood (affective) disorders; and (6) symptoms not due to organic mental disorder or mental retardation.

The DSM-III definition eliminates several entities included in the DSM-II concept. Syndromes that look like schizophrenia but last < 6 mo are called **schizophreniform**. Psychotic syndromes of < 2 wk duration which follow a significant psychosocial stressor are now called **brief reactive psychoses**. Borderline or latent schizophrenia and simple schizophrenia are now diagnosed **borderline** or **schizotypal personality disorders**. Late onset of schizophrenia-like syndromes (eg, the involutional paraphrenias) are diagnosed **paranoid disorder** or **atypical psychosis**. Organic mental disorder or mental retardation and affective disorder are specifically excluded.

The category of **schizoaffective disorder** (see below under differential diagnosis) has been significantly narrowed. Most patients with mixtures of schizophrenic and affective symptoms are better diagnosed as schizophrenics or suffering from mood (affective) disorders (see also Ch. 57).

Subtypes of schizophrenia are described under Course and Diagnosis, below.

Historic Background

Important differences exist among patients with schizophrenia's characteristic cluster of signs and symptoms, and providing a clear demarcation between this behavior and other types of madness has proved difficult. Perceptive, seasoned clinicians from the 17th to the 19th centuries did their best to differentiate what today we call schizophrenia from melancholia, from mania due to fever and that due to wine, from the enfeeblement of the aged, and from brain damage such as that suffered during a war. (The notion of **paranoia** had emerged long before that; its first meaning being simply, "beyond understanding.") Although schizophrenia had many names (stupidity, foolishness, vesania, idiocy, insanity of puberty, monomania, paranoia, etc), early clinicians described the characteristics of family origin, endogenous cause, early onset, remitting or progressive course, bizarre ideation, dissociation of thought and emotion, and social withdrawal, thus moving toward a useful psychiatric classification by using the criteria of symptomatology, course, and outcome.

The concept of dementia praecox was developed from 1896 on, based on the early onset of the tendency toward a deteriorating course. Soon the idea of underlying disturbances in certain psychologic processes, and the distinction between primary and secondary symptoms, were introduced, with attempts to interpret the latter according to freudian psychoanalytic theory. The name "schizophrenia" was coined in 1908, referring to the disconnection or splitting of the psychic functions, believed to be an outstanding symptom of the whole group. It was thought that the illness need not always begin early and could end in various ways, including a so-called social remission; but it was not certain that full recoveries occurred without leaving a scar. No definite pathologic, anatomic, or biologic abnormalities were established. However, the unmistakable disturbances of thought, perception, feeling, and behavior had been recognized. An alternative hypothesis holds that schizophrenia is a recent disease, which explains why more specific descriptions of the disorder were rarely cited before 1800. Although not necessarily incompatible with the view of its ancient origin, this hypothesis claims that some biologic change occurred about 1800, following which a new type of schizophrenia became more common.

Incidence

Schizophrenia occurs worldwide. Using a relatively narrow concept of the disorder, studies of European and Asian populations show the lifetime prevalence to be 0.2% to almost 1%. Higher rates have been found in the USA and USSR, but the criteria used are much broader. Schizophrenia most commonly becomes manifest in late adolescence or early adult life, although paranoid schizophrenia typically has a later onset. Even with available therapy, schizophrenics occupy about 1/2 the hospital beds of mentally ill and mentally retarded patients, and about 1/4 of all available hospital beds. The high prevalence in lower socioeconomic classes has been mainly attributed to social disorganization and consequent stresses, but there is evidence that this association arises partly because some patients in a prepsychotic phase drift down the social scale.

Etiology

We understand little about the etiology of schizophrenia. Most cases are now thought to be caused by a complex interaction between inherited and environmental factors. Current scientific models include those regarding schizophrenia as primarily biologic in origin (genetic, internal environment, or neurophysiologic model), with environmental factors playing only a minor role; and those that consider the cause primarily environmental (ecologic, developmental, or learning model), with the biologic factors playing the minor role. Even in the most advanced biologic model (the genetic), no direct evidence exists. It is based on data that an individual who has a consanguineous relative suffering with schizophrenia has a higher risk of developing an episode, and that the risk varies with the degree of consanguinity. As none of the theories can be shown to be both necessary and sufficient, a vulnerability model is introduced. A genetic predisposition is probably necessary for schizophrenia to occur, but overt manifestations of illness seem to be decided partly by stressful life experiences; eg, faulty patterns of upbringing and disturbed relationships. Those who develop schizophrenia in middle age or later often are unmarried, widowed, or suffer from a serious physical handicap such as deafness.

Attempts to identify the nature of the schizophrenic defect before symptoms appear (eg, the study of a schizophrenic's blood relatives who are not ill, and psychologic studies of eye tracking, reaction time crossover, and span of attention) are under investigation. Other technologies being used to further study how the brain processes information include experimental psychology (masking and dichotic learning), psychometrics (the development of interviewing techniques), and information processing (memory retrieval). Advanced technology in genetics may make it possible to identify certain traits in parallel with the presence of gene maps. There are also new investigations in neuropathology, CT, MRI, positron emission tomography, and cerebral blood flow measurements.

Premorbid personality: Although no specific personality type is seen in all cases, many patients who develop schizophrenia show such traits as hypersensitivity, shyness, unsociability, lack of affect, and paranoid attitudes. Difficulty in personal relationships and social isolation inevitably result. The term **schizoid personality** is used to denote persons with defective capacity to form social relationships; **schizotypal personality** describes those who, in addition to their deficiencies in social relations, show oddities of thinking, perception, communication, and behavior that are not severe enough to meet the criteria for schizophrenia. Schizoid and schizotypal personalities are discussed in Ch. 52.

Recently, a 2-syndrome hypothesis of schizophrenia was introduced, suggesting that there are 2 main types of schizophrenia. **Type 1, or positive schizophrenia,** is characterized by good premorbid adjustment, acute onset, prominent positive symptoms, good response to drug therapy, and hyperdopaminergic transmission. **Type 2, or the negative syndrome,** is characterized by poor premorbid adjustment, insidious onset, prominent negative symptoms, cognitive impairment, structural brain abnormalities, and poor response to treatment. Like most dichotomies, this may be an oversimplification, but its value has been to generate questions as to causes, course, and treatment.

Symptoms and Signs

Thought disorder: Clear, goal-directed thinking becomes increasingly difficult, as shown in a diffuseness or woolliness and circumstantiality of speech. Sudden and incomprehensible changes of subject and obvious flaws in reasoning occur because distraction by fringe associations and the patient's private symbolism determine his thinking as much as does normal logic. "I have always believed in the good of mankind but I know I am not a woman because I have an Adam's apple" seems nonsensical. However, the patient who said this suffered doubts about his sexual identity and believed that a battle for good and evil was raging within him; his implicit identification of women with evil, the switch from mankind to woman (presumably because of the syllable "man"), the search for reassurance by choosing a minor sexual difference because of its symbolism, and the condensation of the themes illustrate the schizophrenic disturbance of thinking. Some schizophrenics report a stoppage of thinking **(thought blocking)** or may claim that their thoughts are **broadcast** or shared with others; delusional interpretations of these experiences (see below) lead to the belief that their minds are being controlled by external agencies. Thinking may be impoverished in many chronic schizophrenics.

Emotional (affective) changes: Blunting and inappropriateness (incongruity) of affect are the most characteristic emotional changes and are obvious and not easily overlooked in severe cases. Minor blunting and incongruity may be difficult to evaluate, since their assessment is subjective and therefore unreliable. Any mood disturbance—depression, excitement, anxiety, elation—may occur, and perplexity is not uncommon in acute schizophrenia.

Perceptual disorders: Auditory hallucinations are the most common, but hallucinations of sight, touch (including sexual sensations), smell, and taste may occur. The auditory hallucinations range from whistling, humming, or machinery sounds to an indirect muttering of voices or clear, complex conversations. Auditory hallucinations can occur in many disorders, but certain types, especially hallucinations of a running commentary on the patient's actions or of voices talking about the patient, strongly suggest schizophrenia.

Delusions: Delusions of persecution are frequent, as are those involving hypochondriacal or religious ideas, jealousy, and sexual identity (particularly homosexuality). Delusions of grandeur are common but also are often found in other disorders, such as in the manic phase of manic-depressive psychosis (see Ch. 57). Delusional interpretations of strange experiences such as thought blocking or broadcasting and depersonalization may lead the patient to believe that telepathy is occurring, that a mechanical device is recording his thoughts and conversation, or that he is under the control of an external agency. The patient suddenly may develop a delusional system that explains in a flash a whole succession of preceding puzzling events that he viewed with ill-defined suspicion, perplexity, or an inexplicable feeling of menace. This type of delusion, almost invariably diagnostic of schizophrenia, may convince the patient of his special significance—that he is the Messiah or the innocent victim in the center of a conspiracy—or provide immovably strong explanations for previous experiences. The delusional system may seem illuminating to the patient but is baffling and incomprehensible to others.

Catatonic signs: Disturbances of movement range from gross overactivity and excitement to marked retardation and even stupor with mutism. Posturing may occur, and the patient may take up a bizarre position (crucifix, or head raised several inches from the pillow) for prolonged periods. Extreme negativism or automatic obedience is sometimes seen. Mannerisms such as a mincing gait, grimaces, or overemphasis of normal movements are more common. Chemotherapy and improved individual management have made severe catatonic symptoms increasingly rare. Catatonic signs are also observed in patients with organic brain disease; eg, carbon monoxide intoxication, cerebral neoplasms.

Violent behavior: Although threats of violence and even minor aggressive outbursts are common

in acute schizophrenic states and relapses, dangerous behavior occurring when the patient obeys commanding voices or attacks his persecutors is uncommon. Occasionally, grotesque violence, with self-mutilation (often of sexual organs) or murderous attacks, may occur. Matricide, the rarest form of murder, is most often perpetrated by schizophrenics, as is filicide. Petty crimes may be committed by a "down and out" chronic schizophrenic patient. The risk of suicide is increased in all stages of schizophrenia.

In addition to violent behavior associated with the psychotic state (including organic brain disease), there are individuals with personality disorders, including the schizoid or schizotypal types, who become severely isolated, depressed, and paranoid and who may seek resolution of their difficulties in an aggressive act (eg, physical attack, murder, assassination) against someone whom they perceive as a single source of their abject state. The victim is usually someone in authority (eg, a parent, teacher, popular idol, or prominent political leader) or a sweetheart, spouse (see Othello syndrome in Ch. 59), or child. In their tormented thinking, these patients appear to seek recognition, love, and honor for their "heroic" act, but at the same time they seem to expect and welcome death as punishment and escape. Hence, the aggressive action usually culminates in suicide.

Nonspecific symptoms: Withdrawal from external reality and failure to coordinate internal drives are frequent findings. There may be abnormalities of psychomotor activities; eg, rocking, pacing, peculiar motor responses, or immobility. The patient may often appear perplexed, eccentrically groomed or dressed, and disheveled. Poverty of speech is common, and ritualistic behavior associated with magical thinking often occurs. The patient may be depressed and exhibit anxiety, anger, or both. There may be ideas of reference and hypochondriacal concerns. Rarely, during a period of excitement, a patient may be confused or disoriented, but usually there is no significant disturbance in the sensorium.

Course and Diagnosis

Even in cases with **acute** onset (commonly of the catatonic or paranoid subtypes) and with an apparent relationship to stressful events in the environment, careful history taking often reveals a prodromal period of weeks or months of increasing withdrawal and disorganization of the previous level of functioning. During the active phase, characteristic symptoms involve psychologic processes (content of thought, language, perception, affect), volition, motor behavior, sense of self, and relationship to the external world. A residual phase often follows the active phase and may be similar to the prodromal phase, but at times with persistent delusional beliefs and emotional blunting.

In order to distinguish schizophrenic disorders from short-term reversible illnesses, DSM-III-R requires that schizophrenia be diagnosed only when continuous signs have lasted for at least 6 mo, and that this period include an active phase of psychotic symptoms with or without a prodromal or residual phase. However, in many patients the deterioration is so gradual that it is difficult to trace back to a specific time when illness supervened in the schizoid personality.

In the early stages of schizophrenia, the patient may become increasingly uneasily aware that his psychologic integrity is impaired. He may worry over his lack of concentration or fear that he is going insane. His personal identity may be threatened by doubts of his sexual gender. He may symbolize his awareness of illness in terms of an internal battle between good and evil or project his feeling of internal dissolution onto the environment as fantasies of the annihilation of the world by some holocaust. The patient's physician as well as family members should constantly be alert to signs of suicide intent.

The onset of schizophrenic behavior in the **adolescent** period often makes it difficult to reach a clear diagnosis. Atypical depressions, anxiety states, identity confusion, and most particularly drug abuse and alcohol may mask, herald, or compound the onset of the psychosis. In the adolescent, when the illness is identified, it is most important to engage those involved in the patient's social network in order that they be properly informed and supported and become ready to cooperate in the care of the patient. These include not only the parents and siblings but also teachers, counselors, employers, etc.

DSM-III-R has classified the course as **subchronic** (< 2 yr), **chronic** (> 2 yr), **subchronic with acute exacerbation**, **chronic with acute exacerbation**, and **in remission**. In the past, schizophrenia was divided into 2 distinct patterns of onset. The first (**reactive**) is the development of illness in a person who has shown satisfactory social functioning but who often possesses an anxious and insecure temperament. This type of illness is frequently precipitated by a traumatic event and has a rapid onset. Patients

with the second pattern (**process type**) have a history of poor social functioning, have few friends, and show occasional bizarre habits. They are described as isolated, shy, and withdrawn (schizoid). There is no distinct precipitating event; the illness begins with a gradual downhill course into withdrawal and isolation.

Certain symptoms commonly cluster together but no clear demarcation exists between **subtypes of schizophrenia**, and individual patients may shift from one to another in successive episodes or even in the same illness. The term **undifferentiated** is used when the episode is characterized by prominent psychotic symptoms not classifiable in any specific subtype, or when it meets the criteria for more than one. Currently, those subtypes of schizophrenia without overt psychotic symptoms (ie, latent, borderline, or simple schizophrenia) are to be diagnosed as **borderline or schizotypal personality disorders**. The emphasis in **hebephrenia (disorganized type)** is on silliness and incongruity of affect and thought disorder with increasing autism (profound withdrawal into the self). Delusions, hallucinations, and other minor catatonic symptoms (eg, mannerisms) are often present, and the personality is severely disorganized. In **catatonia**, movement disorders predominate, with increasing motor agitation or retardation and gross posturing. Autism is extreme. **Paranoid schizophrenia** includes delusions of persecution or grandeur, thought disorder, and hallucinations, but there is less personality disintegration than in other subtypes. In **chronic schizophrenia**, all subtypes tend to have a clinical picture in which blunting of emotion and drive and incoherence or poverty of thought are the dominant features. Delusions, hallucinations, passivity, and catatonic symptoms all may persist, usually with diminished intensity. The diagnostic criteria for **residual type** include a history of at least one previous episode of schizophrenia with chronic psychotic symptoms, and a clinical picture without any prominent psychotic symptoms but continuing evidence of the illness (eg, blunted affect, social withdrawal, and poverty of thought).

Differential diagnosis: Altered states of consciousness are rare in schizophrenia. However, when this occurs accompanied by a clustering of schizophrenic symptoms, it may indicate an organic cerebral etiology caused by toxic (drug, metabolism, infection) or other organic factors. The organic delusional symptoms associated with amphetamines, cocaine, and phencyclidine should be considered particularly. Paranoid disorders are usually distinguished from schizophrenia by the absence of prominent hallucinations, incoherence, or bizarre delusions.

DSM-III-R asserts that affective symptoms are consistent with the diagnosis of schizophrenia and that schizophrenic symptoms are consistent with the diagnosis of affective disorders. The distinction for syndromes with both kinds of symptoms rests upon course. **Schizoaffective disorder** (see also Ch. 57) should be diagnosed whenever the clinician is unable to make a differential diagnosis between schizophrenia and affective disorders, and when there is an episode of affective illness in which preoccupation with mood-incongruent delusions or hallucinations (persecutory delusions, bizarre delusions) dominates the clinical picture and when affective symptoms are no longer present. DSM-III-R's use of the diagnoses of **schizophreniform syndromes, brief reactive psychoses,** and **borderline** or **schizotypal personality disorders** are described in the beginning of this chapter.

Prognosis

Schizophrenia is not necessarily a chronic disorder. About 30% of patients recover completely, and most of the remainder show some improvement. The florid symptoms can nearly always be controlled, but blunting of emotion and drive may remain intractable. Although even minor defects may impair personal relationships and work efficiency, partial remission is compatible with a reasonable life adjustment. With treatment, an active psychosis commonly is controlled within 4 to 8 wk, but residual defects of varying severity may persist for weeks or months before further improvement. Relapse is common unless adequate followup and medication are maintained. Acute exacerbations requiring therapeutic intervention often occur; residual impairment usually increases between episodes. A favorable prognosis is associated with good premorbid personality and adequate social functioning, the presence of precipitating events, abrupt onset, onset late in life, a clinical picture that includes confusion or perplexity, and a family history of affective disorder.

Treatment

The mainstays of treatment are chemotherapy, the development of a therapeutic relationship with a skilled counselor, social support, and graded rehabilitation and retraining. For a first illness or an acute relapse, **hospitalization,** even if involuntary, is usually indicated to ensure a thorough diagnostic study; to stabilize the patient on a suitable chemotherapeutic regimen; to ensure the physical safety of the patient or other persons; to prevent damage to finances, work prospects, or personal relationships; and to relieve the family. Although most states have legal restrictions insisting that hospitalization take place only if the patient is dangerous to himself or to others, the prevailing practice remains dependent on the psychiatrist's clinical judgment of the necessity for hospitalization. However, since schizophrenics are readily susceptible to institutionalism and since family ties are loosened by prolonged separation, hospitalization for more than a few months is harmful unless the severity of the illness makes it essential or it is part of an active rehabilitation program.

Chemotherapy: see Ch. 63.

Electroconvulsive therapy (ECT): In catatonic patients or those with severe depression, elation, or excitement, ECT accelerates the response to antipsychotic drugs; 4 to 10 treatments may be required. Controlled trials comparing ECT with neuroleptics show no advantage for ECT. In essence, ECT has limited usefulness in schizophrenia.

Psychotherapy, counseling, and social management: Working with the patient and his family helps to alleviate distress and problems of work and personal relationships, to establish patterns of readjustment, and to uncover and work out stresses that precipitate schizophrenic episodes. Analytic psychotherapy is not indicated, but establishing a therapeutic relationship with frequent discussions and the therapist's concern and interest is essential. In the initial stages (except rarely when there is no alternative), the therapist should not argue or flatly deny the reality of the patient's psychotic beliefs. Agreeing with the patient, on the other hand, risks compounding and reinforcing such beliefs. A neutral attitude may be achieved by focusing discussions on problems (including the patient's distress) to which the beliefs have given rise. With increasing insight, simple interpretation of certain ideas may be discussed.

Occupational therapy and graded social involvement should be arranged. For those who are more disabled, a comprehensive structured rehabilitation program including employment retraining may be planned. The needs of the family should be considered, and a trained social worker may be helpful.

Primary in the care of chronic schizophrenics is careful control of environmental pressure.

Overstimulation (in the form of high expectancies, high emotional involvement with relatives, or excessive work loads) can cause either a florid exacerbation of symptoms or autistic withdrawal. Understimulation may occur in the home, particularly with overprotective parents, and in the hospital (institutionalism). In evaluating the handicaps of a chronic schizophrenic, it is good practice to assume, in order to avoid therapeutic nihilism, that secondary handicaps from over- or understimulation are present and outweigh the primary defects of the illness. Individual psychotherapy combined with appropriate family and milieu therapy helps foster direct, forthright, and less stressful communication between the patient and his world.

Self-help/mutual-aid groups of spouse, parents, and children have greatly increased in number and contribute to the reduction of shame, guilt, and fear through their concerted efforts to help members support each other, reduce myth and misinformation, and promote hope. The range of treatments that focus on practical help for patients and their families in managing everyday problems includes family management (the patient's family is encouraged to reduce stress in the home as much as possible); hiring neighbors to look after schizophrenics; 24-h crisis teams; and the use of protected environments, in which sheltered jobs and living space for schizophrenics leaving hospitals are made available.

59. DELUSIONAL (PARANOID) DISORDERS

States of heightened self-awareness with a marked tendency to self-reference and projection of the patient's own unconscious ideas to others. In common usage "paranoid" implies persecutory beliefs or attitudes held by the patient.

Paranoid states range imperceptibly from a circumscribed delusional system with no impairment of affect or associative processes, to the more complete disorganization seen in paranoid schizophrenia. This is reflected in inadequate affective responses, increasingly disorganized associations, and symbolization and projection of unconscious mental material as hallucinations.

Etiology

The personality that spawns a paranoid illness reflects a need to shield sensitive portions of inner life, a hunger for recognition, and the fears and guilt feelings these conflicts and strivings evoke. There are 4 main psychologic theories of paranoid phenomena; ie, the shame-humiliation, homosexual, hostility, and homeostatic theories. The **shame- humiliation** theory is considered preferable because of its greater explanatory range and its ability to include the others as special cases. In brief, this theory postulates a concern about inadequacy that, when activated by relevant input, in turn activates the paranoid mode of symbol-processing procedures whose function it is to forestall a threatened perception of humiliation detected by an anticipatory shame signal.

Brief paranoid states: These states, which are often of a psychotic intensity, are reactive illnesses in persons whose personalities are characterized by extreme sensitivity, insecurity, inferiority, and suspiciousness. Isolation from social contact and physical problems (eg, deafness) often are exacerbating factors, and alcoholism is commonly involved. In acute and chronic brain syndromes, the impaired comprehension and dulling of consciousness favor paranoid interpretations and delusions.

The onset generally is quite sudden, and these disorders usually are of < 6 mo duration; they rarely become chronic.

Paranoid psychosis (see also Ch. 52): Typically, a highly elaborated delusional system gradually develops without hallucinations, disorganization of thinking, or other characteristic schizophrenic symptoms. A few patients, however, eventually progress into frank schizophrenic illness. In one form of paranoid psychosis, core symptoms center on some minor real or imagined physical defect. The patient delusionally misinterprets facial expressions or overheard scraps of conversation as confirming his belief that he is discriminated against because of this defect. In other patients, a trivial or illusory asymmetry of face or enlargement of the nose is the focus for a paranoid system. Such patients may trail from specialist to specialist incessantly demanding plastic surgery. Real or imagined slights or injustices may lead to never-ending litigation, or religious fanaticism may insidiously progress to grandiose but encapsulated messianic beliefs.

In one dangerous form of paranoid psychosis, delusional sexual jealousy is the central theme. Jealousy has a complex psychopathology, and morbid jealousy occurs in a variety of conditions, including conjugal paranoia (**Othello syndrome**), which is limited to delusions of jealousy involving the spouse. A primary depression may underlie the illness. The patient's anguish over delusions of his spouse's infidelity is readily converted to rage. The patient may unceasingly make accusations, spy upon or follow his spouse, examine undergarments for seminal stains, and misinterpret simple actions, such as the way a curtain is drawn, as a message to the lover. He may demand confession constantly and assert that forgiveness will ensue. Physical assault is a real danger.

A persecutory delusional system may develop as a result of a close relationship with another person who already has a disorder with persecutory delusions. This type of induction psychosis is a result of sharing the delusions of the dominant person. In the past this disorder has been termed **folie à deux**. In rare instances more than 2 persons may be involved. The prognosis for what is now called **shared paranoid disorder** is a function of the emotional strength of the person in whom the psychosis has been induced.

Symptoms and Signs

Before the psychosis becomes manifest, prodromal symptoms may occur. The patient may have reacted to numerous situations with wounded and bitter pride. He overanalyzes his moods and sensations, may become hypochondriacal, is reserved, and withdraws in disdain from discussing his problems. Gradually, the idea may be born that his failures have been due to the enmity of others, and he sees new and hidden significance in commonplace events, leading to the belief that people deliberately slight him and that his situation is endangered. He experiences vague fears, becomes increasingly resentful, and defends his suspicions vigorously. Hallucinations may or may not occur.

Patients with classic paranoia or reactions closely approximating it probably never recover; however, they do not necessarily deteriorate and may not require hospitalization. If their conduct remains within bounds, society may view them as cranks. However, some patients who at first appear to be suffering from circumscribed paranoid psychoses are later recognized to be schizophrenic.

The history may show that, as a child, the patient needed special appreciation, was moody, resented school and parental discipline, could not form good play adjustments, and was suspicious. While growing up, the rigidity and tendency to pride may have increased, as well as the patient's sensitivity to others' attitudes toward him.

Diagnosis

In contrast to mania, paranoid ideas are more sustained and are supported by a less changeable affect than are manic vacillations. The mental operations are exaggerations of normal mechanisms, and differentiating patients with paranoid psychoses from nonpsychotic patients with extremely paranoid, embittered personalities can be difficult. A patient is psychotic if the reaction is continuous, if his beliefs cannot be corrected, if they tend to spread, and if they are completely illogical and cause major functional impairment. These reactions can be classified as approximating either the paranoid or the schizophrenic pole by evaluating the degree of disturbance in the individual's contact with reality; the more the repressed material comes into consciousness as delusions and hallucinations and the more archaic the form of adjustment, the nearer the reaction approaches schizophrenia. The patient with delusional (paranoid) disorder remains more intact as a person than does the traditional schizophrenic patient (see Ch. 58).

The rapid development of a paranoid illness, particularly in a previously well-adjusted personality, should lead to a very careful clinical assessment and investigations to exclude an underlying organic disorder due to systemic illness (eg, hypothyroidism), brain disease (eg, neurosyphilis), or drug toxicity (eg, amphetamines).

Treatment

The patient should be hospitalized if he is a potential danger to himself or to others. When delusions are directed against specific persons, confinement is often necessary; the greater the expressed hatred, the more imperative is commitment. (See also the discussion of hospitalization under Treatment in Ch. 58.) Establishing a relationship with the patient is a vital step; psychotherapy then will alleviate distress and often modify behavior, even though essential delusional thinking is unaltered. In dealing with paranoid patients, honesty and truthfulness are even more necessary than in approaching other mental sufferers. The patient's concerns should be discussed, and the therapist should try to express an understanding of the patient's point of view, without agreeing with his delusions, belittling them, or strongly contradicting them. Often the patient will follow reasonable suggestions and greatly modify his behavior. The physician may become the patient's one confidant and can help him by being tolerant and combining a philosophic detachment with sympathetic humility, discretion, understanding, warmth, and a sense of humor about his own possible ineptness as well as the patient's peccadilloes. A temporary serenity may be achieved by helping the paranoid patient to reach a calmer environmental adjustment. The physician also can aid in unraveling family problems or irritating work situations.

Antipsychotic drugs (see Ch. 63) are helpful and often minimize symptoms, though complete remission is uncommon even after prolonged drug treatment. In morbid jealousy, neuroleptics are most effective when onset was not insidious. Similarly, antidepressants may, at times, afford some limited benefits. However, it is difficult to persuade patients with this illness to undergo prolonged treatment.

60. SUICIDAL BEHAVIOR
(See also Chs. 46 and 57)

Suicidal behavior includes both completed and attempted suicide. An **attempted suicide** is a suicidal act that was not fatal, possibly because the self-destructive intention was slight, vague, or ambiguous. Most persons who attempt suicide are ambivalent about their wish to die, and the attempt may result from a strong wish to live and a need to communicate a plea for help. When suicide plans and actions appear unlikely to succeed, they are often termed **suicide gestures** and are predominantly communicative in nature. However, a suicide gesture should not be dismissed lightly; it is an important cry for help and requires thorough evaluation and treatment aimed at relief of misery and prevention of further attempts, especially since 20% of those who attempt suicide repeat the attempt within a year and 10% finally succeed. **Completed suicides** differ in many respects from attempted suicides; the differences are discussed below. However, the distinction is not absolute, since attempted suicides also include acts by persons whose determination to die is thwarted only because they are discovered early and resuscitated effectively, and since a suicide attempt may be fatal by miscalculation.

The discussion in this chapter is based on the above categorization. However, a distinction also can be made between **direct destructive behavior** (which usually includes 3 distinctly different groups of phenomena: suicidal thoughts, suicide attempts, and completed suicides) and **indirect self-destructive behavior** (characterized by taking a life-threatening risk without an intention of dying, generally repeatedly, and often unconsciously in such a way that the consequences are ultimately likely to be destructive to the individual). This latter behavior covers a wide variety of phenomena; eg, excessive drinking and drug use, heavy smoking, overeating, neglect of one's health, self-mutilation, polysurgical addiction, hunger strikes, criminal behavior, and deviant traffic behavior.

Incidence

Statistics on suicidal behavior are based mainly on verdicts recorded on death certificates and at inquests, and they underestimate the true incidence. Even so, suicide ranks among the first 10 causes of death for adults in urban communities. It accounts for 10% of deaths between the ages of 25 and 34 and for 30% of deaths among university students. It is the second-ranking cause of death among adolescents (see also SUICIDE IN CHILDREN AND ADOLESCENTS in Ch. 46). Of the approximately 200,000 suicide attempts in the USA each year, 10% are successful. More than 70% of completed suicides are over 40 yr of age, and the incidence rises sharply above age 60, particularly for men. About 65% of attempted suicides are under the age of 40.

Attempted suicides account for about 20% of emergency medical admissions and for 10% of all medical admissions. Women make 2 to 3 times as many suicide attempts as men, but men are generally more successful in their attempts. Adolescent single girls are overrepresented among attempted suicides, and the incidence also is high among single men in their 30s. Several studies have found a higher incidence of suicides among the families of patients who have attempted suicide.

Marriage, for both sexes (particularly a secure relationship), is associated with a significantly low suicide rate; suicide attempts and completed suicide are higher among those alone because of separation, divorce, or spouse's death.

Among blacks, the suicide rate is lower than among whites, but suicide among black women has increased 80% in the last 20 yr. Among **American Indians** the rate has risen in recent years, and in some tribes it is 5 times the national average.

A number of suicides take place in **prisons,** particularly by young men who have not committed violent crimes. Hanging is the usual method, and the suicide is most likely to occur during the first week of imprisonment. Hunger strikes accompanied by suicidal declarations, particularly among political prisoners, occur from time to time. Here, the intention to influence attitudes and behavior of others is overt. Self-injury and death are means to an end rather than goals. **Group suicides,** whether in large numbers or involving only two (as in lovers' or spouse suicides), represent extreme forms of personal identification with others. Suicides in large groups tend to occur in highly emotive settings that overcome the strong drive to self-preservation.

Professional persons, including lawyers, dentists, military men, and physicians, seem to have higher than average suicide rates. The physician rate is largely due to female physicians, whose annual rate of suicide is 4 times that of a matched general population. As for the suicide method, there is a high incidence of overdosage with drugs among both male and female physicians (as compared with the general population), possibly because of easy access and knowledge as to what constitutes a fatal dose. Of the medical specialties, the highest rate is among psychiatrists.

Suicide is less frequent among practicing members of most **religious groups** (particularly Roman Catholics), who are generally supported by their beliefs and are provided with close social bonds protecting against acts of self-destruction. The low rates that have been reported from Catholic countries are only in part due to a tendency of coroners to avoid verdicts of suicide; the rate appears to be actually lower. However, religious affiliation and strong religious beliefs do not necessarily prevent impetuous, unpremeditated suicidal actions that occur in settings of frustration, anger, and despair, especially when associated with delusions of guilt and unworthiness.

Suicide notes are left by about 1 in 6 persons who complete suicide. The notes often refer to personal relationships and events that will follow the patient's death. In the elderly, they often express concern for those left behind, whereas in younger people they may be angry or even vindictive. In attempted suicides, a note indicates premeditation and a serious risk of repeated attempts and, later, completed suicide.

Methods Used in Suicidal Acts

The choice of methods is determined by both cultural factors and the availability of the agent. The methods used also may reflect the seriousness of intention, since some (eg, jumping from heights) make survival virtually impossible, whereas others (eg, drug ingestion) provide a chance of being rescued. However, the use of a method that proves not to be fatal does not necessarily imply that the intention is less serious. A bizarre suicide method suggests an underlying psychosis.

Drug ingestion is the most frequent method used in suicide attempts. The use of barbiturates has decreased, whereas the use of other psychotropic drugs is increasing. Salicylate use has dropped from > 20% of cases to about 10%, with the more frequent use of acetaminophen, which is perceived by the public to be a safe analgesic. However, acetaminophen overdose can be very dangerous (see Ch. 30 and TABLE 145–4).

Two or more methods or a combination of drugs are used in about 20% of attempted suicides, increasing the risk of a fatal outcome, particularly when drugs with serious interactions are combined. Multiple drug ingestion makes it important to determine blood levels of all the possibilities when a patient is seen.

Violent methods such as shooting and hanging are uncommon among attempted suicides. Use of firearms has been the leading method of completed suicide in the USA for males, and the percentage has increased (from 58% in 1970 to 63% in 1980). For females the most frequent method in the past was poisoning, followed by firearms. However, as of 1980, the frequencies for females have reversed (firearms, 39%; poisoning, 27%). Furthermore, suicide rates by the use of firearms vary with the availability of guns and handgun regulations.

Etiology

The psychologic mechanisms leading to suicidal behavior resemble those frequently implicated in other forms of self-destruction, such as alcoholism, reckless driving, self-mutilation, and violent antisocial acts. Suicide is often the final act in a course of self-destructive behavior. Traumatic childhood experiences, particularly the distresses of a broken home or parental deprivation, are significantly more common among persons with a tendency to self-destructive behavior, perhaps because these persons are more likely to have serious difficulties establishing secure, meaningful relationships. Recent studies have shown an association between attempted suicide and the phenomena of battered wives and child abuse, reflecting a cycle of deprivation and violence within the family.

Suicidal acts usually result from multiple and complex motivations. The principal causative factors (see also TABLE 60–1) include **mental disorders** (primarily depression), **social factors** (disappointment and loss), **personality abnormalities** (impulsivity and aggression), and **physical illnesses**. Often, one factor (commonly a disruption in important relationships) is the last straw. An aggressive component often is evident; when its distressing impact is considered, the act appears to be directed at other, significant persons. Homicide followed by suicide provides clear evidence of hostility, as does the high incidence of suicide among prisoners serving terms for violent crimes.

Depression is involved or apparent in over half of all attempted suicides, and although endogenous in some cases, in most the depression is reactive or neurotic. **Social factors** such as marital disharmony, broken and unhappy love affairs, disputes with parents among the young, and recent bereavements (particularly among the elderly) may precipitate the depression. Depression associated with **physical illness** may lead to a suicide attempt, but physical disability, particularly if chronic or painful, is more commonly associated with completed suicide. Physical illness in the elderly, particularly if serious, chronic, and painful, plays an important role in about 20% of suicides.

Among **schizophrenic** patients, suicide sometimes occurs, and in chronic schizophrenia, suicide may result from the episodes of depression to which these patients are prone. The suicide method is usually bizarre and often violent. Attempted suicide is uncommon; it may be the first gross sign of psychiatric disturbance, occurring in the early stages of the illness, possibly when the patient becomes aware of the disorganization of his thought and volitional processes.

Alcohol predisposes to suicidal acts by aggravating the intensity of any depressive mood swing and by lowering self-control. About 30% of patients who attempt suicide have consumed alcohol before the act, and about half of these were intoxicated at the time. Since alcoholism itself, particularly "binge alcoholism," often causes deep feelings of remorse in the intervening periods, alcoholic patients are particularly suicide-prone even when sober. In one follow-up study of alcoholics, 10% of patients committed suicide. Improved treatment programs for alcoholics probably would reduce the suicide rate.

Organic brain disease in its acute form of **delirium** (which may be due to drugs, infection, heart failure, etc) or as **dementia** may be accompanied by emotional lability, when serious violent acts of self-injury may occur during a deep but transient depressive mood swing. Consciousness usually is impaired during the act, and the patient may have only a vague recollection of the event. **Epileptic** patients, especially those with temporal lobe epilepsy, frequently suffer brief but profound episodes of depression, which, together with the availability of drugs prescribed for their condition, put them at a greater-than-normal risk of suicidal behavior.

Individuals with **personality disorders** are prone to attempted suicide, especially emotionally immature persons with a psychopathic personality, who tolerate frustration poorly and react to stress impetuously with violence and aggression. A history of excessive alcohol consumption, drug abuse, or criminal behavior is sometimes found. The large number of attempted suicides among separated or divorced persons may reflect an inability to form mature, lasting relationships and imply reduced social opportunity, loneliness, and depression. The precipitants in such cases are the stresses that inevitably result from the dissolution of even troubled relationships and the burdens of establishing new associations and life-styles. Another important aspect in attempted suicide is the element of "Russian roulette," in which the person decides to let fate determine the outcome. Some unstable persons find excitement in this aspect of such perilous activities as reckless driving, dangerous sports, and other forms of toying with death.

TABLE 60–1. HIGH-RISK FACTORS FOR SUICIDE

Personal and Social Factors	Clinical Features and Symptoms
Male sex	Depressive illness, especially at onset or toward end of illness
Age > 55 yr	
Recent separation, divorce, or widowhood	Marked motor agitation, restlessness, and anxiety
Social isolation with real or imagined unsympathetic attitude of relatives or friends	Marked feelings of guilt, inadequacy, and hopelessness; self-denigration or nihilistic delusion
Impulsive, hostile personality	Severe hypochondriacal preoccupations: delusion or near-delusional conviction of physical disease, eg, cancer, heart disease, or sexually transmitted disease
Personally significant anniversaries	
History of suicide in family, or of affective disorder	
	Command hallucinations
Unemployment or financial difficulties, particularly if causing a drastic fall in economic status	Alcohol or drug abuse
	Physical illness that is chronic, painful, or disabling, especially in patients who have previously enjoyed good health
Previous suicide attempt	
Detailed planning and taking precautions against being discovered	Use of drugs (eg, reserpine) that can cause severe depression

Prevention of Suicide

Any suicide act or threat must be taken seriously. Although some attempted or completed suicides are a surprise and shock even to close relatives and associates, in most cases clear warnings are given, generally to relatives, friends, medical personnel, or volunteers in lay organizations offering a 24-h service to those in distress. Emergency suicide prevention centers attempt to identify the potentially suicidal person, maintain conversation, evaluate the risk, and offer help with immediate problems, usually calling upon others (family, physician, police) for urgent assistance in the crisis and trying to guide the suicidal person to appropriate facilities for follow-up assistance. Although this is a logical approach to helping potentially suicidal individuals, no hard data indicate that it does reduce suicide incidence.

The average physician encounters 6 or more potential suicides in his practice each year. More than half of suicides have consulted their physicians within the previous few months, and at least 20% have been under psychiatric care during the preceding year. Since depressive illness is often involved in suicide, recognition and treatment of depression are the most important contributions a physician can make to suicide prevention. Each depressed patient should be questioned carefully about any thoughts of suicide. The fear that such inquiry, even in a tactful and sympathetic form, may implant the idea of self-destruction in the patient is baseless. The questioning aids the physician in obtaining a clearer picture of the depth of the depression, encourages constructive discussion, and conveys the physician's awareness of the patient's deep despair and hopelessness. The use of rating scales (eg, Beck Depression Inventory) may be helpful in confirming the seriousness of the depressive illness with regard to suicide risk.

Features indicating a possibly high risk of suicide are shown in TABLE 60–1, above. Treatment of depression is outlined in Ch. 57. The risk of suicide is increased early in the treatment of depression, when retardation and indecisiveness are ameliorated but a depressed mood and feelings of gloom still persist. Early results of treatment may, therefore, enable the patient to set about self-destruction effectively in a state of only partially lifted depression. Psychotropic drugs must be prescribed carefully and in controlled amounts. Insomnia may be a symptom of depression, and to treat it with hypnotics without treating the underlying depression is not only ineffective but highly dangerous.

For **dealing with an acute suicide threat** (eg, a patient who calls and declares that he is going to take a lethal dose of a drug or the person who threatens to jump from a height), only general advice can be given. In these situations the desire to die is ambivalent and often transient, and the physician or other person to whom the patient appeals for help must ally himself with the desire to live. The person threatening suicide is in an immediate crisis, and the physician should offer hope that it can be resolved. Emergency psychologic aid may be provided by (1) establishing, a relationship and open communication with the patient; (2) reminding him of his identity (ie, using his name repeatedly) and helping him sort out the problem that has brought on the crisis; (3) offering constructive help with the problem and encouraging the patient to positive action; and (4) involving the patient's family and friends, reminding the patient that others care for him and want to help.

If a patient calls to say that he has already committed a suicidal act (eg, taken a drug or turned on the gas) or is in the process of doing so, his address should be obtained, if possible, and someone else should immediately contact the police to trace the call and attempt a rescue. The patient should be kept talking on the telephone until the police arrive.

A comprehensive follow-up service providing adequate psychiatric and social after-care is, at present, the best means of reducing further suicide attempts and completed suicide. Since many patients who commit suicide have a previous history of suicidal attempts, a psychiatric assessment (see below) is important for *all* patients as soon as feasible after a suicide attempt. This identifies some of the problems that contributed to the act and permits appropriate treatment planning.

Management of Attempted Suicide

Many people who attempt suicide are admitted to a hospital emergency ward in a comatose state. When it is certain that the patient has ingested an overdose of a potentially lethal drug, it is important to (1) remove the poison from the patient, attempting to prevent absorption and expedite excretion; (2) institute symptomatic treatment to keep the patient alive; and (3) administer any known antidote if the specific drug ingested can be firmly identified (see Ch. 145). Every person with a life-threatening self-injury should be hospitalized both to treat the physical injury and to obtain psychiatric assessment. Most patients are well enough to be discharged as soon as the physical injury is treated, but *all should be offered follow-up care* (see below; and under Prevention of Suicide, above).

Psychiatric assessment is made immediately after a suicide attempt, and at this time the patient may deny any problems. Not uncommonly, the severe depression that led to the suicidal act is followed by a short-lived mood elevation, a cathartic effect probably responsible for the finding that further suicide attempts are rare immediately after the initial attempt. Nevertheless, the risk of later, completed suicide is high unless the patient's problems are resolved. The patient needs a secure, strong source of help, which begins when the physician provides sympathetic attention and clear indications of concern and commitment as well as understanding of the patient's troubled feelings.

Steps in the psychiatric assessment are (1) establishment of rapport; (2) understanding the suicide attempt, its background, the events preceding it, and the circumstances in which it occurred; (3) appreciation of the current difficulties and problems; (4) thorough understanding of personal and family relationships, which often are pertinent to the suicide attempt; (5) full assessment of the patient's mental state, with particular emphasis on the recognition of depression, alcohol or drug abuse, and mental illness, which require specific treatment in addition to crisis intervention; and (6) an interview with the spouse, close relative, or friend, and contact with the family physician.

Although the management of suicidal patients can be satisfactorily dealt with by the **involvement of nonmedical personnel** trained in the management of suicidal behavior, it is desirable that the initial assessment be made by a psychiatrist.

Hospitalization: Duration of stay and the kind of treatment required vary. Patients with psychotic illness, organic brain disease, or epilepsy, and some with severe depression whose crisis situation has not resolved, should be admitted to a psychiatric unit for continued supervision until their underlying problems are resolved or can be coped with. The role of the patient's family physician after a suicide attempt is central. If he is not in charge of the case, he should be kept fully informed and given specific suggestions for follow-up care.

Impact of Suicide on Others

Any suicidal act has a marked emotional impact on the associated persons. The completed suicide, especially, leaves physician, family, and friends with strong feelings, which include guilt, shame, and remorse at not having prevented the latest attempt, as well as anger, directed toward the suicide or others. However, the physician must realize that neither he nor the patient's family is omniscient or omnipotent and that the patient's eventual completed suicide was ultimately not preventable. The physician also should recognize that he has the remaining important task of helping the suicide's family and friends deal with their guilt feelings and sorrow.

The impact of attempted suicide on the associated persons is similar in nature to that produced by the completed suicide, but with the important difference that the opportunity remains to resolve these feelings by recognizing and responding appropriately to the "cry for help."

61. PSYCHIATRIC EMERGENCIES

An emergency may be created as much by circumstances as by an event. Behavior that excites comment and action in public may be tolerated at home and regarded as hardly worthy of comment in a psychiatric ward. For the purposes of this chapter the circumstances are those of a general practitioner's office, an emergency ward, or a medical ward. Optimally, the setting should provide privacy, safety, and security for both patient and physician.

Obtaining a good history in an emergency may be impossible, and accounts given by excited relatives or bystanders can be biased or colored by personal involvement in the dramatic and unusual situation. At times, attention to the emotional concerns and needs of family is essential. In some emergencies diagnosis is critical to decision-making, but in others a symptom such as excitement or aggression constitutes the emergency, and diagnosis may have to await its control.

The term **acute psychosis** has been used to characterize certain disorders with impaired capacity to process information. Some cases involve known or knowable organic abnormalities (eg, delirium—see below). Other cases, with unknown causes, are often called **acute functional psychosis** (eg, acute mania or acute schizophrenia)—for their management, see Ch. 57 or Ch. 58.

Panic; Anxiety Attacks
(See also in Ch. 56)

In battle and in periods of civil catastrophe, anxiety is normal, but individuals who are subjected to particularly severe stress or who are especially vulnerable can be incapacitated by terror. They may manifest tremors or dissociative symptoms and bizarre or dangerous behavior. Sedation is valuable, and a tactical withdrawal from the stressful situation for a few days is helpful. Prolonged withdrawal, however, is associated with a considerable risk of chronicity.

In less stressful situations, attacks of acute anxiety occur in susceptible patients. Many anxiety attacks are so brief that the acute phase is over before the patient can reach a doctor. In most cases the anxiety is generalized, but diagnostic problems can arise if various body systems are affected to different degrees, so that cardiovascular manifestations are prominent in one patient and GI symptoms in another. If **overbreathing (hyperventilation)** is the salient feature, the patient may complain of dizziness, lose consciousness, or show signs of tetany.

In everyday circumstances it may be difficult to determine what precipitated an anxiety attack, and advice to separate the patient from the anxiety-provoking situation often is gratuitous. Reassurance sometimes is sufficient to allay the patient's distress, and reassuring relatives and bystanders is helpful. If mild sedation is required, the benzodiazepines (eg, diazepam 5 to 10 mg or oxazepam 15 to 30 mg orally) usually are effective. In more disturbed patients diazepam 10 mg may be given IM or even IV. Major tranquilizers have no advantage over the benzodiazepines in these circumstances. Tricyclic or monoamine oxidase inhibitor (MAOI) antidepressants may prevent the occurrence of panic disorder. Hyperventilation usually will stop if the patient's attention is drawn to it and he is given quiet and supportive reassurance.

Victims of natural disasters or of violence, such as accident, crime, rape, or spouse abuse, require special attention to medical, social, and educational services, provided with concern for individual needs. In addition to the treatment of immediate anxiety (see above), referral to self-help groups and to psychotherapists may be advisable.

Delirium

Delirious patients are a common problem in medical and surgical wards. Acute delirium may be due to toxic drug ingestion (including alcohol); overdose of prescribed medication, particularly anticholinergics; metabolic disorder (including electrolyte imbalance); infection; trauma; seizures; or withdrawal from alcohol and drugs. Acute delirium also may occur as an idiosyncratic reaction to a normal dose of medicine and is not uncommonly seen in situations of intense stress, such as in cardiac care units. It is more common in the elderly.

Difficulties arise when a confused patient with impaired comprehension passively interferes with his medical treatment, or when a patient who becomes paranoid or delusional and begins to hallucinate becomes actively uncooperative and threatens or attacks the nursing staff or dismantles therapeutic equipment. Some patients are elated and overcheerful and disturb the ward by shouting and singing. Others are panic-stricken and may injure themselves in attempts to escape from imaginary persecutors.

Treatment of the cause of the delirium and good nursing care, along with general measures to make the patient comfortable and keep him safe, are needed. For example, keeping lights on during the night and permitting someone known to the patient to stay with him are effective calming maneuvers. Often a major tranquilizer or diazepam administered orally or parenterally must be given urgently; the pharmacologic treatment is similar to that of an excited patient (see below).

Acute Memory Disturbances

Although memory disturbances are most commonly organic, memory loss that presents as an emergency usually is hysterical (see in Ch. 56). Patients with massive dissociation can no longer recall their identity or events of their past; language and knowledge of social customs generally survive. In hysterical pseudodementia, of which the Ganser syndrome is one example, cognitive functions are more profoundly dissociated, and regressive behavior results. In many of these patients a traumatic and often "shameful" event precedes the onset of the dissociation. The patient's memory may return with quiet and persistent interviewing, but hypnosis or abreactive drugs such as amobarbital sodium IV (200 mg slowly infused usually is adequate) may be indicated. Other hysterical symptoms (eg, loss of vision, deafness, muteness, or paralysis) may require similar treatment.

Transient global amnesia creates similar difficulties and may be mistaken for hysterical amnesia. Remote memory is unaffected. There is no treatment for an attack of transient global amnesia; memory is recovered spontaneously in a few hours.

Dementia rarely presents as an emergency but may create one. A solitary patient who has been quietly deteriorating for months or years may be found in a state of indescribable squalor and neglect or may be brought to a doctor's office or emergency ward with no history and no informant. Some patients with AIDS may first present with dementia.

Stupor

Unconsciousness is always an emergency, and in some psychiatric disorders the degree of withdrawal is so substantial that a noncommunicative and unresponsive patient appears unconscious. The symptom of catatonia may be associated with organic brain disease such as carbon monoxide intoxication, encephalitis lethargica, and brain tumors. This condition may also occur in catatonic schizophrenia, severe depression, and hysteria. If a history is available from a friend or relative, earlier characteristic symptoms may indicate the diagnosis, but great care must be taken to ensure that organic causes are not overlooked. Amobarbital sodium IV (200 mg slowly infused usually is adequate) is useful diagnostically in distinguishing hysterical, catatonic, and organic states; may relieve hysterical stupors; and often leads to a temporary remission in catatonic stupor. The technique should be used only by those with specific training and experience. Both catatonic and depressive stupor respond to electroconvulsive therapy.

Excitement, Anger, and Aggression

Although excitement, anger, and their physical concomitant, aggression, occur in a wide range of psychiatric disorders (schizophrenia, mania, psychopathy, and, rarely, in temporal lobe lesions including epilepsy and delirium), the precise diagnosis may be academic if the patient is disturbed and violent. Calm words may not stem the patient's wrath, but meeting his anger with further anger will only aggravate the situation. Violent and potentially violent patients are secured as soon as the diagnosis is made or suspected.

An attempt to persuade the patient to take medication should be made; eg, diazepam 5 to 40 mg or haloperidol 5 to 10 mg orally. However, in most cases a parenteral route will be necessary, despite the patient's verbal and physical objections. This raises medico-legal questions, and physicians should be familiar with local laws and regulations that apply to the management (including commitment) of acutely disturbed patients. Consultation with a psychiatrist or appropriate judicial authority will help protect the patient and the physician. Increasingly, it also appears to be the physician's responsibility to warn and protect threatened third parties. Once the decision to give an injection has been made, adequate forces should be mustered; in all cases security personnel are required. Once the patient has been properly restrained, a major neuroleptic, such as haloperidol 5 to 10 mg IM, should be injected as carefully as it would be in any other individual. The injection may be repeated hourly or more frequently until there is a satisfactory reduction of symptoms, or oversedation or other serious side effects intervene. The patient's vital signs should be carefully monitored. Total dosage varies greatly for different individuals, but failure to respond to 50 mg on the first day calls for reevaluation of the diagnosis. Six to 12 h after control is achieved, the patient may be given haloperidol orally, with the dosage based on the patient's individual needs. With this treatment, side effects (especially acute dystonic reactions) are common. They may be prevented by giving oral benztropine 1 to 2 mg bid. Some

centers are now using fast-acting benzodiazepines, such as lorazepam, instead of a neuroleptic or concomitantly to reduce the neuroleptic dose.

Suicide (see Ch. 60)

Substance Abuse
(See also Ch. 53)

An emergency room presentation is often a complication of substance abuse. Cocaine ("crack") and PCP may result in excitement and aggression; overdose with alcohol, other hypnotic-sedative drugs, or opioids may result in sedation or stupor; withdrawal may lead to discomfort, agitation, or delirium. Misuse or abuse of prescribed medications, as well as substance abuse, are more common in the elderly than is generally realized.

62. ANTIANXIETY DRUGS
(Anxiolytics; "Minor" Tranquilizers; Sedatives)

Anxiolytics, particularly the **benzodiazepines**, are the most widely prescribed psychotropic agents, prescribed more widely by primary care providers than by psychiatrists. Their use peaked in 1974 and has been declining continuously since, probably reflecting concerns of both the public and physicians about claims of excessive use.

It is clear that while these medications are frequently abused (eg, it is common for patients in methadone maintenance programs to test positive for benzodiazepines), the overwhelming majority of patients take these medications at less-than-prescribed doses and do not abuse them. Increasing attempts at regulatory restriction of benzodiazepines raise the question of whether limiting the access of drug abusers justifies the annoyance and stigma placed on the majority of patients who use these medicines briefly and appropriately.

This chapter focuses on benzodiazepines, the anxiolytics of choice for most patients; other drugs for the treatment of anxiety are considered briefly.

Basic Pharmacology of Benzodiazepines

All benzodiazepines are anxiolytics, sedatives, hypnotics, muscle relaxants, and anticonvulsants. Some of the differences in approved indications appear to be related more to

the pivotal studies done to get regulatory approval and to the sponsoring company's marketing plans than to pharmacologic considerations. Benzodiazepines are sometimes used as an adjunct to antipsychotics in an attempt to decrease exposure to dopamine blockers.

Selection of a particular agent should be based on rapidity of onset and duration of action. Thus, the ideal hypnotic should have rapid onset, and the ideal anticonvulsant should have a prolonged half-life ($t_{1/2}$). An anxiolytic used only occasionally, as needed, should have rapid onset, whereas this is relatively less important with continuous use of the anxiolytic. Marketing often does not follow this logic; thus, some drugs carrying hypnotic FDA indications have a slow onset and others have such a long $t_{1/2}$ as to invite accumulation and hangovers the next day. Since all benzodiazepines are hypnotic, alprazolam or lorazepam can also be used for sleep, and flurazepam can be used as an anxiolytic. Since these drugs have so many similarities, the wise practitioner becomes familiar with a few benzodiazepines rather than attempting to know them all.

All benzodiazepines are well absorbed when taken orally. Absorption after IM administration is unpredictable with the exception of lorazepam, the benzodiazepine of choice if IM medications are to be used. **Midazolam**, a benzodi-

TABLE 62–1. PHARMACOKINETICS OF REPRESENTATIVE BENZODIAZEPINES

Parent Generic Compound	Clinically Significant Metabolites	Approximate Dose Equivalence (mg)	Rapidity of Onset
Long-acting			
Chlordiazepoxide (5–30)	Desmethylchlordiazepoxide (5–30) Demoxepam Desmethyldiazepam (36–200)	10	Intermediate
Diazepam (20–100)	Desmethyldiazepam (36–200)	5	Fastest
Clorazepate*	Desmethyldiazepam (36–200)	7.5	Fast
Flurazepam*	Desalkylflurazepam (40–250)	30	Fast
Halazepam*	Desmethyldiazepam (36–200)	15	Intermediate
Prazepam*	Desmethyldiazepam (36–200)	7.5	Slow
Clonazepam (30–60)		2	Intermediate
Quazepam*	Oxoquazepam (25–40) Desalkylflurazepam (36–200)	7.5	Slow
Intermediate-acting			
Alprazolam (12–15)	α-OH-alprazolam Desmethylalprazolam	0.5	Fast
Lorazepam (10–20)		1	Intermediate
Oxazepam (4–15)		15	Slow
Temazepam (8–22)		15	Slow
Ultrashort-acting			
Triazolam (3–5)	α-Hydroxytriazolam	0.5	Fast

* Drug precursors that do not reach the systemic circulation in significant amounts without alteration.
NOTE: The half-life (in hours) for some compounds and metabolites is shown in parentheses.
Modified from Greenblatt DJ, Shader RI, Divol M, et al: "Benzodiazepines: A summary of pharmacokinetic properties." *British Journal of Clinical Pharmacology* 11:11S–16S, 1981; and also adapted from information appearing in Rosenbaum JF: "Current concepts in psychiatry: The drug treatment of anxiety." *New England Journal of Medicine* 306:401–404, 1982; used with permission.

azepine that is not used as an anxiolytic, is available for parenteral use only; it is very short-acting and confined to the induction of anesthesia and for use with invasive procedures such as endoscopy.

TABLE 62–1 lists the basic kinetic profile for most benzodiazepines. Most benzodiazepines have psychoactive metabolites; several are prodrugs for the same metabolites. The notable exceptions—lorazepam, oxazepam, and temazepam—are metabolized by glucuronide conjugation and have lesser potential for drug interactions. They tend to have shorter $t_{1/2}$s, making them better alternatives for elderly patients. The remaining benzodiazepines are metabolized via hepatic oxidation—a slow process, made even more lengthy by age or hepatic injury. Other drugs cleared through this system (eg, alcohol, cimetidine, disulfiram, oral contraceptives) are especially prone to interactions.

The $t_{1/2}$s listed in TABLE 62–1 are reasonable reflections of what will occur with regular use of the medications. Single doses have far shorter durations of action because these drugs are very lipophilic. They readily penetrate the blood-brain

barrier and have very large volumes of distribution. The net effect is that a single dose may have a fairly limited duration of action, whereas regular dosing will lead to a very longlasting effect. These drugs take a long time to reach steady state because of their prolonged $t_{1/2}$s.

Kinetics determine the appropriate role for specific benzodiazepines. Drugs with rapid onset of action make good hypnotics and also are favored by drug abusers. Drugs with a long $t_{1/2}$ are more suited for patients with generalized anxiety disorders. Elderly patients should receive short-acting benzodiazepines; others lead to unacceptable accumulation.

Toxicity of Benzodiazepines

The therapeutic index for benzodiazepines is quite high. Sedation, ataxia, and slurred speech may occur in patients who are overdosed with benzodiazepines. These effects are similar to those of alcohol intoxication. Almost all successful suicides associated with benzodiazepines reflect multiple medications, most typically including alcohol. Treatment of a benzodiazepine overdose is mainly supportive. The primary risk is from respiratory depression. A new drug, flumazenil, can reverse the effects of benzodiazepines after anesthesia or overdose. Another important role may be diagnostic. Patients with CNS depression of unknown cause should respond within minutes to flumazenil 5 mg IV if benzodiazepines are responsible.

There may be subtle cognitive impairment associated with benzodiazepine use; ie, affecting attention, concentration, and motor performance, even when on "therapeutic" dosages. Ultrashort-acting benzodiazepines, such as triazolam, have been associated with a transient anterograde amnesia. These drugs should be used with extra caution in the elderly.

Some patients may experience disinhibition with benzodiazepines, often leading to an increase in dose and further behavioral worsening. This is most likely to occur with cognitively impaired patients.

Benzodiazepines may also induce depression, which is more likely in those with a history of affective disorder.

Benzodiazepine abuse and dependence (see also DEPENDENCE ON ANXIOLYTIC AND HYPNOTIC DRUGS in Ch. 53): Most patients take less drug than prescribed and discontinue the medicine on their own. There are, however, 2 numerically small problem populations—street drug and alcohol abusers and those who take a high enough dose of prescribed medication for a long enough time to become dependent.

Benzodiazepine abuse and street sales tend to be part of a pattern of polysubstance abuse. They are commonly used to prevent the postcocaine "crash" and to augment the effects of opioids. Alcoholics may use benzodiazepines to avert symptoms of alcohol withdrawal. Their street market value is less than that of barbiturates.

There is considerable debate about benzodiazepine dependence. Patients almost never develop tolerance in the sense of needing to escalate dose to maintain effect. Benzodiazepines do not become the central part of patients' lives, and patients do not spend large amounts of time seeking them out. However, serious withdrawal problems can occur after prolonged use of high doses. It is impossible to give any absolute guidelines, but doses > 30 mg/day of diazepam or equivalent taken for > 4 mo should be cause for concern. Abrupt discontinuation after significant exposure may lead to a **withdrawal syndrome** remarkably similar to that associated with alcohol withdrawal, including anxiety, irritability,

tremor, nausea, hypertension, tachycardia, hyperacusis, muscle twitching, hyperreflexia, depersonalization, hallucinations, and major motor seizures. The severity of the withdrawal is correlated with the amount of previous exposure and to the $t_{1/2}$ of the benzodiazepine. Those with a short $t_{1/2}$ tend to expose the patient to frequent troughs, resulting in more severe withdrawal symptoms. Patients exposed to > 1 mo of benzodiazepines should have the drug tapered slowly, proceeding no more rapidly than 10%/day. Very long-acting drugs tend to taper themselves, and many clinicians substitute one of them at the time of discontinuation to ease this problem.

Because alcohol, barbiturates, and benzodiazepines are cross-tolerant, benzodiazepines are substituted for alcohol in the treatment of alcohol withdrawal (see DEPENDENCE ON ALCOHOL in Ch. 53).

An unresolved issue concerns discontinuation of drug in patients taking lower doses. The withdrawal syndrome discussed above represents the end of a continuum; lesser use followed by discontinuation may lead to a very muted version of the difficulties listed. For example, some patients who have been maintained on lower doses might have some anxiety or insomnia only after stopping the medicine, and it may not be possible to say whether this is a recurrence of the symptoms originally treated or a result of benzodiazepine dependence and withdrawal. Clearly, the best approach is to use benzodiazepines intermittently whenever possible, to avoid the development of dependence.

Treatment with Benzodiazepines

Very few patients need continuous treatment. The overwhelming majority of patients need only short-term or intermittent drug treatment. There always should be a simultaneous attempt to address the underlying cause of the anxiety.

The causes of anxiety are many, but ordinary environmental causes should be searched for first; eg, occupational or marital problems, difficulties with child-rearing, etc. Intrapsychic explanations (see below) may be more difficult to ferret out; a mental health professional may be helpful here. Many medical disorders can be significant; eg, hyperthyroidism, arrhythmias, chronic obstructive pulmonary disease, heart failure, abuse of caffeine or other stimulants, alcohol withdrawal, akathisia associated with antipsychotics, complex partial seizures, and pheochromocytoma.

Nongeriatric adults who require a benzodiazepine should probably be treated initially with oral diazepam 5 mg or its equivalent. A list of other agents and their relative potencies is included in TABLE 62–1.

Indications for benzodiazepines in the treatment of anxiety include acute situational stress, generalized anxiety disorder, and panic disorder (see ANXIETY NEUROSIS in Ch. 56 and Panic; Anxiety Attacks in Ch. 61). Prescriptions for acute situational stress should (by definition) be for limited amounts for a limited time. Patients with generalized anxiety disorder more nearly conform to the idea of trait, or continuous, anxiety and may require more chronic treatment. Dosage for these patients should usually begin with diazepam 5 mg orally bid or its equivalent. Adjustments of the dose should not be made until the patient is at steady state, which should be achieved once 4 to 5 t½s have passed (see TABLE 62–1). The dose should only very rarely need to go beyond 40 mg/day of diazepam or equivalent. Panic disorder, if not phobic avoidance, responds either to heterocyclic antidepressants such as imipramine, or to monoamine oxidase **(MAO)** inhibitors, or to high-potency benzodiazepines such as alprazolam. Antidepressants should be taken up to full antidepressant doses. Benzodiazepines typically will require at least 4 mg/day of alprazolam or equivalent. The decision to use a benzodiazepine in this context should not be entered lightly. Discontinuing the medicine will lead to a complicated differential of drug withdrawal vs. symptom reemergence. This is less of an issue when antidepressants are used.

Nonbenzodiazepine Anxiolytics

Antihistamines: These drugs are sedating rather than being true anxiolytics and may result in a sedated but internally agitated patient. They also have considerable potential for inducing delirium owing to their anticholinergic effects. Because of this, these agents are considerably less desirable for the treatment of anxiety.

Antipsychotics (see Ch. 63) exert an antianxiety effect, but *the risks of tardive dyskinesia and neuroleptic malignant syndrome preclude their use for this indication.*

Barbiturates: Prior to the advent of benzodiazepines, these were the agents of choice for the treatment of anxiety. Because of their toxicity, they have been superseded by the benzodiazepines for this indication. They are far more lethal in overdose, withdrawal syndromes are more common and more dangerous, and their abuse liability is higher. Most authorities recommend that their use be confined to anticonvulsant and anesthetic purposes. However, physicians experienced in their use continue to find barbiturates to be effective, safe, and economical when given to selected patients.

β Blockers: The British have long made a distinction between somatic and psychic anxiety. They associate the latter with the cognitive aspects of anxiety and the former with the peripheral, autonomic manifestations. β Blockers do a very reasonable job treating the peripheral manifestations. For some patients this is sufficient; if they do not have the usual autonomic associates of anxiety, they do not experience the full attack. β Blockers do very little to affect the cognitive parts of the disorder, so that while the tremor, the tachypnea, and the palpitations improve, the sense of dread is not altered for most. β Blockers are most clearly effective for those suffering from performance anxiety. Thus, public speakers, musicians, or surgeons may benefit from a single dose of a β blocker prior to the stressful event; eg, propranolol 40 mg orally 1 to 2 h before the performance. β Blockers should not be given to diabetics, to those in heart failure, or to asthmatics.

Buspirone: This recently developed agent's chief advantage over benzodiazepines is its limited toxicity. It does not cause sedation, interact with alcohol, affect the seizure threshold, nor is it a muscle relaxant. Its abuse liability is very low. Since it does not interact with the benzodiazepine receptor, it cannot be directly substituted for a benzodiazepine that has been in long-term use as the patient may experience benzodiazepine withdrawal. It also cannot be used for alcohol withdrawal.

In double-blind trials comparing buspirone and diazepam in chronically anxious patients, the 2 drugs appear to provide comparable benefit. However, a major consideration is that onset of effect with buspirone is not apparent until after 2 wk of treatment. Clinical experience appears to be falling short of the data from the controlled trials. It is not clear whether this reflects different populations or inappropriate use. There has not been much published on patients with more acute anxiety. It would appear that buspirone should be used for the patient with generalized anxiety disorder but is not useful for intermittent, acute anxiety.

Buspirone is typically initiated with a dosage of 5 mg orally tid and increased by 5 mg q 3 to 4 days until the effect is maximized. Doses > 40 mg/day have been associated with dysphoria.

63. ANTIPSYCHOTIC DRUGS
(Neuroleptics)

Since the first clinical use of chlorpromazine in the 1950s, the number of psychiatric beds has fallen by 75%. Other contributory changes (notably the development of the community mental health movement and pressure for deinstitutionalization) are trivial compared with the impact of chemotherapy. Until recently all antipsychotics operated via the same mechanism—blockade of the dopamine receptor. A new drug, clozapine, has a unique, largely unknown mechanism of action, which is associated with both different adverse effects and target symptoms and signs. It offers hope of successfully treating selected, previously refractory, patients (see separate discussion below).

Prescribing practices in antipsychotic dosing go through cyclic changes and seem to be entering a period of increasing conservatism, reflecting heightened awareness of such serious toxic effects as neuroleptic malignant syndrome and tardive dyskinesia.

Mechanism of Action

Except for clozapine, all antipsychotics act by blocking the dopamine receptor. The potency of these agents in blocking the postsynaptic dopamine (D_2) receptor correlates highly with their relative clinical potency, ranging from chlorpromazine on the low end of the spectrum to haloperidol on the high end. More milligrams of a low-potency agent are required to attain equivalent antipsychotic effect to a high-potency agent. This is so predictable that the amount of a drug is often translated into chlorpromazine equivalents. Thus, 1.6 mg of haloperidol represent 100 chlorpromazine equivalents. Since the positive drug effects follow from dopamine blockade, *all conventional antipsychotics are equally efficacious. Drug selection is based upon toxicity* (see TABLE 63–1).

Other receptors are also affected. Many adverse effects of these drugs can be predicted by knowledge of their effects on α-adrenergic, muscarinic, and histamine (H_1) receptors (see TABLE 63–2). **Blockade of H_1 receptors** is associated with weight gain, sedation, and possibly hypotension. **Antimuscarinic (anticholinergic) effects** lead to dry mouth, visual blurring, uri-

nary retention, constipation, tachycardia, and, in vulnerable patients, cognitive dysfunction and delirium. **Alpha$_1$ blockade** may lead to orthostasis. **Dopamine blockade** is associated with extrapyramidal syndromes **(EPS)** and probably with tardive dyskinesia and neuroleptic malignant syndrome (see below).

Since there are variable effects upon other types of receptors, it follows that the toxicity of 2 different agents might be additive, whereas desirable effects can be obtained by simply increasing the dose of one agent. Therefore, *the only indication to prescribe more than one antipsychotic at a time* is when the clinician is loading a patient on a very long-acting depot agent that has not yet had a chance to take effect.

Indications

The most common use of antipsychotics is for schizophrenia, yet these are not antischizophrenia drugs. Some of the symptoms of this disorder, such as apathy and amotivation, respond relatively poorly to conventional antipsychotics; others, such as assaultiveness, hallucinations, delusions, and thought disorder, respond quite well. These symptoms and signs may benefit from antipsychotics whether secondary to mania, schizophrenia, dementia, or drug ingestion. Like most psychotropics, antipsychotics are nonspecific; nonetheless, their indications are listed by diagnostic grouping.

Schizophrenia, schizophreniform disorder, and brief reactive psychoses: Treatment hinges around the phase of the illness.

Acutely agitated patients: These are rare, agitated patients who pose a risk to themselves or others. Rapid tranquilization may be justified to ensure safety for the patient and those around him but will not alter the fundamental course of the illness. High-potency agents, most typically haloperidol, are used. Oral dosing is almost as rapid as IM dosing and should be used unless the patient will not accept oral medication. For an average-sized nongeriatric adult either 10 mg orally or 5 mg IM should be used with doses repeated q 30 min until behavioral control is ob-

TABLE 63-1. COMMONLY USED ANTIPSYCHOTIC DRUGS

Class/Generic Name	Dose (mg) Equivalent	Comments
Phenothiazines		
Aliphatic		
Chlorpromazine	100	The original antipsychotic; the prototypic low-potency agent
Piperidines		
Thioridazine	95	The only agent with an absolute maximum (800 mg/day), owing to pigmentary retinopathy at higher doses; very anticholinergic
Mesoridazine	50	A first-pass metabolite of thioridazine
Piperazines		
Trifluoperazine	5	
Fluphenazine	2	Also available as fluphenazine decanoate and enanthate; these are IM depot forms for which dose equivalents are not available
Dibenzoxazepines		
Loxapine	15	
Dihydroindolones		
Molindone	10	Possibly associated with weight reduction
Thioxanthenes		
Thiothixene	3	Has very high incidence of akathisia
Butyrophenones		
Haloperidol	1.6	The prototypic high-potency drug; decanoate form is available
Diphenylbutylpiperidines		
Pimozide	1.3	Approved only for Tourette's disorder
Clozapine	50	Unique mechanism of action; weekly CBCs are required

Adapted from *A Concise Guide to Somatic Therapies in Psychiatry* by LB Guttmacher. Copyright 1988 by the American Psychiatric Press.

tained. It is most unusual to require > 3 doses. Such regimens are typically well tolerated. Dystonias and other EPS can occur for a day or more after such an aggressive approach, which should be reserved for emergencies.

Antiparkinsonian drugs are prescribed now only when extrapyramidal symptoms become manifest or if the risk of extrapyramidal symptomatology is great (see Adverse Reactions, below). The prophylactic use of antiparkinsonian drugs is indicated when patients have reacted adversely to neuroleptic medication in the past. Usually, antiparkinsonian drugs are given for a short period of time, perhaps < 3 wk, but in some instances with continuing parkinsonism, the use may be extended. Since antiparkinsonian agents are not without potential toxicity, periodic attempts to discontinue them are warranted.

Initial nonacute management: The goal moves from behavioral control to treatment of the more fundamental defect. Primary target symptoms include disorders of communication, stereotypies, hallucinations, delusions, and sleep alterations. Deficit symptoms such as amotivation, disordered affect, and diminished insight and judgment respond more rarely, but they are legitimate targets nonetheless.

The clinical efficacy and side effects of the butyrophenones, thioxanthenes, dihydroindolones, and dibenzoxazepines are the same as those of the phenothiazines. The choice of a specific drug is based largely on which adverse effects the patient will best tolerate. Males with sexual delusions should probably not be placed on low-potency drugs with their increased risk of engendering erectile dysfunction. Catatonic patients should not be placed on high-potency agents, as the differential between an iatrogenic dystonia and catatonia will be quite complicated. Previous response is the best guide to selection

TABLE 63-2. RECEPTOR AFFINITIES OF ANTIPSYCHOTIC DRUGS

Drug	Dopamine Affinity	Standardized Histamine Affinity	Standardized α_1 Affinity	Standardized Muscarinic Affinity
Chlorpromazine	1	1	3	1
Thioridazine	1	1	3	3
Mesoridazine	1	3	3	2
Loxapine	1	3	2	2
Molindone	0/1	0/1	0/1	2
Trifluoperazine	2	0/1	0/1	0/1
Fluphenazine	4		0/1	0/1
Thiothixene	4	0/1	0/1	0/1
Haloperidol	3	0/1	1	0/1
Clozapine	0/1	4	4	4

Based on in vitro receptor binding assays with human brain tissue.

Standardized affinity = $\dfrac{\text{Affinity for the given receptor}}{\text{Dopamine affinity}}$

Scores range from 0 = no effect, to 4 = marked effect.

Adapted from Black JL, Richelson E: "Antipsychotic drugs: Prediction of side-effect profiles based on neuroreceptor data derived from human brain tissue." *Mayo Clinic Proceedings* 62:369-372, 1987; used by permission.

of a medication. The full dosages of antipsychotic medication given to younger patients are liable to cause marked side effects and are rarely required in elderly patients (> 65 yr), who are particularly prone to the full panoply of toxicities, including orthostasis, urinary retention, and parkinsonism. Therefore, caution should be used in arriving at the appropriate, generally lower, dosage. Doses may well be only $^1/_5$ to $^1/_{10}$ of those required by younger patients.

Determining the initial dose is often difficult and hinges on such issues as the patient's age, size, and degree of agitation. Typical initial daily doses are 5 mg of haloperidol, 200 to 300 mg of chlorpromazine, or equivalent given orally. Doses may be divided until steady state is reached. Once this occurs, all of the medicine may be given at bedtime to enhance compliance and to make use of sedation. Dose changes should generally not be made more often than q 3 to 5 days. It may take 6 wk for the maximal impact of any given regimen to become apparent. Generally, doses > 20 mg/day of haloperidol or equivalent offer no advantage, although individual outliers require higher doses. Some data suggest that there is a "therapeutic window" for high-potency agents with a curvilinear response curve showing that either too much or too little of a given agent will not be effective.

While this chapter addresses psychopharmacology, we should not lose sight of the fact that psychopharmacologic treatment alone is not likely to be of benefit. Patients and their families should receive psychoeducational help, psychologic and social supports as discussed under Treatment in Ch. 58.

Maintenance therapy: The goals are to maintain or further the gains achieved during treatment of the acute phase and to prevent relapse. Maintenance with antipsychotic medications is probably best reserved for patients with schizophrenia, in whom they can be invaluable for preventing relapse. Antipsychotics may be effective for some patients with affective disorders, but they are more likely to induce tardive dyskinesia in this population.

It is difficult to know how long to maintain medications. Much of the decision will depend on the relationship between the patient, his family, and his physician. Patients who are likely to report in quickly when they sense the onset of their difficulty can be discontinued more rapidly. Patients who have good insight and reliable premonitory signs can also be maintained for a shorter time. Patients whose episodes begin suddenly and who get themselves into serious difficulties should be maintained longer. Many schizophrenics will not continue to take oral antipsychotic medication. Long-acting depot injections of fluphenazine enanthate or decanoate or haloperidol decanoate are, therefore, often preferred for maintenance treatment, and they reduce the risk of relapse (see below and TABLE 63-6). Depot therapy requires backup facilities. Many special medication clinics have been established, and nurses give defaulting patients their injections at home.

Antipsychotics are highly lipophilic. As a result, patients take a long time to clear them, and noncompliance is often followed by protracted periods when patients do quite well. It is, therefore, often difficult to make the association between discontinuation of the medication and reemergence of symptoms. For the same pharmacokinetic reason, it makes sense to taper the drug slowly. Ideally one would hope that patients will be able to tolerate discontinuation of the drug.

With rapid and complete recovery from an acute episode, drug therapy generally need not be continued for more than 3 to 6 mo after recovery. In more serious forms of illness, drugs should be continued for 2 to 3 yr, and some patients may require antipsychotic medication indefinitely. A rule of thumb of maintenance medication is to continue the patient at $1/3$ to $1/5$ of the dosage required during the acute phase of psychosis. The maintenance phase should be continued for 3 to 6 mo after discharge and tapered slowly for a trial period. A slow taper over several months has the advantage of allowing determination of the precise dose at which symptoms will break through. Periods of stress (family discord, job difficulties, emotional losses, physical illness) may require reinstitution of medication.

Depressive periods due to personal problems or a primary affective swing are not uncommon in otherwise well-controlled schizophrenics and require appropriate counseling and perhaps the prescribing of an antidepressant drug.

Mania: Long-term management should be with one of the thymoleptics such as lithium or carbamazepine. Antipsychotics should not be used routinely for prophylaxis due to the risk of tardive dyskinesia. However, acute manic episodes can be managed with either a thymoleptic such as lithium or an antipsychotic. Combinations of these agents act more quickly than either alone. Typically lithium is taken to blood levels of 1.0 to 1.4 mEq/L for acutely manic patients. Antipsychotic doses are more difficult to predict and should be titrated based on the patient's response.

Psychotic depression: In terms of efficacy, electroconvulsive therapy remains the best treatment for this disorder, followed by the combination of an antipsychotic and an antidepressant, then by either agent alone. Again, every effort should be made to discontinue antipsychotics as rapidly as the patient will tolerate.

Anxiety: Although antipsychotics are reasonably effective anxiolytics, there are safer alternative drugs (see Ch. 62).

Tourette's disorder: Pimozide, a very specific D_2 receptor blocker, associated with QT prolongation, has been approved in the USA for this disorder only. Oral doses typically range from 6 to 10 mg/day, not to exceed 10 mg/day or 0.2 mg/kg/day.

Behavioral dyscontrol associated with delirium and dementia: While antipsychotics are often helpful for the agitation experienced by these patients, they should not be used as a substitute for attempting to understand the origins of the agitation. Antipsychotics are used here purely as symptomatic treatment, but abolition of symptoms should not cause underlying factors, such as congestive heart failure or toxic medication, to be forgotten. Low-potency agents tend to be quite anticholinergic and can worsen patients who are already cognitively compromised. High-potency antipsychotics are to be preferred in the elderly, unless they are suffering from Parkinson's disease. Initial doses should be far lower, probably $1/5$ of those used with younger patients. Every effort should be made for discontinuation once the acute difficulties are resolved.

Treatment of the Refractory Patient

Patients with typical indications who fail to respond should probably be referred to a psychiatrist. Some of the questions that should be considered include the following: (1) Is the diagnosis correct? (2) Is the patient complying with the medication regimen? If not, why not? (3) Is the patient likely to respond to a different agent? This occurs rarely. If a patient fails to respond to an adequate trial of one agent, it is probably wise to switch to a completely different class (eg, from a phenothiazine to a butyrophenone or a thioxanthene). (4) Is the patient absorbing adequate amounts of the drug? Absorption is usually complete, yet one occasionally sees compliant patients who respond to parenteral, but not oral, agents.

A number of laboratories offer antipsychotic blood level measurements. These hold promise

TABLE 63-3. DRUGS FOR THE TREATMENT OF EXTRAPYRAMIDAL SYNDROMES

Class/Generic Name	Usual Dosage	Comments
Anticholinergics		
Benztropine	0.5–2 mg tid	1–2 mg IV for acute dystonia
Biperiden	2 mg daily or tid	
Procyclidine	2.5–7.5 mg tid	
Trihexyphenidyl	1–5 mg tid	2 mg IV for acute dystonia
Antihistamines		
Diphenhydramine	12.5–50 mg tid or qid	25–50 mg IV for acute dystonia
β Blockers		
Propranolol	10–20 mg qid	For akathisia, but not other EPS

for the future, but current technology and understanding do not warrant their use, except as a qualitative assay. Contrary to many laboratories' claims, there are insufficient data to justify discussing "therapeutic" levels. (5) Is there a place for adjunctive or nonpharmacologic treatment? Electroconvulsive therapy still has a role for some nonresponsive schizophrenics (see Ch. 58). Antidepressants, when combined with antipsychotics, may offer additional benefit. Clozapine (see below) should be considered. Nonbiologic interventions, eg, family therapy, behavioral treatment, psychosocial support, should be considered.

Adverse Reactions

Common initial side effects: The **extrapyramidal syndromes (EPS)** that result from the blockade of dopamine receptors include dystonias, parkinsonism, and akathisia. All EPS increase with anxiety, wax and wane, and disappear with sleep. They are all far more likely to occur with high-potency antipsychotics.

Dystonias can involve almost any part of the body but typically include opisthotonus, oculogyric crises, and torticollis. It is important to warn patients of this possibility as dystonias are extremely frightening for the uninformed. They are most common with young males and during the first 5 days after initiation of an antipsychotic or following an increase in the dose. Acute treatment is with either diphenhydramine 25 to 50 mg or benztropine 1 to 2 mg via a syringe slowly IV. These medications may also be given IM, but absorption and onset of action are slower and less predictable than with IV use. Such acute treatment should be followed by prophylactic measures such as lowering the dose of the antipsychotic, switching to a lower potency agent, or continued use of one of the agents listed in TABLE 63-3.

Drug-induced parkinsonism is indistinguishable from the idiopathic variety. Patients may develop masked facies, sialorrhea, festinant gait, cogwheeling, and a 3 cycles/sec tremor. Patients are at highest risk during the first 2 mo of treatment. Prophylactic treatment follows the same principles as for dystonia. Since parkinsonism, like other EPS, can present subtly, it is wise to develop a standardized examination for routine use. One variant is listed in TABLE 63-4.

Some patients have a behavioral form of **akinesia** characterized by amotivation, blunted affect, decreased speech, and apathy that seems to respond to the same measures effective in other EPS. These symptoms are difficult to distinguish from some of the deficit symptoms of schizophrenia and may raise the question of whether the patient is under- or overtreated. Since akinesia is a most subtle form of toxicity, the physician needs to be on the alert for this.

Akathisia is characterized by a sense of restlessness and anxiety. Patients often need to pace. Unlike other forms of EPS, akathisia is often unresponsive to anticholinergics; however, patients often respond well to propranolol.

Treatment with antiparkinsonian drugs is not benign. Anticholinergic agents carry the risks noted above for muscarinic blockade including urinary retention, constipation, failure of visual accommodation, cognitive impairment, and delirium. Dry mouth is very common and generally responds to good hydration and the use of sugarless chewing gums or candies. Since low-potency antipsychotics are often anticholinergic as well, they only rarely require coprescription with an anticholinergic.

Sedation is common with antipsychotics, especially with the low-potency agents. **Orthostatic hypotension** is also more frequent with the low-potency agents and is a common cause of falls among the elderly. Orthostatic vital signs

TABLE 63-4. SUGGESTED EXAMINATION FOR EXTRAPYRAMIDAL SYNDROMES

Observe gait, paying particular attention to arm swing and posture.
0 = Normal; 1 = decreased arm swing; 2 = No. 1 plus obvious rigidity; 3 = stiff gait, arms rigid before abdomen; 4 = stopped, shuffling with propulsion and retropulsion

Physician and patient should stand with arms extended to the side at shoulder height. On a signal, let arms drop.
0 = Normal with loud slap and rebound as they hit the side of the body; 1 = slowed drop, little rebound; 2 = no rebound; 3 = markedly slowed, no slap; 4 = arms fall very slowly as if against resistance

Rotate elbow and wrist, monitoring with other hand. Rate both arms separately for stiffness and cogwheeling. The same procedures can be done for the legs. Rate on a 0 to 4 basis.

Have patient hold out hands. Observe tremor then and at rest.
0 = Normal; 1 = mild finger tremor; 2 = tremor of fingers and hands; 3 = limb tremor; 4 = whole body tremor

Have patient open mouth and raise tongue to assess salivation.
0 = Normal, 1 = pooling with maneuvers above; 2 = occasional problems with speech due to drooling; 3 = as with 2, but frequent; 4 = frank drooling

Physician and patient should place hands on table. Begin to tap index finger as rapidly as possible. Repeat with both hands. Monitor for bradykinesia.
0 = Normal; 1 = mild slowing; 2 = moderate slowing; 3 = severe slowing; 4 = virtually immobilized

Modified from Simpson GM, Angus JWJ: "A rating scale for extrapyramidal side effects." *Acta Psychiatrica Scandinavia* 292(Suppl):11–19, 1970; used by permission. © Munksgaard International Publishers Ltd., Copenhagen, Denmark.

should be monitored routinely, and dosage increases should be made gradually to avoid sudden blockade of the α receptors with the consequent risk of syncope and falls.

Rarer Adverse Reactions

Erectile and ejaculatory disturbances can occur. Retrograde ejaculation is especially a problem with thioridazine. Galactorrhea and gynecomastia may be present, apparently as a function of dopamine blockade and resultant hyperprolactinemia. Antipsychotics may also lead to menstrual irregularities. It is prudent to explicitly remind patients that these drugs do not constitute a reliable form of birth control. Increased appetite and weight gain occur with some frequency but are less likely with molindone than with other agents.

Antipsychotics lower the seizure threshold. It is believed that low-potency agents are especially liable. Photosensitivity can occur and patients can burn severely with little sun exposure. Patients should be warned and a sunscreen recommended. Lenticular and corneal opacities have been reported. The development of pigmentary retinopathy led the FDA to impose an 800-mg/day ceiling on thioridazine. This is the only antipsychotic that has a mandated maximal dose.

Poikilothermia, the loss of ability to regulate internal body temperature in the face of environmental temperature change, can occur. This is most often a problem with the elderly.

Phenothiazines have been associated with cholestatic jaundice, which typically occurs relatively early in the course of treatment. Cross-sensitivity with other agents is unusual.

Neuroleptic malignant syndrome (NMS) is characterized by a decreased level of consciousness, greatly increased muscle tone, and autonomic dysfunction including hyperpyrexia, labile hypertension, tachycardia, tachypnea, diaphoresis, and drooling. Muscle necrosis can be so severe as to cause myoglobinuric renal failure. Laboratory abnormalities include greatly elevated creatinine phosphokinase levels and leukocytosis. NMS is a potentially fatal complication with a mortality of about 10%. Recent data indicate that about 1% of patients exposed to antipsychotics are at risk for developing NMS. It is most common with high-potency agents but has been reported with all antipsychotics. It typically occurs early in the course of treatment but has been reported after 20 yr of exposure. Treatment must include discontinuation of the antipsychotic and is otherwise primarily supportive. Patients should be well hydrated and treated with antipyretics or cooling blankets if hyperthermia is a problem. Arrhythmias should be treated. Low doses of heparin are indicated to decrease the chances of pulmonary emboli. Debate enters as to the wisdom of specific treatment with dan-trolene, levodopa/carbidopa, or bromocriptine. All have their advocates, but there are no con-trolled trials to indicate that any works. Most pa-tients recover on these agents and occasional pa-tients die. The same can be said for supportive treatment alone. Conversely, there is little to indi-cate that any of these medicines makes things worse and they may help.

Tardive dyskinesia (TD) represents the oc-currence of involuntary stereotypical move-ments after prolonged dopamine blockade. It typically involves bucco-oral movements, but any muscle in the body can be affected. The movements are usually choreoathetoid, but more static posturing, classified as tardive dys-tonia, has recently been described as has tardive akathisia. The full range of EPS are seen but are expressed as a delayed consequence of dopa-mine blockade. It may be impossible to distin-guish between TD and EPS on a single examina-tion, but the differing pathophysiology makes it possible to develop a strategy to confirm the di-agnosis.

TD occurs as a result of up-regulation of dopa-mine receptors. Prolonged blockade leads to an increase in numbers of receptors and of the avid-ity with which they bind dopamine. EPS, on the other hand, results from the short-term blockade of these same receptors. Increasing the dose of the antipsychotic will increase the blockade. EPS will then worsen, whereas TD will improve as the denervation hypersensitivity involved in the dis-order will be temporarily overridden. This is not a sensible long-term strategy, as the underlying problem will only get worse. Decreasing the dose will have the opposite effect: in the short range TD will worsen; EPS will improve.

There is currently no effective treatment for TD. Antipsychotics should, whenever possible, be discontinued, but there is nothing beyond this that has proven effective. The tragedy of TD is that it will not always be reversed with drug dis-continuation. There is no reliable means of pre-dicting who will be left with a permanent move-ment disorder. The presence of TD should not lead to an automatic discontinuation of the drug. Many patients prefer the movements to the pos-sibility of relapse. Those who can tolerate clozapine (see below) should probably be switched; those who cannot will need to make an informed decision as to whether or not to con-tinue. If they elect to discontinue the drug, then they should be forewarned that things may worsen in the short run.

The key to management of TD is prevention. The clinician must maintain a watchful eye for early signs of the disorder. The Abnormal Invol-untary Movement Scale is a simple and reliable examination that can be performed during office visits (see TABLE 63–5).

Depot Antipsychotics

Noncompliance with prescribed medication regimens is a major cause of morbidity. Several injectable forms of antipsychotics are available that allow long-term maintenance with injections q 1 to 5 wk (see TABLE 63–6). These agents are best reserved for patients who have demon-strated a history of noncompliance, those who are markedly ambivalent about their medica-tions, or those with ego-syntonic delusional sys-tems that they are reluctant to give up. The re-maining indication is for patients in whom there is a question of malabsorption.

Arriving at the appropriate regimen involves adjusting both dose and duration. These drugs have very long half-lives (especially for haloper-idol decanoate) and require substantially longer to arrive at steady state. During this interim pe-riod it may be necessary to treat the patient with an oral agent. Once steady state is achieved, the dose and the interval between injections can be manipulated. When the antipsychotic effect is in-adequate, the dose can be increased; when the effect is adequate but not sufficiently prolonged, the dosage interval can be decreased.

Clozapine

Clozapine is a new antipsychotic agent that op-erates with an atypical, largely unknown mecha-nism of action. The drug appears to relieve differ-ent target symptoms and also has different ad-verse effects. First marketed in Europe, it was withdrawn after a high incidence of agranulocy-tosis was reported in patients in Finland in 1975. Recent awareness that clozapine-induced gran-ulocytopenia is reversible if identified rapidly has led to unique requirements. There must be a weekly CBC, which is to be continued so long as the drug is prescribed. This process, therefore, requires patients who are sufficiently compliant as to permit weekly phlebotomy.

Clozapine appears to benefit a substantial mi-nority of even the most refractory of schizo-phrenics. Moreover, it appears to target some of the "negative symptoms," such as amotivation, anergia, and impaired judgment, which often re-spond poorly to conventional antipsychotic agents. This occurs in addition to positive effects

Table 63-5. ABNORMAL INVOLUNTARY MOVEMENT SCALE

1. Observe gait on the way into the room.
2. Have patient remove gum or dentures, if ill-fitting.
3. See if patient is aware of any movements.
4. Have patient sit on a firm, armless chair with hands on knees, legs slightly apart, and feet flat on the floor. Now and throughout the examination, look at the entire body for movements.
5. Have patient sit with hands unsupported, dangling over the knees.
6. Ask patient to open mouth twice. Look for tongue movements.
7. Ask patient to protrude tongue twice.
8. Ask patient to tap thumb against each finger for 15 sec with each hand. Observe face and legs.
9. Have patient stand with arms extended forward.

Rate each item on a 0 to 4 scale for the highest severity observed. 0 = None; 1 = minimal, may be extreme normal; 2 = mild; 3 = moderate; 4 = severe. Movements that occur only upon activation merit one point less than those that occur spontaneously.

Facial and oral movements	Muscles of facial expression	0 1 2 3 4
	Lips and perioral area	0 1 2 3 4
	Jaw	0 1 2 3 4
	Tongue	0 1 2 3 4
Extremity movements	Upper	0 1 2 3 4
	Lower	0 1 2 3 4
Trunk movements	Neck, shoulders, hips	0 1 2 3 4
Global judgments	Severity of abnormal movements	0 1 2 3 4
	Incapacitation due to abnormal movements	0 1 2 3 4
	Patient's awareness of abnormal movements (0 = unaware; 4 = severe distress)	0 1 2 3 4

Modified from *ECDEU Assessment Manual for Psychopharmacology* by W Guy. Copyright 1976 by US Department of Health, Education and Welfare.

on the more usual target symptoms (eg, hallucinations, delusions, and aggression). Clozapine is indicated for patients who have not been able to tolerate or who have not responded well to conventional antipsychotics. Since clozapine has minimal to no dopamine blockade, there is little liability for EPS, TD, or NMS.

Clozapine is not benign. Patients frequently become quite sedated. Hypotension and tachycardia can occur and can often be minimized by slow initiation of the drug. Drooling may be so severe as to require discontinuation. The drooling is surprising as clozapine is an extremely potent anticholinergic. A significant number of patients given clozapine will develop a benign hyperthermia early in treatment that is not associated with other signs of infection or with laboratory abnormalities. A more gradual increase in

Table 63-6. DEPOT ANTIPSYCHOTIC DRUGS

Drug*	Dosage/Interval	Single Dose Plasma Half-Life (Days)	Time Until Peak Level After Single Dose (Days)
Fluphenazine decanoate	12.5–50 mg q 1–3 wk	7	1
Fluphenazine enanthate	12.5–50 mg q 1–2 wk	4	2
Haloperidol decanoate	25–150 mg q 1–5 wk	21	7

* Given IM with "Z-track" technique.

dose will typically reverse the temperature increase. Clozapine also lowers the seizure threshold in a dose-related fashion. Weight gain can be significant, especially over the first 6 mo.

The most devastating problem associated with clozapine is the development of agranulocytosis in 1 to 2% of patients. Experience indicates that the diminished WBC count reverses within 2 to 3 wk of discontinuing the drug. *There should be increased scrutiny of any patient with a WBC count < 3500, and treatment should be discontinued for WBCs < 2000 or granulocytes < 1000. Such patients should never be re-exposed to clozapine.* The risk is sufficiently high as to preclude clozapine's being used as a first-line antipsy-

chotic. If there are only limited signs of improvement or if there has been no change within the first several months of treatment, then the drug should be discontinued owing to the continued risk of agranulocytosis.

Clozapine should not be coprescribed with other drugs that depress the WBC count, such as carbamazepine. Concomitant use of benzodiazepines has been associated with respiratory depression.

Clozapine is usually started with 25 mg/day orally and is gradually increased, depending on therapeutic response, to doses of 100 mg tid. The maximum dose is 900 mg, although it is unusual to require > 450 mg.

§5. OTOLARYNGOLOGY

64. CLINICAL EVALUATION OF COMPLAINTS REFERABLE TO THE EARS

Hearing loss, tinnitus, vertigo, earache, and otorrhea are the principal symptoms attributed to the ears. A thorough history should be taken and a physical examination performed with emphasis on the ears, nose, nasopharynx, and paranasal sinuses to evaluate complaints referable to the ears. In addition, the teeth, tongue, tonsils, hypopharynx, larynx, salivary glands, and temporomandibular joint should be examined, since pain and discomfort may be referred from them to the ears. Radiography or CT of the temporal bones is usually indicated in trauma to the ear, possible basal skull fracture, perforation of the tympanic membrane, hearing loss, vertigo, facial paralysis, and otalgia of obscure origin. Measurements of auditory and vestibular functions are of great diagnostic importance in patients with complaints referable to the ears.

HEARING LOSS

Hearing loss caused by a lesion in the external auditory canal or the middle ear is called **conductive**, while that caused by a lesion in the inner ear or the 8th nerve is called **sensorineural**. Conductive and sensorineural hearing loss can be differentiated by comparing the threshold of hearing by air conduction with that by bone conduction (see also DIFFERENTIATION OF SENSORY [COCHLEAR] AND NEURAL [8TH NERVE] HEARING LOSSES, below).

CLINICAL MEASUREMENT OF HEARING
(See also CLINICAL MEASUREMENT OF HEARING IN CHILDREN under SCREENING PROCEDURES FOR INFANTS AND CHILDREN in Ch. 23)

Hearing by air conduction (AC) is tested by presenting an acoustic stimulus, in air, to the ear. A hearing loss or elevation of the threshold demonstrated in this way can be caused by a defect in any part of the hearing apparatus—external auditory canal, middle ear, inner ear, 8th nerve, or central auditory pathways.

Hearing by bone conduction (BC) is tested by placing a sounding source (eg, the oscillator of an audiometer or the stem of a tuning fork) in contact with the head. This causes vibration

throughout the skull, including the walls of the bony cochlea, and stimulates the inner ear directly. Hearing by bone conduction bypasses the external and middle ear while testing the integrity of the inner ear, 8th nerve, and central pathways.

If the air conduction threshold is elevated and the bone conduction threshold is normal, the hearing loss is *conductive*. If air and bone conduction thresholds are elevated equally, the hearing loss is *sensorineural*. Occasionally, a **composite** or **mixed** loss of hearing occurs, with both conductive and sensorineural components. Under these circumstances, both bone and air conduction thresholds are elevated, the air conduction more than the bone.

The Weber and Rinne tuning fork tests are used to differentiate a conductive from a sensorineural hearing loss. For these tests, tuning forks with frequencies of 256, 512, 1024, and 2048 Hz are used. The **Weber tuning fork test** is performed by placing the stem of a vibrating tuning fork on the midline of the head and having the patient indicate in which ear the tone is heard. The patient with a unilateral *conductive* hearing loss hears the tone louder in the affected ear, for reasons that are unclear. By contrast, the patient with a unilateral *sensorineural* loss hears the tone in the unaffected ear, because the tuning fork stimulates both inner ears equally and the patient perceives the stimulus with the more sensitive, unaffected end organ and nerve.

The **Rinne tuning fork test** compares hearing ability by air conduction with that by bone conduction. The tines of a vibrating tuning fork are held first near the pinna (air conduction); then the stem of the still-vibrating fork is placed in contact with the mastoid process (bone conduction), and the patient is asked to indicate which stimulus is louder. Normally, the stimulus is heard longer and louder by air conduction (eg, 40 sec) than by bone conduction (eg, 20 sec), so the ratio is AC>BC. With a conductive hearing loss, this ratio is reversed; the bone conduction stimulus is perceived longer and louder than the air conduction stimulus (BC>AC). With a sensorineural hearing loss, both air and bone conduction perceptions are reduced, but the ratio remains the same (AC>BC).

The **audiometer** is used to quantitate hearing loss. This device delivers acoustic stimuli of specific frequencies (pure tones) at specific intensities so the patient's hearing threshold for each frequency can be determined. The hearing for each ear is measured from 125 or 250 to 8000 Hz by air conduction (using earphones) and by bone conduction (using an oscillator in contact with the head). Hearing loss is measured in decibels (**dB**), which equal 10 times the logarithm of the ratio of the acoustic power of a stimulus required to achieve hearing threshold in a patient to the acoustic power required to achieve threshold in a person with normal hearing. Test results are plotted on graphs called audiograms (see FIG. 64–1). Since intense tones presented to one ear may also be heard in the other ear, the Rinne tuning fork test and audiometry require the use of masking for accurate results. **Masking** is presentation of sound (usually noise) to the ear not being tested so that responses are based on hearing in the ear being tested.

Speech audiometry: The **spondee threshold (ST)**, the intensity at which speech is recognized as a meaningful symbol, is determined by presenting a list of spondaic words (2 syllables equally accented, such as *railroad, staircase, baseball*) at specific intensities, noting the intensity at which the patient repeats 50% of the words correctly. The ST usually approximates the average hearing level at speech frequencies of 500, 1000, and 2000 Hz.

Ability to discriminate the various speech sounds or phonemes is determined by presenting 50 phonetically balanced one-syllable words, containing the phonemes in the same relative frequency as in conversational English, at an intensity of 25 to 40 dB above the ST. The percentage of words correctly repeated by the patient is the **discrimination score**, normally 90 to 100%. This score remains in the normal range in conductive hearing losses but is reduced in sensorineural hearing losses, because analysis of the speech sounds by the inner ear and 8th nerve is impaired. Discrimination tends to be poorer in neural than in sensory hearing losses.

Tympanometry measures the impedance of the middle ear to acoustical energy without any effort expended by the patient. While the patient remains quiet, a sounding source and microphone sealed in the external auditory canal measure the acoustical energy absorbed (passing through) or reflected by the middle ear. In conductive hearing loss, the middle ear absorbs rela-

tively less sound and reflects relatively more sound. Normally the greatest compliance of the middle ear occurs with a pressure in the external auditory canal equal to atmospheric pressure. Increasing or decreasing pressure in the external auditory canal demonstrates various patterns of compliance. With a relatively negative pressure in the middle ear, as in eustachian tube obstruction and middle ear effusion, maximal compliance occurs with a negative pressure in the external auditory canal. With discontinuity of the ossicular chain, as in necrosis or dislocation of the long process of the incus, no point of maximal compliance can be obtained. With fixation of the ossicular chain, as in stapedial footplate ankylosis in otosclerosis, compliance may be normal or reduced. Tympanometry has been used to screen children for middle ear effusions (serous or secretory otitis media), to provide diagnostic clues, and to confirm the type of lesion in patients with conductive hearing losses.

This technique can detect changes in compliance produced by reflex contraction of the stapedius muscle; the acoustic reflex is initiated by presenting to the same or opposite ear a tone about 80 dB above the hearing threshold. The presence or absence of this reflex is important in the topographical diagnosis of facial nerve paralysis. The reflex adapts or decays in neural hearing losses, and the presence or absence of this reflex adaptation or decay, especially below 2000 Hz, aids in differential diagnosis of sensory and neural hearing losses. The acoustic reflex can also confirm voluntary threshold responses.

The minimum comprehensive audiologic assessment includes measurement of pure-tone air and bone conduction thresholds, ST, discrimination, and performance-intensity function for phonetically balanced words; tympanometry; and acoustic reflex testing, including reflex decay testing. Information gained from these procedures helps determine whether more definitive differentiation of a sensory from a neural hearing loss is indicated, as described below.

The patient who cannot or will not respond voluntarily to acoustic stimuli may be evaluated by measuring the cochlear microphonic response and action potentials of the 8th nerve (**electrocochleography**) and by evoked responses from the brainstem and auditory cortex (**auditory brainstem response**) to acoustic stimuli (see under DIFFERENTIATION OF SENSORY [COCHLEAR] AND NEURAL [8TH NERVE] HEARING LOSSES, below). These techniques have been useful in evaluating infants and children suspected of having

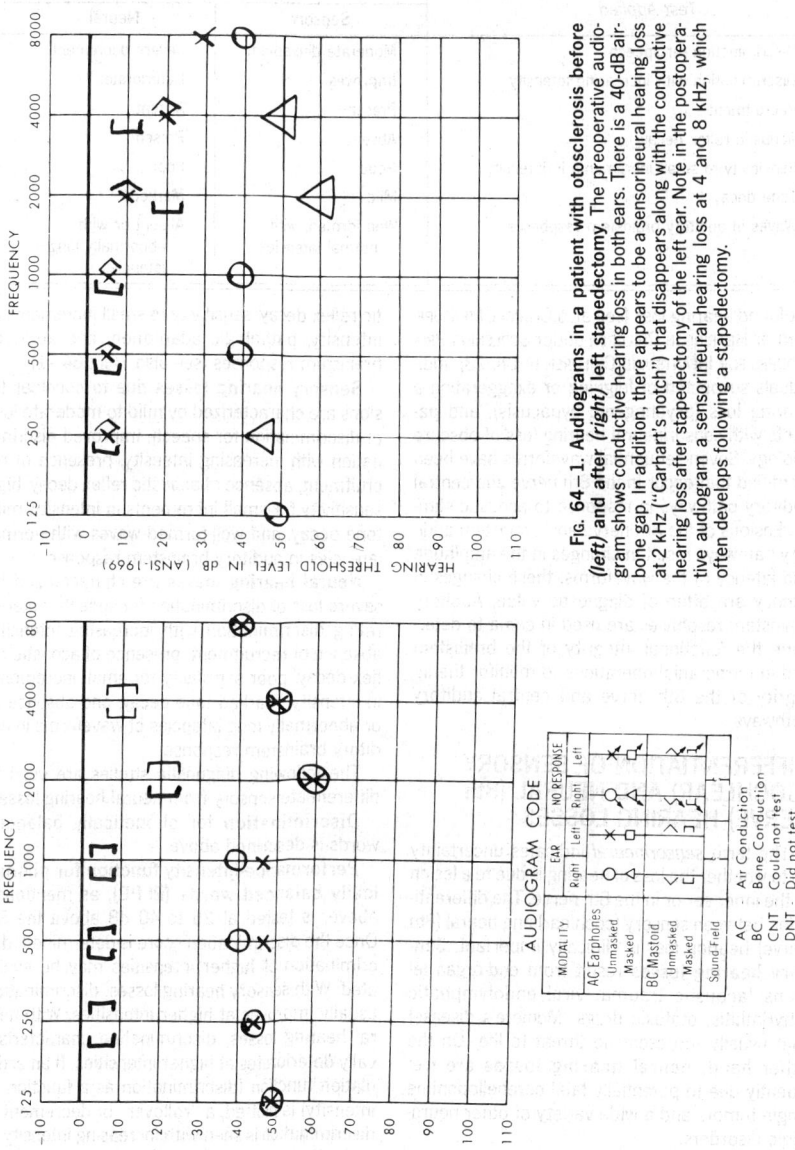

FIG. 64–1. Audiograms in a patient with otosclerosis before *(left)* **and after** *(right)* **left stapedectomy.** The preoperative audiogram shows conductive hearing loss in both ears. There is a 40-dB air-bone gap. In addition, there appears to be a sensorineural hearing loss at 2 kHz ("Carhart's notch") that disappears along with the conductive hearing loss after stapedectomy of the left ear. Note in the postoperative audiogram a sensorineural hearing loss at 4 and 8 kHz, which often develops following a stapedectomy.

AUDIOGRAM CODE

MODALITY	EAR		NO RESPONSE	
	Right	Left	Right	Left
AC Earphones				
Unmasked	◯	✕		
Masked	△	▢		
BC Mastoid				
Unmasked				
Masked	⌐	⌐		
Sound Field	∨	▢		

AC : Air Conduction
BC : Bone Conduction
CNT : Could not test
DNT : Did not test

TABLE 64-1. DIFFERENCES BETWEEN SENSORY AND NEURAL HEARING LOSSES

Test Applied	Type of Hearing Loss	
	Sensory	Neural
Discrimination for speech	Moderate decrement	Severe decrement
Discrimination with increasing intensity	Improves	Deteriorates
Recruitment	Present	Absent
Acoustic reflex decay	Absent	Present
Sensitivity to small increments in intensity	Good	Poor
Tone decay	Mild	Marked
Waves in auditory brainstem responses	Well formed, with normal latencies	Absent or with abnormally long latencies

profound hearing loss (see also CLINICAL MEASUREMENT OF HEARING IN CHILDREN under SCREENING PROCEDURES FOR INFANTS AND CHILDREN in Ch. 23), individuals suspected of feigning or exaggerating a hearing loss (psychogenic hypacusis), and patients with sensorineural hearing loss of obscure etiology. Seven sequential waveforms have been identified that occur in the 8th nerve and central auditory pathways in response to acoustic stimuli. Lesions of the 8th nerve and brainstem auditory pathways result in changes in the amplitude and latency of the waveforms; these changes in latency are often of diagnostic value. Auditory brainstem responses are used in coma to determine the functional integrity of the brainstem and in intracranial operations to monitor the integrity of the 8th nerve and central auditory pathways.

DIFFERENTIATION OF SENSORY (COCHLEAR) AND NEURAL (8th NERVE) HEARING LOSSES

The term *sensorineural* indicates uncertainty as to whether the loss of hearing is due to a lesion in the inner ear or in the 8th nerve. The differentiation between sensory (cochlear) and neural (8th nerve) hearing loss is clinically important. **Sensory hearing losses** result from end-organ lesions (acoustic trauma, viral endolymphatic labyrinthitis, ototoxic drugs, Meniere's disease) that usually represent no threat to life. On the other hand, **neural hearing losses** are frequently due to potentially fatal cerebellopontine angle tumors and a wide variety of other neurologic disorders.

Sensory and neural hearing losses may be differentiated on the basis of tests for discrimination, performance-intensity function for phonetically balanced words (**PI-PB**), recruitment, acoustic reflex decay, sensitivity to small increments in intensity, pathologic adaptation, and auditory brainstem responses (see also TABLE 64-1).

Sensory hearing losses due to cochlear lesions are characterized by mild to moderate loss of discrimination for speech, improved discrimination with increasing intensity, presence of recruitment, absence of acoustic reflex decay, high sensitivity for small increments in intensity, mild tone decay, and well-formed waves with normal latencies in auditory brainstem response.

Neural hearing losses are characterized by severe loss of discrimination for speech, deteriorating discrimination with increasing intensity, absence of recruitment, presence of acoustic reflex decay, poor sensitivity for small increments in intensity, marked tone decay, and absence of or abnormally long latencies of waveforms in auditory brainstem response.

The following diagnostic studies are used to differentiate sensory from neural hearing losses:

Discrimination for phonetically balanced words is described above.

Performance-intensity function for phonetically balanced words (PI-PB), as mentioned above, is tested at 25 to 40 dB above the ST. Once the discrimination score is determined, discrimination at higher intensities may be evaluated. With sensory hearing losses, discrimination usually improves at higher intensities. With neural hearing losses, discrimination characteristically deteriorates at higher intensities. If an articulation function (discrimination as a function of intensity) is plotted, a "rollover" or decrement in discrimination is seen with increasing intensity in patients with an 8th nerve lesion.

Recruitment (*abnormal increase in the perception of loudness or the ability to hear loud sounds normally despite a hearing loss*) can be demonstrated by having the patient compare the loudness of sounds in the affected ear with the loudness of sounds in the normal ear. In sensory hearing losses, the sensation of loudness in the affected ear increases more with each increment in intensity than it does in the normal ear. In neural hearing losses, the sensation of loudness in the affected ear increases no more with each increment in intensity than it does in the normal ear (no recruitment) or increases less with each increment in intensity than it does in the normal ear (decruitment).

Acoustic reflex decay, as mentioned above, adapts or decays with continuous presentation of a tone (particularly below 2000 Hz) over time, mildly in sensory hearing losses and severely in neural hearing losses.

Sensitivity to small increments in intensity can be demonstrated by presenting a continuous tone at a hearing level (dB level above audiometric zero) of 75 dB and increasing the intensity by 1 dB briefly at irregular intervals. The percentage of small increments that the patient can detect yields the short increment sensitivity index (SISI). A high SISI (60 to 100%) is characteristic of sensory hearing losses, while a patient with a neural hearing loss can detect < 30% of the small changes in intensity.

Pathologic adaptation is demonstrated when a patient cannot continue to perceive a constant tone above the threshold of hearing (tone decay). The tone decay is mild in sensory lesions and severe in neural lesions.

Several of these phenomena may be demonstrated with Békésy audiometry, in which the patient can control the intensity of the stimulus. The patient is instructed to press a button when he hears the stimulus, which causes intensity to decrease. When the stimulus is no longer audible, the patient releases the button, and the intensity begins to increase. In this way, the patient traces back and forth across his threshold of hearing. Over the course of 6½ min, the frequency of the test tone may be gradually increased from 100 to 10,000 Hz. Pathologic adaptation, if present, is demonstrated by decay of the response to a continuous presentation of the test stimulus. Decay of the response can be reduced or eliminated by interrupting the tone for ½ sec every second. Testing with continuous and interrupted tone presentations yields 5 patterns of tracings. In the type I pattern, found in normal hearing and in conductive hearing losses, the continuous and interrupted tracings are superimposed. In the type II pattern, the 2 tracings are superimposed up to 1000 Hz. Above this frequency, the threshold for the continuous tones increases by about 20 dB from that for the interrupted tones, and in the higher frequencies the excursions of the continuous tracings become smaller. This pattern is characteristic of sensory hearing losses, as in Meniere's disease, and indicates mild pathologic adaptation. In the type III pattern, the continuous tracing separates sharply from the interrupted tracing at a lower frequency, and excursions of the continuous tracing do not become smaller. This pattern is characteristic of neural lesions, such as acoustic neurinomas, and indicates severe pathologic adaptation. In the type IV pattern, the continuous tracing separates from the interrupted tracing at all frequencies, and excursions of the continuous tracing may or may not become smaller. This pattern indicates active cochlear lesions (such as a recent attack of Meniere's disease) or early neural lesions. In the type V pattern, the apparent thresholds of the continuous and interrupted tones are separated, but the apparent thresholds of the interrupted tones are greater than those of the continuous tones. This pattern occurs in psychogenic or feigned hearing loss.

Auditory brainstem response (ABR) is the most powerful technique for differentiating sensory from neural hearing losses. Five distinct electric waves—generated in the 8th nerve, brainstem, and other regions in response to acoustic stimulation and categorized by Jewett as I, II, III, IV, and V—can be recorded from the head by computer-averaging the responses to many stimuli. Each wave probably emanates from a distinct structure in the auditory pathway, such as the 8th nerve, cochlear nuclei, superior olivary complex, lateral lemniscus, and inferior colliculus. With lesions of the 8th nerve, one or more waveforms may be lost, the latency of the waveforms from the onset of the acoustic stimuli may be increased, and the interwave latencies may be prolonged. With cochlear lesions, the waveforms are easily recognized, and the latency relationships remain normal.

Patients with complaints referable to one cranial nerve, such as the 8th cranial nerve, deserve thorough neurologic evaluation. Emphasis has been placed in this discussion on thorough evaluation of the auditory division of the 8th nerve and its end organ. Further evaluation should include vestibular testing (see below) and MRI of the head using enhancement with gadolinium to demonstrate lesions of the 7th or 8th cranial nerves.

CENTRAL AUDITORY IMPERCEPTION

Lesions of the central auditory pathways (cochlear nuclei, brainstem pathways crossing the midline [trapezoid body, dorsal stria of Held, and stria of von Monakow], superior olivary complex, lateral lemniscus, inferior colliculus, medial geniculate body, auditory radiation, and auditory cortex) characteristically do not result in elevation of pure-tone and spondee thresholds and decreased discrimination for single words. Special tests are required to assess the deficit in auditory function with these lesions. These tests (1) measure discrimination of degraded or distorted connected speech, (2) measure discrimination in the presence of a competing message in the other ear, (3) evaluate the ability to fuse into a meaningful message incomplete or partial messages to each ear, and (4) localize sound in space (median plane localization) when the acoustic stimuli are delivered simultaneously to both ears.

Speech may be degraded or distorted with low-frequency or high-frequency filters, periodic interruptions, or time compression. A loss of discrimination of degraded or distorted connected speech is found in the ear contralateral to a cortical lesion. Likewise, presenting a competing message in the ipsilateral ear results in a loss of discrimination in the ear contralateral to a cortical lesion. Brainstem lesions cause a loss of ability to fuse incomplete messages presented to each ear into a meaningful message and impair the ability to make accurate localizations of sound in space.

TINNITUS

Perception of sound in the absence of an acoustic stimulus. Tinnitus, a subjective experience of the patient, is distinguished from **bruit**, noise that may be heard by the examiner and often by the patient as well.

Tinnitus may be of a buzzing, ringing, roaring, whistling, or hissing quality or may involve more complex sounds that vary over time. It may be intermittent, continuous, or pulsatile (synchronous with the heartbeat). An associated hearing loss is usually present.

The mechanism involved in tinnitus remains obscure. Tinnitus may occur as a symptom of nearly all ear disorders, including obstruction of the external auditory canal as a result of cerumen or foreign bodies, infectious processes (external otitis, myringitis, otitis media, labyrinthitis, petrositis, syphilis, meningitis), eustachian tube obstruction, otosclerosis, middle ear neoplasms such as the glomus tympanicum and glomus jugulare tumors, Meniere's disease, arachnoiditis, cerebellopontine angle tumors, ototoxicity (due to salicylates, quinine and its synthetic analogs, aminoglycoside antibiotics, certain diuretics, carbon monoxide, heavy metals, alcohol, etc), cardiovascular diseases (hypertension, arteriosclerosis, aneurysms, etc), anemia, hypothyroidism, hereditary sensorineural or noise-induced hearing loss, acoustic trauma (blast injury), and head trauma.

Evaluation of the patient with tinnitus requires the minimum comprehensive audiologic assessment described above as well as CT of the temporal bone and MRI of the head. Finding a sensorineural hearing loss indicates the testing described above for differentiating sensory and neural hearing losses. Pulsatile tinnitus requires investigation of the vascular system with carotid and vertebral arteriograms to exclude arterial obstruction, aneurysms, and vascular neoplasms.

Treatment

The patient's ability to tolerate the tinnitus varies. Treatment should be directed toward the underlying disease, since its amelioration may improve the tinnitus. Correction of the associated hearing loss usually results in relief of the tinnitus. Although there is no specific medical or surgical therapy for tinnitus, many patients find relief by playing background music to mask the tinnitus and even go to sleep with the radio playing. A hearing aid for the associated hearing loss often results in suppression of the tinnitus. Some patients benefit from use of a tinnitus masker, a device worn like a hearing aid that presents a noise more pleasant than the tinnitus. Electrical stimulation of the inner ear, as with a cochlear implant, often reduces the tinnitus but is appropriate only for the profoundly deaf.

CLINICAL EVALUATION OF THE VESTIBULAR APPARATUS

Patients with vertigo, difficulty with balance, or a sensorineural hearing loss of unknown etiology should have vestibular function tested. Evaluation of vestibular function centers on thorough history-taking and specific tests that include rapidly alternating movement, finger-to-nose, heel-to-shin, and Romberg tests; gait testing; and electronystagmography **(ENG)** with caloric testing. Since the results in each ear can be compared, caloric tests are more useful clinically than stimulation with acceleration or deceleration in rotational, torsion swing, and lateral swing tests.

Artificial stimulation of the vestibular apparatus produces nystagmus, past-pointing, falling, and autonomic responses such as sweating, vomiting, hypotension, and bradycardia. **Nystagmus**, the most useful response, can be monitored visually or, more reliably, by recording changes in the corneoretinal potential (electronystagmography). Vestibular nystagmus is a rhythmic movement of the eyes. It has a quick and a slow component and may be rotary, vertical, or horizontal. The direction of the nystagmus is determined by the direction of the quick component because it is easier to see. However, the slow component is the more fundamental response to vestibular stimulation, while the quick component is compensatory. The slow component moves in the direction of the movement of the endolymph; past-pointing and falling are also in this direction. The hallucination of movement of the environment is in the direction of endolymphatic flow, and the hallucination of movement of the subject is in the opposite direction.

ENG electronically detects spontaneous, gaze, or positional nystagmus that might not be visually detectable. Eye tracking of a moving target and the response to optokinetic stimulation with a rotating striped drum are conveniently recorded electronically at the time of caloric testing.

Caloric stimulation is produced by irrigating the ears with warm and cool water, which causes convection currents within the endolymph. These currents cause movement of the cupula in the ampulla of the horizontal semicircular canal; the movement is in one direction during cooling and in the opposite direction during warming.

The **Hallpike bithermal caloric test,** an accurate and reproducible measure of vestibular sensitivity, is performed with the patient supine and the head elevated 30° to bring the horizontal semicircular canal into a vertical position. Each ear is irrigated with 240 mL of water delivered in 40 sec, first at 30° C (86° F) and then at 44° C (111° F). The resulting nystagmus is monitored

with the patient gazing straight ahead. Irrigation of the ear with cool water produces nystagmus to the opposite side; warm water produces nystagmus to the same side. A mnemonic device is **COWS** (**C**old to the **O**pposite and **W**arm to the **S**ame).

The duration of the nystagmus, the velocity of the slow component, or the frequency of the nystagmus may be measured. **Canal paresis,** a unilateral reduction or absence of sensitivity, and **directional preponderance,** a relative exaggeration of the nystagmic response in one direction, can be demonstrated. Various combinations of canal paresis and directional preponderance may coexist. The presence of canal paresis, directional preponderance, or combinations of the 2 signals an organic lesion—end organ, 8th nerve, brainstem, or cerebellar—but does not necessarily indicate on which side the lesion is. Occasionally, an important differential point relies on the caloric examination. Acoustic neurinomas frequently show canal paresis or complete lack of response on the side with the neoplasm.

Patients with vertigo should have a minimum comprehensive audiologic assessment and MRI of the head using enhancement with gadolinium, as well as the vestibular evaluation described above.

EARACHE

Pain occurs with infections and neoplasms in the external or middle ear or is referred to the ear from remote disease processes. Even mild inflammation in the external auditory canal produces severe pain. Perichondritis of the pinna produces severe pain and tenderness. Eustachian tube obstruction causes abrupt changes in middle-ear pressure relative to atmospheric pressure that may result in painful retraction of the tympanic membrane. Infection in the middle ear results in painful inflammation of the middle-ear mucous membrane and pain from increased pressure in the middle ear with bulging of the tympanic membrane. The most common cause of earache in children, acute otitis media, requires prompt examination by a physician and antibiotic therapy to prevent serious sequelae. If there is no disease in the ear, the source of referred pain should be sought in those areas receiving sensory supply from the cranial nerves that subserve sensation in the external and middle ear—ie, the trigeminal, glossopharyngeal, and vagus nerves. Specifically, the cause of obscure otalgia should be sought in the nose, paranasal sinuses, nasopharynx, teeth, gingiva, temporomandibular joint, mandible, parotid glands, tongue, palatine tonsils, pharynx, hypopharynx, larynx, trachea, and esophagus. Occult neoplasms in these locations often first make their presence known by pain referred to the ear.

Treatment involves identifying the cause of the pain and providing the therapy appropriate for that disease.

VERTIGO

An abnormal sensation of rotary movement associated with difficulty with balance, gait, and navigation in the environment. The sensation may be subjective: the patient feels he is moving in relation to his environment; or it may be objective: he feels the environment is moving in relation to him. Vertigo results from lesions or disturbances in the inner ear, 8th nerve, or vestibular nuclei and their pathways in the brainstem and cerebellum.

65. EXTERNAL EAR

OBSTRUCTIONS

Cerumen (earwax) may obstruct the ear canal and cause itching, pain, and a temporary conductive hearing loss. It may be removed by irrigation, but rolling the cerumen out of the ear canal with a blunt curet or loop or removing it with a vacuum through a delicate tube is quicker, less messy, and more comfortable for the patient. Irrigation is contraindicated if the patient has a history of otorrhea, perforation of the tympanic membrane, or recurrent external otitis. Allowing water into the middle ear through a perforation may exacerbate chronic otitis media. Cerumen solvents are not recommended because they often do not dissolve the mass and frequently cause maceration of the canal skin and allergic reactions.

Children insert all types of objects into their ear canals, particularly beads, erasers, and beans. A foreign body in the ear canal is best removed by raking it out with a blunt hook. Forceps tend to push smooth objects deeper into the canal. A foreign body lying medial to the isthmus is difficult to remove without injuring the tympanic membrane and ossicular chain. Metal and glass beads can sometimes be removed by irrigation, but a hygroscopic foreign body (eg, a bean) swells when water is added to it, complicating its removal. A general anesthetic should be used when a child is uncooperative or when a mechanical problem could make removal difficult and possibly injure the eardrum or ossicles.

Insects in the canal are most annoying while alive. Filling the canal with mineral oil kills the insect, giving some immediate relief, and facilitates its removal with forceps.

EXTERNAL OTITIS

Infection in the ear canal may be localized (**furuncle**) or diffuse, involving the entire canal (**generalized or diffuse external otitis**). External otitis is more common during the summer swimming season and is often called **swimmer's ear.**

Etiology

Generalized external otitis may be caused by a gram-negative rod such as *Escherichia coli, Pseudomonas aeruginosa,* or *Proteus vulgaris;* by *Staphylococcus aureus;* or rarely, by a fungus. Furuncles are usually due to *S. aureus.* Certain persons (eg, those with allergies, psoriasis, eczema, or seborrheic dermatitis) are particularly prone to external otitis. Predisposing factors include getting water or any of various irritants such as hair spray or hair dye in the ear canal and suffering trauma from cleaning the canal. The ear canal cleanses itself by the movement of desquamated epithelium, like a conveyor belt, from the tympanic membrane outward. The patient's attempts to clean the canal with cotton applicators interrupt the self-cleansing mechanism and promote accumulation of debris by pushing it in the direction opposite the movement of the desquamated epithelium. Debris and cerumen tend to trap water allowed into the canal, the resulting skin maceration sets the stage for invasion of pathogenic bacteria.

Symptoms and Signs

Patients with diffuse external otitis complain of itching, pain, a foul-smelling discharge, and loss of hearing if the canal becomes swollen or filled with purulent debris. Tenderness on traction of the pinna and on pressure over the tragus tends to distinguish it from otitis media. The skin of the external auditory canal appears red, swollen, and littered with moist, purulent debris.

Furuncles cause severe pain and, when draining, brief sanguineous purulent otorrhea.

Treatment

Systemic antibiotics are seldom necessary unless a spreading cellulitis occurs. In **diffuse external otitis**, topical antibiotics and corticosteroids are effective. The infected debris is first gently removed from the canal with suction or dry cotton wipes. A solution containing neomycin sulfate 0.5% and polymyxin B sulfate 10,000 u./mL is effective against the usual gram-negative rods, while the addition of a topical corticosteroid such as 1% hydrocortisone reduces the swelling and allows antibiotic penetration into the depth of the canal; 5 drops are instilled tid for 7 days. External otitis also responds to alteration of the canal's pH with topical 2% acetic acid 5 drops tid for 7 days; the addition of 1% hydrocortisone reduces swelling and enhances the effectiveness of the acetic acid. An analgesic such as codeine 30 mg orally q 4 h is usually necessary for the first 24 to 48 h. If cellulitis is present and extends beyond the ear canal, penicillin G 250 mg orally q 6 h for 7 days is indicated.

Furuncles should be allowed to drain spontaneously, since incision may lead to a spreading perichondritis of the pinna. Topical antibiotics are *ineffective*. Analgesics such as codeine 30 mg orally q 4 h are necessary to relieve the pain. Dry heat also helps relieve pain and hastens resolution.

PERICHONDRITIS

Trauma, insect bites, and incision of superficial infections of the pinna may initiate perichondritis, which causes an accumulation of pus between the cartilage and the perichondrium. The blood supply to the cartilage is provided by the perichondrium. If the perichondrium is separated from both sides of the cartilage, the resulting avascular necrosis leads to a deformed pinna. Septic necrosis also plays a role. The infection tends to be indolent, long-lasting, and destructive. Perichondritis is usually caused by a gram-negative rod. **Treatment:** Wide incision and suction drainage is used to reapproximate the blood supply to the cartilage. Systemic antibiotic

therapy is indicated and should be guided by culture and sensitivity studies; often IV therapy with an aminoglycoside antibiotic and a semisynthetic penicillin is required.

AURAL ECZEMATOID DERMATITIS

Eczema, characterized by itching, redness, discharge, desquamation, and even fissuring leading to secondary infection, frequently involves the pinna and ear canal. Recurrences are common. **Treatment:** Dilute aluminum acetate solution (Burow's solution) is applied as often as required. Itching and inflammation can be reduced with topical corticosteroids. Topical antibiotic therapy as described above for diffuse external otitis may be needed occasionally.

MALIGNANT EXTERNAL OTITIS

Pseudomonas *osteomyelitis of the temporal bone.*

Malignant external otitis occurs mainly in elderly diabetics, beginning as an external otitis caused by *Pseudomonas aeruginosa* and becoming a *Pseudomonas* osteomyelitis of the temporal bone. It is characterized by persistent and severe earache, foul-smelling purulent otorrhea, and granulation tissue in the external auditory canal. Varying degrees of conductive hearing loss may be present. Frequently, facial nerve paralysis occurs. Increased radiodensity develops throughout the air-cell system in the temporal bone and middle ear, as does radiolucency of the temporal bone. Biopsy of the tissue in the ear canal is necessary to differentiate the condition from a malignant neoplasm. The osteomyelitis spreads along the base of the skull and may cross the midline. Surgery is usually not helpful or necessary. Control of the diabetes and prolonged (6 wk) IV therapy with an aminoglycoside antibiotic and a semisynthetic penicillin result in complete resolution in most cases.

TRAUMA

Hematoma

A subperichondrial hematoma may result from blunt trauma to the pinna. The external ear becomes a shapeless, reddish-purple mass when blood collects between the perichondrium and the cartilage. Since the perichondrium carries the blood supply to the cartilage, avascular necrosis of the cartilage may occur. The "cauliflower ear" characteristic of wrestlers and boxers is the consequence of an organized and calcified hematoma. **Treatment:** The clot must be evacuated through an incision, and the skin and perichondrium are reapproximated to the cartilage with suction drainage to keep the cartilage and its blood supply in close approximation.

Lacerations

For lacerations of the external ear that penetrate the cartilage and the skin on both sides, the skin margins are sutured, the cartilage is splinted externally with benzoin-impregnated cotton, and a protective dressing is applied. Sutures should not extend into the cartilage.

Fractures

Forceful blows to the mandible may be transmitted to the anterior wall of the ear canal (posterior wall of the glenoid fossa). Displaced fragments from fractures of the anterior wall may cause stenosis of the canal and must be reduced or removed under general anesthesia.

TUMORS

Sebaceous cysts, osteomas, and keloids may arise in and occlude the ear canal, causing retention of cerumen and a conductive hearing loss. Excision is the treatment of choice.

Ceruminomas arise in the outer third of the external auditory canal. Although these neoplasms appear benign histologically, *they behave in a malignant manner and should be excised widely.*

Basal cell and squamous cell carcinomas frequently develop on the external ear following regular exposure to the sun. Early lesions can be successfully treated with cautery and curettage or irradiation. More advanced lesions involving the cartilage require surgical excision of V-shaped wedges or larger portions of the external ear. Invasion of cartilage makes irradiation therapy less effective and surgery the preferred treatment. Basal cell and squamous cell carcinomas may also arise in or secondarily invade the external auditory canal. Persistent inflammation in chronic otitis media may predispose to development of squamous cell carcinoma. Extensive resection is indicated, followed by radiation therapy. En bloc resection of the external auditory canal with sparing of the facial nerve is performed when lesions are limited to the canal and have not invaded the middle ear.

66. TYMPANIC MEMBRANE AND MIDDLE EAR

The patient with a middle ear disorder may present with one or more of the following complaints: a feeling of fullness or pressure in the ear; constant or intermittent, mild to excruciating pain; otorrhea; diminished hearing; tinnitus; and vertigo. In acute otitis media, systemic symptoms (eg, fever) are commonly present as well. The symptoms may begin with a feeling of fullness and progress serially in additive fashion. Infants and children, especially, may be febrile and present with other prominent systemic manifestations (anorexia, vomiting, diarrhea, lethargy, etc).

The symptoms may result from infection, trauma, or disturbed pressure relationships secondary to eustachian tube obstruction. In determining the cause, the physician should elicit information about antecedent and associated symptoms (eg, rhinorrhea, nasal obstruction, sore throat, URI, and allergic manifestations; headache or other evidence of meningeal involvement; systemic symptoms). The appearance of the external auditory canal and tympanic membrane (see FIG. 66-1) often yields diagnostic clues; the nose, nasopharynx, and oropharynx should also be examined for signs of infection and allergy and for evidence of an underlying disorder—eg, a neoplasm of the nasopharynx.

The function of the middle ear should be evaluated with pneumatic otoscopy, the Weber and Rinne tuning fork tests, tympanometry, and audiologic assessment (see Ch. 64).

TRAUMA

The tympanic membrane may be punctured and the tympanum penetrated by objects placed in the ear canal (eg, cotton applicators) or entering the canal accidentally (eg, twigs on a tree or missiles such as pencils or hot slag). A sudden overpressure (as in an explosion [acoustic trauma], a slap, or swimming and diving accidents) or a sudden negative pressure (as in a kiss over the ear) also can perforate the tympanic

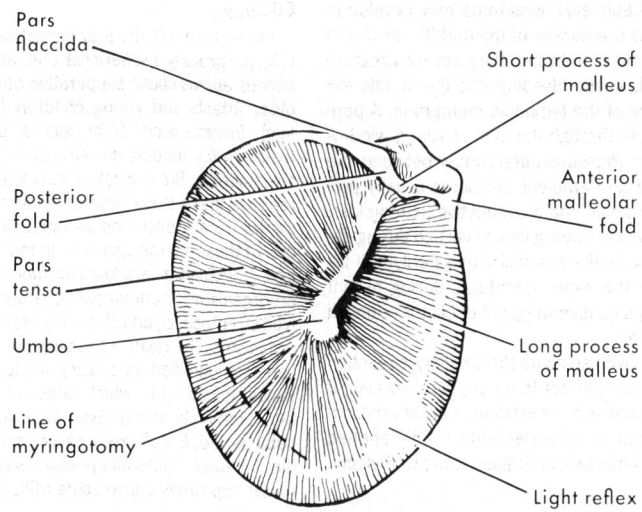

FIG. 66–1. The tympanic membrane (right ear).

Labels on figure:
Pars flaccida
Short process of malleus
Anterior malleolar fold
Posterior fold
Pars tensa
Umbo
Line of myringotomy
Long process of malleus
Light reflex

membrane. Penetration of the eardrum may cause dislocations of the ossicular chain, fracture of the stapedial footplate, displacement of fragments of the ossicles or missile into the inner ear, a perilymph fistula from the oval or round window, or facial nerve paralysis.

Symptoms and Signs

Traumatic perforation of the tympanic membrane results in sudden severe pain followed by bleeding from the ear. A loss of hearing and tinnitus occur. The hearing loss is more severe if there has been a disruption of the ossicular chain or trauma to the inner ear. Vertigo suggests an associated injury to the inner ear, as occasionally a portion of the stapes or a missile is driven into the inner ear. Purulent otorrhea may begin in 24 to 48 h, particularly if water gets into the middle ear.

Treatment

Following perforation, oral penicillin G or V 250 mg q 6 h should be given for 7 days to prevent infection. Aseptic technique is used in examining the ear. If necessary, the displaced flaps of tympanic membrane may be laid in their original positions, under local anesthesia and microscopic control, to facilitate healing. The ear is kept dry, and topical medication with 2% acetic acid 5 drops tid may be administered if the ear becomes infected, but it is not used prophylacti-

cally. Spontaneous closure of the perforation is usual, but if this does not occur within 2 mo, a tympanoplasty is indicated. A persistent conductive hearing loss suggests discontinuity of the ossicular chain; the middle ear should be explored surgically and repaired. A sensorineural hearing loss or vertigo that persists for hours or longer following the injury indicates penetration of the inner ear and requires an exploratory tympanotomy to repair the damage as soon as possible.

BAROTITIS MEDIA
(Aerotitis)

Damage to the middle ear due to ambient pressure changes. During a sudden increase in ambient pressure, as in descent of an airplane or in deep sea diving (see Chs. 120 and 122), gas must move from the nasopharynx into the middle ear to maintain equal pressure on both sides of the tympanic membrane. If the eustachian tube is not functioning properly, as in URI or allergy, the pressure in the middle ear is lower than the ambient pressure, and the relative negative pressure in the middle ear results in retraction of the tympanic membrane; a transudate of blood from the vessels in the lamina propria of the mucous membrane forms in the middle ear. If the difference in pressure becomes great, ecchymosis and subepithelial hematoma may develop in the mucous membrane of the middle ear and in the tympanic membrane. Very severe pressure differentials cause bleeding into the middle ear and rupture of the tympanic membrane. A perilymph fistula through the oval or round window may occur. Pressure differentials between the middle ear and ambient pressures usually produce severe pain and a conductive hearing loss. A sensorineural hearing loss or vertigo during descent suggests the possibility of a perilymph fistula, while the same symptoms during ascent from an aquatic dive suggest bubble formation in the inner ear.

A person with an acute URI or allergic reaction should be advised not to fly or dive. However, if these activities are undertaken, a nasal vasoconstrictor such as phenylephrine 0.25% applied topically 30 min before descent is of prophylactic value.

INFECTIOUS MYRINGITIS
(Bullous Myringitis)

Inflammation of the tympanic membrane secondary to viral or bacterial infections. Vesicles develop in the tympanic membrane in viral infections and in acute bacterial (particularly *Streptococcus [Diplococcus] pneumoniae*) and mycoplasmal otitis media. Pain is sudden in onset and persists for 24 to 48 h. Hearing loss and fever, if present, suggest bacterial otitis media. **Treatment:** Since differentiation of a viral from a bacterial or mycoplasmal otitis is difficult, antibiotic therapy as for acute otitis media is indicated. Pain may be relieved by rupture of the vesicles with a myringotomy knife or by analgesia with a narcotic such as codeine 30 to 60 mg orally q 4 h prn.

ACUTE OTITIS MEDIA

A bacterial or viral infection in the middle ear, usually secondary to a URI. While it can occur at any age, it is most common in young children, particularly from age 3 mo to 3 yr. Microorganisms may migrate from the nasopharynx to the middle ear over the surface of the eustachian tube's mucous membrane or by propagating in the lamina propria of the mucous membrane as a spreading cellulitis or thrombophlebitis.

Etiology

In newborn infants, gram-negative enteric bacilli, particularly *Escherichia coli*, and *Staphylococcus aureus* cause suppurative otitis media. In older infants and young children ($<$ 14 yr of age), *Streptococcus [Diplococcus] pneumoniae*, *Hemophilus influenzae*, Group A β-hemolytic streptococci, *Branhamella catarrhalis*, and *S. aureus* are the causative microorganisms. Viral otitis media usually becomes secondarily invaded by one of these microorganisms. In those $>$ 14 yr of age, *H. influenzae* is a less common causative microorganism; *S. pneumoniae*, Group A β-hemolytic streptococci, and *S. aureus* are the causative organisms. The relative frequency of the microorganisms identified as causing acute otitis media varies according to which ones are epidemic in the community at any given time. After the neonatal period, *E. coli* rarely causes acute otitis media. Likewise, *Klebsiella pneumoniae* and *Bacteroides* spp rarely cause acute otitis media.

Symptoms, Signs, and Complications

The first complaint usually is of persistent, severe earache. Hearing loss may occur. Fever (up to 40.5° C [105° F]), nausea, vomiting, and diarrhea may occur in young children. The tympanic membrane is erythematous and may bulge; landmarks become indistinct, and the light reflex is displaced. Bloody, then serosanguineous, and finally purulent otorrhea may follow spontaneous perforation of the tympanic membrane.

Serious complications include acute mastoiditis, petrositis, labyrinthitis, facial paralysis, conductive and sensorineural hearing loss, epidural abscess, meningitis (the most common intracranial complication), brain abscess, lateral sinus thrombosis, subdural empyema, and otitic hydrocephalus. Symptoms of an impending complication include headache, sudden profound hearing loss, vertigo, and chills and fever.

Diagnosis and Treatment

Diagnosis is usually made on clinical grounds. If myringotomy is performed, exudate obtained during the procedure should be cultured, as should spontaneous otorrhea. Nasopharyngeal cultures may be helpful but do not correlate well with the causative agent.

Antibiotic therapy is indicated for acute otitis media to relieve the symptoms, hasten resolution of the infection, and reduce the chance of labyrinthine and intracranial infectious complications and of residual damage to the hearing mechanism of the middle ear.

Penicillin G or V 250 mg orally q 6 h for 12 days is the drug treatment of choice in patients > 14 yr of age. Amoxicillin 35 to 70 mg/kg/day orally in 3 equal doses q 8 h for 12 days is preferred for those < 14 yr because of the frequency of *H. influenzae* infections. Treatment is continued for 12 to 14 days to ensure resolution and to prevent sequelae. Subsequent therapy depends on cultures, sensitivities, and the clinical course. In penicillin allergy, erythromycin 250 mg orally q 6 h for older children and adults, and a combination of erythromycin 30 to 50 mg/kg/day orally in equally divided doses q 6 h and sulfisoxazole 150 mg/kg/day orally in equally divided doses q 6 h for children < 14 yr, may be given for 12 to 14 days. Sulfonamides are contraindicated in infants < 2 mo of age. Alternatively, trimethoprim and sulfamethoxazole (TMP/SMX) may be used to treat acute otitis media, in infants > 2 mo of age and children: 8 mg/kg/day of TMP and 40 mg/kg/day of SMX in 2 divided doses q 12 h for 10 days, and in adults: 160 mg of TMP and 800 mg of SMX q 12 h for 12 days. In resistant cases, a cephalosporin may be used, such as cefaclor (in children: 20 mg/kg/day in divided doses q 8 h for 12 days, in adults: 250 mg q 8 h for 12 days), cefuroxime (in children < 2 yr of age: 125 mg q 12 h for 12 days, in children 2 to 12 yr of age: 250 mg q 12 h for 12 days, and in adults: 500 mg q 12 h for 12 days), cephalexin (in children: 75 mg/kg/day in 4 divided doses for 12 days, and in adults: 500 mg q 6 h for 12 days), or cefixime (in children: 8 mg/kg/day in 2 divided doses for 12 days, and in adults: 200 mg q 12 h for 12 days).

To improve eustachian tube function, topical vasoconstrictors such as phenylephrine 0.25% 3 drops q 3 h may be instilled into each nasal cavity while the patient is supine with the neck extended. Such therapy should not exceed 5 to 7 days. Systemic sympathomimetic amines such as ephedrine sulfate, pseudoephedrine, or phenylpropanolamine 30 mg orally (for adults) q 4 to 6 h for 7 to 10 days may also be helpful. Antihistamines such as chlorpheniramine 4 mg (for adults) orally q 4 to 6 h for 7 to 10 days may improve eustachian tube function in allergic patients but are not indicated for nonallergic individuals.

Myringotomy should be considered if the tympanic membrane is bulging or if pain, fever, vomiting, and diarrhea are severe or persistent. The patient's hearing, tympanometry, and the appearance and movement of the tympanic membrane should be monitored until there is complete resolution.

SECRETORY OTITIS MEDIA
(Serous Otitis Media)

An effusion in the middle ear resulting from incomplete resolution of acute otitis media or obstruction of the eustachian tube. The effusion may be sterile but usually contains pathogenic bacteria. Secretory otitis media is common in children. The eustachian tube obstruction may be due to inflammatory processes in the nasopharynx, allergic manifestations, hypertrophic adenoids, or benign or malignant neoplasms. The middle ear is normally ventilated 3 to 4 times/min as the eustachian tube opens during swallowing. O_2 is absorbed by the blood in the vessels of the middle ear mucous membrane, and if the patency of the eustachian tube is impaired, a relative negative pressure develops within the middle ear.

Symptoms and Signs

At first, mild retraction of the tympanic membrane occurs, with displacement of the light reflex and accentuation of the landmarks. Then a transudate from the blood vessels in the mucous membrane develops in the middle ear, recognizable by the amber or gray appearance it gives the eardrum and the immobility of the tympanic membrane. An air-fluid level or bubbles of air may be seen through the tympanic membrane; conductive hearing loss occurs. Tympanometry demonstrates maximal compliance with negative pressures in the external auditory canal.

Treatment

Since pathogenic bacteria may have a role in middle ear effusions, a trial of antibiotic therapy as described under ACUTE OTITIS MEDIA, above, is often beneficial and is the first step to consider in therapy. It is effective in relieving eustachian tube obstruction due to bacterial infection and in sterilizing the middle ear.

Systemic sympathomimetic amines such as ephedrine sulfate, pseudoephedrine, or phenylpropanolamine 30 mg orally tid (for adults) may improve eustachian tube function by their vasoconstrictive effect. Antihistamines such as chlorpheniramine 4 mg (for adults) orally q 4 to 6 h may relieve eustachian tube obstruction in allergic patients. Myringotomy may be necessary for aspiration of the fluid and for insertion of a tympanostomy tube, which allows ventilation of the middle ear and ameliorates the eustachian tube obstruction, regardless of the cause. The middle ear may be temporarily ventilated with the Valsalva maneuver or politzerization.

Correction of any underlying condition in the nasopharynx is required. Children may require adenoidectomy, removing lymphoid aggregations on the torus of the eustachian tube and in Rosenmüller's fossa as well as the central adenoid tissue mass, to eradicate persistent and recurrent serous otitis media. Antibiotic therapy should be given to resolve bacterial rhinitis, sinusitis, and nasopharyngitis. Immunologic investigation (see Chs. 33 and 34) is occasionally helpful. Any demonstrated allergen should be eliminated from the patient's environment, or immunotherapy should be tried (see Ch. 34).

ACUTE MASTOIDITIS

Bacterial infection in the mastoid process resulting in coalescence of the mastoid air cells. In acute purulent otitis media, the infection always extends into the mastoid antrum and cells, but progression and destruction of the bony portions of the mastoid process are aborted by suitable antibiotic therapy. The responsible bacteria are the same as those causing acute otitis media. Characteristically, **streptococcal mastoiditis** is preceded by early perforation of the tympanic membrane and profuse otorrhea; **pneumococcal mastoiditis** is likely to be less symptomatic but just as destructive, and advanced coalescence of the mastoid air cells may precede perforation of the tympanic membrane.

Symptoms and Signs

Acute mastoiditis becomes clinically apparent 2 wk or more after the onset of untreated acute otitis media, as one of the cortices of the mastoid process is destroyed. A postauricular subperiosteal abscess may develop as the lateral mastoid cortex is destroyed. Redness, swelling, tenderness, and fluctuation develop over the mastoid process, and the pinna is displaced laterally and inferiorly. An exacerbation of the aural pain, fever, and otorrhea usually occurs. The pain tends to be persistent and throbbing; a creamy, profuse discharge is common. Increasing hearing loss is characteristic.

In acute otitis media, the mastoid air cells are filled with fluid and a soft tissue density may appear on CT, due to purulent fluid, swollen mucous membrane, and granulation tissue in the air cells. In coalescent mastoiditis, cell partitions become indistinct. The individual septum can no longer be seen as the fluid- and tissue-filled air cells coalesce.

Treatment

The initial antibiotic of choice is penicillin. After a sample of the otorrhea is taken for culture and determination of antibiotic sensitivities, penicillin G 1 million u. IV q 6 h is given. Subsequent IV therapy depends on cultures, sensitivities, and the clinical course. Antibiotic therapy should be continued for at least 2 wk.

A subperiosteal abscess calls for complete exenteration of mastoid air cells (mastoidectomy).

CHRONIC OTITIS MEDIA

A permanent perforation of the tympanic membrane.

Chronic otitis media can result from acute otitis media, eustachian tube obstruction, mechanical trauma, thermal or chemical burns, or blast injuries. It can be divided into 2 major categories, depending on the type of perforation: (1) the benign central perforation of the pars tensa and (2) the dangerous attic perforations of the pars flaccida and marginal perforations of the pars tensa.

Some substance of the tympanic membrane remains between the rim of the perforation and the bony sulcus tympanicus in **central perforations** (see FIG. 66–2a). These perforations result in a conductive hearing loss. Exacerbations of chronic otitis media may follow URI or occur when water enters the middle ear during bathing or swimming. They are often caused by gram-negative rods and *Staphylococcus aureus*, resulting in painless, purulent otorrhea, which may be foul-smelling. Persistent exacerbations may produce **aural polyps** (granulation tissue that prolapses from the middle ear through the perforation into the external auditory canal) and destructive changes in the middle ear such as necrosis of the long process of the incus.

Pars flaccida (attic) perforations lead into the epitympanum (see FIG. 66–2b). **Marginal perforations** usually occur in the posterior-superior portion of the pars tensa, and there is no substance of tympanic membrane between the edge of the perforation and the bony sulcus tympanicus (see FIG. 66–2c). Marginal perforations re-

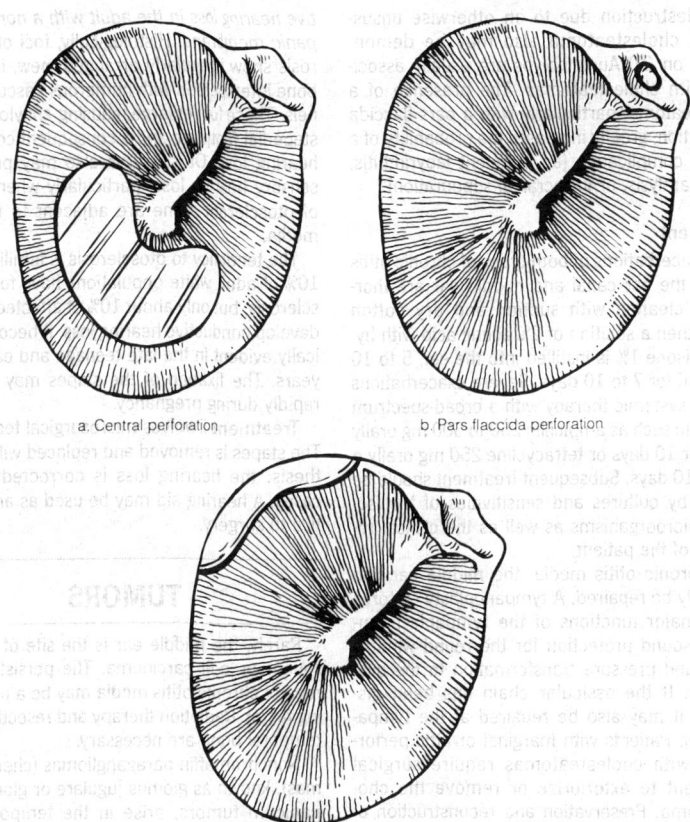

a. Central perforation

b. Pars flaccida perforation

c. Marginal perforation

FIG. 66-2. Perforations of the tympanic membrane (right ear).

sult from an acute necrotizing otitis media that destroys large areas of the tympanic membrane, including the annulus tympanicus and the mucous membrane of the middle ear. These perforations may be associated with a conductive hearing loss, and exacerbations of otorrhea occur as with central perforations. Complications such as labyrinthitis, facial paralysis, and intracranial suppuration are more likely to occur with marginal than with central perforations. Pars flaccida and marginal perforations are frequently associated with **cholesteatomas.**

During the healing of acute necrotizing otitis media, the remaining epithelium of the mucous membrane and the stratified squamous epithelium of the ear canal migrate to cover the denuded areas. Once the stratified squamous epithelium is established in the middle ear, it begins to desquamate and accumulate, resulting in a cholesteatoma. Cholesteatomas may also develop from hyperplasia of the basal layer of the stratified squamous epithelium of the pars flaccida, from progressive retraction of the pars flaccida or the pars tensa, and from squamous metaplasia in the middle ear due to long-standing infection. The desquamated epithelium accumulates in ever-enlarging concentric layers, and collagenases in the epithelium destroy adjacent bone.

Cholesteatomas may be recognized on otoscopic examination by the white debris in the middle ear and the destruction of the external auditory canal bone adjacent to the perforation.

Bone destruction due to an otherwise unsuspected cholesteatoma also may be demonstrated on CT. Aural polyps are usually associated with cholesteatomas. The presence of a cholesteatoma, particularly with a pars flaccida perforation, greatly increases the probability of a serious complication (eg, purulent labyrinthitis, facial paralysis, or intracranial suppuration).

Treatment

In exacerbations of both types of chronic otitis media, the ear canal and middle ear are thoroughly cleaned with suction and dry cotton wipes; then a solution of 2% acetic acid with hydrocortisone 1% is instilled into the ear, 5 to 10 drops tid for 7 to 10 days. Severe exacerbations require systemic therapy with a broad-spectrum antibiotic such as ampicillin 250 to 500 mg orally q 6 h for 10 days or tetracycline 250 mg orally q 6 h for 10 days. Subsequent treatment should be guided by cultures and sensitivities of the isolated microorganisms as well as the clinical response of the patient.

In chronic otitis media, the middle ear can generally be repaired. A tympanoplasty restores the 2 major functions of the tympanic membrane: sound protection for the round window and sound pressure transformation to the oval window. If the ossicular chain has been disrupted, it may also be repaired at the tympanoplasty. Patients with marginal or attic perforations with cholesteatomas require surgical treatment to exteriorize or remove the cholesteatoma. Preservation and reconstruction of the middle ear mechanism is less likely in the presence of cholesteatoma.

OTOSCLEROSIS

*A disease of the bone of the otic capsule and the most common cause of progressive conduc-*tive hearing loss in the adult with a normal tympanic membrane.* Histologically, foci of otosclerosis show irregularly arranged, new, immature bone interspersed with numerous vascular channels. These foci enlarge, causing ankylosis of the stapedial footplate and a consequent conductive hearing loss. Otosclerosis also may produce a sensory hearing loss, particularly when the foci of otosclerotic bone are adjacent to the scala media.

The tendency to otosclerosis is familial. About 10% of adult white populations have foci of otosclerosis, but only about 10% of affected persons develop conductive hearing loss. It becomes clinically evident in the late teenage and early adult years. The fixation of the stapes may progress rapidly during pregnancy.

Treatment involves microsurgical techniques: The stapes is removed and replaced with a prosthesis; the hearing loss is corrected in most cases. A hearing aid may be used as an alternative to surgery.

TUMORS

Rarely, the middle ear is the site of origin of squamous cell carcinoma. The persistent otorrhea of chronic otitis media may be a predisposing factor. Radiation therapy and resection of the temporal bone are necessary.

Nonchromaffin paragangliomas (chemodectomas), known as glomus jugulare or glomus tympanicum tumors, arise in the temporal bone from glomus bodies in the jugular bulb or the medial wall of the middle ear. They produce a pulsatile red mass in the middle ear. The first symptom is often a tinnitus that is synchronous with the pulse. Hearing loss and, later, vertigo develop. Excision is the treatment of choice. Palliation is achieved with radiation therapy for tumors too large to resect.

67. INNER EAR

(See also VERTIGO in Ch. 64 and CONGENITAL SENSORINEURAL HEARING LOSS in Ch. 27)

MENIERE'S DISEASE

A disorder characterized by recurrent prostrating vertigo, sensory hearing loss, and tinnitus, associated with generalized dilation of the membranous labyrinth (endolymphatic hydrops).

The cause of Meniere's disease is unknown, and the pathophysiology is poorly understood. The attacks of vertigo appear suddenly, last from a few to 24 h, and subside gradually. The attacks are associated with nausea and vomiting. The patient may have a recurrent feeling of fullness or pressure in the affected ear, and hearing in that ear tends to fluctuate but progressively worsens over the years. The tinnitus may be constant or intermittent and may be worse before, after, or during an attack of vertigo. Although usually only one ear is affected, both ears are involved in 10 to 15% of patients.

In **Lermoyez's variant** of Meniere's disease, hearing loss and tinnitus precede the first attack of vertigo by months or years, and the hearing may improve with the onset of the vertigo.

Treatment

Treatment is empirical. A number of surgical procedures have been advocated for patients who are disabled by the frequency of vertiginous attacks. Vestibular neurectomy relieves the vertigo, and usually the hearing is preserved. A labyrinthectomy can be performed if the vertigo is sufficiently disabling and the hearing has degenerated to a useless level.

Symptomatic relief of the vertigo may be obtained with anticholinergic agents (eg, atropine 1 to 2 mg orally or scopolamine 0.6 mg orally or IM q 4 to 6 h or by transdermal patch) to minimize vagal-mediated GI symptoms, antihistamines (eg, diphenhydramine, meclizine, or cyclizine 50 mg orally or IM q 6 h) to sedate the vestibular system, or barbiturates (eg, pentobarbital 100 mg orally or IM q 8 h) for general sedation. Diazepam 2 to 5 mg orally q 6 to 8 h is particularly effective in relieving the distress of severe vertigo by sedating the vestibular system.

VESTIBULAR NEURONITIS

A benign disorder characterized by sudden onset of severe vertigo that is persistent at first, then paroxysmal. The disease is thought to be a neuronitis involving the vestibular division of the 8th nerve and to be viral in origin because of its frequent epidemic occurrence, particularly among adolescents and young adults.

The first attack of vertigo is severe, is associated with nausea and vomiting, and lasts for 7 to 10 days. There is persistent nystagmus toward the affected side. The condition is self-limited and may occur as only a single episode, or several subsequent attacks may occur over the next 12 to 18 mo; each subsequent attack is less severe and of shorter duration. There is no associated hearing loss or tinnitus.

The diagnostic evaluation should include an audiologic assessment, electronystagmography with caloric testing, and MRI of the head with

gadolinium enhancement, with particular attention to the internal auditory canals to exclude other diagnostic possibilities, such as cerebello-pontine angle tumor and brainstem hemorrhage or infarction.

Treatment Acute attacks of vertigo may be suppressed symptomatically as in Meniere's disease (see above). With prolonged vomiting, IV fluids and electrolytes may be required for replacement and maintenance.

BENIGN PAROXYSMAL POSITIONAL VERTIGO
(Postural or Positional Vertigo; Cupulolithiasis)

Violent vertigo, lasting < 30 sec and induced by certain head positions. The vertigo occurs when the patient lies on one ear or the other or when he tips his head backward to look up. Nystagmus also occurs, but there is no associated hearing loss or tinnitus. Benign paroxysmal positional vertigo usually subsides in several weeks or months but may recur after months or years.

Etiology

Granular basophilic masses in the cupula of the posterior semicircular canal have been demonstrated. The cupular deposits may represent calcium carbonate derived from the otoliths. Etiologic factors appear to be spontaneous degeneration of the utricular otolithic membranes, labyrinthine concussion, otitis media, ear surgery, and occlusion of the anterior vestibular artery.

Diagnosis

A **provocative test for positional nystagmus** may be performed. The patient is first seated on an examining table; then with his head turned to the side, he quickly assumes the supine position with his head dependent over the end of the table. After a latent period of several seconds, severe vertigo occurs, which is likely to last for 15 to 20 sec and is accompanied by rotary nystagmus. If the left ear is affected, the nystagmus is clockwise when the head is turned to the left; if the right ear, the nystagmus is counterclockwise. When the patient sits up, the response recurs, but the nystagmus is rotary in the reverse direction and is milder. The response fatigues, so that with immediate repetition of the test, the response is diminished.

Positional nystagmus may occur with end-organ or CNS lesions. The latency of the response, the severe subjective sensation, the fatigability of the response, the limited duration, and the direction of the rotary nystagmus distinguish benign paroxysmal positional vertigo from a CNS lesion. The positional nystagmus of CNS lesions lacks latency, fatigability, and the severe subjective sensation. The nystagmus may continue for as long as the position is maintained and may be vertical or changing in direction and, if rotary, is likely to be perverted (ie, not in the anticipated direction).

The diagnostic evaluation should include an audiologic assessment, electronystagmography with caloric testing, and MRI of the head with gadolinium enhancement, with particular attention to the internal auditory canals to exclude other conditions such as acoustic neuroma.

Treatment

The patient is instructed to avoid the provocative position. If benign positional paroxysmal vertigo lasts for as long as a year, it usually can be relieved by dividing the nerve to the posterior semicircular canal of the affected ear at tympanotomy.

HERPES ZOSTER OTICUS
(Ramsay Hunt's Syndrome; Viral Neuronitis and Ganglionitis; Geniculate Herpes)

Invasion of the 8th nerve ganglia and the geniculate ganglion of the facial nerve by the herpes zoster virus, producing severe ear pain, hearing loss, vertigo, and paralysis of the facial nerve.

Vesicles can be seen on the pinna and in the external auditory canal in the distribution of the sensory branch of the facial nerve. Other cranial nerves are often involved, and some degree of meningeal inflammation is common. Lymphocytes may be present in the CSF, and the protein content is often increased. Evidence of a mild generalized encephalitis can be found in many patients. The hearing loss may be permanent, or there may be partial or complete recovery. The vertigo lasts for days to several weeks. The facial paralysis may be transient or permanent.

Treatment

Corticosteroid therapy is the treatment of choice; eg, prednisone 40 mg/day orally for 2 days, then 30 mg/day orally for 7 to 10 days, followed by gradual tapering of the dose. Acyclovir 1 gm orally in 5 divided daily doses for 10 days may also shorten the clinical course. Pain is relieved with codeine 30 to 60 mg orally q 3 to 4 h prn, while the vertigo is effectively suppressed with diazepam 2 to 5 mg orally q 4 to 6 h. Decompression of the fallopian canal, indicated when the nerve excitability declines or electroneurography demonstrates a 90% decrement, occasionally relieves the facial paralysis.

PURULENT LABYRINTHITIS
(Suppurative Labyrinthitis)

Invasion of the inner ear by a bacterium. Purulent labyrinthitis may be secondary to acute otitis media or purulent meningitis. In acute otitis media, the microorganisms may gain access to the inner ear through the oval and round windows; in purulent meningitis, through the cochlear aqueduct. Purulent labyrinthitis is also frequently followed by meningitis as the microorganisms gain access to the subarachnoid space through the cochlear aqueduct.

Purulent labyrinthitis is characterized by severe vertigo and nystagmus. It invariably results in complete hearing loss and, in chronic otitis media and cholesteatoma, is often followed by facial paralysis. **Treatment** includes labyrinthectomy for drainage of the inner ear, radical mastoidectomy, and IV antibiotic therapy appropriate for meningitis.

SUDDEN DEAFNESS

Severe sensorineural hearing loss that usually occurs in only one ear and develops over a period of a few hours or less.

Sudden deafness occurs in about 1/5000 persons every year. Although the sudden onset suggests a vascular cause (embolism, thrombosis, or hemorrhage) by analogy with vascular accidents in the CNS, the evidence supports a viral cause in most cases. Sudden deafness tends to occur in children and in young and middle-aged adults who have no evidence of vascular disease. The histopathologic findings in the temporal bone in sudden deafness are unlike those seen in the inner ear of animals with experimental vascular occlusion or embolization but are similar to those seen in human viral infections of the inner ear that result in sudden deafness—eg, mumps and measles (**viral endolymphatic labyrinthitis**). The viruses of influenza, chickenpox, and mononucleosis; the adenoviruses; and others also produce sudden deafness.

The pathologic findings in individuals with persistent hearing loss due to viral endolymphatic labyrinthitis are similar, regardless of the causative virus. The organ of Corti is missing in the basal turn. Individual hair cells tend to be missing. Ganglion cell populations are reduced in the basal turn. The stria vascularis becomes atrophic. The tectorial membrane is often rolled up and ensheathed in a syncytium. Reissner's membrane may be collapsed and adherent to the basilar membrane.

Perilymph fistulas between the inner and middle ears occasionally occur with severe ambient pressure changes and with strenuous activities like weight lifting. Fistulas in the oval or round windows result in a sudden or fluctuating sensory hearing loss and vertigo. The patient may experience an explosive sound in the affected ear when the fistula occurs. The fistula can be demonstrated by combining the pressure changes in the external ear used in tympanometry with electronystagmography. Nystagmus resulting from pressure changes in the ear canal suggests a perilymph fistula.

Symptoms and Signs

The hearing loss is usually profound, but hearing returns to normal in most patients and partial recovery occurs in others. Tinnitus and vertigo may be present initially, although the vertigo usually subsides in several days. If hearing is going to return, it is likely to do so in 10 to 14 days.

Treatment

Although vasodilators, anticoagulants, low mol wt dextran, corticosteroids, and vitamins have all been advocated, no form of treatment is of proven value. Since micropetechiae and extravasation of blood are characteristic of virus-induced inflammatory reactions, vasodilation and anticoagulation may not be indicated. Furthermore, in an inflammatory reaction, the cochlear blood flow is already increased as much as is beneficial. Although corticosteroids are not of proven value, their use appears rational—eg, prednisone 60 mg/day orally for 2 days, then 40 mg/day orally for 5 to 7 days, followed by a tapering of dosage. Bed rest also seems advisable.

Surgical exploration of the middle ear should be carried out for a suspected perilymph fistula, and the fistula should be repaired with an autogenous graft of fascia.

NOISE–INDUCED HEARING LOSS

Any source of intense noise, such as woodworking equipment, chain saws, internal combustion engines, heavy machinery, gunfire, or aircraft, may damage the inner ear. Exposure to intense noise results in loss of hair cells in the organ of Corti. Individuals vary greatly in susceptibility to noise-induced hearing loss, but nearly everyone will lose some hearing if exposed to sufficiently intense noise for an adequate time. Any noise > 85 dB is damaging. Usually a high-frequency tinnitus accompanies the hearing loss. Loss occurs first at 4 kHz and gradually moves into the lower frequencies with further exposure. In contrast to most sensorineural hearing losses, damage is less at 8 kHz than at 4 kHz. Blast injury, termed acoustic trauma, produces the same kind of sensory hearing loss.

Prevention depends on limiting the length of exposure, reducing the noise at its source, and isolating the person from the sound source. As the intensity of the noise increases, the duration of exposure must be reduced to prevent damage to the inner ear. Noise may be attenuated by wearing ear protectors, eg, plastic plugs in the ear canals or glycerin-filled muffs over the ears. With severe noise-induced hearing loss, a hearing aid is usually helpful.

PRESBYCUSIS

The sensorineural hearing loss that occurs as a part of normal aging. It begins after age 20, first affecting the highest frequencies (18 to 20 kHz) and gradually moving into the lower frequencies; it usually begins to affect the 4- to 8-kHz range by age 55 to 65, although there is considerable variation. Some individuals are severely handicapped by age 60, and some are essentially untouched at 90. Men are affected more often and more severely than women. Stiffening of the basilar membrane and deterioration of the hair cells, stria vascularis, ganglion cells, and cochlear nuclei may play a role in pathogenesis, and presbycusis appears to be related in part to noise exposure.

Speech reading (lipreading), auditory training for making maximum use of nonauditory clues, and amplification with a hearing aid are helpful.

OTOTOXIC DRUGS

Aminoglycoside antibiotics, salicylates, quinine and its synthetic substitutes, and diuretics (ethacrynic acid and furosemide) can be ototoxic. Though affecting both the auditory and vestibular portions of the inner ear, these drugs are particularly toxic to the organ of Corti (cortitoxic). Nearly all ototoxic drugs are eliminated through the kidneys, and renal impairment predisposes to the accumulation of toxic levels. Ototoxic drugs should be avoided in prescribing topical medication for the ear in the presence of a perforated tympanic membrane, since they can be absorbed into the inner ear fluids through the secondary tympanic membrane at the round window.

Streptomycin damages the vestibular portion of the inner ear more readily than the auditory portion. Although vertigo and difficulty with maintaining balance tend to be temporary and eventually completely compensated, severe and permanent loss of vestibular sensitivity may persist, causing difficulty when walking in the dark and Dandy's syndrome (bouncing of the environment with each step). From 4 to 15% of patients who receive 1 gm/day for > 1 wk develop a measurable hearing loss, which usually appears after a short latent period (7 to 10 days) and slowly becomes worse if treatment is continued. Complete, permanent deafness may follow.

Neomycin has the greatest cortitoxic effect of all antibiotics. When large doses are given orally or by colonic irrigation for intestinal sterilization, enough of the drug may be absorbed to affect hearing, particularly if GI ulceration or other mucosal lesions are present. Neomycin should not be used for irrigating wounds or for intrapleural or intraperitoneal irrigation, because massive amounts of the drug may be retained and absorbed, causing deafness. Kanamycin and amikacin are close to neomycin in cortitoxic potential.

Viomycin shows both cochlear and vestibular toxicity. Vancomycin causes hearing loss, especially in the presence of renal insufficiency. Gentamicin and tobramycin have vestibular and cochlear toxic properties in humans and laboratory animals.

Ethacrynic acid given IV has caused profound and permanent hearing loss in gravely ill patients with renal failure who are receiving concomitant aminoglycoside antibiotic therapy. Similarly, transient and permanent hearing loss from IV furosemide has been reported in patients with renal failure or who are receiving concomitant aminoglycoside antibiotics.

Salicylates produce hearing loss and tinnitus that is usually reversible. Quinine and its synthetic substitutes produce a permanent loss of hearing.

Precautions

Ototoxic antibiotics should be avoided in pregnancy. Elderly persons and those with a pre-existing hearing loss should not be treated with ototoxic drugs if other effective drugs are available. If possible, the hearing should be measured before treatment is begun with an ototoxic drug (especially an ototoxic antibiotic) in order to document a preexisting hearing loss. Hearing should be monitored audiometrically while treatment is continued. The highest frequencies are usually affected first, and high-pitched tinnitus or vertigo may develop, though they are not reliable warning symptoms. If renal function is impaired, the dosage of renally eliminated ototoxic drugs should be adjusted so that the blood levels do not exceed those required therapeutically. Peak and trough serum levels of the agent should be monitored to ensure that adequate therapeutic levels have been achieved but not exceeded. Although susceptibility to ototoxic drugs varies somewhat among individuals, hearing can usually be conserved by not exceeding the recommended blood level.

FRACTURES OF THE TEMPORAL BONE

Ecchymosis in the postauricular skin (Battle's sign) suggests a fracture of the temporal bone. Bleeding from the ear following a skull injury is pathognomonic of a temporal bone fracture. The bleeding may be medial to an intact tympanic membrane, may come from the middle ear through a ruptured tympanic membrane, or may come from a fracture line in the ear canal. A hemotympanum gives the eardrum a blue-black color. CSF otorrhea signifies a communication between the middle ear and the subarachnoid space. Longitudinal fractures, which are parallel to the petrous pyramid (80% of cases), extend through the middle ear and rupture the tympanic membrane; they produce facial paralysis in 15% of cases and a profound sensorineural hearing loss in 35%. The middle ear damage may include disruption of the ossicular chain. Transverse fractures (20% of cases) cross the fallopian canal and the cochlea and nearly always produce facial paralysis and a permanent hearing loss. The hearing can be assessed initially with the Weber and Rinne tuning fork tests and subsequently with audiometry. The fracture can usually be demonstrated on CT of the head with special attention to the temporal bone.

Treatment

Penicillin G 1.6 million u. IV q 6 h can be given for 7 to 10 days in an attempt to prevent meningitis. However, this presents a risk in predisposing patients to resistant organisms. Persistent facial paralysis requires decompression of the nerve. Tympanoplasty with repair of the ossicular chain is carried out weeks or months later.

ACOUSTIC NEURINOMA

(Vestibular Schwannoma; Acoustic Neuroma;
8th Nerve Tumor)

Acoustic neurinomas are derived from Schwann cells. They arise twice as often from the vestibular division of the 8th nerve as from the auditory division and account for about 7% of all intracranial tumors.

As the tumor increases in size, it projects from the internal auditory meatus into the cerebellopontine angle and begins to compress the cerebellum and brainstem. The 5th and later the 7th cranial nerves become involved.

Symptoms, Signs, and Diagnosis

A hearing loss and tinnitus are early symptoms. Although the patient complains of dizziness and unsteadiness, true vertigo is not usually present. The sensorineural hearing loss (see Ch. 64) is characterized by greater impairment of speech discrimination than would be expected with a cochlear lesion. Recruitment is absent, and tone decay is marked. Acoustic reflex decay along with absence of waveforms and increase in the latency of the 5th wave in auditory brainstem response testing provide further evidence of a neural lesion. As a rule, caloric testing demonstrates marked vestibular hypoactivity (canal paresis). Early diagnosis is based on the audiologic assessment, particularly auditory brainstem response and MRI with gadolinium enhancement.

Treatment

Small tumors may be removed with microsurgical techniques that allow preservation of the facial nerve, using a middle cranial fossa route to preserve the remaining hearing or a translabyrinthine route if no useful hearing remains. Large tumors are removed by a combined translabyrinthine and suboccipital approach.

HEARING AIDS

Amplification of sound with hearing aids is helpful for persons with conductive or sensorineural hearing losses that are > 30 dB in the speech frequencies. Hearing aids are also helpful to individuals with predominantly high-frequency sensorineural hearing losses and to those with unilateral hearing losses.

Air conduction hearing aids, usually coupled to the ear canal with an airtight seal or open tube, are generally superior to bone conduction hearing aids and are generally used except when there is some contraindication to using an ear mold or tube, as in atresia of the external auditory canal or persistent otorrhea. The **body aid** type, appropriate for profound hearing losses, is the most powerful; it is worn in the shirt pocket or in a body harness and connected by a wire to the earpiece, or receiver, which is coupled to the ear canal by a plastic insert, or ear mold. In infants and young children with hearing loss so profound that determining which ear hears better is impossible, the amplification from the body aid is delivered to both ears by a Y-cord. For moderate to severe hearing losses, a **postauricular or ear-level aid**, which fits behind the pinna and is coupled to the ear mold with flexible tubing, is appropriate. **Eyeglass aids**, which are built into the temple bar of eyeglasses with tubing leading to the ear molds, are usually restricted to individuals who wear eyeglasses continually. The less powerful **in-the-ear aid** is contained entirely within the ear mold and fits less conspicuously into the concha and the ear canal; it is appropriate for mild to moderate hearing losses. **Canal aids** are contained entirely within the ear canal and are cosmetically acceptable to many users who would otherwise refuse amplification. The **CROS aid** (for **C**ontralateral **R**outing **O**f **S**ignals) is used in individuals with monaural hearing; a hearing-aid microphone is placed on the nonfunctioning ear and sound is routed to the functioning ear (either through a wire or miniature radio transmitter), allowing the wearer to hear sounds from the nonfunctioning side and to develop a limited ability to localize sound. If the better ear also has a loss of hearing, both the sound from the poorer side and the sound coming to the better side can be amplified with the **BiCROS aid.**

A **bone conduction aid** is sometimes used in hearing losses in which an ear mold or tube cannot be used, as in atresia of the ear canal or persistent otorrhea. The oscillator is placed in contact with the head, usually over the mastoid, with a spring band over the head, and sound is conducted through the bone of the skull to the cochlea. Bone conduction hearing aids require more power and introduce more distortion than air conduction hearing aids and are less comfortable to wear. Some bone conduction aids can be implanted in the mastoid process, avoiding the discomfort and prominence of the spring band.

In evaluating a patient for a hearing aid, professional advice is required. Selecting the proper hearing aid requires matching the electroacoustic characteristics of the aid with the type of hearing loss on the basis of gain, saturation level, and frequency response. **Gain,** or amplification, refers to the difference between the input and the output of the hearing aid. The more severe the hearing loss, the more gain is generally required. **Saturation level,** the maximum output of the hearing aid regardless of input, is an important consideration for patients with reduced tolerance to sound (as in recruitment). In severe tolerance problems, special circuitry (automatic gain control, or AGC) is available to keep the output of the aid at tolerable levels. **Frequency response** refers to the gain of the aid as a function of frequency. As a general rule, the frequency response should be selected to provide gain consistent with the patient's audiometric configuration. High frequency accentuation can also be achieved by venting the ear mold, which benefits

many individuals with a sensorineural hearing loss that is greater in the high frequencies than in the low frequencies.

COCHLEAR IMPLANTS

Profoundly deaf individuals who cannot be helped by hearing aids in speech reading (lip-reading) or in hearing environmental sounds (doorbells, ringing telephones, alarms, etc) may benefit from a cochlear implant. This electronic device consists of a battery-powered processor that converts sound into modulations of an electric current, an internal and external induction coil system that transmits the electrical impulses through the skin, and an array of electrodes connected to the internal induction coil that stimulates the remaining fibers of the auditory division of the 8th cranial nerve. At mastoid surgery, the electrode array is inserted into the scala tympani of the basal turn of the inner ear. The internal induction coil is implanted into the bone of the skull posterior and superior to the ear; the external conduction coil is held in place on the skin over the induction coil by magnets in the 2 coils.

Cochlear implants help with speech reading by allowing the profoundly deaf to distinguish when a word begins and ends, the intonation of the word, the rhythm of the speech, and some speech percepts. Some cochlear implants even allow minimal discrimination of words *without* visual clues. Cochlear implants allow deaf persons to hear and distinguish environmental sounds and warning signals. They also help deaf persons modulate their voices to make their speech more intelligible to hearing persons.

68. NOSE AND PARANASAL SINUSES
(See also FOREIGN BODIES in Ch. 44)

FRACTURES OF THE NOSE

The nasal bones are fractured more frequently than are other facial bones. The fracture may also include the ascending processes of the maxilla and the septum. The torn mucous membrane results in nosebleed. Soft tissue swelling develops promptly and may obscure the break. Septal hematomas may occur between the perichondrium and the quadrilateral cartilage and may become infected; abscess formation leads to

avascular and septic necrosis of the cartilage, with a saddle deformity of the nose.

Diagnosis

A fracture should be suspected if blunt injury causes bleeding from the nose. Diagnosis can ordinarily be established by gently palpating the dorsum (bridge) of the nose for deformity, instability, crepitus, and point tenderness and is confirmed by x-ray. The most common deformity is deviation of the dorsum of the nose in one direction and depression of the nasal bone and ascending process of the maxilla on the other side.

Treatment

Nasal fractures in adults may be reduced under local anesthesia; children require general anesthesia. The fracture is manipulated into a good position by internal and external traction. A blunt elevator is placed under the depressed nasal bone, and the depressed bone is lifted anteriorly and laterally while pressure is applied to the other side of the nose to bring the nasal dorsum to the midline. The position of the nose may be stabilized by internal packing and external splinting. Septal hematomas must be immediately incised and drained to prevent infection and cartilage necrosis. Septal fractures are difficult to hold in position and often require nasal septal surgery later.

SEPTAL DEVIATION AND PERFORATION

Deviations of the nasal septum from developmental abnormalities or trauma are common but often are asymptomatic and require no treatment. Septal deviation may cause varying degrees of nasal obstruction and predispose the patient to sinusitis (particularly if the deviation obstructs an ostium of a paranasal sinus) and to epistaxis as a result of drying air currents. Treatment of symptomatic deviation of the nasal septum is by septoplasty or nasal septal reconstruction.

Septal **ulcers** and **perforations** may follow nasal surgery, repeated trauma such as picking the nose, and granulomatous infections such as TB and syphilis. Crusting about the margins and repeated epistaxis may result. Small perforations may whistle. Topically applied bacitracin 500 u./gm in a petrolatum base reduces the crusting. Although perforations of the nasal septum may be repaired by using buccal or septal mucous membrane flaps, closing the perforation with a Silastic septal button is a more reliable solution.

EPISTAXIS
(Nosebleed)

Bleeding from the nose occurs secondary to local infections such as vestibulitis, rhinitis, and sinusitis; systemic infections such as scarlet fever, malaria, and typhoid fever; drying of the nasal mucous membrane; trauma (digital, as in picking the nose, or blunt, as in nasal fractures); arteriosclerosis; hypertension; and bleeding tendencies associated with aplastic anemia, leukemia, thrombocytopenia, liver disease, the hereditary coagulopathies, and Rendu-Osler-Weber syndrome (hereditary hemorrhagic telangiectasia—see in Ch. 35).

Treatment

Most nasal bleeding occurs from a plexus of vessels in the anteroinferior septum (Kiesselbach's area). **Bleeding may be controlled by pinching the nasal alae together for 5 to 10 min.** If this fails, the bleeding site must be found. The bleeding point may be cauterized; bleeding can be controlled temporarily by applying pressure over a cotton pledget impregnated with a vasoconstrictor such as phenylephrine 0.25% and a topical anesthetic such as lidocaine 2% until the site is anesthetized. Electrocautery may be used, or silver nitrate in a 75% applicator bead may control bleeding without burning the mucous membrane too deeply.

In epistaxis due to a bleeding tendency, petrolatum gauze is used to apply pressure as atraumatically as possible to the bleeding point. Cautery is not used, since the periphery of a cauterized area may begin to bleed. Attention is directed to identifying and correcting the bleeding disorder.

In arteriosclerosis and hypertension, bleeding is likely to be far posterior in the inferior meatus and may be difficult to control. Ligating the internal maxillary artery and its branches or packing the posterior part of the nasal cavity is required to control the bleeding. The arteries may be ligated with clips under microscopic control, using a surgical approach through the maxillary sinus. To pack the posterior part of the nasal cavity, the choana is obstructed with a postnasal pack made by folding and rolling 4-in. gauze squares into a tight bundle and tying the bundle with 2 strands of heavy silk suture. The ends of one suture are tied to a catheter that has been introduced through the nasal cavity on the side of the bleeding and brought out through the mouth. The catheter is withdrawn from the nose as the pack is placed behind the soft palate into the nasopharynx. The 2nd suture is trimmed below the level of the soft palate so it can be used to remove the pack. (Alternatively, the balloon of a Foley catheter may be inflated in the nasopharynx to obstruct the choana.) The nasal cavity, particularly the posterior part of the inferior meatus, is firmly packed with petrolatum gauze and the first suture is tied over a roll of gauze at the anterior nares to secure the postnasal pack. The packing remains in place for 4 days. An antibiotic such as ampicillin 250 mg orally q 6 h is given to prevent sinusitis and otitis media. Postnasal packing lowers the arterial P_{O_2}, and supplementary O_2 should be given while the packing is in place.

In Rendu-Osler-Weber syndrome, multiple severe nosebleeds may occur from arteriovenous aneurysms in the mucous membrane, resulting in profound and persistent anemia that is not easily corrected with administration of iron. A split-thickness skin graft (septal dermoplasty) reduces the episodes of epistaxis and allows the anemia to be corrected.

Severe epistaxis is often associated with liver disease. Blood may have been swallowed in large amounts and should be eliminated as promptly as possible with enemas and cathartics; the GI tract should be sterilized with nonabsorbable antibiotics (eg, neomycin 1 gm orally qid) to prevent the breakdown of blood and absorption of ammonia.

Need for blood replacement is determined by the Hb level, vital signs, and the central venous pressure.

NASAL VESTIBULITIS

Infection of the nasal vestibule. **Low-grade infections** and **folliculitis** produce annoying crusts, and bleeding occurs as the crusts come away. Bacitracin ointment 500 u./gm applied topically bid for 14 days is effective.

Furuncles of the nasal vestibule are usually staphylococcal; they may develop into a spreading cellulitis of the tip of the nose. Systemic antibiotics should be given along with hot soaks; penicillin G or V is the drug of choice. Furuncles of the central portion of the face should be allowed to drain spontaneously. Since incision and drainage increase the risk of retrograde thrombophlebitis and subsequent cavernous sinus thrombosis, they are **contraindicated.**

RHINITIS

(See also ALLERGIC RHINITIS in Ch. 34)

The most frequent of the acute URIs, characterized by edema and vasodilation of the nasal mucous membrane, nasal discharge, and obstruction.

Acute rhinitis is the usual manifestation of a common cold; it may also be caused by streptococcal, pneumococcal, or staphylococcal infections. **Chronic rhinitis** may occur in syphilis, TB, rhinosclerosis, rhinosporidiosis, leishmaniasis, blastomycosis, histoplasmosis, and leprosy—all conditions characterized by granuloma formation and destruction of soft tissue, cartilage, and bone. Rhinosclerosis also causes progressive nasal obstruction from indurated inflammatory tissue in the lamina propria. These conditions produce nasal obstruction, purulent rhinorrhea, and frequent bleeding. Rhinosporidiosis is characterized by bleeding polyps.

Diagnosis and Treatment

Diagnosis and treatment of **acute bacterial rhinitis** are based on pathogen identification and antibiotic sensitivities. Topical vasoconstriction with a sympathomimetic amine (eg, phenylephrine 0.25%) given q 3 to 4 h for not more than 7 days provides symptomatic relief. Systemic sympathomimetic amines, such as pseudoephedrine 30 mg orally q 4 to 6 h, may be given for vasoconstriction of the nasal mucous membrane.

Diagnosis in **chronic rhinitis** is based on demonstrating the causative microorganism by culture or biopsy. Treatment consists of chemotherapy appropriate to the causative agent.

ATROPHIC RHINITIS

A chronic rhinitis characterized by an atrophic and sclerotic mucous membrane, abnormal patency of the nasal cavities, crust formation, and foul odor. The mucous membrane changes from ciliated pseudostratified columnar epithelium to stratified squamous epithelium, and the lamina propria is reduced in amount and vascularity. Anosmia results, and epistaxis may be recurrent and severe. The cause is unknown, although bacterial infection frequently plays a role. Atrophic rhinitis is differentiated from other forms of chronic rhinitis by the abnormal patency of the nasal cavities, caused by atrophy of the blood vessels and seromucinous glands in the lamina propria.

Treatment is directed toward reducing the crusting and eliminating the odor. Topical antibiotics, such as bacitracin 500 u./gm in a petrolatum base, and topical or systemic estrogens and vitamins A and D may be effective. Occluding or reducing the patency of the nasal cavities, surgically or with a pledget of lamb's wool, decreases the crusting caused by the drying effect of air flowing over the atrophic mucous membrane.

VASOMOTOR RHINITIS

A chronic rhinitis characterized by intermittent vascular engorgement of the nasal mucous membrane, sneezing, and watery rhinorrhea.
The turgescent mucous membrane varies from bright red to a purplish hue. The condition is marked by periods of remission and exacerbation. It appears to be aggravated by a dry atmosphere. The etiology is uncertain, and no allergy can be identified. Vasomotor rhinitis is differentiated from specific viral and bacterial infections of the nose by lack of purulent exudate and crusting. It is differentiated from allergic rhinitis by the absence of an identifiable allergen.

Treatment is empirical and not always satisfactory. Patients benefit from humidified air, eg, from a humidified central heating system or a vaporizer in the workroom and bedroom. Systemic sympathomimetic amines (eg, pseudoephedrine 30 mg orally [for adults] q 4 to 6 h prn) give symptomatic relief but are not recommended for regular long-term use. Topical vasoconstrictors should be **avoided** because the vasculature of the nasal mucous membrane loses its sensitivity to stimuli—eg, the humidity and temperature of the inspired air—which results in vasoconstriction. Vasodilation results, except after application of a strong stimulus such as a topical sympathomimetic amine.

POLYPS

Allergic rhinitis predisposes to polyp formation; polyps may also occur in acute and chronic infections. Nasal polyps form at the site of massive dependent edema in the lamina propria of the mucous membrane, usually around the ostia of the maxillary sinuses. A developing polyp is teardrop-shaped; when mature, it resembles a peeled seedless grape. In acute infections, polyps may regress after the infection resolves. Bleeding polyps occur in rhinosporidiosis. Unilateral polyps occasionally occur in association with benign or malignant neoplasms of the nose or paranasal sinuses.

Treatment: Corticosteroids, such as beclomethasone dipropionate (42 µg/spray) or flunisolide (25 µg/spray) aerosols, 1 or 2 sprays in each nasal cavity bid, sometimes reduce or eliminate polyps, although surgical removal is often still required. Polyps that obstruct the airway or promote sinusitis should be removed, as should unilateral polyps that may be obscuring benign or malignant neoplasms. However, polyps tend to recur unless the underlying allergy or infection is controlled. Following removal of nasal polyps, topical beclomethasone or flunisolide therapy tends to retard recurrence. In severe and recurrent cases, maxillary sinusotomy or ethmoidectomy may be indicated.

WEGENER'S GRANULOMATOSIS

This vasculitis of unknown etiology is characterized by granulomas of the nose and lung and by glomerulitis. Most destructive lesions of bone, cartilage, and soft tissue of the nose and paranasal sinuses are ultimately found on biopsy to be malignant neoplasms, such as lymphoma or carcinoma.

ANOSMIA

Loss of the sense of smell. Anosmia requires thorough evaluation for intranasal and intracranial diseases. Loss of smell occurs when (1) intranasal swelling or other obstruction prevents odors from gaining access to the olfactory area; (2) the olfactory neuroepithelium is destroyed, as in viral infections, atrophic rhinitis, or the chronic rhinitis of granulomatous diseases and neoplasms; or (3) the olfactory nerve fila, bulbs and tracts, or central connections are destroyed, as by head trauma, intracranial surgery, infections, or neoplasms. Head trauma is a major cause of anosmia in young adults; viral infections are a major cause in older adults. Anosmia occurs congenitally in male hypogonadism (Kallmann's syndrome). Most patients with anosmia have normal perception of salty, sweet, sour, and bitter substances, but they lack flavor discrimination, which is largely dependent on olfaction; therefore, they often complain of loss of the sense of taste.

Diagnostic evaluation requires examination of the cranial nerves and upper respiratory tract (particularly the nose and nasopharynx), psychophysical assessment of odor and taste identification and threshold detection, and enhanced

CT of the head to rule out neoplasms and unsuspected fractures of the floor of the anterior cranial fossa.

Treatment for allergic or bacterial rhinitis and sinusitis and removal of nasal polyps and benign neoplasms may result in recovery of the sense of smell. Conditions causing destruction of the olfactory neuroepithelium or its central pathways do not lend themselves to effective therapeutic intervention, although spontaneous recovery frequently follows regeneration of the olfactory neuroepithelium and its central pathways.

SINUSITIS

An inflammatory process in the paranasal sinuses due to viral, bacterial, and fungal infections or allergic reactions.

Etiology and Pathogenesis

Acute sinusitis is caused by streptococci, pneumococci, *Hemophilus influenzae,* or staphylococci and is usually precipitated by an acute viral respiratory tract infection. Exacerbations of chronic sinusitis may be caused by a gram-negative rod or anaerobic microorganisms. In about 25% of cases, chronic maxillary sinusitis is secondary to dental infection.

With a URI, the swollen nasal mucous membrane obstructs the ostium of the paranasal sinus, and the O_2 in the sinus is absorbed into the blood vessels in the mucous membrane. The resulting relative negative pressure in the sinus (vacuum sinusitis) is painful. If the vacuum is maintained, a transudate from the mucous membrane develops and fills the sinus, where it serves as a medium for bacteria that enter through the ostium or through a spreading cellulitis or thrombophlebitis in the lamina propria of the mucous membrane. An outpouring of serum and leukocytes to combat the infection results, and painful positive pressure develops in the obstructed sinus. The mucous membrane becomes hyperemic and edematous.

Symptoms, Signs, and Diagnosis

The symptoms and signs of acute and chronic sinusitis are similar. The area over the involved sinus may be tender and swollen. Maxillary sinusitis causes pain in the maxillary area, toothache, and frontal headache. Frontal sinusitis produces pain in the frontal area and frontal headache. Ethmoid sinusitis causes pain behind and between the eyes and a frontal headache that is often described as "splitting." Pain from sphenoid sinusitis is less well localized and is referred to the frontal or occipital area. Malaise may be present. Fever and chills suggest an extension of the infection beyond the sinuses.

The nasal mucous membrane is red and turgescent; yellow or green purulent rhinorrhea may be present. The seropurulent or mucopurulent exudate may be seen in the middle meatus in maxillary, anterior ethmoid, and frontal sinusitis, as well as in the area medial to the middle turbinate in posterior ethmoid and sphenoid sinusitis.

In acute and chronic sinusitis, swollen mucous membrane and retained exudate cause the affected sinus to be opaque on radiography. Better definition of the extent and degree of sinusitis is obtained with CT. X-rays of the apices of the teeth are required in chronic maxillary sinusitis to exclude a periapical abscess.

Treatment

Improved drainage and control of infection are the aims of therapy in acute sinusitis. Steam inhalation effectively produces nasal vasoconstriction and promotes drainage. Topical vasoconstrictors such as phenylephrine 0.25% spray q 3 h are effective but should be used for a maximum of 7 days; systemic vasoconstrictors such as pseudoephedrine 30 mg orally (for adults) q 4 to 6 h are less reliably effective.

In both acute and chronic sinusitis, antibiotics should be given for at least 10 to 12 days. In acute sinusitis, penicillin G or V 250 mg orally q 6 h is the initial antibiotic of choice, and erythromycin 250 mg orally q 6 h is the second choice. In exacerbations of chronic sinusitis, a broad-spectrum antibiotic such as ampicillin 250 or 500 mg or tetracycline 250 mg orally q 6 h is better. In chronic sinusitis, prolonged antibiotic therapy for 4 to 6 wk often results in complete resolution. The sensitivities of pathogens isolated from the sinus exudate and the patient's response guide subsequent therapy. Sinusitis not responsive to antibiotic therapy may require operative intervention (Caldwell-Luc operation for the maxillary sinuses, ethmoidectomy for the ethmoid sinuses, and sphenoid sinusotomy for the sphenoid sinuses) to improve ventilation and drainage and to remove inspissated mucopurulent material, epithelial debris, and hypertrophic mucous membrane. Chronic frontal sinusitis is managed with an osteoplastic obliteration of the frontal sinuses.

SINUSITIS IN METABOLICALLY OR IMMUNOLOGICALLY COMPROMISED PATIENTS

In patients with poorly controlled diabetes or immunodeficiency from other causes, aggressive and even fatal fungal sinusitis can occur.

Mucormycosis (phycomycosis)—a mycosis due to fungi of the order Mucorales including species of *Mucor, Absidia,* and *Rhizopus*—may develop in poorly controlled diabetics. It is characterized by black, devitalized tissue in the nasal cavity and neurologic signs secondary to retrograde thromboarteritis in the carotid arterial system. Diagnosis is made by the histopathologic demonstration of mycelia in the avascularized tissue, and treatment requires control of the diabetes and IV administration of amphotericin B.

Aspergillosis and **candidiasis** of the paranasal sinuses may occur in the patient who is immunologically compromised as a result of therapy with cytotoxic drugs or from the underlying disease process in leukemia, lymphoma, multiple myeloma, AIDS, and other immunosuppressive diseases. Aspergillosis is characterized by polypoid tissue in the nose and paranasal sinuses. Biopsy and culture of this polypoid tissue are required for diagnosis; aggressive paranasal sinus surgery and IV amphotericin B therapy are advocated as attempts to control these often-fatal infections.

NEOPLASMS

Unilateral bloody nasal discharge and obstruction and facial swelling and numbness indicate cancer of the nose or paranasal sinuses until proved otherwise. **Exophytic papillomas** are squamous cell papillomas having a branching, vascular connective tissue stalk with fingerlike projections on the surface. In the nasal cavity, they often require repeated excision but have a benign course. **Inverted papillomas** are squamous cell papillomas in which the epithelium is invaginated into the vascular connective tissue stroma. They are invasive and behave in a locally malignant manner; excision must involve a large margin of normal tissue, including the bone of the lateral wall of the nasal cavity in a procedure called a lateral rhinotomy.

Other benign tumors that occur in the nasal cavity are fibromas, hemangiomas, and neurofibromas. Fibromas, neurilemomas, and ossifying fibromas occur in the paranasal sinuses.

Squamous cell carcinoma is the most common malignant tumor in the nose and paranasal sinuses; others are adenoid cystic and mucoepidermoid carcinomas, malignant mixed tumors, adenocarcinomas, lymphomas, fibrosarcomas, osteosarcomas, chondrosarcomas, and melanomas. Hypernephroma is the most common metastatic tumor in the paranasal sinuses. Combined irradiation and radical resection give the best survival rates for the primary neoplasms.

69. NASOPHARYNX

(See also ADENOID HYPERTROPHY under BACTERIAL INFECTIONS in Ch. 32 and JUVENILE ANGIOFIBROMA in Ch. 44)

TORNWALDT'S CYST
(Nasopharyngeal Cyst)

A frequently infected cyst found in the midline of the nasopharynx. The cyst is superficial to the superior constrictor muscle of the pharynx and is covered by the mucous membrane of the nasopharynx. If infected, it may cause persistent purulent drainage with a foul taste and odor, eustachian tube obstruction, and sore throat. Purulent exudate may be seen at the opening of the cyst. **Treatment** consists of marsupialization or excision.

NASOPHARYNGEAL CARCINOMA

Squamous cell carcinoma of the nasopharynx occurs in children and young adults. Rare in North America, it is one of the most common cancers in the Orient. The first symptom is often nasal or eustachian tube obstruction; the latter may result in middle ear effusion. Purulent bloody rhinorrhea, frank epistaxis, cranial nerve paralysis due to invasion of the parapharyngeal space and cranial cavity by the tumor, and cervical lymphadenopathy resulting from metastasis are common presenting complaints. **Diagnosis** is by biopsy of the primary nasopharyngeal tumor. Biopsy of the neck metastasis should be avoided until the nasopharynx has been inspected and palpated, and biopsy has been performed on any suspicious lesion there. **Treatment** of the primary tumor is radiation therapy. Radical neck dissection is required for large (> 2 cm at the greatest dimension) or persistent neck masses. The overall 5-yr survival rate is 35%.

70. OROPHARYNX

Retropharyngeal abscess is discussed under BACTERIAL INFECTIONS in Ch. 32.

PHARYNGITIS

Acute inflammation of the pharynx. Usually viral in origin, it may also be due to a Group A β-hemolytic streptococcus, *Mycoplasma pneumoniae*, *Chlamydia pneumoniae*, or other bacteria. It is characterized by sore throat and pain on swallowing. Differentiating viral from bacterial pharyngitis on the basis of physical examination alone is difficult. In both, the pharyngeal mucous membrane may be mildly injected or severely inflamed and may be covered by a membrane and a purulent exudate. Fever, cervical adenopathy, and leukocytosis are present in both viral and streptococcal pharyngitis but may be more marked in the latter. (Pharyngitis in gonorrhea and in other sexually transmitted diseases is discussed in Ch. 21.)

Treatment includes aspirin, to relieve discomfort, and rest. Antibiotic therapy is usually withheld pending positive cultures for Group A β-hemolytic streptococcus. Penicillin G or V 250 mg orally q 6 h for 10 days is indicated for Group A streptococcal pharyngitis, primarily to prevent rheumatic fever. Alternatively, parenteral penicillin G benzathine, erythromycin, or a 1st-generation cephalosporin may be used.

TONSILLITIS

Acute inflammation of the palatine tonsils, usually due to streptococcal or, less commonly, viral infection. Epidemics of viral tonsillitis occur among military recruits. Tonsillitis is characterized by sore throat and pain, most marked on swallowing and often referred to the ears. Very young children may not complain of sore throat but will refuse to eat. High fever, malaise, headache, and vomiting are common.

Diagnosis

The tonsils are edematous and hyperemic. There may be a purulent exudate from the crypts and a membrane—white, thin, nonconfluent, and confined to the tonsil—that peels away without bleeding. The **differential diagnosis** includes diphtheria, Vincent's angina (trench mouth), and infectious mononucleosis. In diphtheria, the membrane is dirty gray, thick, and tough; it bleeds if peeled away and shows *Corynebacterium diphtheriae* on smear and culture. Vincent's angina, characterized by superficial, painful ulcers with erythematous borders, is caused by a fusiform bacillus and a spirochete that are demonstrable on smear. Infectious mononucleosis tonsillitis characteristically is associated with micropetechiae of the soft palate; atypical lymphocytes on smear and a positive Monospot test confirm the diagnosis of mononucleosis.

Treatment

In viral tonsillitis, symptomatic therapy is as for pharyngitis (above). Penicillin G 250 mg orally q 6 h, or penicillin V 125 mg orally q 8 h for children < 6 yr of age, is the treatment of choice in streptococcal tonsillitis and should be continued for 10 days. If possible, the throat should be recultured 5 to 6 days later. Family members' throats should also be cultured initially so that carriers may be treated at the same time. Tonsillectomy should be considered if, despite these precautions, acute tonsillitis repeatedly develops after adequate treatment, or if chronic tonsillitis and sore throat persist or are relieved only briefly by antibiotic therapy.

PERITONSILLAR CELLULITIS AND ABSCESS
(Quinsy)

An acute infection located between the tonsil and the superior pharyngeal constrictor muscle. Peritonsillar abscesses are rare in children but common in young adults. Although usually due to a Group A β-hemolytic streptococcus, peritonsillar infection can also be caused by anaerobic microorganisms such as bacteroides. Severe pain is felt on swallowing; the patient is febrile and toxic, holds his head tilted toward the side of the abscess, and shows marked trismus. The tonsil is displaced medially by the peritonsillar cellulitis and abscess, the soft palate is erythematous and swollen, and the uvula is edematous and displaced to the opposite side.

Treatment

Cellulitis without pus formation responds to penicillin in 24 to 48 h. Initially, penicillin G 1 million u. IV q 4 h is given. If pus is present and does not drain spontaneously, incision and drainage are required. Antibiotic therapy should be continued orally with penicillin G or V 250 mg q 6 h for 12 days. Peritonsillar abscesses tend to recur, and tonsillectomy is indicated (usually performed 6 wk after the acute infection has subsided). With antibiotic therapy, the tonsillectomy can be performed at the time of the acute peritonsillar infection.

PARAPHARYNGEAL ABSCESS

Suppuration of a parapharyngeal lymph node with consequent abscess formation is usually secondary to pharyngitis or tonsillitis and may occur at any age. The abscess is lateral to the superior pharyngeal constrictor muscle and close to the carotid sheath. Pharyngeal inflammation may not be apparent. The anterior cervical triangle is markedly swollen. Penicillin G 150,000 u./kg/day IV in 4 equal doses (for a child) should be given initially and the abscess drained though a cervical, not pharyngeal, incision. Subsequently, penicillin G or V 250 mg orally q 6 h is given to complete 12 days of therapy.

VELOPHARYNGEAL INSUFFICIENCY

Incomplete closure of the velopharyngeal sphincter between the oropharynx and the nasopharynx, resulting in impaired speech and deglutition. The speech is characterized by nasal emission of air and weak oral plosive and fricative articulation.

Normal closure, achieved by the sphincteric action of the soft palate and the superior constrictor muscle, is impaired in patients with cleft palates, repaired cleft palates, congenitally short palates, submucous cleft palates, unusually large nasopharynges, and palatal paralysis.

Diagnosis and Treatment

Regurgitation of solid foods and fluids through the nose denotes gross velopharyngeal insufficiency, but normal speech is a more exacting criterion of competency. Inspection of the palate during phonation may reveal palatal paralysis. Palpation of the midline of the soft palate and transillumination with a flexible nasopharyngolaryngoscope may demonstrate a submucous cleft. A lateral x-ray may demonstrate the congenitally short palate or an unusually large nasopharynx and, if taken during phonation, indicates the degree of insufficiency; cinefluoroscopy during connected speech verifies an inability to maintain velopharyngeal valve closure.

Treatment requires speech therapy and surgical correction by a palatal push-back procedure, pharyngeal flap, pharyngoplasty, or Teflon paste injection of the posterior pharyngeal wall.

CARCINOMA OF THE TONSIL

Squamous cell carcinoma of the tonsil, second in frequency only to carcinoma of the larynx among malignancies of the upper respiratory tract, occurs predominantly in males and is associated with tobacco smoking and ethanol ingestion. Sore throat is the most common presenting complaint, and pain often radiates to the ear on the same side. A metastatic mass in the neck may be the first symptom. **Diagnosis** is made by biopsy. Direct laryngoscopy, bronchoscopy, and esophagoscopy are carried out to exclude a synchronous 2nd primary neoplasm. **Treatment** combines irradiation and surgery, consisting of radical resection of the tonsillar fossa, hemimandibulectomy, and radical neck dissection. The 5-yr survival rate approximates 50%.

71. LARYNX

For discussions of acute laryngotracheobronchitis, see ACUTE EPIGLOTTITIS under BACTERIAL INFECTIONS and CROUP under VIRAL INFECTIONS in Ch. 32.

VOCAL CORD POLYPS

These lesions develop from voice abuse, chronic laryngeal allergic reactions, and chronic inhalation of irritants such as industrial fumes and cigarette smoke. They consist of chronic edema in the lamina propria of the true vocal cord and result in hoarseness and a breathy voice quality. Biopsy of discrete lesions should be performed to exclude carcinoma. Treatment involves surgical removal of the polyp at direct laryngoscopy to restore the voice and attention to the underlying cause to prevent recurrence, including voice therapy if voice abuse is the cause.

VOCAL CORD NODULES
(Singer's Nodules)

These lesions are caused by chronic voice abuse, such as yelling or shouting, or using an unnaturally low fundamental frequency. The nodules are condensations of hyaline connective tissue in the lamina propria at the junction of the anterior $1/3$ and the posterior $2/3$ of the free edges of the true vocal cords. Hoarseness and a breathy voice quality result. Carcinoma should be excluded by biopsy. Treatment involves surgical removal of the nodules at direct laryngoscopy and correction of the underlying voice abuse. Vocal nodules in children usually regress with voice therapy alone.

CONTACT ULCERS

Unilateral or bilateral ulcers of the mucous membrane over the vocal process of the arytenoid cartilage. Contact ulcers are usually due to voice abuse in the form of a sharp glottal attack (abrupt rise in intensity at the onset of phonation). Reflux of gastric contents may also cause contact ulcers. Mild pain on phonation and swallowing and varying degrees of hoarseness result. Biopsy to exclude carcinoma is important. Prolonged ulceration leads to nonspecific granulomas that produce varying degrees of hoarseness.

Treatment consists of prolonged voice rest (6 wk minimum) to heal the ulcers. Patients must recognize the limitations of their voices and learn to adjust their vocal activities to avoid recurrent ulcers. Granulomas tend to recur after surgical removal but respond to voice therapy. Antacids, avoiding eating within 2 h of retiring, and elevating the head of the bed are helpful if gastroesophageal reflux is demonstrated on an upper GI series.

LARYNGITIS

Inflammation of the larynx.

Etiology
The most frequent cause of acute laryngitis is a viral URI. Laryngitis may also occur in the course of bronchitis, pneumonia, influenza, pertussis, measles, and diphtheria. Excessive use of the voice, allergic reactions, and inhalation of irritating substances such as cigarette smoke can cause acute or chronic laryngitis.

Symptoms and Signs
Unnatural change of voice is usually the most prominent symptom. Hoarseness and even aphonia, together with a sensation of tickling, rawness, and a constant urge to clear the throat, may occur. Symptoms vary with the severity of the inflammation. Fever, malaise, dysphagia, and throat pain may occur in the more severe infections; dyspnea may be apparent if laryngeal edema is present. Indirect laryngoscopy discloses a mild to marked erythema of the mucous membrane that may also be edematous. If a membrane is present, diphtheria must be suspected (see DIPHTHERIA under BACTERIAL INFECTIONS in Ch. 32).

Treatment
There is no specific treatment for viral laryngitis. Voice rest and steam inhalations give symptomatic relief and promote resolution of acute laryngitis. Treatment of acute or chronic bronchitis may improve the laryngitis. Treatment of chronic bronchitis may require a broad-spectrum antibiotic such as ampicillin 250 or 500 mg or tetracycline 250 mg orally q 6 h for 10 to 14 days.

VOCAL CORD PARALYSIS

Etiology

Vocal cord paralysis may result from lesions at the nucleus ambiguus, its supranuclear tracts, the main trunk of the vagus, or the recurrent laryngeal nerves. Intracranial neoplasms, vascular accidents, and demyelinating diseases cause nucleus ambiguus paralysis. Neoplasms at the base of the skull and trauma of the neck cause vagus paralysis. Recurrent laryngeal paralysis is caused by neck or thoracic lesions (eg, aortic aneurysm; mitral stenosis; neoplasms of the thyroid gland, esophagus, lung, or mediastinal structures; trauma, thyroidectomy, neurotoxins (lead), neurotoxic infections (diphtheria), or viral illness. Viral neuronitis probably accounts for most cases of idiopathic vocal cord paralysis.

Symptoms and Signs

Vocal cord paralysis results in loss of vocal cord abduction, or adduction and abduction; may affect phonation, respiration, and deglutition; and may result in aspiration of food and fluids into the trachea. The paralyzed cord generally lies 2 to 3 mm lateral to the midline; in recurrent laryngeal nerve paralysis, it may move with phonation but not on inspiration. In **unilateral vocal cord paralysis**, the voice is hoarse and breathy. There is usually no airway obstruction because the normal cord abducts sufficiently. In **bilateral vocal cord paralysis**, the cords are generally within 2 to 3 mm of the midline, and the voice is of limited intensity but good quality. The airway, however, is inadequate, resulting in stridor and dyspnea on moderate exertion.

Diagnosis

The cause must always be sought. The evaluation may include laryngoscopy, bronchoscopy, and esophagoscopy. Neurologic examination; enhanced CT of the head, neck, and chest; thyroid gland scan; and upper GI series are also indicated. Cricoarytenoid arthritis may cause fixation of the cricoarytenoid joint and must be differentiated.

Treatment

In unilateral paralysis, augmenting the paralyzed cord by injecting a Teflon suspension may allow approximation of the cords for voice improvement and prevention of aspiration. Maintenance of an adequate airway is the problem in bilateral paralysis. Tracheostomy may be needed permanently or during URI. An arytenoidectomy with lateralization of the true vocal cord will open the glottis and improve the airway but may adversely affect voice quality.

LARYNGOCELES

Evaginations of the mucous membrane of the laryngeal ventricle. Internal laryngoceles displace and enlarge the false vocal cord, resulting in hoarseness and airway obstruction. External laryngoceles extend through the thyrohyoid membrane, producing a mass in the neck. Laryngoceles are filled with air and can be expanded by the Valsalva maneuver. They tend to occur in musicians who play wind instruments. They appear on CT as smooth, ovoid, low-density masses. Laryngoceles may become infected (laryngopyocele) or filled with mucoid fluid. **Treatment** is excision.

NEOPLASMS

BENIGN

Juvenile papillomas are discussed in Ch. 44. Other benign laryngeal tumors include hemangiomas, fibromas, chondromas, myxomas, and neurofibromas. They may involve any part of the larynx. Removal restores the voice, the functional integrity of the laryngeal sphincter, and the airway.

MALIGNANT

Squamous cell carcinoma, the most common malignant neoplasm of the larynx, is also the most common malignancy of the head and neck. The incidence is higher in males. It is associated with cigarette smoking and ethanol consumption. The true vocal cords (particularly the anterior portion), epiglottis, pyriform sinus, and postcricoid area are common sites of origin. Cordal or glottic carcinoma produces hoarseness early, and all patients with hoarseness lasting > 2 wk should have indirect laryngoscopy. Biopsy of a discrete lesion of the laryngeal mucous membrane should be performed at direct laryngoscopy. Carcinoma of the supraglottic larynx (epiglottis), hypopharyngeal carcinoma (pyriform sinus), and postcricoid carcinoma cause pain and difficulty on swallowing. In the first 2 forms, a metastatic mass in the neck may be the first symptom.

Verrucous carcinoma, a rare variant of squamous cell carcinoma, usually arises in the glottic area. The diagnosis may require multiple biopsies.

Treatment

For **early glottic carcinoma,** radiation therapy or cordectomy results in a 5-yr survival rate of 85 to 95%. For **early cordal carcinoma,** radiation is often preferred, since it usually results in a normal voice. For **advanced carcinoma** with anterior commissure involvement, impaired vocal cord mobility, thyroid cartilage invasion, or subglottic extension, surgery is necessary. A hemilaryngectomy, preserving laryngeal phonation and sphincteric functions, is often possible. More advanced glottic carcinoma requires total laryngectomy. **Early supraglottic carcinoma** can be effectively treated with radiation therapy. For more **advanced supraglottic carcinoma** that does not involve the true vocal cords, a supraglottic partial laryngectomy can be performed to preserve the voice and glottic sphincter. If true vocal cords are involved, a total laryngectomy is required. **Early hypopharyngeal carcinoma** may be managed by an extended partial laryngectomy; more advanced lesions require a total laryngectomy. **Postcricoid carcinoma** requires a total laryngopharyngectomy and replacement of the hypopharynx and cervical esophagus with a free jejunal graft with microvascular anastomoses. For **metastasis to the cervical lymph nodes,** laryngeal surgery is combined with radical or modified radical neck dissection. In **advanced supraglottic and hypopharyngeal carcinoma,** a combination of radiation therapy and surgery is more successful than surgery alone. **Verrucous carcinoma** is treated surgically.

Rehabilitation after total laryngectomy requires developing a new voice by using esophageal speech or creating a tracheoesophageal fistula. **Esophageal speech** involves taking air into the esophagus during inspiration and gradually eructating the air through the pharyngoesophageal junction to produce a sound that is articulated into speech by the pharynx, palate, tongue, teeth, and lips.

A **tracheoesophageal fistula,** created by inserting a one-way valve between the trachea and the esophagus, forces air into the esophagus during expiration to produce a sound that is converted into speech. With this technique, fluids and food may be aspirated into the tracheobronchial tree if the tracheoesophageal valve misfunctions.

An alternative method, using an **electrolarynx** as a sounding source, requires holding the device in place while it produces the sound that is articulated into speech.

72. NEOPLASMS OF THE HEAD AND NECK

Premalignant lesions are discussed in Ch. 111. Neoplasms of specific organs are discussed elsewhere in THE MANUAL. This discussion deals with important general principles of head and neck neoplasms and with the situation in which cervical metastasis is present but the primary neoplasm cannot be determined.

Etiology and Pathogenesis

The most common cancer of the upper respiratory and alimentary tracts is squamous cell carcinoma of the larynx, followed by squamous cell carcinoma of the palatine tonsil and hypopharynx. About 85% of patients with cancer of the head or neck have a history of ethanol and tobacco consumption. Other causes of oral cavity cancer include poor oral hygiene, ill-fitting dental appliances, dipping of snuff, and chewing of tobacco. In India, chewing betel nut is a major cause.

The Epstein-Barr virus plays a role in pathogenesis of nasopharyngeal cancer. Patients who were treated with small doses of radiation therapy 20 or more years ago (for acne, facial hair, enlarged thymus, hypertrophic tonsils, and adenoids) are predisposed to developing thyroid and salivary gland cancer.

Head and neck cancer usually spreads in an orderly fashion, remaining localized to the head and neck for long periods. Local tissue invasion is followed by metastasis to regional lymph nodes. Distant lymphatic metastases tend to occur late. Hematogenous metastases are usually associated with large or persistent tumors and occur in immunosuppressed patients.

Epidemiology

In the head and neck, 90% of cancers are squamous cell (epidermoid) carcinoma; melanomas, lymphomas, and sarcomas make up another 5%. The average age of patients with head and neck cancers is 59 yr; those with sarcomas or cancers of the salivary glands, thyroid, or paranasal sinuses are usually < 59 yr, while those with squamous cell carcinoma of the oral cavity, pharynx, and larynx are generally > 59 yr. Cancer of the nasopharynx is prevalent in immigrant Chinese and slightly less prevalent in first-generation Chinese Americans.

Staging and Prognosis

Head and neck cancers are classified according to size and site of involvement of the primary neoplasm (**T**), number and size of metastases to the cervical lymph nodes (**N**), and evidence of distant metastases (**M**). **Stage I:** The primary neoplasm is ≤ 2 cm at greatest dimension or localized to one anatomic site without regional or distant metastasis ($T_1N_0M_0$). **Stage II:** The primary neoplasm measures 2 to 4 cm at greatest dimension or involves 2 areas within a specific site (eg, larynx) without regional or distant metastasis ($T_2N_0M_0$). **Stage III:** The primary neoplasm is > 4 cm at greatest dimension or involves 3 adjacent areas in a specific head and neck site and/or has an isolated neck metastasis of ≤ 3 cm at greatest dimension (T_3N_0 or $T_{1\text{-}3}N_1M_0$). **Stage IV:** The cancer is massive, invades bone and cartilage, and/or extends outside of its site of origin into another site (eg, oral cavity into oropharynx). Neck metastasis measures > 3 cm; involves multiple ipsilateral, contralateral, or bilateral lymph nodes or is fixed to surrounding tissue; and/or evidence exists of distant metastases ($T_{1\text{-}4}N_{1\text{-}3}M_{0\text{-}1}$).

Exophytic or verrucous-appearing tumors respond to treatment better than infiltrative, ulcerative, or indurated lesions. Cervical or distant metastasis is associated with limited survival. The more poorly differentiated the cancer, generally the greater the chance of regional and distant metastasis. Invasion of muscle, bone, or cartilage reduces cure rates. Perineural spread as evidenced by pain, paralysis, or numbness indicates a highly aggressive neoplasm with a high propensity for persistence.

With appropriate treatment, stage I survival generally approaches 90%; stage II, 75%; stage III, 45 to 75%; and stage IV, < 35%. Overall 5-yr survival is 65% for all patients with local stages II and III squamous cell cancer of the head and neck. The rate drops to ≤ 30% for patients with metastasis to lymph nodes. Patients over age 70 yr often have longer disease-free intervals and better survival rates than younger patients.

Treatment

Stage I neoplasms, regardless of location within the upper respiratory or alimentary tract, respond similarly to surgery or radiation. Usually, radiation therapy is delivered to the primary site and also bilaterally to the cervical lymph nodes if the probability of regional nonpalpable metastasis is > 20%. A 5-yr cure rate of 90% can be expected. Some surgical procedures may be needed to achieve the 90% cure rate. Lesions > 2 cm or with bone or cartilage invasion (with or without regional neck metastasis) require surgery. If lymph node metastases are found or deemed very likely to occur, postoperative radiation to the primary site and cervical lymph nodes bilaterally is necessary. Alternatively, fair survival rates can be attained with radiation with or without chemotherapy. If the cancer recurs, the patient has recourse to surgery. In advanced (most stage II and all stages III and IV) squamous cell carcinoma, a combination of surgery and radiation offers a better chance of cure than treatment with either modality alone. Surgery is more effective than radiation and/or chemotherapy in controlling large primary cancers, while radiation is effective in controlling the periphery of the primary lesion and microscopic or nonpalpable metastases. Radiation therapy may be given pre- or postoperatively, but the latter is usually preferred.

Chemotherapy kills tumor cells at the local site, regional lymph nodes, and distant metastases. Whether adjuvant chemotherapy (in combination with surgery or radiation therapy) increases the cure rate is not known; however, combined therapy does prolong the interval between cancer disappearance and recurrence. Several agents—cisplatin, fluorouracil, bleomycin, and methotrexate—provide useful palliation for pain and reduce neoplasm size in patients who cannot be treated with surgery or radiation therapy.

Adverse effects of treatment: Surgery requires rehabilitation for swallowing and speaking. Radiation produces skin changes, fibrosis, ageusia, xerostomia, and rarely, osteoradionecrosis. Toxic effects of chemotherapy include severe nausea and vomiting, transient hair loss, gastroenteritis, and hematopoietic and immune depression. In cancer excision after chemotherapy or irradiation, the surgeon must remove what was originally involved with the neoplasm before the anticancer therapy was started.

Persisting cancer: *A palpable mass or ulcerated lesion with edema or pain at the primary* *site after therapy* strongly suggests a persistent tumor. Detecting persistence after chemotherapy or radiation therapy is more difficult than after surgery alone; however, persistence after surgery alone is usually more difficult to eradicate than that after radiation and/or chemotherapy. Gallium scan, CT with enhancement, and MRI can sometimes detect persistences or tumors that are $\geq$ 2 cm.

For adequate local control following surgical failure, all scar planes as well as reconstructive flaps must be excised in addition to the cancer. Radiation and/or chemotherapy given after surgical failure is much less effective than when given before or immediately after surgery.

UNKNOWN PRIMARY AND CERVICAL METASTASES

A palpable mass in the neck may represent an infectious, congenital, or neoplastic process. Among neoplasms to be considered are metastasis of carcinoma from the upper respiratory or upper alimentary tract to a lymph node; lymphoma; metastasis of thyroid or salivary gland carcinoma; and metastasis from a distant primary site such as the lung, prostate, breast, stomach, colon, or kidney. About 60% of supraclavicular triangle masses are metastases from distant primary sites. Elsewhere in the neck, in 80% of patients with cancerous cervical adenopathy, the primary carcinoma is found in the

upper respiratory or alimentary tract. Likely sites are the nasopharynx, palatine tonsil, base of tongue, laryngeal surface of the epiglottis, and hypopharynx including the pyriform sinuses.

Diagnosis: Evaluation of a patient with a neck mass should include inspection of the ears, nasal cavities, nasopharynx, oropharynx, hypopharynx, and larynx, as well as palpation of the palatine tonsils, base of the tongue, and thyroid and salivary glands. An upper GI series; thyroid scan; and CT of the head, neck, and chest may be required. Direct laryngoscopy, bronchoscopy, and esophagoscopy with biopsy are indicated for suspicious areas; random biopsy of the nasopharynx, palatine tonsils, and base of the tongue should also be performed when a primary neoplasm has not been identified. If a primary site is not found, the mass may be aspirated with a fine needle for cytologic evaluation, and if necessary, a biopsy should be performed. An excisional biopsy is preferable to an incisional biopsy because it provides better opportunity for diagnosis.

Treatment: Squamous cell carcinoma with cervical metastases from an unknown primary site is treated with radiation therapy to the nasopharynx, palatine tonsils, base of tongue, and both sides of the neck, followed by radical neck dissection if the cervical mass was $\geq$ 2 cm at greatest dimension when radiation therapy began or if the mass persists following radiation therapy.

§6. OPHTHALMOLOGIC DISORDERS

73. CLINICAL EXAMINATION

Since some ocular complaints are nonspecific, a complete history and examination of all parts of the eye and its adnexa (see FIG. 73–1) are necessary to identify the source of the complaint. The patient should be asked about the location and duration of the symptom; the presence and nature of pain, discharge, or redness; and change in visual acuity.

Unless chemicals requiring immediate irrigation have splashed into the eye, the first step in ocular evaluation is to record the visual acuity. Vision is tested by having the patient look at an eye chart 20 ft away; a patient who normally wears glasses should have them on. As each eye is covered alternately, the acuity in the opposite eye is determined. A Snellen notation of 20/40 indicates that the patient sees at 20 ft what the average person sees at 40 ft. Gross inspection of the glasses provides an approximation of the degree of ametropia (eg, nearsightedness, farsightedness, astigmatism). Visual fields and ocular motility may also be determined at this time. The fields can be checked by confrontation examination.

Under a focal light and magnification (eg, provided by a headband loupe or slit lamp), system-atic examination of the eye should proceed. The eyelids are examined for lesions of the margins and subcutaneous tissues. The area of the lacrimal sacs is palpated and an attempt made to express any contents up through the canaliculi and puncta. The lids are then everted, and the palpebral and bulbar conjunctivae and the fornices are inspected for foreign bodies, signs of inflammation (eg, follicular hypertrophy, exudate, hyperemia, or edema), or other abnormalities.

The cornea should be inspected closely. If pain and photophobia make it difficult for the patient to open the eye, topical anesthesia can be accomplished before examination by instilling 1 drop of proparacaine 0.5% or tetracaine. Fluorescein staining with sterile, individually packaged fluorescein strips makes corneal abrasions or ulcers more apparent. The strip is moistened with 1 drop of sterile saline and, with the patient's eye turned upward, is touched to the inside of the lower lid for several seconds. The eye is closed for 5 seconds, then examined under good magnification and cobalt blue illumination. Denuded areas will stain green.

The size and shape of the pupils and their reaction to light and accommodation should be

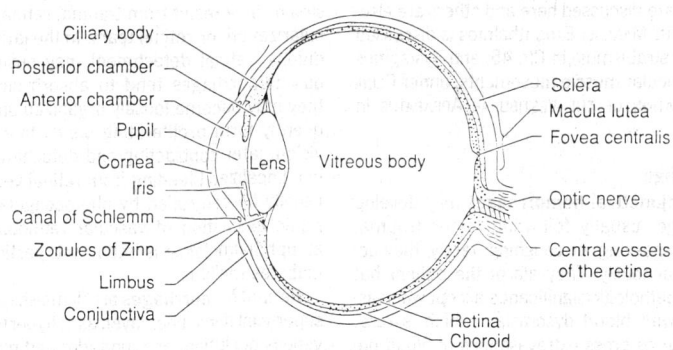

FIG. 73–1. **The eye—cross section.** The **zonules of Zinn** keep the lens suspended, while the muscles of the **ciliary body** serve to focus the lens. The ciliary body also secretes **aqueous humor,** which fills the **posterior chamber,** passes through the pupil into the **anterior chamber,** then drains primarily via the **canal of Schlemm.** The **iris** regulates the light entering the eye by adjusting the size of its central opening, the **pupil.** The visual image is focused on the **retina,** the **fovea centralis** being the area of sharpest visual acuity. Note that the **conjunctiva** ends abruptly at the **limbus.** The **cornea** is covered with an epithelium that differs in many respects from the conjunctival epithelium.

noted. Ocular tension and anterior chamber depth should be estimated before dilation, as mydriasis can precipitate an attack of acute glaucoma if the anterior chamber is shallow.

Ophthalmoscopy is aided by dilating the pupil with 1 drop of tropicamide 0.5% or phenylephrine 2.5% (repeated in 5 to 10 min if necessary); for longer action or wider dilation, cyclopentolate 0.5% or phenylephrine 10% may be used. However, the pupils should not be dilated if the patient has head trauma or is suspected of having acute disease of the CNS. Atropine is not recommended because of its prolonged action. Ophthalmoscopy will disclose opacities of the cornea, lens, and vitreous, as well as retinal and optic nerve lesions. The strength of the ophthalmoscope lens required to bring the retina into focus gives an approximate measure of refractive error. The fundus may show changes due to systemic disease (eg, diabetes mellitus, hypertension).

Other instruments (eg, gonioscope, tangent screen, perimeter) may be needed for precise diagnosis; their use requires special training. The slit-lamp examination is especially helpful in distinguishing corneal lesions. Though other physicians can care for many diseases of the eye, an ophthalmologist should be consulted whenever there is doubt about diagnosis or treatment, especially when the cause of pain or diminished vision is not apparent or when symptoms persist.

Ultrasonography delineates retinal tumors, detachments, and vitreous hemorrhages, even in the presence of opacities of the cornea and lens. Use of ultrasound in ophthalmology started early, with both A- and B-mode techniques. A hand-held B-scanner has simplified ultrasonic examination of the eye and made it possible to do such studies in the ophthalmologist's office. Orbital definition is improved by using higher frequencies (7 to 10 megahertz). Ultrasonography has also been useful in locating metallic and nonmetallic foreign bodies and in determining the axial length of the eye (a measurement needed to calculate the power of an intraocular lens before it is implanted). The most successful application of ultrasonic tissue characterization has been in differentiating between choroidal melanoma and choroidal nevus, metastatic carcinoma, and subretinal hemorrhage. By using a biologic standard, an accuracy of > 90% has been claimed.

74. OCULAR SYMPTOMS AND SIGNS

Some of the more common ocular symptoms and signs are discussed here and others are elsewhere in THE MANUAL: Exophthalmos is discussed in Ch. 76; strabismus, in Ch. 45; and nystagmus and extraocular muscle movements, under CLINICAL EVALUATION OF THE VESTIBULAR APPARATUS in Ch. 64.

Hemorrhage

Subconjunctival hemorrhages may develop at any age, usually following minor trauma, straining, sneezing, or coughing; rarely, they occur spontaneously. They alarm the patient but are of no pathologic significance except when associated with blood dyscrasias, which is rare. They occur as gross extravasations of blood beneath the conjunctiva and are absorbed spontaneously, usually within 2 wk. Topical corticosteroids, antibiotics, vasoconstrictors, and compresses are of no value in speeding reabsorption; reassurance is adequate therapy.

Vitreous hemorrhages, extravasations of blood into the vitreous, produce a black reflex on ophthalmoscopy. They may occur in such conditions as diabetic retinopathy or hypertension or may result from trauma, retinal neovascularization, or retinal tears. In the latter 3 conditions, retinal detachment may ensue. Vitreous hemorrhages tend to absorb slowly, but they may become loosely organized and subsequently form proliferating bands that obscure vision, later contracting and detaching the retina. Localized bleeding from retinal vessels can usually be controlled by photocoagulation. Periodic evaluation of vascular retinopathies by an ophthalmologist is important, particularly in diabetes mellitus.

Retinal hemorrhages are flame-shaped in the superficial nerve fiber layer, as in hypertension or venous occlusion, or round (dot and blot) in the deeper layers, as in diabetes mellitus or septic infarctions. Retinal hemorrhages are always significant, reflecting vascular disease that usually is systemic.

Floaters

Seeing floaters (spots) before one or both eyes is a frequent adult complaint. Floaters are usually most noticeable against a white homogeneous background and seem to move slowly. They result from contraction of the vitreous gel and its separation from the surface of the retina. Since the vitreous gel is denser where it attaches to the optic nerve, floaters are usually more apparent in this area. Though floaters usually are without significance, in a small number of patients they may indicate a tear in the retina. They are more prevalent in highly myopic and older persons, tending to become less noticeable with time. A minute **vitreous hemorrhage** may appear as a brown or red floater. **Retinal detachments** may be preceded by a shower of "sparks" or lightning flashes and may be accompanied by a shower of floaters. Only after the retina actually separates from its underlying structure (the retinal pigment epithelium) does a "curtain" of visual loss move across the visual field. Though floaters are frequently not associated with serious disease, they warrant meticulous examination of the entire retina and media after dilation with a short-acting mydriatic or cycloplegic (eg, cyclopentolate 1%, 1 drop, repeated in 5 to 10 min, or if wider dilation is required and the patient does not have hypertension and is not receiving an oral β blocker, phenylephrine 2.5%, 1 drop, repeated in 5 to 10 min). Examination is done best by indirect ophthalmoscopy, a technique used by most ophthalmologists. Vitreous floaters can be seen with a high plus lens by looking into the red reflex at a distance of 15 to 30 cm (6 to 12 in.). Repeated examinations are warranted if the complaint continues or worsens, if vision is affected, or if apprehension persists. Floaters of recent origin or those accompanied by flashes of light should be evaluated by an ophthalmologist. Disturbance of vision always demands an explanation.

Photophobia

Abnormal visual intolerance to light is common in lightly pigmented persons. Usually it is without significance and may be relieved by wearing dark glasses. It is an important, but nondiagnostic, symptom in keratitis, uveitis, acute glaucoma, and traumatic corneal epithelial abrasions.

Pain

Ocular pain is important and, unless due to an obvious local cause such as a foreign body, acute lid infection, or injury, demands investigation (eg, for uveitis, especially iridocyclitis, or

glaucoma). Sinusitis occasionally causes referred eye pain.

Scotomas

A blind spot in the field of vision is a **negative scotoma.** Frequently it is not noticed by the patient unless it involves central vision and interferes significantly with visual acuity. Negative scotomas noticed by the patient usually are due to hemorrhage or choroiditis. A scotoma found in the same visual field area in each eye is usually a quadrantic or hemianoptic defect resulting from a lesion in the optic pathways. A **positive scotoma,** perceived as a light spot or scintillating flashes, represents a response to abnormal stimulation of some portion of the visual system; eg, as in the migraine syndrome.

Examination of the eyes, including the visual fields, is mandatory to determine the cause of any scotoma. A bilateral scotoma, if not caused by bilateral retinal lesions, demands perimetric examination and neurologic evaluation.

Errors of Refraction

In **emmetropia,** no optical defect exists, and parallel light rays entering the eye focus clearly on the retina. In **ametropia,** an optical defect exists in one or a combination of the following forms: In **hyperopia** (farsightedness), the most common refractive error, the point of focus lies behind the retina, either because the eyeball axis is too short or because the refractive power of the eye is too weak. A convex (plus) lens is used in corrective glasses. In **myopia** (nearsightedness), the image is focused in front of the retina because the axis of the eyeball is too long or the refractive power of the eye is too strong; a concave (minus) corrective lens is used. In **astigmatism,** the refraction is unequal in the different meridians of the eyeball. A cylindric corrective lens (a segment cut from a cylinder) is used that has no refractive power along one axis and is concave or convex along the other axis.

Anisometropia, a significant difference between the refractive errors of the two eyes (usually > 2 diopters), is seen occasionally. When the refractive errors are corrected with lenses, differences in image size **(aniseikonia)** are produced and can lead to difficulties in fusion and even to suppression of one of the images.

Presbyopia, a hyperopia for near vision that develops with advancing age, results from a physiologic change in the accommodative mechanism by which the focus of the eye is adjusted for objects at different distances. Beginning in the teens, the lens substance gradually grows less pliable and eventually cannot change shape (accommodate) in response to the action of the ciliary muscles. As a result, the individual becomes unable to focus well for near vision but usually does not need corrective glasses until he reaches the early to mid-40s.

75.   EYE INJURIES

Trauma to the eye or adjacent structures requires meticulous examination to determine the extent of injury. Vision, range of extraocular motion, depth of anterior chamber, location of lid and conjunctival lacerations and of foreign bodies, and presence of anterior chamber or vitreous hemorrhage or cataract should be determined and recorded in detail for protection of patient, physician, and in industrial cases, employer.

FOREIGN BODIES

1. Conjunctival and corneal foreign body injuries are the most common eye injuries. Seemingly minor trauma can be serious if ocular penetration is unrecognized or if secondary infection follows a corneal abrasion.

Treatment: Adequate light, good anesthesia, and proper instruments are essential to ensure minimal trauma when removing embedded foreign bodies. Fluorescein staining (see Ch. 73) renders foreign bodies and abrasions more apparent. An anesthetic (eg, 2 drops of proparacaine 0.5%) is instilled onto the conjunctiva. Both lids are everted and the entire conjunctiva and cornea inspected with a binocular lens (loupe) or slit lamp. Conjunctival foreign bodies are lifted out with a moist sterile cotton applicator. A corneal foreign body that cannot be dislodged by irrigation may be lifted out carefully on the point of a sterile spud or hypodermic needle, under loupe or slit-lamp magnification. Unless steel or iron foreign bodies are removed immediately, they leave a "rust ring" on the cornea that also requires removal under the light and magnification of the slit lamp.

If the foreign body is tiny, the only treatment is instillation of an antibiotic ointment (eg, erythromycin 0.5% or sulfacetamide sodium 10%). For larger foreign bodies, treatment is the same as for any **corneal abrasion:** dilating the pupil with a short-acting cycloplegic (eg, 1 drop of cyclopentolate 1%); instilling an antibiotic, usually erythromycin or sulfacetamide sodium; and ap-

plying a patch firmly enough to keep the eye closed overnight. Ophthalmic corticosteroid preparations tend to promote the growth of fungi and are **contraindicated.** The corneal epithelium regenerates rapidly; under a patch, large areas heal within 1 to 3 days. Follow-up examination by an ophthalmologist 1 or 2 days after injury is wise, especially if the foreign body was removed with a needle or spud.

2. Intraocular foreign body injuries require immediate **emergency treatment,** and the foreign body that has penetrated the eye must be removed by an ophthalmic surgeon. The pupil is dilated with 2 drops of cyclopentolate 1% to examine the crystalline lens, vitreous, and retina. Antimicrobials are indicated, both systemic and topical; eg, gentamicin 1 mg/kg IV q 8 h (if kidney function is adequate) in combination with cefazolin 1 gm IV q 6 h, and gentamicin 0.3% ophthalmic solution 1 drop hourly. Ointment should be avoided if the globe is lacerated. A patch and a metal shield are placed over the eye to avoid inadvertent pressure that could extrude ocular contents through the penetration site. The patient should not receive anything by mouth in preparation for urgent surgery.

LACERATIONS AND CONTUSIONS

During the first 24 h, **lid contusions (black eye)** should be treated with ice packs to inhibit swelling. The next day, hot compresses may aid absorption of the hematoma. Minor **lid lacerations** may be repaired with fine silk sutures. Lid-margin lacerations are best repaired by an ophthalmic surgeon, since particular care is needed to ensure apposition and avoid a notch in the contour. Major lacerations, especially those involving the lacrimal apparatus, should be repaired by an ophthalmic surgeon.

Trauma to the globe may severely damage internal structures. Hemorrhage into the anterior chamber, laceration of the iris, cataract, dislocated lens, glaucoma, vitreous hemorrhage, orbital-floor fractures, retinal hemorrhage or detachment, and rupture of the eyeball may result. **Emergency treatment** may be needed before care by a specialist. It consists of alleviating pain (eg, with meperidine 50 mg IM q 3 h), keeping the pupil dilated with 2 drops of cyclopentolate 1%, applying protective dressings (including a metal shield), and combating possible infection with local and systemic antimicrobials as for an intraocular foreign body (see above). Traumatized lids should never be opened forcibly, since this could aggravate the injury. If the globe has been lacerated, topical antibiotics should be given in the form of drops only, since ointment could penetrate the globe. Because fungal contamination of open wounds is a danger, corticosteroids are **contraindicated** until after the wounds are closed surgically. Rarely, after a laceration of the globe, the uninjured, contralateral eye becomes inflamed (sympathetic ophthalmia) and may lose vision to the point of blindness.

Anterior chamber hemorrhage (traumatic hyphema) following blunt injury is potentially serious and requires attention by an ophthalmologist. It may be followed by recurrent bleeding, glaucoma, and blood-staining of the cornea. The **immediate treatment** is complete bed rest, binocular bandaging, sedation, and if intraocular pressure rises, a carbonic anhydrase inhibitor (eg, acetazolamide 250 mg to 1 gm/day orally in divided doses). Aminocaproic acid 50 to 100 mg orally q 4 h for 5 days may reduce recurrent bleeding. Products containing aspirin are **contraindicated**. The nonophthalmologist should *not* use miotics or mydriatics in these cases.

Rarely, recurrent bleeding with secondary glaucoma requires evacuation of the blood by an ophthalmologist.

BURNS

Eyelid burns should be cleansed thoroughly with sterile isotonic saline solution, followed by application of petrolatum gauze or an antimicrobial ointment (eg, erythromycin). Sterile pressure dressings are then applied and held by an elastic bandage or stockinet around the head until the surface has healed.

Chemical burns of the **cornea** and **conjunctiva** can be serious and should be treated immediately by copious irrigation with water, 0.9% sodium chloride, or other bland fluids. The eye may be anesthetized with 1 drop of proparacaine 1%, if it is available, but irrigation should never be delayed and should be carried out for 30 min. Pain results from loss of corneal epithelium and chemical iritis, which should be treated by instilling a long-acting cycloplegic (eg, 1% atropine solution), applying an antibiotic ointment, and pressure patching. Prolonged use of topical anesthetics should be avoided. Initially, pain may require codeine 30 to 60 mg orally or meperidine 50 mg IM q 4 h. Severe burns require specialized treatment by an ophthalmologist to save vision and prevent major complications such as iridocyclitis, perforation of the globe, and lid deformities. Patients with significant redness of the eye or loss of normal epithelium should always be seen by an ophthalmologist within 24 h.

76. ORBIT

ORBITAL CELLULITIS

(See also PERIORBITAL AND ORBITAL CELLULITIS under BACTERIAL INFECTIONS in Ch. 32)

Inflammation of the orbital tissues caused by infection that extends from the nasal sinuses or teeth, by metastatic spread from infections elsewhere, or by bacteria introduced via orbital trauma. The most common causes are paranasal sinusitis leading to secondary orbital inflammation and trauma to the eyelid, which becomes infected. Symptoms include extreme orbital pain, exophthalmos, impaired mobility of the eye, lid swelling, chemosis, fever, and malaise. Possible

complications are loss of vision from optic neuritis, thrombophlebitis of the orbital veins resulting in cavernous sinus thrombosis, panophthalmitis, and spread of the infection to the meninges and brain.

Diagnosis and Treatment

The primary locus of infection should be sought. Thorough examination of the skin, nasopharynx, teeth, and oral cavity is helpful, as are x-rays or CT of the sinuses. The conjunctiva, skin, blood, and oral or nasal discharge should be cultured, as indicated. **Treatment** with antibiotics (eg, cephalexin 500 mg orally q 6 h for 14 days for mild cases or cefazolin 1 gm IV q 6 h for 7 days for severe cases) should be started, pending culture results. Incision and drainage are indicated if suppuration is suspected or if the infection does not respond to antibiotic therapy.

CAVERNOUS SINUS THROMBOSIS

A septic thrombosis of the cavernous sinus associated with chronic bacterial sinusitis. The infection may spread from the contiguous sphenoidal or ethmoidal air sinuses, either directly or via the emissary veins. Exophthalmos, papilledema, severe cerebral symptoms (headache, decreased level of consciousness, convulsions), cranial nerve palsies, and a septic temperature curve are present. The prognosis is grave; the mortality rate remains about 30%, despite antibiotic therapy.

Diagnosis and Treatment

Nasal discharge and blood should be cultured; CT scans of the cavernous and air sinuses, orbit, and brain should be performed. Treatment with high-dose IV antibiotics (eg, nafcillin 1 gm q 4 h) should be started, pending culture results. Surgical drainage of the infected air sinus may be indicated, especially if there is no response to the antibiotics in 24 h.

EXOPHTHALMOS
(Proptosis)

Protrusion of one or both eyeballs that results from orbital inflammation, edema, tumors, or injuries; cavernous sinus thrombosis; or enlargement of the eyeball (as in congenital glaucoma *and unilateral high myopia).* In hyperthyroidism, edema and lymphoid infiltration of the orbital tissues may cause unilateral or bilateral exophthalmos. Sudden unilateral onset is usually due to hemorrhage or inflammation of the orbit or accessory sinuses. A 2- to 3-wk onset suggests chronic inflammation or orbital pseudotumor (a nonneoplastic cellular infiltration and proliferation); slower onset suggests neoplasm.

An arteriovenous aneurysm involving the internal carotid artery and the cavernous sinus may produce a pulsating exophthalmos with bruit. Posttraumatic onset is probably due to carotid-cavernous fistula, confirmable by auscultation of the globe. Trauma or infection (especially facial) may cause cavernous sinus thrombosis with unilateral exophthalmos and fever. Unilateral high myopia or meningioma may cause unilateral exophthalmos. Thyroid studies should be performed when the cause is not apparent; if thyroid function is normal, the cause must be sought within the orbit by CT. The degree of exophthalmos can be measured with the exophthalmometer; if it is progressive, exposure of the globe can lead to corneal drying, infection, and ulceration.

Treatment

Etiology determines therapy. Ligation of the involved common carotid artery or selective embolization may be necessary in arteriovenous aneurysm. The exophthalmos of hyperthyroidism may subside when the hyperthyroidism is controlled, but occasionally it follows a relentless course, requiring surgical orbital decompression. Systemic corticosteroids are often beneficial in controlling edema and pseudotumor (eg, prednisone 1 mg/kg orally, given daily for 1 wk, then on alternate days for 5 wk, then gradually reduced to the minimal amount needed to control the proptosis). Tumors must be removed.

77. LACRIMAL APPARATUS

DACRYOSTENOSIS

Stricture of the nasolacrimal duct, often resulting from a congenital abnormality or an infection. Congenital obstruction usually appears between ages 3 and 12 wk as a persistent tearing **(epiphora)** of one eye or, rarely, of both. Epiphora is chronic overflow of tears over the lid margin onto the cheek. Adult patients may complain of tearing but in fact do not have epiphora

unless they or their family members notice the overflow of tears. The later onset and lack of purulent exudate in congenital obstruction differentiate it from neonatal conjunctivitis due to either silver nitrate instillation or bacterial infection. Pressure on the nasolacrimal sac frequently causes a copious reflux of mucus or pus from the punctum. In adults, dacryostenosis with epiphora may result from inflammatory obstruction of the duct due to chronic nasal infection or from severe or chronic conjunctivitis. Fracture of the nose and facial bones may cause mechanical obstruction. Prolonged blockage usually leads to infection of the lacrimal sac (see DACRYOCYSTITIS, below).

Treatment

Congenital dacryostenosis usually resolves spontaneously by age 6 mo. Milking the contents of the lacrimal sac through the nasolacrimal duct with fingertip massage twice daily may speed resolution; antibiotic drops may prevent infection. If resolution is not spontaneous, the punctum should be dilated and the nasolacrimal canal probed. Brief general anesthesia usually is necessary in infants. In **adults**, a local anesthetic such as proparacaine 0.5% is instilled and the punctum is dilated. Isotonic saline is irrigated gently through the nasolacrimal system with a fine, blunt canaliculus needle. (A drop of fluorescein in the saline makes obstruction in the nose easily detectable.) If this fails, lacrimal probing may establish patency. Using probes of increasing size followed by irrigation with sterile isotonic saline may be successful in incomplete obstruction. Complete obstruction requires a surgical opening from the tear sac into the nasal passages.

DACRYOCYSTITIS

Infection of the lacrimal sac. Dacryocystitis is usually secondary to obstruction of the nasolacrimal duct. In infants, it is a complication of congenital dacryostenosis; in others, the duct ob-struction results from nasal trauma, deviated septum, hypertrophic rhinitis, mucosal polyps, hypertrophied inferior turbinate, or residual congenital dacryostenosis.

Symptoms and Signs

Pain, redness and edema about the lacrimal sac, epiphora, conjunctivitis, blepharitis, fever, and leukocytosis are associated with **acute dacryocystitis**; in **chronic dacryocystitis**, slight swelling of the sac may be the only symptom. On pressure, pus may regurgitate through the punctum. The sac may become distended from retained secretions, forming a large mucocele. Recurrent acute inflammations may result in a red, brawny, indurated area over the sac. An abscess, if present, may rupture and form a draining fistula.

Treatment

Acute dacryocystitis is treated by frequent application of hot compresses; cephalexin 500 mg orally q 6 h for mild cases or cefazolin 1 gm IV q 6 h for severe cases; and incision and drainage if an abscess has formed. The systemic antibiotic can be changed after results of culture are available. **Chronic dacryocystitis** may be relieved by dilating the nasolacrimal duct with a probe after using a local anesthetic such as proparacaine or tetracaine 0.5% or cocaine 4%. Contributory nasal or sinus abnormalities should be treated. If conservative treatment fails, nasolacrimal intubation, dacryocystorhinostomy, or removal of the sac may be necessary.

78. EYELIDS

LID EDEMA

Allergies usually produce marked crinkly lid edema of one or both eyes and may be due to topical agents, such as eyedrops (eg, atropine or epinephrine), other drugs, or cosmetics (see OTHER ALLERGIC EYE DISEASES in Ch. 34). Plant allergens can cause lid edema in atopic individuals. Trichinosis produces lid edema that is usually bilateral and resembles the allergic type; the associated fever and other systemic symptoms may not be present initially. An eosinophilia > 10% is characteristic.

In allergic lid edema, removal of the offending cause is often the only treatment needed. Cold compresses over the closed lids may speed resolution; topical corticosteroid creams (eg, triamcinolone 0.1% tid for not more than 7 days) may be needed if swelling persists > 24 h.

BLEPHARITIS

Inflammation of the lid margins with redness, thickening, and often the formation of scales and crusts or shallow marginal ulcers.

Etiology

Ulcerative blepharitis is caused by bacterial infection (usually staphylococcal) of the lash follicles and the meibomian glands. The cause of seborrheic (nonulcerative) blepharitis is often obscure; it may be associated with seborrhea of the face and scalp. Secondary bacterial colonization often occurs on the scales on the lid margin (the portion of the lid from which the eyelashes protrude).

Symptoms and Signs

A foreign-body sensation is common. Itching, burning, and redness of the lid margins, lid edema, loss of lashes, and conjunctival irritation with lacrimation and photophobia may be present. In ulcerative blepharitis, tenacious adherent crusts appear and leave a bleeding surface when removed. Small pustules develop in the lash follicles and eventually break down to form shallow ulcers. During sleep, the lids become glued together by dried secretions. A history of repeated styes and chalazia is common. In the seborrheic type, greasy, easily removable scales develop on the lid margins.

Prognosis and Treatment

Patients should be warned that both types are indolent, recurrent, and stubbornly resistant to treatment. Exacerbations of the seborrheic type are inconvenient and unsightly but not destructive. Repeated attacks of the ulcerative type result in loss of eyelashes, scarring of the lids, and occasionally corneal ulceration.

Ulcerative blepharitis is treated with an antibiotic ointment (eg, erythromycin 0.5% or sulfacetamide sodium 10% qid for 7 to 10 days). Therapy for seborrheic blepharitis is aimed at improved eyelid hygiene and consists of scrubbing the lid margin daily with a cotton swab dipped in a dilute solution of baby shampoo (2 to 3 drops in 1/2 cup of warm water). Occasionally, a topical antibiotic ointment is indicated (erythromycin 0.5% or sulfacetamide sodium 10% tid or qid for 3 to 9 wk). Seborrheic blepharitis also requires attention to the face and scalp (see SEBORRHEIC DERMATITIS in Ch. 90).

HORDEOLUM
(Stye)

An acute localized pyogenic infection of one or more of the glands of Zeis or Moll (external hordeolum) or of the meibomian glands (internal hordeolum, meibomian stye).

Etiology, Symptoms, and Signs

Staphylococci usually are responsible. Styes often are associated with and secondary to blepharitis. Recurrence is common.

External hordeolum usually begins with pain, redness, and tenderness of the lid margin followed by a small, round, tender area of induration. Lacrimation, photophobia, and a foreign-body sensation may be present. Though usually localized, edema may be diffuse. A small yellowish spot, indicative of suppuration, appears in the center of the induration ("pointing"). The abscess soon ruptures, with discharge of pus and relief of pain.

Internal hordeolum involving one of the meibomian glands is more severe. Pain, redness, and edema are more localized. Inspection of the conjunctival side of the lid shows a small elevation or yellow area at the site of the affected gland. Later, an abscess forms, pointing on the conjunctival side of the lid; it sometimes points through the skin. Spontaneous rupture is rare, and recurrence is common.

Diagnosis and Treatment

An external hordeolum is superficial and well localized; it appears to lie at the base of an eyelash. An internal hordeolum is deeper and can be seen through the conjunctiva. If the hordeolum lies near the inner canthus of the lower lid, it must be differentiated from acute dacryocystitis (see in Ch. 77). Successful lacrimal duct irrigation rules out dacryocystitis.

Topical antibiotics are usually ineffective. Suppuration may be aborted in the early stages by systemic antibiotics (eg, dicloxacillin or erythromycin 250 mg orally qid); however, because of the minor nature and short natural history of hordeolum, oral antibiotics are rarely indicated. Pointing is hastened by hot compresses applied for 10 min tid or qid. As soon as suppuration is evidenced by the formation of a central yellow area, the hordeolum should be incised with a sharp, fine-tipped blade and its contents expressed.

CHALAZION

Chronic granulomatous enlargement of a meibomian gland from occlusion of its duct, often following inflammation of the gland.

Symptoms and Signs

At onset, a chalazion may be indistinguishable from a stye, with lid edema, swelling, and irritation. After a few days, however, it resolves, leaving a painless, slowly growing, round mass in the lid. The skin can be moved loosely over the swelling, which may be seen in the tarsus of the lid, generally presenting subconjunctivally as a red or gray mass. When the mass is in the lower lid near the inner canthus, chronic dacryocystitis must be ruled out.

Treatment

Most chalazia disappear after a few months. Hot compresses qid may hasten resolution. Incision and curettage or intrachalazion corticosteroid administration (0.05 to 0.2 mL triamcinolone 10 mg/mL) may be indicated if there is no resolution after 6 wk.

ENTROPION AND ECTROPION

Inversion of the eyelid (**entropion**) *and eversion* (**ectropion**) *can result from aging or from scar formation. Entropion causes irritation as the lashes rub against the globe and may lead to cor-* neal ulceration and scarring. Ectropion is generally the result of tissue relaxation with aging and leads to poor drainage of tears through the nasolacrimal system. Symptoms may include redness, irritation, and epiphora. Both conditions, if persistent, are best treated surgically.

TUMORS

The skin of the eyelids can have both benign and neoplastic growths. **Xanthelasma** is a common, benign type, with yellow-white, flat plaques of lipid material that occur subcutaneously on the upper and lower lids. They need not be removed, except for cosmetic reasons.

Basal cell carcinoma is frequently seen at the lid margins, at the inner canthus, and on the upper cheek. Biopsy establishes the diagnosis. **Treatment** is surgical excision or radiation therapy.

Other malignant tumors are less common; they include squamous cell or meibomian gland carcinoma and melanomas of several types.

79. CONJUNCTIVA

The conjunctiva lines the back of the lid, extends into the space between the lid and the globe, and spreads up over the sclera to the cornea. This tissue can respond to various stimuli with chemosis, hemorrhage, or inflammation. In addition, 2 benign neoplasms of the conjunctiva commonly occur: (1) A **pinguecula** is a raised yellowish-white mass just adjacent to the cornea at either the 3 or 9 o'clock position. It may be unsightly but has no tendency to grow onto the cornea and need not be removed. (2) A **pterygium** is a fleshy growth of conjunctiva onto the cornea and is more often found in hot, dry climates. This growth may spread across and distort the cornea, induce astigmatism, and change the refractive power of the eye. In some cases, removal is indicated to reduce irritation and to prevent changes in vision.

ACUTE CONJUNCTIVITIS

An acute conjunctival inflammation, usually caused by viruses, bacteria, or allergy.

Etiology

Viruses, especially adenoviruses (see under VIRAL INFECTIONS in Ch. 32), bacteria, and allergies (see ALLERGIC CONJUNCTIVITIS in Ch. 34) are the most common causes in populations with good hygiene. Mixed or unidentifiable pathogens may be present. Conjunctival irritation from wind, dust, smoke, and other types of air pollution often is associated; conjunctivitis may also accompany the common cold, exanthems (especially measles), and corneal irritation due to the intense ultraviolet light of electric arcs, sunlamps, and reflection from snow. Acute hemorrhagic conjunctivitis, associated with infection by enterovirus type 70 (see under ENTEROVIRAL DISEASES in Ch. 32), has occurred in outbreaks in Africa and Asia.

Symptoms, Signs, and Diagnosis

TABLE 79–1 indicates prominent symptoms and signs found in acute conjunctivitis. The discharge should be cultured, particularly if it is purulent. Smears should be examined microscopically, stained with Gram stain to identify bacteria and with Giemsa stain to determine the leukocytic response. While cultures can be taken for viral disease, special tissue culture facilities are necessary for growth of the virus.

Lymphoid follicles are present on the undersurface of the lid in viral infection; velvety papillary projections, in allergic disease. The pre-

TABLE 79-1. DIFFERENTIATING FEATURES IN CONJUNCTIVITIS

Etiology	Discharge; Cell Type	Lid Swelling	Node Involvement	Itching
Bacterial	Purulent; polymorphonuclear leukocytes	Moderate	No	No
Viral	Clear; mononuclear cells	Minimal	Yes	No
Allergic	Clear, mucoid, ropy; eosinophils	Moderate to severe	No	Intense

auricular node should be palpated in all cases; it tends to be enlarged and painful in viral conjunctivitis.

Examination of conjunctival scrapings rules out inclusion conjunctivitis, trachoma, and vernal conjunctivitis: in the former 2 (both caused by *Chlamydia*), inclusion bodies are present; in the last, eosinophils are present. Retained corneal or conjunctival foreign bodies and corneal abrasion or ulcer may be ruled out by staining the eye with fluorescein (see Ch. 73) and examining it, under magnification, with a good focal light.

The deep ciliary injection of iritis and of acute glaucoma is readily differentiated, since it is due to fine, straight, deep vessels that radiate from the limbus and are immobile when the conjunctiva is moved. The brick-red conjunctival hyperemia of conjunctivitis is composed of coarse, tortuous, superficial vessels that move with the conjunctiva. Other features that distinguish conjunctivitis from acute iritis and acute glaucoma are given in TABLE 79-2.

Treatment

After examining the patient, the physician must wash hands thoroughly and sterilize instruments to avoid transmitting infection. The patient should be told to use only his own towels. The eyes should be kept free of discharge and not patched. If bacterial infection is suspected, sulfacetamide sodium

TABLE 79-2. DIFFERENTIAL DIAGNOSIS OF CERTAIN ACUTE EYE DISORDERS

Diagnostic Feature	Acute Iritis	Acute Glaucoma	Acute Conjunctivitis
Pain	Moderately severe, photophobia	Very severe, associated with nausea and emesis	Burning but not severe
Vision	Moderately decreased	Considerably decreased	Normal
Intraocular pressure	Usually normal or soft	Increased	Normal
Lacrimation or discharge	Lacrimation	Lacrimation	Mucous or mucopurulent discharge
Hyperemia	Circumcorneal	Circumcorneal and episcleral	Superficial conjunctival hyperemia of globe and eyelids
Cornea	Transparent precipitates may be present on posterior surface	Cloudy	Normal
Anterior chamber	Normal depth	Very shallow	Normal depth
Iris	Dull and swollen	Congested and bulging	Normal
Pupil	Small, irregular	Mid-dilated, unreactive	Normal
Pupillary response to light	Minimal	Minimal	Normal

10% drops or gentamicin 0.3% should be applied qid for 7 to 10 days. This treatment can be used for all forms of conjunctivitis; a poor clinical response after 2 or 3 days indicates that an insensitive bacterium is present or that the cause is viral or allergic. Antibiotic therapy may be modified if necessary when the results of culture and sensitivity studies become available. Corticosteroids should not be used, either separately or with antibiotics, until a causative pathogen is identified or excluded, since herpes simplex virus may be present and may be spread from the conjunctiva to the cornea, with subsequent ulceration and perforation. If allergy is likely on the basis of history and lack of response to antibiotic therapy, topical corticosteroid therapy (eg, prednisolone acetate 0.12% drops tid) can be initiated. With long-term use of corticosteroids, intraocular pressure should be monitored and the lens examined periodically for cataracts.

CHRONIC CONJUNCTIVITIS

A chronic inflammation of the conjunctiva characterized by exacerbations and remissions that occur over months or years. The causal agents, when identifiable, are similar to those of acute conjunctivitis; ectropion, entropion, blepharitis, chronic dacryocystitis, *Chlamydia,* topical drug sensitivity and toxicity, and chronic exposure to irritants are also etiologically associated.

Symptoms and Signs
Symptoms are similar to those of acute conjunctivitis but less severe and include itching, irritation, and a foreign-body sensation; a scant mucoid secretion may be present. The palpebral conjunctiva is reddened, thickened, and velvety. The bulbar conjunctiva may be slightly involved.

Treatment
Specific therapy depends on the cause. Irritating factors must be eliminated. Overtreatment may produce drug sensitivity and should be avoided.

ADULT GONOCOCCAL CONJUNCTIVITIS
(See also NEONATAL CONJUNCTIVITIS under NEONATAL INFECTIONS in Ch. 27)

A rare, severe, purulent conjunctivitis in adults that is acquired from a gonorrheal contact or that occurs as a result of self-inoculation from a gonorrheal genital infection. Usually only one eye is involved. Symptoms similar to those of neonatal conjunctivitis, but more severe, develop 12 to 48 h after exposure; complications include corneal ulceration, abscess, perforation, panophthalmitis, and blindness. Treatment involves a single dose of ceftriaxone 125 to 250 mg IM or amoxicillin 3 gm orally plus probenecid 1 gm orally given as a single dose; bacitracin 500 u./gm, gentamicin 0.3%, or tetracycline 1% ophthalmic ointment instilled into the affected eye q 2 h may also be used. Sexual partners should also be treated.

TRACHOMA
(Granular Conjunctivitis; Egyptian Ophthalmia)

A chronic conjunctivitis caused by Chlamydia trachomatis *and characterized by progressive exacerbations and remissions, with follicular subconjunctival hyperplasia, corneal vascularization, and cicatrization of the conjunctiva, cornea, and lids.*

Epidemiology
The disease is still endemic in poverty-stricken parts of the dry, hot Mediterranean countries and Far East. It occurs sporadically among American Indians and in mountainous areas of the southern USA. It is most contagious in its early stages and is transmitted by eye-to-eye or hand-to-eye contact, by eye-seeking flies, or by sharing contaminated articles (eg, towels, handkerchiefs). The causative organism is a strain of *C. trachomatis* and is related to psittacosis and lymphogranuloma venereum.

Symptoms and Signs
After an incubation period of about 7 days, conjunctival congestion, eyelid edema, photophobia, and lacrimation gradually appear, usually bilaterally. Small follicles develop in the conjunctiva of the upper lids 7 to 10 days later and gradually increase in size and number for 3 or 4 wk, forming yellow-gray semitransparent "sago-grain" granulations surrounded by inflammatory papillae. Pannus formation begins during this stage, with invasion of the upper half of the cornea by loops of vessels from the limbus. The stage of follicular hypertrophy and pannus formation may last from several months to > 1 yr, depending on response to therapy. The entire cornea may ultimately be involved, reducing vision. Rarely, the pannus retrogresses completely

and corneal transparency is restored without treatment.

Unless adequate treatment is given, the cicatricial stage follows. The follicles and papillae gradually shrink and are replaced by scar tissue that often causes entropion and lacrimal duct obstruction. The corneal epithelium becomes dull and thickened, and lacrimation is decreased. Ulcers form in ischemic areas of the pannus. On healing, the conjunctiva is smooth and grayish-white; the extent of residual corneal opacity and vision loss varies. Secondary bacterial infection is common, contributing to scarring and the chronicity of the disease.

Diagnosis

C. trachomatis can be isolated in culture. In the early stage, the presence of minute basophilic cytoplasmic inclusion bodies in Giemsa-stained epithelial conjunctival scrapings differentiates trachoma from acute conjunctivitis. Inclusion bodies are also found in inclusion conjunctivitis, but the developing clinical picture distinguishes this from trachoma. Palpebral vernal conjunctivitis is similar to trachoma in its follicular hypertrophic stage, but eosinophilia and milky flat-topped papillae are present, while basophilic inclusion bodies are not found in the scrapings.

Treatment

Tetracycline or erythromycin ophthalmic ointment, applied bid or qid for 4 to 6 wk, is usually effective. A concomitant course of oral tetracycline or erythromycin is helpful. Lid deformities should be treated surgically.

INCLUSION CONJUNCTIVITIS
(Inclusion Blenorrhea; Swimming Pool Conjunctivitis)

An acute conjunctivitis, known as **neonatal inclusion conjunctivitis** *in the newborn and* **adult inclusion conjunctivitis** *in the adult, caused by a strain of* Chlamydia trachomatis (see Trachoma, above). This organism can persist asymptomatically in the cervix for prolonged periods. As a form of ophthalmia neonatorum, neonatal inclusion conjunctivitis results from passage through an infected birth canal and occurs in 40 to 50% of the newborns exposed to it. Most instances of acute adult inclusion conjunctivitis result from exposure to infected genital secretions.

Symptoms, Signs, and Diagnosis

Neonatal inclusion conjunctivitis usually appears 5 to 14 days after birth as a bilateral, intense papillary conjunctivitis, with lid swelling, chemosis, and mucopurulent discharge. Epithelial-cell inclusion bodies are present in conjunctival scrapings. Adult inclusion conjunctivitis is usually characterized by a unilateral mucopurulent discharge and a marked follicular conjunctivitis. Occasionally, superior corneal opacities and vascularization occur. Preauricular lymph nodes may be swollen on the side of the involved eye.

Treatment

Since at least 50% of infants with neonatal inclusion conjunctivitis also have nasopharyngeal infection and 10% will develop chlamydial pneumonia, treatment is systemic with erythromycin 12.5 mg/kg orally or IV qid for 14 days. The mother and her sexual partner also require treatment.

In adult inclusion conjunctivitis, tetracycline 500 mg orally qid, erythromycin 500 mg orally qid, or doxycycline 100 mg orally bid is given for 3 wk to cure the conjunctivitis and concomitant genital infection. Sexual partners also require treatment (see Ch. 21).

VERNAL KERATOCONJUNCTIVITIS

A bilateral, recurrent conjunctivitis with concurrent corneal epithelial changes, usually allergic in origin, with recurrences in the spring and fall. It is most common in males aged 5 to 20. (See also Allergic Conjunctivitis in Ch. 34.)

Symptoms and Signs

Intense itching, lacrimation, photophobia, conjunctival injection, and a tenacious mucoid discharge containing numerous eosinophils are characteristic. Either the palpebral or the bulbar conjunctiva may be affected. In the **palpebral form**, square, hard, flattened, closely packed, pale-pink to grayish "cobblestone" granulations are present, chiefly in the upper lids. The uninvolved tarsal conjunctiva is milky white. In the **bulbar (limbic) form**, the circumcorneal conjunctiva becomes hypertrophied and grayish. Occasionally, a small, circumscribed loss of corneal epithelium occurs, causing pain and increased photophobia. Symptoms usually disappear during the cold months and become milder over the years.

Treatment

Cromolyn sodium 4% given 6 times a day is a useful maintenance drug for exacerbations. Intermittent applications of a topical corticosteroid (eg, dexamethasone 0.1% drops q 2 h), supplemented (rarely) if necessary by small oral doses, may be required to control itching and photophobia. If topical steroids are used for more than a few weeks, intraocular pressure must be checked routinely.

KERATOCONJUNCTIVITIS SICCA
(Keratitis Sicca; Dry Eyes)

A chronic, bilateral dryness of the conjunctiva and cornea leading to desiccation of the ocular surface.

Symptoms and Signs

As an isolated phenomenon or in association with systemic diseases such as rheumatoid arthritis, systemic lupus erythematosus, or Sjögren's syndrome, dryness of the eyes occurs more commonly in adult women. Initial reduction of tear production leads to burning and irritation. This proceeds to photophobia as the corneal epithelium develops scattered cellular loss, termed superficial keratitis. In its advanced stages, keratinization of the ocular surface occurs, frequently associated with loss of the normal configuration of the conjunctival fornices. In advanced keratoconjunctivitis sicca, ulceration, vascularization, and scarring of the cornea may lead to severe visual disability.

Diagnosis

Diagnosis depends upon the history and examination. If the patient complains of dryness and irritation, particular attention should be paid to the adequacy of the tear meniscus as seen through the slit lamp, as well as the presence or absence of punctate erosion of the conjunctiva and cornea. A **Schirmer test** is done by using standardized strips of filter paper placed, without anesthesia, at the junction between the middle and lateral third of the lower lid. A ≤ 5 mm wet area appearing on the paper within 5 min on 2 successive occasions confirms the diagnosis of dry eye.

Treatment

Frequent use of artificial tears containing methylcellulose or polyvinyl alcohol can be effec-

tive. Most cases are treated adequately throughout the patient's life with such supplementation. Occlusion of the nasolacrimal punctum can be tried before eyelid surgery, but in severe cases partial tarsorrhaphy can reduce loss of tears through evaporation.

EPISCLERITIS

Inflammation of the episcleral tissues, usually localized and recurrent. A red to purplish tender patch is present just under the conjunctiva; a yellow nodule may also be present. The condition usually is self-limited and not associated with systemic disease. **Treatment** usually need not be extensive. However, frequent applications of topical corticosteroid, eg, prednisolone acetate 0.125% drops q 2 h for 5 days and gradually reduced over 3 wk, is usually effective in shortening the attack.

SCLERITIS

An extremely painful, vision-threatening, deep inflammation of the scleral tissues, more purple in appearance than episcleritis. It may be associated with rheumatic disorders. In severe cases, perforation of the globe and loss of the eye may ensue.

Treatment

A systemic corticosteroid (eg, prednisone 1 mg/kg/day) is the initial therapy. When the process is associated with rheumatoid disease or is unresponsive to systemic corticosteroids, systemic immunosuppression with agents such as cyclophosphamide or azathioprine may be warranted. Such treatment requires close monitoring of the hematopoietic, renal, and other organ systems and should be undertaken only in consultation with a specialist experienced in using these drugs.

CICATRICIAL PEMPHIGOID
(Ocular Cicatricial Pemphigoid;
Benign Mucous Membrane Pemphigoid)

A chronic, bilateral, progressive scarring and shrinkage of the conjunctiva with opacification of the cornea. It is an autoimmune disease, in which binding of anticonjunctival basement membrane antibodies results in inflammation. Usually beginning as a chronic conjunctivitis, it progresses to scarring of the eyelid conjunctiva to the globe (symblepharon), trichiasis (inturning eyelashes), keratitis sicca, corneal vascularization and opacification, conjunctival shrinkage and keratinization, and blindness. Oral mucous membrane involvement with ulceration and scarring is common, but skin involvement characterized by scarring bullae and erythematous plaques is uncommon.

Treatment

Tear substitutes and cryo- or electroepilation of the inturning eyelash may increase patient comfort. Systemic immunosuppression with dapsone or cyclophosphamide is indicated for progressive scarring or corneal opacification. Such treatment requires monitoring of the hematopoietic, renal, and other organ systems and should be undertaken only in consultation with a specialist experienced in using these drugs.

80. CORNEA

SUPERFICIAL PUNCTATE KERATITIS

Scattered, fine, punctate loss of epithelium from the corneal surface of one or both eyes. It is often associated with adenovirus, blepharitis, keratitis sicca, trachoma, ultraviolet light exposure (eg, welding arcs, sunlamps), contact lens overwear, systemic drugs (eg, adenine arabinoside), and topical drug or preservative toxicity. Symptoms include photophobia, pain, lacrimation, conjunctival injection, and diminution of vision. An enlarged preauricular node may be present in viral cases. Lesions due to ultraviolet light exposure do not appear until several hours after the exposure; they last 24 to 48 h. Residual vision impairment is rare, regardless of cause.

Treatment

The superficial punctate keratitis of adenovirus resolves spontaneously in about 3 wk. Blepharitis, keratitis sicca, and trachoma require specific therapy (see Chs. 78 and 79). Ultraviolet light exposure and contact lens overwear are treated with short-acting cycloplegics, antibiotic ointment, and patching for 24 h. If superficial punctate keratitis results from a topical drug or preservative, that agent should be discontinued.

CORNEAL ULCER

Local necrosis of corneal tissue due to invasion by bacteria, fungi, viruses, or Acanthamoeba.

Etiology

A staphylococcal, *Pseudomonas*, or pneumococcal infection following trauma, complicating a corneal foreign body, or resulting from contact lens overwear is the usual primary cause. Corneal ulcers also occur as complications of herpes simplex keratitis, chronic blepharitis, conjunctivitis (especially bacterial), trachoma, dacryocystitis, gonorrhea, and acute infectious diseases. Indolent ulcers are considered to be fungal until proved otherwise. Corneal ulcers may also result from disturbances in corneal nutrition secondary to vitamin A or protein malnutrition or from corneal exposure due to eyelid injuries or defective closure of the lids (lagophthalmos).

Symptoms and Signs

Pain, photophobia, and lacrimation are present but may be minimal. The lesion begins as a dull, grayish, circumscribed superficial infiltration and subsequently necroses and suppurates to form an ulcer. This stains green with fluorescein (see Ch. 73 for method) and is readily evident. Considerable ciliary injection is usual, and in long-standing cases blood vessels may grow in from the limbus (pannus). The ulcer may spread to involve the width of the cornea or may penetrate deeply; pus may appear in the anterior chamber (hypopyon).

Ulceration without extensive infiltration may occur in herpes simplex. Fungal ulcerations are densely infiltrated and show occasional discrete islands of infiltrate (satellite lesions) at the periphery.

Complications

The deeper the ulcer, the more severe the symptoms and complications. Corneal ulcers heal with fibrous tissue replacement, causing opaque scarring of the cornea and decreased vision. Iritis, iridocyclitis, corneal perforation with iris prolapse, hypopyon, panophthalmitis, and destruction of the eye may occur with or without treatment. Ulcers caused by fungi are indolent but serious; those caused by *P. aeruginosa* are especially virulent, and those associated with dendritic herpes simplex keratitis may be particularly refractory.

Treatment
Corneal ulcers are emergencies and should be treated only by an ophthalmologist.

HERPES SIMPLEX KERATITIS
(Herpes Simplex Keratoconjunctivitis)

Corneal herpes simplex virus infection, with a spectrum of clinical appearances, commonly leading to chronic corneal inflammation, vascularization, scarring, and loss of vision. The initial infection is usually an undistinguished self-limiting conjunctivitis, generally accompanied by a vesicular blepharitis. Recurrences usually take the form of **dendritic keratitis**, with a characteristic branched lesion of the cornea resembling the veins of a leaf, with knoblike terminals. A foreign-body sensation, lacrimation, photophobia, and conjunctival hyperemia are early symptoms. With multiple recurrences, corneal hypoesthesia or anesthesia, ulceration, and permanent scarring may result. **Disciform keratitis**, a deep, disk-shaped, localized area of corneal edema and haze with accompanying iritis, frequently follows dendritic keratitis and probably represents an immunologic response to the virus. Rarely, direct invasion of the corneal stroma by herpes simplex virus is seen, and occasionally, a recurrent loss of corneal epithelium is seen in patients who have herpes simplex virus without active viral eruption.

Treatment
Trifluridine, vidarabine, and idoxuridine (**IDU**) are specific, though not always effective. The agent, whether an ointment or solution, should be used several times daily. If the epithelium surrounding the dendrite is loose and edematous, debridement by gentle swabbing with a cotton-tipped applicator before beginning drug therapy may speed healing. If healing fails to occur after 7 to 10 days, debridement by gentle swabbing with a cottontipped applicator is indicated. Topical corticosteroids are **contraindicated** in dendritic keratitis but may be effective when used with an antiviral agent in the later stromal or uveitic involvement. Atropine 1% instilled tid is useful in cases with uveitis. Cases that fail to heal after

1 wk and those with stromal or uveal involvement require referral to an ophthalmologist.

OPHTHALMIC HERPES ZOSTER

Involvement of the forehead by herpes zoster may not threaten the globe. However, when the nasociliary nerve is affected, as indicated by medial eyelid or conjunctival involvement or a lesion on the tip of the nose, the eye invariably becomes involved. Marked lid edema, ciliary and conjunctival hyperemia, corneal infiltration, uveitis, glaucoma, and pain all may be present during acute disease. Keratitis accompanied by uveitis may be severe and is followed by scarring. Glaucoma, chronic or recurrent uveitis, and corneal hypoesthesia are common late sequelae.

Treatment
Early treatment with acyclovir 800 mg orally 5 times/day for 10 days reduces ocular complications. Unlike in herpes simplex, keratitis or uveitis in herpes zoster is an indication for corticosteroids without concomitant topical antivirals. Topical therapy (eg, dexamethasone 0.1% instilled q 2 h initially) is usually adequate. The pupil should be kept dilated with atropine 1% or cyclopentolate 0.5 to 1% solution 1 drop tid. Intraocular pressure must be monitored.

In patients > 60 yr of age and in good general health, a brief course of high-dose corticosteroids (eg, prednisone 60 mg/day for 7 days, then 45 mg for 7 days, and then 30 mg for 7 days) may prevent severe postherpetic neuralgia.

PHLYCTENULAR KERATOCONJUNCTIVITIS
(Phlyctenular or Eczematous Conjunctivitis)

A keratoconjunctivitis, usually occurring in children, characterized by discrete nodular areas of inflammation of the cornea or conjunctiva (phlyctenules) and resulting from a hypersensitivity reaction to an unknown antigen. Bacterial proteins from staphylococcal blepharitis and systemic TB have been implicated. The disease is uncommon in the USA.

Phlyctenules appear as crops of small yellow-gray nodules at the limbus, on the cornea, or on the bulbar conjunctiva, persisting from several days to 1 to 2 wk. On the conjunctiva, they ulcerate, but they heal without a scar. When the cornea is affected, severe tearing, photophobia, and pain may be prominent. Frequent recurrence, especially with secondary infection, may lead to corneal opacity and vascularization with loss of vision. **Treatment** with a topical corticosteroid-antibiotic combination is valuable in managing the condition and the primary blepharitis.

INTERSTITIAL KERATITIS
(Parenchymatous Keratitis)

A chronic nonulcerative infiltration of the deep layers of the cornea, with uveal inflammation. It is rare in the USA. Most cases occur in children as a late complication of congenital syphilis. Ultimately, both eyes may be involved. Rarely, acquired syphilis or TB may cause a unilateral form in adults.

Photophobia, pain, lacrimation, and gradual loss of vision are common. The lesion begins in the deep corneal layers; soon the entire cornea develops a ground-glass appearance, obscuring the iris. New blood vessels grow in from the limbus and produce orange-red areas ("salmon patches"). Iritis, iridocyclitis, and choroiditis are common. The inflammation and neovascularization usually begin to subside after 1 to 2 mo. Some corneal opacity may remain, but vision may be impaired even when the cornea clears completely. An ophthalmologist should be consulted for treatment.

PERIPHERAL ULCERATIVE KERATITIS
(Marginal Keratolysis; Peripheral Rheumatoid Ulceration)

A peripheral corneal inflammation and ulceration often associated with active collagen-vascular diseases. Patients often complain of decreased vision, photophobia, and foreign-body sensation. An area of opacification, due to infiltration by WBCs, and ulceration, which stains green with fluorescein (see Ch. 73 for method), is located in the periphery of the cornea. Infectious causes such as bacteria, fungi, and herpes simplex virus must be ruled out by culturing the cornea and eyelid margins. Peripheral ulcerative keratitis is often associated with active and/or long-standing collagen-vascular diseases such as rheumatoid arthritis, Wegener's granulomatosis, and relapsing polychondritis. The high mortality rate of about 40% in 10 yr (mostly from myocardial infarction) in patients with rheu-

matoid arthritis who develop peripheral ulcerative keratitis may be reduced to about 8% in 10 yr with systemic cytotoxic immunosuppression. **Treatment** should be carried out only by an ophthalmologist.

KERATOMALACIA
(Xerotic Keratitis; Xerophthalmia)

A condition associated with vitamin A deficiency and protein-calorie malnutrition, characterized by a hazy, dry cornea that becomes denuded. Corneal ulceration with secondary infection is common. The lacrimal glands and conjunctiva are also affected. Lack of tears causes extreme dryness of the eyes, and foamy Bitot's spots appear on the bulbar conjunctiva. Night blindness may be associated. Antibiotic ointments or sulfonamides (eg, sulfacetamide ophthalmic solution 30% or ointment 10%) are required if secondary infection exists.

KERATOCONUS

A slowly progressive ectasia of the cornea, usually bilateral, beginning between ages 10 and 20. The cone shape that the cornea assumes causes major changes in the refractive power of the eye and necessitates frequent change of spectacles. Contact lenses may provide better visual correction and should always be tried when eyeglasses are not satisfactory. Corneal transplant surgery may be necessary if vision with contact lenses is inadequate, the lenses are not tolerated, or a corneal scar is present.

BULLOUS KERATOPATHY

A condition caused by edema of the cornea, most frequently the result of aging and failure of the corneal endothelium. It is seen occasionally after intraocular operations (eg, for cataract) in which the mechanical stresses further interfere with the process of corneal detumescence.

The fluid-filled bullae on the corneal surface rupture, causing pain and decreased vision. The bullae and swelling of the corneal stroma can be seen on examination.

Treatment, including the use of dehydrating agents (eg, hypertonic saline), soft contact lenses, and corneal transplantation, is best carried out by an ophthalmologist.

81. CATARACT

Developmental or degenerative opacity of the lens.

Developmental or congenital cataracts are discussed under CONGENITAL EYE DEFECTS in Ch. 28.

Juvenile or adult cataract is characterized by progressive, painless loss of vision. The cause may be aging, exposure to x-rays, heat from infrared exposure, systemic disease (eg, diabetes mellitus), uveitis, or systemic medications (eg, corticosteroids).

Symptoms and Signs

The cardinal symptom is a progressive, painless loss of vision. The degree of loss depends on the location and extent of the opacity. When the opacity is in the central lens nucleus (**nuclear cataract**), myopia develops in the early stages, so that a presbyopic patient may discover that he can read without his glasses ("second sight"). Pain occurs if the cataract swells and produces secondary glaucoma.

Opacity beneath the posterior lens capsule (**posterior subcapsular cataract**) affects vision out of proportion to the degree of cloudiness, because the opacity is located at the crossing point of the light rays from the viewed object. Such cataracts are particularly troublesome in bright light.

Diagnosis

Gradual loss of vision beginning in middle age or later is characteristic of glaucoma as well as cataract. Before the pupils are dilated for an ophthalmoscopic examination, increased intraocular pressure and a shallow anterior chamber must be ruled out.

Well-developed cataracts appear as gray opacities in the lens. Examination of the dilated pupil (see Ch. 73) with the ophthalmoscope held about 1 ft away usually discloses subtle opacities. Small cataracts stand out as dark defects in the red reflex. A large cataract may obliterate the red reflex. Slit-lamp examination provides more details about the character, location, and extent of the opacity.

Treatment

Frequent refractions and eyeglass prescription changes help maintain useful vision during cataract development. Occasionally, chronic pupillary dilation (with phenylephrine 2.5 to 10%) is helpful for small lenticular opacities. When useful vision is lost, lens extraction is necessary; it can be accomplished by removal of the lens intact or by emulsification followed by irrigation and aspiration. Age is no contraindication to surgery. Corticosteroids must be given topically and systemically when surgery is needed in the presence of uveitis. Refractive correction is accomplished by intraoperative implantation of an intraocular prosthetic lens, cataract spectacles, or contact lenses.

82. UVEAL TRACT

UVEITIS

Inflammation of the uveal tract (iris, ciliary body, and choroid). Inflammation of the contiguous retina (retinitis), by tradition, is included in the category of uveitis. Uveitis may be anatomically classified as **anterior (iritis and iridocyclitis)**, **intermediate (cyclitis, peripheral uveitis)**, **posterior (choroiditis and retinitis)**, and **diffuse (iritis plus intermediate uveitis plus chorioretinitis)**. Uveitis may be strictly an ocular syndrome, but in about 40% of cases, a complete diagnostic evaluation will disclose an associated systemic disease that may be causally related.

Symptoms and Signs

The symptoms and signs generally are subtle: mainly diminished or hazy vision, black floating spots, or symptoms related to complications of uveitis (glaucoma, cataract, and retinal detachment). Severe pain, redness, and photophobia are classically described but occur only in cases of acute iritis and iridocyclitis. The major signs of acute **anterior uveitis** include pupillary miosis and perilimbal flush (injection adjacent to the limbus). Cells, flare, and keratic precipitates on the corneal endothelium are seen only by means of the biomicroscope (slit lamp). Signs of **intermediate uveitis** include cells in the vitreous, cellular aggregates in the inferior anterior vitreous humor, and exudation and membrane formation overlying the inferior pars plana of the ciliary body. While the vitreal cells and cellular aggregates may be seen with the direct ophthalmoscope, visualization of the membrane over the pars plana usually requires use of the indirect ophthalmoscope (generally used only by ophthalmologists). Signs of **posterior uveitis** often include vitreal inflammatory cells and strands, white fuzzy fundus lesions, and inflammatory sheathing of retinal blood vessels.

The direct damage as well as secondary complications of uveitis are often severe and may develop with alarming rapidity; therefore, when uveitis is suspected, the patient should be referred as soon as possible for ophthalmologic evaluation.

Common Uveitic Syndromes

Common systemic diseases are discussed more fully elsewhere in THE MANUAL. Although therapeutic suggestions are included here, treatment should be attempted only by an ophthalmologist.

Ankylosing spondylitis, a common cause of acute iridocyclitis, is more frequent in males and may be associated with pain, redness, and photophobia in one or both eyes. Typing for HLA-B27 and x-rays of the sacroiliac joint are usually positive. Treatment includes intensive local use of corticosteroid drops as well as mydriatic/cycloplegic drops.

Reiter's syndrome, another common cause of acute iridocyclitis, also is seen mainly in males and is associated with HLA-B27 positivity. Treatment is the same as that for uveitis associated with ankylosing spondylitis.

Juvenile rheumatoid arthritis (JRA) is characteristically associated with a bilateral chronic iridocyclitis. Symptoms are minimal—mainly blurred or diminished vision. This disease occurs primarily in girls with pauciarticular joint disease; 80% demonstrate a positive antinuclear antibody **(ANA)**. Inflammatory exacerbations require treatment with local corticosteroids and mydriatic/cycloplegic therapy.

Pars planitis is a common ocular condition that usually occurs in older children or young adults. The main symptoms of this bilateral vitritis are visual haze and decreased acuity; the latter is usually caused by cystoid macular edema. Treatment, needed only in cases associated with cystoid macular edema, consists of periocular corticosteroid administration.

Toxoplasmosis, the most common cause of posterior uveitis, is usually transmitted congenitally in ocular cases, although the disease may be acquired. The recurrent attacks of acute focal necrotizing retinitis produce diminished and hazy vision. Associated acute secondary iridocyclitis may produce pain, redness, and photophobia. Laboratory testing for antitoxoplasma antibodies by enzyme-linked immunosorbent assay **(ELISA)** or indirect fluorescent antibody is positive but usually only in low titers. Systemic treatment with antitoxoplasmic agents such as pyrimethamine and sulfonamides combined with systemic corticosteroids is often recommended for retinal lesions that threaten the macula.

Cytomegalovirus (CMV) infection, like ocular toxoplasmosis, produces acute necrotizing retinitis secondary to congenitally acquired infection. Symptoms are usually only visual, since secondary iridocyclitis is rare. In adults, CMV retinitis is rare except in patients immunosuppressed for organ transplants or by anticancer treatment or AIDS. Laboratory testing is done for CF antibodies to CMV, and CMV inclusions are occasionally found in urinary sediment. Treatment with the virostatic agent ganciclovir has been effective. Most patients show improvement after a 2-wk course of 5 mg/kg IV bid. Unfortunately, recurrent ocular inflammation is the rule in AIDS cases, and re-treatment or long-term maintenance therapy is usually necessary for continued remission.

Acute retinal necrosis is a severe peripheral retinitis caused by viruses of the herpes family (herpes simplex, herpes zoster, and possibly, CMV). Most cases are unilateral, but about $1/3$ become bilateral within weeks to years of the inflammation in the first eye. Retinal detachment develops in up to 75% of cases but may be prevented by acyclovir IV plus laser treatment. Vitrectomy, diagnostic or therapeutic, may be useful. If the diagnosis is in doubt, retinal biopsy may demonstrate viral capsids. If CMV is demonstrated, treatment with ganciclovir rather than acyclovir is necessary.

Toxocariasis is most common in childhood and usually produces a single, unilateral, peripheral or posterior, retinal granuloma or, occasionally, generalized inflammation of the entire inner eye (endophthalmitis). Uveitis rarely occurs in generalized visceral larva migrans; more often it occurs after only minimal systemic infection with few larvae. The ELISA for *Toxocara* on serum, aqueous, or vitreous samples is usually positive. Treatment is limited to systemic corticosteroids. Anthelmintic agents are not recommended.

Birdshot choroidopathy is a chronic, bilateral, intermediate and posterior uveitis characterized by diffuse vitritis and multifocal areas of choroiditis and frequently complicated by cystoid macular edema. This disease has no known cause, but 80 to 95% of patients carry the HLA-A29 antigen. Periocular or systemic corticosteroids are the mainstay of therapy, although some cases are resistant to these drugs.

Histoplasmosis may be associated with a multifocal choroiditis, peripapillary scarring, and macular hemorrhagic lesions. This is seen especially in patients who have lived in the Ohio, Missouri, and Mississippi river valleys. Since the causal relationship between the fungus and the related ocular findings is tenuous, the term **presumed ocular histoplasmosis syndrome (POHS)** is often used. The uveitis is always noted months to years after acutely acquired systemic histoplasmosis, when the CF test has usually returned to negative. Skin testing with histoplasmin is positive in 80% of cases, and most patients who have macular disease demonstrate presence of the HLA-B7 antigen. Chest x-ray often is useful in showing pulmonary calcifications typical of pulmonary histoplasmosis. Treatment includes systemic and/or periocular corticosteroid injections. Laser photocoagulation may halt the progress of macular disease.

Tuberculosis (TB), although now considered a rare cause, may produce almost any type of uveitis, including a diffuse generalized inflammation of all of the intraocular tissues. Laboratory tests include PPD and chest x-ray. Treatment with antituberculous drugs and systemic corticosteroids is often necessary.

Syphilis (secondary, tertiary, or latent), like TB, is a relatively rare cause of any type of uveitis. Laboratory testing on serum includes the nonspecific Venereal Disease Research Laboratories **(VDRL)** test and the specific fluorescent treponemal antibody absorption **(FTA-ABS)** test, as well as hemagglutination and microhemagglutination tests for *Treponema pallidum* antibodies. Examining the spinal fluid for reagin antibodies is often useful. After the diagnosis has been established, treatment is begun with systemic penicillin or with synthetic or semisynthetic penicillins and corticosteroids.

Behçet's syndrome is rare in the USA. Acute recurrent bilateral iridocyclitis, with pain, redness, photophobia, and severe retinal vasculitis and papillitis, is common. The ocular findings often occur in association with oral and genital aphthae, dermatitis, thrombophlebitis, or other systemic symptoms related to a widely disseminated systemic occlusive vasculitis. Laboratory testing includes biopsy of suspected skin or mucous membrane lesions and search for the HLA-B51 antigen. Treatment with local and systemic corticosteroids may quiet the acute inflammatory episode but is usually ineffective in arresting the relentless progressive damage of the disease. Therefore many authorities recommend immunosuppressive drugs or cyclosporine for this condition.

Sympathetic ophthalmia (SO) is a bilateral granulomatous uveitis that occurs after penetrating injury to one eye. A relatively rare condition, SO is estimated to occur in up to 0.5% of nonsurgical and < 0.01% of surgical penetrating eye wounds. In about 80% of cases, bilateral inflammation appears within 2 to 12 wk after injury; however, rare cases have been reported as early as 1 wk or as late as 20 or 30 yr after the initial injury. SO is believed to be an autoimmune disease in which the injury stimulates the body to begin making antibody to uveal antigens, resulting in diffuse granulomatous inflammation. The uveitis may be mild or severe and is treated with either long-term use of corticosteroids, immunosuppressive agents, or cyclosporine.

Vogt-Koyanagi-Harada (VKH) syndrome, or uveoencephalitis, is much more common in Orientals than in whites. It often begins with bilateral attacks of acute iridocyclitis with pain, redness, and photophobia. Later, severe, diffuse choroiditis may result in serous (inflammatory) detachment of the macular areas, with profound loss of vision. Associated systemic signs include alopecia areata, poliosis, vitiligo, dysacusis, and meningeal headaches. The headaches may be fleeting. Lumbar puncture performed in the course of a headache usually reveals pleocytosis of the spinal fluid—a valuable aid in diagnosis. Treatment with local and systemic corticosteroids or immunosuppressive drugs is often necessary.

Sarcoidosis, a commonly associated disease, may be accompanied by any type of anterior, posterior, or diffuse uveitis. The ocular inflammation often occurs independently of any systemic inflammation, thereby making diagnosis difficult. Useful laboratory tests include biopsy of conjunctival or lacrimal granulomas; serum testing for angiotensin converting enzyme and lysozyme; testing for elevated ESR; chest x-ray for hilar adenopathy; and gallium scan of the head, neck, and chest.

Treatment is limited to use of local, periocular, and systemic corticosteroids.

Reticulum cell sarcoma or **large cell lymphoma,** while not a true uveitis, usually presents as a bilateral vitritis in an older person. The major symptom is hazy, decreased vision. Multiple pale retinal or choroidal lesions may also be seen. The disease is often associated with lymphoma of the brain; usually, the brain is affected first and patients often exhibit personality changes. Lymphoma cells generally can be demonstrated by diagnostic lumbar puncture or vitrectomy. The disease should be suspected in any patient who develops vitritis for the first time at ≥ 50 yr of age. Treatment consists of vitrectomy in combination with radiotherapy. If the brain is involved, cytotoxic agents may be necessary. Prognosis is fairly good if the brain is not involved and fairly poor if it is.

ENDOPHTHALMITIS

Suppurative inflammation involving all the inner layers of the eye, the vitreous, and sclera may result from infection with bacterial or fungal agents. The infection may have been introduced exogenously (by a perforating wound of the eye or intraocular surgery) or endogenously via the bloodstream (from an infective focus elsewhere in the body or from the contaminated needle of an IV drug abuser).

The symptoms and signs of inflammation are often dramatic: severe pain, redness, photopho-bia, and profound loss of vision. Often the fundus cannot be visualized because of inflammation of the vitreous. Early testing of aqueous and especially vitreous aliquots for culture and microscopic examination is recommended.

Treatment *should be as in an emergency,* since delay of a few hours may result in blindness; it consists of administering systemic, periocular, and intraocular broad-spectrum antibiotics (eg, cefazolin or gentamicin). Supplemental corticosteroids usually are needed, and vitrectomy is often necessary.

MALIGNANT MELANOMA OF THE CHOROID

This is the most common primary ocular malignancy. It is rare in blacks. Malignant melanoma usually can be seen with an ophthalmoscope (through a dilated pupil) and appears as a single, round or oval, slightly elevated, gray or nonpigmented lesion. Early detection is important, since prognosis is related to the size of the lesion. If the lesion is small, treatment with lasers or radioactive plaques may cause the tumor to regress and save the eye. Larger tumors require enucleation. If the lesion is ignored, it may exit from the eye via scleral canals and involve the orbit or spread hematogenously to distant organs, especially the liver.

83. RETINA

VASCULAR RETINOPATHIES

Retinal hemorrhage, exudates, edema, ischemia, or infarction due to ocular or systemic vascular disorders.

Arteriosclerotic retinopathy is found in generalized arteriosclerosis and may be associated with hypertension. The walls of the retinal arterioles become thickened, and the changes are reflected on ophthalmoscopy as a widened arteriolar light reflex. As the sclerosis progresses, indentation of the veins at arteriovenous crossings and an increased difference between the sizes of the venous and arteriolar blood columns can be seen. The fine arterioles and veins may become tortuous, and the arteries may appear sheathed.

Hypertensive retinopathy occurs in chronic essential hypertension, malignant hypertension, and toxemia of pregnancy. The fundi show generalized or focal retinal arteriolar constriction in the early stages. As the disease progresses, superficial flame-shaped hemorrhages and small white superficial foci of retinal ischemia (cotton-wool spots) develop. Yellow hard exudates, due to lipid deposition deep in the retina and arising from leaking retinal vessels, are seen later and often produce a star-shaped figure around the macula. The optic disk becomes congested and edematous in severe hypertension, resembling the choked disk caused by brain tumor (**papilledema**—see in Ch. 85).

Treatment

Arteriosclerotic and hypertensive retinopathies can be managed only by medical control of the primary systemic disorder.

CENTRAL RETINAL ARTERY OCCLUSION

Blockage of the central retinal artery produces a painless, sudden, unilateral blindness. The occlusion may be due to embolism (disseminated atherosclerotic plaques, endocarditis, fat emboli, atrial myxoma) or to thrombosis in a sclerotic central artery. Another important cause is cranial arteritis (temporal arteritis). The pupil is semidilated and responds poorly to direct light but constricts briskly when the other eye is illuminated. In acute cases, ophthalmoscopy discloses a pale, opaque fundus with a red fovea (cherry-red spot). The arteries are attenuated and may appear bloodless. An embolic obstruction is sometimes visible; if it is not relieved quickly, retinal infarction occurs and blindness is permanent. If a major branch is occluded rather than the entire artery, fundus abnormalities are limited to that sector of the retina, and a permanent subtotal visual field loss follows unless the occlusion is relieved.

Branch retinal artery occlusion is frequently embolic.

Treatment

Immediate treatment is imperative. Reduction of intraocular tension by intermittent digital massage over the closed eyelids or anterior chamber paracentesis may dislodge an embolus and allow it to enter a smaller branch of the artery, thus reducing the area of retinal ischemia. Inhalation of 5 to 10% CO_2 in O_2 may relieve retinal arterial spasm.

CENTRAL RETINAL VEIN OCCLUSION

Occlusion of the central retinal vein usually appears in elderly patients. Glaucoma, diabetes mellitus, hypertension, increased blood viscosity, or an elevated Hct can be predisposing factors. Occlusion in a young person is uncommon; it may be idiopathic or result from retinal phlebitis. Painless visual loss occurs less abruptly than in arterial obstruction. The retinal veins appear distended and tortuous, the fundus is congested and edematous, and numerous retinal hemorrhages appear. These changes are limited to one quadrant if the obstruction involves only a branch of the vein. Neovascularization of the retina or of the iris (rubeosis iridis) with secondary (neovascular) glaucoma can occur weeks to months after the occlusion. Fluorescein angiography is essential to determine the state of the

circulation. Patients with normal retinal vessel perfusion usually do well; those with poor perfusion are more likely to develop complications.

Treatment

There is no generally accepted medical therapy. Involution of secondary retinal neovascular overgrowth by photocoagulation may decrease vitreous hemorrhages. Secondary neovascular glaucoma requires panretinal photocoagulation.

DIABETIC RETINOPATHY

This major cause of blindness can be particularly severe in persons who have insulin-dependent diabetes mellitus (IDDM); it also occurs frequently with chronic non–insulin-dependent diabetes mellitus (NIDDM). The degree of retinopathy seems more related to the duration of the diabetes than to its stability; retinopathy generally occurs after 10 yr. Two types of diabetic retinopathy are recognized—nonproliferative and proliferative. Nonproliferative retinopathy (also known as background retinopathy) is characterized by increased capillary permeability, microaneurysms, hemorrhages, exudates, and edema. The first signs are often venous dilation and small red dots seen ophthalmoscopically in the posterior retinal pole. The dots are caused by single or clustered capillary microaneurysms that can be demonstrated by fluorescein angiography. Visual symptoms are not encountered until an advanced state is reached. Dot and blot retinal hemorrhages and deep-lying edema and lipid exudates may impair macular function. Macular edema is a common cause of visual impairment in diabetics and may best be detected or confirmed by fluorescein angiography. Soft exudates (cotton-wool spots), which are microinfarcts caused by anoxia (acute vascular deficiency), and hard yellow exudates, usually caused by chronic edema (damaged capillaries), may be found. Both types of exudates may impair normal vision.

Proliferative retinopathy is characterized by new vessel formation (neovascularization within the retina and extending into the vitreous) and scarring, resulting in retinal detachment in advanced disease. The new vessels may extend into the vitreous cavity with subsequent vitreous hemorrhages.

Treatment

Control of the diabetes and blood pressure may be important. Diabetics with IDDM should have thorough annual retinal examinations (generally by an ophthalmologist), beginning 5 yr after diabetes has been diagnosed. Those with NIDDM should have annual examinations beginning at the time of diagnosis. Visual symptoms, including blurred vision; sudden loss of vision in one or both eyes; and black spots, cobwebs, or flashing lights in the field of vision, are indications for ophthalmologic referral at any time.

Panretinal photocoagulation (by xenon arc or argon laser) may diminish or eliminate proliferative retinopathy and neovascularization of the iris. Vitrectomy may be useful in cases of vitreous hemorrhage. Laser treatment is often helpful in slowing progression of background retinopathy.

MACULAR DEGENERATION OF THE AGED

(Age-Related Macular Degeneration [AMD]; Senile Macular Degeneration [SMD])

Atrophy or degeneration of the macula. AMD is a leading cause of visual diminution in the elderly. The condition is without sex predilection but is much more common in white than in black people. No predisposing systemic condition is known, but AMD may be hereditary. Two different forms of AMD can be defined: In **atrophic macular degeneration**, there is pigmentary disturbance in the macular region but no elevated macular scar and no hemorrhage or exudation in the region of the macula; in **exudative macular degeneration**, there is formation of an exudative mound, often surrounded by subretinal and intraretinal hemorrhage. Eventually, this mound contracts and leaves a distinct elevated scar at the posterior pole. Both forms of AMD are often bilateral and are preceded by drusen in the macular region.

Symptoms, Signs, and Diagnosis

A slow or sudden, painless loss of central visual acuity may occur. Occasionally, the first symptom is visual distortion from one eye; this can be tested with an Amsler grid. Funduscopy reveals pigmentary or hemorrhagic disturbance in the macular region of the involved eye; the contralateral eye almost always shows some pigmentary disturbance and the presence of drusen in the macula. Fluorescein angiography may demonstrate a neovascular membrane beneath the retina.

Treatment

If fluorescein angiography shows a neovascular net outside the fovea, it should be treated by appropriate laser photocoagulation. For patients who have lost central vision, low-vision devices are available and low-vision service counseling is advised. Patients with AMD, though often legally blind (< 20/200 vision), have good peripheral vision and useful color vision, and they should be advised that they will not lose all sight.

RETINAL DETACHMENT

Separation of the neural retina from the underlying retinal pigment epithelium.

Although initially detachment may be localized, without treatment the entire retina may detach. **Rhegmatogenous detachment** implies a break through and through in the retina and is seen more frequently in myopia, after cataract surgery, or following ocular trauma. **Nonrhegmatogenous detachments** can be produced by vitreoretinal traction (eg, proliferative retinopathy of diabetes or sickle cell disease) or by transudation of fluid into the subretinal space (eg, severe uveitis, especially in Vogt-Koyanagi-Harada disease, or primary or metastatic choroidal tumors).

Symptoms, Signs, and Diagnosis

Retinal detachment is painless. Premonitory symptoms may include dark or irregular vitreous floaters, flashes of light, or blurred vision. As the detachment progresses, the patient notices a curtain or veil in the field of vision. If the macula is involved, central visual acuity fails drastically.

Any patient with a suspected or established retinal detachment should be seen, on an urgent basis, by an ophthalmologist. Direct ophthalmoscopy may show retinal irregularities and a bullous retinal elevation with darkened blood vessels. Indirect ophthalmoscopy, including scleral depression, is necessary to detect peripheral breaks and detachment.

If a vitreous hemorrhage obscures the fundus, especially in myopia, post-cataract extraction, or eye injury, retinal detachment should be suspected and ultrasonography performed.

Treatment

Rhegmatogenous detachment is treated by finding the retinal holes and sealing them by diathermy or cryotherapy. The eye may be shortened by scleral buckling and by implanting silicone rubber sponges. Fluid may be drained from the subretinal space. Anterior retinal breaks without detachment can be sealed by transconjunctival cryopexy; posterior breaks, by photocoagulation. More than 90% of rhegmatogenous detachments can be reattached surgically.

Nonrhegmatogenous detachments due to vitreoretinal traction may be treatable by intravitreal surgery; transudative detachments due to uveitis may respond to systemic corticosteroid therapy. Primary choroidal neoplasms (malignant melanomas) may require enucleation, though radiation and local resection are used occasionally; choroidal hemangiomas may respond to localized photocoagulation. Metastatic choroidal neoplasms (the usual primary sites are breast, lung, and GI tract) may respond well to radiotherapy.

RETINITIS PIGMENTOSA

A slowly progressive, bilateral, tapetoretinal degeneration. A hereditary pattern is often difficult to establish, but in most cases it appears to be autosomal recessive. It may also be autoso-

mal dominant or, infrequently, X-linked. It may occur as part of a syndrome complex (Bassen-Kornzweig, Laurence-Moon-Biedl).

The retinal rods are affected, producing defective night vision that may become symptomatic in early childhood. A midperipheral ring scotoma (detectable by visual field testing) widens gradually, so that central vision eventually is reduced.

The most conspicuous ophthalmoscopic finding is dark pigmentation in "bone-spicule" configuration in the equatorial retina. The retinal arteries appear narrowed and the disk, in some cases, may have a waxy yellow appearance. Other manifestations can include degenerative vitreous opacities, cataract, and myopia. Congenital hearing loss may be associated.

Diagnosis may be aided by specialized testing (eg, dark adaptation, electroretinography [ERG]). Other retinopathies that can simulate retinitis pigmentosa (eg, syphilis, rubella, chloroquine toxicity) must be ruled out. Family members should be examined as necessary to establish the hereditary mode.

No treatment is effective in slowing the course of the retinal degeneration.

84.   GLAUCOMA

A disorder characterized by increased intraocular pressure that may cause impaired vision, ranging from slight loss to absolute blindness. Primary glaucoma in adults may be of 2 types: (1) chronic open-angle (wide-angle) or (2) acute or chronic angle-closure (closed-angle, narrow-angle, congestive, acute glaucoma attack). Congenital (infantile) glaucoma is also primary (see also under CONGENITAL EYE DEFECTS in Ch. 28). Secondary glaucoma results from preexisting ocular disease, usually uveitis, intraocular tumor, or an enlarged cataract. Prolonged corticosteroid therapy, especially with topical ophthalmic preparations, can produce an increased pressure, particularly in patients with a predisposition, so-called steroid responders. It may be present after 1 wk but usually occurs by the 6th to 8th wk of therapy. The increased pressure usually, but not always, subsides with cessation of therapy. Periodic tonometry is advisable during long-term corticosteroid use to discover early elevated pressure and preclude damage from a severe or prolonged intraocular pressure rise. Absolute glaucoma is the last stage of any form of un-

controlled glaucoma. The eye is blind from progressive atrophy of the optic nerve head. The pupil usually is widely dilated and fixed, the iris atrophied, and the optic disk deeply excavated. Pain is no longer prominent but may recur. The eyeball subsequently degenerates.

A competent gonioscopy examination of the anterior chamber angle is essential for proper diagnosis and classification of the glaucomas.

TABLE 84–1 lists the salient findings and usual treatment for the most common forms of glaucoma. Rarer forms may occur with associated congenital anomalies (eg, Sturge-Weber and Marfan's syndromes) or with vascular or degenerative disorders.

PRIMARY GLAUCOMA

Etiology and Pathogenesis

The causes are unknown. Vasomotor and emotional instability, hyperopia, and especially heredity are among the predisposing factors. The increased intraocular tension is related to an im-

TABLE 84–1. CHARACTERISTICS OF

Type of Glaucoma	Age	Iridocorneal Angle	Cornea	Pupil and Iris
Chronic open-angle glaucoma	Rare in children and young adults; incidence rises from age 30 on	Wide open; may show pigment deposits	Not remarkable	Pupil not dilated; iris may be atrophic late in the course
Angle-closure: acute; glaucoma attack	Any age, but more frequent after age 30	Closed during acute attack; narrow in interim	Cloudy; micro-cystic edema of epithelium frequent	Pupil mid-dilated, fixed; iris appears muddy
Glaucomatocyclitic crisis (Posner-Schlossman syndrome)	Any age from young adulthood on	Narrow (not closed) or wide open	May be clear with keratic precipitates; edema may be present	Pupil not dilated or only slightly dilated
Angle-closure: chronic; recurrent glaucoma attack	Any age	Narrow; closable with peripheral anterior synechiae	Usually cloudy during attack, clear between attacks	Pupil usually dilated during attack, normal between attacks
Congenital (infantile) glaucoma	Birth to first few months of life (usually discovered before age 6 mo)	Closed by membrane	Large in diameter; cloudy	Pupil dilated; iris may show atrophy
Secondary glaucoma	Any age (usually accompanying or following anterior uveitis)	Angle may be blocked by inflammatory debris or pigment	May be cloudy; microcystic edema may be present	Pupil may be narrow; iris may appear muddy
Corticosteroid-induced glaucoma	Any age in suscep-tible individuals (steroid responders) after prolonged ophthalmic use of topical or systemic corticosteroids	Wide open or narrow (not closed)	Usually clear	Pupil reacts; not constricted or dilated

THE COMMON FORMS OF GLAUCOMA

Optic Nerve Head and Visual Field	Intraocular Pressure	Subjective Symptoms	Treatment of Choice
May appear normal or show cupping. Progressive visual field defect if untreated	Elevated slightly (22–30 mm Hg) or markedly (30–45 mm Hg). Usually bilateral	Blurring of vision, frequent change of glasses. Occasional headaches, often ascribed by patient to "nervous tension" or "sinus problems"	*Topical:* Pilocarpine, timolol maleate, betaxolol HCl, levobunolol, metipranolol, epinephrine, dipivefrin, demecarium bromide, echothiophate iodide. *Systemic:* Carbonic anhydrase inhibitors. *Surgical:* Laser trabeculoplasty; subscleral filtering procedure if medication fails
Optic nerve head obscured during attack; may be normal. May show cupping after several attacks. Typical glaucomatous field defects may develop	40–70 mm Hg or even higher. Usually unilateral	Severe head and eye ache, blurred vision, halos around lights, general malaise, nausea, sometimes vomiting (GI symptoms may be misleading, delaying proper diagnosis)	*Topical:* Pilocarpine, timolol maleate. *Systemic:* Osmotic agents, carbonic anhydrase inhibitors. *Surgical:* Laser iridotomy or peripheral iridectomy when eye is quiet
Usually no cupping. *No visual field loss!*	May be ≥ 50 mm Hg. Usually unilateral	Blurred vision, halos around lights, headache. Nausea rare	*Topical:* Corticosteroid drops. *Systemic:* Carbonic anhydrase inhibitors. *Surgical:* Usually contraindicated
As for acute angle-closure glaucoma	Up to ≥ 70 mm Hg during attack; between attacks normal. Usually unilateral	Severe headaches during attacks, blurred vision, halos around lights. Nausea rare.	*Surgical:* Laser iridotomy or iridectomy; filtering surgery if > ½ of iridocorneal angle is permanently closed
Usually hard to evaluate. Later atrophic and may show cupping	Markedly elevated (50–70 mm Hg). Usually bilateral	Not assessable	*Surgical:* Goniotomy, goniopuncture, trabeculotomy
Initially may appear normal; if condition persists, may be cupped or atrophic. Glaucomatous field defect may develop	May be ≥ 50 mm Hg. Usually unilateral	Blurred vision, halos around lights, headache. Nausea rare	*Topical:* Anti-inflammatory management. *Systemic:* Anti-inflammatory management, carbonic anhydrase inhibitors
Initially no cupping; if not treated, cupping may develop. Glaucomatous field defect develops	May be ≥ 50 mm Hg. Frequently unilateral	Blurred vision and halos around lights initially rare; headaches may be present. Blurred vision common in later stages	*Stop corticosteroids. Topical:* Pilocarpine 1 to 4%, timolol maleate 0.25 or 0.5%, betaxolol HCl, demecarium bromide 0.125 or 0.25%, echothiophate iodide. *Systemic:* Carbonic anhydrase inhibitors

balance between production and outflow of the aqueous humor. Obstruction to outflow appears to be mainly responsible for this imbalance. In **chronic open-angle glaucoma,** the anterior chamber and its anatomic structures appear normal, but drainage of the aqueous humor is impeded. In **acute and chronic angle-closure (congestive) glaucoma,** the anterior chamber is shallow, the filtration angle is narrowed, and the iris may obstruct the trabecular meshwork at the entrance of the canal of Schlemm. Dilation of the pupil may push the root of the iris forward against the angle, which may produce angle closure, thus precipitating an acute attack. Eyes with narrow anterior chamber angles are predisposed to acute angle-closure glaucoma attacks of varying degrees of severity.

CHRONIC OPEN—ANGLE GLAUCOMA (COAG)

A disorder characterized by a gradual rise in intraocular pressure, causing slowly progressive loss of peripheral vision and, when uncontrolled, late loss of central vision and ultimate blindness. The most prevalent form of glaucoma, it is common after age 30 but may occur in early childhood. It is usually familial. Rarely, it is unilateral.

Individuals at higher risk of developing COAG are those > 35 yr or those with diabetes (also those with positive glucose tolerance tests), myopia, pigment dispersion syndrome (Krukenberg's spindle), or a family history of glaucoma. Blacks have a 4- to 5-times higher risk of developing COAG than do whites.

Diagnosis

Glaucoma should be suspected in any patient, especially if > 35 yr, who requires frequent spectacle lens changes, has mild headaches or vague visual disturbances, sees halos around electric lights, or has impaired dark adaptation. Since glaucoma can be asymptomatic until irreversible damage has occurred, every routine eye examination (and, optimally, every physical examination) in all adult patients should include tonometry. A single normal reading does not rule out glaucoma, since physiologic pressure shows diurnal variations of about 3 to 4 mm Hg (and even greater). The pressure rise in early glaucoma may be intermittent. A high-normal pressure reading is an indication for frequent follow-up examinations. In suspected cases, a complete glaucoma assessment by a glaucoma subspecialist is indicated.

Cupping of the optic disk is characteristic, but a normal optic disk does not rule out glaucoma, since optic nerve damage develops insidiously and, in some cases, late in the disease. Visual field changes may be subtle, with normal-appearing disks. The earliest changes in the central visual field are a baring of the blind spot and small scotomata above or below fixation, with small and dim visual field targets. Subtle nasal peripheral field defects appear early. The external eye usually appears normal.

Treatment

Most cases can be controlled with eyedrops. The most effective concentration and frequency of administration are determined by trial, starting with the weakest available preparations (eg, pilocarpine 0.5%). Preparations of choice are pilocarpine, timolol maleate, betaxolol, levobunolol, metipranolol, epinephrine, dipivefrin, carbachol (only in patients who are not controlled by or react adversely to pilocarpine), and potent cholinesterase inhibitors such as echothiophate iodide. (CAUTION: *Patients treated with powerful miotics like demecarium, echothiophate, and isoflurophate may develop cataracts or retinal detachment, which must be looked for periodically during treatment.*) Pilocarpine 4% gel (ointment) is used at night to supplement other medication. Carbonic anhydrase inhibitors (eg, dichlorphenamide 50 to 200 mg/day or acetazolamide 125 to 250 mg bid or qid orally) are of value when miotics alone do not control abnormal tension but should be used with great caution. Epinephrine 0.5 to 2%, 1 drop 1 to 2 times/day, may aid control by reducing aqueous production; alternatively, dipivefrin 0.1% solution used once or twice a day may be more effective than epinephrine. The patient should avoid fatigue, emotional upsets, use of tobacco, and drinking large quantities of fluids. Tonometry and charting of visual fields should be performed semiannually or more often when indicated. When medication fails to control intraocular tension or visual fields show progressive defects, laser trabeculoplasty or filtering surgery to improve aqueous drainage should be considered.

ACUTE ANGLE—CLOSURE GLAUCOMA

A disorder characterized by attacks of suddenly increased intraocular pressure, usually unilateral, with severe pain and loss of vision, caused by acute obstruction of aqueous drainage within the eye.

Symptoms and Signs

Prodromal symptoms occur as transitory episodes of diminished visual acuity, colored halos around lights, and pain in the eye and head. At such times, examination shows a somewhat dilated, poorly reacting pupil and shallow anterior chamber in the affected eye. These episodes may last only a few hours and recur at intervals before a typical prolonged attack of acute angle-closure glaucoma. The acute attack is characterized by rapid loss of sight and sudden onset of severe throbbing pain in the eye; the pain radiates over the sensory distribution of the 5th nerve. *Nausea and vomiting are common and may be mistaken for acute GI disease.* Upper lid edema, lacrimation, circumcorneal injection, chemosis of the bulbar conjunctiva, and a somewhat dilated, fixed pupil may be present. The cornea is steamy, the anterior chamber shallow, and the aqueous humor turbid enough to obscure the fundus. Intraocular pressure is increased considerably. (TABLE 79–2 lists findings that distinguish acute glaucoma, iritis, and conjunctivitis.) Symptoms usually subside after medical treatment but may recur. Each acute attack progressively diminishes vision and contracts the visual field. The condition may be bilateral.

Glaucomatocyclitic crisis (Posner-Schlossman syndrome), a recurrent monocular rise in pressure, simulates acute angle-closure glaucoma but is associated with normal anterior chamber depth, keratic precipitates, and other signs of uveitis.

Treatment

Oral glycerin 1 to 2 gm/kg mixed with an equal amount of water (cooled and preferably flavored with lemon) often aborts acute attacks and is excellent initial therapy for reducing elevated intraocular pressure rapidly. Oral carbonic anhydrase inhibitors (eg, acetazolamide 500 mg), if given immediately, generally abort an attack. If not, acetazolamide 500 mg IV and frequent instillation of miotics (eg, pilocarpine 4% q 15 min) for 1 to 2 h are indicated. Once the tension is normal, an oral carbonic anhydrase inhibitor q 6 h can be continued for several doses, together with miotics. If the initial therapy does not reduce the tension, 20% mannitol 500 mL by slow IV drip can be given (unless otherwise con traindicated), to be followed by miotics and a carbonic anhydrase

inhibitor. Surgery, peripheral iridectomy or laser iridotomy, prevents further attacks and is often performed prophylactically on the unaffected eye as well, if by gonioscopy the angle appears to be narrow.

Glaucomatocyclic crisis responds to systemic and topical corticosteroids and carbonic anhydrase inhibitors such as dichlorphenamide or acetazolamide; *surgery is usually contraindicated.*

CHRONIC ANGLE–CLOSURE GLAUCOMA

A disorder characterized by recurrent attacks—usually unilateral, of increased intraocular pressure, pain, and impaired vision—similar to those of acute angle-closure glaucoma but less severe. The causes are similar, but the anterior angle is obstructed gradually, not suddenly. Factors that promote dilation of the pupil may be precipitating causes. The fellow eye frequently becomes involved later. A provocative test for this condition is the **darkroom test** after tonometry, exposing the patient (who must be awake) to 60 min of darkness with the head bent forward in a prone position (best performed leaning on a Mayo table), then promptly measuring the intraocular pressure again. A rise in the pressure of 6 mm Hg during the test is considered positive.

Treatment

One or two drops of pilocarpine 1 or 2% instilled 3 to 6 times/day is the treatment of choice for temporary management. Timolol maleate 1 drop 0.25 or 0.5% solution 1 or 2 times/day can be *added* to aid temporary management; it should not be used without pilocarpine because timolol maleate does not contract the pupil and therefore does not promote removal of the iris from the iridocorneal angle. Oral glycerin or mannitol by IV drip (see ACUTE ANGLE-CLOSURE GLAUCOMA, above) is useful in aborting attacks. Carbonic anhydrase inhibitors are used only during attacks in narrow-angle glaucoma and are **contraindicated** in long-term therapy. Early laser iridotomy or peripheral iridectomy usually prevents further attacks. Permanent damage to the iridocorneal angle may necessitate management of the elevated intraocular pressure, even after successful laser iridotomy or iridectomy.

SECONDARY GLAUCOMA

Glaucoma secondary to an intraocular disorder, usually anterior uveitis.

Etiology and Pathogenesis

Secondary glaucoma is caused by any interference with the flow of aqueous humor from the posterior chamber through the pupil into the anterior chamber to the canal of Schlemm. Inflammatory disease of the anterior segment may prevent aqueous escape by causing complete posterior synechia and iris bombé and may plug the drainage channel with exudates. Other common causes are intraocular tumors, intumescent cataracts, central retinal vein occlusion, trauma to the eye, operative procedures, and intraocular hemorrhage.

Treatment

Secondary glaucoma is best treated by an ophthalmologist; intensive therapy and probably mydriasis are indicated. The underlying cause, usually uveitis, must be treated. Treatment is begun with systemic corticosteroids, and the effect of a mild mydriatic (eg, homatropine 5%, cyclopentolate 1%, or phenylephrine 10%) is tested in the office; atropine 1% bid or tid is given if the mydriasis is successful. If this fails, use of pilocarpine and/or timolol maleate should be considered. A carbonic anhydrase inhibitor or oral glycerin as for acute angle-closure glaucoma may be useful temporarily during the acute phase. Surgical intervention is indicated in iris bombé, tumor, and swollen cataract.

85.   OPTIC NERVE; VISUAL PATHWAYS

PAPILLEDEMA
(Choked Disk)

Swelling of the optic nerve head due to increased intracranial pressure. It is almost always bilateral and occurs with brain tumor or abscess, cerebral trauma or hemorrhage, meningitis, arachnoidal adhesions, pseudotumor cerebri, cavernous or dural sinus thrombosis, encephalitis, space-occupying brain lesions, severe hypertensive disease, and pulmonary emphysema.

Vision is not affected initially and there is no scotoma, but the blind spot is enlarged. The degree of disk elevation is determined by comparing the highest plus lens needed to bring the most elevated portion of the disk into sharp focus with the lens needed to clearly see an unaffected portion of the retina. Engorged and tortuous retinal veins, a hyperemic disk, and retinal hemorrhages about the disk are usually observed. The absence of changes in the arterioles and a normal blood pressure help to differentiate the papilledema of brain tumor from that of hypertension. If the intracranial pressure is not reduced, secondary optic atrophy and loss of vision eventually occur.

PAPILLITIS
(Optic Neuritis)

Inflammation or infarction of that portion of the optic nerve visible ophthalmoscopically. It oc-

curs with foci of inflammation in and about the optic nerve, as part of demyelinating conditions, following a viral illness, with multiple sclerosis, as a result of infarction of a part or all of the optic nerve head in temporal arteritis or other occlusive disease of the ciliary vessels, from tumorous metastasis to the optic nerve head, from certain chemicals (eg, lead, methanol), after bee stings, with meningitis, or from syphilis. It is usually unilateral, though this depends on the etiology. In many cases the cause remains obscure despite thorough evaluation.

Vision loss, varying from a small central or paracentral scotoma to complete blindness and frequently maximal within 1 or 2 days, is the major symptom. Usually, the direct pupillary light reflex is depressed. Ophthalmoscopy discloses hyperemia and/or edema of the disk in the early stages, and more noticeable changes in advanced cases. The retina becomes edematous around the nerve head and its vessels become engorged; a few exudates and hemorrhages may be present near or on the optic nerve head.

A particularly important cause of papillitis in patients over age 60 is **cranial giant cell arteritis (temporal arteritis)**. It may present with papillitis in one eye associated with malaise and an elevated ESR. It can rapidly spread to the other eye and result in bilateral blindness. The diagnosis is confirmed by temporal artery biopsy.

With spontaneous remission or successful removal of the cause early in the course, vision is usually restored; otherwise, postneuritic optic atrophy develops with varying degrees of vision loss, depending on the etiology. **Treatment** with corticosteroids, either systemic (eg, prednisone 60 mg/day or more orally) or retrobulbar (eg, methylprednisolone acetate 20 mg), may be helpful. Treatment of cranial giant cell arteritis with systemic corticosteroids is highly effective.

RETROBULBAR NEURITIS

Inflammation of the orbital portion of the optic nerve, usually unilateral. Multiple sclerosis is responsible for many of the cases; others are due to the same factors that cause papillitis, but idiopathic cases are even more common with retrobulbar neuritis than with papillitis. Rapid loss of vision (similar to that seen with papillitis) and pain on moving the eye are the principal symptoms. In contrast to papillitis, the fundus usually appears normal, though some mild disk hyperemia is seen occasionally. Spontaneous remission, with restoration of normal vision, often occurs in 2 to 8 wk. In some cases a central scotoma and pallor of the temporal portion of the disk remain. Relapses may occur, especially in multiple sclerosis. Each relapse increases the residual visual damage and temporal pallor; optic atrophy and permanent total blindness may result. **Treatment** is the same as for optic neuritis.

TOXIC AMBLYOPIA

A reduction in visual acuity believed to be due to a toxic reaction in the orbital portion of the optic nerve. Toxic amblyopia overlaps with retrobulbar neuritis. It is usually bilateral and most often seen in patients who use alcohol or tobacco excessively. In the former case, malnutrition may be the actual underlying cause. Cases of true tobacco amblyopia are rare. Lead, methanol, chloramphenicol, digitalis, ethambutol, and many other chemicals have also been implicated.

An initially small central or pericentral scotoma slowly enlarges, progressively interfering with vision. It may become absolute and lead to blindness. Abnormalities are not usually seen, but later in the course a temporal disk pallor may develop.

Treatment

Vision may improve when the cause is removed immediately, unless the optic nerve has atrophied. Chelation is indicated in lead poisoning.

OPTIC ATROPHY

Atrophy of the optic nerve, commonly classified as primary or secondary. In **primary optic atrophy**, the disk is white or grayish with sharp edges. The lamina cribrosa is clearly visible in the physiologic cup, and the retina is usually normal. In **secondary optic atrophy**, the disk is dirty white with irregular, indistinct margins and is covered by glial tissue that conceals the lamina cribrosa. Evidence of previous inflammation (such as sheathed vessels) may be seen in the retina.

Visual loss is roughly proportional to the degree of nerve atrophy and can range from little loss of vision to total blindness with no pupillary response to direct light.

Optic atrophy is a sign of chronic optic nerve disease, not a diagnosis in itself; its presence demands search for a cause. Dramatic return of vision can accompany reversal of certain pathologic processes (eg, central vision and visual field may return following decompression of a tumor).

HIGHER VISUAL PATHWAY LESIONS

The site of damage along the optic pathway determines the nature of visual field changes (see Fig. 85–1). Optic nerve lesions cause visual disturbances restricted to the affected eye. Lesions about the chiasm usually affect vision bilaterally. Lesions above or below the chiasm (eg, a pituitary tumor) destroy nerve fibers supplying the inner (nasal) half of both retinas, resulting in defects in the temporal visual fields (**bitemporal hemianopia**). Lesions in the optic tract, optic radiations, or cerebral cortex produce **homonymous hemianopia**, with loss of function in the right or left halves of both visual fields opposite the side affected. This, the most common type of hemianopia, is usually caused by a brain tumor or cerebrovascular accident.

Treatment is that of the primary lesion.

DISORDERS OF OCULAR MOTILITY

THIRD CRANIAL NERVE PALSIES

Partial to complete weakness of the 3rd nerve, resulting in ptosis of the lid and an outwardly turned eye. When the patient attempts to turn the

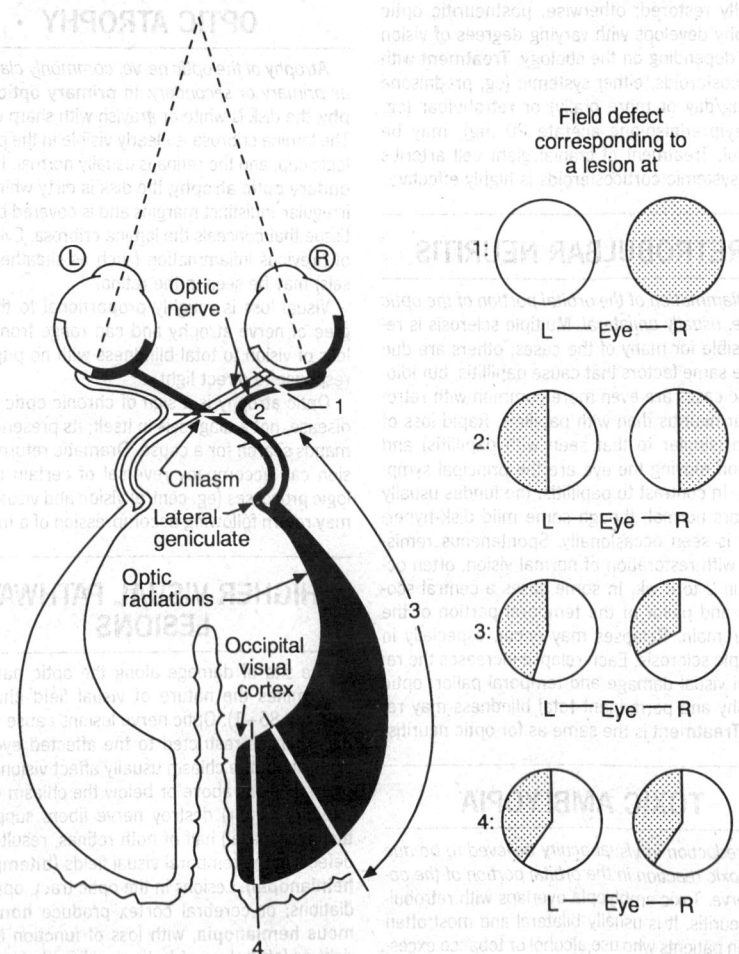

Field defect corresponding to a lesion at

1:

L — Eye — R

2:

L — Eye — R

3:

L — Eye — R

4:

L — Eye — R

FIG. 85-1. Higher visual pathways—lesion sites and corresponding visual field defects.

eye inward, it moves slowly only to the midline. When downward gaze is attempted, the superior oblique muscle causes the eye to rotate inward.

The causes of 3rd cranial nerve palsies are extensive, including most major causes of CNS disease. Thus, diagnostic evaluation should be based on the clinical features of such a palsy in a particular patient. This approach makes better use of diagnostic resources than does an attempt to perform every possible test on every patient.

First, mechanical disorders and myopathies should be distinguished from axon disease. Ex-

ophthalmos or enophthalmos, a history of severe orbital trauma, or an obviously inflamed orbit suggest restrictive orbital disease, which may lead to impaired ocular motility. Myopathies are harder to diagnose but may be suggested by a partial 3rd nerve palsy. The pupil is always spared in a myopathy and usually is spared in diabetes.

A second area of diagnostic importance is the pupil. Completely nonfunctional parasympathetic fibers strongly suggest a process that is anatomically damaging the axons. The most common are aneurysm, trauma, and tumor. If the pupil is completely spared but all other muscles innervated by the 3rd cranial nerve are involved, an ischemic or, less likely, a demyelinative process is likely to be the cause. However, if the pupil is partially involved or not all the extraocular muscles innervated by the 3rd cranial nerve are involved, other criteria must be used.

Third, diagnostic considerations for potentially serious causes of 3rd cranial nerve palsies include involvement of a second cranial nerve, a cranial nerve palsy in a person < 50 yr of age without an apparent medical cause (eg, insulin-dependent diabetes mellitus), and pain that seemingly originates inside the head. (In benign cases, pain should be referred to the eye or eyebrow.)

A thorough clinical examination combined with judicious neuroradiologic scanning and CSF evaluation generally suffices for diagnosing even the most worrisome cases of 3rd cranial nerve palsy. Angiography usually is necessary when the pupil is clearly involved and there is no history of head trauma serious enough to cause a skull fracture.

FOURTH CRANIAL NERVE PALSIES

Weakness of the superior oblique muscle. These palsies are often difficult to detect because this muscle weakness affects vertical eye position predominantly when the eye is turned inward. The patient sees double images, one above and slightly to the side of the other. However, by tilting the head to the side opposite the palsied muscle, the patient may achieve full or almost full ocular motility without double vision.

There are few common identified causes of 4th cranial nerve palsies; many are idiopathic. Closed head trauma without skull fracture is a common cause of both unilateral and bilateral palsies. Aneurysms, tumors, and multiple sclerosis are extremely uncommon causes.

Evaluation of 4th nerve palsies is similar to that of 3rd nerve palsies. Usually, the diagnosis is obvious from the history and physical examination.

SIXTH CRANIAL NERVE PALSIES

Weakness of the abducens nerve. Complete 6th cranial nerve palsies are easy to diagnose. The eye is turned inward; it moves outward sluggishly, reaching the midline at most. However, the diagnostic categories for these palsies are extensive, because the 6th cranial nerve has a long and vulnerable pathway.

Idiopathic cases are common, although many occur in elderly or diabetic patients in whom small vessel disease may be suspected. Such cases should show signs of improvement within 2 mo and no involvement of other cranial nerves.

Of the cases with a determinable etiology, a leading cause is compression of the 6th cranial nerve in the cavernous sinus by tumor originating in the nasopharynx. These cases typically present additionally with severe pain in the head and anesthesia in the distribution of the first division of the 5th cranial nerve.

Anything that can cause shifts of the brain may stretch the 6th cranial nerve because of the acute angle it makes before entering Dorello's canal. This may account for the 6th nerve palsies seen with large brain tumors remote from the nerve, with increased intracranial pressure, and after lumbar puncture.

Other causes include trauma of sufficient violence to cause a basilar skull fracture, infections and tumorous involvement of the meninges, Wernicke's encephalopathy, aneurysm, and multiple sclerosis. In children without evidence of raised intracranial pressure, these palsies can be associated with respiratory infection and thus may be recurrent.

Evaluation of patients often involves differentiating those who should be thoroughly examined from those who can be merely observed with the expectation of spontaneous improvement. Signs that are cause for concern include 6th nerve palsies in persons < 50 yr of age, involvement of any other cranial nerve, pain that persists beyond the first few days of the palsy, and no improvement after 6 wk to 2 mo.

INTERNUCLEAR OPHTHALMOPLEGIA

A weakness or paralysis of eye movements. The coordination of the eyes in horizontal gaze is accomplished by the medial longitudinal fasciculus of the brainstem. This long pathway, which connects the 6th nerve nucleus of one side with the medial rectus subnucleus of the opposite 3rd nerve nucleus, allows coordination of the paired function of abduction of one eye with adduction of the other, thus creating lateral gaze in one direction. Also, the medial longitudinal fasciculus has a number of connections of the vestibular nuclei with the 3rd nerve nucleus.

A lesion that interrupts these fibers weakens the adductive component of lateral gaze (the medial rectus function) but spares the abductive or lateral rectus function. The patient notices a horizontal displacement of images when looking to the side opposite the weak medial rectus and the damaged medial longitudinal fasciculus. This is often associated with nystagmus of the eye turning out, a skew deviation (ipsilateral eye higher than the other), and vertical nystagmus on attempted upward gaze. The medial rectus function in convergence is often preserved.

Unilateral internuclear ophthalmoplegias should be suspected in an isolated palsy of the medial rectus muscle. In the elderly, internuclear ophthalmoplegias are almost always caused by stroke and are usually unilateral. In younger individuals, unilateral or bilateral internuclear ophthalmoplegias are commonly caused by multiple sclerosis. Rare causes are masses external to or within the brainstem, drugs such as naloxone or amitriptyline, SLE, trauma, and the pseudointernuclear ophthalmoplegia of myasthenia gravis.

A still larger lesion involving the medial longitudinal fasciculus and the pontine lateral gaze center of the same side causes the $1^1/_2$ syndrome. Lateral gaze toward the side of the lesion as well as the adductive half of lateral gaze toward the opposite side is paretic. Only abduction of the contralateral eye remains. Causes of this rare condition are multiple sclerosis, infarction, hemorrhage, and tumor.

GAZE PALSIES

Conditions in which the patient cannot perform a conjugate eye movement in one direction, either up, down, right, or left. The most common involve horizontal gaze, although some affect upward and, less commonly, downward gaze.

The anatomic substrates for horizontal gaze are complex, involving stimuli from the hemispheres, the cerebellum, the vestibular nuclei, and the neck, which converge upon the pontine reticular formation. There the various influences are integrated into a final command to the 6th cranial nerve nucleus, which drives the lateral rectus muscle of the same side and the medial rectus muscle of the opposite side, via the medial longitudinal fasciculus.

The most common and devastating alteration of horizontal gaze occurs with lesions of the pons affecting the reticular formation. Such lesions are usually strokes, resulting in a profound loss of lateral gaze ipsilateral to the lesion. Horizontal gaze affected by such a lesion may be resistant to driving forces from any stimuli. In milder cases, weakness of horizontal gaze in that direction may result in a nystagmus or an inability to maintain fixation. Stroke and tumor are the most common causes of horizontal gaze palsy.

Because of its complex anatomy, horizontal gaze could be affected by various lesions in other areas, but a lesion in the contralateral cerebral hemisphere rostral to the frontal gyrus is the next most common cause of a horizontal gaze palsy. In this case, stimuli not dependent upon the hemisphere (eg, cold water caloric stimulation) can still elicit lateral gaze. This lesion can be caused by a stroke and may produce a temporary gaze palsy. Tumor causes a permanent gaze palsy.

The anatomic substrates underlying vertical gaze are less well understood. At least 2 separate oculomotor nuclei inputs influence vertical gaze. One ascends from the vestibular system through the medial longitudinal fasciculus of both sides, affecting both upward and downward gaze. A separate system descends, presumably from the hemispheres, through the pretectum to ultimately reach the 3rd nerve nuclei.

A supranuclear lesion that causes vertical gaze problems is exemplified by **Parinaud's syndrome**, in which a tumor or, less commonly, an infarction of the pretectal region causes a paralysis of upward gaze. Associated findings are pupils that react poorly to light but better to accommodation and convergence-type nystagmus on attempted upward gaze. Less common is paralysis of downward gaze, which is usually seen with bilateral lesions in the mesencephalon under the 3rd nerve nucleus. In both of these cases, stimuli from the vestibular system are still able to drive the eyes upward or downward. This is in contrast to the horizontal gaze system, in which a lesion in the reticular formation can block all stimuli for horizontal gaze. Causes of vertical gaze palsy are chiefly infarction and tumor.

86. CONTACT LENSES

Rigid corneal contact lenses are thin, saucer-shaped disks made of a hard plastic, polymethyl methacrylate **(PMMA)**, that float on the tear layer overlying the cornea. They are 6.5 to 10 mm in diameter and cover part of the cornea. **Soft hydrophilic contact lenses** are about 13 to 15 mm in diameter and cover the entire cornea. Made of poly-2-hydroxyethyl methacrylate

(HEMA) and other flexible plastics, they drape the eye. **Flexible nonhydrophilic lenses** (eg, made of silicone) as well as gas-permeable lenses (rigid) of pure silicone and of silicone and/or fluorocarbon PMMA admixtures are available. They permit increased O_2 transmission to the wearer's cornea.

Contact lenses often provide better visual acuity and peripheral vision than do eyeglasses and are prescribed to correct refractive errors (eg, nearsightedness and farsightedness, astigmatism, presbyopia, anisometropia, aniseikonia, and aphakia after cataract removal) and for keratoconus. Either soft or rigid lenses may be prescribed. Toric rigid and soft contact lenses (similar to cylindrical lenses in spectacles) are used to correct astigmatism; they are very satisfactory in many cases but require special expertise for fitting.

Soft contact lenses are prescribed, usually by an ophthalmologist, for treatment of bullous keratopathy and other corneal disorders ("bandage lenses"). These lenses are also well-tolerated occluders in children who need occlusion therapy (eg, for amblyopia). Prophylactic antibiotic eyedrops may be advisable with a bandage-type soft contact lens. The hydrophilic soft lens as a vehicle for delivering topical medications to the eyes is being studied. Extended wearing of contact lenses, especially for use in aphakia after cataract surgery, is practical but must be strictly monitored by the practitioner. The patient should see the practitioner at least twice a year and should clean the lenses once a week.

Rigid contact lenses require an adaptation period sometimes as long as a week for complete wearing comfort; during this time the wearer gradually increases the daily number of hours the lenses are worn. Wearers usually experience temporary blurring of vision ("spectacle blur"), which should not exceed 2 h, when wearing eyeglasses after removing their contact lenses.

No pain should be present at any time; pain is a sign of an ill-fitting contact lens.

Rigid and soft contact lenses occasionally cause superficial corneal changes (which may be painless) or abrasions accompanied by severe pain, photophobia, and anxiety. Ill effect may be caused by poorly fitting lenses or change in the lens or corneal parameters (swelling of tissues); by wearing the lenses in a harmful (eg, oxygen-poor, smoky, windy) environment; by improperly inserting or removing the lenses; or by small foreign particles (eg, soot, dust) trapped between

the contact lens and the cornea. Discomfort may also occur after removing the lenses, especially after prolonged use (overwearing syndrome). Spontaneous healing may occur in a day or so if the lenses are not worn; in some cases, treatment is required—eg, dilation of the pupil with a mydriatic to prevent posterior synechiae of the iris, topical antibiotic eyedrops or ointments, a firm eye patch, bed rest, and sedation. Recovery usually is rapid, complete, and without vision impairment in most cases. An ophthalmologist should be consulted before the lenses are worn again.

Because of their size, soft lenses are easier for elderly persons to handle. Since soft contact lenses drape over the eye, they are not likely to eject spontaneously (as rigid lenses may), and foreign bodies are less likely to lodge underneath them. Wearing comfort usually is immediate, and a brief or no adaptation period is necessary. Soft lenses apparently do not damage the eye even when the eye is closed for short periods and may thus be better for patients who may become unconscious (eg, epileptics, diabetics). Such patients should carry an emergency card or bracelet that identifies them as contact lens wearers. Soft lenses are brittle when dry and break easily. Rigid lenses are usually somewhat simpler and less time-consuming to care for than are soft lenses, which require special care and handling.

Because most soft lenses are hydrophilic, conventional solutions for rigid contact lenses should not be used with them. Most therapeutic eyedrops can be used with soft lenses.

The manufacturer's instructions for hygiene and handling of either type of lens must be strictly observed by the user. Poor contact lens hygiene may lead to hard-to-reverse inflammatory conditions of the conjunctiva or cornea. *Pseudomonas aeruginosa* and *Acanthamoeba castellani* infections of the cornea, associated with poor contact lens hygiene, require decisive and very active management. Similarly, acute bacterial infections of corneal ulcers associated with poor contact lens hygiene and wearing habits must be treated intensively. Neglected cases may respond poorly or not at all to treatment and could lead to blindness of the affected eye. Conditions that dry the anterior segment of the eye may contraindicate contact lens wear.

Persons susceptible to eye infections, those with a hand tremor or arthritis that interferes with lens insertion or removal, and those who are insufficiently motivated to tolerate the temporary discomfort that may occur while adapting to lenses are unlikely to wear either type of lens successfully. Lenses should not be worn if the eyes are inflamed or infected, during sleep, or when swimming.

Presbyopia can be corrected with contact lenses. In one approach, the nondominant eye is corrected for reading and the dominant eye for distant vision ("monovision"). Rigid and soft bifocal and multifocal contact lenses are also successful but are not popular with practitioners because the fitting procedure is often time-consuming.

§7. DERMATOLOGIC DISORDERS

87. DIAGNOSIS OF SKIN DISEASES

Many skin diseases can be diagnosed by physical examination alone, if one is familiar with the primary and secondary lesions and their arrangement and usual distribution. Except for obviously circumscribed diseases (eg, a plantar wart), the patient should undress for a complete examination, since lesions on some areas are unavailable for self-examination. Good lighting is essential. The oral mucosa, anogenital area, scalp, and nails also often provide clues to the diagnosis. The history may be invaluable for assessing physical findings.

PRINCIPAL TYPES OF LESIONS

Primary Lesions

The earliest skin changes to appear are the most important to recognize and, if necessary, to biopsy.

Macule: *A flat, discolored spot < 10 mm of varied shape* (eg, freckles, flat moles, tattoos, port-wine marks, and the rashes of rickettsial infections, rubella, and rubeola). **Patch:** *A spot similar to a macule > 10 mm.*

Papule: *A solid, elevated lesion usually < 10 mm in diameter.* **Plaque:** *A plateau-like lesion > 10 mm in diameter or a group of confluent papules.* Many cutaneous diseases begin with papules—warts, psoriasis, syphilis, lichen planus, drug eruptions, insect bites, seborrheic and actinic keratoses, some phases of acne, and skin cancers.

Nodule: *A palpable, solid lesion, > 5 or 10 mm in diameter, that may or may not be elevated* (eg, keratinous cysts, small lipomas, fibromas, some types of lymphoma, erythema nodosum, and a variety of neoplasms). Larger nodules (≥ 20 mm) are classified as **tumors.**

Vesicle: *A circumscribed, elevated lesion < 5 mm in diameter containing serous fluid.* **Bulla (blister):** *A vesicle > 5 mm in diameter.* Vesicles or bullae are commonly caused by primary irritants, allergic contact dermatitis, physical trauma, sunburn, insect bites, or viral infections (herpes simplex, varicella, herpes zoster); other causes include drug eruptions, pemphigus, dermatitis herpetiformis, erythema multiforme, epidermolysis bullosa, and pemphigoid.

Pustule: *A superficial, elevated lesion containing pus.* Pustules may result from infection or a seropurulent evolution of vesicles or bullae. Possibilities include impetigo, acne, folliculitis, furuncles, carbuncles, certain deep fungus infections, hidradenitis suppurativa, kerion, pustular miliaria, and pustular psoriasis of the palms and soles.

Wheal (hive): *A transient, elevated lesion caused by localized edema.* Wheals are a common allergic reaction; eg, from drug eruptions, insect stings or bites, or sensitivity to cold, heat, pressure, or sunlight.

Telangiectasia: *Dilated superficial blood vessels,* which may be seen in rosacea or certain systemic diseases (ataxia-telangiectasia, scleroderma) and may result from long-term therapy with topical fluorinated corticosteroids, but for most, the cause is unknown.

Secondary Lesions

These result either from the natural evolution of primary lesions (eg, a vesicle bursts, leaving an eroded area) or from the patient's manipulation of the primary lesion (eg, scratching a vesicle, leaving an eroded or ulcerated area).

Scales: *Heaped-up particles of horny epithelium* (the change may be primary or secondary). The most common scaling rashes are psoriasis, seborrheic dermatitis, superficial fungus infections, tinea versicolor, pityriasis rosea, and chronic dermatitis of any type.

Crust (scab): *Dried serum, blood, or pus.* Crusting occurs in a wide variety of inflammatory and infectious diseases.

Erosion: *Loss of part or all of the epidermis.* Erosion is often seen in infections from herpesviruses and in pemphigus.

Ulcer: *Loss of epidermis and at least part of the dermis.* When ulcers result from physical trauma or acute bacterial infection, the cause usually is apparent. Less obvious causes include chronic bacterial and fungal infections, self-inflicted ulcers, various peripheral vascular diseases and neuropathies, systemic scleroderma, and neoplastic tumors.

Excoriation: *A linear or hollowed-out crusted area, caused by scratching, rubbing, or picking.*

Lichenification: *Thickened skin with accentuated skin markings.* Atopic dermatitis and lichen simplex chronicus (localized scratch dermatitis) are typically associated with lichenification.

Atrophy: *Paper-thin, wrinkled skin.* Atrophy is seen in the aged, in discoid LE, after long-term use of topical highly potent corticosteroids, and after some burns.

Scar: *Fibrous tissue replacing normal skin structures after destruction of some of the dermis.* Scars, like ulcers, may have easily recognized origins (eg, burns or cuts). Others are evolutionary changes (eg, discoid LE).

ARRANGEMENT AND DISTRIBUTION OF LESIONS

Distinctive arrangements of skin lesions may form: The **grouping** of tense vesicles in herpes simplex and zoster, and their linear configuration in the latter, point to the diagnosis. **Annularity** (a tendency to form rings) is typical in granuloma annulare, erythema multiforme, dermatophyte infections, some forms of Lyme disease, and secondary syphilis. **Linearity** is sometimes seen with epidermal nevi, linear scleroderma, and contact dermatitis. Lesions in psoriasis, lichen planus, and flat warts may mimic the shape of trauma to the skin (eg, from scratching, rubbing, or other injury—**the Koebner phenomenon, isomorphic reaction**).

Distribution on the body: Although a disease occasionally does not follow its usual pattern of distribution, some patterns of skin involvement are common.

Acne occurs on the face, neck, chest, and upper back. In "tropical acne" the entire trunk may be involved. **Atopic dermatitis** typically involves the antecubital and popliteal spaces, face, neck, and hands in children and adults. In infants the distribution may be as above but may also be limited to the diaper area or the face. **Erythema multiforme** involves primarily the palms, soles, and mucous membranes but may be widespread. **Erythema nodosum** affects the lower legs, principally on pretibial surfaces. **Lichen planus** occurs on the oral mucosa, flexor surface of wrists, trunk, and genitalia. Lesions may be widespread. **Chronic discoid LE** affects principally the face, scalp, ears, and neck. **Photosensitivity reactions** occur on areas exposed to natu-

ral or artificial light; eg, the V of the neck, the arms below the sleeves, and the face (especially the cheeks and nose). This typical distribution often goes unrecognized and may be confused with contact dermatitis. **Pityriasis rosea** is seen on the trunk and proximal extremities in most cases, with the long axis of oval lesions paralleling the lines of cleavage. Occasionally pityriasis rosea may affect only the extremities and spare the trunk. **Psoriasis** occurs most commonly on extensor surfaces of elbows and knees, scalp, back, anogenital region, and nails, but may appear on flexor surfaces or even on the tip of the penis or on the palms.

SPECIAL DIAGNOSTIC METHODS

Biopsy is essential for diagnosing any obscure dermatosis, particularly a chronic one, and imperative if there is any suggestion of malignancy. A fully developed typical lesion should usually be chosen for biopsy; early lesions are best in vesicular, bullous, or pustular eruptions. The simplest biopsy procedure is to insert a sharp circular punch, 3 mm or more in diameter, well through the dermis, and snip off the base of the plug. An adequate biopsy of some relatively friable lesions (eg, seborrheic keratoses) may be obtained with a sharp curet. For a larger tissue sample, and for deep dermal or subcutaneous lesions, a wedge is removed and the incision sutured. For most small tumors, complete excision with small, normal borders allows microscopic diagnosis and cure with one procedure. All pigmented lesions, including nevi, should be excised deeply enough for histologic evaluation of depth. Superficial biopsies are often inadequate for histologic diagnosis, especially of pigmented lesions. A deep part of the biopsy specimen should be cultured when a mycobacterial or a deep fungal infection is suspected.

Examination of scrapings for fungi: In any suspected superficial fungal infection, the organisms can be demonstrated by microscopic examination of scales taken from the lesion, covered with 20% potassium hydroxide, and warmed gently; broken, misshapen stubs of hairs from a lesion must be examined, since normal hairs will not be infected in tinea capitis. In dermatophyte infections, only hyphae are seen, while in tinea versicolor and candidal infections, both yeast and hyphae are seen; the distinction may be important in selecting specific drug therapy.

Bacterial and fungal cultures: In acute bacterial skin infections, culture and antibacterial sensitivity testing are advised, although treatment should be started promptly. Adequate sampling is essential. With frankly pustular lesions, a swab sample is sufficient; the swab should be placed immediately in broth culture and not allowed to dry out. In chronic infections (eg, TB or deep fungi), where the flora may be mixed and relatively sparse, more ample specimens (including even deep biopsy specimens) must be obtained and special culture media may be needed. Culture of superficial fungal infections will occasionally be positive when the scraping is negative.

Wood's light examination: When the skin is viewed in a darkened room under ultraviolet light filtered through Wood's glass ("black light"), tinea versicolor may fluoresce golden and erythrasma orange-red; scalp hairs in tinea capitis caused by *Microsporum canis* and *Microsporum audouinii* are a light bright green. Most tinea capitis infections are caused by *Trichophyton* species that rarely fluoresce. The earliest clue to a *Pseudomonas* infection, especially in burns, may be a green fluorescence under a Wood's light. The depigmentation of vitiligo can be differentiated from hypopigmented lesions by its ivory-white color on Wood's light examination.

Cytologic examination: The Tzanck test is rapid and reliable (in experienced hands) for diagnosing vesicular eruptions. A smear of cellular material scraped from the base and sides of a vesicle and stained with Wright's or Giemsa stain shows multinucleated giant cells in herpes simplex, herpes zoster, and varicella but not in vaccinia. Virus cultures are more sensitive and are becoming very rapid—an improvement over the more difficult-to-interpret cytologic Tzanck test. If a viral or chlamydial infection is suspected early, vesicle fluid or cervical or urethral material can be put into special transport media for culture in most medical centers. Pemphigus can be diagnosed by finding typical acantholytic cells that have very large nuclei and scant cytoplasm and have lost attachment to each other.

Immunofluorescence (IF) tests: Fluorescence microscopy (see DISORDERS WITH TYPE II HYPERSENSITIVITY REACTIONS in Ch. 34) is an important aid in diagnosing and managing certain skin diseases. The indirect IF test shows that the serum of a patient with pemphigus or bullous pemphigoid contains specific antibodies (Abs) that bind to different areas of the epithelium. In pemphigus, the Ab titer may correlate with the severity of the disease. In the direct IF test, biopsied skin of patients with pemphigus, pemphigoid, dermatitis herpetiformis, herpes gestationis, SLE, and discoid LE shows specific, diagnostic patterns. The direct IF test is more definitive diagnostically for most of these diseases.

Other special diagnostic methods include patch tests used for allergic contact dermatitis (see DISORDERS WITH TYPE IV HYPERSENSITIVITY REACTIONS in Ch. 34) and darkfield examination for syphilis (see Ch. 21).

88. PRINCIPLES OF TOPICAL DERMATOLOGIC THERAPY

Many substances are applied for topical treatment, including absorbents, anti-infectives, anti-inflammatory agents, astringents (drying agents that precipitate protein and shrink and contract the skin), cleansing agents, emollients (skin softeners), and keratolytics (agents that soften, loosen, and facilitate exfoliation of the squamous cells of the epidermis).

Locally acting agents have the following uses: (1) They cleanse, debride, and protect the skin. (2) They destroy causative agents (eg, bacteria, fungi, or protozoa); eradication of specific agents causing skin infections is discussed in the appropriate chapters below. Topical antibiotics are effective in acne, and some newer agents (eg, mupirocin) are effective in the treatment of some superficial skin infections. Topical fungicides, scabicides, and pediculicides are commonly used, as are systemic antibiotics. (3) They attempt to relieve symptoms (eg, pruritus, burning, pain). In addition to analgesics, camphor 0.5 to 3% or menthol 0.1 to 0.2% may be used singly or together in topical creams or ointments. Local anesthetics (eg, lidocaine and dibucaine) are generally not used on the skin because they are ineffective; they are sometimes useful on mucosal surfaces. (4) They reduce inflammation and promote healing.

Topical Formulations

The **vehicle** (base or carrier) for a drug must be selected carefully, since it may alter the effectiveness of the active ingredient. Allergic and irritating reactions (eg, contact dermatitis) may be caused by ingredients of the vehicle as well as by the active agent.

Ointments are oleaginous and contain little if any water; they feel greasy but are generally well tolerated. They are best used to lubricate, especially if applied over hydrated skin; they are preferred for lesions with thick crusts, lichenification, or heaped-up scales, and may be less irritating than a cream on some eroded or open lesions (eg, stasis ulcers). Although messier to use, ointments are usually more potent than creams for delivering a drug to the skin.

Creams, *semisolid emulsions of oil in water or water in oil,* are the mainstay of dermatologic therapy. They are easy to apply and vanish when rubbed into the skin.

Lotions originally were suspensions or dispersions of finely powdered material (eg, calamine) in a water or alcohol base; however, most modern lotions (eg, some corticosteroids) are really oily emulsions. Convenient to apply, lotions cool and dry acute inflammatory and exudative lesions.

Solutions, *homogenous mixtures of 2 or more substances,* are convenient to apply, especially to the scalp. Like lotions, solutions are drying. The most commonly used solvents are ethyl alcohol, propylene glycol, polyethylene glycol, and water.

Agents That Cleanse and Protect

The principal **cleansing agents** are detergents and solvents. Soap is the most popular detergent, but synthetic detergents are also used. Baby-type shampoos are usually well tolerated not only around the eyes but also in cleansing wounds and abrasions; they are useful in psoriasis, eczema, and other forms of dermatitis for removing crusts and scales. However, badly irritated, weeping, or oozing lesions should be cleansed only with water.

Various ingredients often are added to detergents and other skin preparations to enhance or add certain properties. For antidandruff action, zinc dipyrithione or selenium sulfide or tar extracts may be added to a shampoo.

Water is the principal solvent used for cleansing. Using plain **tap-water soaks, baths, or compresses** (made from gauze or old sheets) for 48 to 72 h (changing them q 1 to 2 h) will generally dry, soothe, and cool acute weeping or oozing lesions and often debride them as well. Wet dressings containing aluminum acetate, magnesium sulfate, etc, are seldom better than plain tap water.

Protectants cover the skin: Powders are often used to protect intertriginous areas (ie, between the toes and in the intergluteal cleft, axillae, groin, and inframammary areas). Powders dry macerated skin and reduce friction by absorbing moisture, thereby providing comfort. However, some powders tend to "ball up" and can be irritating when they become moist. Powders may be incorporated into protective creams, lotions, and ointments. Collodion and other films provide a flexible or semirigid continuous coating. Modern moist dressings (hydrophilic polymers) can be applied with a gauze cover. Zinc gelatin (Unna's boot) forms an occlusive dressing. **Sunscreens** help shield the skin from ultraviolet light (see Ch. 113).

Topical Corticosteroids

Corticosteroids, the most effective topical anti-inflammatory agents, are remarkably devoid of major side effects (see TABLE 88–1 for many preparations now available). Itchy, inflammatory dermatoses usually respond favorably to properly used corticosteroids. However, they may worsen some conditions (eg, acne, rosacea, and some fungal infections). Corticosteroids and other preparations are usually prepared for use on the skin as creams, lotions, ointments, or solutions, and less commonly as aerosols and tapes.

Since hydrocortisone 1%, a nonfluorinated preparation, does not induce facial telangiectasia, perioral dermatitis, atrophy, or striae, it is usually preferable to a synthetic corticosteroid for treating facial dermatoses. Although some corticosteroid preparations are available in higher or lower concentrations, the more potent ones should generally be prescribed first. The preparations should be applied sparingly tid, or more frequently for some dermatoses. Newer, very potent topical corticosteroids may be applied less often. For maximum effectiveness, creams should be rubbed in gently until they vanish. Hydrocortisone 0.5% preparations are available without prescription but offer little, if any, benefit. Stronger preparations (eg, hydrocortisone 1%) may be made available soon for nonprescription use.

Intralesional injection of a corticosteroid suspension is a useful method for delivering a high concentration of corticosteroid to a chronic

TABLE 88–1. RELATIVE POTENCY OF SELECTED TOPICAL STEROID PRODUCTS

Potency*	Drug	Form	Strength
I	Augmented betamethasone dipropionate	Cream, ointment	0.05%
	Clobetasol propionate	Cream, ointment	0.05%
	Diflorasone diacetate	Ointment	0.05%
II	Amcinonide	Ointment	0.1%
	Betamethasone dipropionate	Ointment	0.05%
	Desoximetasone	Cream, ointment	0.25%
		Gel	0.05%
	Diflorasone diacetate	Ointment (emollient base)	0.05%
	Fluocinonide	Cream, gel, ointment	0.05%
	Halcinonide	Cream	0.1%
III	Betamethasone dipropionate	Cream	0.05%
	Betamethasone valerate	Ointment	0.1%
	Diflorasone diacetate	Cream	0.05%
	Triamcinolone acetonide	Ointment	0.1%
IV	Desoximetasone	Cream	0.05%
	Fluocinolone acetonide	Ointment	0.025%
	Flurandrenolide	Ointment	0.05%
	Hydrocortisone valerate	Ointment	0.2%
	Triamcinolone acetonide	Cream	0.1%
V	Betamethasone dipropionate	Lotion	0.02%
	Betamethasone valerate	Cream	0.1%
	Fluocinolone acetonide	Cream	0.025%
	Flurandrenolide	Cream	0.05%
	Hydrocortisone butyrate	Cream	0.1%
	Hydrocortisone valerate	Cream	0.2%
	Triamcinolone acetonide	Lotion	0.1%
VI	Betamethasone valerate	Lotion	0.05%
	Desonide	Cream	0.05%
	Fluocinolone acetonide	Solution	0.01%
VII	Hydrocortisone acetate	Lotion, cream, ointment	1.0%

* Potency depends on many factors, including the drug's characteristics and concentration as well as the vehicle in which it is used. The drugs in this table are listed according to their relative potency: Grade I is the most potent.

Adapted from Stoughton RB, Cornell RC: "Review of super-potent topical corticosteroids." *Seminars in Dermatology* 6:72–76, 1987; used with permission from WB Saunders Company; and from *Drug Facts and Comparisons*, 1991 Edition, p 2150, used with permission from Facts and Comparisons, a Division of the JB Lippincott Company, St. Louis.

lesion or to one resistant to topical corticosteroids: The major problem is dermal atrophy, which is usually reversible. In black skin, hypopigmentation may follow injection. Triamcinolone acetonide is the corticosteroid suspension almost always used for intralesional injection. The suspension may be diluted with sterile saline and is usually used at concentrations of 2.5 to 10 mg/mL to minimize risk of local atrophy and hypopigmentation. Higher concentrations should be reserved for treatment of keloids.

Occlusive therapy: Absorption and effectiveness of topical corticosteroids are increased by covering the treated area with a nonporous occlusive dressing. This is used in such conditions as psoriasis, atopic dermatitis, LE, and chronic hand dermatitis. Usually, a polyethylene film (plastic household wrap) is applied overnight over a cream or ointment preparation, since these tend to be less irritating than lotions for occlusive therapy. A plastic tape impregnated with flurandrenolide is especially convenient for treating isolated or recalcitrant lesions. Miliaria, atrophic striae, and bacterial infections may follow occlusive therapy; children and (less often) adults may suffer some pituitary and cortisol suppression after prolonged occlusive treatment of large areas.

The use of topical antibiotics in combination with topical corticosteroids is seldom warranted. The combinations are no more effective than a corticosteroid alone, and allergic contact dermatitis from topical antibiotics, especially neomycin, may complicate the primary problem.

89. PRURITUS
(Itching)

A sensation that the patient instinctively attempts to relieve by scratching.

Etiology, Symptoms, and Signs

Itching may accompany a primary skin disease or may be a symptom of systemic disease—sometimes the only symptom.

Skin diseases in which itching is most severe and lesions apparent include scabies, pediculosis, insect bites, urticaria, atopic dermatitis, contact dermatitis, lichen planus, miliaria, and dermatitis herpetiformis. Dry skin (especially in the elderly) often causes severe generalized itching.

Systemic conditions clearly associated with generalized itching and usually unaccompanied by skin lesions include obstructive biliary disease, uremia (frequently associated with hyperparathyroidism), lymphomas, leukemias, and polycythemia rubra vera. During the later months of pregnancy, itching may occur unaccompanied by primary skin lesions. Many drugs (especially barbiturates and salicylates) can cause pruritus. Unproved associations with generalized itching include hyperthyroidism, diabetes mellitus, and internal cancers of many types. One should be cautious in attributing a psychogenic origin to the generalized pruritus, although pruritus can uncommonly occur on a purely psychogenic basis.

Persistent scratching may produce redness, linear urticarial papules, excoriated papules, fissures, and elongated crusts along scratch lines, and these secondary lesions may obscure the underlying disease. Lichenification and pigmentation may also result from prolonged scratching

and rubbing. On occasion, the patient who complains of severe generalized itching has few signs of scratching or rubbing the skin.

Treatment

First and foremost, the cause of generalized pruritus should be sought and corrected. If no skin disease is readily apparent, an underlying systemic disorder or drug-related cause should be sought.

If feasible, all drugs should be stopped or chemically unrelated drugs substituted. Clothing that is irritating (eg, woolens) or tight should be avoided. Bathing should be minimized, as it may aggravate generalized itching, especially if the patient has dry skin. Emollients (eg, white petrolatum, Eucerin®, or other oil-based products) are good moisturizers, if applied while the skin is still wet. After bathing, the skin should be blotted to remove excess water and emollient applied. Proprietary anesthetics should be avoided. Ultraviolet B to the skin and oral cholestyramine can be helpful in uremia and cholestasis, and at times even when no underlying abnormalities are found. Topical corticosteroids seldom alleviate generalized itching (without dermatitis), but may uncommonly be useful if used with lubricants in elderly patients with dry skin.

If a drug has been adequately ruled out as the cause of the itching, one may prescribe a tranquilizer (eg, hydroxyzine or, for more severe cases, minimal and gradually increasing doses of chlorpromazine or the antidepressant doxepin). If antihistamines are at all helpful, the main reason may be because of their sedative effect.

90. DERMATITIS
(Eczema)

Superficial skin inflammation, characterized by vesicles (when acute), redness, edema, oozing, crusting, scaling, and usually itching. Scratching or rubbing may lead to lichenification.

Here the terms *dermatitis* and *eczema* are used synonymously. Authorities generally disagree about how to distinguish between the two: *Eczematous dermatitis* is often used to mean a vesicular dermatitis, and some still restrict *eczema* to mean chronic vesicular dermatitis.

CONTACT DERMATITIS

An acute or chronic inflammation, often sharply demarcated, produced by substances in contact with the skin.

Etiology

Contact dermatitis may be caused by a primary chemical irritant or may be a type IV delayed hypersensitivity reaction (see Ch. 34).

Irritants may damage normal skin or irritate an existing dermatitis. Weak or marginal irritants (eg, soap, detergents, acetone, or even water) may take several days of exposure to cause clinically recognizable changes. Strong irritants (eg, acids, alkalis, phenol) cause observable changes within a few minutes. The mechanisms by which these irritants damage the skin are unknown.

Allergic contact dermatitis is a delayed hypersensitivity reaction. It takes between 6 and 10 days (in the case of strong sensitizers, eg, poison ivy) to years (for weaker sensitizers) for individuals to become sensitized. Upon reexposure to the sensitizer, itching and dermatitis may appear within 4 to 12 h. Recent studies indicate that Langerhans' cells (a minor subpopulation of epidermal cells) are critical for presentation of allergens to T cells, which thereby become sensitized. Chemical mediators released from keratinocytes and Langerhans' cells may also contribute to sensitivity induction. Patients often find it difficult to believe that they have become allergic to substances they have used for years or to drugs used to treat their dermatitis. However, **ingredients in topical drugs** constitute a major cause of allergic contact dermatitis: antibiotics (penicillin, sulfonamides, neomycin), antihistamines (diphenhydramine, promethazine), anesthetics (benzocaine), antiseptics (thimerosal, hexachlorophene), and stabilizers (ethylenediamine and derivatives). Other commonly implicated substances include **plants** (poison ivy, oak, and sumac; ragweed, primrose); many potential **sensitizers used in the manufacture of shoes and clothing** (tanning agents in shoes; free formaldehyde in durable-press finishes; rubber accelerators and antioxidants in gloves, shoes, underpants, bras, and other wearing apparel);

metal compounds (nickel, chromates, mercury); *p*-phenylenediamine and other **dyes**; and **cosmetics** (depilatories, nail polish, deodorants). Industrial agents capable of producing occupational dermatoses are almost innumerable.

Photoallergic and **phototoxic contact dermatitis** require exposure to light following topical application of certain chemicals. They are manifested as an exaggerated response to sunlight (see polymorphous light eruptions in Ch. 113). Agents commonly responsible for photoallergic contact dermatitis include aftershave lotions, sunscreens, and topical sulfonamides. Phototoxic contact dermatitis is commonly caused by certain perfumes, coal tar, psoralens, and oils used in manufacturing processes. Photoallergic and phototoxic contact dermatitis must be differentiated from photosensitivity reactions to drugs given systemically.

Symptoms and Signs

Contact dermatitis ranges from transient redness to severe swelling with bulla formation; itching and vesiculation are common. Any exposed skin surface that contacts a sensitizing or irritating substance may be involved. Thus, dermatitis may be due to an airborne substance (eg, ragweed pollen, insecticide spray). Typically, the dermatitis is first sharply limited to the site of contact; later it may spread.

The course varies. If the cause is removed, simple erythema disappears within a few days and blisters dry up. Vesicles and bullae may rupture, ooze, and crust. As the inflammation subsides, scaling and some temporary thickening of the skin occur. Continuing exposure to the causative agent or complications (eg, irritation from or allergy to a topical drug, excoriation, infection) may perpetuate the dermatitis.

Diagnosis

Since contact dermatitis may resemble other types of dermatitis, an allergen or irritant should be suspected as the cause or aggravating factor in any puzzling dermatitis. Typical skin changes and a history of exposure facilitate the diagnosis, but identification may require exhaustive questioning and extensive patch testing. The patient's occupation, hobbies, household duties, vacations, wearing apparel, topical drugs, cosmetics, and spouse's activities must all be considered. Knowing the characteristics of topical allergens or irritants, including the typical distribution of lesions, is helpful. The site of the initial lesion is often an important clue.

Patch testing (see DISORDERS WITH TYPE IV HYPERSENSITIVITY REACTIONS in Ch. 34) with a standard group of contact allergens may be helpful if questioning is fruitless. A specialist should select the test concentrations (particularly for industrial agents or cosmetics, in which case an industrial specialist should be consulted). Because the allergen may worsen the eruption in a very sensitive patient and because patch testing may yield ambiguous results during the acute phase of the dermatitis, patch testing is often done after the eruption subsides. A positive patch test reaction does not necessarily identify the agent causing the contact dermatitis. There must be a history of exposure to the test agent in the areas where the dermatitis originally occurred before a definite diagnosis can be made. Moreover, a negative patch test does not rule out contact dermatitis: it may mean only that the offending agent was not included in the tests.

Treatment

Unless the offending agent is removed, treatment may be ineffective or the dermatitis may promptly recur. Patients with photoallergic or phototoxic contact dermatitis should also avoid exposure to light. In the acute phase of dermatitis (eg, that caused by poison ivy), gauze or thin cloths dipped in water and applied to the lesions are soothing and cooling; they should be applied for 30 min, 4 to 6 times/day. Blisters may be drained tid, but the tops should not be removed. An oral corticosteroid (eg, prednisone 60 mg/day) should be given for 12 to 16 days in severe or extensive cases or even in limited cases when there is severe facial inflammation. The prednisone dose can be decreased by 10 to 20 mg q 3 to 4 days. Topical corticosteroids are not helpful in the blistering phase, but once the dermatitis is less acute, a topical corticosteroid cream or, if the dermatitis is very dry, an ointment (see Ch. 88) should be rubbed in gently tid. Antihistamines (except for their sedative effect) and allergen desensitization are ineffective in contact dermatitis.

ATOPIC DERMATITIS

A chronic, itching, superficial inflammation of the skin, frequently associated with a personal or *family history of related disorders (eg, hay fever, asthma).*

Etiology

The cause is unknown. Although the relationship to the dermatitis is not clear, these patients have high levels of cyclic AMP phosphodiesterase in their WBCs. Frequently, numerous inhalants and foods produce wheal-and-flare reactions on scratch or intradermal tests, but these reactions are usually nonspecific. Recent studies suggest that certain foods induce erythema and itching in young individuals. Patients with atopic dermatitis usually have high serum levels of reaginic (IgE) antibodies and peripheral eosinophilia, but the etiologic significance of these findings is unknown. Several studies have reported a defect of T cell regulation that may be associated with increased IgE responses.

Symptoms, Signs, and Course

Atopic dermatitis may begin in the first few months of life, with red, weeping, crusted lesions on the face, scalp, diaper area, and extremities. In older children or adults, it may be more localized and chronic. The course is unpredictable. Although the dermatitis often improves by age 3 or 4 yr, exacerbations are common during childhood, adolescence, or adulthood.

Itching is a constant feature; consequent scratching and rubbing lead to an itch-scratch-rash-itch cycle. In older children and adults, atopic dermatitis typically appears as erythema and lichenification in the antecubital and popliteal fossae and on the eyelids, neck, and wrists. The dermatitis may become generalized. Secondary bacterial infections and regional lymphadenitis are common. Frequent use of drugs, proprietary or prescribed, exposes the atopic patient to many topical allergens, and contact dermatitis may aggravate and complicate the atopic dermatitis, as may the generally dry skin that is common in these patients. Intolerance to primary irritants is common, and emotional stress, environmental temperature or humidity changes, bacterial skin infections, and wool garments commonly cause exacerbations.

Complications

Patients with long-standing atopic dermatitis may develop cataracts while in their 20s or 30s. Herpes simplex may induce a sometimes grave febrile illness (eczema herpeticum) in atopic patients. Therefore, the patient with atopic dermatitis should avoid exposure to patients with clinically active herpes simplex.

Diagnosis

Diagnosis is entirely clinical: It is based on the distribution of lesions, their duration, and often a family history of atopic disorders. Because atopic dermatitis is often hard to differentiate from seborrheic dermatitis in infancy or from primary irritant dermatitis at any age, the physician should see the patient several times before making a definitive diagnosis. The physician must be careful not to attribute all subsequent skin problems to an atopic diathesis.

General Measures of Treatment

1. Offending agents and complex topical drugs should be avoided if possible.

2. Corticosteroid creams or ointments applied tid are the most effective drugs. Because they are expensive, supplemental use of white petrolatum, hydrogenated vegetable oil (as for cooking), or hydrophilic petrolatum (unless the patient is allergic to lanolin) may be advisable. These emollients, applied between corticosteroid applications, help to hydrate the skin, which is important. Prolonged, widespread use of high potency corticosteroid creams or ointments should be avoided in infants, as adrenal suppression (reversible) may ensue. Ineffectiveness of topical steroids can be avoided by interrupting continuous use with simple emollients for a week or more; then steroids may again be effective.

3. Bathing should be minimized if the effect seems deleterious; use of soap on the area of dermatitis should be avoided, since soap and water may be drying and irritating. Oils help to lubricate the skin, and the above-mentioned corticosteroid or emollient ointments should be applied within 3 min after a bath, before the skin is dried, to enhance their emollient effects.

4. For children, an antihistamine (eg, diphenhydramine elixir 25 to 50 mg) may be a useful sedative at bedtime when itching is worst. Doxepin, a dibenzoxepin tricyclic compound, is a very active antihistamine and also has a useful psychotherapeutic effect in itching patients. This agent may be tried, beginning with 10-mg capsules or 5 mg in a calibrated dropper, and increasing the dose slowly as needed and tolerated. Hydroxyzine hydrochloride 25 mg tid or qid (for children, 2 mg/kg/day in divided doses q 6 h or in a single dose) may also be useful.

5. Fingernails should be kept short to minimize excoriations and secondary infections.

6. For secondary infections, an oral penicillinase-resistant penicillin or a cephalosporin 250 mg qid for adults and 25 to 50 mg/kg/day in divided doses for children is advised.

7. If the dermatitis resists home treatment, hospitalization, with its closer psychologic and dermatologic attention and the change in environment, often accelerates improvement.

8. Oral corticosteroids should be considered a last resort. Stunting of growth, osteoporosis, and the other side effects of prolonged systemic corticosteroids are serious hazards when atopic patients take the drug for years, and rebound exacerbations on stopping therapy are frequent. Alternate-day use of corticosteroids may be helpful (eg, for adults, prednisone 20 to 40 mg every other morning); however, severe side effects still occur. The initial dose should be continued for several weeks, then slowly decreased while the patient is encouraged to use topical drugs. A major problem with even starting oral corticosteroids in these patients is that they become dependent on them.

9. Older adults may benefit from psoralen plus high intensity ultraviolet A (PUVA; see under Psoriasis in Ch. 96). PUVA is available in most dermatologic centers. Because of its potential long-term side effects, it is rarely indicated for children or young adults.

SEBORRHEIC DERMATITIS

An inflammatory scaling disease of the scalp, face, and occasionally other areas. Despite the name, the composition and flow of sebum are usually normal.

Symptoms and Signs

Onset in adults is gradual, and the dermatitis usually is apparent only as dry or greasy diffuse scaling of the scalp (**dandruff**) with variable itching. In severe disease, yellow-red, scaling papules appear along the hairline, behind the ears, in the external auditory canals, in the eyebrows, on the bridge of the nose, in the nasolabial folds, and over the sternum. Marginal blepharitis with dry yellow crusts and conjunctival irritation may be present. Seborrheic dermatitis does not cause hair loss.

Neonates (< 1 mo old) may develop seborrheic dermatitis, with a thick, yellow, crusted scalp lesion (**"cradle cap"**), fissuring and yellow scaling behind the ears, and red facial papules. The newborn may also have an associated stubborn diaper rash. Older children may develop thick, tenacious, scaly plaques in the scalp that may measure 1 to 2 cm in diameter.

Genetic and climatic factors seem to affect the incidence and severity of the disease; it is usually worse in winter. The prognosis is better than in atopic dermatitis. Patients with neurologic disease may have severe seborrheic dermatitis. Very rarely, in infants or adults, the condition may become generalized.

Treatment

Therapy depends on the location and severity of the disease. **In adults,** zinc pyrithione, selenium sulfide, sulfur and salicylic acid, or tar shampoo should be used daily or every other day until the dandruff is controlled and twice/week thereafter. A corticosteroid lotion (eg, 0.01% fluocinolone acetonide solution or 0.025% triamcinolone acetonide lotion) should be rubbed into the scalp or other hairy areas bid until scaling and redness are controlled. Hydrocortisone 1% cream rubbed in bid or tid will rapidly improve seborrheic dermatitis of the postauricular areas, nasolabial folds, eyelid margins, and bridge of the nose; the cream is then used once daily if needed. Hydrocortisone cream is best for facial seborrheic dermatitis, as the fluorinated corticosteroids may produce side effects (eg, telangiectasia, atrophy, perioral dermatitis). In some patients, 2% ketoconazole cream (bid for 1 to 2 wk) induces prolonged remissions lasting months. **For infantile seborrheic eczema,** a mild baby shampoo is used daily and a hydrocortisone cream is rubbed in bid. For the thick lesions seen on the scalp of a young child, 10% salicylic acid in mineral oil or a corticosteroid gel is applied at bedtime to affected areas and rubbed in with a toothbrush. The scalp is shampooed daily until the thick scale is gone.

Studies have suggested that topical imidazoles (anti-yeast compounds) may be effective in some patients with seborrheic dermatitis and have focused attention on the possible role of *Pityrosporum ovale* (a common lipophilic yeast normally present in follicles) as a cause for this disease.

NUMMULAR DERMATITIS

Chronic dermatitis characterized by inflamed, coin-shaped, vesicular, crusted, scaling, and usually pruritic lesions.

The etiology of nummular dermatitis is unknown. It is seen most commonly in middle-aged patients and is often associated with dry skin, especially during the winter. Exacerbations and remissions may occur.

Symptoms and Signs

The discoid lesions start as pruritic patches of confluent vesicles and papules that later ooze serum and then form crusts. Lesions are widespread; they are often more prominent on the extensor aspects of the extremities and on the buttocks, but they also appear on the trunk.

Treatment

No treatment is uniformly effective. Oral antibiotics may be given empirically, since many types of bacteria can be cultured and the therapy has been found to decrease the severity of the lesions. Oral cloxacillin or cephalexin 250 mg qid and tap-water compresses are helpful when there is much weeping and pus. Less infected lesions may also improve with tetracycline 250 mg orally qid, which has a beneficial (although not necessarily antibacterial) effect. After the lesions have dried, a corticosteroid cream or ointment should be rubbed in tid and occlusion with a corticosteroid cream under polyethylene film or with flurandrenolide-impregnated tape should be applied at bedtime. When there are few lesions that do not respond to the therapy above, intralesional steroid injections may be beneficial. In more widespread, resistant cases, ultraviolet B radiation alone or ultraviolet A with oral psoralens may be helpful. Occasionally oral corticosteroids are required; a reasonable starting dose is 40 mg of prednisone given every other day to lessen side effects. Long-term use of systemic corticosteroids should be avoided.

CHRONIC DERMATITIS OF HANDS AND FEET

The hands and feet are frequent sites of inflammatory eruptions—the hands because they are subjected to mechanical and chemical trauma; the feet because of the warm, moist conditions in shoes. The eruption commonly becomes chronic and can be crippling at home or at work.

The following primary dermatoses may involve the hands and feet:

1. Contact dermatitis (see above) is common. Many allergens or irritants—caustics, strong soaps, detergents, organic solvents, vacuum cleaner dust, topical drugs—may cause or perpetuate the dermatitis. In any dermatitis of the feet, every effort should be made to obtain patch-test evidence of sensitivity to a component of shoes, since this sensitivity limits the choice of footwear.

2. "Housewives' eczema," a hand dermatitis frequently seen in housewives and other "wet workers," has many causes. It is undoubtedly worsened by washing dishes, clothes, and babies, since repeated exposure to even mild detergents and water or prolonged sweating under rubber gloves may irritate dermatitic skin or may even cause a marginal irritant dermatitis. Occasionally, contact dermatitis that appears urticarial occurs in 10 to 20 min as a reaction to fresh foods.

3. Pompholyx is a chronic condition characterized by deep-seated itchy vesicles on the palms, sides of the fingers, and soles. Scaling, redness, and oozing often follow the vesiculation. The condition is also known as **dyshidrosis**—a misnomer, since sweating may be decreased, normal, or excessive. Though no cause is known in most cases, a primary cause (eg, fungus, contact allergen) should always be sought.

4. Psoriasis localized to the hands presents on the dorsum as the typical thick, silvery, scaling papules or plaques, but palmar lesions are not always characteristic. Though pitted grooves in the nails often indicate psoriasis, they can occur with any dermatitis of the fingers.

5. Recalcitrant pustular eruptions of the palms and soles are characteristically crops of deep-seated sterile pustules of unknown etiology that resist treatment. They may be associated with psoriasis elsewhere.

6. Fungal infection of the feet is common; of the hands, uncommon. Patients with a hand dermatitis should be examined for a fungal infection of the feet, since the latter can produce a nonspecific dermatitis on the hands (**dermatophytid;** see Ch. 92).

Treatment

Treatment should be directed to removing the cause wherever possible. The following general principles are useful if no specific cause is found: (1) A topical corticosteroid cream or ointment applied tid may decrease the itching, but clearing the dermatitis may require overnight occlusive therapy with polyethylene gloves (or nonpermeable plastic bags on the feet) sealed at the wrists (or ankles) with cellophane tape after a 4th application of the cream. (2) Oral cloxacillin or cephalexin 250 mg qid should be given if there is any evidence of secondary infection. (3) Wet chores should be limited to short periods, and white cotton gloves should be worn under rubber gloves. (4) A 14-day course of oral prednisone is needed occasionally, starting with 40 mg/day and slowly decreasing the dose while the patient is taught and encouraged to follow the above routines to decrease the exacerbation that may ensue when the corticosteroid is stopped. (5) If the dermatitis is long-standing and disabling or if benefit from oral corticosteroids is not lasting, short-term hospitalization may be helpful. This removes the patient from the environment, provides intensive therapy, and gives an opportunity for detailed patch testing, cultures, and other diagnostic studies. (6) PUVA delivered to just the hands and feet is often very effective, whatever the cause. (7) Oral retinoids (isotretinoin 40 mg/day) may be a last resort for severe psoriasis or idiopathic pustular eruptions of the hands and, if used with proper precautions, may greatly help these dermatologic cripples.

GENERALIZED EXFOLIATIVE DERMATITIS

A severe, widespread erythema and scaling of the skin.

Etiology

No cause can be determined in most cases. In some patients, the disorder is secondary to certain dermatitides (eg, atopic, psoriatic, pityriasis rubra pilaris, contact); or it may be induced by a systemic drug (eg, penicillin, sulfonamides, isoniazid, phenytoin, or barbiturates) or an irritating topical agent. Exfoliative dermatitis may also be associated with mycosis fungoides or lymphoma.

Symptoms and Signs

The onset may be insidious or rapid. The entire skin surface becomes red, scaly, thickened, and occasionally crusted. Itching may be severe or absent. The characteristic appearance of any primary dermatitis is usually lost. Localized areas of normal skin may be seen when the exfoliative dermatitis is caused by psoriasis, mycosis fungoides, or pityriasis rubra pilaris. Generalized superficial lymphadenopathy is frequently present, and biopsy usually shows benign lymphadenitis.

The patient's temperature may be elevated, or he may feel cold from excessive heat loss, because of the increased blood flow to the skin and exfoliation. These may also cause weight loss, hypoproteinemia, iron deficiency, or even (in patients with borderline cardiac compensation) high-output heart failure.

Diagnosis and Treatment

The disease may be life-threatening, and every attempt must be made to determine the cause. A history or signs of a primary dermatitis may be helpful. Biopsy is usually not helpful, but pemphigus foliaceus or mycosis fungoides may be diagnosed by skin biopsy, or lymphoma by a lymph node biopsy. Sézary syndrome may be diagnosed by a blood smear.

Hospitalization is often necessary. Because drug eruptions and contact dermatitis cannot be ruled out by history alone, all possible drugs, systemic and topical, should be stopped. If possible, essential systemic drugs should be changed to chemically dissimilar ones. Petrolatum applied after tap-water baths gives temporary relief. Subsequent local treatment is the same as for contact dermatitis (see above).

Oral corticosteroids should be used only when topical measures are unsuccessful. Prednisone 40 to 60 mg/day is given; after about 10 days, the drug is given on alternating days. Usually the dose can be further decreased, but if an underlying cause is not found and eliminated, prednisone will be required for long periods.

STASIS DERMATITIS

Persistent inflammation of the skin of the lower legs with a tendency toward brown pigmentation, commonly associated with venous incompetency.

Symptoms and Signs

The eruption is usually localized to the ankle, where erythema, mild scaling, and brown discoloration are seen. Edema and varicose veins are common but by no means always present. Because of the relative lack of symptoms, the condition is often neglected. The usual consequences are increasing edema, secondary bacterial infection, and eventual ulceration. Recent studies have shown perivascular fibrin deposition and abnormal small-vessel vasoconstrictive reflexes that may be the real cause—not venous stasis per se.

Treatment

Leg elevation above the heart to increase venous return and prevent tissue edema, support hose, and topical therapy are necessary. Topical therapy depends on the stage of the process. For acute dermatitis, tap-water compresses should be applied, continuously at first and then intermittently. If the lesion is purulent, a more absorbent hydrocolloid dressing may be the best treatment. When the dermatitis becomes less acute, a corticosteroid cream or ointment should be applied tid or incorporated into zinc oxide paste. Ulcerative lesions are best treated with compresses and bland dressings (eg, zinc oxide paste); various new dressings (eg, DuoDerm®) are very effective. Oral antibiotics are useful when cellulitis is present; topical antibiotics are useless and often cause contact dermatitis. When the edema and inflammation subside, split-thickness skin grafts may be useful. Patients should wear properly fitted support hose when they walk to prevent or decrease edema.

In selected instances, ulcers on ambulatory patients may be healed with an **Unna's paste boot** (zinc gelatin), the less messy **zinc gelatin bandage**, or one of the newer "colloid" dressings: all are available commercially. The Unna's paste boot is being replaced by (more expensive, more effective) absorptive, colloid-type dressings used under elastic support. At first it may be necessary to change the dressing q 2 or 3 days, but as edema recedes and the ulcer heals, once or twice/wk is sufficient. Following healing, an elastic support should be applied before the patient rises in the morning.

Complex or multiple topical drugs or nonprescription remedies should not be used: The skin in stasis dermatitis is vulnerable to direct irritants and to potentially sensitizing topical agents (antibiotics; anesthetics; and vehicles of topical drugs, especially lanolin or wool alcohols).

LOCALIZED SCRATCH DERMATITIS
(Lichen Simplex; Neurodermatitis)

A chronic, superficial, pruritic inflammation of the skin, characterized by dry, scaling, well-demarcated, hyperpigmented, lichenified plaques (thickened skin with accentuated markings) of oval, irregular, or angular shape.

Etiology, Symptoms, and Signs
The disease may have a strong psychogenic component. Allergy appears to play no part. More women are affected than men, with onset usually between ages 20 and 50. The skin lesions are common in Asians and American Indians.

A fully developed plaque has an outer zone of brownish discrete papules and a central zone of confluent papules covered with scales. **Pruritus ani** and **pruritus vulvae** are often instances of circumscribed scratch dermatitis. The involved skin may be only red, moist, and hyperpigmented, or may even appear normal.

The usual course is chronic: From prior irritation or without apparent reason, an area of skin begins to itch recurrently. The principal site is the occipital region; arms or legs, especially ankles, are frequently involved. Vigorous scratching gives transient relief, but the itching recurs. Stress and tension increase the itching, and scratching may become an unconscious habit.

Diagnosis
Diagnosis can usually be made by inspection, but possible underlying causes should be excluded, because generalized itching without apparent skin lesions may occur in patients with a variety of systemic disorders (see Ch. 89). Most

anal and vulvar pruritus is idiopathic but may be due to pinworms, trichomoniasis, hemorrhoids, local discharges or fissures, candidiasis, warts, contact dermatitis, or occasionally psoriasis. Unusual but important causes of anal or vulvar dermatitis are extramammary Paget's disease, Bowen's disease, and lichen sclerosus et atrophicus.

Treatment
It is important for the patient to realize that scratching and rubbing produce the skin changes. The pruritus may be controlled with drugs; topical corticosteroids are the most effective. A cream may be rubbed in, or surgical tape impregnated with flurandrenolide (applied in the morning and replaced in the evening) may be better, since it also prevents scratching. Small areas may be locally infiltrated with a long-acting corticosteroid such as triamcinolone acetonide 2.5 mg/mL (achieved by diluting with saline), 0.3 mL/cm^2 of lesion; this can be repeated q 3 to 4 wk. Oral chlorpromazine or doxepin 10 mg at bedtime, increased to 25 to 50 mg/day if tolerated, may be useful.

Pruritus ani or vulvae is best treated with a hydrocortisone cream tid. Zinc oxide paste can be applied over the cream for protection; it may be removed with mineral oil. Patients should be cautioned not to rub hard with toilet paper after a bowel movement. Pinworms should be eradicated and warts treated. Hemorrhoids or hypertrophic tags should be removed and discharges or fissures corrected surgically if the course is chronic, but this will not always cure the pruritus ani because the cause of itching is frequently unknown.

91. BACTERIAL INFECTIONS OF THE SKIN
(See also Chronic Granulomatous Disease under SPECIFIC IMMUNODEFICIENCIES in Ch. 33)

The specific bacterial cause of a skin infection should be identified (see bacterial and fungal cultures in Ch. 87). Knowledge of the normal skin flora helps to interpret culture reports, since large numbers of bacteria, including micrococci, diphtheroids, and *Propionibacterium acnes*, normally inhabit the skin.

Infection may be the primary cause of a skin lesion or may be superimposed on another skin disease. Primary infections (eg, impetigo, erysipelas) almost always respond promptly to

systemic antibiotics, but secondary infections may clear more slowly. Although *topical* antibiotics are ineffective in most bacterial skin infections and may cause allergic contact dermatitis, a new antibiotic, mupirocin ointment, has been shown to be very effective for some skin infections, particularly staphylococcal- or streptococcal-induced impetigo. Recurrent infections should alert the physician to a possible underlying systemic disorder (eg, diabetes mellitus).

STAPHYLOCOCCAL DISEASES OF THE SKIN

(See also IMPETIGO; ECTHYMA
under BACTERIAL INFECTIONS in Ch. 32)

In the following syndromes, which must be differentiated because some are life-threatening, strains of *Staphylococcus aureus* either cause the syndromes or may be important in their development: **toxic shock syndrome** (see Ch. 8); deep staphylococcal infections, eg, **cellulitis** or **necrotizing fasciitis**; *Staphylococcus epidermidis* **septicemia** (caused by a usually nonpathogenic staphylococcus other than *S. aureus*); and **scalded skin syndrome**, described below, which must be distinguished from **toxic epidermal necrolysis**, described in Ch. 97.

STAPHYLOCOCCAL SCALDED SKIN SYNDROME (SSSS)

(Ritter-Lyell Syndrome)

An acute, widespread erythematous process in which the epidermis peels off. It usually occurs in infants, young children, or immunosuppressed patients.

Etiology

Group II coagulase-positive staphylococci, usually phage type 71 and often resistant to penicillin, elaborate an epidermolytic toxin that splits off the upper part of the epidermis just beneath the granular cell layer. The toxin enters the circulation and affects the skin systemically, as in scarlet fever. SSSS may occur in epidemics in nurseries, with transmission from infant to infant on the hands of personnel. Most frequently, colonized infants are the source, although nursery personnel may be nasal carriers of *S. aureus*. The disease is also seen sporadically in children, usually < 6 yr of age, and in immunosuppressed adults.

Symptoms and Signs

Illness begins with a localized crusted infection (often impetigo-like), most often at the umbilical stump or in the diaper area during the first few days of life. When it occurs sporadically in children aged 1 to 6 yr, it starts with a superficial crusted lesion, frequently around the nose or ear. Within 24 h, tender scarlet areas appear around the crusted area. The red areas may become painful and generalized and may progress rapidly to large, flaccid blisters that are easily broken to produce erosions. The epidermis peels off easily, often in large sheets, when the red areas are touched inadvertently or pushed by the examiner's finger. The disease progresses rapidly to widespread desquamation of the skin within 36 to 72 h and patients may become very ill with systemic manifestations (eg, malaise, chills, and fever). Loss of the protective skin barrier exposes the patient to sepsis and to fluid and electrolyte imbalance. With prompt diagnosis and therapy (see below), mortality rarely occurs.

Diagnosis

Rapid and accurate differential diagnosis is essential, since proper therapy differs drastically in SSSS and toxic epidermal necrolysis (TEN). Age and milieu of the patient help in differential diagnosis; eg, SSSS almost invariably occurs only in infants, young children, and immunocompromised adults and starts with a staphylococcal infection (which may not have been noted). Cultures should be obtained from the skin and nasopharynx. When TEN occurs in older individuals, it is usually due to drugs. Acute onset of a symmetrical erythematous skin eruption associated with systemic signs may suggest a drug hypersensitivity rash, viral exanthem, or scarlet fever, but none of these causes a painful rash. Bullae, erosions, and easily loosened epidermis occur in a number of disorders in which the epidermis is severely damaged: thermal burns, genetic bullous diseases (eg, some types of epidermolysis bullosa), and acquired bullous diseases (eg, pemphigus vulgaris and bullous pemphigoid [see Ch. 98]).

Defining the level of epidermal cleavage is crucial in differentiating SSSS and TEN (see Ch. 97). Either a scraping of the skin (Tzanck test, see Ch. 87) or a frozen section of a fresh specimen will often reveal the level. Biopsy shows cleavage and blister formation within the granular cell (outermost) layer of the epidermis in SSSS, but biopsy in TEN shows blister formation subepidermally (between epidermis and dermis) or at the level of the basal cell.

Treatment

Treatment with systemic penicillinase-resistant antistaphylococcal antibiotics (eg, cloxacillin, dicloxacillin, or cephalexin) must be started as soon as the clinical diagnosis has been made and specimens for cultures have been taken, without waiting for culture reports. In early stages, oral cloxacillin 12.5 mg/kg q 6 h (for infants and children up to 20 kg) and 250 to 500 mg q 6 h (for older children) may be given, but in severe cases methicillin 25 to 50 mg/kg IV or IM should be given q 6 h until improvement is noted; oral cloxacillin 25 mg/kg qid should then be given for at least 10 days. Corticosteroids are contraindicated and topical therapy and patient handling must be minimized. If the disease is widespread and the lesions are weeping, the skin should be treated as if it were burned. Hydrolyzed polymer gel dressings may be very useful and reduce the number of dressing changes. Since the split is high in the epidermis, the stratum corneum is quickly replaced and healing is usually rapid—5 to 7 days after treatment is started. Steps to detect carriers and prevent or deal with nursery epidemics are described in NOSOCOMIAL INFECTION IN THE NEWBORN under NEONATAL INFECTIONS in Ch. 27.

ERYSIPELAS

A superficial cellulitis caused by Group A β-hemolytic streptococci. The face (often bilaterally), an arm, or a leg is most often involved. The lesion is well demarcated, shiny, red, edematous, and tender; vesicles and bullae often develop. Patches of peripheral redness and regional lymphadenopathy are seen occasionally; high fever, chills, and malaise are common. Erysipelas may be recurrent and may result in chronic lymphedema. A nidus of infection may be an interdigital fungal infection of the foot that may require long-term griseofulvin therapy to prevent recurrent erysipelas.

Diagnosis from the characteristic appearance is usually easy. The causative organism is difficult to culture from the lesion, but it may occasionally be cultured from the blood. Direct immunofluorescence using commercially available antibodies may also identify the causative organisms. Erysipelas of the face must be differentiated from herpes zoster; of the arm or hand, from the rare erysipeloid. Contact dermatitis and angioneurotic edema may be mistaken for erysipelas.

Treatment

Penicillin V or erythromycin 500 mg orally qid should be given for at least 2 wk. In acute cases, penicillin G 1.2 million u. IV q 6 h gives a rapid response and should be replaced by oral therapy after 36 to 48 h. In recent cases showing resistance to these antibiotics, cloxacillin or cephalexin has been used. Local discomfort may be relieved by cold packs; aspirin 600 mg, with codeine 30 mg if required, may be given orally for pain.

FOLLICULITIS; FURUNCLES; CARBUNCLES

Folliculitis: *A superficial or deep bacterial infection and irritation of the hair follicles.* It is usually caused by *Staphylococcus aureus*. The acute lesion consists of a superficial pustule or inflammatory nodule surrounding the hair. The condition may follow or accompany other pyodermas. Infected hairs are easily removed, but new papules tend to develop. Folliculitis may become chronic where the hair follicles are deep in the skin, as in the bearded area **(sycosis barbae).** Stiff hairs in the bearded region may emerge from the follicle, curve, and reenter the skin, producing a chronic low-grade irritation without significant infection **(pseudofolliculitis barbae;** see Ch. 95).

Furuncles (boils): *Acute, tender, perifollicular inflammatory nodules resulting from infection by staphylococci.* They occur most frequently on the neck, breasts, face, and buttocks, but are most painful when they occur in skin that is closely attached to underlying structures (eg, on the nose, ear, or fingers). The initial nodule becomes a pustule 5 to 30 mm in diameter, with central necrosis, which discharges a core of necrotic tissue and sanguineous purulent exudate. The condition may be recurrent and troublesome **(furunculosis),** and often occurs in healthy young individuals. Miniature epidemics or clusters have been recorded among teenagers living in crowded quarters with relatively poor hygiene.

Carbuncles: *A cluster of furuncles with spread of infection subcutaneously, resulting in deep suppuration, often extensive local sloughing, slow healing, and a large scar.* Carbuncles develop more slowly than single furuncles and may be accompanied by fever and prostration. They occur most frequently in males and most commonly on the nape of the neck. Diabetes mellitus, debilitating diseases, and old age are predisposing factors, though carbuncles do occur in otherwise healthy persons.

Treatment

The treatment of acute **folliculitis** is similar to that of impetigo. Prompt treatment may prevent development of a chronic infection.

A **single furuncle** is treated with intermittent moist heat to allow the lesion to point and drain spontaneously, since extensive incision may spread the infection. A furuncle in the nose or central facial area should be treated with systemic antibiotics, the selection depending on the results of culture and sensitivity tests. **Multiple furuncles and carbuncles** require culture and sensitivity studies. Usually a penicillinase-resistant penicillin is required, such as cloxacillin 250 mg orally qid, or a cephalosporin in the same dosage. For recurrent **boils**, oral antibiotic therapy continuously for 1 to 2 mo may be advisable.

Clusters of cases are increasing—emphasizing the importance of finding and treating family and friends who may be sources of reinfection for patients. Immunization with staphylococcal vaccines is ineffective. For all bathing, liquid soap containing either chlorhexidine gluconate with isopropyl alcohol or 2 to 3% chloroxylenol may be prophylactic but is not therapeutic.

HIDRADENITIS SUPPURATIVA

An inflammation of the apocrine glands resulting in obstruction and rupture of the ducts with painful local inflammation. Most lesions occur in the axilla or groin, but they may also be found around the nipples or anus. The lesions may be confused with furuncles but tend to be more persistent and are diagnosed primarily by their location and clinical course. Pain, fluctuation, discharge, and sinus tract formation are characteristic. In chronic cases, coalescence of inflamed nodules may cause palpable cordlike bands in the axilla. The condition may become extensive and disabling; if the pubic and genital areas are severely involved, walking may be difficult.

Treatment

Susceptible patients should avoid antiperspirants or other irritants. Early simple cases are treated with rest, moist heat, and prolonged systemic antibiotic therapy as for furunculosis. Intralesional corticosteroids may be effective in isolated lesions. Surgical excision and plastic repair of the affected areas may be necessary if the disease persists. Isotretinoin orally has been effective in some patients. A rather large dosage—2 mg/kg/day—is required, and recurrences are much more common than in acne. Etretinate in a slightly lower dose may also be effective. These drugs must be used with caution (see treatment of acne in Ch. 95).

PARONYCHIAL INFECTIONS

Acute or chronic inflammation of the periungual tissues.

In acute paronychia, the causative organisms—usually micrococci, *Pseudomonas* or *Proteus* sp, but sometimes *Candida albicans* (see Ch. 92)—enter through a break in the epidermis resulting from a hangnail, trauma (eg, from manicuring), or chronic irritation (eg, from excessive exposure to water and detergents). The infection may follow the nail margin ("run-around"), or may extend beneath the nail and suppurate. Rarely, the infection penetrates more deeply into the finger; necrosis of the tendons and further extension of the infection along the tendon sheaths may result. Eventually the chronically infected nail becomes distorted.

Treatment

An acute infection is treated with hot compresses or soaks and, because it is usually of bacterial origin, with a systemic antibiotic. The accumulated debris is painful and should be drained. A purulent pocket should be opened cautiously with the point of a scalpel. Infection extending along the tendon sheaths requires prompt surgical incision and drainage.

In chronic recurrent inflammation, it is important for the hands to remain dry. The subungual debris should be cultured. If *C. albicans* is not present on several cultures, cutting back the nail to the point of its detachment from the underlying skin and applying dilute tincture of iodine (2 drops bid) will help to keep the subungual and paronychial areas dry and free of infection. If *C. albicans* is present, an antifungal lotion (eg, ciclopirox, miconazole) or cream (ketoconazole) should be applied tid to the paronychial and subungual areas after the nail is cut back. As the GI tract is a likely source of contamination with *C. albicans*, oral nystatin 500,000 u. qid may also be advisable. Women should be examined for an accompanying candidal vaginitis, which should also be treated. Grossly distorted nail plates may have to be removed.

ERYTHRASMA

A superficial skin infection caused by Corynebacterium minutissimum, *found most commonly in adults.* The incidence is higher in the tropics and in diabetics.

Erythrasma resembles a chronic fungus infection or intertrigo. In the toe webs, scaling, fissuring, and slight maceration occur, usually confined to the 3rd and 4th interspaces. In the genitocrural region, principally where the thighs contact the scrotum, patches are irregular and pink, later becoming brown with a fine scale. Erythrasma may widely involve the axillae, trunk, and perineum, particularly in obese middle-aged women or in patients with diabetes mellitus.

Differentiation from ringworm is essential. Diagnosis is established readily with a Wood's light, under which erythrasma shows a characteristic coral-red fluorescence.

Prompt clearing follows oral erythromycin or tetracycline 250 mg qid for 14 days, but recurrences 6 to 12 mo later are usual. Antibacterial soaps may also control the infection.

92. SUPERFICIAL FUNGAL INFECTIONS

DERMATOPHYTE INFECTIONS
(Ringworm)

Superficial infections caused by dermatophytes—fungi that invade only dead tissues of the skin or its appendages (stratum corneum, nails, hair). Microsporum, Trichophyton, and Epidermophyton are the genera most commonly involved. Fomites are probably not responsible for transmission. Some dermatophytes produce only mild or no inflammation; in such cases, the organism may persist indefinitely, causing intermittent remissions and exacerbations of a gradually extending lesion with a scaling, slightly raised border. In other cases an acute infection may occur, typically causing a sudden vesicular and bullous disease of the feet or an inflamed boggy lesion of the scalp (kerion) that is due to a strong immunologic reaction to the fungus; the infection is usually followed by remission or cure.

Clinical Types and Diagnosis

Since clinical differentiation of the related dermatophytes is difficult, these infections are conveniently discussed according to the sites involved. Diagnosis is confirmed by demonstrating the pathogenic fungus in scrapings of lesions, either by direct microscopic examination of a potassium hydroxide preparation or by culture (see also SPECIAL DIAGNOSTIC METHODS in Ch. 87).

Tinea corporis (ringworm of the body) is usually caused by a Trichophyton. The characteristic pink-to-red papulosquamous annular lesions have raised borders, expand peripherally, and tend to clear centrally. Differential diagnosis includes pityriasis rosea, drug eruptions, nummular dermatitis, erythema multiforme, tinea versicolor, erythrasma, psoriasis, and secondary syphilis.

Tinea pedis (ringworm of the feet; athlete's foot) is common. Trichophyton mentagrophytes infections begin in the 3rd and 4th interdigital

spaces and later involve the plantar surface of the arch. The toe web lesions often are macerated and have scaling borders; they may be vesicular. Acute flare-ups, with many vesicles and bullae, are common during warm weather. Infected toenails become thickened and distorted. T. rubrum produces scaling and thickening of the soles, often extending just beyond the plantar surface in a "moccasin" distribution. Itching, pain, inflammation, or vesiculation with concomitant itching or pain may be slight or severe. Tinea pedis may be complicated by secondary bacterial infection, cellulitis, or lymphangitis, sometimes of a recurrent nature. Tinea pedis may be confused with maceration (from hyperhidrosis and occlusive footgear), with contact dermatitis (from sensitivity to various materials in shoes, particularly adhesive cement), with eczema, or with psoriasis.

Tinea unguium (ringworm of the nails), a form of onychomycosis, is usually caused by a Trichophyton species. Toenail involvement is common in long-standing tinea pedis; infections of the fingernails are less common. The nails become thickened and lusterless, and debris accumulates under the free edge. The nail plate becomes separated and the nail may be destroyed. Differentiating a Trichophyton infection from psoriasis is particularly important because chemotherapy is specific and prolonged treatment is required.

Tinea capitis (ringworm of the scalp) mainly affects children. It is contagious and may become epidemic. Trichophyton tonsurans infection has become the common cause in the USA; other Trichophyton species (eg, T. violaceum) are common in other parts of the world. T. tonsurans infection of the scalp is subtle in onset and characteristics. Inflammation is low-grade and persistent; the lesions are neither annular nor sharply marginated, and the hairs do not fluoresce under Wood's light. Affected areas of the scalp show characteristic black dots resulting from broken hairs. The fungus, an endothrix, produces chains of arthrospores that can be seen microscopically within the hair. *Trichophyton* species may persist in adults.

Microsporum audouinii and *M. canis*, once predominant, are much less common causes of tinea capitis in the USA. *M. audouinii* lesions are small, scaly, semi-bald grayish patches with broken, lusterless hairs. Infection may be limited to a small area or extend and coalesce until the entire scalp is involved, sometimes with ringed patches extending beyond the scalp margin. *M. canis* and *M. gypseum* usually cause a more inflammatory reaction, with shedding of the infected hairs. A raised, inflamed, boggy granuloma **(kerion)** may also occur; it is followed shortly by healing. Diagnosis of a *Microsporum* infection is facilitated by examining the scalp under Wood's light; infected hairs may fluoresce a light, bright green. The organism is an ectothrix, producing spores to form a sheath around the hair. The sheath can be seen on microscopy. Culture of the fungus is also important in establishing the diagnosis.

Tinea cruris (jock itch), far more common in males, may be caused by various dermatophyte or yeast organisms. Typically, a ringed lesion extends from the crural fold over the adjacent upper inner thigh. Both sides may be affected. Scratch dermatitis and lichenification are often seen. Lesions may be complicated by maceration, miliaria, secondary bacterial or candidal infection, and reactions to treatment. Recurrence is common, since fungi may persist indefinitely on the skin or may repeatedly infect susceptible individuals. Flare-ups occur more often during the summer. Tight clothing or obesity tends to favor growth of the organisms. The infection may be confused with contact dermatitis, psoriasis, erythrasma, or candidiasis. The scrotum is often acutely inflamed in candidal intertrigo, whereas in dermatophyte infections scrotal involvement is usually absent or slight.

Tinea barbae, a mycotic infection of the beard area, is rare. Infections in this area are more commonly bacterial (see FOLLICULITIS in Ch. 91) but may be fungal, especially in agricultural workers. The causative agent is established microbiologically.

Dermatophytids or "id" eruptions are fungus-free skin lesions of various morphology that occur elsewhere on the body during an acute vesicular or inflammatory ringworm infection; they are thought to result from hypersensitivity to the fungus. Vesicular dermatitis of the hands is most commonly due to some other cause (see CHRONIC DERMATITIS OF HANDS AND FEET in Ch. 90).

Treatment

Most skin infections (but not tinea capitis or onychomycosis) respond very well to topical antifungal preparations such as the imidazoles (miconazole, clotrimazole, econazole, ketoconazole) as well as ciclopirox olamine cream and naftifine hydrochloride cream. For resistant cases or those with very widespread involvement, systemic therapy is indicated. **Griseofulvin**, the most widely used systemic antifungal agent, is effective in treating tinea capitis, corporis, pedis, and unguium (onychomycosis) caused by *Trichophyton rubrum, T. schoenleinii, T. mentagrophytes, T. sulfureum, T. verrucosum, T. interdigitalis, Epidermophyton floccosum, Microsporum audouinii, M. canis,* or *M. gypseum;* but it is worthless in candidiasis or tinea versicolor and deep-seated mycoses (eg, histoplasmosis, coccidioidomycosis). The adult dosage is microsize griseofulvin 250 mg orally bid to qid and the drug is best given with a high-fat meal. The ultra-microsize griseofulvin is much better absorbed than the microsize and should be given in a single or divided total dose of 250 to 330 mg for tinea corporis, cruris, or capitis, and in a single or divided total dose of 500 to 660 mg for tinea pedis. Some infections, especially those involving the nails, may require much larger dosage and longer therapy. Headache is the most common side effect. The drug occasionally causes GI distress, photosensitivity, rashes, or leukopenia. Angioedema has been reported. Vertigo and, rarely, transient hearing reduction may occur. Topical imidazoles with oral griseofulvin increase the cure rate. Some of the imidazoles (miconazole, clotrimazole, econazole, ketoconazole) as well as ciclopirox olamine cream and naftifine hydrochloride cream have been found to be only somewhat effective creams for onychomycosis. **Ketoconazole**, an oral imidazole derivative, is also an effective broad-spectrum agent for systemic therapy of candidiasis and some deep fungal infections. Although it is also effective orally for dermatophyte infections, occasional liver toxicity as well as SLE (can be severe or even fatal) limits its use for superficial infections unless safer measures fail (itraconazole, another oral imidazole derivative, is thought to be safer than ketoconazole but is unavailable in the USA).

Tinea corporis: For small-to-moderate lesions, one of the imidazole, ciclopirox, or naftifine creams or lotions should be rubbed in bid until at least 7 to 10 days after lesions disappear. For extensive or resistant tinea corporis, the most effective therapy is oral griseofulvin or oral ketoconazole. Tinea corporis usually responds readily to specific antifungal medication, but may be extensive and resistant to treatment in persons with debilitating systemic diseases.

Tinea pedis: Griseofulvin, the most effective treatment for mycologically proven tinea pedis, should be started even though it may have little immediate effect on the acute inflammatory infection. It is useful to treat chronic infections and prevent acute exacerbations, but clearing may require therapy for many months and is especially difficult, if not impossible, if the toenails are involved. Concomitant topical imidazole or ciclopirox may reduce recurrences.

Good foot hygiene is essential. Interdigital spaces must be dried after bathing, macerated skin rubbed away, and a bland, drying antifungal powder (eg, miconazole) applied. Light permeable footwear is recommended, especially during warm weather; many patients benefit from going barefoot. During acute vesicular flare-ups, bullae may be drained at the margin, but the keratinous tops should not be removed. Tap-water or dilute Burow's solution soaks bid are drying.

Whitfield's tincture (3% salicylic acid and 6% benzoic acid in 70% alcohol solution) or Whitfield's ointment or any of the topical drugs used for tinea corporis may be useful in the subacute or chronic phases. Cure with topical treatment is difficult, but control may be obtained with long-term therapy. Recurrences are common after therapy is discontinued.

Tinea cruris: Topical therapy with a cream or lotion, as in tinea corporis, is often effective. In some cases, griseofulvin orally for 4 to 6 wk may be needed.

Tinea unguium may respond to griseofulvin if treatment is continued until the nail has regrown completely and all infected material is gone. For fingernails, this may require 6 to 12 mo. Treatment of toenails should be discouraged, since 1 to 2 yr may be required, recurrence is usual, and complete cure is unlikely. Preliminary studies suggest that topical ciclopirox (which is uniquely water-soluble) may be effective, with many months of only topical treatment in $1/2$ or more of patients with chronic tinea unguium.

Tinea capitis: Children with *Trichophyton* infection should be given microsize griseofulvin 125 to 250 mg orally bid with meals or milk for at least 4 wk or until all signs of infection are gone. Until the tinea capitis is cured, an imidazole or ciclopirox cream should be applied to the affected child's scalp to prevent spread to other children.

Tinea barbae: Griseofulvin is the best treatment. If the lesions are severely inflamed, a short course of prednisone should be given in addition, starting with 40 mg/day orally (for adults) and tapering the dose over a 2-wk period.

YEAST INFECTIONS

CANDIDIASIS
(Candidosis; Moniliasis)

Candidiasis is usually limited to the skin and mucous membranes; uncommonly, the infection may become systemic and cause life-threatening visceral lesions.

Etiology
Candida albicans is a ubiquitous, usually saprophytic, yeast that can become pathogenic if a favorable environment or the host's weakened defenses allow the organisms to proliferate. Specifically, intertriginous and mucocutaneous areas where heat and maceration provide a fertile environment are the most susceptible sites. Systemic antibacterial, corticosteroid, and immunosuppressive therapy; pregnancy, obesity, diabetes mellitus and other endocrinopathies; debilitating diseases; blood dyscrasias; and immunologic defects increase susceptibility to candidiasis.

Symptoms and Signs
Symptoms vary with the site of the infection. **Intertriginous infections,** the most common, appear as well-demarcated, erythematous, sometimes itchy, exudative patches of varying size and shape. The lesions are usually rimmed with small, red-based pustules and occur in the axillae, inframammary areas, umbilicus, groin and gluteal folds (eg, diaper rash), between the toes, and on the finger webs. **Perianal candidiasis** produces white macerative pruritus ani.

Vulvovaginitis is relatively common, especially during pregnancy or in diabetes mellitus, and appears as a white or yellow discharge with inflammation of the vaginal wall and vulva. Burning, itching, and vaginal discharge are present in varying degrees. **Infection of the glans penis** and the underside of the preputium is less common but may be seen in men with diabetes mellitus or those whose sexual partners have candidal vulvovaginitis. This infection of the glans may be manifested by slightly scaling lesions and/or burning of the glans after coitus.

Oral candidiasis (thrush) appears as creamy white patches of exudate that can be scraped off an inflamed tongue or buccal mucosa (see also under STOMATITIS in Ch. 107). Although oral candidiasis may be seen in normal children and is benign, in young adults it may presage AIDS. **Perlèche,** which appears at the corners of the mouth and is characterized by inflammation with erosion and fissures, may be due to ill-fitting dentures and persistent moisture or to *Candida*, or both.

Candidal paronychia begins around the nail as a painful red swelling that later develops pus. **Subungual infections** are characterized by distal separation of one or several fingernails **(onycholysis)** with white or yellow discoloration of the subungual area.

Defects in cell-mediated immune responses (which, in children, are sometimes genetic) may lead to **chronic mucocutaneous candidiasis (candidal granuloma**—see also in Ch. 33), which is characterized by red, pustular, crusted, and thickened lesions, especially on the nose and forehead. In patients with an immune deficiency, other, more typical, candidal lesions or systemic candidiasis may also be seen.

Diagnosis

Candida can be demonstrated by finding both yeast and pseudohyphae in gram-stained specimens or in potassium hydroxide mounts of scrapings from a lesion. Because *Candida* is a commensal of man, the culture of a species from the skin, mouth, vagina, urine, sputum, or stool should be interpreted cautiously. To confirm the diagnosis, a characteristic clinical lesion, exclusion of other causes, and, at times, histologic evidence of tissue invasion are needed.

Treatment

Topical nystatin, the imidazoles, ciclopirox, and naftifine are all effective against skin and vaginal infections; thus these agents will suppress both dermatophyte and candidal skin infections (for genital infections, see also GENITAL CANDIDIASIS in Ch. 21). A vehicle appropriate to the site of infection must be chosen and frequency of administration should be tid or qid.

When anti-inflammatory and antipruritic actions are desired, equal amounts of the antifungal cream and a low-strength corticosteroid (eg, hydrocortisone) cream can be mixed or each may be applied separately. Recalcitrant or recurrent cases, especially of oral or anogenital candidiasis, benefit from nystatin oral suspension or tablets, 500,000 u. qid dissolved in the mouth (swish and swallow), or clotrimazole troches. When one sexual partner has recurrent candidiasis, both partners should be given a topical anticandidal cream and oral nystatin. For candidal diaper rash, the skin should be kept dry by changing diapers frequently and by generously applying nystatin powder; in severe cases, rubber pants and plastic disposable diaper coverings should be avoided. Oral ketoconazole is effective for many forms (including vaginal) of acute as well as chronic mucocutaneous candidiasis. The hepatic toxicity of oral ketoconazole must be considered and monitored. Treatment of paronychial infections is discussed in Ch. 91.

TINEA VERSICOLOR

An infection characterized by multiple, usually asymptomatic, patches of lesions varying in color from white to brown, and caused by Pityrosporum orbiculare *(formerly* Malassezia furfur*).* It is common in young adults. Tan, brown, or white, very slightly scaling lesions that tend to coalesce are seen on the chest, neck, and abdomen and occasionally on the face. The scaling may not be apparent unless the lesion is scratched. The patient may notice the condition only in the summer, because the lesions do not tan; instead they appear as variously sized white "sun spots." Itching is rare and usually occurs only when the patient is overheated. The condition is diagnosed from the clinical appearance and by finding groups of yeast and short plump hyphae on microscopic examination of scrapings from the lesions. The extent of involvement can be determined by the golden fluorescence or pigment changes under Wood's light. Culture of the organism is difficult without special media and is not needed for diagnosis.

Treatment

Numerous topical therapies are effective in clearing tinea versicolor, including selenium sulfide, the imidazoles, zinc pyrithione, and sulfur-salicylic acid combinations. Selenium sulfide in shampoo form (CAUTION: *Keep out of reach of children*) is applied undiluted and widely to all involved areas, including the scalp, for 3 or 4 days at bedtime and washed off in the morning; the scrotum should be avoided. If irritation occurs, the selenium sulfide should be washed off after 20 to 60 min or treatment should be stopped for a few days. If irritation is too severe, either 2% zinc pyrithione or 2% micropulverized sulfur and 2% salicylic acid in a shampoo base may be applied at bedtime for 2 wk or the topical imidazoles (see Dermatophyte Infections, above) may be applied bid for 2 wk. Oral ketoconazole is also effective, but long-term treatment for this usually trivial disease rarely seems warranted because of the potential toxicity; however, in some studies one 200-mg tablet/day for 1 to 5 days was shown to be effective in eliminating tinea versicolor for several months. The lesions may not become repigmented until the fungus is clear and the patient is exposed again to some sun. Eventual recurrence is almost universal after any treatment because the causative organism is a normal skin inhabitant. The scalp may be the reservoir.

93. PARASITIC INFECTIONS OF THE SKIN

SCABIES
(The Itch)

A transmissible ectoparasite infection, characterized by superficial burrows, intense pruritus, and secondary infection.

Etiology and Incidence

Scabies is caused by the itch mite *Sarcoptes scabiei*. The impregnated female mite tunnels into the stratum corneum and deposits her eggs along the burrow. The larvae hatch within a few days and congregate around the hair follicles. Lesions are thought to result from hypersensitivity to the parasites.

Scabies is transmitted readily, often through an entire household, by skin-to-skin contact with an infected individual; eg, when people sleep together. It is rarely spread by clothing or bedding. However, extensive cleaning or fumigating is unwarranted, since the mite does not live long off the human body.

Symptoms, Signs, and Diagnosis

Marked pruritus is most intense when the patient is in bed. The characteristic initial lesions are burrows seen as fine wavy dark lines a few millimeters to 1 cm long with a minute papule at the open end. The inflammatory lesions occur predominantly on the finger webs, the flexor surface of the wrists, about the elbows and axillary folds, about the areolae of the breasts in females and on the genitals in males, along the beltline, and on the lower buttocks. There may also be numerous nonspecific (uninfected) papules and excoriations over the trunk and extremities. The face is not involved in adults but may be in infants. Patients who have neurologic disorders or various forms of immunodeficiency may have nonpruritic scaling due to infection with myriad mites (particularly on the palms and soles and on the scalp in children).

Burrows may be difficult to find (particularly when the disease has persisted for several weeks) because they are soon obscured by scratching or secondary lesions (eg, urticaria, scratch dermatitis, eczema, or superimposed bacterial infection). Diagnosis can be confirmed by demonstrating the parasite in scrapings taken from a burrow, then mixed with any clear solution (eg, mineral oil, potassium hydroxide, or even water), and examined microscopically.

Treatment

Treatment is curative and may serve as a "therapeutic test" in doubtful cases. The patient should apply 5% permethrin cream to the *entire* body. The cream should remain in contact with the skin for a minimum of 12 h and preferably longer, ie, 24 h. Lindane (γ-benzene hexachloride) 1% cream or lotion is also effective but sometimes irritating. It should be applied over the entire skin surface from the neck down. For infants < 2 yr, permethrin cream or a 5 or 10% sulfur ointment is preferred because of a potential neurotoxicity from absorption of lindane. Contacts, both adults and children (eg, a whole family), should be treated concurrently.

Re-treatment is rarely needed, unless infection is reacquired. A 0.1% fluorinated corticosteroid ointment (see Ch. 88) bid may be used for persistent itching, which may take 1 to 2 wk to subside. Concomitant bacterial infections may require systemic antibiotics but often clear spontaneously when the scabies is cured.

PEDICULOSIS

Infestation by lice may involve the **head** (by *Pediculus humanus capitis*), the **body** (*P. humanus corporis*), or the **genital area** (*Phthirus pubis*). Head lice and pubic (crab) lice live directly on the host; body lice, in the undergarments. Infestation is widespread where overcrowding or inadequate facilities for personal hygiene or clean clothing exist. Body lice are important vectors of organisms that cause epidemic typhus, trench fever, and relapsing fever.

Symptoms, Signs, and Diagnosis

Pediculosis capitis is transmitted by personal contact and by such objects as combs and hats. Without regard to social status, it is common among school children and less common in blacks. Infestation is localized predominantly on the scalp, though it sometimes involves the eyebrows, eyelashes, and beard. Itching is severe, and excoriation of the scalp, sometimes with secondary bacterial infection, may be seen. Moderate discrete posterior cervical adenopathy is frequent. In children, a generalized, nonspecific dermatitis is occasionally caused by lice infesting only the scalp. Diagnosis is simple if infestation is considered and the scalp is inspected, preferably with a magnifying lens. Small, ovoid, grayish-white nits (ova) are seen fixed to the hair shafts, sometimes in great numbers; unlike scales, they cannot be dislodged. Nits mature in 3 to 14 days. Lice may be found (less often than nits) around the occiput and behind the ears.

Pediculosis corporis is uncommon with good hygiene. Nits may be found on the body hairs, but both parasites and ova are easily found in underclothing seams, since body lice primarily inhabit the seams of clothing worn next to the skin. Itching is invariable. Lesions are especially common on the shoulders, buttocks, and abdomen. Inspection may show small red puncta due to bites, usually associated with linear scratch marks, urticaria, or superficial bacterial infection. Furunculosis is an occasional complication.

Pediculosis pubis is usually transmitted venereally. Crab lice ordinarily infest anogenital hairs but may involve other areas, especially in hairy individuals. In all itching dermatoses of the anogenital region, careful inspection should be made for the parasites, which may be few in number. Lice are not easily seen without a diligent search; they resemble the small crusts of scratch dermatitis. Sometimes lice may be seen within small bluish spots on the skin, ordinarily on the trunk. Ova are commonly attached to the skin at the base of the hairs. A sign of infestation is a scattering of minute dark brown specks (louse excreta) on undergarments where they come in contact with the anogenital region. Excoriation and secondary dermatitis, the latter often from self-medication, may develop early.

Treatment and Prevention

Cure is usually rapid with 1% lindane (γ-benzene hexachloride), applied once/day for 2 days in shampoo, cream, or lotion form or as a combination of shampoo followed by the cream or lotion; pyrethrin preparations or 0.5% malathion lotions can be effective, but lindane has neurotoxicity, and all may be irritating or flammable. Application may be repeated in 10 days to destroy surviving nits, but prolonged application of parasiticides should be **avoided**. A safer, more effective and pleasant product, 1% permethrin cream rinse, is now available. Infestation of eyelids and eyelashes may be more difficult to manage; the parasites usually must be removed with forceps. Plain petrolatum applications may kill or weaken the lice on eyelashes. Sources of infestation (eg, combs, hats, clothing, bedding) should be decontaminated by vacuuming, thorough laundering and steam pressing, or dry cleaning. Recurrence is common.

CREEPING ERUPTION
(Cutaneous Larva Migrans)

This disease is caused chiefly by *Ancylostoma braziliense*, the hookworm of the dog or cat. Ova of this parasite are deposited on the ground in dog or cat feces. Larvae persist in warm moist ground or sand and penetrate unprotected skin that contacts the soil. The feet, legs, buttocks, or back is most commonly involved. The haphazard progress of the parasite as it burrows in the epidermis produces a winding, threadlike trail of inflammation. Itching is marked: Scratch dermatitis and bacterial infection may complicate the otherwise typical serpiginous lesion.

Treatment

Applying the oral 10% suspension of thiabendazole topically to all affected areas qid for 7 to 10 days is promptly effective. Topical mebendazole incorporated into cream is said to be effective also, but fewer studies have been done.

94. VIRAL INFECTIONS OF THE SKIN

Herpes simplex and varicella-zoster viruses, although considered viral skin infections, are discussed elsewhere in THE MANUAL.

WARTS
(Verrucae)
(See also GENITAL WARTS in Ch. 21)

Common, contagious, epithelial tumors caused by at least 60 types of human papillomavirus (HPV); some of the tumors can become malignant. (See TABLE 94-1.) Viral warts, which may appear at any age, are most frequent in older children but are uncommon in the aged. Appearance and size depend on their location and on the degree of irritation and trauma to which they are subjected. The course may be variable. Infection may persist as single or multiple lesions, and lesions may develop by autoinoculation. Complete regression after many months is usual with or without treatment, but warts may persist for years and may recur at the same or different sites.

The relative importance of serologic and cell-mediated immunity is not yet clear. Some feel that because wart virus particles are seen only in the outer epithelium (granular layer and beyond), they have little chance to become deep enough to serve as effective antigens. On the other hand, patients with immunosuppression from organ transplants or other causes lack immunity to the virus and get generalized cutaneous infections with many types of virus. This suggests that some types of immune mechanisms are significant. In addition, spontaneous disappearance of multiple warts in immunologically normal people with subsequent development of lifelong immunity needs further explanation.

Differential Diagnosis

Wart viruses are *circular, double-stranded DNA, with about 8000 base pairs.* To qualify as a separate type there must be < 50% of DNA cross-hybridization; subtypes, > 50%. Each type is indicated by a number and, in general, causes certain clinically distinct lesions. Although each DNA is distinctive, most papillomas, including those of bovine origin, also have a common protein antigen that can be shown histologically on fixed tissue with a test that is positive for all types of papillomas and is very useful in diagnosis. When papillomas become malignant, however, they no longer give a positive stain, nor can recognizable papilloma particles be seen with the electron microscope. Oncogenic papilloma DNA can then be found in the cancers by modern molecular hybridization DNA techniques. DNA typing is now available in only a few special research laboratories but is important for prognosis of genital warts and their consequences.

Common warts (verrucae vulgaris), almost universal in the population, are benign. They are sharply demarcated, rough-surfaced, round or irregular, firm, light gray, yellow, brown, or grayish-black tumors 2 to 10 mm in diameter. They appear most often on sites subject to trauma (eg, fingers, elbows, knees, face, scalp) but may spread elsewhere. **Periungual warts** commonly occur around the nail plate.

Plantar warts, common on the sole of the foot, are flattened by pressure and surrounded by cornified epithelium. They may be exquisitely tender and can be distinguished from corns and calluses by their tendency to pinpoint bleeding when the surface is pared away. **Mosaic warts** are plaques of myriad small, closely set plantar warts.

Filiform warts are long, narrow, small growths usually seen on the eyelids, face, neck, or lips. **Flat warts** (smooth, flat, yellow-brown lesions) occur more commonly in children and young adults, most often on the face and along scratch marks through autoinoculation. **Warts of unusual shape** (eg, pedunculated, or resembling a cauliflower) are most frequent on the head and neck, especially on the scalp and bearded region.

Moist or venereal warts (condylomata acuminata) are discussed in Ch. 21.

Treatment

Treatment depends on the location, type, extent, and duration of the lesions, the age of the patient, and the patient's immune status and desire to have the lesions treated.

Most **common warts** disappear spontaneously within 2 yr or with simple nonscarring treatment such as a flexible collodion solution containing 17% salicylic acid and 17% lactic acid ap-

TABLE 94-1. TYPES OF WART VIRUS AND CLINICAL CORRELATIONS

Clinical Form	Types	Clinical Correlations
Common (including palmar, plantar, and periungual)	1, 2, 4, 7	Benign
Flat	3, 10	Benign
Genital (see Ch. 21), also found in mouth, perianal area, bladder, and lung	6, 11	In women, 28% have associated cervical dysplasia with koilocytic cells
	16, 18, 33	Found in > 50% of tumors in women with invasive carcinoma of cervix; type 16 found in 80% of men and women with bowenoid papulosis of external genitals. Lesions usually disappear spontaneously, but future cancers may appear
	6a, b, c, d, e	Buschke-Löwenstein giant condyloma often malignant; also in cervical dysplasia and laryngeal tumors
	Many from 34–58	Most of those associated with cervical intraepithelial neoplasia (see Ch. 10)
Butcher's (meat handler's)	7, 10	Common warts, usually benign
Malignant epidermodysplasia verruciformis	5a, b, 8	Often malignant; sunlight or x-ray therapy cofactors, especially with type 5
Epidermodysplasia verruciformis	1, 2, 3, 4, 7, 9, 10, 12, 14, 17, 18, 19, 20, 23, 24, 25	Most seem benign, except possibly 14, 17, 20
Cutaneous warts in immunosuppressed and transplant patients	8 or others	Often malignant; sunlight a cofactor
Laryngeal papillomas	6, 11, 16, 30	May become malignant; may occur in infants on passage through the vaginal canal and in adults as a consequence of oral-genital sex; may spread to lungs as cancer
Oral papillomatosis (Heck's disease)	13	Benign

plied daily, after gentle peeling, by the patient or parent. Or the physician may freeze the wart (avoiding the surrounding skin) for 15 to 30 sec with liquid nitrogen. This procedure is often curative, but may need to be repeated in 2 to 3 wk. Electrodesiccation with curettage is satisfactory for a solitary lesion or a few lesions, but it may cause scarring. Laser surgery may also be useful but, again, may cause scarring. Recurrence or appearance of new warts close by occurs in about 35% of patients within a year after any treatment, so that scarring methods should be avoided as much as possible.

Plantar warts may require more vigorous maceration with a 40% salicylic acid tape kept in place for several days. While the wart is still damp and soft, the physician debrides it; then it is destroyed by freezing or caustics (eg, 30 to 70% trichloroacetic acid).

In common or even periungual warts, cantharidin 0.7% in flexible collodion is also useful. The physician, using a tiny-tipped applicator and being careful to avoid normal skin, applies the preparation 2 to 3 times (after drying) at one visit and 5 to 10 min later covers the wart with occlusive tape that is left in place for 7 h. The procedure can be repeated in 1 or 2 wk, if necessary. (Cantharidin should not be given to patients for treatment at home.) One of the drawbacks of this treatment is that new warts may appear at the periphery of the treated wart.

Other destructive treatments (eg, CO_2 laser or various acids) will work in many cases; even snipping off **filiform (long single) warts** may be sufficient.

X-ray therapy has no place in treating warts because of its potential to make them more invasive. Ultraviolet exposure is also a potent cocarcinogen in patients with epidermodysplasia verruciformis **(EDV)** or immunosuppression for any reason.

Flat warts can often be treated successfully with daily application of tretinoin (retinoic acid 0.05%), as used in acne. If sufficient peeling does not occur for wart removal, another irritant (eg, 5% benzoyl peroxide) or a 5% salicylic acid cream can be applied sequentially with tretinoin to remove lesions. Spontaneous resolution may follow unprovoked inflammation of the lesions.

Several new methods, whose long-term value and risks are not fully known, are available. One of these, intralesional injection of small amounts of 0.1% solution of bleomycin in saline, often produces necrosis and cures even stubborn plantar warts. However, reports of scleroderma of fingers where warts have been injected with bleomycin suggest caution in spite of its popularity and effectiveness.

Extensive warts, even in hitherto untreatable EDV, have improved or cleared with *oral isotretinoin, or etretinate,* which *must be used by physicians familiar with these drugs and their possible side effects, especially fetal abnormalities if used during pregnancy.*

Interferon, especially interferon-α, intralesionally (3 times/wk for 3 to 5 wk) or IM, has also cleared intractable skin and genital warts.

MOLLUSCUM CONTAGIOSUM

A poxvirus infection characterized by skin-colored, smooth, waxy, umbilicated papules 2 to 10 mm in diameter. A giant single molluscum may grow 2 or 3 times as large.

Transmission is by direct contact, often venereal. Its contagiousness to others varies. The papules may appear anywhere on the skin and often occur as numerous small papules in the genital and pubic area. The lesions are usually asymptomatic, unless secondarily infected, and may be discovered only when the patient is examined for another sexually transmitted disease. They can be diagnosed easily by the characteristic central umbilication or dell, filled with a semisolid white material that, if expressed and Giemsa-stained, shows many large cells containing inclusion bodies. Inclusion bodies alone may be seen. The disease can spread by autoinoculation but after months may disappear spontaneously. Areas of eczematous dermatitis may surround several mollusca, especially in young children; the cause of the dermatitis is unknown.

Treatment, to be successful, usually requires destroying each lesion by freezing, or by removing the central core of the papule with a needle, a comedo extractor, the tip of a #11 scalpel blade, or by cantharidin (as for common warts, above).

95. DISORDERS OF HAIR FOLLICLES AND SEBACEOUS GLANDS

ACNE

A common inflammatory pilosebaceous disease characterized by comedones, papules, pustules, inflamed nodules, superficial pus-filled cysts, and (in extreme cases) canalizing and deep, inflamed, sometimes purulent sacs.

Pathogenesis

The pathogenesis is complex. An interaction between hormones, keratinization, sebum, and bacteria somehow determines the course and severity of acne. It begins at puberty, when the increase in androgens causes an increase in the size and activity of the pilosebaceous glands. The earliest microscopic change is thought to be intrafollicular hyperkeratosis, which leads to blockage of the pilosebaceous follicle with consequent formation of the comedo, composed of sebum, keratin, and microorganisms, particularly *Propionibacterium acnes.* Lipases from *P. acnes* break down triglycerides in the sebum to form free fatty acids **(FFA),** which irritate the follicular wall. Retention of sebaceous secretions and dilation of the follicle may lead to cyst formation. Rupture of the follicle, with release of FFA, bacterial products, and keratin constituents into the tissues, induces an inflammatory reaction that usually results in an abscess that heals with scars in severe cases.

Symptoms and Signs

For therapy and prognosis, acne is best classified as superficial or deep according to the severity of the predominating lesions. Spontaneous remission is the rule, but when this will occur cannot be predicted.

Superficial acne is characterized by comedones, either open (blackheads) or closed (whiteheads); inflamed papules; superficial cysts; and pustules. Large cysts occur occasionally, sometimes after manipulation or trauma to an otherwise uninflamed blackhead. In **deep acne,** deep inflamed nodules and pus-filled cysts, which often rupture and become abscesses, are also present; some of them open on the skin surface and discharge their contents. Scarring is frequent. Lesions are most common on the face, but the neck, chest, upper back, and shoulders may also be affected. The prognosis for healing without scars is good in superficial acne, but clumsy attempts to extrude blackheads or superficial cysts and scratching of ruptured lesions may increase scarring.

Acne is often exacerbated in winter and improved in summer, probably because of the sun's beneficial effect. Diet has little effect, if any; however, if a food is suspected, it should be omitted for several weeks and then eaten in substantial quantities to see if eating it makes any difference. Most such trials prove that the acne is unrelated to food. Acne may cycle with the menses, and it may clear or become worse during pregnancy. In many women who first develop acne in their 20s and 30s, certain cosmetics may act as aggravating agents.

Diagnosis

Diagnosis of acne is usually simple. Comedones are almost always present, and lesions at various stages of development are seen simultaneously. Rosacea may resemble acne, but there are no comedones. Corticosteroid-induced acneiform lesions are usually follicular pustules all in the same stage of development; comedones are absent.

Treatment

Although the disease is almost universal, disfiguring or even mild acne may embarrass adolescents, and some may become withdrawn, using the acne as an excuse to avoid difficult personal adjustments. Supportive counseling for both patient and parents is helpful. Misconceptions about a relationship between acne and diet, athletics, or sex are common and warrant discussion with patients. Some cosmetics aggravate acne (especially those with comedogenic ingredients—eg, isopropyl myristate), and most greasy products should be avoided.

Other treatment depends on the severity of the lesions.

Superficial acne: Although washing several times a day has little effect on lesions, the appearance of an oily face is often improved. Any good toilet soap may be used. Antibacterial soaps are of no benefit, and irritation from abrasive soaps makes it difficult to use the more specific follicular drugs tretinoin or benzoyl peroxide (see below).

Large comedones may be removed carefully once or twice a week, preferably with a Schamberg loop extractor after hot water compresses. The proper technique may be taught to a responsible family member. Many dermatologists doubt the lasting value of such manipulation. Inflammatory lesions should not be opened until they have pointed in a pustule. Picking the crust covering an opened lesion may delay healing for several weeks and produce a pitted scar.

In **superficial pustular acne,** topical clindamycin solution used either alone or with one of the irritants mentioned below is probably the most useful therapy. Sunlight and irritating topical drugs also aid superficial lesions. Sunlight causes mild dryness and slight scaling; it is usually effective, but not always available, and its benefit may be difficult to duplicate with a sunlamp. Topical tretinoin (retinoic acid) in a 0.025, 0.05, or 0.1% cream or liquid, or 0.01 or 0.025% gel, is also often effective. It must be applied cautiously; the liquid should be applied with a cotton-tipped applicator. Tretinoin should be applied nightly (every other night if irritation is excessive), going over the entire affected area *only once*. The eyes, nasolabial folds, and creases of the mouth should be avoided. Exposure to sunlight and use of other drugs often are restricted to prevent severe irritation. Improvement usually requires 3 to 4 wk, and the condition may appear worse at first. Blackheads can be removed easily after a few weeks of treatment. Other topical drugs include 5 to 10% benzoyl peroxide, the best nonprescription topical drug, and various sulfur-resorcinol combinations; they are usually applied bid or one preparation at night and another in the morning. Oral tetracycline (see below) may also be helpful in superficial pustular acne.

Deep acne: Vigorous management is required to reduce residual scarring. Topical treatment is unsatisfactory for severe, deep lesions. Treatment of patients with a few deep lesions is usually a broad-spectrum oral antibiotic: the effect is probably due to reduction of bacterial organisms. The most effective antibiotic with the fewest side effects is tetracycline; 250 mg qid or 500 mg bid (between meals and at bedtime) should be continued for 4 wk and then decreased to the lowest amount that gives a good response. Occasionally the dosage must be increased to 500 mg qid. In patients who do not respond to tetracycline, minocycline 100 mg bid may be tried. Because relapse ordinarily follows short periods of treatment, therapy must be continued for months to years, though as little as 250 or 500 mg/day of tetracycline is often sufficient. Erythromycin in similar dosage may be used if the patient is pregnant. The most common side effect with prolonged antibiotic use is a candidal vaginitis. If local and systemic therapy (see CANDIDIASIS in Ch. 92) do not eradicate this problem, antibiotic therapy for the acne must be stopped. Long-term use of antibiotics may also produce a gram-negative pustular folliculitis, seen around the nose and in the center of the face. This uncommon superinfection may be difficult to clear; the best treatment for this complication is oral isotretinoin (see below).

Oral isotretinoin is the best treatment for patients in whom treatment with antibiotics is unsuccessful or in patients with very severe deep acne. This drug has revolutionized the therapy of acne, *but should be used only by physicians who are thoroughly familiar with its adverse effects.* Since isotretinoin is teratogenic, women taking the drug must use strict contraceptive measures not only 1 mo before and while taking it but also for at least 1 mo after discontinuing the drug. Pregnancy tests before beginning therapy and at monthly intervals are important. The drug is dispensed with warnings against pregnancy. Because severe fetal abnormalities are likely if pregnancy occurs while the woman is taking the drug, discussion and counseling are indicated. The dosage of isotretinoin is usually 1 to 1.5 mg/kg/day for 20 wk. If side effects make this dosage intolerable, it may be reduced to 0.5 mg/kg/day. The most common side effects, seen in about 90% of patients, are dryness of conjunctivae and

mucosae of the genitalia, and chapped lips. Petrolatum is usually beneficial in alleviating some of the symptoms associated with the dryness. Musculoskeletal symptoms, pain or stiffness of large joints or the lower back, may also occur in about 15% of patients. Symptoms often resolve with reduced dosage. Occasionally the drug must be discontinued. CBC, liver function, and triglyceride and cholesterol levels should be determined before treatment. Each, except for the CBC, should be reassessed at 2 wk and then monthly during treatment. Triglyceride levels may increase to a level at which the drug should be discontinued. Liver function is only occasionally affected. Following the 20 wk of therapy, acne may continue to improve. Most patients do not require a second course of treatment; when needed, it should be resumed only after the drug has been stopped for 4 mo. Re-treatment is required more often if the initial dosage is low (0.5 mg/kg/day). With this dosage (which is very popular in Europe) fewer side effects occur, but prolonged therapy is usually required.

For firm lesions, injection of 0.1 mL triamcinolone acetonide suspension 2.5 mg/mL (the 10-mg/mL suspension must be diluted) into an inflamed cyst or abscess is helpful; local atrophy (due to the corticosteroid or to destruction of tissue by the cyst) is usually transient. For isolated, very boggy lesions, incision and drainage is often beneficial but may result in residual scarring.

Dermabrasion for small scars is sometimes useful, but its permanent effect is controversial.

X-ray therapy is not justified. Topical corticosteroids, especially the fluorinated ones, may worsen acne. When other measures fail and acne seems related to the menses, an oral estrogen-progesterone in the usual contraceptive dosage may be tried; therapy for at least 6 mo is needed to evaluate the effect.

ROSACEA

A chronic inflammatory disorder, usually beginning in middle age or later, and characterized by telangiectasia, erythema, papules, and pustules appearing especially in the central areas of the face. Tissue hypertrophy, particularly of the nose **(rhinophyma),** may result. Occasionally, rosacea occurs on the trunk and extremities.

The cause is unknown, but the disease is most common in persons with a fair complexion. Diet probably plays no role in the pathogenesis. Rosacea may resemble acne, but comedones are never present; differential diagnosis also includes drug eruptions (particularly from iodides and bromides), granulomas of the skin, cutaneous LE, and perioral dermatitis.

Treatment

Topical metronidazole gel or broad-spectrum oral antibiotics are usually effective. Tetracycline is the antibiotic preferred because it is most effective and side effects with long-term use are few. A starting dose of 250 mg qid (between meals) should be reduced once a beneficial response is achieved. Often only 250 mg/day or every other day will control the disease. Recalcitrant cases often respond to oral isotretinoin as in acne (see above). Topical fluorinated corticosteroids aggravate rosacea and are contraindicated. Surgical correction may be required for rhinophyma (*a bulbous red nose resulting from neglected rosacea*).

PERIORAL DERMATITIS

A red papular eruption of unknown etiology occurring around the mouth and on the chin. The condition occurs predominantly in women aged 20 to 60. It may superficially resemble acne or rosacea. A zone of normal skin lies between the lesions and the vermilion border of the mouth. Some oily cosmetics, especially moisturizers, may worsen the disorder, as do topical corticosteroids.

Treatment with tetracycline 250 mg qid (between meals) is often effective. The dose should be reduced gradually after 1 mo to the smallest amount that controls the disease. Recalcitrant, disfiguring cases may clear with oral isotretinoin as in acne (see above).

HYPERTRICHOSIS
(Hirsutism)

Excessive hair growth in areas usually not hairy (see also Ch. 6). A familial tendency is common, and occurrence is more frequent in people from the Mediterranean area. An endocrine disorder may be implicated in women and children—most often, adrenal virilism, basophilic adenoma of the pituitary, masculinizing ovarian tumors, and the Stein-Leventhal syndrome. Hirsutism is seen frequently at menopause, with systemic androgenic steroid or corticosteroid therapy, and with some antihypertensive drugs. It also may occur in porphyria cutanea tarda.

Treatment

Any underlying disorder should be treated. The only safe permanent local treatment is destruction of individual hair follicles by electrolysis, a tedious process. Widely used temporary measures include plucking, shaving, and use of epilating wax. Chemical depilatories are acceptable if the directions are followed but may irritate the skin. A hair bleach may mask the condition if the hair is fine. In women with certain types of endocrine abnormalities, one of the new pituitary inhibitors for antiandrogens may be tried. A gynecologic endocrinologist should be consulted.

ALOPECIA
(Baldness)

Partial or complete loss of hair. It may result from genetic factors, aging, or local or systemic disease. (Seborrheic dermatitis and psoriasis, the two dermatoses that affect the scalp most commonly, very rarely produce alopecia.) **Nonscarring (noncicatricial) alopecia** occurs without scarring or gross atrophic changes; **scarring (cicatricial) alopecia** follows scar tissue formation resulting from inflammation and tissue destruction.

Nonscarring Alopecia

Male-pattern baldness is extremely common. It is familial and requires the presence of androgens, but other etiologic factors are unknown. The hair loss begins in the lateral frontal areas or over the vertex. If onset is in the midteens, subsequent baldness is commonly extensive. **Female-pattern alopecia** is not infrequent in women. It is confined ordinarily to thinning of the hair in the frontal, parietal, and crown regions; complete baldness in any area is rare.

Toxic alopecia is usually temporary and may follow, by as long as 3 to 4 mo, a severe, often febrile, illness (eg, scarlet fever). It may also be seen in myxedema, hypopituitarism, or early syphilis, following pregnancy, and with some drugs—particularly cytotoxic agents, thallium compounds, and overdoses of vitamin A or retinoids.

In **alopecia areata,** sudden hair loss in circumscribed areas occurs in individuals who have no obvious skin disorder or systemic disease. Any hairy area may be involved, the scalp and beard most frequently. Rarely, all the body hair may be lost **(alopecia universalis)**. The prognosis is poor if alopecia is extensive, but alopecia confined to a few areas is often reversed in a few months, though recurrences may occur. Antimicrosomal antibodies **(Abs)** and Abs to thyroglobulin, gastric parietal cells, and adrenal cells may be present.

Hair pulling (trichotillomania) is a neurotic habit that usually appears in children; it may remain undiagnosed for a long time. The hairs may be broken off and are of different lengths. Some stubby regrowth may be visible, but the condition is often hard to differentiate from alopecia areata. Biopsy is sometimes helpful.

Scarring Alopecia

If hair loss is due to atrophy or scarring, little regrowth can be expected. In injuries (eg, burns, physical trauma, x-ray atrophy), the cause of the scarring will usually be apparent; if it is not obvious, it should be sought. Cutaneous LE; chronic deep bacterial or fungal infections; deep factitial ulcers; granulomas such as sarcoidosis, syphilitic gummas, or TB; or inflamed tinea capitis (kerion or favus) may produce scarring alopecia. Certain slow-growing tumors may gradually extend in the scalp with resultant scarring. Some rare scarring alopecias are of unknown cause.

Examination should include the entire skin surface and mucous membranes because related lesions will often be found. Biopsy should be done at an area of active inflammatory change, usually at the border of a bald patch. Cultures for bacteria and fungi may be indicated.

Diagnosis

Microscopic examination of plucked hair may differentiate some forms of nonscarring alopecia. Normally 80 to 90% of hairs are in a growing (anagen) phase; the rest are in a resting (telogen) phase. *All* of the hair (about 40 to 60 hairs) from a defined area of the scalp should be plucked, using a strong instrument, and an anagen/telogen count done. Anagen hairs have sheaths attached to their roots, whereas telogen hairs have no sheaths and have tiny bulbs at their roots. Postpartum and post-illness alopecias are characterized by an increased percentage of telogen hairs, whereas alopecias due to thallium or antimitotic drugs are characterized by a normal percentage of telogen hairs. The anagen hair in the latter conditions may break easily because the hair shaft narrows. Alopecia areata is characterized by hairs that look like exclamation points.

Biopsy of the scalp may differentiate various forms of alopecia (eg, alopecia areata and trichotillomania). Either histologic or immunofluorescence examination may delineate LE, lichen planopilaris (lichen planus of the scalp), and scleroderma. Metastatic lesions, which may also produce localized scarring alopecia, are diagnosed by biopsy.

Treatment

No therapy is known for idiopathic male-pattern baldness, though transplants from hairy to bald areas are effective. Minoxidil, an antihypertensive drug, is being used topically in solutions of 2%, although its value is questionable. Significant hair growth is very uncommon.

In alopecia areata, dilute triamcinolone acetonide suspension can be injected intradermally if the lesions are small, but the results may not be lasting. Experimental induction of a mild allergic contact dermatitis has shown some benefit, as have other topical irritants. Although clomipramine has been shown to be of short-term benefit in patients with trichotillomania, behavioral modification may result in long-term benefit or cure.

In scarring alopecia, treatment is directed at eliminating the cause.

PSEUDOFOLLICULITIS BARBAE

Pseudofolliculitis of the beard **(ingrown hairs)** is seen most frequently in black men. The stiff hair tips penetrate the skin before leaving the follicle, or else leave the follicle, curve, and reenter nearby skin, provoking small pustules that are more a foreign-body reaction than an infection. The only consistently effective **treatment** is to have the patient grow a beard. Special razors have been used with varying results. A thioglycolate depilatory may be used every 2 to 3 days but is often irritating. Application of tretinoin (retinoic acid) 0.05% liquid or cream or 10% benzoyl peroxide cream daily or every other day may be effective in mild or moderate cases; they may be irritating and should be used every other day at first, then daily.

KERATINOUS CYST
(Wen; Sebaceous Cyst; Steatoma)

A slow-growing benign cystic tumor of the skin containing follicular, keratinous, and sebaceous material and frequently found on the scalp, ears, face, back, or scrotum. On palpation, the cystic mass is firm, globular, movable, and nontender; it seldom causes discomfort unless infected. Puncture of the cyst produces characteristic cheesy, often fetid, contents formed of epithelial debris and greasy material; soft keratin often predominates, and at times calcium deposits may be found. Secondary bacterial infection with abscess formation occurs. A **milium** is a minute superficial keratinous cyst, usually found on the face or scrotum.

Treatment

For milia, expression of the contents through a tiny stab incision is curative. For larger lesions, the contents are evacuated through a small incision; then the cyst wall is removed through the incision with a curette or hemostat. Surgical excision is also effective. Any large cyst may recur after therapy unless the cyst wall is removed completely. Infected cysts can be incised and drained; a gauze drain is inserted and gradually removed over 7 to 10 days. Oral antibiotics (eg, cloxacillin or erythromycin) may be required.

96. SCALING PAPULAR DISEASES

PSORIASIS

A common chronic, recurrent disease characterized by dry, well-circumscribed, silvery, scaling papules and plaques of various sizes.

Psoriasis varies in severity from 1 or 2 lesions to a widespread dermatosis with disabling arthritis or exfoliation. The cause is unknown, but the thick scaling is probably due to increased epidermal cell proliferation. About 2 to 4% of the white population, and far fewer blacks, are affected. Onset is usually between ages 10 and 40, but no age is exempt. A family history of psoriasis is common and usually reflects genetic factors. Except for the psychologic stigma of an unsightly skin disease, general health is unaffected unless arthritis, intractable exfoliation, or severe, widespread pustulation develops.

Symptoms and Signs

Onset is usually gradual. The typical course is one of chronic remissions and recurrences (or occasionally acute exacerbations) that vary in frequency and duration. Factors precipitating psoriatic eruptions include local trauma (which causes the **Koebner phenomenon** in which lesions appear at the trauma site) and, occasionally, severe sunburn, irritation, topical drugs, chloroquine antimalarial therapy, lithium, β-blockers, interferon-α, and withdrawal of systemic corticosteroids. Some patients (especially children) may have explosive psoriatic eruptions after an acute group A β-hemolytic streptococcal URI.

Psoriasis characteristically involves the scalp (including the postauricular regions), the extensor surface of the extremities (particularly at elbows and knees), the back, and the buttocks.

The nails, eyebrows, axillae, umbilicus, or anogenital region may also be affected. Occasionally the disease is generalized.

The lesions are sharply demarcated, usually nonpruritic, erythematous papules or plaques covered with overlapping silvery or slightly opalescent shiny scales. The lesions heal without scarring, and hair growth is usually unaltered. Papules sometimes extend and coalesce to produce large plaques in bizarre annular and gyrate patterns. Nail involvement may resemble a fungal infection, with stippling, pitting, fraying, or separation of the distal margin and thickening, discoloration, and debris under the nail plate.

Psoriatic arthritis often closely resembles RA and may be equally crippling, but the patient's serum contains no RF. In **exfoliative psoriatic dermatitis,** which may be intractable and may lead to general debility, the entire skin is red and covered with fine scales; at first typical psoriatic lesions may be obscured. **Pustular psoriasis** is characterized by sterile pustules that may be generalized or localized to the palms and soles; typical psoriatic lesions may be absent.

Diagnosis

Diagnosis by inspection is rarely difficult. In psoriasis of the scalp, as elsewhere, the well-defined, dry, heaped-up lesions with large silvery scales are usually distinguished from the diffuse, greasy, yellowish scaling of seborrheic dermatitis. However, psoriasis may be confused with seborrheic dermatitis, squamous cell carcinoma in situ (when on the trunk), secondary syphilis, fungal infections, cutaneous LE, eczema, lichen planus, or localized scratch dermatitis.

Biopsy findings may be typical, but many other skin diseases may have psoriasis-like histologic features that make them difficult to distinguish.

Prognosis and Treatment

The prognosis depends on the extent and severity of the initial involvement—usually the earlier in life it begins, the greater the severity. Acute attacks usually clear up, but complete permanent remission is rare. No therapy assures patients of a cure, but most cases can be well controlled.

Because effective treatments are few, the simplest forms—lubricants, keratolytics, and topical corticosteroids—should be tried first for a limited number of lesions. Exposure to sunlight is recommended, though occasionally sunburn may induce exacerbations. Systemic antimetabolites (eg, methotrexate—see below) should be used only in severe skin or joint involvement. Systemic corticosteroids should not be used because the side effects include severe exacerbations or pustular lesions that may occur during treatment (even with increasing doses) or after therapy has been stopped.

Lubricating creams, hydrogenated vegetable (cooking) oils, or white petrolatum are applied (alone or with corticosteroids, salicylic acid, crude coal tar, or anthralin) bid while the skin is still damp after bathing. Alternatively, crude coal tar ointment or cream may be applied at night and washed off in the morning, followed by exposure to natural or artificial (280 to 320 nm) ultraviolet (UV) light in slowly increasing increments sufficient to produce mild erythema.

Anthralin can be effective as a cream or an ointment, beginning with 0.1% and increasing to 1% if tolerated. Anthralin may be irritating and should not be used in intertriginous areas; it stains sheets and clothing as well as the skin. A new short contact treatment avoids many of these disadvantages: 20 to 30 min after its application, anthralin is washed off by bathing.

Topical corticosteroids may be used as an alternative or adjunct to anthralin or coal tar treatment. As an adjunct they are used bid or tid during the day, and anthralin or coal tar is used at bedtime. Corticosteroids are most effective when used under occlusive polyethylene coverings or incorporated in adhesive tape. This may be applied overnight and a corticosteroid cream rubbed in without occlusion bid or tid during the day. The initial concentration is usually chosen according to the extent of involvement. As lesions improve, the corticosteroid should be applied less often or in a lower concentration to prevent local side effects (atrophy, telangiectases). After about 3 wk, a bland ointment should be substituted for 1 to 2 wk to prevent loss of steroid effectiveness (tachyphylaxis). Triamcinolone acetonide 0.1% (or equivalent—see Ch. 88) is of moderate potency; it is expensive to use corticosteroids because 1 oz (30 gm) of cream is usually needed to cover the entire body. Commercial preparations of lower strength are also available. If potent fluorinated topical corticosteroids are applied to large areas of the body, especially under occlusion, systemic effects can be observed and psoriasis may be aggravated as with systemic corticosteroids. For small, localized lesions, high-potency corticosteroids, left unoccluded, or flurandrenolide-impregnated tape left on overnight and changed in the morning is effective. Relapse after topical corticosteroids is often faster than with other agents. Rest periods, as suggested above, may prevent relapses and unresponsiveness.

Thick scalp plaques may be difficult to treat. A suspension of 10% salicylic acid in mineral oil or Baker's P and S (a phenol and saline preparation readily available over the counter as a solution or shampoo) may be rubbed in at bedtime with a toothbrush and washed out the next morning with a cosmetically acceptable tar shampoo. A shower cap can be worn in bed to enhance penetration and avoid messiness. Nonresidual corticosteroid alcoholic solutions can be applied during the day.

Resistant skin or scalp patches may respond to *local* superficial injection of triamcinolone acetonide suspension diluted with saline to 2.5 mg/mL, the amount depending on the size of the lesion. Injections should not be repeated more often than every 3 wk, and may cause local atrophy. Systemic corticosteroids are usually contraindicated.

Psoralens and high-intensity ultraviolet A (PUVA) therapy is usually highly effective in treating extensive psoriasis. Oral methoxsalen is followed, at a specific interval, by exposure of the skin to long-wave UV light (330 to 360 nm). The dosage of both the methoxsalen and the UV exposure must be individually tailored. Although the treatment is clean and may produce remissions for several months, repeated treatments with intensive light may increase UV-induced skin cancer (especially in those with either prior arsenic or x-ray therapy or a history of skin cancers). With appropriate precautions, adverse effects on eyes and blood seem minimal. Use of oral retinoids with PUVA decreases the dosage of UV light required to induce remissions.

In severe disabling psoriasis (especially severe psoriatic arthritis or widespread pustular or exfoliative psoriasis that is unresponsive to topical agents or PUVA—see above), the most effective treatment is oral methotrexate. Methotrexate seems to act by interfering with the rapid proliferation of epidermal cells. Because the potential toxicity requires monitoring hematologic, renal, and hepatic function and because dosage regimens vary, *methotrexate therapy should be undertaken only by physicians experienced in its use for psoriasis.*

Etretinate or isotretinoin can be particularly effective for pustular psoriasis. Because of its teratogenic potential and long-term retention in the body, women should be warned against becoming pregnant while taking retinoids and for at least 2 yr after etretinate. In several clinical trials, cyclosporine has been shown to be extremely effective. However, it is not approved for treatment of psoriasis because of its many very serious side effects. Topical and systemic vitamin D_3 are also under study.

PITYRIASIS ROSEA

A self-limited, mild, inflammatory skin disease characterized by scaly lesions, possibly due to an unidentified infectious agent. It may occur at any age but is seen most often in young adults. In temperate climates, incidence is highest during spring and autumn.

Symptoms and Signs

A "herald" or "mother" patch, found most commonly on the trunk, usually precedes the generalized eruption by 5 to 10 days. It is slightly erythematous, rose- or fawn-colored, and circinate or oval; it has a scaly, slightly raised border and resembles a superficial ringworm infection. Many similar lesions 0.5 to 2 cm in diameter follow the herald patch and sometimes continue to appear for weeks, usually on the trunk. On the back, their long axes parallel the lines of cleavage, typically radiating from the spinal column in a "Christmas tree" pattern. In blacks the eruption may be primarily papular, with little scaling.

At times, lesions principally affect the arms, with relative sparing of the trunk. The face is involved occasionally. Rarely, lesions become generalized, sometimes giving a scarlatiniform appearance. Systemic symptoms are usually absent, but slight malaise and headache occur rarely; itching is sometimes troublesome. Though the eruption may persist 2 mo or longer, spontaneous remission within 4 or 5 wk is usual. Recurrences are rare.

Differential Diagnosis

Pityriasis rosea must be differentiated from tinea corporis, tinea versicolor, drug eruptions, psoriasis, and, most important, secondary syphilis. A serologic test for syphilis should be strongly considered.

Treatment

No treatment is specific, and usually none is needed. The patient should be reassured that the lesions will clear. Artificial or natural sunlight may hasten involution. Inflamed lesions and itching may be relieved by 0.25% menthol in a vanishing cream base. Prednisone (10 mg orally qid until the itching subsides, then decreased over 14 days) should be used only for severe itching.

LICHEN PLANUS

A recurrent, pruritic, inflammatory eruption characterized by small discrete angular papules that may coalesce into rough scaly patches, often accompanied by oral lesions. Children are affected infrequently.

Etiology

The cause is unknown. Some drugs (eg, arsenic, bismuth, gold) or exposure to certain color-photography developers may cause an eruption indistinguishable from lichen planus. Quinacrine or quinidine taken for long periods may produce hypertrophic lichen planus of the lower legs and other dermatologic and systemic disturbances.

Symptoms and Signs

Onset may be abrupt or gradual. The initial attack persists weeks or months, and intermittent recurrences may be noted for years.

The primary papules are 2 to 4 mm in diameter, with angular borders, a violaceous color, and a distinct sheen in cross-lighting. Rarely, bullae may develop. Moderate to severe, often refractory, itching may be present. The lesions are usually distributed symmetrically, most commonly on the flexor surfaces of the wrists and on the legs, trunk, glans penis, and oral and vaginal mucosa. Lesions are occasionally generalized, but the face is rarely involved. Particularly on the lower legs, the lesions may become large, scaly, and verrucous (hypertrophic lichen planus). During the acute phase, new papules may appear along a site of minor skin injury such as a superficial scratch (the Koebner phenomenon). Hyperpigmentation (and sometimes atrophy) may develop as lesions persist. Rarely, a patchy scarring alopecia of the scalp appears.

The oral mucosa is involved in about 50% of patients, often before cutaneous lesions develop. The cheek mucosa, tongue margins, and mucosa in edentulous areas show asymptomatic ill-defined, bluish-white linear lesions that may be reticulated at first and increase in size in an angular configuration. An erosive form may occur in which the patient complains of shallow, often painful, recurrent oral ulcerations. Long-standing ulcers may result in mouth cancers. Chronic exacerbations and remissions are common.

Diagnosis

Lichen planus is histologically distinctive. Persistent oral or vaginal lichen planus, with thickening and coalescence of the lesions, may sometimes be difficult to differentiate clinically from leukoplakia. Though always indicated, biopsy may not yield specific findings in old lesions.

Widespread erosive oral lesions must be differentiated from those of candidiasis, leukoplakia, carcinoma, aphthous ulcers, herpetic stomatitis, and erythema multiforme. The peripheries of lesions should be examined for short dendritic extensions and characteristic delicate bluish-white lacy patterns.

Treatment

Asymptomatic lichen planus does not require treatment. If a drug or chemical is suspected as the cause, its use should be discontinued. An antihistamine (eg, hydroxyzine 25 mg or chlorpheniramine 4 mg orally qid) may decrease moderate itching through a sedative effect. Localized pruritic or hypertrophic areas may be treated with triamcinolone acetonide suspension diluted with saline to 2.5 to 5 mg/mL and superficially injected into the lesion, using enough to elevate the lesion slightly (not to be repeated more often than every 3 wk); or with occlusive corticosteroid therapy (eg, triamcinolone acetonide 0.1% cream or equivalent under polyethylene wrapping at bedtime, or flurandrenolide-impregnated tape). Tretinoin 0.1% solution with corticosteroids can also be beneficial in treating lichen planus on glabrous skin. It should be applied with a cotton-tipped applicator at night, followed by tid application of a full-strength corticosteroid cream (see Ch. 88). For erosive oral lesions, viscous lidocaine mouthwashes before meals should be tried.

Erosive oral lesions and widespread severely pruritic skin lesions often require a systemic corticosteroid (eg, oral prednisone 40 to 60 mg every morning initially, with the dose decreased by about one third each week). Unfortunately, itching may return after systemic prednisone has been stopped; in this case, a systemic corticosteroid in continued low dosage given every other morning may be tried. Retinoids (see precautions above, under PSORIASIS) have also been reported to be effective.

The disease tends to be self-limiting but may recur after years.

---

97. INFLAMMATORY REACTIONS OF THE SKIN

(See also PRURITIC URTICARIAL PAPULES AND PLAQUES OF PREGNANCY in Ch. 15)

DRUG ERUPTIONS
(Dermatitis Medicamentosa)

An eruption of the skin or mucous membranes after oral or parenteral drug administration. (See also HYPERSENSITIVITY TO DRUGS in Ch. 34 and ADVERSE DRUG REACTIONS in Ch. 138.)

Etiology

Although most drug eruptions occur through unknown mechanisms, many are due to allergic mechanisms: Specific antibodies to the drug or specifically sensitized lymphocytes may develop during a sensitization period that may be as short as 4 or 5 days after initial drug exposure. A later exposure to the drug results in an eruption that may appear within minutes or not for hours or days. Other reactions may be caused by accumulation of a drug (eg, pigmentation from silver), pharmacologic action of a drug (eg, striae or acne from systemic corticosteroids, purpura from excessive anticoagulation), or interaction with genetic factors (eg, porphyria cutanea tarda from estrogens, which induce an enzyme involved in porphyrin metabolism).

Symptoms and Signs

Drug eruptions vary in severity from a mild rash to toxic epidermal necrolysis. Onset may be sudden (eg, urticaria or angioedema after penicillin) or delayed for hours or days (morbilliform or maculopapular eruptions following penicillin or sulfonamides) or even years (exfoliation or pigmentation from arsenic). The lesions may be localized (fixed drug eruptions, oral ulcerations, or dermatitis in light-exposed areas), but many are generalized.

Some drugs produce characteristic eruptions, but reactions may imitate features of practically any dermatosis. Listed below are the patterns seen most often with some typical causative agents. The drugs added most recently are most likely to be the cause, but drugs taken for long periods must also be suspected.

Urticaria (penicillin, aspirin, tartrazine [the dye FD&C yellow No. 5]) is easily recognized by the typical well-defined edematous wheals.

Morbilliform or maculopapular eruptions (almost any drug, especially barbiturates, sulfonamides, ampicillin, and other antibiotics) range in appearance from measleslike to an eruption resembling pityriasis rosea.

Mucocutaneous eruptions (penicillin, barbiturates, sulfonamides, including derivatives used in hypertension and diabetes mellitus) vary from a few small oral vesicles or urticaria-like skin lesions to painful oral ulcerations with widespread bullous skin lesions (see ERYTHEMA MULTIFORME and the Stevens-Johnson syndrome, below).

Acneiform eruptions (corticosteroids, iodides, bromides, hydantoins) resemble acne but lack comedones and usually begin suddenly.

Toxic epidermal necrolysis (barbiturates, hydantoins, penicillin, sulfonamides) is characterized by large areas of loosened, easily detached epidermis that give the skin a scalded appearance (see TOXIC EPIDERMAL NECROLYSIS, below). It may be fatal. A similar condition in infants, young children, and immunosuppressed patients is caused by a specific staphylococcal infection (scalded skin syndrome—see Ch. 91).

Exfoliative dermatitis (penicillin, sulfonamides) is characterized by redness, scaling, and thickening of the entire skin surface; it, too, may be fatal (see in Ch. 90).

Photosensitivity eruptions (phenothiazines, tetracyclines, sulfonamides, chlorothiazide, artificial sweeteners) appear as areas of dermatitis or gray-blue hyperpigmentation (phenothiazines and minocycline) on skin exposed to the sun.

Fixed drug eruptions (phenolphthalein, tetracycline, sulfonamides) are frequently isolated, well-circumscribed, dusky red or purple lesions on the skin or mucous membranes (especially of the genitals) that reappear at the same sites each time the drug is taken.

Lichenoid or lichen-planus–like eruptions (antimalarials, gold, chlorpromazine, thiazides) are angular papules that coalesce into scaly patches (see LICHEN PLANUS in Ch. 96).

Purpuric eruptions (chlorothiazide, meprobamate, anticoagulants) are nonblanching purple macules that vary in size but are usually tiny. Most common on the lower extremities, they may occur anywhere and may indicate a more serious purpuric vasculitis.

Erythema nodosum (sulfonamides, oral contraceptives, iodides, bromides) is described in this chapter, below.

Diagnosis and Treatment

Identification of the causative agent is essential. A detailed history is often required, with persistent inquiry about all drugs, including OTC drugs used for sleep, pain, colds, constipation, and headache, and the use of eyedrops, nosedrops, and suppositories. It is important to remember that some eruptions start after the drug has been stopped (eg, ampicillin), some continue for weeks or months after the drug is stopped, and minute amounts of some drugs may produce a reaction.

Most drug reactions resolve when the offending drug is stopped and require no further therapy. Often, and especially in hospitalized patients who take many drugs, all but life-sustaining drugs must be discontinued and each reinstituted in order of importance at weekly intervals. A physician well versed in the incidence and types of drug eruptions can often withhold the most likely offender and continue the other drugs. When offending or suspected drugs are necessary, chemically unrelated compounds should be substituted when possible.

No laboratory tests are available to aid diagnosis, although lymphocyte transformation and penicillin skin tests are under study. Sensitivity can be confirmed only by readministration of the drug, which may be hazardous.

A lubricant (eg, white petrolatum) may be used for a dry, itching maculopapular eruption. A topical fluorinated corticosteroid ointment (see

Ch. 88) should also be applied in one small area qid and, if effective, applied to the entire eruption. Disabling acute urticaria may require aqueous epinephrine (1:1000) 0.2 mL s.c. or IM, or the slower-acting but more persistent soluble hydrocortisone 100 mg IV, which may be followed by an oral corticosteroid for a short period. For treatment of some serious drug reactions (eg, severe erythema multiforme or the Stevens-Johnson syndrome), see below.

TOXIC EPIDERMAL NECROLYSIS (TEN)

A life-threatening skin disease in which the epidermis peels off in sheets, leaving widespread denuded areas. It most often occurs in adults and usually represents a drug reaction or is idiopathic.

Etiology

In about ¹/₃ of cases, the cause is a drug: Sulfonamides, barbiturates, NSAIDs, phenytoin, allopurinol, and penicillin have been associated with many cases, while numerous other drugs have been implicated in single cases. In about ¹/₃ of cases, the cause is unclear because of noncomitant serious disease (eg, graft-vs.-host disease) and treatment with drugs. In most of the remaining cases, the cause is unknown.

Symptoms and Signs

TEN typically begins with painful localized erythema that disseminates rapidly. At the sites of erythema, flaccid blisters occur or the epidermis peels off. It may peel off in large sheets with gentle touching or pulling. Malaise, chills, myalgias, and fever accompany the denudation. Widespread areas of erosion, including all mucous membranes (eyes, mouth, genitalia) occur within 24 to 72 h and the patient may become gravely ill. Affected areas of skin often look like second-degree burns. Mortality is caused by fluid and electrolyte imbalance, multiorgan sequelae (eg, pneumonia, GI bleeding), and infection.

Diagnosis

Rapid diagnosis is important so that a possibly offending drug can be stopped. Before widespread erythema and epidermal denudation occur, it may be difficult to distinguish TEN from other morbilliform drug eruptions or erythema multiforme and Stevens-Johnson syndrome. TEN is often thought to be a continuum of the latter 2

diseases. Although TEN closely resembles staphylococcal scalded skin syndrome (SSSS), differentiation from SSSS is facilitated by the patient's age, by the clinical setting, and by defining the level of the epidermal split by biopsy, as described under SSSS in Ch. 91.

Treatment

Patients should be hospitalized; excellent nursing care and close observation are essential. *Potentially responsible or suspected drugs should be stopped immediately.* Patients should be isolated to minimize exogenous infection and managed as those with severe burns (see also Ch. 114) by protecting the skin and denuded areas from trauma and infection and replacing fluid and electrolyte losses.

Though their use is controversial, systemic corticosteroids have successfully stopped "allergic" drug reactions, especially early in the course of disease. Some severe cases require from 0.5 to 1.0 gm of methylprednisolone IV for several days to reverse the process. This type of steroid therapy has been associated with many adverse effects and should be given under well-controlled conditions. Corticosteroids often seem to enhance gram-negative or other sepsis (without improving the skin) and increase the mortality rate. Septicemia, which often occurs with pulmonary infections, must be recognized and treated promptly, for it is the most common cause of death. Ophthalmologic consultation is often required, as there may be considerable crusting of the conjunctiva. To prevent phimosis, urologic consultation may also be necessary.

ERYTHEMA MULTIFORME (EM)

(Erythema Multiforme Exudativum or Bullosum)

An inflammatory eruption characterized by symmetric erythematous, edematous, or bullous lesions of the skin or mucous membranes.

Etiology

No cause can be found in > 50% of cases. In the rest, drugs and infectious diseases (eg, herpes simplex [probably the most commonly found causative agent], coxsackie- and echoviruses, *Mycoplasma pneumoniae,* psittacosis, and histoplasmosis) are usually implicated. Vaccinia, BCG, and poliomyelitis vaccines have also induced EM. Almost any drug can cause EM; penicillin, sulfonamides, and barbiturates are the most common causes. The mechanism by which infectious agents or drugs cause the condition is unknown, but it apparently is a hypersensitivity reaction.

Symptoms, Signs, and Diagnosis

Onset is usually sudden, with erythematous macules or papules, or wheals, vesicles, and sometimes bullae, appearing mainly on the distal portion of the extremities, including the palms and soles, and on the face; hemorrhagic lesions of the lips and oral mucosa can also occur (see ORAL ERYTHEMA MULTIFORME in Ch. 107). The skin lesions (target or iris lesions) are symmetric in distribution and often annular, with concentric rings and a central purpura—a grayish discoloration of the epidermis—or vesicle. Itching is variable. Systemic symptoms vary; malaise, arthralgia, and fever are frequent. Attacks that last 2 to 4 wk and recur in the fall and spring for several years are sometimes seen.

Stevens-Johnson syndrome is *a severe form of EM characterized by bullae on the oral mucosa, pharynx, anogenital region, and conjunctiva.* Typical EM lesions may or may not be present elsewhere on the skin. The patient who may be unable to eat or close his mouth properly will drool continually. The eyes may become very painful; conjunctivitis with swelling and pus may make it impossible for the patient to open them. The conjunctival lesions may leave residual corneal scarring. The condition is occasionally fatal.

The skin lesions of EM must be distinguished from bullous pemphigoid and dermatitis herpetiformis; the oral lesions from allergic stomatitis, pemphigus, and herpetic stomatitis.

Treatment

When a cause can be found, it should be treated, eliminated, or avoided. Some cases of EM are associated with mycoplasmal pneumonia and should be treated with a tetracycline. Local treatment depends on the type of lesion. Simple erythema often needs no treatment. Vesicles and bullous or erosive lesions can be treated with intermittent tap-water compresses. Cheilitis and stomatitis of EM may require special care (see ORAL ERYTHEMA MULTIFORME under STOMATITIS in Ch. 107). Systemic corticosteroids (see DRUG ERUPTIONS, above, and Treatment under ORAL ERYTHEMA MULTIFORME in Ch. 107) are not routinely used; however, they have been beneficial in severe EM (if used early) and in chronic EM. Their use is controversial. Some patients, especially those with severe mouth and throat lesions, seem to succumb more readily to fatal respiratory infections if treated with systemic corticosteroids. Intensive systemic antibiotics (as indicated by culture and sensitivity), fluids, and electrolytes may be lifesaving in patients with extensive mucous membrane lesions. If frequent or severe EM is preceded by herpes simplex, acyclovir 200 mg orally 3 or 5 times daily is effective in preventing most attacks, but its long-term effects are unknown.

ERYTHEMA NODOSUM

An inflammatory disease of the skin and subcutaneous tissue characterized by tender red nodules, predominantly in the pretibial region, but occasionally involving the arms or other areas.

Resembling a bruise, the nodules gradually change from pink to bluish to brown. Fever and arthralgia are frequent, hilar adenopathy less frequent. The condition is most common in young adults and may recur for months or years.

Erythema nodosum in children is most commonly caused by URIs, especially from streptococci; in adults, streptococcal infections and sarcoidosis are the most common causes. Less common causes (except in locales where the underlying disease is endemic) include leprosy, coccidioidomycosis, histoplasmosis, primary TB, psittacosis, lymphogranuloma venereum, and ulcerative colitis. The condition can also be a reaction to drugs (sulfonamides, iodides, bromides, oral contraceptives). A prolonged search for systemic infection or causative drug may be required, and in many cases no cause can be determined. An elevated RBC sedimentation rate is the most common laboratory finding.

Treatment

Bed rest helps to relieve painful nodules. If an underlying streptococcal infection is suspected, antibiotic therapy is beneficial (eg, penicillin long-term—at least 1 yr). If symptoms are severe without evidence of underlying infection or drug etiology, aspirin may be helpful, although the lesions often recur. When there are few lesions, intralesional triamcinolone acetonide (2.5 to 5 mg/mL) may provide symptomatic relief. Systemic corticosteroids, often the only means of controlling the lesions, reduce the lesions but may mask an underlying systemic disease.

GRANULOMA ANNULARE

A benign, chronic dermatosis of unknown etiology characterized by papules or nodules that spread peripherally to form a ring with normal or slightly depressed skin in the center. The lesions are yellowish or the color of the surrounding skin, and one or more may be present. They are usually asymptomatic and are usually present on the feet, legs, hands, or fingers. The condition may be seen in children or adults. It is not associated with systemic diseases, except that the incidence of diabetes mellitus is increased among adults with many lesions. In about 5% of cases, exposure to sunlight has brought out showers of lesions. Spontaneous resolution is common. In addition to reassurance and explanation of the benign nature of the disease, high-strength topical corticosteroids under occlusion every night, corticosteroid-containing tape, or intralesional corticosteroids (see Ch. 88) may hasten involution of the disease.

98. BULLOUS DISEASES

(See also HERPES GESTATIONIS in Ch. 15)

PEMPHIGUS

An uncommon, potentially fatal, autoimmune skin disorder characterized by intraepidermal bullae on apparently healthy skin and mucous membranes.

Etiology and Incidence

Pemphigus, rare in children, usually occurs in middle-aged or elderly persons. Foci of high incidence occur in South America, especially Brazil. In the active stage, the serum and skin contain readily demonstrable IgG antibodies (**Abs**) that bind at the site of epidermal damage. These Abs can induce the same pathologic process in vivo and in vitro.

Symptoms and Signs

The primary lesions are bullae of various sizes. They often occur first in the mouth, where they soon rupture and remain as chronic, often painful, erosions for variable periods of time before the skin is affected. On the skin, the bullae typically arise from normal-appearing skin to leave a raw, denuded area and crusting when they rupture later. The extent of both skin and mucosal involvement varies (eg, lesions may occur in the oropharynx and upper esophagus). Itching is usually absent.

In some superficial varieties (eg, pemphigus foliaceus), bullae may not be prominent and usually are absent from the mouth. The process may resemble exfoliative dermatitis, psoriasis, a drug eruption, or many other forms of dermatitis. The lesions may be localized to the face and may suggest a combination of seborrheic dermatitis and cutaneous LE.

Diagnosis

Pemphigus should be suspected in any bullous disorder or chronic mucosal ulceration. It must be differentiated from all other chronic ulcerative oral lesions and from other bullous dermatoses (eg, bullous pemphigoid, benign mucosal pemphigoid, drug eruptions, toxic epidermal necrolysis, erythema multiforme, dermatitis herpetiformis, and bullous contact dermatitis). In pemphigus the epidermis is easily detached from the underlying skin (**Nikolsky's sign**), and biopsy usually shows typical suprabasal epidermal cell separation. In pemphigus foliaceus, the separation occurs within the most superficial part of the epidermis. A Tzanck test (see SPECIAL DIAGNOSTIC METHODS in Ch. 87) is frequently diagnostic when one does a Wright's or Giemsa stain on a smear of cells obtained by scraping the base of a lesion. The acantholytic cells typical of pemphigus are unattached and basal-cell–like, with large centrally placed nuclei and condensed cytoplasm. Direct immunofluorescence (**IF**) tests of perilesional skin or mucous membranes are most reliable and invariably show IgG on the epidermal or epithelial cell surfaces. Indirect IF tests usually show pemphigus Abs in the patient's serum, even when the lesions are localized in the mouth. The Ab titer may correlate with the severity of the disease.

Treatment

The aim of treatment, both immediate and subsequent, is to stop the eruption of new lesions. Specific therapy depends upon the extent and severity of disease: The mainstay is systemic corticosteroids. Some patients with few lesions may respond to low oral doses of prednisone (eg, 20 to 30 mg/day), but most ultimately require higher doses. Patients whose disease is not extensive may be treated as outpatients with a starting oral dose of 60 to 80 mg/day.

Hospitalization and large dosage of corticosteroids are indicated for patients with widespread disease because the condition is potentially fatal if inadequately treated. The initial dose of oral prednisone, 30 to 40 mg bid (or equivalent), should be doubled if new lesions continue to appear after 5 to 7 days. Very high dosages may be necessary to induce the cessation of new lesions. Skin infections should be treated with systemic antibiotics. Reverse isolation procedures may be required. Generous use of talc on patient and sheets may prevent oozing skin from adhering to the sheets, or hydrocolloid dressings may be useful. Silver sulfadiazine cream can be used on erosions to prevent secondary infection.

Corticosteroid dosage should be decreased gradually when no new lesions have appeared for 7 to 10 days, with a total daily dose given every morning at first, then every other morning. The maintenance dosage should be as low as possible. It may be possible, usually after months or years, to discontinue maintenance therapy if no new lesions appear during a trial of several weeks without treatment. Methotrexate, cyclophosphamide, azathioprine, and IM gold have been used successfully, either alone or with corticosteroids, to avoid the undesirable effects of long-term use of corticosteroids, but each carries its own serious risks. Because these drugs are thought to be "steroid sparing," some authorities advocate using one concurrently with a corticosteroid. Plasmapheresis combined with an immunosuppressive to reduce Ab titers has been an effective therapy in a few patients.

BULLOUS PEMPHIGOID

A chronic, benign bullous eruption seen chiefly in the elderly. It is considered an autoimmune disease because Abs directed against the basement membrane zone of the epidermis (the site of histologic damage) are usually found in the serum and skin.

Symptoms and Signs

Characteristic tense bullae develop on normal-appearing or reddened skin, sometimes accompanied by annular, dusky-red, edematous lesions with or without tiny peripheral vesicles. Occasionally, rapidly healing oral lesions are seen. Itching is common, usually without other symp-

toms. As in many other bullous diseases, subepidermal blisters are usually found on biopsy.

Diagnosis

The disease must be differentiated from pemphigus, erythema multiforme, drug eruptions, benign mucosal pemphigoid, dermatitis herpetiformis, and acquired epidermolysis bullosa. Finding serum Abs to the basement membrane zone on an *indirect* immunofluorescence (IF) test is usually diagnostic. Abs or complement, or both, are bound to the basement membrane zone of perilesional skin in the *direct* IF test.

Treatment

The eruption usually improves with oral prednisone 40 to 60 mg every morning. The dose can be tapered slowly to a maintenance level after several weeks. Because of the burden of side effects, occasional new lesions in the elderly should be disregarded (rather than increasing the prednisone dosage, as in pemphigus). In trials, the corticosteroid dosage has been reduced by giving azathioprine adjunctively.

DERMATITIS HERPETIFORMIS

A chronic eruption characterized by clusters of intensely pruritic vesicles, papules, and urticaria-like lesions.

This disease occurs mainly in patients 15 to 60 yr old; rarely in blacks and Orientals. Several immunologic abnormalities have been shown, including IgA deposits in almost all normal-appearing and perilesional skin. Asymptomatic gluten-sensitive enteropathy is found in 75 to 90% of patients and in some of their relatives. There is also an increased incidence of thyroid disease. NSAIDs may exacerbate the disease even when the symptoms are well controlled with sulfone therapy.

Symptoms, Signs, and Diagnosis

Onset is usually gradual. Tiny vesicles, papules, and urticaria-like lesions appear, usually distributed symmetrically on extensor aspects (elbows, knees, sacrum, buttocks, occiput). Vesicles and papules, common on the face and neck, occur in about 1/3 of patients. Itching and burning are severe, and scratching often obscures the primary lesions.

The typical histopathologic picture is seen only in early lesions: In the dermal papillary tips, neutrophils infiltrate microvesicles. Direct IF tests for

IgA deposition in the dermal papillary tips in normal-appearing and perilesional skin are always positive and provide an important diagnostic aid.

Treatment

Dapsone 50 mg orally bid or tid usually relieves symptoms within 1 or 2 days and improves the rash; dramatic relief in itching is seen in 1 to 3 days. If there is no improvement, up to 100 mg qid can be given by increasing the dose weekly. Most patients can be maintained eventually on 50 to 150 mg/day. Although less effective, sulfapyridine may be used as an alternative; initial oral dosage is 2 to 4 gm/day and maintenance dosage is 1 to 2 gm/day. Strict adherence to a gluten-free diet for prolonged periods may control the disease in some patients, obviating or reducing the requirement for drug therapy.

Patients receiving dapsone or sulfapyridine should have a baseline and weekly CBC for 4 wk, then q 2 to 3 wk for 8 wk, and q 12 to 16 wk thereafter, since hematologic changes are the most common side effects. CNS or liver toxicity occurs rarely. If considerable hemolysis occurs or if the patient has significant cardiopulmonary problems due to dapsone therapy, sulfapyridine should be used, as usually it does not induce significant hemolysis.

99. DISORDERS OF CORNIFICATION

ICHTHYOSIS
(Dry Skin; Xeroderma)

Skin texture is genetically determined: Several ichthyotic skin diseases are inherited; ichthyosis is a symptom in several rare hereditary syndromes and in several systemic disorders.

1. **Xeroderma,** the mildest form, is neither congenital nor associated with systemic abnormalities. It usually occurs on the lower legs of middle-aged or older patients, most often in cold weather and in patients who bathe frequently. There may be mild to moderate itching and an associated dermatitis due to detergents or other irritants.

2. The **inherited ichthyoses,** all characterized by excessive accumulation of scale on the skin surface, are classified according to clinical, genetic, and histologic criteria (see TABLE 99—1).

3. Ichthyosis is a characteristic of **Refsum's syndrome** (a hereditary ataxia with polyneuritic changes and deafness), and of **Sjögren-Larsson syndrome** (hereditary mental deficiency and spastic paralysis); both syndromes are autosomal recessive.

4. Asymptomatic ichthyosis occurs in some systemic diseases (eg, leprosy, hypothyroidism, lymphoma, AIDS) and may be an early manifestation. The dry scaling may be fine and localized to the trunk and legs, or it may be thick and widespread. In sarcoidosis, a thick scaling may appear on the legs, and a biopsy usually shows the typical granulomas. In other systemic diseases, biopsy of ichthyotic skin is not diagnostic.

Treatment

In any ichthyosis, an emollient—preferably plain petrolatum or mineral oil—should be applied bid and especially after bathing (for 10 min to hydrate the stratum corneum), while the skin is still wet. Blotting dry with a towel will then remove undesirable excess oil. To remove the scale in ichthyosis vulgaris, lamellar ichthyosis, and sex-linked ichthyosis, a particularly effective agent contains 6% salicylic acid in a gel composed of propylene glycol, ethyl alcohol, hydroxypropylene cellulose, and water. It should be applied bid and at bedtime after hydration of the skin, and covered overnight with an occlusive dressing (eg, thin plastic film or bags). In children, it should be applied only bid and should not be occluded. After scaling has decreased, only occasional application is required. Other useful agents include 50% propylene glycol in water, hydrophilic petrolatum and water (in equal parts), and cold cream and the -hydroxy acids (eg, lactic and pyruvic) in various bases. In lamellar ichthyosis, 0.1% tretinoin (vitamin A acid; retinoic acid) cream is effective.

Soaps should be used only in intertriginous areas. Hexachlorophene products should not be used, because absorption and toxicity are increased.

Patients with epidermolytic hyperkeratosis (bullous ichthyosis) may need long-term cloxacillin 250 mg orally tid or qid or oral erythromycin (in the same dosage) as long as thick intertriginous scaling is present to prevent formation of painful, foul-smelling pustules. Regular use of soaps containing chlorhexidine may also reduce the bacteria. Lubrication may slightly improve ichthyosis

TABLE 99–1. CLINICAL AND GENETIC FEATURES OF SOME INHERITED ICHTHYOSES

Disorder	Inheritance Pattern and Prevalence	Onset	Type of Scale	Distribution	Associated Clinical Findings	Histology
Ichthyosis vulgaris	Autosomal dominant 1:300	Childhood	Fine	Usually back and extensor surfaces; spares flexors; usually many markings on palms and soles	Atopy; keratosis pilaris	May be diagnostic
X-linked ichthyosis	X-linked 1:6000 (males)	Birth or infancy	Large, dark (may be fine)	Prominent on neck and trunk; normal palms and soles	Corneal opacities	May be diagnostic*
Lamellar ichthyosis (nonbullous congenital ichthyosiform erythroderma; "collodion baby")	Autosomal recessive 1:300,000	Birth	Large, coarse	Most of body; thick palms and soles	Ectropion	Diagnostic
Epidermolytic hyperkeratosis (bullous congenital ichthyosiform erythroderma)	Autosomal dominant 1:300,000	Birth	Thick, warty	Most of body; especially warty in flexural creases	Blisters	Diagnostic

*These patients have been shown to have a steroid sulfatase enzyme deficiency.

due to an underlying systemic disease, but remarkable improvement follows if the primary disease can be corrected. The most effective therapies for most of the ichthyoses are oral synthetic retinoids. Etretinate (see precautions under PSORIASIS in Ch. 96) is effective in epidermolytic hyperkeratosis, ichthyosis vulgaris, and X-linked ichthyosis. Isotretinoin is more effective than etretinate in lamellar ichthyosis. The lowest dosage possible should be used. Long-term (≥ 1 yr) treatment with isotretinoin has resulted in bony exostoses in some patients, and other long-term side effects may arise. (CAUTION: *Oral retinoids are absolutely contraindicated in pregnancy.*)

KERATOSIS PILARIS

A common disorder of keratinization in which horny plugs fill the orifices of hair follicles. Multiple small, pointed keratotic papules appear mainly on the lateral aspects of the upper arms, thighs, and buttocks. Facial lesions may also occur, particularly in children. Lesions are most prominent in cold weather and usually improve in the summer. The cause is unknown, but it is often an autosomal dominant inheritance. The problem is chiefly cosmetic. Treatment is usually unnecessary and often unsatisfactory. Hydrophilic petrolatum and water (in equal parts), cold cream, or petrolatum with 3% salicylic acid added may help to flatten the lesions. The 6% salicylic acid gel (described for the treatment of ichthyosis), the buffered lactic acid lotions, or 0.1% tretinoin cream may also be very effective.

CALLUS; CORN
(Tyloma; Heloma)

Callus: *A superficial circumscribed area of hyperkeratosis at a site of repeated trauma.* Corn: *A painful conical hyperkeratosis, found principally over toe joints and between toes.*

Calluses and corns are caused by pressure and friction, usually over a bony prominence. Cal-

luses are usually found on the hands or feet but may occur elsewhere, especially in a person whose occupation entails repeated trauma to a particular area (eg, the mandible and clavicle in a violinist). Corns are pea-sized or slightly larger and occur on the feet. Hard corns occur over prominent protuberances, especially on the toes; soft corns occur between the toes. Corns may ache spontaneously or be tender on pressure.

Diagnosis

A callus may be differentiated from a plantar wart by trimming away the horny skin. A wart (see also in Ch. 94) will appear sharply circumscribed, sometimes with soft macerated tissue or with central black dots resulting from thrombosed capillaries, and paring it will cause pinpoint bleeding. A callus shows only heaped-up keratin, and skin markings are preserved. A corn, when pared, shows a sharply outlined translucent core that interrupts the normal papillary line.

Prophylaxis and Treatment

Prophylaxis is important. Completely eliminating undue pressure on the affected site may not be practicable, but pressure should be reduced and redistributed when possible. For foot lesions, soft, well-fitting shoes are important, and pads or rings of suitable shapes and sizes, moleskin or foam-rubber protective bandages, arch inserts, or metatarsal plates or bars may help to redistribute the pressure.

The hyperkeratotic tissue may be removed with keratolytic agents (eg, 17% salicylic acid in collodion or 40% salicylic acid plasters—taking care to avoid applying the agent to normal skin), or with a nail file. A pumice stone, used while the patient is in a bath, is often most practical. Salicylic acid plasters can be used on calluses anywhere.

Patients with a tendency to calluses and corns may need the regular services of a podiatrist, and those with impaired peripheral circulation, especially if associated with diabetes mellitus, require special care.

100. PRESSURE SORES
(Bedsore; Decubitus Ulcer; Trophic Ulcer)

Ischemic necrosis and ulceration of tissues overlying a bony prominence that has been subjected to prolonged pressure against an external object (eg, bed, wheelchair, cast, splint). It oc-

curs most often in patients with diminished or absent sensation, or who are debilitated, emaciated, paralyzed (eg, from spinal cord injuries or degenerative neurologic diseases), or long bedridden. Tissues over the sacrum, ischia, greater trochanters, external malleoli, and heels are especially susceptible; other sites may be involved, depending on the patient's position. Decubitus ulcers can affect muscle and bone as well as superficial tissues.

Etiology

Intrinsic factors that precipitate pressure sores include loss of pain and pressure sensations (which ordinarily prompt the patient to shift position and relieve the pressure) and the thinness of fat and muscle padding between bony weight-bearing prominences and the skin. Disuse atrophy, malnutrition, anemia, and infection play contributory roles. In a paralyzed extremity, loss of vasomotor control leads to a lowering of tone in the vascular bed and a lowered circulatory rate. Spasticity, especially in patients with spinal cord injuries, can place a shearing force on the blood vessels to further compromise circulation.

The most important of the **extrinsic factors** is pressure. Its force and duration directly determine the extent of the ulcer. Pressure severe enough to impair local circulation can occur within hours in an immobilized patient, causing local tissue anoxia that progresses, if unrelieved, to necrosis of the skin and subcutaneous tissues. The pressure is due to infrequent shifting of the patient's position; friction and irritation from ill-adjusted supports or wrinkled bedding or clothing may be contributory. Moisture, which may result from perspiration or from urinary or fecal incontinence, leads to tissue maceration and predisposes to pressure sores.

Symptoms, Signs, and Course

The stages of decubitus ulcer formation correspond to tissue layers. **Stage 1** consists of skin redness that blanches or disappears on pressure; the skin and underlying tissues are still soft. **Stage 2** shows redness, edema, and induration, at times with epidermal blistering or desquamation. In **stage 3**, the skin becomes necrotic with exposure of fat and drainage from the wound. In **stage 4**, necrosis extends through the skin and fat to muscle; further fat and muscle necrosis characterizes **stage 5**. In **stage 6**, bone destruction begins, with periostitis and osteitis, progressing finally to osteomyelitis, *with the possibility of septic arthritis, pathologic fracture, and septicemia.*

Prophylaxis

The best treatment for pressure sores is prevention. *Pressure on sensitive areas must be relieved.* Unless a full-flotation bed (water bed) is used to provide even distribution of the patient's weight through hydrostatic buoyancy, the bedridden patient's position must be changed at least q 2 h until tolerance for longer periods can be demonstrated (by the absence of redness). Air-filled alternating-pressure mattresses, sponge-rubber "egg-crate" mattresses, and silicone gel or water mattresses decrease pressure on sensitive areas but do not negate the need for position changes q 2 h. A turning (Stryker) frame facilitates turning patients with cord injuries. Protective padding (eg, sheepskin or a synthetic equivalent) at bony prominences should be used under braces or plaster casts, and at potential pressure sites a window should be cut out of the cast. A wheelchair patient must be able to shift his position every 10 to 15 min even if he is using a pressure-relieving pillow. Otherwise, patients in chairs may be more likely to have pressure sores than those who are in bed.

Skin inspection in adequate light is important. Pressure points should be checked for erythema or trauma at least once/day. Able patients, mobile or immobile, and their families must be taught a routine of daily visual inspection and palpation of sites for potential ulcer formation. Exquisite skin care for neurologically damaged parts is necessary to prevent maceration and secondary infection. Lying on a sheepskin helps to keep the patient's skin in good condition and minimize decubiti. Protective padding, pillows, or a sheepskin can be used to separate body surfaces.

Maintaining **cleanliness and dryness** helps to prevent maceration. Bedclothes should be changed frequently, with use of sheets that are soft, clean, and free from wrinkles and particulate matter. Essential hygienic measures include sponging the skin in hot weather and thorough drying after baths. Special efforts are required when patients are incontinent of urine or feces.

Oversedation should be avoided and activity encouraged. Physiotherapy, when practicable, may be carried out by means of passive and active exercises. Hydrotherapy is also valuable. The special activated mattresses mentioned above or ones filled with fluids or tiny spheres seem very useful but are expensive.

A well-balanced diet, high in protein, is important.

Threatened pressure sores (stages 1 and 2) require energetic use of all the above prophylactic measures to prevent necrosis. The area should be kept exposed, free from pressure, and dry. Stimulating the circulation by gentle massage can accelerate healing.

Treatment

The major problem in treating decubitus ulcer is that the ulcer is like an iceberg, a small visible surface with an extensive unknown base, and there is no good method to determine the extent of tissue damage. Ulcers that have not advanced beyond stage 3 may heal spontaneously if the pressure is removed and the area is small. New hydrophilic gels and dressings speed healing.

Stage 4 ulcers require debridement; some may also require deeper surgery. When the ulcers are filled with pus and necrotic debris, application of dextranomer beads or other and newer hydrophilic polymers may hasten debridement without surgery. Conservative debridement of necrotic tissue with forceps and scissors should be instituted. Some debridement may be done by cleansing the wound with 1.5% hydrogen peroxide. Wet dressings of water (especially whirlpool baths) will assist in debriding. The granulation that follows removal of necrotic tissue may be satisfactory for skin grafts to cover small areas.

More advanced ulcers with fat and muscle involvement require surgical debridement and closure. Affected bone tissue requires surgical removal; disarticulation of a joint may be needed. A sliding full-thickness skin flap graft is the closure of choice, especially over large bony prominences (eg, the trochanters, ischia, and sacrum), since scar tissue cannot develop the tolerance to pressure that is needed.

For spreading cellulitis, a penicillinase-resistant penicillin or a cephalosporin is necessary.

Many new dressings and topical agents are being tested and made available for use. No one powder, gel, or dressing is universally superior. The subject is complex; ie, some are wet and lead to *Pseudomonas* infection if used too long, others are painful, all are expensive, and some are of little value. Treatment of skin ulcers requires caution and education about the specific properties and precise method of use of these agents.

101. PIGMENTARY DISORDERS

HYPOPIGMENTATION

A congenital or acquired decrease in melanin production.

Albinism: *A rare autosomal recessive inherited disorder in which melanocytes are present but do not form melanin.* The hair is white, the skin pale, and the eyes pink; nystagmus and errors of refraction are common. Albinos sunburn easily and frequently develop skin cancers. They should avoid sunlight, use sunglasses, and during daylight hours apply on uncovered skin a sunscreen with a sun protection factor (SPF) of ≥ 15.

Vitiligo: *An absence of melanocytes, causing hypopigmented areas, usually sharply demarcated and often symmetric, and varying from 1 or 2 spots to near universality.* The hair in vitiliginous areas is usually white, and the lesions are chalk white under Wood's light. Lesions are prone to sunburn. The cause is unknown; although vitiligo usually is acquired, it is sometimes familial (autosomal dominant, with incomplete penetrance and variable expression) or may follow unusual physical trauma, especially of the head. The association of vitiligo with Addison's disease, diabetes mellitus, pernicious anemia, and thyroid dysfunction, as well as a high incidence of serum antibodies (Abs) to thyroglobulin, adrenal cells, and parietal cells, has led to a postulated immunologic and neurochemical basis. Abs to melanin have been shown in some patients. **Treatment** is for the cosmetic disfigurement. Small lesions may be camouflaged with cosmetic creams or tanning solutions that do not wipe off on clothing and may last for several days. Sunscreens with an SPF ≥ 15 are required to protect against sunburn. Oral and topical psoralens with ultraviolet A (PUVA) have been used, but the treatment is protracted and results vary. Cover-up cosmetics are much more satisfactory for most patients when cure is doubtful.

Postinflammatory hypopigmentation follows healing of certain inflammatory disorders (especially bullous dermatoses), burns, and skin infections, and appears in scars and atrophic skin. The skin may not be ivory-white as in vitiligo, and spontaneous repigmentation may eventually occur. Cover-up cosmetics (eg, leg makeup) or solutions are most satisfactory.

HYPERPIGMENTATION

Increased melanin deposition resulting in hyperpigmentation may be a sign of hormonal changes (eg, in Addison's disease, pregnancy, or use of anovulatory pills). Darkening may also result from increased melanogenesis (eg, in hemochromatosis) or from silver deposits (eg, in argyria).

Melasma (chloasma), dark brown, sharply marginated, roughly symmetric patches of pigmentation on the face (usually on the forehead, temples, and malar prominences), occurs mainly during pregnancy (melasma gravidarum, the "mask of pregnancy") and in women taking anovulatory hormones. It may also occur idiopathically in nonpregnant women and in dark-skinned men. Exposure to sunlight accentuates the pigmentation. In women, the darkening fades somewhat after childbirth, on cessation of the hormone, and with time. Treatment with 2 to 4% hydroquinone in an alcoholic glycol or cream base applied bid may decrease the pigmentation. Hydroquinone should be tested behind one ear for a week before it is used on the face, since it may cause dermatitis. Sequential use of topical 0.1% tretinoin will enhance the effect of hydroquinone. The patient must use an SPF $\geq$ 15 sunscreen over the hyperpigmented areas when outdoors and should avoid excessive exposure to the sun if the bleaching is to work. Only melanosis can be lightened. Dermal pigmentation is unaffected. Long-term application (years) of hydroquinone has, rarely, caused local ochronosis.

102. DISORDERS OF SWEATING

MILIARIA
(Prickly Heat)

An acute inflammatory pruritic eruption due to retained extravasated sweat. Because of duct obstruction and inflammation, sweat fails to reach the skin surface; instead, it is trapped in the epidermis or dermis where it causes irritation (prickling) and often severe itching. The typical minute lesions are vesicular if obstruction is superficial (miliaria crystallina) or red if inflammation is deeper (miliaria rubra). Miliaria is usually seen in warm humid weather, but it may occur in cool weather if the patient is overdressed. Treatment is symptomatic and prophylactic: It includes cooling and drying the involved areas and avoiding conditions that may induce sweating. Air conditioning is ideal. Corticosteroid lotions, sometimes with 0.25% menthol added, are often used; however, any topical therapy is less effective than a change of environment and clothing.

HYPERHIDROSIS

Excessive perspiration due to overactivity of the sweat glands. It may be general or confined to the palms, soles, axillae, inframammary regions, or groin. The skin in affected areas is often pink or bluish white. In severe cases, the skin, especially on the feet, may be macerated, fis-sured, and scaling. Bromhidrosis is *a condition in which there is a fetid odor of the skin caused by decomposition of the sweat and cellular debris by bacteria and yeasts.*

Increased hydration of the skin may be a contributing factor in various skin diseases (fungal or pyogenic infections; contact dermatitis). Generalized hyperhidrosis frequently accompanies fever. An endocrine dysfunction (eg, hyperthyroidism) or, occasionally, a CNS disorder may also cause generalized sweating. The cause of localized hyperhidrosis is unknown; it usually occurs in otherwise healthy individuals. Excessive sweating of the palms and soles may be psychogenic.

Treatment

For generalized hyperhidrosis, the underlying systemic disease must be treated. The hyperhidrosis may be refractory. Side effects make parasympatholytic agents impractical, and the effect of sympathectomy usually is only temporary.

For localized hyperhidrosis, aluminum chloride as a 20% solution of aluminum chloride hexahydrate in absolute ethyl alcohol, applied at night to the dried axillae, palms, or soles and covered tightly with a thin polyethylene film, is usually effective. In the morning, the polyethylene film is removed and the area is washed free of salt. Two applications usually protect the area for 1 wk. If the aluminum chloride under occlusion is irritating, it should be tried without occlusion. In some patients, tap-water iontophoresis (using the Drionic® device) may be effective. A 5% solution of methenamine (available in some countries) in water may also be effective. If the anhydrous aluminum chloride treatment fails, extreme axillary hyperhidrosis may be relieved by excising the concentrated group of glands in the axillary vault.

Bromhidrosis often responds readily to treatment. Scrupulous cleanliness is essential. Daily bathing with a liquid soap containing chlorhexidine and application of an aluminum chlorhydroxy complex preparation (found in most commercial antiperspirants) are usually adequate. Topical antibacterial creams or lotions (eg, clindamycin or erythromycin) may be needed. Shaving the axillary hair may also be necessary.

103. BENIGN TUMORS
(See also WARTS in Chs. 21 and 94 and KERATINOUS CYST in Ch. 95)

MOLES
(Pigmented, Melanocytic, or Nevus-Cell Nevi)

Circumscribed pigmented macules, papules, or nodules composed of clusters of melanocytes or nevus cells.

Almost everyone has a few moles that usually appear in childhood or adolescence: small or large; flesh-colored, yellow-brown, or black; flat or raised; smooth, hairy, or warty; broad-based or pedunculated. During adolescence and pregnancy, more moles may appear and existing ones may enlarge and darken.

About 40 to 50% of malignant melanomas (see also MALIGNANT MELANOMA in Ch. 104) arise from melanocytes in moles; the rest arise from melanocytes in normal skin. The very rare malignant melanomas of childhood arise from large, pigmented moles present at birth. Halo nevi usually resolve spontaneously, but very rarely are melanomas.

Classification of Moles

A **lentigo** is a flat, uniformly pigmented, brown-to-black spot that is due to an increased number of melanocytes at the epidermodermal junction. Lentigines are darker, sparser, and more scattered than freckles, and do not darken or multiply with sun exposure.

Junctional nevi are usually flat but may be slightly elevated. Light brown to nearly black and from 1 to 10 mm in size, they result from clustering of melanocytes at the epidermodermal junction. Moles on the palms, soles, and genitalia are usually junctional.

Compound nevi are usually dark and may be slightly or considerably elevated. Nests of melanocytes occur at the epidermodermal junction and within the dermis.

Intradermal nevi are elevated, flesh-colored to black, and may be smooth, hairy, or warty. Both melanocytes and nevus cells are confined almost entirely to the dermis.

Halo nevi are pigmented moles, usually compound or intradermal nevi, surrounded by a ring of depigmented skin.

Dysplastic nevi (see also below) are irregular, pigmented lesions, ranging from tan to dark brown on a pink background.

Treatment

Since moles are extremely common, but melanomas uncommon, prophylactic removal of moles is not justifiable. However, *a mole should be excised and examined histologically if it enlarges suddenly (especially with an irregular border), darkens or becomes inflamed, shows spotty color changes, or begins to bleed, ulcerate, itch, or be painful.* If the mole is too large for simple complete excision, a biopsy should be deep enough to make an accurate microscopic diagnosis. Extensive surgery—eg, wide primary excision—is inappropriate before an accurate microscopic diagnosis, since many lesions are misdiagnosed clinically as melanomas. Simple excision or biopsy does not increase the likelihood of metastasis should the lesion prove malignant, and it avoids an unnecessary destructive procedure for a benign lesion.

Moles can be removed for cosmetic purposes without fear of subsequent malignant change, but all moles removed should be examined histologically. A hairy mole should be excised completely to prevent hair regrowth.

DYSPLASTIC NEVI

*Pigmented lesions with borders that are usu-
ally irregular and ill-defined; their macular and
papular components have both flat and very
slightly elevated areas.*

Etiology

Dysplastic nevi can be an autosomal dominant
inheritance or may occur sporadically without
detected familial association. **Dysplastic nevus
syndrome** refers to the presence of multiple dysplastic nevi and melanoma in 2 or more first-
degree family members.

Symptoms and Signs

Dysplastic nevi were first recognized because
of their unusual appearance and increased frequency in certain families. Typically, they measure 5 to 12 mm in diameter and are larger than
common moles (see above); color variegations
range from tan to dark brown on a pink background. Although they may appear anywhere on
the body, their relatively more frequent occurrence on covered areas (eg, buttocks, breast,
and scalp) differs from the distribution of common moles. Most individuals have about 10 common moles; those with dysplastic nevi may have
> 100 lesions. Common nevi usually appear by
early adult life, but dysplastic nevi continue to
appear even after age 35.

Diagnosis

Although clinical findings may suggest the diagnosis, criteria for both diagnosis and histologic
findings of dysplastic nevi are still evolving.

The entire skin (including the scalp) of the patient suspected of having one or more dysplastic
nevi should be examined with a biopsy of one or
more atypical-appearing lesions. A family history
should be obtained with special reference to
moles and melanomas or other skin cancer. If
this history suggests melanoma, first-degree relatives should also be examined for melanoma
and dysplastic nevi. Persons with dysplastic nevi
who are from **melanoma-prone families** (*families with 2 or more first-degree relatives having
cutaneous melanomas*) have a high lifetime risk
of developing melanomas (since evidence suggests that melanomas can arise directly from
dysplastic nevi or de novo in presumably normal
skin). It is not known whether the risk of melanoma is increased in individuals who have dysplastic nevi and no family history of melanoma.

Treatment

Lesions suggesting early melanoma should be
excised. The decision to excise such lesions is influenced by their color and progression (see
MOLES, above). Patients with dysplastic nevi
should avoid excessive sun exposure and use
sunscreens with an SPF of 15 or higher (see in
Ch. 101); they should be taught self-examination
to detect changes in existing nevi. To determine
changes in individual lesions, baseline and follow-up color photographs of most of the patient's
body may be used in regular, complete follow-up
examinations.

SKIN TAGS
(Acrochordons)

*Common soft, small, flesh-colored or hyper-
pigmented pedunculated lesions, usually multiple and occurring mainly on the neck, axilla,
and groin.* They are usually asymptomatic but
may become irritated. **Treatment** by freezing
with liquid nitrogen or cutting with a scalpel or
scissors may be done for tags that are irritating
or for cosmetic reasons.

LIPOMAS

*Soft, movable, subcutaneous nodules with
normal overlying skin.* Patients may have one or
many lesions. They occur much more often in
women than men and appear most commonly on
the trunk, nape, and forearms. They are rarely
symptomatic, but pain may occur. **Diagnosis** is
usually made clinically, but a biopsy should be
done if a lesion grows rapidly. Lipomas rarely become malignant. **Treatment** is not usually required, but bothersome lesions may be surgically
excised or removed by liposuction.

ANGIOMAS
(Hemangioma; Vascular Nevus; Lymphangioma)

*Localized vascular lesions of the skin and sub-
cutaneous tissues, rarely of the CNS, that result
from hyperplasia of blood or lymph vessels.*

Angiomas, which occur in about 1/3 of newborn
infants, are usually congenital or appear shortly
after birth. Most disappear spontaneously (**immature hemangiomas**); some persist and create cosmetic problems. Complications may follow overtreatment, posttraumatic ulceration, or

localized tissue hypertrophy from a persistent angioma of the CNS, the face, or an extremity.

Classification and Treatment of Congenital Hemangiomas

1. Nevus flammeus (portwine stain): *A flat, pink, red, or purplish lesion present at birth.* These lesions represent vascular ectasia and are very commonly present in the nuchal area. Nevus flammeus of the trigeminal area may be a component of the **Sturge-Weber syndrome** (*leptomeningeal angiomatosis with intracranial calcification*). A nevus flammeus usually will not fade, though splotchy small red macular lesions in the area above the nose and on the eyelids may disappear in a few months. For **treatment,** the pulsated tunable dye lasers are being used with excellent results in many cases. A nevus flammeus can usually be hidden with an opaque cosmetic cream prepared by a cosmetician to match the patient's skin color.

2. Capillary hemangioma (strawberry mark): *A raised, bright red lesion consisting of proliferations of endothelial cells.* It develops shortly after birth and tends to enlarge slowly during the first several months of life. About 75 to 95% usually involute spontaneously within 5 to 7 yr; regression is usually complete, but at times a brownish pigmentation and scarring or wrinkling of the skin remains. Since spontaneous regression is the usual course, **treatment** is not indicated unless a lesion on or near the eye or a body orifice (eg, urethra, anus) might interfere with function. When treatment is required, oral prednisone 10 mg bid or tid should be given as soon as possible and for at least 2 wk. If resolution starts, the prednisone should be decreased slowly; if not, it should be stopped. Unless complications are life-threatening or vital organs compromised, surgical excision or other destructive procedures should be avoided because these result in more scarring than when the lesion is allowed to involute spontaneously.

3. Cavernous hemangioma: *A raised red or purplish lesion composed of large vascular spaces.* The blood vessels and frequently the lymphatics are often mature, in which case the lesion may contain numerous arteriovenous shunts and vascular malformations. Cavernous hemangiomas rarely involute spontaneously. Partial involution may follow ulceration, trauma, or hemorrhage. **Treatment** must suit the type of lesion. In children, systemic prednisone (as for a capillary hemangioma) occasionally may induce spontaneous resolution. Surgical excision may

be considered, especially if the lesion causes increased growth of an extremity. Small surface nodules may be excised individually or destroyed by electrocoagulation.

Spider angioma (vascular spider): *A bright red, faintly pulsatile lesion consisting of a central arteriole with slender projections like spider legs.* Compression of the central vessel temporarily obliterates the lesion. Vascular spiders are not congenital. One lesion or small numbers that are unrelated to internal disease may be seen in children or adults. Most patients with hepatic cirrhosis develop many vascular spiders that may become quite prominent. Many women develop lesions during pregnancy or while taking oral contraceptives. As spiders are asymptomatic and usually resolve spontaneously about 6 to 9 mo postpartum or after discontinuing oral contraceptives, treatment is not usually required. If resolution is not spontaneous or **treatment** is required for cosmetic purposes, the central arteriole can be destroyed with fine needle electrodesiccation. The superiority of cosmetic results with lasers is not established.

Lymphangiomas: *Elevated lesions composed of dilated, cystic lymphatic vessels; usually yellowish tan but occasionally reddish if small blood vessels are intermingled.* Puncture of the lesion yields a colorless fluid. **Treatment** consists of deep excision.

PYOGENIC GRANULOMA
(Granuloma Telangiectaticum)

A scarlet, brown, or blue-black vascular nodule composed of proliferating capillaries in an edematous stroma. (The term pyogenic granuloma is a misnomer: The lesion, composed of granulation tissue, is neither of bacterial origin nor a true granuloma.) It develops rapidly, often at the site of recent injury, and probably represents a vascular and fibrous response to injury. It must be differentiated from a melanoma or other malignant tumor, which it often resembles. There is no sex or age predilection. The overlying epidermis is thin, and the lesion tends to be friable, bleeds easily, and does not blanch on pressure. The base may be pedunculated and surrounded by a collarette of epidermis. During pregnancy, pyogenic granulomas may become large and exuberant—eg, gingival pregnancy tumors (**telangiectatic epulis**). Pyogenic granulomas sometimes involute spontaneously; if not, a biopsy should be done. **Treatment** consists of removal by excision or electrodesiccation, but the lesions may recur.

SEBORRHEIC KERATOSES
(Seborrheic Warts)

Pigmented superficial epithelial lesions that are usually warty but may occur as smooth papules. The cause is unknown. They occur commonly in middle or old age and most often appear on the trunk or temples; in blacks, especially women, they often occur on the malar part of the face **(dermatosis papulosa nigra)**. Seborrheic keratoses vary in size and grow slowly. Round or oval, flesh-colored, brown, or black, they usually appear "stuck on" and may have a waxy, scaling, or crusted surface. They are not premalignant, and need no **treatment** unless they are irritated, itchy, or cosmetically bothersome. Lesions may be removed with little or no scarring by freezing with liquid nitrogen or CO_2 snow, or by curettage after local injection of lidocaine 1%.

DERMATOFIBROMA
(Fibrous Histiocytoma)

A firm, red-to-brown, small papule or nodule composed of fibroblastic tissue and usually found on the lower legs. Dermatofibromas are common, usually solitary and asymptomatic, but may be multiple and may itch. Their cause is unknown. **Treatment** (excision under local anesthesia) is unnecessary unless there are symptoms: irritation, erosion, sudden enlargement, or other change in surface characteristics.

KERATOACANTHOMA

A round, firm, usually flesh-colored lesion with a characteristic central crater containing keratinous material. Onset is rapid, and within 1 or 2 mo the lesion reaches its full size, which may exceed 5 cm. Common sites are the face, forearm, and dorsum of the hand. Spontaneous involution usually starts within a few months. This lesion is sometimes difficult to differentiate clinically and histologically from squamous cell carcinoma. If there is any doubt about the diagnosis, a lengthwise through-and-through midline or total excisional biopsy should be done. Because spontaneous involution may leave scarring, intralesional injections with fluorouracil or corticosteroids or surgical treatment usually yields better cosmetic results.

KELOID

A smooth overgrowth of fibroblastic tissue that arises in an area of injury or, occasionally, spontaneously. Keloids, more frequent in blacks, are shiny, smooth, often dome-shaped, and slightly pink. They tend to appear on the upper back and chest and deltoid areas, where they may be seen as a consequence of severe acne. **Treatment** with a corticosteroid (eg, triamcinolone acetonide 20 mg/mL, in amounts up to 10 mg/lesion) injected into the base of the lesion monthly (via a Luer-Lok syringe or by jet injection) may flatten the keloid but is often ineffective. Surgical or laser excision followed by intralesional injection of the wound with a corticosteroid can also be tried.

104. MALIGNANT TUMORS

Skin cancers (eg, basal cell and squamous cell carcinomas), the most common malignancies, are usually curable; most arise in sun-exposed areas of skin. The incidence is highest in outdoor workers, sportsmen, and sunbathers and is related to the amount of melanin skin pigmentation; light-skinned persons are most susceptible. Such neoplasms may also develop years after x-ray or radium burns or arsenic ingestion.

Less common malignancies include malignant melanoma, Paget's disease of the nipple or extramammary Paget's (usually near the anus), Kaposi's sarcoma, and cutaneous T cell lymphoma (mycosis fungoides). For different reasons, some of these malignancies are increasing at alarming rates.

BASAL CELL CARCINOMA
(Rodent Ulcer)

The clinical presentation and biologic behavior of basal cell carcinomas are highly variable. They may appear as small, shiny, firm, almost translucent nodules; ulcerated, crusted lesions; flat, scar-like indurated plaques; or lesions difficult to differentiate from psoriasis or localized dermatitis. Most commonly the carcinoma begins as a small shiny papule, enlarges slowly, and, after a few months, shows a shiny, pearly border with prominent engorged vessels (telangiectases) on the surface, and a central dell or ulcer. Recurrent crusting or bleeding is not unusual, and the lesion continues to enlarge slowly. It is common for basal cell carcinomas to alternately crust and heal, which may decrease the concern of both patient and doctor about the importance of the lesion. Basal cell carcinomas rarely metastasize but may be very destructive by invading normal tissues. Rarely, death may ensue because the basal cell carcinoma invades or impinges on underlying vital structures or orifices (eyes, ears, mouth, bone, dura mater). Because of the highly variable appearance of basal cell carcinomas, the differential diagnosis is extensive.

Treatment should be by a specialist after the mandatory biopsy and histologic examination. The clinical appearance, size, site, and histologic findings determine choice of treatment—curettage and electrodesiccation, surgical excision, or occasionally x-ray therapy. Recurrences (about 5%) and morphea-like lesions that have vague borders are treated with **Moh's surgery** (microscopically controlled excision of the tissue). *Topical fluorouracil is now known to be associated with extensive dermal spread under a healed epidermis and should not be used for local treatment of cancer.*

SQUAMOUS CELL CARCINOMA

Squamous cell carcinomas arise from the malpighian cells of the epithelium. Most appear on sun-exposed areas, but they may occur anywhere on the body. A squamous cell carcinoma may develop in normal tissue, in a preexisting **actinic keratosis** or patch of leukoplakia, or in burn scars. The clinical appearance of squamous cell carcinomas is highly variable. The tumor begins as a red papule or plaque with a scaly or crusted surface. It may then become nodular, sometimes with a warty surface. In some, the bulk of the lesion may lie below the level of the surrounding skin. Eventually it ulcerates and invades the underlying tissue. The percentage of squamous cell carcinomas of the skin that metastasize is unknown but is probably quite low. About 1/3 of lingual or mucosal lesions have metastasized before they have been diagnosed. Differential diagnosis includes many types of benign and malignant lesions including basal cell carci-

noma, keratoacanthoma, actinic keratosis, and seborrheic keratosis.

A biopsy is essential. **Treatment** is as for basal cell carcinoma. Squamous cell carcinoma on the lip or other mucocutaneous junction should be excised; at times it is difficult to cure, but in general the prognosis for small lesions removed early and adequately is excellent. As with basal cell carcinoma, recurrences should be treated with Moh's microsurgery.

Bowen's disease (intraepidermal squamous cell carcinoma) is a superficial squamous cell carcinoma in situ. The lesion is solitary or multiple and resembles a localized patch of psoriasis, dermatitis, or dermatophyte infection. It is red-brown and scaly or crusted, with little induration. **Treatment** is as for basal cell carcinoma, although electrodesiccation and curettage may not adequately destroy all of the lesion, as it can extend into hair follicles. Topical therapy with fluorouracil is not curative except for mucosal superficial penile lesions.

Bowenoid papulosis—human papillomavirus-induced lesions that occur as single or, more often, as multiple lesions on the genitalia—are distinct from Bowen's disease.

MALIGNANT MELANOMA
(Melanoma)

A malignant melanocytic tumor arising in a pigmented area: skin, mucous membranes, eyes, and CNS. Malignant melanomas vary in size, shape, and color (usually pigmented), and in their propensity to invade and metastasize. Thus, this neoplasm may spread so rapidly that it will be fatal within months of its recognition, while the 5-yr cure rate of early, very superficial lesions is nearly 100%. Early suspicion by inspection and an adequate biopsy for histologic determination of tumor thickness are the only means of effective management and an optimum prognosis.

Early diagnosis and cure depend upon the patient's consulting a physician early. Because the incidence of melanoma is increasing, vigorous campaigns to alert the public are under way in several areas of the world.

Most malignant melanomas arise from melanocytes in normal skin; about 40 to 50% develop from pigmented moles (see also MOLES and DYSPLASTIC NEVI in Ch. 103). The following danger signals suggest malignant transformation of pigmented nevi: change in size; change in color, especially spread of red, white, and blue pig-

TABLE 104–1. MALIGNANT MELANOMA—5-YR SURVIVAL RELATIVE TO THICKNESS

Depth of Invasion (mm)*	5-Yr Survival (%)
< 0.76	98–100
0.76–1.5	90–94
1.51–2.25	83–84
2.26–3.0	72–77
> 3.0	46

* Assessment of tumor thickness is very difficult if there are histologic signs of regression.

mentation to surrounding normal skin; change in surface characteristics, consistency, or shape; and especially signs of inflammation in surrounding skin. Although melanomas are more common during pregnancy, pregnancy does not increase the likelihood that a mole will become a melanoma. Malignant melanomas are very rare in children but can arise from large pigmented moles (giant congenital nevi) that are present at birth.

Types, Symptoms, and Signs

Four major types of melanoma are described. The prognosis of each type depends largely upon the histologically determined thickness of the melanoma (see TABLE 104–1).

1. **Lentigo-maligna melanoma** arises from lentigo maligna (Hutchinson's freckle or malignant melanoma-in-situ); it appears on the face or other sun-exposed areas in elderly patients as an asymptomatic, large (2 to 6 cm), flat, tan or brown macule with darker brown or black spots scattered irregularly on its surface. In lentigo maligna, both normal and malignant melanocytes are confined to the epidermis; in lentigo-malignant melanoma, the malignant melanocytes invade the dermis. After variable periods, about ⅓ of lentigo malignas develop a progressive malignant focus when cells invade the dermis; therefore, early excision—before the lesion is very large—is recommended. Most other treatment methods usually do not reach deep enough into the involved follicles, which must be removed.

2. **Superficial spreading melanoma** accounts for ⅔ of all melanomas. Usually asymptomatic, it is initially much smaller than the lentigo-maligna melanoma and occurs most commonly on women's legs and men's torsos. The patient seeks help after noting enlargement or irregular coloration: The lesion is usually a plaque with raised, indurated edges, and often shows red, white, and blue spots or small, some-

times protuberant, blue-black nodules. Small surface indentations may be noted. Histologically, atypical melanocytes characteristically invade both dermis and epidermis.

3. **Nodular melanoma** constitutes 10 to 15% of all melanomas. It may occur anywhere on the body and is seen as dark, protuberant papules or a plaque that varies in color from pearl to gray to black. Unless it ulcerates, nodular melanoma is asymptomatic, but the patient usually seeks advice because the lesion enlarges rapidly, often with little radial growth. Occasionally, a lesion contains little if any pigment.

4. **Acrolentiginous melanoma** is uncommon. It arises on palmar, plantar, and subungual skin and has a characteristic histologic picture similar to lentigo-maligna melanoma. It is the most common form of melanoma in blacks.

Differential Diagnosis

Many lesions colored by melanin pigment or blood can be mistaken for malignant melanomas: Among the most common are pigmented basal cell carcinoma, seborrheic keratosis, dysplastic nevus (see DYSPLASTIC NEVI in Ch. 103), blue nevus, dermatofibroma, all types of moles, hematomas (especially on the hands or feet), venous lakes, pyogenic granulomas, and warts. If doubt exists, an excisional biopsy (or, if impossible because of the size or site of the lesion, incisional biopsy) should include the full depth of the dermis and extend slightly beyond the edges of the lesion. By doing step sections, the pathologist can determine the maximal thickness of the melanoma. Definitive radical surgery should not precede a histologic diagnosis.

Diagnostic Criteria

Guidelines for selecting pigmented lesions for excision or biopsy include recent enlargement, darkening, bleeding, or ulceration. However, these features usually indicate that the melanoma has already invaded the skin deeply. Earlier diagnosis is possible if biopsies can be obtained from lesions having (1) variegated colors (eg, brown or black with shades of red, white, or blue), (2) irregular elevations that are either visible or palpable, and (3) irregular borders with angular indentations or notches.

Histologic assessment: Therapy and prognosis largely depend on histologic criteria that define the maximum thickness of the melanoma measured histologically with an optical micrometer. Adequate biopsy specimens are necessary for histologic grading—biopsy should be *excisional* for small lesions and *incisional* for larger lesions. Melanomas arising in the CNS and subungual melanomas are not classifiable by these systems.

The degree of lymphocytic infiltration, which represents the patient's immunologic defense system, may correlate with the level of invasion. Lymphocytic infiltration is maximal in the most superficial lesions; it decreases with deeper levels of tumor cell invasion.

Prognosis and Treatment

The clinical type of tumor is less important to the survival rate than the thickness of the tumor at the time of diagnosis. Thickness is determined by measuring the depth of invasion of melanoma cells from the granular cell layer. Thus, for example, as indicated in TABLE 104–1, survival of patients is greatest when tumors are < 0.76 mm thick and show no signs of histologic regression.

Metastasis of melanoma occurs via both lymphatics and blood vessels. Local metastasis results in the formation of satellite papules or nodules that may or may not be pigmented. Direct metastasis to skin or internal organs may occur, and occasionally metastatic nodules are discovered before the primary lesion is identified. Melanomas arising from mucous membranes have a poor prognosis although they seem quite limited when discovered.

Treatment of melanoma is by surgical excision. The width of margins is still a matter of debate; most experts would agree that for lesions < 1 mm thick, a 1.0 cm lateral tumor-free margin is adequate. **Lentigo-maligna melanoma** and its premalignant precursor, lentigo maligna, are usually treated with wide local excision and, if necessary, with skin grafting. Intensive x-ray therapy is much less effective than surgery. **Nodular** or **spreading melanomas** are usually treated by wide local excision extending down to the fascia. Lymph node dissection is usually rec-

ommended only when there is node enlargement.

Patients with thick melanomas and those with regional or distant metastasis may benefit from consultation with experts in newer forms of therapy. Chemotherapy with dacarbazine (DTIC) or the nitrosoureas (BCNU, CCNU) are being used with limited success. Cis-platinum and others are currently under study. Results using BCG vaccine to alter the patient's immune response have been discouraging, but newer forms of immunotherapy (eg, interleukin-2 and lymphokine-activated killer cells) are promising. Vaccines using melanoma antigen are being studied to measure the patient's antibody response and for possible therapy.

PAGET'S DISEASE OF THE NIPPLE AND EXTRAMAMMARY PAGET'S DISEASE

A rare type of carcinoma that appears as a unilateral dermatitis of the nipple and represents extension to the epidermis of an underlying mammary duct carcinoma. The redness, oozing, and crusting closely resemble dermatitis, but the physician should suspect carcinoma because the lesion is unilateral. Biopsy of the lesion shows typical histologic changes. Paget's disease also occurs at other sites, most often in the groin or perianal area (extramammary Paget's disease). An underlying carcinoma should be sought in all cases. Most cases of extramammary Paget's disease are now thought to arise from apocrine glands. **Treatment** is determined by the surgeon; mastectomy is usual for lesions of the nipple.

KAPOSI'S SARCOMA (KS)
(Multiple Idiopathic Hemorrhagic Sarcoma)

A neoplasm characterized by vascular skin tumors that may appear in 3 distinctive forms. KS lesions originate from multifocal sites in the mid-dermis and extend to the epidermis. Histopathology shows spindle cells and vascular structures admixed to various degrees. The cell of origin in many cases is the endothelial cell shown by specific staining for factor VIII; the tumor cells resemble smooth muscle cells, fibroblasts, and myofibroblasts. An **indolent form** of KS manifests nodular or plaquelike dermal lesions. A **lymphadenopathic form** of KS is disseminated and aggressive, involving lymph nodes, viscera, and occasionally the GI tract. In a form associated with **AIDS** (see in Ch. 20), there may be few lesions or the lesions are widely disseminated in the skin, mucous membrane, lymph nodes, and viscera.

Incidence

Once uncommon, KS was seen most often in eastern Europe, Italy, and the USA, and occurred mainly in the indolent form in men of Italian or Jewish ancestry > 60 yr old. Now, however, KS is endemic in equatorial Africa where it is more aggressive, occurs commonly in children and young men, and accounts for nearly 10% of all malignancies in Zaire and Uganda. Since 1981, the aggressive form of KS has occurred in at least ⅓ of patients with AIDS and has assumed epidemic proportions in the USA and many other countries (see in Ch. 20).

Clinical Manifestations

In older men, KS generally appears first on the toes or legs as purple or dark brown plaques or nodules that may fungate or penetrate soft tissue and invade bone; disseminated lymph node and visceral involvement follow in 5 to 10%.

The **KS lesions associated with AIDS** may be the first notable manifestation of AIDS. As barely elevated pink or red papules or plaques that may be round or oval, they appear first primarily on the upper body or mucosa. They may become widely disseminated on the skin and are associated with visceral lesions and disseminated lymph node involvement.

Treatment and Prognosis

For indolent superficial lesions, freezing, electrocoagulation, or electron beam radiotherapy causes flattening and fading of most lesions. Unresponsive dermal or lymph node disease with lymphedema is treated locally with 10 to 20 Gy (1000 to 2000 rads) of x-ray therapy.

The more aggressive, disseminated form associated with AIDS has been treated with single agent or combination chemotherapy (eg, with etoposide, vincristine, vinblastine, bleomycin, and doxorubicin). Interferon-α effectively slows progression of early lesions and cures others. Intralesion vincristine is also very useful. The course of KS in HIV infection is dictated by the level of immunosuppression, which determines the likelihood of opportunistic infections. Treatment of KS does not help to prolong life in most patients, because infections dominate the clinical course.

§8. DENTAL AND ORAL DISORDERS

105. DENTISTRY IN MEDICINE

MEDICAL—DENTAL CONSULTATION

A dentist should consult a physician when systemic disease is suspected, when a person's ability to withstand general anesthesia or extensive oral surgery must be evaluated, or when an emergency occurs in a dental office.

A physician should consult a dentist on behalf of a child with abnormal growth manifested by peculiar facies, delayed tooth eruption, or gross malformation or malalignment of teeth; or a patient with cleft lip or palate, jaw fracture, oral neoplasm, or newly discovered lump in the neck. Dental consultation is also indicated for obscure facial pain, for unexplained swelling or cellulitis of the neck that might have originated in an infected tooth, or for infection of the parapharyngeal space that might have followed an abscess of a lower posterior tooth. In fever of unknown origin (FUO) or a systemic infection of inapparent cause, the possibility of a dental basis for bacteremia should not be overlooked. Physicians should be familiar with dental procedures and the degree of trauma and risk involved to patients with systemic disease. Dentists who search for oral cancer and who refuse to extract teeth unless valid dental reasons exist are consultants to be prized.

Clarification of the cause of face, head, and neck symptoms often necessitates the pooled knowledge of both physician and dentist. Obscure causes of **face, head, and neck pain** include malocclusion, poorly fitting dental prostheses, disease of the temporomandibular joints, giant cell (temporal) arteritis, unilateral mastication, spasm of the muscles of mastication, and occult cavities in the jawbones. Referred pain may make diagnosis difficult; eg, pain referred to the ear may arise from an inflammation of the gingival flap around a partly erupted mandibular 3rd molar or from the back of the tongue in glossopharyngeal neuralgia. Paresthesias of the lower lip may follow damage to the inferior alveolar nerve during extraction of a mandibular molar, or they could be a rare sign of an oral neoplasm compressing that nerve. Conversely, percussion tenderness in several maxillary teeth may indicate nasal or antral disease adjacent to the root tips.

Patients undergoing oral surgery warrant the same preoperative medical evaluation and postoperative care as those undergoing procedures of comparable scope and severity elsewhere in the body. Oral surgical procedures include simple extractions; removal of impacted teeth; alveoloplasty (cartilage grafts or resection of mucosa with reattachment to deepen the mucobuccal fold so that dentures will fit more securely); repair of jaw fractures; correction of protruding mandibles or retrusive or small jaws; orthognathic surgery (repositioning an area of alveolar bone and its contained teeth) for severe malocclusion; excision of soft tissues, bone cysts, and neoplasms; and surgery on the temporomandibular joint to remedy arthritis, developmental anomalies, or the results of trauma.

DENTAL CARE OF PATIENTS WITH SYSTEMIC DISORDERS

Dental care is occasionally hazardous. Its risks can be minimized by (1) performing elective dental procedures when medical patients are best able to withstand the inherent trauma and (2) encouraging healthy individuals to practice good oral hygiene so that if systemic disease should develop, massive dental treatment in a belated attempt to remedy prolonged neglect would be unnecessary and would not delay medical therapy or cause additional complications.

Routine oral surgery or periodontal treatment puts medical patients at risk when the normal inflammation required for healing is inhibited by such drugs as corticosteroids, immunosuppressive agents used in organ transplantation, and cytotoxic drugs given for cancer. Hemorrhage, delayed healing, local infection, and even septicemia may occur. Dental care should be carried out and time for healing allowed before using such systemic drugs.

People with **bleeding disorders** should be scrupulous about oral hygiene; if caries develops, they should have teeth filled to avoid subsequent extractions. Filling a tooth is almost always a bloodless procedure. Exceptions occur: (1) Deep decay that has entered or almost entered the pulp mandates complete removal of the decayed tooth structure to prevent recurrent caries; the minimal bleeding from the pulp that follows the removal is easily controlled by pressure. (2) Minimal gingival lacerations may occur from instrumentation during preparations for treating interproximal caries. Cavity preparation involving the occlusal surface of a tooth that is not deeply decayed should be completely bloodless.

Suspected **bleeding or coagulation disorders** should be assessed before oral surgery. In patients with acute forms of **leukemia, thrombocytopenia,** or **hepatitis,** extractions should be delayed until the condition improves or stabilizes. Prolonged bleeding following extraction or periodontal procedures may occur in patients with **polycythemia vera** or **macroglobulinemia, disorders of platelet number and function,** and severe **liver disease** with diminished vitamin K–associated plasma coagulation factors or increased fibrinolytic activity. Patients taking aspirin should discontinue the drug for a week before such dental procedures are performed and should not resume taking it until healing occurs. In coagulation disorders, extractions and regional block anesthesia often require pretreatment with the appropriate coagulation factor immediately before, during, and after the oral surgical procedure.

In **leukemia,** oral hygiene is vital because periodontal disease fosters gingival bleeding and probably local tissue infiltration. Infection often follows extraction in disorders with **granulocytopenia.**

Cardiovascular patients may be adversely affected by dental procedures. Following a myocardial infarction, dental procedures should be delayed for 3 mo, if possible, and anticoagulant dosage may need to be temporarily reduced (until prothrombin time is about $1^{1}/_{2}$ times the control value) to avoid undue postextraction bleeding. Individuals with pulmonary or cardiac disease who require inhalation anesthesia for dental procedures should be treated in a hospital. Tooth extraction, scaling (removal of calculus), or other periodontal procedures cause bacteremia; patients with mitral valve prolapse, congenital or rheumatic heart disease, or a prosthetic cardiac valve are predisposed to bacterial endocarditis and should receive antibiotics before and after such dental procedures. It is particularly important for them, as for patients with coagulation disorders, that teeth be filled to avoid extractions and that preventive oral hygiene be practiced to minimize tooth decay and gingivitis.

Epinephrine, used as a vasoconstrictor to potentiate the duration of local anesthetics, may cause arrhythmias or exacerbate hypertension as the exogenous hormone adds to the anxiety or fear-induced endogenous level; cardiac ischemia may result. Sedation or tranquilization is advantageous in fearful cardiovascular patients and facilitates treatment. Electrical equipment such as a cautery, a pulp tester, or even the dental drill can interfere with pacemakers. Such patients and their dentists should be forewarned so that appropriate measures may be taken. The horizontal position of a dental chair may be intolerable to patients with heart failure, and those receiving antihypertensive drugs may develop orthostatic hypotension on arising.

Infections may follow dental procedures such as tooth extraction, particularly of abscessed or periodontally involved teeth. **Bacteremia** may result in endocarditis, mediastinitis, thrombophlebitis of the jugular veins, pneumonia, empyema, meningitis, brain abscess, or cavernous sinus thrombophlebitis. Mediastinitis, thrombophlebitis, a parapharyngeal abscess, or a cellulitis of the floor of the mouth may develop from contiguity with an abscessed tooth, whether or not endodontic treatment (root canal) was performed. Bacteria of oral origin may lodge in the adhesive of prosthetic joints and adjacent tissues, necessitating removal of the implant. Infectious material, such as fragments of teeth or fillings or pus from periodontal infection, may be aspirated and cause a lung abscess. Patients who dissolve illicit drugs in saliva before injecting them IV may disseminate oral bacteria systemically.

Chemotherapy for neoplasms includes drugs (eg, doxorubicin, 5-fluorouracil, bleomycin, dactinomycin, and methotrexate) that cause stomatitis; the severity is often related to the degree of periodontal disease present. Before instituting such drugs, it is advisable to remove calculus (tartar) and improve the health of periodontal tissue to minimize gingival hemorrhage, tissue sloughing, oral pain, and consequent poor food intake. Subsequent proper use of the toothbrush and dental floss will minimize the likelihood of stomatitis.

Prior to radiotherapy of the oral region, patients should have required oral surgery, periodontal treatment, restoration of salvageable teeth, and application of sealants and fluoride treatment (both minimize caries following xerostomia secondary to irradiation and destruction of the salivary glands). Dental work should be completed and healing permitted before radiotherapy begins. *Extraction of teeth from previ-*

ously irradiated tissues is commonly followed by osteoradionecrosis of the jaws, a catastrophic complication (see Osteoradionecrosis in Ch. 128). Thus, extraction should be avoided, if possible, by using dental restorations, dental splints, or endodontic treatment (root canal). Close life-long attention to oral hygiene is necessary to avoid the need for oral or periodontal surgery. Frequent fluoride applications are also indicated for an indefinite period following radiotherapy. Tissue breakdown with persistent ulceration is likely beneath a partial or a complete denture because of scarring and inelasticity of irradiated tissue. The prostheses should be checked and adjusted whenever discomfort is noted.

Extraction of a tooth adjacent to a carcinoma of the gingiva, palate, or antrum facilitates invasion of the alveolus (tooth socket) by the neoplasm. Therefore, extraction should be done only in the course of definitive treatment.

Subcutaneous and mediastinal emphysema rarely may follow use of a high-speed air turbine dental drill or compressed air during a root-canal procedure or in sectioning a tooth or the alveolar bone during an extraction, as air is forced into the alveolus of the bone and then dissects along fascial planes. Acute onset of jaw and cervical swelling with characteristic crepitus on palpation of the swollen skin is diagnostic.

In **endocrine disorders**, tooth extraction is never routine. Dental treatment usually should be postponed until the systemic disease is well controlled. For example, tachycardia may occur in hyperthyroid individuals, accompanying the anxiety often present in dental patients. One exception to postponement is that poorly controlled diabetics may be more easily managed after they receive necessary dental care to improve poor oral hygiene. **Diabetics** are prone to periodontal disease. Following periodontal surgery or extractions, when food intake is limited because of postoperative pain, they may require adjustment of insulin dosage and diet or parenteral fluids. Poorly controlled diabetics, often dehydrated, also have a decreased salivary flow that contributes to caries. Extensive extractions, restorative dentistry, or periodontal surgery should not be done on both sides of the mouth in any one visit, to avoid undue interference with food intake. Patients with **adrenocortical insufficiency** may require supplemental corticosteroids during the stress of major dental procedures. Individuals who have **Cushing's syndrome** or are receiving corticosteroids for a

systemic disease may have delayed wound healing and increased capillary fragility.

An **allergic** individual might, despite previous interrogation, receive an offending antibiotic, local anesthetic, or other medication in conjunction with dental treatment.

In **Bell's palsy**, the natural cleansing action of the lip and cheek on the tooth surfaces of the involved side is lost; without scrupulous oral hygiene and repeated fluoride treatments, unilateral decay will increase.

People with **convulsive disorders** should have fixed (not removable) small dental appliances to prevent swallowing or aspirating them and causing airway obstruction or possibly esophagitis or enteritis due to the foreign body. Tracheoesophageal or enterocolonic fistulas subsequently may develop. Good oral hygiene in **quadriplegics** and individuals with severe upper extremity incoordination or tremor requires conscientiousness on the part of those who care for them. Unexplained fever in such persons may have an oral basis that should be sought.

Hepatitis B virus rarely is transmitted to patients by dentists with antigenemia who are carriers of the disease via open lesions on the dentist's fingers into the alveolus of an extracted tooth or into the patient's mouth and therefore the GI tract. This hazard is diminished if dental personnel with digital lesions, particularly those with a history of hepatitis, wear gloves. In recent years, as autoclaving has become more commonplace for sterilizing dental instruments, the likelihood of transmission of viral hepatitis from an infected patient to a subsequent patient has become less likely but remains a possibility. **Herpes simplex** has been transmitted to patients by a dental hygienist with digital lesions, but this risk can also be minimized by wearing gloves.

Proper instrument sterilization and routine use of gloves, protective eyewear, and masks should make transmission of **AIDS** from a practitioner to a patient (or vice versa) unlikely. Yet, apparent transmission of AIDS from an HIV-infected oral surgeon has been reported. Salivary antibodies would minimize the likelihood of spread from an infected patient.

DENTAL RESTORATIONS AND APPLIANCES

Fillings are inserted after removal of decay. A temporary filling is kept in place for weeks in the hope that the tooth will retain its vitality and deposit secondary dentin to seal a pulp exposure. Silicate, a type of porcelain cement, is used to fill cavities in anterior teeth because it resembles enamel. Plastic resins are also used for the same purpose. The occlusal surfaces of posterior teeth, which bear the brunt of mastication, require stronger materials. The most common ones used, amalgam and gold inlay, can be identified by color. A small, less common filling is gold foil.

If decay is extensive, placing several fillings in one tooth might undermine its structure. To prevent fracture of the natural crown, the dentist removes the decay and fills the sites with cement. Grinding the outer surfaces tapers them so that an artificial **crown**, usually of gold, may be placed. A porcelain jacket crown is used on anterior teeth for its natural appearance. During laryngoscopy, care must be exercised not to dislodge any artificial crowns fixed on anterior teeth.

When teeth are missing, a bridge or partial denture can be made. A **bridge** is usually smaller than a partial denture, but 1 or 2 bridges may be made to cover an entire maxillary or mandibular dental arch. Stress in a bridge is largely borne by abutment teeth (usually on either side of the missing tooth or teeth). Abutment teeth have crowns cemented to them; thus, the bridge is a fixed appliance that is not easily removed. False teeth are soldered to the crowns and to each other. A **partial denture**, typically a removable appliance with clasps that snap over the abutment teeth, may be removed for cleaning. Part of the load of occlusion is borne by the soft tissues underlying artificial teeth, which often are on both sides of the jaw. This appliance is usually used when there are no more natural teeth beyond the tooth or teeth to be replaced.

Complete dentures are removable appliances that help a patient chew solid foods and improve his speech and appearance, but they cannot achieve the efficiency or tactile sensations of good natural dentition.

Recently, some individuals have had partial or complete dentures affixed to submucosal saddles or vertical posts inserted into the jaws to enhance retention. These **dental implants** are not readily removable.

All **removable dental appliances** are generally removed before throat surgery, general anesthesia, or convulsive shock therapy to avoid loss, breakage, aspiration, or swallowing during the procedure. They should be stored in water to prevent dimensional changes that may occur with drying. However, some anesthesiologists believe that leaving the appliance in place aids the passage of an airway tube, keeps the face in a more normal shape so the mask fits better, prevents natural teeth from injuring the opposing gingiva of a completely edentulous jaw, and does not interfere with laryngoscopy.

106. EXAMINATION OF THE ORAL REGION

Examination of the oral region begins with a pertinent history. Knowing the details and frequency of dental visits may alert the physician to a particular dental problem or to a lack of attention to dental care. **Inability to chew food well** suggests insufficient teeth for proper mastication, poorly fitting dental appliances, loose or painful teeth, or disorders affecting the temporomandibular joint **(TMJ)** or the muscles of mastication. **Slight, occasional bleeding** after brushing suggests bristle damage or mild gingivitis; **frequent, spontaneous, or profuse bleeding** may indicate severe gingivitis or a blood dyscrasia. A history of a **single, mild infection** after oral surgery does not necessarily have systemic implications, but **recurring oral and other infections** may indicate agranulocytosis, neutropenia, leukemia, immunoglobulin defects, or disorders of leukocyte function. Immunosuppressed individuals may experience painful reactivation of oral herpes simplex infections with oral ulcerations and consequent interference with food intake. **Root canal treatment**—a common dental procedure for decay that has reached the pulp or for devitalization after trauma—occasionally is associated with osteitis at the tip of the root, which can be the source of a more serious infection that could spread from this site. A history of **sores, lumps, or pain** may indicate disease of teeth and soft tissues. **Medication history** may reveal incompatibilities and duplications. **Abnormal taste sensations** may be due to psychiatric disorders; however, a search for local causes should always be made. A bitter taste may indicate pus originating from a periodontal or alveolar abscess, while a salty taste may indicate bleeding or seepage of tissue fluid from beneath poorly fitting dentures or from inflamed periodontal tissues into the normally sodium-poor oral environment. A sour taste may be caused by an electrolytic reaction between adjacent fillings of dissimilar metals. Correction of such underlying dental problems results in disappearance of the symptom.

The Face

The face and mouth are inspected for marked asymmetry, lesions, or disproportions. An **unusual facial appearance** characterizes many head and neck syndromes of genetic or developmental origin (eg, fetal alcohol syndrome) and often occurs with atypical positioning or malformations of the pinnae or an unusual skull shape, with or without dental abnormalities. An underweight patient may lack teeth or have severe periodontal disease, caries, or poorly fitting dental appliances that interfere with chewing. Not all involuntary weight loss indicates systemic disease in such persons.

Slight facial asymmetry is universal. It may be due to preferential chewing on one side, causing unilateral enlargement of the masticatory muscles; differences in the contour of the dental arches or angulation of the teeth on one side compared with the other; or combinations of these. However, **marked facial asymmetry** occurs in individuals with lipodystrophy, hemiatrophy or hemihypertrophy of the face, or congenital absence of the condyle of the mandible. Awareness of the psychologic trauma of facial malformation should lead to referral for possible facial surgery.

Cheek **contours** depend mainly on the posterior teeth. **Swellings** of the face may be cutaneous (eg, neurofibromas or sebaceous cysts) or may arise from deeper tissues. If one or both cheeks appear swollen, the distention may be in the skin, in the parotid glands (which may be enlarged because of mumps, Sjögren's syndrome, or a tumor), or inside the mouth. An excessively thick denture flange gives the wearer a puffy appearance that disappears on removing the denture and can be remedied by a dentist's grinding down its outer thickness. An abscessed tooth may cause soft-tissue swelling as pus drains from the tooth toward the outer surface of the face or neck. Endodontic (root canal) treatment or extraction promotes drainage and mitigates further spread of infection. Salivary gland and lymph node enlargement is evident on inspection and palpation of the preauricular and submandibular regions.

Fistulas may represent malformations of the embryologic branchial pouches or draining sinuses from abscessed teeth. An abscessed lower molar may drain below the angle of the mandible and eventually leave a depressed scar.

Breath Odor

The physician should wonder why a patient who reeks of mouthwash is self-conscious about his breath. Is it only to camouflage recent ingestion of alcohol, onions, or garlic or use of tobacco, or is it for another reason? Extensive dental caries, periodontal disease, or tonsillitis causes a fetid odor often accompanied by a bad taste. Rhinitis, ozena, or sinusitis also causes halitosis. There are **systemic causes** of bad breath: in liver failure, a mousy odor is present; in uremia, a urinous smell; and in a lung abscess or bronchiectasis, a putrid odor. In diabetic ketosis, acetone is present in the breath.

Lips

Lip movements normally betray emotion as the patient speaks; in scleroderma or Parkinson's disease, the lips are rigid. With a facial nerve paralysis (Bell's palsy), marked asymmetry occurs when the patient talks or smiles. The **vermilion border** (between the mucosa of the lips and the skin of the face) is the site of recurrent infections (cold sores) and carcinoma. **Generalized thickening** of the lips occurs in myxedema, cretinism, and acromegaly. **Localized swellings** may indicate a lymphangioma or hemangioma, the latter causing purplish discoloration as well. Besides cosmetics to camouflage the deformity, more definitive treatment is available (see under ANGIOMAS in Ch. 103). In the absence of anterior teeth, the lips become shorter and more concave. They are attached to the jaws by prominent midline and smaller lateral frena. Other abnormalities are discussed in Ch. 111.

Temporomandibular Joint (TMJ)

The TMJ is palpated laterally and intrameatally for tenderness, range and smoothness of motion, and condylar deformity. As the patient opens his mouth, the examiner notes any limitation or **deviation of jaw movement** indicating abnormality of the 5th cranial nerve or weakness of jaw muscles. Congenital malformation or absence of the TMJ can cause similar signs, and characteristic abnormalities appear on x-ray. Normally the jaw should move symmetrically, and with the mouth open, 3 fingers should fit comfortably between the upper and lower incisors (40 to 50 mm). If less space exists, both articular and nonarticular conditions should be considered in the differential diagnosis, since

TABLE 106-1. RELATIONSHIP BETWEEN DECIDUOUS AND PERMANENT TEETH*

20 Deciduous		32 Permanent	
Symbol	Name	Symbol	Name
A	Central incisor	1	Central incisor
B	Lateral incisor	2	Lateral incisor
C	Canine (cuspid)	3	Canine (cuspid)
D	1st molar	4	1st premolar (bicuspid)
E	2nd molar	5	2nd premolar (bicuspid)
		6	1st molar
		7	2nd molar
		8	3rd molar

* Each quadrant (left or right half of each jaw) contains the teeth listed.

they can produce similar types of dysfunction. The patient may have scleroderma, parotitis, malformation or arthritis of the TMJ, a peritonsillar abscess, or pericoronitis (infection of the gingiva around a partially erupted 3rd molar). Tetanus or a depressed fracture of the zygomatic arch impinging on the coronoid process of the mandible can also impair opening of the mouth. The cervical muscles and muscles of mastication should be palpated for signs of muscular problems (trismus, myofascial pain-dysfunction [MPD] syndrome), which are more common causes of limited jaw movement than are joint problems (ankylosis, disk derangement). An unusually wide opening may indicate a subluxation of the mandible.

By placing the little fingers deeply into the patient's auditory canals, the physician can test the range and smoothness of mandibular condylar motion as the mouth opens and closes.

To assess complaints of ear or facial pain on chewing, the examiner can place a stethoscope in front of each ear as the patient opens and closes his mouth. Clicking or popping sounds indicate an internal disk derangement. A grating noise or crepitus suggests degenerative joint disease. Pain on chewing that does not originate from TMJ or dental abnormalities may be seen in giant cell (temporal) arteritis with ischemia of the muscles of mastication.

Teeth
(See also discussion under GROWTH AND DEVELOPMENT FROM BIRTH THROUGH CHILDHOOD in Ch. 23)

A useful shorthand representation for recording observations is shown in TABLES 106-1 and 106-2. The horizontal line represents the space between the jaws and the vertical line denotes the midline of the face. Another method of identifying teeth is using the letters A to T for the deciduous teeth; eg, in the permanent dentition, numbering begins with the 3rd maxillary right molar and goes to the left across the maxillary arch, then to the right across the mandibular arch to the 3rd mandibular right molar.

Oral hygiene reflects the patient's general attitude toward himself or his physical, psychologic, or economic ability to care for himself. Are teeth decayed or missing? Pain experienced when teeth are tapped with a tongue depressor suggests extensive dental caries or periodontal disease. Severe periodontal disease causes most instances of visibly loose teeth, but rarely, erosion of the alveolar bone by an underlying tumor (eg, ameloblastoma) loosens them. A deeply carious tooth may have an infected or necrotic pulp. A dentist can test the patient's reaction of pain to a weak electrical stimulus to determine whether a tooth is alive. A tooth with decay involving the pulp is a potential source of infection into surrounding alveolar bone. **Calculus (tartar),** if present, is deposited particularly near the orifices of the salivary ducts on the buccal surfaces of the maxillary molars and the lingual surfaces of the mandibular anterior teeth.

The most common motor abnormality of the oral region is probably not Bell's palsy but **bruxism**—the clenching or grinding of teeth that erodes and eventually diminishes the height of dental crowns. Such attrition is common with advancing years; in youth, it often indicates bruxism. The teeth may loosen. Although the patient may be oblivious of his habit, other family members are aware. The treatment requires that the patient consciously try to overcome the habit, perhaps with the help of sedatives or tran-

TABLE 106-2. SHORTHAND REPRESENTATION OF TEETH

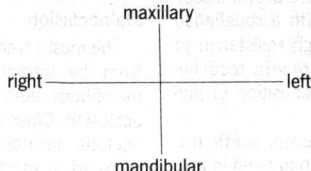

Using the symbol for the tooth from TABLE 106-1,

D̲ represents the mandibular left deciduous 1st molar;

6̲ represents the maxillary right permanent 1st molar.

quilizers and abstinence from alcohol (the latter often aggravates bruxism). A dentist can make a splint to be worn over the teeth to prevent dental injury from the grinding movements. Biofeedback also may be tried.

Maxillary incisor **fractures** are common in children with neurologic disorders who are prone to falls. Malocclusion can result in a front tooth contacting its opponent at an angle that causes the corner of an incisor to be chipped.

Defects in tooth form: Once formed, teeth are never remodeled by systemic influences, only by local ones. Thus, the examiner may find evidence of developmental disorders or endocrinopathies. In **congenital syphilis** the contours of the incisors and 1st molars undergo characteristic changes: The incisors show a constriction at the incisal 3rd, which produces a pegged or screwdriver shape, and a characteristic notch in the central portion of the incisal edge. The 1st molar is dwarfed, with constriction of the occlusal surface and roughening and hypoplasia of the enamel. With hereditary opalescent dentin **(dentinogenesis imperfecta)**, an autosomal dominant trait, the dentin is abnormally formed and teeth are a dull bluish-brown. Such teeth cannot withstand occlusal stresses and rapidly become worn. "Peg" lateral incisors are congenitally narrow but are unassociated with systemic disease. Periapical x-rays show that pituitary dwarfs and congenitally hypoparathyroid individuals have small dental roots, and people with gigantism have large roots. In acromegaly, one sees not only enlargement of the jaws but also hypercementosis of the roots.

Defects in enamel or tooth color: A dead tooth appears gray. Darkening of the teeth and enamel hypoplasia follow **chronic administra-** tion of tetracyclines during the second half of pregnancy or during tooth development in the child. The affected teeth, rather than fluorescing white in ultraviolet light, have a colored fluorescence characteristic of the type of tetracycline given. A dark band may be visible in ordinary light after only 5 days of therapy. A generalized yellowish or brownish discoloration is often seen in smokers. Users of smokeless tobacco develop such changes in the area where the quid is held. The abnormal calcium metabolism associated with **rickets** results in enamel hypoplasia. A rough, irregular band appears around each tooth. The location of the band indicates the area being calcified at the time of abnormal calcification, thus providing an estimate of the age at which the disease occurred and its duration. Such teeth are not unduly susceptible to dental caries. A **high fever** during odontogenesis can also interfere with enamel formation, and a narrow zone of chalky, pitted enamel is visible after the tooth erupts. **Amelogenesis imperfecta**, an autosomal dominant hereditary disease, causes severe enamel hypoplasia. Decalcification of dental crowns occurs with chronic vomiting, as in **bulimia** (the lingual surfaces of the lower anterior teeth being primarily affected), and with **cocaine use.** Chronic snorting followed by salivary dissociation of the drug into the base and hydrochloride, often abetted by massage of the oral mucosa to hasten absorption, results in widespread decalcification of teeth. Development of rampant caries after childhood may indicate chronic use of **marijuana,** which is often accompanied by a craving for sweets and inattention to oral hygiene.

Children who drink water containing > 1 ppm of fluoride during the period of tooth development are likely to develop mottled enamel (**fluorosis**). The enamel changes can range, depending on the amount of fluoride ingested, from irregular whitish opaque areas to severe brown discoloration of the entire crown, with a roughened surface. Such teeth have a high resistance to dental caries. In **congenital porphyria**, teeth fluoresce a reddish color from deposition of pigment in the dentin.

Rampant caries of deciduous teeth frequently indicates that the teeth had been in prolonged contact with a sweetened infant formula, perhaps while the infant napped ("**nursing bottle caries**"). To minimize the prevalence of caries, oral drugs should not be chronically administered to children in a metabolizable sugar-based vehicle.

With age, teeth darken and biting surfaces become worn (**attrition**) so that chewing is less effective. **Gingivae** may **recede**, thus exposing more of the crowns and often even part of the roots. Since a small zone of exposed dentin is sensitive to touch or temperature alterations, noncarious teeth can become painful when enamel and cementum do not quite contact each other. The dentist can desensitize such teeth. Proper keratinization of the oral mucosa requires sex hormones. Hormonal therapy can ameliorate the poorly keratinized, inflamed mucosa commonly found after menopause.

In edentulous jaws of elderly persons, **atrophy of the alveolar process (senile atrophy)** is common. This diminishes the stability of an artificial full denture, particularly the lower one. Oral surgical procedures can improve the situation.

Normal Occlusion

Occlusion should be checked on both sides of the mouth; this can be done by retracting each cheek with a tongue depressor while the patient bites normally. In normal occlusion, the maxillary anterior teeth overlie the mandibular anterior teeth. The outer (buccal) cusps of the maxillary posteriors are external to the corresponding cusps of the mandibular posterior teeth. Since the outer parts of all the maxillary teeth are superficial to the mandibular teeth, the lips and cheeks are displaced from between the teeth so they are not bitten. Furthermore, the lingual (inner) surfaces of the lower teeth are in a smaller arc than that of the upper teeth, confining the tongue and minimizing the likelihood of its being bitten as the teeth occlude. All the teeth should contact their opponents, so that the powerful masticatory forces (which may be > 100 lb in the molar region) are widely distributed. If these forces are applied to only a few teeth, those teeth are likely to loosen.

Malocclusion

The most common **classification** of deviation from the normal contact of the maxillary and mandibular teeth identifies 3 major forms of malocclusion. **Class I:** The upper and lower molars occlude normally, but the anterior teeth are crowded or malpositioned. **Class II:** The lower jaw retrudes and the facial profile is convex. **Class III:** The mandible protrudes.

Etiology: Malocclusion often reflects a disproportion between jaw and tooth size—ie, a jaw so small or teeth so large that the jaw cannot accommodate them all in proper alignment. Other causes are supernumerary, malformed, or missing teeth; delayed eruption or impaction of permanent teeth; ankylosis of the mandible; cleft lip or palate; and rarely, cleidocranial dysostosis or Hurler's syndrome. A frequent cause of acquired malocclusion is loss of teeth with shifting of adjacent teeth and extrusion of opposing teeth unless a bridge or partial denture is worn. Premature loss of deciduous teeth in children often results in approximation of adjacent teeth, causing insufficient space for eruption of the permanent successors. This shift can be prevented by a dental appliance termed a space maintainer. Less frequently, malocclusion results from habits such as thumb- and finger-sucking or tongue-thrusting. Iatrogenic malocclusions can occur from improper dental restorations and appliances, improper fixation of jaw fractures, or a Milwaukee orthopedic back brace, which places constant pressure on the mandible. Rarely, teeth are displaced by an underlying jaw tumor.

Diagnosis and treatment: Malocclusions are corrected primarily for oral health reasons, although the patient often needs help for cosmetic or psychologic reasons. Because early interceptive **orthodontics** usually eliminates a later need for more expensive and difficult techniques, a child should have a dental consultation as soon as malocclusion is suspected. The evaluation includes x-rays of the skull, facial bones, and teeth, and study casts of the teeth. Malocclusion following facial trauma may suggest tooth displacement or fracture, often accompanied by a jaw fracture.

Therapy increases resistance to dental decay, anterior tooth-edge fracture, and periodontal disease, and it improves speaking and mastication.

Occlusion can be improved by selective grinding where teeth or restorations contact prematurely, by aligning teeth properly, or by inserting crowns or onlays to build up teeth that are below the plane of occlusion. Applying a continuous mild force to the teeth by means of orthodontic appliances (braces) moves the teeth by gradually remodeling the alveolar bone. Some patients initially require extraction of 1 or more permanent teeth to obtain enough space for stable alignment. When the final relationship has been achieved, the patient wears a plastic retainer at night until the teeth stabilize in new positions. When it is anticipated that orthodontic treatment may not suffice, surgical correction of jaw abnormalities contributing to malocclusion (orthognathic surgery) is often indicated. Orthodontic treatment of adults is now commonplace.

Oral Mucosa

The patient should be asked to remove dentures so that the underlying soft tissues may be seen. The likelihood of dropping or distorting a dental appliance is greater if the physician attempts to remove it.

With a finger cot for protection against infectious lesions, the examiner palpates the cheek bimanually (with one finger inside and one outside) to delimit lesions. Most people have yellowish, pinhead-size maculae in the buccal mucosa. These are harmless **ectopic sebaceous glands** (Fordyce's granules). Many persons have a thin white line (linea alba) on the buccal mucosa along the occlusal plane. It represents surface keratinization due to accidental, repeated cheek biting over the years.

The **color** of soft tissues can reflect anemia, polycythemia, cyanosis, or jaundice. One looks for generalized inflammation (stomatitis) as well as localized areas of inflammation, ulceration, petechiae, or thickening. Darkly pigmented areas may indicate a racial characteristic, Addison's disease, or very rarely, melanoma. Violaceous Kaposi's sarcoma is a common intraoral finding in AIDS.

Dryness of the mouth may be from dehydration, mouth breathing, or use of diuretics or anticholinergics, or it may reflect salivary gland dysfunction or disease (see Ch. 107). The orifices of the parotid ducts open in the cheek beside the maxillary molars. The sublingual and submandibular salivary gland ducts open on the floor of the mouth behind the lower incisors. When pain or swelling occurs in one of those regions and saliva does not emanate, the duct may be obstructed by a calculus (sialolith).

The **distribution of keratinized and nonkeratinized oral mucosa** can be significant. Keratinized epithelium is on the facial aspect of the lips, the dorsum of the tongue, the gingiva around the base of the dental crowns and adjacent part of the roots of the teeth, and on the hard palate. It is less likely to be damaged by hard food particles than nonkeratinized mucosa that is mobile, as in the cheek, sides of the tongue, soft palate, and floor of the mouth. Keratinized mucosa in these areas is abnormal, and a definite diagnosis must be made. White areas may be seen in the mucobuccal fold in adolescents or others who retain snuff or chewing tobacco there. Such leukoplakias may be precancerous (see Ch. 111). Type 1 herpes simplex eruptions occur on the keratinized mucosa, while the lesions of aphthous stomatitis occur on the nonkeratinized mucosa (see Ch. 107). In some persons, the latter may be a manifestation of cyclic neutropenia.

Gingiva

The gum should be firm and nicely contoured about and adapted to the crowns of the teeth. Pink, stippled tissue should fill the entire interdental space. Keratinized gingiva is present near the crowns. More distant gingiva is nonkeratinized, highly vascular, and continuous with the buccal mucosa. A tongue depressor should express no blood or pus from the gingiva. At the gingival margin, a dark line suggests exposure to lead or some other heavy metal. Gingivitis (see in Ch. 109) is common. Gingival fibromatosis may be idiopathic but is often seen with chronic administration of phenytoin, cyclosporine, or nifedipine. Some patients with regional enteritis have an area of granulomatous gingival hypertrophy that becomes symptomatic with intestinal flare-ups. Widespread gingivitis with only minimal dental calculus (tartar) could indicate a systemic disease (eg, scurvy, diabetes mellitus, leukocyte disorders). Local infection about the teeth predisposes to bacteremia during brushing, dental procedures, and oral surgery.

The Palate

The anterior portion of the hard palate is the site of the incisive papilla adjacent to the central incisors. Behind it are the rugae, firm ridges that keep food from slipping as the tongue crushes the food against them. A person with a cleft palate (see also under Musculoskeletal Defects in

Ch. 28) has a very nasal voice. Normal vocal resonance and articulation involve the anterior teeth, lips, tongue, and palate, as well as the lungs, vocal cords, and pharynx. A very **high palatal vault** is seen in Marfan's syndrome (see under INHERITED DISORDERS OF CONNECTIVE TISSUE in Ch. 42). Punctate areas of inflammation about the ducts of the numerous minor salivary glands of the palate are common, especially in pipe smokers. The boneless soft palate should rise symmetrically when the patient says "ah." The uvula at the far end of the soft palate's midline varies greatly in length among individuals. A very long uvula, associated with very loud snoring, may be present in persons who have obstructive sleep apnea.

Tongue and Floor of the Mouth

As the patient touches the tip of his tongue to his soft palate, one can examine the floor of the mouth and the under surface of the tongue, where cancer often starts. The tongue, having a wide range of **movement**, should be able to twist its tip around the sides of the molar teeth. Normal tongue movement indicates good hypoglossal nerve function, but neuromuscular weakness may prevent its holding a midline position or moving rapidly. For a neurologic evaluation of taste, 0.1 M solutions of NaCl, HCl, sucrose, and urea may be used. The tongue may be **enlarged** in myxedema, amyloidosis, or acromegaly, or if a

rhabdomyoma is present. In edentulous individuals without complete dentures, the tongue tends to broaden.

The **papillae** may be normal or atrophied. The tongue is smooth and pale in pernicious anemia or smooth and fiery red in deficiencies of niacin or riboflavin (see GLOSSITIS in Ch. 107). Oral cancer often occurs on the lateral surface of the tongue (see NEOPLASMS OF SPECIFIC TISSUES in Ch. 111). Oral candidiasis or a slightly elevated white area with a corrugated surface (hairy leukoplakia) may indicate AIDS.

Salivary Glands

Saliva promotes retention of artificial dentures because of its mucin content. Thus, conditions characterized by diminished saliva flow often adversely affect the ease with which dentures may be worn. If natural teeth are present, salivary flow washes away bacteria and food debris, facilitating oral cleanliness. A reduction in flow or decrease in salivary IgA fosters bacterial growth and development of tooth decay. This may be caused by an abnormality of the salivary glands (see in Ch. 107). Contact with a patient's saliva should be avoided, even though the risk of transmitting HIV and hepatitis B virus from saliva may be less than that from blood. The risk might be greater if extensive oral lesions, gingivitis, or periodontitis is present, allowing seepage of serum into the mouth.

107. DISORDERS OF THE LIPS, MOUTH, AND TONGUE

Most diseases affecting the mucous membrane can occur anywhere in the oral mucosa, but they will be mentioned under the most frequent sites. See also Chs. 106 and 111.

LIPS

An acute swelling of the lip may be **angioedema** (see URTICARIA; ANGIOEDEMA under ANAPHYLAXIS in Ch. 34). Brownish-black melanin pigmentation spots in association with GI polyposis occur in the **Peutz-Jeghers syndrome**. **Exfoliative cheilitis** is a chronic desquamation of the superficial mucosal cells; if it persists despite abstention from very hot or irritating foods and alcoholic beverages and despite changes of lip-

stick or dentifrices, triamcinolone acetonide ointment should be tried. A **chancre** has a serosanguineous crust (see SYPHILIS in Ch. 21).

Mucocele (mucous retention cyst), most commonly found on the lower lip, is due to trauma severing the excretory ducts of the accessory salivary glands and permitting the mucin-containing saliva to escape into the tissues. A soft nodule forms. If the nodule is superficial, the overlying epithelium is thinned and assumes a bluish tinge. Treatment is excision.

Tiny painful vesicles characterize 2 common disorders: herpes labialis (**cold sore**), found on the vermilion border of the skin, and recurrent aphthous ulcers (**canker sores**), on the inner aspects of the lips (see also RECURRENT APHTHOUS STOMATITIS and ORAL HERPETIC MANIFESTATIONS in this chapter, below).

Cheilosis (angular cheilitis) is characterized by fissuring and dry scaling of the skin and vermilion surface of the lips and angles of the mouth. The condition is infrequently associated with deficiency of some of the B vitamins, particularly riboflavin and pyridoxine, and frequently accompanies other clinical signs of avitaminosis. One must also consider herpetic involvement, the split papule of syphilis, and the pseudocheilosis or wrinkling at the corners of the mouth accompanying loss of vertical dimension of the face (the distance between the jaws). In edentulous patients, wrinkling can be diminished by inserting dentures that separate the jaws. Loss of skin elasticity with aging normally results in overlapping of the skin at the corners of the mouth, so that saliva pools there and contributes to angular inflammation. Persistent lesions should be cultured to rule out a mycotic infection, particularly candidiasis **(perlèche)**. Mixed infections respond best to a combination of antifungal and anti-inflammatory agents. High doses of vitamin B complex are beneficial if blood tests indicate a deficiency.

BUCCAL MUCOSA
(See also STOMATITIS, below)

Mucosal lesions may cause dentures to hurt or fit poorly. **Koplik's spots** are tiny, grayish-white macules with red margins occurring during the late prodromal and early eruptive stages of measles. **Aspirin burn** is a painful white area of coagulated tissue caused by the local caustic action of aspirin placed against the mucosa to relieve a toothache. Wiping off the white film reveals an inflamed area. **Irritation "fibroma,"** composed of fibrous tissue, is not a true neoplasm. It is usually present opposite the occlusal plane where the patient chronically bites or sucks his cheek. Treatment is excision and breaking the habit or reducing the cusps of offending teeth. **Hereditary hemorrhagic telangiectasia** (see in Ch. 35) is characterized by localized dilated blood vessels in the oral cavity, nasal mucosa, and elsewhere. If bleeding occurs, applying local pressure and an absorbable gelatin sponge ordinarily suffices. If not, a cautery may be used. **Lichen planus** often occurs with cutaneous lesions (see Ch. 96). The mucosa is characteristically netlike and hardened, with papules or erosive areas. Violet atrophic or white hyperkeratotic variations may appear on the dorsum of the tongue. **Bullae** of short duration occur in various mucocutaneous disorders (eg, pemphigus and erythema multiforme), including the severe Stevens-Johnson syndrome. Behçet's syndrome is manifested by oral as well as ocular and genital mucosal ulcers. Herpangina, characterized by vesicles in the posterior part of the mouth, and hand-foot-and-mouth disease, with small ulcerated vesicles, are both due to coxsackieviruses (see in ENTEROVIRAL DISEASES under VIRAL INFECTIONS in Ch. 32).

FLOOR OF THE MOUTH

This area may be the site of a **cellulitis** following extraction of, or root canal treatment on, an abscessed mandibular tooth. Incision, drainage, and aggressive antibiotic therapy (eg, initially 1 gm penicillin V orally, then 500 mg q 6 h for 10 days) are indicated. An extensive sublingual infection, termed **Ludwig's angina,** is very hard to palpation.

An **epidermoid cyst** is an inclusion cyst in the floor of the mouth (usually in the midline) or the mucobuccal fold, which is the junction of the buccal mucosa and the alveolar mucosa. The midline of the floor of the mouth is the most common location for a **dermoid cyst,** which has a doughy feel. All cysts should be excised and carefully examined for evidence of malignancy.

SALIVARY GLANDS

Painless swelling of the parotid glands is often noted in hepatic cirrhosis, in sarcoidosis, in mumps, following abdominal surgery, or in association with neoplasms or infections. The common factors may be dehydration and inattention to oral hygiene. The latter promotes the growth of large numbers of bacteria that in the absence of sufficient salivary flow ascend from the mouth into the duct of a gland. Another cause of a painful salivary gland is **sialolithiasis** (salivary duct stone). The submandibular glands are most commonly affected. Pain and swelling associated with eating are characteristic. Calcium phosphate stones tend to form because of the high pH and viscosity of the submandibular gland saliva, which has a high mucin content. Stones are removed by manipulation or excision.

Autoimmune sialosis is the Mikulicz-Sjögren syndrome, a unilateral or bilateral enlargement of the parotid and/or submandibular glands, and often the lacrimal glands. Occasionally painful, it is associated with xerostomia (dry mouth) due to impaired saliva formation, which is most common in older women.

THE PALATE

Torus palatinus is a common benign overgrowth of bone (osteoma) in the midline of the hard palate where the maxillae fuse. No treatment except reassurance is required unless a dentist wishes to cover the hard palate completely with a denture. If so, surgery is required; the tissue covering a torus is thin and easily traumatized by foods.

A hole in the palate may be a **congenital cleft.** Clefts of the palate or lip occur once in 700 to 800 births. The cleft may vary from involvement of only the soft or hard palate to a complete cleft of both palates, the alveolar process of the maxilla, and the lip. The infant should be referred to a cleft palate team (pediatrician, orthodontist, speech pathologist, plastic surgeon, and psychologist). Causes of **perforating lesions** other than the congenital cleft include salivary gland tumors, the gumma of tertiary syphilis, carcinoma of the palate, and rarely, TB.

In infectious mononucleosis, **petechiae** may occur at the junction of the hard and soft palate. In neutropenia or agranulocytosis, there may be **ulcerations** with little inflammation. Clumps of asymptomatic red **papules** are seen in inflammatory hyperplasia of the palate (pseudopapillomatosis). A denture may irritate such lesions.

The palate may be the site of **Wegener's granulomatosis** (lethal midline granuloma), in which there is destruction of bone with sequestration.

In AIDS, intraoral lesions of **Kaposi's sarcoma (KS)** have a predilection for the palate. They begin as red-to-purple painless macules and progress to painful papules. Local treatment is with radiation therapy or CO₂ laser.

STOMATITIS

An inflammation of the mouth, often a symptom of systemic disease. Fetid breath odor and blood-tinged saliva may accompany any ulcerative lesions of the oral mucosa.

Etiology

Stomatitis may be caused by infection, trauma, dryness, irritants and toxic agents, hypersensitivity, or autoimmune conditions. Infectious agents include streptococci, gonococci, fusospirochetes, *Candida albicans, Corynebacterium diphtheriae, Treponema pallidum, Mycobacterium tuberculosis*, and the viruses of herpes simplex, varicella-zoster, measles, and infectious mononucleosis, as well as coxsackievirus. Stomatitis may also result from avitaminosis, particularly lack of the B vitamins or vitamin C (as in pellagra, sprue, pernicious anemia, or scurvy); or from iron-deficiency anemia with dysphagia **(Plummer-Vinson syndrome)**, agranulocytosis, or leukemia. Lichen planus, erythema multiforme, SLE, Behçet's syndrome, and pemphigus vulgaris frequently present oral mucosa signs. Mechanical trauma from cheek biting, mouth breathing, jagged teeth, orthodontic appliances, ill-fitting dentures, or nursing bottles with nipples that are hard or too long may produce characteristic lesions. Xerostomia resulting from drugs, the aging process, or radiation therapy predisposes the mouth to sensitivity and infection. Generalized stomatitis may follow excessive use of alcohol, tobacco, hot foods, or spices; or sensitization to toothpaste, mouthwash, candy dyes, lipstick, and rarely, acrylic dentures. Phenytoin, iodides, bismuth, mercury, barbiturates, lead, and many other drugs may produce stomatitis. Chemical stomatitis of occupational origin may be due to dyes, heavy metals, acid fumes, or metal or mineral dust. The latter 3 may also cause abrasion of the hard tissues. Mercury causes marked salivation.

Symptoms and Signs

Clinical signs vary widely according to the type of stomatitis present. **Allergic stomatitis** is characterized by an intense, shiny erythema with slight swelling. Itching, dryness, or burning, often present, may be due to sensitivity to foods or to lipstick.

Acute necrotizing ulcerative gingivitis (ANUG) or **Vincent's infection** (see ACUTE NECROTIZING ULCERATIVE GINGIVITIS in Ch. 109) causes ulceronecrotic lesions of the interdental papillae that may extend to the marginal gingivae or produce painful ulcers of the mucous membranes. When associated with HIV infection, the ANUG rapidly becomes destructive.

Candidiasis (thrush), caused by *C. albicans,* is characterized by white, slightly raised patches resembling milk curds that when removed expose a hyperemic area that may bleed slightly. This is the pseudomembranous form. The infection usually begins on the tongue and buccal mucosa and may spread to the palate, gums, tonsils, pharynx, larynx, GI tract, respiratory system, and skin. The mouth usually appears dry. Candidiasis is common in infants; the debilitated; the immunosuppressed; individuals receiving long-term antibiotic, corticosteroid, and antineoplastic therapy; and those with xerostomia. The chronic, erythematous (atrophic) form of candidiasis appears as a generalized redness of the oral mucosa, usually accompanied by diminished taste acuity. A third form (hypertrophic) presents as confluent, white, nonwipeable areas.

Pseudomembranous (or membranous) stomatitis, an inflammatory reaction that produces a membrane-like exudate, may be caused by chemical irritants (eg, gold, iodides) as well as bacteria (streptococci, staphylococci, gonococci, *C. diphtheriae*). Fever, lymphadenopathy, and malaise may occur, or the infection may be localized.

Mucosal lesions accompanying systemic disease include the mucous patches of syphilis; the strawberry, then raspberry, tongue of scarlet fever; Koplik's spots of measles; the ulcers of erythema multiforme; and the smooth, fiery red tongue and painful mouth of pellagra. Hemorrhagic lesions may occur in scurvy and disorders of platelet number and function. Unprovoked bleeding, decreased salivation, and an ammonia-like odor accompany uremic stomatitis.

The **mucocutaneous lymph node syndrome (Kawasaki syndrome)** affects children, causing erythema of the lips and oral mucosa (see KAWASAKI SYNDROME in Ch. 32).

Acrodynia occurs in children and is characterized by oral ulcerations, profuse salivation, and bruxism (see in Ch. 106) with loss of teeth. It is caused by a mercurial toxicity reaction.

Diagnosis

Establishing the cause may be difficult. The history may disclose a systemic disease, a dietary deficiency, or contact with irritants or allergens. Physical examination is obligatory, since it may reveal lesions of other mucous membranes, as in erythema multiforme, candidiasis, or syphilis; lesions of the skin, as in pellagra, pemphigus, lichen planus, or SLE; signs of pulmonary TB, sprue, anemia, or another contributory disease; or a general decrease in exocrine secretions.

Direct smears and cultures from the lesions may disclose a pathogen. Any diphtheria-like membrane should be so examined *promptly.* ANUG usually limits itself to the gingival tissue, differentiating it from primary herpetic gingivo-

stomatitis. Darkfield examination of scrapings from the lesions and STS are indicated in an attempt to rule out syphilis before penicillin is given. In candidiasis, a history of recent antibiotic or corticosteroid therapy is common. To identify *C. albicans,* one should culture and microscopically examine scrapings from suspect lesions in 10% potassium hydroxide hanging drop preparations or methylene blue–stained smears. Blood count, bone marrow examination, gastric analysis, or other laboratory procedures may be indicated.

A solitary, undiagnosed oral lesion of > 1 wk duration that does not respond to treatment must be considered malignant until biopsy proves otherwise.

Treatment

Underlying systemic disorders should be treated specifically. Meticulous oral hygiene is always necessary. **Candidiasis** usually responds to nystatin oral suspension 400,000 u. (4 mL) qid for 10 days as an oral rinse and then swallowed. Clotrimazole 10-mg oral lozenges 5 times a day for 14 days are effective in persistent overgrowths. When compliance is a problem, ketoconazole one 200-mg tablet (for children < 12 yr, $1/4$ tablet) orally once a day is effective. All antifungals should be continued for at least 3 days after symptoms and signs disappear. For oral **bacterial infections,** penicillin V 500 mg orally qid for 10 days is the drug of choice. Large, painful ulcers that prevent eating may be relieved temporarily by rinsing the mouth with 2% lidocaine viscous 15 mL (1 tbsp) before each meal and q 3 h as needed for relief. A mouthwash of $1/2$ tsp sodium bicarbonate in 250 mL (8 oz) warm water qid is soothing and cleansing. Rinsing (and spitting out) after each meal with elixir of dexamethasone 0.5 mg/5 mL (1 tsp) relieves discomfort and promotes healing of nonviral and nonbacterial oral lesions.

RECURRENT APHTHOUS STOMATITIS

Acute painful ulcers on the movable oral mucosa, occurring singly or in groups (canker sores). Minor ulcers, the most common form, are < 1 cm in diameter, last 10 to 14 days, and heal without scarring; major ulcers, > 1 cm in diameter, last weeks to months and heal with scarring. Recurrent attacks are common, with 2 or 3 ulcers during each attack; however, 10 to 15 ulcers are common in some individuals. Women are affected more often than men.

Etiology is unknown, but several factors point toward a localized immune reaction. Deficiencies of iron, vitamin B$_{12}$, and folic acid increase susceptibility. Stress and local trauma are usually the predominant precipitating factors.

Symptoms and Signs

Beginning as a shallow, ovoid erosion with a slightly raised, yellowish border surrounded by a narrow, red, hyperemic zone, the minor aphthous ulcer is covered within 5 to 7 days with a yellowish opaque material composed of coagulated tissue fluids, oral bacteria, and WBCs. The acutely painful phase lasts 3 or 4 days; symptoms then diminish until the lesion heals spontaneously, usually without scarring, in 7 to 10 days. Malaise, fever, and lymphadenopathy may accompany severe attacks. Recurrent attacks vary from one lesion 2 to 3 times/yr to an uninterrupted succession of multiple lesions.

Diagnosis

The mucosal lesion looks distinctive enough to differentiate aphthous stomatitis from primary or recurrent herpetic oral lesions (which may appear concurrently) and from the lesions of erythema multiforme, oral pemphigus, or benign mucosal pemphigoid. Aphthae rarely appear on the immovable mucosa (hard palate, attached gingiva), the prime areas for recurrent intraoral herpetic ulcers. The history and clinical examination exclude herpangina.

Treatment

A topical anesthetic such as 2% lidocaine viscous 5 mL (1 tsp) as an oral rinse q 3 h or before meals provides short-term relief and facilitates eating. A dental protective paste (Orabase®) applied qid prevents irritation of the ulcers by the teeth, dental appliances, and oral fluids. An application of triamcinolone acetonide in emollient dental paste reduces discomfort and promotes healing.

For multiple lesions, tetracycline oral suspension (250 mg qid for 10 days) is held in the mouth for 2 to 5 min to coat the ulcers before swallowing. Children < 8 yr old should not be given systemic tetracycline because of its adverse effect on developing tooth enamel. If treatment is started early after onset, symptomatic relief occurs within a day and new lesions are aborted. Treatment must be repeated for each new attack. Occasionally this therapy results in oral (and vaginal) candidiasis. For severe episodes of minor aphthae or for major aphthae, corticoste-

roid therapy is indicated, both topical and systemic (elixir of dexamethasone 0.5 mg/5 mL [1 tsp] to rinse with [and spit out] after meals and at bedtime for 5 days; prednisone 40 mg/day initially, tapered over 10 days).

ORAL ERYTHEMA MULTIFORME
(See also ERYTHEMA MULTIFORME in Ch. 97)

Acutely painful stomatitis characterized by diffuse hemorrhagic lesions of the lips and oral mucosa and usually associated with constitutional symptoms. Oral, ocular, genital, and dermal lesions can occur concurrently.

Symptoms, Signs, and Diagnosis

Prodromal symptoms may include rhinitis and sinusitis. Multiple vesicles form in the earliest stage. Typical lesions consist of diffuse hemorrhagic eroded areas throughout the mouth; the lips are commonly bloody and crusted, but the gingivae are rarely involved. Extensive oral, conjunctival, and genital lesions may be present, even without dermal eruption.

The patient may have a temperature as high as 40 to 40.6° C (104 or 105° F) during the early stages. Severe constitutional symptoms (fever, malaise, arthralgia) usually persist for 4 or 5 days; as they regress, the typical lesions develop. The constitutional symptoms may be similar to those in allergic stomatitis, pemphigus, and herpetic stomatitis, which must be differentiated. The lesions are a deeper red than the mucous patches of secondary syphilis.

Treatment

Oral lesions in the acute phase may be treated with systemic corticosteroids (prednisone 10 mg orally tid for 5 days) or elixir of dexamethasone 0.5 mg/5 mL (1 tsp) to rinse with and swallow qid for 5 days. Without corticosteroids, the lesions may persist for 3 to 8 wk or longer. When intraoral lesions cause difficulty in eating, a liquid diet is helpful. Dehydration may necessitate IV fluid therapy. A warm mouthwash of 10% sodium bicarbonate solution and anesthetic troches, ointments, or solutions (eg, 2% lidocaine viscous) can be used 5 or 6 times/day. Petrolatum ointment may soothe lip lesions. With treatment, improvement is rapid and lesions usually heal without scarring. Recurrence is not usual.

ORAL HERPETIC MANIFESTATIONS

Acute, painful vesicular eruptions of the oral mucosa or vermilion borders caused by the herpes simplex virus. Primary acute herpetic infection is common in infants and young children and may occur in teenagers and young adults. A history of recent contact with an adult having a herpes simplex eruption is frequent.

In childhood, the initial viral infection usually goes unrecognized unless the stomatitis causes feeding difficulties. After infection, antibody titer remains high throughout life and limits future response to the virus to an occasional recurrent lesion intraorally on the hard palate or extraorally on the vermilion border, often extending to the skin surfaces of the lips. The latter are often called **fever blisters** or **cold sores.** Mild trauma such as that associated with dental treatment, abrasion of the vermilion border, sunburn, food allergy, anxiety, onset of menstruation, or any disease that produces a fever or an increased metabolic rate may precipitate lesions.

Symptoms and Signs

In **primary acute herpetic gingivostomatitis,** multiple shallow ulcers of varying size occur throughout the mouth. The oral ulcerations are preceded by inflamed gingiva resembling acute necrotizing ulcerative gingivitis **(ANUG)** and a 2- to 3-day prodromal period of malaise, fever, and cervical lymphadenopathy. During the first 4 or 5 days, pain may be severe enough to discourage a child from eating and drinking. Although the disease is usually self-limited and symptoms subside in 7 to 10 days, extensive systemic involvement and fatal viremia have occurred in infants and occasionally in older children.

In **recurrent herpes labialis,** patients usually experience a sensation of fullness, burning, and itching before the typical vesicle develops on slightly elevated, erythematous tissue at or near the junction of the vermilion and skin. The greatest extension of the lesion is usually toward the skin. A vesicular lesion may exist for hours before the vesicle breaks and a yellowish, crusted lesion forms. Underlying tissues are not indurated, though varying degrees of edema may be present. Lesions seldom last > 10 days.

Recurrent intraoral herpetic lesions of the hard palate and attached gingiva begin with multiple small vesicles that rupture quickly and unite to form large, superficial ulcerations with irregular margins. A large zone of erythema usually surrounds the ulcers.

Diagnosis

Primary acute herpetic stomatitis must be differentiated from drug eruptions and erythema multiforme, and more rarely in adults, from pemphigus. Allergic forms of stomatitis can usually be suspected from the history. In both erythema multiforme and pemphigus, accompanying skin lesions are common. **Erythema multiforme** (see in Ch. 97) may be discerned by more marked constitutional symptoms and widespread hemorrhagic lesions. In **pemphigus** (see also in Ch. 98), constitutional symptoms usually persist for several weeks, and the patient often recalls a prior episode of large painless bullae without accompanying prodromal symptoms.

Diagnosing the solitary lesion of **herpes labialis** is usually not difficult because of its characteristic appearance and location.

Treatment

In **primary herpetic stomatitis,** a topical analgesic relieves temporary pain; 2% lidocaine viscous 5 mL (1 tsp) as an oral rinse q 3 h or diphenhydramine elixir 5 mL (1 tsp) as an oral rinse q 2 h is used as needed. A sodium bicarbonate mouthwash of 2.5 mL (0.5 tsp) in 250 mL (8 oz) warm water qid soothes and cleanses. Since children tend to decrease fluid intake, they must be watched for dehydration. Supportive therapy consists of increasing fluids and giving diet supplements. Systemic antibiotics may be used to guard against secondary infection.

Recurrent herpetic labialis (lip lesions) can be reduced in frequency by using a sunscreen containing aminobenzoic acid **(PABA)** during sun exposure. *All proposed treatment is more effective if started in the prodromal stage,* ie, at the first symptoms of local change in sensations.

Topically, antiviral agents such as vidarabine or acyclovir ointments discourage spreading and act as lubricants. Applying ice locally reduces swelling. Petrolatum tends to prevent cracking, bleeding, and self-inoculation from manual spread.

Systemic treatment is directed toward improving resistance to the virus. A combination of citrus bioflavonoids 200 mg and ascorbic acid tablets 200 mg tid for 3 days initiated in the prodromal stage may abort or greatly reduce the duration of the lesions. Where frequent recurrences interfere with daily function or nutrition, acyclovir 200-mg capsules 5 times/day will give relief.

Desiccative agents such as alcohol, ether, and chloroform are thought to fractionate the virus, thereby inviting resistant and mutagenic strains.

Corticosteroids can spread the virus, especially on mucosal tissue.

There is no cure for herpes simplex.

TONGUE

Infants may have **mucocutaneous lymph node syndrome (Kawasaki syndrome**—see in Ch. 32), in which there is a bright red tongue and face, edema of the extremities, and thrombocytosis. **Ankyloglossia** (tongue-tie) may be diagnosed if the tip of the tongue cannot contact the alveolar ridge or the tips of the teeth or sweep from one corner of the mouth to the other. To increase mobility of the tongue, the lingual frenum may need cutting. Untreated tongue-tie may affect speech and interfere with mastication and passive cleansing of the teeth. A **burning sensation** is a frequent postmenopausal symptom in association with poor keratinization, or it may be a symptom of diabetic neuropathy; both require treatment of the underlying endocrine disorder. In the absence of physiologic or anatomic abnormalities, depression or an anxiety state should be considered. Amitriptyline 25 mg at bedtime with a weekly increase of dosage is usually effective in 3 to 4 wk.

GLOSSITIS

An acute or chronic inflammation of the tongue.

Etiology

Glossitis may be either a primary disease or a symptom of disease elsewhere. The many and varied causes include the following:

Local: Infectious agents commonly found in the mouth; mechanical trauma (jagged teeth, ill-fitting dentures, oral habits such as tongue-pressing, repeated biting during convulsive seizures); primary irritants (excessive use of alcohol, tobacco, hot foods, spices); or sensitization (by toothpaste, mouthwashes, breath fresheners, candy dyes, and rarely, plastic dentures or restorative materials).

Systemic: Avitaminosis (particularly of the B group, as in pellagra), anemia (pernicious or iron-deficiency), or certain generalized skin diseases (lichen planus, erythema multiforme, aphthous lesions, Behçet's syndrome, pemphigus vulgaris, syphilis).

Symptoms, Signs, and Diagnosis

Clinical manifestations vary widely without strong correlation between the appearance of lesions and the severity of symptoms. Reddened tip and edges of the tongue may indicate incipient pellagra, pernicious anemia, irritation from excessive smoking, or a tooth with a rough surface. In later stages of pellagra, the entire tongue is fiery red, swollen, and often ulcerated. In iron-deficiency and particularly in pernicious anemia, the tongue is pale and smooth. Painful ulcers may indicate primary herpetic or aphthous lesions, pulmonary TB with positive sputum, streptococcal infection, erythema multiforme, or pemphigus vulgaris. Whitish patches suggest candidiasis, the mucous patch of syphilis, lichen planus, leukoplakia, or mouth breathing. Denuded smooth areas, if not painful, may indicate **geographic tongue** (benign migratory glossitis), or if moderately painful, anemia or pellagra; if they are very distressing and persistent, they may be the lesions of **atrophic lichen planus** (slick, glossy, or glazed tongue). **Median rhomboid glossitis**, a localized candidiasis, consists of a rhomboid-shaped smooth, reddish, nodular area on the dorsal surface of the back portion of the middle third of the tongue. **Hairy tongue**, due to a profuse overgrowth of the filiform papillae, is usually asymptomatic and often follows antibiotic therapy, fever, excessive use of O_2-liberating mouthwashes, or a reduction in salivary flow. Brown papillae are usually from tobacco staining or the overgrowth of chromogenic bacteria. Treatment is rectifying the underlying cause and brushing the tongue with a toothbrush. **Hairy leukoplakia**—characterized by white, fixed plaques of viruses on the lateral borders of the tongue—is associated with AIDS.

Severe acute glossitis occasionally results from local infection, burns, or trauma. It may develop rapidly, producing marked tenderness or pain with swelling sufficient to cause protrusion of the tongue and the danger of airway obstruction and suffocation. Mastication, swallowing, and speaking are painful and sometimes impossible. Cervical and submandibular adenitis with evidence of systemic toxicity may be present. Immediate treatment with corticosteroids may be indicated to reduce the edema.

Patients may complain of a painful burning tongue (**glossodynia** and **glossopyrosis**) without obvious clinical evidence of inflammation. Many patients are postmenopausal. Incipient candidiasis, xerostomia, oral habits, anemias, diabetes mellitus, latent nutritional deficiencies, or malignancies should be excluded.

Each case of glossitis deserves study, since the tongue often mirrors disease. History may disclose an irritant, contact allergen, sensitizing drug, deficient diet, or other symptoms of disease. Other mucosal surfaces and the skin should be inspected for evidence of pellagra, erythema multiforme, syphilis, or lichen planus. Studies for an anemia, mild diabetes mellitus, sprue, and syphilis should be performed.

Prognosis

When the cause can be determined and corrected, response is usually prompt but may be delayed in nonspecific or chronic involvement. The patient should be reassured that persistent lesions such as fissured and geographic tongue are innocuous. Aphthous lesions, candidiasis, and hairy tongue often recur periodically. For solitary ulcerations that do not respond to treatment after 1 wk, a biopsy should be performed.

Treatment

General: Specific causative disorders are treated as indicated. Irritants and sensitizing agents are to be *avoided.* A bland or liquid diet, preferably cooled, is given. Meticulous oral hygiene is imperative.

Local: Oral infections call for specific therapy (see STOMATITIS, above). The pain of large lesions that interferes with eating may be relieved temporarily by rinsing with an obtundent mouthwash before each meal; topical anesthetics (lidocaine 5% ointment or 10% spray; benzocaine 2% ointment; dyclonine 0.5% liquid) applied to discrete lesions also give relief and encourage eating. Occasionally, systemic analgesics (aspirin or acetaminophen 650 mg q 4 h) are required. Topical application of triamcinolone acetonide 0.1% in emollient dental paste to specific lesions (except those of viral etiology) tid or qid relieves symptoms and may promote healing.

The patient with painful burning but a clinically normal tongue requires special management. Tests for vitamin B_{12} deficiency should be conducted, especially after menopause. When an emotional basis is diagnosed, reassurance (especially regarding neoplasm) and encouragement are important.

108. DENTAL CARIES AND ITS COMPLICATIONS

TOOTH DECAY

A gradual pathologic disintegration and dissolution of tooth structure by microorganisms, with eventual involvement of the pulp. The principal microorganisms are transmissible and usually are acquired in infancy. Except for the common cold, this is the most prevalent human disorder.

Etiology

The interaction of 3 factors results in dental caries: a susceptible tooth surface, the proper microflora, and a suitable substrate for the microflora. Although several oral acidogenic microorganisms can initiate the carious lesion, laboratory and clinical evidence points to *Streptococcus mutans* as the primary pathogen. Its virulence stems from its ability to synthesize extracellular polysaccharide. Lactic acid, a byproduct of this synthesis, contributes to tooth demineralization. Mono- and disaccharide sugars serve as the principal substrates for the process. The gummy extracellular polysaccharides increase the bulk of dental plaque, facilitating bacterial proliferation and attachment to the tooth surface. **Dental plaque**—a combination of these polysaccharides, microorganisms, salivary glycoproteins, and desquamated mucosal cells—serves as a localized site of acid production.

Dietary carbohydrates play a significant role. The types of carbohydrates and frequency of their ingestion are more important than the amounts consumed. Frequent between-meal snacks, especially of sucrose-containing foods, enhance the carious process; sticky foods that linger are potentially more harmful than non-sticky foods.

Pathogenesis

Dental caries begins on the external crown or exposed root surface of the tooth. Bacterial plaque, not food debris, causes caries. Plaque is not flushed away by the action of oral musculature or saliva. The role of saliva in preventing caries is in its buffering capacity, remineralization effect, and secretory immunoglobulins. Acid action first demineralizes enamel with its high inorganic content; proteolysis of its organic matrix follows. When the carious process reaches the dentin or begins on the root surface, the tooth becomes sensitive to temperature or osmotic changes engendered by foods or by touch. Caries spreads rapidly because of the lower mineral content of dentin and cementum. As demineralization and necrosis of the dentin progress, microorganisms may invade the dentinal tubules. Microbial products preceding the organisms in the dentinal tubules may cause inflammation of the dental pulp before destruction of the surrounding dentin is evident.

Symptoms and Signs

The patient is often unaware of the presence of caries until the lesion is well advanced. Common early symptoms are sensitivity to heat and cold and discomfort after eating sugar-containing foods. A darkened area between anterior teeth or cavitation may be noticed when the carious process has progressed sufficiently. Caries is clinically diagnosed by the dentist when softened enamel or dentin is detected with a sharp instrument. Radiographically, caries appears as a radiolucent area, as do most resin filling materials and bases under metallic restorations. Consequently, radiographic diagnosis must be coupled with a visual examination.

Prophylaxis

Teeth are less susceptible to caries if optimum amounts of fluoride (about 1 mg/day) are ingested while the teeth are developing. Fluoride combines with some of the apatite crystals in the tooth structure to form the less soluble fluorapatite. Maximum benefit accrues when water containing 1 ppm of fluoride is consumed from birth until the permanent dentition completes eruption (age 11 to 13.) Nearly 1/2 the US population still does not have access to optimally fluoridated water. There is no proof that ingesting fluoridated water or fluoride supplements during pregnancy will significantly protect a child's deciduous teeth and permanent 1st molars, although these calcify in utero.

Ingesting excessive fluoride before eruption, while the enamel is forming, may cause permanent mottling of the enamel. Once erupted, teeth cannot develop mottling when exposed to excessive fluoride. During pregnancy, the placenta acts as a barrier against marked increases in fluoride concentration and thus protects the calcifying fetal teeth against mottling.

If the water supply contains less than the optimum amount of fluoride for the local mean maximum air temperature (as prescribed by the Public Health Service Drinking Water Standards), children should receive daily supplements during their tooth-forming years, by using bottled fluoridated water for drinking and cooking or by taking a sodium fluoride tablet.

Applying fluoride compounds to erupted teeth enhances benefits from systemic fluorides in both children and adults; however, it is not a substitute, since the modes of action differ. Periodic applications should be supplemented by daily use of a fluoride-containing dentifrice. Daily use of a mouth rinse containing low fluoride concentrations is also effective for children and adults as prophylaxis against caries. For highly caries-prone patients, custom trays that allow self-application of fluoride gel for 5 min/day are recommended.

Food particles and dental plaque should be removed from all accessible tooth surfaces at least once daily. Mechanical removal is the only effective method currently available. Proper use of a soft-bristled toothbrush removes plaque adequately from all areas except interproximal tooth surfaces and deep pits and fissures of the enamel. Interproximal surfaces, highly susceptible to dental caries, should be cleaned daily with dental floss or tape. Plaque-disclosing tablets or liquids composed of food coloring may be used to check the efficacy of plaque removal. Since fluorides are relatively less effective for preventing pit and fissure caries, sealing enamel pits and fissures with a BIS-GMA–type resin is highly effective in preventing caries and is performed increasingly by dentists. The sealed teeth should be checked annually and the sealant replaced when lost.

Treatment

Although caries may be arrested, destroyed tooth structure cannot regenerate. All affected tooth structure should be removed and replaced with a restorative material. Testing for risk of or susceptibility to caries is recommended for caries-active patients. Such tests include measurements of salivary flow rate and buffering capacity and determination of the colony-forming units (CFU) of S. mutans and Lactobacillus acidophilus. If the CFU is high, treatment with topical fluorides and chlorhexidine mouth rinses is recommended. For details

of filling teeth, see DENTAL RESTORATIONS AND AP-
PLIANCES in Ch. 105.

PULPITIS

*Inflammation of the dental pulp (containing
vascular, connective, and nervous tissue) and of
the adjacent periodontal tissues, resulting in
toothache.*

Etiology and Pathology

Pulpitis may result from thermal, chemical,
traumatic, or bacterial irritation of the pulp.
Pulpal inflammation and infection secondary to
caries is the most frequent cause. Since hard
dentinal walls surround the pulp, an inflammatory reaction usually results in necrosis. The inflammation extends through the apex of the
tooth and involves the periapical tissues (connective tissue of the periodontal membrane and
bone).

Symptoms, Signs, and Diagnosis

In acute suppurative pulpitis, a sharp, throbbing, shooting pain may be intermittent; it is
less intense in pulpitis secondary to mechanical
debridement of a cavity. A distinction must be
made between caries-induced pulpitis, pulpitis
secondary to traumatic occlusion, and dentinal
pain. **Pulpitis pain** may be intense, throbbing,
intermittent, or continuous and usually is more
severe than dentinal pain. The tooth may have
a negative response to an electric pulp test and
be sensitive to percussion and heat. **Dentinal
pain,** derived from irritation of the dentin,
should be suspected when the dentin is exposed, a restoration has recently been placed,
or leakage is present around an existing restoration. The common symptoms of dentinal pain
are sensitivity to cold, to sweet foods, and in
the case of leakage, to pressure when chewing
on the restoration. Any means of protecting the
dentin that results in reduction of symptoms is
usually diagnostic. Intense pain may be difficult
to localize. It may be referred to the opposite
mandible or maxilla or to areas supplied by
common branches of the 5th nerve. X-rays,
pulp testers, percussion, thermal tests, and palpation aid in diagnosis.

Treatment

In early pulpitis, cleansing the cavity to remove food debris and softened dentin, followed by filling the cavity with zinc oxide–eu-

genol cement (clove oil mixed with zinc oxide
powder to form a thick paste), usually affords
temporary relief and prevents food debris from
accumulating. The infected pulpal tissue should
be removed as soon as possible and root canal
therapy instituted, or the tooth should be extracted.

PERIAPICAL ABSCESS
(Dentoalveolar Abscess)

*An acute or chronic suppurative process of the
periapical region.*

Etiology and Pathogenesis

The abscess is secondary to an infection of the
dental pulp usually due to caries. However, it
may occur after trauma to the teeth or from periapical localization of organisms, usually α-hemolytic streptococci or staphylococci.

Symptoms and Signs

Pain is gnawing and continuous. The involved
tooth is painful when percussed, and often the
teeth cannot close without added discomfort.
Hot foods may increase the pain. If treatment is
delayed, the infection may spread through adjacent tissues, causing **cellulitis,** varying degrees
of facial edema, and fever. The infection may extend into osseous tissues or into the soft tissues
of the floor of the mouth. Local swelling and **gingival fistulas** may develop opposite the apex of
the tooth, especially with deciduous teeth. Drainage into the mouth causes a bitter taste. **Abscesses** from lower molars may drain at the angle of the jaw.

A *chronic* periapical abscess usually presents
few clinical signs, since it is essentially a circumscribed area of mild infection that spreads
slowly. In time, the infection may become granulomatous. As the granuloma enlarges, the lesion
may progress to an epithelium-lined cavity and a
periapical cyst results. Persistent periapical
cysts and granulomas may become infected. All
are radiolucent on x-ray examination. Bacteria
may spread via the blood and by contiguity to
involve the brain, cervical, and thoracic structures (see Ch. 105).

Treatment

Extraction or root canal therapy is usually indicated. Even if a fistula is present, drainage
should be instituted by creating an opening
through the tooth crown into the pulp chamber

when extraction or root canal therapy is not immediately performed. If high fever persists, antibiotics (eg, penicillin G or V 250 to 500 mg q 6 h, or erythromycin or a tetracycline 250 mg q 6 h) should be given. Hot saline mouth rinses may encourage pointing. If the swelling becomes fluctuant, it should be drained, usually by intraoral incision. An analgesic (eg, aspirin or acetaminophen 650 mg alone or with codeine 30 to 60 mg orally q 3 to 4 h) is usually needed. Bed rest, a soft diet, and forced fluids may be necessary.

109. PERIODONTAL DISEASE

Inflammation or degeneration of tissues that surround and support the teeth: gingiva, alveolar bone, periodontal ligament, and cementum. Periodontal disease most commonly begins as gingivitis and progresses to periodontitis. If the severity of the disease is disproportionate to the amount of plaque and calculus, **systemic disease** may be present; however, in widespread periodontal disease, local factors are also present. For example, diabetes mellitus, scurvy, leukemia and other disorders of leukocyte number or function, hyperparathyroidism, and osteoporosis aggravate the effects of local factors.

GINGIVITIS

Inflammation of the gingiva, characterized by swelling, redness, change of normal contours, watery exudate, and bleeding. Swelling deepens the crevice between the gingiva and the teeth, and gingival pockets form. Gingivitis is common and may be acute, chronic, or recurrent.

Etiology

The most frequent single cause is poor hygiene, characterized by bacterial plaque (microbial colonies tenaciously attached to the tooth surfaces). Other local factors such as malocclusion, dental calculus (calcified plaque, called tartar), food impaction, faulty dental restorations, and mouth breathing play important secondary roles.

Gingivitis is commonly noted at puberty and during pregnancy and is presumably more severe because of endocrine factors. Gingivitis may be an early sign of a systemic disorder with lowered tissue resistance, eg, primary herpes simplex, hypovitaminosis, leukopenic disorders, allergic reaction, endocrine disturbance (eg, diabetes mellitus), or a debilitating disease. Prolonged ingestion of phenytoin may cause enlargement of the gingiva; the use of birth control pills may increase inflammatory changes; heavy metals (eg, lead and bismuth) may also cause gingivitis. Correcting the factors causing the gingivitis would prevent most periodontal diseases.

Symptoms, Signs, and Diagnosis

Simple gingivitis: The outstanding signs are a band of red, inflamed gingiva along the necks of teeth, edematous swelling of the interdental papillae, and bleeding on minimal injury. Pain is usually absent. The inflammation, sometimes acute in onset, may subside, but without treatment it will persist in chronic form.

Gingivitis of diabetes mellitus: Uncontrolled diabetics have an exaggerated response to gingival irritants; secondary infections and acute gingival abscesses are common. Rapid, progressive periodontal bone loss is a common finding on x-ray examination.

Gingivitis of pregnancy: Mild inflammation of the gingiva may develop in pregnancy; hyperplasia, especially of the interdental papillae, is likely to occur. Pedunculated gingival growths (**pregnancy tumors**) often arise from the papillae in the first trimester, may persist throughout pregnancy, and may or may not subside after delivery. These growths tend to recur if excised before term and may or may not regress following delivery. A similar lesion, **pyogenic granuloma**, is a soft, reddish mass in the interdental gingiva that develops rapidly and then remains static. Treatment is excision. A similar gingivitis may accompany dysmenorrhea.

Desquamative gingivitis is characterized by deep red, painful, easily bleeding gingival tissue. Vesicles may precede the stage of desquamation. Desquamative gingivitis often occurs during menopause. The gingiva is soft because the cornified cells that would resist masticatory trauma are absent. Sequential administration of estrogens and progestins is often beneficial. A similar gingival lesion may be associated with bullous pemphigoid, benign mucosal pemphigoid, or erosive lichen planus, which responds to corticosteroid therapy (see Chs. 96 and 98).

Gingivitis in leukemia: Engorged, edematous, painful, enlarged gingiva that bleeds readily suggests leukemia. This results from reduced tissue resistance, the presence of leukemic infiltrates in the periodontal tissues, and characteristic bleeding abnormalities. The gingiva may become secondarily infected with fusospirochetal organisms, resulting in acute necrotizing ulcerative gingivitis (**ANUG**—see below).

Drug-induced gingivitis: Treatment with phenytoin, cyclosporine, or the calcium channel blockers in the presence of gingival inflammation may cause fibrotic gingival hyperplasia. The interdental papillae enlarge initially. The process may progress until the gingiva is entirely involved and the teeth partially obscured. The hyperplastic tissue is firm and less prone to bleed than in other forms of gingivitis. Excision may provide temporary benefit. A folic acid supplement (3 mg/day) to regain the optimal blood level and meticulous plaque removal help to control the hyperplasia.

Gingivitis in hypovitaminosis: The gingiva in **scurvy** is inflamed, hyperplastic, engorged with blood, and bleeds easily. It may appear as "bags of blood." Petechial and ecchymotic areas may appear on the gingiva and elsewhere in the mouth. Destruction of periosteum and periodontal tissue, resulting in loosened teeth, is common. Gingival changes are not seen in edentulous patients. In **pellagra**, the gingiva is inflamed, bleeds easily, and is subject to secondary infection. The lips are reddened and cracked, the mouth feels scalded, the tongue is smooth and bright red, and tongue and mucosa may show ulcerations.

Pericoronitis: Recurrent episodes of acute inflammation of the gingival flap overlying a partially erupted tooth are common—most often around the 3rd molar; extraction may be considered after the acute process subsides. The gingival flap disappears when the tooth is fully erupted. Treatment is local aqueous irrigation. If the infection is severe, antibiotics may be required; eg, penicillin V 500 mg orally q 6 h for 10 days.

Gingival abscess (parulis) develops from a periapical abscess at the tip of the root of a nonvital tooth. Pus escapes from a sinus that opens on the mucosal surface. A periodontal abscess may drain similarly.

Prophylaxis

Daily removal of plaque with dental floss and a toothbrush, and routine cleaning by a dentist every 3 to 6 mo are essential preventive procedures, especially when systemic conditions predispose to gingivitis.

Treatment

The treatment is to control or correct both plaque and local and systemic factors. Some cases require extensive treatment such as thorough scaling, replacement of overhanging fillings, and correction of poorly contoured restorations. Otherwise, microbial plaque is encouraged to accumulate along the gingival margins. Excision of excess gingiva may be required in specific situations as noted above.

ACUTE NECROTIZING ULCERATIVE GINGIVITIS (ANUG)
(Trench Mouth; Vincent's Infection; Fusospirochetosis)

A noncontagious infection, associated with a fusiform bacillus and a spirochete, that usually begins on the interdental papillae and can affect the marginal and attached gingiva by direct extension. Poor oral hygiene, physical or emotional stress, nutritional deficiencies, blood dyscrasias, debilitating diseases, insufficient rest, and heavy smoking predispose to this disease, which is seen most frequently in young adults.

Symptoms and Signs

Onset, usually abrupt, may be accompanied by malaise. With no secondary infection, there usually is no fever. The chief symptoms are acutely painful bleeding gingiva, salivation, and fetid breath. The ulcerations, usually limited to the marginal gingiva and interdental papillae, have a characteristic punched-out appearance, are covered by a grayish membrane, and bleed on slight pressure or irritation. Swallowing and talking may be painful. Regional lymphadenopathy is often present. Lesions on the buccal mucosa are rare but may appear as diffuse ulcerations covered with an easily removed pseudomembrane. Rarely, lesions occur on the tonsils, pharynx, bronchi, rectum, or vagina.

Diagnosis

The punched-out appearance of the interdental papillae, the interdental grayish membrane, spontaneous bleeding, and pain are pathognomonic. The presence of overwhelming numbers of fusospirochetal forms in stained smears from the lesions confirms the diagnosis. Early differentiation from diphtheria or agranulocytosis is essential when tonsillar or pharyngeal tissues are involved. The differential diagnosis must consider streptococcal or staphylococcal pharyngitis and primary herpetic stomatitis.

Treatment

Gentle but thorough local debridement, oral hygiene, adequate nutrition, high fluid intake, and rest are essential. Using a soft brush and irrigating under low pressure or rinsing the mouth with warm normal saline or 1.5% peroxide solution may be helpful for the first few days. Analgesics may be required during the first 24 h after initial debridement. The patient should avoid irritation (eg, from smoking or from hot or spicy foods) and should have appropriate rest, good nutrition, and high fluid intake. Marked improvement usually occurs within 24 h, and then debridement can be completed. Although the acute stage responds quickly to antibiotic therapy (eg, penicillin G or V, erythromycin, or a tetracycline, 250 mg q 6 h), antibiotics are seldom necessary and should be avoided unless high fever or clinical signs of extension of the infection are present. Poor tissue topography, often produced during the acute phase, may need surgical correction to reduce the possibility of recurrence.

OTHER GINGIVAL DISORDERS

Enlargement of the gingiva occurs frequently during hormonal changes, ie, pregnancy and puberty, particularly where local irritation exists, caused primarily by plaque and calculus. **Idiopathic fibromatosis** is characterized by diffuse enlargement of the gingiva, either smooth or nodular (see also discussion of drug-induced gingivitis, above). The hypertrophied tissue is often removed after the etiologic factors have been controlled.

Gingival **fibromas** often occur near sites of chronic irritation. A **giant cell epulis**, which looks similar, may arise from the periodontal ligament. If the tissue contains such cells, blood chemistry tests for hyperparathyroidism should be performed.

Denture sore mouth, *the painful inflammation under prosthetic appliances,* may result from combinations of candidal infections, poor denture hygiene, and excessive movement of the appliance. Treatment includes improvement of oral and appliance hygiene, rebasement of the appliance or construction of a new one, removal of the appliance for extended periods, soaking the appliance in a cleanser (eg, sodium hypochlorite), and antifungal therapy. The latter may consist of nystatin oral rinses or ointment applied to the tissue surface of the denture or clotrimazole troches 10 mg 5 times/day. Ketoconazole one 200-mg tablet/day may be required. Systemic conditions such as diabetes mellitus and poor nutrition should be ruled out if the inflammation persists.

In thrombocytopenic purpura or disorders of platelet function, gingival petechiae and **hemorrhage** may occur. Localization is predominantly at sites of periodontal disease.

PERIODONTITIS
(Pyorrhea)

Progression of gingivitis to the point that loss of supporting bone has begun. It is the primary cause of tooth loss in adults.

Etiology

Periodontitis results from the same local and systemic factors that cause gingivitis. The duration and severity of these factors as well as the resistance and repair potential of the patient influence the rate of osseous resorption. Faulty occlusion causing an excessive functional load on teeth may contribute to the progress of the disease.

Symptoms, Signs, and Diagnosis

The early symptoms and signs of periodontitis are similar to those of gingivitis. The gingival pockets between the gingiva and the teeth deepen, calculus deposits often enlarge, the gingiva lose their attachment to the teeth, and bone loss begins. The pockets collect debris and allow microbes to proliferate, thus promoting the disease. Destruction of the supporting osseous tissue in varying degree is the earliest evidence seen on x-ray. Loosening of teeth and possible recession of the gingiva follow progressive bone loss; tooth migration is common in later stages. Pain is usually absent unless an acute infection (eg, abscess formation in one or more periodontal pockets) is superimposed on the chronic process.

Treatment
(See also GINGIVITIS, above)

Systemic disorders require correction. Astringent agents, mouthwashes, and antibiotics are of little value in long-term treatment. Dental referral is indicated to correct or eliminate local irritative factors and to instruct in home care that will limit further destruction. If abnormal gingival contour and pockets go uncorrected, surgery will be required. Advanced periodontitis with deep pocket formation and tooth mobility is likely to require extensive periodontal surgery. Splinting of loose teeth and selective reshaping of tooth surfaces to eliminate traumatic occlusion may be necessary. Extractions are often imperative in advanced disease.

JUVENILE PERIODONTITIS
(Periodontosis)

An uncommon widespread degeneration of the periodontal tissues with loss of alveolar bone

resulting in loss of teeth at an early age. It differs from periodontitis in its early-age onset and in associated microbial flora. Typically, there is significant bone loss localized to the 1st molars and incisors during late childhood or the early teens. Specific microorganisms and a hereditary predisposition may be linked to the disease. By early adulthood, typical chronic inflammatory periodontitis may be superimposed on the original juvenile condition. While cause and treatment are not yet definitive, controlling the microbial environment, improving the occlusion, and splinting the teeth may be of value. Periodontal surgery may be necessary to attempt to stabilize the condition.

110. TEMPOROMANDIBULAR JOINT (TMJ) DISORDERS

The TMJ is susceptible to common congenital and developmental anomalies, fractures and dislocations (see Ch. 112), ankylosis, arthritis, and neoplastic diseases. There may also be internal derangements of the intra-articular disk. Nonarticular disorders that affect the area and can mimic true TMJ disease and the muscular disorder known as **myofascial pain–dysfunction (MPD) syndrome** (see below), which may secondarily involve the TMJ, must be considered in differential diagnosis (see Temporomandibular Joint in Ch. 106).

CONGENITAL AND DEVELOPMENTAL ANOMALIES

Agenesis: Congenital absence of the condyloid process results in severe facial deformity. The coronoid process, the ramus, and parts of the mandibular body may also be absent. Abnormalities of the external, middle, and inner ear; the temporal bone; the parotid gland; the muscles of mastication; and the facial nerve are often associated. Without the condyle, the mandible deviates to the affected side and the unaffected side is elongated and flattened. Mandibular skewing results in severe malocclusion. X-rays of the mandible and TMJ show the degree of agenesis and distinguish this condition from others that affect the growing condyle and produce similar facial deformities but are not associated with severe structural loss.

Treatment: Jaw reconstruction by autogenous bone grafting (costochondral graft) should be initiated as soon as possible to limit progression of the facial deformity. Mentoplasty and onlay grafts of bone and cartilage as well as soft tissue flaps and grafts are also frequently used to improve facial symmetry. Orthodontic treatment helps correct malocclusion.

Condylar hypoplasia: This may be developmental in origin but usually results from local injury by trauma, infection, or irradiation during the growth period. Hypoplasia produces facial deformity characterized on the affected side by a short mandibular body, fullness of the face, and deviation of the chin. On the unaffected side, the body of the mandible is elongated and the face appears flat. Malocclusion results from the mandibular deviation. Diagnosis is based on a history of progressive facial asymmetry during the growth period, x-ray evidence of condylar deformity and antegonial notching (a depression in the inferior border of the mandible just anterior to the angle of the mandible), and frequently, a history of trauma.

Treatment: Surgically shortening the normal side of the mandible or lengthening the affected side is usually functionally and aesthetically corrective. Presurgical orthodontic therapy helps to achieve an optimal result.

Condylar hyperplasia: This disorder of unknown etiology is characterized by persistent or accelerated growth at a time when growth should be diminishing or ended. Slowly progressive unilateral enlargement of the mandible causes cross-bite malocclusion, facial asymmetry, and shifting of the midpoint of the chin to the unaffected side. The patient may appear prognathic. The lower border of the mandible is often convex on the affected side. On x-ray, the TMJ may appear normal or the condyle may be symmetrically enlarged and the mandibular neck elongated. The condition is self-limiting. Since chondroma and osteochondroma may produce similar symptoms and signs, they must be ruled out. These grow more rapidly and usually cause asymmetric condylar enlargement.

Treatment: Condylectomy is recommended during the period of active growth, as determined by serial cephalometric x-rays and bone scan. If growth has already stopped, orthodontics and surgical mandibular repositioning are indicated. If the height of the mandibular body is greatly increased, facial symmetry can be further improved by reducing the inferior border.

ANKYLOSIS

Ankylosis of the TMJ is most often a sequel to trauma or infection, though it may accompany RA or be congenital. Chronic, painless limitation of movement occurs. When associated with condylar growth arrest or tissue loss, facial asymmetry is usual (see **condylar hypoplasia,** above). True (intra-articular) ankylosis must be distinguished from false (extra-articular) ankylosis. The latter may be caused by such things as enlargement of the coronoid process, depressed fracture of the zygomatic arch, or scarring from surgery or irradiation. In most cases of true ankylosis, x-rays of the TMJ show loss of normal bony architecture.

Treatment: Forced opening of the jaws is generally ineffective because of bony fusion. Condylectomy can be used if the ankylosis is intra-articular. An ostectomy in the ramus may be needed if the coronoid process and zygomatic arch are also involved. Prolonged use of jaw-opening exercises is essential to maintain the surgical correction.

INTERNAL DISK DERANGEMENT

Internal derangement of the articular disk can be caused by chronic spasm of the lateral pterygoid muscle, trauma, or arthritic changes in the articulating surfaces. Such derangements take 2 forms: anterior disk displacement with reduction during function, which is accompanied by clicking or popping sounds on opening the mouth, and anterior disk displacement without reduction, which is characterized by painful limitation of jaw movement. This clinical distinction is confirmed by MRI, arthrography, or CT scan.

Treatment: Nonsurgical treatment is effective in about 25% of the patients who have anterior disk displacement with reduction. It employs jaw repositioning appliances, nonsteroidal anti-inflammatory drugs, and when there is lateral pterygoid spasm, muscle relaxants, such as diazepam or methocarbamol. For patients with persistent pain and clicking unresponsive to such modalities, the disk can be repositioned surgically.

For anterior displacement of the disk that is not self-reducing, surgical correction by arthrotomy or arthroscopy is indicated. If the disk is in satisfactory condition, it is merely repositioned. Otherwise, it is removed (meniscectomy) and replaced with an alloplastic implant or autogenous graft.

ARTHRITIS

Most forms of arthritis can involve the TMJ; the most common ones, in order of increasing frequency, are infectious, traumatic, rheumatoid, and degenerative (osteoarthritis).

Infectious arthritis may be part of a systemic disease, may arise from direct extension of adjacent infection, or may result from localization of blood-borne organisms from a distant infection. Inflammation and limited jaw movement are present. Early x-rays are negative but bone destruction becomes evident later. Local signs of inflammation, associated with evidence of a systemic disease or an adjacent infection, suggest the diagnosis. In suppurative arthritis, joint aspiration may confirm the diagnosis and identify the causative organism.

Treatment includes antibiotics, proper hydration, control of pain, and restriction of motion. Penicillin G is the drug of choice until a specific diagnosis can be made on the basis of culture and sensitivity testing. Suppurative infections should be aspirated or incised. Once the infection is controlled, jaw-opening exercises are important to prevent scarring and limitation of function.

Traumatic arthritis may be caused by acute injury or excessive opening—eg, during yawning, tooth extraction, or endotracheal intubation. Pain, tenderness, and limitation of motion occur. X-rays are negative except for occasional widening of the joint space due to intra-articular edema or hemorrhage. The diagnosis includes a history of trauma and x-rays negative for fracture. Treatment includes nonsteroidal anti-inflammatory drugs (NSAIDs), heat application, a soft diet, and restriction of jaw movement.

In RA, the TMJ is involved in > 50% of cases, in both adults and children. Pain, swelling, and limited movement are the most common findings. In children, destruction of the condyle results in growth disturbance and facial deformity. Ankylosis may follow in all patients. X-rays of the TMJ are usually negative in early stages, but bone destruction is seen later and may result in an anterior open-bite deformity. The diagnosis is suggested by TMJ inflammation associated with polyarthritis and is confirmed by positive laboratory findings.

Treatment is similar to that for RA of other joints. In the acute stage, NSAIDs are given and jaw function should be limited. When symptoms subside, mild jaw exercises help prevent excessive loss of motion. Surgical correction is necessary if ankylosis develops but should not be undertaken until the condition is quiescent.

Primary degenerative arthritis (osteoarthritis) may involve the TMJ as well as other joints and usually occurs in persons over age 50. Relatively asymptomatic, patients complain only occasionally of stiffness, crepitation, or mild pain. Joint involvement is generally bilateral. X-rays may show flattening and lipping of the condyle. Treatment is symptomatic.

Secondary degenerative arthritis usually occurs in persons aged 20 to 40 after trauma or persistent MPD syndrome (see below) and is characterized by limitation of opening and unilateral pain on motion, joint tenderness, and crepitation. When associated with MPD syndrome, the symptoms intermittently become more severe and some muscles of mastication are tender. X-rays generally show condylar flattening, lipping, spurring, or erosion. The unilateral joint involvement helps to distinguish secondary from primary degenerative arthritis. Treatment is conservative, as for MPD syndrome, though arthroplasty or high condylectomy may be necessary. Intra-articular injection of corticosteroids

may bring symptomatic relief but may harm the joint if repeated often.

NONARTICULAR CONDITIONS MIMICKING TEMPOROMANDIBULAR JOINT DISORDERS

Conditions unrelated to the TMJ that can produce preauricular pain, limitation of jaw movement, or a combination of both include pulpitis, pericoronitis, otitis, parotitis, trigeminal neuralgia, atypical (vascular) neuralgia, temporal arteritis, nasopharyngeal carcinoma, myositis and myositis ossificans, tetanus, scleroderma, depressed fracture of the zygomatic arch, and osteochondroma of the coronoid process. Pain due to these, unlike that in intrinsic TMJ disorders, is usually not exacerbated by finger pressure on the TMJ as the patient opens the mouth.

MYOFASCIAL PAIN–DYSFUNCTION (MPD) SYNDROME

The most common disorder involving the TMJ area, MPD syndrome occurs in women more frequently than in men. Most cases are psychophysiologic in origin and result from tension-relieving jaw-clenching or tooth-grinding habits or a centrally generated increase in masticatory muscle tonus in response to stress. The ensuing muscle fatigue in turn induces spasm of the masticatory muscles, the immediate cause of MPD. Poorly aligned teeth or ill-fitting dentures occasionally contribute to the condition. Secondary degenerative arthritis may involve the joint in the late stages.

Diagnosis is based on clinical findings. Characteristically, the patient complains of unilateral, dull, aching preauricular pain that radiates to the temporal region, the angle of the jaw, and the occiput; tenderness in one or more of the muscles of mastication; jaw limitation; and occasional clicking or "popping" sounds in the joint (see INTERNAL DISK DERANGEMENT, above). Joint pain on awakening may indicate bruxism during sleep. X-rays are usually normal, although secondary degenerative changes are seen occasionally in very late stages. Degenerative arthritis, which causes similar symptoms, must be excluded. Primary degenerative arthritis is usually bilateral. Both primary and secondary degenerative arthritis usually produce x-ray changes in the joint, and secondary degenerative arthritis causes tenderness of the TMJ on lateral or intrameatal palpation; these findings help to distinguish the arthritides from MPD syndrome. However, secondary degenerative arthritis can be a sequela to MPD syndrome, and therefore both conditions can be present simultaneously.

Treatment includes a soft, nonchewy diet; limited use of the jaw; hot, moist applications or diathermy; diazepam 2 to 5 mg qid (the last dose taken at bedtime) as a muscle relaxant and tranquilizer; analgesics (eg, aspirin 650 mg qid) for pain; and use of a biteplate. Clenching or grinding the teeth should be avoided. Possible causative life stresses should be discussed with the patient. Psychologic counseling may be helpful in persistent cases.

111. PRENEOPLASTIC AND NEOPLASTIC LESIONS

Approximately 30,000 new cases of oral cancer (mainly squamous cell) are reported each year in the USA and account for about 5% of cancers in men and 2% in women. More than any other factor, the stage of these cancers determines the prognosis (see Staging and Prognosis in Ch. 72). While oral cancers < 1 cm in diameter are easily cured, most lesions are *not* diagnosed before stage III or IV and ≥ 50% have metastasized to lymph nodes. Therefore, 5-yr survival rates remain at 30 to 40%. This unfortunate situation appears to result from inadequate knowledge of appropriate screening procedures and strongly entrenched misconceptions.

Persons at risk: While screening is easy enough so that all patients can be included, careful attention to those with clearly defined **risk factors** is mandatory; ie, individuals ≥ 40 yr old who smoke cigarettes and those who drink alcoholic beverages regularly. Other less common risk factors are pipe and cigar smoking. Smokeless (chewing) tobacco appears to be related to verrucous carcinoma (a highly differentiated variant of squamous cell carcinoma). Screening has been reported to increase discovery rates of early cancer in these high-risk populations to 1/200 to 250.

Sites at risk: About 90% of oral cancers are detected in only a few high-risk sites: the floor of the mouth, the ventrolateral aspect of the tongue, and the soft palate complex (uvula, soft palate proper, anterior pillar, and lingual aspects of the retromolar trigone). Buccal and labial vestibular carcinoma should be considered in people who use smokeless tobacco.

Misconceptions: Most physicians and dentists have been taught that **leukoplakia** (white lesions) are the most common precancerous lesions in the mouth and that early cancers are white lesions. In fact, < 5% of such lesions ultimately prove to be cancerous. Early, asymptomatic oral cancer appears most often as a **red (erythroplastic) lesion**. These lesions are not precancerous; they are early carcinomas. These areas look like an inflammation, probably as the result of a submucosal round-cell infiltrate that has arisen below the malignant squamous cells in response to the developing neoplasm. When dry, these red lesions appear more granular or slightly abraded. Therefore, they should be dried gently with a piece of gauze and examined carefully under good light. Two distinct types of erythroplastic lesions have been identified: (1) a red, granular lesion (appearing like worn velvet) speckled with islands of keratin (white) or normal mucosa within or peripheral to the red component, and (2) a smooth, nongranular, red lesion with minimal associated keratin, similar to a nonspecific inflammation. Both types may have irregular, ill-defined borders; generally, palpation is not helpful diagnostically, as few are indurated or raised. *Any erythroplastic lesion that does not respond to treatment and persists > 14 days should be considered carcinoma in situ or invasive carcinoma and requires biopsy.* Unfortunately, **squamous cell carcinoma** is not usually diagnosed in its earliest stages and later appears as a deep ulcer, with smooth, indurated, rolled margins, fixed to deeper tissues. Toluidine blue stain may be used as a diagnostic adjunct to clinical impressions. However, biopsy is necessary to diagnose carcinoma.

Other malignancies of the oral cavity are epidermoid carcinoma of the lip, cheek, and tongue; lymphoepithelioma; melanoma; adenocarcinomas of major and minor salivary glands; and myelocytic and lymphocytic leukemias. **Benign lesions that may be found in the oral cavity** include "irritation fibroma," papilloma, granuloma (including pregnancy tumor), the glossitis of avitaminosis, geographic tongue, median rhomboid glossitis, hemangioma and lymphangioma, fibrous hypertrophy of the gingiva, melanosis, myoblastoma, retention cysts (including ranula), xanthomatosis, tori, submandibular duct calculus, hypertrophy of the foliate papillae, radiculodental cysts, and ameloblastoma. Syphilis, erosive lichen planus, benign ulcer, TB, leukoplakia, and dental abscess should also be considered. Exfoliative cytology is useful in screening, but biopsy is essential to establish the diagnosis.

Multiple carcinomas: *Patients with an oral squamous cancer are at high risk (up to 33%) of developing a second primary squamous neoplasm in the mouth, pharynx, larynx, esophagus, or lung.* Therefore, patients identified as having an oral cancer should be screened for cancer in all these sites and reexamined at yearly intervals (eg, examination of mouth and throat, indirect laryngoscopy, chest x-ray).

Treatment

Any recognizable irritation (eg, faulty restorations and prosthetic devices) should be corrected or removed. Tobacco in any form should be eliminated, and mucosal drying agents such as alcoholic beverages and mouth rinses with alcoholic vehicles should be discontinued to prevent the development of second primary cancers.

Treatment of oral neoplasms generally consists of wide local excision for small lesions and en bloc excision of larger lesions in continuity with radical neck dissection if lymph nodes are involved. Radiotherapy alone may be appropriate for certain small or large lesions or may be combined with surgery. Chemotherapy may be used as palliation or as an adjunct to surgery and radiotherapy.

NEOPLASMS OF SPECIFIC TISSUES

Lips, gingiva, and tongue: Smoker's patch is a firm, brownish, keratotic plaque on the vermilion border of the lower lip and is most common in smokers who hold a cigarette or pipe in one location. *Only a biopsy can rule out squamous cell carcinoma.* Cessation of smoking and close observation are recommended even if the lesion is not malignant. **Actinic cheilosis** occurs in adults, especially redheads with fair skin, who spend much time out of doors. The lips are dry with many erosive areas. A person with this *precancerous* lesion should be seen every 3 to 6 mo, avoid prolonged exposure to sunlight, wear a broad-brimmed hat, and use an antiactinic ointment. **Squamous cell carcinoma** usually ap-

pears on the vermilion border of the lower lip as a nonhealing ulcer with a convex, indurated margin, or less commonly, as a keratotic patch. It may be fixed to the underlying tissues. If it is treated early, prognosis is excellent. In **leukemia**, the gingival tissue may be enlarged from infiltration and prone to bleed. **Rhabdomyoma** of the tongue causes a palpable interior mass. It is much rarer than squamous cell carcinoma, which arises in the mucosa.

Cheek: Irritation of the mucosa is commonly seen in the mucobuccal fold, where chewing tobacco or snuff may be habitually retained. The irritation may progress to erythroplakia or leukoplakia and squamous cell carcinoma. A firm, nodular, nonpainful swelling in the cheek covered by normal-appearing mucosa is common, usually resulting from a cheek bite. This "**irritation fibroma**" is considered benign.

Palate: Accessory salivary gland tumor is usually a mixed tumor with both epithelial and mesenchymal components, an adenoid cystic carcinoma, or a mucoepidermoid carcinoma. Typically, it appears as a firm, smooth, painless mass lateral to the midline. Any such swelling that is not bony hard should be considered a salivary gland tumor until a biopsy proves otherwise. When a histologic diagnosis of mucoepidermoid carcinoma or adenocarcinoma of a palatal lesion is made, necrotizing sialometaplasia should be ruled out. This lesion is benign but has histologic and clinical features suggesting malignancy. A **fullness of the palate** can represent extension of a malignant tumor of the lining of the nose or the antrum rather than a primary lesion of the palate. The soft palate may become immobile if a cancer is in the nasopharynx.

Jaws: If not initially detected on x-ray, jaw tumors are diagnosed clinically because their growth causes **swelling** of the face, palate, or alveolar process (the area of the jaw surrounding the teeth). They cause bone tenderness and severe pain originating in the involved bone. **Ameloblastoma**, the most common epithelial odontogenic neoplasm, usually arises in the posterior mandible; it is slowly invasive but rarely metastatic. On x-ray, it typically appears as a multiloculated or soap-bubble radiolucency. **Odontomas**, the most common odontogenic neoplasms, are tumors of the dental follicle or the dental tissues that usually appear in the mandibles of young people; several types include fibrous odontomas and cementomas. An absent molar tooth suggests a composite odontoma.

Other neoplasms include osteogenic sarcoma, giant cell tumor, Ewing's tumor, multiple myeloma, and metastatic tumors.

Salivary glands: The 2 main types of tumors are the benign mixed tumor (pleomorphic adenoma), 60% of which occur in the parotid glands, and mucoepidermoid carcinoma. These tumors occur primarily in major salivary glands, but about 20% are found in accessory salivary glands located mainly in the palate and the buccal mucosa (see above). About 1/6 of tumors in the parotid gland, 1/3 of those in the submandibular gland, almost 1/2 of all palatal tumors, and nearly all sublingual gland tumors are malignant.

Slowly developing parotid swellings may be painless, and the patient complains of a change in appearance; however, acute swelling of the parotid gland is painful because of dense fascia surrounding it. A parotid tumor causes facial paralysis if it compresses or infiltrates the facial nerve, which may also be damaged inadvertently during surgery to remove the tumor. Tumors of the submandibular salivary glands are often painful because of close association with the lingual branch of the trigeminal nerve.

112. DENTAL EMERGENCIES

Emergency dental treatment by a physician is sometimes required when dentists are unavailable, but dental consultation is desirable as soon as possible.

TOOTHACHE AND INFECTION

Pain localized to a particular tooth and provoked by sweets or cold is usually caused by caries that has not yet involved the dental pulp (nerve). Because this type of pain is usually fleeting, the patient should avoid provoking stimuli, use mild analgesics, and seek prompt treatment.

Localized pain that is usually intensified by heat most commonly denotes caries that has reached the dental pulp (see PULPITIS in Ch. 108). Associated periapical inflammation, often present, may be diagnosed by tenderness to percussion. (If all maxillary posterior teeth on one side are sensitive to percussion, maxillary sinusitis should be suspected.) Initial treatment with an analgesic (eg, acetaminophen 325 mg with codeine 30 mg orally q 4 h) and an antibiotic (eg, erythromycin, penicillin V, or a cephalosporin, 250 mg q 6 h) may be indicated until dental therapy can be initiated.

Periapical infection, often accompanied by swelling of contiguous soft tissues, will usually develop from untreated pulpitis. Emergency treatment consists of analgesics and antibiotics, as described above. A periapical abscess that has spread beyond the alveolar bone and is causing swelling and fluctuation in adjacent soft tissue requires incision and drainage; antibiotics alone are inadequate. An intraoral incision is usually appropriate, but a percutaneous incision may be necessary for dependent drainage. To aid in selecting the appropriate antibiotic, a specimen should be cultured. (See also PERIAPICAL ABSCESS in Ch. 108.) Erupting or impacted molar teeth, particularly 3rd molars, can be painful and may cause adjacent soft tissue inflammation that can progress to serious infection; erythromycin, penicillin V, or a cephalosporin, 250 to 500 mg orally qid, should be started. Less common causes of acute perioral swelling include periodontal abscess, infected cysts, antritis, allergy, salivary gland obstruction or infection, peritonsillar infection, or skin infection.

POSTEXTRACTION PROBLEMS

Swelling is normal after intraoral surgical procedures and is somewhat proportional to the degree of manipulation and trauma. If it does not begin to subside by the 3rd postoperative day, infection is likely and an antibiotic (eg, erythromycin, penicillin V, or a cephalosporin, 250 to 500 mg orally qid) should be started.

Postoperative pain, usually moderate, can be controlled with acetaminophen or aspirin 325 mg with codeine 30 mg orally q 4 h.

Postextraction alveolitis (dry socket) is usually peculiar to the removal of mandibular posterior teeth. Typically, the pain begins on the 2nd or 3rd postoperative day, is referred to the ear, and lasts from a few days to many weeks. Alveolitis is best treated with topical analgesic medication; 1/4-in. gauze saturated in eugenol, placed in the socket and changed daily, usually reduces the need for systemic analgesics. Infection is uncommon. Rarely, osteomyelitis may be confused with alveolitis, but osteomyelitis is characterized by fever, local swelling, and later x-ray changes. If osteomyelitis is suspected, an antibiotic such as a cephalosporin should be instituted and the patient referred for definitive care.

Postextraction bleeding usually oozes from small vessels. After removing any superfluous clot with gauze, a pressure dressing (cotton wrapped in gauze or in a tea bag) is applied directly and continuously to the extraction site for 20 to 30 min. This is repeated 2 or 3 times. If the bleeding continues, the site may be anesthetized with 2% lidocaine with 1:100,000 epinephrine by nerve block or infiltration as appropriate, and the socket area sutured under tension, allowing space between the sutures for packing if necessary. Local hemostatic agents such as oxidized cellulose or topical thrombin on a gelatin sponge or microfibrillar collagen may be placed in the socket. If these measures fail, a systemic cause should be sought. Rarely, blood loss may require transfusion.

FRACTURED AND AVULSED TEETH

If a small portion of a crown is fractured and the dental pulp is not exposed, analgesic medication (eg, acetaminophen 650 mg q 4 h) and a topical covering with zinc-eugenol or similar cement are appropriate. If the pulp is exposed or the tooth is mobile, erythromycin, penicillin V, or a cephalosporin, 250 mg q 6 h should also be given. Partially avulsed teeth should be repositioned and stabilized. With any partially or completely avulsed tooth, antibiotic therapy should be prescribed for several days.

Permanent retention of a completely avulsed tooth may be possible *if it is immediately replaced into the socket without washing and with minimal handling.* If debris requires prior washing, use physiologic saline. When replacement is delayed a few minutes or the tooth is washed or handled excessively, it may be retained for a few months to a few years but the prognosis for indefinite retention is poor. Root resorption usually occurs after delayed replacement. Thus, the patient should be instructed to replace the avulsed tooth immediately and seek professional care to stabilize it. If this is not possible, the tooth should be kept moist in saline or in milk and then, if indicated, replaced and stabilized.

FRACTURES OF THE JAW AND CONTIGUOUS STRUCTURES

Fractures of the jaw and contiguous structures are diagnosed primarily by physical examination and x-ray. Fracture should be suspected if there is malocclusion, mobility of the maxillae, discrepancy in the smooth contour of the orbital rims, diplopia, infraorbital anesthesia, tenderness to palpation (particularly over the condyle or condylar neck of the mandible), and restriction or deviation when opening the mouth. A facial fracture is an emergency if there is airway obstruction, uncontrollable hemorrhage, or trauma to the eye or CNS. Routine x-rays usually confirm the diagnosis for fractures of the mandible, but CT scanning may be helpful for midface fractures. *Fracture of a cervical vertebra should be considered when a blow has been sufficient to fracture facial bones.* An oral-maxillofacial surgeon should be consulted for a fractured jaw; otherwise, unrecognized malocclusions may result.

Treatment: Manually holding the mandible in a protruded position or inserting an orotracheal or oropharyngeal airway may be necessary temporarily to maintain an airway. If there is hemorrhage into the oropharynx, an orotracheal airway should be placed or the patient positioned to allow the oropharynx to drain dependently. Until definitive care is available, the jaws usually can be temporarily stabilized and hemorrhage minimized by use of a Barton-type bandage. If a jaw fracture can be treated within the first few hours after injury, closure of lip lacerations is best delayed until the fracture has been reduced.

Fractures through a tooth socket are compound fractures, usually requiring antibiotic prophylaxis (eg, with penicillin V, erythromycin, or a cephalosporin, 250 to 500 mg orally in liquid form q 6 h).

Fractures of the mandibular condyle are usually characterized by preauricular pain, swelling, and limitation of opening. With a unilateral fracture, the jaw deviates to the affected side on attempted opening. Bilateral fracture can produce an anteriorly opened bite. Posterior-anterior and Towne's views of the mandible usually show the fracture on x-ray. **Treatment** is usually intermaxillary fixation for varying periods, but severely displaced, bilaterally fractured condyles may require open reduction and fixation. Jaw-opening exercises are usually used to aid function after fixation is discontinued. In children, some abnormal growth may ensue.

DISLOCATED MANDIBLE

A dislocated mandible will be fixed in a markedly open position with only the most posterior teeth contacting. If the midline is deviated, the dislocation is unilateral rather than bilateral. Injecting a local anesthetic agent (eg, 1% lidocaine 2 to 5 mL) in the joint area and in the area of insertion of the lateral pterygoid muscle may allow the mandible to reduce spontaneously.

Alternatively, or in addition, manual reduction may be necessary. Premedication with diazepam 5 mg IV and a narcotic (eg, for the average healthy adult, meperidine 25 mg IV or 50 mg IM) is desirable. To obtain leverage, the operator should stabilize the patient's head and position the patient so the operator can, with forearms extended, manipulate the jaw. The operator places his thumbs on the external oblique line of the mandible (lateral to the 3rd molar area) and his fingers under the tip of the chin. A rotary motion is used, with the thumbs pressing inferiorly and anteriorly and the fingers pressing superiorly, until the mandible is reseated.

The jaw should be stabilized with a Barton-type bandage to maintain the mandible in the reduced position. The patient should avoid wide opening of the mouth for at least 6 wk. When the patient feels a yawn coming, he should place his fist under his chin to prevent wide opening of the mouth. If this is not the first such dislocation, an oral-maxillofacial surgeon should be consulted.

§9. DISORDERS DUE TO PHYSICAL AGENTS

113. REACTIONS TO SUNLIGHT

The skin responds to excessive sunlight with an acute reaction (sunburn); with chronic changes that may lead to skin cancer after many years; or with an unusual photosensitivity that may be due to the ingestion or application of certain drugs or chemicals, that may be indicative of systemic disease, or that may be idiopathic.

Etiology and Predisposing Factors

Although the sun emits a wide range of ultraviolet (UV) electromagnetic radiation (ie, UVA 320 to 400 nanometers [nm], UVB 280 to 320 nm, UVC 10 to 280 nm), only UVA and UVB reach the earth's surface. The character and amount of such radiation vary greatly with the seasons and with changing atmospheric conditions. Exposure to sunlight depends on multiple factors, eg, clothing, life-style, occupation, and geographic factors including altitude and latitude. Sunburn-producing rays—those below 320 nm—are filtered out completely by ordinary window glass and to a great extent by smoke and smog. Large amounts of sunburn-producing rays may pass through light clouds, fog, or 1 ft of clear water, and many persons unwittingly sustain severe reactions under such conditions or while swimming. Snow, sand, and bright sky enhance exposure by reflecting the rays.

There is increasing concern about depletion of stratospheric ozone, which serves to filter out shorter wavelengths of UV, by man-made chlorofluorocarbons, eg, in refrigerants and aerosols, thereby increasing inadvertent exposure to UVA and UVB.

Following exposure to sunlight, the epidermis thickens and the melanocytes produce melanin at an increased rate, providing some natural protection against further exposure. Furthermore, functional alterations in epidermal Langerhans cells (which are immunologically important) have been identified. Persons differ greatly in their reactivity to sunlight. Uneven melanin deposition occurs in many fairhaired individuals and results in freckling. Pigmentation does not occur in the skin of albinos because of a defect in melanin metabolism, nor in areas of vitiligo because of the absence of melanocytes. Blondes and redheads are especially susceptible and should avoid overexposure. Blacks and other nonwhites are not immune to the effects of the sun and can become sunburned with prolonged exposure. In recent years, "tanning parlors" that utilize artificial light sources to induce tanning without sunburn have become popular. As many such light sources contain some UVB (see below), some long-term deleterious effects should be expected. Other light sources that contain only UVA have also been shown to adversely affect the skin.

ACUTE SUNBURN

Ordinary sunburn results from overexposure of the skin to ultraviolet rays of 280 to 320 nm (UVB). **Symptoms and signs** appear in 1 to 24 h and, except in severe reactions, pass their peak in 72 h. Skin changes range from mild erythema with subsequent evanescent scaling, to pain, swelling, skin tenderness, and blisters from more prolonged exposure. Sunburn affecting the lower legs, particularly the pretibial surfaces, is especially uncomfortable and often slow to heal. Constitutional symptoms (fever, chills, weakness, shock), similar to a thermal burn, may appear if a large portion of the body surface is affected; these may be due to heatstroke or heat exhaustion (see Ch. 115).

Secondary infection and miliaria-like eruptions (see in Ch. 102) are the most common late complications. Following exfoliation, the skin may be hypervulnerable to sunlight for one to several weeks.

Prophylaxis

Simple precautions will prevent most cases of severe sunburn. Initial summer exposure to bright midday sun should not be > 30 min, even in persons with dark brunette skin. In temperate zones, exposure is less hazardous before 10 AM and after 3 PM because sunburn-producing wavelengths are usually filtered out. In winter, the greatest danger of sunburn (and snow blindness) comes during foggy days that may be deceptive and have almost as much UVB as clear days on fresh snow; the danger is increased at high altitude.

Formulations of 5% aminobenzoic acid **(PABA)** or its esters in ethyl alcohol in a gel or in a cream are very effective in preventing sunburn. They take about 30 min to bind strongly to the skin, and therefore should be applied about 30 to 60 min before sun exposure so that wash-off from perspiration or swimming will be minimized. PABA products rarely cause allergic or photoallergic contact dermatitis. Those who cannot tolerate PABA or its esters may use a benzophenone sunscreen. Opaque formulations containing zinc oxide or titanium dioxide physically block and prevent radiation from reaching the skin. When suitably colored with agents such as iron salts, they are cosmetically acceptable. Highly effective, nonopaque lotions containing both a PABA ester and benzophenone are also available. **Sunscreens** are now rated in the USA by the FDA's sun protection factor **(SPF)** numbers; the higher the SPF, the greater is the protection. Sunscreens with SPFs ≥ 15 are usually recommended. Patients with photodrug reactions are rarely protected by these products. Recently, sunscreens have been introduced that are somewhat effective against UVA-induced skin damage.

Treatment

Further exposure should be *avoided* until the acute reaction has subsided. Topical corticosteroids are no more effective than cold tap-water compresses in relieving symptoms. Ointments or lotions containing local anesthetics such as benzocaine and other sensitizing agents should be *avoided.*

Early treatment of extensive and severe sunburn with a systemic corticosteroid (eg, prednisone 20 to 30 mg orally bid for 4 days for adults or teenagers) will decrease the discomfort considerably. (For treatment of heatstroke and heat exhaustion, see Ch. 115.)

CHRONIC EFFECTS OF SUNLIGHT

Chronic exposure to sunlight ages the skin. Wrinkling and elastosis (yellow discoloration with small yellow nodules) and pigment alterations are the most common troubling consequences of long-term exposure. The atrophic effects in some persons may resemble those seen after x-ray therapy. Precancerous keratotic lesions **(actinic keratoses)** are a frequent, disturbing consequence of many years' overexposure. Blondes and redheads are particularly susceptible; blacks are rarely affected. The keratoses are usually hard and sharp on palpation, and gray to dark in color. They should be differentiated from warty brown *seborrheic* keratoses, which increase in number and size with age but occur on covered as well as uncovered areas of the body and are not premalignant.

The incidence of squamous and basal cell carcinoma of the skin in fair, white-skinned persons is directly related to the amount of yearly sunlight in the area. Such lesions are especially common in those who were exposed as children and teenagers and in sportsmen, farmers, ranchers, sailors, and sunworshipers. Malignant melanomas are also increasing in incidence with increasing sun exposure.

Treatment

If there are only a few lesions, cryotherapy, eg, freezing with liquid nitrogen, is the most rapid and satisfactory treatment for actinic keratosis. If there are too many lesions to freeze, actinic keratoses usually respond dramatically to small amounts of 5-fluorouracil **(5-FU)** applied to the affected area nightly. For face lesions, 1% 5-FU in propylene glycol is best; elsewhere (eg, on the arm), 2 or 5% 5-FU cream can be used; if no response is seen on the arms in ≤ 10 days, 0.05% tretinoin solution should be applied a few hours before the 2 or 5% 5-FU application. Treatment is continued for at least 2 wk or until a brisk reaction with redness, scaling, and slight burning is seen, often including patches with no previously detected gross changes. If the reaction is too brisk, application should be suspended for 2 or 3 days. Masking cosmetics can make the treatment more acceptable. Topical 5-FU therapy is free of significant adverse effects but may be disfiguring and painful during treatment. 5-FU should not be used to treat basal cell cancers.

Recently, various therapies including chemical peels, 5-FU, α-hydroxy acids, and tretinoin have been used in attempts to improve the features of chronic sun damage (coarse and fine wrinkling, irregular pigmentation, telangiectasia). Although the beneficial effects of some of these have been widely publicized, there is yet no convincing evidence of sustained improvement or reversibility of tissue pathology.

PHOTOSENSITIVITY REACTIONS

In addition to the acute and chronic effects of sunlight, a variety of unusual reactions may occur after only a few minutes' exposure: eg, areas of erythema or frank dermatitis; urticarial and erythema multiforme–like lesions; bullae; and chronic, thickened, scaling patches.

Numerous factors (many unknown) may contribute to increased photosensitivity: (1) SLE or cutaneous LE—unless the cause is obvious, every patient with pronounced photosensitivity should be studied for these conditions; (2) ingestion of a variety of drugs (eg, sulfonamides, tetracyclines, thiazides, griseofulvin), though sensitivity appears in only a small percentage of patients taking such compounds; (3) external application of or contact with various substances (see also Ch. 90), including toilet waters and bergamot-containing perfumes, sulfonamides, coal tar, soaps containing halogenated salicylanilides, and certain plants (eg, meadow grass, parsley); (4) xeroderma pigmentosum and certain porphyrias, which are less common but serious diseases.

Polymorphous light eruptions are unusual reactions to light that are not associated with systemic disease or drugs, as far as can be determined. Eruptions may be papular or plaque-like, dermatitic, urticarial, or erythema multiforme–like, and appear on sun-exposed areas. They are more common in people from northern climates when first exposed to spring or summer sun than in those who get sun year-round. Direct immunofluorescence of a biopsied lesion and of normal-appearing skin is negative, as opposed to LE, in which the result is usually positive. Diagnosis is by exclusion or by reproduction of the lesions with artificial or natural sunlight when the patient is not using any medication (systemic *or* topical).

Prophylaxis and Treatment

Avoidance of sunlight is important, and the patient should wear protective clothing (eg, hat and long-sleeved shirt) when outdoors on sunny days. Sunscreening preparations (see Acute Sunburn, above) are sometimes helpful. Other treatment is directed to the underlying cause, where possible. Polymorphous light eruptions manifested as papules, plaques, or dermatitis may respond to topical corticosteroids. In this condition or in cutaneous LE, prolonged (2 to 4 mo) administration of hydroxychloroquine 200 to 400 mg/day orally often reduces or completely suppresses photosensitivity and may be tried if treatment is required and sunscreens are not effective. Potential eye toxicity should be watched for by an ophthalmologist, particularly by examining visual fields. PUVA (psoralens plus UVA) is also effective in preventing some cases of polymorphous light eruptions if used before sun exposure but should not be used in LE.

114. BURNS

Tissue injury caused by thermal, chemical, or electrical contact results in protein denaturation, burn wound edema, and loss of intravascular fluid volume due to increased vascular permeability. Systemic effects, such as hypovolemic shock, infection, or respiratory tract injury, are greater threats to life than local effects.

In spontaneous healing, dead tissue sloughs off as new epithelium begins to cover the injured area. With **superficial burns**, regeneration occurs rapidly from uninjured epidermal elements, hair follicles, and sweat glands; little scarring results unless infection occurs. With **deep burns** (destruction of the epidermis and much of the dermis), reepithelialization starts from the edges of the wound, from the scattered remains of integument, or from remaining dermal appendages. The process is slow, and excessive granulation tissue forms before being covered by epithelium. Such wounds generally contract and develop into disfiguring or disabling scars unless treated promptly by skin grafting.

Symptoms, Signs, and Assessment of Burn Injury

The **severity** of the burn is judged by the quantity of tissue involved, represented by the percentage of **body surface area (% BSA)** burned and by the **depth** of the burn. A reasonable classification of burns by severity is the following: small (< 15% BSA); moderate (15 to 49% BSA); large (50 to 69% BSA); and massive (≥ 70% BSA).

The **depth of the burn** may be described as first-, second-, or third-degree. **First-degree** burns are red, very sensitive to touch, and usually moist. There are no blisters, and the surface markedly and widely blanches to light pressure. **Second-degree** burns may or may not have blisters. The bases of the blisters may be erythematous or whitish with a fibrinous exudate. The wound base is sensitive to touch and may blanch to pressure. **Third-degree** burns may, but generally do not, present with blisters. The surface may be white and pliable when pressure is applied, or it may be black, charred, and leathery. Third-degree burns may be pale in color and mistaken for normal skin, but the subdermal vessels do not blanch to pressure. The wound may be bright red because of fixed hemoglobin in the subdermal region. The third-degree burn is generally anesthetic or hypoesthetic. Hairs may be pulled from their follicles easily. Often, the distinction between deep second- and third-degree burns can be made only after 3 to 5 days of observation.

Respiratory tract ventilation injury accompanying thermal burns is due to inhalation of the incomplete products of combustion, which are potent chemical irritants to the respiratory mucosa. Steam inhalation is the only common cause of thermal damage to the lower respiratory tract in alert individuals. However, inhalation of hot gases may thermally damage lower airways in the presence of impaired levels of awareness. Inhalation of hot gases can cause immediate upper airway obstruction; airway edema can produce a more slowly developing upper airway obstruction; and small airway alveolar capillary chemical injury can cause delayed progressive respiratory failure. Increasingly, plastics are major components of combustion material, and toxic products such as cyanide are becoming more important. Symptoms and signs of respiratory tract injuries are described under Initial Treatment of the Burn Victim, below.

In **electrical burns**, injury results from the generation of heat up to 5000° C. Since most of the resistance to electric current is at the point of skin contact with the conductor, electrical burns usually involve the skin and subjacent tissues and may be of almost any size and depth. Progressive necrosis and sloughing are usually greater and involve deeper tissues than the original lesion would indicate. Electrical injury, particularly from alternating current, may cause immediate respiratory paralysis, ventricular fibrillation, or both (see CARDIOPULMONARY RESUSCITATION in Ch. 30).

Chemical burns may be due to strong acids and alkalies, phenols, cresols, mustard gas, or phosphorus. All produce necrosis that may extend slowly for several hours.

About 85% of burns are small and can be treated in outpatient facilities. Criteria establishing when to treat a burn victim as an outpatient are given under OUTPATIENT BURN TREATMENT, below, following a description of the evaluation and inpatient treatment of the more extensively burned patient (> 15% BSA burns in adults, > 10% BSA in small children).

INPATIENT BURN TREATMENT

Initial Treatment of the Burn Victim

Immediate treatment of acute thermal or chemical injury requires that the victim is **removed from the burning process** and (for significant thermal injury) that **O$_2$ is administered**. Removing all smoldering clothing or chemical-laden material will tend to prevent additive injury. Administration of supplemental O$_2$ will tend to raise the blood O$_2$ content and begin to displace carbon monoxide, a potentially lethal oxidation product, which has an extremely high affinity for Hb. Immediate care on arrival at an emergency facility requires establishment of an adequate airway for ventilation and oxygenation, stopping the burning process, replacement of acute plasma volume loss, recognition and management of any associated life-threatening major trauma, diagnosis of metabolic abnormalities, and protection from bacterial contamination.

Ventilation injuries, if severe, can be treated with tracheal (preferably nasotracheal) intubation and mechanical ventilation. **Absolute indications for intubation** include rapid and shallow ventilation with tachypnea of 30 to 40 breaths/min; inadequate ventilation (bradypnea) of < 8 to 10 breaths/min; mechanical airway obstruction from trauma, edema, or laryngospasm; or signs of respiratory failure with arterial pH < 7.2, P$_{O2}$ < 60 mm Hg, or P$_{CO2}$ > 50 mm Hg. **Relative indications for intubation** may include a history of an enclosed space explosion or fire; singed nasal hairs or oral mucosa, erythema of the palate, or soot in the mouth, larynx, or in the sputum; edema associated with a burn of the face or neck; and signs of respiratory distress, eg, nasal flaring, respiratory crowing or stridor, anxiety, agitation, or combativeness. If ventilation mechanics seem adequate, then O$_2$ may be administered by face mask or nasal cannula.

Stopping the burning process involves removing all clothing, especially any smoldering material such as melted synthetic shirts or hot tar-laden material. All chemical agents should first be flushed off the skin with copious amounts of water. **Acid and alkali burns** and burns caused by organic compounds such as **phenols or cresols** should be diluted with copious amounts of water. **Phosphorus burns** should be immersed immediately in water to avoid contact with air. Phosphorus particles are removed gently under water; the wound is then washed with 1% copper sulfate solution to coat any residual particles with a protective film of copper phosphide (these fluoresce and can be readily removed in a darkened room). Care must be taken to avoid excess absorption of copper. Following initial treatment, chemical burns should be treated as thermal burns of comparable size and extent.

Immediate volume replacement: Shock should be *anticipated* in third-degree and extensive second-degree burns involving > 25% BSA of adults or > 30% BSA of children. When hypovolemic shock is present, **volume replacement** should begin immediately with the establishment of a 14- to 16-gauge venous cannula in 1 or 2 peripheral veins. Although central lines may not be necessary initially, their later placement may be difficult because of extensive wound edema. Therefore, if the need for central access is anticipated for fluid or K replacement or for hyperalimentation, a subclavian or internal jugular line should be placed early. If necessary, central or peripheral lines may be placed through burn eschar. A "cutdown" is avoided, since it more likely destroys the vein and precludes its future use, but more importantly, it carries a high risk of infection. Blood should be obtained for determination of Hb, Hct, blood type, and crossmatch.

The immediate resuscitation fluid is lactated Ringer's solution. An initial infusion rate may be estimated after a brief physical examination and initial determination of the extent of injury using the **rule of nines** (see below) or the Lund-Browder chart (see Fig. 114–1). It is anticipated that 2 to 4 mL/kg/% BSA will be required for the first 24 h postinjury. One half of this volume should be given in the initial 8-h period, measured from the time of injury (not from the time of arrival at the emergency facility). The hourly infusion rate should be adjusted, if necessary, after a more detailed physical examination and accurate calculation of fluid requirements (see

below). Continued fluid replacement is determined by careful monitoring of the patient and should be modified to optimize BP, pulse, and urinary output.

Pain from minor burns can usually be relieved by codeine 30 to 60 mg orally or s.c. and aspirin 650 mg orally q 4 to 6 h. In severe burns with peripheral vasoconstriction, morphine 0.1 mg/kg or meperidine 1.0 mg/kg should be given IV q 3 h.

A **tetanus toxoid booster**, 0.5 to 1 mL s.c. or IM, may be given to patients immunized within 4 to 5 yr; otherwise, tetanus immune globulin 250 u. IM should be given (and repeated every 6 wk as necessary), and concomitant active immunization should be started.

Bacterial invasion occurs whenever the epidermis is broken. Dead tissue, warmth, and moisture provide ideal conditions for bacterial growth. Streptococci and staphylococci usually predominate shortly after a burn, and gram-negative bacteria after 5 to 7 days, but mixed flora are always found.

Penicillin G 5 million u. IM or IV is given daily for 3 days as prophylaxis against streptococcal cellulitis.

Long-Range Burn Treatment

Problems and therapeutic solutions should be identified after initial resuscitation. This requires a detailed history and physical examination with a careful evaluation of the injury, calculation of fluids required, monitoring of vital signs and urinary flow to adjust fluid intake, consideration of escharotomies, detection and treatment of metabolic abnormalities, and topical wound care.

History and physical examination: Accurate data about the burn episode usually come from sources such as the ambulance driver, accompanying family member, coworker, police, or firefighter. The following details are important: (1) Where was the patient when the burn occurred? Was he in a closed space? (2) What exactly was he doing when the burn occurred? Was there an explosion? (3) What was the burn source (ie, thermal, electrical, or chemical)? (4) How long was he exposed? (5) What exactly was done to eliminate the burning agent? (6) Did anything happen to him that would suggest additional injuries?

Further history should note allergies, medications, and the presence of heart, pulmonary, or renal disease, diabetes, any other medical or psychiatric disorders (the injury may represent

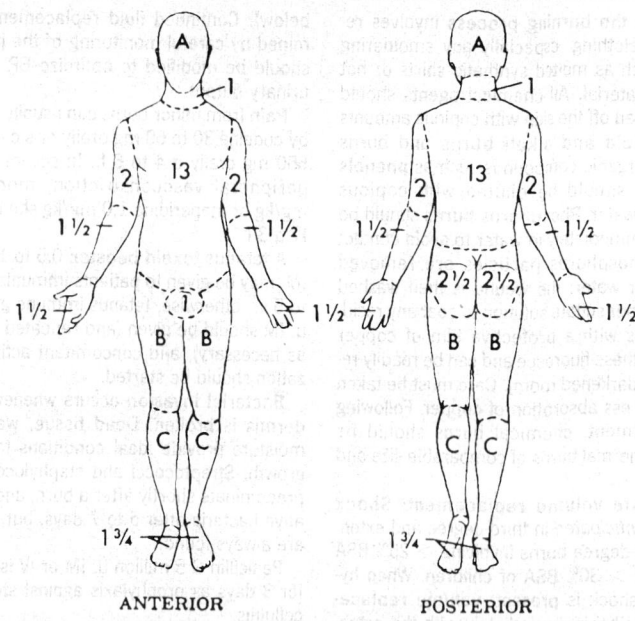

ANTERIOR   POSTERIOR

Relative percentage of body surface areas (% BSA) affected by growth						
	0 yr	1 yr	5 yr	10 yr	15 yr	Adult
A—½ of head	9½	8½	6½	5½	4½	3½
B—½ of 1 thigh	2¾	3¼	4	4¼	4½	4¾
C—½ of 1 lower leg	2½	2½	2¾	3	3¼	3½

FIG. 114−1. Lund and Browder chart for estimating extent of burns. (Redrawn from *The Treatment of Burns*, ed. 2, by CP Artz and JA Moncrief. Philadelphia, WB Saunders Company, 1969; used with permission.)

physical abuse or a suicide attempt), and smoking and drinking habits.

A **complete physical examination** is performed to detect any pulmonary, cardiac, hepatic, neurologic, or renal disease and the extent and severity of injury. This must be done before maturation of burn injuries, when physical findings may be more difficult to discern. A best estimate for height and weight is recorded to allow calculation of the patient's BSA. Often, the height can be measured immediately and preburn weight estimated by a family member. Details of the body surface burned and the estimated depth are recorded on a burn diagram. The area involved is outlined, and its depth indicated by the type or style of the markings. In adults, the extent of the burn (% BSA) is estimated by comparing the burn diagram with the **rule of nines:** head and neck, 9% of BSA; each hand and arm (including deltoid), 9%; each foot and leg as far up as the inferior gluteal fold, 18%; anterior and posterior trunk including buttocks, 18% each; perineum, 1%. **In children,** a more accurate estimate for the % BSA involved may be obtained using the Lund-Browder chart (see FIG. 114−1).

Calculation of volume replacement: The object is to maintain normal physiology as reflected by urine volume, vital signs, mental status, blood electrolytes, and ventilatory function. *The fluid volume needed is related to the extent of the burn.* Most formulas that do not include colloid suggest 2 to 4 mL/kg/%BSA for the first 24 h. Use of colloid (plasma, albumin, etc) and when to start are matters of judgment, and depend on the size of the burn, the patient's age, and concomitant diseases.

Patients with small burns seldom require colloid. Patients with large or massive injuries, young children, elderly patients, and those with cardiac disease will require colloid in the first few hours. The exact volume and rate of crystalloid and colloid administration depend on each patient's response to the fluid delivery. Patients who have inadequate urine output despite administration of a high volume of crystalloid often respond to colloid. Precalculated figures are seldom correct for the total period of resuscitation; formulas are used *only as a guide*.

A general formula that uses colloid during the first 24 h is:
0.5 mL/kg/%BSA of colloid
1.5 mL/kg/%BSA of lactated Ringer's solution
100 mL/h maintenance of lactated Ringer's solution

One half is given in the first 8 h, 1/4 in the second 8 h, and 1/4 in the third 8 h. For the first 4 h, only lactated Ringer's solution is given. The colloid is begun during the second 4 h.

A sample calculation for a 70-kg man with a 40% BSA burn is:
$0.5 \times 70 \times 40 = 1400$ mL of colloid (fresh frozen plasma)
$1.5 \times 70 \times 40 = 4200$ mL of lactated Ringer's solution
2400 mL maintenance of lactated Ringer's solution

Total fluid = 8000 mL fluid over the first 24 h

This should be given by the following schedule:

First 4 h:
1050 mL of lactated Ringer's solution
100 mL/h maintenance of lactated Ringer's solution
Second 4 h:
700 mL of colloid
1050 mL of lactated Ringer's solution
100 mL/h maintenance of lactated Ringer's solution
Second 8 h:
350 mL of colloid
1050 mL of lactated Ringer's solution
100 mL/h maintenance of lactated Ringer's solution
Third 8 h:
350 mL of colloid
1050 mL of lactated Ringer's solution
100 mL/h maintenance of lactated Ringer's solution

Rounding off the calculations, the sample orders would read:
Please administer the following IV solutions:

For the first 4 h:
Lactated Ringer's solution at 360 mL/h
For the second 4 h:
Fresh frozen plasma at 180 mL/h
Lactated Ringer's solution at 360 mL/h
For the second 8 h:
Fresh frozen plasma at 45 mL/h
Lactated Ringer's solution at 220 mL/h
For the third 8 h:
Fresh frozen plasma at 45 mL/h
Lactated Ringer's solution at 220 mL/h

Monitoring: Many parameters must be followed closely to recognize or prevent incipient problems as early as possible. Therefore, it is good procedure to establish a flow chart listing the items discussed here. The goal of fluid replacement is to maintain an adequate BP and a urine output of > 50 to 100 mL/h (0.5 to 1 mL/kg/h) in an adult or 1 mL/kg/h in a child while avoiding circulatory overload. An indwelling Foley catheter should be placed to monitor urine output. **Insufficient therapy** can be recognized by a decline in urine volume, an increase in hemoconcentration, and symptoms of shock. **Excess therapy** (resulting in pulmonary edema and congestive failure) should be prevented by monitoring the pulse, respiration, BP, and neck vein distention or the central venous pressure. The lung bases should be auscultated frequently for rales.

Patients with preexisting cardiovascular-renal disease present a special problem. Fluid, electrolyte, and colloid administration should be limited to amounts sufficient to produce minimal adequate urinary output (25 mL/h), and the patient should be watched for signs of circulatory overload.

Pulse, BP, temperature, ECG, and arterial blood gases should be monitored in the elderly, in patients with severe burns, or in those with preexisting disease. Most cardiac arrhythmias are caused by hypovolemia, hypoxia, acidosis, or hyperkalemia. These metabolic disorders should be evaluated and corrected before cardiac drugs are used. Ventricular tachycardia and fibrillation are exceptions requiring immediate treatment while underlying metabolic abnormalities are evaluated. Silver nitrate 0.5%, used as a topical antibacterial agent, is hypotonic and leaches Na and Cl and some K from the tissues into the wet dressing. Losses may result in severe **hypona-**

tremia, hypochloremia, and hypochloremic alkalosis.

Serum K is aggressively maintained above 4 mEq/L. **Hypokalemia** is common in the early resuscitation period for 3 reasons: (1) Many patients present with depleted K stores secondary to prior diuretic therapy; (2) K is not generally included in the early vigorous fluid replacement; (3) some K is lost into the hypotonic 0.5% silver nitrate dressings.

Hypoalbuminemia results from the combination of dilutional effects of crystalloid replacement therapy and enhanced loss of protein into the subeschar edema fluid. Colloid solution is continued throughout the resuscitation period at rates previously described in order to maintain albumin levels at about 2.5 gm/dL and a total protein > 5 gm/dL. Most serum Ca is reversibly bound to albumin. **Hypocalcemia** may therefore be a result of hypoalbuminemia. The ionized fraction of serum Ca is usually normal but should be measured periodically. Replacement Ca, phosphate, and Mg are given daily.

Generalized poor tissue perfusion, a result of hypovolemia or cardiac failure, results in **metabolic acidosis**. Blood pH < 7.2 should be treated with sodium bicarbonate IV. Focal poor tissue perfusion can result from a constricting eschar or fascia that should be treated with escharotomy and fasciotomy (see also escharotomies and operative management, below).

Myoglobinuria can result from ischemic constrictions of muscle, crush injuries, or deep thermal or electrical burns of muscle, and should be treated initially by maintenance of a urinary output of 100 mL/h in adults and > 1 mL/kg/h in children. Initial management consists of an osmotic diuresis, giving mannitol 12.5 gm IV q 4 to 8 h or more frequently as necessary until the myoglobinuria clears. In severe myoglobinuria, the urine should be alkalinized with 50 mEq sodium bicarbonate IV q 4 to 8 h as necessary, with frequent monitoring of both serum and urine pH. The goal is a urinary pH > 8. **Hemoglobinuria** may result from erythrocyte destruction following burns and is treated identically to myoglobinuria. *Both myoglobinuria and hemoglobinuria may result in renal tubular necrosis if not promptly and accurately managed.*

Hb is determined q 3 to 4 h for the first 72 h, and therapy is regulated to avoid Hb levels > 16 or < 11 gm/dL. Hct should be maintained above 30%.

Body temperature should be closely followed because hypothermia occurs frequently in the extensively burned patient. Those with rectal temperatures < 97° F (36° C) are treated by warming the resuscitation fluids. Rewarming patients from temperatures < 91° F (33° C) may be associated with fatal arrhythmias. These patients should be warmed slowly and monitored continuously (see Ch. 116).

Escharotomies: Indications for escharotomies are liberal in circumferential third-degree burns, eg, the loss of a previously palpable pulse, or a nonpalpable pulse in a single extremity with easily palpable pulses in the remaining extremities. Peripheral ischemia is suspected when a single extremity is cooler than the others and has a poor capillary refilling time; Doppler ultrasound is confirmatory. A tense eschar is released even in the presence of Doppler pulses if peripheral ischemia is strongly suspected. With injuries to the skin that do not involve deeper tissue, the depth of the escharotomy incision extends only through the dermis, excluding the hypodermis or fat. The incision should extend well beyond the tense region of eschar to ensure complete release. Some apparent full-thickness eschars may retain partial pain sensation, making the releasing incision painful. Anesthesia may be obtained with 1% lidocaine.

Topical wound care: Under aseptic conditions, the burned surface is washed with water, cultured, treated with the appropriate topical agent, and covered with sterile dressings. Common topical agents include 0.5% silver nitrate solution, mafenide acetate, and 1% silver sulfadiazine. To use silver nitrate, the wounds are covered with up to 8 layers of cotton roll bandages and the silver nitrate is poured over the dressing at 2-h intervals. This keeps the dressing moist and the concentration of the silver nitrate at the skin at about 0.5%. A lower concentration probably is not bactericidal. A higher concentration, which is a result of evaporation, can further burn the skin. Both the mafenide and silver sulfadiazine are applied directly as a cream and then may be covered with a few layers of cotton rolls; residual agent should be removed before applying fresh material. Following topical applications of silver nitrate, patients may develop excessive Na losses, hypokalemia, hypochloremia, alkalosis, or methemoglobinuria. Mafenide acetate cream applied topically inhibits carbonic anhydrase activity and may produce compensated metabolic acidosis and, occasionally, proximal renal tubular acidosis. Silver sulfadiazine should be used with caution in patients with sensitivity to sulfonamides and has been associated with hematologic abnormalities.

Operative management: Excision or removal of the burn eschar creates a clean wound bed that can be covered with grafting material. In the absence of excisional therapy, deep second- or third-degree burns separate and slough wound eschar over a period of time, leaving a raw wound bed. Excision is best done during the first 1 to 4 days after the burn (early excision). This removes devitalized tissue, avoids subeschar sepsis, and allows early wound closure, which shortens hospitalization and improves the functional result.

It should be determined (1) which areas will not be expected to heal in 3 wk and therefore need excision and (2) in what sequence these areas should be excised. Any deep second-degree and all third-degree burns should be excised. If the extent of injury is large and there is a question of patient survival, the largest areas of involvement should be removed first. This most expeditiously reduces the volume of open burn wound. The areas most likely to be treated initially are the back, chest, and abdomen, which are also the most successful for graft acceptance. At a single sitting, no more than 30% BSA should be excised, including donor sites. When the issue is not survival but cosmesis or optimization of functional result, then hands, upper extremities, feet, and lower extremities are excised first and in that order. The face should be conservatively excised, retaining as much of the soft tissues as possible.

Excision results in a burn wound bed that requires closure with graft material. Available graft materials are (1) autografts, the patient's own skin; (2) allografts, viable skin usually from cadaver donors; and (3) xenografts, skin from porcine sources. Autografts can be transplanted as either sheet or meshed grafts. A sheet graft is a solid piece of skin. Mesh grafts are used when donor skin is scarce, but not in burns < 20% BSA; small incisions are made at regular intervals in the sheet of donor skin with a skin meshing instrument that permits the graft to cover a larger area. Meshed grafts heal with an uneven gridlike appearance, and some wounds heal with excessive hypertrophic scarring. Autografts are histocompatible and therefore are not rejected. Sufficient autograft material is not available in burns > 50% BSA. However, autograft may be taken from the same donor site region repeatedly at 14-day intervals, which expands the

autograft supply in time. Both allografts and xenografts are temporary and will be rejected in as early as 10 to 14 days. They must be replaced with autograft, but their use is lifesaving in massive burns.

Physical and occupational therapy: Positioning, exercising, splints, and pressure garments help preserve function and appearance as burn wounds heal. Body surfaces with high skin tension and movement, eg, the face, joints, upper legs, and chest, are most susceptible to formation of scars and contractures.

Splints to prevent contractures and keep specific joints in the position of function should be applied as soon as possible after admission. They must be fitted properly, and constantly assessed in the early stages of treatment, to avoid constriction of the extremity that may result in increasing edema. Later, as edema subsides, the splints often need to be remodeled for a closer fit. In extensive burns, splints are worn continuously until the area is grafted and shows substantial healing. Joints are also maintained in functional positions throughout convalescence with dressings and blanket rolls.

With extensive burns, the total body position is considered. The **neck** is extended using soft foam pads fashioned to conform to the skull. The **axilla** is flexed about 30 to 60° with arm troughs and should be abducted. The **elbow** is positioned and splinted at extension or slight flexion. The **wrist** is slightly extended 20 to 30°. The **metacarpophalangeal joints** are flexed at 90°. The **proximal and distal interphalangeal joints** are extended completely to decrease the stretch of the dorsal skin over them and the possibility of ischemic necrosis. The **thumb** is in slight apposition to the palm. The **hips** should be abducted and are prevented from external rotation by lateral extensions of the ankle splints. The **ankle** is splinted at 90° dorsiflexion to stretch the Achilles tendon.

Joints are put through active and passive range of motion exercises once or twice a day before grafting, to preserve function. Both exercise and positioning become easier as the initial edema subsides. After skin grafting, the grafted part is usually kept immobile for 5 to 10 days, awaiting graft stability before starting postoperative exercises.

Nutrition: Aggressive metabolic support is indicated in patients with > 20% BSA burn, preinjury malnutrition, complications such as sepsis or associated injury, and a weight loss > 10% of the premorbid weight. This support begins 1 to 2 days after the fluid resuscitation phase of burn therapy.

Oral feeding is preferred because of fewer complications and lower cost, but anorexia, facial burns, or dysphagia may make it difficult or impossible. If oral feeding is inadequate but GI motility and absorption are normal, then **enteral (tube) feedings** are used as a supplemental or total caloric source. **Parenteral nutrition** is indicated in those patients with prolonged gastric and colonic ileus related either to the burn wound, repeated operations, or sepsis. Complications are more likely in parenteral than in enteral nutrition.

OUTPATIENT BURN TREATMENT

Superficial burns involving a small body surface area and without inhalation injury may be treated in outpatient facilities. The general criteria are (1) first- and superficial second-degree burns of < 15 to 20% BSA (adults) or < 10% BSA (small children), (2) moderate to deep second-degree burns involving < 10% BSA, and (3) third-degree burns of < 1% BSA. The patient is admitted if a wound is not expected to heal spontaneously in 3 wk or less. Admission is planned either at the first visit or at follow-up a few days later. Patients are more likely to be admitted if (1) the face, hand, perineum, or feet are involved with the deeper aspects of the burn, (2) poor compliance with elevation and dressing changes is anticipated, or (3) the patient's age is < 2 yr or > 70 yr.

Outpatient burn treatment requires a history and physical examination as described above, including recorded estimates of the depth and extent (% BSA) of the burn; cleansing, debriding, splinting, and positioning the wound; topical and systemic therapy; instruction on home care; and arrangement for outpatient follow-up.

Wound cleaning, removing the burning agent, and debridement: Small burns should immediately be immersed in cold water, if possible. Chemical wounds should be copiously irrigated with water. The burn wound should be cleaned with soap and water. All debris should be carefully removed. For deeply embedded dirt, the wound may be anesthetized with a local infiltration of 1 to 2% lidocaine and scrubbed with a stiff brush and soap.

The blisters of the burn wound should be sharply debrided away if they are already broken or are likely to be broken. If burn depth is in question, blisters should be removed and the wound base examined for full thickness injury.

Topical therapy: Once the wound is clean, a topical agent (eg, silver sulfadiazine cream) may be applied. One layer of the cream is applied with sterile technique, using a sterile tongue blade as an applicator, and the wound is covered with gauze roll bandages.

Splinting and positioning: If the burn involves a joint and is at least of second-degree depth, splinting is required (see also above). The hand is splinted by wrapping each finger individually with cotton roll gauze over the hand and wrist in a figure-8 pattern. The palm should receive extra padding to maintain the metacarpophalangeal and interphalangeal joints in slight flexion. The wrist or elbow may be splinted by using an arm sling. The lower extremities are not usually splinted in outpatient care.

The most important therapeutic maneuver is elevation of the extremity, especially in patients with a lower extremity or hand burn. The extremity should be placed above heart level at all times except for brief periods of ≤ 20 min during the day. Bed rest with elevation is difficult to achieve as an outpatient, and with lower extremity injuries hospital admission is often required.

Medications: Patients with burns of second degree or more are often given penicillin V 1 to 2 gm/day orally in 4 divided doses as prophylaxis for streptococcal cellulitis over the first few days. Erythromycin 1 to 2 gm/day orally in 4 divided doses may be used in patients with a penicillin allergy. Active immunization against tetanus is given as described under INPATIENT BURN TREATMENT, above. Analgesia is prescribed as necessary.

Home care instructions: The patient should be advised (1) to keep the wound clean and dry; (2) to keep the wound elevated; (3) to change the dressing twice daily as directed, and to clean the wound completely with water to remove all the residual topical medication before applying a new layer; (4) to take the antibiotics as directed; and (5) when and where to return for follow-up.

Outpatient follow-up visits are required to (1) monitor compliance with wound care; (2) debride the wound; (3) examine for cellulitis; (4) further assess the burn depth; (5) evaluate and arrange for ambulatory, occupational, and physical therapy; and (6) consider excisional therapy.

The first follow-up visit is usually within 24 to 48 h after the burn or immediately if signs of sepsis occur. Subsequent outpatient visits are q 24 to 72 h, as necessary, depending upon the severity of the burn depth and the ability of the patient to care for the wound.

115. HEAT DISORDERS

HEATSTROKE AND HEAT EXHAUSTION

Mild to grave reactions to high temperature due to inadequate or inappropriate responses of heat-regulating mechanisms.

Etiology

Exposure to high ambient temperature may lead either to excessive fluid loss and hypovolemic shock **(heat exhaustion)** or to failure of heat loss mechanisms and dangerous hyperpyrexia **(heatstroke)**. Prolonged exposure (> 2 to 3 wk) and excessive sweating, especially if accompanied by vomiting or diarrhea, lead to dehydration; sodium, potassium, and magnesium depletion; and hypovolemia. High ambient humidity, by decreasing the cooling effect of sweating, and prolonged strenuous exertion with increased heat production by muscle increase the risk of heat illness. Age, obesity, chronic alcoholism, debility, and many drugs (eg, anticholinergics, antihistamines, phenothiazines, numerous psychotropic drugs, alcohol, and cocaine) increase susceptibility to heat illness, particularly heatstroke. Though stemming from the same cause, heatstroke and heat exhaustion are sharply different (see TABLE 115–1).

Prophylaxis

Common sense is the best preventive; strenuous exertion in a very hot environment, inadequately ventilated space, or heavy, insulating clothing should be avoided; fluid and electrolytes (often lost imperceptibly in very hot, very dry air) should be replaced by continuous oral fluids slightly salty to taste (ie, near isotonic). Sometimes, exertion in a hot environment cannot be avoided; every effort should then be made to replace lost fluid and salt and to keep the skin temperature cool by evaporation. Salt tablets occasionally cause gastric distress and are less desirable than lightly salted beverages and foods. Potassium, magnesium, and calcium depletion are a hazard only when heat exposure is prolonged (see above).

HEATSTROKE
(Sunstroke; Hyperpyrexia; Thermic Fever; Siriasis)

Symptoms and Signs

An abrupt onset is sometimes preceded by prodromal headache, vertigo, and fatigue. Sweating is usually but not always decreased, and the skin is hot, flushed, and usually dry. The pulse rate increases rapidly and may reach 160 to 180; respirations usually increase, but BP is

TABLE 115–1. DIFFERENTIATION BETWEEN HEATSTROKE AND HEAT EXHAUSTION

	Heatstroke	Heat Exhaustion
Cause	Inadequacy or failure of heat loss mechanism	Excessive fluid loss leading to hypovolemic shock
Warnings	Headache, weakness, sudden loss of consciousness	Gradual weakness, nausea, anxiety, excess sweating, syncope
Appearance and signs	Hot, red, dry skin; little sweating; hard, rapid pulse; very high temperature	Pale, grayish, clammy skin; weak, slow pulse; low BP; faintness
Management	Emergency cooling by wrapping or immersing in cold water or ice; immediate hospitalization	As for simple syncope: head down, replace lost salt and water (usually orally, rarely IV)

seldom affected. Disorientation may briefly precede unconsciousness or convulsions. The temperature climbs rapidly to 40° or 41° C (104° or 106° F) and the patient feels as if burning up. Circulatory collapse may precede death; after hours of extreme hyperpyrexia, survivors are likely to have permanent brain damage.

Diagnosis and Prognosis

Hot, dry, flushed skin, high body temperature, and rapid pulse in a person exposed to a hot environment are usually enough to distinguish heatstroke from food, chemical, or drug poisoning. Any drugs (see under Etiology, above) that might have precipitated the episode should be considered. Heatstroke is a *serious emergency* and unless promptly and energetically treated, results in convulsions and death or permanent brain damage. Core temperature of 41° C (106° F) is a grave prognostic sign; temperature a degree higher is often fatal. Old age, debility, or alcoholism worsens the prognosis.

Treatment

Heroic measures should be instituted immediately. If distant from a hospital, the patient should be wrapped in wet bedding or clothing, immersed in a lake or stream, or even cooled with snow or ice while waiting for transportation. WARNING: *The temperature should be taken every 10 min and not allowed to fall below 38.3° C (101° F) to avoid converting hyperpyrexia to hypothermia.* In the hospital, more exact control measures are instituted and the core temperature is monitored continuously to avoid hypothermia. Stimulants and sedatives including morphine are avoided; diazepam or a barbiturate may be given IV if convulsions are not otherwise controllable. Electrolyte determinations should guide IV therapy. Bed rest is desirable for a few days after severe heatstroke, and temperature lability may be expected for weeks.

HEAT EXHAUSTION
(Heat Prostration, Collapse, or Syncope)

Symptoms and Signs

Because of excessive fluid loss, this disorder gives adequate warning by increasing fatigue, weakness, anxiety, and drenching sweats, leading to circulatory collapse with slow thready pulse; low or imperceptible BP; cold, pale, clammy skin; and disordered mentation followed by a shock-like unconsciousness. **Syncope,** a mild form of heat exhaustion precipitated by standing for a long time in a hot environment, is due to pooling of blood in heat-dilated vessels in the lower extremities. Temperature is usually below normal and the picture is that of simple syncope. Heat exhaustion gives adequate warning by increasing fatigue.

Diagnosis and Prognosis

Heat exhaustion causing vasomotor collapse is more difficult to differentiate from insulin shock, poisoning, hemorrhage, or traumatic shock than is heatstroke. Hyperventilation syndrome should be easily detected and not confuse the diagnosis. Usually, the history of heat exposure, failure of hydration, absence of other apparent cause, and response to treatment are sufficient for diagnosis. The condition is usually transient, and the prognosis is good unless circulatory failure is prolonged.

Treatment

Heat exhaustion requires restoration of normal blood volume and assurance of adequate brain perfusion. The patient should be placed flat or with head down. Small amounts of cool, slightly salty fluids should be given orally every few minutes to restore normovolemia. Isotonic saline IV, cardiac stimulants, or plasma volume expanders (albumin, dextran) are seldom needed but should be given cautiously to avoid overloading an embarrassed circulatory system.

HEAT CRAMPS

Severe cramps of striated muscle resulting from excessive sweating due to exertion and/or high ambient temperatures.

Etiology

Heat cramps are due to excessive loss of sodium and occasionally potassium and magnesium (see above) during strenuous activity at high atmospheric temperatures ($> 38°$ C [100° F]). They are common in manual laborers (eg, engine room personnel, steel workers, and miners), in mountaineers or skiers overdressed against the cold, and in those not acclimatized to hot, dry climates where excessive sweating is almost undetected because of rapid evaporation.

Symptoms and Signs

Onset is often abrupt, with muscles of the extremities affected first. Severe pain and carpopedal spasm may incapacitate the hands and feet. Often episodic, the cramping makes the muscles feel like hard knots. When the cramps affect only the abdominal muscles, the pain may simulate an acute abdomen. Vital signs are usually normal. The skin may be either hot and dry or clammy and cool, depending on the humidity.

Prophylaxis and Treatment

In most instances, heat cramp is prevented and also rapidly relieved by drinking fluids or eating foods containing sodium chloride. If the patient cannot take food or drink orally, 0.9% sodium chloride IV may be necessary. Sodium chloride tablets are often used for prophylaxis but can cause stomach irritation, and overdose may lead to edema. Awareness of the problem is usually sufficient to prevent it.

116. COLD INJURY

(Frostnip; Frostbite; Accidental Hypothermia; Exposure;
Immersion or Trench Foot; Chilblains; Pernio)

Injury by cold causing structural and functional disturbances of small blood vessels, cells, nerves, and skin; or generalized lowering of body temperature.

Etiology

Exposure to damp cold (temperatures around freezing) causes **frostnip** and **immersion (trench) foot**. Exposure to dry cold (temperatures well below freezing) causes **frostbite** and **accidental hypothermia**. Loss of body heat is by conduction (wet clothing, contact with metal), convection (windchill), and radiation. Susceptibility to cold injury is increased by dehydration; drug or alcohol excess; impaired consciousness; exhaustion; hunger; anemia; impaired circulation due to cardiovascular disease, constricted vessels, or polycythemia; and in very young or elderly persons.

Hypothermia occurs when the body cannot sustain normal temperature. Windchill, wet or inadequate clothing, substance abuse, or debility may cause dangerous hypothermia even though ambient temperature is no lower than 10 to 15° C (50 to 60° F). As shivering ceases, the body becomes unable to warm itself and the core temperature falls (see also ACCIDENTAL HYPOTHERMIA in Ch. 124).

Pathology

Ice crystals may form within or between cells, interfering with the sodium pump, thus rupturing cell walls; RBCs clump, and platelet microemboli form to cause thromboses; neurovascular impulses shunt blood, often sacrificing an injured part to save the whole. Any or all of these events may produce mild to severe injuries. **Dry cold injury** is usually superficial: the hard carapace of dry gangrene is often only a few millimeters thick over healthy tissue. **Wet gangrene** is often complicated by infection and tends to be deeper. **Immersion** or **trench foot** causes physiologic aberrations such as edema, blotchy cyanosis, increased sweating, and paresthesias, rather than tissue loss. The pathology of long-lasting symptoms from mild cold injury (**chilblains**) is unknown.

Symptoms, Signs, and Diagnosis

Frostnip manifests as firm, cold, white areas on face, ears or extremities. Peeling or blistering (as from sunburn) may occur in 24 to 72 h, and occasionally mild hypersensitivity to cold persists. In **immersion** or **trench foot**, the extremity is pale, edematous, clammy, cold, and numb; tissue maceration and infection are likely. Increased sweating, pain, and hypersensitivity to temperature change may persist for years due to autonomic disturbance. In **frostbite**, the area is cold, hard, white, and anesthetic; on warming it becomes blotchy red, swollen, and painful. Depending on the extent of injury, the area may recover normally or deteriorate to soft wet gangrene or to the black carapace of dry gangrene. In **hypothermia**, the falling core temperature leads to lethargy, clumsiness, mental confusion, irritability, hallucinations, slowed or arrested respiration, and slowed, irregular, and finally arrested heartbeat. A victim should not be considered dead until "warm and dead." Recovery has occurred even when core temperature was 26° C (79° F). Rectal temperature below 34° C (93° F) will help to differentiate hypothermia from cardiac disease, diabetic coma or hyperinsulinism, CVA, or substance abuse that may also be present. Ordinary clinical thermometers will not accurately indicate core temperature in hypothermia; a special low temperature thermometer is available from Becton Dickinson, Stanley Street, Rutherford, NJ 07070 (201-460-2000).

Prophylaxis

Preventive measures, though obvious, are often ignored. Several layers of warm clothing, and protection against wetting and wind, are important even though weather may not seem to threaten cold injury. Gloves and socks should be kept as dry as possible, and insulated boots that do not impede circulation are essential in very cold weather. Warm head covering is particularly important, since 30% of heat loss is from the head. Ample fluids and food are important to sustain metabolic heat production. Being alert for and warming cold numb parts may prevent damage. As the body cools, shivering, exertion, warm clothing, and hot drinks may prevent hypothermia.

Treatment

Frostnip is treated by warming with an unaffected hand or a warm object. **Frostbitten** extremities should be warmed rapidly in water that is tolerably hot to the hand of the attendant, being careful not to scald the anesthetized tissues. If the victim must walk some distance to care, a difficult decision is faced: Thawed tissue is further damaged by any trauma; however, the longer a part remains frozen, the greater the ultimate damage. It may be wiser to thaw the foot and to walk carefully on it. Refreezing after thawing compounds the problem. Attention should be given to warming the whole body as well. Warm drinks, warm dry clothing, and snuggling with a warm companion will help provide heat to the chilled extremities. If the decision in the field is to not thaw the tissue, the frozen member should be carefully cleaned and dried and wrapped loosely in sterile compresses whenever possible. A broad-spectrum antibiotic should be started.

In the hospital, extremities should be warmed in large containers of water kept at 38 to 43° C (100 to 110° F) while overall assessment is made. Many interventions have been used to restore microcirculation, decrease microembolization, and minimize cell damage. Of these, antibiotics and tetanus toxoid (to control or prevent infection), ibuprofen (to decrease platelet clumping), hydration, restoration of normal electrolyte levels, and early physiotherapy seem most effective. Reserpine (0.5 mg) may be given into the brachial or femoral artery of the affected extremity to dilate vessels and decrease sludging; pit viper venom is preferred by European doctors.

After warming, extremities should be kept dry, open to air, and as sterile as practicable. Phenoxybenzamine 10 mg/day orally, increasing by 10 mg/day at 4- to 6-day intervals, may decrease tissue loss. Oxygen is helpful only at altitude. Chemical or surgical sympathectomy is rarely needed. Nutrition and morale require special attention. Surgery should be delayed as long as possible, since the ominous black carapace often will be shed, leaving viable tissue; "Freeze in January, operate in July" remains a valid adage. Whirlpool baths followed by gentle drying, rest, and time are the best long-term management. No treatment for the prolonged symptoms following immersion foot or frostbite is known.

In hypothermia, when shivering stops and lethargy and other symptoms increase, *a major emergency is imminent.* The victim is often found unconscious some distance from shelter. At the scene, further heat loss should be prevented and rapid assessment made. If the patient is conscious, warming by any means available may proceed while evacuation is planned. If unconscious, many factors must be considered, and there is debate whether warming should precede or follow removal to hospital. If a pulse is detectable, however faint, transport is preferred, preventing further heat loss and taking extreme care to avoid jarring or sudden motion, which may trigger ventricular arrhythmia to which the cold heart is prone. If no pulse is detectable, cardiopulmonary resuscitation takes priority, but it may be difficult to restore sinus rhythm. Ventricular tachycardia or fibrillation may occur. Some authorities prefer to control fluids, pH, and oxygenation before resuscitation, providing this can be accomplished rapidly. Unconscious hypothermic victims cannot generate enough heat to warm spontaneously and must be warmed externally.

In the hospital, blood should be drawn immediately for Hct and electrolyte determinations. Rapid warming by total immersion in a tub of water kept at 45 to 48° C (113 to 118° F) is preferred. Inhalation of warm moist air or oxygen, heating pads, or thermal blankets should be used while the bath is prepared. In desperate cases, peritoneal dialysis with large volumes of warm saline may be lifesaving. Acidosis can be expected during warming, and pH, K, and Na levels should be monitored q 2 h until consciousness and rectal temperature of at least 35° C (95° F) are present. The ECG should be monitored to detect arrhythmia.

117.   RADIATION REACTIONS AND INJURIES

The harmful effects—acute, delayed, or chronic—produced in body tissues by exposure to ionizing radiations.

Etiology

Harmful sources of ionizing radiation once were limited primarily to high-energy x-rays used for diagnosis and therapy and to radium and other naturally occurring radioactive materials (eg, radon). Present sources include nuclear reactors, cyclotrons, linear accelerators, alternating gradient synchrotrons, sealed cobalt and cesium sources for cancer therapy, and numerous other artificially produced radioactive materials for use in medicine and industry.

Accidental escape of large amounts of radiation from reactors has occurred several times. The most publicized accident in the USA was that involving the nuclear power plant at Three Mile Island in Pennsylvania on March 28, 1979. More recently, on April 26, 1986, a major accident occurred in the nuclear power complex at Chernobyl in the Ukraine, USSR, resulting in > 20 deaths and a large number of injuries due to radiation. Significant radiation was also detected in most of Eastern Europe and parts of Western Europe, Asia, and the USA. This event may have been unique because of the differences in design of Russian reactors and the lack of a containment vessel. Radiation exposure from nuclear reactors during the first 40 yr of nuclear energy use, up to 1985 (not including Chernobyl), resulted in 35 serious exposures (whole body irradiation ≥ 1 sievert [Sv]) with 10 deaths; none were associated with power plants. The Three Mile Island accident did not result in any major radiation exposure. Estimated doses received ranged from 0.73 mSv at 0 to 1 mile from the plant to 0 to 0.2 mSv at 10 to 20 miles. Doses received by the population in the immediate area of the Chernobyl plant were considerably higher. TABLE 117–1 puts these doses in perspective. Nuclear power generators in the USA must meet stringent federal standards that limit effluent radioactivity to extremely low levels. Although background radioactivity in the earth and in its atmosphere increased after the years of atmospheric nuclear weapons testing, it appears to have stabilized at present levels.

Ionizing radiation—whether as x-rays, neutrons, protons, α or β particles, or γ rays—acts either directly or by secondary reactions to produce biochemical lesions that initiate a series of histologic changes and physiologic symptoms

TABLE 117–1. ANNUAL WHOLE–BODY RADIATION
DOSE–EQUIVALENT RATES IN THE USA

Source	Average (mSv/yr)	Percentage of Total
Natural background (cosmic, terrestrial, internal)	0.82	44.6
Medical radiation		
X-rays	0.77	41.8
Radiopharmaceuticals	0.14	7.6
Fallout (weapons testing)	0.04–0.05	2.4
Nuclear industry	< 0.01	< 0.5
Research	<< 0.01	<< 0.5
Consumer products	0.03–0.04	1.9
Airlines		
Travel	0.005	0.3
Transport of radiopharmaceuticals	0.0001	0.005
	1.84	100%

Modified from "The Effects on Populations to Low Levels of Ionizing Radiation," 1980, with permission of the National Academy Press, Washington, DC.

TABLE 117-2. CONVERSION OF RADIATION UNITS

SI Units	Conventional Units	
1 gray (Gy)	100	rad
10 milligray (mGy)	1	rad
1 milligray	100	millirad (mrad)
1 centigray (cGy)	1	rad
1 microgray (µGy)	0.1	millirad
1 sievert (Sv)	100	rem
1 centisievert (cSv)	1	rem
10 millisievert (mSv)	1	rem
1 millisievert	100	millirem (mrem)
1 microsievert (µSv)	0.1	millirem

and signs that vary with the radiation dose and its duration.

The biologic effect of a given dose of radioactivity is also dependent on the rate at which it is administered. A single rapid dose of radioactivity may be fatal, while the same dose given over a period of weeks or months may be tolerated with little measurable acute effect. Relationships between the degree of damage and the healing or death of a cell are quite complex. In addition to the early somatic effects of large doses (observable within days), changes in the DNA of rapidly proliferating cells may be manifested as a disease or as a genetic effect in offspring many years later.

Radiation usually is characterized in the lay press as low level (0.2 to 0.3 gray [Gy]) or high level. Medical doses are usually < 0.05 Gy and frequently < 0.01 Gy.

Total dose and dose rate determine somatic or genetic effects. Commonly used units of measurement are the roentgen, the gray, and the sievert. The **roentgen (R)** is a measure of quantity of x or γ ionizing radiation in air. The **gray (Gy)** is the amount of energy absorbed in any tissue or substance from exposure and applies to all types of radiation. The R and the centigray (cGy) are nearly equivalent for practical purposes. The **sievert (Sv)** is used in describing the observation that some types of radiation, such as neutrons, may produce more biological effect for an equivalent amount of absorbed energy; thus the Sv is equal to the Gy times a constant called the "quality factor." For x and γ radiation, the Sv is equal to the Gy. The Gy and the Sv have replaced the rad and the rem in the scientific nomenclature. In SI units, the **gray (Gy)** is equal to 100 rads, and the **sievert (Sv)** is equal to 100 rem (see TABLE 117-2).

The **dose rate** is the radiation dose/unit of time. From the very low dose rates of unavoidable background radiation (about 1 to 2 mGy/yr), where no effect can be detected, the probability of measurable effects increases as the dose rate and/or total dose increases. An observable effect becomes quite certain after a single dose of several Gy, but may require higher doses if given at a low dose rate or intermittently. Large doses have immediate somatic effects, while low doses have potential for late somatic and long-term genetic effects. The effects of radiation exposure on an individual are cumulative.

The **body area** exposed is also important. The entire human body can probably absorb up to 2 Gy without fatality; however, as the whole-body dose approaches 4.5 Gy the death rate will approximate 50% (ie, LD$_{50}$), and a total whole-body dose of > 6 Gy received in a very short time will almost certainly be fatal. By contrast, tens of Gy delivered over a long period of time (eg, for cancer treatment) can be tolerated by the body when small volumes of tissue are irradiated. **Distribution of the dose** within the body is also important. For example, protection of bowel or bone marrow by appropriate shielding permits survival of the exposed individual from what would otherwise be a fatal whole-body dose. Recent advances in bone marrow transplantation have improved the prospects for survival at higher radiation doses.

Pathophysiology

Tissues vary in response to immediate radiation injury, in descending order of sensitivity: (1) lymphoid cells, (2) gonads, (3) proliferating bone marrow cells, (4) bowel epithelial cells, (5) epidermis, (6) hepatic cells, (7) epithelium of lung alveoli and biliary passages, (8) kidney epithelial cells, (9) endothelial cells (pleura and peritoneum), (10) nerve cells, (11) bone cells, (12) muscle and connective tissue. Generally, the more rapid the turnover of the cell, the greater the radiation sensitivity.

If the absorbed dose of radiation is sufficiently high, necrosis of any living cell will occur. Large but sublethal doses may produce disturbances in cell proliferation: the rate of mitosis is decreased, and DNA synthesis is slowed or cells may become polyploid. These and other ill-defined effects of radiation are reasonably inevitable after significant doses in tissue categories 1 to 4, above.

Diminished cell production in tissues that normally undergo continual renewal (eg, enteric mucosa, marrow, gonads) results in dose-dependent progressive hypoplasia, atrophy, and eventually fibrosis. Some cells, injured but still capable of mitosis, may be so damaged that they will pass through 1 or 2 generative cycles, producing abnormal progeny (eg, giant metamyelocytes and hypersegmented neutrophils) before they die. Most of our estimates of the effects of very low exposure (< 100 mGy) are usually obtained by linear extrapolation from studies of higher doses. Some workers postulate a threshold effect, citing experiments in which animals subjected to extremely low levels of increased radiation actually had *prolonged* survival compared to animals receiving radiation from background sources only. Regardless, there are very few objective data documenting the somatic and genetic effects of doses of radiation < 100 mGy.

Symptoms and Signs

The disruption of cell renewal systems and direct injury of other tissues produce clearly defined clinical syndromes:

1. Acute radiation syndromes can be divided into cerebral, GI, and hematopoietic categories, depending on dose, dose rate, area of the body, and time after exposure.

The **cerebral syndrome**, produced by extremely high total body doses of radiation (> 30 Gy), is always fatal and consists of 3 phases: a prodromal period of nausea and vomiting; then listlessness and drowsiness ranging from apathy to prostration (possibly due to nonbacterial inflammatory foci in the brain or to radiation-induced toxic products); and, finally, a more generalized component characterized by tremors, convulsions, ataxia, and death within a few hours.

The **gastrointestinal syndrome** (≥ 4 Gy) occurs when the total body dose of radiation is smaller but still high. It is characterized by intractable nausea, vomiting, and diarrhea that lead to severe dehydration, diminished plasma volume, vascular collapse, and death. The GI syndrome

results from the initial "toxemia" due to necrosis of tissue and is perpetuated by progressive atrophy of the GI mucosa. Bacteremia also occurs. Ultimately, the intestinal villi are denuded, with massive loss of plasma into the intestine. Regeneration of GI epithelial cells may be possible after large doses of radiation; massive plasma replacement and antibiotics during the first 4 to 6 days will keep patients alive until this occurs. However, even if the patient does survive, the respite is temporary, since hematopoietic failure will ensue within 2 or 3 wk.

The **hematopoietic syndrome** (2 to 10 Gy), characterized by anorexia, apathy, nausea, and vomiting, may be maximal within 6 to 12 h. Symptoms subside completely within 24 to 36 h after exposure. During this period of relative well-being, lymph nodes, spleen, and bone marrow begin to atrophy, leading to pancytopenia. This atrophy results from direct killing of radiosensitive cells and from inhibition of new cell production. In the peripheral blood, lymphopenia commences immediately, becoming maximal within 24 to 36 h. Neutropenia develops more slowly. Thrombocytopenia may be prominent within 3 or 4 wk.

Increased susceptibility to infection (by both saprophytic and pathogenic organisms) develops owing to (1) a dose-dependent decrease in circulating granulocytes and lymphocytes, (2) a dose-dependent impairment of antibody production, (3) impairment of granulocyte migration and phagocytosis, (4) decreased ability of the reticuloendothelial system to kill phagocytized bacteria, (5) diminished resistance to spread in subcutaneous tissues, and (6) hemorrhagic areas (due mainly to the thrombocytopenia) of the skin and bowel that encourage entrance and growth of bacteria.

With acute total body radiation > 6 Gy, hematopoietic or GI malfunction will be fatal; with doses < 6 Gy, survival probability is inversely related to total dose.

2. Acute "radiation sickness" following therapeutic irradiation (particularly of the abdomen) in a small proportion of patients is characterized by nausea, vomiting, diarrhea, anorexia, headache, malaise, and tachycardia of varying severity. The discomfort subsides within a few hours or days; its cause is not understood.

3. Delayed effects may be intermediate or late. *Intermediate effects:* Prolonged or repeated exposure to low-dose rates from internally deposited or external sources of radiation may produce amenorrhea, decreased fertility in both sexes, decreased libido only in the female, anemia, leukopenia, thrombocytopenia, and cataracts. More severe or highly localized exposure causes loss of hair, skin atrophy and ulceration, keratosis, and telangiectasia, and ultimately may cause squamous cell carcinomas. Osteosarcomas may appear years after ingestion of radioactive bone-seeking nuclides such as radium salts.

Serious injury to exposed organs occasionally occurs after extensive radiotherapy for cancer. Renal functional changes include a decrease in GFR and tubular function. Acute onset of clinical manifestations may occur after extremely high doses (after a latent period of 6 mo to 1 yr) and may include proteinuria, renal insufficiency of varying degree, anemia, and hypertension. When cumulative kidney exposure is > 20 Gy in < 5 wk, radiation fibrosis and oliguric renal failure will occur in about 37% of cases. The remainder will develop variable changes over a prolonged time. Large accumulated doses to muscles may result in painful myopathy with atrophy and calcification. Very rarely, these changes are followed by a neoplastic change, usually a sarcoma. Radiation pneumonitis and subsequent pulmonary fibrosis may be severe when lung metastases are irradiated, and can be fatal after a cumulative dose of > 30 Gy if treatment is not spread over a sufficient period. Radiation pericarditis and myocarditis have been produced by extensive mediastinal radiotherapy. Catastrophic myelopathy may develop after a segment of the spinal cord has received cumulative doses > 50 Gy. Following vigorous therapy of abdominal lymph nodes (for seminoma, lymphoma, or ovarian carcinoma), chronic ulceration, fibrosis, and perforation of the bowel may develop. Skin erythema and ulceration were observed fairly often during the era of orthovoltage x-ray therapy, but the high-energy photons from modern cobalt-60 units and linear accelerators penetrate deeply into tissues and have virtually eliminated these complications.

Late somatic and genetic effects: Radiation alters the "information system" of proliferating somatic and germ cells. With somatic cells this may result in somatic disease—eg, cancer (leukemia, thyroid, skin, bone) or cataracts—or, as suggested by animal models, in nonspecific shortening of life. Leukemia from substantial radiation in humans has been observed. It is *postulated* that there is no "threshold" dose for leukemia, and that the incidence increases with dose.

Thyroid carcinoma has been observed 20 to 30 yr after x-ray therapy for adenoid and tonsillar hypertrophy, and x-ray treatment for nonmalignant conditions is now considered inappropriate except in highly unusual situations. However, several large studies have failed to show increased thyroid cancer in persons receiving up to 80 mGy to the thyroid delivered by radioisotopes.

With germ cell exposure, mutations are increased. When mutations are perpetuated by procreation, animal studies indicate that an increasing number of genetic defectives will be expressed in the course of generations. Although this has not been demonstrated in man, the possibility presents serious medical, ethical, and philosophic problems with respect to unborn generations. It imposes a moral obligation to limit radiation exposure to that which is absolutely necessary for valid diagnostic or therapeutic purposes and to strictly control occupational exposure. The potential harm, however, should be kept in perspective. Some investigators believe that no measurable effects will occur below a certain threshold, while others insist that any radiation is potentially harmful. The long-term probability of a measurable genetic or somatic effect appearing in a given individual is estimated to be 10^{-2}/Gy.

Diagnosis and Prognosis

When a person is receiving therapeutic radiation or has been exposed during a radiation accident, etiology is obvious. Prognosis depends on dose, dose rate, and body distribution. Serial hematologic and bone marrow studies to gauge the severity of marrow injury provide additional prognostic information.

When the cerebral or GI syndromes are present, the diagnosis is simple but the prognosis is grave. Death occurs with the cerebral syndrome within hours to a few days; with GI symptoms in 3 to 10 days; and with hematopoietic symptoms in 8 to 50 days. In the latter, death may occur from a supervening infection in 2 to 4 wk or from massive hemorrhage between 3 and 6 wk.

In chronic cases, where external exposure is either unknown or overlooked, a diagnosis may be difficult or impossible. A search for possible occupational exposure is required. In institutions licensed by federal or state governments, records of exposure to radiation are maintained. Serial chromosome studies can be performed to watch for types and frequency of chromosomal abnormalities that are likely to occur after significant radiation, but that may have preexisted or been induced by nonradiation sources. Periodic examination for early cataracts is appropriate in chronic radiation exposure of the eye, especially from neutrons.

Alleged radiation exposure is difficult to evaluate, since emotional or psychologic factors tend to predominate. Unless the individual has received a documented external or internal dose, exact diagnosis is probably impossible. Normal hematologic values and the absence of objective clinical illness would permit reassurance of the patient and others concerned.

Prophylaxis

Many drugs and chemicals increase survival rate in animals if given prior to irradiation; eg, sulfhydryl compounds. However, none are currently of practical value in man. The only way to minimize fatal or serious overexposure is the rigorous enforcement of protective measures and adherence to the maximum permissible dose (MPD) levels. These values are listed in *Basic Radiation Protection Criteria*, NCRP Report No. 39, published by the National Council on Radiation Protection and Measurements (P.O. Box 30175, Washington, DC 20014).

Treatment

Contamination of the skin by radioactive materials should be immediately removed by copious water irrigation and special chelating solutions containing EDTA when available (Radiac Wash®). Small puncture wounds must be treated vigorously to remove contamination. Irrigation and debridement are indicated until the wound is free of radioactivity. Ingested material should be removed promptly by induced vomiting or lavage if exposure is recent. If radioiodine is inhaled or ingested in large quantities, the patient should be given Lugol's solution or saturated solution of potassium iodide to block thyroid uptake for days to weeks, and diuresis should be promoted. Monitoring of exposed patients is mandatory, using hand-type rate-meter probes or sophisticated whole-body counting. Urine should be analyzed for non-γ-emitting radionuclides if exposure to these agents is suspected. Radon breath analysis can be done in cases of suspected radium ingestion.

Since the **acute cerebral syndrome** is uniformly fatal, treatment is palliative and directed toward combating shock and anoxia, relieving pain and anxiety, and giving sedation for control of convulsions.

Symptoms of **radiation sickness due to therapeutic irradiation of the abdomen** can be diminished by an antiemetic (eg, prochlorperazine 5 to 10 mg orally or IM qid) and may be prevented by prior administration. Attention to nutrition and fluid balance through close cooperation between radiotherapist and referring physician is mandatory. Most difficulties can be avoided or minimized by careful planning of overall management (eg, dose, time interval between treatments, supportive therapy).

Gastrointestinal syndrome: After modest exposure, antiemetics and sedation may suffice. If oral feeding can be started, a bland diet is tolerated best. Fluid, electrolytes, and plasma, by appropriate routes, may be required in large volumes. The amount and type will be dictated by blood chemistry (especially electrolytes and proteins), blood pressure, pulse, fluid exchange, and skin turgor.

Management of the **hematopoietic syndrome,** with its potentially lethal factors of infection, hemorrhage, and anemia, is similar to that of marrow hypoplasia and pancytopenia from any cause. Antibiotics, fresh blood, and platelet transfusions are the main therapeutic aids. Rigid asepsis during all skin-puncturing procedures is mandatory, as is strict isolation to prevent exposure to pathogens.

Concurrent antineoplastic chemotherapy or use of other marrow-suppressing drugs, unless strongly indicated because of some preexisting clinical condition or sudden complication, should be *avoided* because of the potential for further suppression of bone marrow.

Bone marrow transplants have proved helpful in genetically identical animals. If a dose > 2 Gy is suspected, tissue typing and search for a compatible bone marrow should be made. If an identical twin is available, a marrow transplant will increase the probability of survival. If granulocytes and platelets continue to decrease at a constant rate and fall to < 500 and 20,000/μL, respectively, homotransplantation of marrow should be considered, though the likelihood of success is small and the transplant may be followed by a potentially fatal immunologic graft-vs.-host reaction.

In dealing with **late somatic effects due to serious chronic exposure,** removal of the patient from the radiation source is the first step. With radium, thorium, or radiostrontium deposition in the body, prompt administration of oral and parenteral chelating agents (EDTA) will increase excretion. However, in the late stages these agents are useless. Radiation ulcers and cancers require surgical removal and plastic repair. Radiation-induced leukemia is treated like any similar spontaneous leukemia. Anemia is corrected by whole-blood transfusion. Thrombocytopenic bleeding may be reduced by platelet transfusions. However, these measures are of only temporary value since the probability is slight that an extensively damaged bone marrow will regenerate. No effective treatment for sterility, or for ovarian and testicular dysfunction, except for hormonal supplementation, has been devised.

118. ELECTRIC SHOCK

Injury caused by an electric current passing through the body. The electricity may be atmospheric (lightning) or man-made; ie, from high-voltage transmission or low-voltage lines. Potential injuries include physiologic aberrations and burns.

Pathogenesis

Factors that determine the form and severity of injury (which may range from a minor burn to death) include (1) the type and magnitude of current, (2) the resistance of the body at the point of contact, (3) the current pathway, and (4) the duration of current flow.

The **type and magnitude of current** have a profound influence upon the injury sustained. In general, **direct current (DC)**, which has zero frequency (although it may be intermittent or pulsating), is less dangerous than **alternating current (AC)**, the type generally used in the USA. The effects of AC on the body depend largely on the frequency; low-frequency currents, 50 to 60 Hz (cycles/sec), are the common variety and are usually more dangerous than high-frequency currents and 3 to 5 times more dangerous than DC of the same voltage and amperage. DC tends to cause a convulsive contraction, often forcing the victim away from further current exposure. AC, 60 Hz, causes muscle tetany, often "freezing" the hand to the circuit as the fist clenches the current source and may result in prolonged exposure with severe burns if the voltage is high. *Generally, the higher the voltage and the amperage, the greater the damage from either type of current.* Both AC and DC may affect the body either by altering physiologic functions (involuntary muscular contractions and seizures, ventricular fibrillation, respiratory arrest due to CNS injury or muscle paralysis, etc) or by producing thermal, electrochemical, or other damage (burns, necrosis of muscle and other tissue, hemolysis, coagulation, dehydration, vertebral and other skeletal fractures, muscle and tendon avulsion,

etc). Electric shock often causes a combination of these effects.

The **threshold of perception** for DC entering the hand is about 5 to 10 milliamperes **(mA)**; for AC, 60 Hz (household current), about 1 to 10 mA. The maximum current that can cause contraction of the flexor musculature of the arm but still permit the subject to release his hand from the current source is termed the "let-go" **current**. For DC, this value is about 75 mA; for AC, about 15 mA and varies with muscle mass. A low-voltage (110 to 220 v) 60-Hz AC current traveling through the chest for a fraction of a second may induce **ventricular fibrillation** at currents as low as 60 to 100 mA; about 300 to 500 mA of DC are required. If the current has a direct pathway to the heart (eg, via a cardiac catheter or pacemaker electrodes), much lower currents (< 1 mA, AC or DC) can produce fibrillation.

Body resistance (measured in ohms/cm^2) is concentrated primarily in the skin and varies directly with the skin's condition. Dry, well-keratinized, intact skin has an average resistance of 20,000 to 30,000 ohms/cm^2, whereas the resistance of moist, thin skin is about 500 ohms/cm^2. If the skin is punctured (eg, from a cut or abrasion, or by a needle), or if current is applied to moist mucous membranes (eg, mouth, rectum, vagina), the resistance may be as low as 200 to 300 ohms/cm^2. A thickly calloused palm or sole may have a resistance of 2 to 3 million ohms/cm^2. As current passes through the skin, much energy may be dissipated at the surface if the skin resistance is high, and large surface burns can result at both the entry and exit points with charring of tissues in between (heat = amperage^2 × resistance). Tissues are also burned internally, depending on their resistance; nerves, blood vessels, and muscles conduct electricity more readily than denser tissues, eg, fat, tendon, and bone. If the skin resistance is low, the patient may have few, if any, extensive burns but may still suffer cardiac arrest if the current reaches the heart.

The **pathway of current** through the body can be crucial in determining injury. Conduction from arm to arm or between an arm and a foot at ground potential is much more dangerous than contact between a leg and ground, since the current may traverse the heart. Electrical injuries to the head may cause seizures, intraventricular hemorrhage, respiratory arrest, ventricular fibrillation or asystole, or, as a late effect, cataracts. The most common entry point for electricity is the hand, followed by the head. The most common exit is the foot. Lightning rarely, if ever, has entry and exit wounds.

The **duration of current flow** through the body is important. While the heart is vulnerable to small currents at relatively low voltages, in general, the amount of injury to the body is directly proportional to the duration of exposure because tissue breakdown occurs with longer durations, allowing internal current flow. Heat is produced by current flow through tissues, causing severe burns, protein coagulation, vascular thrombosis, and tissue necrosis.

When a victim freezes to a circuit (see "let-go" current, above), he may suffer severe burns. Conversely, a lightning victim rarely suffers external or internal burns, despite the higher voltage, because the extremely short duration of current is not enough to cause skin breakdown. It "flashes over" the victim, producing little internal damage other than electrical short-circuiting of systems (heart—asystole, brain—confusion and loss of consciousness).

Symptoms and Signs

The effects and clinical manifestations of electrical injuries depend on the complex interaction of the factors discussed above. Electricity can startle a person and cause him to fall down or be thrown. It may cause severe, spastic contraction of the muscles with accompanying fractures, dislocations, and loss of consciousness. Both respiratory paralysis (apnea) and cardiac arrhythmias or arrest may occur. Sharply demarcated electrical burns may be present on the skin and extend well into deeper tissues.

High voltage may cause coagulation necrosis of internal tissues between entry and exit points of the current. Massive edema may follow as the veins coagulate and the muscles swell. Hypotension, fluid and electrolyte disturbances, and severe myoglobinuria may cause acute renal failure. Dislocations, fractures, and blunt injuries may be present from powerful muscle contractions or falls secondary to the electric shock.

"Bathtub accident" victims (typically, a wet [grounded] individual who contacts a 110-v circuit) may show no burns but suffer cardiac arrest.

Lightning rarely leaves entry or exit wounds and seldom causes muscle damage or myoglobulinuria. Coma and other neurologic sequelae may be present but usually resolve within hours or days. Death is most frequently due to cardiopulmonary arrest and its sequelae.

Prevention

Prevention of electrical injuries entails proper design, installation, and maintenance of all electric devices. Education and compliance, as well as common sense and respect in dealing with electricity, are essential. Any electric device that touches or may be touched by the body and has life-threatening potential should be properly grounded and incorporated in circuits containing fail-safe equipment. **Ground-fault circuit breakers**, which trip at current leakage to ground levels of as low as 5 mA, are excellent safety devices and are readily available. With lightning, common sense, use of proper protection devices, and seeking appropriate shelter in storms are essential.

Treatment

Treatment consists of (1) separating the patient from the current source, (2) reestablishing vital functions immediately, and (3) giving supportive care as required.

Contact between the victim and the current source can be broken either by **shutting off the current** or by **removing the person from contact with it.** The best method is to cut off the source, if it can be done rapidly (eg, throwing a circuit breaker or switch, disconnecting the device from its electrical outlet); otherwise, the victim must be removed from the source. *For low voltage* (110 to 220 v), the rescuer should first ensure that he himself is well insulated from ground, and then should use an insulating material (eg, cloth, dry wood, rubber, leather belt) to pull the person free. *If it is suspected that higher voltage lines are involved, it is best to leave the victim alone until the power can be shut off.* High and low voltage lines are not always easily differentiated, particularly outdoors.

Once it has been established that it is safe to touch the victim, **a rapid examination for vital** functions should be performed (eg, radial, femoral, or carotid pulses; respiratory function; level of consciousness). Airway stabilization is the first priority. If spontaneous respiration is not observed or cardiac arrest has occurred, immediate resuscitation is required. Heart-lung resuscitation techniques are detailed under CARDIOPULMONARY RESUSCITATION in Ch. 30. The treatment of shock and other manifestations of massive burns is discussed in Ch. 114.

Once vital functions have been reestablished, the full nature and extent of the injury must be evaluated (see Pathogenesis, above) and treated. A search for dislocations, fractures, and cervical-spine and blunt injuries should be made. If myoglobinuria is present, fluid loading is essential, and mannitol or furosemide may be indicated to increase renal flow.

Lightning injuries are usually superficial, but victims may require cardiac resuscitation, monitoring, and supportive care. Fluid restriction is the rule because of potential brain edema. After being struck by lightning, patients without vital signs for 15 min or even longer have been revived by CPR, although this is unusual.

Tetanus prophylaxis is required for any burn. An ECG, cardiac enzymes, CBC, and a urinalysis especially for myoglobin are baseline determinations for all electrical injuries. Other tests may be indicated as necessary. Any suggestion of cardiac damage, arrhythmias, or chest pain requires monitoring for at least 24 h. Any deterioration in the level of consciousness mandates a CT scan to rule out intracranial hemorrhage.

Children and Lip Burns

Toddlers who suck on extension cords can get burns to the mouth and lips. These may cause not only cosmetic deformities but growth problems of the teeth, mandible, and maxilla. Victims should be referred to a pedodontist or oral surgeon familiar with their evaluation and continuing long-term care. An added danger is that of labial artery hemorrhage when the eschar separates 7 to 10 days postinjury, which occurs in 10% of cases.

119. MOTION SICKNESS

A disorder caused by repetitive angular and linear acceleration and deceleration and characterized primarily by nausea and vomiting. Sea-, air-, car-, train-, swing-, and space-sickness are specific forms. Prevention is easier than treatment.

Etiology

Excessive stimulation of the vestibular apparatus by motion is the primary cause. Individual susceptibility varies greatly. Afferent pathways from the labyrinth to the vomiting center in the medulla are undefined, but motion sickness occurs only when the 8th nerve and cerebellar vestibular tracts are intact. Visual stimuli (eg, a moving horizon), poor ventilation (fumes, smoke, and carbon monoxide), and emotional factors (eg, fear, anxiety) commonly act in concert with motion to precipitate an attack. Motion sickness in space travel is referred to as the **space adaptation syndrome**; weightlessness or zero gravity is an etiologic factor. This syndrome is a major problem in the efficiency of astronauts in the first few days of space flight, but adaptation occurs over several days.

Symptoms and Signs

Cyclic nausea and vomiting are characteristic. They may be preceded by yawning, hyperventilation, salivation, pallor, profuse cold sweating, and somnolence. Aerophagia, dizziness, headache, general discomfort, and fatigue may also occur. Once nausea and vomiting develop, the patient is weak and unable to concentrate. With prolonged exposure to motion, individuals may adapt and gradually return to well-being. However, symptoms may be reinitiated by more severe motion or by recurrence of motion after a short respite.

Prolonged motion sickness with vomiting may lead to arterial hypotension, dehydration, inanition, and depression. Motion sickness can be a serious complication in patients who are ill from other causes.

Prophylaxis and Treatment

Susceptible individuals should minimize exposure by positioning themselves where there is the least motion (eg, amidships or, in airplanes, over the wings). A supine or semirecumbent position with the head braced is best. Reading should be avoided. Keeping the axis of vision at an angle of 45 above the horizon will reduce susceptibility. Avoiding visual fixation on waves or other moving objects is helpful to some. A well-ventilated cabin is important, and going out on deck for a breath of fresh air is helpful. Alcoholic or dietary excesses before or during travel increase the likelihood of motion sickness. Small amounts of fluids and simple food should be taken frequently during extended periods of exposure; if the exposure is short, as in air travel, food and fluids should be avoided. In the space adaptation syndrome, movement aggravates the symptoms.

Prophylactic drugs should be given before nausea and vomiting occur. One hour before departure, susceptible individuals may be given diphenhydramine, meclizine, or cyclizine 50 mg orally; promethazine 25 mg or diazepam 5 to 10 mg orally; or scopolamine HBr 0.6 mg orally to minimize the vagally mediated GI symptoms. A smaller dose of scopolamine can be delivered via a dermal patch applied 4 h before departure from which 0.5 mg is released over 3 days. If emotional factors are significant, phenobarbital 15 to 30 mg may be given orally 1 h prior to departure. Sedation with pentobarbital 100 mg orally to induce light sleep may be helpful if alertness is not required. However, sedation should be mild enough to allow mental clarity when the passenger arrives at the destination. All dosages should be appropriately modified for prolonged exposure. After vomiting begins, medication must be given rectally or parenterally to be effective. With prolonged vomiting, IV fluids and electrolytes may be required for replacement and maintenance.

120. MEDICAL ASPECTS OF AIR AND FOREIGN TRAVEL

Commercial aviation safely transports millions of passengers each year but imposes a variety of potential medical stresses. While absolute prohibitions on flying exist for very few medical conditions, planning and precautions are necessary for some patients. Commercial pilots undergo rigorous screening and physical examinations, and accidents due to their illness or to substance abuse are extremely rare.

General aviation, a rapidly growing area for business and recreational flying, also presents a number of potential health hazards. The Federal Aviation Administration (FAA) requires periodic medical examination of private pilots by specially designated physicians, but most of these approximately 1 million pilots licensed in the USA receive their medical care from private practitioners. Of the > 4000 accidents that occur each year in general aviation, most happen in recreational aircraft and are often related to the injudicious use of alcohol or drugs. The physician may counsel his pilot patient in these matters, caution about side effects of medications (eg, antihistamines), and provide current tetanus immunization.

Aircraft of all types present increasing environmental health hazards in terms of urban noise and air pollution, occasional large-scale disasters, and toxic contamination in agricultural areas. For patients living near large airports, continuous high-level noise and air pollution can aggravate a wide variety of medical conditions. Local disaster facilities near airports should be prepared to provide initial management of major trauma and burns of air crash survivors. Physicians in agricultural communities should know the toxic manifestations of the chemicals used in aerial spraying that may accidentally contaminate farm workers or nearby populated areas (see Ch. 145).

Clinical Manifestations

Major problems imposed on the air traveler relate to (1) changes in barometric pressure, (2) decreased O_2 tension, (3) turbulence, (4) circadian dysrhythmia, and (5) psychologic stress.

Changes in barometric pressure: Modern jet aircraft, including the supersonics, maintain cabin pressure equivalent to between 5000 and 8000 ft. At such altitudes, free air in body cavities tends to expand by about 25% and may aggravate certain medical conditions. The occasional accidental loss of cabin pressure and the fact that some airplanes are unpressurized must be kept in mind. Upper respiratory inflammation or allergy may obstruct eustachian tubes or sinus ostia, resulting in barotitis media (see Ch. 66) or barosinusitis (see also Ch. 68). Frequent yawning or closed-nose swallowing during descent, decongestant nasal sprays, and antihistamines taken before or during flight often prevent or relieve these conditions. Children are particularly susceptible to barotitis media and should be given oral fluids or feedings during descent to encourage swallowing (chewing gum or hard candy is more effective than eating). Facial pain of dental origin may occur with air pressure changes. Air travel is *contraindicated* in patients with pneumothorax or potential for its development (eg, large pulmonary blebs or cavities) and in those in whom air or gas is trapped and even modest expansion may cause pain or stress tissue (eg, incarcerated bowel or recent [< 10 days] laparotomy). Patients with a colostomy should wear a large bag and expect frequent filling.

Decreased O_2 tension: Cabin pressure at a 7500-ft altitude-equivalent results in a Pa_{O_2} of about 70 mm Hg, which is well tolerated by healthy travelers. Problems may arise, however, in a number of conditions, including moderate or severe **pulmonary disease** (eg, asthma, emphysema, cystic fibrosis), **heart failure, anemia** with a Hb < 8.5 gm/dL, severe **angina pectoris, sickle-cell disease** (but not trait, see Ch. 35), and some **congenital heart diseases.** Patients with these conditions usually can fly safely with specially designed continuous O_2 equipment, which must be provided by the airline; 72 h advance notice is required (all commercial aircraft carry O_2 for use during an in-flight emergency). Patients recovering from **myocardial infarction** may fly when stable, often within 10 to 14 days. Ankle edema is common on long flights and should not be confused with increased heart failure. **Hypertension** is affected by psychologic stress of flight and may be controlled by a mild preflight tranquilizer. Smoking can aggravate mild hypoxia and should be avoided. The impact of alcohol may be increased by fatigue and hypoxia. In general, anyone able to walk 100 yd or climb one flight of stairs and whose disease is stable should tolerate normal cabin conditions without additional O_2.

Turbulence may cause air sickness (see Ch. 119) or injury and can occur at any time. Passengers should keep their seat belts fastened at all times while seated.

Circadian dysrhythmia ("jet lag"): Rapid travel across multiple time zones creates many biologic and psychologic stresses; after long trips, travelers should plan on 24- to 48-h rest upon arrival and avoid major commitments or decisions during this adjustment period. A gradual shift in sleeping and eating patterns (a high-protein, low-calorie intake is recommended) before departure may partly alleviate the problem. Some therapeutic regimens require alteration to compensate for circadian dysrhythm, eg, diabetics using long-acting insulin may need to change to regular insulin until they have adjusted to the destination time, available food, and activity. Other medication schedules may require adjustment based on elapsed rather than local time.

Psychologic stress: Fear of flying and claustrophobia are psychologic and not influenced by logic or reason; hypnosis and behavioral modification psychotherapy have reduced the fear of flying in some. Fearful passengers may benefit from mild sedation before and during flight. Hyperventilation may provoke unconsciousness or tetany-like convulsions or may simulate cardiovascular disease; physician-passengers may be asked to volunteer Good Samaritan services in such in-flight situations. Psychotic tendencies may become more acute and troublesome in flight, and patients with violent or unpredictable tendencies must be accompanied by an attendant and be appropriately sedated.

Other considerations: (1) **Thrombophlebitis** (with delayed risk of deep vein thrombosis) is a possibility for anyone sitting for long periods, especially pregnant patients and those with venous disease; frequent (q 1 to 2 h) walks around the cabin and short-movement exercises should be practiced while seated. (2) **Dehydration** may develop because of very low cabin humidity, but can be avoided by adequate intake of fluids and avoidance of alcohol. (3) **Wired jaw:** Maxillofacial injury immobilized by fixed wires, unless fitted with a special quick-release device, is a contraindication to air travel since air sickness may result in aspiration of vomitus. (4) **Pacemakers and metal prostheses:** Newer models of pacemakers are effectively shielded from interference from security devices; older units may be affected. Battery life sufficient for the length of travel should be ensured. The metal content of pacemakers and of metal orthopedic prostheses and braces may trigger a security alarm; a physician's letter should be carried to avoid security difficulties. (5) **Communicable disease:** Patients with any communicable disease that may endanger others in a crowded aircraft are not acceptable as passengers. International immunization requirements change frequently; current information may be obtained from local or state health departments. **(6) Contact lens** wearers should instill artificial tears frequently to avoid corneal irritation resulting from low cabin humidity. **(7) Medications and records:** The experienced traveler carries on his person essential medications sufficient to ensure continued therapy in the event of lost baggage, theft in hotels, delayed arrival, or local unavailability. Patients who must carry narcotics or unusually large amounts of any medication should have a verifying letter from their physician to avoid possible security or customs complications. A summary of a patient's medical record (including ECG) may be invaluable if a patient becomes ill away from home. Patients subject to disabling illness (eg, epilepsy) or who are at high risk should wear a medical identification bracelet or necklace (eg, as provided by Medic-Alert Foundation, Turlock, CA 95380). A recent dental checkup and carrying extra glasses and hearing-aid batteries are wise precautions. **(8) Uncomplicated pregnancy** through the 8th mo is acceptable; high-risk patients must be individually evaluated if travel is planned. Acceptance during the 9th mo usually requires a physician's written approval dated within 72 h of departure and indicating delivery date. Seat belts should be worn across the thighs. Thrombophlebitis is a specific risk when sitting for long periods (see above). **(9) Children:** Infants $<$ 7 days of age are not accepted for travel. For children with chronic disease (eg, congenital heart disease, chronic lung disease, anemia), the same precautions apply as for adults. **(10) The elderly and the handicapped:** There is no upper age limit, and airlines make all reasonable efforts to accommodate patients with handicaps. Wheelchair and litter patients can often be accommodated on commercial aircraft; otherwise, air ambulance service is necessary. Some airlines will accept patients requiring special equipment (IV fluids, respirators, etc) provided appropriate personnel accompany the patient and arrangements have been made in advance. **(11) Special foods,** including low-sodium, low-fat, and diabetic diets, are usually available upon advance request.

Further advice regarding air travel may be obtained from the medical department of major airlines or from the FAA Regional Flight Surgeon. Special arrangements (eg, O_2, wheelchair, etc) can be made through regular reservations clerks, but at least 72 h advance notice is usually required.

Foreign travel may involve significant difficulties in case of illness. Millions travel abroad yearly; about 1 in 30 requires emergency care. Many insurance plans, including Medicare, are not valid in foreign countries; overseas hospitals often require a substantial cash deposit, regardless of insurance. A variety of travel insurance plans, including some that will arrange for emergency evacuation, are available through travel agents and some major credit card companies. Directories listing English-speaking physicians in foreign countries are available from several organizations (eg, International Association for Medical Assistance to Travelers, 417 Center Street, Lewiston, NY 14092); US consulates may also assist in obtaining emergency medical services. *Fielding's Traveler's Medical Companion,* by Graber and Siegel, Fielding/Morrow, 1990, has valuable information for persons traveling abroad, including those with special health needs. Information is available 24 h/day on a wide variety of foreign travel risks from the US State Department's Citizen's Emergency Center, 202-647-5225.

Travel in developing countries can be additionally hazardous. Motor vehicle accidents, especially at night, are the leading cause of traveler injury and death. Drinking only bottled water or carbonated beverages will reduce the risk of acquiring water-borne disease; ice cubes and tap water should not be ingested in any amount (showering or brushing teeth). Only hot foods or peeled fruits should be consumed; salads, dairy products, and shellfish transmit disease.

Chemoprophylaxis, insect repellant, and mosquito netting are essential precautions in malarial areas. Many countries require special immunizations, some of which must be given 2 to 4 wk before departure. "Health Immunization for International Travel," a booklet containing immunization and chemoprophylaxis requirements, is published annually by the Centers for Disease Control **(CDC),** Atlanta, GA (Government Printing Office publication #HE 20.7315:988). The most up-to-date information is available from the CDC's Travelers' Health Section, 404-332-4559, or from Immunization Alert, 203-487-0611.

Some tropical diseases become evident months after a traveler has returned home; a travel history is useful in patients who present with puzzling illnesses.

121.   NEAR-DROWNING

Pathophysiology

Near-drowning victims, because of aspiration or laryngospasm, usually sustain significant hypoxemia, with the consequent danger of respiratory failure and hypercapnia. Acute reflex laryngospasm may result in asphyxia without aspiration of water. Aspiration of fluid and particulate matter may cause chemical pneumonitis, damaging cells lining the alveoli, and may impair alveolar secretion of surfactant, resulting in patchy atelectasis.

The perfusion of nonaerated, atelectatic areas of the lungs leads to intrapulmonary shunting of blood and aggravates hypoxemia; the more fluid aspirated, the greater the surfactant loss, atelectasis, and hypoxemia. Aspiration of large quantities of water may cause sizable areas of atelectasis, resulting in stiff noncompliant lungs and respiratory failure. Respiratory acidosis with hypercapnia and hypoxemia can occur. A concomitant metabolic acidosis may also result from tissue hypoxia. Hypoxemia and tissue hypoxia often result in pulmonary edema and even cerebral edema. On x-ray, pulmonary edema may simulate atelectasis and the 2 conditions may coexist.

The mammalian **diving reflex** in cold water allows survival after long periods of submersion. The diving reflex, first identified in seagoing mammals, slows the heartbeat and constricts the peripheral arteries, shunting oxygenated blood away from the extremities and the gut to the heart and brain. In cold water, the O_2 needs of the tissues are reduced, extending the possible time of survival.

Respiratory insufficiency is more critical than changes in electrolytes and blood volume, which vary in magnitude depending on the type and volume of aspirated fluid. **Sea water** may cause a mild elevation of Na and Cl, but the levels are rarely life-threatening. By contrast, aspirating large quantities of **fresh water** can cause a sudden increase in blood volume, profound electrolyte imbalance, and hemolysis. Victims may succumb to the effects of these changes—asphyxia and possibly ventricular fibrillation—at the scene of the tragedy. Cardiac arrest, usually preceded by fibrillation, causes many of the deaths attributed to drowning. However, current belief is that the pulmonary edema following near-drowning is a direct result of hypoxemia and analogous to pulmonary edema of high altitude, ie, noncardiogenic pulmonary edema.

Prevention

Eating and drinking shortly before swimming should be avoided. Children require proper supervision at beaches and near pools or ponds. All swimmers should be accompanied by an experienced swimmer or swim only in guarded areas. Nonswimmers and small children should wear flotation jackets when in boats or playing near bodies of water. Children should be taught to swim as early as possible, and adults and children over 12 should be familiar with the basics of resuscitation. All swimming pools should be adequately fenced ($\geq$ 4 ft in height). Infants, children, the debilitated, and the elderly should not be left unattended in bathtubs.

Treatment

The key factors for surviving submersion without permanent injury appear to be duration of submersion, water temperature, age of the individual (the diving reflex is more active in children), and speed of resuscitation efforts. Survival depends more on the prompt correction of hypoxemia and acidosis (ventilatory insufficiency) than correction of electrolyte imbalance, the goal being to prevent pulmonary and cerebral edema due to tissue hypoxia.

If near-drowning takes place in very cold water, the victim may be hypothermic. Because of the diving reflex and the reduced metabolic needs associated with hypothermia, vigorous attempts should be made to resuscitate victims (especially children), even if they have been submerged for periods up to 1 h or longer. The management of hypothermia is discussed in Ch. 116.

Emergency mouth-to-mouth resuscitation should begin immediately if the victim is apneic—in the water, if necessary. If heart beat and carotid pulse cannot be detected, closed chest cardiac massage (see CARDIOPULMONARY RESUSCITATION in Ch. 30) is initiated as soon as artificial ventilation is started. Mechanical ventilators, which supply higher inspired O_2 concentrations, should be used if available. Electrical defibrillation may be necessary.

Time should not be wasted in attempts to drain water from the lungs in a fresh-water victim, because the hypotonic fluid passes rapidly into the circulation. Sea water, being hypertonic, draws plasma into the lung, and the Trendelenburg position may promote drainage.

Hospitalization is mandatory for all victims. Resuscitation should continue during transport, regardless of the patient's condition. Consciousness is not synonymous with recovery, since *delayed death from hypoxia can occur.*

Initial emphasis in the hospital continues to be intensive pulmonary care to achieve adequate arterial blood gas and acid-base levels. Required measures range from simple O_2 administration for a spontaneously breathing patient to continuous ventilatory support of an apneic patient by tracheal intubation with a cuffed tube connected to a mechanical ventilator. Sodium bicarbonate IV is usually indicated, since metabolic acidosis almost invariably accompanies the tissue and cellular hypoxia. Further bicarbonate administration, ventilatory support, and proper inspired O_2 concentrations are determined by monitoring blood gases. High supplemental levels of O_2 inhalation must be continued until the arterial blood gas studies indicate that lesser O_2 concentrations are adequate.

Frequent manual hyperinflation of the lungs is indicated to reexpand atelectatic alveoli. β_2-Agonists by inhalation or injection help to reduce bronchospasm. Since near-drowning with fluid aspiration is a form of aspiration pneumonitis, corticosteroids and antibiotics may be considered, depending on the individual case.

Fluid and electrolyte solutions are required to correct significant electrolyte imbalance. A large quantity of fluid may be extravasated into the lungs in sea water immersion, producing a reduced blood volume that may be reflected by lowered central venous pressure; infusion of volume expanders may be indicated. Fluid restriction is usually not advisable, since the pulmonary and cerebral edema caused by hypoxia are related to direct pulmonary epithelial damage or osmotic gradients rather than to circulatory overload as in congestive heart failure. RBC replacement to increase the O_2-carrying capacity of the blood, and forced diuresis to facilitate excretion of the free plasma Hb may be necessary if there is significant hemolysis.

The patient who develops acute respiratory distress syndrome requires mechanical ventilation. Positive end-expiratory pressure (PEEP) may help to maintain patency of alveoli, prevent alveolar collapse, and expand collapsed alveoli. Pulmonary care may be necessary for hours or days, depending on the arterial blood gas and pH analyses. Permanent brain damage from hypoxemia and tissue hypoxia may be a residual problem in some cases. Cerebral resuscitation measures and the role of neurologic classification for brain injury require further study. The following measures may be beneficial but carry intrinsic risks: hyperventilation, hyperoxygenation with hyperbaric chambers (see Ch. 128), hypothermia, barbiturate coma, and steroids. Acetazolamide IV has been effective in relieving cerebral edema due to hypoxia.

122. MEDICAL ASPECTS OF DIVING AND WORK IN COMPRESSED AIR

Serious errors in diagnosis and treatment may occur when illness arises from diving or other activities involving **increased environmental pressure.** Diving with **scuba** (self-contained underwater breathing apparatus) has grown enormously as a popular sport and in commercial and scientific applications. As a result, many individuals are now potential victims of conditions that were once confined to deep sea divers and construction workers in tunnels or caissons.

A patient with almost any disorder that develops during, or especially following, exposure to increased pressure could have decompression sickness or gas embolism and urgently need recompression. Physicians who see such patients must have a high index of suspicion and be ready to seek advice. This chapter provides basic information. For full coverage, see *The Physi-*

cian's Guide to Diving Medicine (PGDM), Undersea and Hyperbaric Medical Society, 9650 Rockville Pike, Bethesda, MD 20814. The **Divers Alert Network (DAN),** coordinated by the Duke University Medical Center, Durham, NC, provides consultation at any hour **(919-684-8111).**

DEPTHS AND PRESSURES

Increased pressure at depth results from the weight of water, just as barometric pressure on land reflects the weight of the atmosphere above. Pressures in diving are often expressed in units of depth or atmospheres absolute (**atm abs; ATA**). A diver at 33 ft (10 m) in sea water is exposed to a pressure of 14.7 psi, 760 mm Hg, or one atmosphere (atm) greater than the barometric pressure at the surface. The **total pressure** at 33 ft, 2 atm abs, includes both the weight of the water and the barometric pressure at the surface. Every additional 33 ft of descent adds 1 atm of pressure. In a caisson or tunnel, compressed air is used to exclude water from the work site, and the interior pressure reflects the pressure of water outside.

Pathophysiologic Effects of Increased Pressure

Medical problems caused by exposure to increased pressure involve one or more of the following mechanisms:

1. Local differences in pressure ("squeeze"): When external pressure on the body increases with depth, the pressure of gas in the lungs and airways increases accordingly. If the eustachian tubes can be opened normally (eg, by swallowing or yawning), pressure in the middle ear can be kept equal to the increasing external pressure. If a structural anomaly, allergic or vasomotor rhinitis, or URI prevents such equalization, the excess external pressure is exerted directly on the eardrum. The external pressure is also fully transmitted to all blood vessels of the body, including those in the mucosa of the middle ear where, if the pressure remains lower than the external pressure, the capillaries may dilate, leak, and rupture. If edema fluid and extravasated blood do not occupy enough space to equalize the pressure, the eardrum may rupture. Middle ear infection often follows such injury (**barotitis media**—see also Ch. 66).

Barotrauma by the same mechanism may also occur in the paranasal sinuses. It is signaled by local pain or, in sphenoid sinus squeeze, by pain referred to the occiput, vertex, or frontal area. Mucosal congestion causing inability to equalize pressure in the ears or sinuses may respond to local or systemic decongestants, but persistent efforts to dive without free equalization of pressure will usually produce some injury.

Any rigid or semirigid airspace attached to the body can also become the site of local squeeze. Face masks are equalized by air from the nose, but goggles and some diving suits can cause discomfort, local hemorrhage, and tissue damage. Ear plugs form a closed space in the auditory canal and must *not* be used in diving.

2. Compression and expansion of gas: Boyle's Law indicates that the volume of a given mass of gas changes inversely with the absolute pressure; eg, 1 L of air at the surface (1 atm abs) is compressed to ½ L at 33 ft of depth (2 atm abs).

Equalization of pressure in body airspaces during descent must compensate for such compression. Compression of lung gas limits the safe depth of a "breath-hold" dive, but breathing from a diving helmet or scuba regulator compensates for compression of gas in the respiratory system.

Changes in pressure and gas volume in the middle ear can produce **vertigo** by at least 3 different mechanisms. (1) If the eardrum ruptures when a diver is bareheaded in cold water, the effect is like that of a **caloric test** (see in Ch. 64) and can produce severe and potentially disastrous vertigo, disorientation, nausea, and vomiting. (2) Unequalized pressure differences in the middle ear may affect the inner ear via the round window and produce **alternobaric vertigo,** a possible cause of the disequilibrium sometimes experienced by divers upon starting ascent. (3) **Perilymph fistula,** with leakage of perilymph through the round or oval window, is an uncommon but serious cause of vestibular disorder, and requires prompt surgical repair. It can be confused with inner-ear decompression sickness when it becomes evident following a dive.

Compression of gas at depth produces **increased gas density** proportional to the pressure in atm abs. Since a scuba diver normally breathes at about the same rate and tidal volume at depth as during comparable work at the surface, the number of gas molecules respired per minute at depth increases in proportion to the pressure. Thus at 2 atm abs it is twice that at the surface. Not only does the diver's air supply duration decrease proportionately, but breathing becomes increasingly difficult at greater depths because of the gas-flow limitations of the diver's airways and breathing apparatus. Respiratory limitation can accentuate overexertion, respiratory exhaustion, and general fatigue—potentially significant problems of diving even under ideal conditions.

Life-threatening complications can arise from the expansion of pulmonary gas on ascent. If a diver inspires even a single breath of air or other gas at depth and then fails to let it escape freely on ascent, the expanding gas may overinflate the lungs. Possible consequences include **pneumothorax, mediastinal and subcutaneous emphysema,** and **gas (air) embolism;** the latter is an extreme emergency and a leading cause of death among scuba divers (see below and TABLE 122–1).

3. Partial-pressure effects: The partial pressure of a gas is determined by the concentration of the gas and the ambient pressure, eg, the concentration of O_2 in air is about 21%, and the par-

TABLE 122–1. CONDITIONS REQUIRING RECOMPRESSION

	Decompression Sickness	Gas Embolism
Symptoms and signs	Extremely variable; three main types (singly or in combination): 1. Bends—pain, most often in or near a joint 2. Neurologic involvement of almost any type or degree 3. Chokes—respiratory distress followed by circulatory collapse *(extreme emergency)*	Common: unconsciousness, often with convulsion Less common: milder cerebral manifestations (mediastinal and subcutaneous emphysema and/or pneumothorax may also be present) *Assume that any unconscious diver has gas embolism and seek recompression promptly*
Onset and immediate course	Gradual or sudden onset during decompression or as long as 24 h after dives* deeper than 30 ft (or hyperbaric exposures beyond 2 atm abs) (Also possible in exposure to low pressure, as at altitude)	Sudden onset during or shortly after 1. Ascent, *even from a few feet of depth* 2. Decompression from any increased pressure 3. Any accident or procedure that could permit gas to enter circulation
Proximate cause	Usual: Diving or hyperbaric exposure beyond "no-stop limits" and without proper decompression stops Occasional: 1. Dive or pressure exposure within "no-stop limits" or with appropriate decompression stops 2. Low-pressure exposure, as in loss of cabin pressure in aircraft at altitude	Usual: Breath-holding or airway obstruction during ascent or reduction of pressure Other: Entry of free gas into cardiovascular system during heart surgery or other medical/surgical procedure
Mechanism	Excess dissolved gas forms bubbles in blood or tissue upon reduction of external pressure. Bubbles produce local mechanical effects or circulatory impairment	Usual: Overinflation of lungs causes entry of free gas into pulmonary vessels followed by embolization of the brain by bubbles Other: Pulmonary, cardiac, or systemic circulatory obstruction by free gas from any source
Immediate management	Essential emergency care (airway, hemostasis, CPR, etc) Prompt transport to nearest suitable chamber Horizontal position 100% O_2 by close-fitting mask Fluids orally if conscious, otherwise IV	

*Repetitive dives are frequently involved

tial pressure of O_2 in air at surface (1 atm abs) is about 0.21 atm. The concentration of O_2 in air remains the same at depth, but the partial pressure reflects the increasing pressure and compression of the gas. At 2 atm abs, the number of O_2 molecules per unit volume is twice what it is at the surface, and the partial pressure is double.

The physiologic effects of gases are related to their partial pressure and change according to depth. Toxic effects appear as the partial pressure of O_2 increases. **Pulmonary oxygen toxic-**ity can cause lung damage with extended exposure to a P_{O_2} above 0.6 atm (equivalent to 60% O_2 at surface or 30% O_2 at 33 ft). **Oxygen convulsions** may occur, especially in working dives, if the P_{O_2} approaches or exceeds 2 atm (eg, 100% O_2 at 33 ft or 50% O_2 at 99 ft).

Increased partial pressures of N_2 produce **nitrogen narcosis**, a condition resembling alcohol intoxication. In divers who breathe air, this effect becomes noticeable at 100 ft or less. It is generally incapacitating at about 10 atm abs (300 ft), where it produces an anesthetic effect resembling that of 30% nitrous oxide at sea level. (**Helium** lacks this anesthetic property and is used in place of N_2 as the diluent for O_2 in deep diving.)

Partial pressures of O_2 and CO_2 in alveolar gas are modified by the pressure of depth in **breath-hold diving** and in underwater swimming without breathing apparatus. The impulse to return to the surface and resume breathing depends largely upon CO_2 buildup in the body. A breath-holding diver may hyperventilate beforehand to extend time underwater; this blows off CO_2 but adds little to stores of O_2, and may then cause **unconsciousness from hypoxia** without warning before P_{CO_2} rises enough to become an effective stimulus.

Diving to a significant depth during the breath-hold complicates the situation by elevating the P_{O_2} and permitting extended O_2 uptake at depth. A diver who has "pushed the limits" under those circumstances may lose consciousness when alveolar P_{O_2} falls to a low level on ascent. This phenomenon is probably responsible for many unexplained drownings among spearfishing competitors and others who do extensive breath-hold diving. The term **shallow-water blackout** is sometimes applied, but it is best reserved for its original meaning: unconsciousness from CO_2 buildup in rebreathing types of scuba. (**Hypoxia** is also a potential problem in rebreathing units if O_2 is displaced by excess N_2.)

Carbon dioxide poisoning: In normal individuals on land, hyperpnea or breathlessness usually provides ample warning of increased CO_2 in inspired gas. Such a response may be more the exception than the rule under water, especially where high P_{O_2} and exertion are also factors. Some individuals develop spontaneous CO_2 **retention** through an inadequate increase in pulmonary ventilation during exertion. Whatever the source, abnormally high P_{CO_2} per se can cause **loss** or **impairment of consciousness** at depth and can also increase the likelihood of O_2 **convulsions** and augment the severity of **nitrogen narcosis**. The tendency to retain CO_2 may be suspected in divers who frequently experience post-dive headaches or pride themselves on low air-use rates.

Carbon monoxide (CO) poisoning from contaminated air can cause incapacitation or death in divers. It should be suspected in any diver who complains of nausea or headache or shows weakness, clumsiness, or mental changes. "Cherry-red" skin is not a reliable sign. Usual sources of CO in divers' air are a compressor intake too close to engine exhaust or "flashing" of lubricating oil in a malfunctioning compressor. Divers' air must be tested periodically for CO and other contaminants. (See also Ch. 128.)

Inert-gas uptake in the blood and tissues occurs whenever the partial pressure of gases such as N_2 is increased. When the pressure is subsequently reduced by ascent, bubbles may form with various consequences (see TABLE 122–1 and DECOMPRESSION SICKNESS, below).

4. Pressure per se: Certain neuromuscular and cerebral abnormalities comprise the **high pressure neurologic syndrome (HPNS)**, which is seen in deep diving and may appear at about 600 ft on descent. HPNS is attributed to hydrostatic pressure without reference to gas compression or partial pressures. It has no evident medical importance at shallower depths.

5. Complicating factors in diving include poor visibility, currents requiring excessive effort, and cold. **Hypothermia** can develop rapidly in water, and early effects may include crucial loss of judgment and dexterity. Cold water can trigger fatal **cardiac arrhythmias** in susceptible individuals. **Hypoglycemia** is a hazard in insulin-dependent diabetics and probably in those who indulge in alcohol while neglecting adequate food intake. **Drugs**, including medications as well as **alcohol** and other drugs of abuse, may have unanticipated effects at depth.

CONDITIONS REQUIRING RECOMPRESSION

GAS EMBOLISM
(Air Embolism)

A disorder resulting from overinflation of the lungs by expanding pulmonary gas during reduction of surrounding pressure (eg, ascent from depth in diving), generally characterized by early loss of consciousness and/or other CNS manifestations, and attributed to cerebral gas emboli originating in the lungs. (See TABLE 122–1.)

Etiology

Overinflation of the lungs is the usual cause of **arterial gas embolism**. This accident occurs most commonly because of breath-holding during ascent from a scuba dive. Running out of air at depth is a common precipitating event. Even swimming-pool depths are sufficient to cause gas embolism if the individual has access to any source of air or gas and takes even a single breath underwater. Gas inspired at any depth expands on ascent and, if not allowed to escape freely, overinflates the lungs and elevates alveolar pressure, resulting in escape of gas into pulmonary veins returning blood to the heart. If this gas reaches the carotid arteries, embolization of cerebral vessels is almost inevitable.

Symptoms, Signs, and Diagnosis

Prompt loss of consciousness, with or without convulsions or other cerebral manifestations, is a typical consequence of gas embolism. A diver who loses consciousness during or very shortly after ascent *must be assumed to have gas embolism and should be recompressed very promptly* (see RECOMPRESSION TREATMENT, below). Milder symptoms and signs, ranging from behavioral changes to hemiparesis, are sometimes seen.

Overinflation of the lungs also can produce mediastinal and subcutaneous emphysema, alone or with gas embolism. Pneumothorax is less frequent but more consequential. Hemoptysis or bloody froth suggests pulmonary injury. Iatrogenic arterial gas embolism is not unknown. For example, it may be suspected when a patient fails to regain consciousness after heart surgery.

Emergency Treatment

The patient must be transported to a suitable chamber for recompression without any delay for nonessential procedures. Transport by air may be justified if it will save a significant amount of time, but exposure to reduced pressure at altitude must be minimized. Authorities formerly recommended the Trendelenburg position when gas embolism was suspected. Lifesaving emergency measures take precedence where indicated (eg, attention to the airway, control of bleeding, CPR), but these, together with administration of a maximal concentration of O_2 and fluid therapy, can usually be carried out during transport. Recompression treatment is discussed below.

DECOMPRESSION SICKNESS
(Caisson Disease; The Bends)

A disorder resulting from reduction of surrounding pressure (as in ascent from a dive, exit from a caisson or hyperbaric chamber, or ascent to altitude), attributed to formation of bubbles from dissolved gas in blood or tissues, and usually characterized by pain and/or neurological manifestations. (See TABLE 122-1.)

Pathophysiology

A diver or compressed-air worker breathing air under increased ambient pressure takes up additional quantities of O_2 and N_2 in solution in the blood and tissues. O_2 is utilized continuously, but N_2 (or any other "inert" gas present) leaves the body only via the reverse of its entry through the lungs and circulation. Gradients of partial pressure govern uptake and elimination of the gas, but the degree of supersaturation (excess of blood or tissue gas pressure over ambient pressure) is crucial in determining whether significant bubble formation occurs in the body during or after ascent.

The consequences of bubble formation from dissolved gas are known as decompression sickness, caisson disease, or the bends (see TABLE 122-1). Although "the bends" refers strictly to painful manifestations, it is often used as a synonym for decompression sickness.

Consequential bubble formation can usually be avoided by (1) restricting the uptake of gas, as by limiting the depth and duration of dives to a range that does not require decompression stops on ascent: "no-decompression (no-stop) limits" or (2) using an air decompression table such as that in the *US Navy Diving Manual* (obtainable from the Superintendent of Documents, US Government Printing Office, Washington, DC 20402). The table provides a pattern of ascent that normally allows excess inert gas to escape harmlessly. Decompression sickness seldom occurs after dives within appropriate no-stop limits or when adequate decompression tables are followed; but the diver's account of depth, duration, and decompression procedure is not necessarily reliable. Many divers incorrectly believe that large "safety factors" are built into US Navy diving tables and do not follow them accurately. Newer no-stop limits, tables, and diver-carried decompression computers are claimed to have a greater margin of safety, but they can also be misused. Divers are urged to observe carefully the depths and times of no-stop limits, to ascend at the specified rate, and to make a safety stop of a few minutes around 15 ft (5 m).

Repetitive dives are a major source of difficulty. Some divers are unaware that an excess of inert gas remains in the body after every dive and increases with each subsequent exposure. If the interval between dives is < 12 h, special repetitive dive tables (eg, as provided by the *US Navy Diving Manual*) must be used.

Few decompression tables have been tested for adequacy in females or in older divers; such persons should use them with caution. Dives conducted at **altitude** and **flying after diving** require special procedures or precautions. Spending 24 h at the surface before going to altitude is usually recommended.

Symptoms and Signs

Local pain (the bends) is present in a large proportion of cases of decompression sickness, but it is often accompanied by neurologic abnormalities. In divers, pain is most commonly reported in or near an arm joint. In compressed-air workers, joints of the leg are more often affected. The pain is characteristically hard to describe and often poorly localized. "Deep" and "like something boring into the bone" are expressions sometimes used. Sharp, clearly localized pain is sometimes reported. At first, pain may be mild or intermittent, but it may increase steadily and can become very severe. Local inflammation and tenderness are often absent and the pain may not be affected by motion.

Neurologic manifestations may accompany pain or be present independently. They are much more common following dives with scuba than in "hard-hat" diving or caisson work. Currently, the proportion of neurologic problems reported among cases of decompression sickness exceeds 50%. The spinal cord is especially vulnerable, and many divers are unaware of the dire significance of seemingly minor manifestations such as weakness or numbness in the extremities.

Neurologic symptoms and signs are exceedingly variable. They range from mild paresthesia to major cerebral problems. Vestibular involvement may produce severe vertigo and may be difficult to differentiate from **perilymph fistula** (perilymph leakage through a torn round or oval window). Spinal cord lesions leading to paraplegia are a particular hazard, and delay in treatment may render the condition irreversible.

The condition known as **the chokes**, or **respiratory decompression sickness**, is rare in occurrence but grave in significance. It arises from massive bubble-embolization of the pulmonary vascular tree. Some cases resolve spontaneously, but rapid progression to circulatory collapse and death is not uncommon without prompt recompression. Substernal discomfort and coughing on deep inspiration or inhalation of tobacco smoke are often early manifestations of chokes. In animal studies, chokes are strongly associated with exposure to **altitude** soon after diving. Chokes and other serious manifestations appearing at altitude are not necessarily cured

by return to ground level and may require prompt chamber recompression.

Other manifestations of decompression sickness include **itching**, skin **rash**, and exceptional **fatigue**. These have not customarily been treated by recompression, but they are sometimes forerunners of much more serious problems. Divers complaining of them should at least be kept under observation. One hundred percent O_2 by mask may relieve such symptoms. **Cutaneous edema** is a rare occurrence and probably reflects obstruction of lymphatic channels by bubbles. It deserves recompression if progressive or persistent. **Mottling** ("marbling") of the skin is uncommon but may precede or accompany conditions that require recompression. **Abdominal pain** may reflect bubble formation at the site; but, especially in the form of **girdle pain**, it can be an important warning of spinal cord involvement.

Late effects of decompression sickness include **dysbaric osteonecrosis** (a form of *aseptic bone necrosis*). This is much more common in compressed-air workers than in divers, but divers are not immune. Prolonged or closely repeated exposures presumably entail the greatest risk. Lesions adjacent to articular surfaces are most common in the shoulder and hip and can cause great damage to the joint with chronic pain and severe disability. Bone necrosis is an insidious hazard because it becomes symptomatic or is detected by x-ray months or years after the responsible insult, which may be a single improper decompression.

Permanent neurologic defects, eg, **paraplegia,** are frequently attributable to delayed or inappropriate treatment of early signs of spinal cord involvement. In some instances, the initial damage may be too severe to remedy even with prompt and well-chosen treatment. However, repeated treatments with **hyperbaric oxygen** (see in Ch. 128) appear to assist in recovery. The prognosis is very much more favorable in spinal cord injury from decompression sickness than from other forms of cord trauma.

Emergency Treatment

Decompression sickness requires recompression. *Transport to a suitable recompression facility takes precedence over any procedure that can be conducted during transport or postponed without serious risk to life.* Transport should not be delayed even in cases that appear mild, since more serious manifestations may develop. O_2 in maximal concentration should be administered by close-fitting mask. Shock may develop, especially in severe cases with delayed treatment. Adequate fluid intake should be ensured and both intake and output recorded along with the vital signs.

RECOMPRESSION TREATMENT
(See also Ch. 128)

Recompression is imperative in both decompression sickness and gas embolism and should be accomplished as soon as possible to avoid serious and lasting injury. Its objective is to compress bubbles to asymptomatic size, redissolve them, and restore adequate O_2 to affected tissues. Regardless of the distance to a chamber or length of delay, it is likely to be beneficial. Unnecessary recompression involves far less risk than palliative treatment prescribed in the hope that the problem will subside without recompression.

Recompression in the water *must not* be attempted except in remote areas where specific arrangements for such treatment have been made. Divers themselves, and medical facilities and rescue and police units in popular diving areas, should know the location of the nearest suitable chamber, the means of reaching it rapidly, and the most appropriate source of consultation by telephone. In the absence of such local forethought, the Divers Alert Network (DAN) number (919-684-8111) is invaluable.

When a physician recommends recompression but cannot be sure that the patient will receive proper treatment in a suitable chamber, signed and witnessed acknowledgment of the recommendation should be obtained. What constitutes a "suitable" chamber is debatable. Many cases can be treated successfully in one-person hyperbaric chambers available in many areas; however, the need for hands-on access to the patient or for greater pressure capability often cannot be foreseen and may be vital.

The need for recompression is established by the fact that the individual has been exposed to increased pressure and has symptoms or signs suggestive of decompression sickness or gas embolism. Details of the history, physical examination, and laboratory findings usually add little of value. Sometimes, a conclusive diagnosis cannot be made without a trial of recompression. At some point, at least before leaving maximum treatment pressure, a careful neurologic examination is important to identify any defect that might require modifying the course of treatment.

Failure to provide prompt and appropriate treatment of decompression sickness or gas embolism entails totally unacceptable risk of serious and lasting injury.

Tables for treatment and guidelines for their selection and use are found in the *US Navy Diving Manual* and the *PGDM* (see above). The main difference in treatment between gas embolism and decompression sickness is that tables specifically designed for the former include an excursion to 6 atm abs with the aim of rapid compression of cerebral bubbles. Otherwise, treatment of both conditions normally relies upon breathing O_2 at pressures < 3 atm abs.

The US Navy treatment tables achieve a high percentage of success in cases of decompression sickness that follow ordinary diving with air as the breathing medium. Dives involving unusual gas mixtures or extraordinary depths or durations may require special therapeutic procedures.

Medical adjuncts to recompression: Patients will sometimes need medical or surgical procedures in addition to recompression. If it is impossible to provide both simultaneously, recompression takes precedence over any measure that can be postponed without serious risk to life. Intensive care, when required, can be provided in a well-equipped chamber.

Adequate fluid intake with monitoring is important. If IV fluids are required, 0.9% sodium chloride is generally preferred. The possibility of bladder paralysis and need for catheterization should be kept in mind. Periodic measurement of Hct is desirable, and measurement of central venous pressure and circulating blood volume may be necessary in severely ill patients.

Corticosteroids (eg, dexamethasone sodium phosphate 20 to 40 mg IV, then 4 mg IM q 6 h) may be useful in curbing inflammation from decompression sickness and in controlling CNS edema. Additional measures for reducing brain/cord swelling are indicated when CNS manifestations are present, especially if the response to recompression is inadequate or delayed.

Sedatives and narcotics may obscure symptoms and cause respiratory insufficiency. They should be avoided before and during treatment or used in minimum effective dosage when urgently needed.

EVALUATION OF FITNESS FOR DIVING

Although asked to judge the fitness of individuals for diving or related pursuits, physicians usually cannot bar anyone from diving and function largely as advisors. It is advisable not only to explain unwelcome findings and their implications but to make them a matter of record with signed acknowledgment by the individual concerned.

Physical and psychologic fitness for diving is discussed in detail in the *PGDM* (see above), but uniform standards have not been established. A few self-evident considerations can be cited:

1. Divers must be able to take care of themselves over a wide range of conditions. Diving can involve unusually **heavy exertion**, even for individuals who do not plan to participate in any arduous underwater activities. Air cylinders are heavy, currents can necessitate strenuous swimming, etc. Divers should be free of any significant cardiac or pulmonary disease and possess normal to superior **aerobic capacity**. Gross **obesity** is often associated with poor exercise tolerance and increased susceptibility to decompression sickness. **Physical handicaps** must be assessed in terms of the individual's ability to aid a "diving buddy" as well as to function as a diver with minimal assistance himself.

Rigid **age limits** are inappropriate, but older aspirants deserve special scrutiny, especially in **cardiopulmonary fitness.** Family history and coronary risk factors should be considered. Certain **cardiac arrhythmias**, including some that are acceptable in other sports, should rule out diving even in younger people. **Patent foramen ovale** allows bubbles to escape filtration in the lungs and may explain cases of cerebral decompression sickness or apparent gas embolism. It must be ruled out before the individual dives again. A history of serious injury to an extremity or of peripheral vascular disease suggests increased susceptibility to musculoskeletal decompression sickness (the bends).

2. Divers must be able to equalize pressure uneventfully in all body air spaces. Pulmonary conditions that involve air trapping may cause gas embolism on ascent. *Absolute contraindications* include lung cysts, asthma, emphysema, and a history of pneumothorax. Chronic nasal congestion, perforated eardrum, and certain otologic operations are *contraindications*. Diving should be avoided during respiratory infections and exacerbations of vasomotor or allergic rhinitis. Habitual air-swallowing and a tendency toward regurgitation have unfavorable implications.

3. Divers must not be subject to impairment of consciousness, alertness, or judgment. Such lapses, even if momentary, can lead to underwater mishaps endangering the diver and companions. Epilepsy, syncope, insulin-dependent diabetes, and alcohol or drug abuse are incompatible with diving. Medications that cause drowsiness or reduce alertness are undesirable and may potentiate N_2 narcosis. Lack of emotional stability is perilous for a diver and associates. It is suspected when motivation seems inappropriate or when the history suggests accident-proneness or impulsive behavior.

Women have taken up scuba diving in large and increasing numbers, and present knowledge suggests that, with few possible exceptions, fit and healthy women can dive as safely as men. Some studies have suggested that women are more susceptible to decompression sickness and should be even more conservative about **decompression** than men. Another exception concerns **pregnancy,** with the likelihood that diving increases the incidence of birth defects and fetal death. Safe limits of exposure cannot be specified with confidence, so diving is best avoided by women who are, or may be, pregnant.

Evaluation of professional divers and others at unusual risk warrants special procedures including pulmonary function testing, stress electrocardiography, audiometry, and bone x-rays.

Adequate diver training is an absolute necessity for safe diving, and the physician should emphasize its importance. Courses under the auspices of national organizations are widely available.

123.   HIGH—ALTITUDE ILLNESS

(Acute Mountain Sickness [AMS]; High-Altitude Pulmonary Edema [HAPE]; High-Altitude Cerebral Edema [HACE]; Soroche; Puna; Mareo)

Syndromes due to decreased O_2 at high altitudes.

Etiology, Pathology, and Pathophysiology

Atmospheric pressure decreases as altitude increases, but the percentage of O_2 in air remains constant; thus, the partial pressure of O_2 decreases with altitude and at 18,000 ft (5500 m) is about $1/2$ that at sea level. About 20% of persons ascending above 9000 ft (2700 m) in < 1 day will develop symptoms and signs of altitude illness in which the dominant form may vary. Persons who have had one attack are slightly more susceptible to another under similar conditions, but there is great variation between and even within individuals. Children under 6 yr and women premenstrually may be especially vulnerable. Very rapid ascent (as in unpressurized aircraft, balloons, or a decompression chamber) causes a different form of hypoxic illness.

Hypoxia stimulates breathing, which increases tissue oxygenation but also causes respiratory alkalosis, which contributes to the symptomatology until it is partially compensated by loss of HCO_3 in urine. Hypoxia may impair the O_2-dependent "sodium pump," resulting in the accumulation of Na and water within, and the movement of K out of cells; it is thought that the resultant swelling of cells is the basic pathophysiology of altitude illnesses. ADH secretion is increased by hypoxia in some individuals, causing further water retention. The roles of atrio-natriuretic peptide (ANP), aldosterone, and renin-angiotensin remain unclear.

No specific pathology has been demonstrated in AMS. Hypoxia from any cause increases pulmonary vascular resistance and pulmonary artery pressure; systemic resistance and arterial pressure are little changed. Cerebral blood flow is decreased by hypercapnia and increased by hypoxia; consequently, it varies with the balance between arterial CO_2 and O_2. Its role in symptomatology is unclear. In HACE, the CSF pressure may be elevated, but the fluid is normal. CT brain scans of patients with HAPE and HACE often show diffuse cerebral edema, and edema and hemorrhages are found on autopsy. In HAPE, interstitial edema precedes frank alveolar edema. The fluid resembles plasma, and HAPE is considered to be a high-pressure edema with increased microvascular permeability. Platelet and fibrin emboli and venous thromboses often occur in cerebral, pulmonary, and peripheral vessels. Stretching of distended pulmonary arterioles releases biologically active substances (arachidonic acids, prostaglandins, thromboxanes), which may cause the distended capillaries to leak, causing blood-stained, sometimes grossly bloody sputum. Discrepancy between perfusion and ventilation in portions of the lung is considered the most likely pathophysiology in HAPE. Endocrine glands are normal, though their function is often altered. Liver, kidneys, and heart are normal, and passive congestion is not seen.

Symptoms, Signs, and Diagnosis

The various forms of altitude illness are not separate entities but a continuum in which now one, now another may dominate. **Acute mountain sickness (AMS)** is the most common and may appear at altitudes as low as 6500 ft (2000 m). It is characterized by headache, fatigue, nausea, dyspnea, sleep disturbance, and rapid, forceful heartbeat. Exertion aggravates the symptoms. Unless dehydration is severe or hyperventilation is excessive, AMS usually subsides within a few days. Laboratory studies are nonspecific and rarely required for diagnosis.

High-altitude pulmonary edema (HAPE) is less common but more serious, usually developing 24 to 96 h after rapid ascent above 9000 ft (2700 m). Long time high-altitude residents, returning after a brief stay at low altitude appear to be at a slightly greater risk, as are children. HAPE is characterized by increasing dyspnea; irritative cough that becomes productive of frothy, often bloody sputum; weakness; ataxia; and later coma. Cyanosis, tachycardia, and low-grade fever are common, and together with fine and coarse rales (often audible without a stethoscope) may lead to a misdiagnosis of pneumonia. Even a minor respiratory infection appears to increase the risk of HAPE. Chest x-ray shows Kerley lines and patchy edema quite unlike that seen in heart failure. Atrial pressure is normal, but pulmonary artery pressure is even greater than that found in normal subjects during hypoxia. HAPE may worsen rapidly, and coma and death may occur within hours.

The absence of one pulmonary artery is a rare congenital anomaly that greatly increases the risk of HAPE, even as low as 5000 ft (1500 m), probably because of the resulting mismatch between perfusion and ventilation. Persons who develop HAPE repeatedly or at unusually low altitude should be studied for unsuspected pulmonary artery pathology.

High-altitude cerebral edema (HACE) is believed present to some degree in all forms of altitude illness. The severe form presents with ataxia, headache, mental confusion, and hallucinations. Coma and death may develop within a few hours of the first symptoms; gait ataxia is a reliable early warning sign. Stiff neck is not seen and papilledema is not necessary for diagnosis. HACE must be differentiated from other causes of coma (eg, infection, vascular accident, ketoacidosis) by history, absence of significant fever or paralysis, and by normal blood and CSF studies.

Retinal hemorrhages appear as low as 9000 ft (2700 m) in severe cases; they are common above 16,000 ft (5000 m). They are usually asymptomatic unless in the macular region and clear rapidly without sequelae. Cotton-wool spots occur rarely. Splinter hemorrhages beneath nail beds are often seen above 16,000 ft (5000 m), but nosebleed is rare.

Peripheral or facial edema may be due to altitude or to strenuous exertion. **Thrombophlebitis** may occur at extreme altitude, especially with dehydration and inactivity. **Transient dimmed vision** or even **total blindness** is a rare complication at very high altitude.

Prophylaxis

Altitude illness is best prevented by slow ascent, taking 2 days from sea level to 8000 ft (2500 m) and 1 day for every 2000 ft (600 m) above this. Physical fitness and climbing experience, though they enable greater exertion for less O_2 consumption, do not protect against any form of altitude illness. Strenuous effort should be avoided for several days, but bed rest is less beneficial than mild exercise. Because of great individual variation, those going to altitude should learn how fast they can ascend without symptoms; a climbing party should be paced at the rate of its slowest member.

Water loss is greatly increased by overbreathing the dry air at altitude, and dehydration with some degree of hypovolemia aggravates symptoms. Drinking much more water than usual is important, but additional salt should be avoided. Alcohol seems to worsen AMS. Frequent small meals, high in easily digested carbohydrates (fruits, jams, starches), improve altitude tolerance and are recommended for the first few days.

Acetazolamide is an effective prophylactic for AMS. Recent work suggests that 50 to 125 mg orally q 8 h is protective without causing diuresis. It is administered on the day ascent is started and for 2 days after reaching altitude; sustained-release capsules (500 mg) are also available. Acetazolamide inhibits carbonic anhydrase and allows increased ventilation and better O_2 transport with less alkalosis; it halts **periodic breathing** (almost universal during sleep at altitude), thus preventing sharp falls in blood O_2. Low-flow O_2 during sleep accomplishes the same but is inconvenient. Analogs of acetazolamide offer no advantage. Aspirin may relieve headache and possibly decrease the risk of HAPE by preventing platelet emboli. Prochlorperazine 10 mg orally q 6 h, a popular preventive in Europe, has not been widely used in the USA. Antacids are worthless. Dexamethasone 4 mg orally q 6 h minimizes symptoms of AMS, perhaps by the eupho-

ria it causes, but is not recommended for prevention because of side effects. Pentoxifylline is used in some countries to improve cerebral function at altitude.

Acclimatization: Persons exposed to altitude gradually develop an integrated series of responses that restore tissue oxygenation toward normal. Full acclimatization takes more time the higher the altitude, and above 18,000 ft (5500 m) deterioration is more rapid and there are no permanent residents. **Major features of acclimatization** include sustained hyperventilation with persistent partially compensated alkalosis, normal or low cardiac output, increased RBC mass, and increased tolerance for anaerobic work. After many generations at altitude, different populations have acquired slightly different strategies of acclimatization. Acetazolamide 125 mg bid is widely used to enhance acclimatization but controlled studies are lacking; abrupt cessation has led to HAPE and HACE.

Treatment

AMS seldom requires treatment other than fluid, analgesics, light diet, mild activity, and (rarely) descent. Acetazolamide 250 mg orally q 4 h is helpful in AMS and HAPE. When **HAPE** is suspected, bed rest and O_2 may be tried, but if the condition worsens, *immediate descent is essential.* Although morphine is effective, respiratory depression may outweigh its value. Digitalis, phlebotomy, and limb tourniquets are of no value since heart failure is not at fault. Furosemide (20 to 40 mg orally q 2 h or 20 mg slowly IV) has been effective. (CAUTION: *Brisk diuresis may cause hypovolemic shock, since the patient is often already dehydrated; oral fluid replacement is essential.*) In hospital, treatment is based on ruling out other causes of pulmonary disease; adequate oxygenation, perhaps by intubation and positive end-expiratory pressure (PEEP); bed rest; judicious diuresis; postural drainage; and antibiotics, if superimposed infection is suspected. Placing the victim in a large bag in which the pressure is then increased, thus simulating descent, has proved as effective as supplementary O_2. Nifedipine lowers pulmonary artery pressure and improves HAPE; it may cause hypotension and at present its value is debated; sustained-release capsules are available. When promptly treated, recovery from HAPE is usual within 24 to 48 h. Persons who experience one episode of HAPE are likely to have another and should be warned. Dexamethasone 8 mg IV q 4 h is used to treat **severe HACE,** though its effect is not dramatic. **Retinal hemorrhages** require no treatment, generally resolving during stay at altitude.

A syndrome called **subacute chronic mountain sickness** has been described in troops stationed for several weeks at 21,000 ft; it is due to right-sided heart failure and improves slowly with descent and appropriate treatment.

Chronic mountain sickness (CMS or Monge's disease) is an uncommon condition that affects longtime altitude residents; it is characterized by fatigue, dyspnea, aches and pains, excessive polycythemia, and thromboembolism. CMS resembles **alveolar hypoventilation** (formerly called pickwickian syndrome) and both are thought caused by an inadequately sensitive respiratory center. The victim should descend to sea level; recovery is slow, and return to altitude may cause recurrence. Repeated phlebotomy has been helpful but is not the most desirable management. Intermittent upper airway obstruction, sleep apnea, or chronic snoring at sea level may mimic CMS.

§10. SPECIAL SUBJECTS

124. GERIATRIC MEDICINE

Geriatric medicine (geriatrics) is an interdisciplinary approach to management of sickness and disability in the elderly. Gerontology studies the changes of normal aging as distinguished from disease effects. Most age-related biologic functions peak before age 30; some show subsequent gradual linear decline, have no practical implications for daily activity, but can become critical in periods of great stress. Thus, disease, rather than normal aging, is the prime determinant of functional loss in old age. Physiologic processes that decline with age include renal blood flow and creatinine clearance, maximum heart rate and thus cardiac output with exercise, glucose tolerance, vital capacity of the lung, lean body mass, and cellular immunity. But many liver functions and total lung capacity remain the same across the age spectrum, and secretion of ADH in response to osmolar stimuli actually increases with age.

Many of the decrements previously reported as due to aging are attributable to life-style, behavioral, dietary, and environmental influences that are modifiable; eg, in healthy but previously sedentary older people, declines in V_{O_2MAX}, muscle strength, and glucose tolerance can be partially reversed by aerobic exercise. The effects of pure aging may be far less dramatic than previously thought, and healthier, more vigorous aging may be accessible for many individuals.

Studies on aging are difficult because, as people age, healthy subjects become harder to find. Cross-sectional studies, which compare individuals of different ages, are relatively easy to do but may be less useful than longitudinal studies, in which long-term monitoring compares the same persons to their younger selves. Such studies are difficult because of the time factor and drop-out rate.

Caring for an elderly person with multiple interacting diseases—and often difficult socioeconomic circumstances—demands high diagnostic, analytic, synthetic, and interpersonal skills of the physician. Often the physician's familiarity with patient behavior, history, satisfaction, fears, and aspirations underlies early recognition of disease and interventions that may involve life-style adjustments. Knowing the patient through a thorough life history and mental status test is very important. First signs of physical illness, often reversible, commonly are mental or emotional, tending to confirm the stereotype of "senility" and deterring proper diagnosis and treatment if casually accepted.

DEMOGRAPHY AND HEALTH CARE DELIVERY

Americans > 65 yr were, at the turn of the century, 4% of the population; currently, they are $> 12\%$ (32 million, with a net gain of $> 1000/$ day). It is estimated that in 2030, when the large cohort of post–World War II baby boomers will reach age 80, there will be > 70 million Americans (1:5) over age 65, and the "over 85s" are expected to experience the highest percentage increase of all.

More recent cohorts of elderly persons are reaching age 65 in better health than their predecessors. Old age, in its conventional but erroneous image as "severe debilitation after age 65," is more aptly applied to the post-80 or -85 population (the old-old population), which is mostly female because women outlive men. Maximum human life span (currently estimated at 110 to 120 yr) has increased modestly compared with the major increase in average life expectancy during this century. Although the elderly are an increasingly healthy and active group, many problems emerge, especially after age 75. Burdens of multiple diseases are complicated by social disadvantage, emotional vulnerability, and poverty (as individuals outlive their resources and supportive age peers).

Today a 65-yr-old man has a 13-yr life expectancy; if he lives to 75, he has 9 more years ahead of him. A 65-yr-old woman will live > 18 yr on the average, and at age 75 she can expect to live 12 more years. Overall, women live about 8 yr longer than men, probably the result of genetic, biologic, and environmental factors. Survival differences have not narrowed, despite women smoking more and moving into traditionally male job markets, and women will probably always outlive men.

Caring for increasing numbers of old and infirm citizens makes extraordinary demands on traditional health care systems; the strains increase disproportionately, since the elderly, having more illness and complicating psychosocial sequelae, use more medical and social supportive services. Though only 12% of our population, the elderly account for > 40% of our acute hospital bed days, buy > 30% of all prescription (and 40% of over-the-counter) drugs, and spend 30% of our > 600 billion dollar health budget (> 50% of the federal health budget). Nursing home care cost $21 billion in 1980 and an estimated $50 billion in 1990. As early as 1972, nursing home beds began to outnumber acute hospital beds. Of the 1.5 million nursing home beds in America, 90% are occupied by people > 65 yr, yet < 5% of Americans > 65 yr live in nursing homes or other institutions.

Other ways of looking at the same data give a different perspective. Among the "over 65s," 40% will spend time in a nursing home before death, and of those surviving beyond age 80, > 50% will die there. Nursing home beds in America outnumber acute hospital beds, but twice as many dependent elderly live in the community as in nursing homes, and 25% of the community-dwelling elderly have no living relatives. A segment of our > 65 population is institutionalized or at high risk for institutionalization (especially in the absence of community services). These approximately 6 million older Americans consume a disproportionate share of health resources. Special attention to their health care needs could add quality and years to their lives while restraining cost increases.

Studies done in the early 1950s in Scotland examined the response of older people to illness; they illustrate *qualitatively* different health care demands. Each patient had a doctor responsible for continuing outpatient care, the doctor's office was conveniently located, and care was free to the patient. Although this system appeared adequate, startling numbers of people were identified with multiple medical problems that were *unknown to the responsible physician*. The problems unearthed by screening with history, physical examination, and simple laboratory tests were not esoteric. Common treatable conditions, such as B_{12}- or iron-deficiency anemia, heart failure, GI bleeding, uncontrolled diabetes mellitus, active TB, foot disease interfering with mobility, oral disorders interfering with eating, correctable hearing and vision defects, and a high incidence of dementia and depression, often go undiagnosed in the elderly. Important characteristics of disease in old age include the following:

1. Elderly patients tend to conceal legitimate complaints pointing to serious treatable diseases. Many elderly, as well as young people, believe that old age is a time of sickness and disability, and that not feeling well is a natural part of aging. Elderly persons with symptoms tend to report them only to family members, who at least half the time do not pursue the symptoms further. The prevalence of depression, combined with the cumulative losses of old age and the discomfort of illness, reduces interest in regaining health. Impaired cognition impedes the patient's complaining and reduces the physician's diagnostic searching. Today's old people grew up when hospitals were places for dying, and are reluctant to seek care.

2. The phenomenon of multiple disorders in the elderly complicates diagnosis and treatment. In one study, an average of 6 diseases was found among several thousand older people, and the primary physician was unaware of half of the diagnoses. Disease in one organ system stresses another weakened system that can begin a concatenation of deteriorations, passing multiple points of no return, leading to infirmity, dependence, and, if uninterrupted, death. Active case-finding surveillance mechanisms for the aging must be added to our current passive health care system. Alert early intervention may prevent compounding and improve the quality of life through relatively minor maneuvers.

3. Disorders often present atypically (see DISORDERS WITH UNUSUAL PRESENTATIONS IN THE ELDERLY, below).

4. "Predeath," *a period of dependency due to immobility, incontinence, or impaired cognition* (frequently in combination), precedes nearly 3/4 of deaths in old age. This period, often spent in hospitals or nursing homes, is strongly age-related and approaches 3 mo in the group > 85 yr. The cost, in human suffering and in money, is substantial. Immobility, incontinence, and cognitive impairment are clarions of serious underlying disease that demand prompt evaluation and specific treatment to avoid prolonged dependency.

BASIC PRINCIPLES IN CARING FOR THE ELDERLY

Predictable hazards for aged hospitalized patients include (1) nighttime confusion or "sundowning," (2) falls, (3) fractures with no identifiable trauma, (4) sudden appearance of decubiti, (5) fecal impaction and urinary retention, (6) falling victim to diagnostic and therapeutic endeavors, (7) prolonged convalescence, and (8) loss of home while hospitalized.

There is a special need to identify. multiple concomitant pathologic processes. Treating one disorder without treating associated ones may accelerate decline. Common conditions coexist in the elderly (eg, anemia, heart failure, angina pectoris, venous and arterial insufficiency in the legs, diabetes mellitus, osteoporosis, osteoarthritis, frail gait, chronic constipation, chronic renal failure, urinary precipitancy, chronic pain, sleep disturbance, depression, cognitive impairment, and multiple drug regimens with poor compliance—see Compliance, below). When multiple problems coincide, bed rest, surgery, drugs, and other treatments may be disastrous if not well integrated and scrupulously monitored.

Disorders in old age can be divided into 2 broad groups—those seen commonly *only* in the elderly and those that also occur in other age groups but present *with unusual features* or *without usual features* in the elderly.

DISORDERS COMMON ONLY IN THE ELDERLY

Problems usually restricted to the elderly include normal pressure hydrocephalus, accidental hypothermia, and urinary incontinence (these are discussed below). Other disorders common only in the elderly are diabetic hyperosmolar nonketotic coma; stroke; polymyalgia rheumatica—giant cell arteritis; decubitus ulcers; metabolic bone disease; degenerative osteoarthritis; hip fracture and its rehabilitation; dementia; falling; prostatic carcinoma; monoclonal gammopathies; chronic lymphatic leukemia; angioimmunoblastic lymphadenopathy with dysproteinemia (lymphoma); TB (especially miliary); herpes zoster; basal cell carcinoma; and parkinsonism. Separate discussions elsewhere in THE MANUAL are listed in the index.

NORMAL PRESSURE HYDROCEPHALUS (NPH)

Cerebral ventricular dilation with normal lumbar CSF pressure, presenting with a characteristic clinical syndrome of dementia, apraxia of gait, and urinary incontinence. Previously considered common, NPH is a rare cause of dementia in the elderly. Etiology may be attributed to previous surface inflammation of the brain, usually from subarachnoid hemorrhage or diffuse meningitis, presumed to result in scarring of the arachnoid villi over the brain convexities where CSF absorption usually occurs. Supporting data are meager, however, and many elderly NPH patients have no history of predisposing disease.

Clinical Manifestations

The syndrome classically consists of dementia, incontinence, and apraxia of gait, associated with ventricular dilation and normal CSF pressure (recent studies suggest a highly variable picture, but gait disorder is usually most prominent). Typically, there is neither motor weakness nor staggering, but rather what has been described as the "slipping clutch" phenomenon in which initiation of gait is hesitant, but eventually walking occurs. Many patients with a variety of other gaits have been described. NPH has also been described in association with various psychiatric manifestations that are not distinctive, and it should be considered in the differential diagnosis of any new psychiatric illness in old age.

Treatment

Shunting CSF from the dilated ventricles sometimes results in clinical improvement, but the longer the disease has been present, the less likely shunting will be curative. Radiographic or pressure measurements do not predict response to shunting.

ACCIDENTAL HYPOTHERMIA (AH)
(Hypothermia)
(See also Ch. 116)

Unexpected fall of body temperature to $< 35°$ C (95° F). AH in the elderly, as a common winter event, was noted 25 yr ago in Britain. The afflicted are at high risk for a potentially fatal clinical syndrome mimicking stroke or metabolic derangement. Studies suggest that thousands of elderly people die each year in Great Britain from AH, but one American study could not find lowered temperature among high-risk community-dwelling elders in Maine during the winter. The wide range of estimates can be explained by the lack of definitive pathologic evidence of hypothermia death. Stated simply, most dead people are cold; therefore, death cannot confidently be attributed to AH postmortem. Temperatures of elderly patients entering hospitals in Britain during winter months were accurately recorded using a low-reading thermometer, disclosing that $> 3.5\%$ of patients > 65 yr had body temperatures $< 35°$ C. Lack of central heating or indoor plumbing was not a risk factor for these patients. If these data are extrapolated, nearly 50,000 elderly Americans may be entering hospitals each winter with occult hypothermia.

Etiology and Pathogenesis

Elderly people with borderline low temperatures have age-related autonomic defects producing low peripheral resting blood flow, a nonconstrictor vasomotor response to cold, and easily provoked orthostatic hypotension. These defects are exacerbated by phenothiazines, especially chlorpromazine, and correlate with hypothermia risk.

The provocative cold stress does not have to be prolonged exposure to severe cold; rather, these aged patients may become hypothermic while in their mildly cool homes (as warm as 18.3° C [65° F]), though most episodes are initiated by temperatures < 18.3° C. Besides inadequate environmental heating in the winter, contributory factors include diminished perception of cold and poor heat conservation mechanisms. AH takes many hours to several days to develop. Body temperature, once falling below 35° C, continues to fall slowly and insidiously, terminating in death if the environment is unaltered. The overall mortality rate is about 50%, but survival is largely determined by the presence and severity of complicating disease.

Predisposing factors include a variety of drugs (eg, neuroleptics, sedatives and hypnotics, tranquilizers, alcohol), heart failure, hypothyroidism, hypopituitarism, uremia, Addison's disease, starvation, ketoacidosis, pulmonary infection, sepsis, brain injury, and any immobilizing illness.

Symptoms and Signs

As body temperature drops, the patient proceeds from fatigue, weakness, incoordination, apathy, and drowsiness to an acute confusional state that, when body temperature falls below 32.2° C (90° F), progresses to stupor and coma. Hallucinations, combativeness, and resistance to aid may be seen. While hands and feet of many people are cold to the touch in winter, these patients also have cold abdomens. Shivering and pallor are strikingly absent, respirations are shallow and infrequent, slow pulse and low BP with a host of atrial and ventricular arrhythmias are common, and the face may be puffy and pink. The ECG may show a **characteristic J wave** early—a small positive deflection following the QRS complex in the left ventricular leads—which is found in no other condition. Unfortunately, it only appears in slightly < 50% of hypothermic patients. More commonly, the ECG shows base-line oscillation produced by a **fine rapid muscle tremor** that is often mistaken for electrical interference or voluntary motion. This fine trembling is usually not grossly apparent but probably is the elderly hypothermic patient's physiologic equivalent of shivering. Neurologic signs of tremor, ataxia, pathologic and depressed reflexes, coma, seizures, and a marked increase in muscle tone may all occur. If temperature fall is uninterrupted, death usually occurs between 29.4 and 23.9° C (85 and 75° F) from cardiac standstill or ventricular fibrillation.

General metabolic effects of hypoxia and tissue necrosis are the rule; though, if the patient survives, low temperature may delay the onset of many complications (most commonly pancreatitis, pulmonary edema, pneumonia, metabolic acidosis, renal failure, and gangrene of the extremities).

Diagnosis

Knowledge of AH, a high index of suspicion, and a low-reading thermometer are required. The standard clinical thermometer reads from 34.4 to 42.2° C (94 to 108° F) and is rarely shaken down below 35.6° C (96° F). A low-reading thermometer, registering 28.9 to 42.2° C (84 to 108° F), is available (see Symptoms, Signs, and Diagnosis in Ch. 116). Health personnel caring for the elderly must be oriented to look for low body temperature, since the usual custom is to document only normal or elevated temperatures when evaluating a patient.

Treatment

Slow spontaneous rewarming, which allows body temperature to return to normal gradually (not faster than 0.6° C [1° F]/h) by conserving heat still being produced by the hypothermic patient, is recommended. *More rapid rewarming has often resulted in irreversible hypotension.* Heat conservation is achieved with blankets or more sophisticated insulating materials in a warm room. Careful monitoring and anticipation of common complications are essential to successful treatment (see also Treatment in Ch. 116).

URINARY INCONTINENCE

The involuntary loss of urine while awake or asleep is a malodorous social stigma, commonly concealed by its embarrassed victim with a mountain of absorbent pads. An estimated 10 million Americans are incontinent, at a cost of $10 billion/yr. The prevalence ranges from 10 to 30% in people > 65 yr at home, reaches 50% in those hospitalized, and is even higher in the chronically institutionalized elderly. As much as 25% of nursing time in geriatric hospitals is consumed dealing with incontinence. Such patients require a 200% increase in allotted nursing time to deal with linens and pads and nearly 600% more time to be bathed satisfactorily, compared with the nursing required by continent peers.

The causes of urinary incontinence may be transient or established. More than ⅔ of patients can be cured or significantly improved by treatment.

DISORDERS WITH UNUSUAL PRESENTATIONS IN THE ELDERLY

The characteristic symptoms and signs of many disorders are frequently absent in old age and are often replaced with one or more nonspecific manifestations, such as refusal to eat or drink, falling, incontinence, dizziness, acute confusion, increasing dementia, weight loss, and failure to thrive. Depression is the most common affective disorder in the "over 65" population, but is no more common than in younger persons. Organic psychoses, other affective disorders, paranoid states, hypochondriasis, and suicide (eg, stopping eating, drinking, or essential medications) become more common with age; all may present atypically.

Diseases that are especially likely to be diagnostic enigmas in the elderly are drug intoxication, alcoholism, myxedema, myocardial infarction, pulmonary embolism, pneumonia, malignant disease (especially of colon, lung, and breast), acute abdomen, and thyrotoxicosis, which is discussed illustratively below.

OCCULT HYPERTHYROIDISM

Apathetic and masked hyperthyroidism are 2 variant thyrotoxic syndromes lacking the readily recognizable usual symptoms and signs. Although > 50% of thyrotoxic patients are aged 40 to 60 yr, 15% are > 65 yr. Occult hyperthyroidism is found in 1 to 2% of newly hospitalized patients > 65 yr in Great Britain. Forty percent of these patients show no goiter, and > 50% show no eye signs or tachycardia. The classic constellation of diffuse goiter, eye signs, and thyroid bruit occurs in only 20% of older thyrotoxic patients. One explanation of the paucity of classic findings in the elderly is that their diminished physiologic reserve is depleted quickly by hypermetabolic stress. T_3 toxicosis is uncommon in the elderly.

Symptoms and Signs

Masked hyperthyroidism is the more common of the 2 syndromes (65 to 70%). The usual features of multisystem involvement in thyrotoxicosis are absent, and symptoms and signs referable to a single organ system, most often the heart, dominate the clinical picture. Heart failure poorly responsive to digitalis, atrial fibrillation with slow ventricular response, other fixed or paroxysmal arrhythmias, cardiomegaly, and palpitations are common. GI involvement can include constipation, weight loss with anorexia, and hepatomegaly. Psychiatric manifestations include confusion, psychomotor retardation, chronic depression, and apparent "senile" dementia. Increased bone calcium turnover is reflected in elevated serum calcium, bone pain, osteoporosis, and frequent fracture.

Apathetic hyperthyroidism occurs in 10 to 15% of aged thyrotoxics. Apathy and inactivity replace the usual hyperkinesis and dominate the clinical picture even though there may be associated cardiac or other organ system findings. These patients look extremely old and wizened, but with treatment rapidly lose wrinkling and become more youthful-looking. They have been described as having a "characteristic senile appearance" of mild chronic illness, but when afflicted with an acute illness or stress, they "quietly and peacefully sink into coma and die an absolutely relaxed death without activation."

Laboratory values are generally the same for older and younger adults, but T_3 levels decline 10 to 20% in euthyroid elderly. **Treatment** is usually effective with radioactive iodine, but up to 50% of the patients need temporary prior and subsequent pharmacologic thyroid suppression.

DRUG THERAPY IN THE ELDERLY

Elderly patients, in or out of the hospital, are more than twice as susceptible to adverse drug reactions as younger patients. These reactions are likely to be more serious and extend hospitalization longer than for a younger patient. Old people at home take nearly 3 times as many drugs as the general population, with women taking twice as many as men. The average older person receives 18 prescriptions annually and spends 20% of "disposable income" on drugs. When the prevalence of intellectual and visual impairment in the elderly is juxtaposed to the similar size, shape, and color of many medicines, errors in administration seem inevitable. More than 50% of elderly patients do not take their drugs as prescribed, and about 25% of them make errors likely to result in drug-induced illness (see Compliance, below).

Elderly patients are more susceptible to the adverse and toxic effects of most drugs, and the aged often bear the brunt of reflexive prescribing for uninvestigated symptoms. Changes with aging in body composition, and in drug distribution, metabolism, excretion, and response, make the elderly more vulnerable to adverse reactions. Since most clinical trials and pharmacologic studies have been performed in younger people, drug treatment standards thus developed and applied to the elderly are often hazardous. Recently, formal guidelines for trials in older individuals of drugs intended for use in elderly patients have been established.

Physiologic data demand that extreme care be used in selecting drugs and dosages to treat old people. An indicated drug should not be withheld because of a patient's age, but extra care is required in prescribing for and supervising the elderly.

Drug absorption can be influenced by numerous changes in the aging GI tract. Decline of gastric acid secretion, decreased mesenteric blood flow, shrinkage of total surface area of the gut, and decline of active transport mechanisms tend to decrease absorption and result in a lower serum level of an orally administered drug. Decreasing motility, largely due to higher pH of gastric contents, makes absorption more complete and thus elevates serum levels. The net effect of these factors is small, so that blood levels for most drugs in the elderly are not predictably influenced by differences in absorption.

Body composition changes occurring with age collaborate to make blood levels of drugs higher after standard doses. Weight declines, but body fat increases modestly (5 to 20%) in men and women. Lean body mass relative to total weight and total body water both decline, resulting in more drug/wt of metabolically active tissue, and a smaller volume of distribution with standard doses of water-soluble drug (fat-soluble drugs have an increased volume of distribution). Serum albumin falls in many chronic disease states, so that the many drugs that bind substantially to protein are less bound and thus more active. Such changes in body composition combine to make toxic accumulation of drugs more likely in the elderly.

Metabolism, largely by liver enzymes, accounts for inactivation of many drugs. The overall pattern with age is a decrease in inducible microsomal enzymes involved in redox mecha-

nisms **(Phase I reactions)** and an increase in hydrolytic enzymes. **Phase II reactions** (conjugation, acetylation) are unchanged. Many drugs have an increased half-life and thus a prolonged clearance (eg, aminopyrine, diazepam, amobarbital, propranolol, acetaminophen, chlordiazepoxide), but phenytoin is cleared more rapidly, and isoniazid and ethanol show no change. Smoking and alcohol consumption have more influence on hepatic metabolism of drugs than does aging.

Decline in kidney function is a major factor in producing elevated blood levels of drugs in the elderly. Average renal blood flow falls nearly 1%/yr after age 30, resulting in about a 30 to 40% decrease in most elderly persons. Diminished renal blood flow is reflected by a similar fall in GFR, urea, and creatinine clearance. However, serum creatinine, the commonly used measure of renal function, rises little or not at all, largely because of decreased muscle mass and creatinine production in the elderly. Similarly, BUN rises far less than expected because of diminished protein intake in old age. Therefore, creatinine clearance is a far more reliable indicator of drug-clearing capacity of the aging kidney, and is generally predictable by an age-creatinine clearance nomogram for individuals free of renal disease (see Fig. 130-1). A small subset of elderly individuals shows little or no change in renal function with age.

Changes in the aging brain reduce reserve capacity and make cognitive decline a particularly high-risk early event when elderly patients accumulate high blood levels of many drugs. Tissue sensitivity to some drugs increases, producing greater effects from standard doses.

Compliance

Compliance problems and the degree of noncompliance among elderly patients are about the same as those of other age groups. However, there is less margin for error, as older persons are generally more sensitive to medications. A large number of elderly people have been shown to decrease their dose of several types of medications in order to decrease adverse reactions, and so exemplify the concept of **"intelligent noncompliance"** (see also Ch. 139). To improve compliance, prescribers can follow a number of straightforward rules, eg, keeping the regimen simple and communicating clearly. The patient and the family members or care givers must understand the dose and regimen as well as the desired therapeutic outcome and potential adverse effects. The dose of medication should be adjusted on the basis of outcome.

125. AIDS FOR THE DISABLED PATIENT

The family providing long-term home care for a bedridden or partially disabled patient requires guidance in routine nursing care as well as instruction in more complicated procedures. Personnel from the Visiting Nurse Association or the local Board of Health can provide invaluable instruction and assistance.

The **ambulatory, partially disabled patient** and his family must learn together, at the outset of treatment, methods of ambulation, safety measures, and any ongoing treatments. The patient optimally should be able to direct and be responsible for any measures that he cannot manage for himself. Family members should be helped to acquire a proficiency that makes them relatively secure, and they should feel free to ask questions.

Equipment

A **wheelchair** must have brakes and be compatible with the patient's disability, size, weight, and activity, so that a stable sitting position without contractures is maintained; selection guidelines are available from manufacturers, distributors, and physical therapy departments. **Crutches** are measured and adjusted with the patient standing against a wall or supported by a chair. In use, the top bar should be 2 in. below the anterior axillary fold and the tips 6 to 8 in. ahead of and to each side of the toes, so that the crutches and legs form a supporting tripod. The patient's weight is borne on the hand pieces, which should be adjusted to allow a 15° angle at the elbow.

A **cane** should provide 25° of elbow flexion. To walk correctly with a cane, the patient stands in a normal walking position with the cane held on the side opposite to the weak leg. With his weight on the cane and the weak leg, he moves the good leg forward. Then he puts his weight on the good leg and moves the cane and the weak leg forward. An alternative method is to place the cane a step ahead of his feet, move the weak leg forward, shift his weight to the cane and the weak leg, and then move the good leg forward.

Building Modifications

Stairs should have a 10 in. deep tread, be ≤ 7 in. high, preferably have a snub nose, and have at least one **railing**, which should be 32 in. high and extend 18 in. beyond the top and bottom steps. Door resistance should be of 1 to 2 lb, and handles should be of the lever type (not knobs). **Wheelchair access** requires 32-in. doorways; a space 60 × 60 in. for turns; and **ramps** with a nonskid surface, a grade of 1 in./ft (8.33%), and railings 48 in. apart, 32 in. high, extending 1 ft beyond the ramp at top and bottom. A small wheelchair elevator is useful for outside accessibility when space prohibits a ramp. A seat-type elevator may be installed on an inside stairway.

Toilet bars should be 1½ in. in diameter, 33 in. above and parallel to the floor, and 1½ in. from the wall. Bars that can be attached to the toilet are available commercially. An elevated toilet seat may aid in wheelchair transfers. Two **tub grab-bars** are needed: one parallel to the tub and 4 in. above the tub surface, and the other vertical to the tub starting 9 in. from the tub surface. Both should be 1½ in. from the wall. **Shower grab-bars** should reach from the floor to head height (minimally knees to head) and be 1½ in. from the wall. A number of tub or shower seats, removable or built-in, are available. Roll-in shower chairs are available, and a "telephone" shower-head allows greater independence for the severely disabled.

Kitchen requirements include counters 26¼ to 26½ in. from the floor (or waist high), a stove with controls at the front, an oven at chair-arm height, and a sink that is open below and with the pipes flush to the wall to allow a chair to roll under. Faucet handles should be of the lever type, preferably wing, and operable by gross movement of the hand or arm. Placement of the fixture at the side rather than at the back of the sink may allow greater ease of function.

---

126. NUCLEAR MEDICINE

The medical application of unsealed radioactive materials for diagnosis and therapy.

Radionuclides emit electromagnetic radiation as gamma rays **(photons)**. These can be eas-

ily detected, quantitated, and localized within the body accurately and noninvasively with modern instrumentation. Radionuclides may be administered orally, parenterally, or through intracavitary routes and usually deliver significantly lower doses of radiation than alternative radiographic techniques.

Radionuclides decay at unique and characteristic rates (half-life) to more stable states, emitting gamma rays that are specific for a given radionuclide. The measurement of the energy spectrum of radiation emitted by a radioactive element and of the half-life of that element permit its accurate identification in microgram quantities (tracer dose), without exposing the patient to any pharmacologic toxicity; eg, a tracer dose of ^{131}I may be given safely to a patient with known iodine sensitivity. Patients with a history of contrast media sensitivity can be studied safely with alternative nuclear medicine techniques.

Many nuclides emit negatively charged beta particles (electrons) as well as gamma rays that are useful in certain forms of in vitro analysis such as radioimmunoassay, but they cannot be used diagnostically in vivo because they are not measurable externally and they yield significant radiation to the patient (their entire energy is absorbed by the tissue in which they localize). Other forms of radiation include alpha particles (helium nuclei ejected from the nucleus) which, because of their relatively heavy mass and energy, are associated with the highest radiation dose and lowest penetrability.

Another form of particle emission is the positron. This positively charged particle is emitted from the nucleus and on encountering an electron is annihilated, with the resultant production of 2 gamma rays of characteristic energy (511 KeV) that are emitted at 180° from each other, permitting very accurate localization and quantitation. Many of the naturally occurring elements that are vital constituents of organic matter, including carbon, oxygen, and nitrogen, can be made radioactive and capable of detection by positron emission tomography (PET), a valuable method for evaluating normal and abnormal biochemical processes. Since most positron emitters have very short half-lives requiring on site production, PET has been mainly a research technique. However, an increasing number of clinical centers are being established. Single photon emission tomography (SPECT) is a related technique that uses a tomographic principle for imaging conventional radionuclides. Clinical use of this technique has become widespread; eg, by imaging a tomographic slice of activity, diagnosis may be improved by eliminating interference from parts of an organ overlying a suspected lesion.

Radioactive isotopes (radioisotopes) may be utilized as simple salts of an element, eg, sodium radioiodine, or they may be chemically bound to another molecule to produce a labeled compound (radiopharmaceutical). These substances generally behave physiologically and biochemically identically to the stable nonradioactive form; eg, radioactive ^{131}I behaves identically in the body to nonradioactive or stable ^{127}I. This property makes the use of Lugol's solution beneficial in people who have been exposed accidentally to radioiodine. By saturating the thyroid with a large amount of nonradioactive iodine, thyroid uptake of the radioactive form is reduced. Alternatively, small amounts of radioiodine (^{123}I, ^{131}I) may be used to measure thyroid function in the radioactive iodine uptake test. If radioiodine is attached to a molecule such as albumin, the molecule continues to behave as albumin, but its fate and location in the body may be easily traced.

Therapy has not been a prominent part of nuclear medicine practice, with the major exception of radioiodine treatment of benign and malignant thyroid disease. Radiophosphorus is used in some hematologic disorders and colloidal chromic phosphate P 32 has been of help in ascites secondary to malignancy. Recently, a number of radionuclides have been introduced for use in metastatic malignancy to bone, including strontium 89 and rhenium 186 and appear to be highly effective in reducing bone pain. Problems relate to the difficulty of delivering an adequate amount of radioactive material to the target organ without excessively exposing the rest of the body. Therapeutic use of some radioactive materials overlaps slightly with the practice of radiotherapy, in which radioactive materials also may be used in the form of sealed sources.

A major potential application of nuclear medicine in cancer therapy is the development of monoclonal antibodies. By placing a radioactive label on an antibody specific for tumor tissue, the aim is to deliver large amounts of radiation directly to the tumor while minimizing damage to normal tissues. This area is under intensive investigation.

RADIATION DETECTION

The growth of nuclear medicine depends on improved methods for radiation detection and the synthesis of radiopharmaceuticals for studying specific organs. The earliest practical clinical radiation detector was the scintillation probe. A probe consists of a carefully prepared crystalline block of sodium iodide doped with minute traces of thallium that make it highly sensitive to gamma radiation, which is absorbed by the crystal, resulting in the emission of an equivalent amount of visible light. A light-sensitive photocathode behind the crystal can detect and convert light to an electrical current, which is then amplified and used to quantitate the amount and energy of the gamma radiation.

The **scintillation camera**, a device with imaging capabilities, combines a number of photomultiplier tubes behind a very large crystal. It utilizes a sophisticated electronic system to analyze not only the number of gamma ray events in the crystal and their energy but also their location within the crystal. Lead collimators allow radioactivity to reach the crystal only at 90° to its surface. Each site in the body corresponds, therefore, to only one site on the crystal. If a radiopharmaceutical is concentrated in a specific organ, it will provide an image that can be interpreted both morphologically and physiologically (based on the time activity relationships of the accumulation and disappearance of the tracer and its mechanism of uptake and metabolism or excretion).

Gamma camera studies appear as rather simple images but contain a large amount of data, which a computer can process and display in a variety of forms including time activity curves. The computer can also display and modify portions of the image.

RADIATION DOSIMETRY

Nuclear medicine procedures depend on internally distributed radioactive material (radiopharmaceutical or radionuclide) usually following IV, oral, or inhalation administration. **Units of radioactivity** commonly in use in the USA are the microcurie (**μCi**) and millicurie (**mCi**), which are being replaced by the becquerel (**Bq**). One mCi equals 37 MBq (37 × 10^6 Bq), and one μCi equals 37 KBq. The dose of radioactivity administered should be differentiated from the **radiation absorbed dose (rad)**, which refers to *the radiation energy imparted to the exposed tissues* (one **gray [Gy]** equals 100 rads). The implications of radiation dosimetry, along with a table to illustrate relative commonly encountered doses (TABLE 117–1), are given in Ch. 117. TABLE 126–1 may be used to gain a perspective of the radia-

tion dosimetry involved in common nuclear medicine procedures.

With an IV urogram, the skin may receive 33 mGy; with an IV cholangiogram, 290 mGy. Skin doses are of concern in radiographic procedures but are usually negligible in isotope procedures.

RADIOPHARMACEUTICALS

A wide variety of mechanisms are used to deliver radiopharmaceuticals to the organ of interest. They may depend upon active transport from the blood to the target organ; eg, the thyroid, which traps radioiodine, and the kidneys, which selectively concentrate ^{131}I-labeled orthoiodohippurate. Phagocytosis is relied upon for imaging of the liver and spleen, where macrophages remove particulate matter such as technetium Tc 99m–sulfur colloid. Cell sequestration can be used to image the spleen by damaging ^{99m}Tc-labeled RBCs with heat, thereby making them susceptible to splenic uptake. Capillary blockade (*trapping of radioactive particles within the capillaries*) is used for pulmonary imaging. Other approaches include exchange diffusion, in which a radioactive element such as xenon 133 gas is inhaled and an image of the ventilation of the lungs is obtained by the diffusion of the gas throughout the inspired air. Physicochemical adsorption is the probable basis for skeletal imaging, in which ^{99m}Tc phosphonates are trapped in bone through exchange with normal bone constituents in the hydration shell. Compartmental localization takes advantage of normal barriers within the body; eg, the diffusion of ^{99m}Tc-labeled albumin is restricted within the vascular system. Newer approaches include the use of compounds such as radioiodinated estrogens that are taken up by specific receptor sites and provide an index of the quantity and activity of receptor sites in a given area. Radiolabeled monoclonal antibodies promise to further improve radiopharmaceutical localization.

The major physical characteristics of many of the commonly used radionuclides are shown in TABLE 126–2.

SPECIFIC ORGAN–IMAGING PROCEDURES

Although the diagnoses of specific diseases and disorders are discussed in their appropriate sections of THE MANUAL, an overview of nuclear medicine procedures follows:

TABLE 126–1. RADIATION DOSE TO THE PATIENT IN RADIONUCLIDE STUDIES*

Radiopharmaceutical	Target Organ	Milligray (mGy)
^{57}Co-Vitamin B$_{12}$ (Schilling test)	Total body	0.80
^{99m}Tc-Pertechnetate (thyroid scan)	Thyroid	1.5
^{99m}Tc-Diphosphonate (bone scan)	Bone	4.5
^{99m}Tc-Sulfur colloid (liver scan)	Liver	10.0
^{99m}Tc-Albumin aggregated (lung scan)	Lung	4.0
^{99m}Tc-DTPA (kidney scan)	Kidney	1.5
^{123}I-Iodide (RAI)	Thyroid	6.5
^{131}I-Iodide (RAI)	Thyroid	42.0
^{123}I-Hippuran (kidney scan)†	Kidney	3.0
^{131}I-Hippuran (kidney scan)	Kidney	3.0

RAI = radioactive iodine.
* Calculated from the usually administered dose; 1 mGy equals 100 mrads.
† The dose of ^{123}I-Hippuran is 3 to 4 times larger than that of ^{131}I-Hippuran.

Thyroid: The best known and understood test in nuclear medicine is the **thyroid uptake**, based on the concentration of radioiodine by the thyroid for incorporation into thyroid hormone. Several important points bear on this test. Radioiodine thyroid tests should not be ordered for in vivo evaluation of thyroid function prior to in vitro testing that yields accurate information without exposing the patient to radiation. When morphologic information, in addition to functional information, is required (eg, to evaluate thyroid nodules and other forms of neoplastic disease), a **thyroid scan** is necessary, but it carries a significantly larger radiation burden than the uptake alone; therefore, the combination of an uptake and scan should *not* be ordered routinely.

Liver and spleen: Unfortunately, due to the great variety of space-occupying diseases that may affect the liver, no single test is uniformly successful in identifying disease. A liver scan with ^{99m}Tc–sulfur colloid provides morphologic and functional information about the state of the reticuloendothelial system. For instance, in patients with severe liver disease, a "colloid shift" may be seen, in which more than the normal amount of colloid is taken up by the bone marrow and spleen because of reduced liver function. Similarly, uptake of colloid by the spleen provides information about the functional integrity of that organ. No simple guidelines exist for deciding between ultrasound, CT scanning, and nuclear medicine techniques for liver and spleen studies. These tests are useful in a variety of overlapping conditions, and consultation with specialists should be sought in choosing a first line of investigation.

Biliary scanning has been improved by the introduction of iminodiacetic acid derivatives that are easily labeled with ^{99m}Tc. These compounds are actively concentrated and secreted by the liver, providing morphologic and physiologic information about the integrity of the biliary tract and the gallbladder. They are particularly valu-

TABLE 126–2. SOME COMMONLY USED RADIONUCLIDES

Substance	Half-Life	Photon Energy (KeV)	Beta Emission
^{99m}Tc	6 h	140	No
^{131}I	8.05 days	364	Yes
^{123}I	13 h	159	No
^{67}Ga	78 h	90–390	Yes
^{133}Xe	5.3 days	80	Yes
^{81m}Kr	13 sec	190	No
^{111}In	2.8 days	170, 250	No
^{201}Tl	73 h	70, 135, 167	No

KeV = kiloelectron-volts; Tc = technetium; I = iodine; Ga = gallium; Xe = xenon; Kr = krypton; In = indium; Tl = thallium.

able in the diagnosis of acute cholecystitis when failure to visualize the gallbladder occurs, providing evidence of the functional deficit. These agents also provide information about bile production and flow, gallbladder emptying, and postoperative leaks or obstructions.

Stomach: Agents in which ^{99m}Tc is incorporated into food are increasingly being used to evaluate gastric motility and emptying and as an adjunct to other evaluations of hiatal hernia. The test can also be used to evaluate therapeutic interventions (eg, the administration of bethanechol in gastroesophageal reflux).

Intestines: GI bleeding can be localized very precisely angiographically but can be diagnosed with ^{99m}Tc-labeled RBCs.

Lung perfusion scanning, with ^{99m}Tc-labeled microspheres to visualize the distribution of pulmonary arteriolar blood flow, and **ventilation scanning,** using radioactive gases or aerosols, are very useful to detect pulmonary embolism. Lung scanning also can be used to evaluate pulmonary function and to evaluate agents that improve pulmonary function, but these applications have not achieved widespread use.

Urogenital: Radiopharmaceuticals can be used to measure GFR (technetium Tc 99m DTPA), renal plasma flow (orthoiodohippurate I 131, technetium Tc 99m mertiatide [Tc-MAG₃]), renal perfusion (technetium Tc 99m pertechnetate), and renal morphology (technetium Tc 99m DMSA, technetium Tc 99m glucoheptonate). These studies are reliable, safe, and useful in patients who have known contrast media sensitivity or underlying renal insufficiency. The tests offer morphologic and functional information, whereas IV urography and arteriography offer mainly morphologic information. Radionuclide renography coupled with diuretics is especially valuable in distinguishing nonobstructive from obstructive dilation of the urinary tract. The use of the angiotensin-converting enzyme inhibitor captopril provokes significant changes in the renogram if renovascular hypertension is present and has become a routine application. Tracer techniques can provide images of the kidneys in severe renal failure and can be used to evaluate ureteral reflux and to differentiate torsion of the testicle from epididymitis.

Adrenal gland: ^{131}I-labeled 19-iodocholesterol can be used for adrenal cortex imaging in diseases such as primary hyperaldosteronism. ^{131}I-labeled benzylguanidine permits adrenal medulla imaging for diseases such as pheochromocytoma. These techniques also offer potential for therapeutic as well as diagnostic use in adrenal diseases.

Bone and joint diseases are major subjects for radionuclide techniques (for therapeutic use in bone metastases, see above). ^{99m}Tc-labeled phosphonates are highly sensitive to changes in bone turnover and therefore are very useful for detecting early bone and joint abnormalities and are more sensitive than x-ray, which can only detect relatively extensive changes in bone composition. Bone surveys should be carried out only with radionuclides, since they expose the patient to much less radiation and have a higher sensitivity than x-rays.

Brain: Although cisternography still is used in selected patients with dementia, hydrocephalus, or suspected CSF leak, the role of nuclear medicine in brain and other neurologic diseases has been replaced largely by CT scanning and MRI. Newer agents that specifically measure brain receptors or are related to cerebral blood flow are achieving increasing use. Recently, ^{123}I-tofetamine HCl and ^{99m}Tc-HMPAO have been approved for brain imaging. These compounds are blood flow–related, lipid-soluble imaging agents used with single photon emission tomography for early evaluation of stroke.

Vascular: Peripheral blood flow can be measured with radioactive xenon or sodium and can be estimated by muscle uptake of thallium. In addition, images of the aorta can be obtained to evaluate renal perfusion, aortic aneurysm, superior vena caval syndrome, and related conditions. These are simple screening tests that often may obviate the need for angiography.

Total body scanning is useful in a few situations; eg, in suspected bone disease and in the detection of an unknown infection site. Gallium 67 uniquely localizes in infection sites. Alternatively, indium 111–labeled WBCs can be used in whole body scanning to seek infection. Gallium 67 can also be used in suspected cases of interstitial nephritis, where its uptake is intense, and in diagnosing sarcoidosis and *Pneumocystis carinii* in patients with AIDS, in whom abnormal pulmonary uptake occurs.

Transplantation: Radioisotopes have been used in managing liver, lung, pancreas, and kidney transplantation. Their greatest use is in providing a very sensitive method for detecting renal transplant rejection, which is visually characterized by severely decreased perfusion and function, often in spite of continued urine production. Acute tubular necrosis in transplant recipients is characterized by modest perfusion reduction, better uptake of iodohippurate than in rejection, and virtual anuria. Kidney transplants also may concentrate ^{99m}Tc–sulfur colloid during rejection.

127. SPORTS MEDICINE

More than 10 million sports injuries are treated each year in the USA. Yet only in the past few years have physicians begun to receive training in the recently established principles of sports medicine. These principles, outlined below, can be applied to the treatment of all musculoskeletal injuries.

Many of the factors that increase an athlete's risk of injury are associated with similar injuries in nonathletes. Tennis elbow can be caused by carrying a suitcase, turning a screwdriver, or opening a stuck door; runner's knee can be caused by excessive pronation while walking; and plantar fasciitis can be caused by stiff-soled shoes. Physicians who do not treat athletes will see many patients with injuries of the types described below.

TREATMENT OF ACUTE INJURIES

Immediate treatment for almost all acute athletic injuries is Rest, Ice, Compression, and Elevation (RICE). Rest is instituted immediately to minimize hemorrhage, injury, and swelling. Ice causes dermal vasoconstriction and helps limit inflammation and reduce pain. Compression and elevation help limit edema.

The injured part should be elevated. A bag that is chemically cooled or filled with chipped or crushed ice (which will conform better than ice cubes to body contours) should be placed on a towel over the injured part. An elastic bandage should be wrapped over the ice bag and around the injured part, loosely enough to permit blood flow. After 10 min, the wrapping and the ice bag should be removed, but the injured part should be kept elevated. After a further 10 min, the ice bag and the wrapping should be replaced. Ten minutes with and without ice should be alternated for 60 to 90 min. This procedure can be repeated several times during the first 24 h.

Pathophysiology of ice application: Cold **limits swelling** by vasoconstriction and reduction in capillary permeability. It helps to limit pain by reducing impulse transmission from pain receptors. It **limits muscle spasm** by reducing impulse transmission from tendon receptors to muscles (5° C reduction in skin temperature can significantly reduce muscle spasm). It **limits tissue destruction** by decreasing cellular metabolism.

Prolonged application of ice, however, can cause vasodilation, increased swelling, pain, and tissue destruction. When ice is first applied, surface blood vessels constrict, and skin temperature drops from its normal of around 32° C (90° F). When it reaches about 15° C (59° F), hypothalamic-induced vasodilation occurs, and the skin turns red, feels hot and itchy, and may become painful (**hunting response**); this promotes edema (by increasing fluid exudation from damaged blood vessels) and tissue damage (by markedly increasing the release of oxidants and free radicals). This rebound vasodilation occurs about 9 to 16 min after ice is applied and lasts 4 to 8 min following its removal. Therefore, *ice should be removed if vasodilation occurs or after 10 min*, but can be reapplied 10 min after removal.

The principles of diagnosis and further management of acute injuries are similar to those for chronic injuries (see below).

CHRONIC WEAR–AND–TEAR INJURIES

Etiology

Just as a chain will break at its weakest link, every athlete has tissues susceptible to injury because of inherent weakness or biomechanical factors. Without correction, there is a high risk of repeated injury, because specific motions are performed repeatedly in all sports. Some individuals are unusually susceptible; eg, those with exaggerated lumbar lordosis (at risk of back pain when they swing a baseball bat), or those with excessive pronation of their feet (at risk of knee pain when they run long distances). The pain will usually disappear when activity is stopped but

TABLE 127–1. ALTERNATE SPORTS FOLLOWING AN INJURY

Site of Injury	Alternate Sports
Lower leg and foot	Bicycling, swimming, skating, skiing, rowing
Upper leg	Jogging in place, jogging on a trampoline, swimming, rowing (sometimes)
Lower back	Bicycling, swimming
Shoulder and arm	Jogging, skating, skiing

will recur each time the same work load is reached.

Overuse: The most common cause of injury is overuse of muscles or joints. The injury is exacerbated by failure to stop exercising when sustained pain occurs. Overuse may result from **poor training methods,** eg, by not allowing $\geq$ 48 h recovery from a hard workout, whether the person is a competitive athlete or merely exercising for fitness.

Every time muscles are stressed by an intense workout, some fibers are injured and some use up their available glycogen, which is their main energy source. Since only uninjured fibers or those with adequate glycogen can function properly, vigorous exercise demands the same work from fewer fibers, increasing the likelihood of injury. It takes $\geq$ 48 h for fibers to heal and even longer for the glycogen to be replaced. If exercisers insist on working out every day, they should alternate sports that stress different parts of their bodies (see TABLE 127–1).

Most training methods emphasize **the "hard-easy principle,"** exercising intensely on one day and at a more relaxed pace on the next. Many weightlifters alternate intense workouts on one day with no workout on the next. A runner may run at a 5 min/mile pace on one day and a 6- to 8-min pace on the next. If an athlete trains twice/day, each hard workout should be followed by at least 3 easy ones. Only swimmers can take a hard and an easy workout each day. Presumably, the buoyancy of the water helps protect their muscles and joints.

Biomechanical factors: Muscles, tendons, and ligaments may be injured when they are too weak for the exercise (they can be strengthened by appropriate resistance exercises, using progressively heavier weights). Bones can be weakened by insufficient calcium, estrogen (in women), or resistance exercise. Joints are more likely to be damaged when supporting muscles and ligaments are weak.

Structural abnormalities can stress certain parts unevenly; eg, unequal leg lengths place greater force on the hip and knee of the longer leg. Many roads are slanted a few degrees toward the sides to facilitate drainage; eg, if an athlete always runs against traffic, the right leg will usually strike higher ground than the left, transmitting greater force to the right hip and increasing the risk of pain or injury at this site.

By far, the most common biomechanical factor that causes foot, leg, and hip injuries is excessive **pronation** (*rolling in of the feet after they strike the ground*) while running. Pronation helps to prevent injuries (by distributing the force of impact with the ground) but, when excessive, can cause injuries through exaggerated medial twisting of the lower leg, resulting in foot, leg, and knee pain. The ankles of such people are so flexible that the arches touch the ground while walking and running, giving the appearance of a very shallow or absent arch. Following pronation, the foot rolls back toward the lateral plantar aspect (**supination**), then is raised up on the toes just before stepping off the ground and shifting weight to the other foot.

A foot with a very high arch is called **cavus.** Many people who appear to have a cavus foot have normal arches but rigid ankles, so that they pronate very little. Their feet usually are poor shock absorbers, increasing the risk of developing small cracks in the bones of their feet and legs.

Principles of Diagnosis

Following a physical examination and a history with particular focus on occupational and recreational activities, specialist referral for a variety of further tests may be considered, including plain x-rays, stress x-rays under general anesthesia, CT, MRI, arthroscopy, electromyography, and computer-aided physiologic testing.

Principles of Treatment

Acute aspects of the injury should be addressed first (including pain management and rest of the injured part, eg, by splinting). Muscle relaxants (eg, diazepam, cyclobenzaprine, chlorzoxazone, methocarbamol, metaxalone, or carisoprodol) may also be considered. Local corticosteroids may be helpful (see below). Surgery may be necessary.

Local corticosteroid injections (peri- or intra-articular) can relieve pain and reduce swelling and are a useful adjunct to analgesics and rest. However, they also inhibit fibroblast function and collagen deposition and thus can delay healing. Corticosteroid injections markedly reduce tendon blood supply, which can cause necrosis, and can therefore increase the risk of rupture. Injection should be close to the tendon, not into the tendon itself. Injected weight-bearing tendons are weaker than noninjected tendons for as long as 15 mo. Repeated intra-articular injections can cause cartilage to lose its hyaline luster and become soft and fibrillated; occasional injections may avoid this.

The patient should avoid the activity or sport until healing occurs. If possible, exercise that does not stress the injured part or cause pain should be encouraged, eg, by choosing an appropriate alternative sport (see TABLE 127–1). Such exercise will offset the tendency toward loss of fitness, because complete inactivity causes muscle atrophy, with reduced strength and endurance. Every week of rest usually requires ≥ 2 wk of exercising to reach preinjury fitness level.

Risk of injury recurrence should be minimized by addressing the cause. An appropriate training program should be instituted (see above).

Excessive pronation is often treated with shoe inserts (orthotics). They can be flexible, semirigid, or rigid, and can extend proximal to the metatarsal heads, or proximal to or beyond the toes. Most orthotics for serious runners are semirigid and extend proximal to the toes.

Orthotics must be placed in appropriate shoes. Good running shoes should have a rigid heel counter to control the rearfoot, a saddle to prevent the foot from slipping medially over the orthotic and pronating excessively, and a padded collar to restrict the ankle from rolling inward excessively. They must also allow space for the orthotic, which usually reduces shoe width by one letter grade; eg, a D width becomes a C.

Principles of Prevention

Warming up: Muscles should not be exercised vigorously until they have been exercised at a relaxed pace for a few minutes. Resting muscle temperature is around 36.7° C (98° F); a few min-

utes of exercise can raise it to around 38° C (101° F), making the muscle more pliable, stronger, and resistant to injury. Active warm-up by exercise, preferably by performing a sport at a relaxed pace, prepares muscles for competition more effectively than passive heating with warm water, a heating pad, ultrasound, or infrared lamp.

Stretching can help to improve performance, elongating muscles so they can develop greater torque; however, controlled studies have not shown prevention of injuries. Stretching should be done after a warm-up or after exercise. To avoid direct injury, athletes should never stretch further than they can hold for a count of 10.

Cooling down (gradually slowing down before stopping the exercise) can help prevent dizziness and even syncope. If the athlete exercises vigorously and stops suddenly, blood can pool in the dilated leg veins, causing dizziness and even fainting. Cooling down maintains increased circulation and helps to clear lactic acid from the bloodstream. It has never been shown to prevent next-day muscle soreness, which is caused by damage to the muscle fibers.

COMMON SPORTS INJURIES

In the following discussions, treatment is directed toward correcting the cause and preventing recurrence. A selection of the more common injuries is described. Since each injury can be caused by many different factors, this section should serve only as a broad outline, subject to the experience and judgment of the treating physician. In some instances, surgery may be indicated in place of the treatments described.

METATARSAL STRESS FRACTURES

Runners push off from their toes, putting great stress on the metatarsal heads. The 1st metatarsal is usually immune to fracture because it is much thicker and stronger than the others. The 5th metatarsal is relatively immune because the major force of "toeing off" comes from the first 2. The 2nd, 3rd, and 4th metatarsals are unusually susceptible because of their thin diaphyses.

Risk factors include a cavus foot, training shoes with inadequate shock-absorbing qualities, markedly increasing the intensity or volume of training, and amenorrhea. Many women with irregular periods lack sufficient estrogen, which can cause bone demineralization and increased susceptibility to fractures; exercise does not pre-

TABLE 127-2. BUCKET HANDLE EXERCISE

The athlete should:

1. Wrap a towel around the handle of an empty water bucket.
2. Sit on a table that is high enough to prevent the feet from touching the ground.
3. Place the bucket handle over the front part of the shoe.
4. Slowly raise the front part of the foot by flexing the ankle, then slowly extending it. This is done 10 times, followed by a few seconds rest, then 2 more sets of 10.
5. To increase the resistance, add water to the bucket, but not so much that it hurts to do the exercise.

Modified from Mirkin G, Shangold M: *The Complete Sports Medicine Book for Women.* New York, Simon & Schuster, 1985, p 96; used by permission of The Miller Press.

---

vent demineralization caused by estrogen lack. Exercise-associated irregular periods are caused most often by estrogen lack secondary to inadequate food intake rather than to the exercise itself.

Symptoms, Signs, and Diagnosis

Patients usually present with forefoot pain, often during a long or intense workout, which disappears within seconds of stopping exercise. On successive exercising, the pain returns earlier than previously, ultimately becoming so severe that it may prohibit exercise and persist even with the patient lying in bed. Palpating the swollen area causes pain at the fracture site. An x-ray usually is not sensitive enough to diagnose the fracture until a callus forms 2 to 3 wk after the injury. Often a technetium diphosphonate bone scan is necessary for diagnosis.

Treatment

Treatment includes stopping all sports that require running; trying alternate sports (see TABLE 127-1); wearing sports shoes with adequate shock-absorbing qualities; and, after healing, running on grass or other soft surfaces. Casts are rarely needed; if applied, they should be left on for only 1 to 2 wk because they can cause significant muscle atrophy and delay rehabilitation. Healing usually takes 3 to 12 wk (it may take longer in elderly and in debilitated patients). Women with recurrent stress fractures and oligomenorrhea or amenorrhea may need to be treated with calcium, estrogen, and progesterone.

SHIN SPLINTS

ANTEROLATERAL SHIN SPLINTS

The anterior compartment muscles (tibialis anterior, extensor hallucis longus, and extensor digitorum longus) hold the forefoot up during foot descent and contract eccentrically immediately after the heel strikes the ground. They are opposed by the much larger gastrocnemius and soleus muscles, which pull the forefoot down. The tremendous force of eccentric contractions can damage the anterior compartment muscles.

Symptoms and Signs

Pain occurs in the anterior compartment muscles, at first only immediately after the heel strikes the ground during running. If running is continued, the pain will occur throughout each step, eventually being felt constantly. By the time advice is sought, there is usually severe point tenderness over the anterior compartment muscles.

Treatment

Treatment includes stopping running, trying an alternate exercise (see TABLE 127-1), stretching the calf muscles, and doing exercises to strengthen the anterior compartment muscles after they start to heal; eg, the bucket handle exercise in 3 sets of 10 every other day (see TABLE 127-2).

POSTEROMEDIAL SHIN SPLINTS

Etiology

The main function of the posteromedial compartment muscles is to supinate the foot and raise and evert the heel just before "toeing off." Increased traction on the muscles is caused by excessive pronation and by running on banked tracks or crowned roads (exacerbated by wearing shoes that do not effectively restrict pronation). Excessive pronation causes the arch to drop lower than normal, increasing the force necessary to lift the arch during supination.

Symptoms, Signs, and Diagnosis

Pain usually starts in the posteromedial compartment muscles, 2 to 20 cm above the medial

TABLE 127–3. TOE RAISES AND OUTWARD ROLLS

Toe Raises

The athlete should stand up, slowly rise up on the toes, then slowly descend back on the heels. This should be done 10 times, followed by 1 min of rest, then 2 more sets of 10. When this exercise feels easy, progressively heavier weights should be held in the hands.

Outward Rolls

The athlete should stand up, slowly roll the ankles outward (evert the heels) so that the medial part of the bottom of the foot is raised off the ground, then slowly lowered to touch the ground again. Three sets of 10 should be done.

malleolus. It becomes more severe when the athlete rises up on his toes or everts the foot. If he continues running, the pain then moves forward to involve the medial aspect of the tibia, and can then move up the medial side of the tibia, to reach within 5 to 10 cm of the knee.

Pain location and severity depend on injury progression. First, there is a tendinitis of the muscles of the deep posterior compartment (flexor hallucis longus, flexor digitorum longus, and tibialis posterior). If the athlete continues to run, the pain may progress into the muscle bodies themselves; then traction on the tibialis posterior tendon can lift the muscle from its bony origin, causing subperiosteal hemorrhage and periostitis. With continued traction, part of the tibia can be torn away.

Treatment

Treatment is to stop running until it causes no pain, choose an alternate exercise (see TABLE 127–1), wear shoes with rigid heel counters and special arch supports to limit pronation, avoid future running on banked tracks and crowned roads, and strengthen the injured posteromedial muscles (see TABLE 127–3).

If the flexor digitorum longus and tibialis posterior muscles are avulsed from their attachments to the posterior aspect of the tibia, they may not reattach to the bone. Treatment includes long-term avoidance of running and, possibly, surgical reattachment. Although considered experimental, salmon calcitonin 100 IU/day by s.c. injection can sometimes heal shin splints unresponsive to other measures. Sometimes, no treatment is effective.

POPLITEUS TENDINITIS

The popliteus muscle arises from the lateral face of the lateral femoral condyle and inserts into the triangular area in the back of the tibia. Together with the anterior cruciate ligament, it limits forward femoral displacement. Downhill

running and excessive pronation tend to exaggerate forward femoral displacement and so increase forces on the popliteus tendon.

Symptoms, Signs, and Diagnosis

Tenderness of the popliteus tendon is accentuated by downhill running. Diagnosis requires the athlete to sit with the lateral side of the heel of the injured leg resting on the knee of the other leg. Point tenderness is felt just anterior to the fibular collateral ligament.

Treatment

The patient should wear shoes with a varus wedge (*hard triangular-shaped wedge placed on the medial half of the space between the heel and body of the shoe*) or orthotic to limit pronation. A good alternate sport is bicycling. Running should be avoided until it can be done without pain, and downhill running should especially be avoided for the first few weeks.

ACHILLES TENDINITIS

The Achilles tendon has 2 major functions during running. The calf muscles (1) lower the forefoot to the ground after heelstrike; and (2) raise the heel during "toeing off." Achilles tendinitis is caused by a force on the tendon greater than its inherent strength.

Most runners land on their heels with their forefoot still 2 in. from the ground. Running fast and up and down hills places extra force on the Achilles tendon. **During downhill running,** the forefoot strikes the ground with greater force than on level ground, since it drops further and has more distance to accelerate. **During uphill running,** the heel is much lower than the forefoot, so it takes a much greater force by the calf muscles to raise the heel before toeing off.

A **soft heel counter** allows excessive movement of the heel in the shoe. The rearfoot is not as stable and the Achilles tendon has to pull on a wobbly insertion. This places uneven force on the tendon and increases its chance of being torn. **Stiff-soled shoes** that do not bend just behind the first metatarsophalangeal joint place great stress on the Achilles tendon just before toeing off. **Biomechanical factors** include excessive pronation, landing too far back on the heel (check running shoes for the site of major heel wear), genu varum, tight hamstrings and calf muscles, a cavus foot, tight Achilles tendons, and varus deformities of the heel.

Symptoms and Signs

The Achilles tendon does not have a true synovial sheath but is surrounded by a paratenon (*fatty areolar tissue that separates the tendon from its sheath*). The early pain of Achilles tendinitis is caused by injury to the paratenon rather than to the tendon itself. Pain is greater when the patient gets up in the morning and often feels better with continued walking (as the tendon moves more freely inside the paratenon). Similarly, pain increases when exercise is begun and often feels better as exercise continues. The Achilles tendon is tender when squeezed between the fingers.

If pain is ignored and running is continued, the inflammation spreads to the tendon, which is eventually replaced by mucoid degeneration and fibrosis. Pain is then constant, exacerbated by movement, and decreases as exercise continues.

Treatment

The athlete should stop running; try an alternate exercise (see TABLE 127–1); reduce tension on the tendon by placing a heel lift in the shoes, by stretching the hamstring muscles as soon as this does not cause pain, and by using shoes with soles that bend easily just behind the first metatarsophalangeal joint; improve rearfoot control by inserting orthotics in shoes with tight, stiff heel counters; and do exercises to strengthen the Achilles tendon when it will not hurt to do so. Ask the patient to perform toe raises (see TABLE 127–3) and to avoid fast uphill and downhill running when running is resumed. Hill training may begin after the tendon heals.

PATELLOFEMORAL STRESS SYNDROME
(Runner's Knee)

A condition in which the patella articulates against the femur, instead of following its normal tracking between the femoral condyles.

There are many causes of runner's knee: patella alta (*a congenitally high-riding patella*); plicae (*fibrous bands attached to the patella*); tight hamstrings; tight heel cords; tightness of the vastus lateralis, iliotibial tract, and lateral retinaculum; weakness of the vastus medialis; and Q angle (*the angle between the patella tendon and the long axis of the thigh*) > 15°.

The most common treatable cause is a combination of excessive pronation and lateral pulling of the patella. During pronation, the lower leg twists medially, while 3 quadriceps pull the patella laterally (one, the vastus medialis, pulls the patella medially). The 3 lateral-pulling quadriceps cause the patella to rub against the femur.

Symptoms, Signs, and Diagnosis

There is often pain anteromedial and anterolateral to, and behind, the patella during running. Usually, it first occurs only when the patient runs downhill, but later it occurs during all running, and eventually even when not running (especially when walking down steps).

If the patella faces upward when the patient sits with the knee bent at 90°, patella alta is usually present.

Treatment

This includes stopping running until it can be done without pain, riding a bicycle if it does not cause pain (otherwise, rowing or swimming), stretching the hamstrings and quadriceps, placing store-bought arch supports in both walking and exercise shoes (if the pain continues, custom-made orthotics may be necessary), and exercising to strengthen the vastus medialis, which pulls the patella medially (see TABLE 127–4).

POSTERIOR FEMORAL MUSCLE STRAIN
(Hamstring Tear)

The quadriceps muscles flex the hip and extend the knee during running and jumping. They are opposed by the weaker hamstrings, which extend the hip and flex the knee and should be ≥ 60% as strong as the quadriceps on isotonic testing; otherwise, simultaneous contraction of the hamstrings and quadriceps can cause a hamstring tear.

Symptoms and Signs

A hamstring tear usually presents as acute pain in the posterior aspect of the thigh when the posterior femoral muscles are contracted suddenly and violently; eg, when a sprinter takes off

TABLE 127-4. EXERCISES TO STRENGTHEN THE VASTUS MEDIALIS

The athlete should stand up with both knees straight.

The quadriceps should be contracted and the patella raised. This position should be held for a count of 10 and then the muscles relaxed. This should be repeated frequently throughout the day.

The athlete should sit on the floor with both knees straight and legs far apart. The toes should be pointed as far laterally as possible, then the injured leg slowly raised and lowered. The knee should be kept straight. Three sets of 10 should be done every other night.

The athlete should sit on the floor with 2 pillows under the knee so that it is flexed at 135°. A 5-lb weight should be placed on the ankle, then the foot slowly raised, the knee straightened, and the foot slowly lowered. Three sets of 10 should be done. Progress is made by increasing the weight, not the number of repetitions.

Modified from Mirkin G, Shangold M: *The Complete Sports Medicine Book for Women.* New York, Simon & Schuster, 1985, p 101; used by permission of The Miller Press.

from the starting blocks, or a high jumper takes off from the pit.

Treatment

This includes RICE for the acute injury (see TREATMENT OF ACUTE INJURIES, above); reassurance; stopping running and jumping; trying jogging in place, rowing, or swimming (if no pain); and strengthening the injured hamstring muscles after they have started to heal (see TABLE 127-5).

LUMBAR STRAIN
(Weightlifter's Back)

Etiology

Any great force can tear the muscles and tendons of the lower back. This occurs commonly in sports that require pushing or pulling against great resistance; eg, snatching a heavy weight from the ground in weightlifting or pushing against an opposing lineman in football. It also

occurs in sports that require sudden twisting of the back; eg, turning to dribble after snagging a rebound in basketball, or swinging a bat in baseball or a club in golf.

Risk factors include an exaggerated lumbar lordosis, a forward-tipped pelvis (bottom to top), inflexible and weak paraspinal muscles, tight inflexible hamstrings, weak abdominal muscles, and intrinsically weakened lumbar structure; eg, arthritis, spondylolysis, spondylolisthesis, disk rupture, spinal stenosis, tumor, or Scheuermann's epiphysitis.

Symptoms and Signs

While twisting, pushing, or pulling, the athlete experiences sudden lumbar pain. At first, he often can continue playing, but 2 or 3 h later, continued bleeding stretches the torn muscles and tendons, and the resulting muscle spasm causes severe pain, aggravated by virtually any back movement. The athlete usually prefers to remain

TABLE 127-5. EXERCISES TO STRENGTHEN HAMSTRING MUSCLES

To strengthen the hamstrings, primarily the top (after a high hamstring tear):

The athlete should attach a 5-lb weight to the foot, lie on a bed, face down, with the lower body off the bed from the waist down. The toes should touch the floor. Keeping the knee straight, the leg should be slowly raised and lowered. Three sets of 10 should be done every other day. As strength increases, heavier weights should be used.

To strengthen the hamstrings, primarily the bottom (after a low hamstring tear):

The athlete should attach a 5-lb weight to the foot on the injured side, then stand up on the other foot. The weighted foot should be slowly raised toward the buttocks by bending the knee and then lowered toward the floor by straightening the knee. Three sets of 10 should be done every other day. As strength increases, heavier weights should be used.

Modified from Mirkin G, Shangold M: *The Complete Sports Medicine Book for Women.* New York, Simon & Schuster, 1985, p 102; used by permission of The Miller Press.

perfectly still in the fetal position, with knees bent and lumbar spine arched posteriorly (ie, trunk flexed).

On physical examination, there may be point tenderness or diffuse spasm and tenderness in the lumbar region, aggravated by any movement, particularly bending forward. (CAUTION: *Point tenderness on the lumbar spine associated with markedly increased pain on extension should be checked for spondylolysis [a fracture of the pars interarticularis].*)

Treatment

As soon as possible after the injury, the patient should be treated with rest, ice, and compression (see TREATMENT OF ACUTE INJURIES, above—elevation is not practicable for injuries to the trunk). Once healing begins, most people benefit from exercises to strengthen the abdominal muscles and to stretch and strengthen the back muscles; a rowing machine is excellent, provided it does not cause pain.

Exaggerated lumbar lordosis tends to increase forces on the muscles and ligaments that support the back. The degree is largely determined by the tilt of the pelvis. Exercises that tilt the top of the pelvis backward help decrease lumbar lordosis. Thus, the rectus abdominus muscles should be shortened by resistance training, and the hamstring and quadriceps muscles should be elongated by stretching.

Long-term treatment may include pelvic tilts to flatten the lumbar lordosis, abdominal curls to strengthen the abdominal muscles, sitting trunk flexions to stretch the lumbar spine, back-strengthening exercises, the swan to improve lumbar flexibility, anterior hip stretches for the rectus femoris, and single leg lifts to stretch the hamstrings and arch the lumbar spine (see TABLE 127–6).

LATERAL EPICONDYLITIS
(Backhand Tennis Elbow)

Etiology

This is an overuse syndrome caused by continued stress on the grasping muscles (extensor carpi radialis brevis and longus) and supination muscles (supinator longus and brevis) of the forearm, which originate on the lateral epicondyle of the elbow. First, there is pain in the extensor tendons when the wrist is extended against resistance. With continued stress, the muscles and tendons hurt even at rest, and there is progression to subperiosteal hemorrhage, periostitis,

calcification, and spur formation on the lateral epicondyle.

During a backhand return, the elbow and wrist are extended, causing the extensor tendons, particularly the extensor carpi radialis brevis, to be damaged when they roll over the lateral epicondyle and radial head. Contributing factors are poor backhand technique and weak shoulder and wrist muscles. Other factors include using a too-tightly-strung racket, using too small a handle, hitting heavy wet balls, and hitting "off-center" on the racket.

Symptoms, Signs, and Diagnosis

The first symptom is pain along the lateral epicondyle when the patient hits a backhand shot. Often this is ignored and exercise is continued. Eventually, the pain becomes constant and can extend from the lateral epicondyle to the wrist.

On examination, if the patient is asked to extend his fingers against resistance when the elbow is held straight, pain will occur along the common extensor tendon. Alternatively, the patient sits on a chair with the arm resting on a table. The hand is held palm downward, and the elbow is straight. The examiner places a hand firmly on top of that of the patient, who is asked to try to raise the hand by bending the wrist. The same pain will occur.

Treatment

Treatment is to avoid any activity that hurts on extending or pronating the wrist, and to substitute any exercise that does not cause pain, eg, jogging, cycling, basketball (even racquetball or squash, as the force of the ball on the racket is less than in tennis). With healing, exercises to strengthen the wrist extensors can be started (see TABLE 127–7). Generally, exercises to strengthen the wrist flexor pronators (see TABLE 127–8) are also recommended.

MEDIAL EPICONDYLITIS
(Forehand Tennis Elbow;
Baseball Elbow; Suitcase Elbow)

Forceful wrist flexion and pronation can damage the tendons that attach to the medial epicondyle; eg, serving in tennis (with too heavy a racket, heavy balls, an undersized grip, a spin serve, or having too much tension on the strings, together with weak shoulder and hand muscles), pitching in baseball, throwing the javelin, and carrying a heavy suitcase. If the athlete contin-

TABLE 127–6. LUMBAR EXERCISES

The pelvic tilt (to flatten lumbar lordosis)

The athlete should:
1. Lie on the back with knees bent and heels on the ground.
2. Place the weight on the heels.
3. Lower the small of the back so that it touches the ground and raise the bottom part of the pelvis up about ½ in. from the ground (by rolling the bottom of the pelvis upward).
4. Contract the belly muscles.
5. Hold this position for a count of 10 and repeat 20 times. This should be done daily.

Back-strengthening exercises—a rowing machine can be used

Abdominal curls (to strengthen abdominal muscles)

The athlete should:
1. Lie on the back with knees bent.
2. Put the hands across the abdomen.
3. While keeping the shoulders on the ground, slowly raise the head.
4. Slowly raise the shoulders 10 in. from the ground and then slowly lower them.
5. Do 3 sets of 10.
6. When this exercise becomes too easy, wrap a weight in a towel and hold it behind the neck. The weight should be increased as strength improves.

Back-stretching exercises

The athlete should:
1. Sit on the floor with knees straight and legs as far apart as possible.
2. Place both hands on the same knee.
3. Slowly move both hands down that leg toward the ankle. The athlete should stop if it hurts and go no farther than a position that can be held comfortably for 10 sec.
4. Slowly release and do the other leg. The exercise should be repeated 10 times.

Back-flexibility exercises

The swan (forcibly extending spine can worsen many back conditions, so it should be done with caution and stopped if painful)

The athlete should:
1. Lie on the belly with elbows bent and hands touching the ears.
2. Raise the shoulders and legs from the ground at the same time. The knees should not be bent. If it hurts, the exercise should be stopped immediately.
3. Hold this position for a count of 10 and repeat 20 times. This exercise should be done daily.

Quadriceps-stretching exercises

Anterior hip stretch

The athlete should:
1. Stand up with one foot on the ground, and the knee of the other leg bent at 90°.
2. Hold the front of the ankle of the bent leg in the same-sided hand.
3. Pull the ankle backward, while the knees are kept touching.
4. Hold for a count of 10.
5. Repeat for the other leg.
6. Repeat 10 times.

Single leg lifts with arched spine

The athlete should:
1. Lie on the back with knees bent at 90° and both heels on the ground.
2. While keeping the knee bent, grab one knee in both hands and bring it to the chest.
3. Hold the knee on the chest to count of 10; slowly lower that leg and repeat with the other leg.
4. Repeat 10 times.

Modified from Mirkin G, Shangold M: *The Complete Sports Medicine Book for Women.* New York, Simon & Schuster, 1985, pp 105–107; used by permission of The Miller Press.

TABLE 127–7. EXERCISES TO STRENGTHEN THE WRIST EXTENSORS (FOR BACKHAND TENNIS ELBOW)

The athlete should:
1. Sit on a chair next to a table.
2. Place the forearm on the table, palm facing down, elbow straight, with the wrist and hand hanging over the edge.
3. Hold a 1-lb weight in the hand.
4. Slowly raise and lower the hand by bending and straightening the wrist.
5. Do this exercise 10 times, rest 1 min, and then do 2 more sets of 10 (it should be stopped immediately if pain is felt and tried again 2 days later; _the exercise should be repeated every other day_).
6. As the exercise becomes easier, the hand weight should be increased.

Next, the athlete should:
1. With palm downward, wind up a 1-lb weight that is attached by a rope to a piece of wood that has the diameter of a broomstick.
2. Do this 10 times, but stop if pain is felt; _the exercise should be repeated every other day_.
3. Gradually increase the weight. The number of times that the weight is rolled up should not be increased.

Modified from Mirkin G, Shangold M: _The Complete Sports Medicine Book for Women._ New York, Simon & Schuster, 1985, p 109; used by permission of The Miller Press.

ues to stress the wrist flexors, the tendon can be pulled from the bone, causing subperiosteal hemorrhage, periostitis, spur formation, and tearing of the medial collateral ligament.

Symptoms, Signs, and Diagnosis

The patient complains of pain in the flexor pronator tendons (that attach to the medial epicondyle) and in the medial epicondyle when the wrist is flexed or pronated against resistance or when a hard rubber ball is squeezed.

To confirm the diagnosis, the patient sits in a chair with his arm from the elbow to the wrist resting on a table. The hand is supinated, and the patient is asked to try to raise his fist by bending the wrist, while the examiner holds it down. Pain will be elicited on the medial epicondyle and in the flexor pronator tendons.

Treatment

The patient should avoid performing any activity that hurts on flexing or pronating the wrist and

TABLE 127–8. EXERCISES TO STRENGTHEN WRIST FLEXOR PRONATORS (FOR FOREHAND TENNIS ELBOW)

The athlete should:
1. Sit on a chair next to a table.
2. Place the forearm on the table, palm facing up, with the wrist and hand hanging over edge.
3. Hold a 1-lb weight in the hand.
4. Slowly raise and lower the hand by bending and straightening the wrist.
5. Do this exercise 10 times, rest 1 min, and do 2 more sets of 10. If pain is felt, the exercise should be stopped immediately and tried again the next day.
6. As the exercise becomes easier, increase the weight.

Next, the athlete should:
1. With palms facing up, wind a 1-lb weight that is attached by a rope to a piece of wood that has the diameter of a broomstick.
2. Do this exercise 20 times. Stop if pain is felt; gradually increase the weight. The number of repetitions should not be increased.

Finally, (several times a day, and whenever convenient) the athlete should gently squeeze a soft sponge ball and then relax.

Modified from Mirkin G, Shangold M: _The Complete Sports Medicine Book for Women._ New York, Simon & Schuster, 1985, p 109; used by permission of The Miller Press.

TABLE 127−9. EXERCISES TO STRENGTHEN THE SHOULDERS

Downward lat pulls

The lat machine has a weight on the floor. A rope is attached to the weight and passes over a pulley
$\geq$ 1 ft over the head. The rope then comes down toward the head and is attached to a bar that is
held in the hands.

The athlete should:
1. Hold the bar over the head with the elbows bent.
2. Pull the bar down toward the head and slowly let the weight raise the bar up again.
3. Do 3 sets of 10 repetitions every other day.
4. As strength improves, increase the weight, not the number of repetitions.

Upright rows

The athlete should:
1. Hold a barbell in the hands with the thumbs held medially, in front of the quadriceps. The back
   should be kept straight.
2. Slowly raise the barbell by raising and bending the elbows, then slowly lower the barbell.
3. Do 3 sets of 10.
4. As strength improves, increase the weight, not the number of repetitions.

Bench press (CAUTION: *This should be started with a very light weight because the injured muscles are
being stressed.*)

The athlete should:
1. Lie on the back with a special bench or strong friend to help lift the weight from himself when
   finished with this exercise.
2. Hold the barbell in the hands with the thumbs held medially.
3. Slowly raise the weight from the chest and then slowly lower it.
4. Do 3 sets of 10, stopping immediately if pain is felt.
5. As strength improves, increase the weight.

should try an alternative sport, as for lateral epicondylitis, above. Later, he should learn how to hit the ball by applying more force from the wrist and shoulders and do exercises to strengthen the muscles in the hand, wrist, elbow, and shoulder (see TABLE 127−8). Generally, exercises to strengthen the wrist extensors (see TABLE 127−7) should also be done.

ROTATOR CUFF TENDINITIS
(Swimmer's Shoulder; Tennis Shoulder;
Pitcher's Shoulder; Shoulder Impingement
Syndrome)

The **rotator cuff** (supraspinatus, subscapularis, and teres major) holds the humeral head tightly in the glenoid fossa of the scapula. Tearing and inflammation of the tendons of these muscles often occur in sports requiring the arm to be moved over the head repeatedly; eg, pitching in baseball; moving the arm forward when swimming the free style, backstroke, and butterfly; lifting a heavy weight over the head in weightlifting; and serving in racket sports. Reaching forward causes the humeral head of the anteriorly flexed shoulder to abut the acromium and coracoacromial ligament, which in turn is rubbed

by the tendon of the supraspinatus. Chronic irritation can cause subacromial bursitis, inflammation of the tendons, and tearing of the rotator cuff. If exercise continues in spite of the pain, the lesion progresses to a periostitis and then avulsion of the tendons from their attachments on the humeral tuberosities.

Symptoms, Signs, and Diagnosis

Initially, pain occurs only when the athlete participates in any sport that requires him to hold his arm over his head and forcibly bring it forward (see above for examples). Later, pain may occur when the arm is moved forward to shake hands. Usually, pain will be elicited by pushing things away, with little or no pain on pulling objects in.

To palpate the rotator cuff, abduct the arm backward and away from the body in internal rotation with the elbow straight. The patient will complain of tenderness over the tendons, especially when the arm is raised above the shoulder, but often not when the arm is held down by the side. Severe pain is caused by adduction of the arm across the chest. Shoulder abduction will be weak, usually due to underuse atrophy of the deltoid. An arthrogram is usually not sensitive enough to diagnose a partial tear of the rotator cuff but can demonstrate a complete tear.

Treatment

First, the injured tendons should be rested and the uninjured shoulder muscles strengthened. The patient should avoid exercises that push

things away and do ones that bring things toward him, provided there is no pain; eg, upright rows and downward "lat pulls" (see TABLE 127–9).

Surgery may be necessary if the injury is particularly severe, if there is a complete tear of the rotator cuff, or if the tendons do not heal within 1 yr.

128. HYPERBARIC OXYGEN THERAPY
(HBO Therapy)

A medical treatment in which the patient is entirely enclosed in a pressure chamber breathing 100% O_2 at > 1 atmosphere pressure. Either a monoplace chamber pressurized with pure O_2 or a larger multiplace chamber pressurized with compressed air where the patient receives pure O_2 by mask, head tent, or endotracheal tube may be used.

To locate hyperbaric facilities in the USA, Canada, and the Caribbean area in an emergency, call the **Divers Alert Network (DAN)** at Duke University, **919-684-8111.**

Contraindications and indications approved by the Committee on Hyperbaric Oxygenation of the Undersea Medical Society are presented below.

CONTRAINDICATIONS

An **absolute contraindication** to HBO therapy is untreated pneumothorax, because with decompression the intrapleural air may double or triple in volume as normal atmospheric pressure is approached. If pneumothorax occurs in the multiplace chamber under pressure, it must be relieved surgically before decompression. In the monoplace chamber, a McSwain dart or other chest tube is made ready, the chamber is decompressed not taking longer than 1 min, and the chest tube inserted as the patient emerges. Other absolute contraindications include the concomitant administration of doxorubicin or cisplatin as chemotherapeutic agents for cancer. HBO and doxorubicin given together has caused death in rats (probably from cardiac toxicity), and cisplatin with HBO weakens the tensile strength of healing wounds in mice. Disulfiram blocks the production of superoxide dismutase, a protective antioxidant, and is also contraindicated in conjunction with HBO.

Premature infants *are susceptible to retrolental fibroplasia, and therefore HBO is contraindicated.* Full-term babies may be safely treated

with HBO. Babies may require papoose restraints, and young children may need mild sedation. Concerns that HBO treatment of **pregnant women** might stimulate premature closure of the patent ductus in the fetus have been mitigated by research in the Soviet Union in which women in all stages of pregnancy, when treated with HBO, produced normal children. The chamber is used if there is an overriding need to treat a pregnant patient; eg, in carbon monoxide poisoning (where the fetus suffers much more than the mother) or gas gangrene.

Relative contraindications: A history of **spontaneous pneumothorax** requires readiness to manage complications, as noted above. **Previous thoracic surgery** is a concern, as air trapping that could cause ruptured lung and air embolism are possibilities. Any pulmonary lesion may increase the possibility of air trapping, but patients with pneumonia and severe inhalation pneumonitis have been treated. In severe emphysema with CO_2 intoxication, removal of the hypoxic drive may cause respiratory arrest. **Upper respiratory infections** may make it difficult for the patient to equalize pressure in the ears and sinuses; decongestants are indicated. If the patient has a **history of middle ear surgery** for the treatment of otosclerosis, a wire or plastic strut might be displaced if the patient cannot equalize pressure in the ears; tympanostomy tubes may be needed. **Seizure disorders** may increase susceptibility to O_2 seizures, and additional premedication (eg, with diazepam) may be advisable. **Uncontrolled high fever** may predispose to O_2 seizures and should be reduced before placing the patient in the chamber. **Respiratory viral infections** may tend to worsen with HBO. Such an infection is a reason to temporarily interrupt daily treatment of some chronic illnesses. In **congenital spherocytosis**, RBCs are fragile, and high O_2 partial pressures may cause severe hemolysis. A **history of optic neuritis**, even if not active, has sometimes been associated with blindness following HBO treatment. Although rare, treatment should be halted immediately if the patient complains of a sudden change in vision.

Side Effects

O_2 seizures may occur, particularly when therapy is given at $>$ 2.4 atmospheres absolute (ATA). Some patients are idiosyncratically susceptible to high O_2 partial pressures. O_2 seizures cease when the O_2 is withdrawn; there are no known sequelae. The incidence of seizure is low, being reported at 1.3/10,000 treatments. Pulmonary O_2 toxicity, consisting of substernal chest pain, cough, and patchy atelectasis, may occur but is not seen if treatment protocols are adhered to.

After 20 or 30 treatments in the chamber, some patients complain of numb fingers, usually in the ulnar distribution; but this sensation disappears within 4 to 6 wk after therapy.

Serous otitis may result from daily HBO but usually is a minor problem; treatment is with decongestants.

A change in the refractive power of the lens is one of the most common side effects. Myopia, particularly in the elderly, tends to become worse, but presbyopes report an improvement in visual acuity, especially when reading. The original refractive state usually returns within 4 to 6 wk after therapy. The only cases in which visual acuity has not returned to pretreatment status are those with preexisting lenticular opacities. It has been suggested, but not proved, that preexisting cataracts mature more rapidly with HBO.

INDICATIONS

Carbon Monoxide (CO) Poisoning

Automotive exhaust, home heating, and industrial exposure are the most common sources. Fumes from paint strippers containing methylene chloride are metabolized to CO in the body and can cause severe symptoms. The diagnosis cannot be made unless one suspects exposure, especially in any afebrile individual or family group exhibiting flu-like symptoms. Headache, nausea, vomiting, weakness, and collapse often are followed by coma and death. Cherry-red coloration of the skin is rare and an unreliable diagnostic sign. The percentage of carboxyhemoglobin in the blood likewise does *not* correlate

with the prognosis and very often does not correspond to the patient's clinical condition, which is caused by tissue toxicity (disruption of cellular metabolism and an increase in products of lipid peroxidation—the latter is blocked by HBO).

Criteria for hyperbaric treatment: Unconsciousness, neurologic symptoms or signs, depression of the ST segment on the ECG, or a carboxyhemoglobin level $>$ 40% are indications for HBO therapy. Evaluation of mental status is much more important than the carboxyhemoglobin level, and severity of acidosis is a good indication of the severity of the poisoning. The sooner HBO is initiated, the better. In one large study of 250 cases of severe poisoning, those patients treated within 6 h experienced a 13.5% mortality, while 30.1% of those treated later died. All had received 100% O_2 before HBO. Patients with long CO exposures have a worse prognosis. If a hyperbaric chamber is located in the patient's hospital, treatment may be started at a lower carboxyhemoglobin level (25%) in the absence of other symptoms and signs. In the obtunded patient, treatment is indicated, even if the CO level is zero, if it is certain that CO poisoning caused the problem. The patient should be transferred to the nearest HBO facility—in the community (if available) or via air if practical. Despite reports of good results, the use of HBO in CO poisoning is not universally accepted.

Treatment: One hundred percent O_2 is given by tight-fitting mask (eg, aviator mask, anesthesia mask) or an endotracheal tube. Plastic "rebreather" masks commonly used in emergency rooms rarely deliver $>$ 50 to 60% O_2 and *should not routinely be used in the treatment of CO poisoning.* Acidosis and arterial pH are corrected to $\geq$ 7.15, and it is important to supplement potassium (K) if needed. Low K is frequently seen, and arrhythmias can result from the vigorous administration of HCO_3 in hypokalemia.

In a monoplace chamber, the patient is treated for 90 min. If residual symptoms persist, re-treatment can be carried out in 6 to 12 h. In the multiplace chamber, the patient is taken to 3 ATA and treated with two to three 23-min periods of 100% O_2 by mask, with 5-min "air breaks" in between. This is accomplished by removing the mask in the multiplace chamber or decompressing to the surface in the monoplace chamber for this brief period. If the monoplace chamber is equipped with a mask supplied with compressed air, the patient (if capable) may don the mask for air breaks in lieu of decompression. Treatment can then be continued at 1.9 ATA. In severe cases, US Navy Decompression Sickness Treatment Table 6 may be used from the onset. This provides at least 4 h of O_2 breathing at pressures starting at 2.8 ATA. In a conscious patient who cannot equalize his middle ear, myringotomy is indicated; it is optional in the unconscious patient but should not delay definitive treatment. Patients with a markedly impaired sensorium should be restrained, as they may awaken combative (diazepam IV may be used to manage them).

Decompression Sickness and Gas (Air) Embolism
(See Conditions Requiring Recompression in Ch. 122)

Air embolism also is seen in the hospital setting secondary to surgery, IV therapy, lung biopsy, ventilator accidents, renal dialysis, and arterial catheterization. It is also seen following oral inflation of the vagina with air during pregnancy (see discussion of HBO in pregnancy under Contraindications, above), and in victims escaping from submerged vehicles.

Gas Gangrene
The use of HBO in gas gangrene, despite good animal studies and large clinical series, is not universally accepted.

Clostridium perfringens is the most common cause of gas gangrene, although another one or more anaerobic organisms are usually present. Pathogenesis is primarily mediated by α-toxin, a lecithinase, which dissolves RBCs (producing hemolysis and hematuria) and severely damages muscle, cell membranes, and renal tubules. Gas gangrene myonecrosis can produce profound shock that responds only to whole blood or packed cells. Death may ensue within 6 h of the diagnosis unless immediate corrective action is taken. HBO therapy, if available, must be carried out early in the course of the disease. If the patient with truncal gangrene is first treated in the chamber > 24 h after the diagnosis is made, the mortality falls to 75%; if treated within 24 h, the mortality falls to < 20%. When a limb is involved, mortality may be > 9% if HBO treatment is delayed > 24 h, but it approaches zero if instituted within 24 h, regardless of the type or time of surgery. If the syndrome progresses despite HBO therapy, amputation or major debridement must be carried out. The prognosis is especially grave in the elderly compromised host with gangrene of the abdomen or trunk. After the patient is no longer toxic, all necrotic material should be immediately removed surgically.

Surgery requiring general anesthesia should be deferred until after the first HBO treatment is given, for the following reasons: (1) Surgery entails delay in giving HBO treatment, during which the α-toxin damages all the organs of the body. (2) A general anesthetic given to a patient in septic shock vastly increases the morbidity and mortality. (3) A cleaner line of demarcation between the viable and necrotic tissue appears after 2 or more HBO treatments, often making possible less disfiguring surgery and even the salvage of entire limbs. (4) After surgery, large open debrided areas that constantly ooze blood and serum complicate fluid balance and subsequent chamber treatment.

HBO given at a pressure of 3 ATA in the multiplace chamber or 2.5 ATA in the monoplace chamber probably inhibits production of α-toxin when the tissue P_{O_2} rises to high levels. Circulating α-toxin is fixed and deactivated in the tissues within about 30 min. Treatment is for 90 min.

In severely ill, febrile patients, the risk of convulsion can be diminished if an air break (see Treatment of CO poisoning, above) of 5 min is provided in the middle of the 90-min treatment. Usually, 3 treatments are given in the first 24 h, followed by 2 treatments in the ensuing two 24-h periods, making a total of 7 treatments. Fewer treatments may be given if the patient's signs of toxicity disappear, but up to 10 treatments may be necessary.

Crush Injury and Compartment Syndrome
Crush or degloving injuries (stripping of the skin and flesh from the bones, usually of the hands or feet as seen in wringer or industrial roller injuries) can interrupt both large vessels and the continuity of capillary beds. Large vessels must be repaired surgically, but the ischemic anoxia associated with decreased capillary flow may benefit from HBO treatment. Edema soon forms, increasing the distance O_2 must diffuse from functioning capillaries. This often creates a vicious circle and causes complications such as compartment syndrome and frank sloughing of compromised tissue. HBO preserves ATP in the cell membranes, preventing water loss into the interstitial space.

Treatment: With a globally hypoxic limb, edema formation can be reduced by 50% if HBO treatment is initiated within about 8 h, assuming that damaged large vessels have been surgically repaired. HBO treatment reduces blood flow in muscle about 20%, reduces edema, and increases the amount of O_2 in physical solution in the plasma. Tissues receive abundant O_2, even though functioning capillaries may be sparse, thereby reducing tissue necrosis by about 50% in severely compromised compartments. Thus, HBO is most valuable in impending compartment syndrome but remains an adjunct to fasciotomy in established compartment compromise. Treatments are usually continued for 3 to 5 days.

Compromised Skin Grafts and Flaps

Most skin grafts and flaps will take without the adjunctive use of HBO therapy, but there is a 28% improvement in take in HBO-treated groups. Failing full-thickness flaps must be treated early at the first signs of cyanosis or failure to take; treatment is continued bid for 3 to 7 days, depending on graft appearance. In the compromised host in whom previous split-thickness grafts have failed, graft take can often be achieved using HBO therapy to produce granulation tissue adequate for grafting and for 3 days bid following grafting.

Mixed Soft Tissue Infections

Most infections respond to adequate debridement and antibiotics, but in patients with peripheral ischemia (tissue P_{O_2} 30 mm Hg), leukocyte killing cannot take place and HBO can play a role. In one study, when HBO was used as an adjunct in necrotizing fasciitis, mortality and the number of debridements required for infection control were significantly reduced. Treatment daily or bid establishes granulation tissue to aid control of infection. If *Bacteroides* is the causative organism, initial HBO therapy should follow a gas gangrene protocol (see above). However, in treating the diabetic foot, an ankle arterial pressure (measured by Doppler) > 75 mm Hg is necessary or HBO will not be of value. Additionally, transcutaneous P_{O_2} measurements may be helpful. If transcutaneous P_{O_2} readings are > 40 mm Hg, healing with closure of the wound can probably be achieved using HBO therapy. If readings < 40 mm Hg rise to levels of $\geq$ 1000 when the patient is placed in the chamber at 2.4 ATA, healing will most likely occur. Otherwise, amputation is probably indicated.

Burns
(See also Ch. 114)

Deep second-degree burns may deteriorate to full-thickness loss, and HBO may be considered

to reduce hypoxia and edema formation. HBO therapy reduces edema secondary to vasoconstriction and results in a 35% reduction in fluid requirement within the first 24 h. *To be effective, HBO therapy must be started within 24 h of the burn, preferably as soon as possible.* HBO therapy will aid in the treatment of concomitant smoke inhalation and CO or cyanide poisoning (see Smoke Inhalation, below). Additionally with HBO, Curling's ulcer rarely appears, hypertrophic scarring and contracture are reduced, and burn encephalopathy is rare.

Mafenide must be carefully removed before starting HBO therapy as it produces a peripheral vasodilation that, when coupled with the central vasoconstriction caused by HBO, produces worse results than either HBO or mafenide used alone. Silver sulfadiazine may be used. HBO is administered for 90 min q 8 h for the first 24 h, and then bid until all wounds are covered with epithelium or securely grafted. Burn therapy otherwise is as described in Ch. 114, but the necessity of controlling acidosis when HBO is used is especially important. It is recommended that 10 mEq of bicarbonate be added to each liter of Ringer's solution. In order to avoid pulmonary O_2 toxicity, HBO is discontinued if the patient requires supplemental O_2 of $\geq$ 40% outside the chamber. Tangential excision is used with HBO but can be delayed 3 to 4 days, and grafting is carried out as soon as there is uniformly healthy granulation tissue. HBO should be used only in established burn centers in accordance with rigid protocols.

Smoke Inhalation
(See also Ch. 114)

Smoke inhalation usually consists of CO and/or cyanide poisoning combined with a severe chemical pneumonitis. (Modern building construction materials yield significant amounts of cyanide.) Bronchospasm and pulmonary edema typically worsen over the first 24 to 36 h, mandating that smoke inhalation patients be observed and have blood gases monitored for at least 24 h prior to discharge. HBO treatment in smoke inhalation is adjunctive to respiratory care. HBO rapidly clears carboxyhemoglobin from blood and provides O_2 dissolved in plasma, while counteracting the tissue toxic effects of both CO and cyanide.

Initial therapy should be as for Carbon Monoxide Poisoning, above. Ventilatory support may be necessary, but early HBO treatment can reduce the need for intubation.

Soft Tissue Radiation Necrosis

Six to 18 mo following local radiation of tissue, medium-sized blood vessels begin to progressively sclerose, sharply limiting blood supply and causing profound tissue ischemia. Induration and fibrosis ensue and, if a break develops in the integument, infection usually supervenes and prevents healing. Wounds tend to enlarge when WBCs can no longer kill bacteria because of a fall in the tissue P_{O_2} to < 30 mm Hg. This problem is most common following radiation of head and neck tumors but also can be a serious problem in the abdomen and other areas.

Treatment: Prior to HBO therapy, surgery was the only treatment. Extirpation of the irradiated area and use of vascularized soft tissue grafts to close the defect are often successful. When this is not possible, because of the presence of critical structures (eg, the carotid artery), surgery should *not* be attempted until there has been adequate pretreatment with HBO to establish the necessary granulation tissue to support a graft.

In the hyperbaric chamber, tissue P_{O_2} will rise to 75 to 80% of normal after 18 to 30 treatments, as vascular granulation tissue develops. Skin grafts then may be applied, and HBO therapy is performed bid for at least 3 days following surgery and then once a day as necessary. Using pretreatment HBO, spontaneous closure of orocutaneous fistulas has been reported, and infections can be controlled when the P_{O_2} rises sufficiently. Wounds tend to be stable and do not exhibit long-term deterioration following adequate HBO treatment.

Osteoradionecrosis

Bone necrosis caused by irradiation.

This condition most commonly involves the mandible secondary to radiation for head and neck tumors. Supervoltage x-ray results in aseptic degeneration, due to loss of viable osteoblasts and osteoclasts. Most cases of osteoradionecrosis of the jaw originate from tooth extraction, required because radiation caries develop with subsequent infection. The trauma of tooth removal causes a breakdown of gum tissue and subsequent progressive infection. Exposed bone is often visible and there is evidence of infection with pus formation, but the disorder is not a form of osteomyelitis. The infection is invariably periosseous in origin. Granulation tissue cannot form to bridge over dead bone, and the infection continues despite meticulous wound care and antibiotics; the resolution rate is only about 8% without the use of HBO.

Prevention: When tooth extraction is necessary, it is best to give 20 preoperative HBO exposures on a once-a-day basis 5 or 6 days a week. Postoperatively, the patient is treated daily 10 more times with HBO. Perioperative antibiotics are used as appropriate. Even in patients who have received > 60 Gy (6000 rads) to the jaw area, osteoradionecrosis is prevented in about 92%.

Treatment: If only a small patch of bone is exposed and x-ray reveals that radiation damage has not extended throughout the corpus of the mandible (a **Stage I** lesion), the patient is treated with HBO 30 times on a once-a-day basis while meticulous wound care is given. If the mucosa closes over the bone within 30 treatments, HBO is continued for 60 treatments total. Should the lesion not heal within 30 treatments, the lesion is classified as **Stage II**, and an alveolar sequestrectomy is performed with a watertight closure of the mucosa. Up to 30 more treatments are given.

X-ray evidence of total involvement of the mandible, an orocutaneous fistula, an extensive area of denuded bone, a pathologic fracture, or dehiscence of a Stage II lesion is classified as a **Stage III** lesion. Thirty daily treatments are given, followed by resection of the mandible back to bleeding bone; the mandibular nerve is preserved, and any orocutaneous fistulas are closed. Following operation, the position of the jaw is maintained with an external acrylic arch bar, and 10 to 20 additional HBO treatments are given. Ten weeks later, following transcutaneous insertion of a bone graft, $\geq$ 10 additional HBO treatments are given to ensure take of the graft. About 94% of the cases will achieve freedom from pain, reestablishment of an intact mucosa, and normal shape and function with sufficient alveolar height to support dentures.

Chronic Refractory Osteomyelitis
(See also Ch. 42)

When osteomyelitis does not resolve with surgery and antibiotics, there is often generalized host compromise due to another underlying disorder or local ischemic compromise of the wound. In the center of osteomyelitic wounds, P_{O_2} is often < 20 mm Hg, preventing leukocytes from killing bacteria, and preventing fibroblast activity from producing collagen and scar formation. HBO treatment aims to produce O_2 levels in the infected area $\geq$ 30 mm Hg. Normally, only refractory osteomyelitis that fails to respond to surgery and antibiotics is considered for HBO therapy, but osteomyelitis of the skull and of the sternum are exceptions. The skull is an exception because of its close proximity to the brain (with possible spread of infection) and because of the risk of disfigurement if ablative surgery becomes necessary. With osteomyelitis of the sternum (a common complication of the sternum-splitting approach used for cardiac surgery), HBO may be considered, if locally available, at the first indication of infection, as movement of the sternum caused by breathing can render eradication of persistent infections extremely difficult.

Treatment: HBO therapy is adjunctive to adequate saucerization, sequestrectomy, and IV antibiotic therapy. If the wound has been refractory for < 2 yr, arrest of about 85% of the infections can be anticipated; later, the arrest rate may fall to 50%.

Treatment is given once a day and continued for 10 days after all drainage ceases and there is no further evidence of infection. After 30 treatments, if the wound continues to drain, it is wise to repeat the x-ray to see if a sequestrum has become evident. Occasionally, 40 to 60 treatments may be necessary.

Exceptional Blood Loss Anemia

In certain instances of blood loss (eg, in Jehovah's Witnesses who refuse blood products for religious reasons) and in cases of severe hemolysis or a rare blood type for which no adequate cross-match may be obtained, blood transfusions may not be possible. Patients with as little as 1 gm of Hb have been salvaged when HBO has been used. Enough O_2 can be physically dissolved in plasma at 3 ATA to support life, and there appears to be no inhibition of erythropoiesis when HBO is used intermittently. However, platelet loss is a major problem, and continued bleeding is often difficult to control.

HBO may be required as often as every other hour, with 1 h spent at pressures up to 2.5 ATA. More commonly, 1 or 2 h spent at 2 ATA suffices, with a surface interval of from 2 to 6 h. Initial treatment frequencies are determined by signs of ischemia, eg, substernal pain or ischemic bowel. Later, the best indicator is the ECG; inverted T waves indicate hypoxemia. Treatment is continued for up to 10 days with gradually lengthening intervals between treatments to bid or tid.

Actinomycosis

Most *Actinomyces israelii* infections respond to surgery and antibiotics. However, in rare refractory cases or those in which ablative surgery to eradicate the infection involves critical structures (eg, the middle ear), HBO may be indicated; O_2 has a direct effect on this organism. The patient is treated on a gas gangrene protocol (see Gas Gangrene, above).

129. HOSPICE MEDICINE

Specialized palliative care of patients with terminal illness.

Hospice is a specialized program that provides skilled care and support to both patient and family. Its goal is to enhance the quality of life through relief of physical, emotional, social, and spiritual pain. It condones neither euthanasia nor prolongation of dying.

Hospice care usually covers the last 6 mo of life and is appropriate for all ages and all terminal illness, although most patients have an incurable malignancy. A patient is considered terminal when curative measures are judged ineffective and remission is improbable. Factors that help estimate remaining life span include tumor type, extent of metastases, disease progression, change in the Karnofsky scale of activities of daily living, emotional and physical withdrawal, reduced level of nutrition, and progression of symptoms. Hospice care can be provided in the home (the most common site in the USA), hospital, cancer center, nursing home, or free-standing hospice facility.

Providing patients with truthful information about their illness allows them choice and control in determining how best to live the remainder of their lives. While patients need not acknowledge that they are terminal, they must accept that their illness is without cure and that hospice care is palliative. Patients should not be given false hope. Prognostic information should be provided in a compassionate and loving manner, preferably by a person who is trusted and understands the individual family dynamics. Denial, as a coping mechanism, should not be discouraged unless it interferes with necessary decisions.

When curative therapies are terminated and palliative care is accepted by patient and family, the emphasis is on relief of pain and other symptoms, while providing the patient and family with maximum self-determination. Noncurative interventions may reduce tumor size and prolong life, but should be avoided when the primary considerations of symptom relief and patient comfort are not met.

Somatic or visceral pain is treated with nonsteroidal anti-inflammatory drugs, opioids, and drug combinations to provide maximum relief with minimal side effects. Traditional concerns about narcotic addiction are not applicable. Pain relief is provided on a regular, around-the-clock basis. A prn dosing schedule, permitting "breakthrough" pain, is ill-advised. Prevention of other symptoms (eg, constipation and debilitating nausea) is emphasized.

Antibiotics are used when they offer additional life with quality. Enteral feedings (nasogastric tube, gastrostomy) and parenteral feedings (hyperalimentation, IV fluids) are discouraged. Decreased intake of food and fluids is a natural part of the dying process and is usually without discomfort. Good oral hygiene can add to the patient's comfort. For chronic progressive anemia, intermittent transfusions of packed RBCs on an outpatient basis may be helpful if symptomatic improvement results. Massive hemorrhage as a terminal event can be treated with opioids and skilled nursing care. Radiation therapy may provide excellent palliation of symptoms secondary to malignancy. Bone metastases are particularly responsive (see also Ch. 126 on the use of radionuclides in bone metastases). Radiation may be given in larger doses over a shorter time, since complications are unlikely to present in the patient's lifetime.

Chemotherapy should usually be completed prior to hospice admission. Patients may often demonstrate no further response to chemotherapy or may refuse further treatment. Hormonal therapies (eg, corticosteroids, estrogens, antiestrogens) are usually continued.

Surgery may be indicated. The general condition of the patient and the impact on the quality of life must always be the primary consideration. Bowel obstruction not related to the primary malignancy (eg, due to adhesions) may justify surgical intervention. Femoral fracture may be managed by open reduction and internal fixation if the patient is able to return to an ambulatory status or if stabilization of the fracture contributes to the patient's well-being. Intensive care in the traditional sense is usually not appropriate. Intensive nursing care can be provided in the home, when appropriate.

Maladaptive emotional responses are treated with anxiolytic and antidepressive medications and with short-term psychotherapy.

All members of the hospice team (attending physician, hospice physician, nurse coordinator, psychosocial worker, volunteer, chaplain, and pharmacist) provide expertise. Issues of grief and loss are addressed both during the living-dying period, and after death with family and friends during the period of bereavement.

130. LABORATORY MEDICINE

"**Normal laboratory values**" are mean values in a healthy population $\pm$ 2 standard deviations (SD); ie, 5% of results from normal individuals may be labeled as abnormal. Since each test is independent of the others, *the probability of a normal individual having completely normal results is relatively low;* eg, when a sequential multiple analyzer (SMA) is used, one abnormal test result is expected in almost $1/2$ the patients having an SMA-12 and in $2/3$ of patients having an SMA-20. Determination of values is further complicated by sex, age, diet, malnutrition, drugs, latent disease, time of day, and position of the patient when the specimen is drawn. An increase in plasma volume occurs when changing from the standing to the supine position, which will reduce the plasma concentrations of nondiffusible substances. Automated methods tend to be more subject to errors, eg, a trace of a previous sample remaining in the instrument.

Artifactual errors include high serum potassium due to cellular release, eg, following prolonged tourniquet constriction; low serum glucose in patients with high leukocyte counts; low serum sodium or high plasma Hb in patients with hyperlipidemia; and high serum creatinine in patients with diabetic ketoacidosis because of interference of acetoacetate in the automatic assays.

The **sensitivity** of a test depends on the proportion of patients with a disease in whom the test is positive (ie, percentage *positive in disease*). The **specificity** of the test depends on the

TABLE 130–1. OPERATING CHARACTERISTICS OF DISCRIMINATING TESTS USED IN DIAGNOSING ANEMIA

Test	Sensitivity (%)	Specificity (%)	Disease
RDW > 15	87–100	66	Iron-deficiency anemia
Ferritin < 12	65–97	99	Iron-deficiency anemia
Transferrin < 16	95	70–95	Iron-deficiency anemia
Reticulocyte count	62–90	99 (> 10%)	Hemolysis
Coombs' test	90	?95	Autoimmune hemolytic anemia
MCHC > 36	?100	100*	Hereditary spherocytosis
Splenomegaly	100	?	Hereditary spherocytosis
MCV > 105	11	95	Vitamin B_{12} or folic acid deficiency
MCV < 100	100	?40–50	Iron-deficiency anemia
MCV < 80	100	?	Thalassemia
Hemosiderin (urine)	100	?	Paroxysmal nocturnal hemoglobinuria

* Provided that artifacts are excluded.

MCHC = mean corpuscular hemoglobin concentration; MCV = mean corpuscular volume; RDW = red cell distribution width.

From Djulbegovic B, Hadley T, Pasic R: "A new algorithm for diagnosis of anemia." *Postgraduate Medicine* 85(5):119–130, 1989; used with permission.

proportion of disease-free patients in whom the test is negative (ie, percentage *negative in health*). TABLE 130–1 shows the sensitivity and specificity of test procedures for the evaluation of anemia. Often ≥ 2 tests are required to evaluate a diagnostic possibility. TABLE 130–2

TABLE 130–2. HYPOTHETICAL DATA COMPARING ULTRASOUND AND CT SCAN IN DIAGNOSIS OF PANCREATIC CARCINOMA

Test	Sensitivity %	Specificity %
Ultrasound (A)	80	60
CT scan (B)	90	90
A or B positive*	98	54
A and B positive†	72	96

* If a positive result is accepted as *either* test A or B positive, then (1) combined sensitivity = the percentage of patients with carcinoma identified by test A (sensitivity, A) plus the percentage of the remaining patients with carcinoma identified by test B (100% − sensitivity, A × sensitivity, B) = 80+ (20 × 90%) = 98%, and (2) combined specificity = the percentage of patients without carcinoma in whom *both* tests are negative = specificity, A × specificity, B = 90% × 60% = 54%.

† If a positive result requires that *both* tests be positive, then (1) combined sensitivity = sensitivity, A × sensitivity, B = 80% × 90% = 72%, and (2) combined specificity = the percentage of patients without carcinoma identified by test A (specificity, A) plus the percentage of the remaining patients without carcinoma identified by test B (100% − specificity, A × specificity, B) = 60% + (40% × 90%) = 96%.

From Griner PF, Mayowski MD, Mushlin MD, Greenland P: "Selection and interpretation of diagnostic tests and procedures." *Annals of Internal Medicine* 94(4):553–570, 1981; used with permission.

TABLE 130-3. EFFECT OF AGING ON LABORATORY PARAMETERS

Increased	Unchanged	Decreased
Serum copper	Hemoglobin	Serum calcium
Serum ferritin	RBC count	Serum iron
BUN	WBC count	Serum phosphorus
Serum creatinine*	Serum vitamin A	Serum thiamine
Serum alkaline phosphatase	Leukocyte zinc	Serum zinc
Serum immunoglobulin M	Serum pantothenate	Serum 1,25-dihydroxyvitamin D
Serum immunoreactive parathormone	Serum riboflavin	Serum vitamin B_6
Serum cholesterol	Serum carotene	Serum vitamin B_{12}
Serum uric acid	ESR	Plasma vitamin C
Monoclonal gammopathy		Serum selenium
Serum fibrinogen		Plasma gammatocopherol (vitamin E)
Serum norepinephrine		T_3 when age $>$ 75 yr
Serum triglycerides		Serum testosterone
Serum glucose		Dihydroepiandrosterone
		Serum albumin
		Creatinine clearance†

* May be normal, even when renal function is abnormal—see text.
† See also FIG. 130-1.

presents hypothetical data comparing ultrasound and CT scan used individually and together to diagnose pancreatic carcinoma. When either test is positive, combined sensitivity is higher than either alone, but specificity is lower. When both tests are positive, the combined specificity is higher, but sensitivity is lower.

There is progressive decline in cardiac, pulmonary, renal, and metabolic function with age, but these occur at somewhat different rates. The declines correlate with changes in laboratory parameters (see TABLE 130-3). However, only relatively mild changes can be attributed to age alone, and not every elderly patient will show change.

Certain screening tests are very useful. Fasting blood glucose is useful and relatively inexpensive for the diagnosis of diabetes mellitus. Total cholesterol (TC) determined by a reliable laboratory is helpful in assessing risk for coronary artery disease. HDL cholesterol determination may also be required for a more accurate risk assessment. If triglycerides (TG) are also determined,

LDL cholesterol can then be calculated, using the following formula:

$$LDL = TC - HDL - \frac{TG}{5}$$

Serum creatinine is a useful screen for renal disease, except in the older patient, in whom measuring creatinine clearance is required because the age-related decline in muscle mass and consequent fall in creatinine production may result in normal serum creatinine levels even in the presence of renal disease (see FIG. 130-1).

Certain other tests commonly used for screening are not very useful. Abnormal total serum protein is not very sensitive for any of the conditions with which it is associated. A number of treatable diseases are associated with elevation of alkaline phosphatase. Routine screening of electrolytes is not indicated in the absence of clinical symptoms, history of vomiting or diarrhea, or history of drug ingestion. It has been

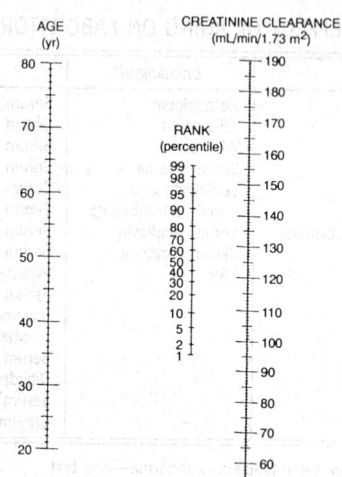

FIG. 130–1. Nomogram for determination of age-adjusted percentile rank in creatinine clearance of normal men. A straight line connecting the subject's age with his observed creatinine clearance intersects the rank scale at his percentile rank. (From *Aging—Its Chemistry*, edited by A Dietz. Washington, DC, American Association for Clinical Chemistry, 1980, p 8; used with permission.)

estimated that most screening tests yield < 5% unanticipated and potentially important findings.

The reliability of laboratory tests is closely related to disease prevalence. When prevalence is high, a positive result tends to confirm the diagnosis; when low, a normal result tends to exclude the diagnosis. For example, using a test with sensitivity and specificity of 94%, and with a 1% disease prevalence, the probability of disease with an abnormal test result is only 16%. Extreme values are more predictive than minimally abnormal ones.

TABLES 130–4 and 130–5 list commonly measured biochemical values and the effects of various diseases upon them.

TABLE 130–4. COMMON TESTS AND THEIR DISEASE ASSOCIATIONS

Laboratory Test	Increase	Decrease
Acid phosphatase	Prostatic carcinoma, postprostatic massage, prostatitis, myocardial infarction, excess platelet destruction, bone disease, liver disease	
Alanine aminotransferase (ALT or SGPT)	Hepatitis, cirrhosis, liver metastases, obstructive jaundice, infectious mononucleosis, hepatic congestion, pancreatitis, renal disease, ethanol ingestion	Pyridoxine (vitamin B_6) deficiency

(Continued)

TABLE 130–4. COMMON TESTS AND THEIR DISEASE ASSOCIATIONS *(Cont'd)*

Laboratory Test	Increase	Decrease
Albumin	Dehydration, diabetes insipidus	Overhydration, malnutrition, malabsorption, nephrosis, hepatic failure, burns, multiple myeloma, metastatic carcinomas
Alkaline phosphatase	Bone growth, bone metastases, Paget's disease, rickets, healing fracture, hyperparathyroidism, hepatic disease, obstructive jaundice, hepatic metastases, pulmonary infarction, heart failure, pregnancy	Pernicious anemia, hypoparathyroidism, hypophosphatasia
α-Fetoprotein	Hepatoma, testicular tumor, hepatitis	
Amylase	Pancreatitis, GI obstruction, mesenteric thrombosis and infarction, macroamylasemia, parotitis, mumps, renal disease, ruptured tubal pregnancy, lung carcinoma, acute ethanol ingestion, postoperative abdominal surgery	Marked pancreatic destruction
Aspartate aminotransferase (AST or SGOT)	Myocardial infarction, heart failure, myocarditis, pericarditis, myositis, muscular dystrophy, trauma, hepatic disease, pancreatitis, renal infarct, eclampsia, neoplasia, cerebral damage, seizures, hemolysis, ethanol	Pyridoxine (vitamin B_6) deficiency, terminal stages of liver disease
Bilirubin	Hepatic disease, obstructive jaundice, hemolytic anemia, pulmonary infarct, Gilbert's disease, Dubin-Johnson syndrome, neonatal jaundice	
Calcium	Hyperparathyroidism, bone metastases, myeloma, sarcoidosis, hyperthyroidism, hypervitaminosis D, malignancy without bone metastases, milk-alkali syndrome	Hypoparathyroidism, renal failure, malabsorption, pancreatitis, hypoalbuminemia, vitamin D deficiency, overhydration
Cholesterol	Hypothyroidism, obstructive jaundice, nephrosis, diabetes mellitus, pancreatitis, pregnancy, familial factors	Hyperthyroidism, infection, malnutrition, heart failure, malignancies, severe liver damage (due to chemicals, drugs, hepatitis)
HDL cholesterol	Vigorous exercise, increased clearance of triglyceride (VLDL), moderate ethanol consumption, insulin, estrogens	Starvation, obesity, cigarette smoking, diabetes mellitus, hypothyroidism, liver disease, nephrosis, uremia
Creatine kinase	Myocardial infarction, muscle disease, burns, chest trauma, collagen-vascular disease, meningitis, drugs (eg, lovastatin), burns, status epilepticus, brain infarction, hyperthermia, postoperative increase	

(Continued)

TABLE 130-4. COMMON TESTS AND THEIR DISEASE ASSOCIATIONS *(Cont'd)*

Laboratory Test	Increase	Decrease
Creatinine	Renal failure, urinary obstruction, dehydration, hyperthyroidism, diet, muscle disease	Aging
Glucose	Diabetes mellitus, IV glucose, thiazides, corticosteroids, pheochromocytoma, hyperthyroidism, Cushing's syndrome, acromegaly, brain damage, hepatic disease, nephrosis, hemochromatosis, stress (eg, emotion, burns, shock, anesthesia), acute or chronic pancreatitis, Wernicke's encephalopathy (vitamin B_1 deficiency), epinephrine, estrogens, ethanol, phenytoin, propranolol, chronic hypervitaminosis A	Excess insulin, insulinoma, Addison's disease, myxedema, hepatic failure, malabsorption, pancreatitis, glucagon deficiency, extrapancreatic tumors, early diabetes mellitus, postgastrectomy, autonomic nervous system disorders, idiopathic leucine sensitivity, enzyme diseases (von Gierke's disease, fructose intolerance), oral hypo-glycemic medications (factitious), malnutrition, alcoholism
Lactate dehydrogenase (LDH)	Myocardial infarction, pulmonary infarction, hemolytic anemia, pernicious anemia, leukemia, lymphoma, other malignancies, hepatic disease, renal infarction, seizures, cerebral damage, trauma, sprue	
Lipase	Same as amylase (except not in parotitis, mumps), macroamylasemia	
Magnesium	Renal disease, excess Mg (IV or po)	Diarrhea, malabsorption, renal tubular acidosis, acute tubular necrosis, chronic glomerulonephritis, drugs (diuretics, antibiotics), aldosteronism, hyperthyroidism, hypercalcemia, uncontrolled diabetes, nutritional deficit
Phosphorus	Renal failure, hypoparathyroidism, diabetic acidosis, acromegaly, hyperthyroidism, high phosphate intake (IV or po), vitamin D intoxication, lactic acidosis, cell lysis, leukemia, volume contraction, spurious, prolonged refrigeration of sample, heparin sodium contamination, hyperbilirubinemia, hyperlipidemia, dysproteinemia	Hyperparathyroidism, osteomalacia, rickets, Fanconi's syndrome, cirrhosis, hypokalemia, excess IV glucose, respiratory alkalosis, dietary deprivation, P-binding antacid, alcoholism, gout, hemodialysis
Potassium	Hyperkalemic acidosis, diabetic acidosis, hypoadrenalism, hereditary hyperkalemia, hemolysis, myoglobinuria, K-retaining diuretic, ACE inhibitors, large exogenous K load, renal tubular defect, thrombocytosis	Cirrhosis, malnutrition, vomiting, metabolic alkalosis, diarrhea, nephrosis, diuretics, hyperadrenalism, familial periodic paralysis, ectopic ACTH excess, β-hydroxylase deficiency

(Continued)

TABLE 130–4. COMMON TESTS AND THEIR DISEASE ASSOCIATIONS *(Cont'd)*

Laboratory Test	Increase	Decrease
Sodium	Dehydration, diabetes insipidus, excessive salt ingestion, diabetes mellitus with diuresis, diuretic phase of acute tubular necrosis, hypercalcemic nephropathy with diuresis, "essential" hypernatremia due to hypothalamic lesions	Excess antidiuretic hormone, nephrosis, hypoadrenalism, myxedema, heart failure, diarrhea, vomiting, diabetic acidosis, diuretics, adrenocortical insufficiency, spurious (serum osmolality is normal or increased—avoid by using direct-reading potentiometry with ion-selective electrode); hyperlipidemia (serum Na decreases by 1 mmol/L per every 4.6 gm/L increase in lipid), hyperglycemia (serum Na decreases 3 mEq/L per every 100 mg/dL increase of serum glucose), mannitol, hyperproteinemia (eg, multiple myeloma)
Total protein	Multiple myeloma, myxedema, lupus, sarcoidosis, diabetes insipidus, dehydration, collagen disease	Burns, cirrhosis, malnutrition, nephrosis, malabsorption, overhydration, GI protein loss
Triglyceride	Nephrosis, cholestasis, pancreatitis, cirrhosis, diabetes mellitus, hepatitis, dietary excess, hereditary	Malnutrition
Urea nitrogen	Renal disease, dehydration, GI bleeding, leukemia, heart failure, shock, postrenal azotemia, any obstruction of urinary tract (BUN:creatinine > 10:1), acute myocardial infarction	Hepatic failure, overhydration, pregnancy, acromegaly, diet, IV feedings only
Uric acid	Gout, renal failure, diuretic therapy, leukemia, lymphoma, polycythemia, acidosis, psoriasis, hypothyroidism, eclampsia, multiple myeloma, pernicious anemia, tissue necrosis, inflammation, 25% of relatives of patients with gout, cancer chemotherapy (eg, nitrogen mustards, vincristine, mercaptopurine), hemolytic anemia, sickle cell anemia, high-protein weight-reduction diet, lead poisoning, Lesch-Nyhan syndrome, polycystic kidneys, calcinosis universalis and circumscripta, hypoparathyroidism, sarcoidosis, elevated serum triglycerides	Uricosuric drugs, allopurinol, Wilson's disease, large doses of vitamin C, Fanconi's syndrome, xanthinuria

ACE = angiotensin converting enzyme; VLDL = very low density lipoprotein.
Based on material appearing in *Interpretation of Diagnostic Tests*, ed. 4, by J Wallach. Boston, Little, Brown and Company, 1986, pp 41–96; used with permission.

TABLE 130–5. URINE AND BLOOD CHANGES IN ELECTROLYTES, pH, AND VOLUME IN VARIOUS CONDITIONS

Measurement	Pulmonary emphysema	Congestive heart failure	Excessive sweating	Diarrhea	Pyloric obstruction	Dehydration	Starvation	Malabsorption	Salicylate intoxication	Primary aldosteronism	Adrenal cortical insufficiency	Diabetes insipidus	Diabetic acidosis	Thiazide administration	Renal tubular acidosis	Chronic renal failure	Acute renal failure
Blood sodium	N	N or D	D	D	D	I	N	D	N	I	D	N or I	D	D	D	D	D
Potassium	N	N	N	D	D	N	D	D	N or D	D	I	N	N or I	D	D	N or D	I
Bicarbonate	I	N	N	D	I	N or D	D	N or D	D	I	N or D	N	D	D	D	D	D
Chloride	D	D	D	D	D	I	N	N	I	D	D	I	D	D	I	D or N	I
Volume	N or I	I	N	D	D	D	N or D	D	N	N	D	D	D	D	D	V	I
Urine sodium	D	D	D	D	D	I	N or I	D	I	D	I	N	I	I	I	I	D
Potassium	N	N	N	N or D	N	I	I or N	D	N or I	I	N or D	N	I	I	I	I	D
pH	D	N	N	D	I	D	D	N or D	I	N or D	N or I	N	D	N or I	I	I	N or I
Volume	N	D	N	D	D	D	I	N	N	I	N or D	I	I	I	I	V*	D

* Usually increased.
N = normal; D = decreased; I = increased; V = variable.
Adapted from *Interpretation of Diagnostic Tests*, ed. 4, by J Wallach. Boston, Little, Brown and Company, 1986; used with permission.

NORMAL VALUES

TABLE 130–6 lists reference values for selected clinical laboratory tests. They reflect methods used at the Massachusetts General Hospital and published in *The New England Journal of Medicine*. Système international **(SI)** units are given in addition to conventional units. These international units have been used in the European literature for many years. Increasingly, the American literature is doing the same. The benefits include scientific standardization in reporting and the use of molar concentrations, which are more meaningful because they represent relative combining power of chemical species.

TABLE 130–6. NORMAL LABORATORY VALUES IN THE MASSACHUSETTS GENERAL HOSPITAL
BLOOD, PLASMA, OR SERUM VALUES

Determination	Reference Range		Minimal mL Required	Note
	Conventional	SI		
Acetoacetate plus acetone	Negative		1 – B	
Aldolase	1.3 – 8.2 u./L	22 – 137 nmol·sec^{-1}/L	2 – S	Use unhemolyzed serum
Ammonia	12 – 55 µmol/L	12 – 55 µmol/L	2 – B	Collect in heparinized tube; deliver *immediately* packed in ice
Amylase	53 – 123 u./L	884 – 2050 nmol·sec^{-1}/L	1 – S	
Ascorbic acid	0.4 – 1.5 mg/dL	23 – 85 µmol/L	7 – B	Collect in heparinized tube before any food is given
Bilirubin	Direct: up to 0.4 mg/dL Total: up to 1.0 mg/dL	Up to 7 µmol/L Up to 17 µmol/L	1 – S	
Blood volume	8.5 – 9.0% of body wt in kg	80 – 85 mL/kg		
Calcium	8.5 – 10.5 mg/dL (slightly higher in children)	2.1 – 2.6 mmol/L	1 – S	
Carbamazepine	4.0 – 12.0 µg/mL	17 – 51 µmol/L		
Carbon dioxide content	24 – 30 mEq/L	24 – 30 mmol/L	1 – S	Fill tube to top
Carbon monoxide	Less than 5% of total hemoglobin		3 – B	Fill tube to top
Carotenoids	0.8 – 4.0 µg/mL	1.5 – 7.4 µmol/L	3 – S	Vitamin A may be done on same specimen
Ceruloplasmin	23 – 43 mg/dL	1.5 – 2.9 µmol/L	2 – S	
Chloramphenicol	10 – 20 µg/mL	31 – 62 µmol/L	0.2 – S	
Chloride	100 – 108 mmol/L	100 – 108 mmol/L	1 – S	
Copper	Total: 70 – 150 µg/dL	11 – 24 µmol/L	1 – S	
Creatine kinase (CK)	Female: 10 – 79 u./L Male: 17 – 148 u./L	167 – 1317 nmol·sec^{-1}/L 283 – 2467 nmol·sec^{-1}/L	1 – S	
CK isoenzymes	5% MB or less		0.2 – S	
Creatinine	0.6 – 1.5 mg/dL	53 – 133 µmol/L	1 – S	
Ethanol	0 mg/dL	0 mmol/L	2 – B	Collect in oxalate and refrigerate
Glucose	Fasting: 70 – 110 mg/dL	3.9 – 5.6 mmol/L	1 – P	Collect with oxalate-fluoride mixture
Iron	50 – 150 µg/dL (higher in males)	9.0 – 26.9 µmol/L	1 – S	

(Continued)

TABLE 130–6. NORMAL LABORATORY VALUES IN THE MASSACHUSETTS GENERAL HOSPITAL (Cont'd)
BLOOD, PLASMA, OR SERUM VALUES (Cont'd)

Determination	Reference Range		Minimal mL Required	Note
	Conventional	SI		
Iron-binding capacity	250–410 μg/dL	44.8–73.4 μmol/L	1–S	
Lactic acid	0.5–2.2 mmol/L	0.5–2.2 mmol/L	2–B	Collect with oxalate-fluoride mixture; deliver immediately packed in ice
Lactic dehydrogenase	45–90 u./L	750–1500 nmol·sec⁻¹/L	1–S	Unsuitable if hemolyzed
Lead	50 μg/dL or less*	Up to 2.4 μmol/L	2–B	Collect with oxalate-fluoride mixture
Lipase	4–24 u./dL	667–4001 nmol·sec⁻¹/L	1–S	
Lipids Cholesterol Triglycerides	120–220 mg/dL 40–150 mg/dL	3.10–5.69 mmol/L 0.4–1.5 gm/L	1–S 1–S	Fasting Fasting
Lipoprotein electrophoresis (LEP)			2–S	Fasting; do not freeze serum
Lithium	0.5–1.5 mEq/L	0.5–1.5 mmol/L	1–S	
Magnesium	1.5–2.0 mEq/L	0.8–1.3 mmol/L	1–S	
5'-Nucleotidase	1–11 u./L	17–183 nmol·sec⁻¹/L	1–S	
Osmolality	280–296 mOsm/kg water	280–296 mmol/kg	1–S	
Oxygen saturation (arterial)	96–100%	0.96–1.001	3–B	Deliver in sealed heparinized syringe packed in ice
Pco₂	35–45 mm Hg	4.7–6.0 kPa	2–B	Collect and deliver in sealed heparinized syringe
pH	7.35–7.45	Same	2–B	Collect without stasis in sealed heparinized syringe; deliver packed in ice
Po₂	75–100 mm Hg (dependent on age) while breathing room air Above 500 mm Hg while on 100% O₂	10.0–13.3 kPa	2–B	
Phenobarbital	15–50 μg/mL	65–215 μmol/L	1–S	
Phenylalanine	0–2 mg/dL	0–120 μmol/L	0.4–S	
Phenytoin	Therapeutic level: 5–20 μg/mL	19.8–79.5 μmol/L	1–S	

Phosphatase (acid) Prostatic	0-0.8 u./L	0-13.3 nmol·sec⁻¹/L	1-S	Must always be drawn just before analysis or stored as frozen serum; avoid hemolysis

Test	Conventional	SI	Specimen	Comments
Phosphatase (acid) Prostatic	0-0.8 u./L	$0-13.3$ nmol·sec^{-1}/L	1-S	Must always be drawn just before analysis or stored as frozen serum; avoid hemolysis
Phosphatase (alkaline)	13-39 u./L; infants and adolescents up to 104 u./L	$217-650$ nmol·sec^{-1}/L; up to 1.26 μmol·sec^{-1}/L	1-S	
Phosphorus (inorganic)	3.0-4.5 mg/dL (infants in 1st year up to 6.0 mg/dL)	$1.0-1.5$ mmol/L	1-S	
Potassium	3.5-5.0 mEq/L	$3.5-5.0$ mmol/L	1-S	Serum must be separated promptly from cells
Primidone	Therapeutic level: 4-12 μg/mL	$18-55$ μmol/L	1-S	
Procainamide	4-10 μg/mL	$17-42$ μmol/L	1-S	
Protein: Total	6.0-8.4 gm/dL	$60-84$ gm/L	1-S	Globulin equals total protein minus albumin
Albumin	3.5-5.0 gm/dL	$35-50$ gm/L	1-S	Quantitation by densitometry
Globulin	2.3-3.5 gm/dL	$23-35$ gm/L	1-S	
Electrophoresis	% of total protein			
Albumin	52-68			
Globulin:				
α₁	4.2-7.2			
α₂	6.8-12			
β	9.3-15			
γ	13-23			
Pyruvic acid	0-0.11 mEq/L	$0-0.11$ mmol/L	2-B	Collect with oxalate-fluoride; deliver *immediately* packed on ice
Quinidine	1.2-4.0 μg/mL	$3.7-12.3$ μmol/L	1-S	
Salicylate	100-200 mg/L	$724-1448$ μmol/L	2-P	
Sodium	135-145 mEq/L	$135-145$ mmol/L	1-S	
Sulfonamide	5-15 mg/dL		2-P	
Transaminase (AST or SGOT) (ALT or SGPT)	7-27 u./L 1-21 u./L	$117-450$ nmol·sec^{-1}/L $17-350$ nmol·sec^{-1}/L	1-S	
Urea nitrogen (BUN)	8-25 mg/dL	$2.9-8.9$ mmol/L	1-S	
Uric acid	3.0-7.0 mg/dL	$0.18-0.42$ mmol/L	1-S	
Vitamin A	0.15-0.6 μg/mL	$0.5-2.1$ μmol/L	3-S	

(Continued)

TABLE 130–6. NORMAL LABORATORY VALUES IN THE MASSACHUSETTS GENERAL HOSPITAL *(Cont'd)*
URINE VALUES

Determination	Reference Range Conventional	Reference Range SI	Minimal Quantity Required	Note
Acetone plus acetoacetate (quantitative)	0	0 mg/L	2 mL	
Amylase	0–375 u./L	0–6251 nmol-sec^{-1}/L		
Calcium	300 mg/day or less	7.5 mmol/day or less	24-h specimen	Collect in special bottle with 10 mL of concentrated HCl
Catecholamines Epinephrine Norepinephrine	< 20 μg/day < 100 μg/day	< 109 nmol/day < 590 nmol/day	24-h specimen	Collect with 10 mL of concentrated HCl (pH should be 2.0–3.0)
Chorionic gonadotropin	0	0 arb. u.	First morning voiding	
Copper	0–100 μg/day	0–1.6 μmol/day	24-h specimen	
Coproporphyrin	50–250 μg/day Children < 80 lb (36 kg): 0–75 μg/day	80–380 nmol/day 0–115 nmol/day	24-h specimen	Collect with 5 gm of sodium carbonate
Creatine	< 100 mg/day or < 6% of creatinine. In pregnancy, up to 12%. In children < 1 yr, may equal creatinine; in older children, up to 30% of creatinine	< 0.75 mmol/day	24-h specimen	Order serum creatinine also
Creatinine	15–25 mg/kg/day	0.13–0.22 mmol·kg^{-1}/day	24-h specimen	
Cystine or cysteine	0	0	10 mL	Qualitative
Hemoglobin and myoglobin	0		Freshly voided sample	Chemical examination with benzidine
5-Hydroxyindole-acetic acid	2–9 mg/day (women lower than men)	10–45 μmol/day	24-h specimen	Collect in special bottle with 10 mL of concentrated HCl
Lead	*0.08 μg/mL or 120 μg or less/day*	*0.39 μmol/L or less*	*24-h specimen*	Collect in special bottle with 10 mL of concentrated HCl
Phosphorus (inorganic)	Varies with intake; average 1 gm/day	32 mmol/day	24-h specimen	
Porphobilinogen	0	0	10 mL	Use freshly voided urine
Protein: Quantitative	< 165 mg/24 h	< 0.16 gm/day	24-h specimen	

Determination	Conventional			SI		Minimal mL Required	Note
Steroids:							
17-Ketosteroids		mg/day			μmol/day	24-h specimen	Not valid if patient is receiving meprobamate
	Age	Male	Female	Male	Female		
	10	1–4	1–4	3–14	3–14		
	20	6–21	4–16	21–73	14–56		
	30	8–26	4–14	28–90	14–49		
	50	5–18	3–9	17–62	10–31		
	70	2–10	1–7	7–35	3–24		
17-Hydroxy-steroids	3–8 mg/day (women lower than men)			8–22 μmol/day as tetrahydrocortisol		24-h specimen	Keep cold; chlorpromazine and related drugs interfere with assay
Sugar:							
Quantitative glucose	0			0 mmol/L		24-h or other timed specimen	
Urobilinogen	Up to 1.0 Ehrlich u.			To 1.0 arb. u.		2-h specimen (1–3 PM)	
Uroporphyrin	0–30 μg/day			< 36 nmol/day		See Coproporphyrin	
Vanillylmandelic acid (VMA)	Up to 9 mg/24 h			Up to 45 μmol/day		24-h specimen	Collect as for catecholamines

SPECIAL ENDOCRINE TESTS

Determination	Reference Range		Minimal mL Required	Note
	Conventional	SI		
Steroid hormones				
Aldosterone	Excretion: 5–19 μg/24 h	14–53 nmol/day	5/day	Keep specimen cold
	Supine: 48 ± 29 pg/mL	133 ± 80 pmol/L	3–S,P	Fasting, at rest, 210-mEq Na diet
	Upright: (2 h) 65 ± 23 pg/mL	180 ± 64 pmol/L		Upright, 2 h, 210-mEq Na diet
	Supine: 107 ± 45 pg/mL	279 ± 125 pmol/L		Fasting, at rest, 110-mEq Na diet
	Upright: (2 h) 239 ± 123 pg/mL	663 ± 341 pmol/L		Upright, 2 h, 110-mEq Na diet
	Supine: 175 ± 75 pg/mL	485 ± 208 pmol/L		Fasting, at rest, 10-mEq Na diet
	Upright: (2 h) 532 ± 228 pg/mL	1476 ± 632 pmol/L		Upright, 2 h, 10-mEq Na diet
Cortisol	8 AM: 5–25 μg/dL	0.14–0.69 μmol/L	1–P	Fasting
	8 PM: < 10 μg/dL	0–0.28 μmol/L	1–P	At rest
	4-h ACTH test: 30–45 μg/dL	0.83–1.24 μmol/L	1–P	20 u. ACTH IV/4 h
	Overnight suppression test: < 5 μg/dL	< 0.14 nmol/L	1–P	8 AM sample after 0.5 mg dexamethasone at midnight
	Excretion: 20–70 μg/24 h	55–193 nmol/day	2–day	Keep specimen cold

(Continued)

TABLE 130–6. NORMAL LABORATORY VALUES IN THE MASSACHUSETTS GENERAL HOSPITAL (Cont'd)
SPECIAL ENDOCRINE TESTS (Cont'd)

Determination	Reference Range Conventional	SI	Minimal mL Required	Note
Dehydroepiandro-sterone (DHEA)	Male: 0.5–5.5 ng/mL	1.7–19 nmol/L	2–S,P	
	Female: 1.4–8.0 ng/mL	4.9–28 nmol/L		Adult
	0.3–4.5 ng/mL	1.0–15.6 nmol/L		Postmenopausal
Dehydroepiandro-sterone sulfate (DHEAS)	Male: 151–446 µg/mL	3.9–11.4 µmol/L	2–S,P	
	Female: 84–433 µg/mL	2.2–11.1 µmol/L		Adult
	1.7–177 µg/mL	0.04–4.5 µmol/L		Postmenopausal
11-Deoxycortisol	Responsive: > 7.5 µg/dL	> 0.22 µmol/L	1–P	8 AM sample preceded by metyrapone 4.5 gm orally/24 h or by single 2.5-gm dose orally at midnight
Estradiol	Male: < 50 pg/mL	< 184 pmol/L	5–S,P	
	Female: 23–361 pg/mL	84–1325 pmol/L		Adult
	< 30 pg/mL	< 110 pmol/L		Postmenopausal
	< 20 pg/mL	< 73 pmol/L		Prepubertal
Progesterone	Male: < 1.0 ng/mL	< 3.2 nmol/L	5–S,P	
	Female: 0.2–0.6 ng/mL	0.6–1.9 nmol/L		Follicular phase
	0.3–3.5 ng/mL	0.95–11 nmol/L		Midcycle peak
	6.5–32.2 ng/mL	21–108 nmol/L		Postovulatory phase
Testosterone	Adult male: 300–1100 ng/dL	10.4–38.1 nmol/L	1–P	AM sample
	Adolescent male: > 100 ng/dL	> 3.5 nmol/L		
	Female: 25–90 ng/dL	0.87–3.12 nmol/L		
Unbound testosterone	Adult male: 3.06–24 ng/dL	106–832 pmol/L	2–P	AM sample
	Adult female: 0.09–1.28 ng/dL	3.1–44.4 pmol/L		
Polypeptide hormones				
ACTH	15–70 pg/mL	3.3–15.4 pmol/L	5–P	Place specimen on ice and send promptly to laboratory. Use EDTA tube only
Calcitonin	Male: 0–14 pg/mL	0–4.1 pmol/L	5–S	Test done only on known or suspected cases of medullary carcinoma of the thyroid
	Female: 0–28 pg/mL	0–8.2 pmol/L		
	> 100 pg/mL in medullary carcinoma	> 29.3 pmol/L		
Follicle-stimulating hormone	Male: 3–18 mu/mL	3–18 arb. u.	5–S,P	Same sample may be used for LH
	Female: 4.6–22.4 mu/mL	4.6–22.4 arb. u.		Pre- or postovulatory
	13–41 mu/mL	13–41 arb. u.		Midcycle peak
	30–170 mu/mL	30–170 arb. u.		Postmenopausal
Growth hormone	< 5 ng/mL	< 233 pmol/L	1–S	Fasting, at rest
	Children: > 10 ng/mL	> 465 pmol/L		After exercise
	Male: < 5 ng/mL	< 233 pmol/L		
	Female: Up to 30 ng/mL	0–1395 pmol/L		
	Male: < 5 ng/mL	< 233 pmol/L		After glucose load
	Female: < 5 ng/mL	< 233 pmol/L		
Insulin	6–26 µu/mL	43–187 pmol/L	1–S	Fasting
	< 20 µu/mL	< 144 pmol/L		During hypoglycemia
	Up to 150 µu/mL	0–1078 pmol/L		After glucose load

Polypeptide hormones (cont'd)				
Luteinizing hormone	Male: 3–18 mu./mL Female: 2.4–34.5 mu./mL 43–187 mu/mL 30–150 mu/mL	3–18 arb. u. 2.4–34.5 arb.u. 43–187 arb.u. 30–150 arb.u.	5–S,P	Pre- or postovulatory Midcycle peak Postmenopausal
Parathyroid hormone	< 25 pg/mL	< 2.94 pmol/L	5–P	Keep blood on ice, or plasma must be frozen if it is to be sent any distance; AM sample
Prolactin	2–15 ng/ml	0.08–6.0 nmol/L	2–S	EDTA tubes, on ice; normal diet
Renin activity	Supine: 1.1 ± 0.8 ng/mL/h Upright: 1.9 ± 1.7 ng/mL/h Supine: 2.7 ± 1.8 ng/mL/h Upright: 6.6 ± 2.5 ng/mL/h Diuretics: 10.0 ± 3.7 ng/mL/h	0.9 ± 0.6 (nmol/L)h 1.5 ± 1.3 (nmol/L)h 2.1 ± 1.4 (nmol/L)h 5.1 ± 1.9 (nmol/L)h 7.7 ± 2.9 (nmol/L)h	4–P	Low Na diet
Somatomedin C (Sm-C, ICF-1)	0.08–2.8 u./mL 0.9–5.9 u./mL 0.34–1.9 u./mL 0.45–2.2 u./mL	0.08–2.8 arb.u. 0.9–5.9 arb.u. 0.34–1.9 arb.u. 0.45–2.2 arb.u.	2–P	Low Na diet Prepubertal During puberty Adult males Adult females
Thyroid hormones				
Thyroid-stimulating hormone (TSH)	0.5–5.0 μu./mL	0.5–5.0 mu./L	2–S	
Thyroxine-binding globulin capacity	15–25 μg T₄/dL	193–322 nmol/L	2–S	
Total triiodothyronine by radioimmuno-assay (T₃)	75–195 ng/dL	1.16–3.00 nmol/L	2–S	
Reverse diiodothyronine (rT₃)	13–53 ng/ml	0.2–0.8 nmol/L	2–S	
Total thyroxine by radioimmuno-assay (T₄)	4–12 μg/dL	52–154 nmol/L	1–S	
T₃ resin uptake	25–35%		2–S	
Free thyroxine index (FT₄I)	1–4	0.25–0.35	2–S	EDTA plasma

(Continued)

TABLE 130–6. NORMAL LABORATORY VALUES IN THE MASSACHUSETTS GENERAL HOSPITAL (Cont'd)

HEMATOLOGIC VALUES

Determination	Reference Range Conventional	Reference Range SI	Minimal mL Required	Note
Coagulation factors				
Factor I (fibrinogen)	0.15–0.35 gm/dL	4.0–10.0 μmol/L	4.5–P	Collect in vacuum tube containing sodium citrate
Factor II (prothrombin)	60–140%	0.60–1.40	4.5–P	Collect in plastic tubes with 3.8% sodium citrate
Factor V (accelerator globulin)	60–140%	0.60–1.40	4.5–P	Collect as for factor II
Factor VII-X (proconvertin-Stuart)	70–130%	0.70–1.30	4.5–P	Collect as for factor II
Factor X (Stuart factor)	70–130%	0.70–1.30	4.5–P	Collect as for factor II
Factor VIII (antihemophilic globulin)	50–200%	0.50–2.0	4.5–P	Collect as for factor II
Factor IX (plasma thromboplastic cofactor)	60–140%	0.60–1.40	4.5–P	Collect as for factor II
Factor XI (plasma thromboplastic antecedent)	60–140%	0.60–1.40	4.5–P	Collect as for factor II
Factor XII (Hageman factor)	60–140%	0.60–1.40	4.5–P	Collect as for factor II
Coagulation screening tests				
Bleeding time	3–9.5 min	180–570 sec		
Prothrombin time	< 2-sec deviation from control	< 2-sec deviation from control	4.5–P	Collect in vacuum tube containing 3.8% sodium citrate
Partial thromboplastin time (activated)	25–38 sec	25–38 sec	4.5–P	Collect in vacuum tube containing 3.8% sodium citrate
Whole-blood clot lysis	No clot lysis in 24 h	0/day	2.0 whole blood	Collect in sterile tube and incubate at 37°C
Fibrinolytic studies				
Euglobin lysis	No lysis in 2 h	0 (in 2 h)	4.5–P	Collect as for factor II
Fibrinogen split products	Negative reaction at > 1:4 dilution	0 (at > 1:4 dilution)	4.5–S	Collect in special tube containing thrombin and aminocaproic acid
Thrombin time	Control ± 5 sec	Control ± 5 sec	4.5–P	Collect as for factor II

"Complete" blood count			
Hematocrit	Male: 45–52% Female: 37–48%	0.45–0.52 0.37–0.48	1–B	Use EDTA as anticoagulant; the 7 listed tests are performed automatically on the Ortho ELT 800, which directly determines cell counts, Hb (as the cyanmethemoglobin derivative), and MCV, and computes Hct, MCH, and MCHC. MCV = mean corpuscular volume MCH = mean corpuscular hemoglobin MCHC = mean corpuscular hemoglobin concentration
Hemoglobin	Male: 13–18 gm/dL Female: 12–16 gm/dL	8.1–11.2 mmol/L 7.4–9.9 mmol/L		
Leukocyte count	4300–10,800/μL	4.3–10.8 × 10⁹/L		
Erythrocyte count	4.2–5.9 million/μL	4.2–5.9 × 10¹²/L		
MCV	86–98 μm³/cell	86–98 fl (femtoliter)		
MCH	27–32 pg	1.7–2.0 pg/cell		
MCHC	32–36%	0.32–0.36		
ESR	Male: 1–13 mm/h Female: 1–20 mm/h	1–13 mm/h 1–20 mm/h	5–B	Use EDTA as anticoagulant
Erythrocyte enzymes				
Glucose-6-phosphate dehydrogenase	5–15 u./gm Hb	5–15 u./gm	9–B	Use special anticoagulant (ACD solution)
Pyruvate kinase	13–17 u./gm Hb	13–17 u./gm	8–B	Use special anticoagulant (ACD solution)
Ferritin (serum) Iron deficiency	0–12 ng/mL (borderline: 13–20)	0–4.8 nmol/L (borderline: 5.2–8)		
Iron excess	> 400 ng/L	> 160 nmol/L		
Folic acid Normal	> 3.3 ng/mL	> 7.3 nmol/L	1–S	
Borderline	2.5–3.2 ng/mL	5.75–7.39 nmol/L	1–S	
Haptoglobin	40–336 mg/dL	0.4–3.36 gm/L	1–S	
Hemoglobin studies				
Electrophoresis for abnormal Hb			5–B	Collect with anticoagulant
Electrophoresis for A₂ Hb	1.5–3.5% (borderline: 0.3–3.5%)	0.015–0.035 (borderline: 0.03–0.035)	5–B	Use oxalate as anticoagulant
Fetal Hb	< 2%	< 0.02	5–B	Collect with anticoagulant
Met- and sulf-Hb	0	0	5–B	Use heparin as anticoagulant
Serum Hb	0–3 mg/dL	1.2–1.9 μmol/L	2–S	Any anticoagulant
Thermolabile Hb	0	0	1–B	Collect as for factor II
Lupus anticoagulant	0	0	4.5–P	

(Continued)

TABLE 130–6. NORMAL LABORATORY VALUES IN THE MASSACHUSETTS GENERAL HOSPITAL (Cont'd)
HEMATOLOGIC VALUES (Cont'd)

Determination	Reference Range		Minimal mL Required	Note
	Conventional	SI		
LE (lupus erythematosus) cell preparation				
Hargraves method	0		5–B	Use heparin as anticoagulant
Barnes method	0		5–B	Use defibrinated blood
Leukocyte alkaline phosphatase: Qualitative method	Males: 33–188 u. Females (off contraceptive pill): 30–160 u.	33–188 u. 30–160 u.	Smear-B	
Muramidase (lysozyme)	Serum: 3–7 μg/mL Urine: 0–2 μg/mL	3–7 mg/L 0–2 mg/L	1–S 1–U	
Osmotic fragility of erythrocytes	Increased if hemolysis occurs in > 0.5% NaCl; decreased if hemolysis is incomplete in 0.3% NaCl		5–B	Use heparin as anticoagulant
Peroxide hemolysis	< 10%	< 0.10	6–B	Use EDTA as anticoagulant
Platelet count	150,000–350,000/μL	150–350 × 10⁹/L	0.5–B	Use EDTA as anticoagulant. Counts are performed on Clay Adams Ultraflow. Low counts are confirmed by hand counting
Platelet function tests				
Clot retraction	50–100%/2 h	0.50–1.00/2h	4.5–P	Collect as for factor II
Platelet aggregation	Full response to ADP, epinephrine, and collagen	1.0	18–P	Collect as for factor II
Platelet factor 3	33–57 sec	33–57 sec	4.5–P	Collect as for factor II
Reticulocyte count	0.5–2.5% red cells	0.005–0.025	0.1–B	
Vitamin B₁₂	205–876 pg/mL (borderline: 140–204)	150–674 pmol/L (borderline: 102.6–149)	12–S	

CEREBROSPINAL FLUID VALUES

Determination	Reference Range		Minimal mL Required	Note
	Conventional	SI		
Bilirubin	0	0 μmol/L	2	
Cell count	0–5 mononuclear cells		0.5	
Chloride	120–130 mEq/L	120–130 mmol/L	0.5	20 mEq/L higher than serum chloride
Colloidal gold	0000000000–0001222111	same	0.1	
Albumin	Mean: 29.5 mg/dL ± 2 SD: 11–48 mg/dL	0.295 gm/L 0.11–0.48	2.5	
IgG	Mean: 4.3 mg/dL ±2 SD: 0–8.6 mg/dL	0.043 gm/L 0–0.086		
Glucose	50–75 mg/dL	2.8–4.2 mmol/L	0.5	30–50% less than blood glucose
Pressure (initial)	70–180 mm of water	70–180 arb. u.		
Protein: Lumbar Cisternal Ventricular	15–45 mg/dL 15–25 mg/dL 5–15 mg/dL	0.15–0.45 gm/L 0.15–0.25 gm/L 0.05–0.15 gm/L	1 1 1	

MISCELLANEOUS VALUES

Determination	Reference Range		Minimal mL Required	Note
	Conventional	SI		
Carcinoembryonic antigen (CEA)	0–2.5 ng/mL	0–2.5 μg/L	20–P	Must be sent on ice
Chylous fluid				Use fresh specimen
Digitoxin	9–25 μg/L	11.8–32.8 nmol/L	1–S	Medication with digitoxin or digitalis
Digoxin	0.9–2.0 ng/mL	1.15–2.56 nmol/L	1–S	
Gastric analysis	Basal: Females 2.0 ± 1.8 mEq/h Males 3.0 ± 2.0 mEq/h Maximal: (after histalog or gastrin) Females 16 ± 5 mEq/h Males 23 ± 5 mEq/h	0.6 ± 0.5 μmol/sec 0.8 ± 0.6 μmol/sec 4.4 ± 1.4 μmol/sec 6.4 ± 1.4 μmol/sec		

(Continued)

TABLE 130-6. NORMAL LABORATORY VALUES IN THE MASSACHUSETTS GENERAL HOSPITAL *(Cont'd)*
MISCELLANEOUS VALUES *(Cont'd)*

Determination	Reference Range Conventional	Reference Range SI	Minimal mL Required	Note
Gastrin-I	0–200 pg/mL	0–95 pmol/L	4–P	Heparinized sample
Immunologic tests				
α-Fetoglobulin	Undetectable in normal adults		2–S	
α 1–Antitrypsin	85–213 mg/dL	0.85–2.13 gm/L	10–B	Send to laboratory promptly
Antinuclear antibodies	Negative at a 1:8 dilution of serum		2–S	
Anti-DNA antibodies	Negative at a 1:10 dilution of serum		50–u	
Bence-Jones protein	Abnormal if present		10–B	Must be sent on ice
Complement, total hemolytic	150–250 u./mL			
C3	Range: 83–177 mg/dL	0.83–1.77 gm/L	2–S	
C4	Range: 15–45 mg/dL	0.15–0.45 gm/L	2–S	
Rheumatoid factor	< 60 IU/mL		10 mL clotted blood	Fasting sample preferred
Immunoglobulins				
IgG	639–1349 mg/dL	6.39–13.49 gm/L	2–S	
IgA	70–312 mg/dL	0.7–3.12 gm/L	2–S	
IgM	86–352 mg/dL	0.86–3.52 gm/L	2–S	
Viscosity	1.4–1.8 relative viscosity units		10–B	Expressed as the relative viscosity of serum compared with water
Iontophoresis	Children: 0–40 mEq Na/L	0–40 mmol/L		Value given in terms of sodium
	Adults: 0–60 mEq Na/L	0–60 mmol/L		
Stool fat	< 5 gm in 24 h or < 4% of measured fat intake in 3-day period	< 5 gm/day	24-h or 3-day specimen	
Stool nitrogen	< 2 gm/day or 10% of urinary nitrogen	< 2 gm/day	24-h or 3-day specimen	
Synovial fluid				
Glucose	Not < 20 mg/dL lower than simultaneously drawn blood sugar	See blood glucose	1 mL of fresh fluid	Collect with oxalate-floride mixture
D-Xylose absorption	5–8 gm/5 h in urine (40 mg/dL in blood after 2 h of ingestion of 25 gm D-xylose)	33–53 mmol (2.7 mmol/L)	5–U	Administer 25 gm of D-xylose orally
			5–B	

* Blood lead levels much lower than this are of concern in children. For discussion, see Ch. 30.
SI = Systeme International d'Unites; P = plasma; B = blood; S = serum; U = urine.
Modified from *The New England Journal of Medicine* 314(1):39–49, January 2, 1986, and 315(25):1606, December 18, 1986; used with permission of The Massachusetts General Hospital and *The New England Journal of Medicine.*

131. READY REFERENCE GUIDES

Milligram-Milliequivalent Conversions

The **milliequivalent (mEq)** expresses the chemical activity, or combining power, of a substance relative to the activity of 1 mg of hydrogen. Thus, 1 mEq is represented by 1 mg of hydrogen, 23 mg of sodium, 39 mg of potassium, 20 mg of calcium, and 35 mg of chlorine. Conversion equations are as follows:

$$mEq/L = \frac{(mg/L) \times valence}{formula\ wt}$$

$$mg/L = \frac{(mEq/L) \times formula\ wt}{valence}$$

(NOTE: formula wt = atomic or molecular wt)

The mEq is roughly equivalent to the **milliosmole (mOsm)**, the unit of measure of osmolality or tonicity. Normally, the body fluid compartments each contain about 280 mOsm/L of solute.

TABLE 131–1. METRIC SYSTEM

Weight:

1 kilogram (kg)	= 1000 grams (10^3 gm)
1 gram (gm)	= 1000 milligrams (10^3 mg)
1 milligram (mg)	= 1000 micrograms (10^{-3} gm)
1 microgram (μg)	= 1000 nanograms (ng) (10^{-6} gm)
1 millimicrogram (mμg)	= 1000 picograms (pg) (10^{-9} gm)

Volume:

1 liter (L)	= 1000 milliliters (mL)
	= 1000 cubic centimeters (cc)

TABLE 131–2. METRIC–NONMETRIC EQUIVALENTS (approximate)

Liquid:		Weight:	
30 mL	= 1 fluid ounce	65 mg	= 1 grain (gr)
250 mL	= 8+ fluid ounces	28.35 gm	= 1 ounce (oz)
500 mL	= 1+ pint	1 kg	= 2.2 pounds (lb)
1000 mL	= 1+ quart	**Linear:**	
(1 liter)		1 millimeter (mm)	= 0.04 inch (in.)
		1 centimeter (cm)	= 0.4 inch
		2.5 centimeters	= 1 inch
		1 meter (m)	= 39.37 inches

TABLE 131–3. HOUSEHOLD NONMETRIC–METRIC EQUIVALENTS
(approximate)

1 teaspoon (tsp)	=	4 mL
1 teaspoon, medical	=	5 mL
1 dessert spoon	=	8 mL
1 tablespoon (tbsp)	=	15 mL = ½ fluid ounce
1 cup	=	240 mL = 8 fluid ounces

TABLE 131–4. ATOMIC WEIGHTS OF SOME COMMON ELEMENTS
(approximate)

Hydrogen (H)	= 1	Magnesium (Mg)	= 24
Carbon (C)	= 12	Phosphorus (P)	= 31
Nitrogen (N)	= 14	Chlorine (Cl)	= 35.5
Oxygen (O)	= 16	Potassium (K)	= 39
Sodium (Na)	= 23	Calcium (Ca)	= 40

TABLE 132–5. CENTIGRADE–FAHRENHEIT EQUIVALENTS

Centigrade°	Fahrenheit°	Centigrade°	Fahrenheit°
Freezing (water at sea level):		Pasteurization (holding),* 30 min at:	
0	32	62.8	145.0
Clinical range:		Pasteurization (flash),* 15 sec at:	
36.0	96.8	71.7	161.0
36.5	97.7	Boiling (water at sea level):	
37.0	98.6		
37.5	99.5	100.0	212.0
38.0	100.4		
38.5	101.3		
39.0	102.2		
39.5	103.1	Conversion	
40.0	104.0	To convert °F to °C, subtract 32, then multiply by	
40.5	104.9	$5/9$ or 0.555	
41.0	105.8	To convert °C to °F, multiply by $9/5$ or 1.8, then	
41.5	106.7	add 32.	
42.0	107.6		

* According to the Food and Drug Administration Code of Federal Regulations, 1991.

132. CROSS–CULTURAL ISSUES IN MEDICINE
(Folk Medicine; Ethnomedicine)

As immigration from developing to developed nations increases, physicians are likely to encounter patients with a great variety of "unscientific" indigenous medical beliefs and practices **(ethnomedicine)**, which may seem foreign, irrational, or simply wrong and an impediment to delivering health care; this need not be so.

Contemporary biomedicine is a highly refined form of folk medicine. It is the traditional practice in industrialized Western nations, carries tremendous emotional and intellectual weight, and is based on empiric science; folk medicine is equally dependent on empiric observation.

People who have been immersed in ethnomedicine throughout their lives often feel threatened or intimidated by biomedicine. When physicians reject their traditional beliefs, patients may avoid necessary biomedical attention. Thus, optimal care may be achieved by combining biomedicine and ethnomedicine. This requires cross-cultural tolerance and an understanding of key ethnomedical concepts.

Health, disease, and illness are fundamental concepts of biomedical care. **Health** is *an existential state of bio-organic, emotional, and spiritual harmony.* **Disease** is *an abnormal state of health,* caused by inherent dysfunction, or invasion by or exposure to some foreign agent. **Illness** is *the individual experience of disease.* These definitions vary in different cultures.

Health is generally defined either in experiential or functional terms. **Experiential health** is *the individual idea of health* (the individual's sense of accommodation and reaction to the socially prescribed scenario), while **functional health** is *the socially defined concept of health* (the ability to fulfill socially predicated roles and obligations, eg, work, parenting). The two are interdependent and often commingled, with **individual health** being *able to do what the individual wants, even though those wants are defined by culture.* Patient descriptions of their state of health may be based on any of these definitions, necessitating some physician probing. For example, a young Egyptian man presents with hematuria caused by schistosomiasis. To him, hematuria (male menstruation) may be considered "normal" if it does not interfere with lifestyle; ie, he believes he is in good health. Alternatively, the patient may be physically sound but unable to perform culture-bound duties and therefore may consider himself ill. For example, in some areas of Mexico, insufficient money to meet social obligations (from poverty or overspending) may be considered due to "money illness."

Disease may be defined as the result of organ or social dysfunction or as a sense of individual or social unease. However, physical and social processes tend to overlap.

Social problems can be considered manifestations of illness with a clear folk cause. Indeed, organic illness may be interpreted to signify an underlying social problem; eg, an immigrant family from a rural background moves to an urban setting in the USA. The youngest daughter develops abdominal cramps, vomiting, and fever. Rather than seek medical attention, the family may try to determine a folk cause, such as a breach of some taboo or failure to maintain ritual obligations. The family is more likely to atone for such perceived lapses of behavior than seek medical therapy.

Immigrants may subscribe to a **humoral theory** of disease and medicine (probably the most universal pattern, prevalent among cultures from Africa, India, Southeast Asia, China, Japan, Mexico, and Central and South America). Usually, health is perceived as a state of balance between "hot and cold" elements. Treatment may require **opposites** (hot conditions require cold medicine), **analogs** (hot conditions require hot medicine), or **some combination.** "Temperature" of medicines is based on a variety of characteristics; eg, some Middle Eastern cultures consider oral contraceptives hot since they stop menstrual flow (dry the womb), while other cultures use color (blue pills are cold). Thus, when prescribing drugs, is the form, color, or method of application acceptable? If not (as noncompliance will often result), can an alternative be pre-

scribed? If the patient is concerned about the color, explaining that the color makes the pill seem better to most patients in the USA (or other developed country) or that under the coating the medicine is a neutral color may induce patient cooperation.

Aside from ideas of causality, **folk ideas of contagion** can be important in treating patients and preventing further illness. In many areas of the world, folk practitioners have incorporated germ theory into their causal repertoire, but this should not imply Western knowledge of *germ-based* contagion. In Mexico, for example, some practitioners claim that germs cause disease, yet they engage in nonsterile practices (eg, recycling hypodermic needles, sharing unwashed utensils with sick parties, allowing patently ill persons to prepare food) because they believe that if God or spirits want one to fall ill, nothing can be done. Contagion involves the transfer of some essence from one entity to another, often by modes that seem magical. In a sense, this is justified, since magic deals with the unseen world. Spirits and gods, germs and viruses are equally invisible to the unaided eye, and a specialist must manipulate technologies to reveal them (whether it involves transmitted light microscopy or trance states). Once the causal agent is identified, treatment can begin. Thus, the approach in traditional and biomedical technologies is similar in form if not in content.

Major differences in content between folk and biomedical concepts (**ethnophysiology**) can affect health care delivery. For example, as with hematuria in certain Egyptian communities, *Ascaris* infection is considered quite normal in some places and even essential to digestion of food. This is analogous to the nutritional role of certain members of the GI microflora in biomedicine. Thus, eradication may be culturally unfeasible and would be resisted. Indeed, if an infected patient is made acutely ill by the worms, it may be considered due to his no longer being a good host. The patient wants to placate the worms; the physician wants to eradicate them. Some middle ground must be found; eg, if the patient has become a bad host, perhaps the worms need an incentive—in the form of a helminthicide—to move elsewhere.

Ethnophysiologic ideas may also dictate suitable food and medicines and prevent weakened and debilitated patients from taking necessary drugs. For example, an anemic patient is weak and therefore (by folk logic) has a weak stomach. He may refuse to take iron supplements in tablet form because the pill is hard, therefore hard to digest. In such a case, liquid supplements should be prescribed.

Folk ideas about strength extend to **fertility.** For example, in some areas of South Asia, strength of the egg is believed to wane during the course of the menstrual cycle. This idea makes intercourse desirable from 4 to 16 days after menstruation, and couples will abstain from sexual relations after the 16th day for fear of engendering a "weak" child. Where this practice precludes fertility, the couple often cannot be induced to engage in intercourse outside this "window of strength."

Many ideas about strength involve **blood.** Many cultures (especially the Middle East and Mexico) hold that humans have a fixed amount of blood, making it often hard to solicit blood for transfusion or examination. Little can be done except to bargain with the donor or patient. However, the patient often will gratefully accept a transfusion (blood may be more valuable than gold). Alternatively, he may reject a transfusion because of questionable moral, spiritual, or ethnic characteristics of the donor that are believed to be contagious. Explanations must be individualized.

Perhaps the most frustrating aspect of cross-cultural medicine is the phenomenon of **culture-bound syndromes.** These have no clear analog in biomedicine and most commonly involve folk concepts of causality. **Supernatural causation** (eg, witchcraft, spirit attack, soul loss, breach of taboo) or **natural causation** (eg, hot/cold imbalance, heavy/light food ingestion) or some combination are the usual factors. These syndromes may seem farfetched and magical but can (and often do) cause death. Many have presentations that, in some ways, mimic recognized biomedical disease.

Spirit disease is *a disorder of the soul or spirit.* A foreign spirit force (eg, ghost) enters the body; some portion of the patient's soul is lost or stolen **(susto);** or the disease is retribution for broken taboos, in which the soul of the individual is severely traumatized, resulting in illness.

Spirit disease is quite common in African, Asian, Latin American, and native North American groups. Typical biomedical symptoms include seizure, trance states, amenorrhea, fever, lethargy, and malaise. Folk symptoms include fear, laziness, and general misfortune.

Often, no biomedical explanation is found and these disorders can prove refractory to standard biomedical therapies. Folk therapy consists of determining the type of spirit disease, its "causative and operative agents," and the appropriate steps to restore proper social or religious balance.

Presumed causality dictates acceptable therapy. An immigrant from rural Latin America who has experienced a fright may suffer from soul loss (susto). This can manifest as lethargy, anxiety, fever, and malaise. Thus, a susto victim may appear to be suffering from nutritional deficiencies, anemia, or even shock, but treatment of these will not alleviate the underlying problem. In another example of susto, a person may fall victim to a magical projectile (an imagined invisible intrusion into the body, which may cause systemic or local reactions, or both). A suppurative sore may be blamed on such a projectile. Antibacterial therapy will promote a remission, but infection will recur until the offending object is "removed" by a folk specialist. Surgical excision is not the answer.

Spirit disease (susto is one of many) and spirit deaths may have analogs in biomedicine. Labeled psychogenic illness or psychogenic death, these conditions reflect the **"giving up/given up" syndrome,** in which patients who feel helpless and hopeless develop a withdrawal-depression that may be a precipitating factor in organic disease or even lead to death. If spirit and psychogenic ailments are analogous, the two systems of medical practice have common ground.

For the physician to cope with culture-bound syndromes, humoral medicine, and "odd" ideas of physiology, the key is tolerance and acceptance of cultural variation without judgment (**cultural relativism**). While physicians are not expected to know the details of the many folk modalities used around the world, some factors are universal, allowing a common approach. In the course of patient and family interviews, one should find out the country of origin, the sort of medicine practiced, and whether the patient interacts with a community of other immigrants. If so, there may be folk (traditional) therapists in that community, offering the possibility of conjoint therapy. Allowing the patient to benefit from a belief in traditional medical practices can be therapeutic and may allow needed biomedical treatment.

If the goal is the maintenance of or a return to health, all available mechanisms should be used. If an immigrant patient presents with an atypical syndrome or if an apparently recognizable syndrome proves refractory to standard therapy, ask the patient what would be done in his native country. If he states that a traditional therapist would be visited, consider referring him to one and even making contact with that practitioner (establishing good rapport can lead to mutual patient referral, with improved patient care). This requires mutual trust and respect between practitioners and is facilitated by a relativistic rather than a judgmental attitude.

§11. CLINICAL PHARMACOLOGY

133. DRUG INPUT AND DISPOSITION

Drugs are compounds almost always foreign to the body. As such, they are not continually being formed and eliminated as are endogenous substances. The processes of inputting, distributing, and eliminating drugs are therefore of paramount importance in determining the onset, duration, and intensity of effect.

DRUG ABSORPTION

The process of drug movement from the site of administration toward the systemic circulation.

Drug product: *The actual dosage form of a drug, consisting of the drug itself plus other ingredients formulated into a usable medicine; eg, as a tablet, capsule, or solution.* Drug products are formulated for administration by a variety of routes, including oral, buccal, sublingual, rectal, parenteral, topical, and inhalational. The physicochemical properties of drugs, their formulations, and the routes of administration are important in absorption. A prerequisite to absorption of any drug is that it be able to enter into solution. The solid drug product (eg, tablet) must undergo disintegration and deaggregation, and the active ingredients must undergo dissolution before the drug can be absorbed.

Except when given IV, a drug must traverse several semipermeable cell membranes before reaching the general circulation. These membranes act as biologic barriers that selectively inhibit the passage of drug molecules. Cell membranes are composed primarily of a bimolecular lipid matrix, containing mostly cholesterol and phospholipids, in which are embedded globular protein macromolecules of random size and composition. The membrane proteins may be involved in transport processes and may also function as receptors for cellular regulatory mechanisms. Membrane lipid provides stability to the membrane and determines its permeability characteristics.

Processes

The processes by which drugs move across a biologic barrier include passive diffusion, facilitated diffusion, active transport, and pinocytosis.

Passive diffusion: *Transport across a cell membrane in which the driving force for movement is the concentration gradient of the solute.* Most drug molecules are transported across a membrane by simple diffusion from a high concentration area (eg, GI fluids) to a low concentration area (eg, blood) without expenditure of energy. The net rate of diffusion is directly proportional to this net gradient and depends upon lipid solubility, degree of ionization, molecular size, and the area of the absorptive surface. Since the drug is rapidly removed by the systemic circulation and distributed into a large volume, the concentration of drug in blood is initially low compared with that at the site of administration. The resulting large concentration gradient serves as the driving force for absorption. However, since the cell membrane is lipoidal in nature, drugs that are lipid soluble diffuse more rapidly than drugs that are relatively lipid insoluble. Furthermore, small molecules tend to penetrate membranes more rapidly than do large ones.

Most drugs exist as weak organic acids or bases in both nonionized and ionized forms in an aqueous environment. The nonionized fraction is usually lipid soluble and diffuses readily across cell membranes. The ionized form cannot penetrate the cell membrane easily because of its low lipid solubility. The charged groups on the surface of the cell membrane may also impede passage of the ionized form. Thus, the combination of low lipid solubility and high electrical resistance can make penetration of the ionized form so slow that what does penetrate may be attributed mainly to the nonionized form.

Consequently, equilibrium in the distribution of a weak electrolyte across a membrane is determined by the pK_a of the substance and the pH gradient when a pH gradient exists. The extent of ionization of a weak electrolyte on the 2 sides of a membrane differ—for a weak acid, the higher the pH, the lower the ratio of nonionized to ionized fractions. Consider the partitioning of a weak acid (eg, pK_a 4.4) between plasma and gastric fluid. In plasma (pH 7.4) the ratio of nonionized to ionized forms is 1:1000; in gastric fluid (pH 1.4) the ratio is reversed, ie, 1000:1. When the weak acid is given orally, a large concentration gradient is established between the stomach and the plasma, a condition favorable to diffusion through the gastric mucosa. At equilibrium, the concentrations of nonionized drug in the stomach and in the plasma are equal because it is the only chemical species that can penetrate the membranes. In contrast, the concentration of ionized drug in the plasma at equilibrium will be approximately 1000 times greater than that in the gastric lumen. For a weak base with a pK_a of 4.4, the situation is reversed. Thus, weakly acidic drugs (eg, aspirin) theoretically should be more readily absorbed from an acid medium (gastric lumen) than weak bases (eg, quinidine). However, regardless of pH, most drug absorption occurs in the small intestine as discussed under Oral Administration, below.

Facilitated diffusion: For certain molecules (eg, glucose), the rates of penetration are greater than expected from their low lipid solubility and the concentration gradients present. It is postulated that a "carrier component" combines reversibly with the substrate molecule at the cell membrane exterior and that the carrier-substrate complex diffuses rapidly across the membrane with release of the substrate at the interior surface. This carrier-mediated diffusion process is characterized by **selectivity** and **saturability**. The carrier mechanism accepts for transport only those substrates having a relatively specific molecular configuration, and the process is limited by the availability of carrier. No expenditure of energy is required by this process; substrate is not transported against a concentration gradient.

Active transport: In addition to selectivity and saturability, active transport *requires energy expenditure by the cell, and substrates may accumulate intracellularly against a concentration gradient.* Active transport processes appear to be limited to agents with structural similarities to normal body constituents. These agents are usually absorbed from specific sites in the small intestine. Active transport processes have been identified for various ions, vitamins, sugars, and amino acids.

Pinocytosis refers to *the engulfing of particles or fluid by a cell.* The cell membrane invaginates, encloses the particle or solute, and then fuses again, forming a vesicle that later buds off within the interior of the cell. This mechanism also requires the expenditure of energy. Pinocytosis probably plays a minor role in drug transport.

Oral Administration

Because the oral route of administration is the most common, absorption usually refers to the transport of drugs across the membranes of the epithelial cells within the GI tract. Absorption after oral administration is confounded by differences down the alimentary canal in the luminal pH; surface area per luminal volume; perfusion of the tissue, bile, and mucus flow; and the epithelial membranes. The faster absorption of acids in the intestine compared with the stomach appears to contradict the hypothesis that the nonionized form of a drug more readily crosses membranes. The discrepancy can be reconciled by the greatly increased surface area and a greater permeability of the membranes in the small intestine.

Gastric emptying and intestinal transit time: Because the absorption of virtually all compounds is faster from the small intestine than from the stomach, the rate of gastric emptying is a controlling step. Food, especially fatty foods, slows gastric emptying, which explains why some drugs are recommended to be taken on an empty stomach when a rapid onset of action is desired. The extent of absorption may be enhanced by food if the drug is poorly soluble (eg, griseofulvin) or reduced if degraded in the stomach (eg, penicillin G). Drugs that affect gastric emptying (eg, parasympatholytic agents) also affect the rate of absorption of other drugs.

The rate of transit down the intestines can also influence drug absorption. This is particularly true for drugs that are absorbed by a facilitated transport process (eg, the B vitamins), are dissolved slowly (eg, griseofulvin), or are too polar to cross the membranes readily (eg, many antibiotics).

Absorption from solution: Drug given orally in solution may be absorbed along the entire alimentary canal, but to do so it must pass through various fluids and tissues and survive encounters with several enzyme systems. The **oral mucosa** has a thin epithelium and a rich vascularity that favors drug absorption, but solutions are in contact too briefly for absorption to be appreciable.

The **stomach** has a relatively large epithelial surface, but because of the mucous layer and the relatively short time a drug spends there, the extent and rate of absorption depend on how long the drug remains in the stomach. For some drugs, eg, penicillin G, physiologic processes that delay gastric emptying increase the degradation of the drug in the stomach and profoundly decrease systemic absorption. The acidic environment of the stomach favors the absorption of weak acids that are largely lipid soluble and nonionized.

The **small intestine** presents the largest GI surface area for absorption; however, its environment varies. In the duodenum the pH is 4 to 5, but the intraluminal pH becomes progressively more alkaline farther along the alimentary canal (eg, the pH of the lower ileum is about 8). The GI flora may inactivate certain drugs, reducing their absorption and bioavailability. Decreased blood flow (eg, in shock) may lower the concentration gradient across the intestinal mucosa and decrease absorption by passive diffusion. (Decreased peripheral blood flow also alters drug distribution and metabolism.)

In contrast to the small intestine, the **large intestine** has no villi. Nevertheless, molecules that escape absorption in the small intestine may be absorbed here, albeit less efficiently.

Absorption from solid dosage forms: Most orally administered drugs are in the form of tablets or capsules primarily for convenience, economy, stability, and patient acceptance. They must disintegrate and dissolve before absorption can occur. **Disintegration** greatly increases the surface area of the drug in contact with the GI fluids, thereby promoting dissolution. Disintegrants and other excipients (eg, diluents, lubricants, surfactants, binders, and dispersants) are often added during manufacturing to facilitate these processes. Factors capable of varying or retarding disintegration of solid dosage forms include excessive pressure applied during the tableting procedure and special coatings applied to protect the tablet from the digestive processes of the gut. Hydrophobic lubricants (eg, magnesium stearate) may bind to the active drug and reduce its bioavailability. Surfactants increase the wetability, solubility, and dispersibility of the active drug and thereby increase its dissolution rate.

The **dissolution rate** determines the availability of the drug for absorption. When slower than the absorption process itself, dissolution becomes the rate-limiting step, and overall absorption can be altered by manipulating the drug or the dosage formulation. Factors that affect the dissolution rate include salt form, particle size, crystal form, and hydration states; eg, the Na salts of weak acids (eg, barbiturates and salicylates) dissolve faster than their corresponding free acids regardless of the pH of the medium. Reduction of particle size is frequently used to increase the surface area of a drug and is effective in increasing the rate and extent of GI absorption of a drug for which absorption is normally rate-limited by slow dissolution. Certain drugs exhibit polymorphism, existing in

amorphous or various crystalline forms. Chloramphenicol palmitate exists in 2 polymorphs, but only one form gives sufficient dissolution and absorption to be of clinical value. A hydrate is formed when one or more water molecules combine with a drug molecule in crystal formation. The solubility of such a solvate may be markedly different from the nonsolvated form; eg, anhydrous ampicillin has a greater rate of dissolution and in vivo absorption than its corresponding trihydrate.

Food can delay the stomach's emptying and the entry of drug particles into the intestine. Giving drugs with food may reduce (eg, increased degradation of penicillin by stomach acid), enhance (eg, the poorly soluble drug griseofulvin given after a high-fat meal), or have little or no effect on the extent of absorption.

Parenteral Administration

Direct placement of a drug into the bloodstream (usually IV) ensures complete delivery of the dose to the general circulation. However, administration by a route that requires drug transfer through one or more biologic membranes to reach the bloodstream precludes a guarantee that all of the drug will eventually be absorbed. IM or s.c. injection of drugs bypasses the skin barrier, but the drug must penetrate the capillary walls. Because the capillaries tend to be highly porous, the perfusion (blood flow/gram of tissue) is a major factor in the rate of absorption. Thus, the injection site can markedly influence a drug's absorption rate; eg, the absorption rate of diazepam injected IM into a site with poor blood flow can be much slower than that following an oral dose.

Absorption may be delayed or erratic when salts of poorly soluble acids and bases are injected IM; eg, the parenteral form of phenytoin is a 40% propylene glycol solution of the Na salt with a pH of about 12. When the solution is injected IM, the propylene glycol is absorbed and the tissue fluids, acting as a buffer, decrease the pH, producing a shift in the equilibrium between the ionized and free acid forms of the drug. The poorly soluble free acid then precipitates. Subsequently, dissolution and absorption occur very slowly (over 1 or 2 wk).

Absorption via the lymphatic system contributes little to the total absorption of drug molecules because the flow of lymph is relatively slow. However, lymphatic absorption may be significant in the case of larger molecules (eg, insulin) or highly lipid-soluble drugs (eg, griseofulvin).

Controlled-Release Dosage Forms

Controlled-release dosage forms are designed to reduce the frequency of dosing and to maintain more uniform plasma drug concentrations, thus providing a more uniform pharmacologic effect. Additionally, greater patient convenience (less frequent administration) may improve compliance with the prescribed regimen. Ideally, suitable drugs for such dosage forms are those that require frequent dosing because of a short biologic half-life and a short duration of effect.

Oral controlled-release dosage forms are often designed to maintain therapeutic concentrations of drug for 12 h or more. They generally release a normal therapeutic dose of drug initially, and subsequently release sustaining amounts more slowly. Reduction of the absorption rate can be achieved in various ways; eg, by coating the drug particles with wax or related water-insoluble material, by embedding the drug in a matrix from which it is released slowly during transit through the GI tract, or by complexing the drug with ion-exchange resins.

Topical controlled-release dosage forms have been designed to provide drug release for extended periods; eg, clonidine diffusion through a membrane provides controlled drug delivery over a period of 1 wk, and nitroglycerin-impregnated polymer bonded to an adhesive bandage provides controlled drug delivery over a period of 24 h. Drugs for transdermal delivery must have suitable skin penetration characteristics and high potency.

Many nonintravenous parenteral preparations have been formulated to provide sustained blood levels. In some cases, insoluble salts (eg, penicillin G benzathine) injected IM may provide activity for several weeks or a month. For other drugs, suspensions or solutions in nonaqueous vehicles are formulated; eg, insulin may be injected in crystalline suspensions for prolonged action. Amorphous insulin, with a high surface area for dissolution, has an intermediate onset and duration. The procaine salt of penicillin is poorly soluble and slowly absorbed when injected IM.

BIOAVAILABILITY

The rate at which and the extent to which the active moiety (drug or metabolite) enters the general circulation, thereby gaining access to the site of action.

While the physicochemical properties of a drug govern its absorptive potential, the properties of the dosage form can also be a major determinant of its bioavailability. Hence, the concept of equivalence among drug products is important in clinical decisions. **Chemical (pharmaceutical)** equivalence refers to *drug products that contain the same compound in the same amount and that meet current official standards;* however, inactive ingredients in the drug products may differ. **Bioequivalence** refers to *chemical equivalents that, when administered to the same individual in the same dosage regimen, result in equivalent concentrations of drug in blood and tissues.* Therapeutic equivalence refers to *2 drug products that, when administered to the same individual in the same dosage regimen, provide essentially the same therapeutic effect or toxicity; they may or may not be bioequivalent.*

The concept of bioavailability relates to the efficiency of the dosage formulation as an extravascular drug delivery system and permits comparison of drug products for relative availability or bioequivalence. It includes consideration of both the amount and rate of absorption into the systemic circulation following extravascular administration, although the term generally refers to the extent of input only. Bioavailability depends upon a number of factors, including how a drug product is designed and manufactured, its physicochemical properties, and factors that relate to the physiology and pathology of the patient.

Although a drug may be absorbed completely, its rate of absorption may also be important. It may be too slow to attain a therapeutic blood level in an acceptable period of time or too rapid, resulting in toxicity from high drug levels just after each dose.

Causes of Low Values of Bioavailability

When a drug rapidly dissolves from a drug product and readily passes across membranes, absorption from most sites of administration tends to be complete. This is not always the case for drugs given orally. Before reaching the vena cava, a drug must move down the alimentary canal and pass through the gut wall and liver, which are common sites of drug metabolism; thus, the drug may be metabolized before it can be measured in the general circulation. This cause of a decrease in drug input is called the **first-pass effect.** A large number of drugs show low bioavailabilities owing to extensive first-pass metabolism. In many instances, the extraction is so complete that the bioavailability is virtually zero (eg, isoproterenol, norepinephrine, phenacetin, and testosterone).

The 2 other most frequent causes of low bioavailability are an insufficient time in the GI tract and the presence of competing reactions. Ingested drug is exposed to the entire GI tract for no more than 1 to 2 days and to the small intestine for only 2 to 4 h, unless gastric emptying is considerably delayed. If the drug does not dissolve readily or if the drug is incapable of penetrating the epithelial membrane (highly ionized and polar), there may be insufficient time at the absorption site. Not only is the bioavailability low in this case, but it tends to be highly variable. In addition, individual variations in age, sex, activity, genetic phenotype, stress, disease (eg, achlorhydria, malabsorption syndromes), and previous GI surgery can alter and further increase variability in drug bioavailability.

Reactions that compete with absorption can reduce bioavailability. These include complex formation (eg, tetracycline complexes with polyvalent metal ions), hydrolysis by gastric pH or digestive enzymes (eg, penicillin and chloramphenicol palmitate hydrolysis), conjugation in gut wall (eg, sulfoconjugation of isoproterenol), adsorption to other drugs (eg, digoxin and cholestyramine), and metabolism by luminal microflora.

Estimation of Bioavailability

Bioavailability considerations are encountered most commonly for orally administered drugs. The bioavailability value is determined by measuring either the concentration of drug in plasma or the amount excreted unchanged in urine.

Differences in the bioavailability of various pharmaceutical formulations of a given drug have clinical significance. Differences between individuals and even within the same individual at different times make its assessment difficult. Such assessment is further complicated because bioavailability of a preparation in man does not always correlate with laboratory tests (eg, tablet dissolution rate) or with studies in animals.

Poor bioavailability is most commonly seen with oral dosage forms of poorly water-soluble, slowly absorbed drugs. Slow or incomplete absorption is often associated with capricious results, since more factors affect bioavailability in this situation than when drugs are rapidly and completely absorbed. Therapeutic problems are encountered most frequently during long-term therapy when a patient who is stabilized on one pharmaceutical formulation receives a nonequiv-

alent substitute. Clinically important examples of ineffective therapy or toxicity resulting from substitution of nonequivalent dosage forms have been noted previously for several drugs, eg, digoxin and phenytoin.

Sometimes therapeutic equivalence may be achieved despite differences in bioavailability; eg, the margin between an effective concentration of penicillin and its toxic level is so wide that the prescribed dosage usually achieves a blood concentration far above the minimum effective level. Moderate blood concentration differences due to bioavailability differences in penicillin products might therefore not affect therapeutic effect or safety. In contrast, bioavailability differences would be important for a drug with a relatively narrow range between therapeutic and toxic levels.

Assessment of bioavailability from plasma concentration–time data usually involves 3 measurements: the maximum (or peak) plasma drug concentration, the time of occurrence of maximum plasma drug concentration, and the area under the plasma concentration–time curve (see Fig. 133–1). The plasma drug concentration increases with the rate and extent of absorption; the peak is reached when the rate of drug removal equals the rate of absorption. The slower the absorption, the later the time when the peak is reached.

Bioavailability determinations based on the peak plasma concentration can be misleading, since drug removal begins immediately upon entry into the bloodstream. The peak plasma concentration time is related to the absorption rate and is the most widely used general index of the rate. The **area under the concentration curve (AUC)** is the most important measurement of bioavailability. It is directly proportional to the total amount of unchanged drug in the body. To determine AUC accurately, blood must be sampled at frequent intervals and over a length of time sufficient to observe virtually complete elimination. Drug products may be considered bioequivalent in both extent and rate of absorption if their plasma-level curves are essentially superimposable. Two drug products that have similar AUCs but different shapes of plasma concentration–time profiles are equivalent in *extent* but are absorbed at different *rates*.

Single vs. Multiple Doses

Multiple dosing permits evaluation of bioavailability. This procedure has advantages; eg, it may more closely represent the usual clinical sit-

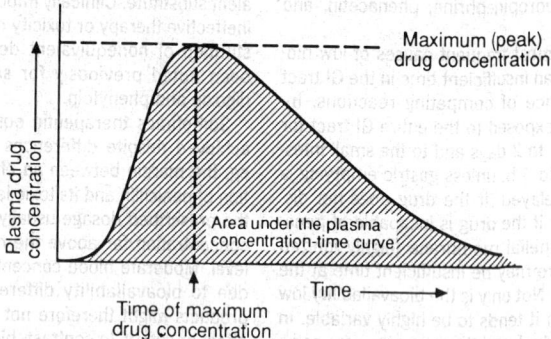

Maximum (peak) drug concentration

Area under the plasma concentration-time curve

Time of maximum drug concentration

Time ⟶

FIG. 133—1. Representation of the plasma concentration—time relationship after a single dose of a hypothetical drug.

uation; also, plasma levels higher than those following a single dose are usually achieved, facilitating drug analyses. After repetitive dosing at a fixed-dosing interval for 4 or 5 elimination half-lives, the blood concentration should approximately reach steady state. The extent of absorption can then be analyzed by measuring the AUC during one of the dosing intervals, but the AUC over a full 24-h period is probably preferred because of diurnal variations in physiologic functions and because the dosing intervals and absorption rates may not be the same throughout the day.

For drugs that are primarily excreted unchanged in the urine, bioavailability may be estimated by measuring the total amount of drug excreted. Ideally, urine should be collected over a period of 7 to 10 elimination half-lives for complete recovery of the drug and to evaluate the extent of absorption. Comprehensive bioavailability studies utilize both plasma and urinary excretion data.

DRUG DISTRIBUTION

After a drug enters the general circulation, it distributes throughout the body's tissues. Distribution is generally uneven because of differences in binding in tissues, regional variations in pH, and differences in the permeability of cellular membranes.

The rate of entry of a drug into a tissue depends upon the rate of blood flow to the tissue, the tissue mass, and the partition characteristics of the drug between blood and tissue. Richly vascularized ar-

eas achieve equilibrium with blood (rates in and out are the same) more rapidly than do poorly perfused areas, unless diffusion across membrane barriers is the rate-limiting step. After **distribution equilibrium** is attained, the concentrations of drug in tissues and extracellular fluids are reflected by the plasma concentration. Metabolism and excretion occur simultaneously with distribution, making the process dynamic and complex. The measurement of the extent of drug distribution is described in Ch. 134, while factors affecting drug distribution are discussed below.

Dilution Space

The volume of fluid into which a drug appears to be distributed or diluted is called the **apparent volume of distribution**. Every drug is distributed in the body in a unique manner. Some prefer to go into fat, others remain in the ECF, while still others are bound avidly to specific tissues, as occurs frequently in liver or kidney. The apparent volume of distribution does not provide information on the specific pattern of distribution, but it does provide a reference for the concentration expected for a given dose and, conversely, the dose required to achieve a given concentration.

Typical values of volume of distribution are shown in TABLE 133—1.

Many acids (eg, warfarin and salicylic acid) are highly protein bound and thus have a small volume of distribution. Many bases (eg, amphetamine and meperidine) are avidly taken up by the tissues and thus have a volume of distribution that is larger than the volume of the entire body. This seeming paradox is the result of the definition of the "apparent" volume of distribution.

TABLE 133–1. VOLUMES OF DISTRIBUTION OF SELECTED DRUGS

Drug	L/70 kg	Drug	L/70 kg
Warfarin	8	Quinidine	189
Aspirin	12	Amitriptyline	581
Gentamicin	18	Pentamidine	1,500
Theophylline	35	Chloroquine	15,000
Acetaminophen	66	Quinacrine	40,000
Procainamide	133		

Binding Components

The extent of the distribution of drugs into tissues depends on binding to plasma proteins and tissue components.

Plasma protein binding: Drugs are transported in the bloodstream partly in solution (as free drug) and partly bound to various blood components (eg, plasma proteins and blood cells). The major determinant of the ratio of bound to free drug in plasma is the reversible interaction between a drug molecule and a molecule of the protein to which it binds, an interaction governed by the Law of Mass Action. Many plasma proteins can interact with drugs. Albumin, α_1-acid glycoprotein, and lipoproteins are the most important ones. Acidic drugs are generally bound more extensively to albumin, while basic drugs often are more extensively bound to either one or both of the latter 2 proteins. TABLE 133–2 gives examples of the extent of drug binding to plasma proteins.

Because only the unbound form is available for passive diffusion to the extravascular or tissue sites where pharmacologic effects occur, plasma protein binding influences the distribution and apparent relationship between pharmacologic activity and plasma (total) drug concentration. As free drug leaves the circulation, the remaining protein-bound form (eg, sulfonamides) may be confined largely to the plasma compartment, serving as a depot that can release more drug as it is removed from the circulation by distribution, metabolism, and excretion. As the dose of a drug increases, the number of sites occupied approaches a limit, the number of sites totally available for binding. The binding is then said to show **saturability.** This kinetic behavior is the basis of displacement interactions among drugs (see DRUG INTERACTIONS in Ch. 137).

The fraction unbound (ratio of unbound and total concentrations) is often more useful than the fraction bound. The unbound drug is believed to be more closely related to drug at the active site and, therefore, to the drug's effects. The fractions unbound for the representative drugs are also given in TABLE 133–2.

Tissue Binding

The **substances to which drugs bind** in tissue are highly varied. Often these substances are not proteins. Furthermore, they may be very specific, as is the case for the binding of chloroquine to nucleic acids. Tissue binding usually involves an association of drug with a macromolecule within an aqueous environment. Another kind of association that results in apparent tissue binding is **partitioning of drug into body fat.** Because fat is poorly perfused, the equilibration time is long for this tissue.

Drug reservoir: Accumulation of drugs in tissues or body compartments can prolong drug action because the tissues serve as depots. As the plasma level declines, stored drug is released into the circulation, prolonging the sojourn of drug in plasma and the drug action. The location of the active site and the relative differences in tissue distribution can also be important. The anesthetic thiopental is an example of a drug in which storage in tissue reservoirs shortens the drug effect initially but later may prolong it. Thiopental is highly lipid soluble and rapidly distributes to the brain following a single IV injection. After a few minutes of drug buildup in brain, the tissue concentration declines in parallel with that in plasma, and the termination of anesthesia ends rapidly as the drug distributes to more slowly perfused tissues of the body. Thus, following a single dose, anesthesia is terminated rapidly because of a redistribution of drug. However, if drug levels are followed long enough, a third phase of distribution, which represents slow release of drug from fat, can be distinguished. With continued administration of thiopental, large amounts can

TABLE 133-2. EXTENT OF BINDING OF SELECTED DRUGS IN HUMAN PLASMA

Drug	% Bound	% Unbound
Warfarin	99.5	0.5
Diazepam	99	1
Furosemide	96	4
Dicloxacillin	94	6
Propranolol*	93	7
Phenytoin	89	11
Quinidine*	71	29
Lidocaine*	51	49
Digoxin	25	75
Gentamicin	3	97
Atenolol	~0	~100

* Significant binding to α_1-acid glycoprotein and/or lipoproteins.

accumulate and be stored in fatty tissue; these tissues can then act as a reservoir for the drug and prolong its anesthetic action.

Some drugs accumulate in cells in higher concentrations than those in ECF. Such accumulation most commonly involves binding of drugs with protein, phospholipids, or nucleic acids. Antimalarial agents such as chloroquine are notorious for total intracellular binding and can reach intracellular concentrations in eye and liver tissue that are thousands of times higher than those in plasma. The stored drug is in equilibrium with that in plasma and moves into the plasma as the drug is eliminated from the body, but its rate of release is sometimes too slow to produce and maintain a plasma concentration that produces pharmacologic effects. Consequently, this type of storage represents a site of loss (and possible local toxicity) rather than a depot for continued systemic drug action.

Passage of drugs into the CNS takes place in the capillary circulation and the CSF. Although the brain receives a large proportion of the cardiac output (about 1/6), distribution of drugs to brain tissue is restricted. While some lipid-soluble drugs (eg, thiopental) do enter and exert their pharmacologic effects rapidly, many drugs, particularly the more water-soluble agents, enter the brain slowly. The endothelial cells of the brain capillaries, which appear to be more tightly joined to one another than are those of other capillary beds, contribute to the slow diffusion of water-soluble substances. Another important barrier to water-soluble substances is the close approximation of the glial connective tissue cells (astrocytes) to the basement membrane of the capillary endothelium. The capillary endothelium and the astrocytic sheath together are referred to as the **blood-brain barrier**. They confer permeability characteristics on the brain different from those of other tissues in that the barrier is associated with the capillary wall and not the parenchymal cell. Thus, polar compounds are unable to enter the brain but can access the interstitial fluids of most other tissues.

Drugs may enter the ventricular CSF directly via the choroid plexus, gaining access to brain tissue by passive diffusion from the CSF. The choroid plexus is also a site of active transport of organic acids (eg, penicillin) from CSF to blood.

The major **factors determining the rate** of drug penetration into the CSF or into other tissue cells include the extent of protein binding, the degree of ionization, and the lipid-water partition coefficient of the compound. The penetration rate into the brain is slow for highly protein-bound drugs; for the ionized form of weak acids and bases, penetration can be so slow as to be virtually nonexistent. Differences in pH between the plasma and brain compartments may appreciably influence the distribution ratio of drugs between the compartments through an ion-trapping effect. Under normal conditions there is a small pH difference between plasma (pH 7.4) and CSF (pH 7.3).

For other tissues of the body, perfusion is a major determinant of the drug distribution rate. The CNS is so well perfused that permeability is generally the major factor. However, for poorly perfused tissues (eg, muscle and fat), distribu-

TABLE 133-3. EXAMPLES OF DRUGS WITH
THERAPEUTICALLY IMPORTANT METABOLITES

Drug	Metabolite
Acetohexamide	Hydroxyhexamide
Aspirin*	Salicylic acid
Amitriptyline	Nortriptyline
Chloral hydrate*	Trichloroethanol
Chlordiazepoxide	Desmethylchlordiazepoxide
Codeine	Morphine
Diazepam	Desmethyldiazepam
Flurazepam	Desethylflurazepam
Glutethimide	4-Hydroxyglutethimide
Imipramine	Desipramine
Lidocaine	Desethyllidocaine
Meperidine	Normeperidine
Phenacetin*	Acetaminophen
Phenylbutazone	Oxyphenbutazone
Prednisone*	Prednisolone
Primidone*	Phenobarbital
Procainamide	N-acetylprocainamide
Propranolol	4-Hydroxypropranolol

* Prodrugs; metabolites are primarily responsible for their therapeutic effects.

tion is greatly prolonged, especially if the tissue has a high affinity for the drug.

DRUG ELIMINATION

The sum of the processes of drug loss from the body. Removal of drugs from the body occurs by **metabolism** and **excretion**.

METABOLISM

The process of chemical alteration of drugs in the body. The liver is the principal, but not the sole, site of drug metabolism. Some metabolites are pharmacologically active (see TABLE 133–3). When the substance administered is inactive and an active metabolite is produced, the administered compound is called a **prodrug**. Metabolic reactions may be classified as nonsynthetic and synthetic.

Classification

In **nonsynthetic reactions**, the drug is chemically altered by either (1) oxidation, (2) reduction, (3) hydrolysis, or (4) a combination of these

processes. These reactions usually represent only the first stage of biotransformation; metabolic products formed may subsequently undergo a synthetic reaction prior to elimination. The metabolites of nonsynthetic processes may be pharmacologically active. Most oxidation and reduction reactions are catalyzed by the microsomal enzyme systems in the endoplasmic reticulum of the liver. Hydrolysis reactions and a few oxidative and reductive reactions are mediated by nonmicrosomal enzyme systems.

Examples of drugs metabolized by nonsynthetic reactions include amphetamine, chlorpromazine, imipramine, meprobamate, phenacetin, phenobarbital, phenytoin, procainamide, quinidine, and warfarin.

In **synthetic reactions** (or **conjugations**), the parent drug, or intermediate formed by nonsynthetic reactions, combines with an endogenous substrate, such as an amino acid or glucuronic acid, to yield an addition or conjugation product. Metabolites formed from synthetic reactions are usually biologically inactive and, because they are more polar, are more readily excreted by the kidney (in urine) and the liver (in bile) than those derived from nonsynthetic reactions. Although the synthetic products are often pharmacologically inert, such is not always the case.

Several synthetic reactions are frequently encountered. **Glucuronidation,** the most common synthetic reaction, is the only one that takes place in the liver microsomal enzyme system. Glucuronides are eliminated in the urine and secreted in the bile. Examples of drugs metabolized this way are salicylic acid, morphine, meprobamate, and chloramphenicol. **Amino acid conjugation** with glutamine and glycine produces conjugates that are readily excreted in the urine but are not extensively secreted via bile. **Acetylation** is the primary metabolic pathway for sulfonamides. Other drugs that are acetylated include hydralazine, isoniazid, and procainamide. **Sulfoconjugation** is the reaction between phenolic or alcoholic groups and inorganic sulfate, which is partially derived from sulfur-containing amino acids such as cysteine. The sulfate esters formed are polar and readily excreted in the urine. **Methylation** is a major metabolic pathway for inactivation of some catecholamines. Other compounds that are methylated are niacinamide and thiouracil.

Changes with Age

Neonates have partially developed liver microsomal enzyme systems and, consequently, have difficulty with the metabolism of many drugs (eg, hexobarbital, phenacetin, amphetamine, and chlorpromazine). The experience with chloramphenicol in neonates highlights the serious consequences that can occur because of slower conversion to the glucuronide. Equivalent mg/kg doses of chloramphenicol that are well tolerated by older patients can result in serious toxicity in neonates (the gray baby syndrome) and are associated with prolonged and elevated blood levels of chloramphenicol. Elderly patients often show a reduced ability to metabolize drugs. The reduction varies depending on the drug and is not as severe as that in neonates. (See DRUG THERAPY IN THE ELDERLY in Ch. 124.)

Individual Variation

Variability among individuals (see also Ch. 137) makes it difficult to predict the clinical response to a given dose of a drug. Some patients may metabolize a drug so rapidly that therapeutically effective blood and tissue levels are not achieved; in others, metabolism may be so slow that toxic effects result with usual doses.

For example, plasma phenytoin levels vary from 2.5 to > 40 mg/L in different persons given the same dose. Some of this variability is due to differences in the amount of the key enzyme, cytochrome P-450, available in the liver, and to differences in the affinity of the enzyme for the drug. Genetic factors play a major role in determining these differences. Concurrent disease states, particularly chronic liver disease, drug interactions, especially those involving induction or inhibition of metabolism, and other factors also contribute.

Capacity Limitation

Drugs are metabolized by enzymes that share the kinetic property of having an upper limit on the rate at which they can catalyze a reaction. Thus, the rate of metabolism by any metabolic pathway is expected to show a capacity limitation. At therapeutic concentrations, usually only a small fraction of the enzyme sites is occupied. Occasionally, most of the enzyme sites are occupied. Under these circumstances the rate of metabolism does not increase in proportion to the drug concentration. The result is capacity-limited metabolism. Examples of compounds showing these properties are phenytoin and alcohol.

EXCRETION

The process by which either a drug or a metabolite is eliminated from the body without further change in its chemical form. The kidney is the major organ of excretion and is responsible for eliminating water-soluble substances. The biliary system also excretes certain drugs and metabolites. Although drugs may also be eliminated via other pathways (eg, intestine, saliva, sweat, breast milk, and lungs), the overall contribution of these routes is generally small. An exception is the excretion of volatile anesthetics via the lung in expired air. Although elimination via breast milk may not be important to the mother, it may be to the suckling infant.

RENAL EXCRETION

Glomerular filtration and tubular reabsorption: About $^1/_5$ of the plasma reaching the glomerulus is filtered through pores in the glomerular endothelium; the remainder passes along the efferent arterioles to the renal tubules. Drugs bound to plasma proteins are not filtered; only unbound drug appears in the filtrate. The principles that govern renal tubular reabsorption of drugs are those of any transmembrane passage.

Polar compounds and ions are unable to diffuse back into the circulation and are excreted unless a specific transport mechanism for their reabsorption exists, eg, as there is for glucose, ascorbic acid, and the B vitamins.

Effects of urine pH: Although the glomerular filtrate that enters the proximal tubule has the same pH as plasma, the pH of voided urine varies from 4.5 to 8.0, and this may markedly affect the rate of drug excretion. Since the nonionized forms of nonpolar weak bases and weak acids tend to be reabsorbed readily from tubular urine, acidification of the urine increases reabsorption (ie, decreases excretion) of weak acids and decreases reabsorption of weak bases (ie, are excreted more rapidly). The opposite is true for alkalinization of urine.

These principles may be applied in some cases of overdosage to enhance the elimination of weakly basic or acidic drugs. With the weak acids phenobarbital or aspirin, for example, alkalinization of the urine increases their excretion. Conversely, acidification may accelerate the urinary elimination of certain bases, such as methamphetamine. The overall extent to which changes in urinary pH alter the rate of drug elimination depends upon the contribution of the renal route to total elimination, as well as the polarity (of nonionized form) and the degree of ionization of the molecule.

Tubular secretion: Mechanisms for active tubular secretion exist in the proximal tubule and are important in the elimination of many drugs; eg, penicillin, mecamylamine, and salicylic acid. This process is energy-dependent and may be blocked by metabolic inhibitors. The secretory transport capacity can be saturated at high concentrations, and each substance has its own characteristic maximum secretion rate, termed **transport maximum.** Anions and cations are handled by separate transport mechanisms. Normally, the anion secretory system eliminates metabolites that have been conjugated with glycine, sulfate, or glucuronic acid. The various anionic compounds compete with one another for secretion. This tendency can be used therapeutically; eg, probenecid blocks the normally rapid tubular secretion of penicillin, resulting in higher plasma penicillin concentrations for a longer time. Organic cations also compete with each other but usually not with anions.

BILIARY EXCRETION

Drugs and their metabolites that are extensively excreted in the bile are transported across the biliary epithelium against a concentration gradient, requiring an active secretory process. This mechanism may become saturated by high plasma concentrations of a drug (transport maximum), and substances with similar physicochemical properties may compete for excretion via the same mechanism.

Biliary elimination is enhanced by a mol wt > 300 (smaller molecules are generally secreted only in negligible amounts); the presence of both polar and lipophilic groups; and conjugation, particularly with glucuronic acid. Biliary excretion is only occasionally a major route of drug elimination.

When a drug undergoes biliary secretion and reabsorption from the intestine, it completes an **enterohepatic cycle.** Drug conjugates that are secreted into the intestine also undergo enterohepatic cycling when the conjugate is hydrolyzed and the drug reabsorbed. Biliary excretion is a route of elimination from the body only to the extent that the enterohepatic cycling is incomplete, ie, when all the secreted drug is not reabsorbed from the intestines.

134. KINETIC PRINCIPLES OF DRUG ADMINISTRATION
(Pharmacokinetics)

The study of the time course of a drug and its metabolites in the body following drug administration by any route.

Drugs are administered to achieve a therapeutic objective. This usually requires the attainment and maintenance of a pharmacologic response, which in turn requires an appropriate concentration of drug at the site of action. The appropriate concentration and the dosage needed to achieve it depend upon the patient's clinical state, the severity of the condition being treated, the presence of other drugs and concurrent disease, and other factors.

TABLE 134–1. BASIC PHARMACOKINETIC PARAMETERS AND THEIR DEFINING RELATIONSHIPS

Relationship		Parameter		
Absorption				
1. Rate of absorption	=	Absorption rate constant	×	Amount remaining to be absorbed
2. Amount absorbed	=	Bioavailability	×	Dose
Distribution				
3. Amount in body	=	Volume of distribution	×	Plasma drug concentration
4. Unbound drug concentration in plasma	=	Fraction unbound	×	Plasma drug concentration
Elimination				
5. Rate of elimination	=	Clearance	×	Plasma drug concentration
6. Rate of renal excretion	=	Renal clearance	×	Plasma drug concentration
7. Rate of metabolism	=	Metabolic clearance	×	Plasma drug concentration
8. Rate of renal excretion	=	Fraction excreted unchanged	×	Rate of elimination
9. Rate of elimination	=	Elimination rate constant*	×	Amount in body

* Another conceptually useful parameter is biologic half-life. Its relationship to the elimination rate constant is half-life = 0.693/(elimination rate constant).

The pharmacologic response observed relative to the concentration at the active site depends upon the **pharmacodynamics** of the drug, while the attainment and maintenance of the appropriate concentration are a function of the **pharmacokinetics** of the drug. The former is concerned with how a drug acts on the body; the latter deals with how the body acts on a drug.

Because of individual differences, successful therapy requires planning drug administration according to each patient's needs. Traditionally, this has been accomplished by empirically adjusting dosage until the therapeutic objective is met. This method is frequently inadequate because of delays or undue toxicity. An alternative approach is to initiate drug administration according to the expected absorption and disposition (distribution and elimination) of the drug in a patient and to adjust dosage by monitoring the plasma drug concentration, a reflector of drug at the active site, in addition to drug effects. This approach requires knowledge of the drug's pharmacokinetics as a function of age and weight, and the kinetic consequences of the presence of renal, hepatic, cardiovascular, or a combination of diseases.

To identify and quantitate the variables in pharmacokinetics, isolation of the input and disposition processes is helpful. Absorption, distribution, and elimination and the factors affecting them are described in Ch. 133.

BASIC PHARMACOKINETIC PARAMETERS

The pharmacokinetic behavior of most drugs may be summarized by parameters that relate variables to each other (see TABLE 134–1). The parameters are constants, although their values may differ from patient to patient and in the same patient under different conditions.

Bioavailability and Absorption Rate Constant

The extent of drug absorption into the general circulation is expressed by the **bioavailability**, as defined in Ch. 133, the fraction of a dose reaching the plasma site of measurement. The speed of absorption is often expressed by the **absorption rate constant,** provided absorption follows Relationship 2 in TABLE 134–1. Changes in these 2 parameters influence the maximum (or peak) concentration, the time at which the maximum concentration occurs, and the area under the concentration-time curve after a single oral dose. In chronic drug therapy, bioavailability is the more important measurement because it relates to the average level obtained, whereas the degree of fluctuation is related to the absorption rate constant.

Volume of Distribution and Unbound Fraction

The **apparent volume of distribution** and the **fraction unbound** in plasma are the 2 most widely used parameters for drug distribution. The volume of distribution is useful because it allows estimation of the dose required to achieve a given concentration and, conversely, the concentration achieved on administering a given dose. The unbound fraction is useful because it relates the measured total concentration to the unbound concentration, which is presumably more closely associated with drug effects. It is a particularly useful parameter when plasma protein binding is altered, eg, in hypoalbuminemia, renal disease, hepatic disease, and displacement interactions.

Clearance, Renal Clearance, and Fraction Excreted Unchanged

The rate at which a drug is eliminated from the body is proportional to the plasma concentration, Relationship 5, TABLE 134–1; the parameter relating the two is clearance. The parameters relating rates of renal excretion and metabolism to the plasma concentration are **renal clearance,** Relationship 6, and **metabolic clearance,** Relationship 7, respectively. Because the rate of elimination is the sum of the rates of renal excretion and extrarenal elimination, usually metabolism, it follows that

Total clearance = Renal clearance + Extrarenal (metabolic) clearance

The ratio of the rate of renal excretion to the rate of total elimination, also the ratio of renal clearance to (total) clearance, is the **fraction excreted unchanged,** Relationship 8, TABLE 134–1. This parameter is useful in assessing the potential effect of renal and hepatic diseases on drug elimination.

The rate of extraction of a drug from the blood in an eliminating organ, such as the liver, cannot exceed the rate of its presentation to the organ. Thus, clearance has an upper limit. When high extraction exists, elimination is limited by drug delivery and hence by blood flow to the organ. Furthermore, when the eliminating organ is the liver or gut wall and a drug is given orally, a portion of the dose administered may be lost on its requisite passage through the tissues enroute to the general circulation. This is called the **first-pass effect;** it applies to metabolism in the gut wall as well as in the liver. Thus, whenever a drug is highly extracted (high clearance) in either of these locations, the bioavailability is low due to first-pass elimination, sometimes precluding oral administration or resulting in an oral dose much larger than an equivalent parenteral dose. A large first-pass effect is shown by a number of drugs, such as alprenolol, hydralazine, isoproterenol, lidocaine, meperidine, morphine, nifedipine, nitroglycerin, propranolol, and verapamil.

Elimination Rate Constant and Half-life

The **elimination rate constant** relates the rate of elimination to the amount of drug in the body. As the rate of elimination equals clearance times plasma drug concentration (Relationship 5, TABLE 134–1) and the amount of drug in the body equals volume of distribution times plasma drug concentration (Relationship 3), it follows that

$$\text{Elimination rate constant} = \frac{\text{Clearance}}{\text{Volume of distribution}}$$

Expressed in these terms, the elimination rate constant is a function of how a drug is cleared from the blood by the eliminating organs and how the drug distributes throughout the body.

Half-life (elimination) is a convenient parameter. It is the time required for the plasma drug concentration or the amount in the body to decrease by 50%. For most drugs, the half-life remains constant regardless of how much drug is in the body. It is related to the elimination rate constant by

$$\text{Half-life} = \frac{0.693}{\text{Elimination rate constant}}$$

Mean Residence Time

Another measure of elimination is mean residence time **(MRT),** *the average time a drug molecule resides within the body after rapid administration of a single IV dose.* Like clearance, its

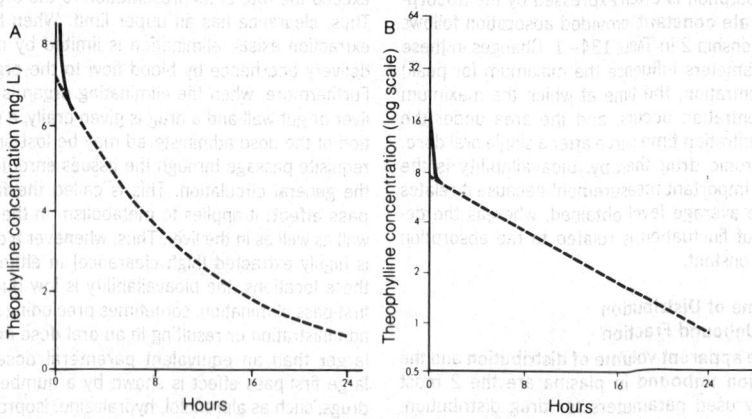

FIG. 134–1. Decline of the plasma theophylline concentration in Patient A following the IV administration of a single 320-mg dose of aminophylline. Shown on linear (A) and semilogarithmic (B) plots. Key: observation (——); prediction from parameter values given (----).

value is independent of dose administered. MRT is calculated from the relationship

$$MRT = \frac{AUMC}{AUC}$$

where the **AUMC** is the area under the first moment of the plasma concentration–time curve, and **AUC** is the area under the plasma concentration–time curve. For a drug with one-compartment characteristics, as in the example given in TABLE 134–1, MRT is equal to the reciprocal of the elimination rate constant.

Indexes of Internal Exposure

The exposure to a drug can be assessed either following a single dose or during chronic administration. After a single dose, the dose itself is one measure, but the time the drug is in the body is not included. A more useful index of internal exposure is the product of dose and MRT:

Exposure (single dose) = Dose • MRT

This is equivalent to

Exposure (single dose) = V • AUC

where **V** is the apparent volume of distribution. Thus, the AUC becomes a practical measure of exposure after a single dose.

Following chronic administration, exposure is better expressed by the average amount in the body. It follows then that

Exposure (chronic) = Rate of input • MRT

This is equivalent to

Exposure (chronic) = V • C_{ss}

Thus, the steady-state plasma concentration (C_{ss}) becomes a practical measure of chronic exposure. C_{ss} and AUC are useful, except when V is altered as can occur in hypoalbuminemia. Then the product of MRT and dose (or bioavailability [F] • dose, if given extravascularly) or MRT and rate of input (F• dose/τ, if given orally on a fixed-dose, fixed-interval [τ] regimen) may be the more reliable.

DRUG ADMINISTRATION

Pharmacokinetic parameter values are obtained experimentally. When these values are known, the kinetics of a drug can be predicted. The kinetic consequences of administering a drug as a single IV dose, by constant-rate infusion, as an oral dose, and in multiple doses are described below using the drug theophylline as an example. The metabolism of this drug shows concentration dependence in some individuals, especially children; however, for illustrative purposes, consider a 70-kg individual (Patient A) whose metabolism is concentration independent. The patient's parameter values are bioavailability, 1.0; absorption rate constant, 1.0

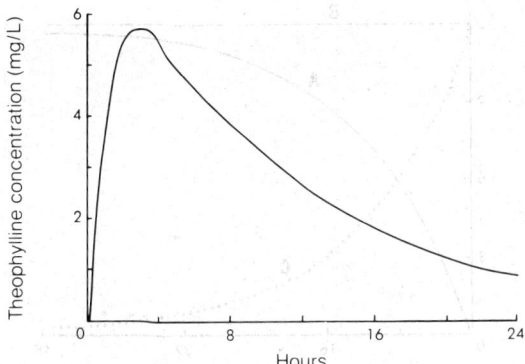

Fig. 134-2. Time course of the plasma theophylline concentration following the oral administration of a single 300-mg dose of aminophylline to Patient A.

h^{-1}; volume of distribution, 0.5 L/kg; clearance, 43 mL/h per kg; and half-life, 8 h.

Single Dose

Intravascular: The expected time course of theophylline in plasma following the IV administration of a single 320-mg dose of aminophylline (hydrous form is 80% theophylline) to Patient A is shown in Fig. 134-1 with both linear and semilogarithmic plots. The predicted initial plasma concentration is 7.3 mg/L (dose of theophylline [256 mg]/volume of distribution [L/kg × 70 kg]). The subsequent decline is estimated from the half-life; every 8 h the concentration decreases by a factor of 2.

The discrepancy between the observed (solid line) and the predicted (dashed line) concentration-time profiles within the first 2 h is explained by the time required to distribute drug throughout the body. This is often called the **distribution phase** and explains why single doses of many drugs, including aminophylline, must be administered by a short-term infusion over 5 to 10 min or more.

Extravascular: The predicted concentration of theophylline in this patient after a single 300-mg oral dose of aminophylline (anhydrous form is often used orally; it is 85% theophylline) is shown in Fig. 134-2. Several points are pertinent: (1) The time course is different from that of a single IV dose (see Fig. 134-1) because time is required to absorb the drug; however, the area under the curve is the same because this drug is virtually totally available. (2) The more rapid the absorption, the closer the curve is to that of the

IV dose. (3) At the peak concentration, absorption is not complete; here, the rate of absorption is simply equal to the rate of elimination.

Constant Rate of Input

The expected plasma concentration of theophylline on IV infusion of aminophylline to Patient A at a constant rate of 45 mg/h is shown in Curve A of Fig. 134-3.

Plateau concentration: The plasma concentration of theophylline and the amount of drug in the body rise until the rate of elimination equals the rate of infusion. The plasma concentration and the amount of drug in the body are then at steady state—having reached a plateau level. From Relationships 5 and 9, Table 134-1, it follows that

Rate of infusion = Clearance × Plateau
plasma drug concentration

and

Rate of infusion = Elimination rate constant
× Plateau amount of drug in body

Thus, the plateau plasma concentration is controlled only by the clearance value and the rate of infusion; the plateau amount of drug in the body is determined only by the elimination rate constant and the rate of infusion.

Time to reach plateau: The time required to accumulate theophylline in the body depends on the half-life of the drug. This is demonstrated in Fig. 134-3 by the administration of a single dose (530 mg) of aminophylline to attain a concentration of 12 mg/L, followed immediately by an infusion of 45 mg/h of aminophylline to maintain the

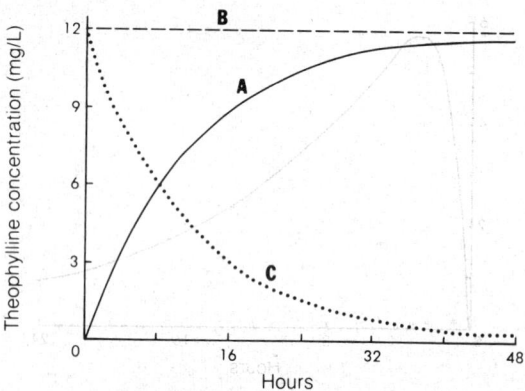

Fig. 134-3. Time course of the plasma theophylline concentration following the constant-rate IV infusion of 45 mg/h of aminophylline without (——, Curve A) and with (·····, Curve B) the administration of an IV loading dose of 530 mg of aminophylline to Patient A. Curve C shows drug remaining from the loading dose.

level, Curve B of Fig. 134–3. Drug from the loading dose disappears as shown in Curve C, with ½ remaining at one half-life, ¼ at 2 half-lives, and so on. The amount of drug in the body from the infusion, therefore, increases (Curve A) so that ½ of the plateau amount is present at one half-life, ¾ at 2 half-lives, etc.

If the infusion were stopped at 48 h, the post-infusion curve would resemble Curve C but would be displaced in time. The important principle is that the time frame for both accumulation and disappearance of drug is determined by the half-life. In Patient A, without a loading dose, aminophylline must be infused for at least 32 h (4 half-lives in the patient) for the concentration to approach the plateau value. Measuring a plasma concentration after this time would then provide an estimate of theophylline clearance.

The principles above for an IV infusion apply to any constant-rate input; eg, there are a number of devices used for transdermal, intraocular, oral, and intrauterine delivery of drugs at a constant rate. The plateau plasma concentration and the time to reach the value depend on the clearance and half-life values, respectively, as for IV infusions. Bioavailability may also be a factor.

Multiple Dosing

Drug accumulation: On repetitively administering 300 mg of aminophylline orally q 6 h to Patient A, the theophylline concentration increases as shown in Curve A of Fig. 134–4. As with IV infusion, the average concentration at

plateau depends upon the clearance, and the time required to accumulate the drug is a function of the half-life. Here, however, the levels fluctuate because of intermittent dosing. The kinetic consequence of an altered clearance of theophylline is demonstrated by Curves B and C. Curve B is the time course of plasma theophylline concentration in Patient B, who has heart failure and whose clearance is only 21.5 mL/h per kg (about half that of Patient A). On administering 300 mg of aminophylline q 6 h to Patient B, the drug accumulates to values about double those of Patient A. Furthermore, the time to reach the plateau levels is twice as long, a result of a 16-h half-life in Patient B.

Plasma concentrations of 10 to 20 mg/L are usually associated with optimal theophylline therapy. Above 20 mg/L the probability of toxicity increases. Thus, Patient B is at risk of developing toxicity (nausea, vomiting, CNS stimulation, seizures) that could have been averted, with prior knowledge of decreased metabolism in heart failure, by decreasing the dosage. The slow metabolism also might have been detected by plasma concentration monitoring.

Dosage regimens: The requirement of Patient B for theophylline would probably be met with 200 mg aminophylline q 8 h (25 mg/h). However, because of the long half-life and the slow accumulation in this individual, rapid attainment of a therapeutic concentration (and response) cannot be achieved without administering a load-

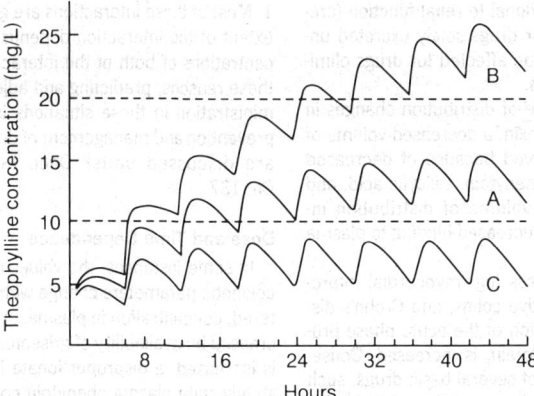

FIG. 134–4. Accumulation of theophylline on orally administering 300 mg of aminophylline every 6 h. Curve A: in Patient A. Curve B: in Patient B, whose clearance is $1/2$ that of Patient A. Curve C: in Patient C, whose clearance is twice that of Patient A. The dashed lines are the usual therapeutic limits and represent the *therapeutic window*.

ing dose. The loading dose of aminophylline required (volume of distribution × desired theophylline concentration × factor to convert theophylline into aminophylline) is about 500 mg:

$$\left(35\ L \times \frac{12\ mg}{L} \times \frac{100\ mg\ aminophylline}{85\ mg\ theophylline} \right)$$

Curve C of FIG. 134–4 shows the time course of theophylline in a young, otherwise healthy, asthmatic adult (a heavy smoker). The clearance in this patient is 86 mL/h per kg and the half-life is 4 h. Administration of 300 mg aminophylline q 6 h (50 mg/h) would probably be ineffective. The need for more drug could have been anticipated. Measurement of a plasma concentration, just before the next dose, would support this need. However, administration of aminophylline to this patient would be difficult because of the short half-life, high clearance, and large dosage requirements (100 mg/h). This is an example of a patient for whom the use of prolonged-release type of dosage form may be indicated. Because absorption is more or less sustained, 600 mg q 6 h is reasonable, since widely fluctuating levels would be avoided.

VARIABILITY IN PARAMETER VALUES

Many of the variables affecting pharmacokinetic parameters have been recognized and can be taken into account to tailor drug administration to an individual patient's needs; although even with dosage adjustment, sufficient variability usually remains to require careful monitoring of drug response and, in many cases, of plasma drug concentration.

Age and Weight

For some drugs, changes in pharmacokinetics with age and weight are well established. In children and young people (6 mo to 20 yr), renal function appears to correlate well with body surface area. Thus, for drugs primarily eliminated unchanged by renal excretion, clearance varies with age according to the change in surface area. In persons over age 20, renal function decreases about 1%/yr. Taking these changes into account permits tailoring of dosage of these drugs to age. Body surface area also has been found to correlate with metabolic clearance in children, although exceptions are common. For neonates and young infants, both renal and hepatic functions are not fully developed and no generalization, except for the occurrence of rapid change, can be made.

Disease

Renal function impairment: The renal clearance of most drugs appears to vary directly with creatinine clearance, regardless of the renal disease present. The change in (total) clearance depends upon the contribution of the kidneys to total elimination. Thus, (total) clearance is expected to be proportional to renal function (creatinine clearance) for drugs solely excreted unchanged and not to be affected for drugs eliminated by metabolism.

Sometimes volume of distribution changes in renal failure. For digoxin, a decreased volume of distribution is observed because of decreased tissue binding. For phenytoin, salicylic acid, and many other drugs, volume of distribution increases because of decreased binding to plasma proteins.

In physiologic stress (eg, myocardial infarction, surgery, ulcerative colitis, and Crohn's disease) the concentration of the acute phase protein, α_1-acid glycoprotein, is increased. Consequently, the binding of several basic drugs, such as propranolol, quinidine, and disopyramide, to this protein is increased. The volume of distribution of these drugs is decreased accordingly.

Hepatic disease produces changes in metabolic clearance, but good correlates or predictors of the changes are unavailable. Dramatically reduced drug metabolism has been associated with hepatic cirrhosis. Reduced plasma protein binding is often observed in this disease because of lowered plasma albumin. Acute hepatitis, with elevated serum enzymes, is usually not associated with altered drug metabolism. Heart failure, pneumonia, hyperthyroidism, and many other diseases also alter the pharmacokinetics of drugs.

Drug Interactions

Drug interactions can cause changes in pharmacokinetic parameter values and, therefore, in drug response. Interactions are known that affect each of the parameters in Table 134–

1. Most of these interactions are graded, and the extent of the interaction depends upon the concentrations of both of the interacting drugs. For these reasons, predicting and adjusting drug administration in these situations is difficult. The prevention and management of drug interactions are discussed under Drug Interactions in Ch. 137.

Dose and Time Dependence

In some instances, the values of the pharmacokinetic parameters change with dose administered, concentration in plasma, or time; eg, a decreased bioavailability of griseofulvin as the dose is increased, a disproportionate increase in the steady-state plasma phenytoin concentration on increasing its dosing rate, and a decrease in plasma carbamazepine concentration during its chronic administration. The decreased bioavailability of griseofulvin is due to the drug's low solubility in the GI tract. Phenytoin shows a concentration (dose) dependency because the metabolizing enzymes have a limited capacity to eliminate the drug, and the usual rate of administration approaches the maximum rate of metabolism. Carbamazepine shows time dependence because it induces its own metabolism.

Although relatively less common, dose and time dependencies introduce variability into the kinetics and response to several drugs. Other causes of dose- and time-dependent kinetics are saturable plasma protein and tissue binding (eg, phenylbutazone), saturable secretion in the kidney (eg, high-dose penicillin therapy), and saturable metabolism during the first pass through the liver (eg, propranolol).

135.   MONITORING DRUG TREATMENT

Once a therapeutic objective is defined and a drug and dosage regimen are chosen for a patient, drug therapy is conventionally managed by monitoring the incidence and intensity of both therapeutic and undesirable effects.

MONITORING RESPONSES

Although preferable, a direct measure of therapeutic effect is not always possible. For many

drugs alternative end points are used, eg, prothrombin time for oral anticoagulants, rosette inhibition test for immunosuppressive agents, blood or urine glucose for hypoglycemic drugs, and serum uric acid for uricosurics. Signs of toxicity are also used, eg, tinnitus and nystagmus in therapy with salicylate and phenytoin, respectively. Because minor toxicities do not always occur before more severe toxicities and because of the inherent undesirability of toxic reactions, this procedure clearly has limitations.

MONITORING DRUG IN PLASMA

Plasma drug concentration monitoring is an alternative procedure that can provide a more facile and rapid estimation of dosage requirements than by observing drug effects alone. For some drugs it is routinely useful; for others it can be helpful in certain situations. In all circumstances, it should be thought of as additional information to help guide therapy. Furthermore, an individual trained in clinical pharmacokinetics is required to optimize the information obtainable from such monitoring.

A plasma drug concentration may be useful in the initiation as well as in the maintenance of drug therapy. The basic idea is to achieve and maintain a target concentration or range of concentrations. Such monitoring helps reduce toxicity when the probability and severity of toxicity are closely related to the plasma concentration. Plasma concentration then serves as an intermediate therapeutic end point to help prevent toxicity.

INDICATIONS FOR MONITORING

A strategy for drug administration may be developed entirely around the plasma drug concentration, but this approach must be placed in perspective with all methods of monitoring. Certain criteria have been established, some related to the drug and others to the circumstances of its use. A few of the criteria are absolutely necessary; others are only relatively important. However, most of them must be met for the strategy to be effective.

Criteria Related to the Drug

1. The intensity and probability of therapeutic or toxic effects must correlate quantitatively with the plasma level.

2. The objective of the regimen must be to attain and maintain a therapeutic effect. This usually requires maintenance of plasma concentration within a limited range. Drugs for which only acute or intermittent effects are desired are therefore excluded. Tolerance also diminishes the potential for applying the method.

3. When readily assessed therapeutic end points are lacking, plasma concentration monitoring becomes particularly attractive; eg, in antiepileptic therapy, for which the therapeutic end point is the absence of seizures.

4. The probability of a therapeutic problem is greater for a drug with a narrow range between those concentrations giving the desired response and those producing toxicity; ie, a drug with a low margin of safety or a low therapeutic index.

5. Prior knowledge of the therapeutic concentrations and the pharmacokinetic parameters of a drug is essential for plasma concentration monitoring to be effective. Furthermore, knowledge of the conditions in which these concentrations and parameters are likely to be altered is also important. However, this requirement is relative; by monitoring the concentration, adjustments in dosage can be made.

6. A sensitive, accurate, and specific assay for the drug must be available; the results must be available quickly enough to permit prudent therapeutic decisions. The half-life of the drug is an index of this "turn-around" time, as it is the time frame of accumulation on multiple dosing and of disappearance on discontinuing the drug.

7. Interindividual differences and, in certain conditions, intraindividual differences in the pharmacokinetics of drugs are principal reasons for monitoring plasma concentrations. Drugs with poor and erratic absorption and those that are primarily metabolized, in contrast to those mostly excreted unchanged, are often candidates for monitoring. The larger the variability in the absorption and disposition of the drug, the greater is the need for monitoring it.

TABLE 135–1 lists drugs for which plasma level monitoring is now commonly used as well as the respective plasma concentrations usually associated with optimal therapy—the **therapeutic window** (see below).

Criteria Related to the Situation

For some drugs, plasma level monitoring is not *routinely* suggested, but it may be helpful in situations where a therapeutic problem is anticipated or presented; eg, when there is a high probability of encountering a therapeutic failure because of the patient's clinical status. For a patient with GI disease or with a gastric resection, an orally administered drug known to have poor bioavailability may be a candidate for monitoring. Similarly, the presence of renal, hepatic, thyroid, or cardiovascular disease may also suggest monitoring. For drugs that are primarily excreted unchanged, the presence of renal disease requires special attention, particularly if renal function is severely impaired or is variable with time.

The concurrent administration of several drugs, especially those known to interact phar-

TABLE 135-1. COMMONLY MONITORED DRUGS AND THEIR
THERAPEUTIC PLASMA CONCENTRATIONS

Drug	Plasma Concentration Usually Associated with Optimal Therapy (mg/L)	
Amikacin	12-25*	< 10†
Digitoxin	0.01-0.03‡	
Digoxin	0.0006-0.002‡	
Gentamicin	4-12*	< 2†
Lithium	0.7-2.0 (mEq/L)§	
Phenobarbital**	10-30	
Phenytoin	7-20	
Procainamide††	4-8	
Quinidine	1-4	
Theophylline	10-20	
Tobramycin	4-12*	< 2†

* Concentration obtained 30 min after the end of a 30-min infusion.
† Concentration just before the next dose.
‡ Often expressed in units of ng/mL: digitoxin, 10-30 ng/mL; digoxin, 0.6-2.0 ng/mL.
§ Usual units are given.
** When used as an anticonvulsant.
†† Concentration of active metabolite, N-acetylprocainamide, is also monitored.

macokinetically, is also a situation in which plasma monitoring should be considered (see DRUG INTER-ACTIONS in Ch. 137). Finally, plasma concentration monitoring may be useful where noncompliance is likely to occur (see Ch. 139).

Presence of a therapeutic problem: The lack of a response at usual or even higher dosages or a toxic reaction at customary or lower dosages are therapeutic problems. Appropriately planned plasma levels may help explain whether noncompliance, poor absorption, altered metabolism, or an unusual pharmacodynamic resistance or sensitivity to the drug is the cause of the problem.

TABLE 135-2 is an illustrative list of additional drugs for which situations may arise in which monitoring may be useful. As more clinical pharmacokinetic information becomes available, the status of these drugs and those in TABLE 135-1 will undoubtedly change.

COMPLICATING FACTORS

The occurrence of active metabolites is one of the major limitations of plasma monitoring. The antiarrhythmic agent procainamide, for example, forms an active acetylated metabolite, N-acetylprocainamide, by a hepatic enzyme that

shows genetic differences. Procainamide is partially excreted unchanged, while the metabolite is almost entirely handled by the kidneys. Thus, in patients who are rapid acetylators and who have compromised renal function, the correlation between response and procainamide concentration is expected to differ from that observed in patients who are slow acetylators and have normal renal function. The concentration of both the drug and its metabolite should be monitored, especially in the presence of renal disease.

Delay in the response to a given drug concentration: The effects of digoxin on the heart exemplify a delay caused by the time required to distribute drug to the active site. Therefore, digoxin concentrations should not be measured within 6 h of a dose, even after IV administration, as the plasma concentration will not reflect the concentration at the active site. An observed response that is an indirect measure of the actual drug effect may be another cause of delay; eg, the measurement of serum uric acid concentrations following the administration of a uricosuric agent and the determination of the one-stage prothrombin time following the use of an oral anticoagulant.

TABLE 135–2. ADDITIONAL DRUGS AND SITUATIONS FOR WHICH
PLASMA CONCENTRATION MONITORING IS USEFUL*

Drug	Plasma Concentration Usually Associated with Optimal Therapy (mg/L)†	Situations Suggesting Monitoring of Drug Concentration
Ethosuximide	25–75	Question of compliance; drug is coadministered with other anticonvulsants and source of toxicity is desired
Lidocaine	1.4–6.0	Patient has chronic hepatitis; infusion of drug is prolonged
Methotrexate		In high-dose therapy, concentration is used as a measure of potential toxicity and of requirement for citrovorum factor rescue
Nortriptyline	0.05–0.15 (50–150 ng/mL)	Inadequate patient response; plasma concentrations above 0.15 are less effective
Propranolol	0.02–0.2 (20–200 ng/mL)	Question of compliance or low availability; patient has chronic hepatitis
Primidone‡	8–12	Question of compliance; drug is coadministered with other anticonvulsants and source of toxicity is desired
Salicylates§	100–300 (10–30 mg/dL)	Patient has impaired hearing or is receiving high-dose antacid therapy that increases urine pH

* Selected examples of situations are given.
† For each drug the therapeutic window is defined in terms of the concentration at the time of sampling. Usually a trough concentration is measured. When concentration units other than mg/L are commonly used, they are so noted.
‡ Metabolized to phenobarbital. The concentration of phenobarbital should also be monitored.
§ Metabolism and protein binding are dose dependent. Serum albumin must be considered in the interpretation of a salicylate concentration. Therapeutic window refers to the anti-inflammatory use of the drug.

THE THERAPEUTIC WINDOW

The range of plasma concentrations with a high probability of therapeutic success. Although generally applicable, the therapeutic window of a typical population is sometimes inappropriate for an individual patient. Higher or lower than usual values may then be appropriate depending on the condition's severity.

For drugs that are bound to plasma proteins and in situations in which an alteration in binding is anticipated, the total concentration (bound + unbound) must be adjusted to give the desired unbound concentration. Conditions that reduce binding to albumin (to which many acidic drugs bind) include end-stage renal disease, cirrhosis, hypoalbuminemia, severe burns, and pregnancy. Binding to α_1-acid glycoprotein and lipoproteins (proteins to which many basic drugs bind) has been observed to be increased during stress and decreased in chronic hepatic disease. In these cases, adjustment of the therapeutic window is accomplished by estimating the fraction unbound in plasma in the patient and comparing it to the usual fraction unbound. Thus,

$$\text{Adjusted concentration} = \frac{\text{Usual fraction unbound}}{\text{Anticipated fraction unbound}} \times \text{Usual concentration}$$

For example, the fraction unbound for phenytoin is increased from 0.1 to about 0.25 in severe renal disease. Therefore, the usual therapeutic window, 7 to 20 mg/L, becomes 3 to 8 mg/L after adjustment.

EVALUATION OF A MEASURED CONCENTRATION

In contrast to usual clinical laboratory tests, the interpretation of plasma drug concentrations requires the application of pharmacokinetic principles. The subsequent presentation is illustrative.

Collection of Pertinent Information

The history of drug administration, the clinical status of the patient, and a firm knowledge of the clinical pharmacokinetics of the drug are re-

TABLE 135–3. COLLECTION OF PERTINENT DATA

History of drug administration
  Drug, dosage, dosage forms, routes of administration, times of administration, compliance (inpatient or outpatient)

Time of sampling (relative to dose)

Present and previous (if any) plasma drug concentrations

Clinical status of patient
  Weight, age, sex, condition being treated, concurrent disease states (especially cardiovascular, hepatic, and renal diseases)

Laboratory data
  Renal function (serum creatinine, creatinine clearance, BUN)
  Hepatic function (prothrombin time, serum albumin, serum bilirubin, hepatic enzymes in blood)
  Protein binding (plasma proteins and albumin)

Concurrent drug therapy
  Drug interactions
  Assay interferences

Active metabolites

Assay method (accuracy, sensitivity, and specificity)

Usual pharmacokinetic parameters associated with type of patient in question
  Bioavailability, absorption rate constant, volume of distribution, unbound fraction in plasma, renal clearance, hepatic clearance

quired (see TABLE 135–3). The drug administration history, including doses, times of dosing, and times of sampling, is mandatory, as are the age and weight of the patient.

The need for other information (eg, renal, hepatic, and cardiovascular functions; serum proteins; active metabolites; assay methods) varies with the drug and the situation. An ability to estimate renal function from a serum creatinine measurement is also important.

Interpretation of Data

After collecting the information needed, including the present and any previous plasma concentrations, 2 approaches may be taken. One is to compare the observed value with that predicted from known information. This approach is helpful in identifying problems such as noncompliance, low or high bioavailability, or unusually slow or rapid elimination. The other approach is to determine the pharmacokinetic parameters of the drug in the individual, a particularly useful analysis in determining an individual patient's dosage requirements. Whether the measured value is a good estimate of the minimum, average, or maximum concentration at steady state on a fixed-dose, fixed-dosing-interval regimen, or is a nonsteady-state value obtained shortly after starting the drug or following an unequal dosage schedule, must be immediately established from the dosing history and the time of sampling.

Steady state: A value that represents an estimate of the average steady-state concentration on a fixed-dose, fixed-dosing-interval regimen is handled most readily. This requires a plasma sample obtained after dosing for at least 3 half-lives. Furthermore, the fluctuation of the concentration within a dosing interval must be small, especially if the sample is obtained just before the next dose. This condition is satisfied if the dosing interval is < 1 half-life; eg, for the daily administration of digoxin (half-life of ≥ 2 days). The observed concentration can then be compared with the expected concentration.

The predicted average concentration (C_{av}) is a function of the expected values of bioavailability (F), clearance (CL), and the rate of administration (D/τ, dose/dosing interval), that is,

$$C_{av} \text{ (expected)} = \frac{F}{CL} \text{ (expected)} \cdot \frac{D}{\tau} \quad (1)$$

If the ratio of concentrations, observed to predicted, is > 1, either the input is greater or the elimination is slower than expected, or both. The converse is true for a ratio < 1. Thus, there is a set of explanations consistent with either observation.

Causes of either an altered input or an altered elimination are summarized in TABLE 135–4. Perhaps the most common cause is the difference between how the patient takes the drug and how he is supposed to or is believed to take it—a

TABLE 135–4. CAUSES OF AN UNEXPECTED STEADY–STATE PLASMA CONCENTRATION

Factor Involved	Concentration Ratio > 1*	Comment	Concentration Ratio < 1*	Comment
Compliance	Noncompliance— taking more than directed	Probably less frequently a cause than taking less than directed	Noncompliance— taking less than directed	A very frequent problem
Bioavailability	Higher than usual	An explanation only if bioavailability is usually low	Lower than usual	A more frequent problem for drugs that are usually poorly absorbed
Renal clearance	Lower than usual	A valid explanation for drugs whose major route of elimination is renal excretion. May be due to altered pH, inhibition of secretion, or simply decreased renal function	Greater than usual	Not a frequent explanation. May occur because of altered urine pH or flow. The renal route must usually be or become the major route of elimination
Hepatic clearance	Lower than usual	An explanation for drugs whose major route of elimination is metabolism or biliary secretion. May be due to competitive inhibition by another drug, decreased blood flow, hepatic disease, or may be genetic in origin	Greater than usual	An explanation if hepatic elimination is or becomes the major route of elimination. May be due to enzyme induction or activation or may be genetic in origin
Plasma protein binding	Greater than usual	Not usually an explanation	Less than usual	May be a result of displacement, hypoalbuminemia, hepatic and/or renal disease

* Observed concentration divided by expected concentration.

compliance problem. Bioavailability is a factor that needs to be considered only for drugs in which its value is low or variable or where malabsorption is suspected. Renal and hepatic clearances may explain altered elimination depending on the major route of drug elimination. Plasma protein binding is a concern for highly bound drugs because clearance depends upon it.

Fluctuation: The dosage regimens of many drugs result in considerable fluctuation in the plasma concentration. The dosing interval may be comparable to or greater than the half-life, or the regimen may be similar to a 9−1−5−9 regimen in which the drug is taken q 4 h for 4 doses followed by a 12-h interval. In either case, if there is much fluctuation it must be considered.

For drugs in which the regimen involves considerable fluctuation, the preferred time of sampling is usually just before the next dose. The trough concentration, C, expected at the end of a fixed-dosing interval, τ, following the administration of a fixed dose, D, under steady-state conditions, is

$$C = \frac{F \cdot D \cdot e^{\left[-\frac{CL}{V} \cdot \tau\right]}}{V\left(1 - e^{\left[-\frac{CL}{V} \cdot \tau\right]}\right)} \quad (2)$$

where e is the natural logarithm base (approximately 2.718), CL is total clearance, V is the apparent volume of distribution, and F is the bioavailability. Again, the observed concentration may be compared to the value predicted from the expected values of the parameters.

A maximum concentration, from a sample obtained soon after an IV dose or at the peak time after an oral dose, is often unreliable. Either absorption or distribution, or both, may take time to be complete; they also often vary with time and among patients.

When absorption and distribution are rapid, eg, after the IM administration of the aminoglycosides, measurement of plasma concentration soon after the dose and close to the peak has been found to be useful. Under these conditions, the peak concentration can be estimated from

$$C_{peak} = \frac{F \cdot D}{V\left(1 - e^{\left[-\frac{CL}{V} \cdot \tau\right]}\right)} \quad (3)$$

or from the relationship

$$C_{peak} = C + F \cdot D/V \quad (4)$$

where $F \cdot D/V$ is the increment of change in the concentration on adding $F \cdot D$ to the body.

Nonsteady state: A plasma sample may be obtained at a time when the drug has not fully accumulated or after an erratic pattern of previous doses and dosing intervals. Steady-state principles cannot be applied in these circumstances; however, other methods may be used.

Estimation of Parameter Values

For adjusting dosage in an individual patient, the most useful procedure is to estimate the value of clearance and sometimes the values of the volume of distribution and half-life from the monitored concentrations. Clearance is the most valuable parameter, because it is needed to predict the dosage required to achieve a given concentration and the converse.

From a steady-state value: When a concentration is a good estimate of an average steady-state concentration, bioavailability is not variable, compliance is assured, and the patient is on a fixed-dose fixed-interval dosage regimen, clearance is readily estimated from:

$$CL = \frac{F \cdot D/\tau}{C_{av}} \quad (5)$$

a rearrangement of equation 1. For example, if a digoxin concentration of 1.2 µg/L were obtained on chronically administering 0.125 mg IV (F = 1.0) per day to a patient, the clearance would be 104 L/day. From equation 1, then, a concentration of 1.4 µg/L, a value near the middle of the usual therapeutic window, would be expected.

Clearance may be calculated from the relationship:

$$CL = \frac{V}{\tau} \cdot \ln\left[\frac{F \cdot D}{V \cdot C} + 1\right] \quad (6)$$

when a trough concentration is obtained under steady-state conditions, large fluctuations are anticipated (dosing interval >> half-life), and the drug is given IV or absorption is rapid. For example, gentamicin is a drug whose concentration fluctuates extensively because the usual half-life and dosing interval are 2 and 8 h, respectively. If a steady-state trough gentamicin concentration of 3 mg/L were obtained in a 70-kg patient on an IV regimen of 80 mg q 8 h, the clearance would be 2.0 L/h (F = 1, V = 0.25 L/kg, ln = natural

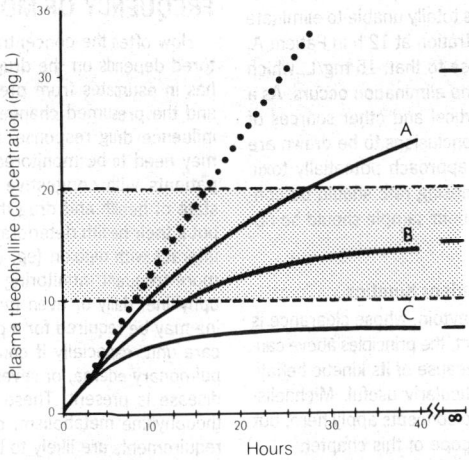

FIG. 135−1. Plasma theophylline concentrations in 3 patients with different clearance rates.

logarithm). One's confidence in the estimate depends on several factors, including variability in the values of V and F, assay errors, and the assumptions above.

The dosage required to achieve a given average concentration can then be computed from the clearance and bioavailability estimates as follows:

$$D/\tau = \frac{CL}{F} \cdot C_{av} \qquad (7)$$

In the example of digoxin above, the daily oral dose required to achieve a concentration of 1.4 μg/L is 0.25 mg. For gentamicin, the 12-h IV dose required to maintain an average concentration of 3 mg/L, from equation 5, is then 72 mg. The peak, equations 3 or 4, and trough, equation 2, are then 5.5 and 1.4 mg/L, respectively.

From a nonsteady-state value: Clearance may also be estimated from a nonsteady-state concentration. As an example, consider the interpretations that would be given to theophylline concentrations obtained in 3 different 70-kg patients 12 h after starting an IV infusion of 42.5 mg/h (aminophylline, 53 mg/h). Clearance is highly variable for theophylline, whereas the volume of distribution is relatively constant (0.5 L/kg). On infusing the drug in Patients A, B, and C who have clearances of 20, 40, and 80 mL/h per kg, respectively, the plasma concentration rises as shown in FIG. 135−1. The plasma concentra-

tion in Patient A reaches toxic levels, but it takes > 24 h of infusion. The concentration in Patient B approaches a steady-state value within the therapeutic window. The values for Patient C remain subtherapeutic.

For a plasma sample obtained 12 h after starting an infusion, the concentration in Patient C is close to a steady-state value and clearance is reasonably estimated using the steady-state approach. The concentrations in Patients A and B are not near the steady-state, but the levels do provide some information. The concentration expected at this point in time may be calculated from the values of clearance, CL, and volume, V, using the relationship

$$C = \frac{R}{CL} \cdot \left(1 - e^{-\left[\frac{CL}{V} \cdot t \right]} \right) \qquad (8)$$

where R is the rate of infusion, and t is the duration of the infusion. The steady-state concentration is R/CL.

The observed concentration in Patient B is identical to that calculated, indicating that a steady-state concentration of about 15 mg/L will be approached. For Patient A, however, the observed value of 12 mg/L is above that expected at this time. A steady-state concentration in the potentially toxic range is possible, but one has little confidence in estimating what the value will be. The reason for the lack of confidence is indicated by the dotted line in FIG. 135−1. This line represents the increase in the plasma concentration in a patient who is totally unable to eliminate the drug. The concentration at 12 h in Patient A, about 12 mg/L, is close to that, 15 mg/L, which would be observed if no elimination occurs. As a consequence of analytical and other sources of error, the only valid conclusions to be drawn are that the patient may approach potentially toxic levels, a decrease in dosing rate should be considered, and a subsequent sample should be obtained.

Concentration-Dependent Kinetics

For a drug, like phenytoin, whose clearance is concentration dependent, the principles above cannot be applied. Yet, because of its kinetic behavior, monitoring is particularly useful. Michaelis-Menten enzyme kinetic concepts apply here, but they are beyond the scope of this chapter.

FREQUENCY OF MONITORING

How often the concentration should be monitored depends on the drug, the confidence one has in estimates from previous measurements, and the presumed change in those factors that influence drug response. For example, digoxin may need to be monitored only occasionally in patients with congestive heart failure whose state of health and drug therapy remain stable; but if their health deteriorates or drugs known to interact with digoxin (eg, quinidine) are added, more frequent monitoring is indicated. For theophylline, daily or even more frequent monitoring may be required for a patient in an intensive care unit, especially if congestive heart failure, pulmonary edema, or severe constrictive airway disease is present. These conditions decrease theophylline metabolism; consequently, dosage requirements are likely to be less than normal.

136. PHARMACODYNAMICS

The study of the biochemical and physiologic effects of drugs and their mechanisms of action.

MECHANISMS OF DRUG ACTION

MEMBRANE INTERACTION

Certain drugs produce pharmacologic responses by interacting with cell membranes.

General anesthetics: General anesthetics are believed to act by causing membranes of central neurons to expand (to become more disordered). Proteins in membranes and in Na channels may be altered, diminishing Na^+ influx; this inhibits depolarization and cellular activity is reduced. In support of this theory, anesthetized animals have been shown to recover rapidly from general anesthesia when placed in a hyperbaric chamber to reverse the membrane effect. **Local anesthetics:** Procaine and related drugs act similarly. Upon application to peripheral nerves, conduction ceases. If toxic doses are applied, resulting in systemic absorption, local anesthetics can also inhibit central neurons.

RECEPTOR INTERACTION

The mechanisms by which many drugs exert their therapeutic effects have been estimated classically by studying their effects on physiologic functions at different anatomic loci, both in vivo and in vitro. Few if any drugs show absolute specificity, but most act in a relatively selective manner; eg, atropine inhibits the actions of acetylcholine on exocrine glands and smooth muscles, but not on skeletal muscle. The characteristic actions of many such selective drugs are a consequence of their physicochemical interaction with biochemical components of the organism (ie, drug recognition sites), conventionally termed **receptive substances** or **receptors**. Among the drug and hormonal receptors that have been isolated, structurally identified, and reconstituted to functional responsiveness in cellular membranes are cholinergic, nicotinic and muscarinic, α- and β-adrenergic subtypes, benzodiazepine, and the insulin family of receptors. The binding characteristics of drugs (ie, **ligands**) to their complementary receptors as determined in vitro can reveal important aspects of their behavior at cellular and subcellular levels. Also, it is understood that "nonspecific" drug-binding occurs; ie, not all molecular sites at which drugs bind are properly designated as receptors.

Drug-receptor theory, grounded in the Law of Mass Action, is somewhat comparable to kinetic analyses of enzyme-substrate interaction and inhibition. Many drug mechanisms can be studied and categorized within this reference frame (eg, aspirin—prostaglandin synthetase inhibitor, neo-

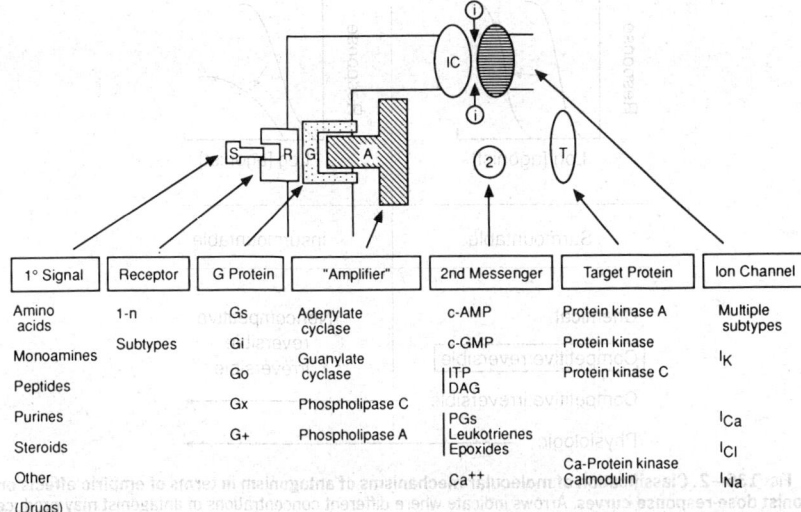

1° Signal	Receptor	G Protein	"Amplifier"	2nd Messenger	Target Protein	Ion Channel
Amino acids	1-n	Gs	Adenylate cyclase	c-AMP	Protein kinase A	Multiple subtypes
Monoamines	Subtypes	Gi	Guanylate cyclase	c-GMP	Protein kinase	I_K
Peptides		Go		ITP DAG	Protein kinase C	
Purines		Gx	Phospholipase C	PGs		I_{Ca}
Steroids		G+	Phospholipase A	Leukotrienes Epoxides		I_{Cl}
Other				Ca^{++}	Ca-Protein kinase Calmodulin	I_{Na}
(Drugs)						

FIG. 136–1. Scheme illustrating multiple components of cellular hormonal and drug receptor mechanisms throughout the body. Each ligand (physiologic substrate or exogenous drug) has recognition binding sites that may exist in multiple receptor subtypes. Activated receptors directly or indirectly regulate ion conductances and/or other intracellular functions (eg, secretion/contraction). In many cases, the activated receptor acts within the cell membrane through guanine nucleotide–binding proteins (G proteins), which, in turn, activate a second messenger–synthesizing enzyme ("signal amplification"). The several different second messengers act intracytoplasmically to regulate target proteins such as protein kinases. These enzymes then act on preferred substrates, according to cell type, to evoke the physiologic (or pharmacologic) effect. (Adapted from Bloom EF: "Neurotransmitters: Past, present, and future directions." *FASEB Journal* 2:32–41, 1988; used with permission.)

stigmine—cholinesterase inhibitor, deprenyl—monoamine oxidase B inhibitor, digitalis—Na⁺/K⁺ ATPase inhibitor, etc). Drug **occupation theory** assumes that a pharmacologic response emanates only from those receptors occupied by an appropriate ligand; ie, there is direct proportionality between receptor occupancy and ultimate tissue response or effect. Contemporary **rate** and **allosteric** theories address kinetic processes ("onset/offset" rates) of ligand-receptor occupancy, associated activation states ("active/inactive") of receptors, and the lack of apparent proportionality between ligand-receptor occupancy and ultimate tissue or organ response. Thus, current theoretic models consider variations in signal transduction efficiency, and the existence of "spare" receptors and partial agonists (see below). Receptors are recognized as dynamic cellular elements under external chemical and hormonal influences as well as continuous intracellular regulatory control. Receptor **up-**

regulation and **down-regulation** bear relevance to clinically important drug-related adaptational phenomena variously described as **desensitization, tachyphylaxis, tolerance, and acquired resistance**.

Drug actions involve several complex mechanisms: (1) a physiologic function of a tissue (eg, contraction, secretion) may be subserved by multiple receptor-mediated mechanisms, and consequently modulated by dissimilar molecular stimuli; (2) several intermediate steps (eg, receptor-coupling and second messenger substances) may be interposed between the initial drug-receptor interaction and "ultimate" tissue or organ response; and (3) the efficiency of stimulus-response mechanisms and receptor density can vary from tissue to tissue (see FIG. 136–1).

Inherent concepts in drug receptor theory are those of **affinity**, reflecting the probability of the drug occupying a receptor at any given instant, and **intrinsic efficacy, intrinsic activity,** or sim-

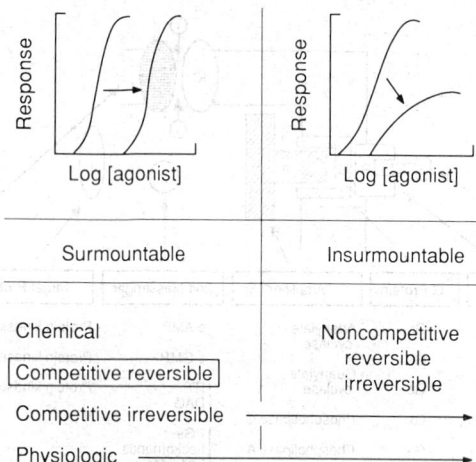

Fig. 136–2. Classification of molecular mechanisms of antagonism in terms of empiric effects on agonist dose-response curves. Arrows indicate where different concentrations of antagonist may produce both surmountable antagonism and insurmountable antagonism. (From *Pharmacologic Analysis of Drug-Receptor Interaction* by TP Kenakin. New York, Raven Press, 1987, p 207; used with permission.)

ply **efficacy,** terms attempting to express the association between drug-occupancy conditions and activation-state of the receptors, ie, the capacity to excite. **Agonist** drugs are defined as *those whose interaction with receptors initiates a response culminating in modified cellular activity (ie, increasing or decreasing it).* Agonists must possess the characteristics of affinity and intrinsic efficacy. Typical examples include endogenous substances (acetylcholine, histamine, norepinephrine) and many drugs such as morphine, phenylephrine, and isoproterenol. Many other classes of important drugs interact selectively with receptors but do not initiate the sequence of events leading to an observed effect. These drugs are **antagonists;** they possess affinity but lack intrinsic efficacy. This agonist-antagonist dualism is complicated by the fact that structural analogs of agonist molecules frequently exhibit a mixture of agonist and antagonist properties; such drugs are referred to as **partial agonists** or low-efficacy agonists. For example, isoproterenol is a full or strong agonist, and prenalterol a partial agonist for β-adrenergic receptors.

According to receptor theory, full agonists can evoke a maximal tissue response even when they occupy only a fraction of the total receptor population, suggesting the presence of receptor reserve (ie, spare receptors).

FIG. 136–2 shows mechanistic aspects of drugs exhibiting antagonist properties. Antagonists can be classified as **reversible** or **irreversible,** depending on their kinetics of interaction with receptors. Reversible antagonists readily dissociate from their receptor; irreversible antagonists form a stable chemical bond with the receptor (eg, alkylation), or only slowly dissociate **(pseudoirreversible antagonism).** If the antagonist binds to the same locus (recognition site) on the receptor as an agonist, the term **competitive antagonism** is used. For example, naloxone, which is structurally similar to morphine, has little or no morphine-like activity but blocks the expected effects when given before or after morphine. More morphine is needed to overcome the competition, resulting in the characteristic parallel shift to the right of the dose-response curve. Thus, in the presence of a competitive antagonist the agonist's maximal effect may be achieved, but only at very high concentrations. Such conditions are called **surmountable** antagonism. Noncompetitive antagonists may bind to a site on the receptor distinct from the agonist recognition site, thereby preventing agonist activation of the receptor through allosteric or other mechanisms. Finally, the antagonist may chemically inactivate ("neutralize") the agonist, or it may interfere with some cellular process subse-

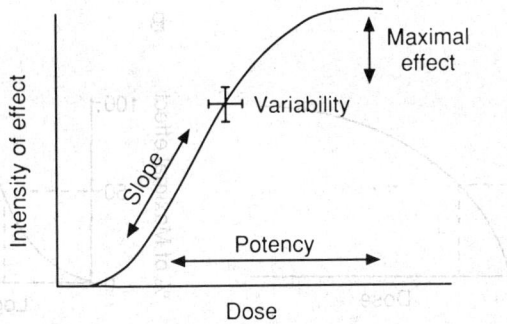

Fɪɢ. 136–3. **The log dose-effect relationship.** Representative log dose-effect curve, illustrating its four characterizing variables. (From Nies AS: "Principles of therapeutics," in *Goodman and Gilman's The Pharmacological Basis of Therapeutics*, ed. 8, edited by AG Gilman, TW Rall, AS Nies, P Taylor. New York, Pergamon Press, 1990, pp 62–83; used with permission.)

quent to agonist-receptor activation, thus evoking **physiologic** or **functional antagonism.**

CHEMICAL INTERACTION

Some drugs provide a therapeutic effect by reacting directly with endogenous or exogenous substances.

Antacids (eg, aluminum hydroxide, magnesium hydroxide) combine with HCl to yield relatively inactive products. They neutralize excess gastric acidity and are of benefit in treating gastric irritation and related disorders. Sodium bicarbonate as a powder (eg, baking soda) should *never* be used as an antacid; in some patients, a large volume of CO_2 was produced which re-

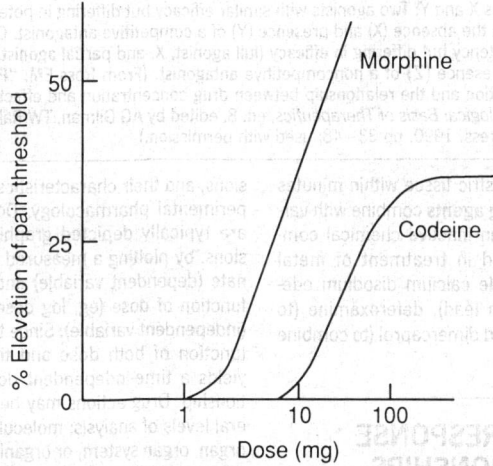

Fɪɢ. 136–4. **Schematic representation of dose-response curves for analgesic action of morphine and codeine.** (From Jenden DJ: "Biologic variations and the principles of bioassay," in *Essentials of Pharmacology*, ed. 3, edited by JA Beven and JH Thompson. New York, Harper & Row, 1983, p 93; used with permission.)

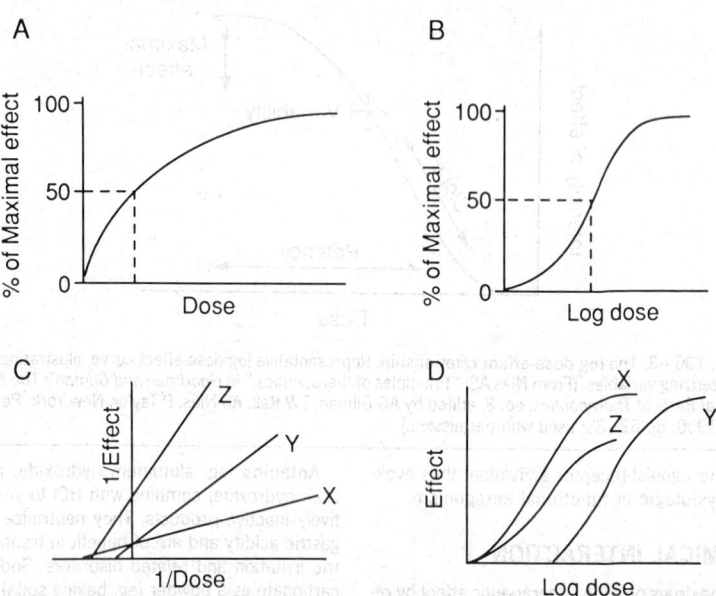

FIG. 136–5. **Different representations of dose-effect curves.** *A,* The ideal relationship between the concentration (dose) of a drug and the magnitude of response to it. When plotted on a linear scale of dose, a hyperbolic curve results. *B,* A sigmoidal dose-effect curve results when the magnitude of effect observed is plotted vs. the logarithm of drug dose. *C* and *D,* Representative double-reciprocal plots (*C*) and log dose-effect curves (*D*). Curves X and Y: Two agonists with similar efficacy but differing in potency (X more potent than Y), or an agonist in the absence (X) and presence (Y) of a competitive antagonist. Curves X and Z: Two agonists with similar potency but differing in efficacy (full agonist, X, and partial agonist, Z) or an agonist in the absence (X) and presence (Z) of a noncompetitive antagonist. (From Ross EM: "Pharmacodynamics: Mechanisms of drug action and the relationship between drug concentration and effect," in *Goodman and Gilman's The Pharmacological Basis of Therapeutics,* ed. 8, edited by AG Gilman, TW Rall, AS Nies, P Taylor. New York, Pergamon Press, 1990, pp 33–48; used with permission.)

sulted in tearing of gastric tissue within minutes of ingestion. **Chelating agents** combine with various metals to form an inactive chemical complex or chelate. Used in treatment of metal poisoning, they include calcium disodium edetate (to combine with lead), deferoxamine (to combine with iron), and dimercaprol (to combine with arsenic).

DOSE–RESPONSE RELATIONSHIPS

The correspondence between the amount of an administered drug and the magnitude of the evoked reaction. Knowledge of dose-response relationships helps in making therapeutic deci-

sions, and their characteristics are a basis of experimental pharmacology. Dose-response data are typically depicted graphically in 2 dimensions, by plotting a measured effect on the ordinate (dependent variable) and the dosage or a function of dose (eg, log dose) on the abscissa (independent variable). Since the drug effect is a function of both dose and time, this practice yields a time-independent dose-response relationship. Drug actions may be quantified at several levels of analysis: molecular, cellular, tissue, organ, organ system, or organism. Thus, the conditions of study, as well as the mathematical approach to data analysis, determine the precise means of defining the drug-induced effect and preclude the existence of any single characteristic relationship between the intensity of drug effect and drug dosage. Effects are frequently presented as maxima, recorded at time of peak-effect, or under steady-state conditions (eg, during continuous IV infusion).

Fig. 136-3 illustrates 4 variable features of a hypothetical dose-effect curve: (1) potency (location of curve along the dose axis), (2) maximal efficacy or ceiling effect (greatest attainable response of the system under measurement), (3) slope (change in response per unit dose), and (4) biologic variation (variation in magnitude of response among test subjects in the same population given the same dose of drug).

Fig. 136-4 shows a comparison of morphine and codeine with respect to their differing potencies and maximal efficacies, using eleva-tion in pain threshold as the common pharmacologic effect. The dose-response curves show that more codeine than morphine is needed to achieve the same degree of analgesia. Thus, morphine has greater biologic activity per dosing equivalent and is more potent than codeine. In addition, no matter how much codeine is given, there is a point beyond which no practical increased effect will occur. Thus, morphine is not only more potent than codeine, but it also has a higher maximal efficacy or ceiling effect.

Several different methods of graphing dose-response relationships, and brief descriptions of their interpretive utility, are shown in Fig. 136-5.

137. FACTORS AFFECTING DRUG RESPONSE

PHARMACOGENETICS

A pharmacogenetic reaction is *a variation in drug response caused by hereditary factors.* Many of these effects are unexpected and can be adverse; when they occur in a small number of individuals, they are termed **idiosyncratic.** Pharmacogenetic responses may be classified as either direct or indirect.

Direct Pharmacogenetic Response

Only a few clinical examples have been identified that link an unusual pharmacologic effect directly to genetic alterations in the function of a particular tissue or receptor site.

Reduced warfarin activity: Certain individuals exhibit substantially lower anticoagulant activity following usual therapeutic doses of warfarin; a dose up to 20 times greater than normal may be necessary to produce the desired pharmacologic effect. Since biotransformation is not abnormal in such cases, this familial effect may be due to a reduction in binding affinity of warfarin to its receptor.

Malignant hyperthermia: After receiving a combination of muscle relaxant (usually succinylcholine) and inhalation general anesthetic (most frequently halothane), certain patients (about 1:20,000) undergo a life-threatening elevation in body temperature. Muscular rigidity is often the first sign; others (in addition to hyperthermia) include tachycardia and other arrhythmias, acidosis, and shock. The mechanism appears related to halothane-induced potentiation of Ca activity in skeletal muscle (sarcoplas-mic reticulum); in susceptible patients, this tissue is hyperreactive to Ca. As a result, Ca-induced biochemical reactions are accelerated, causing extreme muscle contractions and an elevated metabolic rate. Since this rapidly progressive reaction is often fatal, *treatment must be initiated immediately.* Surgery and anesthesia should be discontinued as rapidly as possible; corrective therapy includes administration of dantrolene (IV), management of metabolic acidosis, and core and surface cooling. Muscle biopsy and elevated CK levels may be used to identify other sensitive members of the same family.

Indirect Pharmacogenetic Response

An altered rate of biotransformation or an abnormally low enzyme level can produce unexpected changes in therapeutic and toxic effects of drugs; this is the major mechanism by which pharmacogenetic responses appear. Nonhereditary factors such as smoking, acute or chronic use of alcohol and other drugs (eg, cimetidine, phenobarbital), diet, health status, and environment (eg, air pollution) can also influence drug metabolism. See also DRUG ELIMINATION in Ch. 133 and DRUG INTERACTIONS, below.

Reduced biotransformation: Adverse reactions to certain drugs develop more frequently and at lower therapeutic doses in patients with this type of enzymatic alteration.

Acetylation: In about 50% of the US population, hepatic *N*-acetyltransferase is hypoactive (slow acetylators). As a result, isoniazid and certain other drugs (eg, hydralazine, phenelzine, procainamide, sulfamethazine) are slowly metabolized by this enzyme. Slow acetylators tend to be more susceptible to adverse reactions associated with these medications, eg, peripheral neuritis (isoniazid), lupus erythematosus (hydralazine, procainamide), sedation and nausea (phenelzine).

Hydrolysis: Persons with plasma **pseudocholinesterase deficiency** (about 1:2500) have a decreased ability to inactivate succinylcholine, resulting in prolonged paralysis of the respiratory muscles when conventional doses are administered. Prolonged apnea may require mechanical ventilation.

Oxidation: About 5 to 10% of whites in North America and Europe exhibit a decreased oxidative biotransformation of debrisoquin (guanethidine-like compound used in clinical studies to detect slow oxidation). Reduced hydroxylation of various drugs has been correlated with an unusually large therapeutic response (eg, abnormally high degree of β receptor blockade with metoprolol or timolol) or greater toxicity than expected (eg, excessive CNS depression with nortriptyline or phenytoin). Other drugs that appear to be affected by this metabolic difference include tricyclic antidepressants (eg, amitriptyline, desipramine) and an antitussive agent (dextromethorphan).

Accelerated biotransformation: Patients with an increased biotransformational capacity will require therapeutic doses larger than usual; they may also be more susceptible to certain toxic effects.

Acetylation: While almost half of the US population exhibits reduced N-acetyltransferase activity (see above), the remainder are rapid acetylators. These patients require, on a daily basis, larger or more doses of isoniazid in order to obtain the desired therapeutic response and are also more likely to develop hepatotoxicity as a result of acetylhydrazine accumulation.

Oxidation: Alcohol dehydrogenase (**ADH**) is an important enzyme in the biotransformation of alcohol, oxidizing it to acetaldehyde. Apparently, about 85% of the Japanese population has an atypical ADH which operates about 5 times faster than normal; other Asian groups may exhibit this same phenomenon. Consumption of alcohol by such persons leads to accumulation of acetaldehyde, resulting in extensive vasodilation, facial flushing, and compensatory tachycardia.

Enzyme deficiency: Insufficient levels of various enzymes may result in higher rates of drug-induced toxicity.

Glucose-6-phosphate dehydrogenase (G6PD): This enzyme is essential for those RBC reduction reactions which maintain cellular integrity. Patients with **G6PD deficiency** (including about 10% of blacks) are at increased risk of developing hemolytic anemia when given oxidant drugs such as antimalarials (eg, chloroquine, pamaquine, primaquine), aspirin, probenecid, or vitamin K.

Glutathione synthetase: This enzyme is found in erythrocytes and hepatocytes. Similar to G6PD deficiency (see above), lack of RBC glutathione synthetase results in development of hemolytic anemia after administration of oxidant drugs. When hepatocytes have low levels of this enzyme, patients are at increased risk of liver damage following administration of drugs such as acetaminophen and nitrofurantoin.

DRUG INTERACTIONS

Alteration of the effects of one drug by the prior or concurrent administration of another (drug-drug interactions); alteration of the effects of a drug by food (drug-food interactions). The effects of one of the drugs are usually increased or decreased. Desired interactions are achieved with combination therapy (eg, in the treatment of hypertension, asthma, certain infections, and malignancy), in which 2 or more drugs are used to increase therapeutic effects or reduce toxicity. Unwanted interactions can cause adverse drug reactions (**ADRs**) or therapeutic failure.

Since it is often difficult to predict the *clinical significance* of known or suggested drug interactions, the possibility of problems developing must be viewed in perspective. If an interaction appears likely, therapeutic alternatives should be considered; but a patient should not be denied needed therapy solely because of the possibility.

The mechanisms of drug interactions are usually pharmacodynamic or pharmacokinetic. Although the majority are pharmacodynamic, most of the literature deals with the pharmacokinetic type.

PHARMACODYNAMIC INTERACTIONS

Pharmacodynamic interactions include the concurrent administration of drugs having the same (or opposing) pharmacologic actions and alteration of the sensitivity or the responsiveness of the tissues to one drug by another. Many of these interactions can be predicted from a knowledge of the pharmacology of each drug. By monitoring the patient clinically, deviations from the expected effect often can be quickly detected and the dosage adjusted accordingly (see Ch. 135).

Drugs with Opposing Pharmacologic Effects

Interactions resulting from the use of 2 drugs with opposing pharmacologic effects should be among the easiest to detect, but various factors may preclude early identification of such antagonism. For example, thiazides and certain other diuretics may elevate blood glucose levels. When a diuretic is prescribed for a diabetic who takes insulin or an oral hypoglycemic agent, the hypoglycemic action of the antidiabetic drug may be partially counteracted, necessitating a dosage adjustment.

Drugs with Similar Pharmacologic Effects

An example of this type of interaction is the increased CNS-depressant effect that often occurs when persons taking antianxiety agents, antipsychotic agents, antihistamines, or other drugs having depressant effects drink alcoholic beverages. Many people risk these combinations without serious difficulty, but they can be lethal. Combining drugs with CNS-depressant activity increases the risks of excessive sedation and dizziness. Older patients are especially susceptible and are at increased risk of falls and injuries, eg, hip fractures.

Excessive anticholinergic effects are common with the concurrent use of drugs such as an antipsychotic agent (eg, chlorpromazine), an antiparkinsonian drug (eg, trihexyphenidyl), and a tricyclic antidepressant (eg, amitriptyline). In some individuals, particularly elderly patients, this additive effect may result in an atropine-like delirium that could be mistakenly interpreted as a worsening of psychiatric symptoms or the presence of dementia. Distinguishing between the symptoms of the conditions being treated and the effects of drug therapy may be difficult but is essential. Concurrent use of drugs with anticholinergic activity may also result in dry mouth and associated dental complications, blurring of vision, and hyperpyrexia in patients exposed to high temperature and humidity. In the elderly, they increase the risks of memory impairment and of decreased self-care capacity.

Commonly, a patient may unknowingly take several different products that contain the same nonsteroidal anti-inflammatory drug. An arthritic patient, using prescribed ibuprofen (often at dosage levels at or near the recommended maximum), may purchase an OTC ibuprofen product for pain or discomfort not associated with the arthritis, not knowing that the 2 products contain the same drug and increase the risk of adverse effects.

Interactions at Receptor Sites

The enzyme monoamine oxidase (MAO) metabolizes catecholamines such as norepinephrine. Norepinephrine accumulates within the adrenergic neurons when MAO is inhibited. Drugs that cause a release of these greater-than-usual amounts of norepinephrine can bring about exaggerated responses, including severe headache, hypertension (possibly a hypertensive crisis), and cardiac arrhythmias. Such an interaction may occur between MAO inhibitors (eg, isocarboxazid, phenelzine, tranylcypromine, pargyline) and indirectly acting sympathomimetic amines. While most sympathomimetic amines (eg, amphetamine) are available only by prescription, others (eg, ephedrine, phenylephrine, phenylpropanolamine), known to interact with MAO inhibitors, are present in many popular OTC cold, allergy, and diet remedies. Patients taking MAO inhibitors should avoid using such products.

Serious reactions (hypertensive crises) have occurred in patients being treated with MAO inhibitors following the ingestion of foods and beverages having a high tyramine content, including certain cheeses, alcoholic beverages, concentrated yeast extracts, broad-bean pods, and pickled herring. Tyramine is metabolized by MAO, which is present in the intestinal wall and the liver; this enzyme protects against the pressor actions of amines in foods. When the enzyme is inhibited, unmetabolized tyramine can accumulate, releasing norepinephrine from adrenergic neurons.

The antineoplastic drug procarbazine and the anti-infective drug furazolidone (or probably its metabolite) can also inhibit MAO, and the same warnings apply to these drugs as to other MAO inhibitors. With furazolidone, however, the enzyme inhibition usually does not occur within the first 5 days of therapy, and the course of treatment is often completed within that time. The new antiparkinsonian agent, selegiline, selectively inhibits MAO, type B. When used in the recommended dosage, selegiline is unlikely to interact with other drugs and tyramine-containing foods. However, if the dosage is increased, its selectivity diminishes and the risk of interactions increases.

PHARMACOKINETIC INTERACTIONS

Pharmacokinetic interactions are more complicated and difficult to predict because the interacting drugs often have unrelated actions; the interactions are mainly due to alteration of absorption, distribution, metabolism, or excretion, which changes the amount and duration of a drug's availability at receptor sites. The *type* of response expected from the interacting drugs is *not* changed, only the *magnitude* and *duration*. Thus, a pharmacokinetic interaction represents an altered effect of one, or possibly both, of the participating drugs and is predictable from a knowledge of what the individual drugs can do. Such interactions may be detected by patient-monitoring procedures (see Ch. 135). A change in blood drug levels usually occurs, and useful information may be obtained by measuring these levels.

Alteration of Gastrointestinal Absorption

Interactions that involve a change in drug absorption from the GI tract are of variable importance. Overall drug absorption may be reduced and its therapeutic activity compromised, or absorption may be delayed though the same amount of drug is eventually absorbed. Delayed drug absorption is undesirable when a rapid effect is needed to relieve acute symptoms, such as pain.

Alteration of pH: Many drugs are weak acids or weak bases, and the pH of the GI contents can influence absorption. Since the nonionized (more lipid-soluble) form of a drug is more readily absorbed than the ionized form, acidic drugs are usually more readily absorbed from the upper regions of the GI tract, where they are primarily in a nonionized form. Although changes in absorption might be predicted for many acidic and basic drugs, clinically important interactions are uncommon.

An acidic medium is required to adequately dissolve ketoconazole following oral administration. Therefore, an antacid, anticholinergic agent, histamine H_2 receptor antagonist, or omeprazole should not be given simultaneously; if one or more of these agents is needed, it should be given at least 2 h after ketoconazole is administered.

Complexation and adsorption: Tetracyclines can combine with metal ions (eg, Ca, Mg, Al, and Fe) in the GI tract to form poorly absorbed complexes. Thus, certain foods (eg, milk) or drugs (eg, antacids, products containing Mg, Al, and Ca salts, or Fe preparations) can significantly decrease tetracycline absorption. Absorption of doxycycline and minocycline is influenced to a lesser extent by food or milk, and either drug might be preferred when gastric irritation occurs or appears likely. However, aluminum-containing antacids will decrease the absorption of these tetracyclines. The increase in pH of the GI contents probably also contributes to the reduction of the tetracycline absorption.

Antacids also markedly reduce the absorption of fluoroquinolone derivatives (eg, ciprofloxacin), probably as a result of the metal ions complexing with the drug. Antacids should not be used simultaneously or < 2 h (or preferably, an even longer period) after ciprofloxacin.

Complexation can be expected with cholestyramine and colestipol. In addition to binding with and preventing reabsorption of bile acids, these agents can bind with drugs in the GI tract, having the greatest affinity for acidic drugs, eg, thyroid hormone or warfarin. To minimize the possibility of such an interaction, the interval between taking cholestyramine or colestipol and another drug should be as long as possible (preferably, at least 4 h).

Some antidiarrheals (eg, those containing kaolin and pectin), as well as antacids, may adsorb other drugs, resulting in decreased absorption. Such interactions have not been thoroughly evaluated, but their potential suggests that the interval between taking these preparations and another drug should be as long as possible.

Alteration of motility: By *increasing* GI motility, metoclopramide or a cathartic may hasten the passage of drugs through the GI tract, resulting in decreased absorption, particularly of drugs that require prolonged contact with the absorbing surface and those that are absorbed only at a particular site along the GI tract. Similar problems can occur with enteric-coated and sustained-release formulations.

By *decreasing* GI motility, anticholinergics may either reduce absorption by retarding dissolution and slowing gastric emptying, or increase absorption by keeping a drug for a longer period of time in the area of optimal absorption.

Effect of food: Food may delay or reduce the absorption of many drugs. Food often slows gastric emptying, but it may also affect absorption by binding with drugs, by decreasing their access to absorption sites, by altering their dissolution rates, or by altering the pH of the GI contents.

Food in the GI tract will reduce the absorption of many antibiotics. Although there are exceptions (eg, penicillin V potassium, amoxicillin, doxycycline, minocycline), it is generally recommended that penicillin and tetracycline derivatives, erythromycin stearate and formulations of erythromycin base that are not enteric coated, as well as several other antibiotics, be given at least 1 h before meals or 2 h after meals to achieve optimal absorption. Food has also been reported to decrease the absorption of many other therapeutic agents including astemizole, captopril, and penicillamine, and it is important that these drugs be administered apart from meals.

Although food does not significantly alter the activity of theophylline, when the drug is given in an immediate-release formulation, there has been considerable variation among the timed- or controlled-release formulations with respect to their potential to interact with food. For example, when one controlled-release formulation was taken < 1 h before a high fat-content meal, there was a significant increase in theophylline absorption and peak serum levels, as compared to administration in the fasting state. If information is insufficient to assess the potential for a particular theophylline formulation to interact with food, the drug should preferably be administered apart from meals.

Alteration of Distribution

Displacement of drugs from protein-binding sites may occur when 2 drugs capable of protein binding are given concurrently, especially when they are capable of binding to the same sites on the protein molecule (competitive displacement). Since the number of plasma or tissue protein-binding sites is limited, drugs can displace one another. Although the protein-bound fraction of a drug is not pharmacologically active, an equilibrium exists between the bound and unbound fractions. As the unbound or free drug is metabolized and excreted, the bound drug is gradually released to maintain the equilibrium and pharmacologic response. The risk of interactions from protein displacement is significant primarily with drugs that are highly protein bound (> 90%) and have a small apparent volume of distribution, especially during the first few days of concurrent therapy.

Both phenylbutazone and warfarin are extensively bound to plasma proteins, especially albumin, but phenylbutazone has a greater affinity for the binding sites. When the 2 drugs are taken concurrently, fewer binding sites are available for warfarin, thus increasing the amount of free anticoagulant and the risk of hemorrhage. Phenylbutazone also inhibits the metabolism of warfarin, resulting in continued enhancement of its anticoagulant effect.

The binding of acidic drugs to serum albumin has been studied most extensively; however, binding of basic drugs to α_1-acid glycoprotein is also important.

Alteration of Metabolism

Stimulation of metabolism: Many drug interactions result from the ability of one drug to stimulate the metabolism of another by increasing the activity of hepatic enzymes involved in their metabolism (enzyme induction). In this manner, phenobarbital increases the rate of metabolism of coumarin anticoagulants such as warfarin, resulting in a decreased anticoagulant response. The dose of the anticoagulant must be increased to compensate for this effect, but this is potentially dangerous if the patient discontinues the phenobarbital without appropriately reducing the anticoagulant dose. The use of alternative sedatives (eg, the benzodiazepines) eliminates this risk. Phenobarbital also accelerates the metabolism of other drugs such as steroid hormones. Enzyme induction also is caused by other barbiturates and by various therapeutic agents (eg, carbamazepine, phenytoin, and rifampin).

Disturbed calcium metabolism and osteomalacia are associated with the use of anticonvulsants such as phenobarbital and phenytoin. Reduced serum calcium levels are caused by vitamin D deficiency, resulting from enzyme induction by the anticonvulsants. This risk is greatest when the patient's dietary intake of vitamin D is borderline.

Pyridoxine can antagonize the activity of the antiparkinsonian drug levodopa by accelerating the conversion of the levodopa to its active metabolite, dopamine, in the peripheral tissues. In contrast to levodopa, dopamine cannot cross the blood-brain barrier, where it is required for the antiparkinsonian effect. In patients receiving both levodopa and carbidopa (a decarboxylase inhibitor), the addition of pyridoxine does not reduce the action of levodopa.

Studies show that the efficacy of certain drugs (eg, chlorpromazine, diazepam, propoxyphene, theophylline) may be decreased in individuals who smoke heavily, because of increased hepatic enzyme activity from the action of polycyclic hydrocarbons found in cigarette smoke.

Inhibition of metabolism: One drug may inhibit the metabolism of another, causing its prolonged and intensified activity. For example, disulfiram, used in the treatment of alcoholism, inhibits the activity of aldehyde dehydrogenase, thus inhibiting the oxidation of acetaldehyde, an oxidation product of alcohol. This results in the accumulation of excessive acetaldehyde and causes the characteristic disulfiram effect following the consumption of alcohol (see under Treatment in DEPENDENCE ON ALCOHOL in Ch. 53). Disulfiram also enhances the activity of warfarin and phenytoin, presumably by inhibiting their metabolism.

Allopurinol reduces the production of uric acid by inhibiting the enzyme xanthine oxidase. However, xanthine oxidase is involved in the metabolism of such potentially toxic drugs as mercaptopurine and azathioprine; when the enzyme is inhibited, the effect of these 2 agents can be markedly increased. Therefore, when allopurinol is given concurrently, a *reduction* to about $1/3$ to $1/4$ the usual dose of mercaptopurine or azathioprine is advised.

Cimetidine inhibits oxidative metabolic pathways and is likely to increase the action of other drugs that are metabolized via this mechanism (eg, carbamazepine, phenytoin, theophylline, warfarin, and certain benzodiazepines). Most benzodiazepines (eg, diazepam) are metabolized via oxidative mechanisms; however, lorazepam, oxazepam, and temazepam undergo glucuronide conjugation and their action is not affected by cimetidine. Although ranitidine also binds, to a limited extent, to the hepatic oxidative enzymes, it appears to have less affinity for the enzymes than does cimetidine and, as a consequence, clinically significant interactions with ranitidine are less likely to occur. Studies of the newer agents famotidine and nizatidine suggest that they are not likely to inhibit oxidative metabolic pathways and to interact with other drugs via this mechanism.

Erythromycin has been reported to inhibit the hepatic metabolism of agents such as carbamazepine and theophylline, thereby increasing their effects. The fluoroquinolones (eg, ciprofloxacin) also increase the activity of theophylline, presumably by the same mechanism.

Alteration of Urinary Excretion

Alteration of urinary pH: Urinary pH influences the ionization of weak acids and bases and thus affects their reabsorption and excretion. A nonionized drug more readily diffuses from the glomerular filtrate into the blood. More of an acidic drug is nonionized in an acid urine than in an alkaline urine, where it primarily exists as an ionized salt. Thus, more of an acidic drug (eg, a salicylate) diffuses back into the blood from an acid urine, resulting in prolonged and perhaps intensified activity. The risk of a significant interaction is greatest in patients who are taking large doses of salicylates (eg, for arthritis). Opposite effects are seen for a basic drug like dextroamphetamine. When the urinary pH was maintained at about 5 in one study, 54.5% of a dose of dextroamphetamine was excreted within 16 h, compared to a 2.9% excretion when the pH was maintained at about 8.

Alteration of active transport: Probenecid increases the serum levels and prolongs the activity of penicillin derivatives, primarily by blocking their tubular secretion. Such combinations have been used to therapeutic advantage. For example, probenecid improves the effectiveness of penicillin and its analogs when used in single-dose regimens in the treatment of gonorrhea.

Significantly greater serum digoxin levels are found when quinidine is administered concurrently than when digoxin is given alone. Quinidine appears to reduce the renal clearance of digoxin, although other nonrenal mechanisms are probably also involved in this interaction.

A number of nonsteroidal anti-inflammatory drugs (NSAIDs) have been reported to increase the activity and toxicity of methotrexate. There have been reports of fatal methotrexate toxicity in patients also receiving ketoprofen, and it has been suggested that ketoprofen inhibited the active renal tubular secretion of methotrexate. However, other mechanisms probably also contribute to an increase in serum methotrexate concentrations. Most of the patients were receiving high-dose methotrexate therapy for neoplastic disorders; however, caution should also be exercised in patients receiving lower doses, particularly since there is an increased use of low-dose methotrexate regimens in patients with rheumatoid arthritis who are also taking an NSAID.

PRINCIPLES OF MANAGEMENT

The following general points concerning drug interactions warrant emphasis:

1. The drugs for which interactions are most significant clinically are those with potent effects, low safety margins, and a steep dose-response curve; eg, warfarin, digoxin, cytotoxics, hypotensives, and hypoglycemic agents.

2. It may be difficult to distinguish a drug interaction from pathophysiologic factors affecting the response to therapy.

3. Potentially expected interactions may not occur; individual factors, such as dose and patient metabolism, determine the events.

4. When drug effects are closely monitored, an interaction usually requires a change of dosage or therapy and does not result in significant adverse effects.

5. In the displacement-from-protein-binding types of interaction, one fact is often overlooked. Any displacement alters the relationship between total and unbound drug and thus complicates the clinical interpretation of total drug levels in the blood. Total plasma concentrations of highly bound and displaceable drugs do not have the same meaning in the presence of displacing drugs as in their absence. Awareness of this becomes more important as blood levels are used increasingly to aid in the therapeutic control of patients on a variety of drugs.

To minimize the incidence and clinical consequences of drug interactions, the prescriber should (1) know the patient's total drug intake, including agents prescribed by others and all OTC medications; (2) prescribe as few drugs in as low doses for as short a time as needed; (3) know the effects, both wanted and unwanted, of all the drugs used (since the spectrum of drug interactions is usually contained within these effects) and, where possible, use drugs for which the dosage range permits a considerable margin of error; (4) observe and monitor the patient for the drugs' effects, particularly after any alteration in therapy (some interactions, eg, metabolic effects depending on enzyme induction, may take a week or more to appear); and (5) consider drug interactions as possible causes of any unanticipated troubles. If unexpected clinical responses do occur, blood levels of drugs being taken should be measured, if possible; the literature or someone with specific knowledge of drug interactions should be consulted; and, most importantly, the dose of the drug should be altered until the desired effect is obtained. If this fails, the drug should be changed to one that will not interact with other drugs being taken.

138. DRUG TOXICITY

(See also DRUGS IN PREGNANCY under PRENATAL CARE in Ch. 14, and DRUGS IN LACTATING MOTHERS under MANAGEMENT OF THE NORMAL NEWBORN in Ch. 23)

PRECLINICAL AND CLINICAL EVALUATION OF TOXICITY

Before a drug is approved for general clinical use by the FDA, preclinical and clinical data showing substantial evidence of safety and efficacy are required by law. Drug studies proceed through various phases, as follows.

Preclinical Investigation (Animal Studies)

Animal toxicity studies must precede human drug exposure. While the FDA has not proposed specific guidelines for the conduct of particular animal toxicity studies, they have issued regulations (Good Laboratory Practices) governing the way animal studies are performed and documented. Two main principles are involved in all animal toxicity testing. First, the effects of chemicals in laboratory animals, when properly qualified, are applicable to man. Second, the use of high doses in experimental animals is a necessary and valid method to discover possible toxicity in man. Because the number of animals used in toxicity studies is relatively small and interest is in detecting the low-incidence toxic response, larger doses must be given in order to validate the extrapolation to man.

Animal studies used to determine or define the safety of a drug include studies of acute, subchronic, and chronic toxicity in several animal species. **The initial acute toxicity studies** are to determine the **median lethal dose (LD50)**, the toxic symptoms developed by the animals, and the time that they appear. At least 3 species of animals, one not a rodent, are usually used, and acute toxicity is usually determined by more than one route of administration. In recent years the number of animals used in determining LD50s has been reduced, with a corresponding reduction in their precision. It has been recognized that this precision is not necessary in the overall assessment of toxicity of drugs in humans. These initial studies give an indication of species differences, nature of the toxic effects, time periods, and dosages at which they will be elicited. The LD50 alone, however, has little predictive value unless accompanied by longer-term studies using measures of toxicity other than death.

Subchronic toxicity studies are conducted in at least 2 animal species and usually consist of daily administration of the test drug for up to 90 days. In each species, at least 3 dose levels are used, varying from the expected therapeutic doses to levels high enough to produce toxicity. Ideally, the drug is administered by the route to be used in human trials. Physical and laboratory examinations are performed throughout the observation period. At the termination of the study, the animals are sacrificed and pathologic examinations conducted to determine the target organs of toxicity.

Chronic toxicity studies are carried out in at least 2 species, one of which is not a rodent. These studies usually last for up to the lifetime of the animal (ie, 2 yr in a rodent or longer in a nonrodent), but their length will depend on the intended duration of administration of the drug to humans. Three dose levels are again used, varying from low level or nontoxic to a greater-than-therapeutic dose level, high enough to produce a toxic response on chronic administration. Again, laboratory tests and observations are made at intervals throughout the period of drug administration. Some animals may be sacrificed periodically for gross and histologic postmortem examination. The results of these tests determine chronic organ toxicity and whether the drug is potentially carcinogenic.

Additionally, extensive reproduction experiments are carried out in rats and rabbits to detect any alterations in the reproductive cycle or any teratogenic effects on the unborn. These more specialized animal tests and the longer chronic toxicity studies may be conducted concurrently with the initial studies in human subjects, particularly when the drug is intended only for short-term human use.

There is a growing interest in the use of in vitro toxicity tests, which provide more rapid, cost-effective predictive tests for drug toxicity. The greatest emphasis has been in the area of mutagenicity, with the most popular test being the Ames bioassay. A chemical shown to be a mutagen would also have the potential to be a carcinogen in mammalian experimentation. Although they are not yet recognized and accepted as substitutes for animal testing and are used only as supportive information in the regulatory process, in vitro toxicity tests are employed by the pharmaceutical industry to focus on specific chemical compounds for further in vivo and pharmacologic development. These in vitro methods will most likely play an increasing role in drug development.

Clinical Investigation (Human Studies)

The data from preclinical animal toxicity studies are submitted in the form of an application for an investigational new drug (IND) and must be approved by the FDA before clinical studies can begin.

Clinical studies of new drugs, prior to approval by the FDA for marketing, are conducted in 3 phases. The widespread general use of the drug and postmarketing surveillance of drug use can be regarded as a 4th phase. Some adverse effects of drugs cannot be discerned in animals; eg, dizziness, nausea, headaches, ringing in the ears, heartburn, and depression. It has been estimated that $\geq$ 50% of undesirable drug effects seen most frequently can be ascertained only during human trials.

Phase 1 represents the first administration of a new drug to man. Informed consent is a prerequisite, as are certain legal requirements; eg, submitting the results of animal studies, information about product composition and manufacture, the intended clinical study protocol, approval from the local Institutional Review Board (IRB), and information about the training and experience of the investigators to the FDA, whose permission is required to initiate the study. These investigational drug studies are performed under a permit from the FDA known as an investigational new drug exemption permit. A small number of closely monitored subjects, mainly healthy volunteers, are usually involved. Initially, each receives a single dose of the drug to determine a safe dose range and assess pharmacokinetic data. The primary objective of this necessarily cautious phase of the investigation is to determine a safe and tolerated dosage in humans; however, observation of toxicity, if it occurs, and of absorption, metabolism, and excretion may also be made during Phase 1.

Phase 2 begins after satisfactory preliminary evidence regarding safety has been obtained. It involves the supervised administration of the drug to patients for treatment of, or prophylaxis against, the disease or symptoms for which the drug is intended. These studies usually are conducted in randomized clinical trials comparing the new drug with the prototype drug, if any, for a particular indication. Often this is the first opportunity to observe the effect of long-term administration of the drug to humans. These are the most crucial tests in the development and evaluation of a new drug, since the decision to proceed with extensive trials in large populations must be made on the basis of the data obtained in a relatively small number of patients.

Phase 3 begins after the initial phases have provided reasonable evidence of safety and efficacy. It consists of more widespread clinical trials that may move from the realm of clinical investigators to practicing physicians. These studies yield data on which the sponsor and the FDA can base a decision that the drug is safe and effective for its intended use. As many as 150 clinicians may participate in these studies, and the patients under their supervision usually number > 1500 and may even exceed 3000. Phase 3 extends up to the time the drug is released for general use.

There are no definitive rules on what constitutes safety and efficacy. These quantities must be judged in relation to the specific clinical conditions for which the drug is to be used and to alternative therapeutic modalities. When sufficient data have been collected to justify continued use of the drug, a **New Drug Application (NDA)** is submitted. Usually at least 4 yr or more have elapsed between the time the drug was selected on the basis of the original pharmacologic screen and the date of completion and filing of the NDA.

Phase 4 is the study of the actual use of the drug in medical practice and, though often not recognized as a phase of clinical investigation, is a most important one from a clinical standpoint. The preclinical and clinical investigations are relatively insensitive and are only capable of detecting adverse reactions with a frequency of > 1:1000 administrations. It is obvious that with many drug therapies a frequency of 1:10,000 or 1:50,000 may be clinically relevant and can only be determined with postmarketing surveillance that occurs after approval of the NDA. New therapeutic or toxic effects may be discovered, including rare or long-term effects that were not discernible in small numbers of patients. The sponsor's claims of drug efficacy and safety that are to appear in brochures and advertising are reviewed and approved by the FDA. Reports concerning current clinical studies must be sent to the FDA periodically during this phase of clinical investigation; specifically, reports are due every 3 mo during the 1st yr, every 6 mo during the 2nd yr, and annually thereafter. These reports must also include information about the quantity of drug distributed and copies of mailing pieces, labeling, and advertising. The manufacturer must also notify the FDA of any unexpected side effects, injury, and toxic or allergic reactions. Thus, the FDA is responsible for ensuring that drugs are safe and effective before being marketed, and for their continued surveillance thereafter.

ADVERSE DRUG REACTIONS (ADRs)

These embody *a wide variety of toxic drug reactions, dose- or non-dose-related, that occur in therapeutic situations.* The term usually excludes nontherapeutic overdosage (eg, accidental exposure or attempted suicide) or failure of the drug to have its intended effect (ie, lack of efficacy).

The practicing physician plays an important role in documenting ADRs, particularly those associated with newly marketed drugs. These should be reported even though a physician may not be able to attribute a causal role to the adverse reaction. It is only through active use of this **FDA Adverse Drug Reaction monitoring program**, which acts as an early warning signal, that unexpected adverse effects can be elucidated and investigated further. In addition to the alert physician, other potential useful sources include nurses, pharmacists, and other health care practitioners.

ADRs are usually classified as **mild** (no antidote, therapy, or prolongation of hospitalization necessary); **moderate** (requires a change in drug therapy, although not necessarily cessation of the drug, and may prolong hospitalization or require special treatment; **severe** (potentially life-threatening, requires discontinuation of the drug and specific treatment of the adverse reaction); and **lethal** (directly or indirectly contributes to the death of the patient).

The incidence of ADRs varies widely, from about 1 to 30%. Admission to a hospital because of an ADR has been shown to account for 3 to 7% of all admissions. Most prospective studies in hospitalized patients (excluding the mildly ill) show ADRs of 10 to 20%. About 10 to 20% of these are severe. The incidence of deaths due to ADRs is unknown; rates of 0.5 to 0.9% of medical patients have been suggested, but these include many patients with serious and complex diseases.

The incidence and severity of drug toxicity can also be influenced by patient variables such as age, sex, disease, genetic factors, and geographic factors; and by drug-related factors such as type of drug, route of administration, duration of therapy, dosage, and bioavailability. The extent to which misprescribing and patient compliance errors contribute to the incidence of ADRs is not clear.

The most commonly reported causes of drug-related deaths are (1) **gastrointestinal hemorrhage and peptic ulceration** (corticosteroids, aspirin, other anti-inflammatory drugs, anticoagulants); (2) **other hemorrhages** (anticoagulants, cytotoxic agents); (3) **aplastic anemia** (chloramphenicol, phenylbutazone, gold salts, cytotoxic agents; (4) **hepatic damage** (chlorpromazine, isoniazid); (5) **renal failure** (analgesics); (6) **infection** (corticosteroids, cytotoxic drugs); and (7) **anaphylaxis** (penicillin, antisera). Allergy is an important factor in nonfatal drug reactions, but it is less important as a cause of death.

Dose-Related, Predictable Drug Reactions

Although individuals vary considerably in their responsiveness to a particular drug effect, most drug toxicity is related to the amount of drug taken; the nature of the toxic manifestations is determined by the properties of the drug molecule. Previous contact with the drug is not necessary for the development of toxicity. Dose-related reactions can occur as side effects or overdosage toxicity, as defined below.

Side effects are *predictable pharmacologic effects that occur within therapeutic dose ranges and are undesired in the given therapeutic situation.* Side effects may be useful under certain circumstances. For example, the drowsiness produced by an antihistamine may be considered a "side effect" in the treatment of an allergy during the day, whereas the sedative-hypnotic effect may contribute to the desired overall therapy in the treatment of the allergy and associated insomnia at bedtime.

Overdosage toxicity is *the predictable toxic effect that occurs with dosages in excess of the therapeutic range for a particular patient.* It overlaps with side-effect toxicity to some extent, especially in drugs with a small therapeutic index. The severity of the reaction is usually dose-related (eg, hemorrhage with oral anticoagulants or convulsions due to local anesthetic agents). Some overdosage toxicity may occur because of drug accumulation caused by the patient's ineffective renal elimination or hepatic metabolism of the offending drug.

Non-Dose-Related, Unpredictable Effects

Drug allergy: Allergic reactions depend on altered reactivity of the patient as a result of prior contact with a drug that functions as an antigen or allergen. They are not dose-related; the symptoms and signs that develop are determined by antigen-antibody interactions and are largely independent of the pharmacologic properties of the drug. Allergic reactions are not completely unpredictable; a careful clinical history and appropriate skin tests may suggest those at risk. This subject is discussed in greater detail under HYPERSENSITIVITY TO DRUGS in Ch. 34 (see also DRUG ERUPTIONS in Ch. 97).

Idiosyncrasy is an imprecise term that has been used as a classification for unexpected and peculiar adverse reactions occurring in a small percentage of individuals exposed to a drug. Idiosyncratic reactions are not related to a drug's known pharmacologic effects and are not obviously allergic in nature, eg, the aplastic anemia which may occur with chloramphenicol. Idiosyncrasy has been defined by some as *a genetically determined abnormal reactivity to a drug,* but not all idiosyncratic reactions have a pharmacogenetic cause. The term idiosyncrasy may become obsolete as specific mechanisms of ADRs become elucidated (see PHARMACOGENETICS in Ch. 137). For example, hemolysis occurring in individuals taking certain drugs (eg, antimalarials) can no longer be considered idiosyncratic because a genetic predisposition (G6PD deficiency) can be detected in the laboratory, and hemolysis is therefore predictable and dose-related.

Management and Prevention

Prevention of ADRs requires familiarity with the drug used and awareness of the potential reactions to it. Mild ADRs can often be recognized before serious effects develop.

If an ADR occurs, the type and any precipitating factors (eg, digitalis toxicity occurring from hypokalemia due to concurrent diuretic therapy) must be determined if possible. With dose-related ADRs, dose modification or attention to precipitating factors may suffice; increasing the rate of drug elimination is rarely necessary. With non-dose-related ADRs, the drug usually should be withdrawn and re-exposure avoided.

CARCINOGENESIS

A carcinogen is a *chemical or physical agent that has the potential of producing neoplasia.*

Chemical carcinogens are defined by their ability to produce tumors as measured by (1) development of types of tumors not seen in the controls (ie, unique); (2) an increased incidence of tumor types occurring in the treated animals compared to controls; (3) an occurrence of tumors earlier than in the controls; and (4) an increased multiplicity of tumors in individual animals. It is generally accepted that environmental or nutritional factors account for as much as 90% of human cancers. The factors include smoking, dietary habits, and exposure to sunlight, chemicals, and drugs. Genetic, viral, and radiation factors are estimated to cause the remaining 10%. Most carcinogenic effects of chemicals have a long latency period; 20 to 30 yr is not unusual prior to the development of tumors. Such delayed effects are rarely detected in early clinical trials of new drugs. Chemicals capable of producing cancer in laboratory animals have diverse structures, suggesting a high likelihood that numerous mechanisms are involved in the induction of cancer. Carcinogenesis is believed to be a multistep process, with most carcinogens being unreactive compounds (procarcinogens or secondary carcinogens) that are converted in the body to primary carcinogens.

It has been proposed that carcinogens be divided into those that are genotoxic and those that are epigenetic. **Genotoxic agents** *function as electrophilic reactants and directly alter DNA, thus producing or initiating an abnormal cell.* Genotoxic compounds include all direct acting and primary carcinogens as well as many procarcinogens or secondary carcinogens. The **epigenetic agents** include *those carcinogens for which there is no evidence of genotoxicity.* To date, identified drug-carcinogens fall primarily into the epigenetic classification. This category includes some solid state carcinogens, many hormones and immunosuppressants, and the group of compounds called cocarcinogens and promoters (which are not carcinogens per se but potentiate the effects of a carcinogen). Promotion involves increased growth and development of dormant or latent tumor cells; the time from initiation to the development of the tumor probably depends on the presence of such promoters.

Detection of low incidence of carcinogenic potential is a serious problem during the evaluation phase of new drugs. For example, it is normal for 100 animals to be used in any given dose or study, and the incidence of tumor development would have to exceed 4% to be statistically signif-

icant. A 4% incidence of tumors would be extremely high for most drug categories.

Drugs with a high carcinogenic potential should be avoided, but therapeutic decisions depend upon benefit-risk assessments. For example, though alkylating chemotherapeutic agents are potent carcinogens in a variety of animals, it would be illogical to withhold them from a patient with a potentially lethal disease. (The situation is analogous to exposure to x-rays, which also have carcinogenic potential.)

Very few drugs are in use for which there is good evidence of carcinogenesis in humans. Oral contraceptives appear rarely to cause hepatic adenomas, which are benign in terms of their own growth but are extremely vascular and can cause fatal hemorrhage. An association between reserpine and carcinoma of the breast has been claimed by some workers on the basis of case-control studies, but it has not been confirmed by others in cohort studies. There is convincing evidence that some nondrug chemicals are carcinogens. This evidence includes the associations between aflatoxins and hepatoma, vinyl chloride and liver hemangiosarcoma, coal tars and skin cancer, cigarette smoke and lung carcinoma, and aniline dyes and bladder tumors.

Short-term mutagenicity testing is developing into a reasonably accurate method of detecting potential carcinogens prior to large-scale human exposure and holds promise of becoming an even better predictor of human carcinogenicity.

BENEFIT—TO—RISK RATIO

In every therapeutic endeavor, risks must be weighed against benefits for each particular clinical situation and patient. Drug therapy is justified only if the possible benefits outweigh the possible risks after considering the qualitative and quantitative impact of using a drug and the likely outcome if the drug is withheld. This decision depends on adequate clinical knowledge of the patient, of the disease and its natural history, and of the drug and its potential adverse effects.

Although the term "benefit-to-risk *ratio*" is convenient and often used, *for individual patients numerical predictions of benefit or risk do not exist,* and the mathematical division (to obtain a ratio) is never performed. A more accurate term is benefit-to-risk analysis. The following factors must be taken into account.

Patient factors: Age, sex, presence or capability of pregnancy, occupation, social circumstances, genetic traits, etc, may change the magnitude of risks and benefits by influencing the course and severity of the disease or the response to medication. Examples include the poor prognosis of very young or old patients with pneumonia that requires aggressive therapy, the sensitivity of the fetus to drugs that may be relatively safe for a nonpregnant woman, and industrial exposure to organophosphates or genetic cholinesterase deficiency resulting in increased sensitivity to depolarizing muscle relaxants. A 60-yr-old patient with atherosclerosis, poor cerebral blood flow, and a BP of 200/120 mm Hg requires different therapy than would an otherwise healthy young patient with the same BP.

Disease factors such as the course, duration, mortality, and morbidity influence risks and benefits of treatment. It makes little sense to treat a self-limiting disease causing little debility, such as herpes labialis, with a potent systemic drug such as cytarabine; whereas such therapy may be justified in herpetic encephalitis, which is otherwise usually fatal.

Drug factors include the frequency, severity, and predictability of adverse reactions, the relationship of such reactions to dosage, the means by which they can be prevented or treated, and the availability of alternative drugs or therapies. For example, penicillin anaphylaxis is rare, but it is potentially fatal and may sometimes be avoided by taking an adequate history and doing appropriate skin tests. If anaphylaxis occurs when one is prepared for it, successful treatment is possible. Penicillin, therefore, should not ordinarily be withheld in streptococcal pharyngitis for fear of anaphylaxis. On the other hand, aplastic anemia due to chloramphenicol is also fatal and relatively rare, but it is unpredictable and often irreversible. Therefore, although chloramphenicol is also effective against streptococcal pharyngitis, safer alternatives exist, and its use here is not justified. However, for a serious disease such as *Hemophilus influenzae* meningitis, few alternative drugs exist and chloramphenicol therapy may be justified.

A drug's efficacy should also be known, including the predictability of a favorable response, whether the effect is symptomatic or curative, the relationship to dosage, and the duration of the beneficial effect. Acute myeloid leukemia in children responds to aggressive combination chemotherapy and is justified. However, use of aggressive chemotherapy is debatable in such malignancies as gastric carcinoma, in which response is poor and chemotherapy may increase morbidity.

Judicious use of drug combinations may increase benefits and reduce risks; eg, the use of adrenergic blocking agents with a thiazide diuretic and potassium supplements in the treatment of hypertension.

139. PATIENT COMPLIANCE

The degree to which patients adhere to a treatment plan.

The more common problems of patient compliance are discussed here. Compliance in children is discussed in Ch. 25; compliance in the elderly is discussed under BASIC PRINCIPLES IN CARING FOR THE ELDERLY in Ch. 124.

Even the most thorough and well-designed therapeutic regimen will fail without patient compliance. Depending on the variable studied and the strictness of definition, 15 to 95% of patients have been found to be noncompliant. Overall, probably $1/3$ to $1/2$ of patients make some error with their medications—incorrect dose, inaccuracies of timing, adding unprescribed medications, or not taking medication. Capricious or irregular dosing exposes a patient to the risks of medication without concomitant therapeutic benefit. Whereas most patients occasionally default or make errors, some never stray and others continually fail to comply.

It is difficult to identify patients who do not take their medications as prescribed. The same patient may act differently depending on the treatment, disease, adverse effects, or other factors in his life. In dealing with noncompliance, *the prescriber must discuss it with the patient and ascertain why the patient is not following the prescribed treatment.* The cause for noncompliance may be remediable with such a discussion, or the therapeutic regimen may need to be modified.

Patient factors in noncompliance: Age, sex, race, and educational level are not predictors of compliance. "Forgetfulness" is the most frequently cited reason, but it is not really an explanation. It may be a rationalization to cover unconscious or partly conscious concerns about the patient's health status, his diagnosis, and the taking of medication. Commonly, there is fear of adverse effects, of addiction, of the disease state that treatment implies, and of loss of independence. For example, patients with hypertension have an asymptomatic disease and must cope with medical advice from physicians, public health advertisements, and well-intentioned friends regarding their risks of stroke, heart attack, and renal disease. Many deal with the resultant anxiety by denying illness, a prominent sign of which is neglecting to take medication. In other cases, medications may be stopped because symptoms and signs decrease or disappear. Although medications account for a small fraction of total personal health care expenditures, some patients decrease the dose or the duration of treatment to save money. More rarely, a patient may not fill the prescription at all for financial or other reasons.

Medication factors in noncompliance: Complex regimens with frequent dosing or many medications increase errors in dosage times, scheduling with meals, etc. A regimen of once or twice/day dosing is more easily followed correctly; compliance appears to be roughly equal with these 2 schedules. However, missing a dose of a once/day medication results in 24 h without medication. The key aspect of scheduling for good compliance is avoiding midday, out-of-the-house doses. If preparations look alike, patients may confuse them and inadvertently repeat or omit doses. Other factors include adverse effects (real or imagined), unpleasant tastes or smells, and precautions imposed by therapeutic regimens (eg, no alcohol or cheese).

Disease factors in noncompliance: Certain illnesses, such as chronic diseases with day-to-day fluctuation in symptoms (or without symptoms), seem more likely to lead to compliance problems. When a medication causes more symptoms than the disease under therapy (eg, hypertension), noncompliance or defaulting is more likely.

The physician's role in improving patient compliance: Making a correct diagnosis and designing a simple, effective therapeutic regimen start the therapeutic process and help to increase the likelihood of compliance. Directions to the patient must be clear, precise, and tailored to the vagaries and necessities of the patient's life and the disease process. Adverse effects should be discussed in a general way. Prescribers should urge patients to mention undesired or unexpected effects to the physician prior to stopping medication. Inappropriate termination of the therapeutic regimen may be prevented if the physician explains features of the plan such as the delay associated with the onset of the benefit characteristic of some drugs, eg, antidepressants. Asking about adherence to the regimen and the reasons for any problems may help to correct noncompliance and is necessary, since patients often do not volunteer such information. The belief that education promotes rational choices and improves compliance is not supported by hard evidence. Dealing specifically with patient factors that underlie noncompliance is far more effective. Trust—in the personal physician, in the prescribed therapy, or perhaps in medical science in general—appears most crucial to patient compliance. Explaining the purpose of the components in the regimen and the beneficial and adverse effects of a medication, as well as its shape, color, and dosage schedule, are educational; but, more importantly, they may help create a relationship of trust.

The pharmacist's and nurse's role in improving compliance: Nurses and pharmacists may detect compliance problems. Information that patients do not discuss with physicians may be transmitted to less threatening figures and can be relayed to the physician; eg, by the pharmacist who notes that the patient cannot pay for a full prescription or does not obtain refills. Illogical or incorrect prescriptions, which can decrease compliance, may be noted by a pharmacist and corrected in consultation with the prescriber. Nurses and pharmacists may instruct patients on their medications, especially prior to discharge from the hospital. By reviewing the physical characteristics of medications, directions, side effects, drug interactions, precautions, specific patient concerns, and the necessity for each medication, they can uncover misunderstandings and fears and enhance the patient's knowledge.

Patients may not take medications for valid and important reasons. "Intelligent noncompliance" (where the patient discontinues or decreases the dose of medication based on a correct interpretation of the clinical situation) may decrease adverse effects and improve the therapeutic outcome. Too often, however, the therapist does not know of these efficacious maneuvers. If the patient can act as a therapeutic monitor, reporting desirable and detrimental effects, the physician can better adjust therapy, exploring dose-effect relationships or discontinuing unneeded drugs.

140. PLACEBOS

Putatively inactive substances used in controlled studies for comparison with presumed active drugs or prescribed for relief of symptoms or to meet a patient's demands. A placebo may be any therapeutic maneuver, including surgical and psychologic techniques, or medication in any form (eg, oral, parenteral, topical); this discussion is limited to drugs.

The term placebo harks back to the 116th Psalm in the Hebrew Bible. Through a number of translation errors, the Vulgate (Latin) version came to contain the word "placebo" (I shall please). Over the centuries, the term was applied to the Vespers for the Dead, derisively to servile flatterers and toadies, and to laments sung at funerals by professional mourners.

In 1785, the word placebo first appeared in a medical dictionary as "a commonplace method or medicine." Two editions later, the placebo had become a "make-believe medicine," allegedly inert and harmless. We now know that placebos may have profound effects, both good and bad.

The Binary Nature of Placebo Effects

The medical literature is replete with reports on the power of the placebo to help patients with anxiety, tension, melancholia, schizophrenia, pain of all sorts, headaches, cough, insomnia, seasickness, chronic bronchitis, the common cold, arthritis, peptic ulcer, hypertension, nausea, senile dementia, etc. But the placebo is not only able to help, it has also been associated with side effects including nausea, headache, dizziness, sleepiness, insomnia, fatigue, depression, numbness, hallucinations, itching, vomiting, tremor, tachycardia, diarrhea, pallor, rashes, hives, ataxia, and edema, to name a few.

This remarkable list of *subjective and objective* changes, both desirable and unwanted, becomes more understandable and is put into perspective once one recognizes that there are 2 components of the **placebo effect**. One is the anticipation (usually optimistic) of results because of the expectations associated with medication. One can call this "suggestibility," "faith," "hope," or whatever.

The 2nd component, spontaneous change, is at times even more important. If a placebo has been taken before spontaneous improvement, it may be given credit for the result; conversely, if someone spontaneously develops a headache or a rash after taking a placebo, the latter may be blamed.

The "Placebo Reactor"

Studies to determine whether certain personality characteristics correlate with responses to placebos have disagreed extravagantly. This is not surprising, since some investigators call a "placebo reactor" one who gets benefit from placebos, and others use the term for people who report side effects from placebos. It seems unlikely that the same personality traits would predispose to such different responses.

It is probably more accurate to talk about a spectrum of "placebo reactivity" than about "placebo reactors," since virtually anyone is suggestible under some circumstances. However, some people seem more prone to influence than others. We can only speculate, but these differences at times may relate to the recipient's personality; eg, dependent personalities, who want to please their physicians, may be more likely to report beneficial effects, and histrionic personalities may be more likely to note any effect, good or bad (see also Ch. 52). Probably the most important factors are those that relate to specific attitudes toward the illness, medication, and physician. For example, when a patient with acute pain has a favorable attitude toward medicines and is given a placebo by a concerned and confident physician, a better response may occur than when a patient with chronic pain who views drugs as dangerous chemicals is given a placebo by a gruff physician who appears uncertain.

Placebo addicts: At least 2 patients have been reported who were addicted to placebos. One consumed 10,000 placebos in 1 yr. The other showed many of the characteristics of a true drug addict: a tendency to increase the dose, inability to stop the "medicine" without psychiatric help, a compulsive desire to take the tablets, and an abstinence syndrome when deprived of the tablets.

Use in Research

Difficulty in sorting out the 2 components of the placebo response does not detract from the utility of the placebo as a control in clinical trials, where its effects must be subtracted from the overall results in much the same way as a "blank" serves the chemist in negating "background noise" in a chemical assay. Whatever the relative importance of suggestibility and spontaneous change, the test drug must perform better than the placebo to justify its being marketed. In some studies (eg, comparison with a new drug to relieve angina pectoris), relief with placebo commonly exceeds 50%, presenting a significant challenge to demonstrate effectiveness of the active test drug.

Use in Therapy

There is a placebo factor in every therapeutic maneuver; therefore, effects attributed to drugs will vary from patient to patient and physician to physician, depending on placebo reactivity. Patients with a "positive" orientation to drugs, physicians, nurses, and hospitals are more likely to respond favorably to placebos than are patients with a "negative" orientation. The latter may deny benefit or complain of untoward effects. A positive placebo effect is more likely when both patient and physician believe that therapeutic benefit will result. Thus, an active agent with no accepted pharmacologic effect on the process being treated (eg, vitamin B_{12} in a patient with arthritis) may provide a favorable response, or a mildly active agent (eg, a vasodilator in a patient with intermittent claudication) may have an enhanced effect.

With deliberate placebo use (which is rare in current clinical practice, as opposed to research trials), there are several additional major **hazards:** (1) Since the physician is deceiving the patient, there may be an adverse effect on the physician-patient relationship. At the very least, the physician must be more guarded, lest his deception be discovered. Should it be discovered, the patient will lose face and feel betrayed, and his confidence in the physician will be impaired. (2) The physician may misinterpret the patient's response; particularly pernicious is the unwarranted conclusion that a positive response means that the patient's symptoms are not based on somatic illness or are neurotically exaggerated. When other physicians or nurses are involved in the deception (as in a group practice or hospital setting), the potential for adversely modifying the attitudes and behaviors of any or all of the others toward the patient and the potential for discovery are increased. Considering the availability of a host of drugs that have at least the potential to alleviate most of the complaints seen in practice and the danger of damaging or destroying a physician-patient relationship with placebo use, placebos qua placebos are rarely (if ever) indicated.

Today, physicians may prescribe vitamin "tonics" or B_{12} injections that are often tantamount to placebos, although they rarely prescribe lactose tablets or "sterile hypos." For example, most young physicians pick up patients from another physician who has left practice. Such patients who have taken B_{12} or other vitamins as a "tonic" with great faith and perceived benefit for many years, often feel ill and can become seriously upset if denied their "medicine." Based on cultural or psychologic sets, some patients seem to require and obtain benefit from either an unrequired medication or a particular dosage form (eg, by injection when an oral agent should suffice).

141. NEUROTRANSMISSION

A nerve cell or neuron has 2 major distinguishing functions—propagation of the action potential along the axon, and transmission of the signal from one nerve or cell structure to elicit a response (eg, nerve impulse, muscle contraction). While impulses conducted along an axon are caused by the movement of Na and K ions across the membrane and are electrical in nature, the transmission of impulses from one neuron to another neuron or to a non-neuronal cell is chemical and depends upon the action of certain **neurotransmitters (NTs)** on specific receptors.

A particular neuron generates the same action potential following each stimulus and conducts it at a fixed speed along the axon. Thus, nerve propagation is basically an "all or none" response and is not subject to modulation. Drugs either do not affect propagation or abolish it completely (eg, local anesthetics). Only a few diseases alter the structure of the nerve (eg, multiple sclerosis) and interfere with propagation.

In contrast, transmission via NTs is a highly complex and sensitive process. Synaptic relationships in the periphery involve neuron-neuron or neuron-effector interactions. In the CNS, more complex arrangements exist. Functional contact between 2 neurons may occur between axon and cell body, axon and dendrite, cell body and cell body, or dendrite and dendrite. Neurotransmission can be increased or decreased to accommodate any physiologic situation. Many neurologic

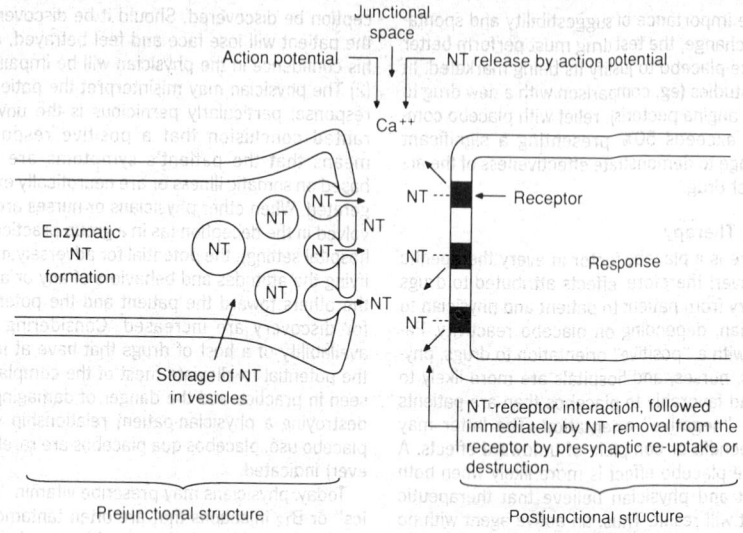

Fig. 141 – 1. Schematic representation of neurotransmission.

and psychiatric diseases are caused by a pathologic over- or underactivity of neuronal transmission. Many drugs can modify neurotransmission to cause adverse effects (eg, hallucinogens) or to correct pathologic conditions (eg, antipsychotic drugs—see below).

The development and maintenance of the cells of the nervous system depend on certain proteins. These neurotrophic factors include nerve growth factor, brain-derived neurotrophic factors, and neurotrophin-3.

Basic Principles of Neurotransmission

Neurotransmission involves (1) synthesis and storage of the NT in the prejunctional nerve structure; (2) release of the NT from the nerve terminal; (3) interaction of the NT with a specific postjunctional structure (receptor); (4) rapid termination of the NT-receptor interaction; and (5) destruction of NT or re-uptake into the terminal (see FIG. 141 – 1).

The nerve cell body, which contains the nucleus and DNA, has the enzymes that are involved in the synthesis of most NTs. These enzymes act on precursor molecules that are taken up by the neuron to form the NT.

Storage of the NT occurs at the nerve terminal in distinct vesicles. These NT molecules are usually bound to specific proteins in the presence of ATP and certain cations. The amount of NT in one vesicle (usually several thousand molecules) is termed a quantum.

Some NT molecules are constantly extruded from the terminal, but the amounts are insufficient to elicit a significant physiologic response. However, an action potential arriving at the terminal and the activation of calcium cause the simultaneous release of NT molecules from many vesicles by fusing the walls of these vesicles to that of the nerve terminal and forming an opening through which the NT molecules are expelled into the synaptic cleft (exocytosis).

To keep the quantities of NT in the terminals relatively constant and independent of nerve activity or inactivity, formation of NTs is tightly regulated. Regulation of NT amounts varies among neurons but is achieved through increased or decreased precursor uptake or activity of NT synthesizing or destroying enzymes. Also, stimulation or blockade of postsynaptic receptors can decrease or increase presynaptic NT synthesis.

The quanta released from these vesicles diffuse across the cleft and bind briefly to receptors, causing activation and a physiologic response. Depending on the receptor, this interaction can be excitatory (eg, initiation of a new action potential) or inhibitory (eg, inhibition of the development of a new action potential). The response of non-neuronal structures (skeletal, smooth or cardiac muscle cells, and glands) may also be stimulatory or inhibitory.

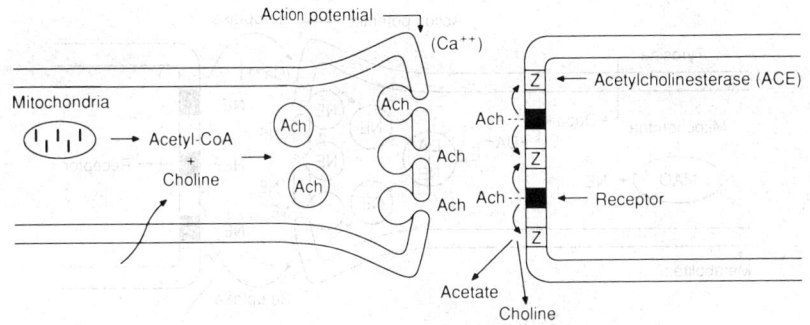

FIG. 141–2. Schematic representation of a cholinergic junction.

To ensure rapid, consecutive activation of the same receptors ("Morse code"), the NT-receptor interaction is very brief **(termination)**. The NT is quickly "pumped" back by active processes (re-uptake) into the nerve terminals, destroyed by enzymes located near the receptors, or diffused into the surroundings **(destruction)**.

Major Neurotransmitters

A neurotransmitter **(NT)** is defined as *a chemical that is selectively released from a nerve terminal by an action potential, interacts with a specific receptor on an adjacent structure, and elicits a specific physiologic response.* The following criteria must be satisfied before a chemical can qualify as an NT: (1) the chemical must be present in the nerve terminal; (2) the chemical must be released from the nerve terminal by an action potential; (3) the chemical when applied experimentally to the receptor must produce the identical effect. Although evidence exists from in vitro and animal studies that certain chemicals function as NTs, little such evidence is available for human nerve tissue. Thus, all the NTs discussed below should be understood as being putative in humans.

Most NTs derive from **amino acids** (or related compounds such as choline). Certain neurons synthesize only one, neuron-specific NT; others have been shown to synthesize 2 or more NTs. Some neurons modify amino acids to form the "amine" transmitters (eg, norepinephrine, serotonin, acetylcholine); others combine amino acids to form "peptide" transmitters (eg, endorphins, enkephalins); and still other neurons use amino acids unchanged or synthesized as transmitters. A few NTs are not related to amino acids.

Acetylcholine (Ach), the major NT of the motoneurons, autonomic preganglionic fibers, postganglionic cholinergic (parasympathetic) fibers, and many neurons in the CNS (basal ganglia, motor cortex), is synthesized from choline and mitochondrially derived acetyl-coenzyme A by the enzyme choline acetyltransferase **(CAT)**. Upon release, Ach stimulates cholinergic receptors of adjacent structures. This interaction is rapidly terminated by hydrolysis of Ach to choline and acetate by the enzyme acetylcholinesterase **(ACE)** found adjacent to the receptors. Ach levels are regulated by the activity of CAT and by choline uptake (see FIG. 141–2).

Dopamine (DA) is the NT of some peripheral nerve fibers and of many central neurons (eg, substantia nigra, midbrain, hypothalamus). The amino acid tyrosine is taken up by dopaminergic neurons, converted by the enzyme tyrosine hydroxylase to 3,4-dihydroxyphenylalanine **(dopa)**, decarboxylated by the enzyme aromatic L-amino acid decarboxylase to DA, and stored in vesicles. After release, DA interacts with dopaminergic receptors and is then "pumped" back by active processes (re-uptake) into the prejunctional neurons. DA levels are held constant by changes in tyrosine hydroxylase activity and the enzyme monoamine oxidase **(MAO)**, which is localized in nerve terminals and metabolizes dopamine. DA is metabolized to several metabolites, including specifically homovanillic acid.

Norepinephrine (NE) is the NT of most postganglionic sympathetic fibers and many central neurons (eg, locus ceruleus, hypothalamus). NE synthesis, like that of DA, also starts with the precursor tyrosine but continues as DA is hydroxyl-

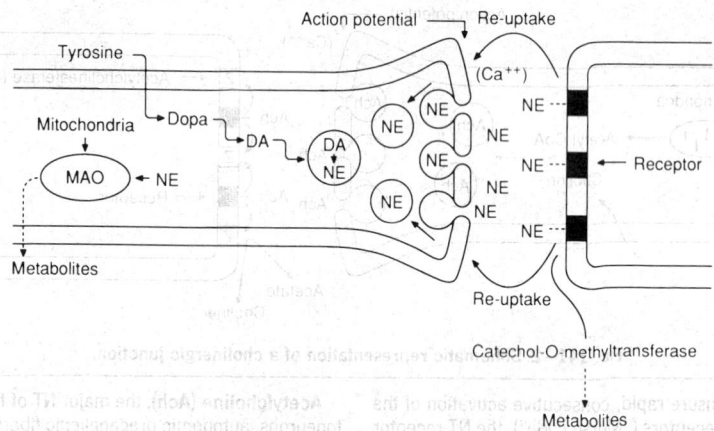

FIG. 141–3. Schematic representation of an adrenergic junction.

ated by dopamine-β-hydroxylase to form NE, which is stored in vesicles. Upon release, NE interacts with adrenergic receptors. This action is terminated largely by the re-uptake of NE back into the prejunctional neurons (see FIG. 141–3). Tyrosine hydroxylase and MAO regulate intraneuronal NE levels. Metabolism of NE occurs via MAO and catechol-O-methyltransferase to inactive metabolites (eg, normetanephrine, 3-methoxy-4-hydroxyphenylethylene glycol, 3-methoxy-4-hydroxymandelic acid).

Serotonin (5-HT) is the NT of many central neurons (eg, raphe nucleus). Its synthesis begins with the uptake of tryptophan into serotonergic neurons. Tryptophan is hydroxylated by the enzyme tryptophan hydroxylase to 5-hydroxytryptophan, and then decarboxylated to serotonin (5-hydroxytryptamine) by the enzyme aromatic L-amino acid decarboxylase. Levels of 5-HT are controlled by the uptake of tryptophan and intraneuronal MAO. Metabolism occurs mainly via MAO to 5-hydroxyindoleacetic acid.

γ-Aminobutyric acid (GABA) causes mostly inhibitory responses in the CNS and is found in many areas (eg, basal ganglia, cerebellum). GABA is derived from glutamic acid, which is decarboxylated by glutamic acid decarboxylase. After interaction with its receptors, GABA is actively "pumped" back into the neuronal terminals. It is metabolized by a GABA-transaminase.

β-Endorphin (β-End) is a polypeptide and is the transmitter of many central neurons (eg, hypothalamus, amygdala, thalamus, locus ce-

ruleus). In the cell body, amino acids are assembled by several enzymes into a large polypeptide, called pro-opiomelanocortin. This polypeptide is transported down the axon and is cleaved by specific peptidases into fragments, one of which is β-End containing 31 amino acids. After release and interaction with peptidergic (opioid) receptors, it is hydrolyzed by peptidases into smaller, inactive peptides and amino acids.

Methionine-enkephalin and **leucine-enkephalin** are small peptides present in many central neurons (eg, globus pallidus, thalamus, caudate, central gray). Their synthesis is similar to that of endorphin in that larger precursor peptides are formed in the cell body (proenkephalin) and split by specific peptidases in the axon into smaller peptides. Two of the fragments are the enkephalins both having 5 amino acids but either methionine or leucine as the terminal amino acid. After release and interaction with peptidergic (opioid) receptors, the enkephalins are hydrolyzed by other peptidases into smaller, inactive peptides and amino acids.

Dynorphins are a group of 7 peptides with similar amino acid sequences and are present in the same areas as are the enkephalins. These peptides are derived from prodynorphin and are hydrolyzed after receptor activation.

Substance P is a peptide and the transmitter of many central neurons (eg, dorsal root ganglia, basal ganglia, hypothalamus). Its synthesis and fate are similar to those of the other peptide NTs.

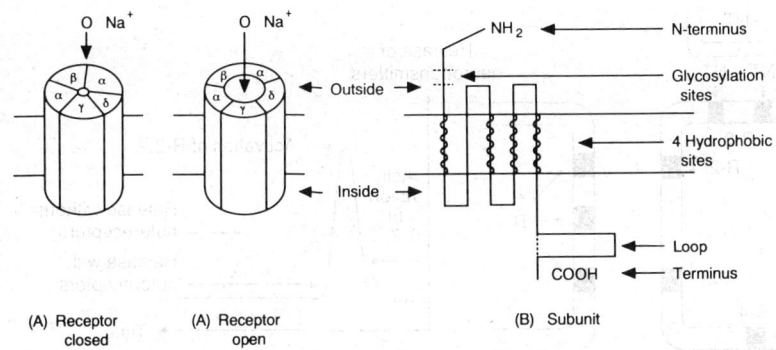

FIG. 141–4. Schematic representation of the nicotinic receptor (closed and open, A) and one of its subunits (B).

Glycine, glutamate, and aspartate are NTs used directly by certain neurons without change (although glycine might also be synthesized from serine). Aspartate is mainly present in the cortex, glutamate in the cerebellum and spinal cord, and glycine in the interneurons of the spinal cord. Glutamic and aspartic acid cause excitatory responses, while glycine is inhibitory.

Other neurotransmitters, whose roles in neurotransmission have not been as firmly established, include epinephrine, histamine, vasopressin, vasoactive intestinal peptide, carnosine, bradykinin, cholecystokinin, bombesin, somatostatin, corticotropin-releasing factor, neurotensin, and others.

In addition to these amino acid–related NTs, some NTs are different, eg, adenosine.

Major Receptors

A receptor is a small binding or recognition site with a specific molecular configuration on a cell surface or within the cell structure, which causes a physiologic response upon stimulation by an NT or other chemical, such as a drug or toxin. Some receptors cause inhibitory (eg, relaxation of a muscle) or excitatory (eg, initiation of nerve impulse or contraction of a muscle) responses. Usually, movement of Na^+ depolarizes and is stimulatory, whereas movement of Cl^- hyperpolarizes and is inhibitory. Ion channel receptors can be classified into receptors that are part of the channel (eg, nicotine, GABA, glycine, and glutamate receptors) or second messenger receptors that are activated by a second messenger to affect the channel (eg, adrenergic, mus-

carinic, serotonergic, and dopaminergic receptors). A neuron might carry hundreds or thousands of the same or different receptors. Not all of these receptors are functional; many are dormant.

NT-stimulated receptors are protein complexes that are arranged across the membrane. Second messenger receptors are usually monomeric, whereas the ion channel receptors consist of different proteins (subunits). A schematic representation of the nicotinic receptor and one of its subunits is shown in FIG. 141–4. Receptors are continuously synthesized in the cell body, transported to the respective sites, stored in the membrane, actively incorporated into the membrane ("externalization," "activation"), and after use degraded. Their half-lives range from days to weeks. The number of receptors and their affinity for specific NT molecules is not constant but will vary. Receptors that are continuously stimulated by NTs or drugs (agonists) become hyposensitive ("down-regulation"), whereas receptors that are not stimulated by their NT or are blocked by drugs (antagonists) become hypersensitive ("up-regulation"). This is mostly done by changes in affinity and, more often, numbers of receptors. The result of such altered receptors is a decreased or increased physiologic response of the effector cell.

Up-regulation or down-regulation of receptors plays a major role in the development of tolerance and physical dependence (pharmacodynamic tolerance or dependence). Withdrawal is usually a rebound phenomenon due to an altered receptor affinity and/or density.

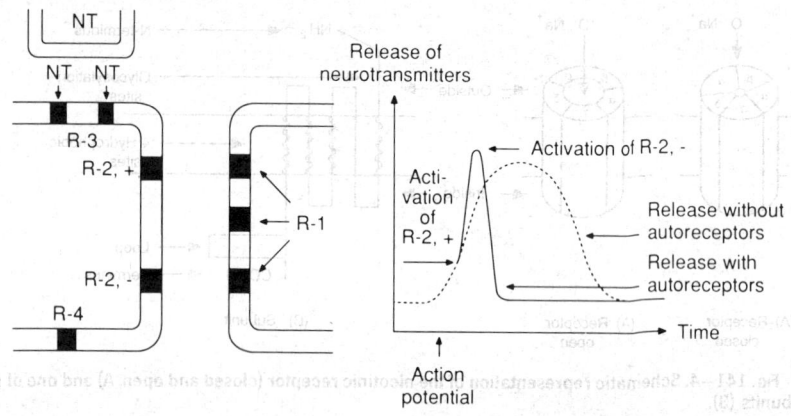

FIG. 141—5. Schematic representation of different receptor sites and the action of auto-receptors.

Most NTs interact primarily with the **post-synaptic receptor (R-1)** to produce a physiologic response in the adjacent structure. However, receptors are also located on presynaptic neurons and control the release of a specific NT. These receptors can be divided into different classes. The **autoreceptors (R-2)** respond only to released NT and are of 2 types: (R-2, +) that increase the release of NT, and (R-2, −) that inhibit the release of NT. These autoreceptors cause a brief, intense release of the NT as shown in FIG. 141—5. **Presynaptic receptors (R-3)** opposite impinging neurons can increase or inhibit the release of an NT. In addition, **receptors for neuromodulators (R-4)** or substances that are not released from nerve terminals (eg, steroids, prostaglandins) can modulate the release of the NT. However, the following discussion centers mostly on postsynaptic receptors.

Receptors always interact physiologically with their respective NT; eg, Ach released from cholinergic neurons all over the body interacts with all cholinergic receptors to produce a response. However, not all cholinergic receptors are identical. Such differences reveal themselves by the action of chemicals or drugs; eg, muscarine preferentially stimulates cholinergic receptors located on effector cells innervated by postganglionic cholinergic (parasympathetic) fibers, whereas nicotine preferentially stimulates those cholinergic receptors located on skeletal muscle cells, autonomic ganglia, and the adrenal medulla. For this reason, the first receptors are called muscarinic and the latter, nicotinic. The discovery of subclasses allows for the more se-

lective action of drugs; ie, drugs can be developed that will not stimulate all cholinergic receptors, but only those of the muscarinic *or* nicotinic type. This results in a more selected therapeutic approach. Some major receptor classes and their respective subclasses are described below.

Cholinergic receptors can be divided into nicotinic N_1 (adrenal medulla, autonomic ganglia) and N_2 (skeletal muscle) receptors as well as muscarinic M_1 (autonomic system, striatum, cortex, hippocampus) and M_2 (autonomic system, heart, intestinal smooth muscle, hindbrain, cerebellum) receptors. Receptors are composed of 5 subunits (2 α's, β, γ, and δ) which surround an ion channel. The α unit contains the primary recognition site for Ach or cholinergic drugs.

Adrenergic receptors can be divided into α_1 (postsynaptic in the sympathetic system) and α_2 (presynaptic in the sympathetic system and postsynaptic in the brain) receptors, as well as β_1 (heart) and β_2 (other sympathetically innervated structures) receptors.

Dopaminergic receptors can be classified as D_1, D_2, and D_3 receptors. D_1 receptors activate adenylate cyclase via stimulatory G-proteins, whereas D_2 receptors inhibit this enzyme via inhibitory G-proteins. D_1 receptors are more frequent than D_2 receptors (4:1), but both receptors are formed in the same brain areas (eg, limbic region, basal ganglia). The D_3 receptor does not seem to affect adenylate cyclase and is more localized in the limbic areas. In addition, isoforms of the individual receptors have been detected.

GABA receptors can be divided into GABA$_A$ receptors activating chloride channels, or GABA$_B$ receptors potentiating adenosine 3',5'-cyclic phosphate (cAMP) formation. The GABA$_A$ receptor consists of several distinct polypeptides (α, β, γ, δ), with the recognition site for GABA located on the β subunit. This site can be influenced by other sites that bind benzodiazepines (eg, benzodiazepine binding increases GABA binding), barbiturates, picrotoxin, or muscimol. There are also subpopulations of the GABA$_A$ receptors which show differential sensitivity to GABA and benzodiazepines.

Serotonin (5-HT) receptors can be divided into 5-HT$_1$, 5-HT$_2$, and 5-HT$_3$ receptors. The 5-HT$_1$ receptor consists of 4 subtypes: 5-HT$_{1A}$ to 5-HT$_{1D}$. 5-HT$_{1A}$ receptors are found pre- and postsynaptically in the raphe nucleus and hippocampus and modulate adenylate cyclase. 5-HT$_2$ receptors are found in the 4th layer of the cortex and are involved in the hydrolysis of phosphoinositide (see below). 5-HT$_3$ receptors are found presynaptically in the nucleus tractus solitarius.

Glutamate receptors (excitatory) can be subclassified as N-methyl-D-aspartate (affecting the flow of Na$^+$, K$^+$, Ca^{++}), quisqualate (Na$^+$, K$^+$), and kainate (Na$^+$, K$^+$) receptors.

Endorphin-enkephalin or opioid receptors can be divided into μ_1 and μ_2 (sensorimotor integration, analgesia), δ (motor integration, cognitive function), and κ_1 and κ_2 (water balance regulation, analgesia, food intake). All receptors are inhibitory in nature, are often located presynaptically, and seem to be coupled to G-proteins.

Second Messenger Systems

Second messenger systems are complexes of regulatory (eg, G-proteins) and catalytic (eg, adenylate cyclase, phospholipase C) proteins, which are activated by NTs (first messengers) to form specific chemicals or second messengers (eg, cAMP, inositol triphosphate or IP$_3$, diacylglycerol or DAG). The second messenger produces the physiologic response (eg, initiation of nerve impulse, muscle contraction). There are many such systems.

Adenylate cyclase—cAMP is perhaps the best known second messenger system. Here, the first messenger (NT, hormone) binds to the receptor activating a stimulatory G-protein (Gs) by displacing guanosine diphosphate (GDP) with guanosine triphosphate (GTP). G-proteins consist of α, β, and γ subunits; the α unit binds the gua-

nine nucleotide and provides specificity for receptors. The activated protein amplifies the signal of the first messenger and activates adenylate cyclase. This enzyme converts adenosine triphosphate (ATP) to cAMP, which activates specific phosphorylating enzymes or protein kinases to produce the physiologic response. The action of cAMP is terminated by the enzyme phosphodiesterase. In addition to the stimulatory G-protein, inhibitory G-proteins (Gi) exist. By activation of a different receptor and this Gi, adenylate cyclase is inhibited (see FIG. 141–6). In each category, different G-proteins have been identified (eg, Gs$_1$, Gs$_2$, Gs$_3$ and Gi$_1$, Gi$_2$, Gi$_3$). In addition, other G-proteins have been classified as Go, whose function is still unknown.

Another system, the phosphoinositide system, generates 2 second messengers, IP$_3$ and DAG. Upon receptor stimulation and G-protein activation, phospholipase C is stimulated, which hydrolases membrane phosphatidyl inositol 4,5-biphosphate into IP$_3$ and DAG. IP$_3$ releases calcium from intracellular stores, and DAG activates protein kinase C. Effects on ion channels or phosphorylation of specific proteins causes the physiologic effects. The actions of these messengers are then terminated by specific enzymes.

Pathology of Neurotransmission

Defects in the processes of NT synthesis, storage, release, and degradation or changes in the number and affinity of receptors lead to altered neurotransmission and can result in clinical pathology. Some clinical conditions, their established or proposed defects in neurotransmission, and drug therapies are listed in TABLE 141–1.

Pharmacology of Neurotransmission

Most drugs that affect the nervous system modulate the neurotransmission process. Correction of the neurotransmission defect that causes the disease therefore constitutes the mechanism underlying the drug's therapeutic effect. Interference with other, normal NT processes constitutes the mode of action of the side effects.

Drugs can increase or decrease the synthesis, storage, release, or degradation of a specific NT, usually in all neurons in the body and brain (see TABLE 141–2). Such drugs, therefore, are not selective in their action on a specific organ; eg, ephedrine increases the release of NE from all NE-containing neurons, and the released NE stimulates all adrenergic receptors in the body.

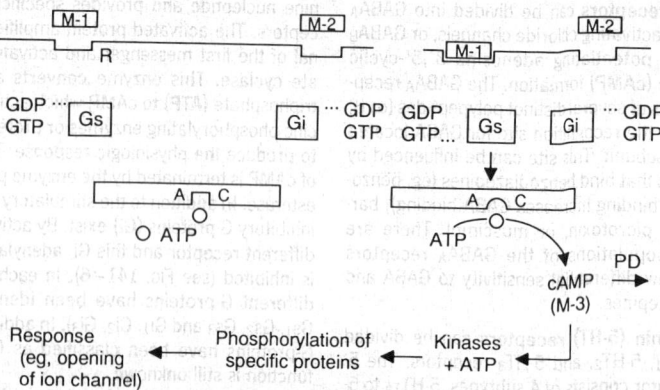

FIG. 141-6. Schematic representation of the formation and action of adenosine 3',5' cyclic phosphate (cAMP). M-1 = stimulatory neurotransmitter; R = receptor; M-2 = inhibitory neurotransmitter; Gs = stimulatory G-protein; Gi = inhibitory G-protein; GDP = guanosine diphosphate; GTP = guanosine triphosphate; AC = adenylate cyclase; cAMP = M-3; Response = modulation of ion channels, activation of kinases, and phosphorylation of cell components; PD = phosphodiesterase, which destroys cAMP.

In contrast, certain drugs can rather selectively stimulate (agonists) or block (antagonists) specific receptors and can be more selective (concentration dependent) in their effects; eg, the sympathomimetic drug phenylephrine will activate α-adrenergic but not β-adrenergic receptors.

TABLE 141-1. SELECTION OF DISEASES AND POISONINGS ASSOCIATED WITH CERTAIN DEFECTS IN NEUROTRANSMISSION

Disease/Disorder	Proposed Abnormality in Neurotransmitter (NT) System and Putative Mode of Action of Therapeutic Drugs
Schizophrenia	Overactivity of the dopaminergic system, perhaps due to increased D_2 receptor density. Antipsychotic drugs block DA receptors and reduce dopaminergic overactivity to normal state.
Depression	Reduction of NE levels in presence of reduced 5-HT levels, accompanied by increased number of β-adrenergic and serotonergic receptors. Antidepressant drugs down-regulate receptors either directly or indirectly by increasing NT levels (inhibition of re-uptake system or MAO blockade).
Mania	Increase in NE levels in presence of reduced 5-HT levels, accompanied by decreased number of adrenergic receptors. Lithium reduces NE release and reduces second messenger synthesis; up-regulation of receptors.
Anxiety	Reduction in the action of the inhibitory NT GABA, perhaps due to imbalance of endogenous inhibitors or stimulators of the GABA receptor. Benzodiazepines increase GABA binding and inhibitory activity and reduce anxiety.
Myasthenia gravis	Destruction of Ach receptors at neuromuscular junction due to autoimmune reactions. "Anticholinesterases" inhibit acetylcholinesterase, increase Ach levels at junction, and stimulate remaining receptors for increased muscle activity.
Huntington's disease (chorea)	Major neuronal damage in cortex and striatum with proposed reductions in levels of GABA, Ach, and cholecystokinin receptors and overactivity of DA system. Initial damage may be caused by excessive stimulation of cells by excitatory amino acid NTs. No specific therapy.

(Continued)

TABLE 141–1. SELECTION OF DISEASES AND POISONINGS ASSOCIATED WITH
CERTAIN DEFECTS IN NEUROTRANSMISSION *(Cont'd)*

Disease/Disorder	Proposed Abnormality in Neurotransmitter (NT) System and Putative Mode of Action of Therapeutic Drugs
Parkinson's disease	Loss of neurons in substantia nigra and other areas with reduction in levels of DA and methionine-enkephalin, allowing the Ach system to become overactive. L-dopa increases levels of DA, amantadine increases DA release, and bromocriptine stimulates DA receptors. Anticholinergic drugs reduce activity of the cholinergic system.
Alzheimer's disease	Loss of brain cells in cortex and hippocampus, some of which synthesize and utilize Ach. No specific drug therapy.
Epilepsy	Sudden synchronous firing at high frequency of localized groups in certain brain areas, perhaps caused by a reduction of the inhibitory activity of GABA. Phenytoin stabilizes neuronal membranes and reduces excessive NT release, phenobarbital enhances GABA binding, and valproic acid increases GABA levels.
Eaton-Lambert syndrome	Degeneration and atrophy of terminal motor axons with reduction in Ach release. Guanidine increases release of Ach.
Autism	Possible hyperserotonemia, which occurs in 30 to 50% with no evidence of central 5-HT abnormalities. No specific drug therapy.
Pain	Involves a variety of initiators (eg, bradykinins, prostaglandins) and NTs in the neuronal pain pathways; the latter can be stimulatory (eg, substance P which transmits nerve impulses) or inhibitory (eg, enkephalins, endorphins which interfere with nerve impulses). Nonsteroidal analgesics inhibit prostaglandin synthesis and reduce pain impulse formation; narcotic analgesics stimulate enkephalin/endorphin receptors and reduce pain impulse transmission.
Drug-induced disorders (eg, pseudo-parkinsonism)	Pseudoparkinsonism results from a reduced dopaminergic system due to acute blockage of dopaminergic receptors by antipsychotic drugs. Anticholinergic drugs reduce cholinergic activity and restore balance between both systems. Tardive dyskinesia results from hypersensitive DA receptors due to chronic blockade by antipsychotic drugs.
Injury associated with prolonged seizures, trauma, or hypoxia-ischemia	Injury causes excessive stimulation of adjacent cells by glutamate, leading to neuronal death and loss. No specific drug therapy.
Poisonings	Botulism—inhibition of Ach release from motoneurons by toxin from *Clostridium botulinum*. No specific drug therapy.
	Organophosphates—inhibition of acetylcholinesterase and marked increase in levels of Ach in synaptic cleft. Pralidoxime removes toxin from enzyme, and atropine protects receptors from high levels of Ach.
	Mushroom poisoning—*Amanita muscaria*: inhibition of anticholinesterase and blockade of Ach receptors by isoxazole derivatives. *Inicybe, Clitocybe*: stimulation of muscarinic receptors by muscarine and related compounds. Atropine protects muscarinic receptors.
	Snake venoms (*Bungarus multicinctus*)—blockade of Ach receptors at neuromuscular junction by α *Bungarus* toxin.

DA = dopamine; NE = norepinephrine; 5-HT = serotonin; GABA = γ-aminobutyric acid; Ach = acetylcholine; MAO = monoamine oxidase.

TABLE 141–2. EXAMPLES OF DRUG ACTION ON NEUROTRANSMISSION AND THE RESULTING EFFECTS

Process	Drug	Result (Response)
NT synthesis (↑)	L-dopa	↑ DA
	Tryptophan	↑ 5-HT
NT synthesis (↓)	Metyrosine	↓ NE
NT storage (↓)	Reserpine	↓ NE, ↓ 5-HT
NT release (↑)	Ephedrine	↑ NE
	Carbachol	↑ Ach
	Amphetamine	↑ NE, DA
NT release (↓)	Lithium	↓ NE, DA
NT uptake (↓)	Cocaine	↑ NE*
	Imipramine (tricyclic antidepressants)	↑ NE*, 5-HT*
NT metabolism (↓)	Phenelzine (MAO inhibitors)	↑ NE, 5-HT
	Neostigmine (anticholinesterases)	↑ Ach*
Receptor activity (↑)	Phenylephrine	↑ α₁
	Clonidine	↑ α₂†
	Epinephrine	↑ β₁, β₂, α
	Metaproterenol	↑ β₂
	Neostigmine (anticholinesterases)	↑ Ach* (nicotinic)
	Pilocarpine	↑ Muscarinic
	Diazepam‡ (anxiolytics)	↑ GABA
	Buspirone	↑ 5-HT₁A (presynaptic)
	Morphine (certain analgesics)	↑ Opioid (enkephalin-endorphin, μ)
Receptor activity (↓)	Phentolamine	↓ α₁, α₂
	Prazosin	↓ α₁
	Yohimbine	↓ α₂
	Propranolol	↓ β₁, β₂
	Metoprolol	↓ β₁
	Atropine	↓ Muscarinic
	Trimethaphan	↓ Nicotinic (ganglia)
	d-Tubocurarine	↓ Nicotinic (neuromuscular junction)
	Chlorpromazine (antipsychotics)	↓ DA (D₂ >> D₁)
	Diphenhydramine (antihistamines)	↓ H₁
	Cimetidine (H₂ blockers)	↓ H₂
	Methysergide	↓ 5-HT (all)
	Ketanserin	↓ 5-HT₂

NT = neurotransmitter; DA = dopamine; 5-HT = serotonin; NE = norepinephrine; Ach = acetylcholine; GABA = γ-aminobutyric acid; MAO = monoamine oxidase.
* In the synaptic or junctional space, acute effect.
† Dose and time dependent.
‡ Acts on a regular or modular component of the GABA receptor and increases GABA binding and activity.

142. PROSTAGLANDINS, THROMBOXANES, AND LEUKOTRIENES

Prostaglandins (PGs) are a group of cyclic fatty acids with diverse and potent biologic activities affecting cell function in every organ system. The parent compound, prostanoic acid, contains a 20-carbon chain with a cyclopentane ring. Variations in the number and position of the double bonds and hydroxyl groups determine the physiologic activities of the different PGs. The important substitutions are on the cyclopentane ring.

PGs are referred to as PG_1 or PG_2 depending on whether there are one or 2 double bonds in the aliphatic side chain. The PG_2s are the most common.

PGs are formed from dietary essential fatty acids (principally arachidonic acid) esterified to phospholipids and in some instances to triglycerides. The rate-limiting step in the formation of the products of arachidonic acid (referred to as the arachidonic acid cascade) appears to be the Ca-dependent release of free arachidonic acid from the membrane phospholipid pool by phospholipases A_2 and/or C. Following release, arachidonic acid is converted to PGs, thromboxanes (TXs), and leukotrienes (LTs). In the first pathway, PG cyclooxygenase catalyzes the initial step yielding the endoperoxides PGG_2 and PGH_2, a reaction that is inhibited by aspirin, indomethacin, and other nonsteroidal anti-inflammatory drugs (NSAIDs). This enzyme activity results in the formation of PGA_2, PGE_2, PGD_2, and $PGF_{2\alpha}$. Unstable PGI_2 is formed by the action of prostacyclin synthetase; unstable thromboxane A_2 (TXA_2) by the action of thromboxane synthetase. Both of these biologically active compounds are converted to the stable metabolites 6-oxo-PGF_1 and thromboxane B_2, respectively. Metabolism of PGs to inactive compounds occurs primarily in the lungs, renal cortex, and liver with metabolite excretion in the urine.

In the 2nd pathway of arachidonic metabolism, 5-lipoxygenase results in the formation of a series of LTs, A_4, B_4, C_4, D_4, E_4, and F_4 (through the intermediate 12-hydroxyperoxyarachidonic acid), which have potent proinflammatory and bronchoconstrictor properties.

BIOLOGIC ACTIONS

Reproductive System and Neonatology

PGE and PGF induce luteolysis, decrease progesterone secretion, stimulate the gravid uterus to contract at all stages of pregnancy, and act at the hypothalamic-pituitary level as mediators of luteinizing hormone releasing factor (LRF) on luteinizing hormone (LH) secretion.

Effects on the ovulatory cycle: It is thought that during the secretory phase of the ovulatory cycle progressively larger amounts of estradiol produced by the maturing follicle increase $PGF_{2\alpha}$, which is probably secreted by the oviduct and delivered directly to the ovary. $PGF_{2\alpha}$ reduces luteal blood flow and inhibits progesterone synthesis; this effect may be mediated through the hypothalamic-pituitary axis, and prostaglandin antagonists inhibit it.

Dysmenorrhea: Many symptoms of dysmenorrhea (abdominal cramping, headache, etc) have been ascribed to the actions of PGs on the uterus and/or GI tract, and treatment with PG synthetase inhibitors (indomethacin, ibuprofen, naproxen, etc) has proved quite successful (see PRIMARY DYSMENORRHEA in Ch. 5).

Effects on the uterus: Endogenous $PGF_{2\alpha}$ is present in amniotic fluid, and its plasma concentration rises steadily during pregnancy, reaching high levels immediately prior to delivery. This results in decreased progesterone, an increased uterine sensitivity to oxytocin, and the onset of labor. PGE_2 and/or $PGF_{2\alpha}$ are believed to be essential to normal parturition, although the precise agents responsible for the onset of labor remain unknown. This is supported by the fact that PG synthesis inhibition with NSAIDs at term delays the onset of labor, resulting in postdatism and postmaturity. PGE_2 and to a lesser extent $PGF_{2\alpha}$ are also essential to cervical effacement and dilation, being synthesized by cervical cells.

Parturition and pregnancy termination: For the induction of labor at term or in postdate pregnancy, PGE_2 (and to a lesser extent $PGF_{2\alpha}$) has been administered orally, IV, intra-amniotically, and intravaginally. The most beneficial effects are obtained with the instillation of PGE_2 gel (0.5 to 2.5 mg) into the vagina or, preferably, into the portio vaginalis of the cervix. This results in cervical "ripening" and dilation with enhancement of the onset of labor spontaneously or with the aid of oxytocin. Nausea, vomiting, and diarrhea are uncommon with either intracervical or vaginal PGE_2 instillation. IV administration of PGs alone appears to offer little advantage over IV oxytocin for labor induction.

Although PGs induce labor at all stages of pregnancy, current usage in abortion is restricted to pregnancy termination during the second trimester. Commonly used routes include injection of $PGF_{2\alpha}$ into the amniotic sac, IM injection of 15-methyl $PGF_{2\alpha}$, extra-amniotic instillation of PGE_2 (via catheter between uterine wall and fetal membranes), and by suppository. Side effects and success rates are discussed in Ch. 4.

Effects on the fetus and newborn: Ductally synthesized PGE_2 plays a critical role in maintaining patency of the ductus arteriosus in the fetus during pregnancy. After delivery, fetal pulmonary arterial pressure falls with ensuing closure of the ductus arteriosus, which is associated with a decreased ductal synthesis of PGE_2. Treatment of systemic illnesses with NSAIDs during late pregnancy results in postmature infants and a high incidence of premature closure of the ductus arteriosus, with resultant pulmonary hypertension and right ventricular hypertrophy. Thus, *NSAIDs are contraindicated during the latter stages of pregnancy.*

Patent ductus arteriosus (PDA) and congenital heart disease with right-sided obstruction (pulmonary stenosis and atresia) and left-sided outflow obstruction (coarctation, transposition, aortic stenosis, etc): see under CONGENITAL HEART DISEASE in Ch. 28.

Cardiovascular-Renal Systems

The kidney possesses PGA_2 and PGE_2, which are potent vasodilating compounds with a putative *anti*hypertensive function. These PGs, as well as the more recently discovered PGD_2 and PGI_2, also have important effects on renal blood flow, Na and water excretion, and renin release.

Renal blood flow and sodium and water excretion: PGA, PGE, PGD, PGG, PGH, and PGI all increase renal blood flow and natriuresis. This natriuretic action may be due to nonspecific renovasodilation as is observed with any renovasodilator (eg, acetylcholine, bradykinin). Similarly, the PG precursor arachidonic acid produces a rise in deep cortical and inner medullary flow accompanied by Na and water loss; these actions are inhibited by indomethacin. Loop diuretics (eg, ethacrynic acid, furosemide) also increase renal blood flow, natriuresis, and urinary PGE excretion, suggesting that they act through PG release. In fact, inhibition of PG synthesis with indomethacin almost completely abrogates the natriuretic and antihypertensive effects of furosemide. Caution must be observed in utilizing diuretics in combination with NSAIDs for the treatment of edematous states such as cirrhosis, heart failure, and in essential hypertension where refractoriness to such antihypertensive diuretics may be observed.

PGs probably do not directly maintain resting blood flow, but they act to oppose renal vasoconstriction due to angiotensin, norepinephrine, sympathetic nervous stimulation, and renal artery occlusion by providing an offsetting vasodilatory action. This is important in diseases such as lupus nephritis, where renal blood flow becomes partially dependent on PG synthesis and release. Administration of NSAIDs to such patients results in a marked deterioration of renal function. Thus, NSAIDs should be administered cautiously in patients with compromised renal blood flow, particularly those in renal failure.

Studies have shown a rise in plasma PGA and urinary PGE during volume depletion induced by low Na intake, diuretics, or hemodialysis. A major role of the renal PGs in such volume-depleted states is to counteract the antinatriuretic and prohypertensive effects of the renin-angiotensin-aldosterone axis. The rise in PGE_2 production in this instance is believed to be secondary to a direct stimulatory effect of angiotensin II on PG synthesis (see FIG. 142-1).

PGEs may attenuate vasopressin-stimulated adenyl cyclase and the accompanying increase in water movement. Aspirin, indomethacin, or meclofenamate can increase vasopressin-stimulated water reabsorption and maximal urinary osmolality. Thus PGE_2, which is normally secreted by the collecting duct cells, may be a physiologic antagonist of vasopressin acting at the site of vasopressin-induced water movement in the collecting duct cell.

Renin release and blood pressure regulation: Arachidonic acid, PGA_1, PGA_2, PGE_1, PGE_2, and PGI_2 all stimulate renin production. PG synthesis inhibition results in marked renin reduction and partial inhibition of the natriuretic and antihypertensive effects of loop diuretics, which suggests that volume depletion leads to a reduction in renal blood flow that triggers PG release, leading to an increase in renin, angiotensin II, and aldosterone. Theoretically, volume depletion such as that resulting from a low Na intake or diuretic therapy should not lower BP as is clinically observed, since there is a marked activation of the renin-angiotensin-aldosterone axis under these conditions. Possibly the rise in plasma, renal, or local vascular PGs offsets the vasoconstricting effects of angiotensin II, thus lowering BP (see FIG. 142-1). The fact that indomethacin and aspirin increase BP in normotensives and hypertensives when plasma renin activity is markedly decreased supports this contention and suggests that inhibition of the vasodepressor PG system allows pressor mechanisms such as the renin-angiotensin system to act unopposed, even at lower plasma concentrations. Clinically, this has important connotations in **Bartter's** syndrome (see Ch. 41) where hyperreninemia, hyperaldosteronism, and hypokalemic alkalosis have been shown to be associated with increased plasma and urinary levels of PG, all of the above being temporarily reversed by PG synthesis inhibition with aspirin or indomethacin. However, it is now believed that this syndrome is

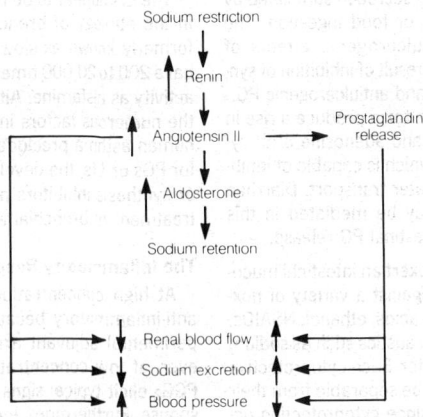

FIG. 142–1. Hypothetical schema whereby volume depletion may lead to renin-angiotensin release and physiologic antagonism of angiotensin II, antinatriuretic, and hypertensive actions. (From Lee JB: "Prostaglandins and the renin-angiotensin axis." *Clinical Nephrology* 14:159–163, 1980. Published by Dustri-Verlag, West Germany; used with permission.)

not the result of a primary PG excess, but is the result of a defect in chloride transport in the thick ascending limb.

In summary, the evidence supports an antihypertensive function for renal and systemic PGs at least during volume depletion by antagonizing the vasopressor activity of the renin-angiotensin or the adrenergic nervous systems.

Hypertension: The first PG given to a hypertensive human was PGA_2. When given IV, the total calculated peripheral resistance fell as the result of direct peripheral arteriolar vasodilation and a fall in BP associated with a reflex baroreceptor-mediated increase in cardiac output. Subsequently, PGA_1 was shown to have the same mechanism of action as PGA_2. However, following infusion of PGA_1, the BP did not fall immediately; rather, there was an initial increase in renal blood flow and in Na, K, and water excretion. Later, when the BP fell to normotensive levels, there was a return to control levels. Thus, normotension induced by PGAs is associated with normal renal blood flow and normal Na and water excretion, in contrast to antihypertensive agents that compromise renal blood flow. The initial natriuresis and diuresis are associated with about a 10% fall in plasma volume, which is in part responsible for the hypotensive action of PGA. PGA_1 and PGA_2 appear to act as ideal antihypertensives, reversing many of the known abnormalities in patients with essential hyperten-

sion. They favorably influence total peripheral resistance, renal resistance, cardiac output, baroreceptor activity, plasma volume, and Na and water balance. To date, however, no clinical trials of oral PGA have been undertaken for the treatment of hypertension.

Nephrosis, cirrhosis, and heart failure: PG synthesis inhibition with indomethacin and other NSAIDs has been shown to decrease the proteinuria of the nephrotic syndrome. However, this has occurred with a concomitant suppression of GFR, and the use of NSAIDs in edematous states should be undertaken with great caution; *acute irreversible renal failure has been observed.* This occurs because under conditions of intravascular volume depletion (eg, in edema), renal blood flow is PG-dependent, and eradication of renal PGs by NSAIDs allows vasoconstrictor influences such as angiotensin II to act unopposed, leading to acute renal failure.

Diabetes insipidus: Since PGE_1 inhibits vasopressin but not cAMP water reabsorption in the collecting duct and since NSAIDs enhance vasopressin-stimulated water reabsorption and maximal urinary osmolality, the use of aspirin, indomethacin, and other PG synthetase inhibitors may be beneficial in patients with diabetes insipidus.

Gastrointestinal System

Gastric secretion and intestinal absorption: PGE_1, PGE_2, and PGA_1 and their 16,16-dimethyl analogs inhibit gastric HCl secretion stimulated by histamine, pentagastrin, or food ingestion. The hyperchlorhydric and ulcerogenic effects of NSAIDs are probably the result of inhibition of synthesis of antichlorhydric and antiulcerogenic PG.

Both PGE_1 and cholera toxin produce a rise in mucosal adenyl cyclase and adenosine 3':5'-cyclic phosphate (cAMP) which is capable of inhibiting intestinal Na and water transport. Diarrhea due to cholera toxin may be mediated in this manner by increased intestinal PG release.

Cytoprotection: PGs exert an intestinal mucosal "protective" action against a variety of noxious stimuli including bile acids, ethanol, NSAIDs, bacterial endotoxin, and caustics such as sodium hydroxide and boiling water. Such cytoprotective action of PGs appears to be separable from their antisecretory activities, since cytoprotection occurs with a much lower dose than antisecretory activity and many nonsecretory PGs exert intestinal mucosal protective effects.

Clinical considerations of PGs revolve around the endogenous role and therapeutic potential of PGs in peptic ulcer disease and necrotizing enterocolitis in the neonate. Recently, **misoprostol** (a synthetic methyl analog of PGE_1) was approved for clinical use during NSAID administration to prevent GI bleeding and ulceration. The recommended dosage is 100 to 200 μg orally qid. Noteworthy side effects are nausea, abdominal pain, and diarrhea. The many complex factors involved in peptic ulceration preclude any conclusions as to the clinical superiority of PGs over standard peptic ulcer regimens.

Respiratory System

PGE_1 and PGE_2 relax human bronchiolar smooth muscle and increase pulmonary blood flow; PGD_2, $PGF_{2\alpha}$, and LTs C and D contract bronchiolar smooth muscle and inhibit the bronchodilating effect of isoproterenol. This suggests that pulmonary synthesis and release of PGE may be significant in increasing pulmonary blood flow in response to hypoxia. Furthermore, some bronchial asthma may be caused by a reduced PGE:PGF ratio, leading to bronchial constriction. In certain prone individuals (estimated to be 10% of the adult asthma population), NSAIDs provoke or aggravate the asthmatic attack, suggesting an inhibition of pulmonary vasodilator PGE_2 production with a resultant decrease in the $PGE_2/PGF_{2\alpha}$ ratio. PGE produces bronchial dilation by different mechanisms than isoproterenol, since PGE is devoid of β-adrenergic stimulation.

The LTs appear to be more significant than PGs in the etiology of bronchial asthma. They were formerly known as slow-reacting substance and have 200 to 20,000 times the bronchoconstrictor activity as histamine. Although the complexity of the numerous factors involved in the genesis of human asthma precludes an oversimplified role for PGs or LTs, the development of LT antagonist or synthesis inhibitors may hold promise in the treatment of bronchial asthma.

The Inflammatory Response

At high concentrations PGs are considered anti-inflammatory because they ameliorate experimental adjuvant arthritis in animals. However, at low concentrations, PGEs, PGD_2, and PGG_2 elicit typical signs of the inflammatory response. Furthermore, increased amounts of PGs are present in local areas of inflammation. PG synthetase activity is inhibited by NSAIDs, and many of their actions are attributed to this inhibition.

PGs also may play a role in systemic inflammatory reactions. Pyrogen-induced fever, which has been associated with an increased PGF_2 content in the third ventricle, can be reduced by prior administration of a PG synthetase inhibitor, eg, indomethacin or aspirin. The analgesic effect of NSAIDs in headache may be mediated by inhibition of PG synthesis, since PGE produces severe headaches in man. In rheumatoid arthritis, large amounts of PGs and LTs in the synovium may contribute to inflammation and to periarticular bone demineralization from their Ca resorptive actions.

LTs are now viewed as the major pathophysiologic mediators of the inflammatory response, since they are much more potent than the PGs with regard to increasing vascular permeability, adhesion of leukocytes to the vessel wall, and edema production. Inhibitors of LT synthesis are being developed for possible anti-inflammatory applications.

The greatest **clinical application** in inflammatory disorders is the use of PG synthesis inhibitors in rheumatoid arthritis, osteoarthritis, acute bursitis and tendinitis, and allied inflammatory disorders.

Hematologic Effects

PGE_1 is a potent inhibitor of platelet aggregation, while PGE_2 stimulates platelet aggregation; both actions are mediated through cAMP. Although platelets normally contain PGE_2, which is

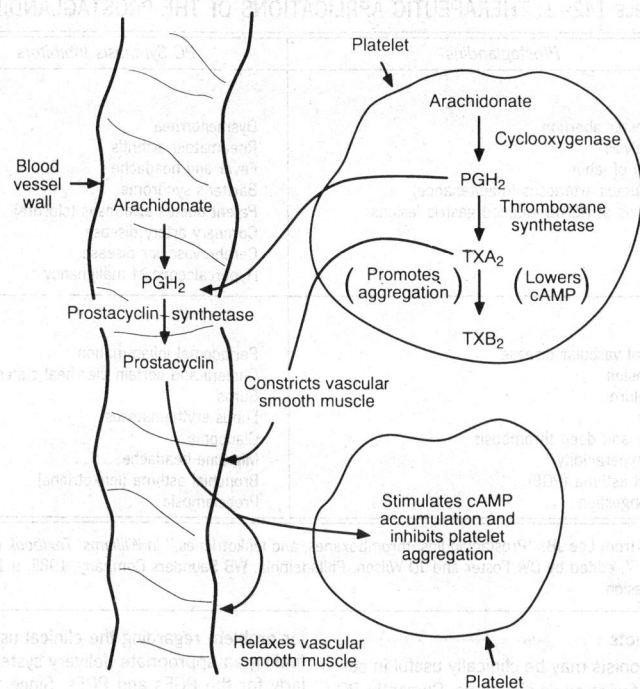

Platelet

Arachidonate

Cyclooxygenase

PGH₂

Thromboxane
synthetase

Blood
vessel
wall

Arachidonate

TXA₂

$\left(\begin{array}{c}\text{Promotes}\\ \text{aggregation}\end{array}\right)$ $\left(\begin{array}{c}\text{Lowers}\\ \text{cAMP}\end{array}\right)$

PGH₂

TXB₂

Prostacyclin synthetase

Prostacyclin

Constricts vascular
smooth muscle

Stimulates cAMP
accumulation and
inhibits platelet
aggregation

Relaxes vascular
smooth muscle

Platelet

Fig. 142–2. Model of human platelet homeostasis. (From Gorman RR: "Modulation of human platelet function by prostacyclin and thromboxane A₂." *Federation Proceedings* 38(1):83–88, 1979; used with permission of the Federation of American Societies for Experimental Biology.)

released during clotting, the major compounds involved in the clotting process are PGI₂ (prostacyclin) and thromboxane A₂ (TXA₂). PGI₂ is synthesized ubiquitously in blood vessel walls from arachidonate derived from either the vessel wall or the platelet. It is the most potent of all inhibitors of platelet aggregation and has vascular dilatory properties as well. Conversely, TXA₂, a potent platelet aggregator and vasoconstrictor, is synthesized primarily by the platelet.

Following endothelial damage, platelets adhere to the subendothelial connective tissue, releasing catecholamines, serotonin, ADP, and TXA₂, which promote platelet aggregation through a decrease in platelet cAMP formation. TXA₂ is thought to be the main compound in this platelet-aggregating process; it has a very short half-life and breaks down into the stable thromboxane B₂ (TXB₂). Conversely, once an interaction between the platelet and the vessel wall takes place, PGG₂ is converted to PGI₂, which

inhibits platelet aggregation (see Fig. 142–2). Whether physiologic or pathologic clot formation ensues appears to depend on the relative amount of PGI₂ vs. TXA₂ production. The net effect of aspirin appears to be on the anticlotting activity, since inhibition of TXA₂ synthesis occurs during the entire platelet lifetime and its effects on vascular PGI₂ synthesis is shorter lasting. This probably explains the beneficial effects of aspirin on thrombotic processes; ie, a prolonged bleeding time. Low-dose daily aspirin administration (81 to 325 mg) is widely used for preventive therapy in patients with angina, postmyocardial infarction or stroke, and in patients with incipient risks for these catastrophes (abnormal plasma lipids, smokers, positive family history, etc).

From the above considerations, it is an obvious clinical corollary that aspirin (and other NSAID) treatment should be avoided in hypoprothrombinemia, oral anticoagulant therapy, and other bleeding diatheses.

TABLE 142–1. THERAPEUTIC APPLICATIONS OF THE PROSTAGLANDINS

Prostaglandins	PG Synthesis Inhibitors
Current	
Midtrimester abortion	Dysmenorrhea
Hemodialysis	Rheumatoid arthritis
Induction of labor	Fever and headache
Patent ductus arteriosus (maintenance)	Bartter's syndrome
Prophylaxis of NSAID-induced gastric lesions	Patent ductus arteriosus (closure)
	Coronary artery disease
	Cerebrovascular disease
	Hypercalcemia of malignancy
Potential	
Peripheral vascular disease	Periodontal inflammation
Hypertension	Cholera and certain diarrheal states
Heart failure	Burns
Infertility	Lupus erythematosus
Coronary and deep thrombosis	Glaucoma
Gastric hyperacidity	Migraine headache
Bronchial asthma (PGE)	Bronchial asthma (leukotriene)
Nasal congestion	Preeclampsia

Modified from Lee JB: "Prostaglandins, thromboxanes, and leukotrienes," in *Williams' Textbook of Endocrinology*, ed. 7, edited by DW Foster and JD Wilson. Philadelphia, WB Saunders Company, 1985, p 1359; used with permission.

Ocular Effects

PG antagonists may be clinically useful in certain forms of wide-angle glaucoma. Currently, PG inhibition with indomethacin in patients undergoing corneal or lens transplant is used as an effective method of reducing the degree and incidence of postoperative macular edema. Similarly, NSAIDs have been utilized successfully in the treatment of ocular inflammatory diseases such as uveitis.

POTENTIAL THERAPEUTIC APPLICATIONS

TABLE 142–1 summarizes the current and potential therapeutic applications of the PGs. A major problem regarding the clinical use of PGs is finding an appropriate delivery system, particularly for the PGEs and PGFs. Since these compounds are metabolized during circulation through the lungs and appear to function as local hormones, their use would be limited if given orally or parenterally. However, PGA and PGI compounds are not degraded in the lungs, and may have a role as oral systemic antihypertensive agents.

In general, unique delivery systems that can provide local delivery are required for clinical use; eg, the intrauterine administration of PGE or PGF for abortion. Aerosol delivery of a PGE preparation may be feasible in bronchial asthma, and oral administration of PGA or PGE may have value for inhibition of HCl secretion.

143. CALCIUM ANTAGONISTS
(Calcium Channel Blocking Agents; Calcium Blockers; Calcium Channel Antagonists; Calcium Entry Blockers)

Calcium antagonists inhibit Ca ion movement into cells. Three drugs in this class, **diltiazem, nifedipine,** and **verapamil,** are well established in the management of a variety of cardiovascular disorders. This chapter deals primarily with them. A second generation of Ca antagonists has been introduced offering the potential advantage of greater vascular selectivity with small effects on the heart. These are discussed, including **nicardipine** and **nimodipine,** which have recently been approved by the FDA.

Pharmacology

Although all Ca antagonists belong to the same pharmacologic class, they are heterogeneous compounds with different chemical structures and varying potencies for blocking Ca slow channel mediated processes of the cardiovascular system. Their differences allow the rational choice of an agent for a particular clinical situation. The primary sites of action include cardiac muscle, the cardiac electrophysiologic system, and systemic and coronary arterial smooth muscle cells. The cardiac effects include a decrease in myocardial contractility, a decrease in the rate of the sinus node pacemaker and suppression of atrioventricular (**A-V**) nodal conduction, and a decrease in resistance in the coronary and systemic arterial systems through vasodilation. Ca antagonists have the ability to block ergonovine-mediated coronary constriction. Each agent, however, possesses a distinct pharmacodynamic profile of action (see TABLE 143–1).

Diltiazem is produced in both oral and IV forms (although the latter is not available in USA) and is approved for the management of angina pectoris and hypertension. Diltiazem has also been shown to be effective in the management of certain supraventricular arrhythmias, although it has not been approved for such usage. It is well absorbed following oral administration, but the bioavailability is only 40 to 50% with extensive first-pass hepatic metabolism and should be used with caution in patients with significant hepatic insufficiency. Therefore, the initial response can be variable and may not reflect the effect of a given dose with chronic use. Following administration of diltiazem tablets, the onset of action is 30 to 60 min with peak effect at about 2 to 3 h. The half-life of diltiazem is $3\frac{1}{2}$ to 7 h, and consequently it is most effective in a tid to qid regimen. The sustained-release formulation allows once-daily administration for the management of hypertension. The active metabolite is desacetyldiltiazem, which possesses 40 to 50% of diltiazem activity but typically makes up only 10 to 20% of the parent compound in plasma.

Diltiazem decreases the sinus node pacemaker and slows conduction through the A-V node; these effects are less pronounced than for verapamil. Diltiazem is less potent as a peripheral and coronary dilator than nifedipine or verapamil and possesses less negative inotropic effects (verapamil has the most negative inotropic effects—see below).

Nifedipine is approved for the management of angina and is an effective antihypertensive agent. It is rapidly and well absorbed from the GI tract following oral administration and undergoes significant first-pass metabolism with a bioavailability of about 50%. Metabolic products are inactive. The half-life is 3 to 4 h, and thus it is most effective when administered tid to qid. The onset of action is about 20 min, with peak effects at 30 min after oral administration. Nifedipine is available as a liquid within a capsule formulation; biting the capsule permits the liquid to be absorbed sublingually. Where rapid effects are warranted, this provides an onset of action in 3 to 5 min.

Nifedipine is the most potent peripheral arterial dilator compared with diltiazem and verapamil. It does not affect A-V nodal conduction, but it may increase heart rate due to reflex baroreceptor stimulation of the sympathetic nervous system from peripheral vasodilation. This increase in heart rate tends to augment contractility and thereby counteract weak direct negative inotropic properties noted with in vitro preparations.

Verapamil is approved for the treatment of angina, hypertension, and certain supraventricular arrhythmias. Like other Ca antagonists, it is rapidly and almost completely absorbed after oral administration. The half-life is variable between 3 and 7 h (increasing to $4\frac{1}{2}$ to 12 h with chronic therapy). The onset of action is 30 min with peak effects at 1 to 2 h. It is typically administered tid. A sustained-release formulation allows once-daily administration for the management of essential hypertension. First-pass metabolism is more extensive than for diltiazem and nifedipine, with an initial bioavailability as low as 20%. With chronic administration, liver metabolism decreases and bioavailability increases. In addition to alterations in liver metabolism over time, the pharmacology of verapamil is more complex because it exists as 2 stereoisomers, an active *l*-form and an inactive *d*-form. Stereoselective first-pass metabolism of the active *l*-form can lead to significantly higher initial concentrations of the inactive *d*-isomer. Consequently, plasma levels may be misleading. Optimal therapeutic effects of a given dose may require several dosing intervals.

TABLE 143–1. DOSAGE AND PHARMACOKINETICS OF SELECTED CALCIUM ANTAGONISTS

Drug	Dose	GI Absorption	Onset of Action	Peak Effect	Plasma Half-life	Active Metabolite
Diltiazem	30–90 mg orally tid or qid 5–10 mg (0.075–0.15 mg/kg) IV, repeat at 30 min as needed	80–90%	30–60 min	2–3 h	3.5–7 h	Desacetyldiltiazem (40–50% of parent activity)
Nicardipine	20–40 mg orally tid	> 90%	< 30 min	0.5–2 h	8.6 h	None
Nifedipine	10–40 mg orally tid or qid 10–20 mg sublingually	90%	20 min 3–5 min	30 min	3–4 h	None
Nimodipine	60 mg orally q 4 h × 21 days	> 90%	45–60 min	1 h	1–2 h	None
Verapamil	80–160 mg orally tid 5–10 mg (0.075–0.15 mg/kg) IV, repeat at 30 min as needed	90%	30 min	1–2 h	3–7 h (4.5–12 h)*	Norverapamil (20% of parent activity)

* Half-life increases with chronic therapy.

Both verapamil and diltiazem have significant electrophysiologic effects on the heart. They decrease the rate of the sinus node pacemaker and slow conduction across the A-V node. Verapamil is less potent than nifedipine as a peripheral arterial dilator. Conversely, it possesses the most significant negative inotropic properties compared with the other agents.

Therapeutic Indications

Hypertension: Vascular smooth muscle cells are dependent on Ca influx for maintaining normal or heightened vascular tone. Blockade of Ca influx into vascular smooth muscle cells causes arterial relaxation. Thus, the antihypertensive mechanism of Ca antagonists works by directly decreasing peripheral vascular resistance.

The 1988 report of the Joint National Committee on Treatment of High Blood Pressure lists Ca antagonists as effective, well-tolerated, safe first-line agents for treating mild to moderate hypertension. Preliminary data suggest that Ca antagonists do not affect blood glucose, lipids, or uric acid levels. Sustained-release preparations of Ca antagonists are gaining in popularity, as they should improve compliance in outpatients. Although not approved for use in patients with hypertensive emergencies, a number of recent reports suggest that nifedipine 10 to 20 mg sublingually is effective in early therapy of such patients. However, most will require a short-acting, IV agent that will allow rapid titration of BP (ie, sodium nitroprusside, nitroglycerin, labetalol, or trimethaphan camsylate).

The spectrum of pharmacologic actions of Ca antagonists provides flexibility in individualizing antihypertensive therapy, particularly in patients who present with complicating associated conditions. Since diltiazem, nifedipine, and verapamil possess coronary dilator properties and block coronary spasm, they are generally well suited for the management of hypertension in patients with coronary artery disease. However, nifedipine can cause a baroreceptor-mediated reflex tachycardia in some patients, altering myocardial O_2 demand in the setting of restricted O_2 supply; therefore, caution is required in patients with myocardial ischemia.

Diuretics and β blockers can adversely affect glucose homeostasis and lipid metabolism in patients with diabetes mellitus. The Ca antagonists provide a safe and effective alternative to the management of hypertension in diabetic patients.

In patients with obstructive pulmonary disease, β blockers are contraindicated as primary agents for treating coexisting hypertension. Diuretics can produce electrolyte imbalances, and β blockers have the potential for increasing airways obstruction. Ca antagonists do not alter electrolytes or airways resistance and thus simplify antihypertensive therapy in these patients.

The diverse effects of Ca antagonists are not always an advantage in patients with coexisting problems; eg, they do not have an established role in the management of hypertension in patients with heart failure. In this setting, it is extremely important to lower systemic vascular resistance while preserving ventricular function. Both diltiazem and verapamil possess significant negative inotropic properties, and nifedipine is not as effective as the angiotensin-converting enzyme inhibitors. Some of the 2nd-generation Ca antagonists may prove to have a role here.

Myocardial ischemic syndromes: Patients with ischemic syndromes can present with a variety of manifestations including stable angina, progressive anginal symptoms (unstable angina), variant angina, myocardial infarction, or sudden death. The underlying pathophysiologic possibilities are diverse, but most patients have occlusive atherosclerotic coronary artery disease and develop myocardial ischemia in situations of increased O_2 demand. Also, coronary spasm may play an important role in producing myocardial ischemia with or without associated atherosclerotic coronary artery disease.

Ca antagonists possess a variety of properties that are additive in decreasing or protecting against myocardial ischemia and are established as either first-line or adjunctive therapy. They block coronary spasm and decrease coronary vascular resistance. Systemic vascular resistance is decreased through peripheral arteriolar dilation, reducing left ventricular wall stress and myocardial O_2 consumption. In addition, the negative inotropic and chronotropic effects diminish myocardial O_2 demands.

Diltiazem, nifedipine, and verapamil are useful in managing **chronic stable angina**, providing beneficial effects on all significant markers for myocardial ischemia. The number of symptomatic and asymptomatic episodes of ischemia is reduced, and treadmill exercise time to onset of anginal symptoms is increased.

The salutary effects of the Ca antagonists on **unstable angina** are the same as noted above for stable angina. In this setting, they can be used in combination with nitrates and β blockers after consideration of the clinical situation and the patient profile.

About 60% of episodes of myocardial ischemia occur without symptoms, and about 80% of transient ischemic events are not precipitated by alterations in heart rate or BP. These observations suggest that coronary artery spasm reducing myocardial blood flow may play a prominent role in causing transient ischemic episodes. Although not all physicians agree about the need to treat **silent myocardial ischemia**, Ca antagonists can dilate coronary vasculature and block provoked coronary constriction.

The use of Ca antagonists in the setting of an **acute** infarction is under active investigation. They are effective in treating some patients with recurrent pain. Prophylactic therapy following a transmural myocardial infarction has not proved to reduce mortality or the incidence of reinfarction. A recent report indicates that patients with an initial non-Q-wave myocardial infarction without pulmonary congestion and normal ventricular function demonstrate a beneficial prophylactic response to diltiazem with respect to early reinfarction, although the mechanism for this effect has not been defined.

Although the Ca antagonists are effective in treating myocardial ischemia, they do not have an established role in primary therapy for ventricular arrhythmias induced by ischemia—ectopy, tachycardia, or fibrillation.

Arrhythmias: The use of Ca antagonists to treat arrhythmias is primarily confined to those in whom the A-V node is an integral part of their pathophysiology. These fall into 3 general categories: (1) atrial fibrillation or flutter, usually with a rapid ventricular response; (2) paroxysmal supraventricular tachycardia due to reentry within the A-V node; and (3) reciprocating tachycardia with an accessory pathway directly connecting atrial and ventricular tissue and using a circuit with antegrade conduction (orthodromic) over the A-V node.

The primary effects of certain Ca antagonists on the cardiac electrophysiologic system are slowing of the sinus node pacemaker, prolongation of conduction across the A-V node, and increase in the refractoriness of the A-V node. Effects on the A-V node tend to predominate. Nifedipine does not directly affect the A-V node, but it can produce a baroreceptor-mediated reflex sinus tachycardia and is thus *not* used for arrhythmia management. While a number of studies suggest that IV diltiazem is effective in treating atrial fibrillation and flutter, it has not

been approved for this use. Most clinical experience has involved the use of verapamil as an antiarrhythmic agent.

Verapamil is also effective in controlling the ventricular response in patients with atrial fibrillation or flutter. The IV form is used for urgent situations. The rapid onset of this effect (3 to 5 min) is a significant advantage over parenteral digoxin (20 to 30 min) when rapid control of the ventricular response is needed. The oral form is useful for chronic therapy. Verapamil is *contraindicated* in the presence of significant left ventricular dysfunction or hypotension. Verapamil is not very effective in converting atrial fibrillation to sinus rhythm. Occasional patients with atrial flutter will convert to atrial fibrillation. Cardioversion should be performed in any situation of hemodynamic instability instead of attempting medical management.

A-V nodal reentry tachycardia is due to a circuit consisting of 2 functionally different pathways within the node. Typically, bidirectional conduction and differences in the speed of conduction and refractoriness between the 2 pathways are the components that permit a properly timed early impulse to trigger the arrhythmia. Verapamil terminates reentry by prolonging conduction over the circuit and by increasing refractoriness. The conversion rate of this arrhythmia approaches 90% in an outpatient population. With the introduction of IV adenosine, verapamil is rapidly becoming the treatment of choice.

In patients with Wolff-Parkinson-White syndrome, verapamil should be used *only* to terminate a reentry tachycardia, in which antegrade conduction is over the A-V node and retrograde conduction is over the accessory pathway. Again, the mechanism of termination is prolongation of conduction across the A-V node coupled with an increase in refractoriness of the A-V node. Verapamil has not been well studied in patients with Wolff-Parkinson-White syndrome and antidromic tachycardia. Verapamil does not affect conduction or refractoriness of the accessory pathway and is *contraindicated* in patients with Wolff-Parkinson-White syndrome and atrial fibrillation/flutter because it can accelerate the ventricular response by shifting atrial impulse conduction from the A-V node to the accessory pathway.

In general, extreme caution is warranted in the use of verapamil to treat wide-complex tachycardias. Although it can effectively treat certain supraventricular arrhythmias associated with aberrant conduction, devastating consequences can occur in patients if ventricular tachycardia is misinterpreted as supraventricular tachycardia.

Newer Calcium Antagonists

Recently, a number of 2nd-generation Ca antagonists have become available with indications similar to those mentioned above. Nicardipine, isradipine, nitrendipine, and felodipine possess vascular selectivity with little direct cardiac effect. A 5th agent, nimodipine, demonstrates selectivity for the cerebral vasculature.

Nicardipine is approved for the management of hypertension and chronic stable angina pectoris; it can be used alone or in combination with other agents. Nicardipine is a potent peripheral vasodilator with preferential effects on the coronary circulation. It has little electrophysiologic effect; however, it can produce a reflex tachycardia from the decrease in BP. Following oral administration, nicardipine is almost completely absorbed, with plasma levels detected at 20 min; peak plasma levels are reached between 30 min and 2 h, with a mean of 1 h. As with the other dihydropyridines, there is extensive first-pass hepatic metabolism. The plasma half-life is 2 to 4 h, requiring tid dosing. Nicardipine has minor negative inotropic effects on the heart; however, it may lead to increased heart failure in patients with severe left ventricular dysfunction.

Nimodipine is approved for use to improve neurologic deficits due to cerebral vasospasm following subarachnoid hemorrhage in patients in good neurologic condition. This agent is highly lipophilic, probably accounting for its ability to cross the blood-brain barrier and its consequent cerebrovascular selectivity. It is rapidly and almost completely absorbed following oral administration, with peak plasma concentrations reached within 1 h. There is extensive first-pass hepatic metabolism. The terminal elimination half-life is 8 to 9 h; however, earlier elimination rates are significantly more rapid and equivalent to a half-life of approximately 3 h. As a result, dosing is required at 4-h intervals. Therapy should be started within 96 h of the event and continued for 21 days. Nimodipine is only available in capsule form. If the patient is unable to swallow, the contents of the capsule can be extracted into a syringe with an 18-gauge needle, emptied into a nasogastric tube, and washed with 30 mL of 0.9% sodium chloride.

Isradipine is effective for the management of hypertension and angina. There is extensive first-pass hepatic metabolism as with all agents in this subclass of Ca antagonists. Peak plasma levels occur in 1 to 2 h, and there are no active metabolites. The half-life is 6 to 8 h, allowing for bid dosing. Isradipine is highly selective for peripheral and coronary vasculature. It has little effect on the A-V node or myocardial contractility. There is some selective suppression of sinus node function. As a result it produces significant peripheral vasodilation without a reflex tachycardia. This agent may provide greater flexibility in the management of angina and hypertension in patients with heart failure or conduction system abnormalities.

Nitrendipine is an effective antihypertensive agent. Peak plasma levels are reached in 1 to 2 h. A long half-life of 8 to 12 h allows once-daily dosing. It is a potent peripheral arterial dilator and in clinical doses does not produce cardiac electrophysiologic effects, but it can cause a reflex tachycardia that may precipitate ischemia in patients with coronary artery disease. Clinical experience will define the role of this drug in the management of hypertension relative to other agents.

Felodipine is approved for the treatment of hypertension; it can be used as a single agent and is also compatible with other antihypertensive agents. The antihypertensive effect of felodipine is through peripheral vasodilation, and there is no effect on the cardiac conduction system. Although felodipine has not demonstrated significant negative inotropic effects in preliminary studies in patients with mild to moderate heart failure, its safety in patients with heart failure has not been established. A reflex increase in heart rate commonly occurs and is most noticeable during the first week of therapy. The increase in heart rate typically declines over time to levels of 5 to 10 beats/min elevation over baseline with chronic therapy. Following oral administration, felodipine is almost completely absorbed and undergoes extensive first-pass hepatic metabolism. A reduction in BP is noted within 2 to 5 h. The mean plasma half-life is between 11 and 16 h, which allows once-daily administration. Caution is advised when using felodipine in patients > 65 yr of age or in patients with impaired liver function because of the potential for elevated plasma levels.

Adverse Reactions

The pharmacologic profiles of diltiazem, nifedipine, and verapamil predict their major side-effect profiles (see TABLE 143–2). The most

TABLE 143–2. COMMON ADVERSE REACTIONS OF
SELECTED CALCIUM ANTAGONISTS

Diltiazem		Nicardipine		Nifedipine	
Side Effect	Incidence (%)	Side Effect	Incidence (%)	Side Effect	Incidence (%)
Headache	12.0	Flushing	9.7	Dizziness	27.0
Dizziness	7.0	Headache	8.2	Headache	23.0
Nausea	1.3	Pedal edema	8.0	Flushing	25.0
Dependent edema	6.0	Dizziness	6.9	Dependent edema	7.0
Rash	1.0	Asthenia	5.8	Tinnitus	6.0
A-V block	7.6	Increased angina	3.0	Nausea	11.0
Bradycardia	6.0	Palpitation	3.0	Nasal congestion	6.0

Nimodipine		Verapamil	
Side Effect	Incidence (%)	Side Effect	Incidence (%)
Hypotension	3.8	Constipation	7.3
Headache	1.2	Dizziness	3.3
Nausea	1.2	Nausea	2.7
Bradycardia	1.0	Headache	2.2
		Hypotension	2.5
		A-V block	2.0
		Heart failure	1.8

important side effects are direct extensions of their therapeutic actions. Diltiazem is usually well tolerated and has the lowest incidence of side effects. Negative inotropic and chronotropic effects are mild compared with those of verapamil. The effects on the A-V node are less than for verapamil, and peripheral vasodilator effects are less pronounced than those of nifedipine.

The predominant cardiovascular effect of nifedipine is peripheral vasodilation. Its cardiac side effects are secondary to the decrease in systemic vascular resistance; eg, reflex tachycardia and possible exacerbation of myocardial ischemia.

Since verapamil's major effects are on the cardiac conduction system and myocardial contractility, potential side effects are high-grade A-V block and heart failure. Constipation is also a common problem and may be particularly troublesome in the elderly.

Adverse Drug Interactions

Adverse drug interactions with Ca antagonists typically fall into 3 general categories. **Adverse pharmacokinetic** interactions commonly occur when there is an alteration in the metabolism of one agent due to a second agent. This is usually manifested by an altered plasma level of one of the agents. **Adverse hemodynamic interactions** often occur when a Ca antagonist is used with a second agent possessing similar actions,

such as combination therapy with an antihypertensive agent. Ca antagonists also have the potential for adverse **electrophysiologic interactions** when used with other agents that affect myocardial conduction. In certain clinical situations, drug interactions can provide therapeutic advantages over single-agent therapy; however, unwanted responses can result when the physician is unaware of potential interactions. The drugs listed below are commonly used in patients receiving Ca antagonists. This list is not a complete guide of possible drug interactions, and the physician should consult other reference sources for more information.

β-Adrenergic blocking agents: Verapamil and diltiazem can exacerbate the suppressive effects of certain β blockers on heart rate, A-V conduction, and myocardial contractility. When used in combination, close monitoring of the patient and these parameters is warranted. Other Ca antagonists are generally well tolerated.

Digitalis: Verapamil has been reported to significantly increase digitalis levels in patients on chronic combination therapy. This effect is more pronounced in patients with liver dysfunction. Isolated reports have noted elevated digitalis levels with both nifedipine and diltiazem, while other studies failed to identify this change. Monitoring of digitalis levels is recommended when used in combination with any of these agents. Nicardipine and nimodipine have not been shown to alter digitalis levels during chronic therapy.

Cimetidine: Plasma levels of nifedipine, diltiazem, and nicardipine are significantly elevated with cimetidine therapy. Patients taking ranitidine have demonstrated smaller and nonsignificant changes in diltiazem and nifedipine levels. Verapamil and nimodipine have not been well studied.

Cyclosporine: Posttransplant patients receiving cyclosporine present a special clinical situation. Adequate plasma levels of cyclosporine are important in controlling organ rejection, while significantly elevated plasma levels can lead to devastating side effects. Consequently, the physician must be aware of potential adverse drug interactions. Significant increases in cyclosporine levels can occur with both nicardipine and verapamil. Diltiazem has been shown to increase cyclosporine levels; however, conflicting data exist. Isolated reports also indicate that nifedipine may increase cyclosporine levels. Careful monitoring of cyclosporine levels is warranted when cyclosporine is used in combination with Ca antagonists.

144. SOME TRADE NAMES OF GENERIC (NONPROPRIETARY) DRUGS

Most prescription drugs placed on the market are given trade names (also called proprietary, brand, or specialty names) to distinguish them as being produced and marketed exclusively by a particular manufacturer. In the USA these names are usually registered as trademarks with the Patent Office and confer on the registrant certain legal rights with respect to their use. A trade name may be registered as representing a product containing a single active ingredient (with or without additives) or one containing 2 or more active ingredients.

A drug marketed by several companies may have several trade names. Drugs manufactured in one country and marketed in many countries may have different trade names in each country.

Throughout this book we have used nonproprietary or "generic" names whenever possible. However, since trade names are found in many publications and are used extensively in clinical medicine, as a convenience to our readers, we have included a list of most of the drugs mentioned throughout THE MANUAL, in alphabetic order, followed by many of their trade names (see TABLE 144–1).

With few exceptions, we have limited the trade names in this list to those marketed in the USA.

This list is by no means all-inclusive and no effort has been made to list every trade name in current use for each drug. A few are investigational and may subsequently be released as approved new drugs. The inclusion of a drug in this list does not indicate approval or disapproval of its use in any category, nor does it imply efficacy or safety of its action.

Finally, the reader must keep in mind that many drugs are marketed almost exclusively by their official nonproprietary name and that the inclusion of a trade name in this list does not indicate its endorsement by this book nor its preference as the product of choice.

Constant changes in information resulting from new research and clinical experience, reasonable differences in opinion among authorities, and the unique aspects of individual clinical situations require that physicians exercise their own best judgments in the choice and use of a drug. In particular, physicians are advised to check the product information included in each package of drug that they plan to administer or prescribe, especially if the drug is one that is unfamiliar or is used only infrequently, or is one in which the effective therapeutic levels are close to the toxic levels.

TABLE 144–1. SOME TRADE NAMES OF COMMONLY USED GENERIC DRUGS

Generic Name	Trade Names	Generic Name	Trade Names
Acebutolol	SECTRAL	Acetohexamide	DYMELOR
Acetaminophen	DATRIL, TYLENOL	Acetohydroxamic acid	LITHOSTAT
Acetazolamide	DIAMOX	Acetophenazine	TINDAL

(Continued)

TABLE 144–1. SOME TRADE NAMES OF COMMONLY USED GENERIC DRUGS (Cont'd)

Generic Name	Trade Names	Generic Name	Trade Names
Acetylcysteine	MUCOMYST	Buspirone	BuSPAR
ACTH	See Corticotropin	Busulfan	MYLERAN
Acyclovir	ZOVIRAX	Butorphanol	STADOL
Adenosine	ADENOCARD	Calcifediol	CALDEROL
Albuterol	PROVENTIL, VENTOLIN	Calcitonin-human	CIBACALCIN
Allopurinol	ZYLOPRIM	Calcitonin-salmon	CALCIMAR
Alprazolam	XANAX	Calcitriol	ROCALTROL
Amantadine	SYMMETREL	Capreomycin	CAPASTAT
Amikacin	AMIKIN	Captopril	CAPOTEN
Amiloride	MIDAMOR	Carbamazepine	TEGRETOL
Aminocaproic acid	AMICAR	Carbenicillin	GEOPEN, PYOPEN
Aminophylline	SOMOPHYLLIN	Carbenicillin indanyl	GEOCILLIN
Amiodarone	CORDARONE	sodium	
Amitriptyline	ELAVIL, ENDEP	Carbidopa-levodopa	SINEMET
Amoxapine	ASENDIN	Carbinoxamine	CLISTIN
Amoxicillin	AMOXIL, LAROTID	Carboprost	PROSTIN/15M
Amoxicillin/clavulanate	AUGMENTIN	tromethamine	
potassium		Carmustine	BiCNU
Amphotericin B	FUNGIZONE	Cefaclor	CECLOR
Ampicillin	AMCILL, OMNIPEN,	Cefadroxil	DURICEF, ULTRACEF
	POLYCILLIN, PRINCIPEN	Cefamandole	MANDOL
Amrinone	INOCOR	Cefazolin	ANCEF, KEFZOL,
Anisotropine	VALPIN		ZOLICEF
Anthralin	ANTHRA-DERM	Cefixime	SUPRAX
Asparaginase	ELSPAR	Cefonicid	MONOCID
Astemizole	HISMANAL	Cefoperazone	CEFOBID
Atenolol	TENORMIN	Ceforanide	PRECEF
Auranofin	RIDAURA	Cefotaxime	CLAFORAN
Azathioprine	IMURAN	Cefotetan	CEFOTAN
Azlocillin	AZLIN	Cefoxitin	MEFOXIN
Aztreonam	AZACTAM	Ceftazidime	FORTAZ, TAZIDIME,
Baclofen	LIORESAL		TAZICEF
Beclomethasone	BECLOVENT, VANCERIL	Ceftizoxime	CEFIZOX
dipropionate		Ceftriaxone	ROCEPHIN
Benzene hexachloride,	See Lindane	Cefuroxime	CEFTIN, KEFUROX,
gamma			ZINACEF
Benzonatate	TESSALON	Cephalexin	KEFLEX
Benzquinamide	EMETE-CON	Cephapirin	CEFADYL
Benztropine mesylate	COGENTIN	Cephradine	ANSPOR, VELOSEF
Benzylpenicilloyl-	PRE-PEN	Chenodiol	CHENIX
polylysine		Chloral hydrate	NOCTEC
Beta carotene	SOLATENE	Chlorambucil	LEUKERAN
Betamethasone	CELESTONE	Chloramphenicol	CHLOROMYCETIN
Betamethasone	UTICORT	Chlordiazepoxide	LIBRIUM
benzoate		Chlorhexidine	HIBICLENS
Betamethasone valerate	VALISONE	Chlormezanone	TRANCOPAL
Betaxolol	BETOPTIC, KERLONE	Chlorotrianisene	TACE
Bethanechol chloride	DUVOID, URECHOLINE	Chlorpheniramine	CHLOR-TRIMETON,
Bisacodyl	DULCOLAX		TELDRIN
Bitolterol	TORNALATE	Chlorpromazine	THORAZINE
Bleomycin	BLENOXANE	Chlorpropamide	DIABINESE
Bretylium	BRETYLOL	Chlorthalidone	HYGROTON
Bromocriptine	PARLODEL	Cholestyramine	QUESTRAN
Brompheniramine	DIMETANE	Cimetidine	TAGAMET
Bumetanide	BUMEX	Ciprofloxacin	CIPRO
Bupropion	WELLBUTRIN	Cisplatin	PLATINOL

(Continued)

TABLE 144–1. SOME TRADE NAMES OF COMMONLY USED GENERIC DRUGS *(Cont'd)*

Generic Name	Trade Names	Generic Name	Trade Names
Clemastine	TAVIST	Diphenhydramine	BENADRYL
Clindamycin	CLEOCIN	Diphenidol	VONTROL
Clofazimine	LAMPRENE	Diphenoxylate with	LOMOTIL
Clofibrate	ATROMID-S	atropine	
Clomiphene	CLOMID	Dipivefrin	PROPINE
Clonazepam	KLONOPIN	Dipyridamole	PERSANTINE
Clonidine	CATAPRES	Disopyramide	NORPACE
Clotrimazole	LOTRIMIN, MYCELEX	Disulfiram	ANTABUSE
Cloxacillin	TEGOPEN	Divalproex	DEPAKOTE
Clozapine	CLOZARIL	Dobutamine	DOBUTREX
Colestipol	COLESTID	Docusate sodium	COLACE
Corticotropin (ACTH)	ACTHAR	Dopamine	INTROPIN
Cortisol	CORTEF, HYDROCORTONE,	Doxepin	ADAPIN, SINEQUAN
	SOLU-CORTEF	Doxorubicin	ADRIAMYCIN
Cosyntropin	CORTROSYN	Doxycycline	VIBRAMYCIN
Co-trimoxazole	See Trimethoprim-	Dronabinol	MARINOL
	sulfamethoxazole	Droperidol	INAPSINE
Cromolyn sodium	INTAL, NASALCROM,	Echothiophate iodide	PHOSPHOLINE IODIDE
	OPTICROM	Edrophonium	TENSILON
Cyclandelate	CYCLOSPASMOL	Enalapril	VASOTEC
Cyclizine	MAREZINE	Encainide	ENKAID
Cyclobenzaprine	FLEXERIL	Epoetin alfa	EPOGEN
Cyclopentolate	CYCLOGYL	Ergocalciferol	DELTALIN, DRISDOL
Cyclophosphamide	CYTOXAN	Erythromycin	E-MYCIN, ERYTHROCIN,
Cycloserine	SEROMYCIN		ILOSONE
Cyclosporine	SANDIMMUNE	Esmolol	BREVIBLOC
Cyproheptadine	PERIACTIN	Ethacrynic acid	EDECRIN
Cytarabine	CYTOSAR-U	Ethambutol	MYAMBUTOL
Dacarbazine	DTIC-DOME	Etidronate disodium	DIDRONEL
Dactinomycin	COSMEGEN	Etoposide	VePESID
Danazol	DANOCRINE	Etretinate	TEGISON
Dantrolene	DANTRIUM	Factor IX complex	KONYNE, PROPLEX
Daunorubicin	CERUBIDINE	(human)	
Deferoxamine	DESFERAL	Famotidine	PEPCID
Demeclocycline	DECLOMYCIN	Fenfluramine	PONDIMIN
Desipramine	NORPRAMIN, PERTOFRANE	Fenoprofen	NALFON
Desmopressin	DDAVP	Fentanyl	SUBLIMAZE
Dexamethasone	DECADRON, HEXADROL	Flecainide	TAMBOCOR
Dexchlorpheniramine	POLARAMINE	Fluconazole	DiFLUCON
Dextromethorphan	DELSYM, BENYLIN DM	Flucytosine	ANCOBON
Diazepam	VALIUM	Fludrocortisone	FLORINEF
Diazoxide, IV	HYPERSTAT	Flumethasone pivalate	LOCORTEN
Diazoxide, oral	PROGLYCEM	Flunisolide	AEROBID, NASALIDE
Diclofenac sodium	VOLTAREN	Fluocinolone acetonide	FLUONID, SYNALAR
Dicloxacillin	DYNAPEN, DYCILL,	Fluocinonide	LIDEX
	PATHOCIL	Fluoxetine	PROZAC
Dicyclomine	BENTYL	Fluoxymesterone	HALOTESTIN, "ORA-
Diethylpropion	TENUATE, TEPANIL		TESTRYL"
Diflunisal	DOLOBID	Fluphenazine	PERMITIL, PROLIXIN
Digitoxin	CRYSTODIGIN, PURODIGIN	Flurandrenolide	CORDRAN
Digoxin	LANOXIN	Flurazepam	DALMANE
Dihydrotachysterol	HYTAKEROL	Flurbiprofen	ANSAID, OCUFEN
Diltiazem	CARDIZEM	Furosemide	LASIX
Dimercaprol	BAL	Ganciclovir	CYTOVENE
Dinoprost	PROSTIN F2 ALPHA	Gemfibrozil	LOPID
Dinoprostone	PROSTIN E2	Gentamicin	GARAMYCIN

(Continued)

TABLE 144–1. SOME TRADE NAMES OF COMMONLY USED GENERIC DRUGS *(Cont'd)*

Generic Name	Trade Names	Generic Name	Trade Names
Glipizide	GLUCOTROL	Loperamide	IMODIUM
Glyburide	DIABETA, MICRONASE	Lorazepam	ATIVAN
Gold sodium thiomalate	MYOCHRYSINE	Lovastatin	MEVACOR
Griseofulvin	GRIFULVIN, GRISACTIN, FULVICIN	Loxapine	LOXITANE
		Lypressin	DIAPID
Guaifenesin	HYTUSS, ROBITUSSIN	Mafenide	SULFAMYLON
Guanethidine	ISMELIN	Maprotiline	LUDIOMIL
Halazepam	PAXIPAM	Mazindol	MAZANOR, SANOREX
Haloperidol	HALDOL	Mebendazole	VERMOX
Haloprogin	HALOTEX	Mechlorethamine	MUSTARGEN
Hydralazine	APRESOLINE	Meclizine	ANTIVERT, BONINE
Hydrochlorothiazide	ESIDRIX, HydroDIURIL, ORETIC	Meclofenamate	MECLOMEN
		Medroxyprogesterone	PROVERA
Hydrocortisone	See Cortisol	Mefenamic acid	PONSTEL
Hydromorphone	DILAUDID	Megestrol acetate	MEGACE
Hydroquinone	ELDOPAQUE, ELDOQUIN	Melphalan	ALKERAN
Hydroxychloroquine	PLAQUENIL	Menadiol	SYNKAYVITE
Hydroxyprogesterone caproate	DELALUTIN	Menotropins	PERGONAL
		Meperidine	DEMEROL
Hydroxyurea	HYDREA	Mephenytoin	MESANTOIN
Hydroxyzine	ATARAX, VISTARIL	Meprobamate	EQUANIL, MILTOWN
Ibuprofen	MOTRIN, RUFEN	Mercaptopurine	PURINETHOL
Idoxuridine	DENDRID, HERPLEX, STOXIL	Mesalamine	ROWASA
		Mesoridazine	SERENTIL
Ifosfamide	IFEX	Metaproterenol	ALUPENT, METAPREL
Imipenem/cilastatin	PRIMAXIN	Metaraminol	ARAMINE
Imipramine	PRESAMINE, TOFRANIL	Methadone	DOLOPHINE
Indapamide	LOZOL	Methamphetamine	DESOXYN
Indomethacin	INDOCIN	Methandrostenolone	DIANABOL
Ipratropium bromide	ATROVENT	Methdilazine	TACARYL
Iron dextran	IMFERON	Methenamine hippurate	HIPREX, UREX
Isoetharine	BRONKOSOL	Methenamine mandelate	MANDELAMINE
Isoniazid	INH, NYDRAZID		
Isopropamide iodide	DARBID	Methicillin	STAPHCILLIN
Isoproterenol	ISUPREL	Methimazole	TAPAZOLE
Isosorbide dinitrate	ISORDIL, SORBITRATE	Methocarbamol	ROBAXIN
Isotretinoin	ACCUTANE	Methotrimeprazine	LEVOPROME
Kanamycin	KANTREX	Methoxsalen	OXSORALEN
Ketoconazole	NIZORAL	Methsuximide	CELONTIN
Ketoprofen	ORUDIS	Methyldopa	ALDOMET
Ketorolac	TORADOL	Methylphenidate	RITALIN
Labetalol	NORMODYNE, TRANDATE	Methylprednisolone	MEDROL
Lactulose	CEPHULAC, CHRONULAC	Methyltestosterone	METANDREN, ORETON
Levallorphan	LORFAN	Methysergide	SANSERT
Levamisole	ERGAMISOL	Metoclopramide	REGLAN
Levarterenol bitartrate	See Norepinephrine	Metolazone	DIULO, ZAROXOLYN
Levodopa	DOPAR, LARODOPA	Metoprolol	LOPRESSOR
Levothyroxine (T$_4$)	SYNTHROID	Metronidazole	FLAGYL
Lidocaine	XYLOCAINE	Metyrapone	METOPIRONE
Lincomycin	LINCOCIN	Mexiletine	MEXITIL
Lindane	KWELL	Mezlocillin	MEZLIN
Liothyronine (T$_3$)	CYTOMEL	Miconazole	MICATIN, MONISTAT
Liotrix	EUTHROID, THYROLAR	Minocycline	MINOCIN
Lisinopril	PRINIVIL	Minoxidil	LONITEN
Lithium carbonate	LITHANE, LITHONATE	Misoprostol	CYTOTEC
Lomustine	CeeNU	Mitomycin	MUTAMYCIN

(Continued)

TABLE 144–1. SOME TRADE NAMES OF
COMMONLY USED GENERIC DRUGS *(Cont'd)*

Generic Name	Trade Names	Generic Name	Trade Names
Mitotane	LYSODREN	Phenelzine	NARDIL
Molindone	MOBAN	Phenmetrazine	PRELUDIN
Moxalactam	MOXAM	Phenobarbital	LUMINAL
Nadolol	CORGARD	Phenoxybenzamine	DIBENZYLINE
Nafcillin	UNIPEN	Phensuximide	MILONTIN
Nalbuphine	NUBAIN	Phentermine	IONAMIN
Nalidixic acid	NegGRAM	Phentolamine	REGITINE
Naloxone	NARCAN	Phenylbutazone	AZOLID, BUTAZOLIDIN
Naltrexone	TREXAN	Phenylephrine	NEO-SYNEPHRINE
Nandrolone	DURABOLIN	Phenytoin	DILANTIN
Naproxen	NAPROSYN	Phytonadione	KONAKION, MEPHYTON
Neostigmine	PROSTIGMIN	Pindolol	VISKEN
Niclosamide	NICLOCIDE	Piperacillin	PIPRACIL
Nifedipine	PROCARDIA	Piperazine	ANTEPAR, BRYREL
Nimodipine	NIMOTOP	Pipobroman	VERCYTE
Nitrofurantoin	FURADANTIN, MACRODANTIN	Piroxicam	FELDENE
		Plicamycin	MITHRACIN
Nitroprusside	NIPRIDE	Pralidoxime	PROTOPAM
Nizatidine	AXID	Prazepam	CENTRAX
Norepinephrine bitartrate	LEVOPHED	Praziquantel	BILTRICIDE
		Prazosin	MINIPRESS
Norfloxacin	NOROXIN	Prednisolone	DELTA-CORTEF, HYDELTRASOL
Nortriptyline	AVENTYL		
Nystatin	MYCOSTATIN, NILSTAT	Prednisone	DELTASONE, METICORTEN
Octreotide	SANDOSTATIN	Primidone	MYSOLINE
Omeprazole	PRILOSEC	Probenecid	BENEMID
Oxacillin	BACTOCILL, PROSTAPHLIN	Probucol	LORELCO
Oxamniquine	VANSIL	Procainamide	PRONESTYL, PROCAN SR
Oxandrolone	ANAVAR	Procaine	NOVOCAIN
Oxazepam	SERAX	Procarbazine	MATULANE
Oxybutynin	DITROPAN	Prochlorperazine	COMPAZINE
Oxymetazoline	AFRIN, DURATION	Procyclidine	KEMADRIN
Oxymetholone	ANADROL	Promazine	SPARINE
Oxytocin	PITOCIN, SYNTOCINON	Promethazine	PHENERGAN
Pancrelipase	COTAZYM, ILOZYME	Propantheline	PRO-BANTHINE
Pancuronium	PAVULON	Proparacaine	OPHTHETIC, OPHTHAINE
Papaverine	CERESPAN, PAVABID	Propiomazine	LARGON
Paramethadione	PARADIONE	Propoxyphene	DARVON, DOLENE
Paramethasone	HALDRONE	Propranolol	INDERAL
Pargyline	EUTONYL	Protriptyline	VIVACTIL
Paromomycin	HUMATIN	Pseudoephedrine	SUDAFED
Penicillamine	CUPRIMINE	Pyrantel pamoate	ANTIMINTH
Penicillin G benzathine	BICILLIN, PERMAPEN	Pyridostigmine	MESTINON
Penicillin G potassium	PENTIDS	Pyrimethamine	DARAPRIM
Penicillin G procaine	DURACILLIN, WYCILLIN	Pyrvinium pamoate	POVAN
Penicillin V	PEN-VEE, V-CILLIN	Quinacrine	ATABRINE
Penicilloyl-polylysine	See Benzylpenicilloyl-polylysine	Quinethazone	HYDROMOX
		Quinidine	CARDIOQUIN, QUINAGLUTE, QUINIDEX, QUINORA
Pentamidine isethionate	NEBUPENT, PENTAM 300		
Pentazocine	TALWIN		
Pentobarbital	NEMBUTAL	Ranitidine	ZANTAC
Pentoxifylline	TRENTAL	Ribavirin	VIRAZOLE
Pergolide	PERMAX	Rifampin	RIFADIN, RIMACTANE
Perphenazine	TRILAFON	Ritodrine	YUTOPAR
Phenacemide	PHENURONE	Secobarbital	SECONAL
Phenazopyridine	PYRIDIUM	Selenium sulfide	SELSUN

(Continued)

TABLE 144–1. SOME TRADE NAMES OF COMMONLY USED GENERIC DRUGS *(Cont'd)*

Generic Name	Trade Names	Generic Name	Trade Names
Silver sulfadiazine	SILVADENE	Tolazoline	PRISCOLINE
Simethicone	MYLICON, SILAIN	Tolbutamide	ORINASE
Somatrem	PROTROPIN	Tolmetin	TOLECTIN
Somatropin, biosynthetic	HUMATROPE	Tolnaftate	TINACTIN
		Tranylcypromine	PARNATE
Spectinomycin	TROBICIN	Trazodone	DESYREL
Spironolactone	ALDACTONE	Tretinoin	RETIN-A
Stanozolol	WINSTROL	Triacetin	ENZACTIN
Streptokinase	KABIKINASE, STREPTASE	Triamcinolone	ARISTOCORT, KENA-CORT, KENALOG
Streptozocin	ZANOSAR		
Sucralfate	CARAFATE	Triamterene	DYRENIUM
Sulfamethoxazole	GANTANOL	Triazolam	HALCION
Sulfasalazine	AZULFIDINE	Triclofos	TRICLOS
Sulfinpyrazone	ANTURANE	Trientine	CUPRID
Sulfisoxazole	GANTRISIN	Trifluridine	VIROPTIC
Sulindac	CLINORIL	Trifluoperazine	STELAZINE
Suprofen	PROFENAL	Triflupromazine	VESPRIN
Tamoxifen	NOLVADEX	Trihexyphenidyl	ARTANE, TREMIN
Temazepam	RESTORIL	Trimeprazine	TEMARIL
Terbutaline	BRETHINE, BRICANYL	Trimethadione	TRIDIONE
Terfenadine	SELDANE	Trimethaphan	ARFONAD
Testolactone	TESLAC	Trimethobenzamide	TIGAN
Testosterone cypionate	DEPO-TESTOSTERONE	Trimethoprim	PROLOPRIM, TRIMPEX
Testosterone enanthate	DELATESTRYL	Trimethoprim-sulfamethoxazole	BACTRIM, SEPTRA, COMOXOL
Tetanus immune globulin (human)	HYPER-TET		
Tetracycline	ACHROMYCIN V, TETRACYN, TETREX	Trimipramine	SURMONTIL
		Tripelennamine	PBZ
Theophylline	ELIXOPHYLLIN, THEO-DUR, THEOPHYL	Triprolidine	ACTIDIL
		Tromethamine	THAM
Thiabendazole	MINTEZOL	Tropicamide	MYDRIACYL
Thiethylperazine	TORECAN	Valproic acid	DEPAKENE
Thioridazine	MELLARIL	Vancomycin	VANCOCIN
Thiothixene	NAVANE	Vasopressin	PITRESSIN
Thyrotropin	THYTROPAR	Verapamil	CALAN, ISOPTIN
Ticarcillin	TICAR	Vidarabine	VIRA-A
Timolol maleate	BLOCADREN, TIMOPTIC	Vinblastine	VELBAN
Tobramycin	NEBCIN	Vincristine	ONCOVIN
Tocainide	TONOCARD	Warfarin	COUMADIN, PANWARFIN
Tolazamide	TOLINASE	Zidovudine	RETROVIR

§12. POISONING; VENOMOUS BITES AND STINGS

145. POISONING

(See also Ch. 30)

Some general principles for diagnosing and treating poisoning are discussed first. Highlights of symptoms and treatment for individual chemicals and drugs or groups of substances follow alphabetically.

Poisoning due to bacterial or other toxins in food is discussed under BOTULISM in Ch. 32. Venomous bites and stings are dealt with in Ch. 146. Alcoholism and drug dependence are discussed in Ch. 53. Drug reactions are discussed in Chs. 34, 97, and 138.

GENERAL PRINCIPLES OF TREATMENT

Diagnosis

Worldwide, > 9 million natural and synthetic chemicals have been identified; fortunately, fewer than 3000 cause > 95% of accidental and deliberate poisonings. Identifying a poison and accurately assessing its potential toxicity are critical to a physician's successful management of poisoning. Otherwise, the physician must rely on simple general supportive treatment unless a specific "toxidrome" (toxicologic symptom complex) is pinpointed. Increasingly, physicians are depending on local or regional Poison Control Centers for technical information, particularly concerning ingredient data (toxic potentials) and consultations.

Poisoning should be considered in the differential diagnosis of any unexplained symptoms or signs, especially in children < 5 yr. Similarly, in the young adult, any disparity between expected history and clinical findings should suggest poisoning. Recently, poisonings among the elderly (especially medication mix-ups), among hospitalized patients (drug errors), among workers exposed to occupational chemicals, and as a result of environmental pollution have been increasingly recognized. Often the type and speed of onset of the total clinical picture will confirm or refute a suspicion of poisoning. Occasionally, the absence of a specific finding will be as important as its presence. Any pertinent history should be secured and the person and premises in-

spected for traces of drugs, ie, imprint identifications on solid medication forms, alcohol, etc, particularly for the unconscious patient.

> Ingredients, first aid measures, and antidotes often printed on product containers may be inaccurate or out of date. Information about household and industrial chemicals can be obtained through poison centers in all parts of the USA and Europe. Consultation with the centers is encouraged. The name of the nearest center is often listed under Emergency Numbers in the local telephone directory, or is available from the operator.

Immediate Care

1. Determine adequacy of cardiac and respiratory function and begin resuscitation if needed (see CARDIOPULMONARY RESUSCITATION in Ch. 30).

2. Determine quickly what has happened. If possible, identify the substance ingested, its route of entry into the body, and its toxicity potential. *Save any containers and appropriate specimens of the product or of emetic returns.* Determine the need for medical care, recognizing that many substances (see TABLE 145–1) need no further treatment. At all times, recall that overtreatment also may be a hazard and is expensive.

3. Unless contraindicated, immediately dilute and remove the toxic substance from the body suface. A person who has ingested a toxic substance may also have spilled it on the skin and may be inhaling fumes as well.

Ingested poison: Emesis will usually remove more of the toxic substance than will gastric lavage. Immediately induce vomiting with ipecac syrup 15 to 30 mL (1 to 2 tbsp) for children and adults, taken with water or soft drinks (orally: 15 mL/kg for infants; 1 qt [1 L] for adults). The dose of ipecac may be repeated in 15 to 30 min if necessary. If ipecac is not available, give soapy water, anionic or nonanionic detergent (hand-

TABLE 145–1. SUBSTANCES GENERALLY NONTOXIC WHEN INGESTED*

Ball-point inks (amount in 1 pen)	Magnesium silicate (antacid)
Barium sulfate	Matches
Bathtub toys (floating)	Methylcellulose
Blackboard chalk (calcium carbonate)	Modeling clay
Candles (insect-repellent type may be toxic)	Paraffin, chlorinated
Carbowax (polyethylene glycol)	Pencil lead (graphite)
Carboxymethylcellulose (dehydrating material	Pepper, black (except inhaled in mass)
packed with drugs, film, etc)	Petrolatum
Castor oil	Polyethylene glycols
Cetyl alcohol	Polyethylene glycol stearate
Crayons (children's: marked A.P., C.P., or	Polysorbate (Tweens®)
C.S. 130–46)	Putty
Detergents, anionic and nonionic	Red oil (turkey-red oil, sulfated castor oil)
Dichloral (herbicide)	Silica (silicon dioxide)
Dry cell battery	Spermaceti
Glycerol	Stearic acid
Glyceryl monostearate	Sweetening agents
Graphite	Talc (except when inhaled)
Gums (acacia, agar, ghatti, etc)	Tallow
Hormones	Thermometer fluid or mercury
Kaolin	Titanium oxide
Lanolin	Triacetin (glyceryl triacetate)
Lauric acid	Vitamins, children's multiple (with or without
Linoleic acid	iron)
Linseed oil (not boiled)	Vitamins, multiple without iron
Lipstick	

* Substances listed here may, however, be present in combination with phenol, petroleum distillate vehicles, or other toxic chemicals. Since manufactured products may be changed in their composition, this table is intended only as a guide, and prudence requires that a poison center be consulted for up-to-date information.

washing liquid detergent) plus water, and try to induce vomiting by inserting a finger or blunt instrument into the patient's throat to stimulate the gag reflex. Avoid being bitten. Place a child in the head-down position. Save a portion of the vomitus for analysis. (CAUTION: *Do not induce vomiting if the patient is comatose, is having convulsions [or is likely to], or has ingested petroleum distillates or corrosive substances. Emesis of petroleum distillates is rarely indicated unless some other compound that requires evacuation [eg, parathion] has been dissolved in the distillates.*)

When **gastric lavage** is carried out (*do not use lavage if the patient is convulsing or if the ingested substance is corrosive*), use the largest tube appropriate for the patient. For comatose or sedated patients > 2 yr, use a cuffed endotracheal tube to prevent aspiration. For those < 2 yr, no cuff is needed on the endotracheal tube because of the snug fit. Have the patient in a head-low position. For adults, physiologic (0.9%) sodium chloride solution or tap water may be used; for children, 0.45% sodium chloride solution is recommended. Introduce lavage fluids in 20- to 30-mL aliquots and remove the stomach

contents by siphon or syringe after each instillation. Continue the rinsing procedure until washings return free of toxin. After the return is clear, instill a specific antidote if one is available; otherwise instill a slurry of activated charcoal (see below).

The use of **cathartics** remains controversial; some evidence suggests that they may actually enhance absorption rather than promote excretion. If a cathartic is used, it is best limited to sodium sulfate 30 gm dissolved in 250 mL water, with proportionally reduced amounts for children, or sorbitol/charcoal solutions (but use no more than 2 doses).

When taken internally, **activated charcoal** with its molecular configuration and large surface area adsorbs significant amounts of many poisons, precluding their absorption from the gut. The earlier the charcoal is used, the more effective it is. From 5 to 10 times the amount of charcoal as that of the poison suspected of being ingested should be used. For children < 5 yr, the usual dose is 10 to 25 gm; for older children and adults, 50 to 100 gm. Charcoal is administered as a slurry (20 to 200 gm in water), preferably by stomach tube. It should not be administered before or immediately after syrup of ipecac has been given because ipecac induces vomiting; remember that 30% of patients vomit after charcoal administration alone. Charcoal is especially effective when the patient is already symptomatic and when the compound is re-excreted into the gut (eg, glutethimide). Increasingly, charcoal is being accepted as the primary technique of management in the emergency room.

Specific antidotes: While not numerous, specific antidotes are remarkably effective—eg, naloxone in opioid overdoses, atropine in organophosphate encounters, methylene blue for methemoglobinemia, acetylcysteine for acetaminophen, Digibind® for digoxin. A poison center should be contacted to determine if new specific antidotes have been developed, particularly for new drugs.

Inhaled poison: The patient should be removed from the contaminated environment, his respiration supported, and other personnel protected from contamination.

Skin and eye contamination: Contaminated clothing (including shoes and socks) should be removed. The skin should be thoroughly washed and the eyes flushed with water (see also Chs. 75 and 114). Helpers should be protected from contamination.

CNS stimulation by the poison may require **sedation.** Usually, diazepam or a barbiturate is used. In pure amphetamine poisoning, chlorpromazine is the drug of choice. To terminate convulsions, diazepam (5 to 10 mg for adults; 0.1 to 0.2 mg/kg for children) is given slowly IV. Phenobarbital (100 to 200 mg for adults and 4 to 7 mg/kg for children) may be used IV or IM to either terminate or prevent the recurrence of a convulsion. The patient should be kept oxygenated. Refractory seizures very rarely require general anesthesia; the above measures usually are satisfactory to control the hypoxic and cardiovascular consequences of convulsions.

Continuing Care

Symptomatic and supportive treatment depends on symptoms and signs and on anticipation of the clinical course, based upon identification of the poison. Continuation of the appropriate measures already begun and attempts to enhance the excretion of poison already absorbed are basic considerations. Stimulants are unlikely to be effective and are generally *contraindicated. Severe CNS depression* requires support of the circulation and ventilation. Endotracheal intubation and, rarely, tracheostomy may be necessary. In suspected or known narcotic poisoning, naloxone should be used (see DEPENDENCE OF THE OPIOID TYPE in Ch. 53).

Cerebral edema is common in poisonings due to sedatives, carbon monoxide, lead, and other CNS depressants. A 20% mannitol solution (5 to 10 mL/kg) is given slowly IV over a 30- to 60-min period. Corticosteroids are also used (dexamethasone 1 mg/m^2 of BSA q 6 h by IV drip). Intracranial monitoring with hyperventilation to alter the degree of cerebral edema is enjoying less widespread use. The use of barbiturate coma in cerebral edema associated with hypoxic episodes was advocated in the past but has fallen from favor.

Renal failure may occur in poisoning, and dialysis may be required. Elimination of poisons sometimes can be hastened either by augmenting normal excretory pathways or by using artificial means such as dialysis or perfusion, depending upon the nature of the poisoning, the availability of the facilities, and the condition of the patient. Flushing out the poison by simply increasing urine volume is rarely helpful. Alkalinization or acidification of the urine can occasionally be helpful (eg, in acute salicylate ingestions, giving 2 to 3 mEq/kg of sodium bicarbonate IV will augment excretion significantly). In general, weak acids are captured in alkalinized urine and weak bases in acidified urine.

Hemo- and **peritoneal dialysis** have been augmented by the development of "**lipid dialysis**," aimed at removal of lipid-soluble substances from the blood, and **hemoperfusion,** to provide an even more rapid and efficient clearance of toxic substances from the blood. However, these techniques are useless if the involved substance has a large apparent volume of distribution—ie, if it is stored in fatty tissue (eg, digitalis and tricyclic compounds) or is extensively bound to tissue protein. In select circumstances these techniques may be effective, but in many instances their yield is negligible. Thus, while digoxin is rapidly cleared from the blood via hemoperfusion, such a small amount (3 to 5%) of the total body digoxin is in the blood that hemoperfusion is ineffective. Tricyclic antidepressants are also largely confined to other than the vascular compartment, and the use of hemoperfusion for overdoses is likewise not warranted. TABLE 145−2 lists some representative toxic substances that are dialyzable.

TABLE 145–2. SOME DIALYZABLE TOXIC SUBSTANCES*

Alcohols	Chloramphenicol	Meprobamate
Aminoglycoside antibiotics	Chlorates	Methaqualone
Amphetamines	Chlordiazepoxide	Methyprylon
Aniline	Chromic acid	Monoamine oxidase inhibi-
Barbiturates	Diphenhydramine	tors
γ-Benzene hexachloride	Ethchlorvynol (lipid)	Paraldehyde
(lindane)	Ethinamate	Penicillins
Boric acid	Ethylene glycol	Phenytoin (diphenylhy-
Bromides and other halides	Glutethimide (lipid)	dantoin)
Calcium	Lithium	Potassium
Camphor	Metals (arsenic, copper,	Salicylates
Cephaloridine	iron, lead, magnesium,	Sodium
Chloral hydrate	strontium, zinc)	Tetracycline
		Theophylline
		Thiocyanates

* NOTE: Only in unusual circumstances is dialysis or hemoperfusion actually clinically useful.

TABLE 145–3. CHELATION THERAPY*

Edetate calcium disodium (calcium disodium edathamil; CaNa₂-EDTA)
Toxic substances:

Cadmium	Copper salts	Radium	Vanadium
Chromium	Lead	Selenium	Zinc
Cobalt	Manganese	Tungsten	Zinc salts
Copper†	Nickel	Uranium	

Dosage: Dilute to 3% (or less) for IV use
Give 25 to 35 mg/kg IV slowly (over 1 h) q 12 h for 5 to 7 days
Interrupt for 7 days, then repeat

Dimercaprol (BAL)
Toxic substances:

Antimony	Bismuth	Chromium trioxide†	Mercury
Arsenic	Chromates†	Copper salts	Nickel
Bichromates†	Chromic acid†	Gold	Tungsten
			Zinc salts

Dosage: Use 10% BAL in oil; give IM only
1st day: 3 to 4 mg/kg q 4 h
2nd day: 2 mg/kg q 4 h
3rd day: 3 mg/kg q 6 h
Then 3 mg/kg q 12 h every 10 days until recovery

Penicillamine
Toxic substances:

Bichromates	Chromic acid	Copper salts	Nickel
Cadmium	Chromium trioxide	Lead	Zinc salts
Chromates	Cobalt	Mercury†	

Dosage: 15 to 20 mg/kg orally bid

Succimer (meso 2,3-dimercaptosuccinic acid, DMSA)—see also TABLE 30–4
Toxic substance: Currently FDA-approved for lead in children
whose blood lead levels exceed 45 μg/dL
Dosage: 10 mg/kg q 8 h for 5 days
Then 10 mg/kg q 12 h for 14 days

NOTE: Neither iron nor thallium salts are chelated effectively by the above agents, but each has its own chelating agent (see Iron and Thallium salts in TABLE 145–4).

* Dosages depend on type and severity of poisoning.
† Chelator of choice.

Chelating agents are useful in treating poisoning by many metals and other toxic substances. The most commonly used agents, the toxic substances that they effectively chelate, and the usual doses required are given in TABLE 145–3.

Prevention

Widespread, voluntary, and now mandatory use of child-resistant containers (safety caps) has produced a dramatic decline in poisoning deaths, from about 500 deaths in the USA among children < 5 yr of age in 1959 to some 32 in 1989. Labeling of household products and prescription items, use of drug imprints on solid medication forms, improved monitoring of toxic exposures within industry and throughout the environment, widespread public and professional education programs such as that built around the **Mr. Yuk Program®** or that of the American Association of Poison Control Centers, and intense community-wide efforts to make syrup of ipecac available in each home and to make each home aware of the nearest poison center's phone number are examples of successful and effective activities aimed at preventing poisoning.

SPECIFIC POISONS

TABLE 145–4 lists the special toxicology for individual agents or groups of substances having related actions or similar treatment. However, the inclusion of a substance under a particular heading (eg, toluene under benzene) does not necessarily indicate that the toxicity is similar; it indicates that they are chemically related or that one substance may be found as an ingredient or impurity of another.

TABLE 145–4. SPECIFIC POISONS: SYMPTOMS AND TREATMENT

Poison	Symptoms	Treatment
Acetaminophen (see also ACETAMINOPHEN POISONING in Ch. 30)	Early: Often asymptomatic; mild nausea, vomiting, diaphoresis, pallor; beginning signs of hepatotoxicity; oliguria. Later (at 24–48 h): Nausea & protracted vomiting, right upper quadrant pain, jaundice, coagulation defects, hypoglycemia, encephalopathy, hepatic failure; renal failure, myocardiopathy may occur	Emesis; gastric lavage and/or charcoal. Monitor plasma drug levels for prognosis: if > 160–200 μg/mL at 4 h, hepatic damage may occur; if > 300 μg/mL at 4 h, hepatic damage is almost certain. If given before 18 h, oral acetylcysteine (Mucomyst®) 140 mg/kg to start and 70 mg/kg q 4 h for 4 to 18 doses has been effective in preventing significant hepatotoxicity
Acetanilid Aniline (indelible) inks Aniline oils Chloroaniline Phenacetin (acetophenetidin)	Cyanosis due to formation of methemoglobin & sulfhemoglobin, dyspnea, weakness, vertigo, anginal pain, rashes & urticaria, vomiting, delirium, depression, respiratory & circulatory failure	(1) Inhalation: Give O₂; support respiration. Blood transfusion. For severe cyanosis, methylene blue 1–2 mg/kg IV (2) Skin: Remove clothing & wash area with copious soap & water; then as in (1) (3) Ingestion: Give ipecac emetic; if this fails, gastric lavage and/or charcoal; then as in (1)
Acetic acid: see Acids and alkalis		
Acetone Ketones Model airplane glues, cements Nail polish remover	Inhalation: Bronchial irritation, pulmonary congestion & edema, decreased respirations, dyspnea, drunkenness, stupor, ketosis Ingestion: As above except direct pulmonary effect	Remove from source; evacuate stomach except for small amounts; support respiration; give O₂ & fluids; correct metabolic acidosis
Acetonitrile Cosmetic nail adhesive	Converted to cyanide, with usual symptoms & signs	Manage as for cyanide
Acetophenetidin: see Acetanilid		
Acetylene gas: see Carbon monoxide		

TABLE 145–4. SPECIFIC POISONS: SYMPTOMS AND TREATMENT *(Cont'd)*

Poison	Symptoms	Treatment
Acetylsalicylic acid: see ASPIRIN AND OTHER SALICYLATE POISONING in Ch. 30		
Acids & alkalis (see also specific acids & alkalis by name, and INGESTION OF CAUSTICS in Ch. 30)		
Acids Acetic Hydrochloric Nitric Phosphoric Sulfuric (some drain or toilet bowl cleaners, some dishwasher detergents)	Corrosive burns from inhalation, skin contact, eye contact, & ingestion; local pain. In general, alkali is more damaging to the GI tract Drooling & stridor are suggestive of damage	Skin or eye: Flush with water for 15 min Ingestion: Dilute with water or milk; *do not stimulate vomiting*; consider gastric lavage if large amounts of alkali granules have been consumed Hospitalize; give opiates for pain; treat shock if present; endoscopy is recommended; tracheostomy may be needed; for verified esophageal burns, give antibiotics & dexamethasone 1 mg/m² BSA q 6 h or equivalent for 2–3 wk
Alkalis Ammonia water (ammonium hydroxide) Potassium hydroxide (potash) Sodium hydroxide (caustic soda, lye) Carbonates of the above Detergent powders Some drain or toilet bowl cleaners; some dishwasher detergents	NOTE: Even in the absence of mouth lesions, strong alkalis (pH > 10.5–11.0) can burn the esophagus; esophagoscopy is advised	
Airplane glues, cements (model-building): see Acetone; Benzene; Petroleum distillates		
Alcohol, ethyl (ethanol) Brandy, whiskey, & other liquors	Emotional lability, impaired coordination, flushing, nausea & vomiting, stupor to coma, respiratory depression	Emesis; gastric lavage; support respiration; IV glucose to prevent hypoglycemia, dialysis if blood levels > 300–350 mg/dL; generous fluid administration as serum alcohol increases serum osmolarity
Alcohol, isopropyl Rubbing alcohol	Dizziness, incoordination, stupor to coma, gastroenteritis, hypotension; *no retinal injury*	Emesis; gastric lavage; IV glucose; correct dehydration & electrolyte changes; dialysis
Alcohol, methyl (methanol, wood alcohol) Antifreeze Paint solvent Solid canned fuel Varnish	Very toxic: 60–250 mL (2–8 oz) fatal in adults; 8–10 mL (2 tsp) in children. Latency period 12–18 h; headache, weakness, leg cramps, vertigo, convulsions, dimness of vision, decreased respiration	Combat acidosis with IV sodium bicarbonate; give 10% ethanol/5% dextrose solution IV; initially, a loading dose of 0.7 gm/kg of ethanol to impede methanol metabolism is infused over 1 h followed by 0.1–0.2 gm/kg/h to maintain a blood ethanol level of 100 mg/dL; investigate use of 4-methylpyrazole (currently pending FDA approval); *hemodialysis*
Aldrin: see DDT		
Alkalis: see Acids & alkalis		
Aminophylline Caffeine Theophylline	Wakefulness, restlessness, anorexia, vomiting, dehydration, convulsions; with hypersensitivity, immediate vasomotor collapse may occur. Adults are more susceptible than children	If ingested, use emetic or charcoal (avoid emesis if seizures are imminent). Stop medication; obtain theophylline blood level; phenobarbital or diazepam for convulsions; give parenteral fluids; maintain BP; if serum level > 50–100 mg/dL, consider dialysis; consider using a β blocker, eg propranolol, if patient is nonasthmatic

TABLE 145–4. SPECIFIC POISONS: SYMPTOMS AND TREATMENT *(Cont'd)*

Poison	Symptoms	Treatment
Amitriptyline: see Tricyclic antidepressants		
Ammonia gas	Irritation of eyes & respiratory tract; cough, choking; abdominal pain	Flush eyes with tap water for 15 min. *No gastric lavage or emetic.* If severe, positive pressure O_2 to manage pulmonary edema; support respiration
Ammonia water: see Acids & alkalis		
Ammoniated mercury: see Mercury		
Ammonium carbonate: see Acids & alkalis		
Ammonium fluoride: see Fluorides		
Ammonium hydroxide: see Acids & alkalis		
Amobarbital: see Barbiturates		

Amphetamines
    Amphetamine sulfate, phosphate
    Dextroamphetamine
    Methamphetamine
    Phenmetrazine
	Increased activity, exhilaration, talkativeness, insomnia, irritability, exaggerated reflexes, anorexia, dry mouth, arrhythmia, anginal chest pain, heart block, psychotic-like states and inability to concentrate or sit still	Emesis, lavage, or charcoal may be effective long after ingestion because of recycling via gastric mucosa
		Sedate with chlorpromazine 0.5–1 mg/kg IM or orally q 30 min as needed; reduce external stimuli; hypothermia; combat cerebral edema; hemodialysis. Use of β blockers may be helpful in nonasthmatics

Amyl nitrite: see Nitrites		
Aniline: see Acetanilid		
Ant poison: see DDT (chlordane); Thallium salts		
Antidepressants: see Tricyclic antidepressants		
Antifreeze: see Alcohol, methyl; Ethylene glycol		
Antihistamines	Excitation or depression, drowsiness, nervousness, disorientation, hallucinations, tachycardia, arrhythmias, hyperpyrexia, delirium, convulsions	Ipecac emesis (avoid emesis if seizures are imminent), gastric lavage, charcoal; support respiration/BP; control seizures with diazepam; physostigmine 0.5–2.0 mg (adults), 0.02 mg/kg (children) IM or IV (slowly) only after all else fails. (CAUTION: *Seizures* [see Physostigmine])
Antimony: see Arsenic & antimony		

Antineoplastic agents
    Methotrexate
    Mercaptopurine
    Vincristine
	Effects on hematopoietic system, nausea, vomiting	Emesis > lavage; supportive care; "leucovorin rescue"; observe for post-acute problems (beyond 24–48 h)

Arsenic & antimony
    Antimony compounds
        Stibophen
        Tartar emetic
    Arsenic
        Donovan's solution
        Fowler's solution
        Herbicides
        Paris green
        Pesticides
	Throat constriction, dysphagia; burning GI pain, vomiting, diarrhea; dehydration; pulmonary edema; renal failure; liver failure	Emesis; gastric lavage, then a demulcent; chelation with penicillamine; BAL if patient cannot take oral medication; hydration; treat shock, pain; sorbitol or saline cathartic (sodium sulfate 15–30 gm in water)

Arsine gas	Acute hemolytic anemia	Transfusions; diuresis

TABLE 145–4. SPECIFIC POISONS: SYMPTOMS AND TREATMENT (Cont'd)

Poison	Symptoms	Treatment
Aspirin: see ASPIRIN AND OTHER SALICYLATE POISONING in Ch. 30		
Atropine: see Belladonna		
Automobile exhaust: see Carbon monoxide		
Barbiturates Amobarbital Meprobamate Pentobarbital Phenobarbital Secobarbital	Headache, confusion, ptosis, excitement, delirium, loss of corneal reflex, respiratory failure, coma	Empty stomach up to 24 h after ingestion. If immediately after, use ipecac emetic; if sedated, use lavage and charcoal with cuffed endotracheal tube. Good nursing care; support respiration, give O_2; correct any dehydration. Rarely dialysis, especially for long-acting barbiturates where alkalinization hastens excretion
Barium compounds (soluble) Barium acetate carbonate chloride hydroxide nitrate sulfide Depilatories Fireworks Rodenticides	Vomiting, abdominal pain, diarrhea, tremors, convulsions, hypertension, cardiac arrest	To precipitate barium in stomach, give 60 gm sodium or magnesium sulfate orally. Then emesis or gastric lavage. Control convulsions with diazepam; atropine s.c., IM, or IV 0.5–1.0 mg (adults), 0.01 mg/kg (children) for colic; sublingual nitroglycerin 1/100–1/50 for hypertension; O_2 for dyspnea & cyanosis; quinidine 100–300 mg (adults), 6 mg/kg (children) to prevent ventricular fibrillation; correct hypokalemia
Belladonna Atropine Hyoscyamine Hyoscyamus Scopolamine (Hyoscine) Stramonium	Dry skin & mucous membranes; pupils dilated; flushing, hyperpyrexia; tachycardia, restlessness; coma; respiratory failure; convulsions	Emesis or charcoal; support respiration. May need to catheterize bladder. Physostigmine 0.5–2.0 mg (adults), 0.02 mg/kg (children) IM or IV (slowly) may reverse peripheral and central effects, but use only for severe problems. (CAUTION: Seizures [see Physostigmine])
Benzene Benzol Hydrocarbons Model airplane glue Toluene Toluol Xylene	Dizziness, weakness, headache, euphoria, nausea, vomiting, ventricular arrhythmia, paralysis, convulsions; with chronic poisoning, aplastic anemia, leukemia	If sizeable ingestion ($> 0.5–1$ mL/kg), emesis or cautious gastric lavage. Give O_2; support respiration; monitor ECG—ventricular fibrillation can occur early. Control seizures with diazepam. Blood transfusion for severe anemia. Do not give epinephrine
γ-Benzene hexachloride BHC Hexachlorocyclohexane Lindane	Irritability, CNS excitation, muscle spasms, atonia, clonic & tonic convulsions, respiratory failure, pulmonary edema	Emesis immediately after ingestion; gastric lavage; diazepam for convulsions. Avoid all oils—they promote absorption. Charcoal hemoperfusion prn
Benzin, benzine: see Petroleum distillates		
Benzodiazepines Dalmane® Librium® Valium®	Sedation to coma, particularly if accompanied by alcohol	Emesis; lavage; supportive care; suicidal precautions. IV flumazenil antidotes benzodiazepine overdose (CAUTION: if tricyclics are involved, seizures are a risk).
Benzol: see Benzene		
BHC: see γ-Benzene hexachloride		
Bichloride of mercury: see Mercury		
Bichromates: see Chromic acid		

TABLE 145–4. SPECIFIC POISONS: SYMPTOMS AND TREATMENT *(Cont'd)*

Poison	Symptoms	Treatment
Bishydroxycoumarin: see Warfarin		
Bismuth compounds	Poorly absorbed. Ulcerative stomatitis, anorexia, headache, rash, renal tubular damage	Ipecac emesis; gastric lavage; respiratory support; BAL (see TABLE 145–3, Chelation Therapy)
Bitter almond oil: see Cyanides		
Bitter almond oil, artificial: see Nitrobenzene		
Bleach, chlorine: see Hypochlorites		
β blockers	Hypotension, bradycardia, seizures, cardiac arrhythmias	Monitor closely, evacuate stomach. If symptomatic, initiate glucagon 3–5 mg IV or in saline; consider cardiac pacing
Borates Boric acid	Nausea, vomiting, diarrhea, hemorrhagic gastroenteritis, weakness, lethargy, CNS depression, convulsion, "boiled lobster" skin rash, shock	Ipecac emesis; gastric lavage; remove from skin; prevent or treat electrolyte changes & shock; control convulsions. Rarely, dialysis for severe poisoning
Boric acid: see Borates		
Brandy: see Alcohol, ethyl		
Bromates: see Chlorates		
Bromides	Nausea, vomiting, rash (may be acneiform), slurred speech, ataxia, confusion, psychotic behavior, coma, paralysis	Ipecac emesis, gastric lavage for acute ingestion; stop use as medication; promote mild diuresis by hydration & sodium chloride IV; ethacrynic acid is specifically useful. Hemodialysis only if severe
Bromine: see Chlorine		
Bulan: see DDT		
Cadmium Solder	Severe gastric cramps, vomiting, diarrhea; dry throat, cough, dyspnea; headache; shock, coma; brown urine, renal failure ("ouch-ouch disease")	Ipecac emesis; gastric lavage with milk or albumin; respiratory support; hydration; intermittent positive pressure breathing (IPPB) for pulmonary edema. Give edetate calcium disodium (see TABLE 145–3, Chelation Therapy), *not* BAL
Caffeine: see Aminophylline		
Calomel: see Mercury		
Camphor Camphorated oils	Camphor odor on breath, headache, confusion, delirium, hallucinations, convulsions, coma	Ipecac emesis (avoid emesis if seizures are imminent), charcoal, or gastric lavage. Prevent & treat convulsions with diazepam; support respiration. Lipid dialysis is still being explored
Canned fuel, solid: see Alcohol, methyl		
Cantharides Cantharidin Spanish fly	Skin and mucous membranes irritated, vesicles; nausea, vomiting, bloody diarrhea; burning pain in back and urethra; respiratory depression; convulsions, coma; abortion, menorrhagia	Avoid all oils; ipecac emesis; support respiration; treat convulsions; maintain fluid balance; no specific antidote
Carbamates	Usually less intense than those for organophosphates	See management of organophosphates, except for pralidoxime (2-PAM)

TABLE 145−4. SPECIFIC POISONS: SYMPTOMS AND TREATMENT *(Cont'd)*

Poison	Symptoms	Treatment
Carbolic acid: see Phenols		
Carbon bisulfide: see Carbon disulfide		
Carbon dioxide	Dyspnea, weakness, tinnitus, palpitations	Respiratory support; O_2
Carbon disulfide Carbon bisulfide	Garlic-breath odor, irritability, weakness, manic depression, narcosis, delirium, mydriasis, blindness, parkinsonism, convulsions, coma, paralysis, respiratory failure	Wash skin; emesis; gastric lavage; O_2; diazepam sedation; support respiration & circulation

Carbon monoxide
  Acetylene gas
  Automobile exhaust
  Carbonyl iron
  Coal gas
  Furnace gas
  Illuminating gas
  Marsh gas
	Toxicity varies with length of exposure, concentration inhaled, respiratory & circulatory rates. Symptoms vary with % carboxyhemoglobin in blood. Headache, vertigo, dyspnea, confusion, dilated pupils, convulsions, coma	100% O_2 by mask; respiratory support if needed; obtain carboxyhemoglobin level immediately. *Avoid all stimulants.* Hyperbaric O_2 appears to be effective if carboxyhemoglobin is $>$ approx. 25%; primary value may be at level of cytochrome (see Ch. 128)

Carbon tetrachloride
  Cleaning fluids
    (nonflammable)
	Nausea, vomiting, abdominal pain, headache, confusion, visual disturbances, CNS depression, ventricular fibrillation, renal injury, hepatic injury	Wash from skin; emesis or gastric lavage; give O_2; support respiration; monitor renal & hepatic function & treat appropriately. *Avoid alcohol, epinephrine, ephedrine*

Carbonates (ammonium, potassium, sodium): see Acids & alkalis		
Caustic soda: see Acids & alkalis		
Chloral hydrate Chloral amide	Drowsiness, confusion, shock, coma; respiratory depression; renal injury, hepatic injury	Ipecac emesis; gastric lavage; respiratory support; look for concomitant ingestions

Chlorates
  Bromates
  Nitrates
  Permanent wave
    neutralizers
	Vomiting, nausea, diarrhea, cyanosis (methemoglobin), toxic nephritis, shock, convulsions, CNS depression, coma, jaundice	Ipecac emesis; gastric lavage; transfusion for severe cyanosis; *do not use methylene blue for chlorates or bromates.* Treat shock; O_2; consider dialysis for complex cases

Chlordane: see DDT		
Chlorinated lime: see Chlorine		

Chlorine (see also Hypochlorites)
  Bromine
  Chlorinated lime
  Chlorine water
  Tear gas
	Inhalation: Severe respiratory & ocular irritation, glottal spasm, cough, choking, vomiting; pulmonary edema; cyanosis
	Ingestion: Irritation, corrosion of mouth & GI tract, possible ulceration or perforation; abdominal pain, tachycardia, prostration, circulatory collapse
		Inhalation: O_2; respiratory support; watch for & treat pulmonary edema
		Ingestion: Ipecac emesis; gastric lavage; treat shock

Chloroaniline: see Acetanilid		

Chloroform
  Ether
  Nitrous oxide
  Trichloromethane
	Drowsiness, coma; with nitrous oxide, delirium	Inhalation: Respiratory, cardiac, and circulatory support
		Ingestion: Ipecac emesis; gastric lavage; observe for renal and hepatic damage

TABLE 145–4. SPECIFIC POISONS: SYMPTOMS AND TREATMENT *(Cont'd)*

Poison	Symptoms	Treatment
Chlorophenothane: see DDT		
Chlorothion: see Organophosphates		
Chlorpromazine: see Phenothiazine		
Chromates: see Chromic acid		

Chromic acid
  Bichromates
  Chromates
  Chromium trioxide
	Corrosive due to oxidation. Ulcer and perforated nasal septum; severe gastroenteritis; shock, vertigo, coma; nephritis	Milk or water to dilute; BAL (or penicillamine) for severe symptoms; fluids & electrolytes, with caution, to support renal function

Chromium: see TABLE 145–3, Chelation Therapy		
Chromium trioxide: see Chromic acid		
Cimetidine; ranitidine	Slight dryness & drowsiness; can alter metabolism of concomitant drugs	No specific antidotal treatment available: maintain a focus on metabolism of other drugs
Clonidine	Sedation; periodic apnea; hypotension	Emesis; lavage; supportive care; tolazoline IV & dopamine drip; naloxone 5 µg/kg up to 2–20 mg, repeated as necessary
Coal gas: see Carbon monoxide		
Cobalt: see TABLE 145–3, Chelation Therapy		
Cobaltous chloride: see Nitrogen oxides		
Cocaine	Stimulation, then depression; nausea & vomiting; loss of self-control, anxiety, hallucinations; sweating; respiratory difficulty progressing to failure; cyanosis; circulatory failure; convulsions	Emetic early; charcoal or gastric lavage; if needed, IV propranolol, with extreme caution, for arrhythmias, diazepam for excitation; O_2 respiratory & circulatory support. Observe for myocardial or pulmonary disorder (usually occurs prior to emergency room arrival)
Codeine: see Narcotics		
Copper: see TABLE 145–3, Chelation Therapy		

Copper salts
  Cupric sulfate, acetate, subacetate
  Cuprous chloride, oxide
  Zinc salts
	Vomiting, burning sensation, metallic taste, diarrhea, pain, shock, jaundice, anuria, convulsions	Emesis; gastric lavage; penicillamine or BAL (see TABLE 145–3, Chelation Therapy); electrolyte & fluid balance; respiratory support; monitor GI tract; treat shock, control convulsions; monitor for hepatic & renal failure

Corrosive sublimate: see Mercury		
Creosote; cresols: see Phenols		

Cyanides
  Bitter almond oil
  Hydrocyanic acid
  Nitroprusside
  Potassium cyanide
  Prussic acid
  Sodium cyanide
  Wild cherry syrup
	Tachycardia, headache, drowsiness, hypotension, coma, convulsions, death; venous blood bright red; *very rapidly lethal* (1–15 min)	*Speed essential.* Remove from source if inhaled; immediate emesis or lavage, amyl nitrite inhalation, 0.2 mL (1 ampule) 30 sec of each min, 100% O_2, support respiration; 10 mL 3% sodium nitrite 2.5–5 mL/min IV (in child: 10 mg/kg) then 25–50 mL 25% sodium thiosulfate at 2.5–5 mL/min IV; repeat the above if symptoms recur. Use Lilly cyanide kit

DDD: see DDT		

TABLE 145–4. SPECIFIC POISONS: SYMPTOMS AND TREATMENT *(Cont'd)*

Poison	Symptoms	Treatment
DDT (chloro-phenothane) Aldrin Bulan Chlordane Chlorinated organic insecticides DDD Dieldrin Dilan Endrin Heptachlor Methoxychlor Prolan Toxaphene	Vomiting (early or delayed); paresthesias, malaise; coarse tremors, convulsions; pulmonary edema, ventricular fibrillation, respiratory failure	Emesis; gastric lavage if not convulsing, or charcoal; diazepam or phenobarbital to prevent & control tremors & convulsions; avoid epinephrine & sudden stimuli; parenteral fluids; monitor for renal & hepatic failure
Deodorizers, household: see Naphthalene; Paradichlorobenzene		
Depilatories: see Barium compounds		
Desipramine: see Tricyclic antidepressants		
Detergent powders: see Acids & alkalis		
Dextroamphetamine: see Amphetamines		
Diazinon: see Organophosphates		
Dicumarol: see Warfarin		
Dieldrin: see DDT		
Diethylene glycol: see Ethylene glycol		
Dilan: see DDT		
Dinitrobenzene: see Nitrobenzene		
Dinitro-o-cresol Herbicides Pesticides	Fatigue, thirst, flushing; nausea, vomiting, abdominal pain; hyperpyrexia, tachycardia, loss of consciousness; dyspnea, respiratory arrest. Also absorbed through skin	Emesis; gastric lavage; fluid therapy; O₂; anticipate renal & hepatic toxicity; no specific antidote. Rinse skin with detergents
Diphenoxylate with atropine	Lethargy, nystagmus, pinpoint pupils, tachycardia, coma, respiratory depression (NOTE: toxicity may be delayed up to 12 h)	Ipecac emesis, gastric lavage; activated charcoal; naloxone; admit all children for observation if ingestion is verified
Dipterex: see Organophosphates		
Dishwasher detergents: see Acids & alkalis		
Diuretics, mercurial: see Mercury		
Doxepin: see Tricyclic antidepressants		
Drain cleaners: see Acids & alkalis		
Endrin: see DDT		
Ergot derivatives	Thirst, diarrhea, vomiting, lightheadedness, burning feet; convulsions, hypotension, coma, abortion; gangrene of feet; cataract	Ipecac emesis; gastric lavage; benzodiazepine or short-acting barbiturate for convulsions; papaverine 60 mg IV, 1–2 mg/kg IV for children

TABLE 145–4. SPECIFIC POISONS: SYMPTOMS AND TREATMENT *(Cont'd)*

Poison	Symptoms	Treatment
Eserine: see Physostigmine		
Ethanol: see Alcohol, ethyl		
Ether: see Chloroform		
Ethyl alcohol: see Alcohol, ethyl		
Ethyl biscoumacetate: see Warfarin		

Ethylene glycol
  Diethylene glycol
  Permanent antifreeze
	Eye contact: iridocyclitis
	Ingestion: Inebriation but no alcohol odor on breath; nausea, vomiting; carpopedal spasm, lumbar pain; oxalate crystalluria; oliguria progressing to anuria & acute renal failure; respiratory distress, convulsions, coma
		Flush eyes
		Ingestion: Emesis; gastric lavage, support respiration, correct electrolyte imbalance (anion gap); give ethanol (see Alcohol, methyl); hemodialysis

Explosives: see Barium compounds (fireworks); Nitrogen oxides		
Ferric salts: see Iron		
Ferrous gluconate, ferrous sulfate: see Iron		
Fireworks: see Barium compounds		

Fluorides
  Ammonium fluoride
  Hydrofluoric acid
  Rat poisons
  Roach poisons
  Sodium fluoride
  Soluble fluorides generally
	Inhalation: Intense eye, nasal irritation; headache; dyspnea, sense of suffocation, glottal edema, pulmonary edema, bronchitis, pneumonia; mediastinal & subcutaneous emphysema from bleb rupture
	Skin & mucosa: Superficial or deep burns
	Ingestion: Salty or soapy taste; in large doses: tremors, convulsions, CNS depression; shock; renal failure
		Inhalation: O_2, respiratory support; prednisone for chemical pneumonitis (adults 30–80 mg/day in divided doses); manage pulmonary edema
		Skin: Copious flushing with cold water; debride white tissue; inject 10% calcium gluconate locally or intra-arterially & apply magnesium oxide paste
		Ingestion: Ipecac emesis; gastric lavage—leave aluminum hydroxide gel, calcium, or magnesium hydroxide or chloride in stomach; IV glucose & saline; 10% calcium gluconate, 10 mL IV (1 mL/kg in child); monitor for cardiac irritability; treat shock & dehydration

Formaldehyde
  Formalin
  (NOTE: May contain methyl alcohol)
	Inhalation: Irritation of eyes, nose, respiratory tract; laryngeal spasm & edema; dysphagia; bronchitis, pneumonia
	Skin: Irritation, coagulation necrosis; dermatitis, hypersensitivity
	Ingestion: Oral & gastric pain, nausea, vomiting, hematemesis, shock, hematuria, anuria, coma, respiratory failure
		Inhalation: Flush eyes with saline; O_2; support respiration
		Skin: Wash copiously with soap & water
		Ingestion: Give water or milk to dilute; treat shock; correct acidosis with sodium bicarbonate; support respiration; observe for perforations

Fowler's solution: see Arsenic & antimony		
Fuel, canned: see Alcohol, methyl		
Fuel oil: see Petroleum distillates		
Furnace gas: see Carbon monoxide		

TABLE 145–4. SPECIFIC POISONS: SYMPTOMS AND TREATMENT *(Cont'd)*

Poison	Symptoms	Treatment
Gamma benzene hexachloride: see γ-Benzene hexachloride		

Gas
  Acetylene, automobile exhaust, coal, furnace, illuminating, marsh: see Carbon monoxide
  Ammonia: see Ammonia gas
  Nerve: see Organophosphates
  Sewer, volatile hydrides: see Hydrogen sulfide
  Tear: see Chlorine		

Gasoline: see Petroleum distillates		
Glues, model airplane: see Acetone; Benzene; Petroleum distillates		
Glutethimide	Drowsiness, areflexia, mydriasis, hypotension, respiratory depression, coma	Ipecac emesis; gastric lavage, activated charcoal; support respiration, maintain fluid & electrolyte balance; hemodialysis may help; treat shock
Gold salts: see TABLE 145–3, Chelation Therapy		
Guaiacol: see Phenols		
Halogenated hydrocarbons: see DDT		
H₂ blockers	Minor GI problems; may alter the concentration level of other drugs	Nonspecific supportive measures
Heptachlor: see DDT		
Herbicides: see Arsenic & antimony; Dinitro-o-cresol		
Heroin: see Narcotics		
HETP (hexaethyl tetraphosphate): see Organophosphates		
Hexachlorocyclohexane: see γ-Benzene hexachloride		
Hormones—single acute oral overdose—no toxicity		
Hydrides, volatile: see Hydrogen sulfide		
Hydrocarbons: see Benzene		
Hydrocarbons, halogenated: see DDT		
Hydrochloric acid: see Acids & alkalis		
Hydrocyanic acid: see Cyanides		
Hydrogen chloride, fluoride: see Nitrogen oxides		

Hydrogen sulfide
  Alkali sulfides
  Phosphine
  Sewer gas
  Volatile hydrides
	"Gas eye" (subacute keratoconjunctivitis), lacrimation & burning; cough, dyspnea, pulmonary edema; caustic skin burns, erythema, pain; profuse salivation, nausea, vomiting, diarrhea; confusion, vertigo; sudden collapse & unconsciousness	Give O₂, support respiration; amyl nitrite & sodium nitrite as for cyanide (*no thiosulfate*)

Hyoscine, hyoscyamine, hyoscyamus: see Belladonna		

Hypochlorites
  Bleach, chlorine
  Javelle water
	Usually mild pain & inflammation of oral & GI mucosa; cough, dyspnea, vomiting; skin vesicles	Usual 6% household preparations require little except milk dilution; treat shock; esophagoscopy only if concentrated forms have been ingested

Illuminating gas: see Carbon monoxide		

1161

TABLE 145-4. SPECIFIC POISONS: SYMPTOMS AND TREATMENT *(Cont'd)*

Poison	Symptoms	Treatment
Imipramine: see Tricyclic antidepressants		
Indelible markers: see Acetanilid—usually no problem		
Ink, aniline: see Acetanilid—usually no problem		
Insecticides: see DDT; Organophosphates; Paradichlorobenzene; Pyrethrum		
Iodine	Burning pain in mouth & esophagus; mucous membranes stained brown; laryngeal edema; vomiting, abdominal pain, diarrhea; shock, nephritis, circulatory collapse	Give milk, starch, or flour orally; gastric lavage; fluid & electrolytes; treat shock; tracheostomy for laryngeal edema
Iodoform Triiodomethane	Dermatitis; vomiting; cerebral depression, excitation; coma; respiratory difficulty	Skin: Wash with sodium bicarbonate or alcohol Ingestion: Emetic or gastric lavage; respiratory support
Iron Carbonyl iron: see Carbon monoxide Ferric salts Ferrous salts Ferrous gluconate Ferrous sulfate Vitamins with iron (NOTE: Children's chewables with iron are remarkably safe)	Vomiting, upper abdominal pain, pallor, cyanosis, diarrhea, drowsiness, shock; concern if > 40–70 mg/kg of elemental iron ingested	Ipecac emesis, gastric lavage; if serum iron > 400–500 mg/dL at 3–6 h, give deferoxamine 1 gm IV (maximal rate of 15 mg/kg/h) or 1–2 gm IM q 3–12 h (urine turns red within 2 h; if no color change, no further dose is needed); for shock, give deferoxamine 1 gm IV (maximal rate 15 mg/kg/h); exchange transfusion
Isoniazid (INH)	CNS stimulation, seizures, obtundation, coma	Emesis; lavage; diazepam sedation; pyridoxine (mg for mg INH ingested) up to 200 mg slowly IV for seizures, repeat prn; NaHCO₃ for acidosis
Isopropyl alcohol: see Alcohol, isopropyl		
Javelle water: see Hypochlorites		
Kerosene: see Petroleum distillates		
Ketones: see Acetone		
Lead Lead salts Solder Some paints & painted surfaces	Acute inhalation: Insomnia, headache, ataxia, mania, convulsions Acute ingestion: Thirst, burning abdominal pain, vomiting, diarrhea, CNS symptoms as above Lead encephalopathy: see LEAD POISONING in Ch. 30	See LEAD POISONING in Ch. 30
Lead, tetraethyl	Vapor inhalation, skin absorption, ingestion: CNS symptoms—insomnia, restlessness, ataxia, delusions, mania, convulsions	Supportive treatment; eg, diazepam, chlorpromazine, fluid & electrolytes; eliminate the source
Lime, chlorinated: see Chlorine		

TABLE 145-4. SPECIFIC POISONS: SYMPTOMS AND TREATMENT *(Cont'd)*

Poison	Symptoms	Treatment
Lindane: see γ-Benzene hexachloride		
Liquor: see Alcohol, ethyl		
Lithium salts	Nausea, vomiting, diarrhea, tremors, drowsiness, renal failure, diabetes insipidus	Acute: Emesis; diazepam—consider dialysis Chronic: Reduce dose; supportive therapy
Lye: see Acids & alkalis		
Lysergic acid diethylamide (LSD)	Confusion, hallucinations, hyperexcitability—coma. Flashbacks	Supportive therapy; diazepam; chlorpromazine (50-100 mg IM in adults)
Malathion: see Organophosphates		
Manganese: see TABLE 145-3, Chelation Therapy		
Marsh gas: see Carbon monoxide		
Meperidine: see Narcotics		
Meprobamate: see Barbiturates		
Mercurial diuretics: see Mercury		
Mercuric chloride: see Mercury		
Mercury All mercury compounds Ammoniated mercury Bichloride of mercury Calomel Corrosive sublimate Diuretics Mercuric chloride Mercury vapor Merthiolate	Acute: Severe gastroenteritis, burning mouth pain, salivation, abdominal pain, vomiting; colitis, nephrosis, anuria, uremia. Skin burns from alkyl & phenyl mercurials Chronic: Gingivitis, mental disturbance, neurologic deficits Mercury vapor: severe pneumonitis	Gastric lavage, activated charcoal; give penicillamine (or BAL)—see TABLE 145-3, Chelation Therapy; maintain fluid & electrolyte balance; hemodialysis for renal failure; observe for GI perforation Skin: Scrub with soap & water Lungs: Supportive care
Merthiolate: see Mercury—usually no problem		
Metaldehyde	Nausea, vomiting, retching, abdominal pain, muscular rigidity, hyperventilation, convulsions, coma	Emesis, if not spontaneous; supportive therapy; diazepam
Metals	Symptoms vary with metals; see specific metals	See TABLE 145-3, Chelation Therapy
Methadone: see Narcotics		
Methamphetamine: see Amphetamines		
Methanol: see Alcohol, methyl		
Methoxychlor: see DDT		
Methyl alcohol: see Alcohol, methyl		
Methyl salicylate: see ASPIRIN AND OTHER SALICYLATE POISONING in Ch. 30		
Mineral spirits: see Petroleum distillates		
Model airplane glues, solvents: see Acetone; Benzene; Petroleum distillates		
Morphine: see Narcotics		
Moth balls, crystals, repellent: see Naphthalene; Paradichlorobenzene		
Nail polish remover: see Acetone		

TABLE 145–4. SPECIFIC POISONS: SYMPTOMS AND TREATMENT *(Cont'd)*

Poison	Symptoms	Treatment
Naphtha: see Petroleum distillates		
Naphthalene (see also Paradichlorobenzene) Deodorizer cakes Moth balls, crystals, repellent cakes	Contact: Dermatitis, corneal ulceration Inhalation: Headache, confusion, vomiting, dyspnea Ingestion: Abdominal cramps, nausea, vomiting; headache, confusion; dysuria; intravascular hemolysis; convulsions. Hemolytic anemia in persons with G6PD deficiency	Contact: Remove clothing if formerly stored with naphthalene moth balls; flush skin and eyes Ingestion: Ipecac emesis, gastric lavage; blood transfusion for severe hemolysis; alkalize urine for hemoglobinuria; control convulsions
Naphthols: see Phenols		
Narcotics (see also Ch. 53) Alphaprodine Codeine Heroin Meperidine Methadone Morphine Opium Propoxyphene	Pinpoint pupils, drowsiness, shallow respirations, spasticity, respiratory failure	*Do not give emetics.* Gastric lavage, charcoal, respiratory support. Naloxone 5 μg/kg IV to awaken & improve respiration; if patient does not respond, give 2–20 mg naloxone (dosage may need to be repeated as often as 10–20 times); fluids IV to support circulation
Neostigmine: see Physostigmine		
Nerve gas agents: see Organophosphates		
Nickel: see TABLE 145–3, Chelation Therapy		
Nicotine: see Tobacco		
Nitrates: see Chlorates		
Nitric acid: see Acids & alkalis		
Nitrites Amyl nitrite Butyl nitrite Nitroglycerin Potassium nitrite Sodium nitrite	Methemoglobinemia, cyanosis, anoxia, GI disturbance, vomiting, headache, dizziness, hypotension, respiratory failure, coma	Ipecac emesis, gastric lavage; O_2; for methemoglobinemia, 1% methylene blue 1–2 mg/kg slowly IV; when > 40% methemoglobin, transfusion with whole blood
Nitrobenzene Artificial bitter almond oil Dinitrobenzene	Bitter almond odor (suggests cyanides), drowsiness, headache, vomiting, ataxia, nystagmus, brown urine, convulsive movements, delirium, cyanosis, coma, respiratory arrest	See Acetanilid
Nitrogen oxides (see also Chlorine, Hydrogen sulfide, Sulfur dioxide) Air contaminants that form atmospheric oxidants; liberated from missile fuels, explosives, agricultural wastes Cobaltous chloride Fluorine Hydrogen chloride Hydrogen fluoride	Delayed onset of symptoms with nitrogen oxides unless heavy concentration; other irritant gases give warnings—local burning in eye, nasal, pharyngeal mucous membranes. Fatigue, cough, dyspnea, pulmonary edema; later, bronchitis, pneumonia	Bed rest; O_2 as soon as symptoms develop; for excessive pulmonary foam: suction, postural drainage, tracheostomy; to prevent pulmonary fibrosis: prednisone 30–80 mg/day (adults) and dexamethasone 1 mg/m^2 BSA (children) have been used
Nitroglycerin: see Nitrites		

TABLE 145–4. SPECIFIC POISONS: SYMPTOMS AND TREATMENT *(Cont'd)*

Poison	Symptoms	Treatment
Nitrous oxide: see Chloroform		
Nortriptyline: see Tricyclic antidepressants		
Oil of wintergreen: see ASPIRIN AND OTHER SALICYLATE POISONING in Ch. 30		

Oils
  Aniline: see Acetanilid
  Fuel, lubricating: see Petroleum distillates		

OMPA (octamethyl pyrophosphoramide): see Organophosphates		
Opiates: see Narcotics		

Organophosphates
  Chlorothion
  Demeton
  Diazinon
  Dipterex (trichlorfon)
  HETP (hexaethyl
    tetraphosphate)
  Malathion
  Nerve gas agents
  OMPA (octamethyl
    pyrophosphor-
    amide)
  Parathion
  Systox
  TEPP (tetraethyl
    pyrophosphate)
	Nausea, vomiting, abdominal cramping, excessive salivation; increased pulmonary secretion, headache, rhinorrhea, blurred vision, miosis; slurred speech, mental confusion; breathing difficulty, frothing at mouth, coma. Absorbed through skin, via inhalation, or orally	Remove clothing, flush & wash skin. Empty stomach; atropine: adults 2 mg, children 0.01 mg/kg IV or IM q 15–60 min, if no signs of atropine toxicity, repeat as needed; pralidoxime chloride (PAM): adults 1–2 gm, children 20–40 mg/kg, IV over 15–30 min, repeat in 1 h if needed; O_2; support respiration; correct dehydration. *Do not use morphine or aminophylline.* Attendant should avoid self-contamination

Oxalates: see Oxalic acid		

Oxalic acid
  Ethylene glycol
  Oxalates
	Burning pain in throat, vomiting, intensive pain; hypotension, tetany, shock; glottal & renal damage; oxaluria	Give milk or calcium lactate; careful gastric lavage if at all; 10% calcium gluconate 10–20 mL IV; pain control, saline IV for shock; demulcents by mouth; watch for glottal edema & stricture

Paint solvents: see Mineral spirits (under Petroleum distillates); Turpentine		
Paints: see Lead		

Paradichlorobenzene
  Insecticide
  Moth repellent
  Toilet bowl deodorant
	Abdominal pain, nausea, vomiting, diarrhea, seizures, tetany	Ipecac emesis, gastric lavage; fluid replacement; diazepam for seizure control

Paraldehyde	Paraldehyde odor on breath, incoherent, pupils contracted, respirations depressed, coma	Ingestion: Ipecac emesis, gastric lavage; support respiration, O_2
Paraquat	Immediate: GI pain and vomiting; within 24 h: respiratory failure	Emesis, fuller's earth plus Na_2SO_4; limit O_2; call poison center or manufacturer
Parathion: see Organophosphates		
Paris green: see Arsenic & antimony		
Pentobarbital: see Barbiturates		
Permanent wave neutralizers (bromates): see Chlorates		
Pesticides: see Arsenic & antimony; Barium compounds; DDT; Dinitro-*o*-cresol; Fluorides; Organophosphates; Paradichlorobenzene; Phosphorus; Pyrethrum; Thallium salts; Warfarin		

TABLE 145–4. SPECIFIC POISONS: SYMPTOMS AND TREATMENT *(Cont'd)*

Poison	Symptoms	Treatment
Petroleum distillates (see also HYDROCARBON POISONING in Ch. 30)		
Asphalt Benzine (benzin) Fuel oil Gasoline Kerosene Lubricating oils Mineral spirits Model airplane glue Naphtha Petroleum ether Tar	Vapor inhalation: Euphoria; burning in chest; headache, nausea, weakness; CNS depression, confusion; dyspnea, tachypnea, rales Ingestion: Burning throat & stomach, vomiting, diarrhea; pneumonia, only if aspiration has occurred Aspiration: Early acute pulmonary changes	Since major problems are consequential to aspiration, as opposed to GI absorption, in most instances no gastric evacuation is warranted; gastric lavage only with rapid- onset depression from large amounts ingested; arterial blood gas levels to monitor care; supportive care for pulmonary edema; O_2, respiratory support
Petroleum ether: see Petroleum distillates		
Phenacetin: see Acetanilid		
Phencyclidine (PCP)	"Spaced-out," unconscious; hypertension	Quiet environment; prolonged gastric lavage; propranolol & diazepam
Phenmetrazine: see Amphetamines		
Phenobarbital: see Barbiturates		
Phenols Carbolic acid Creosote Cresols Guaiacol Naphthols	Corrosive. Mucous membrane burns; pallor, weakness, shock; convulsions in children; pulmonary edema; smoky urine; respiratory, cardiac, & circulatory failure	Remove clothing, wash external burns. Lavage with water, activated charcoal. *Do not use alcohol or mineral oil.* Demulcents; pain relief; O_2; support respiration; correct fluid imbalance; watch for esophageal stricture (rare)
Phenothiazine Chlorpromazine Prochlorperazine Promazine Trifluoperazine (etc)	Extrapyramidal tract symptoms (ataxia, muscular & carpopedal spasms, torticollis), usually idiosyncratic; overdose results in dry mouth, drowsiness, coma, hypothermia, respiratory collapse. Leukopenia, jaundice, coagulation defect, skin rashes	Ipecac emesis, charcoal, or gastric lavage; diphenhydramine 2–3 mg/kg IV or IM for extrapyramidal symptoms; diazepam for convulsions; warm patient. Avoid levarterenol & epinephrine; dialysis is of no benefit
Phenylpropanolamine	Nervousness, irritability, *hypertension* plus other sympathomimetic effects	Supportive therapy; diazepam; treat hypertension with phentolamine (Regitine® 5 mg) or nitroprussides
Phosphoric acid: see Acids & alkalis		
Phosphorus (yellow or white) Rat poisons Roach powders (NOTE: Red phosphorus is unabsorbable & nontoxic)	3 Stages of symptoms: 1st—Garlicky taste; garlic odor on breath; local irritation, skin & throat burns, nausea, vomiting, diarrhea 2nd—Symptom-free 8 h to several days 3rd—Nausea, vomiting, diarrhea, liver enlargement, jaundice, hemorrhages, renal damage, convulsions, coma Toxicity enhanced by alcohol, fats, digestible oils	Protect patient & attendant from vomitus, gastric washing, feces. If phosphorus is imbedded in skin, keep patient's body submerged in water. Gastric lavage copiously—some still recommend potassium permanganate (1:5000) or cupric sulfate (250 mg in 250 mL water); mineral oil 100 mL (to prevent absorption) & repeat in 2 h; combat shock; vitamin K_1 IV; transfusion with fresh blood
Physostigmine Eserine Neostigmine (Prostigmin®) Pilocarpine Pilocarpus	Dizziness, weakness, vomiting, cramping pain; pupils dilated, then contracted	Atropine sulfate 0.6 to 1 mg (adults), 0.01 mg/kg (children) s.c. or IV with repeat doses prn. (CAUTION: *Using physostigmine to counter anti-cholinergics is associated with a 15% seizure rate*)

TABLE 145–4. SPECIFIC POISONS: SYMPTOMS AND TREATMENT *(Cont'd)*

Poison	Symptoms	Treatment
Pilocarpine, pilocarpus: see Physostigmine		
Potash: see Acids & alkalis		
Potassium bichromate, potassium chromate: see Chromic acid		
Potassium carbonate: see Acids & alkalis		
Potassium cyanide: see Cyanides		
Potassium hydroxide: see Acids & alkalis		
Potassium nitrate: see Chlorates		
Potassium nitrite: see Nitrites		
Potassium permanganate	Brown discoloration & burns of oral mucosa, glottal edema; hypotension; renal involvement	Gastric lavage, demulcents; maintain fluid balance
Prochlorperazine: see Phenothiazine		
Prolan: see DDT		
Promazine: see Phenothiazine		
Propoxyphene: see Narcotics		
Propranolol	Confusion and seizures	Emesis; lavage; supportive care; diazepam sedation; pacemakers and glucagon (0.05 mg/kg stat plus 2–5 mg/h) have been effective
Prostigmin®: see Physostigmine		
Protriptyline: see Tricyclic antidepressants		
Prussic acid: see Cyanides		
Pyrethrum Pyrethrin	Allergic response (including anaphylactic reactions, skin sensitivity) in sensitive people. Otherwise low toxicity, unless vehicle is a petroleum distillate (see that entry)	For sizeable ingestion, emesis if patient is alert; otherwise, endotracheal tube & gastric lavage; wash skin well
Radium: see TABLE 145–3, Chelation Therapy		
Rat poison: see Barium compounds; Fluorides; Phosphorus; Thallium salts; Warfarin		
Resorcinol (resorcin)	Vomiting, dizziness, tinnitus, chills, tremor, delirium, convulsions, respiratory depression, coma	Emetic or gastric lavage; support respiration
Roach poison: see Fluorides; Phosphorus; Thallium salts		
Rodenticides (rat poison): see Barium compounds; Fluorides; Phosphorus; Thallium salts; Warfarin		
Rubbing alcohol: see Alcohol, isopropyl		
Salicylates: see ASPIRIN AND OTHER SALICYLATE POISONING in Ch. 30		
Salicylic acid: see ASPIRIN AND OTHER SALICYLATE POISONING in Ch. 30		
Scopolamine: see Belladonna		
Secobarbital: see Barbiturates		
Selenium: see TABLE 145–3, Chelation Therapy		
Sewer gas: see Hydrogen sulfide		

TABLE 145-4. SPECIFIC POISONS: SYMPTOMS AND TREATMENT *(Cont'd)*

Poison	Symptoms	Treatment
Silver salts Silver nitrate (NOTE: Chloride, bromide, iodide, & oxide salts are usually benign)	Stain on lips (white, brown, then black); gastroenteritis, shock, vertigo, convulsions	Gastric lavage with saline (0.9% sodium chloride) solution; control pain; control convulsions with diazepam
Smog: see Sulfur dioxide		
Soda, caustic: see Acids & alkalis		
Sodium carbonate: see Acids & alkalis		
Sodium cyanide: see Cyanides		
Sodium fluoride: see Fluorides		
Sodium hydroxide: see Acids & alkalis		
Sodium nitrite: see Nitrites		
Sodium salicylate: see ASPIRIN AND OTHER SALICYLATE POISONING in Ch. 30		
Solder: see Cadmium; Lead		
Stibophen: see Arsenic & antimony		
Stramonium: see Belladonna		
Strychnine	Restlessness, hyperacuity of hearing, vision, etc; convulsions from minor stimuli, complete muscle relaxation between convulsions; perspiration; respiratory arrest	Isolate & restrict stimulation to prevent convulsions. Activated charcoal orally; control convulsions with IV diazepam, curariform drugs; support respiration; acid diuresis with ammonium chloride or ascorbic acid; gastric lavage *after* convulsions are controlled
Sulfur dioxide Smog	Respiratory tract irritation; sneezing, cough, dyspnea pulmonary edema	Remove from contaminated area, give O_2; positive pressure breathing, respiratory support
Sulfuric acid: see Acids & alkalis		
Syrup of wild cherry: see Cyanides		
Systox: see Organophosphates		
Tar: see Petroleum distillates		
Tartar emetic: see Arsenic & antimony		
Tear gas: see Chlorine		
TEPP: see Organophosphates		
Tetraethyl lead: see Lead, tetraethyl		
Thallium salts (formerly used in: Ant poison Rat poison Roach poison)	Abdominal pain (colic), vomiting (may be bloody), diarrhea (may be bloody), stomatitis, excessive salivation; tremors, leg pains, paresthesias, polyneuritis, ocular & facial palsy; delirium, convulsions, respiratory failure; loss of hair about 3 wk after poisoning	Ipecac emesis, gastric lavage; treat shock, control convulsions with diazepam; chelation therapy is still experimental. Contact local poison center for latest information.
Theophylline: see Aminophylline		

TABLE 145-4. SPECIFIC POISONS: SYMPTOMS AND TREATMENT *(Cont'd)*

Poison	Symptoms	Treatment
Thyroxine	Most are asymptomatic; rarely, increasing irritability progressing to thyroid storm in 5–7 days	Emesis; observation at home; diazepam; consider antithyroid preparations and propranolol *only* if actual symptoms occur
Tobacco Nicotine	Excitement, confusion, muscular twitching, weakness, abdominal cramps, clonic convulsions, depression, rapid respirations, palpitations, collapse, coma, CNS paralysis, respiratory failure	Ipecac emesis, gastric lavage; activated charcoal; support respiration, O_2; diazepam for convulsions; wash skin well if contaminated

Toilet bowl cleaners, deodorizers: see Acids & alkalis; Paradichlorobenzene

Toluene, toluol: see Benzene

Toxaphene: see DDT

Trichlorfon: see Organophosphates

Trichloromethane: see Chloroform

Tricyclic antidepressants Amitriptyline Desipramine Doxepin Imipramine Nortriptyline Protriptyline	Anticholinergic effects (eg, blurred vision, urinary hesitation); CNS effects (eg, drowsiness, stupor, coma, ataxia, restlessness, agitation, hyperactive reflexes, muscle rigidity, & convulsions); CVS effects (tachycardia & other arrhythmias, bundle branch block, impaired conduction, congestive heart failure). Respiratory depression, hypotension, shock, vomiting, hyperpyrexia, mydriasis, & diaphoresis may also be present	Symptomatic & supportive; emesis (avoid emesis if seizures are imminent), charcoal, gastric lavage; monitor vital signs & ECG; maintain airway & fluid intake. Sodium bicarbonate as a rapid IV injection (0.5–2 mEq/L), repeat periodically to maintain blood pH > 7.45, precludes development of arrhythmias. Diazepam controls most CNS problems; only if symptoms persist should physostigmine salicylate (slowly IV) be used to reverse both CNS and cardiac manifestations of overdosage—adults: 2 mg with repeat of 1–4 mg prn at 20- to 60-min intervals; children: 0.5 mg repeated prn at 5-min intervals to maximum 2 mg

Trifluoperazine: see Phenothiazine

Triiodomethane: see Iodoform

Tungsten: see TABLE 145-3, Chelation Therapy

Turpentine Paint solvent Varnish	Turpentine odor; burning oral & abdominal pain, coughing, choking, respiratory failure; nephritis	Emesis (alert patient) if > 1–4 oz, gastric lavage; support respiration; O_2; control pain; monitor renal function

Vanadium: see TABLE 145-3, Chelation Therapy

Varnish: see Alcohol, methyl; Turpentine

Verapamil; nifedipine; diltiazem	Nausea, vomiting, mental confusion, bradycardia, hypotension	Emesis; atropine has reversed bradycardia; avoid β agonists

Vitamins—single acute oral ingestion of isolated or multiple dose form—no toxicity

Warfarin Bishydroxycoumarin Dicumarol Ethyl biscoumacetate Superwarfarins	Single ingestion not serious, multiple overdoses result in coagulopathy; even with "super" drugs, most are uneventful	For hemorrhagic manifestations, vitamin K_1 till prothrombin time is normal, transfusion with fresh blood if necessary

Wax, floor: see Carbon tetrachloride

Whiskey: see Alcohol, ethyl

TABLE 145—4. SPECIFIC POISONS: SYMPTOMS AND TREATMENT *(Cont'd)*

Poison	Symptoms	Treatment
Wild cherry syrup: see Cyanides		
Wintergreen oil: see ASPIRIN AND OTHER SALICYLATE POISONING in Ch. 30		
Wood alcohol: see Alcohol, methyl		
Xylene: see Benzene		
Zinc: see TABLE 145—3, Chelation Therapy		
Zinc salts: see Copper salts		

146. VENOMOUS BITES AND STINGS

POISONOUS SNAKES

In the USA, about 25 species of snakes are venomous or have toxic salivary secretions. These include the **pit vipers** (Crotalidae), the **coral snakes** (Elapidae), and a few species of Colubridae. TABLE 146—1 lists some medically important snakes of the USA and their usual geographic distribution.

Epidemiology

Although > 45,000 people/yr are bitten by all snakes in the USA, < 8000 cases of snake venom poisoning are reported. Fewer than 15 fatalities/yr occur, mostly in children or the elderly, in untreated or undertreated cases, or in members of religious sects who handle venomous serpents. Rattlesnakes account for about 70% of venomous snake bites and for almost all the deaths. Most other venomous snake bites are by copperheads and, to a lesser extent, cottonmouths. Coral snakes inflict < 1% of all bites. Imported snakes found in zoos, schools, snake farms, and amateur and professional collections account for about 15 bites/yr.

Chemistry, Pharmacology, and Pathology

Snake venoms are complex mixtures, chiefly proteins, many having enzymatic activity. Although the enzymes contribute to the deleterious effects of the venom, some of the more important toxic components are smaller polypeptides, which can be more toxic than the crude venom. Most venom components appear to interact with specific chemical and physiologic receptor sites.

Envenomation may be further complicated by the release of autopharmacologic substances (eg, histamine, serotonin) that can make diagnosis and treatment difficult. *Arbitrary grouping of snake venoms into categories such as "neurotox-* *ins," "hemotoxins," and "cardiotoxins" is pharmacologically superficial and can lead to grave errors in clinical judgment.* A so-called neurotoxin venom can produce marked cardiovascular changes or direct hematologic effects. The so-called hemotoxin venoms can also produce changes in the nervous system or in vascular dynamics. A patient with snake venom poisoning must be considered a victim of a complex poisoning.

Rattlesnake and many other viper venoms produce local tissue damage, blood cell changes, coagulation defects, blood vessel injury, changes in vascular resistance, and neurologic defects. The Hct may fall rapidly, although hemoconcentration may occur during very early stages. Thrombocytopenia is common, and the coagulation profile is often abnormal. Pulmonary edema may be present in severe poisoning, and bleeding may occur in the lungs, peritoneum, kidneys, and heart. Renal failure may occur because of a critical deficit in glomerular filtration secondary to hypotension or because of the effects of hemolysis. Proteinuria, hemoglobinuria, and myoglobinuria are common in severe cases of some rattlesnake bites. Although cardiac dynamics may be disturbed, the early cardiovascular collapse seen in an occasional patient bitten by a rattlesnake is due chiefly to a sharp fall in circulating blood volume. This appears to be caused by a loss of blood plasma and protein through the vessel walls and by blood pooling. Most North American crotalid venoms produce relatively minor changes in neuromuscular transmission, but Mojave rattlesnake venom may cause serious neurologic deficits.

Most elapid venoms cause changes in neuromuscular transmission, in nerve conduction, and, to a much lesser extent, in the CNS. Some

TABLE 146–1. SOME MEDICALLY IMPORTANT

Snakes	Wash, Ore, Idaho	Calif, Nev	Ariz, NM	Tex
Pit vipers (Crotalidae)				
Cottonmouths and Copperheads (*Agkistrodon*)				
Cottonmouths (*A. piscivorus*)				X
Copperheads (*A. contortrix*)				X
Rattlesnakes (*Crotalus*)				
Eastern diamondback (*C. adamanteus*)				
Western diamondback (*C. atrox*)		X	X	X
Sidewinder (*C. cerastes*)		X	Ariz	
Timber (*C. horridus*)				X
Rock (*C. lepidus*)			X	X
Speckled (*C. mitchelli*)		X	Ariz	
Black-tailed (*C. molossus*)			X	X
Twin-spotted (*C. pricei*)			Ariz	
Red diamond (*C. ruber*)		Calif		
Mojave (*C. scutulatus*)		X	X	X
Tiger (*C. tigris*)			Ariz	
Western (*C. viridis*)				
Prairie (*C.v. viridis*)	Idaho		X	X
Grand Canyon (*C.v. abyssus*)			Ariz	
Southern Pacific (*C.v. helleri*)		Calif		
Great Basin (*C.v. lutosus*)	Ore, Idaho	X	Ariz	
Northern Pacific (*C.v. oreganus*)	X	X		
Ridge-nosed (*C. willardi*)			Ariz	
Massauga and Pigmy Rattlesnakes (*Sistrurus*)				
Massauga (*S. catenatus*)			X	X
Pigmy (*S. miliarius*)				X
Coral snakes (Elapidae)				
Sonoran coral snake (*Micruroides euryxanthus*)			X	
Eastern coral snake (*Micrurus fulvius*)				X

Certain groups of adjoining states are treated here as units. The symbol X indicates that distribution of the species is widespread within the unit. Restriction of a species to a part of a unit is indicated appropriately.

elapid venoms also cause local tissue damage and necrosis, blood changes, and severe renal complications.

Symptoms, Signs, and Diagnosis

Venomous snake bites are medical emergencies requiring immediate attention and considerable judgment. Before any treatment is begun, it must be determined whether the snake was venomous and whether envenomation occurred, since a venomous snake may bite and *not* inject venom (no poisoning occurs in about 20 to 30% of pit viper bites and in about 50% of cobra and certain other elapid bites). When no envenomation occurs, or if the bite is inflicted by a nonvenomous snake, it should be treated as a puncture wound.

Although the identity of the offending snake can be suggested by the fang marks, *these should never be relied on for positive identification.* Typical fang-mark patterns are based on the anatomy of the snake's jaw and laboratory studies and may not be seen under field conditions. Rattlesnakes may leave 1 or 2 fang marks, as well as other teeth marks; single fang punctures are very common. Bites by nonvenomous snakes usually show multiple teeth marks.

Numerical grading of rattlesnake bites is sometimes described in the literature, but it is more practical to describe cases as minor, moderate, or severe, depending on *all* the symptoms, signs, and laboratory findings rather than on just 1 or 2 symptoms (eg, swelling and pain). Bites by the Mojave rattlesnake, for example, may cause

SNAKES OF THE UNITED STATES

Mont, Mich, Wis, Minn, SD, ND, Neb, Iowa, Wyo, Utah, Colo	Kan, Okla, Ark, Mo	Tenn, Ky, Ill, Ind, Ohio	NC, SC, Ga, Ala, Miss, La	Fla	Pa, NJ, Md, Del, Va, WVa, NY, New England
Neb, Iowa	X	Tenn, Ky, Ill	X	X	Va
Neb, Iowa	X	X	X	X	X
			X	X	
Okla, Ark			X	X	
Utah					
Minn, Wis, Neb, Iowa	X	X	X	X	
Not Mich, Minn, Wis	Kan, Okla				
Utah					
Mich, Wis, Minn, Neb, Iowa, Colo	Not Ark	Ill, Ind, Ohio			NY, Pa
	Not Kan	Tenn	X	X	
	Ark		X	X	

Adapted from *Snake Venom Poisoning* by FE Russell. Port Washington, NY, Scholium International, 1983; used with permission.

only minimal edema, local tissue changes, and pain, and therefore be graded as 1, yet this snake's venom lethal index is the highest of the North American snakes. In the presence of minimal symptoms and signs, insufficient antivenin may be given and a poor, even fatal, outcome may ensue following the bite of this snake.

Pit viper envenomation: Symptoms and signs vary considerably depending on the species of snake, the amount of venom injected, and other factors. If there is evidence of poisoning soon after a bite, the possible consequences must not be underestimated.

Bites by rattlesnakes, cottonmouths, and copperheads usually cause immediate swelling, edema, and pain. Contrary to popular opinion, severe pain is not a constant finding; it may even be mild or absent. Usually, however, some pain immediately follows envenomation, and swelling and edema appear within 10 min—they are rarely delayed > 20 to 30 min. By the time the patient arrives at the physician's office, a diagnosis of crotalid bite with envenomation can usually be made (or envenomation excluded) on the basis of fang marks, swelling and edema, pain, and, in bites by some species, tingling or numbness periorally or in the fingers or toes, a metallic or rubbery taste in the mouth, and certain other findings.

Untreated, the edema progresses rapidly and may involve the entire extremity within hours. There may be lymphangitis and enlarged, tender, regional lymph nodes. Skin temperature over the injured part and body temperature are usually elevated, although the patient may complain of chills. Weakness, a rapid and weak pulse, syncope, sweating, nausea, and vomiting may be present. BP often drops and shock may develop early. Respiratory distress may occur, particularly following bites by the Mojave rattlesnake; muscle fasciculations, spasms, and weakness are common, but true paralysis is rare. The patient may complain of headache, blurred vision, ptosis, and marked thirst.

Ecchymosis is common in moderate or severe rattlesnake poisoning and may begin to appear over the bite area within 3 to 6 h. It is severe following bites by the eastern and western diamondbacks and the prairie and Pacific rattlesnakes, less severe following copperhead and Mojave rattlesnake bites. The skin may appear tense and discolored; vesicles usually appear in the bite area within 8 h, often becoming blood-filled. These changes are usually superficial, since North American rattlesnake bites tend to be limited to dermal and subcutaneous tissues. Necrosis is common around the bite area in untreated cases, and surrounding superficial blood vessels may be thrombosed. Most venom effects reach their peak before the 4th day.

There may be hemorrhage from the gums, hematemesis, melena, and hematuria. Bleeding and clotting times are prolonged. The prothrombin time (PT), partial thromboplastin time (PTT), and fibrinogen values may be abnormal, and platelet counts may fall sharply in moderate or severe envenomations. In most cases, a sharp rise in the packed cell volume is an early finding, although in severe cases hemolysis may cause a rapid fall in the Hct.

Coral snake envenomation: Pain and swelling are absent or minimal and often transitory. Paresthesia is often noted around the bite, and some weakness of the part may become evident within several hours. Muscular incoordination may develop, and the patient may complain of marked weakness and lethargy. There may be increased salivation, difficulties in swallowing and phonation, and visual disturbances. Respiratory distress and failure may ensue. In fatal cases, shock, leading to cardiovascular and respiratory failure, usually precedes death.

Laboratory Tests

In all but trivial cases, a CBC (including platelets), coagulation profile (PT, PTT, fibrinogen), blood typing, and urinalysis are essential. Other tests, such as ESR, serum electrolytes, BUN, creatinine, and RBC fragility tests, may be useful. An ECG is indicated in all severe cases. Coagulation defects are not uncommon in snake venom poisoning and may vary considerably with the species of snake involved.

Treatment

Pit viper: If the patient is within 30 to 40 min of a medical facility, he should be put at rest, reassured, kept warm, and transported there as quickly as possible. The injured part should be loosely immobilized in a functional position just below heart level, and all rings, watches, and constrictive clothing removed. If the patient is > 40 min from medical care, single incisions can be made through the fang marks (no longer than $1/4$ in. and no deeper than $1/8$ in.) within the first 5 min. Suction, using Sawyer's extractor, applied directly over the incisions or even over the fang punctures is of value if applied within a few minutes of the bite and continued for 30 to 60 min. The wound should be cleansed and covered with a sterile dressing.

Antivenin is generally required in about 55 to 60% of crotalid bites in the USA. When needed, a skin test for horse serum sensitivity should be performed as described in the antivenin brochure. If the patient is mildly sensitive to horse serum and the poisoning is serious, diphenhydramine IV may be indicated before giving the antivenin. When a patient is 3+ or 4+ sensitive and life or limb is at stake, the patient should be carefully monitored by a physician, and antivenin given with caution. The technique for this procedure has been described in the literature, and consultation can be obtained by calling (602) 626-6016. A tourniquet, O_2, epinephrine, and other drugs and equipment for treating anaphylaxis should be available during any antivenin therapy.

The amount of Antivenin (Crotalidae) Polyvalent® to be given depends on many factors, the most important being the severity and progression of the symptoms and signs. In minimal rattlesnake poisoning, 50 to 80 mL (5 to 8 vials) of antivenin (reconstituted) will usually suffice; moderate cases may require 80 to 130 mL (8 to 13 vials); severe cases may need 150 mL (15 vials) or more. Water moccasin poisoning usually requires lesser doses, and in copperhead bites antivenin is usually required only for children and the elderly. Reconstituted antivenin should be diluted in sterile 0.9% sodium chloride or 5% dextrose and given by IV drip in most cases. If IM injection is necessary, it should be given in the buttocks. Absorption time, however, will be 4 to

6 h longer. *Never inject antivenin into a toe or finger.* Measuring the circumference of the extremity at 3 points increasingly proximal to the bite and recording the measurements every 15 to 30 min provides one guide to antivenin dosage. If additional antivenin is needed, it is added to the IV drip and given over 3 to 4 h. Antivenin is of less value the longer its administration is delayed; however, it can be effective, particularly for clotting defects, even after 24 h. IV fluids should be kept to a minimum, except when shock or hypovolemia is present.

Antitetanus therapy should be given when indicated, and a broad-spectrum antimicrobial should be administered in serious cases. Signs of hypovolemic shock, often with concomitant lysis of RBCs and platelet destruction, require fluid and blood component replacement; eg, plasma or albumin for hypovolemia and packed cells or whole blood for decreased RBC mass. Severe defects of hemostasis—ie, abnormal clotting or lysis of cells or clots, or a disturbance of platelet activity—require replacement with specific clotting factors, fresh frozen plasma, or platelets.

At the first sign of respiratory distress, O_2 should be given and mechanical support provided. Tracheal intubation or tracheostomy may be indicated, particularly if trismus, laryngeal spasm, or excessive salivation is present. Mild sedation with diazepam (which may reduce analgesic requirements) or midazolam is indicated in all severe bites when respiratory failure is not a problem. Aspirin or codeine may be used for moderate pain, and meperidine or morphine if the pain is severe. Cooling (10° to 15° C) may reduce pain, but an extremity should *never* be iced for an extended period, as the impaired circulation may lead to amputation.

Surgical debridement of blebs, bloody vesicles, or superficial necrosis, if present, should be carried out between the 3rd and 10th days and may need to be done in stages. The injured part should be soaked in 1:20 Burow's solution tid for 15 min. O_2 bubbled through the solution at the same time may be of value.

Corticosteroids are of little or no value during the acute stages of poisoning and may be contraindicated, except in treating anaphylactic crisis; they are not a substitute for fluids and catecholamines in snake venom shock. Local infiltration of 0.5 mL of 0.05-M EDTA in 0.9% sodium chloride around the bite area may reduce some of the local necrotizing effects of the venom if carried out within 20 min of the bite. All cases of snake bite, whether venomous or nonvenomous, should be observed for at least 6 h.

Follow-up care: Fasciotomy should be discouraged. It is usually unnecessary and reflects the use of insufficient or no antivenin during the first 12 h of the poisoning. Fasciotomy may be necessary, however, when there is clear evidence of severe vascular embarrassment, as demonstrated by measurements of compartment pressures over several hours. Within 2 days of the injury, a complete evaluation should be made of joint motion, muscle strength, sensation, and girth measurements. To avoid contractures, immobilization is interrupted by frequent periods of gentle exercise, progressing from passive to active. Follow-up care also includes sterile whirlpool treatment, debridement as indicated, and daily cleansing of the wound with 3% hydrogen peroxide followed by 15-min soaks in 1:20 Burow's solution. A polymyxin-bacitracin-neomycin ointment can be applied at bedtime. Daily exposure to continuous flowing O_2 while the part is immobilized in a plastic bag may be of value. The lesion should be covered with a sterile dressing and a loose bandage when the patient is supine, and a reasonably firm bandage when the patient is ambulatory.

Coral snake: The general principles noted above for pit viper envenomation should also be considered in coral snake bites, but incision and suction and other such first aid measures are of little value. Three vials of antivenin (*Micrurus fulvius*) should be given when a diagnosis of probable coral snake envenomation has been established. If symptoms develop, 3 to 5 additional vials may be indicated. The physician should contact a poison control center, zoo, or Wyeth Laboratories for the nearest source of this antivenin. In severe cases, cardiopulmonary and intensive care may be indicated.

Imported species: The local zoo is the first place to call when dealing with a bite by an imported venomous snake. Most zoos maintain a list of consulting physicians as well as the *Antivenin Index*, which lists the location and number of vials of antivenin available for imported species. Poison control centers in major cities also maintain listings for antivenins. Federal regulations on the use of foreign-prepared antivenins, however, indicate that it is prudent to contact a local public health officer before giving these antisera.

In all serious envenomations, particularly in children and the elderly, it is wise to consult with a poison control center; eg, the center at the University of Arizona (602) 626-6016, where trained physicians are on 24-h call.

POISONOUS LIZARDS

Only 2 lizards—the Gila monster (*Heloderma suspectum*) found in Arizona and Sonora and adjacent areas, and the beaded lizard *(H. horridum)* of Mexico—are known to be venomous. Their venom, somewhat similar to those of some snakes, contains hyaluronidase, phospholipase A, and one or more salivary kallikreins.

Symptoms and signs following poisoning include localized pain, swelling and edema, ecchymosis, lymphangitis, and lymphadenopathy. Systemic manifestations may develop in moderate or severe poisonings, including weakness, sweating, thirst, headache, and tinnitus. In severe cases, there may be cardiovascular collapse. The findings and clinical course are generally similar to those of a mild to moderate case of western diamondback rattlesnake bite.

Treatment consists of supportive measures similar to those recommended above for pit viper envenomation. No specific antiserum is commercially available.

SPIDERS

With the exception of 2 small groups, all spiders are venomous. Fortunately, the fangs of most species are too short or fragile to penetrate the skin. Nevertheless, at least 60 species in the USA have been implicated in bites on humans. Species that are dangerous include the widow spiders, *Latrodectus mactans* and related species; the brown or violin spider, *Loxosceles reclusa* (sometimes called the brown recluse) and related species; the jumping spiders, *Phidippus* sp; the tarantulas, *Rheostica* and *Pamphobeteus* sp; the trap-door spiders, *Bothriocyrtum* and *Ummidia* sp; the so-called banana spiders, *Phoneutria* and *Cupiennius sallei, Lycosa* (wolf spider), and *Heteropoda;* the crab spider, *Misumenoides aleatorius;* the running spiders, *Liocranoides* and *Chiracanthium;* the orbweavers, *Neoscona vertebrata, Araneus* sp, and *Argiope aurantia* (orange argiope); the running or gnaphosid spiders, *Drassodes;* the green lynx spider, *Peucetia viridans;* and the comb-footed or false black widow, *Steatoda grossa. Pamphobeteus, Cupiennius,* and *Phoneutria* are not na-

tive to the USA but may be brought into the country on produce or other materials.

The incidence of spider bites in the USA is unknown. Fewer than 3 fatalities/yr occur in the USA, usually in children.

Chemistry and Pharmacology

Only a few spider venoms have been studied in any detail. Black widow venom consists chiefly of proteins, a few of which are enzymatic. The lethal fraction appears to be a peptide that markedly affects neuromuscular transmission. Brown or violin spider venom consists of at least 10 or 12 proteins. Its enzyme activity is greater than that of *Latrodectus* venom, but no fraction of *Loxosceles* venom has been isolated that produces the entire sequence of events that give rise to the unusual necrotic lesion characteristic of *Loxosceles* bites. Polymorphonuclear leukocyte infiltration plays a major role in the poisoning, but the mechanism is not understood. Tarantula venom contains approximately 12 proteins, of which at least one affects cardiovascular function; however, it is highly unlikely that the bite of one tarantula would produce a harmful cardiac effect in a human. Tarantulas native to the USA are not considered dangerous.

Symptoms and Signs

Widow spiders: A *Latrodectus* bite usually gives rise to a sharp pinprick-like pain, followed by a dull, sometimes numbing pain in the affected extremity, and by cramping pain and some muscular rigidity in the abdomen or the shoulders, back, and chest. Associated manifestations may include restlessness, anxiety, sweating, headache, dizziness, ptosis, eyelid edema, skin rash and pruritus, respiratory distress, nausea, vomiting, salivation, weakness, and increased skin temperature over the affected area. Blood and CSF pressures are usually elevated in the more severe cases in adults.

Brown or violin spiders: A *Loxosceles* bite may cause little or no immediate pain, but some localized pain develops within an hour or so. The bite area becomes erythematous and ecchymotic and may itch. There may also be generalized pruritus. A bleb forms, often surrounded by either an irregular ecchymotic area or a more target-like lesion. The lesion may appear as a bull's eye; the central bleb becomes larger, fills with blood, ruptures, and leaves an ulcer over which a black eschar forms and eventually sloughs, leaving a large tissue defect, which may include muscle. Pain can be severe and involve the entire injured area. Systemic symptoms and signs may develop, including nausea and vomiting, malaise, chills, sweats, hemolysis, thrombocytopenia, and kidney failure; death is a rare sequela.

Differential Diagnosis

Far more common than spider bites are flea, bedbug, tick, mite, and biting fly bites; these are often mistaken for spider bites. Some arthropod bites may give rise to bullous lesions that rupture and ulcerate, resembling those produced by the violin and certain other spiders. Numerous reports of necrotic or gangrenous arachnidism attributed to *L. reclusa*, particularly in areas where this species is not found, are probably caused by spiders other than *Loxosceles* or more probably by other arthropods. Every attempt should be made to capture and identify the offending animal. Some cases of so-called brown recluse bites are misdiagnoses of epidermal necrolysis, erythema chronicum migrans, erythema nodosum, Lyell's syndrome, chronic herpes simplex, etc.

Treatment

Black widow spider: No first aid measures are of value. An ice cube may be placed over the bite to reduce pain. All patients < 16 yr or > 60 yr, or who have hypertensive heart disease, or who have symptoms and signs of severe envenomation, should be hospitalized and, when symptomatic treatment is unsuccessful, should be given 1 vial (6000 u.) of Antivenin (*Latrodectus mactans*)® IV in 10 to 50 mL of 0.9% sodium chloride after the appropriate skin test. One vial is usually sufficient and is usually given over 3 to 15 min. Children may require respiratory assistance. Vital signs should be checked frequently during the first 12 h following the bite. In the elderly, acute hypertension may require nitroprusside treatment.

For muscle pain and spasms, 10 mL of 10% calcium gluconate may be given slowly IV. Several doses at 4-h intervals may be necessary. In adults, a relaxant, particularly methocarbamol or dantrolene sodium given IV, is sometimes effective; diazepam 10 mg orally tid has had varying degrees of success. Meperidine 50 to 100 mg, or morphine 6 to 16 mg s.c. or IM q 6 h, may provide relief. Hot baths may afford relief in mild cases.

Brown or violin spider: A piece of ice can be placed over the bite area. Excision of the bite in proven cases of envenomation seen within several hours of the bite is finding less favor today. Also, in the past, persons bitten by this spider (or by an unidentified species) who developed a skin lesion within 12 h that increased in size during the next 12 h received a corticosteroid such as dexamethasone 4 mg IM q 6 h during the acute phase, then in decremental doses in accordance with standard practice. This protocol is still favored by many physicians. Presently, diaminodiphenylsulfone and acetyltrimethylcolchicinic acid are being evaluated. An antivenin has been prepared in the USA but is not yet commercially available.

Ulcerating lesions should be cleansed daily with 3% hydrogen peroxide, soaked in 1:20 Burow's solution tid for 15 min, and debrided as needed. Polymyxin-bacitracin-neomycin ointment can be applied at bedtime. O_2 applied to the lesion several times a day through an improvised face mask or plastic bag may be of some value. Most bites require only local treatment.

BEES, WASPS, HORNETS, ANTS

Stings by insects of the order Hymenoptera are common throughout the USA. While it may take over 100 bees to inflict a lethal dose of venom in most adults, one sting can cause a fatal anaphylactic reaction in a hypersensitive person. There are 3 to 4 times more deaths in the USA from bee stings than from snake bites. In the few fatalities that have resulted from multiple bee stings, death has been attributed to acute cardiovascular collapse.

In the South, particularly the Gulf region, stings by the **imported fire ants**, *Solenopsis richteri* and *S. invicta*, account for many thousands of stings each year. As much as 40% of the population in infested urban areas may be stung each year, and at least 30 deaths have been attributed to these insects. The fire ant sting usually results in immediate pain and the development of a wheal-and-flare lesion, which often resolves within 45 min and gives rise to a sterile pustule at the sting site. This breaks down within 30 to 70 h. The lesion sometimes becomes infected and can lead to sepsis. In some cases, an edematous, erythematous, and pruritic lesion, rather than pustules, develops. Anaphylaxis following fire ant stings probably occurs in less than 1% of patients. Some patients do not associate the sting, which can be minor, with the development of anaphylactic manifestations. Mononeuritis and seizures have also been reported to occur following fire ant stings.

Fire ant venom is 95% alkaloid, having hemolytic, cytolytic, antimicrobial, and insecticidal properties. As venom alkaloids do not appear to induce allergic reactions, the 3 or 4 small aqueous protein fractions are probably responsible for the allergic response. The venom of bees contains, among other components, peptides and nonenzymatic proteins (eg, apamin, melittin, and/or kinins), enzymes (eg, phospholipase A and B, and hyaluronidase), and amines (eg, histamine and 5-hydroxytryptamine).

Treatment

The stingers of many Hymenoptera may remain in the skin and should be removed by teasing or scraping rather than pulling. An ice cube placed over the sting will reduce pain; an antihistamine-analgesic-corticosteroid balm is often useful. Persons with known hypersensitivity to such stings should carry a kit containing an antihistamine and aqueous epinephrine in a prefilled syringe when in endemic areas. Desensitization is advised and can be carried out using insect whole-body antigens or, preferably, whole-venom antigens in the case of bee and vespid stings. Following initial immunotherapy, maintenance doses may need to be carried out for up to 5 yr. In fire ant stings, the maintenance dose should be carried out indefinitely in those persons who are continually exposed to the insect. (See also Ch. 34.)

OTHER BITING ARTHROPODS

Among the more common biting and sometimes bloodsucking arthropods in the USA are the ticks and mites; sand, horse, and deer flies; mosquitoes; fleas; lice; bedbugs; kissing bugs; and certain water bugs. The composition of the saliva of these arthropods varies considerably, and the lesions produced by bites vary from a small papule to a large ulcer with swelling and acute pain. Dermatitis may also occur. Most serious bites are complicated by sensitivity reactions or infection. In hypersensitive persons, bites can be fatal.

Treatment

The offending arthropod should be quickly removed. For ticks and some of the bugs, this is best accomplished by direct application of a petroleum product or other irritant to the animal or

by slowly withdrawing the arthropod while twisting it slowly with forceps. Care should be taken not to leave the capitulum in the wound, as it may induce chronic inflammation or migrate into deeper tissues and give rise to a granuloma. The bite should be cleansed, and an antihistamine-analgesic-corticosteroid balm should be applied. Serious hypersensitivity reactions should be treated as described in Ch. 34.

TICKS AND MITES

Ticks are vectors of many diseases. In addition to the reactions noted above, ticks are also involved in poisonings. In North America, some species of *Dermacentor* and *Amblyomma* cause **tick paralysis**. Symptoms and signs include anorexia, lethargy, muscle weakness, incoordination, nystagmus, and ascending flaccid paralysis. Bulbar or respiratory paralysis may develop. The bite of some *Ornithodorus* ticks (pajaroello), found in Mexico and southwestern USA, causes local vesiculation, pustulation with rupture, ulceration, and eschar, with varying degrees of local swelling and pain. Similar reactions have been observed following the bites of other ticks.

Mite infestations are quite common and are responsible for "**chiggers**" (*intensely pruritic dermatitis caused by the mite larva, or chigger*), various forms of scabies, demodicidosis, and a number of other diseases. The bites produce varying degrees of local tissue reaction, with or without sensitization.

Treatment

Treatment of tick paralysis is symptomatic. O_2 and respiratory assistance may be needed. An antitoxin is under study. Pajaroello tick lesions should be cleansed, soaked in 1:20 Burow's solution, and debrided when necessary. Corticosteroids are of value in severe reactions. Infections are common during the ulcer stage but rarely require more than local antiseptic measures.

Mite infestations may be treated as described under SCABIES in Ch. 93.

CENTIPEDES AND MILLIPEDES

Some of the larger centipedes of the genus *Scolopendra* can inflict a painful bite, with some localized swelling and erythema. Lymphangitis and lymphadenitis are common. Necrosis is rare and infection almost unknown. Symptoms and signs seldom persist for > 48 h. Millipedes do not bite but when handled may secrete a toxin that can cause local skin irritation and, in severe cases, tissue changes. Some non-US species can spray a highly irritating repugnant secretion that may cause severe conjunctival reactions.

Treatment

An ice cube will control the pain of most centipede bites. Toxic secretions of millipedes should be washed from the skin with copious amounts of soap and water; alcohol should not be used. A topical corticosteroid should be applied if a skin reaction develops. Eye injuries require immediate irrigation and the application of a corticosteroid-analgesic ointment.

SCORPIONS

All North American scorpions except *Centruroides exilicauda (sculpturatus)* are relatively harmless, their stings usually causing no more than some localized pain with minimal swelling, some lymphangitis with regional lymph gland swelling, and increased skin temperature and tenderness around the wound. Some localized tissue reaction may occur. *C. exilicauda* is found in Arizona, New Mexico, and the California side of the Colorado River. Its sting causes some immediate pain and sometimes numbness or tingling over the involved part. Swelling is not usually present. Children become tense and restless and display abnormal and random head, neck, and eye movements. In adults, tachycardia, hypertension, increased respirations, weakness, and motor disturbances may predominate. Respiratory difficulties may occur in both children and adults, often complicated by excessive salivation.

Treatment

The stings of most North American scorpions require no specific therapy. Placing an ice cube over the wound reduces pain, or an antihistamine-analgesic-corticosteroid balm can be applied over the injury at 4-h intervals. Hypertension can be controlled with diluted nitroprusside, 3 μg/kg/min IV, as directed by the manufacturer. Labetalol, 0.25 mg/kg IV over a 3-min period and repeated q 15 min as necessary and according to the manufacturer's recommendations, is an alternative hypertensive agent. Muscle spasms usually respond to calcium gluconate. Complete bed rest is indicated, and no food is given for the first 8 to 12 h. Antivenin should be used in all

unresponsive, severe cases and, particularly, in children. Information on its availability and use may be obtained from the Arizona Poison Control System at (602) 626-6016.

MARINE ANIMALS

Stingrays once caused about 750 stings/yr along North American coasts, but the present incidence is unknown. The venom is contained in the one or more spines located on the dorsum of the animal's tail. Injuries usually occur when the unwary victim treads on the fish while wading in ocean surf, bay, or slough. The pressure provokes the fish to thrust its tail upward and forward, driving the dorsal spine (or spines) into the victim's foot or leg. The integumentary sheath surrounding the spine is ruptured and the venom escapes into the victim's tissues, causing immediate severe pain. While often limited to the area of injury, the pain may spread rapidly, reaching its greatest intensity in < 90 min, and often persists (if untreated), though gradually diminishing over 6 to 48 h. Syncope, weakness, nausea, and anxiety are common and may be due, in part, to peripheral vasodilation. Lymphangitis, vomiting, diarrhea, sweating, generalized cramps, inguinal or axillary pain, and respiratory distress have been reported. The wound is usually jagged, bleeds freely, and is often contaminated with parts of the integumentary sheath. The edges of the wound are often discolored, and some localized tissue destruction may occur. Generally, there is some swelling and edema. Open wounds are subject to infection.

Mollusks include the cones, octopuses, and bivalves. *Conus californicus* is the only dangerous cone found in North American waters. Its sting produces localized pain, swelling, redness, and numbness. The bites of North American octopuses are rarely serious.

Echinoderms contain several classes known to be venomous. Certain **sea urchins** have venom organs (globiferous pedicellariae) with calcareous jaws capable of penetrating human skin, but injuries from these are rare. Far more common are injuries by sea urchin spines, which can break off in the skin and give rise to local tissue reactions. If not removed they may migrate into deeper tissues, causing a granulomatous nodular lesion, or they may wedge against bone or nerve. Joint and muscle pains and dermatitis may also occur.

Coelenterates (Cnidaria) include the corals, sea anemones, jellyfishes, and hydroids (the Portuguese man-of-war is a colonial hydroid). Many possess a highly developed stinging unit (the nematocyst) that can penetrate the skin. These are particularly abundant on the animal's tentacles, and a single tentacle may fire thousands of nematocysts into the skin following contact. The lesions vary with the type of coelenterate involved. Generally, the initial lesions appear as small papular eruptions in one or several discontinuous lines, at times surrounded by an erythematous zone. The papules develop rapidly, and the area becomes red and raised. Pain may be severe, and itching is common. The papules may vesiculate and proceed to pustulation and desquamation. Systemic manifestations include weakness, nausea, headache, muscle pain and spasms, lacrimation and nasal discharge, increased perspiration, changes in pulse rate, and chest pain that increases on respiration. In North American waters, the Portuguese man-of-war has caused deaths.

Treatment

Stingrays and most other fish stings: Injuries to an extremity should be irrigated with the salt water at hand. An attempt should be made to remove the integumentary sheath if it can be seen in the wound. The extremity should then be submerged in water as hot as the patient can tolerate without injury for 30 to 90 min. The wound should again be examined for remnants of the sheath and debrided. The appropriate antitetanus agent should be given, and the injured extremity kept elevated for several days. An antimicrobial agent may be necessary, and the wound closed surgically.

If the initial first aid measures are delayed, the wound may be anesthetized locally with lidocaine; regional blocks may offer relief. Meperidine IM may need to be used for pain. The primary shock that sometimes immediately follows stingray injuries usually responds to simple supportive measures.

Mollusks: The treatment of *Conus* stings and octopus bites is largely empirical. Local measures appear to be of little value. Local injection

of epinephrine and subsequent use of neostigmine have been suggested. Severe *Conus* stings may require mechanical ventilation and measures to combat shock.

Echinoderms: Pedicellariae stings are treated by washing the area and applying an antihistamine-analgesic-corticosteroid balm. Sea urchin spines should be removed immediately. A bluish discoloration at the site of entry may help in locating the spine, which may sometimes be seen by xeroradiogram. Vinegar dissolves most superficial spines, and soaking the wound in vinegar several times/day and covering the area with a wet vinegar compress may be sufficient; surgery is seldom necessary at this point. If a small incision needs to be made to extract the spine, care must be taken as it is very fragile. In time, a spine may migrate into deeper tissues and require surgical removal.

Coelenterates: Various remedies for coelenterate stings have been advocated. In some parts of the world, no treatment is advised except the local application of ammonia or vinegar. In the USA, the local application of meat tenderizers (eg, papain) has been popular. Sodium bicarbonate, boric acid, lemon or fig juice, alcohol, and many other agents have also been espoused, and it may be that merely changing the pH of the skin alleviates some of the localized pain. The following procedures are suggested: ocean water (not fresh water) is poured over the injured areas; the tentacles are removed, preferably with an instrument or a gloved hand; the area is soaked in 50% vinegar for 30 min; flour or baking powder is then poured over the wound area and scraped off with a sharp knife; the area is rinsed, soaked again in vinegar, and a topical antihistamine-analgesic-corticosteroid balm applied.

More serious cases may require O_2 or respiratory assistance. Painful muscle spasms may be relieved with 10 mL of 10% calcium gluconate given IV. Meperidine is preferred for severe pain. IV fluids and epinephrine may be needed in the few cases in which shock develops. An antivenin for the stings of certain Australian species of coelenterates is available, but it is of no value for stings of North American species.

INDEX

Page numbers followed by *f* indicate FIGURE; by *t*, TABLE

A

T

NOTES

NOTES

NOTES

NOTES

NOTES

NOTES

NOTES

NOTES